A TEXTBOOK OF
HISTOLOGY

BLOOM AND FAWCETT

A TEXTBOOK OF HISTOLOGY

DON W. FAWCETT, M.D.
Hersey Professor of Anatomy, Emeritus
Harvard Medical School
Boston, Massachusetts
Senior Scientist
International Laboratory of Research
on Animal Diseases
Nairobi, Kenya, Africa

TWELFTH EDITION

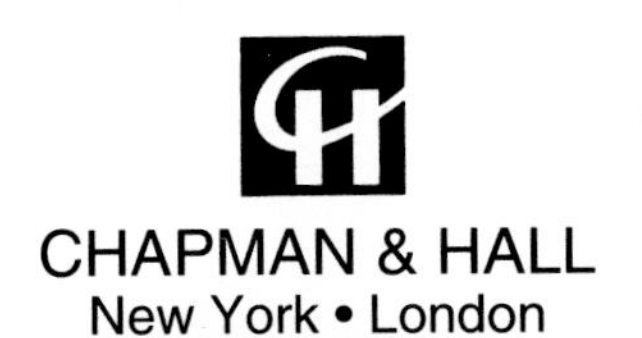
CHAPMAN & HALL
New York • London

This edition published by
Chapman & Hall
One Penn Plaza
New York, NY 10119

Published in Great Britain by
Chapman & Hall
2-6 Boundary Row
London SE1 8HN

Printed in the United States of America

Library of Congress Cataloging in Publication Data

Fawcett, Don Wayne, 1917-
Bloom and Fawcett, a textbook of histology / by Don W. Fawcett and Elio Raviola. — 12th ed.
p. cm.
Rev. ed. of: A textbook of histology / Don W. Fawcett 11th ed. 1986.
Includes bibliographical references and index.
ISBN 0-412-04691-1
1. Histology. I. Bloom, William, 1899- . III. Raviola, Elio, 1932- . III. Fawcett, Don Wayne, 1917- . Textbook of histology. IV. Title. V. Title: Textbook of histology.
[DNLM: 1. Histology. QS 504 F278b 1993]
QM551.F34 1993
611'.018—dc20
for Library of Congress 93-14568
CIP

British Library Cataloguing in Publication Data available

Please send your order for this or any Chapman & Hall book to **Chapman & Hall, 29 West 35th Street, New York, NY 10001, Attn: Customer Service Department.** You may also call our Order Department at 1-212-244-3336 or fax your purchase order to 1-800-248-4724.

For a complete listing of Chapman & Hall's titles, send your requests to **Chapman & Hall, Dept. BC, One Penn Plaza, New York, NY 10119.**

Contents

Preface

A firm foundation in histology continues to be essential to an understanding of the function of tissues and organs and for recognizing and interpreting their changes in disease. The content of other texts on histology is largely confined to description of the microscopic structure of the body. A unique feature of this book is a section on histophysiology in each of the chapters on the organs. This makes the book more interesting to medical students and expands their appreciation of the relevance of this subject to their future careers.

The book has been more thoroughly revised in this 12th edition than it was in recent editions. Outmoded interpretations have been removed and much new material has been added. A hundred or more old, or redundant, illustrations have been removed and 120 new figures have been added.

This textbook has a long history. In the period of political turmoil that followed the Russian revolution, the distinguished histologist, Alexander Maximov, and his wife and step-son, escaped over frozen Lake Ladoga to Finland. They subsequently made their way to America and Professor Maximov joined the faculty of the University of Chicago, where he continued to work on an unfinished textbook of histology. The text, in Russian, was still unfinished at the time of his death in 1928. It was completed by Dr. William Bloom, with the assistance of several of his colleages at the University of Chicago, and was published by the W. B. Saunders Company in 1930 as the Maximov and Bloom *Textbook of Histology*. The stated objective of the book was to provide students with a description of the microscopic structure of the body and the morphological evidence of its functions, introducing as much information on physiology as seemed desirable in a textbook for medical, dental, and veterinary students. The successful first edition was followed by revised editions in 1934, 1938, 1942, 1948, 1952, and 1957. The book evidently met a real need, for it was widely used throughout this country, and students abroad have benefitted from Spanish, Polish, Italian and Japanese translations.

In the 1950s and 1960s the electron microscope extended the range of visible structure down to the level of macromolecules, and autoradiography, immunohistochemistry, X-ray diffraction and other new methods rapidly expanded our knowledge of the structural basis of cell and organ function. Dr. Bloom asked me to join him in incorporating some of this new information into an 8th edition of the book, which was published in 1962 as the Bloom and Fawcett *Textbook of Histology*. Although Dr. Bloom's knowledge and wisdom have been greatly missed since his death in 1972, I have tried in the 10th and 11th editions to maintain the goals and standards he set.

The effort to understand complex living organisms by studying their smallest components has continued, and we are now in a period dominated by research on the molecular basis of cell function. A large fraction of contemporary research is now being done on cell lines that can be grown in tissue culture, on the questionable assumption that isolated cells function in vitro exactly as they do in association with other cell types in the more complex environment of the tissues and organs. Valuable biochemical information on the genome and the intracellular biosynthetic pathways is certainly being gained from such studies, but regrettably, the current preoccupation with the molecular level of cell organization has led some schools to shorten their courses in histology in order to make more curricular time available for courses in molecular biology and genetics. In other schools, the course in histology has been dropped and its content interwoven with that of pathology, physiology and clinical medicine in so-called integrated curricula. The demand for a large book on histology has therefore declined. At some time in the future, I believe that the pendulum will swing back from research on single cell types, isolated in vitro, and there will again be greater interest in the complex interactions of the many different cell types in their normal environment in whole animals. When this comes to pass, I hope this book will be a valuable reference for a generation of graduate students, postdoctoral fellows, and junior faculty who have mastered molecular biology but learned very little histology in their basic training.

I am very grateful to Dr. Elio Raviola who has participated in revision of the chapters on the immune system and the lymphoid organs, and to Dr. Jay Angevine who has thoroughly revised the chapter on the nervous system.

A TEXTBOOK OF HISTOLOGY

1 THE CELL

The living substance of plants and animals is described by the general term *protoplasm,* and the smallest unit of protoplasm capable of independent existence is the *cell.* The simplest plants and animals consist of a single cell. Higher animals can be thought of as a complex society of interdependent cells of many kinds that are specialized to carry out the functions essential for survival and reproduction of the animal as a whole. Cells serving the same general function are bound together by varying amounts of extracellular matrix to form *tissues* (bone, muscle, etc.). Two or more tissues are combined to form larger functional units called *organs* (skin, kidney, lung, etc.). Several organs having interrelated functions constitute an *organ system,* for example, the respiratory system (comprised of the nose, larynx, trachea, and lungs) or the urinary system (made up of the kidneys, ureters, urinary bladder, and urethra).

Although the term *histology* suggests that it is a branch of morphological science primarily concerned with the tissues, its province is much broader, encompassing the study of all of the many cell types and extracellular components of the body and the varying patterns in which the cells are associated to form the functional units of the organs. Histology can be considered synonymous with *microscopic anatomy.* Its limits were formerly defined by the resolving power of the light microscope, but the introduction of the electron microscope greatly extended the boundaries of the field. It now embraces the study of biological structure at all levels from the lower limit of direct visual inspection down to the structure of large molecules. The development of ingenious *histochemical* and *immunocytochemical* methods has made it possible to identify the intracellular sites of specific enzymatic activities and even to localize small peptides, and the antigenic portions of larger molecules, by their binding of specific antibodies that have been labeled to make them visible with the microscope. By such methods, certain functions can be localized in histological sections, or within intact cells, with greater precision than is possible with the disruptive techniques necessary for biochemical analysis.

THE CELL

There are hundreds of microscopically distinguishable cell types in the body, but all have certain structural features in common. This chapter describes the structural components of cells, in general, leaving an account of the distinctive identifying features of particular cell types to later chapters.

The cell is partitioned into two major compartments, the *nucleus* and the surrounding *cytoplasm,* which are easily distinguished by their form and staining characteristics. The formed components within these compartments are assigned to one of two categories, *organelles* or *inclusions,* based on certain assumptions as to their function. Organelles are components found in all cells and are considered to be *metabolically active* internal organs carrying out specific essential functions (Fig. 1–1). Inclusions, on the other hand, are *metabolically inert* accumulations of cell products, such as pigment deposits, or stored metabolites, such as lipid and carbohydrate. Organelles are regarded as essential, whereas inclusions are dispensable and often temporary constituents of cells. This distinction between organelles and inclusions is still useful, but assignment of cell components to these categories was made at a time when too little was known about their ultrastructure and function to make valid judgments as to whether they were metabolically active or inert, essential or dispensable. As our knowledge of cell biology has progressed, the list of cell organelles has lengthened and the traditional classification of some structures as inclusions has become debatable. For example, melanosomes, pigment granules formerly considered to be inert, have now been found to have a

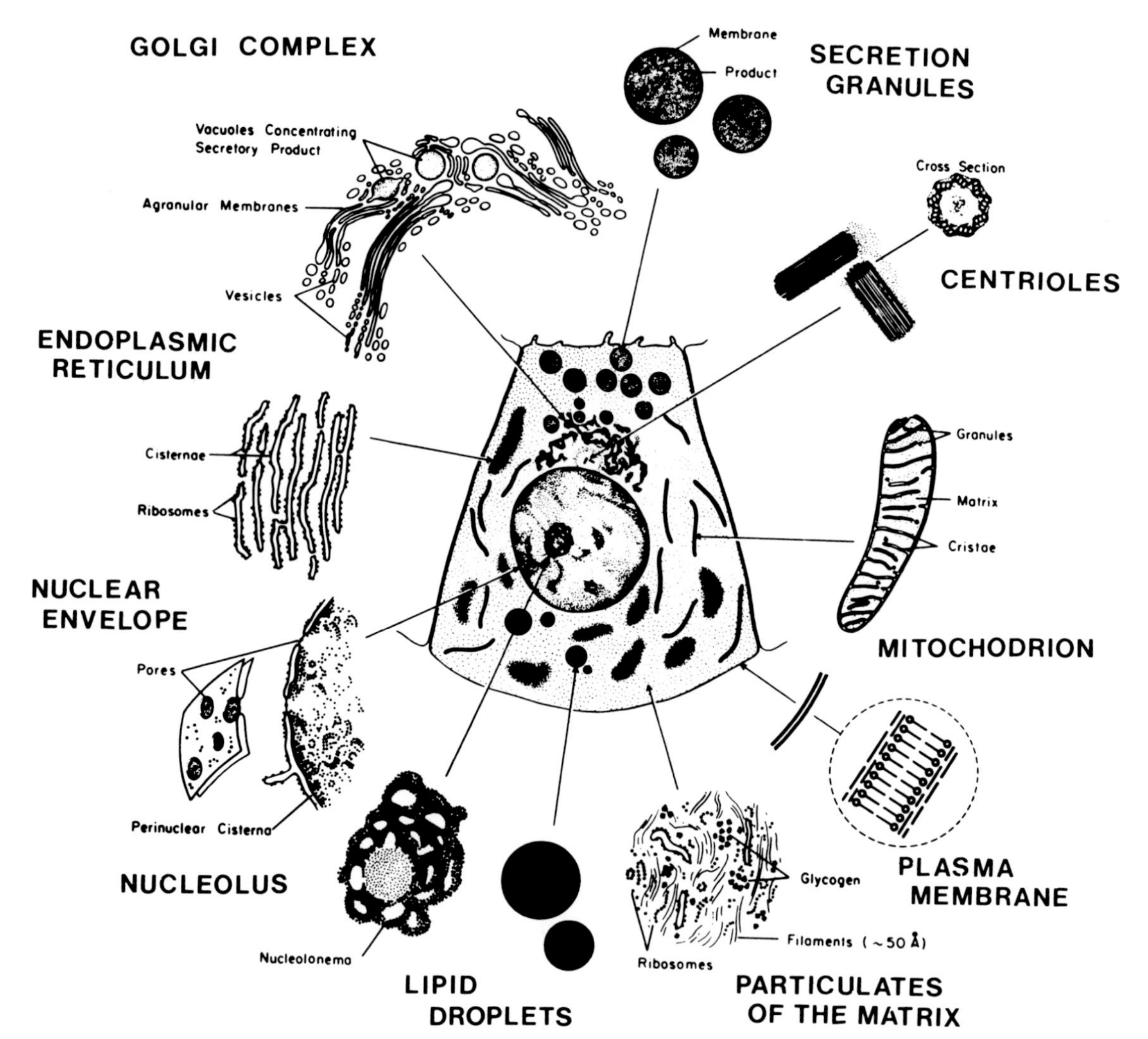

Figure 1–1. In the center, a depiction of the cell and its organelles as they appear with the light microscope. Around the periphery are drawings of the same components as these appear in electron micrographs. The substructure of the plasma membrane, encircled, is not directly visualized, but represents the bimolecular layer of phospholipids inferred from indirect methods of analysis.

highly organized internal structure and to have enzymatic activities that require their reclassification as an organelle. Similarly, secretory granules, formerly considered to be simply stores of cell product, are now found to be bounded by an enzymatically active membrane and, therefore, qualify as organelles.

The electron microscope has revealed a number of fibrillar elements in the cytoplasm that escaped detection with the light microscope. These are neither organelles nor inclusions, but are grouped together in a third category of cell components, the *cytoskeleton.*

The organelles visible with the light microscope (mitochondria, Golgi complex, ergastoplasm) were interpreted as solid granular or lamellar structures, but the electron microscope has shown that these, and newly described organelles, have a complex structure and all are bounded by membranes composed of lipid and protein. Most of the physiologically important processes take place at surfaces and interfaces, and the demonstration of the extensive compartmentation of the cytoplasm by membranes has been an important contribution of modern ultrastructural studies of the cell. The partitioning of the cytoplasm achieved by membrane-bounded organelles enhances the efficiency of countless chemical reactions by amplifying the area of the physiologically active interfaces within the cell. It also facilitates control of cell metabolism by enabling the cell to maintain a separation of enzymes and their substrates at some times, and, at other times, permitting their controlled interaction by varying the permeability of a particular membrane or the rate of active transport across it. If there were unlimited diffusion and interaction within the cell, it would be impossible to maintain the high degree of chemical heterogeneity characteristic of the cytoplasm. Enzymes would attack their substrates and all of the potential interactions of the countless chemical constituents of the cytoplasm would race out of control. This does not occur. The cell is able to regulate its metabolic processes and to hold in reserve a large repertoire of unexpressed biochemical reactions. It can activate each of these at the appropriate time and control its rate to conform to the varying needs of the whole organism. That this is possible is due in large measure to the segregation of biochemical processes in the membrane-bounded organelles of the cytoplasm.

CELL MEMBRANE

All cells are bounded by a *cell membrane* (plasma membrane, plasmalemma). This is not resolved in thin sections viewed with the light microscope, but in electron micrographs, it appears as a thin dense line, 8.5 to 10 nm in thickness around the periphery of the cell. Its appearance at low magnification gives no hint of the complexity of its molecular organization or the diversity of its functions. It contains local specializations for cell attachment and cell-to-cell communication. Its permeability properties permit diffusion of ions and gases in solution into and out of the cell, but prevent passive entry of most larger molecules.

In micrographs of high magnification, the membrane appears as two electron-dense lines (2.5–3.0 nm) separated by an electron-lucent intermediate zone (3.5–4.0 nm) (Fig. 1–2). Except for minor differences in thickness, all membranes of the cell have this same appearance. They consist of a bimolecular layer of mixed phospholipids with their hydrophilic portions at the outer and inner surfaces of the membrane and their hydrophobic chains projecting toward the middle of the bilayer. The two dense lines, seen in electron micrographs of osmium-fixed tissue, are due to deposition of the heavy metal in the hydrophilic ends of the phospholipid molecules, whereas the intervening pale zone represents their unstained hydrocarbon chains. Cholesterol and varying amounts of proteins, glycoproteins, and glycolipids are intercalated in the phospholipid bilayer (Fig. 1–3). The position of the integral proteins within the membrane depends on the location of hydrophilic and hydrophobic regions along the length of the molecule. The majority are transmembrane proteins that have nonpolar regions traversing the hydrophobic interior of the membrane and polar regions, at either end of the molecule, exposed on its outer and inner surfaces. The lipid bilayer behaves as a two-

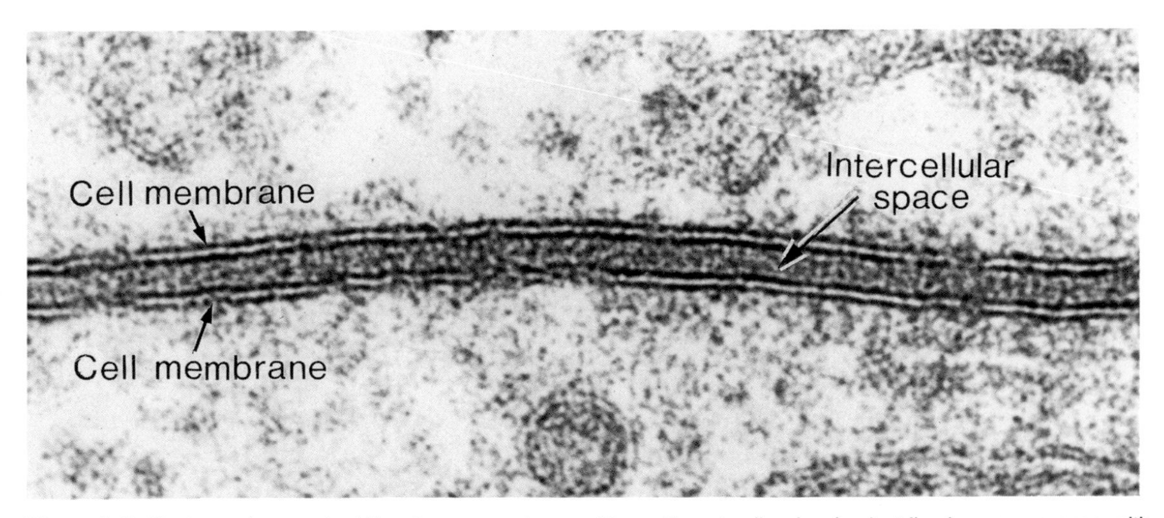

Figure 1–2. Electron micrograph of the plasma membrane of two adjacent cells, showing its trilaminar appearance, with two dense layers and a light intermediate layer. The intercellular space is occupied by material rich in carbohydrate, consisting, in part, of the glycocalyx of the apposed membranes.

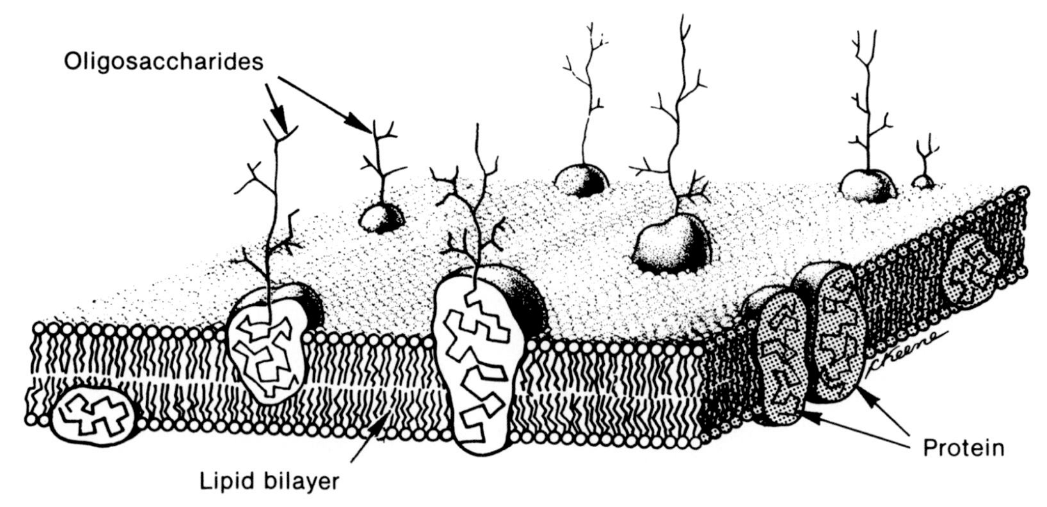

Figure 1–3. Schematic drawing of the fluid mosaic model of the cell membrane. Globular protein molecules are positioned in the lipid bilayer at different depths depending on the distribution of their hydrophilic and hydrophobic regions. Some extend through the bilayer (transmembrane proteins). The lipid bilayer is fluid and the integral proteins are free to diffuse laterally within the plane of the membrane if not resisted by binding to peripheral proteins in the underlying cytoplasm. Terminal oligosaccharides of the glycoproteins extend outward contributing to the surface coat or glycocalyx.

dimensional viscous solution, within which the proteins can move about if they are not bound to filaments in the underlying cytoplasm. The lipid constituents of the membrane are largely responsible for its form and its permeability properties, whereas receptors, ion pumps, and enzymatic activities reside in its proteins.

The integral proteins of the plasma membrane are not visible in electron micrographs of tissue sections, but they can be studied in tissues prepared by the freeze–fracture method. In this procedure, tissue is rapidly frozen in liquid Freon and then fractured under vacuum, by impact of a blade cooled to −196°C. The plane of fracture follows the path of least resistance through the hydrophobic region of the lipid bilayers and, thus, cleaves the membranes in half (Fig. 1–4). A replica of the exposed surface is then made by evaporation of a heavy metal, such as platinum, from a source at an acute angle to the fracture surface. Carbon is then deposited uniformly over this surface by evaporation from a separate electrode directly over the specimen, forming a stable replica of all irregularities on the fracture face. The tissue is then digested away and the replica is recovered for examination with the electron microscope.

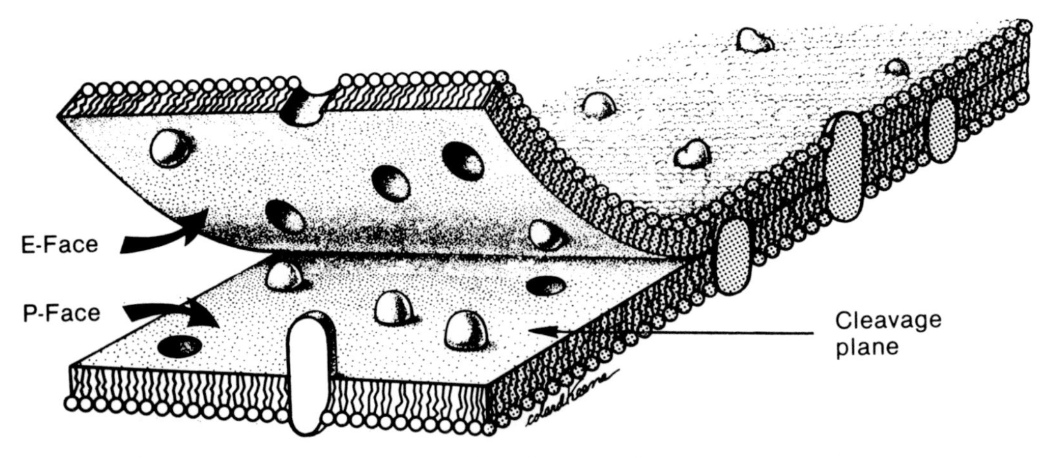

Figure 1–4. In the freeze–fracture method of study, the fracture plane follows the hydrophobic region of the membrane, exposing two fracture faces—the E-face, the inwardly facing outer half, and the P-face, the outwardly facing inner half, which usually contains the majority of the integral protein particles.

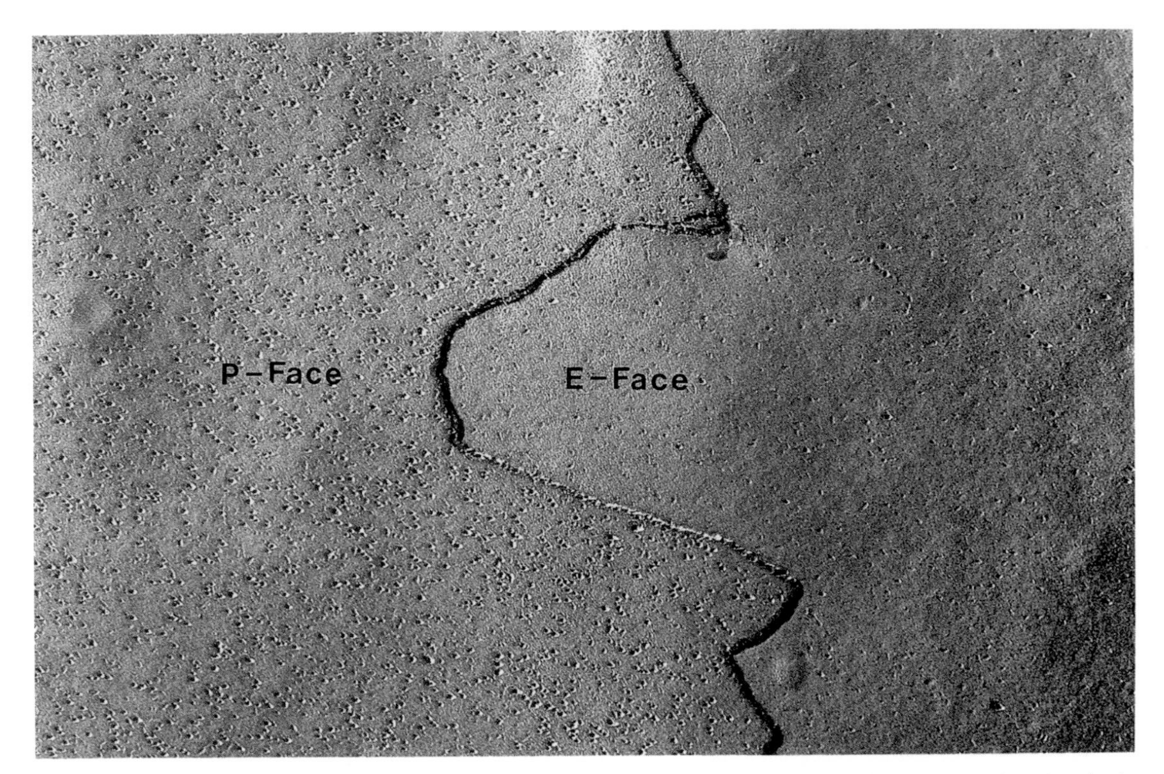

Figure 1–5. A freeze–fracture preparation of the plasma membrane of two adjacent cells. The fracture plane has broken across from one to the other, exposing the E-face of one and the P-face of the other.

In such preparations, the cleaved cell membrane presents two distinct appearances. The outwardly facing inner half-membrane, called the *P-face,* shows numerous randomly distributed 6–9-nm convexities that are replicas of the membrane proteins (Fig. 1–5). The inwardly directed outer half-membrane, called the *E-face,* is relatively smooth but may show shallow depressions, corresponding, in their distribution, to the convexities on the opposing P-face that represent the protein molecules of the membrane. In the various intracellular membranes, the concentration of particles observed by this method correlates well with the protein content of the same membranes as determined by biochemical analysis. Because many enzymes are membrane proteins, it is not surprising that the concentration of intramembrane particles is greater in organelles that have a high degree of metabolic activity.

The seemingly random distribution of particles within the plasma membrane gives a misleading impression of uniformity of membrane function over the entire cell. It is known, however, that the luminal, lateral, and basal membranes of epithelial cells differ in their enzymatic activities. Although the proteins are able to move laterally within the lipid bilayer, translocation of proteins from the apical to the basolateral domain of epithelial cells is prevented by a circumferential tight-junction between adjoining cells that constitutes a barrier to diffusion between these two domains, and therefore serves to maintain their distinctive properties. It is possible that movement of some transmembrane proteins is also prevented by their binding to cytoskeletal elements in the underlying cytoplasm.

The lipid bilayer is permeable to water, oxygen, nitrogen, and certain small uncharged polar molecules. It has very low permeability to larger uncharged molecules and to all charged molecules. Entry of these substances into cells depends on active transport by integral proteins of the membrane. Some of the transmembrane proteins transport glucose and amino acids; others form channels permitting passive diffusion of certain ions; and still others function as pumps, moving sodium, potassium, hydrogen, and calcium into and out of cells against a concentration gradi-

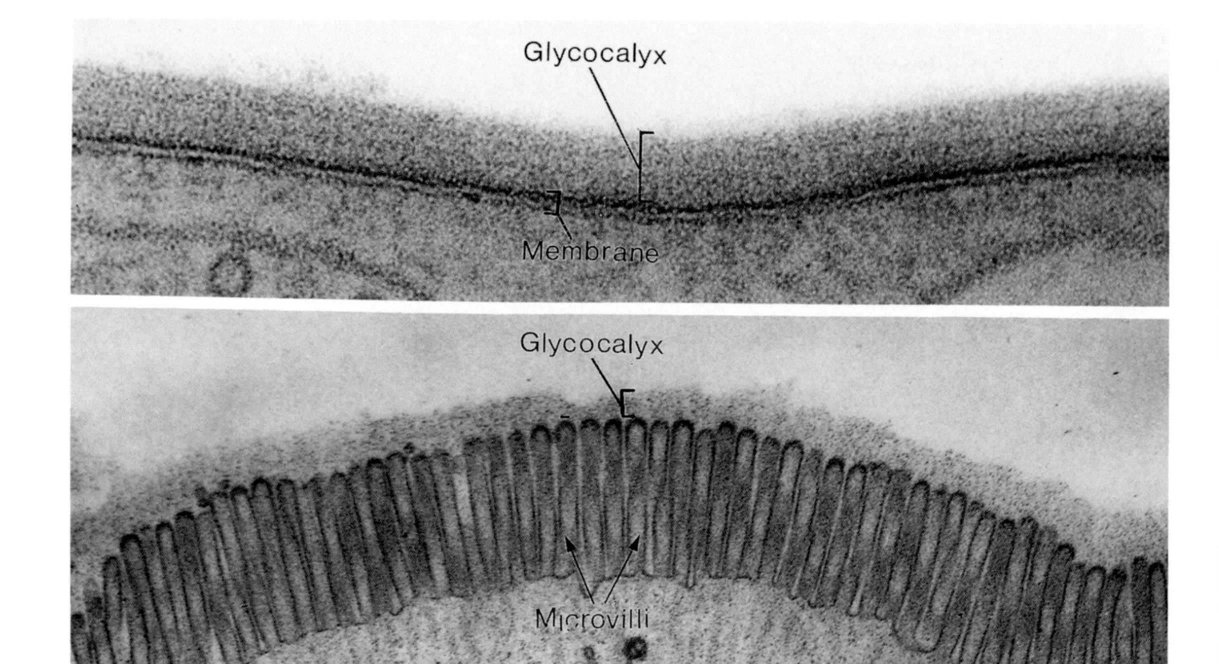

Figure 1–6. (A) A high-magnification micrograph of the plasma membrane and the unusually thick glycocalyx on an insect cell. (B) A low-magnification micrograph of the brush border of an intestinal epithelial cell, showing the glycocalyx on the tips of the microvilli.

ent. Such pumps maintain, in the cytoplasm, stable concentrations of ions that are essential for normal cell function.

Other transmembrane proteins are *receptors* that enable the cell to recognize and bind specific molecules. There are receptors for neurotransmitters, hormones, and certain essential nutrients. Receptors for the neurotransmitter, acetylcholine, contain an ion channel that opens upon ligand binding, and the resulting ion flux through the channel induces a response in the cell. Receptors for hormones form a complex that induces an associated membrane protein to generate a messenger molecule that diffuses into the cytoplasm to trigger the cells response. After ligand binding, other receptors for specific macromolecules needed by the cell aggregate into a small area of membrane that invaginates and pinches off, carrying the ligand into the cytoplasm in a small vesicle. This process, called *receptor-mediated endocytosis,* will be discussed more fully later in this chapter.

The membrane proteins include proteoglycans, molecules consisting of a core protein bearing multiple glucosaminoglycan side-chains that are linear polymers of disaccharide subunits. A lipophilic segment of the core protein spans the lipid bilayer, whereas the portion of the long molecule bearing the carbohydrate side-chains projects from the outer surface of the membrane. The carbohydrate-rich chains of many such molecules form a surface coat on the cell, called the *glycocalyx* (Fig. 1–6). Such a coat is present on all cells, but it is especially conspicuous on the coherent layer of cells that form the epithelium lining the gastrointestinal tract. In electron micrographs, the glycocalyx appears as a mat of delicate branching polysaccharide filaments. The chemical properties of this coat endow it with a high degree of selectivity with respect to the substances that can bind to the cell surface. Ionized carboxyl and sulfate groups on the polysaccharides have a strong negative charge and avidly bind cationic ferritin and the dyes Alcian-blue and ruthenium-red which are commonly used to stain the glycocalyx.

Organogenesis during embryonic life requires recognition and adhesion of like cells, and in postnatal life, immunological defenses require recognition between unlike cells. The specificity of these cell interactions may be provided by a stereochemical fit between complimentary molecules on membranes of the two cells. Carbohydrates offer a greater structural diversity for recognition than proteins. As few as four different monosaccharides can form very great numbers of distinct tetrasaccharides. Thus, the sequence of glycosidic subunits of the large polysaccharides projecting from the cell membranes can present an infinite variety of molecular configurations as a basis for cell recognition. Recent studies suggest that cell–cell recognition during histogenesis involves modulation of a relatively small number of integral membrane proteins now called *cell-adhesion molecules* (CAMs). An increasing number of these are being identified. Among them are, one for brain cells and muscle (N-CAM), one for liver cells (L-CAM), and one responsible for adhesion of glial cells to neurons (NG-CAM). These consist of a polypeptide chain linked to a carbohydrate such as sialic acid.

In addition to the widely distributed adhesion molecules that are of submicroscopic dimensions, there are local specializations of the membranes of epithelial cells for cell attachment or cell-to-cell communication. In these, membrane particles are closely aggregated to form distinct plaques or circumferential bands that are visible in micrographs of freeze–fracture preparations. These so-called *junctional complexes* will be discussed more fully in the following chapter on epithelia.

NUCLEUS

The nucleus, the largest organelle of the cell, is centrally situated and usually round or ellipsoidal, but, in some cell types, it may be deeply infolded or lobulated. In stained tissue sections, irregular clumps of *chromatin* of varying size may be scattered throughout the nucleoplasm, but they tend to adhere to the inner aspect of the nuclear membrane. Chromatin consists of nucleic acids and associated histone proteins that strongly bind hematoxylin and other basic dyes. The principal nucleic acid of chromatin *deoxyribonucleic acid* (DNA) can be specifically stained with the Feulgen reaction. A portion of the DNA that is inactive is *condensed,* and therefore stainable, whereas other portions that are being transcribed are in an *extended* state and are not visible with the microscope (Fig. 1–7). The nucleus also

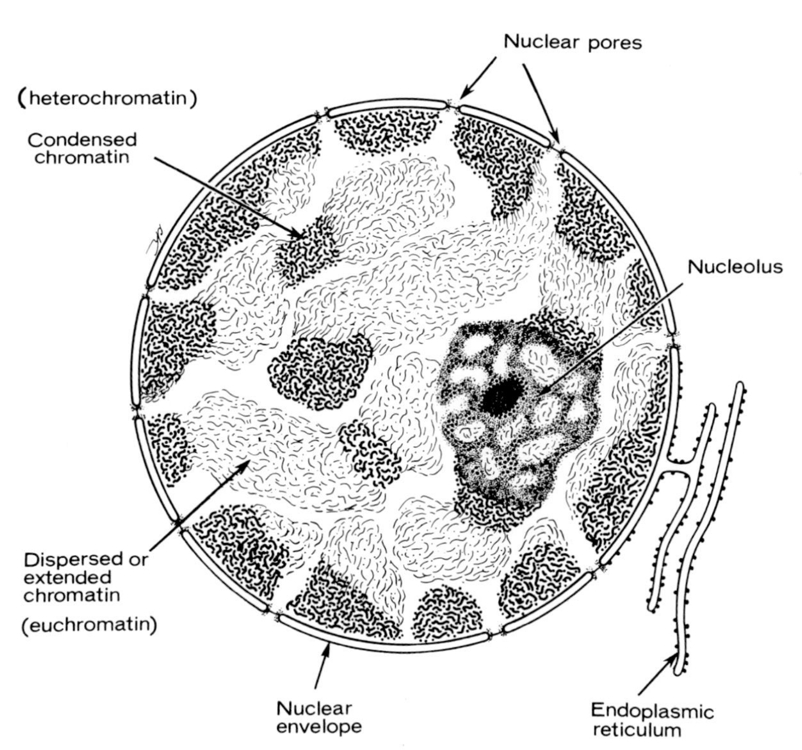

Figure 1–7. Schematic interpretation of the state of the chromatin in the interphase nucleus. The condensed portions of the chromosomes (heterochromatin) are relatively inactive. The extended or uncoiled segments (euchromatin) are the sites of active transcription. Also shown is the nuclear envelope consisting of a perinuclear cisterna which is often continuous with the endoplasmic reticulum in the cytoplasm.

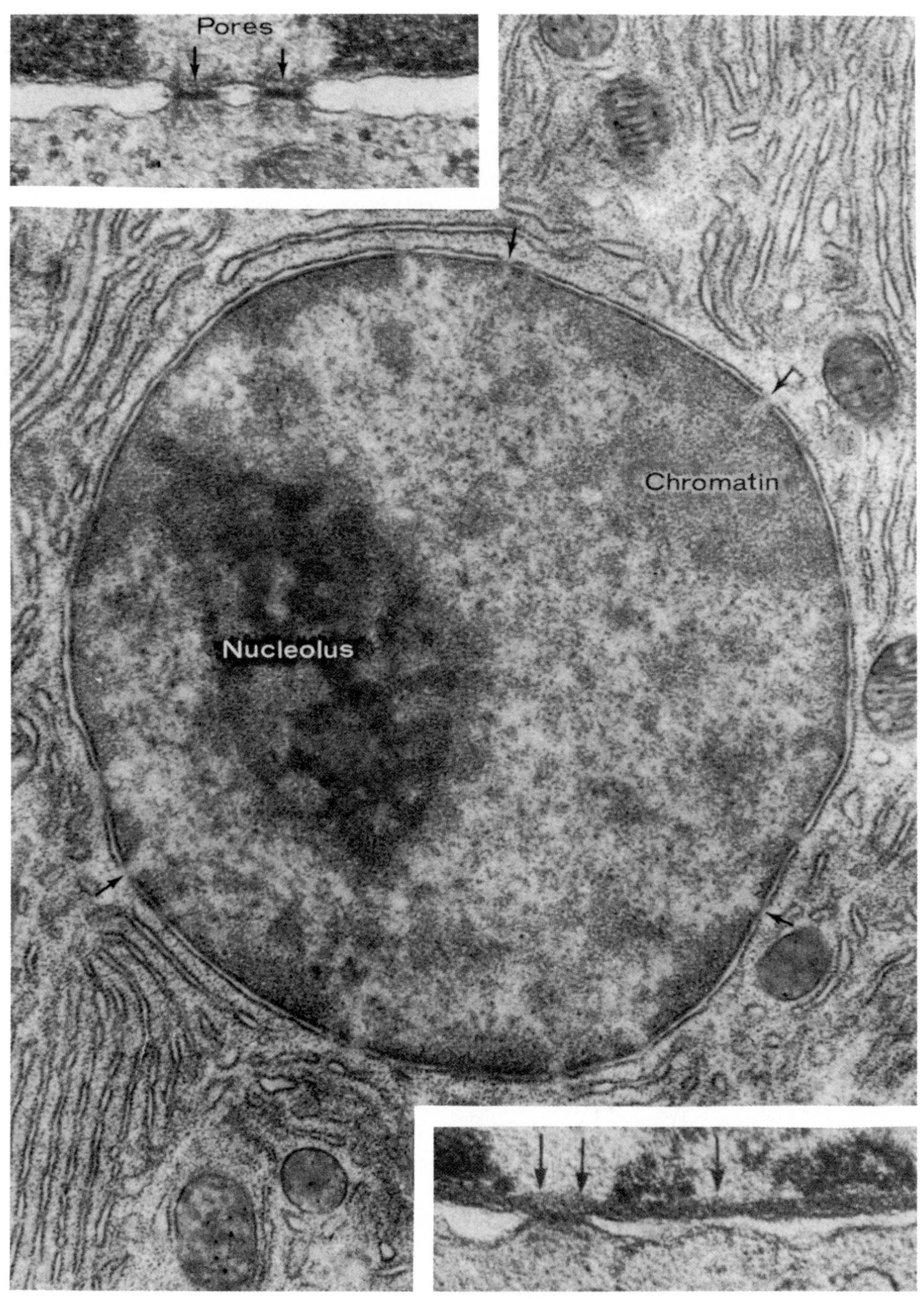

Figure 1–8. Micrograph of a typical nucleus showing a prominent nucleolus and large aggregations of heterochromatin against the nuclear membrane, which is traversed by pores (at arrows). Inset upper left: two nuclear pores and their pore diaphragms. Inset lower right: the fibrous lamina present on the inner aspect of the nuclear envelope.

contains one or two *nucleoli* that consist mainly of ribonucleoprotein and these are unstained by the Feulgen reaction.

The nucleus is the archive of the cell, the repository of its genetic material. Encoded in the sequence of nucleotides in its long DNA molecules is the information necessary for synthesis of all of the integral proteins and the secretory products of the cell. The synthetic activities of the cell are directed by informational macromolecules formed on the template of DNA in the nucleus and transported to the cytoplasm to direct protein synthesis.

NUCLEAR ENVELOPE

The nucleus is bounded by a *nuclear envelope* that participates in the organization of the chromatin and controls the movement of macromolecules between the nucleoplasm and the surrounding cytoplasm. Its structure was not resolved with the light microscope but it was assumed to be a membrane. The electron microscope reveals that it consists of two parallel membranes separated by a 10–30-nm space, the *perinuclear cisterna*. The outer membrane may have small granules (ribosomes) adhering to its outer surface and it is often continuous with membrane-bounded tubular elements extending throughout the cytoplasm (the endoplasmic reticulum). At many sites around the circumference of the nucleus, the inner and outer membranes of the nuclear envelope are continuous with one another, around circular *nuclear pores* that serve as avenues of communication between the nucleoplasm and the cytoplasm (Fig. 1–8). The pores are not always uniformly distributed (Fig. 1–9), and their number varies from a few dozen to several thousand in cell types that are metabolically very active.

In thin sections, the pores appear to be closed by a thin *pore diaphragm* (Fig. 1–8, inset). Negatively stained preparations of the isolated nuclear envelope reveal several nonmembranous structures associated with the pores. Attached to the membrane at the inner

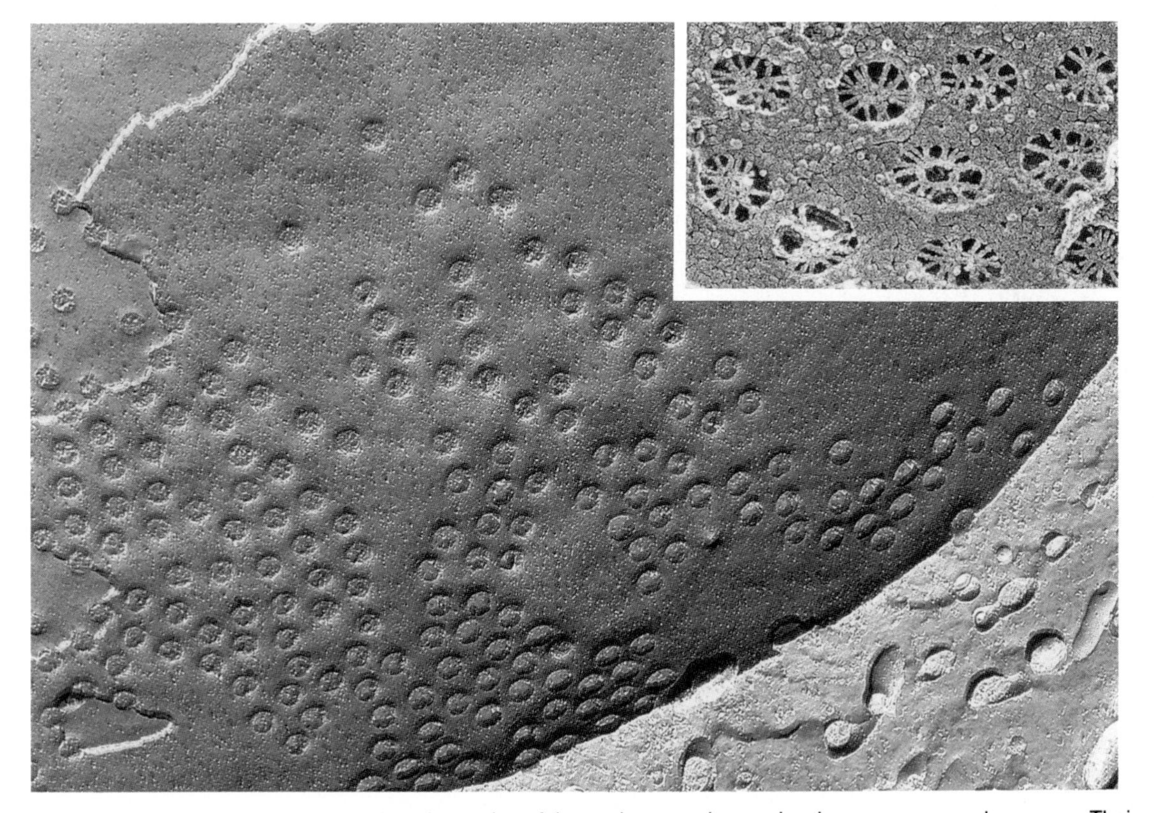

Figure 1–9. A freeze–fracture preparation of a portion of the nuclear membrane showing numerous nuclear pores. Their number and distribution changes as the cell differentiates or changes its activity. (D.W. Fawcett and H.E. Chemes. 1979. Tissue and Cell 11:147). Inset: nuclear pores as they appear with a different method of preparation (courtesy of E. Bearer and L. Orci).

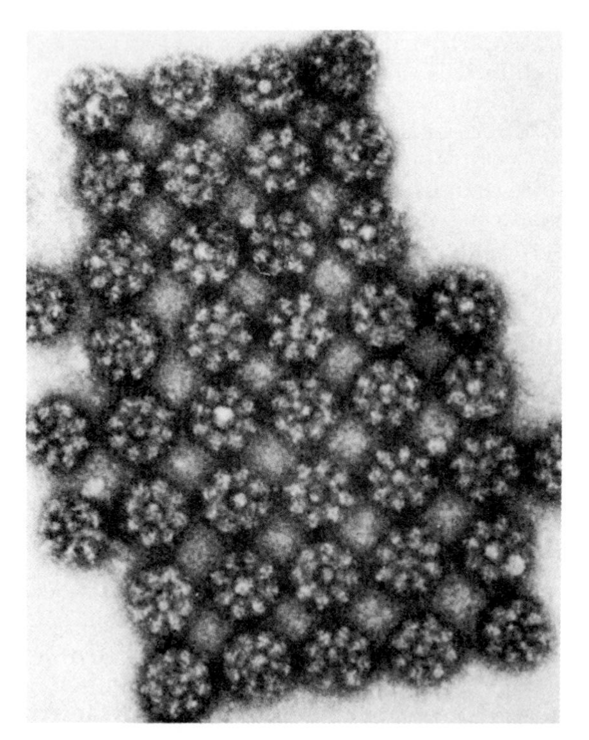

Figure 1–10. Negatively stained preparation of the nuclear pore complexes isolated from an amphibian oocyte (P.N.T. Unwin. 1982. J. of Cell Biol. 93:63.

and outer rims of the pore are particles arranged in two distinct coaxial rings, about 120 nm in diameter. Each ring is composed of eight subunits 15–20 nm in diameter (Figs. 1–10 and 1–11). Projecting inward from these subunits are eight radially arranged *spokes* that converge at what appears to be a *central granule* or *plug*. The eight subunits of the rings, their radial spokes, and connecting links form a structural framework that imposed on the pore an octagonal symmetry around an axis perpendicular to the plane of the nuclear envelope. The term *nuclear pore complex* is now used to include both the membranous and nonmembranous constituents of this structure. The spokes and central granule are evidently responsible for the specious appearance of a pore diaphragm in micrographs of low magnification. The central granule and the radial spokes are obviously the principal barrier to movement through the pores, but the complex seems to have a central channel that acts as a molecular sieve with an effective diameter of 10 nm.

In the two-way traffic between nucleoplasm and cytoplasm, molecules less than 10 nm in diameter pass through the pores by passive diffusion, but larger molecules require an energy-dependent transport mechanism. Newly synthesized proteins that enter the nucleus, and ribonucleoproteins that leave it, are of a size that would require an opening 20 nm or more in diameter. Transport of such molecules appears to depend on their possession of a signal sequence of amino acids that targets them to the nuclear envelope. It is speculated that binding of the signal sequence to the nuclear pores may trigger opening of the channel from 10 nm to more than 20 nm to permit mediated transport of such large molecules. Much remains to be learned about how this gating of the pores works. If a monoclonal antibody to the nuclear pore complex is injected into the cytoplasm, it completely inhibits nucleocytoplasmic transport of ribosomal and transport RNAs, but does not interfere with diffusion of small molecules. Three glycoproteins, designated *nucleoporins,* have been identified as components of the pore complex, but their exact location and function in facilitating transport remain unclear. A lectin that binds to one of these nucleoporins completely inhibits transport into the nucleus.

A continuous meshwork of fine filaments is interposed between the inner nuclear mem-

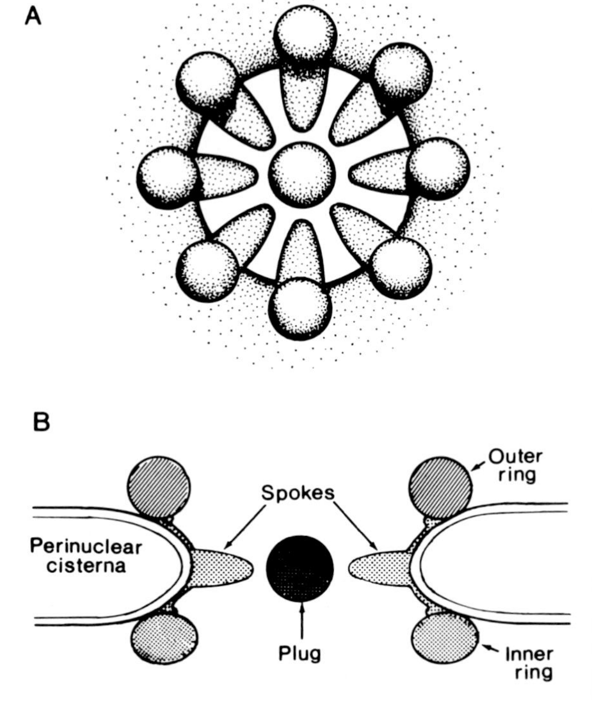

Figure 1–11. Diagrammatic representation of the nuclear pore complex (A) viewed from the cytoplasmic surface and (B) in thin sections. The nuclear lamina on the inner surface of the envelope is not depicted.

brane and the peripheral heterochromatin (Fig. 1–8, inset). This *nuclear lamina* varies in thickness (30–100 nm) in different cell types, and in the same cell type in different species, but it seems to be a ubiquitous adjunct to the nuclear envelope. Its filaments are polymers of polypeptides called *lamins* that range in mass from 60 to 75 kilodaltons (kD). *A-type* and *B-type* lamins are distinguished on the basis of their location and chemical properties. Those of the A-type are located mainly on the inner aspect of the nuclear lamina. The B-type predominate near its outer surface and are responsible for its binding to integral membrane proteins that are specific to the inner nuclear membrane.

When the nuclear envelope disintegrates during cell division, the lamins are disassembled into monomeric form, permitting nuclear membrane dissolution. At telephase of mitosis, reconstruction of the nuclear membrane takes place by fusion of membrane-limited vesicles that are adherent to the telophase chromosomes. The concurrent self-assembly of the lamins into a continuous nuclear lamina plays an important role in this process. If antibodies to lamins are injected into cells during mitosis, the daughter cells are able to complete cytokinesis but are not able to form normal nuclei. The chromatin remains condensed and inactive and nucleoli are not reconstituted. Thus, it appears that the lamins are involved in the functional organization of the interphase nucleus.

CHROMATIN

Deoxyribonucleic acid (DNA), the genetic material of the nucleus, resides in the chromosomes. These are not identifiable, as such, in the nondividing *interphase nucleus,* but in cells preparing to divide, they become visible as basophilic rod-like or thread-like structures 3–6 μm in length and 0.5–0.8 μm in diameter. During reconstitution of the nucleus after cell division, some segments of the chromosomes remain condensed and are visible as clumps of chromatin at the periphery (Fig. 1–8). Other segments of the chromosomes become uncoiled and dispersed in the nucleoplasm. In this loosely packed state, the DNA and associated protein have little affinity for basic dyes and in electron micrographs are indistinguishable from other granular or flocculent components of the nucleoplasm. The stainable, electron-dense portions of the interphase chromosomes constitute the *heterochromatin* of the nucleus, whereas the dispersed portions that are not microscopically identifiable are the *euchromatin.* Only a fraction of the total complement of units of heredity (genes) is actively involved, at any given time, in directing protein synthesis. This portion is in the euchromatin, whereas the *genes* that are not being expressed are in the heterochromatin. The numerous cell types in the body differ greatly in their synthetic activities and, accordingly, in the proportion of their DNA that is in the active extended form. The pattern of heterochromatin in the nucleus, therefore, differs from cell type to cell type and provides one of the criteria for cell-type identification.

The appearance of chromatin in histological sections gives no hint of the high degree of order that would be expected from genetic considerations, and progress in understanding its organization has been relatively recent. In electron micrographs of thin sections, heterochromatin seems to be made up of closely packed 20–30-nm subunits, but whether these are small granules or cross sections of highly convoluted fibrils is not apparent. However, if isolated nuclei are disrupted and their content spread on the surface of water, the dispersed chromatin can be picked up on specimen grids, dried, and examined directly with the electron microscope. In such preparations, the chromatin appears as a tangle of 30-nm fibrils. With higher shearing forces, these can be further extended, and then they appear as a beaded strand of regularly spaced discoid subunits, called *nucleosomes,* connected by a thin filament 4 nm in diameter (Fig. 1–12). More detailed analysis is beyond the reach of microscopy and has depended on X-ray crystallographic and biochemical studies. These have identified the thin filament connecting the nucleosomes as a double-stranded DNA molecule and have shown that the core of the nucleosome is an octomer of two molecules each, of four histones (H_4, H_3, H_2A, and H_2B). A segment of the DNA molecule is coiled around each nucleosome with straight spacer segments of DNA, of varying length, between successive nucleosomes (Fig. 1–13). An additional histone H_1, is associated with the connecting segments of the DNA molecule. In condensed chromatin of the intact cell nucleus, the beaded filaments are believed to be helically coiled to form the 30-nm fibrils. The granular appearance of heterochromatin in electron micrographs is probably attribut-

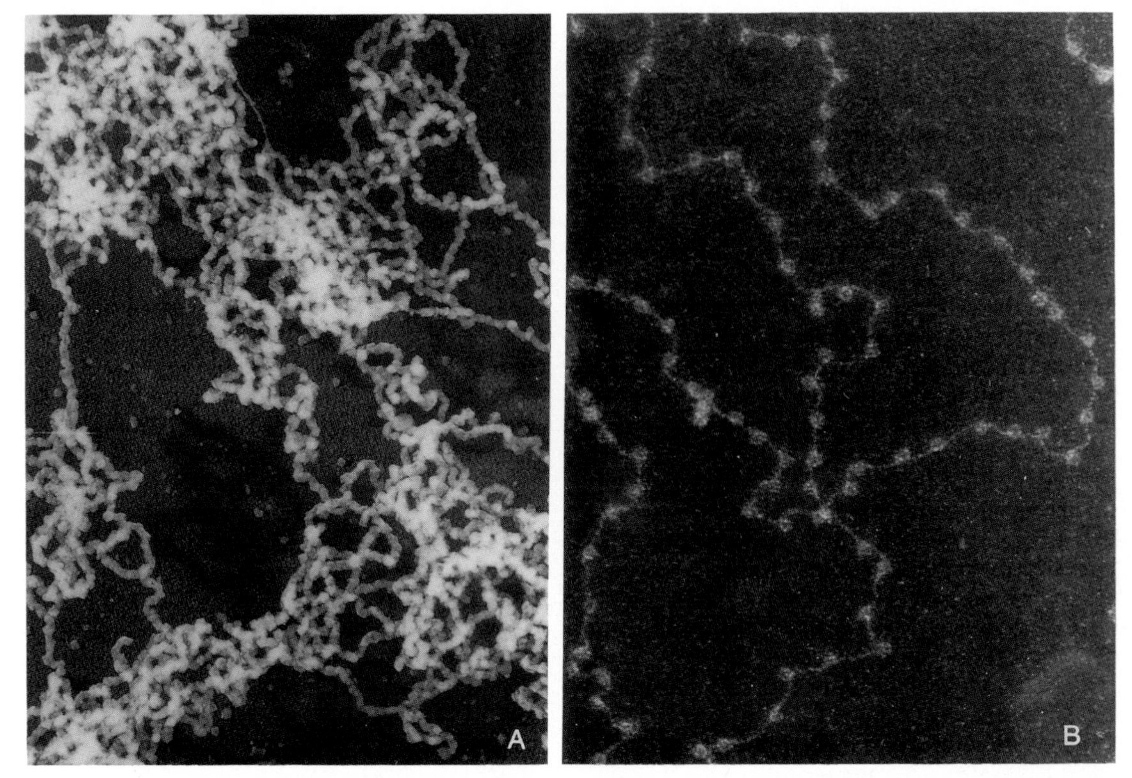

Figure 1–12. (A) Chromatin from a salamander erythrocyte, spread on water, fixed in formalin, critical-point dried, and shadowed with carbon-platinum. It appears as a tangled mass of 20–30-nm fibrils (Micrograph courtesy of H.Ris). (B) If chromatin fibrils are extended sufficiently by shear forces, the fibrils uncoil and appear as delicate beaded strands of nucleosomes connected by segments of double-stranded DNA. (Micrograph courtesy of A. Olins.)

able to closely packed transverse and oblique sections of these fibrils. The configuration of the euchromatin is largely conjectural, but it is assumed that in these portions of the chromosomes, the 30-nm fibrils have uncoiled and extended, exposing the DNA to facilitate expression of its genes.

In dividing cells, all of the chromatin condenses and is organized into a number of chromosomes that is characteristic of each animal species. Electron micrographs of thin sections provide little insight into their substructure, but when isolated from cells in division and studied in whole mounts, chromosomes are found to be made up of a 30-nm fibril forming closely spaced loops arranged radially around an axial scaffold of structural protein (Fig. 1–14). The fibril is thought to be formed by supercoiling of the 10-nm coiled filament of DNA and nucleosomes observed in dissociated chromatin from interphase nuclei. If isolated chromosomes are treated with dextran sulfate and heparin to extract the histones, the 30-nm fibril straightens, uncoils, and spreads in a broad halo around the axial scaffold. Examined at high magnification, this halo appears as an elaborate labyrinthine pattern traced by a continuous, highly tortuous 4-nm filament of DNA, devoid of associated nucleosomes (Fig. 1–15).

The DNA molecule consists of two polynucleotide chains intertwined in an antiparallel double helix. Each strand is a linear polymer of nucleotide subunits, each of which consists of a phosphate group, a pentose sugar (deoxyribose), and an organic base. The bases are of four kinds: adenine, cytosine, guanine, and thymidine. These project toward, and are linked to, complementary bases on the other strand. The genetic information in the DNA molecule is encoded in the sequence of bases along the polynucleotide chains. The unit of heredity, the *gene,* is a sequence of bases in the DNA that contain the information necessary for the synthesis of a nucleic acid or a protein. In directing protein synthesis, this information is first *transcribed* from DNA to a *messenger ribonucleic acid* (mRNA), which is a linear polymer of the nucleotides adenylate, cytodylate, guanylate, or urodylate. Along the

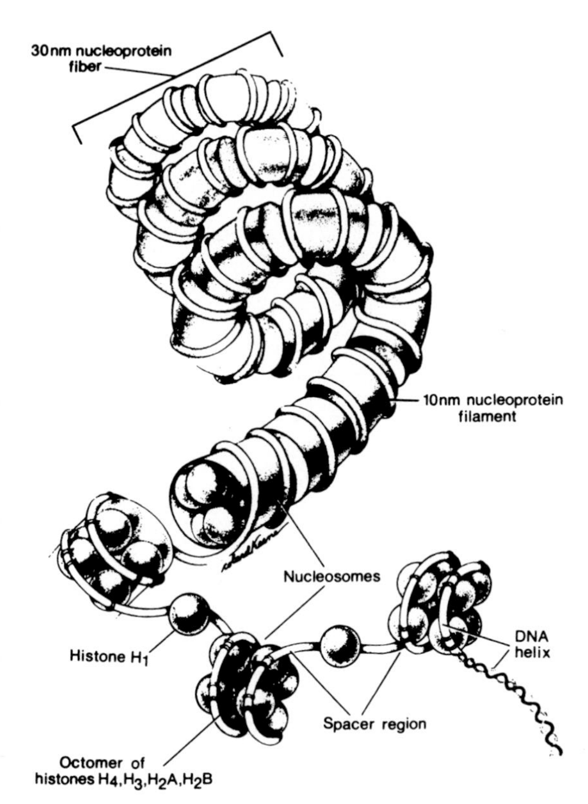

Figure 1–13. Diagram of a 30-nm chromatin fiber showing its postulated helical structure around a central channel. In the lower part of the figure, the fiber is drawn out to maximal extension to illustrate the nucleosome core of histones with the RNA double helix wrapped around it. Successive nucleosomes are joined by spacer segments of DNA and their associated histones. (Redrawn after R. Bradbury. 1978. La Recherche 9:644; and A. Worcel and C. Benyaj. 1978. Cell 12:88 from Amer. Scientist 66:704).

length of the mRNA molecule, specific sets of three successive nucleotides, called *codons,* designate each of the 20 amino acids that are the building blocks of proteins. Messenger RNA is transported to the cytoplasm for *translation,* in which the sequence of its nucleotides determines the order in which amino acids are assembled in the synthesis of a specific protein. Two other ribonucleic acids, *ribosomal ribonucleic acid* (rRNA) and *transfer ribonucleic acid* (tRNA) are transcribed in the nucleus and transported to the cytoplasm to play essential roles in protein synthesis that will be discussed later.

Each chromosome is believed to contain a single very long molecule of DNA. The total length of the DNA in the human diploid genome is estimated to be 1.8 m, containing 10^8 to 3×10^8 nucleotide base pairs. The several orders of coiling and supercoiling described above achieve nearly a 10,000-fold reduction in length, making it possible to pack a very large amount of genetic information into a nucleus that is only 6 μm in diameter. How this orderly process of DNA compaction is controlled at each cell division, so as to maintain a consistent chromosomal form and the same arrangement of genes along their length, still defies explanation.

NUCLEOLUS

The nucleolus is visible in the living cell as a rounded refractile body usually eccentrically placed in the nucleus. In histological sections, it is deeply stained by basic dyes due to its content of ribonucleoprotein. It is usually unreactive with the Feulgen reaction for deoxyribonucleoprotein, but it is often surrounded by an intensely stained rim of *nucleolus-associated chromatin.* In electron micrographs, the nucleolus appears as a three-dimensional network of anastomosing dense strands, bounding electron-lucid interstices that are occupied by material indistinguishable from the surrounding nucleoplasm. This network, called the *nucleolonema* or *pars granulosa,* is made up of 15-nm ribonucleoprotein particles in a matrix of fine filaments. Rounded areas with a lower density and a fibrillar texture are found at two or more sites within the nucleolus (Fig.

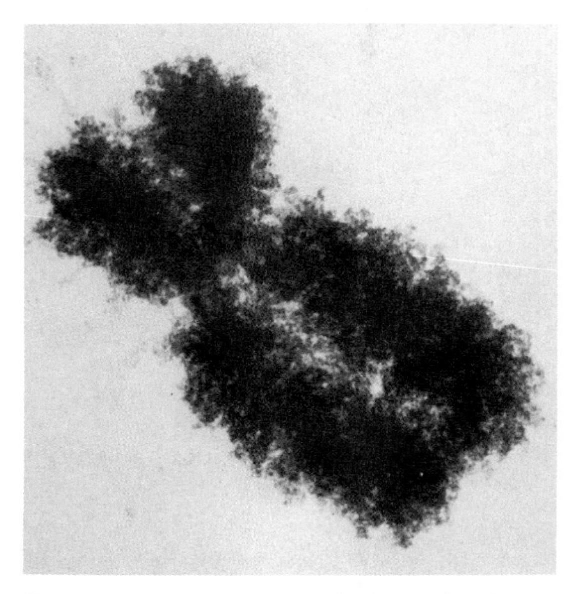

Figure 1–14. Electron micrograph of unsectioned metaphase chromosome from a cultured cell showing the chromatids, primary constriction, and what appear to be closely packed loops of filaments radially arranged around the long axis of the chromatids. (Micrograph courtesy of H. Ris.)

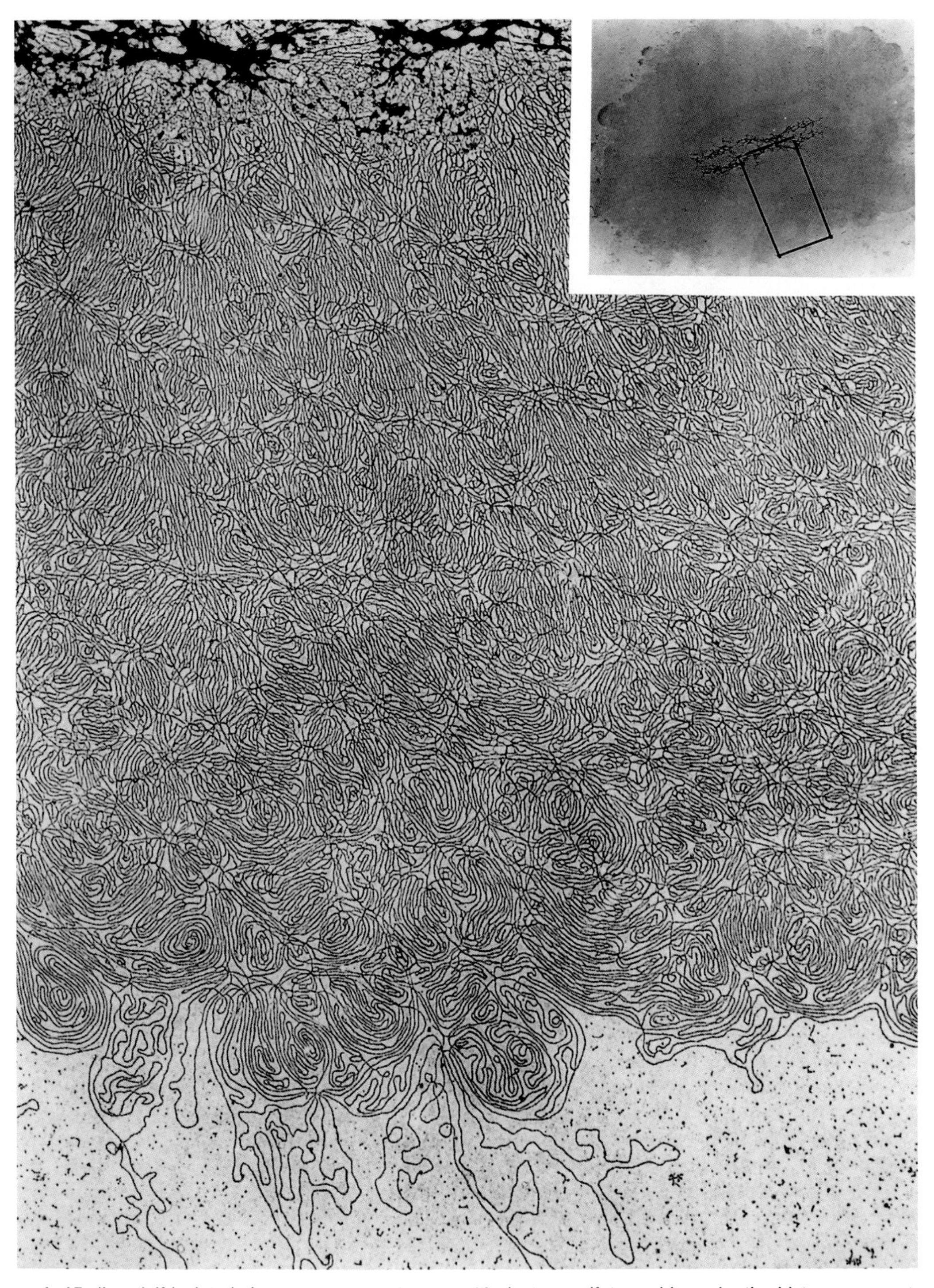

Figure 1–15. (Inset) If isolated chromosomes are treated with dextran sulfate and heparin, the histones are extracted, permitting the DNA to uncoil, forming a broad halo around the core structural proteins. If an area such as that in the rectangle is examined at higher magnification, the halo is revealed as a labyrinthine pattern of 4-nm filaments of DNA. (Micrograph from J.R. Paulsen and U.K. Laemmli. 1977. Cell 12:817).

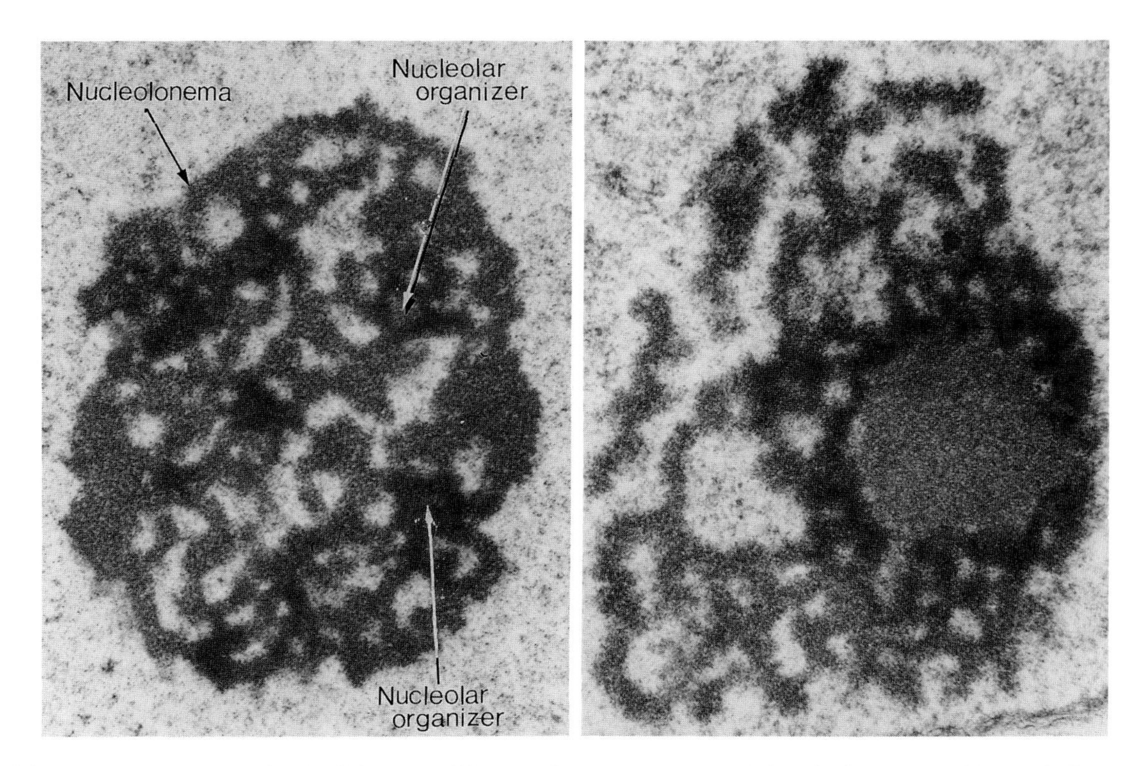

Figure 1–16. Examples of nucleoli from two different cell types, showing variations in the pattern of the nucleolonema and in the number and size of the nucleolar organizer regions.

1–16). These so-called *fibrillar centers* contain the *nucleolar-organizer regions* of those chromosomes possessing nucleolar genes. Immediately surrounding each of these paler areas is a rim of electron-dense filaments referred to as the *pars fibrosa* or *dense fibrillar component* of the nucleolus. The size of the nucleolus and the pattern of its nucleolonema may differ considerably from one cell type to another and in different functional states of the same cell type. It is largest in cells that are very active in protein synthesis.

Nucleolar genes code for *ribosomal RNA* and it appears that their transcription occurs in the fibrillar centers of the nucleolus, whereas the early steps in the processing of RNA-precursor molecules and RNA-protein assembly takes place in the surrounding dense fibrillar component. The resulting ribonucleoprotein particles accumulate in the pars granulosa, where later steps of maturation of the ribosomal subunits are carried out. The ribosomal proteins are believed to be synthesized in the cytoplasm and targeted to their intranuclear site of assembly by nuclear-localization-signal sequences on the molecules. The completed ribosomal subunits are then transported through the nuclear pores into the cytoplasm where they carry out their function.

Most of the events described above are not accessible to morphological study, but it has been possible to isolate from amphibian oocytes DNA-containing transcriptionally active nucleolar genes. In a remarkable electron micrograph of such a preparation (Fig. 1–17), one can see multiple RNA-precursor molecules radiating from the isolated segment of the genome in a Christmas-tree-like configuration, with the transcripts quite short near the start and steadily progressing to full-length completed molecules at the other end.

The nucleolus disappears during cell division and is reformed in the daughter cells during reconstruction of their nuclei. Nucleoli initially develop from each of several, nucleolus-organizing regions in the set of chromosomes, but their subsequent coalescence usually reduces the number of nucleoli in the interphase nucleus to one or two, but larger numbers may be found in polyploid cells.

The protein synthetic activities of the cytoplasm are dependent on the functional integrity of the nucleolus. Its destruction by a laser beam results in cessation of incorporation of RNA precursors into the ribosomes on which protein synthesis depends. In a mutant of the African clawed fog *Xenopus,* which lacks nucleoli, embryonic development is arrested

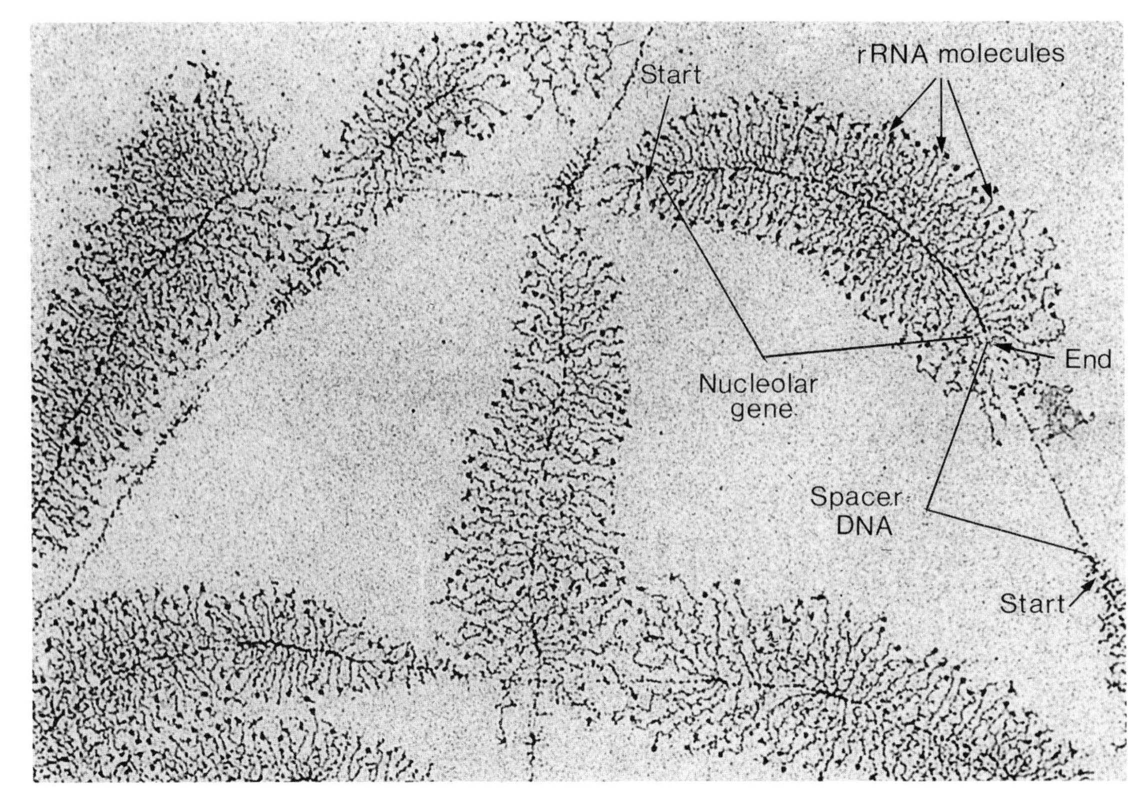

Figure 1–17. Micrograph of a dissociated amphibian nucleolar core, showing rRNA–precursor molecules radiating from nucleolar genes. (Micrograph courtesy of O. Miller and C. Beatty. 1969. Science 164:164).

at a very early stage due to the inability of the cells to synthesize rRNA.

NUCLEAR MATRIX

Considerable progress has been made in studying isolated condensed chromosomes, but relatively little is known about the form and disposition of the chromosomes in the interphase nucleus. It has been suggested that there may be a karyoskeletal network of fibrils in the interior of the nucleus on which the chromosomes are arranged. After deoxyribonuclease digestion of the chromatin from resinless sections, and extraction with nonionic detergents, a network of relatively thick fibrils, coated with adherent residues of the nucleoplasm, has been reported. Further treatment with high-ionic strength salt solutions strips away adherent material and leaves behind a network of thin, branching, 8–10-nm filaments composed of RNA and protein. The view has been advanced that the chromosomes, and other components of the nucleoplasm, may be organized around these *core filaments*. However, it is possible that the network revealed may be a product of the procedures required for its demonstration and not a true reflection of the architecture of the nucleoplasm in vivo. The notion of an internal karyoskeleton anchored to the fibrous lamina at the periphery of the nucleus has not gained general acceptance.

CYTOPLASM

The principal metabolic activities and the various specialized functions of the cell are carried out in its extranuclear portion, the *cytoplasm,* which contains several kinds of *cell organelles* that carry out different functions that are essential to cell metabolism. The majority of the organelles are membrane-bounded elements that have a highly characteristic form and internal structure. They are suspended in a semifluid cytoplasmic matrix called the *cytosol.* A coarse network, consisting of bundles of fine filaments that traverse the cytoplasm and attach to the cell membrane, provide internal support and help to maintain the normal shape of the cell. These, together with slender straight microtubules, constitute the *cytoskeleton*. We proceed now to a description of the cell organelles.

ENDOPLASMIC RETICULUM

In the cytoplasm of nearly all cell types, there is an extensive system of membrane-bounded canaliculi called the *endoplasmic reticulum*. This organelle is not ordinarily visible in histological sections, but if intact cells in tissue culture are stained with a lipophilic, nonionic, fluorescent dye, it appears as a lace-like network throughout the cytoplasm (Fig. 1–18). Its continuity is less evident in electron micrographs of thin sections, where it is represented by branching tubular profiles of varying length. The tubules may be locally expanded into broad flat saccules called *cisternae* (Fig. 1–19). These are often closely spaced in parallel arrays (Fig. 1–20).

Two morphologically and functionally distinct regional differentiations of the organelle are identified: the *rough endoplasmic reticulum* bearing small dense particles on the outer surface of its limiting membrane; and the *smooth endoplasmic reticulum,* which lacks adherent particles. The two forms are continuous, but their relative proportions vary in different cell types. The rough or granular reticulum is most abundant in glandular cells that secrete protein. The 20–25-nm particles associated with the rough form of endoplasmic reticulum are called *ribosomes*. Despite their small size, they are complex structures consisting of ribonucleic acid and 20 or more proteins. At high magnifications, a larger and a smaller subunit can be resolved in each ribosome, and it is the larger subunit that is bound to the membrane of the reticulum. Clusters of ribosomes are also found free in the cytoplasmic matrix. Both bound and free ribosomes are sites where amino acids are assembled in the synthesis of proteins. To carry out this function, the ribosomes must be associated with a molecule of *messenger RNA* (mRNA) which contains the information determining the sequence in which the amino acids are assembled to form polypeptides. Ribosomes usually occur in clusters of 10 or more linked together by their common attachment to a long molecule of mRNA. Such units of several ribo-

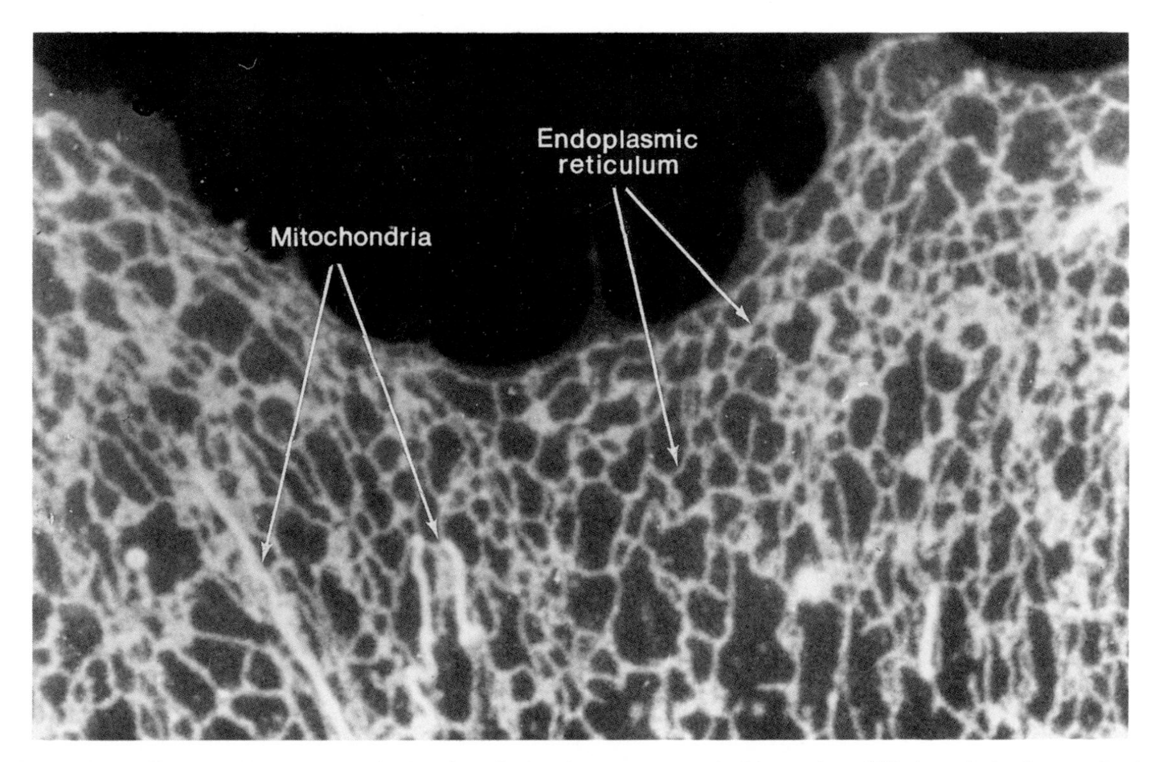

Figure 1–18. The continuity of the endoplasmic reticulum is not apparent in thin sections. This is a photomicrograph of a portion of a thin intact tissue culture cell stained with a lipophilic cationic fluorescent dye. The reticulum appears as a lace-like network of tubular elements. (Photomicrograph courtesy of M. Teresaki.)

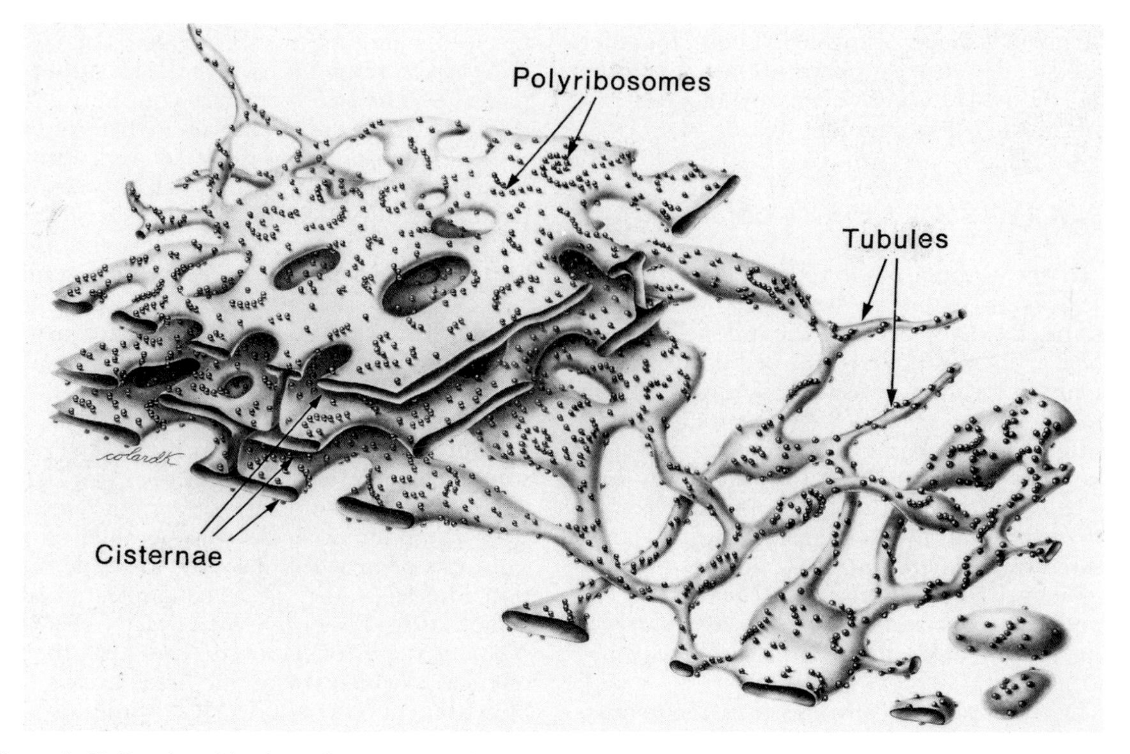

Figure 1–19. Drawing of the three-dimensional configuration of the rough endoplasmic reticulum. It consists of branching and anastomosing tubular elements and expanded saccules called cisternae. Polyribosomes occur in spirals or rosettes on the outer surface of its limiting membrane.

somes bound to the same strand of mRNA are called *polyribosomes* or *polysomes.* As amino acids are added to their ends, the forming polypeptide chains elongate vectorially from the larger subunit of each ribosome, extending through the underlying membrane of the rough endoplasmic reticulum and into its lumen. When the polypeptides have attained their full length, they are released from their respective ribosomes and are then free within the rough endoplasmic reticulum (RER). Small vesicles containing the newly synthesized protein pinch off from the endoplasmic reticulum and are transported to a second organelle, the Golgi complex, where they are concentrated and packaged into secretory granules for export from the cell. All intrinsic proteins of the cytoplasm and nucleoplasm are also synthesized on polyribosomes either on the reticulum or free in the cytoplasmic matrix. The intracellular pathway taken by secretory proteins will be considered in greater detail in a later chapter, Glands and Secretion.

Most of our knowledge of the mechanisms of protein synthesis has been based on biochemical studies on centrifugal fractions of homogenized cells. The cell fraction principally involved was found to be the *microsome fraction,* which consisted of vesicular fragments of the rough endoplasmic reticulum that was broken up during cell homogenation. If the microsome fraction was treated with lipid solvents to remove the membranes, further centrifugation at high speeds yielded a *ribosome fraction,* and protein synthesis could be induced, in vitro, by the addition of messenger RNA and cofactors to this fraction.

In the late 1800s, cytologists described coarse clumps of material in the basal cytoplasm of secretory epithelial cells that stained intensely with basic dyes. The amount of this material, which they called the *ergastoplasm,* changed in different phases of the secretory cycle. A strongly basophilic cytoplasm and a prominent nucleolus came to be regarded as defining features of secretory cells producing a product rich in protein. With the development of suitable histochemical staining methods and ultraviolet absorption techniques, the basophilic material of such cells was identified as ribonucleoprotein. In the 1940s, the electron microscope revealed an abundance of rough endoplasmic reticulum in secretory

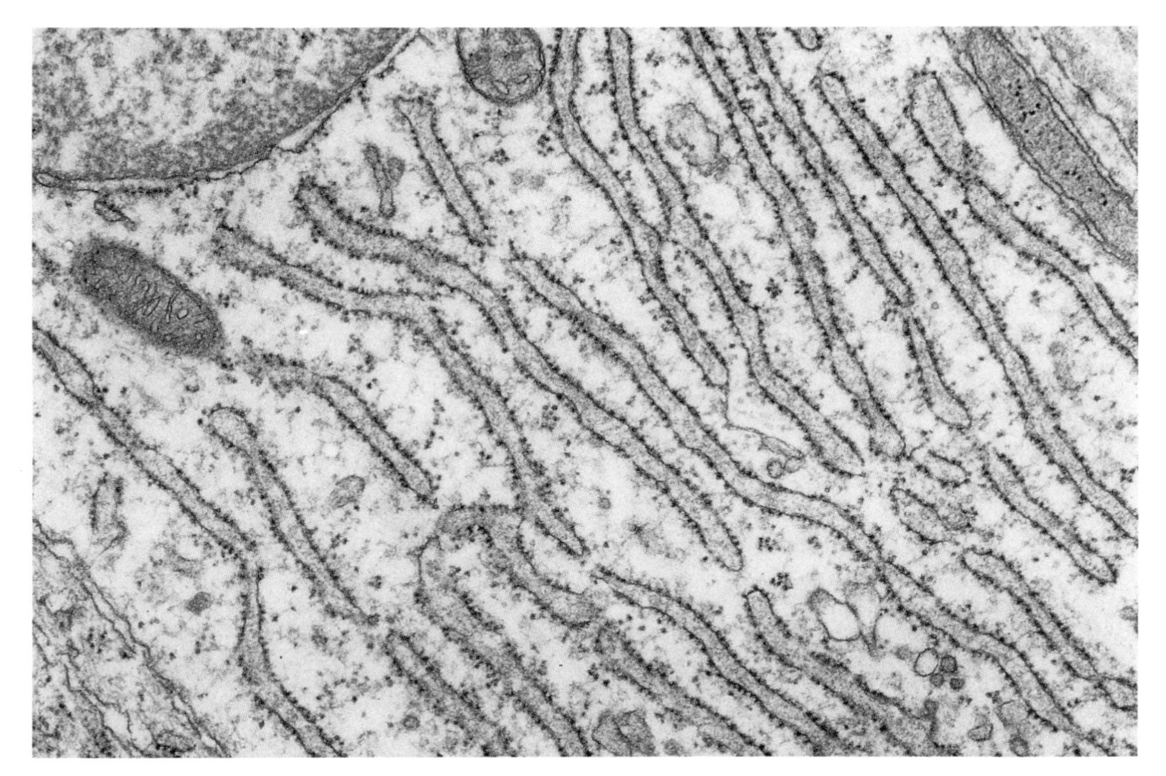

Figure 1–20. Micrograph of several cisternae of rough endoplasmic reticulum, bearing ribosomes on its limiting membrane and products of protein synthesis in its lumen. (Micrograph courtesy of H. Warshawsky.)

cells and isolated ribosomes were found to bind basic dyes. It then became clear that aggregations of rough endoplasmic reticulum correspond to the ergastoplasm of classical cytologists and that the basophilia of the cytoplasm of cells, in general, is largely attributable to their content of ribosomes.

The smooth endoplasmic reticulum is less extensive than the rough, in most cell types, and usually takes the form of a close-meshed network of branching tubules (Fig. 1–21). Smooth-surfaced cisternae are rarely observed. The smooth reticulum is involved in the synthesis of fatty acids and other lipids. It is found in greatest abundance in cells of steroid-secreting endocrine glands. In the liver, it plays an important role in the synthesis of the lipid component of very-low-density lipoproteins that are carriers of cholesterol in the blood. It is also the principal site of detoxification and metabolism of lipid-soluble exogenous drugs. Chronic administration of such drugs induces a marked hypertrophy of the smooth endoplasmic reticulum of the liver. Striated muscle contains a specialized form of smooth reticulum, the *sarcoplasmic reticulum*, which forms networks around all of the myofibrils of the myocytes. Its principal function is the sequestration of calcium ions that control muscle contraction.

ANNULATE LAMELLAE

The term *annulate lamellae* describes an organelle that is relatively uncommon. It consists of stacks of parallel lamellae or cisternae containing many pores that are similar to those of the nuclear envelope (Fig. 1–22). The cisternae are spaced 80–100 nm apart and are often continuous, at their ends, with tubules or cisternae of the rough endoplasmic reticulum. In surface view, the pores are 70–80 nm in diameter and closely spaced in hexagonal array. The interlamellar cytoplasm often contains small densities that have a fibrillar substructure.

Annulate lamellae tend to occur in rapidly dividing cells, especially germ cells, and in a few other cell types in the early stages of their differentiation. Because they contain pores resembling those of the nuclear envelope, they were formerly thought to arise by delamination from the nuclear membrane. It is now considered more likely that they arise as pre-

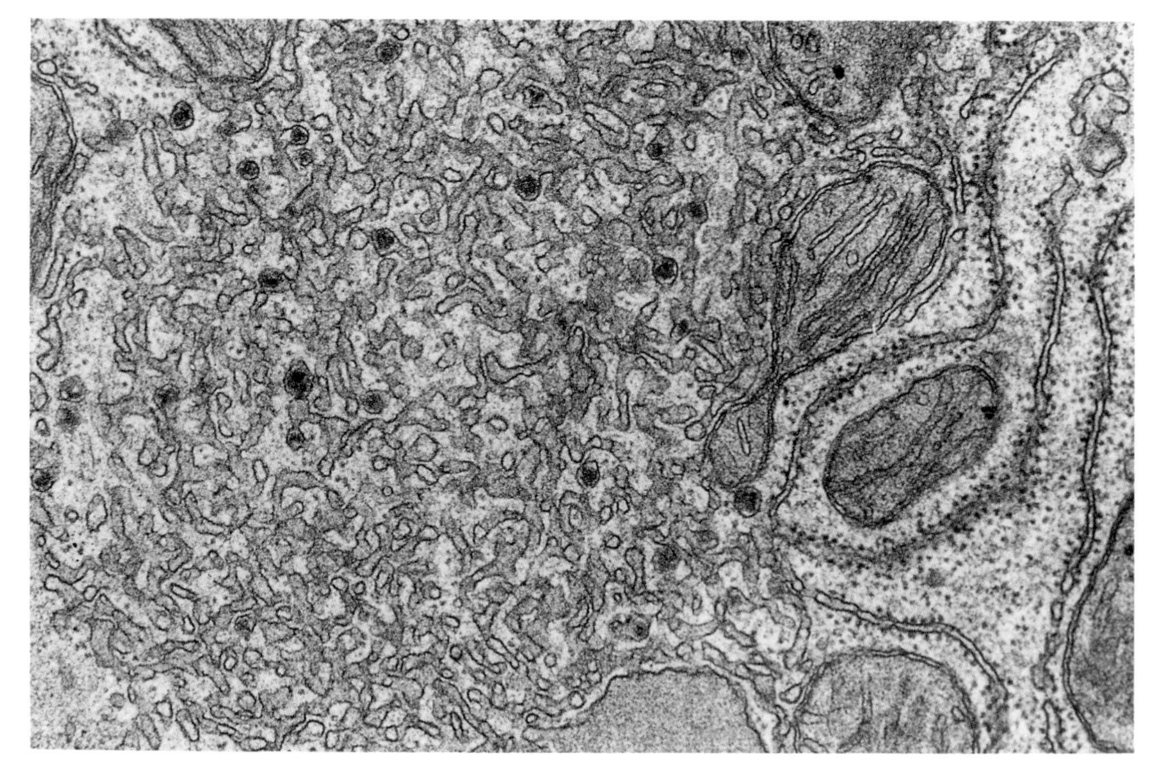

Figure 1–21. Micrograph of a small area of liver cell cytoplasm showing a tight-meshed network of tubular elements of smooth endoplasmic reticulum. Some contain small droplets of very-low-density lipoprotein. (Micrograph courtesy of R. Bolender.)

cursors of the nuclear envelope in cells preparing to divide. If present in excess, those not incorporated in the nuclear envelope during the next cell division may persist for some time and then break down.

Despite their morphological similarity to the nuclear envelope, the possibility remains that the two structures are unrelated. Annulate lamellae do not react positively with labeled antibody to the lamins that form the fibrous lamina of the nuclear envelope. Conversely, an antibody believed to be specific for annulate lamellae fails to cross-react with the nuclear envelope. The origin and functional significance of annulate lamellae remain obscure.

GOLGI COMPLEX

The *Golgi complex* (Golgi apparatus) is a major organelle found in nearly all cells. It is an essential organelle in the secretory pathway and is most conspicuous in those cell types that produce a large volume of secretion. Proteins synthesized in the endoplasmic reticulum are transported to the Golgi complex for further processing, concentration, and packaging in secretory granules for discharge from the cell. In addition to its function in the processing of secretory proteins, the Golgi complex control the traffic in small vesicles involved in the recycling of membrane between organelles, and from the cytoplasm to the surface for renewal of the cell membrane.

The Golgi complex is not seen in routine histological preparations but it can be revealed by silver or osmium impregnation in classical staining methods developed in the 1800s. It can also be identified with histochemical procedures for localizing some of its enzymes. In electron micrographs, it appears as stack of 4 to 10 parallel cisternae (Figs. 1–23 and 1–24). The lumen of these cisternae is narrow throughout most of their length but tends to be slightly expanded at their ends. Although the complex is quite variable in form, its two or three stacks of cisternae are often curved, with a convex outer surface and a concave inner surface. These correspond to the arciform structures called *dictyosomes* by early cytologists.

Functional polarity is evident in the organization of the Golgi complex. The convex sur-

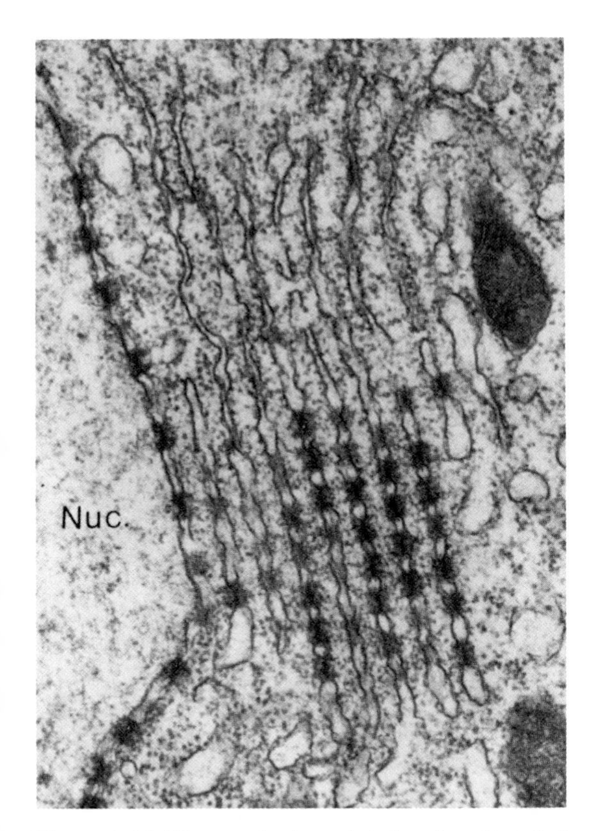

Figure 1–22. Micrograph of annulate lamellae. Note their close resemblance to the nuclear envelope at the left of the figure (Nuc). The lamellae are continuous above with cisternae of rough endoplasmic reticulum. (Micrograph courtesy of S. Ito.)

face, to which secretory protein is transported from the endoplasmic reticulum, is called the *cis-face* of the organelle, and the opposite side is the *trans-face*. There is considerable difference in the cisternae along the cis–trans axis. The first element at the cis-face is highly fenestrated and, in reconstructions from serial sections, it appears as a network of anastomosing tubules, rendering somewhat inappropriate its description as a flat saccule or cisterna. The succeeding elements are true cisternae, but they may have a central fenestration in register with similar opening in the overlying and underlying cisternae. The resulting discontinuity in the stack of cisternae may contain a few small vesicles. Similar vesicles are commonly found around the periphery of the stacks of cisternae. The transport of material from the cis- to the trans-face of the organelle is believed to depend on vesicles budding off from one cisterna and fusing with the next in the stack. Near the trans-side of the Golgi, the lumen of the cisternae tends to be wider and may contain precipitated protein. The terminal cisterna on that side of the organelle often has distended segments forming *condensing vacuoles* that are precursors of secretory granules. Other portions of the terminal cisterna are highly fenestrated, forming a specialized region of the organelle, called the *trans-Golgi network* (Fig. 1–23).

Based on the distribution of enzymes revealed by histochemical staining methods, the Golgi complex is thought to have three functionally distinct compartments through which proteins pass in sequence. The highly fenestrated initial cisterna has the unique property of being heavily stained by prolonged exposure to osmium and is designated the *cis-compartment.* The next few cisternae that react positively for nicotinamide adenine dinucleotide phosphatase (NADPase), and *N*-acetyl glucosamine transferase (AGT), form the *intermediate compartment,* and a number of succeeding cisternae that stain for thiamine pyrophosphatase (TTPase), sialyl transferase (ST), and galactosyl transferase (GT) constitute the *trans-compartment.* In most secretory cells, glycoproteins synthesized in the endoplasmic reticulum undergo only minor posttranslational modification in the Golgi, involving removal of mannose groups from certain oligosaccharides and the addition of *N*-acetylglucosamine in the intermediate compartment, followed by the addition of galactose and sialic acid in the trans-compartment. However, in cartilage cells producing matrix proteoglycans, the Golgi complex has a major synthetic role, adding to the core protein up to 10 times its weight in glycosaminoglycan polysaccharides.

The endoplasmic reticulum synthesizes a very great number of different proteins. Some of these are for export as secretory products, but many others are destined to be incorporated into structural components of the cell. One of the more challenging problems in cell biology has been to discover how the various proteins are sorted and delivered to their respective destinations. It is now known that specific chemical groups are added to the proteins in the reticulum and modified in their journey through the Golgi complex, and these groups label the proteins for separate packaging and serve to "address" them to the appropriate sites within the cell. The sorting takes place at the trans-face of the Golgi complex. There, certain proteins are condensed into secretory granules, others are packaged in smooth-surfaced small vesicles, and still others are enclosed in vesicles having a bristle-like coating. The majority of the vesicles appear to arise

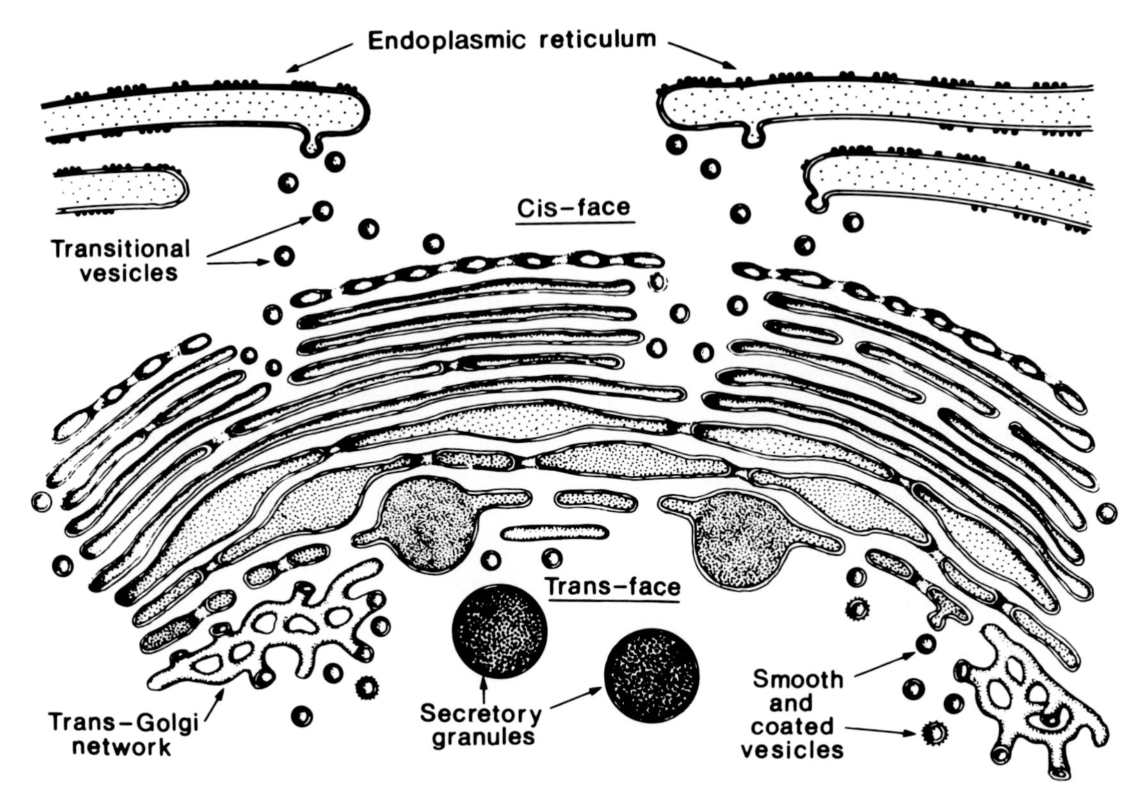

Figure 1–23. Schematic representation of the components of the Golgi complex and its relation to the rough endoplasmic reticulum. It is considered to have three compartments, the cis-, intermediate, and trans-compartments.

from the trans-Golgi network. The secretory granules move to the cell surface for exocytosis. There is suggestive evidence that the coated vesicles transport newly synthesized enzymes to late endosomes and then to lysosomes. The smooth vesicles may be involved either in constitutive secretion or in membrane recycling.

The network of tubules associated with the terminal cisternae of the Golgi complex was identified some 30 years ago as a potential site of biogenesis of the lysosomes and was assigned the acronym GERL to indicate its close relation to the Golgi (G), its continuity with the endoplasmic reticulum (ER), and its role in lysosome formation (L). In later studies, its continuity with the reticulum was not confirmed. This network of anastomosing tubules is now considered to be an integral part of the Golgi complex and a major site of exit of materials from it. The acronym GERL has now fallen into disfavor and has been replaced by the term *trans-Golgi network.*

There is strong evidence that, after newly synthesized lysosomal enzymes have been transferred from the endoplasmic reticulum to the Golgi, specific oligosaccharide chains rich in mannose are phosphorylated in the 6-carbon position. This modification evidently serves as a label, enabling these enzymes to bind to mannose-6-phosphate receptors. These receptors and their ligands are found to be concentrated in the trans-Golgi network where they are packaged in small vesicles that fuse specifically with the membrane of developing lysosomes. The signals and the sorting mechanisms are not yet known for the many other proteins that are processed in the Golgi complex.

MITOCHONDRIA

Slender rods 0.4–0.8 μm in diameter and 4–9 μm in length can be seen in thin living cells examined with the phase contrast microscope. These *mitochondria* are quite flexible, changing shape as they slowly move about in the cytoplasm. Their function is to provide the energy required for the biosynthetic and motor activities of the cell. Mitochondria may be randomly distributed in the cytoplasm or concentrated near sites of high energy utilization. Their numbers range from a few to sev-

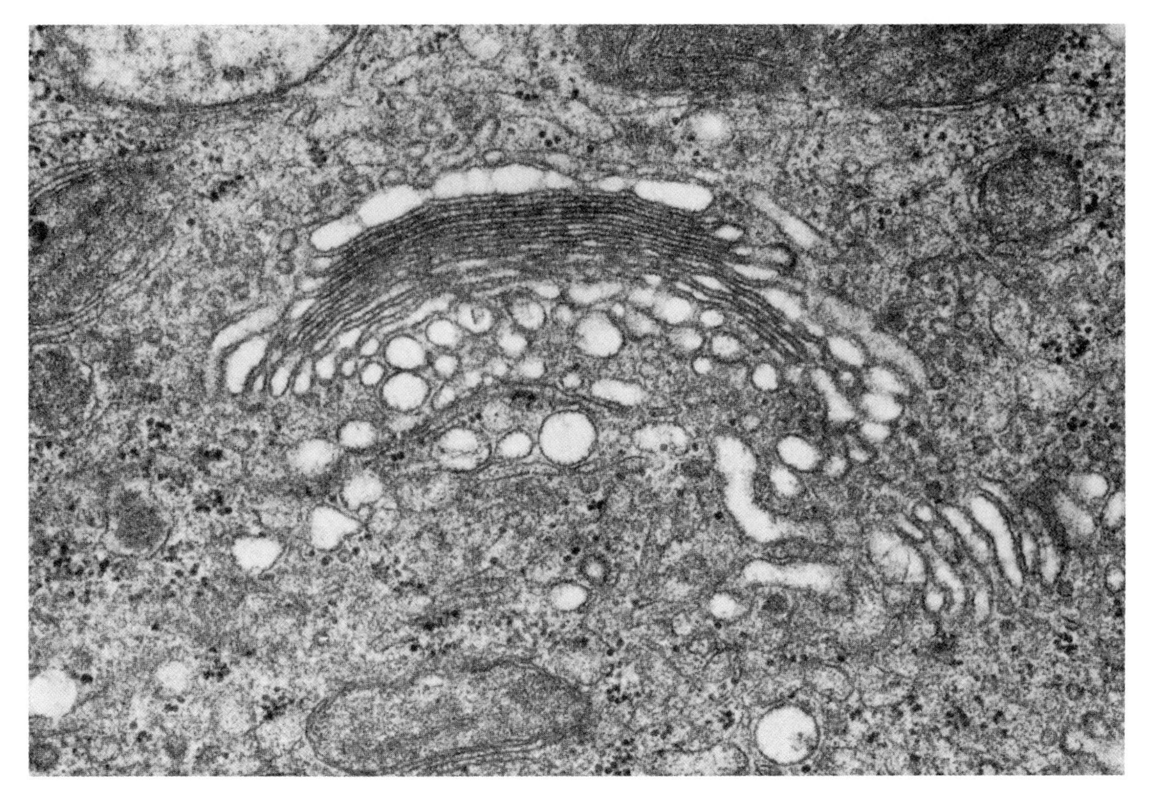

Figure 1–24. Micrograph of the Golgi complex of a cell in the epithelium of the vas deferens. (Micrograph courtesy of D. Friend.)

eral hundred depending on the size and energy needs of the various cell types.

In electron micrographs, a mitochondrion is limited by a smooth-contoured *outer membrane* about 7 nm thick and a slightly thinner *inner membrane*. The inner membrane runs parallel to the outer membrane, except where it forms thin folds that project into the interior of the organelle. These are called the *cristae mitochondriales* (Fig. 1–25). This plication of the inner membrane is a device for increasing the area of this enzyme-rich membrane. The number of cristae per mitochondrion is much greater in cells with high-energy requirements than in those having a lower rate of metabolism. In a few cell types, the cristae mitochondriales are tubular instead of slender folds of the inner membrane (Fig. 1–26).

The mitochondrial membranes bound two compartments: a large *intercristal space*, comprising all of the area within the inner membrane, and a smaller *membrane space*, consisting of the narrow cleft between the outer and inner membranes and extending inward between the two leaves of the cristae. These latter extensions are sometimes referred to as the *intracristal spaces*, but they are not functionally distinct from the rest of the membrane space. The membrane space is only 10–20 nm across and appears empty, for it apparently contains no protein precipitable by chemical fixatives. The larger intercristal space is occupied by a moderately electron-dense *mitochondrial matrix*. In negatively stained preparations of mitochondria that have been isolated and broken open, the inner membrane is studded with numerous minute particles called the *inner membrane subunits*. These consist of a globular head, about 10 nm in diameter, connected to the membrane by a slender stem 3 to 4 nm thick and about 5 nm long. In conventional electron micrographs, these subunits are not visible and the inner and outer membranes look alike. However, they differ in chemical composition and physiological properties. The outer membrane contains a protein that forms transmembrane channels that are freely permeable to small particles. The inner membrane is relatively impermeable and has a higher content of protein than any other membrane in the cell.

Dense, more-or-less spherical *matrix gran-*

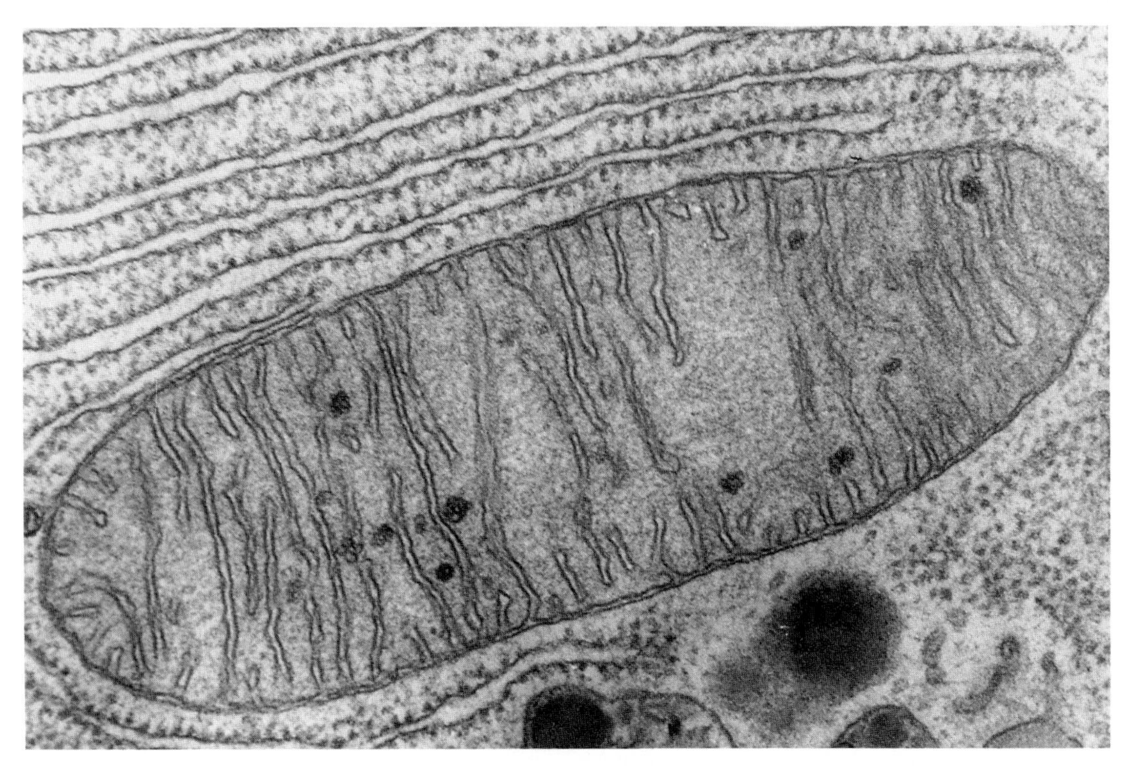

Figure 1–25. Electron micrograph of a typical mitochondrion from the pancreas of a bat, showing the cristae, matrix, and matrix granules. (Micrograph courtesy of K.R. Porter.)

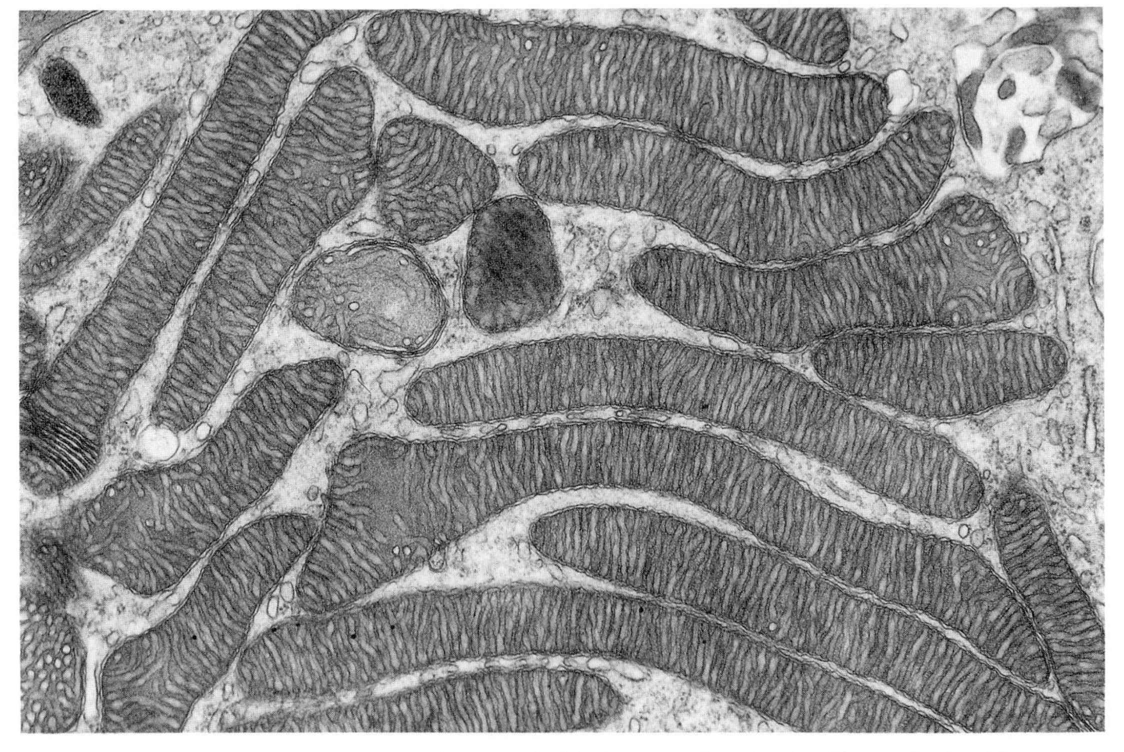

Figure 1–26. Electron micrograph of mitochondria in a cell of the hamster adrenal cortex. These mitochondria are unusual in containing large numbers of cristae that are tubular instead of lamellar.

ules, 30 to 50 nm in diameter may be found anywhere in the intercristal space but are often located near the cristae. Their density tends to obscure their internal structure, but in very thin sections, they appear to contain multiple minute compartments separated by relatively thick septa. Their composition and function continue to be subjects of controversy. When calcium or other divalent cations are present in high concentration in the fluid bathing isolated mitochondria, the size and density of the matrix granules are increased. This led to the suggestion that they may be involved in regulation of the internal concentration of ions in the matrix. This interpretation has been weakened by X-ray microanalysis which failed to reveal calcium in the matrix granules of mitochondria in most tissues. There is, at present, no convincing evidence that mitochondrial matrix granules, in tissues other than cartilage and bone, are involved in calcium sequestration in vivo. Their ultrastructure, and their affinity for osmium, suggest that their major component is lipid and biochemical analysis of centrifugal fractions enriched in matrix granules indicates that they are composed of phospholipoprotein. At present, their function is purely conjectural.

Mitochondria are self-replicating organelles, with a limited life span, that maintain their numbers by a form of division that resembles the binary fission of bacteria. Indeed, mitochondria are believed to have evolved from symbiotic bacteria very early in the evolution of unicellular organisms, at a time when the Earth's atmosphere was poor in oxygen and most of the organisms depended on anaerobic fermentation of organic molecules. It is speculated that a small bacterium that had evolved the ability to utilize oxygen, invaded a larger anaerobic cell type and a symbiotic relationship developed, in which the aerobic symbiont generated energy in return for protection and nutrients supplied by the larger host cell. With the passage of time, the interdependence of the two increased and the parasite became an indispensable cell organelle, passed on by the host cell to its progeny. Mitochondria retain a mode of division in which elongation of a centrally situated crista forms a partition across the organelle and opposing folds of the outer membrane then extend between the leaves of the partition to meet and fuse, completing the separation of the two halves—a mode of division resembling that of the ancestral symbiotic bacterium and of many modern bacteria (Fig. 1–27).

Mitochondria possess their own DNA and ribosomal, transfer, and messenger RNAs. At very high magnifications, their DNA can be seen as lose aggregations of slender filaments in electron-lucent areas of the mitochondrial matrix. When isolated from centrifugal fractions of mitochondria and examined in negatively stained preparations, it closely resembles the DNA of bacteria, consisting of a double helix of naked DNA in the form of a circle with a circumference of about 5.5 μm (Fig. 1–28). It differs from DNA of the nucleus in its circular form and much lower molecular weight. Although mitochondria have their own genome, they are not self-sufficient. Their DNA contains only about 15,000 nucleotides and, thus, has a very limited coding capacity. It encodes the RNA of mitochondrial ribosomes, which are visible as 12-nm granules distributed throughout the matrix, and for transfer RNAs, but its messenger RNAs code for only a few components of the respiratory enzyme complexes of the inner membrane. Nuclear DNA encodes the rest of the inner membrane proteins, those of the outer membrane and those of the matrix. These proteins are all synthesized in the cytoplasm and imported into the mitochondria. All enzymes needed to replicate DNA and transcribe it into RNA also depend on nuclear genes. Thus, in evolving from free-living bacteria, mitochondria have given over to the nucleus and cytoplasm of the host cell the coding and synthesis of most of their proteins. However, it is interesting that mitochondrial protein synthesis is blocked by antibacterial antibiotics that do not affect protein synthesis elsewhere in the cell.

The principal biochemical activity of mitochondria is *oxidative phosphorylation*—the oxidation, by molecular oxygen, of metabolites of the nutrients (glucose and fatty acids) that the cell receives from the blood. The energy thus generated is used to synthesize *adenosine triphosphate* (ATP) from *adenosine diphosphate* (ADP) and inorganic phosphate. ATP released from the mitochondria, into the cytoplasm, is an ubiquitous store of energy that is needed for transport across membranes for all synthetic processes and for the mechanical work involved in motor activities of the cell. On demand, a high-energy phosphate bond in ATP is split, instantly releasing energy and converting ATP to ADP. ATP is then regenerated from ADP, by the mitochondria, using phosphoric acid and energy derived from cell nutrients. Mitochondria can be regarded as the powerhouses of the cell.

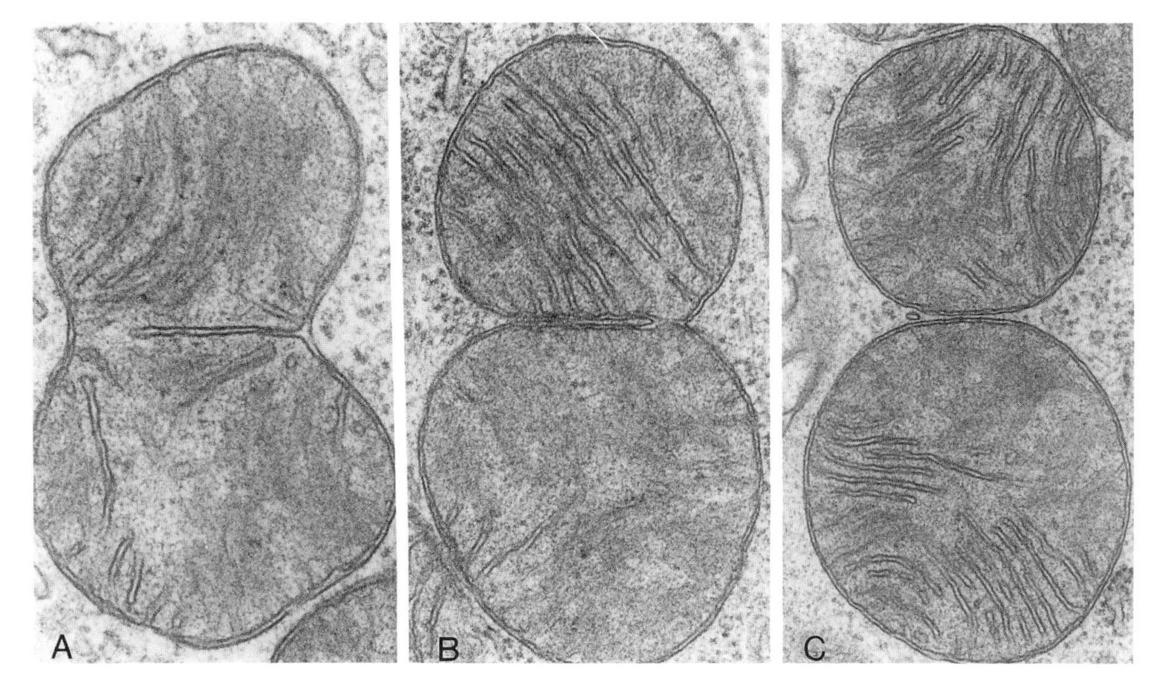

Figure 1–27. Micrographs of successive stages (A–C) in the division of a mitochondrion. (Micrograph courtesy of T. Kanaseki.)

LYSOSOMES

Lysosomes range in number from a few to several hundred per cell, in different cell types. They were not recognized as a true cell organelle by classical cytologists because they do not have consistent form or tinctorial properties with traditional staining methods. Attention was drawn to them by histochemical reactions for acid hydrolases and by electron microscopic images. They are so heterogeneous that no single description encompasses all of their variations, but, in general, they are round, ovoid, or highly irregular, electron-dense bodies 0.25–0.8 μm in diameter (Fig. 1–29). Their interior may appear homogeneous or may consist of dense granules of varying size in a less-dense matrix. They may contain crystals or concentric systems of lamellae, interpreted as myelin forms of phos-

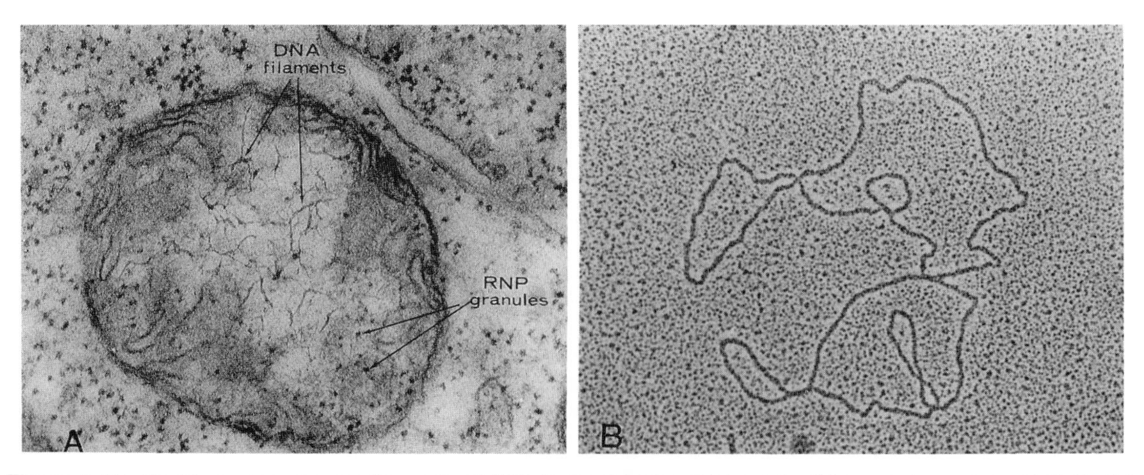

Figure 1–28. (A) Micrograph showing filaments of DNA in the mitochondrial matrix. (Micrograph courtesy of H. Swift.) (B) DNA isolated from mitochondria of a Xenopus oocyte. Mitochondrial DNA occurs in the form of circles 5–6 μm in contour length. (Micrograph courtesy of I.B. Dawid and D.R. Wolstenholme.)

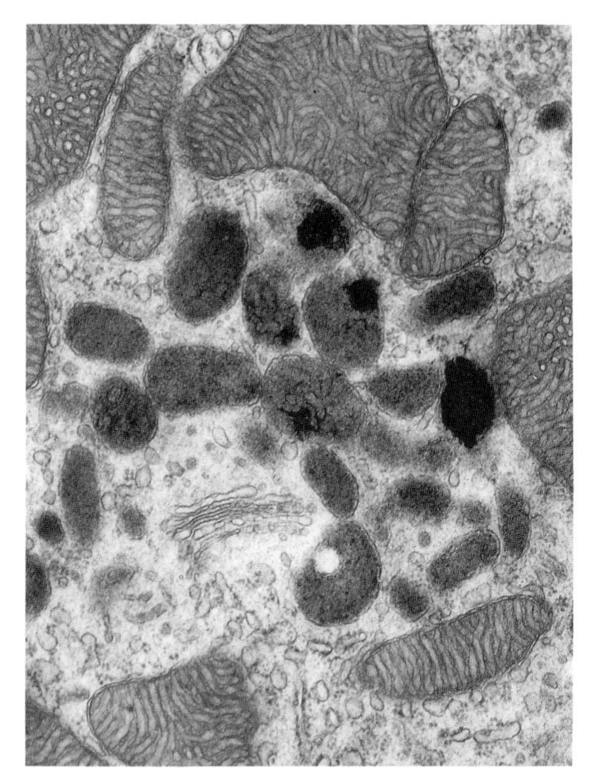

Figure 1–29. Micrograph of a group of lysosomes in the Golgi region of a cell of the adrenal cortex.

pholipid. Lysosomes cannot be confidently identified, as such, by morphological criteria alone. Histochemical demonstration of acid phosphatase or other hydrolases in their interior is required for verification.

Forty or more hydrolytic enzymes have now been reported to occur in lysosomes. These include proteases, glycosidases, nucleases, phosphatases, phospholipases, and sulfatases. The pH optima of nearly all of these enzymes are in the acid range. The lysosomes are now regarded as an intracellular digestive system capable of degrading nearly all naturally occurring chemical constituents of cells. In the normal cell, these potentially damaging enzymes are safely contained within the limiting membrane of the lysosome. However, in certain pathological conditions, the permeability of this membrane may be altered, allowing enzymes to escape and digest or lyse the cell.

Cell digestion by lysosomes is not limited to disease states. Programmed death of certain cells is a normal event in the embryonic development of some organs. In postnatal life, certain organs may undergo a massive regression, as in the mammary gland after weaning or in the endometrium of the uterus in menstruation. In these normal events, the lysosomal membranes are altered permitting escape of acid hydrolases that break down the cells no longer needed.

Lysosomes play their most important role in the defense of the organism against bacterial invasion. Lysosomes are abundant in polymorphonuclear leukocytes of the blood and in tissue macrophages which are cell types specialized for *phagocytosis*—the ingestion and intracellular digestion of bacteria and other foreign particulate matter. When bacteria are engulfed by these cells they are taken into the cytoplasm in a membrane-bounded *phagocytosis vacuole* or *phagosome*. Lysosomes then gather around this vacuole and their membranes fuse with its membrane, releasing into its interior hydrolytic enzymes that destroy the ingested bacterium (Fig. 1–30).

The lysosomes of the cell are also involved in the elimination of cell organelles in reorganizations of the cytoplasm associated with changes in physiological activity. Mitochondria or endoplasmic reticulum that are present in excess are enveloped in a membrane to form an *autophagic vacuole*. Lysosomes then fuse with this vacuole releasing enzymes that digest its contents (Fig. 1–31). This process of controlled degradation of organelles in a healthy cell is called *autophagy* to distinguish it from *heterophagy* which is the digestion of exogenous material taken into the cell.

Owing to the substrate diversity of the lysosomal enzymes, digestion of the content of autophagic and heterophagic vacuoles is usually quite complete; however, undigestible residues, in small amounts, may persist in membrane-bounded *residual bodies*. These may coalesce into larger masses that are variously designated as *wear-and-tear pigment, lipochrome pigment,* or *lipofuchsin pigment*. Where abundant, these may be visible with the light microscope as irregularly shaped, yellow or brown masses in the cytoplasm. The development of the concept of lysosomes as intracellular digestive organelles has led to a proliferation of redundant terms. To simplify the terminology, it has been suggested that *primary lysosome* be used to describe those that have not yet become engaged in digestive activity and that the term *secondary lysosome* be applied to any vacuolar structure that is the site of current or past digestive activity. The latter term would thus encompass autophagic and heterophagic vacuoles and the enzymatically inactive residual bodies and lipofuchsin pigment deposits.

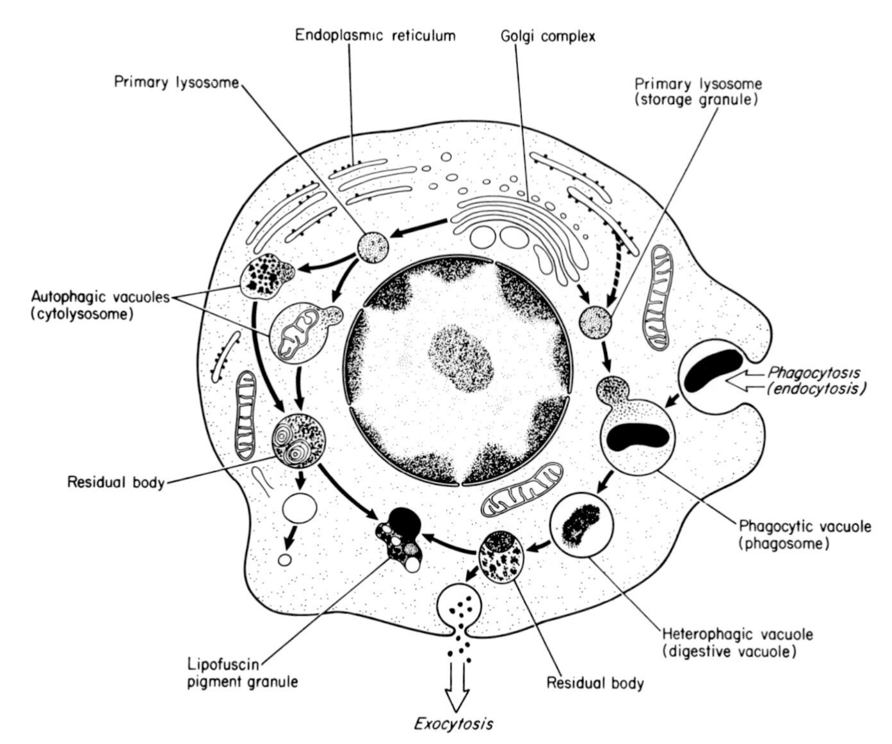

Figure 1–30. Schematic depiction of the role of lysosomes in heterophagy (lower right) and in autophagy (upper left). Bacteria are taken up by phagocytosis in endocytic vacuoles. Primary lysosomes fuse with these vacuoles and their enzymes digest their contents. In autophagy, membranes may be formed around excess organelles or inclusions and lysosomes then fuse with these vacuoles. The end products of both processes may be recognized as residual bodies or lipofuchsin pigment deposits.

The origin of lysosomes has long been controversial, but recent research indicates that lysosomal enzymes are synthesized, together with secretory and other proteins, in the endoplasmic reticulum and transported in vesicles to the Golgi complex. There mannose residues on enzymes destined to be incorporated in lysosomes are phosphorylated. They then bind to mannose-6-phosphate receptors in the membrane of the trans-Golgi network, from which they are transported in small vesicles targeted to developing lysosomes. Uncertainty persists as to the origin of the structures with which these vesicles fuse to form lysosomes. This will be discussed later in this chapter in the section on endocytosis.

Although lysosomes usually carry out their digestive function intracellularly, there are a few situations in which lysosomal enzymes are released from cells. Osteoclasts, cells specialized for the remodeling of bone, secrete enzymes into a sealed cavity between the cell and the underlying bone to digest the bone matrix. Also, at sites of acute inflammation, where leukocytes are actively phagocytizing bacteria, lysosomes may fuse with a forming phagosome before its complete closure and enzymes may escape, destroying collagen and elastin in the surrounding connective tissue. It is now realized that some of the damage to kidneys, joints, and lungs following protracted inflammation is a consequence of this leakage of acid hydrolases from activated phagocytic cells that were mobilized for defense against invading bacteria.

Clinical interest in lysosomes has been stimulated by the discovery that a number of uncommon "storage diseases" of children are due to an inherited inability to synthesize certain lysosomal enzymes. In the absence of a particular lysosomal enzyme, its normal substrate accumulates in large membrane-bounded inclusions, which are, in effect, autophagic vacuoles that are unable to digest their content. Massive accumulations of such material in the cells of the liver, and other organs, seriously affects their functions and leads to early death.

PEROXISOMES

In early electron microscopic studies of the liver, 0.2–1.0-μm membrane-limited bodies

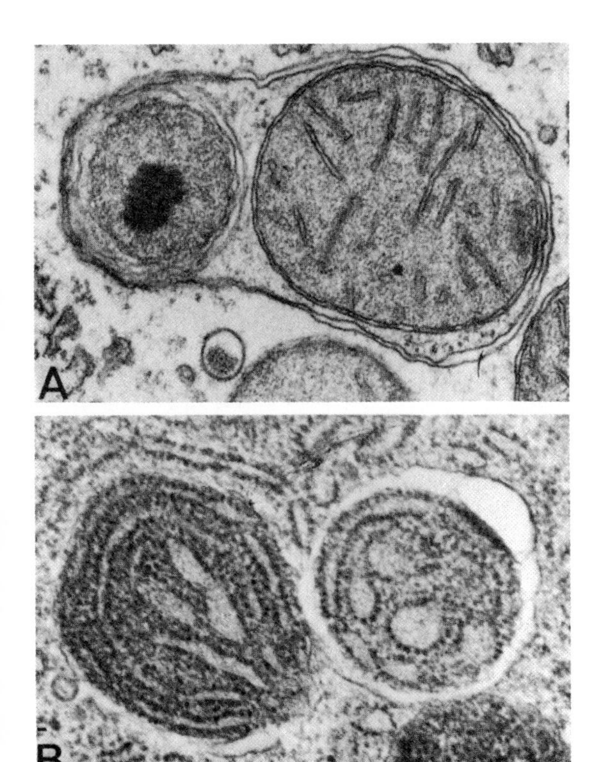

Figure 1–31. Examples of autophagic vacuoles. (A) A peroxisome and a mitochondrion enclosed in the same vacuole. (B) Elements of the endoplasmic reticulum in two adjacent autophagic vacuoles.

of lower density than lysosomes were observed and tentatively called *microbodies.* A decade later, with the development of centrifugation procedures of improved resolution, it was possible to separate these from a crude lysosomal fraction and to study their biochemical properties. They were found to lack hydrolases, but to contain *urate oxidase, D-amino acid oxidase* and *catalase.* They are able to β-oxidate very-long-chain fatty acids producing H_2O_2 as a byproduct. Administration of drugs used to lower the lipid and cholesterol content of the blood results in a 10-fold increase in the content of β-oxidative enzymes in liver peroxisomes. To counter the potential toxic effects of H_2O_2 produced in the cells as a byproduct of β-oxidation, their catalase breaks down hydrogen peroxide to water and oxygen. Peroxisomes have been found to contain more than 40 enzymes. Although they generate energy by oxidation of their substrates, peroxisomes differ from mitochondria, in that, they are unable to store energy in the form of ATP for subsequent use by the cell. It has been suggested that the energy generated by their oxidation of fatty acids is dissipated as heat and may contribute to the maintenance of body temperature. The metabolic interaction of reactions within the peroxisomes with pathways in the surrounding cytoplasm is extensive, necessitating the transport of a variety of metabolites across their membrane. The functions of peroxisomes in cell metabolism are still incompletely understood.

Peroxisomes are present in nearly all cell types and they number in the hundreds in metabolically active cells such as those of the liver. In electron micrographs of cells in several animal species, there is a denser region of the peroxisome, called the *nucleoid,* which is eccentrically situated in an otherwise homogeneous gray matrix. The nucleoid is a paracrystalline array of minute tubules of urate oxidase. Peroxisomes of birds and primates lack this enzyme and do not have a nucleoid.

Clinical interest in peroxisomes rests on the finding that there are several inherited diseases in which there is either deficiency of a single enzyme (X-linked adrenoleukodystrophy) or defects in peroxisome formation and deficiency of several enzymes (Zellweger syndrome).

CENTROSOME AND CENTRIOLES

In suitably stained cells, one can usually find a *centrosome,* a small, more-or-less spherical area with a texture differing slightly from that of the surrounding cytoplasm. In its center are two short rods, the *centrioles.* In addition to the centrioles, it may also contain a variable number of small dense bodies called *centriolar satellites.* In some epithelia, the centrosome and its pair of centrioles are located in the supranuclear cytoplasm partially surrounded by the Golgi complex. In other epithelia, the centrioles are found in the apical cytoplasm, immediately beneath the plasma membrane.

The centrioles are cylindrical structures about 0.2 μm in diameter and 0.5–0.7 μm in length, with an electron-dense wall surrounding an electron-lucent central cavity. Embedded in the wall are nine evenly spaced triplet microtubules. Viewed in cross section, each triplet is set at an angle of about 40° to its respective tangent. This oblique orientation of the triplets results in a pattern resembling the vanes of a turbine (Fig. 1–32, inset). The three subunits of each triplet are designated A, B, and C, with subunit A nearest to the axis of the centriole. Short fibers connect subunit A of each triplet to subunit C of the adjacent triplet. The long axes of the two centrioles are usually perpendicular to one another.

In preparation for cell division, the two cen-

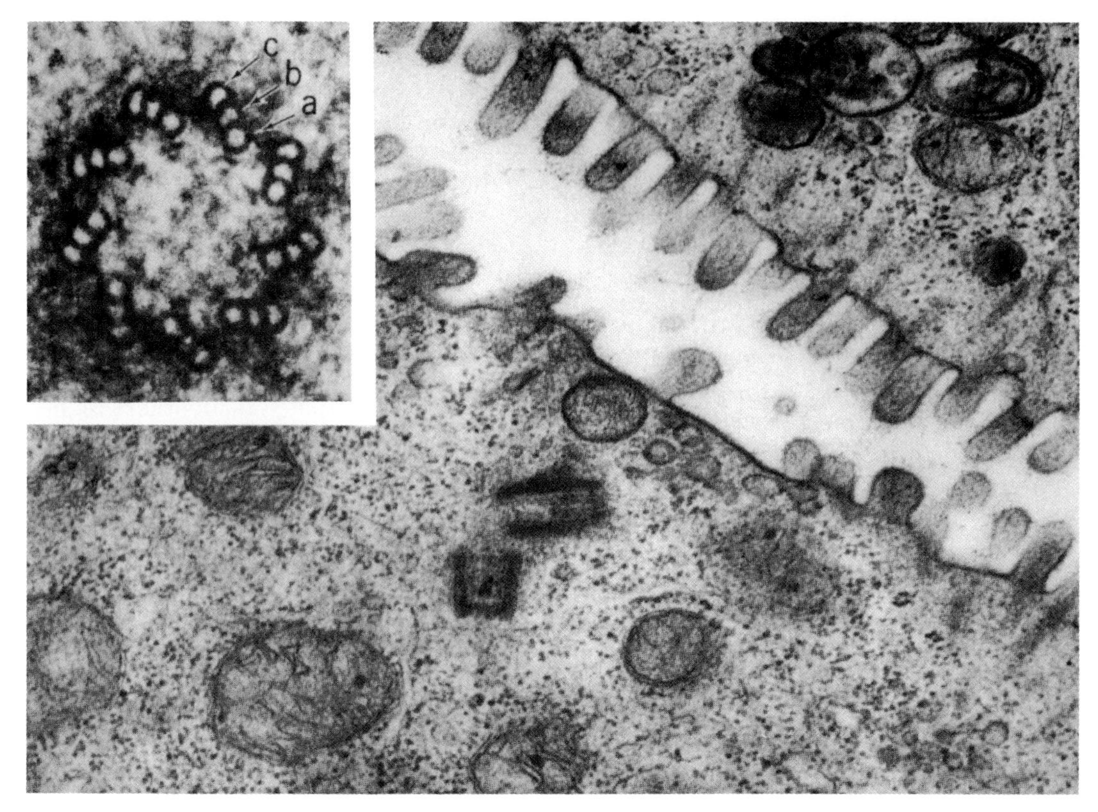

Figure 1–32. Micrograph of a diplosome near the surface of an epithelial cell. The long axes of the two centrioles are usually perpendicular. (Micrograph courtesy of S. Sorokin.) The inset shows a centriole in cross section at higher magnification. Its wall is composed of nine triplet microtubules. (Micrograph courtesy of J. André.)

trioles replicate. Centrioles do not replicate by division. Instead, a new centriole develops in end-to-side relationship to a specific region on the wall of the preexisting centriole, but separated from it by a narrow electron-lucent space. The anlage of the new centriole, called the *procentriole,* is an annular condensation of dense material having the same diameter as a centriole, but initially devoid of microtubules. It elongates by progressive accretion of material to its end, and there is a concurrent polymerization of tubulin to form the triplets within its wall. When its development is complete, the newly formed centriole separates from the parent centriole, but maintains its perpendicular orientation to it (Fig. 1–33). After replication, the two members of the original diplosome move apart, and each, together with its newly formed daughter centriole and other components of the centrosome, move to opposite poles of the cell. There, the centriolar satellites seem to serve as *microtubule organizing centers,* becoming sites of nucleation of the microtubules that will form the *mitotic spindle.* The centrosome is rich in tubulin, but it is not yet clear which of its components is responsible for initiating microtubule formation. Two unique biochemical components of pericentriolar cytoplasm have been identified: a calcium-binding 20 kD protein, called *centrin,* and an unnamed, related 165 kD protein. Their functional significance is yet to be determined. The centrioles themselves are evidently not essential for mitosis because acentriolar divisions are not uncommon in plant cells. The association of centrioles with the poles of the spindle, in animal cells, may have evolved as a device for ensuring that both daughter cells receive a pair.

In the differentiation of ciliated epithelial cells, a proliferation of centrioles precedes the development of the cilia. They accumulate in large numbers beneath the apical plasma membrane where each serves as a *basal body,* initiating tubulin polymerization that results in formation of the axoneme of a cilium. The basal bodies of the cilia usually have a short lateral projection, the *basal foot.* These are aligned in the same direction in the rows of cilia. Cross-striated *rootlets* develop on the

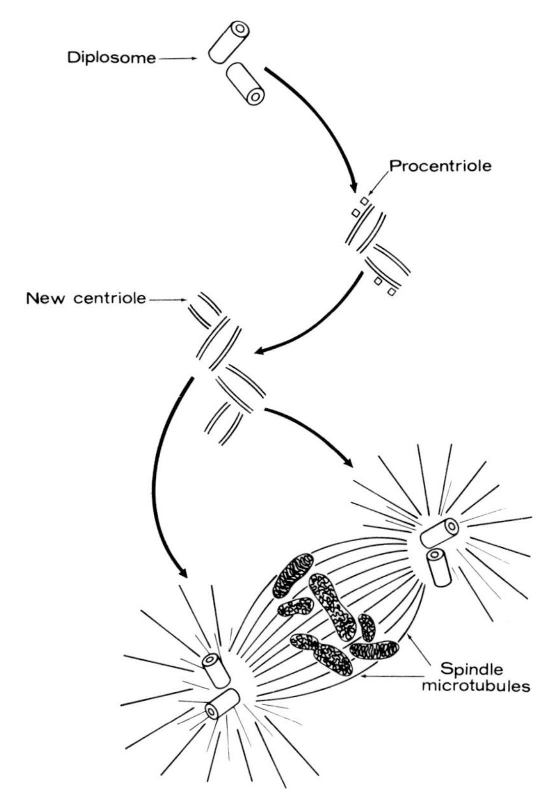

Figure 1–33. Before the onset of cell division, each member of the diplosome becomes a site of nucleation of a new centriole. Its anlage, the procentriole, is a ring-like structure devoid of microtubular elements. It elongates by accretion to its distal end and microtubules assemble within its wall. Each member of the original diplosome, together with its newly formed daughter centriole, migrate to opposite poles of the division figure.

lower end of the basal bodies and extend a short distance down into the apical cytoplasm. The basal feet and the rootlets evidently serve to stabilize the bases of the cilia.

The capacity of the centrioles for self-duplication has long fostered the speculation that they might contain DNA. Recently, a DNA probe, cloned from a biflagellate green alga, has been reported to localize in the basal bodies of the flagella, providing suggestive evidence for the existence of centriolar DNA, but this needs further verification.

CYTOPLASMIC INCLUSIONS

In addition to the *organelles,* which are essential active participants in the biochemical processes of cell metabolism, there are other passive components of the cytoplasm that represent stored nutrients, inert by-products of metabolism, or accumulations of endogenous or exogenous pigment. These are called *cytoplasmic inclusions.* Organelles are bounded by a membrane; inclusions usually are not.

GLYCOGEN

Animal cells store carbohydrate in the form of a polymer of D-glucose, called *glycogen.* As needed, this is depolymerized to yield glucose, which is a major energy source for metabolic processes and which also supplies short carbon chains that are reused in the synthesis of various constituents of protoplasm. The principal sites of carbohydrate storage in the body are the liver and muscle, but the cells of many other tissues contain small amounts of glycogen. It is not visible in routine histological preparations but, when present in abundance, it can be stained with the periodic-acid Schiff reaction. Glycogen is visible in electron micrographs as 20–30-nm dense granules that are slightly irregular in outline. In liver, these so-called *beta particles* form slightly larger aggregates called *alpha particles* (Fig. 1–34). These may occur anywhere in the cytoplasm but they tend to be more concentrated in areas rich in smooth endoplasmic reticulum. The membranes of this organelle are reported to contain the enzyme glycogen phosphorylase, that breaks down glycogen to glucose, and glucose-6-phosphatase, one of several enzymes involved in the degradation of glucose (glycolysis). Glycogen is normally confined to the cytoplasm, but in diabetes and in a rare glycogen-storage disease, it may also accumulate in the nucleus.

LIPID

Although most of the lipid stores of the body are in the adipose tissue which is specialized for this function, many other cell types contain a few small lipid droplets, consisting mainly of triglycerides that are liquid at body temperature. In histological sections, lipids have been extracted, during specimen preparation, by the solvents used for tissue dehydration, and only round clear vacuoles are left behind. However, in tissues fixed in glutaraldehyde and osmium tetroxide, the lipid is preserved as spherical globules stained gray or black, depending on the degree of unsaturation of their constituent fatty acids (Fig. 1–35).

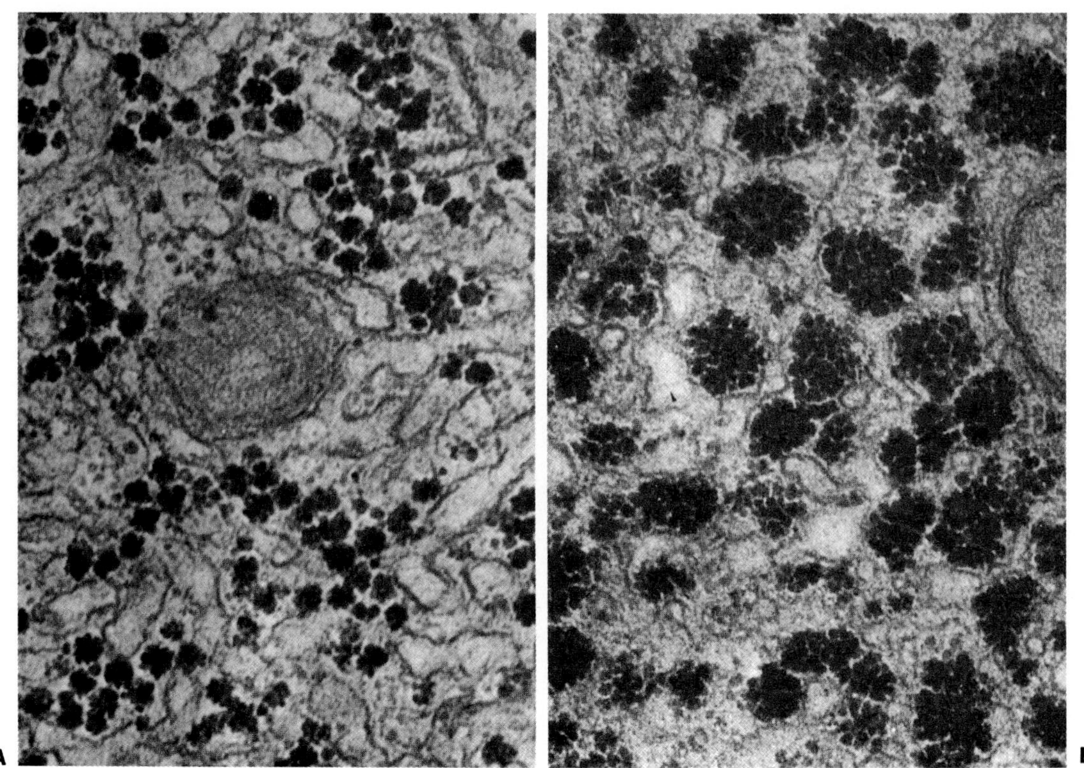

Figure 1–34. Micrographs of liver glycogen of two different species at the same magnification. In the salamander liver (A) the particles are considerably smaller than in the hamster (B). In both, the particles are aggregates of smaller subunits.

Lipid serves as an energy source and provides short carbon chains that can be used by the cell for synthesis of membranes and other lipid-rich structural components. The smooth endoplasmic reticulum is the site of synthesis of lipid, lipoproteins, and steroid derivatives of cholesterol. Multiple small lipid droplets are common in the cytoplasm of steroid-secreting endocrine glands. In adipose cells, specialized for lipid storage and release, lipid occurs in a single very large droplet that occupies over 90% of the cell volume.

PIGMENT

Cell types with a relatively long life span, such as those of cardiac muscle and certain cells of the brain, often contain deposits of a yellow-brown pigment *lipofuscin* (Fig. 1–36). This pigment represents the accumulated undigestible residues of lysosomal activity and arises by coalescence of residual bodies, defined earlier in this chapter. These masses of pigment are bounded by a membrane but they have no demonstrable enzymatic activity, and are, therefore, classified as inclusions, rather than organelles.

The most abundant pigment in the body is *hemoglobin,* the oxygen-carrying pigment of the red blood cells. At the end of their limited life span, these cells are phagocytized by macrophages in the spleen and liver and the hemoglobin is broken down in lysosomes to *hemosiderin* and *bilirubin.* Bilirubin is returned to the blood and excreted, but hemosiderin accumulates in the phagocytic cells resulting in a distinct brown color of certain areas of the spleen. The amount of this pigment is greatly increased in diseases in which there is an accelerated destruction of red blood cells. Hemosiderin can be distinguished from other pigments of similar color by its staining reaction for iron. In electron micrographs, hemosiderin appears as dense masses of 9-nm particles of *ferritin,* an iron-storing protein.

The pigmentation of the skin and hair is due to *melanin,* synthesized in cells called melanocytes. Melanin is bound to the structural protein of *melanosomes,* dense ellipsoidal granules in their cytoplasm. The pigment is actively synthesized in these granules from the amino-acid tyrosine via a colorless intermediate product dihydrophenylalanine. Because the melanosomes actively synthesize this pigment, they are regarded as organelles of the melanocyte. However, some of the melanin produced is transferred to the cytoplasm of neighboring skin cells (keratinocytes) in synthetically inactive granules that qualify as cytoplasmic inclusion of these cells. Melanin also occurs in neurones of the substantia nigra in the brain and in the pigment epithelium of the retina.

CRYSTALS

The least common of the inclusions are crystals that may occur free in the cytoplasm or within the lumen of expanded segments of the rough endoplasmic reticulum. Most of these have not been isolated and characterized chemically, but their staining and solubility properties suggest that they may be a storage form of protein. Large *crystals of Reinke* may be found in the cytoplasm, and rarely in the nucleus, of the interstitial cells of the human testis, but not in those of other species. Fusiform *crystals of Charcot-Böttcher* are occasionally observed in the Sertoli cells of the human testis. In humans, there seems to be no excretory pathway for excess iron stored in the form of ferritin and, as mentioned above, it accumulates in granular aggregates of hemosiderin but it does not crystallize. However, *crystals of ferritin* are common in the intestinal cells of insects. *Crystals of guanine* occur in the skin cells of amphibians. The eye-shine of cats and other nocturnal species is due to precisely oriented intracellular crystals in the tapetum lucidum of the retina.

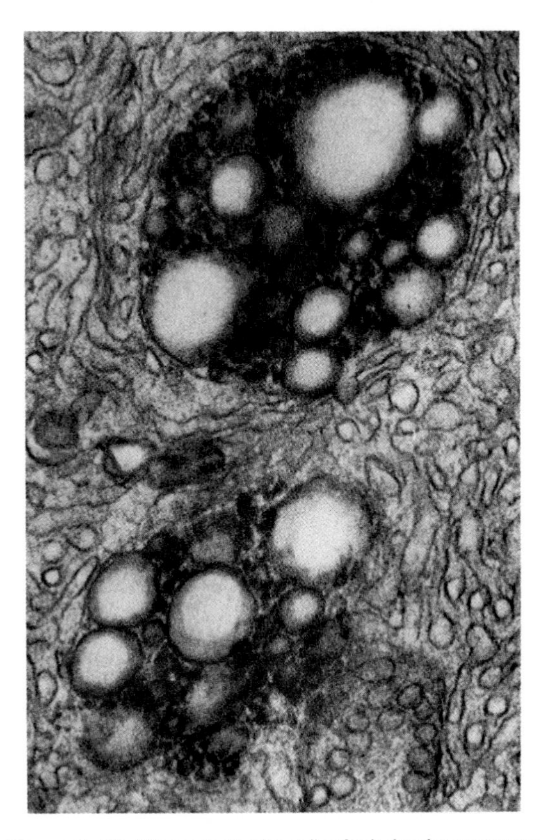

Figure 1–36. Micrograph of two lipofuchsin pigment granules in a cell from the human adrenal cortex.

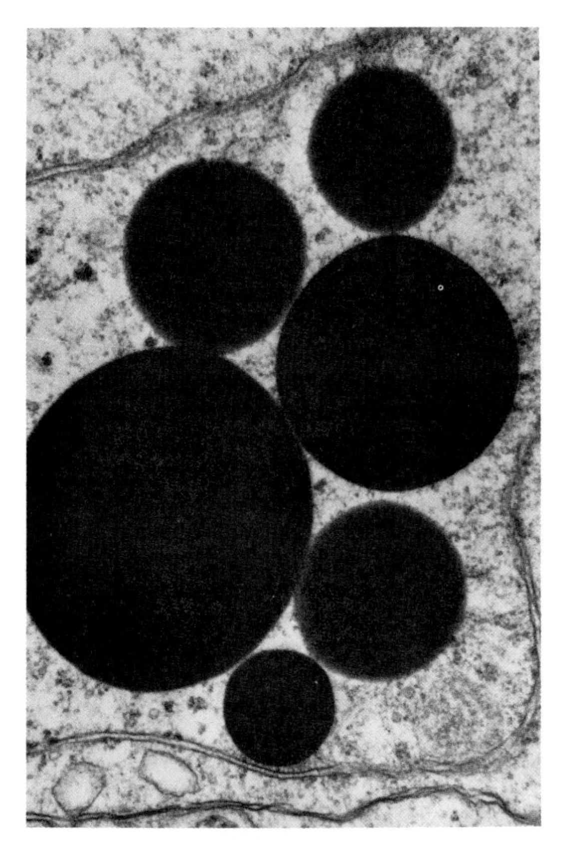

Figure 1–35. Lipid droplets in an electron micrograph of an osmium-fixed cell. After glutaraldehyde fixation, they are not blackened and often appear a pale gray.

Although crystalline inclusions are rare in normal cells, viruses often form crystalline nuclear or cytoplasmic inclusions in infected cells.

CYTOSKELETON

The gel-like consistency of cytoplasm is due, in part, to a three-dimensional lattice of filaments that form a structural framework commonly referred to as the *cytoskeleton*. Its principal components are *microfilaments* and *intermediate filaments*, but these are supplemented by straight, slender *microtubules*. The

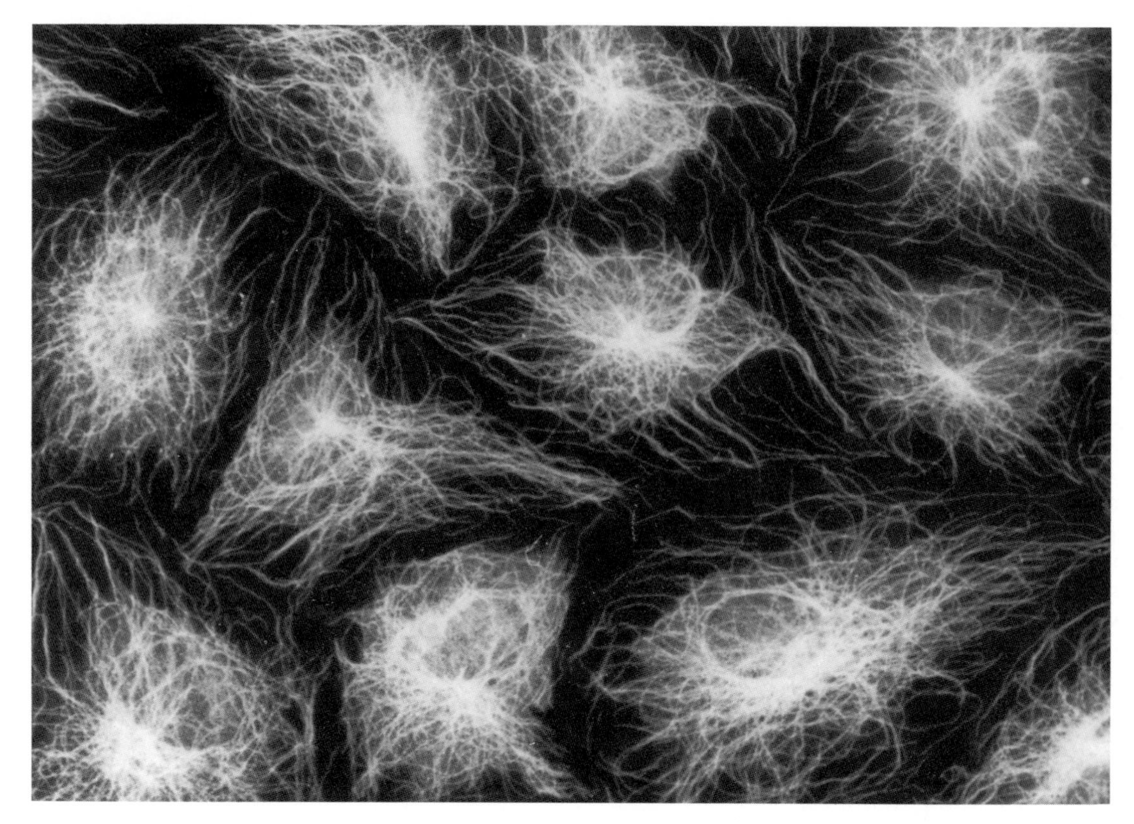

Figure 1–37. Photomicrograph of several cells in tissue culture that have been stained with a fluorescent antibody to tubulin. Microtubules are seen radiating from the cell center throughout the cytoplasm. (Photomicrograph courtesy of R.O. Hynes. 1978. Cell 13:151.)

filaments are detectable in histological sections, only when they occur in relatively coarse bundles. Their distribution can, however, be studied with the light microscope in thinly spread whole cells in tissue culture that have been stained with fluorescent antibodies to polypeptide subunits specific for each class of filaments.

The three-dimensional organization of the cytoskeleton cannot be studied with satisfaction in electron micrographs because only relatively short segments of the filaments and microtubules are included in the ultrathin sections required. Its architecture can be seen better in thin-tissue culture cells that have been quick-frozen in liquid helium, then dried from the frozen state and rotary shadowed with platinum. In electron micrographs of such preparations, the individual filaments and microtubules are resolved and their interrelations can be studied. It becomes apparent that the stability of the cytoskeleton depends on interconnections between its filaments that are maintained by specific cross-linking proteins. The cytoskeleton is involved in changes of cell shape, stabilization of cell attachments, the distribution of cell organelles, and in cell motility.

MICROTUBULES

Microtubules are about 25 nm in diameter with a wall 9 nm thick and a 15-nm lumen. The wall is made up of 13 protofilaments of *tubulin,* a protein of 50,000 molecular weight (MW) that occurs in two forms, *β-tubulin* and *α-tubulin.* Heterodimers of these two tubulins are the units that polymerize end-to-end to form the protofilaments in the wall of the microtubules. Microtubules may be several microns in length but they can be followed in electron micrographs for only a short distance before they go out of the plane of section.

Microtubules may occur anywhere in the cytoplasm and in any orientation, but the majority tend to radiate from the centrosome which appears to be the *microtubule organizing center* of the cell (Fig. 1–37). The *centriolar satellites* are believed to serve as nucleation sites

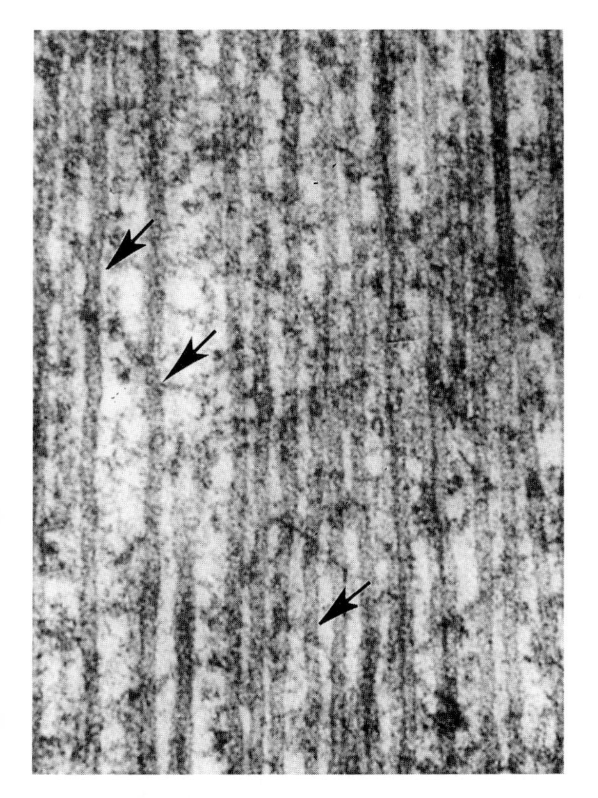

Figure 1–38. A small area of cytoplasm containing multiple microtubules shown here in longitudinal section. Such arrays of microtubules occur in the male germ cells during their elongation to form spermatozoa.

for polymerization of tubulin. Before cell division, when the centrioles replicate and move to opposite poles of the cell, highly ordered arrays of microtubules are generated to form the mitotic spindle. The exact role of these microtubules in the subsequent movement of the chromosomes is still debated.

The microtubules are ephemeral structures in dynamic equilibrium with a large reserve of soluble tubulin in the cytoplasm. The number in the cytoplasm varies from cell type to cell type and at different times in the same cell. They can be rapidly disassembled and reassembled in a new pattern to meet the cytoskeletal requirements of a change in cell shape. In elongating, they preferentially add subunits at one end (the *plus end*) and may simultaneously depolymerize at the other end (the *minus end*), returning subunits to the cytoplasmic pool. Microtubules of different degrees of stability may coexist in the same cell, with some turning over with a half-life as short as 10 min, whereas others are more stable, having a half-life of several hours.

When tubulin is extracted from cells, about 15% of this fraction always contains several other proteins that have been designated *microtubule-associated proteins* (MAPS). One or more of these are believed to form the short lateral projections that can be seen with the electron microscope, at regular 32-nm intervals along the length of the microtubules. These may form cross-links where microtubules are associated laterally (Fig. 1–39). The function of some of the other MAPS has recently been clarified.

Microtubules have an important role in directing the movement of organelles and small vesicles from place to place in the cytoplasm. A microtubule-associated protein, *kinesin,* is a motor responsible for movement of vesicles along microtubules. One end of this molecule is bound to the vesicle while a binding site on the other end undergoes cyclic interaction with the microtubule that moves the vesicle toward its plus end (Fig. 1–40). To achieve two-way traffic, another MAP called *dynein* moves vesicles toward the minus end. Yet an-

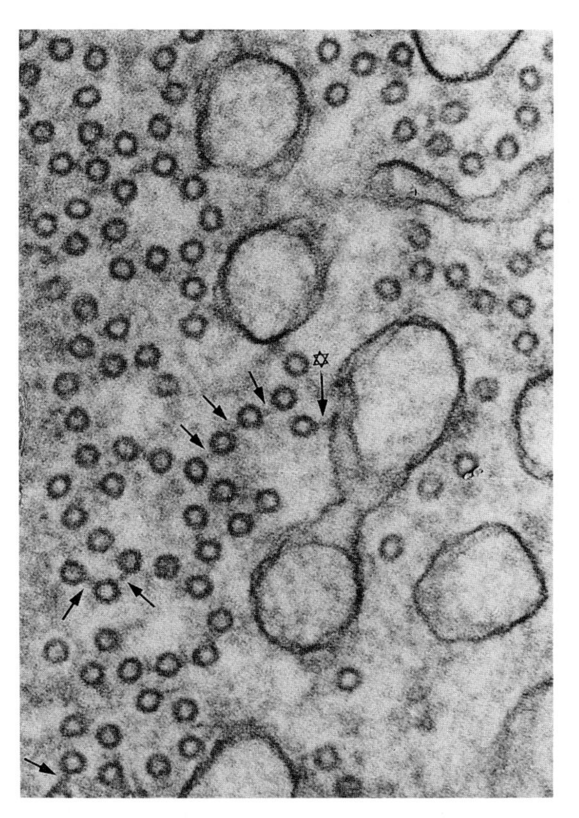

Figure 1–39. Micrograph of a cross section of an array of microtubules involved in elongation of the cell and transport of vesicles during differentiation of a male germ cell. A microtubule associated protein (MAP) can be seen linking microtubules to one another (arrows) and to a vesicle (*).

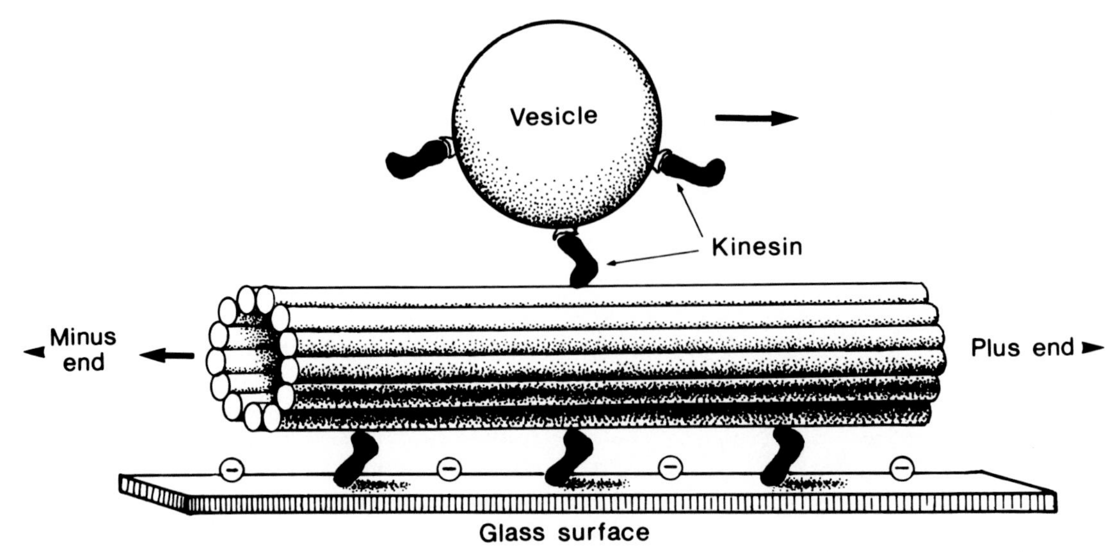

Figure 1–40. Schematic representation of how kinesin generates movement of vesicles and organelles along microtubules. Movement is unidirectional, with vesicles moving toward the plus end. In vitro, microtubules also move along a glass surface bearing a negative charge, with their minus end leading. (Redrawn after Vale et al. 1985. Cell 40:559.)

other MAP, *dynamin,* is a 100 kD polypeptide that forms the regularly spaced cross-bridges between neighboring microtubules. In the growth cones of elongating nerve axons, where microtubules occur in bundles, it serves as a motor for sliding some microtubules of the bundle with respect to others, resulting in elongation of the bundle.

In the cilia of epithelial cells and the flagellum of spermatozoa, tubulin forms stable *doublet microtubules* composed of one complete microtubules with 13 protofilaments (subunit-A), joined to one that is C-shaped in cross section, and has only 10 protofilaments (subunit-B) (Fig. 1–41). As described earlier, the wall of centrioles and basal bodies is made up of nine short *triplet microtubules,* each consisting of one complete microtubule and two that are C-shaped in section (Fig. 1–41). No movement occurs between the centriolar triplets, but the beating of cilia and flagella depends on the sliding of nine doublets of the axoneme with respect to one another. Evenly spaced pairs of short lateral projections, called *arms,* extend from subunit A of each doublet to subunit B of the next. The arms of the doublets are composed of *axonemal dynein,* a microtubule-associated protein that is the motor for ciliary motion. Thus, cells have four microtubule-based motors, kinesin, cytoplasmic dynein, axonemal dynein, and dynamin. There may be others yet to be discovered.

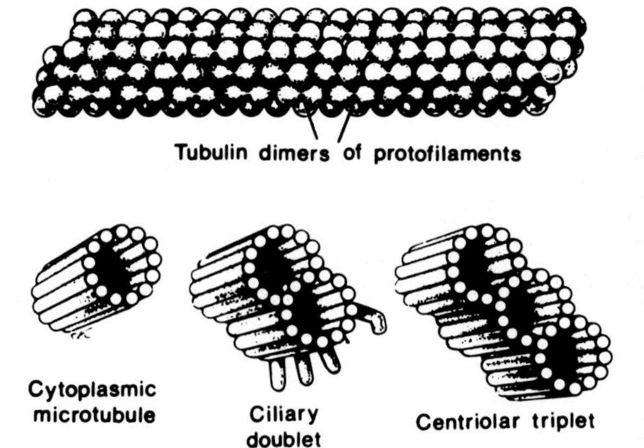

Figure 1–41. Drawing of the arrangement of linear polymers of tubulin that form the protofilaments in the wall of the microtubule. Below are the three configurations in which the protofilaments may be assembled: singlet microtubules in the cytoplasm, doublets in ciliary and flagellar axonemes, and triplets in the wall of the centriole.

MICROFILAMENTS

The microfilaments of the cytoskeleton are about 7 nm in diameter and of variable length. They consist of globular subunits of a 42 kD protein, *G-actin,* polymerized to form two identical strands that are helically coiled around one another to form a filament (*F-actin*). Present in nearly all cells, actin filaments contribute to the viscoelastic and contractile properties of the cytoplasm. They are most abundant in the *ectoplasm* (cortex) of the cell, a gel-like peripheral zone of cytoplasm immediately beneath the cell membrane. In this zone, the actin filaments are cross-linked in a three-dimensional meshwork from which the organelles are excluded. In the more fluid *endoplasm,* they are less abundant but may aggregate in bundles that terminate at the cell membrane. The larger of these bundles are visible in living cells with the light microscope and have been called *stress fibers,* although there is little evidence that this is an appropriate term.

Actin constitutes 10–15% of the total protein of cells, but, at any given time, only about half of it is in the form of F-actin. The filaments are formed, as needed, by polymerization from a pool of soluble G-actin. During a change in cell shape, they depolymerize, returning subunits to that pool, and then repolymerize into filaments with a different orientation. Under appropriate conditions, G-actin extracted from cells will polymerize into filaments, in vitro.

Microfilaments are not ordinarily resolved with the light microscope but the distribution of actin in the cell can be revealed by using a fluorescein-labeled anti-actin antibody. Actin filaments are visible in electron micrographs, but in lower than normal concentrations because they tend to be extracted by prolonged exposure to conventional fixatives. Better preservation of all components of the cytoskeleton can be achieved by rapid freezing of tissue culture cells in liquid helium, followed by freeze-drying and rotary-shadowing with carbon and platinum. With this method, actin filaments are present in the cytoplasm in greater numbers than in routine preparations (Figs. 1–42, 1–43).

Locomotion of cells depends on interaction of actin filaments with the actin-binding protein *myosin.* In muscle, which is specialized for contraction, the myosin forms highly ordered arrays of relatively thick filaments that interdigitate with actin filaments. Shortening of the muscle involves sliding of the thin actin filaments with respect to the thicker myosin filaments. In cells other than muscle, myosin is present in a much lower ratio to actin and it does not form microscopically identifiable filaments. The mode of interaction of actin and myosin in non-muscle cells is still poorly understood. It is speculated that myosin molecules may form very short bipolar filaments that bind to actin; then, triggered by calcium ions and ATP, the myosin may change its configuration in such a way as to exert traction on the actin filaments.

The deployment of actin filaments in the cytoplasm is influenced by a number of actin-binding proteins. *Profilin* binds to G-actin monomer, preventing polymerization and, thus, helps to maintain a supply of monomer that can be drawn on as needed to form new actin filaments. *Capping protein* binds to the end of an actin filament, limiting further increase in its length. Another protein, *fimbrin,* rigidly binds adjacent actin filaments, in parallel, to form bundles. Another, *filamin,* forms flexible links between intersecting microfilaments, stabilizing a three-dimensional network. Still another, *gelsolin,* is able to insert itself between subunits of a filament, breaking it into shorter segments. Two other actin-binding proteins, *vinculin* and *α-actinin,* mediate the binding of actin filaments to the cell membrane at intercellular junctions and at the cell base.

INTERMEDIATE FILAMENTS

Early studies of the cytoskeleton concentrated upon the microtubules (24 nm) and the microfilaments (7 nm), but it soon became apparent that the cytoplasm of most cells contains another major category of filaments about 10 nm in diameter (Fig. 1–44). Because their diameter fell between microfilaments and microtubules, they were called *intermediate filaments.* When isolated from various cell types and analyzed, they proved not to be a single entity but a family of ultrastructurally similar, but biochemically distinct, filaments composed of subunits differing widely in molecular weight. Five major classes of intermediate filaments are now distinguished by immunocytochemical methods: *keratin, vimentin, desmin, neurofilaments,* and *glial filaments.*

Keratin filaments are characteristic of epithelial cells and are not found in cells of mesenchymal origin. They are most abundant in the stratified squamous epithelium of the skin, where they occupy a large fraction of the cytoplasm in the fully differentiated superficial cells. The so-called tonofilaments described by early light microscopists are bundles of keratin filaments. In other epithelial cells, they often form a network around the nucleus with bundles radiating to the periphery where they terminate in local specializations of the membrane for cell-to-cell attachment. Unlike microfilaments and microtubules, which are in dynamic equilibrium with a pool of mono-

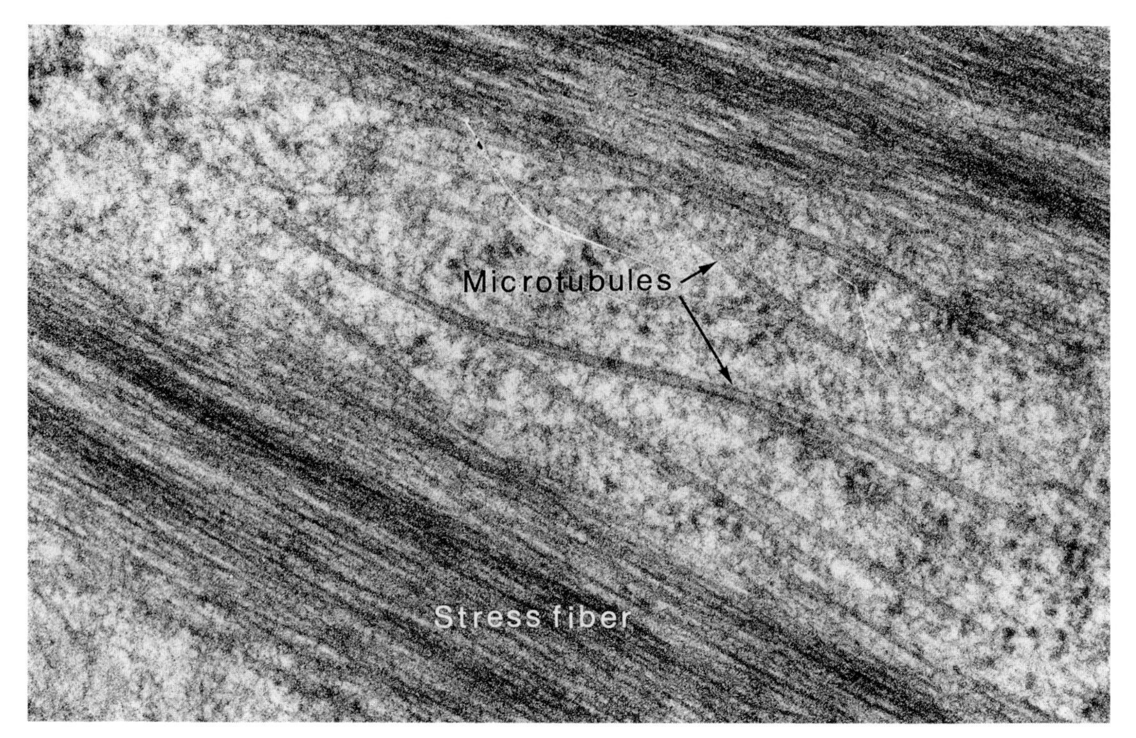

Figure 1–42. Micrograph of a small area of fibroblast cytoplasm, prepared by quick-freezing in liquid helium and freeze substitution. Portions of two stress fibers, made up predominantly of actin filaments course diagonally across the field. Between them are a few microtubules. (Micrograph courtesy of J. Heuser and M. Kirschner. 1980. J. Cell Biol. 86:212.)

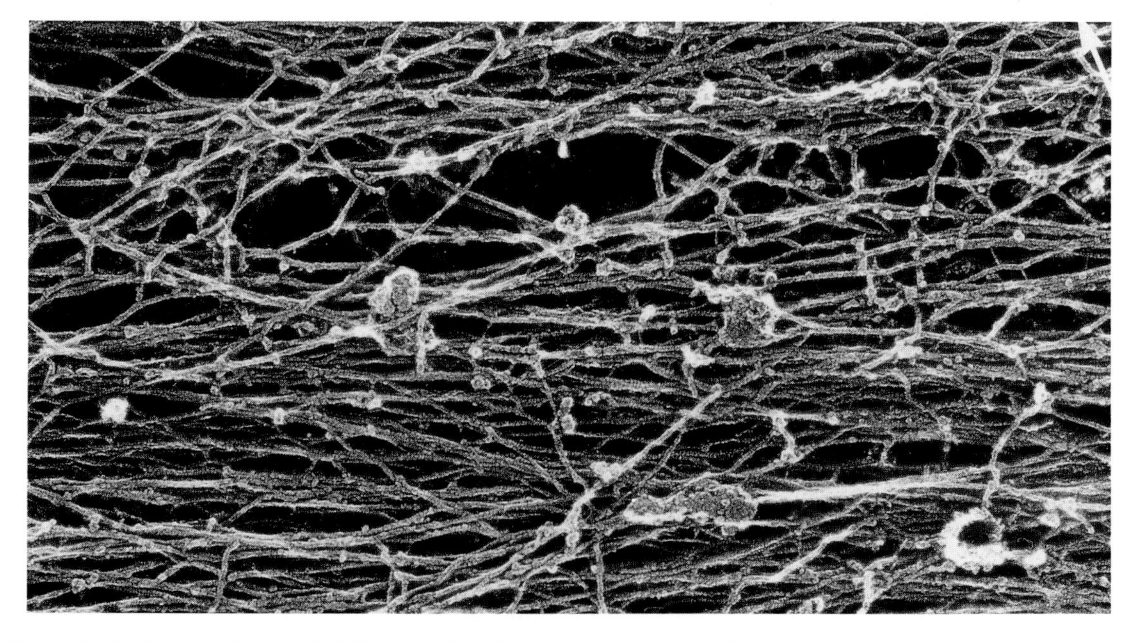

Figure 1–43. A rotary-shadowed platinum replica of a segment of a stress fiber extracted with Triton. The stress fiber is composed mainly of actin filaments. 70,000 × (Micrograph courtesy of J. Heuser and M. Kirschner. 1980. J. Cell Biol. 86:212).

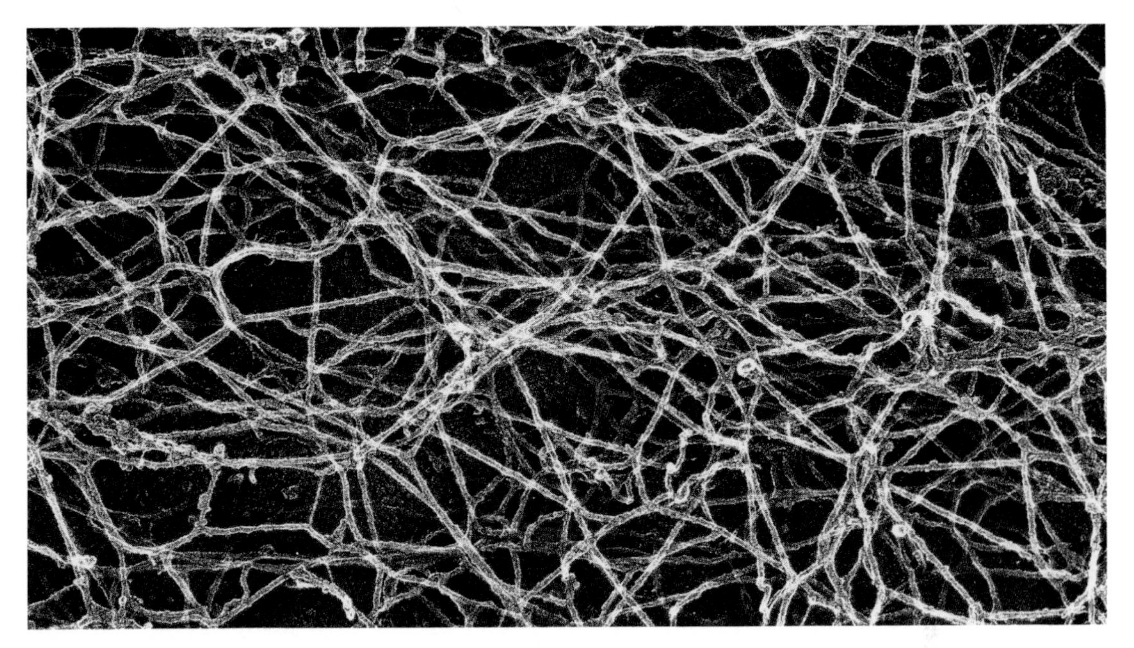

Figure 1–44. Micrograph of a small area of the cytoskeleton found within the cytoplasmic matrix after extraction of the actin. The rich network of filaments remaining is composed of the intermediate filament protein, vimentin. (Micrograph courtesy of J. Heuser and M. Kirschner. 1980. J. Cell Biol. 86:212).

mers, keratin filaments do not undergo rapid assembly and disassembly. Their function is mainly mechanical, stabilizing the shape of the cell and strengthening its attachment to other cells and to the basal lamina.

Keratins isolated from various cell types are not a single compound but are members of a complex multigene family of proteins made up of six or seven 40–70 kD polypeptide subunits in different combinations. Although all keratin filaments are similar in their ultrastructure, those in different epithelia, and indeed in different stages of differentiation of the same cell type, may differ in the proportions of their several polypeptide subunits.

Intermediate filaments of the 53 kD acidic protein *desmin* are characteristic of smooth, striated, and cardiac muscle. They are not a conspicuous component of striated muscle, but they form a loose network around, and between, the contractile elements. They appear to keep the sarcomeres of neighboring myofibrils in register across the width of the muscle fiber. They also link the Z-bands of peripheral myofibrils to the sarcolemma. Desmin filaments are more abundant in smooth muscle cells, where they are aggregated into thin bundles that link together the dense bodies at the sites of convergence of actin filaments and to dense plaques on the inner aspect of the plasma membrane. This cytoskeleton of desmin filaments transmits the pull of the contractile proteins and ensures a uniform distribution of tensile force throughout the smooth muscle cell.

In fibroblasts, and other mesenchymal derivatives, the intermediate filaments consist of the 58 kD protein, *vimentin*. They may associate in bundles or may be randomly oriented in a loose network throughout the cytoplasm. This meshwork of vimentin filaments can be seen in rapid-freeze freeze-dry preparations (Fig. 1–44).

Neurofilaments are a conspicuous feature of the perikaryon, dendrites, and axon of neurons. They are made up of three major polypeptides of 210 kD, 160 kD, and 68 kD. Neurofilaments are oriented parallel to the long axis of the nerve axon. They provide internal support and may help to maintain the gelated state of the axoplasm. This latter function is inferred from the observation that when the contents of the axon are expressed, the axoplasm is a firm gel, but it rapidly becomes a sol in the presence of calcium ions that trigger proteolytic degradation of the neurofilaments.

Glial filaments are the intermediate filaments of the non-neural cells of the central nervous system: astrocytes, oligodendrocytes, and microglial cells. They consist of the 51 kD *glial fibrillary acidic protein* and have the same function in these cells as the neurofilaments in neurons.

Just as there are several actin-binding polypeptides associated with the microfilaments, there are a number of polypeptides associated with the intermediate filaments: *filaggrin, plectin,* and *synamin.* Filaggrin, found in epidermal cells, binds to keratin filaments, causing them to aggregate into bundles. Plectin seems to be preferentially located at sites of intersection of vimentin intermediate filaments and is probably responsible for their linkage into a cytoskeletal network. Synamin is found in muscle, where it may have a similar role.

Separation of morphologically identical intermediate filaments into five separate classes on the basis of differences in their polypeptide subunits may seem to be splitting hairs, but it has practical application in pathology. Immunofluorescent-specific antibodies against subunits of each kind of intermediate filament are now available and they have become valuable reagents for distinguishing cell types in pathological conditions, in which morphological criteria alone are insufficient for identification. For example, in malignant tumors, the cells may become so altered that it is difficult to determine the tissue of origin. In such cases, immunocytochemical identification of the type of intermediate filament in their cytoplasm often makes it possible to determine whether a tumor is of epithelial, mesenchymal, neural, or glial origin.

CYTOPLASMIC MATRIX

Opinion has varied as to whether the cell organelles are suspended in a viscous fluid or in a gelated cytoplasmic matrix. In either interpretation, it is difficult to envision how the movements of organelles and vesicles that is observed in living cells could take place through dense networks of filaments extending throughout the cytoplasm. Some insight into this problem has been gained by studies combining video-enhanced light microscopy with electron microscopy of rapidly frozen, freeze-dried, and rotary-shadowed cells. These have led to the concept that the cytoplasm has two functional domains. In a central domain around the nucleus, Brownian motion of small particles and directed movements of organelles are observed in living cells. In a peripheral domain, no such movements occur except along narrow radial extensions of the central domain. Tubulin-specific ligands stain the central domain and actin-specific ligands stain the outer domain. In electron micrographs, the outer domain (the ectoplasm) consists of a dense meshwork of actin microfilaments, whereas the central domain (the endoplasm) containing microtubules, vesicles, and the organelles is traversed by a few supporting bundles of intermediate filaments but is otherwise relatively free of filamentous components. The dynamism of the cytoplasm in the living cell evidently involves directed movement of vesicles and organelles along microtubules in a fluid central domain, whereas the maintenance cell shape and its modification depends mainly upon the actin-rich outer domain.

CELL ACTIVITIES

Having described the principal structural components of cells, it will facilitate explanation of the function of the tissues and organs, in later chapters, if a few activities that are common to most cell types are briefly discussed here. Among these are cell division, endocytosis, exocytosis, cell locomotion, and cell death.

CELL DIVISION

Growth, repair, and renewal in all multicellular organisms depend on the formation of new cells by the division of preexisting cells. There are two mechanisms of cell division, *mitosis,* which occurs in *somatic cells,* and *meiosis,* which is confined to the developing *germ cells* in the ovary and the testis. The two have many features in common, but they differ in the behavior of the chromosomes during the early stages of division. An understanding of both is fundamental to the science of genetics because many inherited disorders are attributable to abnormal behavior of the chromosomes during cell division.

Chromosomes are flexible rod-like structures that become visible when all of the chromatin of the cell nucleus reverts to the condensed (heterochromatic) state. The number of chromosomes in cells is constant and characteristic for each species. In the somatic cells of the human, that number is 46, which is referred to as the *diploid* number (Fig. 1–45). The germ cells have half as many, 23, the *haploid* number. In the fusion of sperm and ovum during fertilization, the union of their respective haploid sets of chromosomes restores the diploid number in the resulting *zy-*

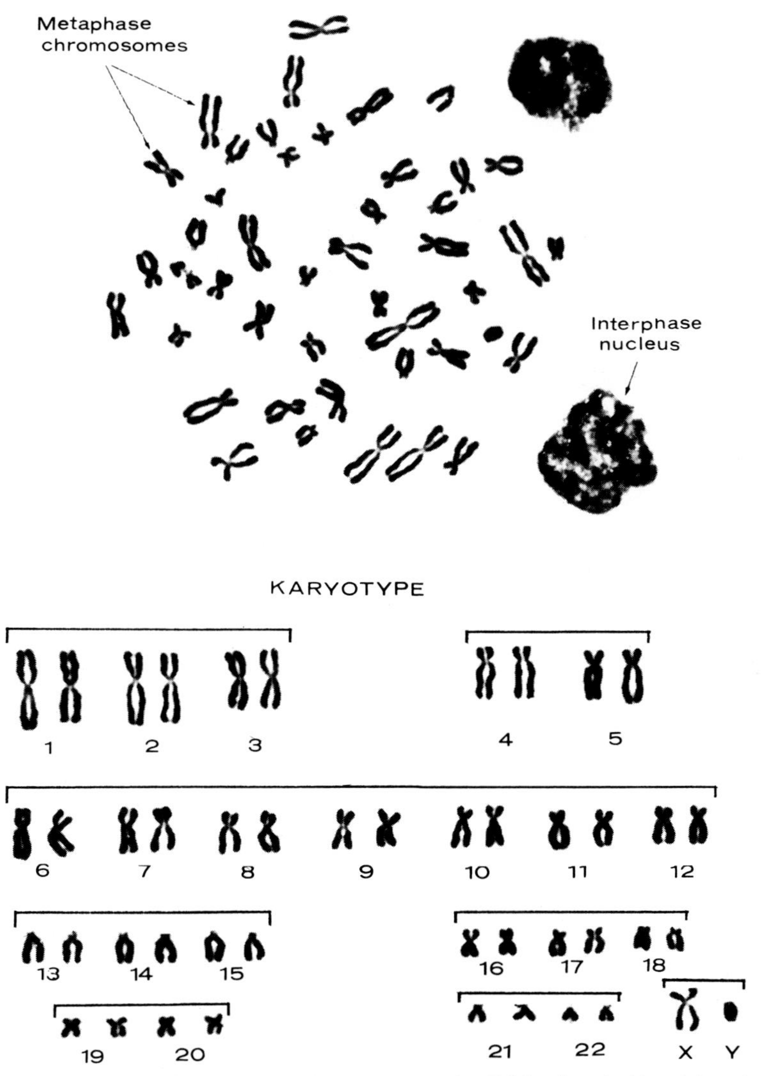

Figure 1–45. Photomicrograph of human metaphase chromosomes of a dividing lymphoblast (above). Below: the human karyotype constructed by cutting out the chromosomes from such a photograph and arranging them in groups according to their size, and the location of the primary constriction. The 22 pairs of autosomes are identified by number, and the sex chromosomes by *X* and *Y*. (Photomicrograph courtesy of H. Lisco and L. Lisco.)

gote. A few cell types that contain more than two sets of chromosomes are said to be *polyploid.* Cells exhibiting departures from the diploid number that do not involve whole sets of chromosomes are described as *aneuploid.*

Each chromosome in a haploid cell has its own distinctive size and shape. A diploid cell has two chromosomes of each kind, forming *homologous pairs,* one member of the pair having been contributed by the sperm and the other by the ovum at conception (Fig. 1–45). In males, one pair, the *sex chromosomes,* differs from the other 22 pairs in that one of its members, the *Y-chromosome,* is shorter than its partner, the *X-chromosome.* In meiotic division of the developing germ cells, the homologous pairs separate, one member going to each daughter cell. Therefore, the human male produces, in equal numbers, spermatozoa containing a Y-chromosome and spermatozoa containing an X-chromosome. Thus, in the human, the male is the *heterogametic sex* with a chromosome complement designated 44XY. The female is the *homogametic sex* (44XX) and produces ova, all of which contain an X-chromosome. Fertilization of such an ovum by a 22X spermatozoon results in a female offspring (44XX), whereas fertilization by a 22Y spermatozoon results in a male (44XY).

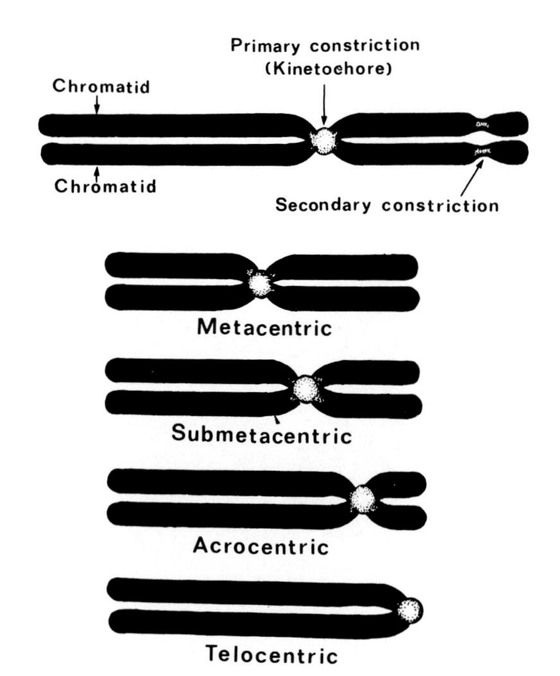

Figure 1–46. Diagram presenting the descriptive terms applied to chromosomes based on the location of the primary constriction or kinetochore.

MITOSIS

Mitotic division results in two daughter cells possessing identical copies of the genome of the parent cell. Before the onset of division, the DNA is replicated so that the cell enters mitosis with twice the normal diploid complement. Division extends over a period of 30–60 min in mammals, but may take considerably longer in cold-blooded vertebrates. The period between successive episodes of cell division is called *interphase.* The sequence of events in mitosis is divided into four stages: *prophase, metaphase, anaphase,* and *telophase.*

During interphase, only the nucleolus and a few clumps of condensed chromatin can be seen in the nucleus. Except for these condensed (heterochromatic) segments, the chromosomes are in an extended (euchromatic) state and are not identifiable in sections. After replication, and some condensation, of the DNA in preparation for division, the chromosomes become visible in both living and fixed material as slender thread-like structures in the nucleus (Fig. 1–47E). The appearance of chromosomes marks the beginning of prophase. Throughout this stage, they continue to condense, becoming shorter and thicker. Each consists of two parallel strands called *chromatids,* joined to one another at the *centromere,* a constricted segment common to both strands. At this site, there is a trilaminar disc, the *kinetochore,* consisting of two dense layers separated by a paler middle layer. Concurrent with these events, the centrioles replicate and migrate to opposite poles of the cell. This is followed by a breakdown of the nuclear envelope which marks the end of prophase.

Metaphase begins with the alignment of the chromosomes in the same plane in the middle of the cell to form the *equatorial plate* (metaphase plate). This orderly assembly of the chromosomes is associated with the development of the *mitotic spindle,* a fusiform array of microtubules, some of which extend from the centrioles to the chromosomes on the equatorial plate, whereas others extend from pole to pole.

An early event in anaphase is the separation of the single kinetochore of each pair of chromatids into two, so that each chromatid has its own. The sister chromatids, no longer bound together by a shared kinetochore, are then free to move to opposite poles of the spindle as separate chromosomes. The mechanism of the poleward movement of the chromosomes has long been a subject of controversy. The traditional view that they were "pulled" toward the poles by the "chromosomal fibers" of the spindle was abandoned when ultrastructural studies revealed that the spindle consists of microtubules which have no contractile properties. The kinetochore of each chromosome attaches to one or more spindle microtubules. Ingenious experiments have shown, to the satisfaction of most, that the chromosomes do not move along the microtubules. To account for their movement to the poles, it is postulated that the microtubules shorten, during anaphase, by depolymerization at one end or the other. The bulk of evidence favors depolymerization at the kinetochore end. Dynein has recently been found to be associated with the kinetochore which raises the possibility that the chromosome may be moved by a dynein motor, concurrently with depolymerization at that end of the microtubules. Chromosomal movements at anaphase would thus be analogous to the transport of vesicles along microtubules, but with the additional feature of concurrent depolymerization of the microtubules.

At telophase, the chromosomes are clustered at the spindle poles, and soon thereafter, segments of a nuclear envelope are formed around them. The chromosomes then uncoil, losing their stainability except in those regions

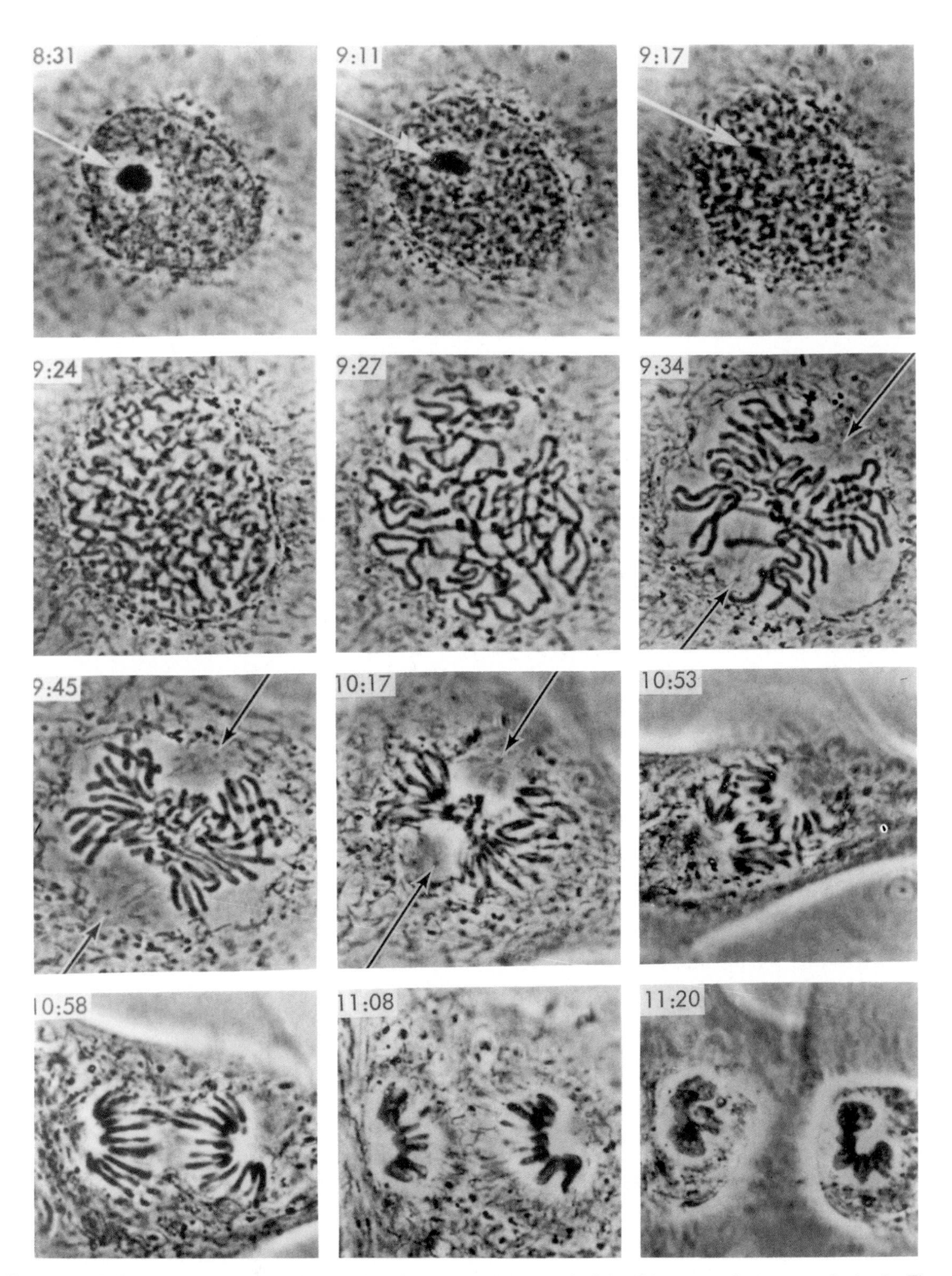

Figure 1–47. Phase-contrast photomicrographs of an amphibian mesothelial cell in successive stages of mitosis. The large white arrow points to the nucleolus; black arrows indicate the centrioles. A to E, prophase; F to H, metaphase; I to K, anaphase; L, telophase. The duration of 3 h shown here is much longer than required for mitosis in warm-blooded vertebrates.

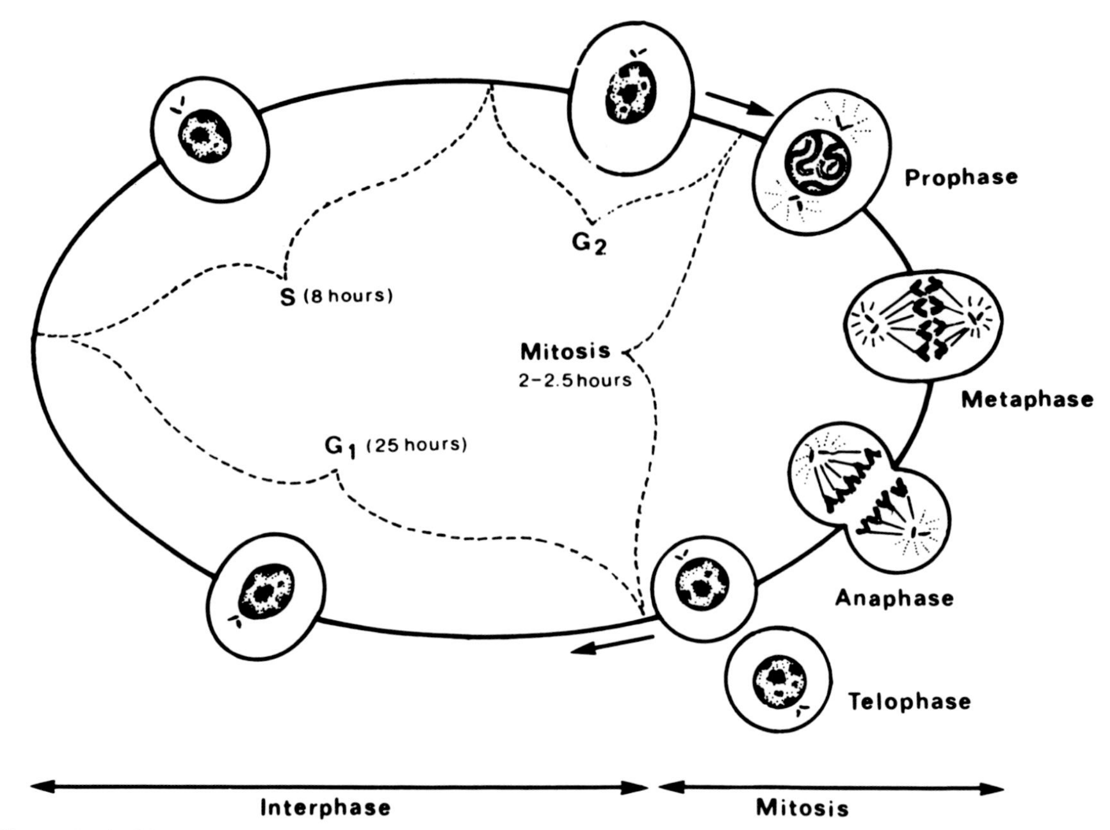

Figure 1–48. Diagram showing the phases of the cell cycle and their approximate duration in proliferating bone cells with a cycle length of 25 h. Cycle length varies greatly among different cell types. (Redrawn from L.C. Junquiera and J. Carneiro. 1983. Basic Histology. Lange Medical Publishers.)

destined to remain condensed as the heterochromatin of the interphase nucleus. At the conclusion of these changes, *karyokinesis* is complete. Nucleoli are reformed and the initially discontinuous segments of nuclear envelope coalesce to form a complete perinuclear cisterna. While reconstitution of the nuclei is in progress, there is a constriction of the cytoplasm midway between them. This *cleavage furrow* deepens until it encounters the microtubules of the spindle. For a short time, the daughter cells remain connected by a slender cytoplasmic bridge occupied by residual spindle microtubules that are bound together at their midpoint by dense amorphous material, forming the so-called the *midbody*. After a brief delay, the microtubules depolymerize and the intercellular bridge is sundered at one side of the midbody and the two halves are retracted into the cytoplasm of the daughter cells to complete *cytokinesis*.

In the cells of females, one of the X-chromosomes remains condensed during interphase and can be identified as a small clump of intensely staining heterochromatin, usually located adjacent to the nuclear envelope. This *sex chromatin* or *Barr body* is not found in the nuclei of males. This sexual dimorphism of the interphase nuclei makes it possible to identify the sex of an individual by examining squamous epithelial cells scraped from the inside of the mouth. This simple test is useful in the differential diagnosis of certain abnormalities of sexual development.

MEIOSIS

Meiosis is a kind of cell division occurring only in the development of ova and spermatozoa. It consists of two successive divisions with only one replication of the chromosomes. In the first division, the members of each homologous pair separate and go to opposite poles, thereby reducing the number of chromosomes in the daughter cells by half. The second division involves replication of each chromosome and separation of the two chromatids so formed. The four cells resulting from the two meiotic divisions have half the normal diploid number of chromosomes, and the gametes that develop from them are, therefore, haploid. After union of the male and female gametes at fertilization, the diploid number of chromosomes is restored in the cells of the zygote.

Meiosis is characterized by a very long prophase, which is divided into five stages. In the earliest of these, called *leptotene,* the chromosomes become visible in the nucleus as long thin single strands. In the second, *zygotene,* homologous chromosomes begin to come together in close lateral apposition, with corresponding sites along their length in register. This pairing is called *synapsis.* In the ensuing *pachytene* stage, the chromosomes coil, becoming shorter and thicker. Because of their very close apposition, in this stage the homologous chromosomes may give the erroneous impression that they are a single chromosome. However, in the succeeding *diplotene* stage, they separate along their length and it becomes apparent that each of them has replicated and is double stranded. Each chromosome pair, or bivalent, now consists of four chromatids. At certain points along their length, homologous chromatids cross one another, break, and the fragments recombine at these sites so that segments have been exchanged. These sites of segment interchange are called *chiasmata* and are the basis for what geneticists call *crossing-over,* an important mechanism for ensuring genetic diversity. Shortening and thickening of the chromosomes continues and they tend to clump together in the center of the nucleus. The nucleolus that has persisted throughout the early stages of prophase fragments and later disappears.

At metaphase, the nuclear membrane breaks down and a spindle is formed, as in mitosis. The bivalents gather in alignment on the equatorial plate. Their kinetochore does not divide, as it does in mitosis. Consequently, in anaphase of the first meiotic division, it is whole chromosomes, not sister chromatids, that separate and move to opposite poles. Thus, the daughter cells of this division contain half the diploid number of chromosomes. In teleophase, nuclei are briefly reconstituted, but they soon proceed to the second division, which is very much like mitosis. The chromatids separate, the kinetochores divide, and the sister chromatids move apart to opposite poles. The two meiotic divisions thus result in four cells, all of which have haploid nuclei. Because the reduction in chromosome number occurs in the first division, it is commonly called the *reduction division* and the second is called the *equational division.*

The biological significance of meiosis is twofold. It ensures constancy of chromosome number from generation to generation by producing haploid male and female gametes, and it creates genetic diversity by crossing-over of the chromosomes. After meiosis, the chromosomes are genetically different from the preexisting chromosomes due to the exchange of segments in prophase of the first division. The randomness of the distribution of the homologues to the daughter nuclei during reduction division contributes further to the genetic diversity of the gametes.

The discovery, in 1959, that the cells of children with the common congenital disorder *Down's syndrome* (mongolism) have an extra chromosome stimulated intense interest in the examination of human chromosomes and led to the identification of a number of other disease states that are associated with visible chromosomal abnormalities. Therefore, it has become important for students of medicine to have some knowledge of chromosomal morphology and behavior during cell division. Chromosomal analysis has now become a routine procedure on the obstetrical and pediatric services of hospitals. It is often possible to detect congenital anomalies before birth by examining the chromosomes of cells aspirated from the amniotic cavity (amniocentesis).

Because chromosomes are accessible for analysis only at metaphase of mitosis, a dependable source of dividing cells is required for cytogenetic analysis. White blood cells are separated by centrifugation from a blood sample and grown in culture for a few days after their exposure to a phytohemagglutinin that stimulates proliferation of lymphocytes. The cultures are then treated with colchicine that blocks formation of the mitotic spindle, arresting cell divisions at metaphase. This procedure permits accumulation of cells at the stage most favorable for chromosomal analysis.

Successful cytogenetic analysis requires that the 23 chromosomes be individually identifiable. Differences in length and position of the centromere are useful criteria. If the centromere is in the middle, and the arms are of about equal length, the chromosome is classified as *metacentric.* If the centromere is between the midpoint and one end, the chromosome is described as *submetacentric.* If it is near one end, it is *acrocentric,* and if it is at the very end, it is classified as *telocentric* (Fig. 1–46). As an aid to cytogenetic studies of any given species, the chromosomes are cut out of an enlarged photomicrograph. The homologous chromosomes are identified, juxtaposed, and arranged in groups on the basis of differences in length, and position of the centromere. Such an ordered arrangement of chromosomes is referred to as the *karyotype* of the species under study.

The human karyotype consists of seven groups with the members of each arranged in order of decreasing size (Fig. 1–45). Group-A includes large metacentric chromosomes numbered 1–3; group-B includes large submetacentrics, 4 and 5; group-C contains shorter metacentrics 6–12 and the X-chromosome; group-D, medium-sized acrocentrics 13–15; group-E, small submetacentrics 16–18; group-F small metacentrics 19 and 20, and group-G contains the smallest of the acrocentrics, 21 and 22 and the Y-chromosome of the male. Some cytogeneticists prefer to set the X- and Y-chromosome apart as a separate group instead of including them with the autosomes, according to their size (Fig. 1–45).

Within the groups, identification of individual chromosomes by number is facilitated by staining them with a fluorescent quinacrine compound that brings out a characteristic pattern of cross-banding that adds another criterion for identification. The genes are known to be arranged in linear order along the chromosomes, and although they cannot be seen with the microscope, the location of a particular gene (gene locus) can sometimes be described in relation to one of the stainable bands characteristic of that chromosome.

Cytogenetic anomalies of clinical significance may involve *aneuploidy* of one or more chromosomes; loss of a portion of a chromosome (*deletion*), or transfer of a segment to a nonhomologous chromosome (*translocation*). For example, in *Down's syndrome* there is an extra chromosome 21 (*trisomy-21*) due to failure of one member of that homologous pair to move to the appropriate spindle pole in meiotic division during gametogenesis. *Turner's syndrome* is an example of aneuploidy in which loss of an X-chromosome (44XO) results in a phenotypic female whose ovaries are vestigial and usually devoid of germ cells. An extra X-chromosome in a phenotypic male (44XXY) results in *Klinefelder's syndrome,* characterized by underdevelopment of the testes, sterility, and breast development (gynecomastia).

ENDOCYTOSIS

The cells of the body are surrounded by extracellular fluid derived from the blood and they must extract from this fluid the molecules that they need as nutrients and as precursors for synthesis of intrinsic components and products for export. Ions and small water-soluble molecules, such as glucose, and amino acids flow or are pumped through minute protein-lined channels that traverse the cell membrane. Larger molecules are taken up by *endocytosis,* an active process of ingestion in membrane-bounded invaginations of the cell membrane that close at their neck, forming a vesicle or vacuole that moves into the cytoplasm. The uptake of fluid and solutes in small vesicles is called *pinocytosis* (drinking by cells). The ingestion of solid matter by extending processes that envelope and draw the particle into the cytoplasm is called *phagocytosis* (eating by cells).

PHAGOCYTOSIS

Phagocytosis is not an activity common to all cells but it is highly developed in the white blood cells and tissue macrophages, which are specialized for defense of the organism against bacterial invasion. Such cells are referred to by the collective term *phagocytes.* Ingestion is initiated by binding of a bacterium, or an inanimate particle, to receptors on the cell surface. This stimulates mobilization of actin and myosin in the ectoplasm underlying the site of contact, and cell processes, called *pseudopodia,* are formed. These slowly elongate as their membrane advances over the surface of the bacterium in a zipper-like process of binding of ligand to receptors. When the leading ends of the enveloping pseudopodia meet on the other side, their membranes fuse and the bacterium is drawn into the cytoplasm in a vacuole bounded by a detached portion of the cell membrane (Fig. 1–49). Lysosomes then fuse with the vacuole and their acid hydrolases digest its contents. Macrophages also have thin, undulating, fin-like *lamellipodia* extending from their surface. Bacteria may bind to these preexisting processes and be engulfed and drawn into the cytoplasm without the necessity of forming blunt pseudopodia to envelope the particle.

Ingestion of bacteria depends on their having a surface that will bind to the membrane of the phagocyte. Some pathogenic bacteria

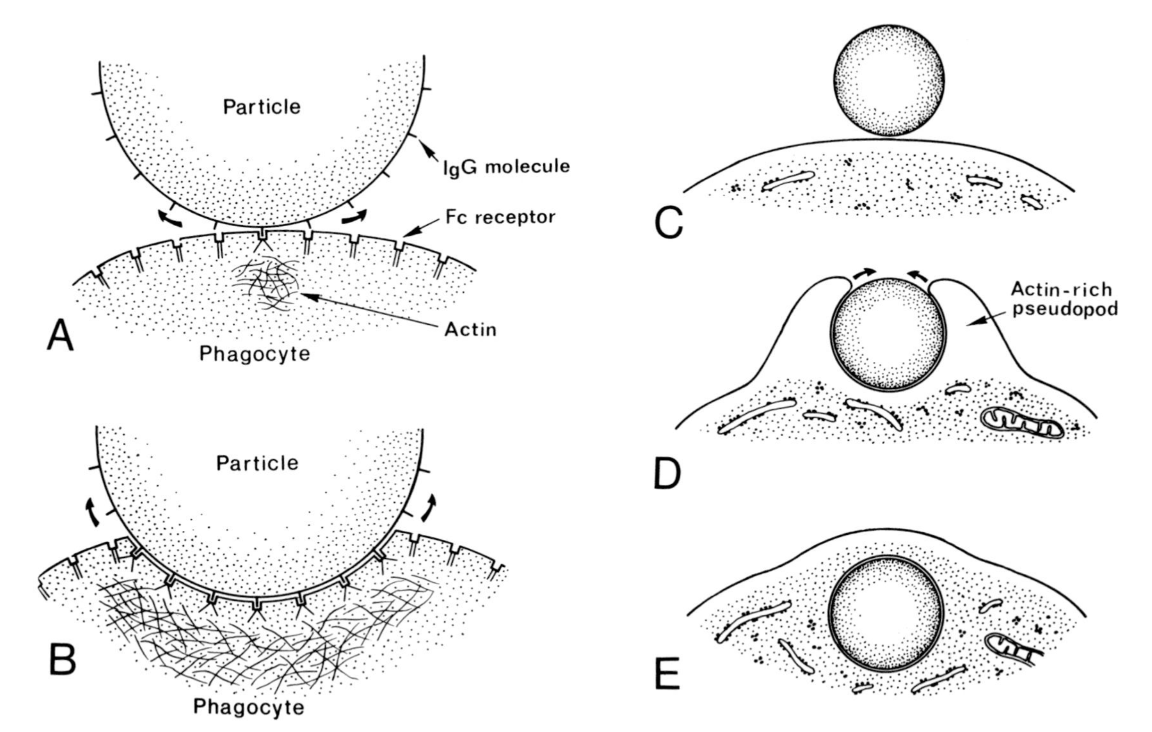

Figure 1–49. Schematic representation of the mechanism of phagocytosis. In the attachment phase, ligands on the surface of the particle bind to receptors on the phagocyte membrane. Progressive circumferential binding spreads from the site of initial contact, zippering the membranes together. This triggers polymerization of actin in the underlying cytoplasm and extension of engulfing pseudopods that bring the phagocyte membrane into contact for binding around the entire circumference of the particle. When the pseudopods meet and fuse, interiorization is complete.

have a protective carbohydrate capsule that resists binding. However, this defensive strategy can be circumvented if there are specific *antibodies* to that organism in the blood of the host. These will coat the capsule and the bacterium will then bind to receptors for antigen–antibody complexes that are normally present in the membrane of phagocytes. Another serum protein called *complement* coats foreign objects nonspecifically and facilitates their binding to complement receptors. Phagocytes take up many particles other than bacteria. The binding of such inanimate foreign particles to phagocytes appears to depend on their surface charge and other properties that are not yet understood.

PINOCYTOSIS

Pinocytosis is exhibited, to varying degree, in nearly all cell types. Thin lamellipodia may envelope and interiorize sizable droplets of extracellular fluid (0.5–1.5 μm). This process of *macropinocytosis* can be observed with the phase contrast microscope in some living cells, in vitro, but the more common *micropinocytosis*, in which fluid and solutes are taken up in minute vesicles (80–90 nm), can be detected only in electron micrographs (Fig. 1–50). The volume of fluid continuously taken up by micropinocytosis is not generally appreciated because profiles of these small membrane invaginations are not abundant in micrographs owing to the thinness of the sections used. However, scanning micrographs of the cytoplasmic surface of isolated membranes reveal that there may be 50 or more pinocytosis vesicles per square micron (Fig. 1–51). In most cells, the fluid taken in is used by those cells, but in the capillary endothelium, fluid and solutes may be transported across the vessel wall from the lumen to the basal surface of the cells, where they fuse with the membrane and discharge their content. This process, called *transcytosis,* is an important mechanism for moving solutes from the blood to the extracellular spaces.

In *fluid-phase pinocytosis,* the vesicles formed are smooth surfaced and they contain ions and molecules in the same concentration as in the extracellular fluid. The process is therefore *nonselective.* There is another form, *receptor-mediated pinocytosis,* that is a highly *selective*

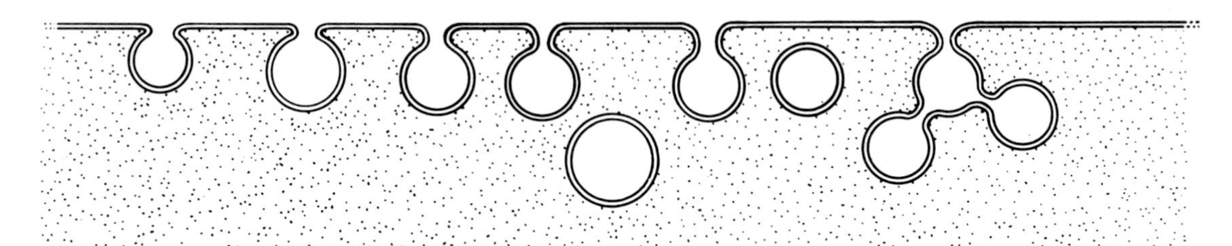

Figure 1–50. In fluid-phase micropinocytosis, minute invaginations of the cell membrane detach and move into the cytoplasm as smooth vesicles. In some epithelia, they may transport substances across the cell. In endothelium, chains of communicating vesicles may form transient channels from lumen to cell base. This form of pinocytosis is nonselective.

process for uptake of specific proteins, including hormones and other regulatory molecules. Its selectivity depends on the presence of specific receptors in the portion of the membrane that is invaginated. To date, more than 25 such receptors have been identified. After binding of molecules to their specific receptors, the ligand–receptor complexes aggregate in shallow indentations of the membrane called *coated pits.* Their coat consists of large molecules of a 180 kD protein, *clathrin,* that becomes associated with the cytoplasmic domain of the receptor molecules and polymerizes to form a cage-like lattice on the cytoplasmic surface of the pit. As polymerization of the clathrin progresses, the pit deepens and ultimately constricts at its neck to form a *coated vesicle* that is then free in the cytoplasm (Figs. 1–52 and 1–53). The spiny clathrin cage around these vesicles serves to distinguish them from the smooth vesicles formed in fluid-phase pinocytosis.

After interiorization of the ligand–receptor complexes in coated vesicles, the clathrin coat is depolymerized and multiple vesicles fuse with preexisting vacuoles in the cytoplasm, forming structures called *endosomes.* These membrane-bounded transient organelles are irregular in outline and often have short tubular extensions. Those in the peripheral cytoplasm are designated *early endosomes* and others, deeper in the cytoplasm, are *late endosomes.* Labeled ligands taken up by receptor-mediated endocytosis appear first in coated vesicles, then in early endosomes and finally in late endosomes. A lower pH in the early endosome, results in dissociation of the ligands from their receptors and leaves them free in the lumen. Portions of the endosome membrane, containing the unoccupied receptors, then bud off in small vesicles that return to the cell membrane and fuse with it. Receptors are thus recycled, returning to the cell membrane within a few minutes of their being interiorized in coated vesicles.

The late endosomes are a prelysosomal compartment in the endocytotic pathway. Opinion is divided as to whether early endosomes move deeper in the cytoplasm and mature into late endosomes, or whether they remain in the peripheral cytoplasm while their content is transported to late endosomes by carrier vesicles that move along microtubules. The late endosomes differ from the early endosomes in their larger size, greater content of internal membranes, their lower pH, and their positive histochemical reaction for acid phosphatase. Their limiting membrane contains receptors for mannose-6-phosphate which serves as a marker targeting newly synthesized acid hydrolases to the endosomes. The possibility that late endosomes lose their mannose-6-phosphate receptors and undergo condensation to form lysosomes has been considered, but the volume of endocytosis in some cells is such that conversion of all late endosomes to lysosomes would result in far greater numbers of lysosomes than are observed. Much remains to be learned about the endocytic pathway and its relation to the lysosomes. It is the prevailing view that late endosomes fuse with lysosomes and their ligands are broken down by acid hydrolases and the products exported into the cytoplasm (Fig. 1–54). Endocytosis goes on continuously with interiorization and recycling of large amounts of membrane. In some epithelial cells, the number of coated vesicles formed is estimated to be in excess of a thousand per minute.

A couple of examples may contribute to a better understanding of how the endocytic pathway works. Cholesterol is needed by cells as a major component of their membranes. Cholesterol synthesized and stored in the liver is released into the blood in the form of large, spherical, low-density lipoprotein particles (LDL) which have a core of some 1500 cholesterol molecules. The particles have a specific binding protein on their surface that is recognized by receptors on the surface of cells. The

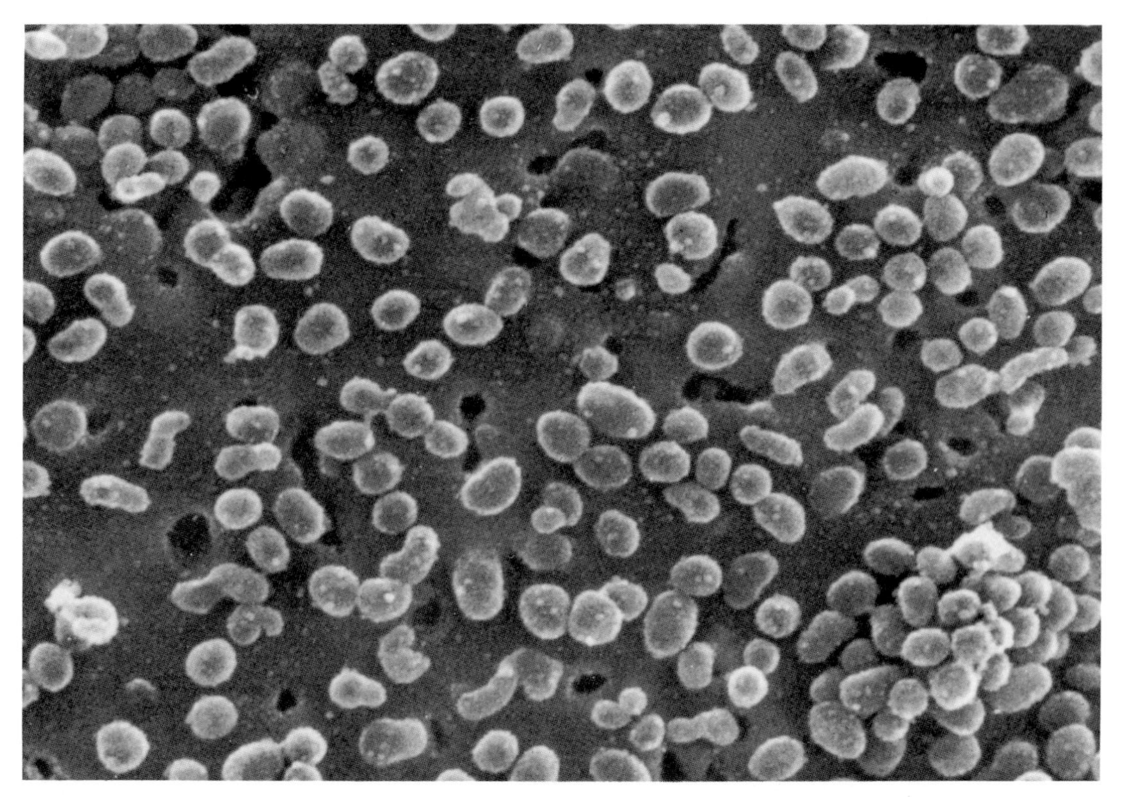

Figure 1–51. A scanning electron micrograph of the cytoplasmic face of a mesothelial cell plasma membrane showing large numbers of pinocytosis vesicles. Thin sections of cells include relatively few such vesicles and, therefore, fail to give a true picture of their abundance. (Micrograph courtesy of T. Inoue and H. Osatako. 1989. J. Submicros. Cytol. Pathol. 21:215)

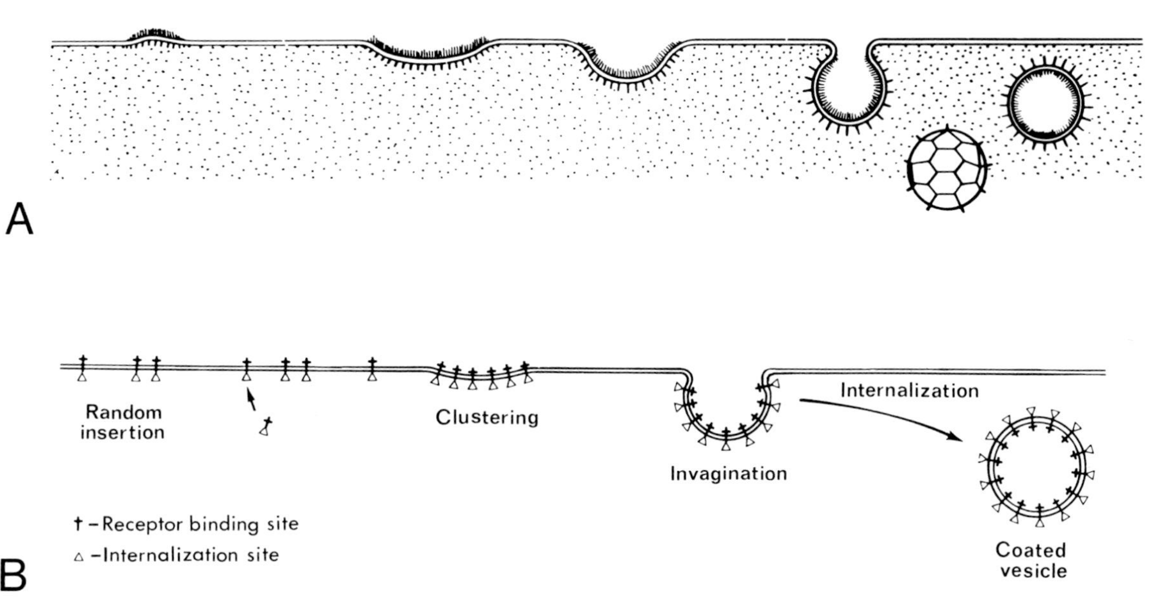

Figure 1–52. (A) In receptor-mediated pinocytosis, the vesicles are lined by a thin, carbohydrate-rich coat and their cytoplasmic surface is enclosed in a basket-like lattice of clathrin. (B) In the current interpretation of this, transmembrane receptors are thought to be randomly distributed in the membrane. Binding of specific macromolecules caused clustering of the receptors, and this portion of the membrane then forms a coated pit that subsequently separates from the membrane as a coated vesicle. (Redrawn and modified from Goldstein et al. 1979. Nature 279:679.)

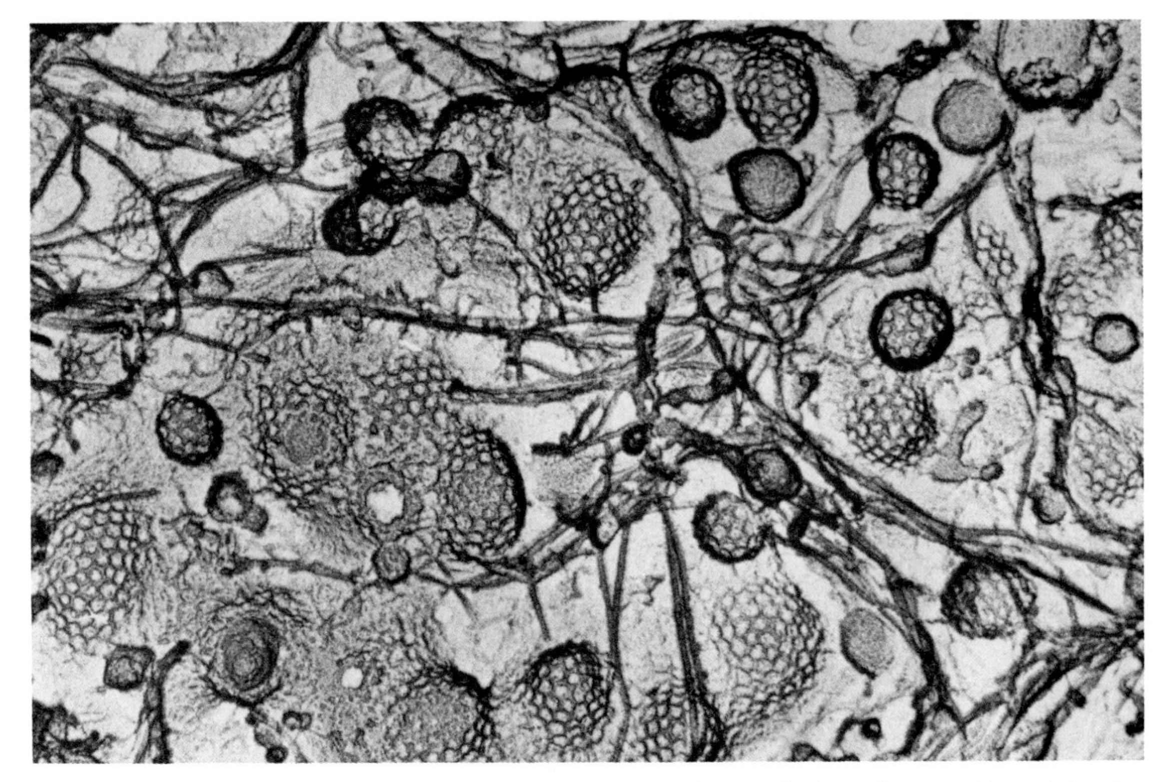

Figure 1–53. Electron micrograph of the cytoplasmic side of the plasmalemma of a liver cell prepared by rapid-freezing, fracturing, and deep etching. Filaments of the cortical cytoplasm are visible, as well as the clathrin lattice of many forming coated pits and vesicles. (Micrograph courtesy of N. Hirokawa and J. Heuser.)

particles are interiorized by receptor-mediated endocytosis and the resulting endosomes fuse with lysosomes. The hydrolytic enzymes of the lysosomes degrade the binding protein and split fatty acids from cholesterol, releasing fatty acid and cholesterol into the cytoplasm for incorporation in new membrane. In another example, iron, which is required by most cells, is brought to them from the intestine or the liver by a carrier molecule, transferrin. This molecule, carrying two ferric ions, binds to specific receptors on the cell and is taken up by receptor-mediated pinocytosis and transferred to an endosome where the acid pH dissociates the ferric ions, making them available to the cell. In this case, the carrier molecule is not degraded but is subsequently secreted from the cell, as apotransferrin, to recirculate in the blood and transport more iron. Because it is known that each transferrin molecule carries two ferric ions, it has been possible to quantitate the number of transferrin receptors on the cell type used in these experiments and the time required for recycling of the carrier. That cell type was calculated to possess 150,000 ferrotransferrin receptors and it takes only 16 min from binding to secretion of the apotransferrin.

EXOCYTOSIS

The term *exocytosis* refers to the release of cell products into the extracellular compartment. After the secretory product has traversed the Golgi complex of a glandular cell, it is concentrated to form spherical secretory granules bounded by a membrane. These may be stored, for some time, in the apical cytoplasm, and then, in response to neural stimulus, they move to the surface and their membrane fuses with the plasmalemma, permitting outflow of their contents. The secretory product thus leaves the cell without creation of a breach in its membrane. The excess membrane added to the plasmalemma during exocytosis is subsequently removed by endocytosis in small vesicles that are believed to be recycled to the Golgi complex. Stimulus-dependent exocytosis is called *regulated secretion* and is characteristic of cells specialized for synthesis and release of a large volume of

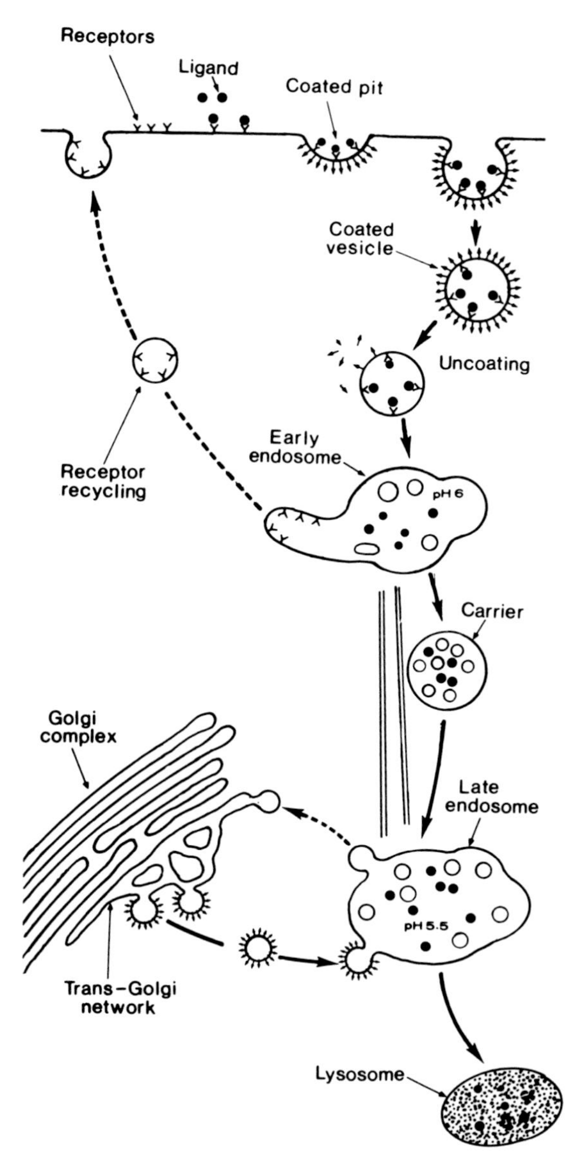

Figure 1–54. Schematic representation of the endocytic pathway. Aggregation of receptors in coated pits; formation of coated vesicles; fusion of vesicles to form endosomes; recycling of receptors to the plasma membrane; transport to late endosome which receives acid hydrolases from the trans-Golgi network; fusion of late endosomes with lysosomes.

secretion. Other cell types produce a product that is not concentrated into conspicuous secretory granules but is released continuously in small vesicles that fuse with the plasma membrane. This is called *constitutive secretion.* The vesicles involved are morphologically indistinguishable from pinocytosis vesicles and this form of secretion went unrecognized until the synthesis and release of cell products could be traced, in studies employing radiolabeled precursors. Since then, constitutive secretion has been found to be widespread among cell types that, previously, were not considered secretory.

CELL LOCOMOTION

Locomotion is required during embryonic development for movement of cells from their origin to the sites of organogenesis, and in postnatal life, migration of cells is often necessary to adapt to changes in their environment or to respond to injury. All cells are capable of some degree of motility, but where they are in close contact, their movements may be limited to changes in the configuration of their free surface or to changes in shape associated with mitosis. However, during repair after injury, even relatively sessile epithelial cells flatten and migrate to cover a denuded area of basal lamina. When cells that normally show very little movement are removed from their in vivo environment and cultured in vitro, they are stimulated to proliferate and migrate over the floor of the culture vessel. There are other cell types that do not adhere to one another, in vivo, to form compact organs but remain solitary and are continually migrating through the connective tissues.

Analysis of the mechanism of cell motility has been one of the more challenging problems in cell biology. Most of the research has concentrated on the type of locomotion exhibited by freely migrating cells, such as the leukocytes of the blood and macrophages of the connective tissues. This is described as *amoeboid locomotion* because of its resemblance to the movements of amoeba, a protozoan in which locomotion has been very thoroughly studied. It has been the traditional view that amoeboid locomotion depends on a gel–sol transformation at the front, and a contraction of the cell body at the rear. The resulting flow of endoplasm toward the area unsupported by a gelated ectoplasm forms a pseudopodium projecting in the direction of movement. As the pseudopodium elongates, a recurrent flow of cytoplasm from its tip gels at its base, advancing the anterior margin of the ectoplasm. The wall of the pseudopodium in this region, thus, becomes the anterior portion of the wall of the cell body, as the nucleus and organelles are moved into it by forward streaming of the endoplasm, propelled by contraction of the trailing end of the cell. The cell slowly moves forward as new pseudopodia are formed, attach to the substrate, and are gradually incorporated into the cell body. The contraction of the tail end was attributed to interaction of actin and myosin filaments as in skeletal muscle. This traditional explanation lost some of its thrust when electron micrographs failed to reveal any myosin filaments comparable to those of muscle. But it may still be viable, because it has recently been found that one kind of myosin can form submicroscopic nonfilamentous bipolar units with their heads forming short lateral projections that bridge the gap between myosin and adjacent actin filaments. It is speculated that repeated cycles of bridge-forming and bridge-breaking by these myosin units may move the actin filaments during contraction of the ectoplasm at the posterior end of the cell.

Cells that do not migrate through the tissues have a different mode of locomotion. For example, fibroblasts in cell culture flatten with their leading edge closely applied to the substrate. No pseudopodia are formed, but they slowly glide over the surface at a rate of about 1 cm a day. Carbon particles applied to their surface can be seen to slowly move from the leading edge to the trailing end of the cell. This anteroposterior movement is attributed to membrane removal by endocytosis at the trailing end and membrane insertion by exocytosis at the leading edge. Improbable as it may seem, quantitative studies indicate that endocytosis results in removal of about 2% of the cell membrane per minute and it is calculated that a fibroblast could take up an amount of membrane equal to its entire surface area every 50 min. In a fibroblast that is not moving, endocytosis is randomly distributed over its surface and no anteroposterior flow of membrane can be demonstrated. However, in motile cells, endocytosis appears to be concentrated in the trailing end of the cell. The membrane interiorized there is thought to be recycled by exocytosis at its leading edge. It is assumed that the resulting anteroposterior flow of membrane would have a propulsive action comparable to the lower half of the tread on a tank or caterpillar tractor. Much remains to be learned about what triggers this form of locomotion, how exocytosis is directed to the leading edge, and the mechanism of binding of the membrane to the substrate.

CHEMOTAXIS

The wandering of amoeboid cells generally appears to be random, but under certain circumstances they exhibit *chemotaxis*—a directional migration along a gradient of a diffusible substance, from an area of low concentration to an area of higher concentration. A number of substances have been identified that are chemotactic for leukocytes and macrophages. Some of these are secreted by other cell types and some are products of bacteria. The leukocytes have receptors for these, and upon binding of a chemotactic agent to their receptors, the leukocytes change their direction and migrate up the gradient to its source. Chemotaxis plays a very important role in the body's response to invasion by bacteria. Macrophages are initially mobilized at the site by chemotactic bacterial products, but they, in turn, secrete substances that are attractants for neutrophil leukocytes and monocytes, inducing them to assemble at the site and join the battle against the bacteria. Just how the chemotactic agent determines the direction of their migration is not known.

MOVEMENT WITHIN CELLS

Considerable movement occurs within cells that are not in motion. Organelles are redistributed, vesicles are constantly moving to and from the surface, and chromosomes move to the poles in dividing cells. How these movements are generated was long a mystery, but, in recent years, a number of motor molecules have been identified that may be involved. Dynein and kinesin that move vesicles and organelles along microtubules were briefly discussed earlier in the chapter. A great deal of investigative attention is now being directed to the new form of myosin, *myosin-I,* which appears to consist of the globular head of conventional myosin (myosin-II) without the alpha-helical, coiled-coil tail that permits assembly into filaments. Myosin-I bound to actin has been found to be capable of moving adjacent actin filaments in vitro and, therefore, has the potential for producing limited contraction in vivo. It has also been shown to move vesicles along actin filaments. Membrane-bound myosin-I might be able to move the cell membrane with respect to actin filaments in the underlying ectoplasm and, thus, play a role in cell movement, and it is conceivable that it can also move receptor proteins and their ligands within the lipid bilayer to sites of assembly for receptor-mediated endocytosis. It is speculated that myosin-I motor units, in vivo, may have a variety of very short tails with binding properties that may determine in which of the above activities they participate. Thus, it is increasingly apparent that multiple force-transducing molecules are available for the movements observed within living cells. Myosin-I seems to be involved in actin filament-based movements, whereas cytoplasmic dynein and kinesin are the motors for microtubule-based movement.

CELL DEATH

Dying cells are often observed in tissue sections. Two distinct processes of cell death can be recognized, *necrosis* and *apoptosis*. Necrosis may result from mechanical injury, exposure to toxins, or anoxia due to impairment of the blood supply. The changes observed include swelling, clumping of the chromatin, pale staining of the cytoplasm, and deteriorization of the organelles, followed by lysis with release of the cell contents which are then phagocytized by macrophages.

Apoptosis, on the other hand, is not a result of injury but is an active form of cell death, initiated by the cell on the basis of information from the environment, from its developmental history, and from its genome. The many different kinds of cells in the body have normal life spans ranging from a few days to 80 years or more. Death of certain cells is a normal and essential part of morphogenesis in embryonic life. In the adult, programmed elimination of cells of limited life span is common. Cells die in great numbers in the periodic involutional changes occurring in organs that are cyclically dependent on trophic hormones. The massive death of thymocytes in response to corticosteroids is an example. The cytological changes associated with apoptosis differ from those of necrosis. There is an early condensation of chromatin and degradation of DNA due to activation of endonucleases. The cells do not swell. Instead, the cell volume decreases and the cell membrane and the organelles remain intact. The cell ultimately fragments into several membrane-bounded globules that are phagocytized by neighboring cells. Neutrophils and macrophages are not involved in the terminal stages of this process to same extent that they are where cells are undergoing necrosis.

The biochemical mechanisms involved in apoptosis are still not completely understood. An increase in intracellular calcium apparently activates endonucleases that fragment the DNA. It is evident that this form of cell death is an active process because it can be prevented by compounds that inhibit protein synthesis. In insects, many new polypeptides are synthesized when cell death is triggered. In another invertebrate, several genes have been identified that are involved in apoptosis. There is also evidence suggesting that the cell membrane is altered in the process in a manner that marks the resulting globular fragments of the cell for phagocytosis.

BIBLIOGRAPHY

GENERAL

Brachet, J. and E. Mirsky (1974–1976). The Cell: Biochemistry, Physiology, Morphology. Vols. I–IV. New York, Academic Press.

Busch, H.B., ed. 1974. The Cell Nucleus. 3 Vols. New York, Academic Press.

Darnell, J., H. Lodish, and D. Baltimore. 1986. Molecular Cell Biology. Scientific Books. New York.

Fawcett, D.W. 1979. The Cell, 2nd Ed. Philadelphia, W.B. Sauders Co.

Watson, J.D., ed. Organization of the Cytoplasm. Cold Spring Harbor Symp. Quant. Biol. 46:1982.

CELL MEMBRANE

Bretscher, M.S. 1985. The molecules of the cell membrane. Sci. Am. 226:30.

Edelman, G.M. 1983. Cell adhesion molecules. Science 219:450.

Fry, C.F. 1972. The structure of cell membranes. Sci. Am. 226:30.

Hendler, R.W. 1971. Biological membrane ultrastructure. Physiol. Rev. 51:66.

Ito, S. 1965. The surface coat of enteric microvilli. J. Cell Biol. 27:475.

Marchesi, V.T., H. Furthmayr, and M. Tomita. 1976. The red cell membrane. Annu. Rev. Biochem. 45:667.

Rambourg, A.M., M. Neutra, and C.P. Leblond. 1966. Presence of a cell coat rich in carbohydrates at the surface of cells in the rat. Anat. Rec. 154:41.

Robertson, J.D. 1981. Membrane structure. J. Cell Biol. 91:189s.

Sharon, N. and H. Lis. 1989. Lectins as cell recognition molecules. Science 246:227.

Singer, S.J. 1974. Molecular organization of membranes. Annu. Rev. Biochem. 43:805.

Singer, S.J. and G.L. Nicholson. 1972. The fluid mosaic model of the structure of cell membranes. Science 175:720.

Steck, T.L. 1974. The organization of proteins in human red blood cell membranes. J. Cell Biol. 62:1.

NUCLEAR ENVELOPE

Aaronson, R.P. and G. Blobel. 1974. On the attachment of the nuclear pore complex. J. Cell Biol. 62:746.

Benvente, R. and G. Kohne. 1986. Involvement of the nuclear lamins in post-mitotic reorganization of the chromatin. J. Cell Biol. 103:1847.

Davis, L. and G. Blobel. 1986. Identification and characterization of a nuclear pore complex protein. Cell 46:699.

Dingwall, C. and R.A. Laskey. 1986. Protein import into the cell nucleus. Annu. Rev. Cell Biol. 2:367.

Dworetsky, S.I. and C.M. Feldherr. 1988. Translocation

of RNA-coated gold particles through the nuclear pores of oocytes. J. Cell Biol. 106:575.

Fawcett, D.W. 1966. On the occurrence of a fibrous lamina on the inner aspect of the nuclear envelope in certain cells of vertebrates. Am. J. Anat. 119:129.

Featherstone, C.M., K. Darby and L. Gerace. 1988. A monoclonal antibody against the nuclear pore complex inhibits nucleocytoplasmic transport of protein and RNA in vivo. J. Cell Biol. 107:1289.

Feldherr, C.M. and S.I. Dworetsky. 1988. The pore complex in nucleocytoplasmic exchange. Cell Biol. Internat. Reports 12:791.

Francke, W.W. 1974. Structure, biochemistry and functions of the nuclear envelope. Internat. Rev. Cytol. (Suppl. 4):72.

Gerace, L. and B. Burke. 1988. Functional organization of the nuclear envelope. Annu. Rev. Cell Biol. 4:335.

Maul, G.C. 1977. The nuclear and cytoplasmic pore complex structure, dynamics, distribution, and evolution. Int. Rev. Cytol. (Suppl. 6) 76.

Senior, A. and L. Gerace. 1988. Integral membrane proteins specific to the inner nuclear membrane and associated with the nuclear lamina. J. Cell Biol. 107:2029.

Unwin, P.N. and R.A. Milligan. 1982. A large particle associated with the perimeter of the nuclear pore complex. J. Cell Biol. 93:63.

CHROMATIN

Hozier, J., M. Renz, and R. Niels. 1977. The chromosome fiber: evidence for an ordered superstructure of nucleosomes. Chromosoma 62:301.

Kornberg, R. 1977. Structure of chromatin. Annu. Rev. Biochem. 467:931.

Olins, D.A. and A.L. Olins. 1978. Nucleosomes: the structural quantum of chromosomes. Am. Scientist 66:704.

Worcel, A. and C. Benyajati, 1977. Higher order coiling of DNA in chromatin. Cell 12:83.

CHROMOSOMES

Gall, J.G. 1956. On the submicroscopic structure of chromosomes. Brookhaven Symp. Biol. 8:17.

Laemmle, U.K., S.M. Cheng, K.W. Adolf, et al. 1977. Metaphase chromosome structure: the role of nonhistone proteins. Cold Spring Harbor Symp. Quant. Biol. 42:35.

Marsden, M.P. and U.K. Laemmli. 1979. Metaphase chromosome structure: evidence for a radial loop model. Cell 17:849.

Ris, H. and D. Kubai. 1970. Chromosome structure. Annu. Rev. Genetics 4:263.

Stubblefield, E. 1973. The structure of mammalian chromosomes. Internat. Rev. Cytol. 35:1.

NUCLEOLUS

Brown, D.D. and J.B. Gurdon. 1964. Absence of RNA synthesis in the anucleolate mutant of *Xenopus laevis*. Proc. Nat. Acad. USA 51:39.

Ghosh, S. 1976. The nucleolar structure. Internat. Rev. Cytol. 44:1.

Hay, E.D. 1967. The fine structure of the nucleolus in normal and mutant *Xenopus* embryos. J. Cell Sci. 2:151.

Jordan, E.G. 1978. The Nucleolus, 2nd Ed. Oxford, Oxford University Press.

Miller, O.L. 1966. Structure and composition of peripheral nucleoli of salamander oocytes. Nat. Cancer Inst. Monographs 23:53.

Perry, R.P. 1964. Role of the nucleolus in ribonucleic acid metabolism and other cellular processes. Nat. Cancer Inst. Monographs 18:325.

Sommerville, J. 1985. Organizing the nucleolus. Nature 318:410.

CYTOPLASMIC ORGANELLES

Mitochondria

Ernster, L. and G. Schatz. 1981. Mitochondria: a historical review. J. Cell Biol. 91:227s.

Grivell, L.A. 1983. Mitochondrial DNA. Sci. Am. 248:60.

Hinkle, P.C. and R.E. McCarty. 1983. How cells make ATP. Sci. Am. 238:104.

Lehninger, A.L. 1964. The Mitochondrion. New York. W.B. Benjamin.

Palade, G. 1953. An electron microscopic study of mitochondrial structure. J. Histochem. Cytochem. 1:188.

Reich, E. and D.J. Luck. 1966. Replication and inheritance of mitochondrial DNA. Proc. Nat. Acad. Sci. USA 55:1600.

Sinclair, J.H. and B.V. Stevens. 1966. Circular DNA filaments from mouse mitochondria. Proc. Nat. Acad. Sci. USA 56:508.

Whittaker, P.A. and S.M. Danks. 1979. Mitochondria: Structure. Function, and Assembly. New York, Longman.

Rough Endoplasmic Reticulum and Ribosomes

Alberts, B., D. Bray, J. Lewis et al. 1983. The endoplasmic reticulum. *In* Molecular Biology of the Cell, p. 335. New York, Garland Publishing.

Jamieson, J.D. and G.E. Palade. 1977. Production of secretory proteins in animal cells. *In* B.R. Brinkley and K.R. Porter, eds. International Cell Biology 1976–1977. New York, Rockefeller University Press.

Lake, J.A. 1971. The ribosome. Sci. Am. 245:84.

Palade, G.E. 1955. A small particulate component of the cytoplasm. J. Biophys. Biochem. Cytol. 1:59.

Palade, G.E. and K.R. Porter. 1954. Studies on the endoplasmic reticulum. I. Its identification in cells in situ. J. Exp. Med. 100:641.

Porter, K.R. 1953. Observations on a submicroscopic basophilic component of the cytoplasm. J. Exp. Med. 97:727.

Siekevitz, P. and P.C. Zamecnik, 1981. Ribosomes and protein synthesis. J. Cell Biol. 91:53s.

Smooth Endoplasmic Reticulum

Cardell, R., R.S. Bodenhausen, and K.R. Porter. 1967. Intestinal triglyceride absorption in the rat. J. Cell. Biol. 34:123.

Jones, A.L. and D.W. Fawcett. 1966. Hypertrophy of the agranuilar reticulum in hamster liver induced by phenobarbital. J. Histochem. Cytochem. 14:215.

Porter, K.R. and G.E. Palade. 1958. Studies on the endoplasmic reticulum. III. Its form and distribution in striated muscle cells. J. Biophys. Biochem. Cytol. 3:269.

Remmer, H. and H.J. Merker. 1963. Effect of drugs on the formation of smooth endoplasmic reticulum and drug metabolizing enzymes. Ann. N.Y. Acad. Sci. 123:79.

Golgi Complex

Bearns, H.W. and R.G. Kessel. 1968. The Golgi apparatus, structure and function. Internat. Rev. Cytol. 23:209.

Brown, W.J. and M. Farquhar. 1984. The mannose-6-phosphate receptor for lysosomal enzymes is concentrated in cis-Golgi cisternae. Cell 38:295.
Farquhar, M.G. 1985. Progress in unraveling pathways of Golgi traffic. Annu. Rev. Cell Biol. 1:447.
Farquhar, M.G. and G.E. Palade. 1981. The Golgi apparatus 1954–1981, from artefact to center stage. J. Cell Biol. 91 (Suppl.):77.
Griffiths, G. and K. Simons. 1986. The trans-Golgi network: Sorting at the exit site of the Golgi complex. Science 234:438.
Ichikawa, M., A. Ichikawa, and T. Tanabe. 1982. High resolution analysis of the three-dimensional structure of the Golgi apparatus in rapid frozen, substitution fixed gerbil sublingual gland acinar cells. J. Electron Microsc. 31:397.
Jamieson, J.D. 1971. Role of the Golgi complex in the intracellular transport of secretory proteins. *In* F. Clementi and B. Ceccarelle, eds. Advances in Cytopharmacology. Vol. 1. New York, Raven Books.
Lingappa, V. 1989. Intracellular traffic of newly synthesized proteins. J. Clin. Invest. 83:739.
Neutra, M. and C.P. Leblond. 1969. The Golgi apparatus. Sci. Am. 220:100.
Rambourg, A., Y. Clermont, L. Herma, and D. Segretain. 1987. Tridimensional architecture of the Golgi apparatus and its components in mucous cells of Brunner's glands of the mouse. Am. J. Anat. 179:95.
Rambourg, A., Y. Clermont and L. Hermo. 1979. Three dimensional architecture of the Golgi apparatus in Sertoli cells of then rat. Am. J. Anat. 154:466.
Rothman, J.E. 1985. The compartmental organization of the Golgi apparatus. Sci. Am. 253:74.
Whaley, W.G. 1975. The Golgi Apparatus. New York, Springer-Verlag.

Lysosomes

Alberts, B., D. Bray, J. Lewis et al. Lysosomes and peroxisomes. *In* Molecular Biology of the Cell. p. 367. New York, Garland Publishing.
Allison, A. 1967. Lysosomes and disease. Sci. Am. 217:62.
DeDuve, C. and R. Wattiaux. 1966. Function of lysosomes. Ann. Rev. Physiol. 28:435.
Hirsch. J.G. 1962. Cinematographic observations on granule lysis in polymorphonuclear leukocytes during phagocytosis. J. Exp. Med. 116:827.
Kolodny, E.H. 1976. Lysosomal storage diseases. N. Eng. J. Med. 294:1217.
Weissman, G., R.B. Zurier, P.J. Spieler, and I.M. Goldstein. 1971. Mechanisms of lysosomal enzyme release from leukocytes exposed to immune complexes and other particles. J. Exp. Med. 134:149s.

Peroxisomes

DeDuve, C. and P. Baudhuin. 1966. Peroxisomes. Physiol. Rev. 46:323.
Fahimi, H.D. 1968. Cytochemical localization of peroxidase activity in rat hepatic microbodies. J. Histochem. Cytochem. 16:547.
Novikoff, P.M. and A.B. Novikoff. 1972. Peroxisomes in absorptive cells of mammalian small intestine. J. Cell Biol. 53:532.

Annulate Lamellae

Kessel, R.G. 1983. The structure and function of annulate lamellae. Internat. Rev. Cytol. 82:181.
Kessel, R.G. 1989. Annulate lamellae—from obscurity to spotlight. Electron Microsc. Rev. 2:257.

Centrioles

Berns, M.W., J.B. Rattner, and S. Brenner. 1977. The role of the centriolar apparatus in animal cell mitosis: a laser-microbeam study. J. Cell. Biol. 72:351.
Brinkley, B.R. 1985. Microtubule organizing centers. Annu. Rev. Cell. Biol. 1:145.
MacIntosh, J.R. 1983. The centrosome as an organizer of the cytoskeleton. Mod. Cell Biol. 2:115.
Peterson, S.P. and M.W. Berns. 1980. The centriolar complex. Internat. Rev. Cytol. 64:81.
Sorokin, S. 1968. Reconstruction of centriole formation and ciliogenesis in mammalian lungs. J. Cell Sci. 3:207.

CYTOPLASMIC INCLUSIONS

Glycogen

Biava, C. 1963. Identification and structural forms of human particulate glycogen. Lab. Investig. 12:1179.
Revel, J.P., L. Napolitano, and D.W. Fawcett. 1960. Identification of glycogen in electron micrographs of thin tissue sections. J. Biophys. Biochem. Cytol. 8:575.
Revel, J.P. 1964. Electron microscopy of glycogen. J. Histochem. Cytochem. 12:104.

Lipid

Napolitano, L. 1963. The differentiation of white adipose tissue. J. Cell Biol. 18:663.
Senior, J.R. 1964. Intestinal absorption of fats. J. Lipid Res. 5:495.

Pigment

Bjorkerud, S. 1963. The isolation of lipofuscin granules from bovine cardiac muscle. J. Ultrastr. Res. (Suppl.) 5:5.
Fitzpatrick, T.B. and G. Szabo. 1959. The melanocyte: cytology and cytochemistry. J. Investig. Dermatol. 32:197.
Mann, D.M. and P.O. Yates. 1974. Lipochrome pigments—their relationship to aging in the human nervous system. I. Lipofuscin content of nerve cells. Brain 97:481.
Szabo, G. 1969. The biology of the pigment cell. *In* E.B. Bittar and N.F. Bittar, eds. Biological Basis of Medicine, Vol. 6. New York, Academic Press.

CYTOSKELETON

Microtubules

Burnside, B. 1975. The form and arrangement of microtubules: An historical primarily morphological review. Ann. N.Y. Acad. Sci. 253:14.
Fujiwara, K. and L.G. Tilney. 1975. Substructural analysis of the microtubule and its polymeric forms. Ann. N.Y. Acad. Sci. 253:27.
Koshland, D.E., T.J. Mitchison, M.W. Kirschner. 1988. Poleward chromosome movement driven by microtubule depolymerization in vitro. Nature 331:499.
McNiven, M.A. and K.R. Porter. 1986. Microtubule polarity confers direction to pigment transport in chromatophores. J. Cell Biol. 103:1547.
Mitchisen, T. and M. Kirschner. 1984. Microtubule assembly nucleated by isolated chromosomes. Nature 312:232.
Olmsted, J.B. and G.B. Borisy. 1973. Microtubules. Annu. Rev. Biochem. 42:507.
Vale, R.D., B.J. Schnapp, T.S. Reese, and M.P. Sheetz. 1985. Movement of organelles along filaments disso-

ciated from the axoplasm of the squid giant axon. Cell 40:449.
Vale, R.D., T.S. Reese, and M.P. Scheetz. 1985. Identification of a novel force-generating protein, kinesin, involved in microtubule based motility. Cell 42:39.

Filaments

Bridgeman, P.C. and T.S. Reese. 1984. The structure of the cytoplasm in directly frozen cultured cells. I. Filamentous meshworks and the cytoplasmic ground substance. J. Cell Biol. 99:1655.
Franke, W.W., B. Appelhaus, E. Schmel, and C. Freudenstein. 1979. The organization of cytokeratin filaments in the intestinal epithelium. Eur. J. Cell. Biol. 19:255.
Heuser, J.E. and M.W. Kirschner. 1980. Filament organization revealed in platinum replicas of freeze-dried cytoskeletons. J. Cell Biol. 86:212.
Hirokawa, N., L.G. Tilney, K. Fujiwara, and J.E. Heuser. 1982. Organization of actin, myosin, and intermediate filaments in the brush border of intestinal epithelial cells. J. Cell. Biol. 94:425.
Pollard, T.D. 1977. Cytoplasmic contractile proteins. *In* B.R. Brinkley and K.R. Porter, eds. International Cell Biology 1976–1977. New York, Rockefeller University Press.
Pollard, T.D. 1981. Cytoplasmic contractile proteins. J. Cell Biol. 91:1568.
Shelanski, M.L. and R.K. Liem. 1979. Neurofilaments. J. Neurochem. 33:5.
Skalli, O. and R.D. Goldman. 1991. Recent insights into the assembly, dynamics, and function of intermediate filament networks. Cell Motil. Cytoskel. 19:67.
Steinert, P.M., J.C. Jones, and R.D. Goldman. 1984. Intermediate filaments. J. Cell Biol. 99:22s.
Steinert, P. and A.D. Perry. 1985. Intermediate filaments. Conformity and diversity of expression and structure. Ann. Rev. Cell Biol. 1:41.

CELL DIVISION AND THE CELL CYCLE

Bajer, A. and J. Mole-Bajer. 1971. Architecture and function of the mitotic spindle. Adv. Mol. Biol. 1:231.
Baserga, R. and F. Weibel. 1969. The cell cycle of mammalian cells. Internat. Rev. Exp. Pathol. 7:1.
Inoue, S. 1981. Cell division and the mitotic spindle. J. Cell Biol. (Suppl.) 93:131.
Leblond, C.P. and B.E. Walker. 1956. Renewal of cell populations. Physiol. Rev. 36:255.
Mazia, D. 1964. The cell cycle. Sci. Am. 250:54.
Mitchison, T. and M. Kirschner. 1984. Microtubule assembly nucleated by isolated centrosomes. Nature 312:232.
Rappaport, R. 1972. Cytokinesis in animal cells. Internat. Rev. Cytol. 31:301.
Saxton, W.M. and J.R. McIntosh. 1987. Interzone microtubular behavior in late anaphase and telophase spindles. J. Cell Biol. 105:875.
Vallee, R. 1990. Dynein and the kinetochore. Nature 345:206.

CELL ACTIVITIES

Cell Motility

Allen, R.A. 1981. Cell motility, J. Cell Biol. (Suppl.) 93:148.
Bretscher, M.J. 1987. How animal cells move. Sci. Am. 257:72.
Warrick, D. and J. Spudich. 1987. Myosin structure and function in cell motility. Annu. Rev. Cell Biol. 3:379.

Endocytosis

Allison, A.C. and P. Davies. 1974. Mechanisms of endocytosis and exocytosis. Symp. Soc. Exp. Biol. 28:419.
Anderson, R.G. and J. Kaplan. 1983. Receptor mediated endocytosis. *In* B.H. Satir, ed. Modern Cell Biology, Vol. 1. New York, Alan R. Liss.
Goldstein, J.L., R.G. Anderson, and M.S. Brown. 1979. Coated pits, coated vesicles, and receptor mediated endocytosis. A Review. Nature 279:679.
Heuser, J. and L. Evans. 1980. Three dimensional visualization of coated vesicle formation in fibroblasts. J. Cell. Biol. 84:560.
Hirsch, J.G. 1965. Phagocytosis. Annu. Rev. Microbiol. 19:339.
Pearse, B.M. 1976. Clathrin: a unique protein associated with the intracellular transfer of membrane by coated vesicles. Proc. Nat. Acad. Sci. USA 73:1255.
Rothman, J.E. and S.L. Schmid. 1986. Enzymatic recycling of clathrin from coated vesicles. Cell 46:5.
Silverstein, S.C., R.M. Steinman, and Z.A. Cohn. 1977. Endocytosis. Ann. Rev. Biochem. 46:669.

Apoptosis

Waring, P., F.J. Kos, and A. Mullbacher. 1991. Apoptosis or programmed cell death. Medicinal Res. Rev. 11:219.
Wyllie, A.H., J.F. Kerr, and A.R. Currie. 1980. Cell death: The significance of apoptosis. Internat. Rev. Cytol. 68:251.

2

EPITHELIUM

Although cells, in general, have most of the organelles described in the previous chapter, many have a distinctive shape and are associated with each other and with extracellular components to form five *basic tissues* specialized for different functions: *epithelium, connective tissue, blood, muscle,* and *nervous tissue.* This chapter, and the four following, will define the identifying characteristics of these tissues, and later chapters will describe the patterns in which these basic tissues are combined to form the larger functional units called *organs.*

An epithelium consists of contiguous cells, in apposition over a large portion of their surface. In its simplest form, epithelium consists of a single layer of identical cells covering an external surface or lining an internal cavity. The cells rest on a continuous extracellular layer, called the *basal lamina,* consisting of a meshwork of fine filaments. A primary function of such simple epithelia is to form a boundary layer that can control the movement of substances between the external environment and the internal milieu, or between compartments within the body. To serve this barrier function, the intercellular spaces must be sealed to prevent free diffusion across the epithelium, and the activities of the cells must be coordinated so that the entire epithelium functions as a unit. To these ends, there are specializations of the lateral cell surfaces that seal the intercellular spaces and others that permit the spread of signaling molecules from cell to cell in the plane of the epithelium.

All of the cells may be specialized for secretion of a product into the lumen of a duct or into a body cavity, or only a few may be secretory and the majority may bear motile cilia to move a film of fluid or mucus over the surface of the epithelium. In the more complex epithelia on the exterior of the body, the cells form multiple layers with those near the surface differentiated to resist abrasion and dehydration. The many kinds of epithelium in the body are specialized for a host of different functions.

ORIGINS OF EPITHELIUM

Two of the three primary germ layers of the early embryo, the *ectoderm* and the *endoderm,* are epithelia, and most of the epithelial organs of the body are derived from these germ layers. The ectoderm gives rise to the corneal epithelium and the epidermis of the skin, which together cover the entire surface of the body. Invagination and proliferation of this covering epithelium gives rise to tubes or solid cords that form the glandular appendages of the skin, the sudoriparous, sebaceous, and mammary glands. Epithelium of endodermal origin lining the embryonic alimentary tract gives rise to the intestinal glands, liver, and pancreas. All of the *exocrine glands* of the adult communicate via ducts with the epithelium of an internal cavity or external surface from which they developed in embryonic life. The ductless *endocrine glands* lose their connection with the epithelium from which they arose.

There are a few organs containing epithelia that arise from the third germ layer, the *mesoderm.* Among these are the kidney and the male and female reproductive tracts. The continuous layer of cells lining the blood and lymph vessels, the peritoneal cavity, and other serous cavities are also of mesodermal origin. Although these are, in all respects, typical epithelia, it is customary to refer to the lining of serous cavities as *mesothelium* and the lining of blood and lymph vessels, as *endothelium.*

CLASSIFICATION OF EPITHELIA

Several categories of epithelium are assigned different names to lend precision to the description of the tissues and organs by histologists and pathologists. They are classified according to the number of cell layers, the shape of the cells, and the specializations of their free surface. An epithelium made up

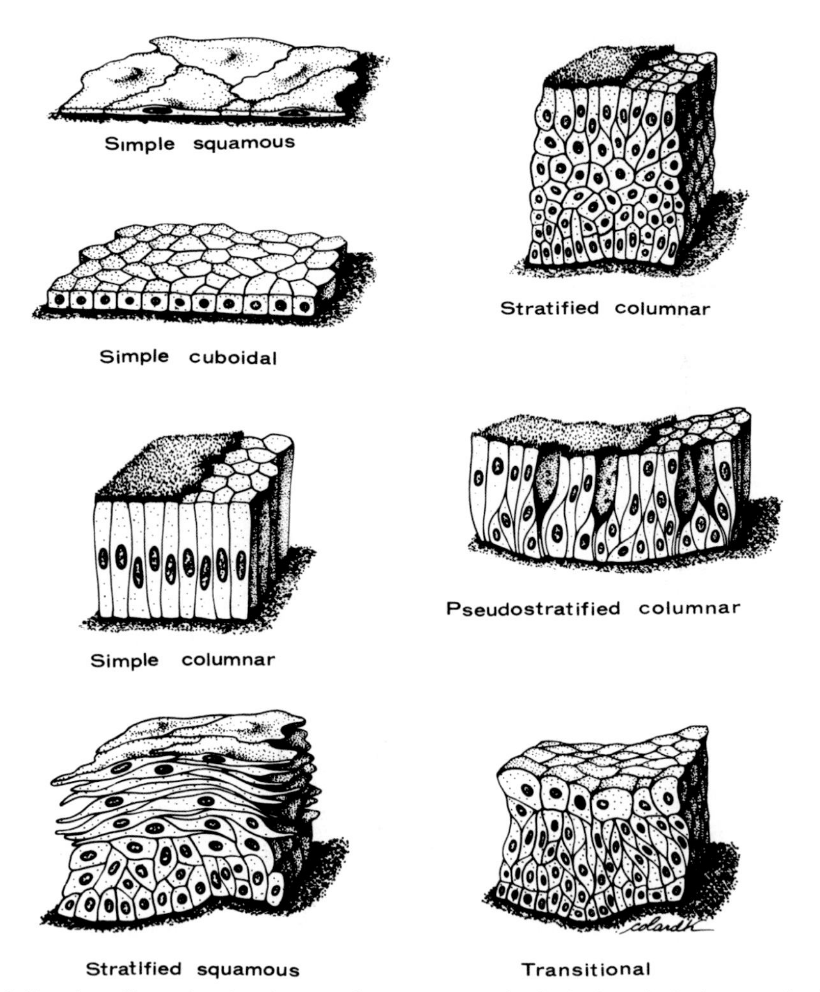

Figure 2–1. Drawings illustrating the shape and arrangement of cells in the principal types of epithelium.

of a single layer of cells is called a *simple epithelium,* and if there are multiple layers, it is a *stratified epithelium.* The modifiers *squamous, cuboidal,* or *columnar* are added to these designations to indicate the shape of the cells of the uppermost layer. Thus, a single layer of flat cells is a *simple squamous epithelium;* a single layer of tall prismatic cells is a *simple columnar epithelium.* The corresponding multilayered epithelia are *stratified squamous epithelium* and *stratified columnar epithelium* (Fig. 2–1). If the cells have cilia on their free surface, this is noted in the classification of the epithelium, as in *ciliated simple columnar epithelium.*

SIMPLE SQUAMOUS EPITHELIUM

When simple squamous epithelium is examined in surface view after staining the cell boundaries with silver nitrate, it presents a tile-like pattern of closely adherent cells that are polygonal in outline (Fig. 2–2). In sections perpendicular to the plane of the epithelium, the cells are thin and fusiform or rectangular in profile. Because of the large area of the flattened cells, the plane of section will pass through the nucleus of only some of the cells.

Simple squamous epithelium is found lining the pulmonary alveoli; the parietal layer of Bowman's capsule, and in the thin segments of Henle's loop in the kidney; in the rete testis; on the inner aspect of the tympanic membrane in the middle ear; and elsewhere. The endothelium lining the blood and lymph vessels is also a simple squamous epithelium.

SIMPLE CUBOIDAL EPITHELIUM

In vertical section, this epithelium appears as a row of square or rectangular profiles (Fig. 2–3), and in surface view, as a mosaic of polygonal cell outlines much smaller than those of

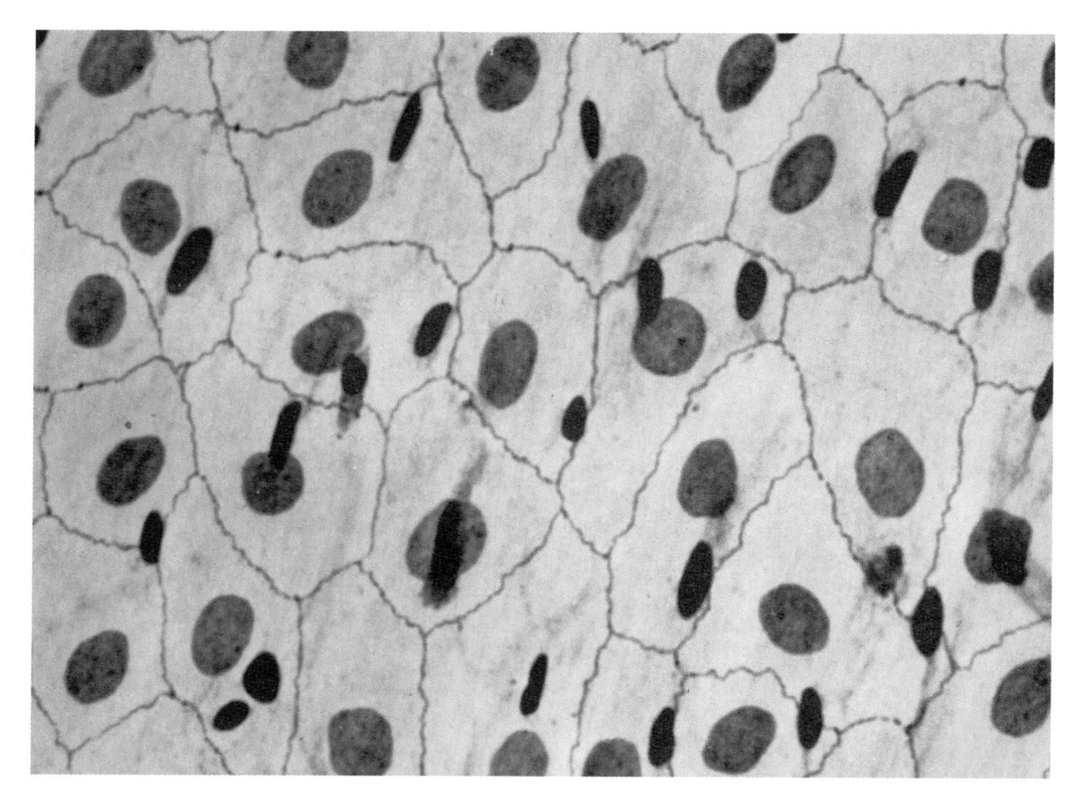

Figure 2–2. A thin spread of guinea pig mesentery, treated with silver nitrate and subsequently stained. The limits of the simple squamous mesothelial cells have been blackened by the silver, revealing their polygonal outlines. The large nuceoli are those of the mesothelial cells. The darker ellipsoidal nuclei are those of fibroblasts beneath the mesothelium.

squamous epithelium. Simple cuboidal epithelium is found lining the follicles of the thyroid gland; on the surface of the ovary; in the choroid plexus; on the capsule of the lens; in the pigment epithelium of the retina; and in the ducts of many glands. The secretory acini of many glands can also be included in this category, but these cells tend to be more pyramidal than cuboidal.

SIMPLE COLUMNAR EPITHELIUM

In simple columnar epithelium, the cells have rectangular outlines with their long axis perpendicular to the basal lamina. The height of the cells may be only slightly more than in cuboidal epithelium, but more often they are tall and slender and, hence, columnar in form (Fig. 2–4A–E), and their nuclei all tend to be

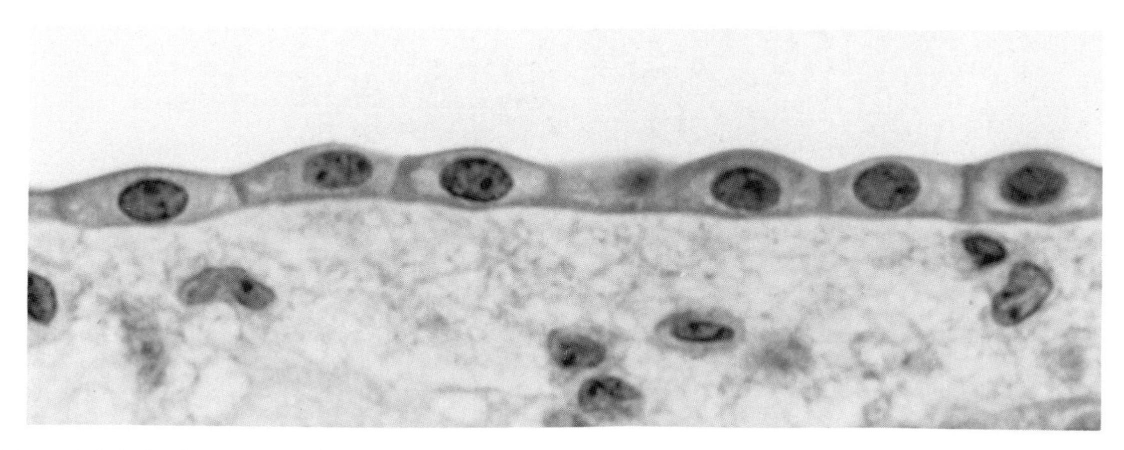

Figure 2–3. Epithelium of a collecting duct of the dog kidney. The cells are flattened to form a relatively thick squamous epithelium. In other species, they may be cuboidal.

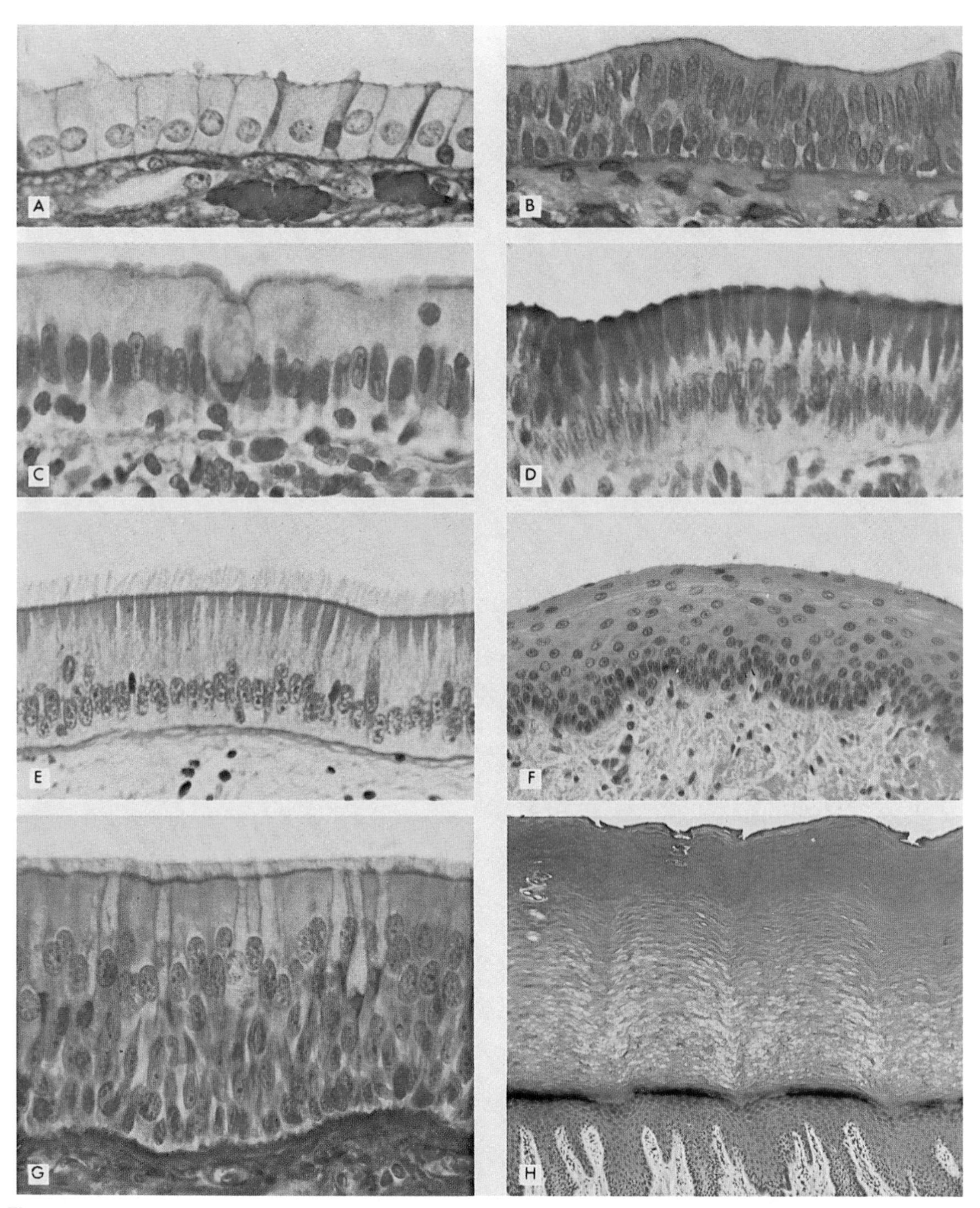

Figure 2–4. Photomicrographs of various types of epithelium. (A) A simple low columnar epithelium from the papillary duct of the dog kidney. (B) Stratified columnar epithelium from a large duct of the salivary gland. (C) Simple columnar epithelium from the intestinal mucosa of a cat. The epithelium has a striated border. (D) Simple columnar epithelium of mucous-secreting cells from the stomach. The mucus is stained a deep magenta. (E) Simple ciliated columnar epithelium from the typhlosole of a mollusc. Note the long cone of ciliary rootlets extending from the basal bodies downward into the cytoplasm. (F) Stratified squamous epithelium from the esophagus. (G) Ciliated pseudostratified columnar epithelium from the human trachea. (H) Keratinized stratified squamous epithelium of the epidermis of the sole of the foot. Note the very thick superficial stratum of devitalized, fully keratinized cells.

aligned at the same level. Epithelium of this kind lines the digestive tract from the cardia of the stomach to the anus and is found in the larger excretory ducts of some glands. Ciliated simple columnar epithelium (Figs. 2–4E and 2–5) is found lining the uterus and oviducts; in the pulmonary bronchi; in the paranasal sinuses; and in the central canal of the spinal cord.

STRATIFIED SQUAMOUS EPITHELIUM

In this relatively thick stratified epithelium, the cells vary in shape from the base to the free surface (Fig. 2–4F and 2–6). The cells on the basal lamina have rounded or beveled upper ends. Those above this layer are irregularly polyhedral, becoming increasingly flattened toward the surface, and in the superficial layers they are thin squamous cells.

Stratified squamous epithelium is found in the epidermis of the skin; lining the oral cavity, the epiglottis, and esophagus; on the conjunctiva and cornea; and in the vagina and distal portion of the urethra. Where it occurs on the surface of the body, the superficial layers of cells lose their nuclei and the cytoplasm is largely replaced by the scleroprotein, keratin. The cells become dry, devitalized scales. Such an epithelium is called a *keratinized stratified squamous epithelium* (Fig. 2–4H). On most inner surfaces, the superficial cells are viable nucleated cells resembling those of the deeper layers except for their greater degree of flattening. In these unexposed sites, the cells contain keratin but it is not present in excess, so the epithelium is (inappropriately) described as *nonkeratinizing stratified squamous epithelium* (Fig. 2–4F).

STRATIFIED COLUMNAR EPITHELIUM

In this uncommon type of epithelium, the superficial cells are columnar and the basal cells are cuboidal with a rounded upper end. In some examples, one or more rows of polygonal cells are interposed between the basal cells and the columnar cells. Stratified columnar epithelium is found in the fornix of the conjunctiva; in the cavernous urethra; in the

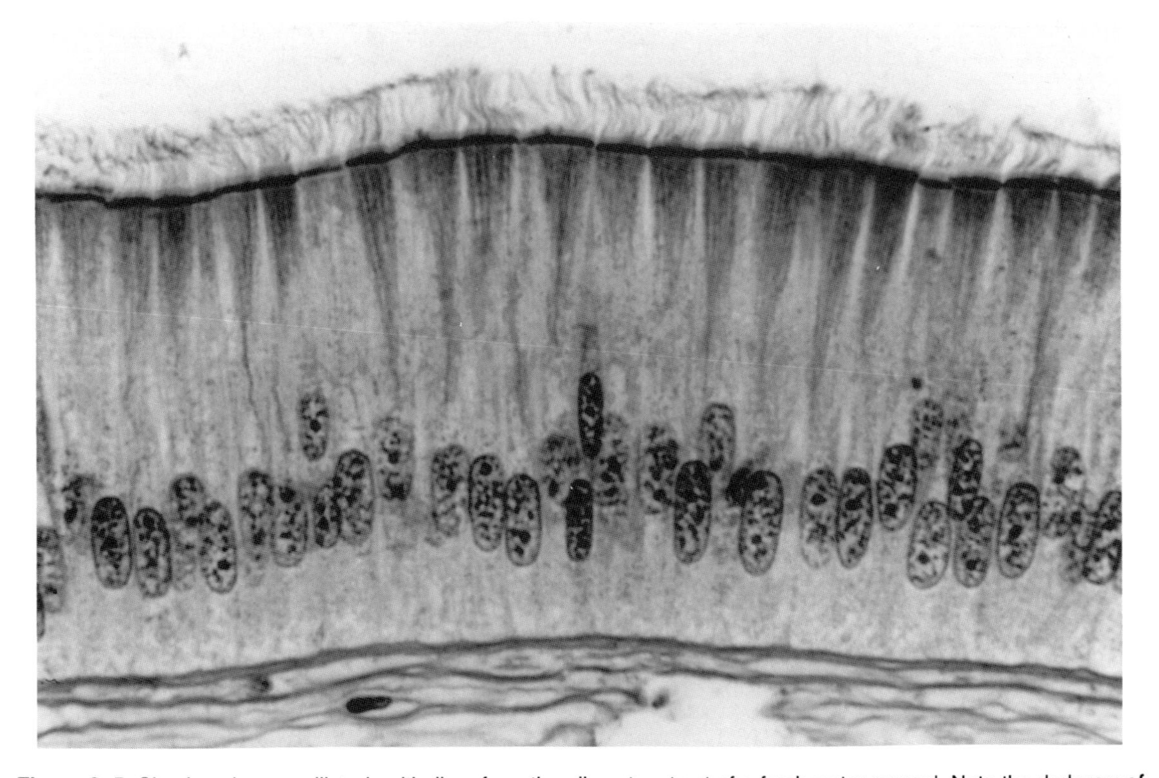

Figure 2–5. Simple columnar ciliated epithelium from the alimentary tract of a fresh water mussel. Note the dark row of ciliary basal bodies beneath the free surface and the cones of fibrous rootlets extending downward into the cytoplasm. Observe also the distinct "basement membrane" on which the epithelium rests.

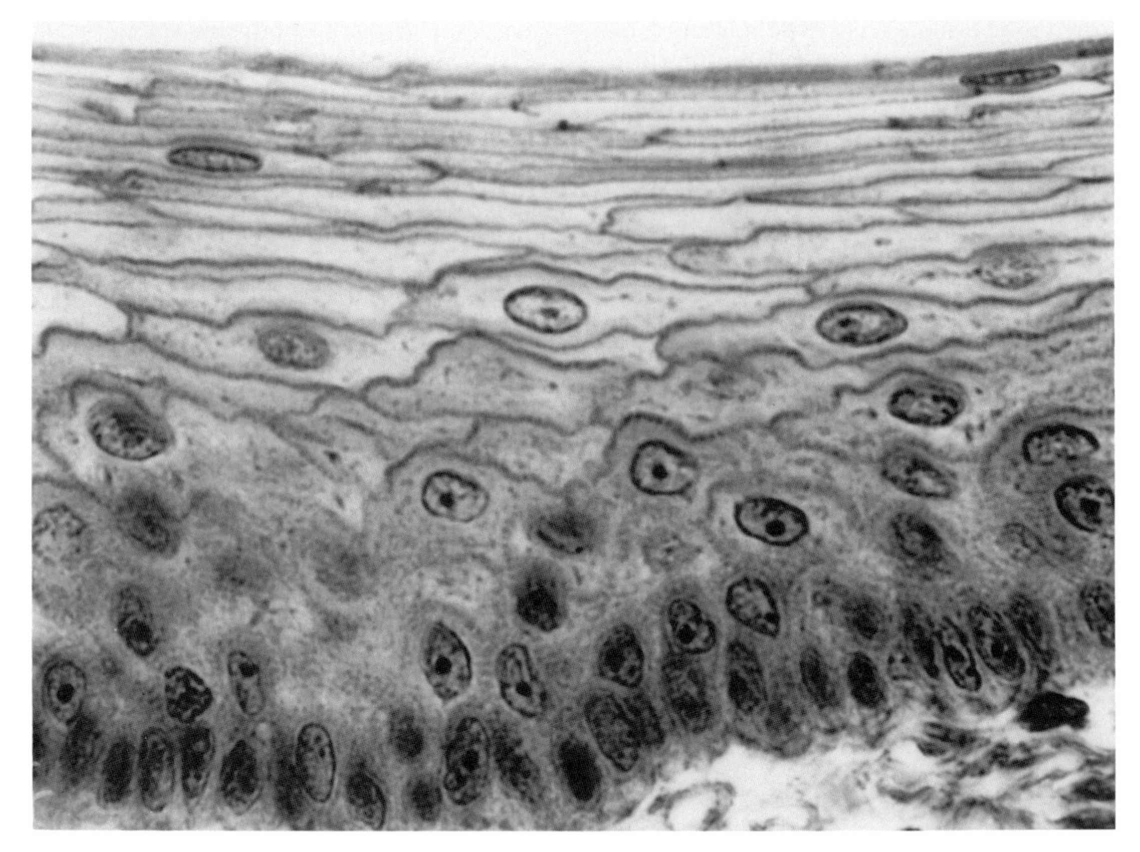

Figure 2–6. Photomicrograph of stratified squamous epithelium from the gingiva of a kitten. Observe the darker-staining cuboidal cells of the basal layer and the progressive flattening of cells in the more superficial layers.

pharynx; in small areas of the anal mucous membrane; and in the large excretory ducts of some glands (Figs. 2–4B and 2–7). Ciliated stratified columnar epithelium is found on the nasal surface of the soft palate; in the larynx; and transiently in the fetal esophagus.

PSEUDOSTRATIFIED COLUMNAR EPITHELIUM

In stratified epithelia, only the lower layer of cells is in contact with the basal lamina. In pseudostratified columnar epithelium, all cells are in contact with the basal lamina but only a portion of them reach the surface (Fig. 2–4G). The cells are quite variable in shape. Some have fairly broad attachment at their base but narrow rapidly and extend upward only part way to the surface. Other taller cells extend through the entire thickness of the epithelium, but are widest near the free surface and narrow to a slender process that passes downward to the basal lamina, between the broader basal cells. Because the nuclei are in the wider part of cells of both shapes, they are found aligned at two levels in the epithelium, creating a false impression of cell stratification—hence, the descriptive term *pseudostratified* epithelium. Epithelium of this kind occurs in the urethra of the male and in the excretory duct of the parotid gland. Ciliated pseudostratified columnar epithelium lines the greater part of the trachea and primary bronchi of the respiratory tract (Fig. 2–4G); the auditory tube; part of the tympanic cavity; and the lacrimal sac.

TRANSITIONAL EPITHELIUM

This epithelium was originally interpreted as intermediate between columnar and stratified squamous epithelium. The name has persisted, although its implication of transition from one type of epithelium to another is quite inappropriate. Transitional epithelium occurs mainly in the urinary bladder. This

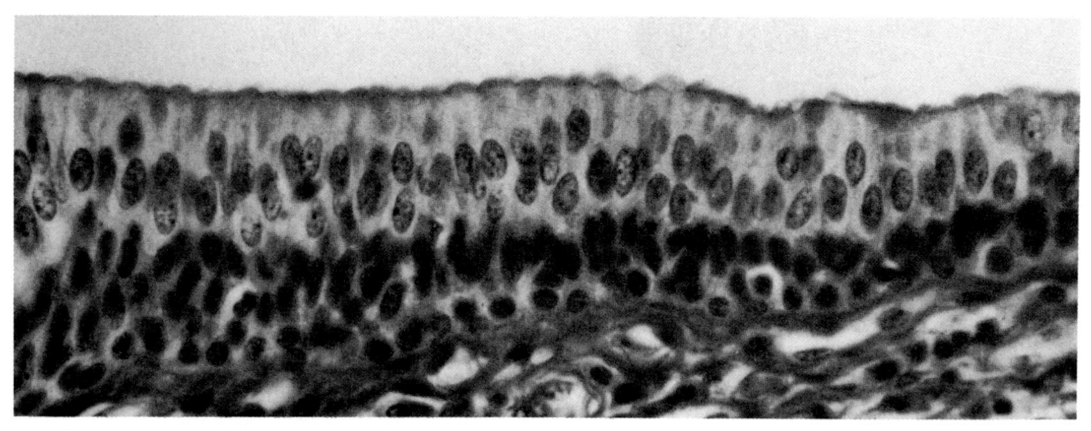

Figure 2–7. Photomicrograph of stratified columnar epithelium from the human male urethra. Note the columnar form of the superficial layer of cells and the multiple layers of nuclei that are not attributable to obliquity of the section.

organ undergoes major changes in volume with filling and emptying, and its appearance, in histological sections, varies greatly depending on its degree of distension at the time of fixation. In the empty, contracted bladder, it has many cell layers (Fig. 2–8). The cells at the base have a cuboidal or low columnar shape. Above these are several layers of polyhedral cells and the superficial cells are very much larger, with a characteristic rounded free surface. During filling of the bladder, the relationships of the cells in the epithelium change; in the distended state, there are usually only two layers: a superficial layer of very large squamous cells overlying a layer of smaller, more-or-less cuboidal cells. Transi-

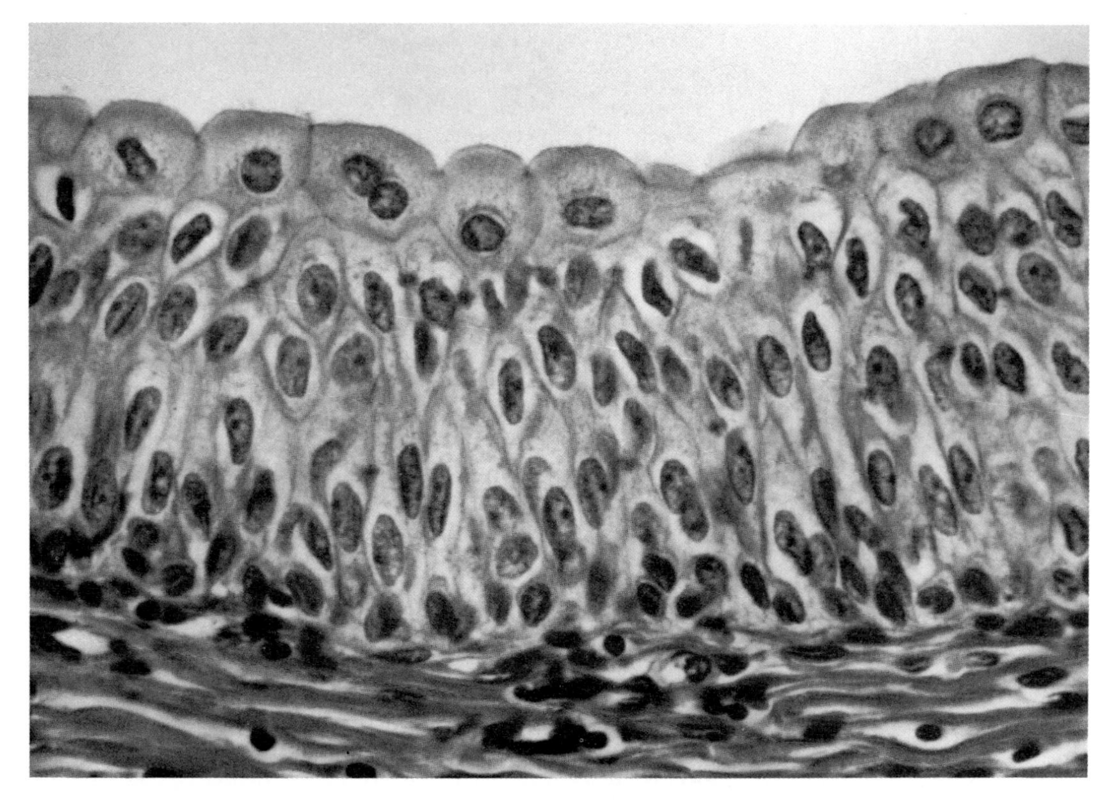

Figure 2–8. Photomicrograph of stratified transitional epithelium from the renal pelvis of a monkey, showing the characteristic superficial layer of large rounded cells that are often binucleate.

tional epithelium is found throughout the urinary tract from the renal calyces to the urethra. *Uroepithelium* might be a better descriptive term than transitional epithelium.

In adult mammals, the type of epithelium characteristic of each organ in the body is normally constant. However, in pathological conditions, an epithelium may change from one type to another, a change called *metaplasia*. For example, in chronic inflammation of the bronchi, the ciliated pseudostratified epithelium may become transformed to stratified squamous epithelium, a change called *squamous metaplasia*. This transformation can be induced experimentally. If one nostril is surgically closed, the enhanced evaporative loss of water resulting from increased ventilation through the open nasal passage will cause its ciliated pseudostratified epithelium to transform into stratified squamous epithelium.

The classification of epithelia presented above applies mainly to the tissues of higher vertebrates. Additional categories would be necessary to describe adequately the patterns of cell association found in some of the epithelia of lower vertebrates and invertebrates.

EPITHELIAL POLARITY

The cells of epithelia are structurally and functionally *polarized* to carry out the vectorial functions of secretion or absorption and to regulate the transepithelial traffic in ions and solutes necessary to maintain a concentration gradient between the external environment and the body fluids, or between compartments within the body. Polarity is evident in the specializations that amplify the area of the free surface; in the supranuclear location of the centrosome and Golgi complex; and in the accumulation of secretory products in the apical cytoplasm. At the ultrastructural level, polarity is expressed in the sealing of the intercellular clefts by tight junctions located on the cell boundaries near the free surface, and in other specializations for attachment or cell-to-cell communication that are confined to the lateral cell surfaces (Fig. 2–9).

The plasma membrane of nonpolarized cells is of uniform biochemical composition over the entire surface; however, in epithelial cells, polarity is expressed at the submicroscopic level in the segregation of certain membrane proteins and lipids in functionally distinct domains: the *apical domain* and the *basolateral domain*. The apical membrane is especially rich in glycolipids and cholesterol and contains H^+-ATPase, hydrolytic enzymes, ion channels, and transport proteins for specific nutrients. It is also the site of release of products of the regulated secretory pathway. The basolateral domain, on the other hand, contains Na^+/K^+-ATPase, anion channels, receptors for hormones, and neurotransmitters, and it is the principal site of constitutive secretion. The basal portion of the basolateral domain also contains binding sites for molecular constituents of the basal lamina.

To maintain these regional differences in membrane composition, newly synthesized membrane proteins are sorted in the trans-Golgi network on the basis of specific signal sequences and segregated in separate vesicles for transport to, and fusion with, the appropriate surface domain. Mixing of components of the apical and basolateral domains is prevented by the tight junctions that encircle the apical pole of the cells. Movement of membrane proteins is further restricted by their binding to the cytoskeleton of the underlying ectoplasm.

CELL COHESION AND COMMUNICATION

A fundamental property of epithelial cells is their maintenance of extensive lateral contact to form continuous sheets of cells. Before the advent of the electron microscope, epithelial cell cohesion was attributed to a hypothetical adhesive, called intercellular cement. This interpretation was based on the observation that if an epithelium was immersed in a silver nitrate solution, and subsequently exposed to sunlight, the cell boundaries were clearly revealed by intercellular deposition of metallic silver (Fig. 2–2). A similar delineation of the cell outlines was observed in preparations stained with the periodic-acid–Schiff reaction, suggesting that a major component of the intercellular adhesion was carbohydrate in nature. When the electron microscope became available, it did little to lend credence to the concept of an intercellular cement. The membranes of contiguous epithelial cells were found to be only 15–20 nm apart, and the content of this space was of very low electron density and devoid of resolvable structure. Electron micrographs did reveal conspicuous local junctional specializations that were desig-

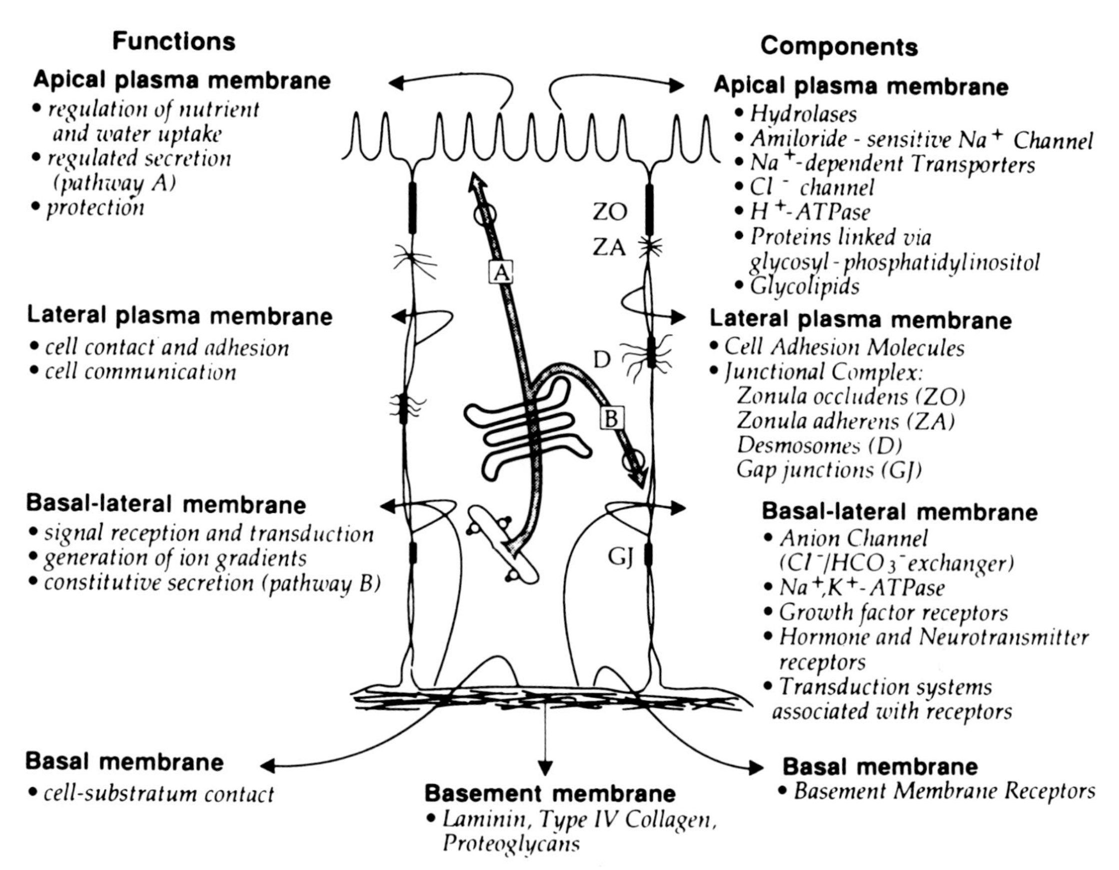

Figure 2–9. Diagrammatic presentation of the polarity of columnar epithelial cells as expressed in biochemically and functionally distinct apical, lateral, and basal domains of the plasma membrane. (From Rodriguez-Boulan and Nelson. 1989. Science 245:718.)

nated the *zonula occludens, zonula adherens, desmosomes,* and *gap junctions.* In the years that followed, these became the focus of investigative attention as the principal structures responsible for epithelial cell cohesion (Fig. 2–10).

ZONULA OCCLUDENS OR TIGHT JUNCTION

In appropriately stained vertical sections of columnar epithelium examined with the light microscope, a fusiform dark spot is seen on each lateral cell boundary, just below the free surface. In subtangential horizontal sections, this structure appears as a dark band outlining the apex of the cell. These structures were formerly called *terminal bars* and were erroneously interpreted as local deposits of intercellular cement that served to seal the intercellular spaces. Electron micrographs disclosed two distinct junctional specializations at this level, the *zonula occludens* (tight junction) and the *zonula adherens* immediately below it (Fig. 2–10). At the zonula occludens, the membranes of adjoining cells converge and are in very close proximity for a distance of 0.1–0.3 μm. In this short segment, the membranes fuse at from two to four points, diverging slightly between sites of fusion. Freeze–fracture preparations of this region reveal a variable number of thin intramembranous strands or fibrils that are more-or-less parallel but interconnected to form a loose network on the inner half-membrane (the P-face). A corresponding pattern of shallow grooves is found on the outer half-membrane (the E-face) (Fig. 2–11). The number of rows of these fibrils corresponds to the number of sites of membrane fusion seen in thin transverse sections of the junction. Along each line of fusion, in the tight junction, the membranes evidently share a single junctional fibril. The

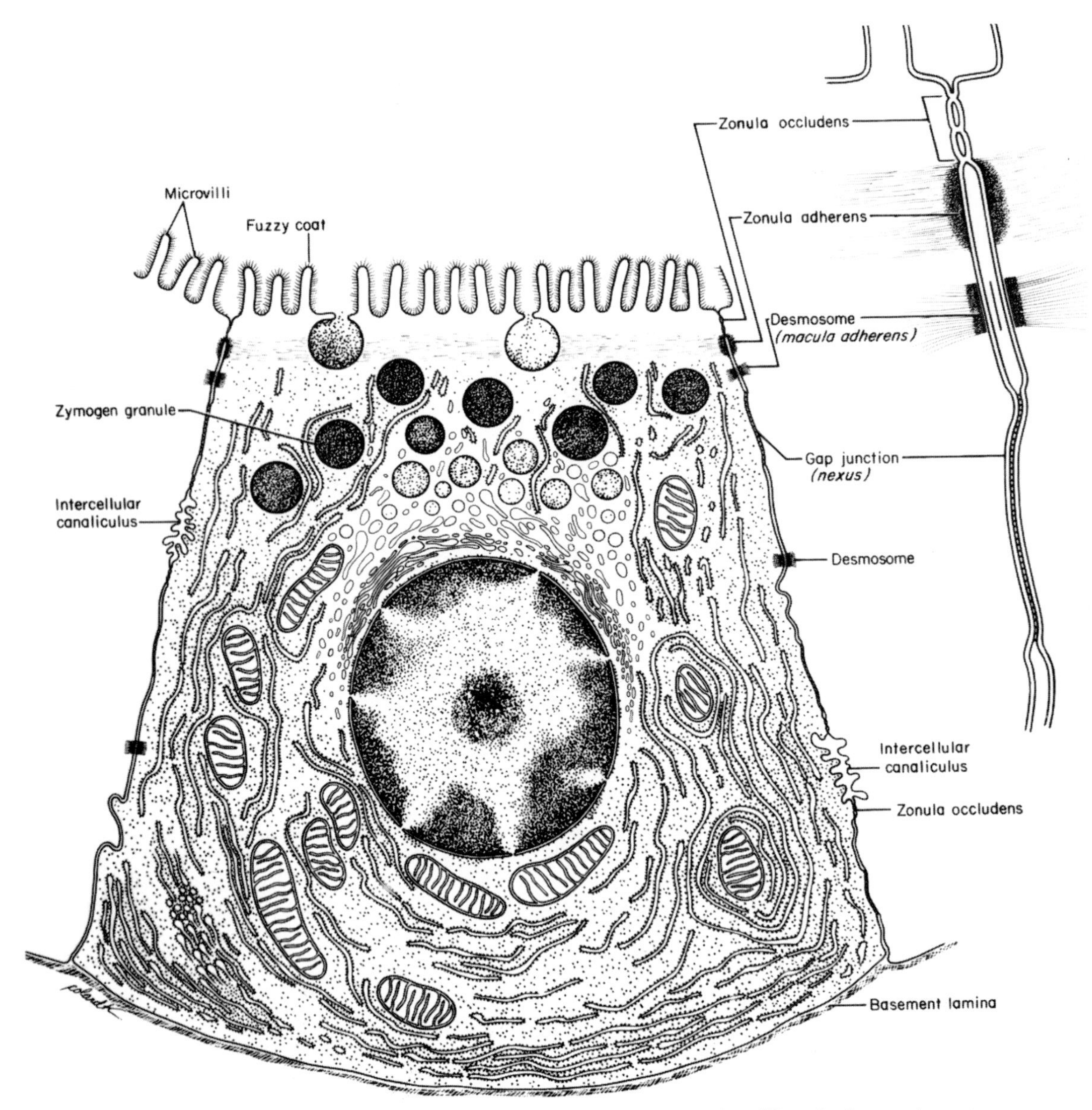

Figure 2–10. Drawing of a typical epithelial cell, illustrating the basal lamina, microvilli on the free surface, desmosomes on the lateral surfaces, and a juxtaluminal junctional complex. The latter consists of a zonula occludens, zonula adherens, and macula adherens. In addition, a gap junction is depicted near the junctional complex. (Drawing from Hay, E. *In* R.O. Greep, ed. Histology. 2nd ed. New York, McGraw-Hill Book Co.)

fibrils are believed to be attached directly or indirectly to the underlying cytoskeleton, which may explain their preferential association with the P-face in freeze–fracture replicas.

The chemical nature of the junctional fibrils is not known. They appear to develop by aggregation and alignment of integral membrane proteins. Two other membrane proteins of high molecular weight, designated *ZO-1* and *cinqulin,* are exclusively associated with the zonula occludens. Both seem to be components of the junction, with ZO-1 localized immediately adjacent to the sites of membrane fusion and cingulin distributed more diffusely. Their function is unknown.

Cell attachment is stronger at the zonula occludens than elsewhere on the lateral boundaries, but this mechanical function is probably of less physiological significance than the role of this junction as a permeability barrier, blocking the paracellular passage of large and small molecules. Its efficiency varies in different epithelia, some being classified as

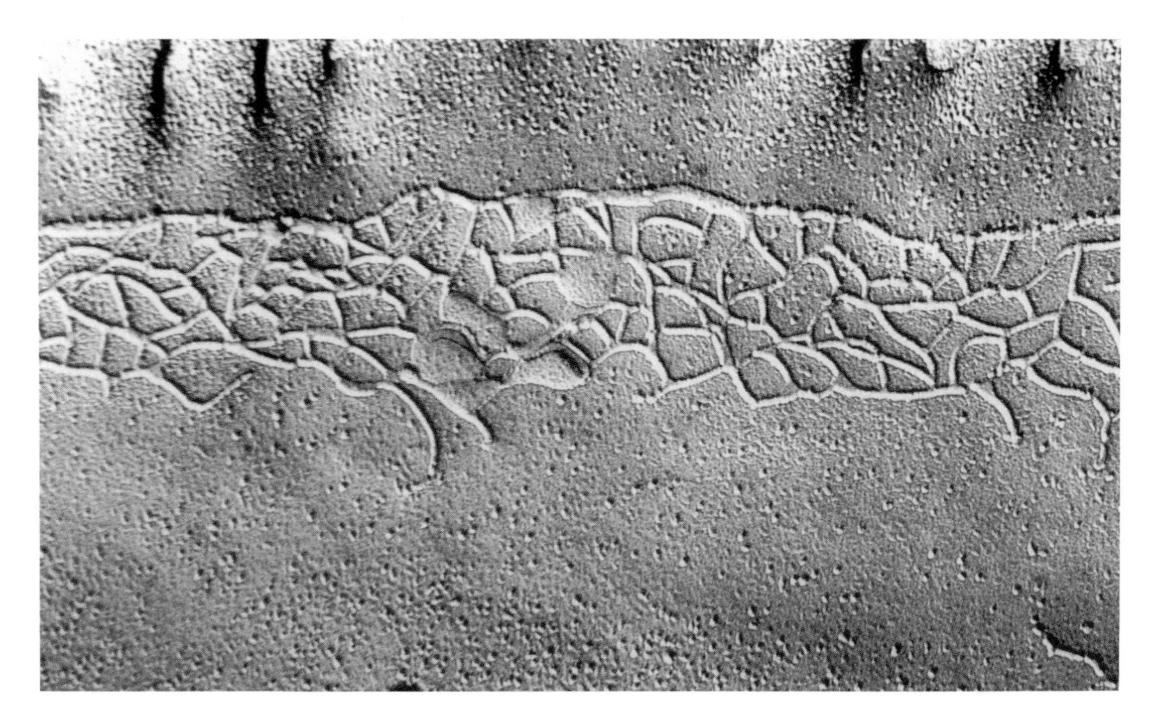

Figure 2–11. Electron micrograph of a freeze-fracture replica of a zonula occludens in intestinal epithelium. A reticular pattern of anastomosing strands is seen on the P-face of the cleaved lateral cell membrane just below the brush border. (Micrograph courtesy of J.P. Revel.)

"leaky" and other as "tight," and these differences depend in large measure on the number and pattern of linear membrane fusions in the zonula. In epithelia that are relatively permeable, the rows of junctional fibrils are few and may show short discontinuities. In tight epithelia, there are usually multiple rows of continuous junctional fibrils that completely close the paracellular route, ensuring that solutes traverse the epithelium via the transcellular route, involving active transport mechanisms of the apical and basolateral membranes. As mentioned above, the occluding junctions also constitute a barrier to diffusion of integral membrane proteins between the apical and basolateral domains of the plasmalemma. If epithelial cells are prevented from establishing such junctions, they are unable to maintain the distinctive biochemical properties of these domains.

THE ZONULA ADHERENS

The *zonula adherens* is a band-like specialization of the membrane and subjacent cytoplasm that encircles the apex of adjoining cells, below the tight junction, and strongly bonds the cells together. In this junction, the opposing membranes are 15–20 nm apart and the intercellular space is occupied by material of low electron density that may exhibit an exceedingly fine transverse striation. Freeze–fracture preparations reveal no intramembranous components that distinguish this zone from other regions of the cell membrane. In sections, the most conspicuous feature of the zonula adherens is a plaque-like dense area of cytoplasm closely applied to the junctional membrane of adjacent cells. At high magnification, these subplasmalemmal densities are resolved as a mat of fine filaments. This band of microfilaments around the apex of the cells generally has rather ill-defined inner limits but, in some epithelia, it appears to be continuous with the *terminal web,* a thin transverse zone of cytoplasm rich in actin filaments, crossing the cell a short distance below its free surface. Freeze–fracture preparations reveal no intramembranous components that distinguish this junctional zone from other regions of the cell membrane.

Immunocytochemical studies have localized *actin* and the actin-associated proteins, *α-actinin* and *vinculin* in the subplasmalemmal dense band of the zonula adherens. These may be involved in the cross-linking and binding of microfilaments of the band to the junctional membrane. A 135 kD glycoprotein, specific for adherens junctions, has been localized in the membranes or the interspace between them. This has been called *adherens junction-specific cell adhesion molecule* (A-CAM). The antibody to this molecule is reported to prevent development of this type of junction.

The zonula adherens is clearly a major site of epithelial cell cohesion. Its association with the actin-rich terminal web and other elements of the cytoskeleton in columnar epithelia having a brush border suggests that it may also have a role in stabilizing this specialization of the free surface. The staining of the dense band of the zonula adherens was probably the basis for descriptions of "terminal bars" in such epithelia, in the early histological literature.

MACULA ADHERENS OR DESMOSOME

The third component of the junctional complex of epithelia is the *macula adherens*. Unlike the zonula occludens and zonula adherens, the maculae adherentes do not form a continuous band encircling the cell apex, but are separate plaques arranged in a row around the cell, just below the zonula adherens. These plaques correspond to dots or fusiform thickenings of the cell boundaries that were seen with the light microscope and called *desmosomes,* a term still widely used. These structures may also be found scattered over the lateral surfaces of epithelial cells, away from the junctional complex. In electron micrographs, they are bipartite structures consisting of a subplasmalemmal dense plaque 10–15 nm thick on the cytoplasmic side of the opposing membranes (Fig. 2–12). The intercellular cleft, at these sites, is 15–20 nm wide and a thin dense line is often seen midway between the opposing membranes. With intense heavy-metal staining, a delicate transverse striation may also be detected. Intermediate filaments in the cytoplasm converge on the desmosomes and terminate in a satellite zone of moderate density on the inner aspect of the dense plaque. Thus, desmosomes are not only sites of cell attachment but they also contribute to the structural stability of the epithelium as a whole by linking the cytoskeleton of adjoining cells. The integrity of the desmosomes is calcium dependent. If exposed to a calcium chelating agent, the two halves of the desmosome separate and the cells dissociate.

Seven or more biochemical components of the desmosome have been identified. Three of these are glycoproteins: *desmoglein-I* (165 kD), *desmocollin-I* (130 kD), and *desmocollin-II* (115 kD). Four are nonglycosylated proteins: *desmoplakin-I* (250 kD), *desmoplakin-II* (215 kD), *pakoglobin* (83 kD), and a 75 kD *basic polypeptide*. The small size and electron density of the maculae adherentes has made localization of these components difficult, but the desmocollins seem to be located in the intercellular cleft and are probably adhesive proteins. Desmoglein appears to be present both in the intercellular cleft and in the dense plaque. The desmoplakins, pakoglobin, and the 75 kD component occur principally in the plaque, but desmoplakins are also localized in the in-

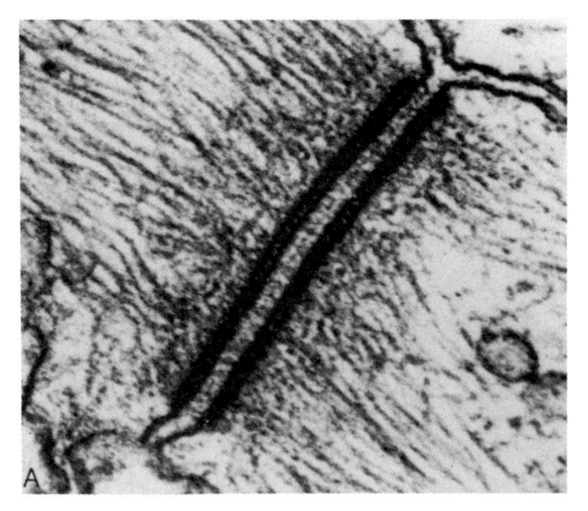

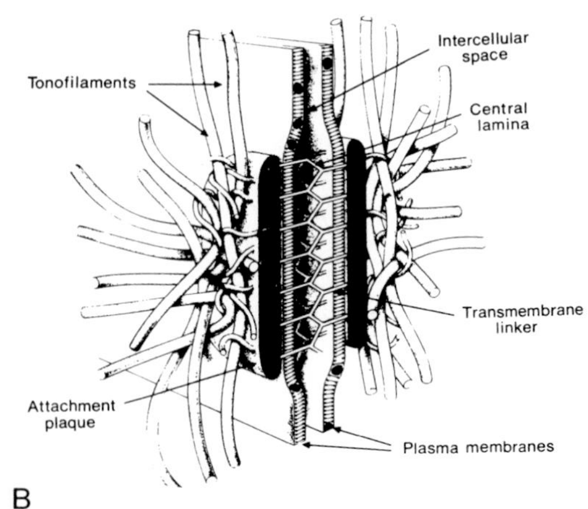

Figure 2–12. (A) Electron micrograph of a desmosome from amphibian epidermis showing the attachment plaque and tonofilaments forming recurving loops in the adjacent cytoplasm. (Micrograph courtesy of D. Kelly.) (B) Schematic representation of the structure of the desmosome. (Redrawn after Staehelin, L.A. and B.E. Hill. 1978. Sci. Am. 238:146.)

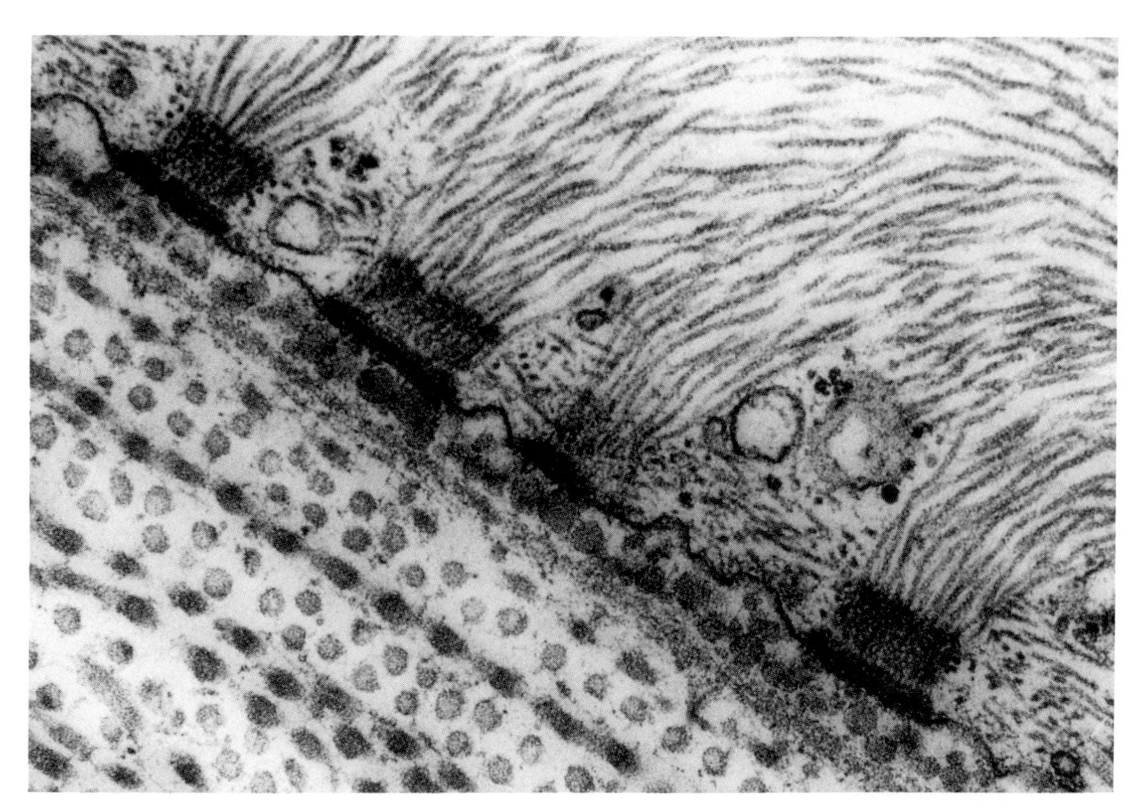

Figure 2–13. Electron micrograph of hemidesmosomes along the base of an amphibian epidermal cell. Note the tonofilaments converging on the hemidesmosomes. At the lower left are cross sections of collagen fibers in the connective tissue underlying the epithelium. (Micrograph courtesy of D. Kelly.)

ner zone in which the intermediate filaments are anchored.

Stratified squamous epithelium is somewhat atypical in that junctional complexes are not found. Zonulae occludentes and zonulae adherentes are lacking in the superficial cell layer. Instead, this epithelium is rendered impervious to substances in solution by the deposition of lipid in the intercellular spaces. However, desmosomes are exceptionally abundant in the deeper layers of the epithelium. They occur where short processes of the cells meet end-to-end. Evidently, the formation of a dense plaques in one cell induces the formation of its counterpart in the adjoining cell, resulting in a symmetrical, bipartite desmosome. Between the desmosomes, the intercellular spaces are widened to form a labyrinthine system of *interfacial canals.* At the basal surface of stratified squamous epithelium, there are numerous *hemi-desmosomes,* binding the epithelium to the underlying basal lamina (Fig. 2–13).

In addition to scattered desmosomes on the lateral cell boundaries of columnar epithelia, occasional, less-conspicuous junctional specializations, called *puncta adherentes,* may be found. These lack the clearly defined dense plaque typical of desmosomes. Instead, there is a very small subplasmalemmal density in which thin cytoplasmic filaments terminate. Desmoplakins are not demonstrable in these, but α-actinin and vinculin can be detected. These minute punctate junctions are believed to serve mainly as sites of attachment for the actin-based contractile system of the cytoplasm and are probably of little significance for maintaining cell cohesion.

THE NEXUS OR GAP JUNCTION

A region of intimate cell contact that went undetected with the light microscope is the *gap junction* or *nexus* which permits passage of small molecules between cells, coordinating the activities of an epithelium. In section, these junctions bear some resemblance to a tight junction but there is no actual fusion of the membranes. The intercellular cleft is

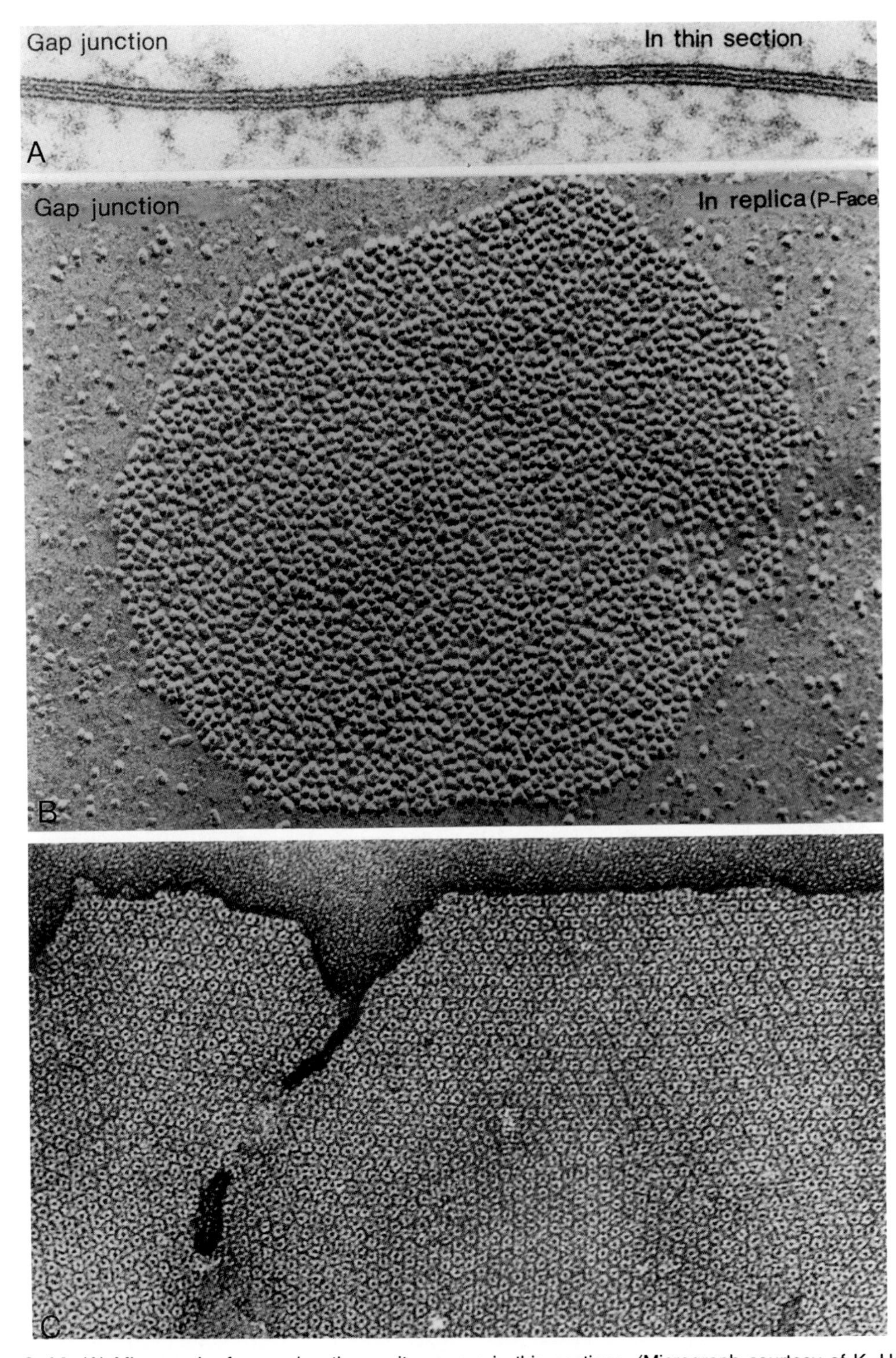

Figure 2–14. (A) Micrograph of a gap junction as it appears in thin sections. (Micrograph courtesy of K. Hama.) (B) Freeze–fracture replica of the P-face of a gap junction. (Micrograph courtesy of D. Albertini.) (C) Isolated gap junctions as they appear in negatively stained preparations. The connexons have a central dot representing the 1.5–2.0 nm central channel. (Micrograph courtesy of B. Gilula.)

narrowed to ~3 nm and is of constant width throughout (Fig. 2–14A). In favorable sections, minute structures, called *connexons,* can be seen bridging the gap. In freeze–fracture replicas of the P-face of the membranes, the junction appears as a round area of closely packed particles (Fig. 2–14B). When isolated and negatively stained with an electron opaque probe, such as lanthanum, the connexons of the gap junction, appear as hexagonally packed annular units with a center-to-center spacing of 9 nm (Fig. 2–14C). They are cylindrical in form and ~7.5 nm in length with a wall made up of six rod-like subunits around a central pore 1.5–2.0 nm in diameter. Connexons in the opposing membranes of the junction are in register and project ~1.5 nm into the intercellular space, where they are linked end-to-end. Their central pores, thus, form a continuous hydrophilic channel connecting the cytoplasm of contiguous cells. Ions, cyclic AMP, amino acids, and other molecules smaller than 2 nm in diameter pass freely through the channels (Fig. 2–15). The electrical coupling of cells throughout an epithelium is attributed to the flow of ions through these channels. Junctions of this kind are also abundant in smooth and skeletal muscle where they provide low-resistance pathways through which excitation passes rapidly between the cellular units permitting muscle to function as though it were a syncytium.

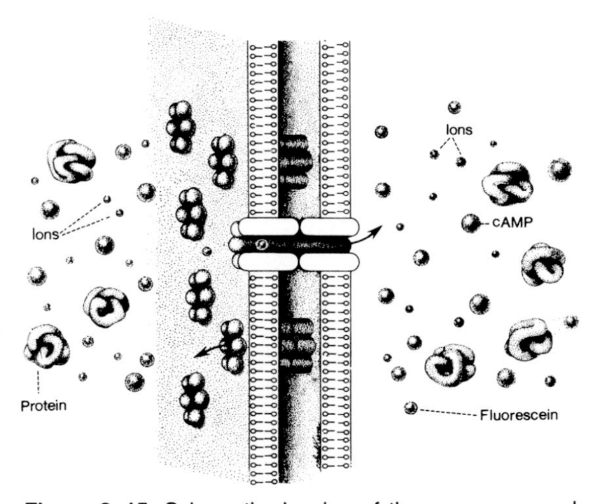

Figure 2–15. Schematic drawing of the connexons and their subunits in a portion of a gap junction. The hydrophilic pores through the connexons permit passage of ions and small molecules, such as AMP or the dye fluorescein, but exclude larger molecules. (Redrawn after Tagawa, B. and T. Lowenstein. 1975. *In* G. Weismann and R. Caiborne, eds. Biochemistry Cell Biology and Pathology. New York, H.P. Publishing Co.)

The permeability of gap junctions is affected by pH and the concentration of free calcium ions. An influx of calcium, due to cell injury, causes a change in the configuration of the subunits in the wall of the connexons that results in closure of their channels. This may be beneficial in preventing the spread of damage from the injured cell to other viable cells.

CELL ADHESION MOLECULES OR INTEGRINS

Interest in submicroscopic devices for cell cohesion has been revived in recent years by the extraction and chemical characterization of a family of surface glycoproteins that are called *integrins* or *cell adhesion molecules* (ICAMs). Some of these bind to other cells, whereas others bind to components of the extracellular matrix. Sixteen or more integrins have been identified to date and designated by letters and numerals that are meaningful only to specialists who are familiar with their biochemistry. Some are cell-type specific; others occur on many different cell types.

These membrane proteins are believed to play an essential role in mutual recognition and aggregation of cells of the same type during embryonic development, and in epithelial cell cohesion and attachment to substrate in postnatal life. Little is known about how the extracellular domain of these proteins recognizes and binds to its counterpart on an adjoining cell. It is known that the adhesive properties of the principal class of epithelial ICAMs, called *cadherins,* are dependent on the presence of calcium. Chelation of calcium results in dissociation of an epithelium, and these adhesion molecules seem to be a prerequisite for the development of other cohesional devices because specific blocking of their function prevents formation of the junctional complexes described earlier.

The ligands for the integrins that bind to the extracellular matrix include fibronectin, laminin, and collagens. Cells secrete these extracellular components and then attach to them via the integrins in the cell membrane. These molecules also appear to be essential for cell migration during tissue repair. For example, the keratinocytes of the skin do not normally have an integrin binding to fibronectin, but during healing of a skin wound, such an integrin is expressed on their surface and is believed to facilitate their migration over the fibronectin-rich wound matrix to restore epithelial continuity.

THE BASAL SURFACE

The base of most epithelia is smooth contoured, but in transporting epithelia, such as those of the kidney tubules, the membrane at the cell base may be deeply infolded, partitioning the basal cytoplasm into numerous narrow alcoves occupied by mitochondria. Such amplification of the cell base serves to increase the area of the membrane engaged in pumping ions to generate an osmotic gradient to move water across the epithelium.

At the boundary between the epithelium and the underlying connective tissue, there is a thin supporting layer, traditionally called the *basement membrane.* Because it is not a lipid bilayer like the membranes of cells, the term *basal lamina* is now preferred. A similar layer surrounds smooth and striated muscle fibers and certain other sessile cells of mesenchymal origin. The term *external lamina* is applied to the layer completely surrounding these cell types.

In electron micrographs, two zones are distinguishable within the basal lamina: the *lamina lucida,* a pale zone of very low density immediately adjacent to the basal cell membranes of the epithelium, and the *lamina densa,* an outer zone of greater density exposed to the underlying connective tissue (Fig. 2–16). The two are generally of similar thickness (40–50 nm), but in exceptional cases, the lamina densa may be considerably thicker. It consists of a meshwork of randomly oriented and interwoven 4-nm filaments. Little substructure is resolved in the lamina lucida, but in some preparations, it is traversed by very fine strands that extend from the cell membrane to the lamina densa.

The principal chemical constituents of the basal lamina are *type-IV collagen, laminin,* and *proteoglycans.* Type-IV collagen occurs exclusively in the basal lamina and consists of three α-chains retaining a terminal peptide that prevents their assembly into the cross-striated fibers characteristic of other forms of collagen. The chains of type-IV collagen are cross-linked to form the resilient three-dimensional meshwork of the basal lamina. The large glycoprotein, laminin (900 kD), is localized mainly in the lamina lucida. Its molecules are adherent to specific receptors in the basal membrane of the cells at one end, and to the collagen of the lamina densa at the other end. The proteoglycans of the lamina densa include heparan sulfate, which gives the lamina a strong anionic charge that may contribute to its function as a selective

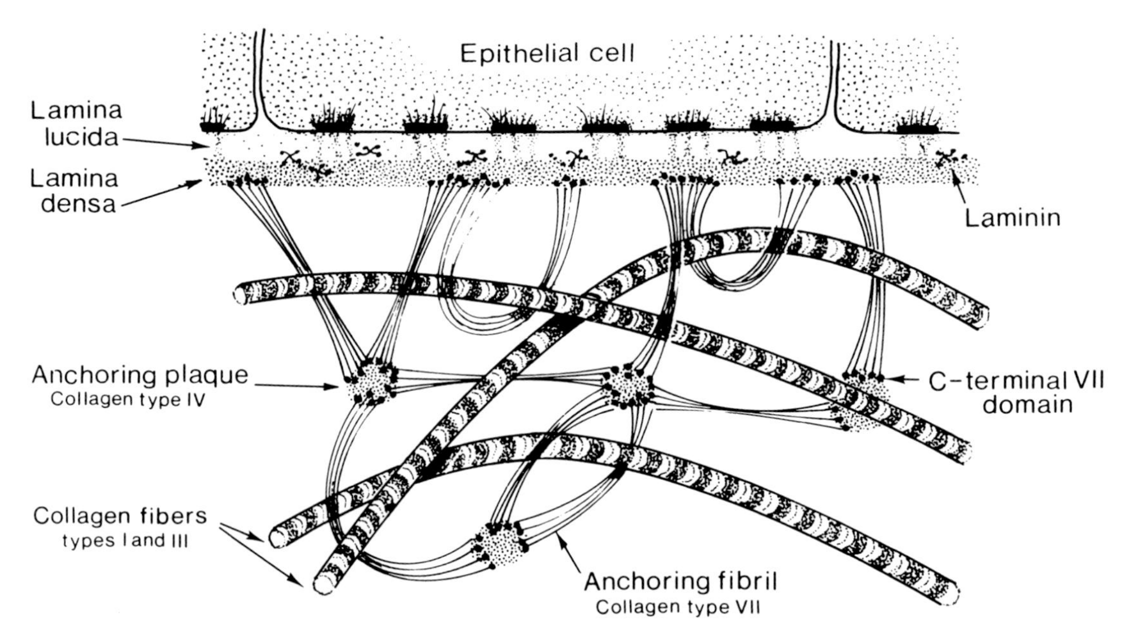

Figure 2–16. Diagram of the anchoring fibril network beneath an epithelium. It is believed that the anchoring fibrils are composed of lateral aggregates of type-VII procollagen molecules aligned in nonstaggered array. The fibrils originate in the basal lamina and insert into anchoring plaques consisting of type-IV collagen. (Redrawn after Keene, D.R., et al. 1987. J. Cell Biol. 104:611.)

filter. *Fibronectin* can be detected on the side of the basal lamina away from the cells and it may be involved in its attachment to reticular fibers of the underlying stroma. Slender *anchoring fibers* of type-VII collagen course downward from the basal lamina, looping around collagen fibers in the subjacent connective tissue and terminating in *anchoring plaques,* dense bodies in the extracellular matrix that have a substructure similar to that of the lamina densa and contain both type-IV and type-VII collagen (Fig. 2–16). Anchoring fibers are abundant beneath the stratified squamous epithelium of the epidermis, especially in those areas of the skin subject to frictional stress. They are less common in epithelia in the interior of the body.

The primary function of the basal lamina is to support the epithelium. The meshwork of type-IV collagen in the lamina densa has considerable tensile strength and enough flexibility to permit stretching and recoil of epithelia lining hollow organs that are subject to changes in volume. In repair after injury to an epithelium, the persisting basal lamina provides a substrate that guides the migration of new cells from the margins of the wound to restore epithelial continuity.

The basal lamina also serves as a passive molecular sieve or ultrafilter. This is apparent in the kidney, where urine is formed as an ultrafiltrate of the blood passing through the glomerular capillaries. The basal lamina of the capillary endothelium is the filter holding back molecules on the basis of their size, shape, and electrostatic charge. The pore size of the filter is determined, in part, by the fine mesh of type-IV collagen in the lamina densa. The charge-dependent selectivity of the filter is attributed to the polyanionic chains of the associated proteoglycans, which have large spheres of hydration, leaving little space occupied by free water that would permit passage of macromolecules.

SPECIALIZATIONS OF THE FREE SURFACE

STRIATED BORDER

Absorptive columnar epithelia often have a refractile free border that exhibits fine vertical striations, under the light microscope. In electron micrographs, this *striated border* or *brush border* is found to consist of slender, cylindrical, membrane-bounded cell processes 1–2 μm long and 80–90 nm in diameter, called *microvilli* (Fig. 2–17). These are closely packed in parallel array with some 60 per square micrometer of epithelial surface. They result in a 15–30-fold increase in the area of cell membrane exposed to the lumen. Delicate branching filaments, projecting from the membrane at the tips of the microvilli, form a coat, or *glycocalyx,* on the luminal surface of the epithelium (Fig. 2–17). These fine filaments are terminal oligosaccharides of integral membrane proteins. Staining histological sections with a histochemical method for carbohydrates renders the glycocalyx visible with the light microscope.

The interior of each microvillus contains a bundle of 25–35 actin filaments that are attached to the membrane at the tip of the villus and extend down into the apical cytoplasm, where they are anchored in a zone of transversely oriented filaments, called the *terminal web* (Fig. 2–18). The actin filaments are cross-linked by a polypeptide called *villin,* and at intervals of 33 nm along their length, short filaments extend laterally, linking the core bundle to the membrane of the microvillus. It was formerly thought that the core filaments might interact with myosin in the apical cytoplasm to shorten the microvilli, but they are now believed to have a purely supportive function, stiffening the microvilli and helping to maintain their parallel orientation.

Biochemical analysis of brush borders isolated from intestinal epithelium has shown that their membrane is rich in enzymes that carry out the terminal stages of digestion of carbohydrates. This border is, therefore, a specialization for increasing both the digestive and absorptive efficiency of the epithelium by greatly amplifying the area of membrane exposed to nutrients in the intestinal lumen. In epithelia that are not engaged in absorption or transport, microvilli are few in number and irregularly oriented, and generally lack cores of actin filaments.

STEREOCILIA

A tuft of long, slender processes can be seen, with the light microscope, on cells of the pseudostratified columnar epithelium of the epididymis. The individual processes in these tufts resemble microvilli but they are very much longer (Figs. 2–19 and 2–20). Because

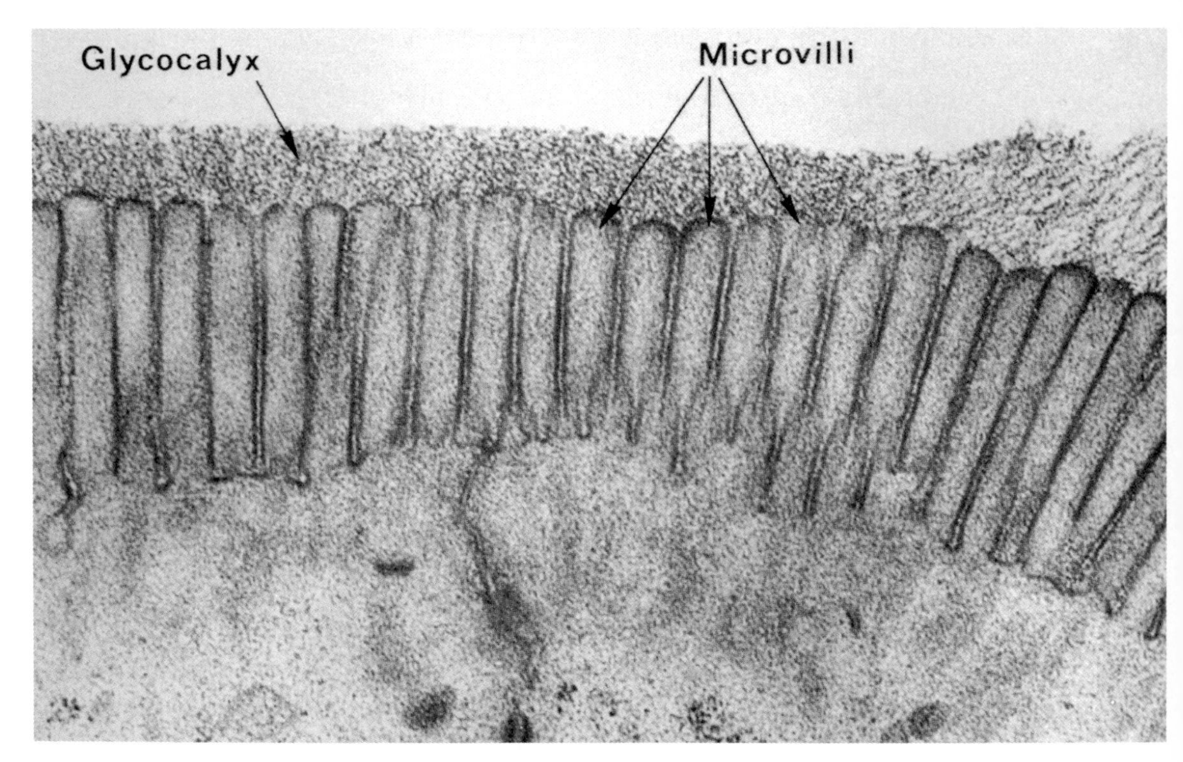

Figure 2–17. Electron micrograph of the brush border of an intestinal epithelial cell, showing the closely-packed microvilli. The layer on the tips of the microvilli is the glycocalyx, a mat of fine filaments that are terminal oligosaccharides of membrane glycoproteins. (Micrograph courtesy of S. Ito.)

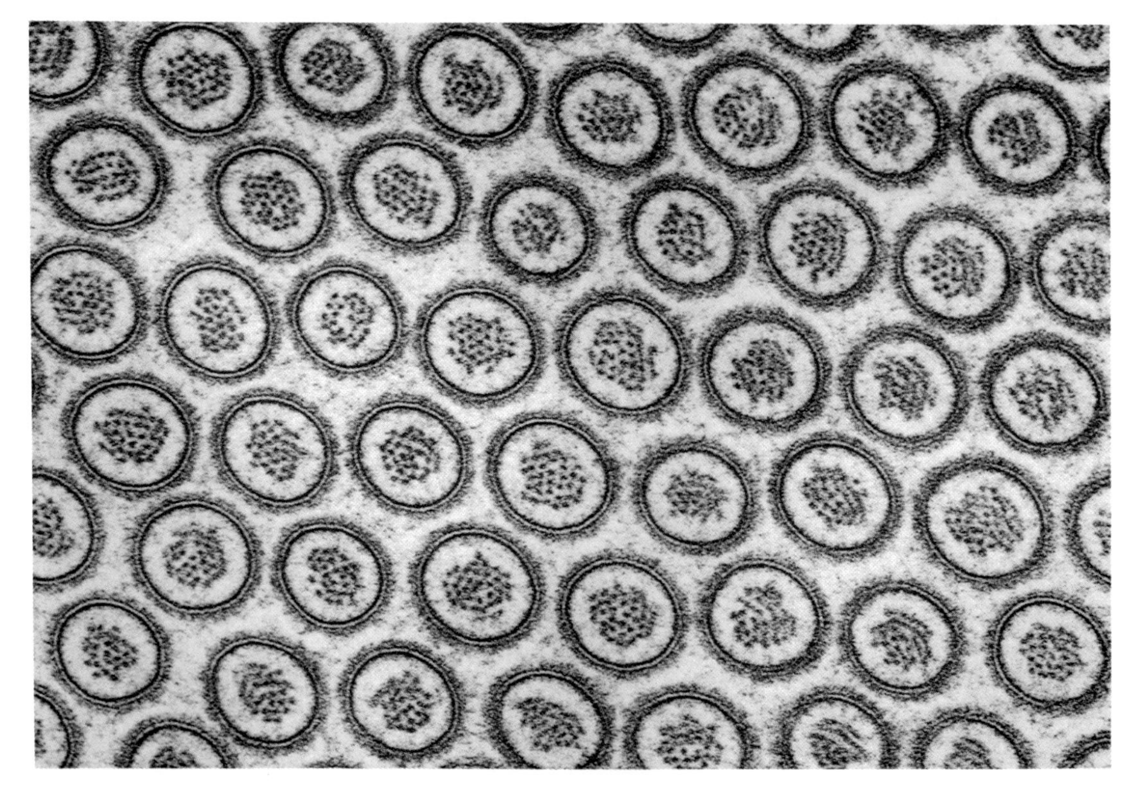

Figure 2–18. Micrograph of a transverse section through some of the microvilli of the brush border on an intestinal epithelial cell. Note the relatively thin glycocalyx on the sides of the microvilli and the bundle of actin filaments in their core. (Micrograph courtesy of A. Ichikawa.)

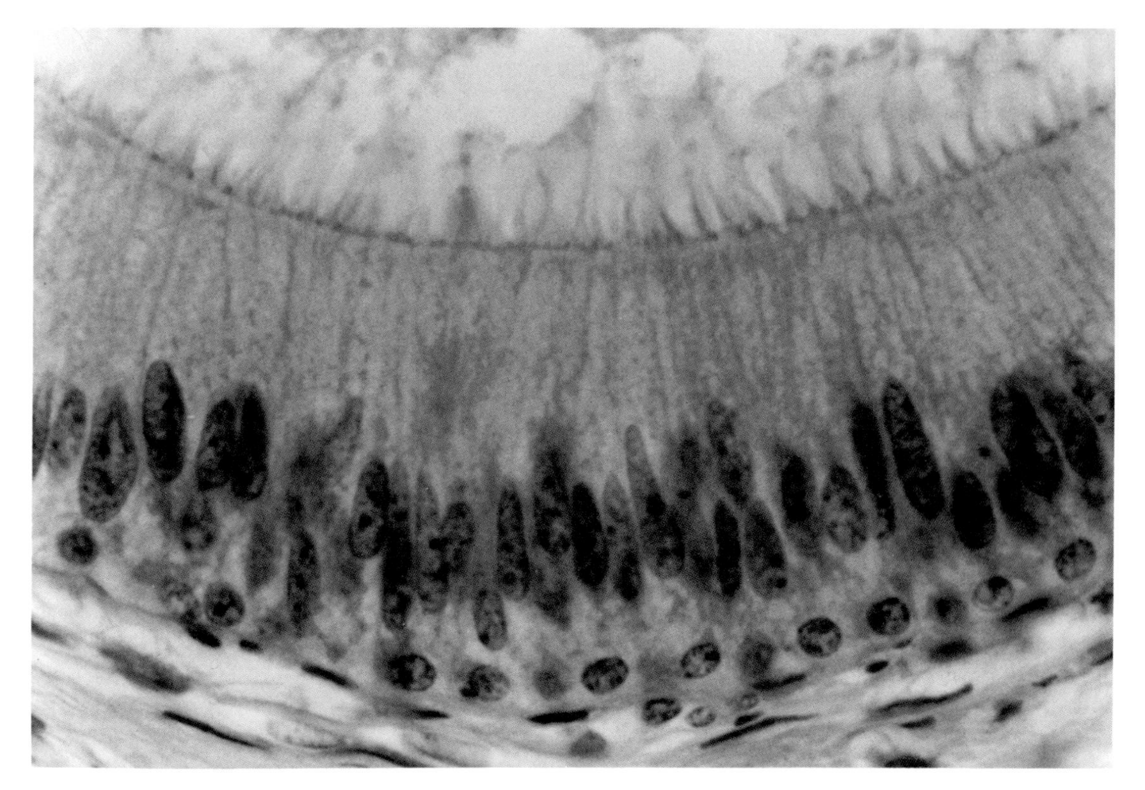

Figure 2–19. Photomicrograph of pseudostratified columnar epithelium of the human epididymis. Note the tufts of long flexible stereocilia projecting from each cell.

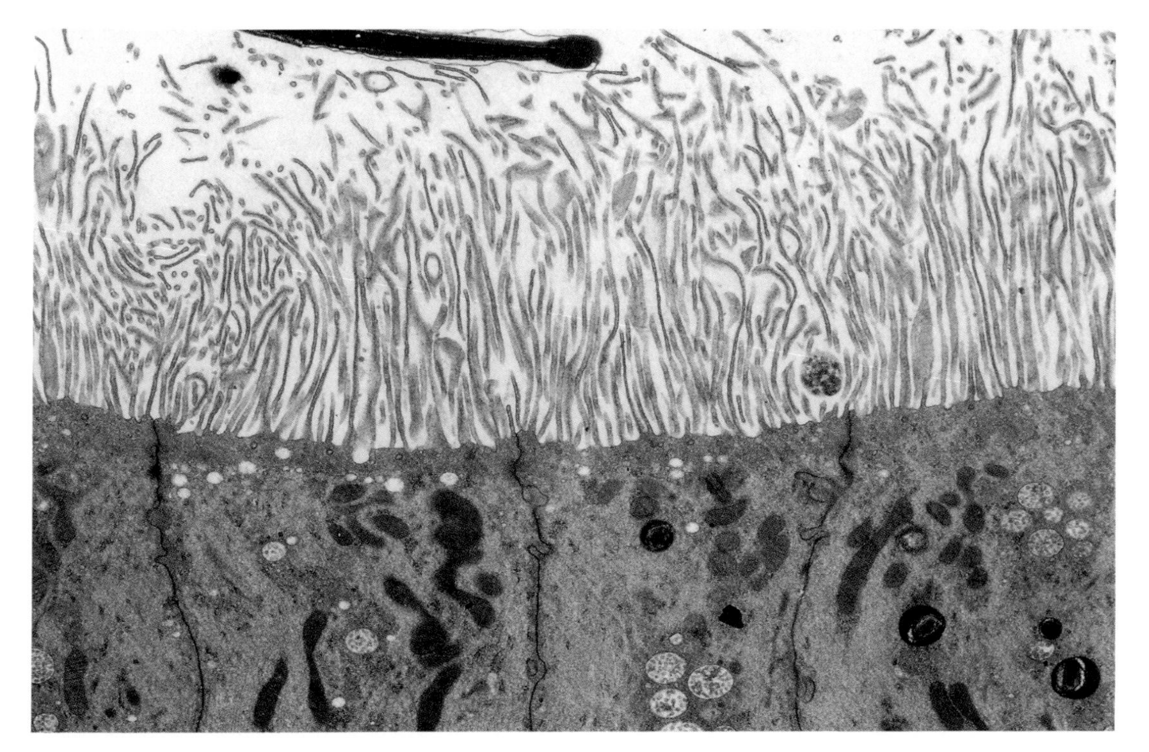

Figure 2–20. Electron micrograph of the apical region of four cells of the ductus epididymidis, illustrating the slender stereocilia which are much longer and less highly ordered than the microvilli of a brush border.

they are nonmotile, they are called *stereocilia* to distinguish them from the motile *kinocilia* on other epithelia. In electron micrographs, they have a core bundle of actin filaments that extends into the apical cytoplasm, but it is less well organized than in microvilli of intestinal absorptive cells. The stereocilia are parallel at their base but become sinuous and entwined nearer their tips. Their function is not entirely clear, but this epithelium is known to absorb 90% of the original volume of fluid secreted by the testis, and the increased surface provided by the stereocilia no doubt contributes to the efficiency of the epithelium in concentrating the seminal plasma during its passage through the epididymal duct.

A highly regular array of stereocilia is found on the hair cells of the inner ear. These are narrow at their base and wider at their free ends and may be 100 μm in length. Their interior is packed with actin filaments, making them rigid processes. When they are mechanically stimulated by sound, they slide past one another, bending only at their narrow base. Ion channels opened by their displacement generate an electrical signal that is conveyed to the central nervous system. These atypical stereocilia are, therefore, essential to the auditory process. Stereocilia are found only on the epididymal epithelium and the hair cells of the inner ear.

KINOCILIA

Cells that are specialized for transport of fluid or a film of mucus over the surface of an epithelium have *cilia* on their free surface that execute rapid to-and-fro oscillations. They are 7–10 μm in length, 0.2 μm in diameter, and are visible in histological sections (Fig. 2–5), but their arrangement in rows and their shape are more apparent in the three-dimensional images afforded by the scanning electron microscope (Fig. 2–21).

When observed on living cells, the cilia beat rapidly in a constant direction. If the rate of beat is slowed down in cinematographic studies, each cilium is observed to stiffen on the more rapid forward or *effective stroke* and to bend on the slower *recovery stroke*. All of the cilia on an epithelium may beat synchronously in an *isochronal rhythm*, but, more commonly, they have a *metachronal rhythm*, in which the successive cilia in each row start their beat in sequence so that each is slightly more advanced in its cycle than the cilium behind it in that row. This sequential activation of the cilia results in the formation of waves that sweep slowly over the surface of the epithelium. When viewed from above, this activity is reminiscent of the waves that run before the wind across a field of wheat, but the metachronal waves on ciliated epithelia are constant in direction and have a very regular periodicity. The effect of this coordinated activity of the cilia is to move a blanket of mucus slowly over the epithelium or to propel fluid or particulate matter through the lumen of a tubular organ.

No internal structure is discernible in cilia with the light microscope, but electron micrographs reveal a core complex called the *axoneme,* consisting of longitudinal microtubules that are constant in number and arrangement. Two single microtubules are in the center of the axoneme with nine doublet microtubules uniformly spaced around them (Figs. 2–22 and 2–23). The central microtubules are identical to those in the cell cytoplasm, consisting of 13 protofilaments. The peripheral doublet microtubules consist of one complete microtubule, *subunit-A,* with a circular cross section, and an incomplete microtubule, *subunit-B,* which has a C-shaped cross section. Together, these two units have a figure-eight cross section with a segment of the wall of subunit-A closing the defect in the wall of subunit-B (Fig. 2–23). Subunit-B of the doublet consists of only 10 protofilaments and shares three with subunit-A. A *radial spoke* extends from subunit-A of each doublet toward the central pair, and neighboring doublets appear to be connected by flexible links of *nexin* between subunit-A of one doublet and subunit-B of the next (Fig. 2–24). On each doublet, there are short *arms* of dynein that project from subunit-A toward subunit-B of the next doublet. These are spaced at 24-nm intervals along the entire length of the doublet. The outer and inner arms diverge slightly and are directed clockwise from the point of view of an observer looking along the axoneme from base to tip. At the base of each cilium, there is a *basal body* having a fine structure identical to that described above for the centrioles. The central microtubules of the axoneme terminate at the base of the cilium, but the peripheral doublets are continuous with the two inner subunits of the triplet microtubules in the wall of the basal body.

The structure of the axoneme is now known in considerable detail, but the exact mechanism by which the active stroke of ciliary beat is produced is still not completely understood.

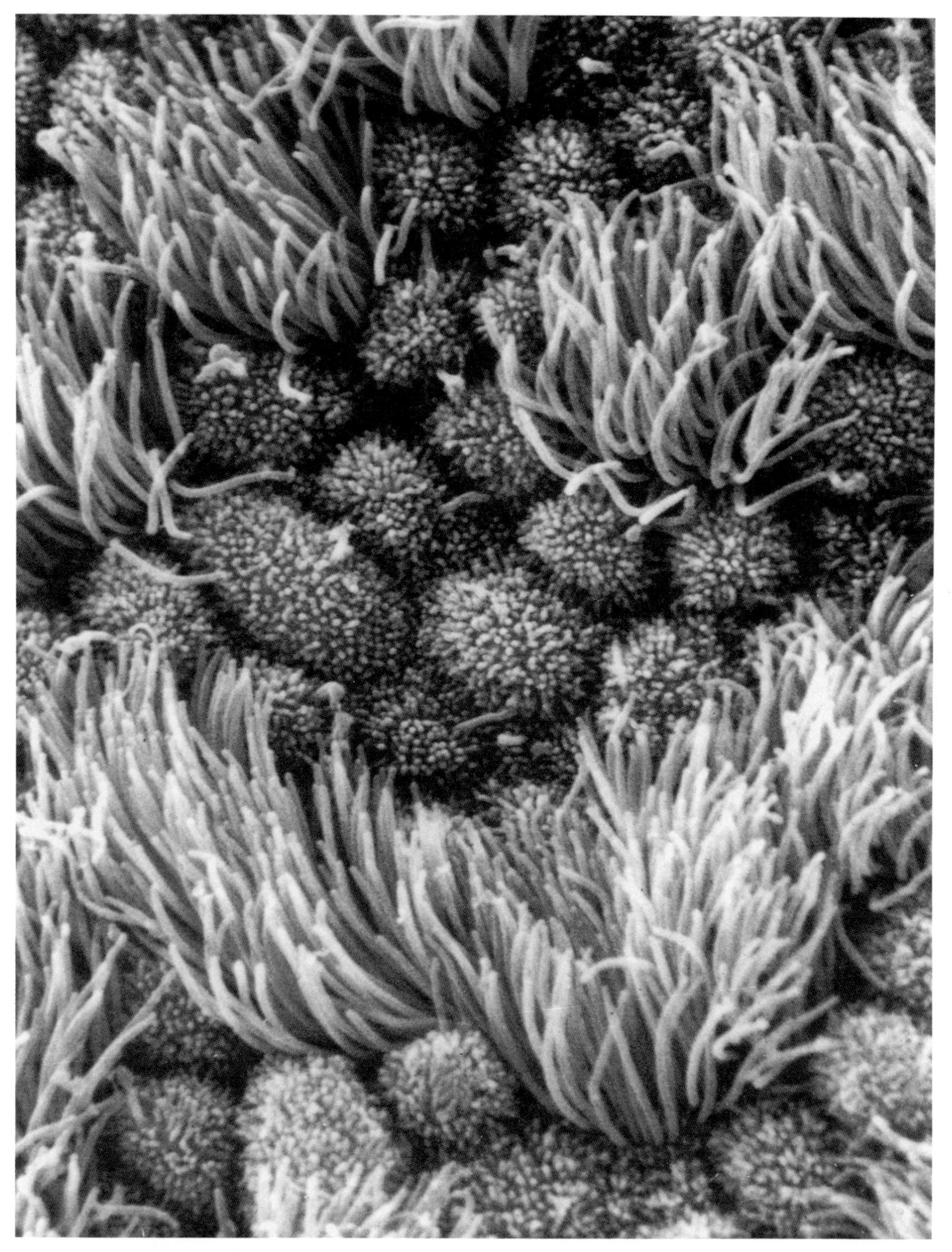

Figure 2–21. A scanning electron micrograph of the luminal surface of the human oviduct, showing the apical ends of ciliated cells and nonciliated cells. The latter bear short microvilli. (Micrograph from Gaddum-Rosse, P., R. Blandau, and R. Tiersch. 1973. Am. J. Anat. 138:269.)

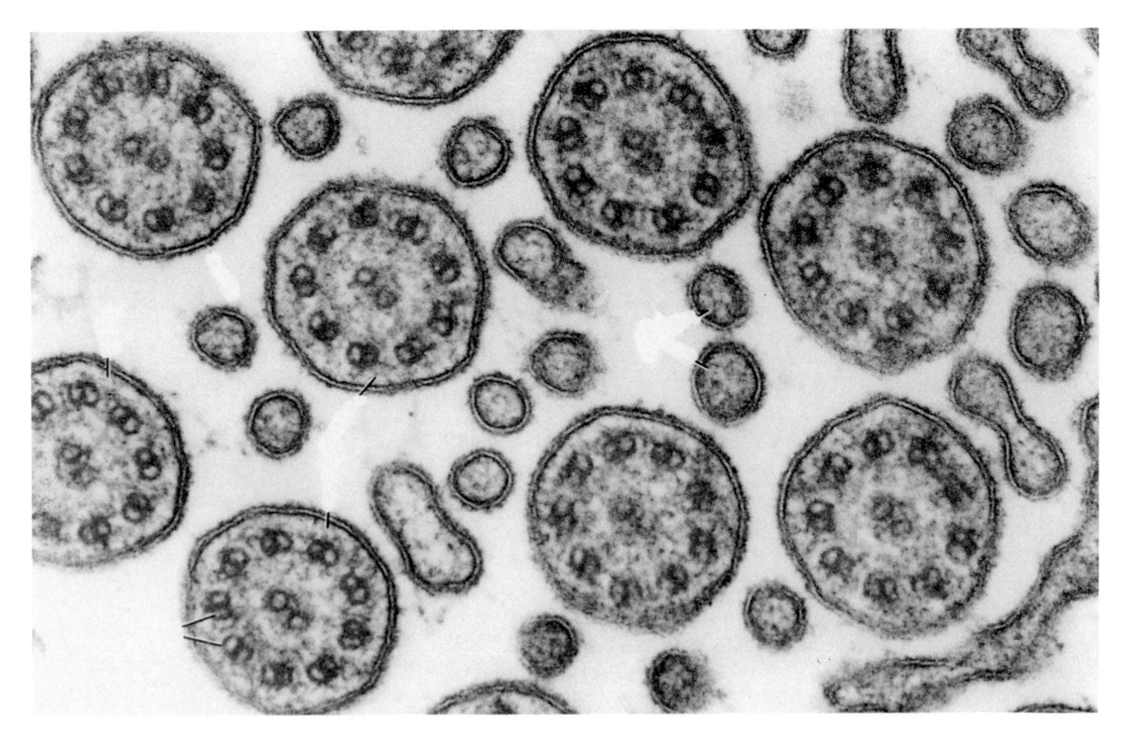

Figure 2–22. A micrograph of a thin section cut parallel to the surface of the tracheal epithelium, affording a comparison of the cross-sectional appearance of the cilia and the intervening microvilli. (Micrograph from Simionescu, M. and N. Simionescu. 1976. J. Cell Biol. 70:608. Reproduced by permission of Rockefeller Institute Press.)

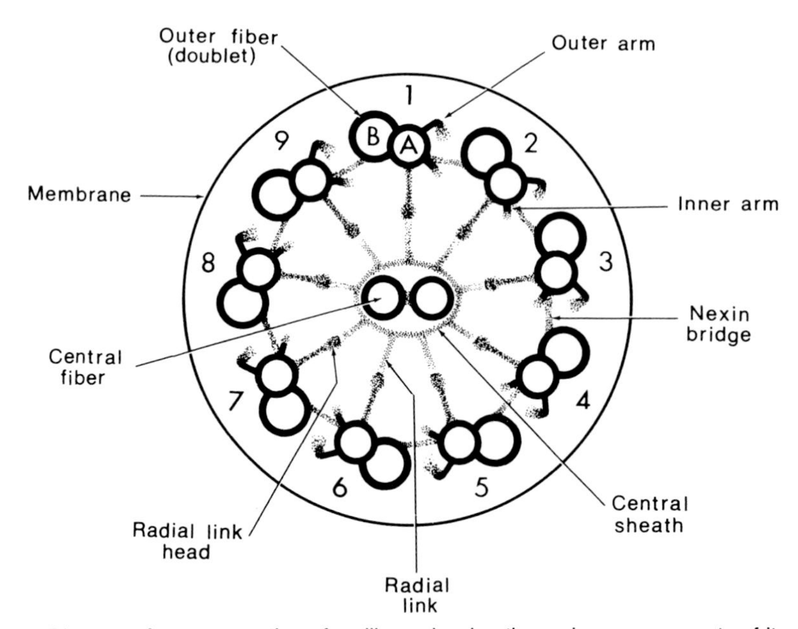

Figure 2–23. Diagram of a cross section of a cilium, showing the various components of its axoneme.

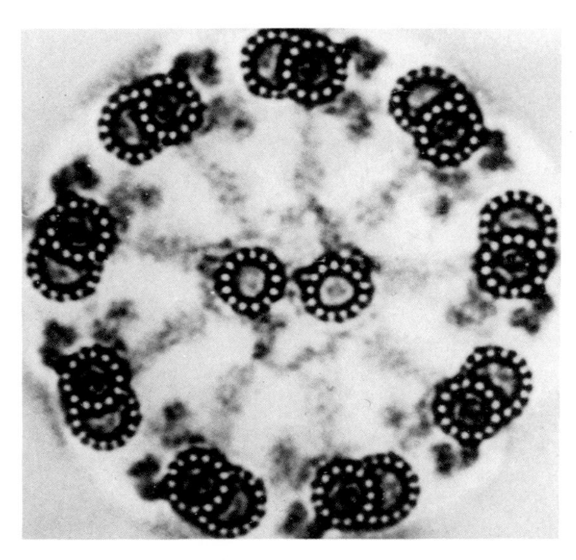

Figure 2–24. A computer-enhanced electron micrographic image of the axoneme of a rat sperm flagellum, in cross section. The protofilaments of the A-and B-submicrotubules and the dynein arms are clearly shown. (Micrograph courtesy of A.B. Afzelius.)

Isolated axonemes will beat, in vitro, if ATP is added, and ATPase activity is known to reside in the dynein arms. If isolated dynein arms are exposed to the axonemes from which they were removed, they will reattach at the proper sites and motility in response to ATP is restored. Thus, the dynein arms are the motors of ciliary beat. Binding of ATP apparently causes them to attach transiently to a specific protofilament of the adjacent doublet and they change their conformation in such a way as to move that doublet toward the tip of the cilium. Upon hydrolysis of ATP, the arms detach and then reattach at a lower site on the adjacent doublet. Rapid repetition of this cycle of attachment and detachment evidently results in the sliding of the doublets with respect to one another. The sliding of the doublets is believed to be converted to bending of the axoneme by restraints imposed by the radial spokes. To account for the alternation in direction of ciliary bending, it is suggested that the dynein arms on doublets 1 to 4 are active during the effective stroke and that those on doublets 6 to 9 then become active, bending the cilium in the opposite direction, during the recovery stroke. This switching of activity from one set of doublets to the other results in a to-and-fro motion of the cilium. The location of the hypothetical switch or oscillator is unknown, but it is speculated that it may reside in the central pair of microtubules and their associated structures.

The interpretation that ciliary motion depends on dynein-generated sliding of doublet microtubules derives indirect support from in vitro experiments in which dynein added to cytoplasmic microtubules bridges the gaps between them and causes them to slide with respect to one another. Further evidence for the essential role of dynein is found in humans with *Kartagener's syndrome,* a rare congenital disorder in which dynein arms are lacking on the doublets of the axoneme, resulting in immotile cilia and flagella and consequent infertility and an inability to clear the upper respiratory tract of mucus. The speculation that the radial spokes may be involved in converting microtubule sliding to bending gains some support from studies on a mutant protozoan in which only these components of the axoneme are lacking, but the cilia fail to bend.

In the differentiation of a ciliated epithelium, formation of the basal bodies precedes the formation of cilia. The basal bodies were thought, by classical cytologists, to arise exclusively from successive divisions of the cell's centrioles. More recent studies of ciliogenesis indicate that basal bodies can arise de novo, without participation of the centrioles. They develop around small spherical dense bodies, called *deuterosomes* or *procentriole organizers.* These serve as nucleation sites for assembly of multiple annular *procentrioles* arranged radially around each organizing site (Fig. 2–25). The ring-like procentrioles then lengthen by polymerization of tubulin at their ends to form the nine triplet microtubules that become the major structural component of their wall. The basal bodies so formed then dissociate from the deuterosomes and become arranged in rows beneath the apical plasma membrane, where each gives rise to a cilium. Two members of each triplet in the wall of the basal body become sites of tubulin polymerization to form the doublet microtubules of the axoneme of the developing cilium. The basal bodies, thus, serve as templates during ciliogenesis, imposing on the axoneme the ninefold radial symmetry expressed in the arrangement of triplet microtubules in their wall. Elongation of the axoneme is rapid, reaching its full length in less than 50 min. A root-like appendage may develop at the lower end of each basal body to stabilize the base of the cilium.

FLAGELLA

Flagella are not a common constituent of epithelia, but they are considered here be-

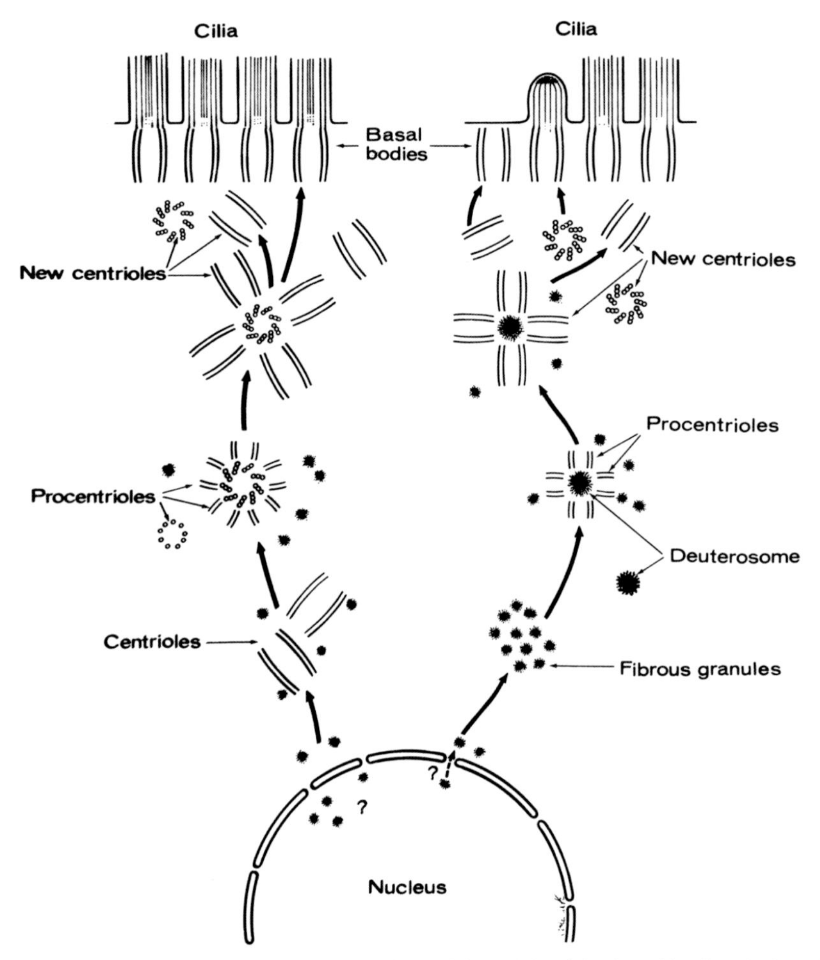

Figure 2–25. Schematic depiction of alternative interpretations of the origin of the basal bodies during ciliogenesis. New basal bodies may form around one or both of the preexisting centrioles as indicated on the left, or they may arise, de novo, from fibrogranular precursors coalescing around organizing centers called procentriole organizers or deuterosomes, as shown at the right. The latter mechanism probably accounts for most of basal bodies formed.

cause of their similarity to cilia. Their internal structure is the same, but they are very much longer, reaching lengths of 15–200 μm. They usually occur singly or in pairs on free-swimming cells such as spermatozoa or protozoa. On protozoa, they are located at the anterior pole of the cell and they have an undulatory motion in which waves of bending are propagated along the flagellum, pulling the organism through its fluid medium. The spermatozoa of most multicellular animals are propelled by a flagellum that extends posteriorly and moves the cell body forward (Fig. 2–26). In marine invertebrates, the internal structure of the sperm flagellum is identical to that of a cilium, but in higher forms, where the flagellum may reach a length of hundreds of micrometers, there is an additional row of nine dense longitudinal fibers peripheral to the nine doublets of the axoneme. (See Chapter 31.)

Epithelial cells of mammals may occasionally have a single very short flagellum, sometimes shorter than a cilium. Its significance is unknown and it is not certain that all of them are motile. They may be found on certain cells of the renal tubules; in the ducts of some glands; in the rete testis; and on nonciliated cells of the uterine epithelium. It is not clear what function they could have, other than simple agitation of the fluid in the lumen of these organs, and certainly some of them have incomplete axonemes and are not motile. Still more puzzling is the fact that single short flagella are often observed on the epithelial cells of organs that have no lumen. They are occasionally observed on the cells of the anterior lobe of the hypophysis, on cells of the islets

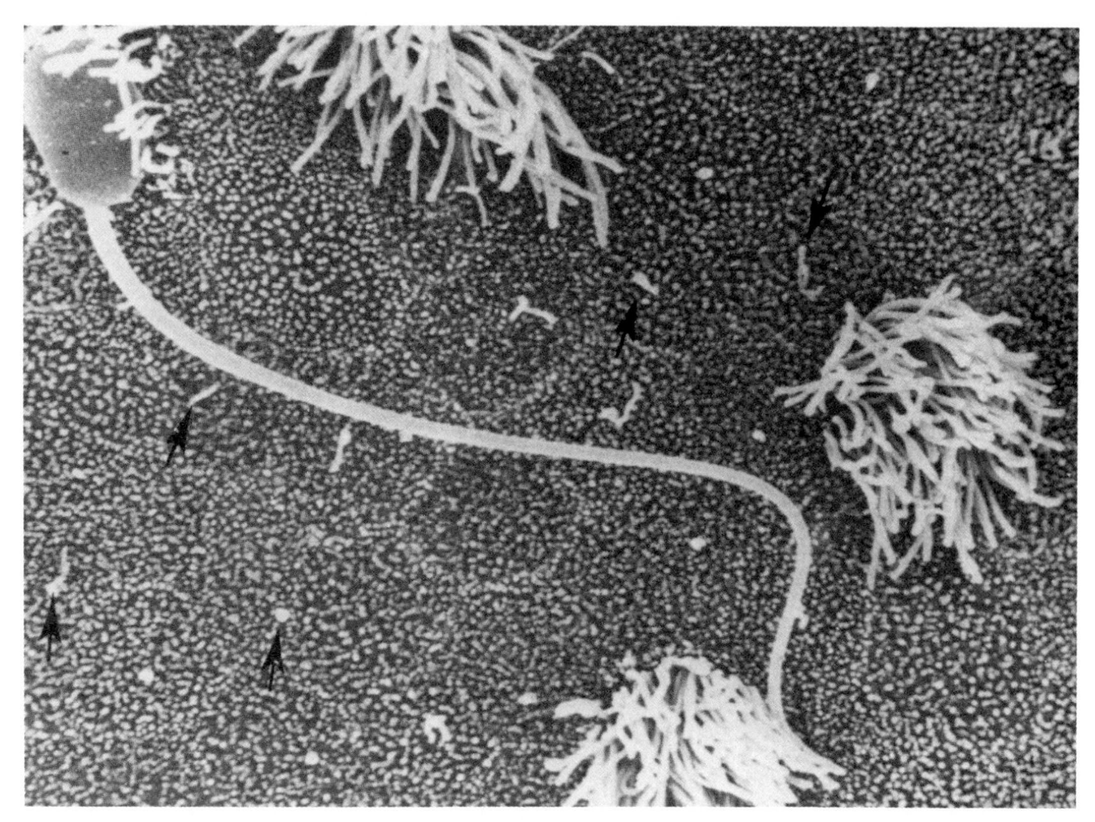

Figure 2–26. Scanning micrograph of a spermatozoon on the surface of the uterine epithelium. The illustration permits comparison of the length of the sperm flagellum with that of the cilia on three ciliated epithelial cells in this field. Each of the nonciliated cells has a centrally placed vestigial cilium (at arrows). (From Motta, P., P. Andrews, and K.R. Porter. 1977. Microanatomy of Cell and Tissue Surfaces. Philadelphia, Lea & Febiger.)

of Langerhans of the pancreas, and on the amacrine cells of the retina. In these instances, the vestigial flagellum projects into the intercellular clefts or into the connective tissue stroma where their movement would serve no purpose. Abortive flagella have been reported on smooth muscle cells and on the stromal cells of the endometrium. Some of these have a normal-appearing axoneme, whereas others lack the central pair of microtubules and surely are not motile. Because some sensory receptors, such as the retinal rods and cones, and olfactory neurones possess modified cilia or flagella, it has been suggested that the nonmotile flagella on a wide variety of cell types might also have a sensory function. To date, there is no experimental evidence to support this conjecture.

RENEWAL AND REGENERATION

Epithelium on the surface of the body is subject to frequent injury. In the skin, the superficial cells of the stratified squamous epithelium undergo keratinization and die. The layer of dead cells provides some degree of protection for the viable cells deeper in the epithelium. The fully keratinized dead cells are continually desquamated and replaced by division of cells at the base of the epithelium, that keratinize as they move to the surface of the epithelium.

In the digestive tract, damaged cells and cells at the end of their limited life span are continually exfoliated at the tips of the intestinal villi and are replaced by division of cells in the crypts. Here the rate of cell loss and cell division is so great that the epithelium covering the villi is completely replaced every few days. On the other hand, in the respiratory tract the epithelial cells are quite long lived, cell degeneration is relatively rare, and the rate of epithelial renewal is quite slow. In all epithelia there are provisions for cell replacement.

During the healing of a wound, the cells at the margins of the defect flatten into a thin sheet that spreads to fill the gap in the epithelium. Cell division begins somewhat later, at the margins of the wound, to provide the additional cells necessary to restore the epithelium to its normal thickness.

BIBLIOGRAPHY

JUNCTIONAL SPECIALIZATIONS

Boyer, B. and J.P. Thiery. 1989. Epithelial cell adhesion mechanisms. J. Mol. Biol. 112:97.

Brightman, M.W. and T.S. Reese. 1969. Junctions between intimately apposed cell membranes in vertebrate brain. J. Cell Biol. 40:648.

Cowin, P., H. Kapprell, W.W. Franke, J. Tamkun, and R.O. Hynes. 1986. Pakoglobin: A protein common to different kinds of intercellular junctions. Cell 46:1063.

Farquhar, M.G. and G.E. Palade. 1963. Junctional complexes in various epithelia. J. Cell Biol. 17:375.

Gilula, N.B., O.R. Reeves, and A. Steinbach. 1972. Metabolic coupling, ionic coupling, and cell contacts. Nature 235:262.

Kelly, D. 1966. Fine structure of desmosomes, hemidesmosomes and an adepidermal globular layerin developing newt epidermis. J. Cell Biol. 28:51.

Kelly, D.E. and A.M. Kuda. 1981. Traversing filaments in desmosomal and hemidesmosomal attachments: Freeze-fracture approaches toward their characterization. Anat. Rec. 199:1.

Lowenstein, W.R. 1972. Cellular communication through membrane junctions. Arch. Int. Med. 129:299.

Musil, L.S. and B.A. Goodenough. 1990. Gap junctional communication and the regulation of connexin expression and function. Curr. Opinion Cell Biol. 2:875.

Pirbazari, M. and D.E. Kelly. 1985. Analysis of desmosomal intramembrane particle populations and cytoskeletal elements: Detergent extraction and freeze-fracture. Cell Tissue Res. 241:341.

Staehelin, A. 1974. Structure and functions of intercellular junctions. Internat. Rev. Cytol. 39:191.

Staehelin, A. 1974. Structure and functions of intercellular junctions. Internat. Rev. Cytol. 39:191.

Suhrbier. A. and D. Garrod. 1986. An investigation of the molecular components of desmosomes in epithelial cells of five species of vertebrates. J. Cell Sci. 81:221.

Volk, T. and B. Geiger. 1986. A-CAM: A new 135-kD receptor of intercellular adherens junctions. I. Immunoelectron microscopic localization and biochemical studies. Cell Biol. 103:1441.

EPITHELIAL POLARITY

Achler, C., D. Filmer, C. Merte, and D. Drenckhahn. 1989. Role of microtubules in polarized delivery of apical membrane proteins to the brush border of intestinal epithelium. J. Cell Biol. 109:179.

Gumbiner, B. 1990. Generation and maintenance of epithelial polarity. Curr. Opinion Cell Biol. 2:881.

Handler, J.S. 1989. Overview of polarity. Ann. Rev. Physiol. 51:729.

Matlin, K.S. 1986. The sorting of proteins to the plasma membrane in epithelial cells. J. Cell Biol. 103:256.

Misek, D.M., E. Bard, and E. Rodriguez-Boulan. 1984. Biogenesis of epithelial cell polarity. Intracellular sorting and vectorial ectocytosis of an apical plasma membrane protein. Cell 31:357.

Mostov, K., G. Apodaca, B. Aroeti, and C. Okamoto. 1992. Plasma membrane protein sorting in polarized epithelial cells. J. Cell Biol. 116:577.

Rodriguez, E. and W.J. Nelson. 1989. Morphogenesis of the polarized epithelial cell phenotype. Science 245:718.

Simons, K. and S.D. Fuller. 1985. Cell surface polarity in epithelia. Ann. Rev. Cell Biol. 1:242.

Vega-Salas, D.E., P.J. Salas, and E. Rodriguez-Boullan. 1988. Exocytosis of vacuolar apical compartment: A cell–cell contact controlled mechanism for establishment of the apical plasma membrane domain in epithelial cells. J. Cell Biol. 107:1717.

BASAL LAMINA

Aumailley, M. and R. Timpl. 1986. Attachment of cells to basement membrane collagen type IV. J. Cell Biol. 103:1569.

Clermont, Y. and L. Hermo. 1988. Structure of the complex basement membrane underlying the epithelium of the vas deferens in the rat. Anat. Rec. 221:482.

Hay, E.D. and J.P. Revel. 1963. Auytoradiographic studies of the origin of the basement lamina in Amblystoma. Dev. Biol. 7:152.

Kanwar, Y.S. and M.G. Farquhar. 1979. Presence of heparan sufate in the glomerular basement membrane. Proc. Nat. Acad. Sci. USA 76:1303.

Kefalides,N.A., A. Alper, and C.C. Clark. 1979. Biochemistry and metabolism of basement membranes. Internat. Rev. Cytol. 61:167.

Pierce, G.B., T.F. Beals, J. Sri Ram, and A.J. Midgley. 1964. Basement membranes. IV. Epithelial origin and immunoilogical cross-reactions. Am. J. Pathol. 45:929.

Pierce, G.B., A.R. Midgley, and J. Sri Ram. 1963. Histogenesis of the basement membrane. J. Exp. Med. 117:339.

Terranova, V.P., C.R. Rao, T. Kalbic et al. 1980. The role of laminin in attachment of epithelial cells to basement membrane collagen. Cell 22:719.

Timpl, R., H. Rohde, P. Gehron-Robey et al. 1979. Laminin—a glycoprotein from basement membrane. J. Biol. Chem. 254:9933.

SPECIALIZATIONS OF THE FREE SURFACE

Afzelius, B.Q. 1976. A human syndrome caused by immotile cilia. Science 193:317.

Fawcett, D.W. 1961. Cilia and Flagella. *In* J. Brachet and E. Mirsky, 1961. Eds. The Cell: Biochemistry, Physiology, Morphology. Vol II. New York, Academic Press.

Fawcett, D.W. and K.R. Porter. 1954. A study of the fine structure of ciliated epithelia. J. Morphol. 94:221.

Gibbons, I.R. and A.J. Rowe. 1965. Dynein: a protein with adenosine triphosphatase activity from cilia. Science 149:424.

Ito, S. 1965. The surface coat of enteric microvilli. J. Cell Biol. 27:475.

Pedersen, H. and H. Rebbe. 1975. Absence of arms on the axoneme of immobile human spermatozoa. Biol. Reprod. 12:541.

Satir, P. 1985. Switching mechanisms in the control of ciliary motility. Mol. Cell Biol. 4:1.

Sleigh, M.A. 1971. Cilia. Endeavour 30:11.

Warner, F.D. and P. Satir. 1974. The structural basis of ciliary bend formation. Radial spoke positional changes accompanying microtubule sliding. J. Cell Biol. 63:35.

REGENERATION AND RENEWAL

Bertalanffy, F.D. and K.P. Nagy. 1961. Mitotic activity and renewal rate of the epithelial cells of the human duodenum. Acta Anat. 45:362.

Leblond, C.P. and B.E. Walker. 1956. Renewal of cell populations. Physiol. Rev. 36:255.

Leblond, C.P. 1964. Classification of cell populations on the basis of their proliferative behavior. Natl. Cancer Inst. Monogr. 14:119.

Lipkin, M., P. Serlock, and B. Bell. 1963. Cell proliferation kinetics in the gastrointestinal tract of man. Gastroenterology 45:721.

Messier, B. and C.P. Leblond. 1960. Cell proliferation and migration as revealed by radioautography after injection of tritiated-thymidine into rats and mice. Am. J. Anat. 106:247.

3

GLANDS AND SECRETION

Secretion is the process by which small molecules are taken up and transformed, by intracellular biosynthesis, into a more complex product that is then actively released from the cell. The energy-consuming chemical reactions involved in secretion are not to be confused with the passive *excretion* of the end products of metabolism, which requires little energy and may take place by simple diffusion. Groupings of cells specialized for secretion are called *glands*. Two major categories of glands are distinguished on the basis of the path of release of their products. Those that deliver their secretion into a system of ducts opening onto an external or an internal surface are called *exocrine glands*. Those that release their product into the blood or lymph for transport to target tissues in another part of the body are called *endocrine glands*.

Secretion was formerly thought to be a function limited to epithelia and to cells that contained a secretory product stored in granules visible with the light microscope. With the development of the electron microscope and autoradiographic methods for tracing the uptake of precursors and the release of cell products, it became evident that many nonepithelial cells synthesize and release substances into their immediate environment, without the accumulation of microscopically visible secretory granules in their cytoplasm. Cells of mesenchymal origin, such as fibroblasts, osteoblasts, and chondrocytes, were found to secrete components of the surrounding extracellular matrix.

In the past two decades, it has been found that a number of cell types, widely dispersed in the tissues and organs, secrete molecules that mediate cell-to-cell communication. Secretions of this kind are collectively called *cytokines*. If the signaling molecules simply diffuse to cells in the immediate vicinity, their effect is described as *paracrine*. If they act back upon the cell producing the secretion, they are said to have an *autocrine* effect, and if the signaling molecules are carried in the blood to distant target cells, their effect is described as *endocrine*.

A distinction is now made between two modes of secretion. In one, called the *regulated secretory pathway*, glandular cells concentrate and store their product in membrane-bounded granules until a neural or hormonal signal for its release is received. In the other, called the *constitutive secretory pathway*, the product is transported directly to the cell surface in small vesicles that go undetected with the light microscope. In the latter mode of secretion, the product is not appreciably concentrated and is not stored while awaiting an external stimulus for its discharge, but is released as rapidly as it is produced.

EXOCRINE GLANDS

REGULATED SECRETORY PATHWAY

The traditional interpretation of the secretory process was based on light microscopic studies on the changes in glandular cells after their stimulation. The number of secretory granules in the cytoplasm was observed to decrease concomitantly with an increase in outflow of secretion from the ducts of the gland. After depletion of the granules, the basophilic component of the cytoplasm (the ergastoplasm) became more prominent, the Golgi complex enlarged, and the nucleus and nucleolus increased slightly in volume. Therefore, each of these organelles was thought to be involved, in some way, in the synthetic activities of the cell. As new secretory granules began to accumulate in the cells, it was noted that they first appeared very close to the Golgi complex and this organelle was thought to be the site of concentration of material synthesized elsewhere in the cytoplasm.

Since 1940, electron microscopic and biochemical studies have substantiated these classical observations and have defined more precisely the respective roles of the various cell

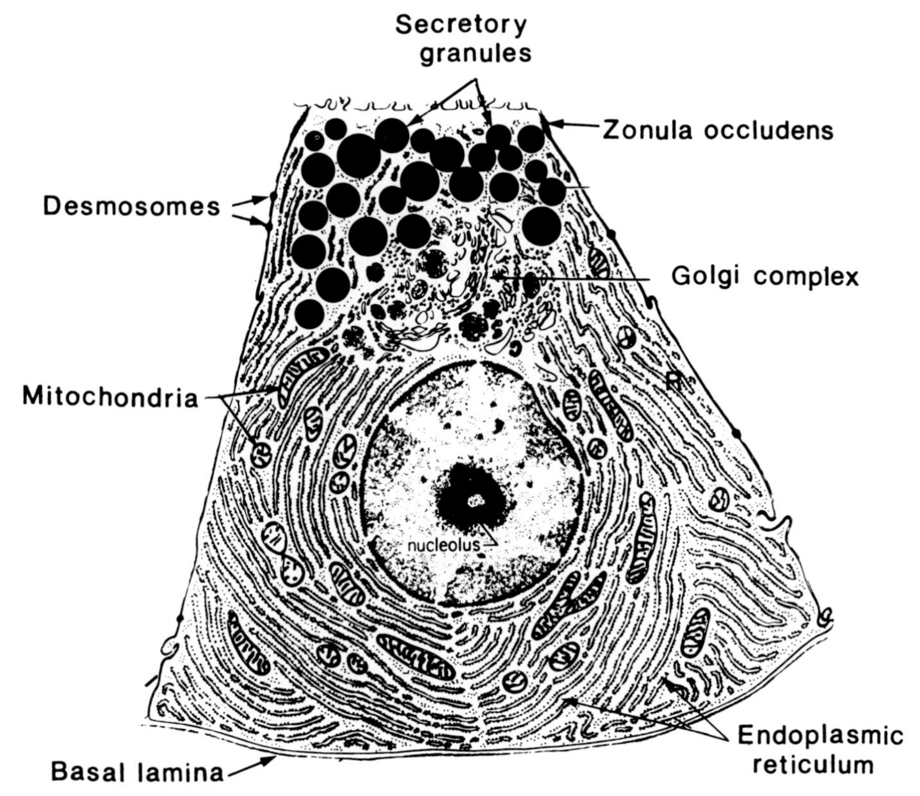

Figure 3–1. Drawing of the fine structure of a pancreatic acinar cell, a typical protein-secreting cell of an exocrine gland.

organelles in the secretory process. The glandular cell type most thoroughly studied has been the pancreatic acinar cell (Fig. 3–1), which secretes several essential digestive enzymes. The description of the intracellular pathway of protein synthesis, that will follow, is based largely on studies of this cell, but it also applies to other glandular cells producing a secretion rich in proteins.

The chemical nature of the secretory product is determined in the nucleus, where the information or "blueprint" for construction of each protein is encoded in the sequence of nucleotides in a segment of the DNA of the chromosomes. The cell components that utilize this information for protein synthesis reside in the cytoplasm. The specific protein synthesized depends on which nucleotide sequence (gene) in the DNA is exposed and available for *transcription* at that time. Transcription involves intranuclear synthesis of *messenger RNA* (mRNA), using the exposed sequence of nucleotides as a template. Concurrently, another ribonucleic acid, *ribosomal RNA*, is transcribed from a nucleotide sequence in DNA closely associated with the nucleolus, and in that organelle, it is combined with protein to form *ribosomal nucleoprotein* (rRNA). This passes through the nuclear pores into the cytoplasm, where it forms *ribosomes*, small particulates that are the sites of *translation* of the information encoded in messenger RNA to form molecules of the protein secretory product.

In the cytoplasm, each of the many ribosomes produced in the nucleus becomes associated with an *initiation site* at one end of a long molecule of mRNA. After attachment, the ribosome slowly moves along the length of the mRNA "reading," in each successive set of three nucleotides (*codons*), the instructions that determine the sequence of assembly of the several kinds of amino acids that will make up the protein. Each amino acid subunit to be incorporated in the protein is brought to the assembly site on the ribosome by a molecule of *transfer RNA* (tRNA) that is specific for that amino acid. The tRNA molecule, carrying its specific amino acid, recognizes, and binds to, the appropriate complimentary site on the mRNA molecule. Its amino acid is then inserted into the nascent polypeptide chain, and the tRNA molecule is released. The ribosome then moves along the mRNA molecule to the

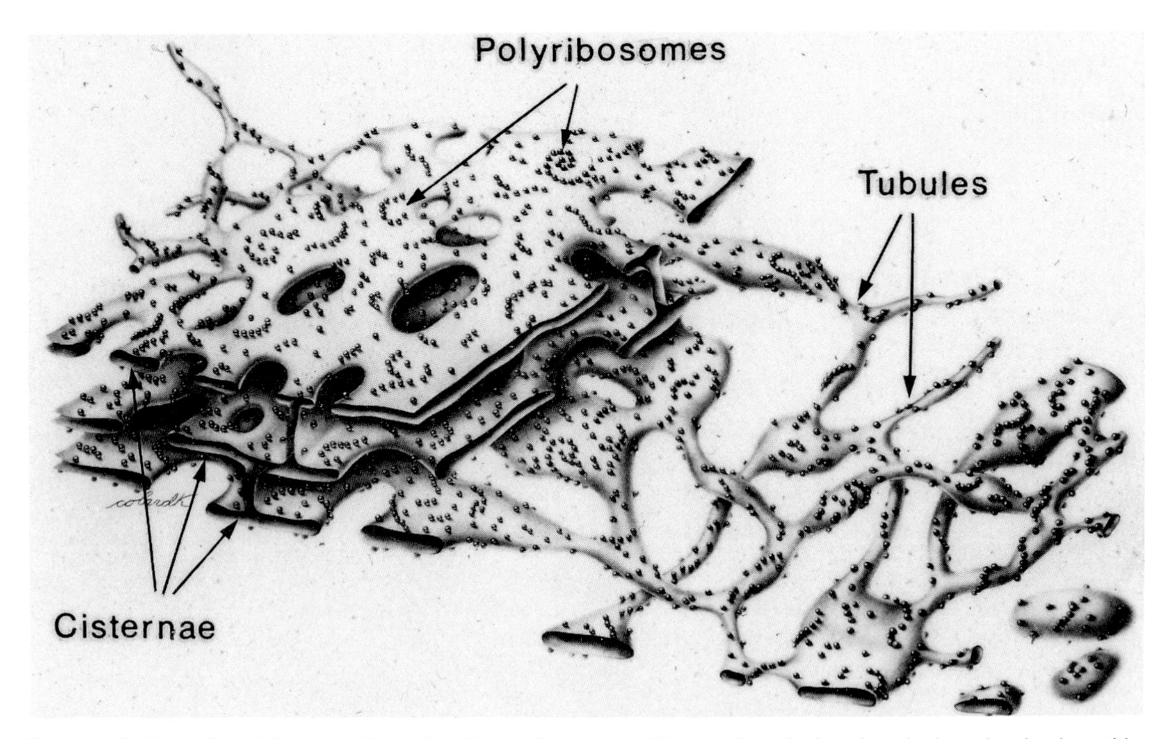

Figure 3–2. A drawing of the three-dimensional form of a portion of the rough endoplasmic reticulum showing branching and anastomosing tubules continuous with fenestrated cisternae that are often in parallel array. Polyribosomes, in spiral or circular configuration, are attached to the outer surface of the membrane.

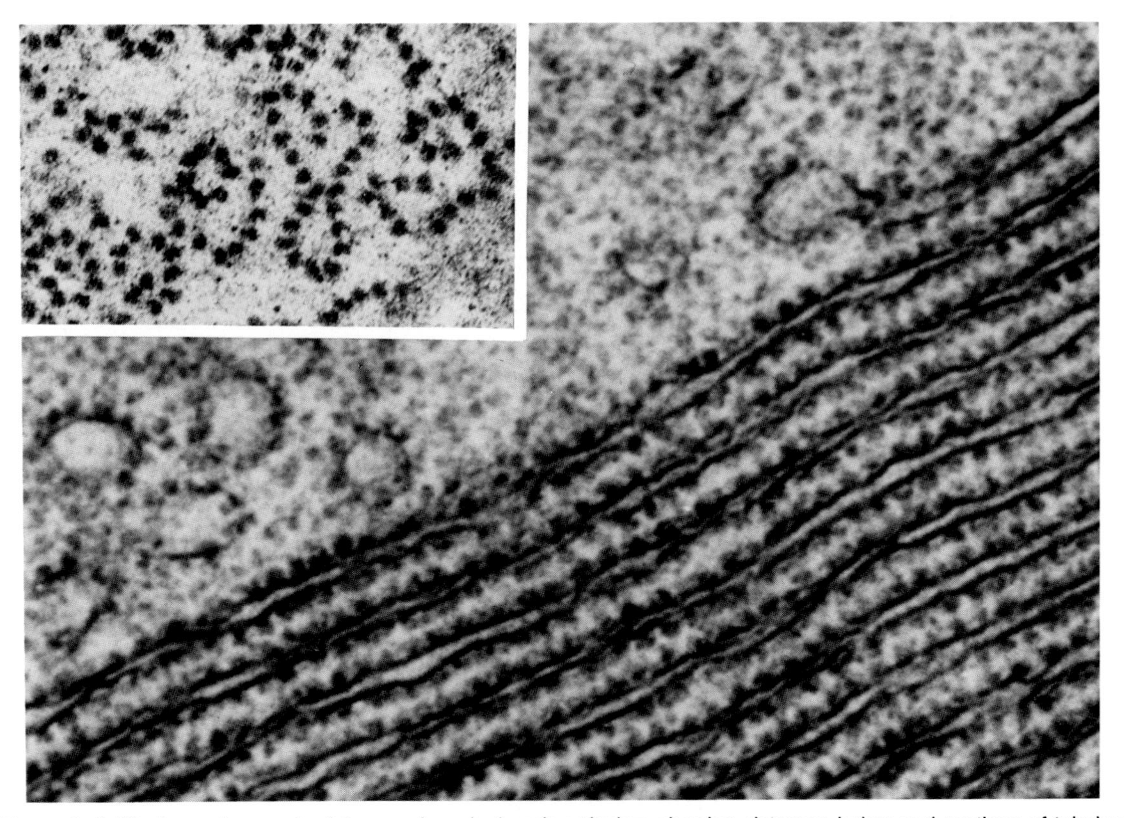

Figure 3–3. Electron micrograph of the rough endoplasmic reticulum showing cisternae below and sections of tubules above, both bearing ribosomes on their outer surface. The inset is a surface view of a small area of a cistern showing polyribosomes, each consisting of multiple ribosomes associated with a long molecule of messenger RNA.

next codon, and the process is repeated with insertion of one amino acid after another until the entire message has been read and a molecule of secretory protein has been assembled. Other ribosomes, in turn, attach to the initiation site, vacated by the first ribosome, and they follow along after it, each reading the same codons and assembling another molecule of the same secretory protein. Several ribosomes, thus, become associated with same mRNA molecule forming a chain of interconnected ribosomes (Fig. 3–4). In electron micrographs, these chains, called *polyribosomes* or *polysomes,* are found either free in the cytoplasm or attached to the limiting membrane of the endoplasmic reticulum (Figs. 3–2, and 3–3). The free polysomes are generally involved in the synthesis of protein constituents of the cell, while those attached to the endoplasmic reticulum are engaged in synthesis of secretory proteins for export from the cell. In glandular cells, the vast majority of the ribosomes are associated with the reticulum.

The messenger RNAs for secretory proteins have a special sequence of nucleotides, the *signal codons,* that are lacking on the messenger RNAs for integral proteins. When these codons are read, the resulting *signal peptide* binds to a *signal receptor particle.* This particle serves as an adapter, binding the ribosome and the signal peptide to *ribosome receptor proteins* in the membrane of the endoplasmic reticulum (Fig. 3–5). Interaction of the signal receptor particle and signal sequence with the membrane is believed to cause aggregation of ribosome receptor proteins of the membrane in a configuration that forms a transmembrane channel, through which the lengthening polypeptide chain of the secretory protein extends into the lumen of the reticulum. When elongation of the chain has advanced the signal sequence into the lumen of the reticulum, a *signal peptidase* on the inner surface of its membrane cleaves off the signal sequence (Fig. 3–5). When the entire message has been translated and the synthesis of the secretory polypeptide is terminated, the ribosome separates from the reticulum and the transmembrane channel is obliterated by lateral diffusion of the ribosome receptor proteins in the membrane.

Thus, the occurrence of a signal sequence

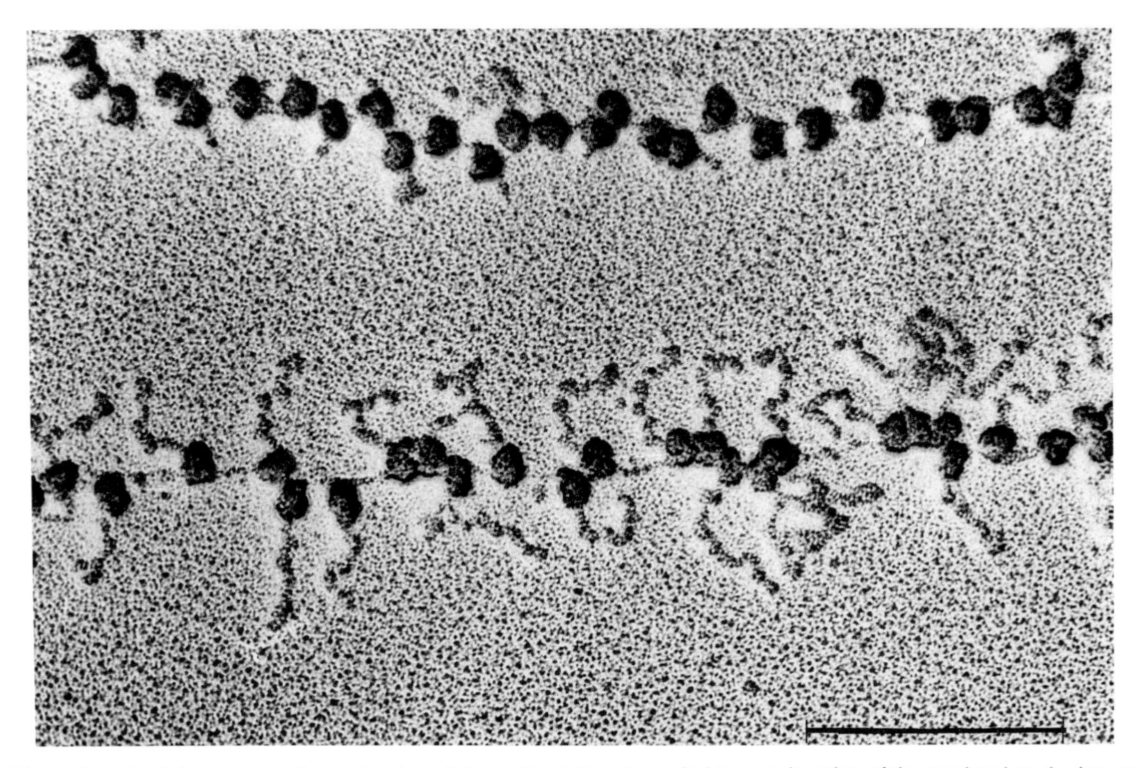

Figure 3–4. In Chironomus salivary gland, protein synthesis is not coupled to translocation of the product into the lumen of the endoplasmic reticulum. It is possible, therefore, to isolate translation units such as those shown in this remarkable electron micrograph. Clearly visible is the long, thin molecule of mRNA, the associated ribosomes, and emerging nascent polypeptide chains. (Micrograph courtesy of E. Kiseleva.) Bar = 0.2 um.

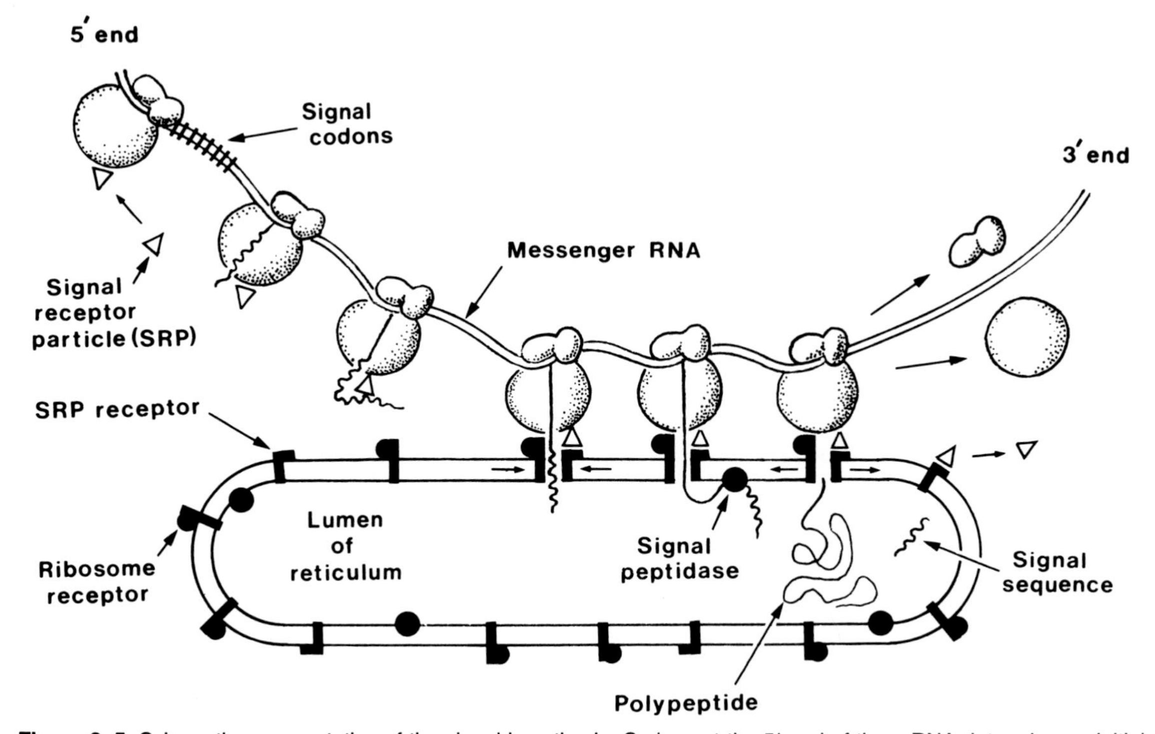

Figure 3–5. Schematic representation of the signal hypothesis. Codons at the 5′ end of the mRNA determine an initial amino acid sequence called the "signal." When the nascent polypeptide chain emerges from the ribosome, its signal sequence binds to a *signal recognition protein* (SRP). This, in turn, binds to an *SRP receptor* in the membrane. Interaction of *ribosome receptor* and *SRP receptor* forms a transmembrane pore, through which the lengthening polypeptide chain is translocated into the lumen of the reticulum. The signal segment of the polypeptide is subsequently cleaved off by a *signal peptidase* located at the inner aspect of the limiting membrane of the reticulum. (Redrawn after Blobel, G. 1976–77. *In* Internat. Cell Biol. 320; and Walter, P. and G. Blobel. 1981. J. Cell Biol. 91:557.

on the messenger RNA molecule and the presence in the cytoplasm of signal recognition molecules capable of binding to the membrane of the endoplasmic reticulum ensures that the molecules destined for secretion become segregated in the lumen of the endoplasmic reticulum. There, the newly formed polypeptides undergo posttranslational modification and are then moved to a ribosome-free *transitional region* of the reticulum, where they are incorporated in small vesicles that bud off from the reticulum. These *transport vesicles*, each containing a small quantity of the newly synthesized protein, move to, and fuse with, the flat saccule or cisterna at the cis-face of the Golgi complex.

There is no continuity between successive cisternae of the Golgi complex, and there has been some debate as to how the product of protein synthesis traverses this organelle. It is the prevailing view that it is transported in small vesicles that bud off from the edges of each cisterna and fuse with the next one in the stack of cisternae (Figs. 3–6 and 3–7), but the paucity of images of such vesicles forming, or in transit, remains puzzling. The cisternal subunits of the Golgi complex appear to be relatively stable structures for histochemical methods demonstrate consistent differences in the enzymatic activities of the cis-, intermediate-, and trans-cisternae. Those at the cis-face often remain unstained, whereas intermediate cisternae exhibit nicotinamide adenine dinucleotide phosphatase, and the trans-cisternae display acid phosphatase, thiamine pyrophosphatase, nucleoside diphosphatase, and galactosyltransferase activity. During transport through the Golgi complex, the product received from the endoplasmic reticulum is further modified. In the case of glycoprotein secretions, glycosylation, begun in the reticulum, is continued by glycosyltranferases in the trans-Golgi cisternae. Similarly, the synthesis of sulfated glycoproteins and sulfated glycosaminoglycans is completed by sulfotransferases in these Golgi membranes.

In the cisternae near the cis-face of the Golgi, the product is evidently rather dilute because these cisternae appear empty in electron micrographs, due to extraction of their content during specimen preparation. But the product undergoes a 20–25% concentration in its transit through the Golgi, and cisternae near the trans-face often have a content of appreciable density (Fig. 3–7). When the processing of the product is complete, the cisterna at the trans-face of the organelle breaks up into segments that round up and fuse with one another to form larger *condensing vacuoles*. With further concentration of their content, these become the *secretory granules* of the cell and move to the apical cytoplasm (Fig. 3–8). Their designation as "granules" is probably inappropriate in its implication that they are solid. It is more likely that their content is a viscous fluid, and the term secretory vacuole might be more accurate.

When a glandular cell is stimulated, the secretory granules that have accumulated in its apical cytoplasm move individually to the cell surface where their limiting membrane fuses with the cell membrane at the point of contact, permitting their content to flow out (Fig. 3–8). As the secretory vacuole is emptied, its membrane is incorporated into the cell membrane. Thus, in the process of *exocytosis*, the product leaves the cell without creating any discontinuity in the cell membrane. The excess plasma membrane resulting from exocytosis is recycled by invagination and separation of small vesicles that return to the Golgi complex.

The biosynthetic events that have taken some time to describe here actually proceed quite rapidly. When tritium-labeled amino acids are injected into a small animal, the label can be detected in the endoplasmic reticulum of the pancreatic acinar cells in 5 min and in forming secretory granules in 12 min. The total transit time for exportable protein is estimated to be less than 50 min. In constitutive secretion, the sequence of events is the same, but there is little or no concentration of the product in the Golgi complex and no storage of the product.

Glandular cells that use the regulated secre-

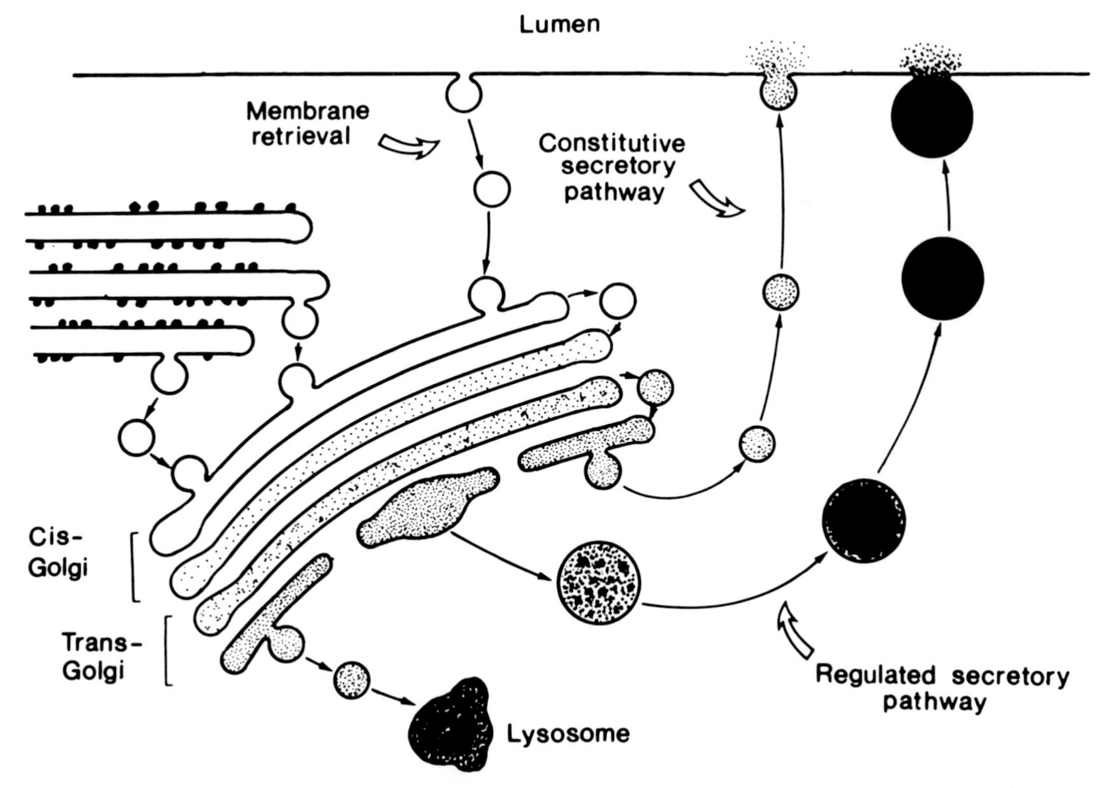

Figure 3–6. Schematic representation of the regulated secretory pathway in which the product is stored in secretory granules until a neural or hormonal stimulus is received, and the constitutive pathway, in which the product is released at the cell surface as rapidly as it is formed. Intrinsic proteins, such as the enzymes of the lysosomes, go directly to their intracellular site. Sorting of proteins and their packaging in vesicles for translocation along these three different pathways takes place in the trans-Golgi.

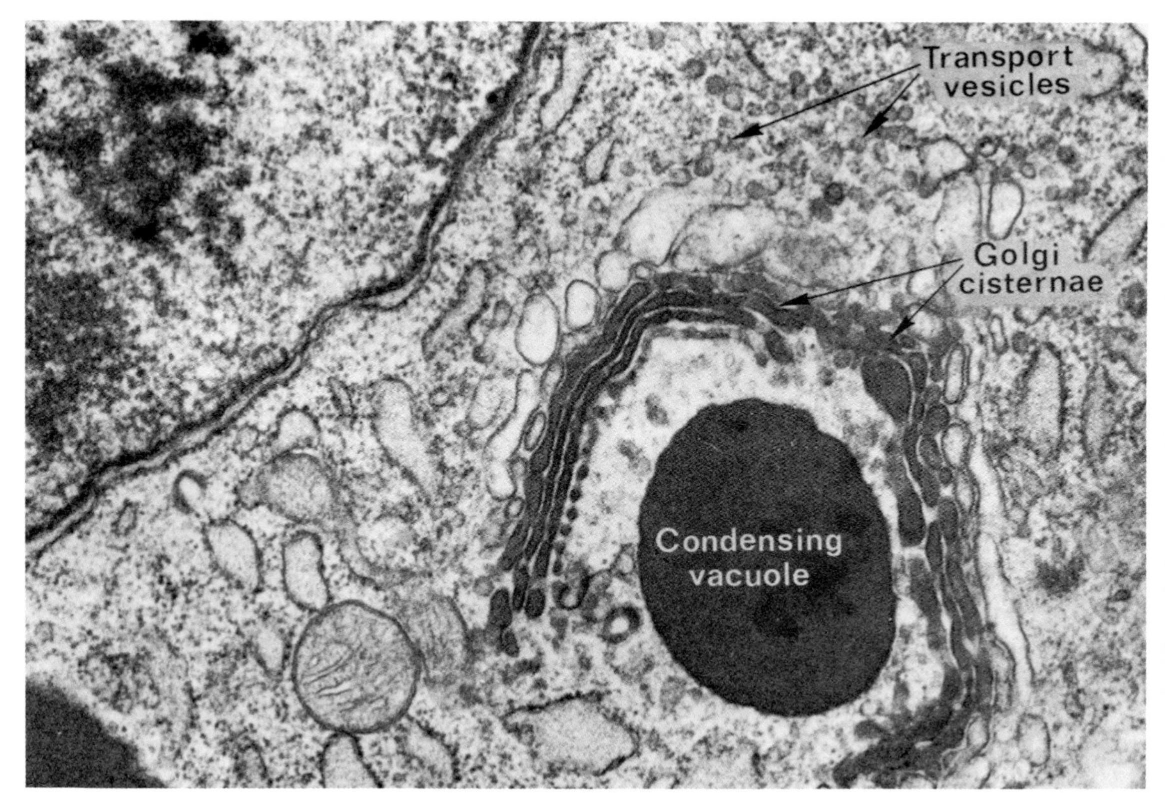

Figure 3–7. Micrograph of the Golgi region of an actively secreting glandular cell showing transport vesicles and concentration of the product in the trans-cisternae of the Golgi. A large condensing vacuole is present in the concavity of the Golgi.

tory pathway for products exported from the cell also synthesize lysosomal enzymes and integral proteins for insertion into the plasmalemma. The concurrent synthesis of multiple proteins with different destinations requires a mechanism for intracellular sorting. The trans-Golgi network is believed to be the site where specific receptors recognize signal sequences on the various proteins that permit sorting and routing of the vesicles to their proper destinations (Fig. 3–6).

MECHANISMS OF PRODUCT RELEASE

Three mechanisms by which cells discharge their secretory products have long been recognized: *merocrine*, *apocrine*, and *holocrine secretion*. *Merocrine secretion* was defined as release of product with the cell membrane remaining intact. The light microscope did not reveal how this was accomplished, but it was assumed that the secretion either diffused through an intact membrane or that whole secretory granules escaped through transient discontinuities in the plasmalemma. The ultrastructural observations on exocytosis have shown that the product is released without creating discontinuities in the membrane. Merocrine secretion is now understood to consist of discharge by fusion of the limiting membrane of secretory granules or vesicles with the cell membrane followed by outflow of their content.

Apocrine secretion by an epithelial cell was thought to involve constriction and pinching off of a portion of the apical cytoplasm containing the secretory granules. Membrane continuity was believed to be restored at the site of constriction and the cell survived to reaccumulate secretion. This mode of secretion is uncommon and has not been thoroughly studied. The mammary gland was regarded as the classical example of apocrine secretion. Electron micrographs have now confirmed that some cytoplasm is indeed lost in this type of secretion, but certainly less than was envisioned by light microscopists. One or more lipid droplets surrounded by a thin film of cytoplasm and a portion of the cell membrane project from the apex of the cell. This is then pinched off by constriction at its base.

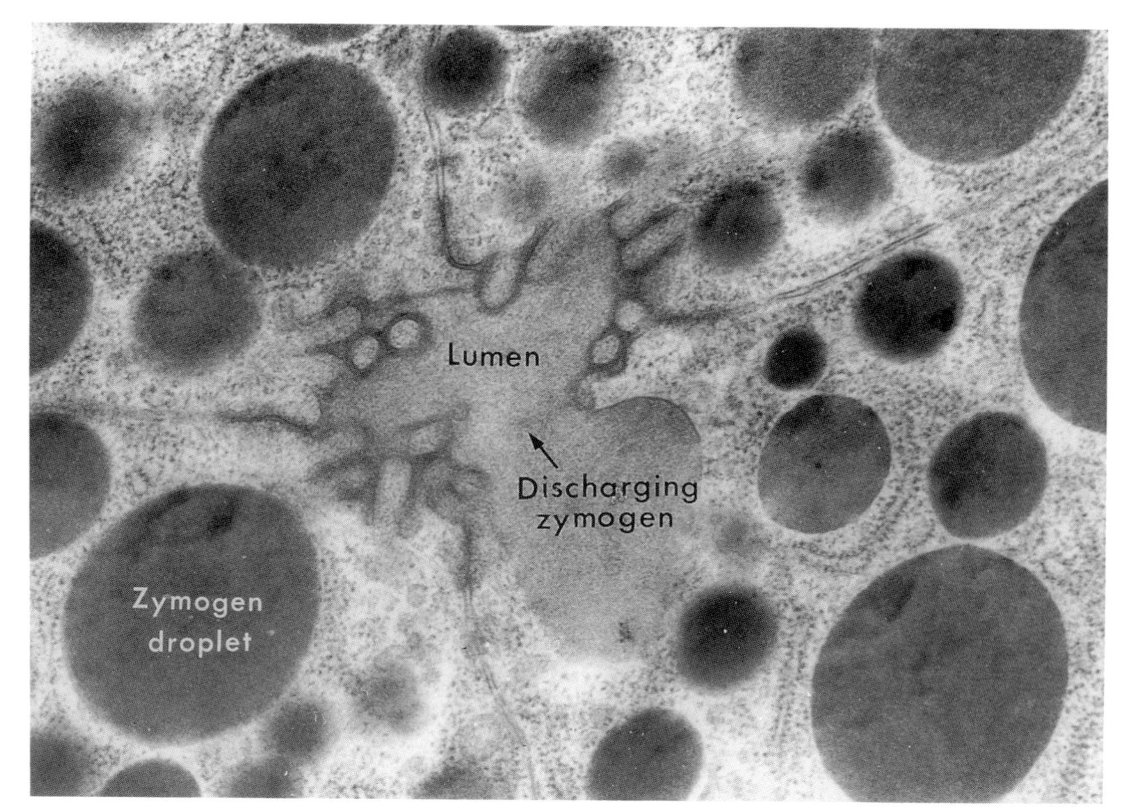

Figure 3–8. Electron micrograph of the lumen of an acinus and the apical portions of four acinar cells. Large, dense zymogen droplets or granules are found in the cell apex. The limiting membrane of one of these has fused with the cell membrane and its contents are being discharged into the lumen.

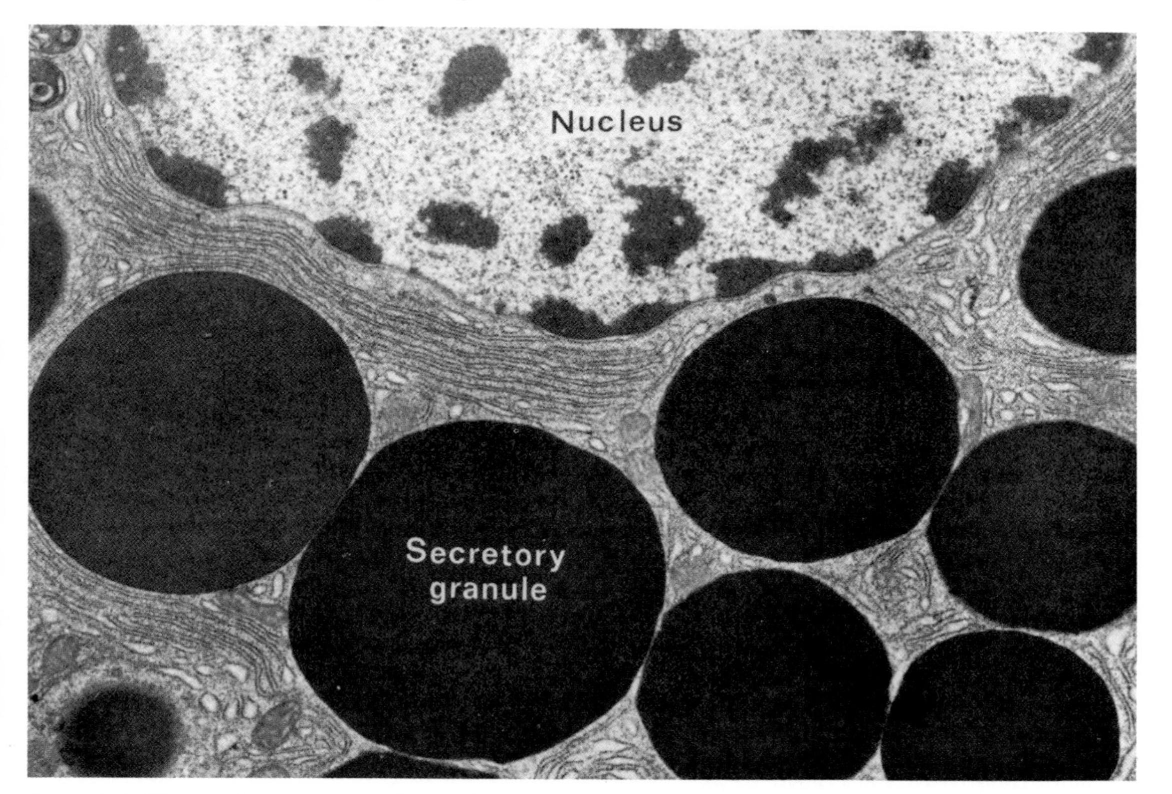

Figure 3–9. Micrograph of the juxtanuclear region of a glandular cell showing multiple condensed secretory granules.

A globular membrane-bounded portion of the cell is, thus, cast off without creating a breach in the cell membrane and the cell survives to reaccumulate cytoplasm and product.

Holocrine secretion consists of the bulk release of whole cells or discharge of their cytoplasm into the excretory ducts of the gland. The classical example of holocrine secretion was in the sebaceous glands of the skin, where the cells break down with an outpouring of cytoplasm and accumulated lipid-rich secretion. The release of spermatozoa from the seminiferous epithelium has been regarded, by some, as a form of holocrine secretion in which intact living cells are the product, but this unique example rather stretches the definition of holocrine secretion.

Although the traditional terms merocrine, apocrine, and holocrine secretion have required some redefinition on the basis of ultrastructural observations, they are still widely used.

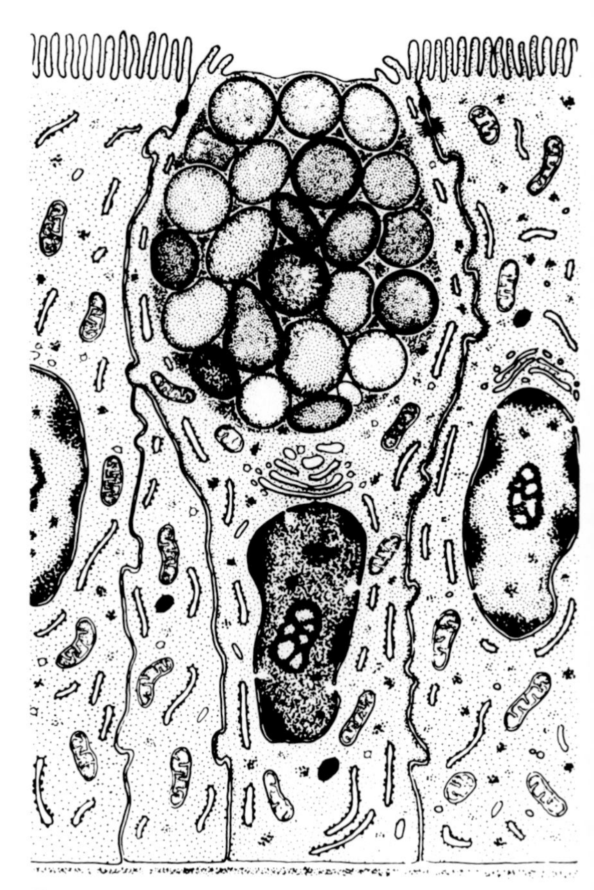

Figure 3–10. Drawing of an intestinal goblet cell. The stored mucus often depresses the nucleus farther toward the base of the cell and may deform it.

CLASSIFICATION OF EXOCRINE GLANDS

Exocrine glands may be *unicellular* or *multicellular*. The multicellular glands are further classified as *tubular, alveolar, tubulo-alveolar,* or *saccular*, according to the geometry and organization of their epithelium.

UNICELLULAR GLANDS

The most common example of a unicellular gland is the *mucous cell*, or *goblet cell*, often found scattered among the columnar cells of the epithelium in the respiratory and digestive tracts. It secretes *mucin*, a glycoprotein which, upon hydration, forms the viscous solution called *mucus*. A fully differentiated cell of this type has an expanded apical end filled with pale-staining droplets of *mucigen* and a basal end containing a somewhat compressed nucleus and a small amount of deeply basophilic cytoplasm. The name goblet cell is descriptive of the form of the cell which has, at the apex, an expanded, cup-shaped rim of cytoplasm, called the *theca*, filled with secretory droplets, and a slender base resembling the stem of a goblet (Fig. 3–10). In histological sections, the mucigen droplets are seldom resolved as separate entities because they tend to swell and coalesce during specimen preparation. They are preserved in a more life-like state by rapid freezing followed by freeze-substitution. The contents of the theca stain intensely with the periodic-acid–Schiff reaction for carbohydrate owing to their high polysaccharide content.

In electron micrographs, the individual mucin droplets are enveloped by a membrane that is often broken during specimen preparation. The nucleus is usually displaced downward and deformed by the accumulated secretory droplets in the theca. A well-developed Golgi complex is located between the nucleus and the mucigen droplets in the theca. Cisternae of rough endoplasmic reticulum are deployed parallel to the lateral surfaces, in the paranuclear and basal cytoplasm, which also contains many free ribosomes.

Mucus is produced via the regulated secretory pathway. Tracer studies using ^{35}S- or ^{3}H-glucose show them to be incorporated in the supranuclear region, indicating that the Golgi complex is the principal site of glycosylation and sulfation of the very large glycoproteins characteristic of mucus. Mucus secretion proceeds continuously but is accelerated by chemical irritation or by parasympathetic nerve stimulation. Goblet cells retain their characteristic shape throughout their short life span, which is about four days in intestinal epithelium.

MULTICELLULAR GLANDS

The simplest form of multicellular gland is an epithelium in which all, or most, of the cells are secretory. Examples are the surface epithelium of the gastric mucosa and the epithelium lining the uterine cavity. In other organs, clusters of mucus-secreting cells gather together to form *intrapithelial glands* that lie entirely within the epithelium, but are arranged around a small lumen that serves as their duct (Fig. 3–11). Examples are found in the pseudostratified epithelium of the nasal mucosa, in the epithelium of the urethra, and that of the ductuli efferentes of the testis.

Other multicellular glands develop as tubular invaginations of an epithelium and grow downward into the connective tissue of the lamina propria. Their secretory product reaches the surface of the epithelium through a short duct made up of nonsecretory cells. In some such glands, the surface area available for exocytosis is increased by slender intercellular *secretory canaliculi* between the cells. The wall of these canaliculi is opposing grooves in the lateral surfaces of neighboring secretory cells. They may branch, but they always terminate blindly above the basal lamina. Short microvilli often project into their lumen. Examples include the bile canaliculi of the liver. A unique example of an *intracellular secretory canaliculus* is found in the parietal cells of the gastric mucosa. These are tubular invaginations of the apical plasma membrane that extend deep into the cytoplasm and conduct the acid secretion to the cell surface. The surface area of these canaliculi is increased by many microvilli.

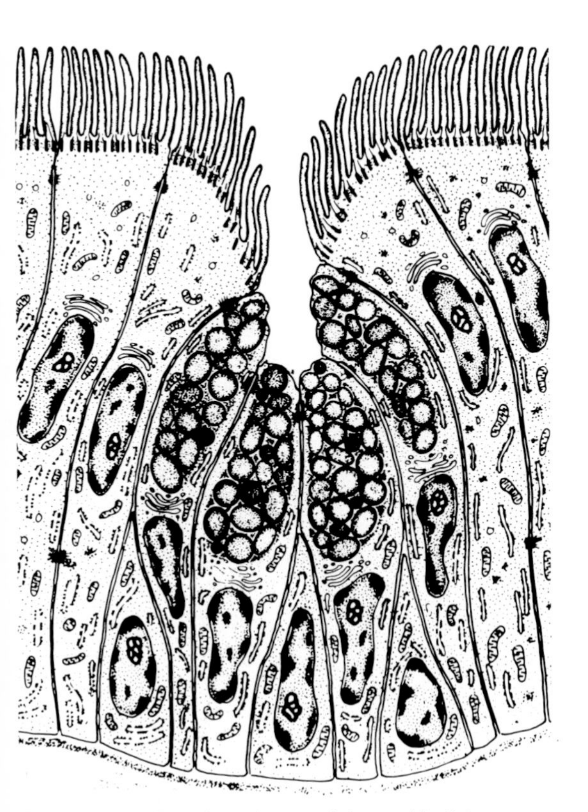

Figure 3–11. Drawing of a small intraepithelial mucous gland in the ciliated epithelium of the respiratory tract.

SIMPLE EXOCRINE GLANDS

A classification of glands has evolved that may seem unnecessarily complex, but it permits more precise description of the many patterns of cell association in the body. A *simple exocrine gland* is one in which the secretory portion is connected to a surface epithelium by an *unbranched* duct (Fig. 3–12). Glands fulfilling this criterion are further categorized on the basis of the configuration of their secretory portion. Thus, they may be described as *simple tubular, simple coiled tubular, simple branched tubular*, and *simple acinar*.

Simple tubular glands are usually a straight tubule opening directly onto an epithelial surface without a duct (Fig. 3–12a). Examples are glands of the intestinal mucosa. In a *simple coiled tubular gland*, the secretory portion is a coiled tubule connected to the surface by an unbranched excretory duct (Fig. 3–12b); the sweat glands of the skin are an example. In *simple branched tubular glands*, the terminal secretory portions bifurcate and there may be a short unbranched excretory duct, as in some glands of the oral cavity, esophagus, and duodenum. An excretory duct may be absent as in the glands of the gastric and uterine mucosae. In acinar or alveolar glands, the terminal secretory portion is expanded into a bulbous or bottle-shaped structure. If a single acinus is associated with an unbranched duct it is called a *simple acinar gland*, but if several acini are clustered around the duct, it is a *simple branched acinar gland* (Figs. 3–12f and 3–12g).

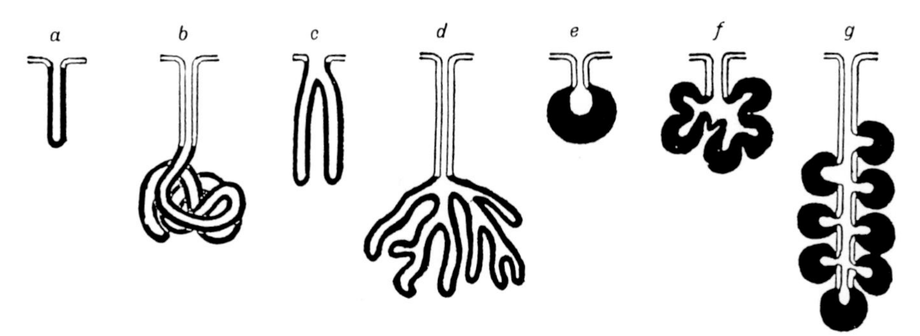

Figure 3–12. Diagrams of various forms of simple exocrine glands. (a) Simple tubular; (B) simple coiled tubular; (c) and (d) simple branched tubular; (e) simple alveolar; (f) and (g) simple branched alveolar. Secretory portions black; ducts double-contoured.

COMPOUND ACINAR GLANDS

Many of the larger glands are classified as *compound exocrine glands* which indicates that the duct *branches* repeatedly. Such a gland can be thought of as consisting of numerous simple glands at the end of an arborescent system of ducts of progressively diminishing caliber (Fig. 3–14). The aggregations of acini on separate main branches of the duct system may appear as distinct lobes or lobules.

The secretory units of the smallest lobules in *compound tubular glands* are tubules that are more-or-less coiled and usually branched. In this category are the larger mucous glands of the oral cavity; the glands of the stomach; and the duodenal glands (Fig. 3–14); and the bulbourethral glands. In *compound acinar*

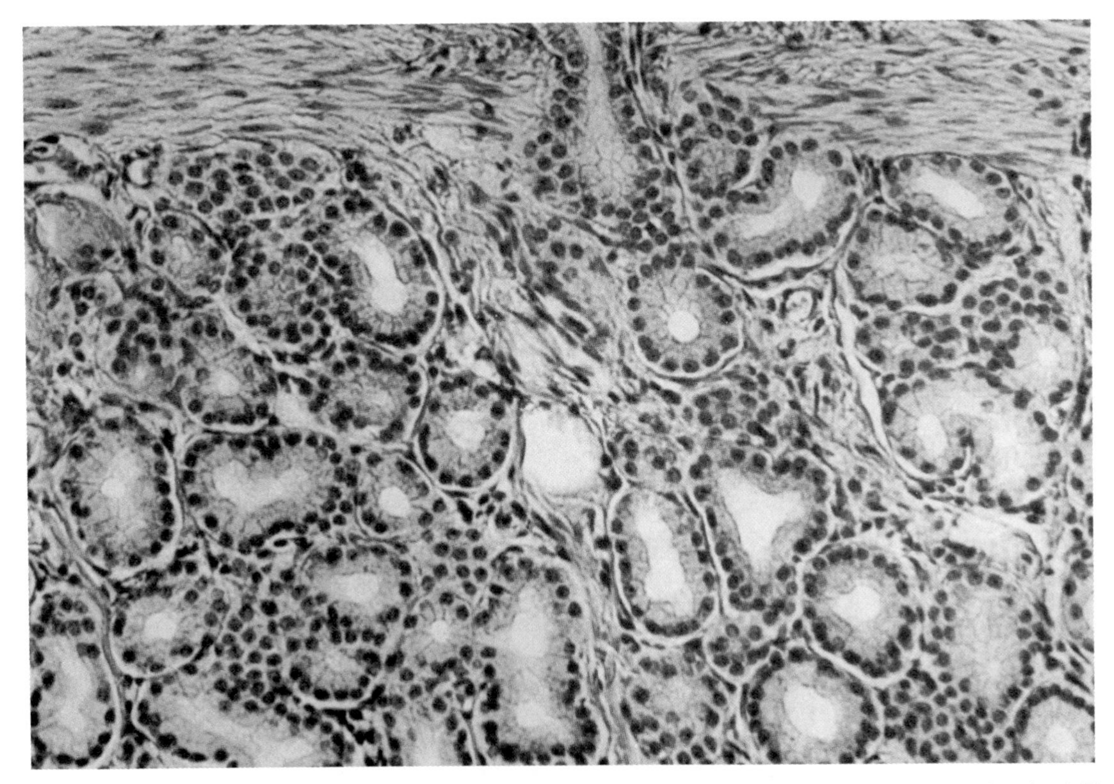

Figure 3–13. Photomicrograph of an intestinal submucosal gland, an example of a simple branched tubular gland. The duct seen penetrating the overlying muscularis mucosae is unbranched, but the secretory portion branches repeatedly. The branches are seen here mainly in cross section.

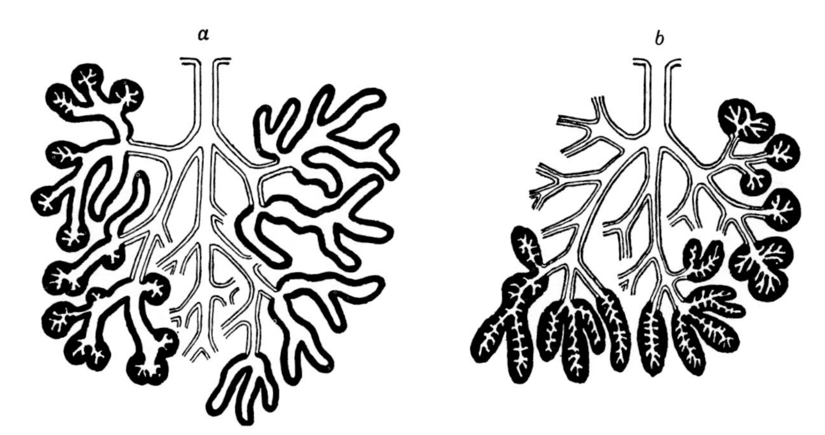

Figure 3–14. Diagram of compound exocrine glands. (A) Mixed compound tubular (right) and tubuloacinar (left); (B) compound acinar. Secretory portions black; ducts double-contoured.

glands, the terminal portions are bulbous or pear-shaped structures made up of pyramidal cells around a very small lumen. Quite commonly, however, secretory cells form the walls of short tubules having a number of acini along their sides and at their blind end. Such glands are more precisely described as *compound tubuloacinar glands*. Examples are the salivary glands and the pancreas (Figs. 3–14 and 3–15). Some would also include the prostate and mammary glands, but others prefer to assign these to a separate category, *compound saccular glands*, because of the greater size and relatively large lumen of their secretory units. In the mammary gland, prostate, and lacrimal gland, the duct system does not converge on a single main duct. Instead, several medium-sized ducts open separately on a restricted area of an epithelial surface.

Compound glands may be more simply clas-

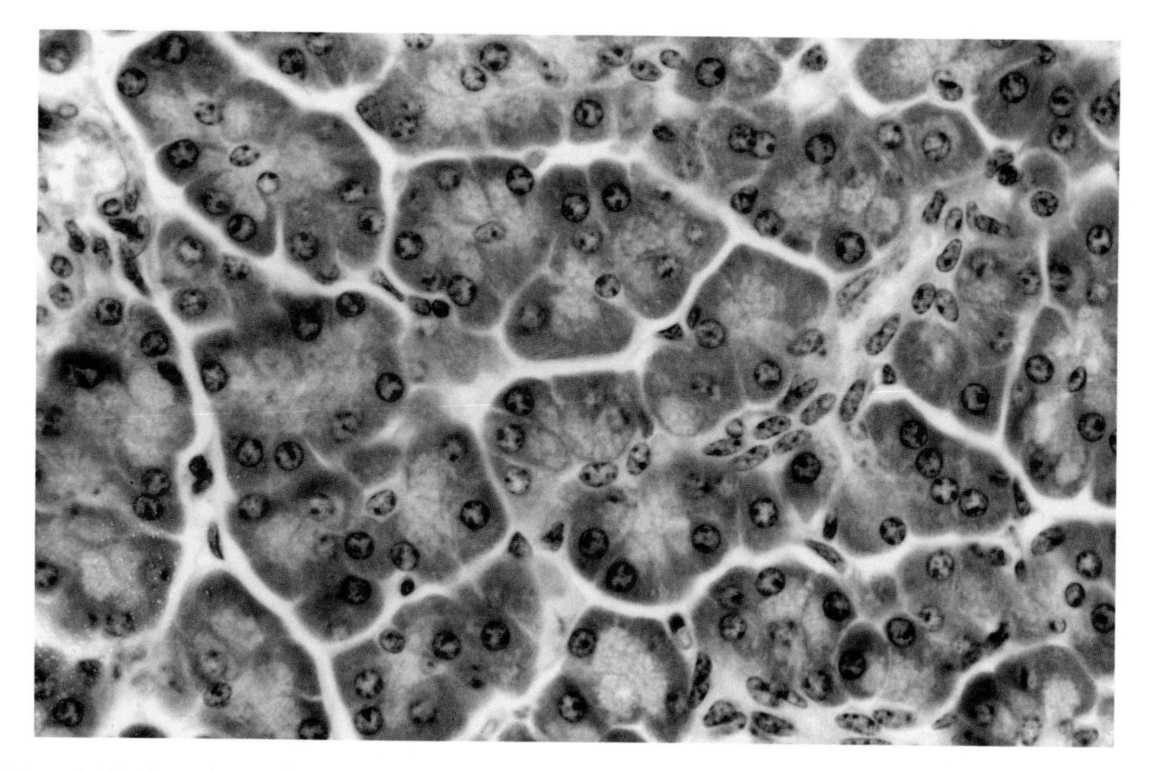

Figure 3–15. Photomicrograph of the pancreas, a compound tubuloacinar gland. At the right of the figure is a longitudinal section of a small duct, which branches to the several acini clustered around it.

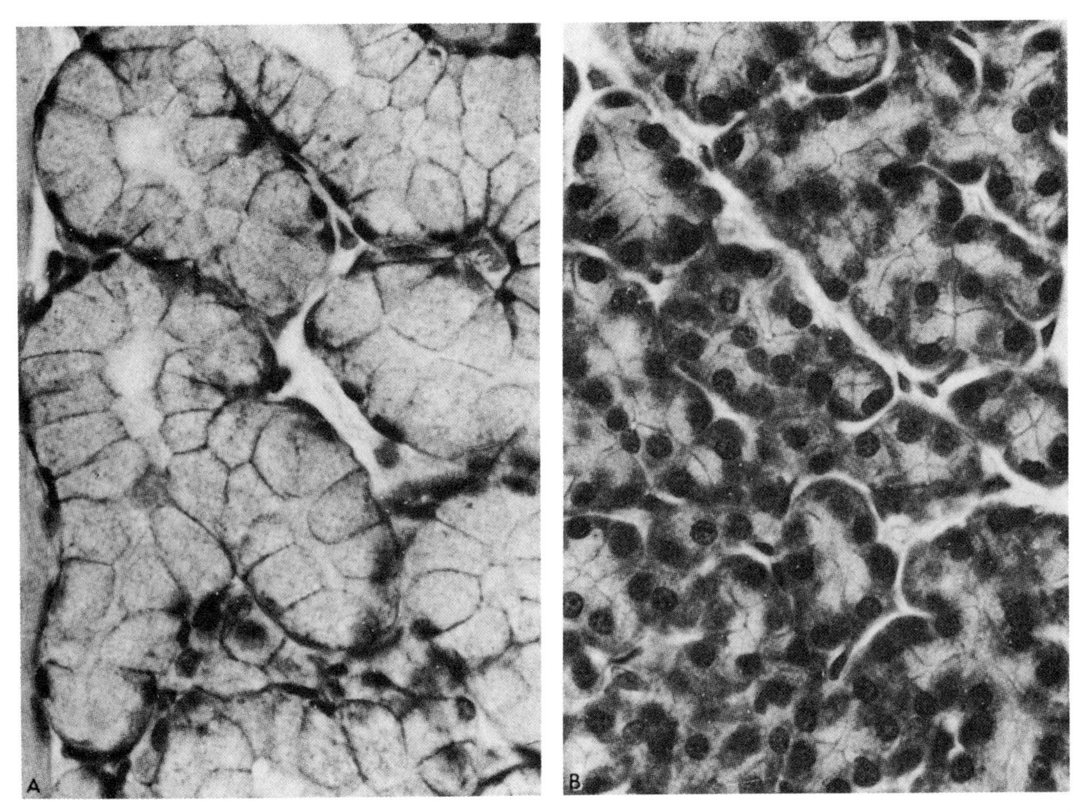

Figure 3–16. Photomicrographs illustration the contrasting appearance of a mucous gland (A) and a serous gland (B). Both are from the tongue.

sified according to the nature of their secretions. Thus, they may be designated *mucous glands, serous glands,* or *mixed glands.* Mucous glands secrete a viscous fluid rich in mucopolysaccharides that have a protective or lubricating function (Fig. 3–16A). Serous glands produce a watery secretion often rich in enzymes (Fig. 3–16B). Mixed glands contain both mucous and serous cells. The mucous cells often make up the bulk of the gland with flattened serous cells forming crescentic caps, called *serous demilumes,* over the ends of the acini. The cells of the demilunes communicate with the lumen via intercellular secretory canaliculi (Figs. 3–17 and 3–18).

ORGANIZATION OF LARGE EXOCRINE GLANDS

The pancreas, which is typical of large exocrine glands, is enclosed in a condensation of connective tissue forming its *capsule.* Septa of connective tissue extend inward from the capsule dividing it into grossly recognizable subdivisions called *lobes.* These, in turn, are partitioned by thinner septa into smaller units called *lobules* (Fig. 3–19). These are made up of the microscopic subunits called *acini* or *alveoli.* Dense connective tissue from the septa penetrates only a short distance into the lobules before giving way to a delicate network of reticular fibers that surrounds the terminal ducts and acini of the gland. The connective tissue components of a gland are referred to as its *stroma* and its epithelial portion is called the *parenchyma.*

The branching system of ducts within the gland carries its secretion to the lumen of the intestine. Groups of acini are drained by *intercalary ducts.* These converge on *intralobular ducts* which, in turn, join larger *interlobular ducts* in the septa between lobules. Several of these join to form a few *lobar ducts* which converge and join to form the *main duct.* The lining of the smallest ducts is squamous epithelium, becoming cuboidal in larger ducts (Fig. 3–20) and low columnar in the main duct. The secretion may be somewhat modified in its passage through the duct system by removal of water and electrolytes and by addition of products of the lining epithelium.

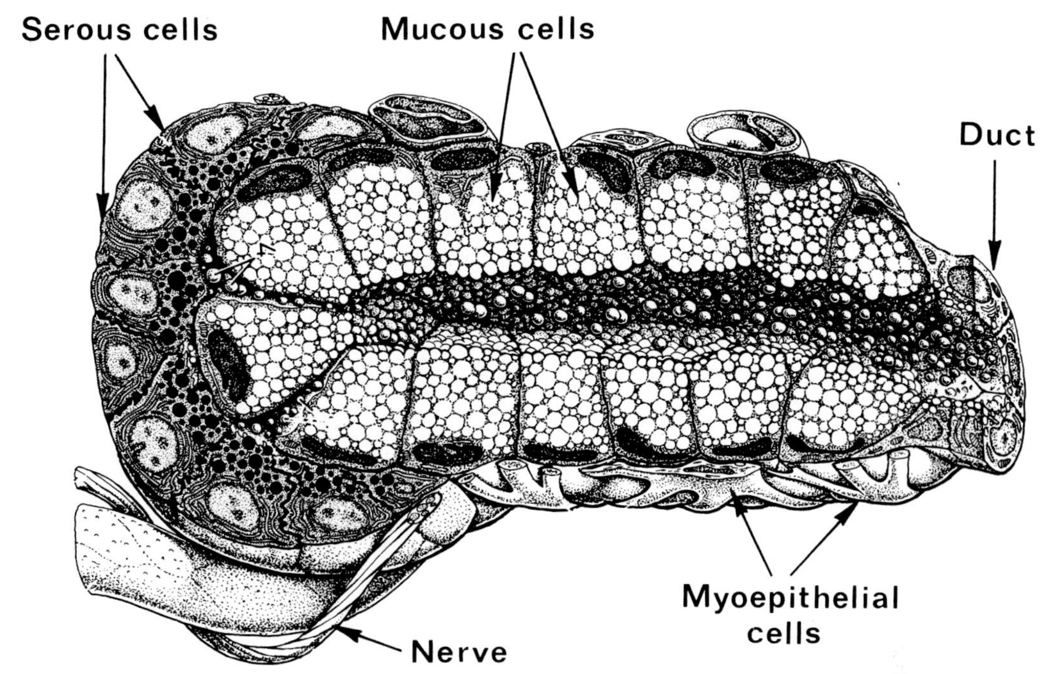

Figure 3–17. Drawing of the end-piece of a tubuloacinar salivary gland, showing the mucous cells and the so-called serous demilune forming a cap over the end of the acinus of mucous cells. (Modified from Krstic, 1978. Gewebe des Menschen und Saugetiere. Heidelberg, Springer-Verlag.)

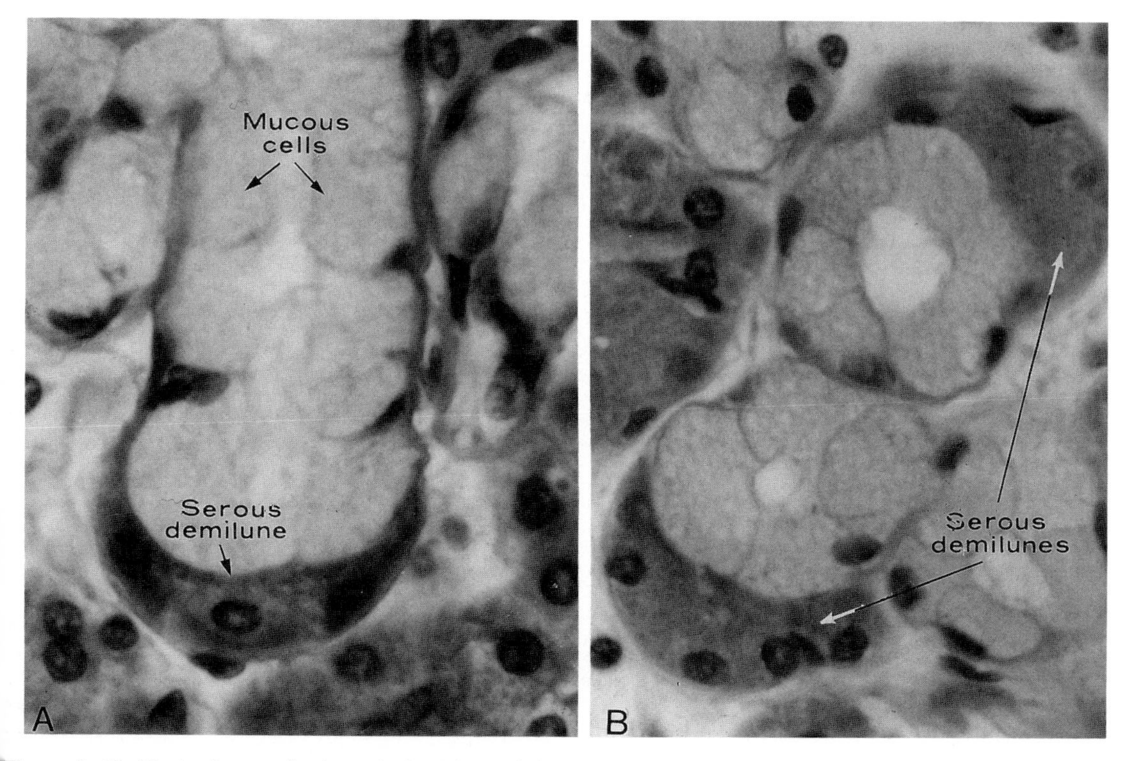

Figure 3–18. Photomicrograph of terminal portions of the submandibular gland. This is a mixed gland. Some of the terminal elements consist entirely of mucous cells, whereas others have crescentic caps of serous cells, described as serous demilunes. This relationship is better seen in longitudinal section (A) than in transverse sections of the acini (B).

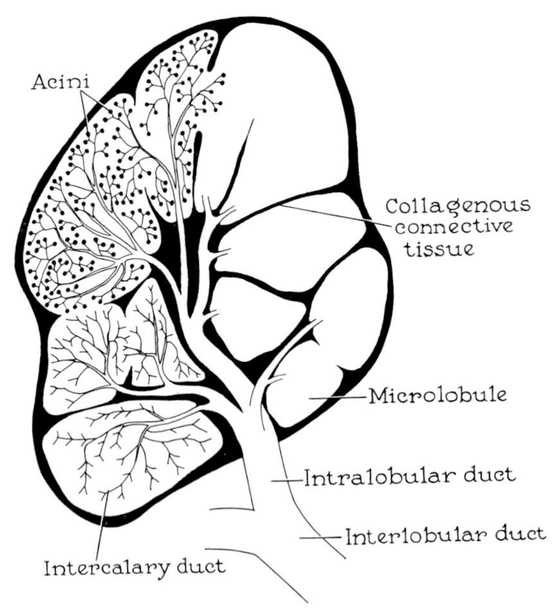

Figure 3–19. Diagram of the duct system within a lobule of a compound tubuloacinar gland. Collagenous connective tissue stroma (in black) partially surrounds the lobule and extends between smaller subdivisions. The main duct to the acinus is a branch of an interlobular duct. The interlobular duct, in turn, branches into intralobular ducts of several orders. These are continuous with very small terminal intercalary ducts that end in the secretory acini.

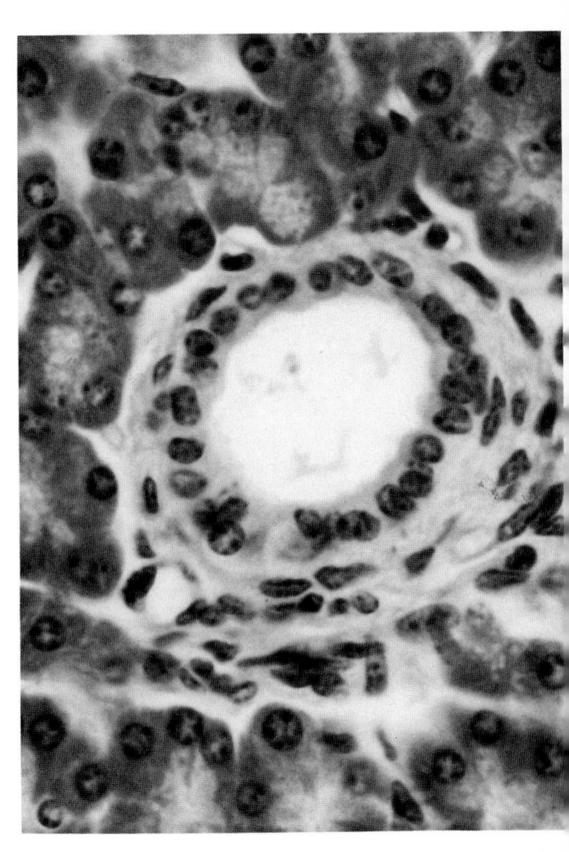

Figure 3–20. Cross section of an intralobular duct of the pancreas showing its lining of cuboidal epithelium.

CONTROL OF EXOCRINE SECRETION

Many glands secrete continuously at a low rate, but under certain conditions they are stimulated to secrete a larger volume of their product. The regulation of secretion varies greatly from gland to gland. In some, stimulation is solely by the autonomic nervous system. In others, the stimulus for secretion is hormonal, and in still others, there is a dual mechanism. For example, it is well known that the sight or smell of food will induce enhanced gastric secretion of acid, mucus, and digestive enzymes. The final common path for these psychic stimuli is the vagus nerves. Their effects on the gastric mucosa are abolished by severance of the these nerves. On the other hand, food placed in the stomach also initiates gastric and pancreatic secretion, even if the food was not previously seen, smelled, or tasted. Stimulation of secretion, in this case, depends on intrinsic nerves and on locally produced hormones. Intrinsic nerves in the gastric mucosa release the neurotransmitter acetylcholine that stimulates release of the hormone, gastrin, and this, in turn, activates secretion by the gastric glands.

There are no morphological criteria by which the histologist can determine whether a given gland is stimulated by hormones, but nervous control can be inferred from the finding of nerve endings in close contact with the base of the glandular cells. In the pancreas, numerous nerve endings can be found beneath the basal lamina in contact with the exocrine cells. Physiological studies have shown that these cells are also responsive to the hormone *gastrin* produced in the gastric mucosa and to *secretin* and *cholecystokinin,* hormones secreted by the duodenum. Thus, secretion by the pancreas is controlled by multiple factors, whereas some other glands are controlled solely by the nervous system.

ENDOCRINE GLANDS

In the course of evolution, three mechanisms developed for integrating the function of the various tissues in multicellular organisms. It is speculated that the earliest to appear was simple diffusion of chemical signals from one group of cells to others at a limited distance from the source. This primitive mechanism was too slow, and too poorly controlled, to meet the needs of larger metazoa and it was supplemented by development of a system of nerve cells with the capacity to respond to external stimuli and to conduct a signal over long cell processes (axons). Later, with the development of a circulatory system in larger animals, these two integrative systems were supplemented by development of ductless glands (*endocrine glands*) synthesizing chemical signals (*hormones*) that were carried in the blood to act on distant *target organs*. Such chemical signals have a longer latent period because they are distributed in the blood, but they have the advantage that they can produce more sustained effects than signals carried by nerves. Although they probably evolved sequentially, all three integrative mechanisms are represented in contemporary mammals: short-range diffusion of chemical signals (cytokines); distribution of chemical signals in the blood (hormones): and conduction of action potentials along nerve axons.

Most of the endocrine glands arise, in the embryo, as tubular evaginations or solid outgrowths from epithelia lining cavities, but later in development, they lose their connection with the surface from which they originated. Their anlagen are penetrated by blood vessels that form a dense network of capillaries around the cords or follicles of endocrine cells. This intimate relation between the cells and the capillaries facilitates delivery of their hormones into the blood. Endocrine glands are usually separate organs, but two are incorporated within large exocrine glands. The *islets of Langerhans*, the endocrine component of the pancreas, are small groups of cells scattered throughout the exocrine portion of the gland. In the testis, the *Leydig cells*, secreting male sex hormones, are located in the interstitial tissue between the seminiferous tubules, which are the exocrine portion of that organ. In these mixed glands, the exocrine portion secretes into a system of ducts, whereas the endocrine portion releases its product into the blood for transport to distant target cells. The liver is unique in that its cells have both endocrine and exocrine functions. Bile is secreted into intercellular tributaries of a duct system, and other products are released into the blood flowing through the sinusoids of the organ.

The principal endocrine glands are the *hypophysis, thyroid, parathyroid, pancreas, adrenals, pineal, testes, ovaries*, and *placenta*. These are so diverse in their tissue architecture that they do not lend themselves to classification on the basis of their histological organization. Although one cannot describe cytological features common to all endocrine glands, one can assign them to groups on the basis of the chemical nature of their hormones. These include modified amino acids, peptides, proteins, glycoproteins, and steroids.

POLYPEPTIDE-SECRETING ENDOCRINE GLANDS

Endocrine cells secreting peptides and proteins share many of the ultrastructural features of protein-secreting exocrine glands described earlier in the chapter, but the rough endoplasmic reticulum is less extensive, a finding consistent with the smaller volume of their secretion. The acinar cells of the pancreas produce over a liter of enzyme-rich digestive juice per day, whereas the output of peptide or glycoprotein secreting endocrine glands would be measured in milligrams or micrograms.

The *beta cells* of the pancreatic islets that secrete the hormone *insulin* are representative of this category of endocrine cells. In electron micrographs, they contain a few meandering profiles of rough endoplasmic reticulum, a small Golgi complex, and numerous secretory granules 200–300 nm in diameter. The granules tend to accumulate at the vascular pole of the cell, but they may be found anywhere in the cytoplasm (Figs. 3–21 and 3–22). In the human, insulin may form pleomorphic crystals in the matrix of the granules, but in other mammalian species, the content of the granules is uniformly dense and homogeneous. Except for minor differences in size, this same description would apply to the secretory granules of the *alpha cells* of the pancreas that secrete *glucagon*; to the thyrotroph, somatotroph, and corticotroph cells of the hypophysis that secrete *growth hormone, thyroid-stimulating hormone, gonadotrophic hormone*, and *adrenocorticotrophic hormone*. In all of these cell types, the intracellular pathway of secretion involves synthesis of hormone on the ribosomes, its segregation in the reticulum, followed by processing and concentration in the Golgi complex, and storage in membrane-bounded secretory granules.

The thyroid gland is exceptional in that its product, *thyroglobulin*, is stored extracellularly. Its cells are arranged in a simple cuboidal epi-

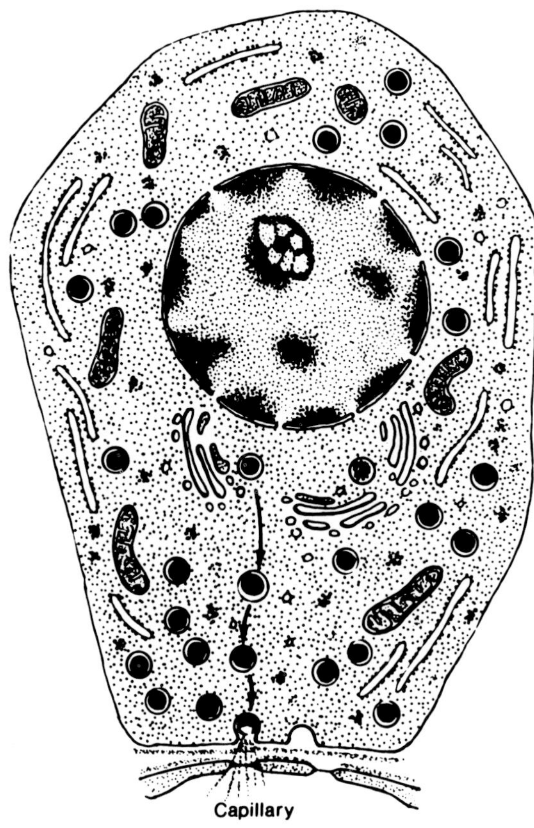

Figure 3–21. Drawing of a polypeptide-secreting endocrine cell. During secretion, the granules move to the cell surface and their limiting membrane coalesces with the cell membrane. The exteriorized granule disintegrates and the hormone diffuses into the blood through the fenestrated endothelium of a neighboring capillary or sinusoid.

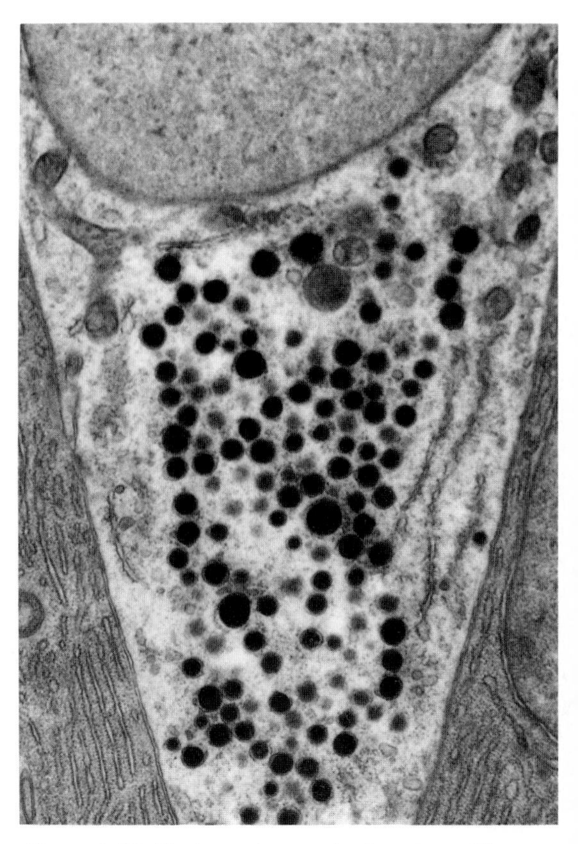

Figure 3–22. Electron micrograph of a polypeptide-secreting endocrine cell of the pancreas illustrating its pale cytoplasm and relatively small secretory granules.

thelium bounding spherical follicles of varying size. The cells have a relatively extensive endoplasmic reticulum having cisternae that are often distended with thyroglobulin, the glycoprotein precursor of thyroid hormone (Fig. 3–23). This substance is packaged in the Golgi complex in sizable vesicles that do not accumulate in the cytoplasm but move directly to the apical cell membrane to discharge their content into the follicle. When thyroid hormone is needed to control metabolism, thyroglobulin is taken up from the lumen by endocytosis and hydrolyzed. The hormone liberated is released into the perifollicular capillaries.

STEROID-SECRETING ENDOCRINE GLANDS

The steroid-secreting endocrine cells of the ovary, testis, and adrenal gland are similar in their ultrastructure, and quite different from protein-secreting cells. They have little rough endoplasmic reticulum and few free ribosomes. Their most characteristic feature is a very extensive smooth endoplasmic reticulum, which forms a close-meshed network of branching and anastomosing tubules (Figs. 3–24 and 3–25). The juxtanuclear Golgi complex is large, but has no associated secretory granules. The numerous mitochondria vary in size and shape and have an unusual internal structure, with tubular or vesicular amplifications of the internal membrane instead of the usual lamellar or foliate cristae found in other cell types. The cytoplasm also contains small numbers of lysosomes, peroxisomes, and lipid droplets. Deposits of lipochrome pigment are common.

Steroidogenic cells store very little hormone but do accumulate the precursor, cholesterol. Lipid droplets in the cytoplasm contain cholesterol esters as well as triglycerides. In some species, steroidogenic cells take up cholesterol from the blood, whereas in other species, they

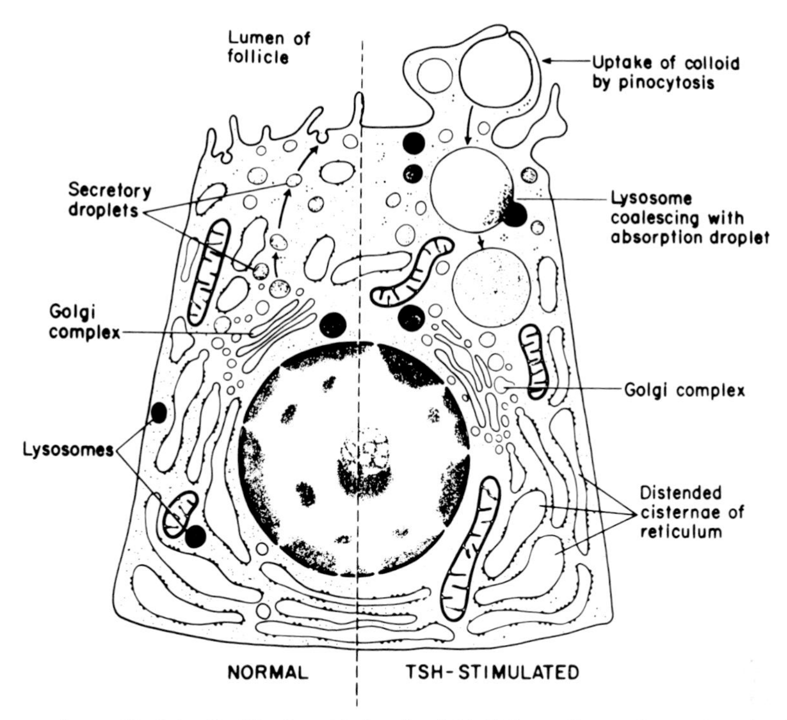

Figure 3–23. Diagram of an epithelial cell of the thyroid showing (at left) the pathway of secretory droplets from the Golgi to the cell surface for release and extracellular storage. The right half of the figure depicts the ultrastructure of a TSH-stimulated cell in which droplets of colloid are being taken up from the lumen of the follicle by pinocytosis and then coalescing with lysosomes, resulting in degradation of thyroglobulin and diffusion of thyroxin into perifollicular capillaries.

synthesize most of the cholesterol they use for the synthesis of steroid hormones. The enzymes for this synthesis reside in the abundant smooth endoplasmic reticulum. In the synthesis of adrenal steroids, there is an additional step that takes place in the mitochondria. Little is known about how the cholesterol is moved back and forth between the reticulum and the mitochondria.

There is little or no storage of hormone in these cells and their abundant smooth reticulum is no doubt a specialization providing the enzymes necessary for rapid synthesis of steroid on demand. Steroid-secreting cells respond very rapidly to stimulation. The blood level of the circulating adrenal hormone, *cortisol*, increases two to four times within 30 min of administration of adrenocorticotrophic hormone. The observation that the lipid content of these cells diminishes on stimulation is interpreted as evidence of depletion of stored precursor cholesterol during enhanced steroid production. It is not yet known what role is played by the conspicuous Golgi complex, but the fact that it increases in size in response to stimulation of the cell by trophic hormone would seem to indicate that it is involved in some way in the secretory process. Upon entry into the circulation, the duration of action of the chemical signals released by endocrine cells varies greatly. The half-life of different hormones ranges from a few minutes to several days. Inactivation or degradation of the hormone may take place in the target organ or in the liver or kidney.

RECEPTORS AND MECHANISM OF HORMONE ACTION

Hormones circulating in the blood reach all parts of the body. Their selective action on specific target cells depends on the presence of *receptors* in the membranes of those cells that have a high affinity for the hormone. Receptors for peptide and catecholamine hormones are integral protein molecules of the cell membrane and the responsiveness of the target cells is a function of the number of available receptors. Their number varies in different cells but may be on the order of 10,000 to 15,000. They are not static components of the plasmalemma, but are in a dynamic state of turnover, with a prepro-

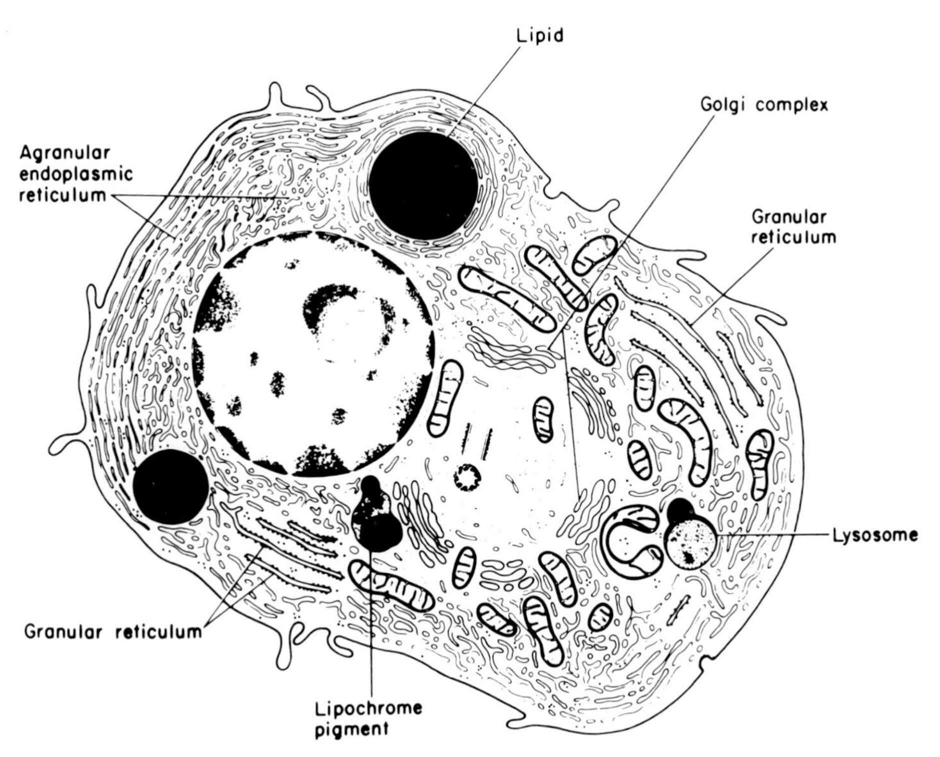

Figure 3–24. Schematic drawing of the ultrastructure of a steroid-secreting cell. Notable features are a large Golgi complex and a very extensive smooth endoplasmic reticulum.

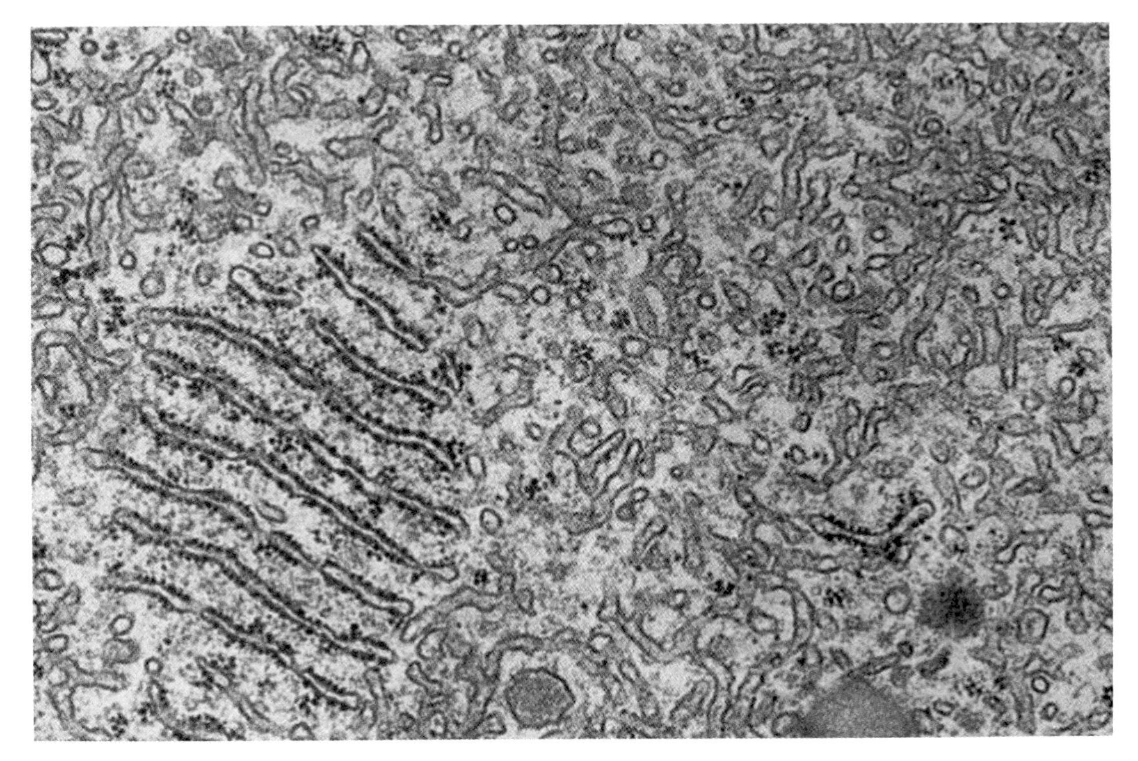

Figure 3–25. Electron micrograph of a small area of cytoplasm from a cell of the human fetal adrenal cortex, a steroid-secreting organ. A few cisternae of granular reticulum are present, but most of the cytoplasm is occupied by branching tubules of smooth endoplasmic reticulum. (Micrograph courtesy of N.S. McNutt.)

grammed rate of synthesis and insertion into the membrane. Their number can change with the state of cell differentiation and can be influenced by exposure to unphysiological levels of the specific hormone (homospecific regulation). The action of one hormone on a cell can induce the appearance of receptors for another hormone (heterospecific regulation).

The mechanism by which hormones elicit a response in their target cell has been a subject of intensive investigation and much remains to be learned. Our present understanding of the process is based largely on early studies of the release of glucose from the liver in response to the hormone epinephrine. The binding of the hormone to a receptor in the membrane results in a conformational change in the receptor and in another membrane protein (G-protein) that leads to activation of the enzyme adenylate cyclase (AC), which catalyzes the formation of cyclic adenosine monophosphate (cyclic AMP) from adenosine triphosphate (ATP). Accumulation of cyclic AMP in the cytoplasm results in activation of phosphorylases that break down glycogen, releasing glucose into the blood stream (Fig. 3–26). It was soon discovered that a similar train of events occurs after binding of other hormones. This led to the *second messenger* concept. Briefly stated, this holds that the *first messenger*, the hormone, binds to a receptor on a target cell and activates adenylate cyclase, resulting in the formation of a *second messenger*, cyclic AMP, which sets in motion a cascade of reactions leading to the specific physiological response. It has since been found that the same mechanism applies to the hypophyseal hormones adrenocorticotropin, thyrotropin, and the gonadotropins. In all cases in which this mechanism is operative, the action of the hormone can be duplicated by exposure of the target cells to exogenous AMP.

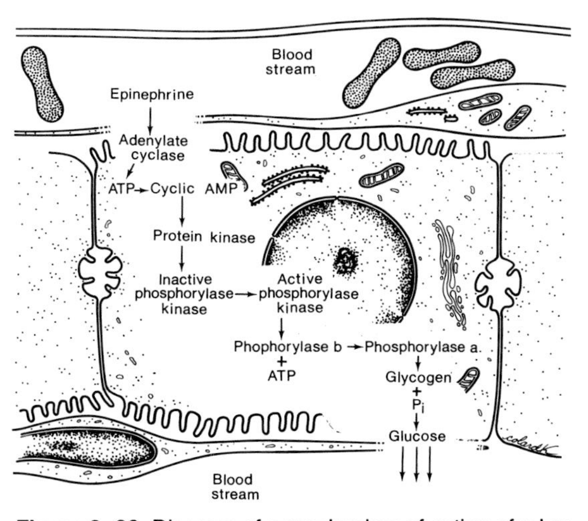

Figure 3–26. Diagram of a mechanism of action of a hormone on the liver. The hormone epinephrine (first messenger) carried to the liver cell membrane in the blood activates the enzyme adenylate cyclase in the membrane, causing it to convert ATP in the cytoplasm into cyclic AMP (second messenger). This then activates a protein kinase, which activates a second kinase. This initiates a four-step sequence that converts glycogen to glucose, which then passes out into the blood in the hepatic sinusoids.

A satisfactory explanation of the remarkable diversity of responses by various target cells, to the same second messenger, is still being sought. However, the cyclic AMP appears to act by controlling the activity of protein kinases that catalyze the transfer of phosphate from ATP to protein. The varying cellular responses thus seem not to depend on the control system but on distinctive proteins available in different cell types and their varied biological activities when phosphorylated.

Unlike protein hormones, steroid hormones do not bind to receptors on the cell surface, but diffuse through the lipophilic cell membrane and bind to receptors located in the nucleus. Binding results in a change in the receptor that enables the hormone–receptor complex to bind to a specific site on the DNA, activating gene transcription that initiates synthesis of the appropriate mediator of the cell's response.

Much remains to be learned about the mechanism of hormone action, but enough is known to explain some congenital defects that were previously very puzzling. Children inheriting the condition called *testicular feminization* have the male complement of chromosomes (46XY) but fail to develop male genitalia and normal testicular function because the tissues are unresponsive to the steroid hormone *dihydrotestosterone*. It is found that receptors for this hormone are completely absent in some of these patients. In others, they are present, but the hormone–receptor complex formed in the nucleus is abnormal and is unable to activate gene transcription. Comparable receptor anomalies are responsible for *familial male pseudohermaphroditism*.

Endocrine disturbances may arise in adults as a consequence of production, by the immune system, of antibodies that bind to receptors of specific target organs. Patients with *Grave's disease* (thyrotoxicosis) often have an abnormal immunoglobulin in their blood serum that binds to receptors for thyrotrophic hormone and activates adenylcyclase, resulting in continuous stimulation of the thyroid cells to produce excess thyroid hormone. By competing with thyrotrophic hormone for receptors, the immunoglobulin overrides the normal control mechanisms that govern thyroid function. Similarly, some cases of *diabetes* are attributable to an abnormal immunoglobulin that competes with insulin for receptor sites. In this condition, the immunoglobulin does not induce a second messenger and acts by blocking insulin binding.

RELATION TO THE VASCULAR SYSTEM

A common feature of endocrine glands is their great vascularity. They are so organized that nearly every cell is in close relation to one or more vessels of a rich vascular bed. In some glands, the vessels are typical capillaries, whereas in others, they are better described as sinusoids. The latter are generally larger than true capillaries and often irregular in outline, conforming to the shape of the spaces they occupy among the plates or cords of cells that make up the parenchyma of the gland. Whether the vessels are capillaries or sinusoids, their wall is very thin and often fenestrated. It offers no significant barrier to diffusion of the hormone into the blood.

The course of the blood vessels after leaving the gland can have special relevance to its function. For example, the releasing factors produced in the hypothalamus are carried to responding target cells immediately downstream in the anterior lobe of the pituitary gland. Another example of a physiologically important path of drainage from an endocrine gland is found in the adrenal. This gland consists of an outer cortex which secretes steroid hormones and an inner medulla which secretes the catecholamines, epinephrine and norepinephrine. No capsule or other barrier separates the two zones and the blood flows centripetally, first supplying the cortex and then flowing inward to the medulla. In has now been found that a relatively high concentration of cortical steroids is necessary for induction and maintenance of an enzyme in the cells of the medulla that is essential for synthesis of catecholamines. This condition is met by the flow of blood, carrying corticosteroids, from the cortex directly to the medulla. Thus, local "downstream" effects of hormones can be as important as the effects they exert at a distance via the general circulation.

Although in most endocrine glands the hormones are released directly into the blood, recent studies show that lymphatics may also be important pathways for egress of hormone from the gland. This is especially true of the perifollicular lymphatics of the thyroid and the lymphatics of the testis. The lymph ultimately enters the blood vascular system and mixes with the blood for wider distribution.

INTERACTION OF CONTROL MECHANISMS

Some endocrine glands respond to small changes in the concentration of specific ions or metabolites in the extracellular fluid, and their hormones serve to maintain the constancy of the internal environment. For example, a rise in blood glucose concentration stimulates the beta cells of the endocrine pancreas to release the hormone *insulin*. This acts on the liver and other cells to increase their uptake of glucose. The resulting lowering of the concentration of blood glucose acts back on the beta cells to reduce their output of insulin. Such an interaction, in which, release of a hormone brings about a change that acts back on the endocrine gland to decrease its rate of secretion is called *negative feedback* and is the commonest mechanism for controlling the activity of endocrine glands.

Neural and endocrine control mechanisms may be combined, as in the suckling reflex. Stimulation of sensory nerve endings in the nipples, by a suckling infant, generates nerve impulses carried via afferent neural pathways to the spinal cord and then to the brain. There the stimulus is relayed to neurosecretory cells of the hypothalamus that release the hormone *oxytocin* at their terminations in the posterior lobe of the pituitary gland. This hormone, carried in the blood to the mammary gland, stimulates contraction of myoepithelial cells around the acini of the gland, resulting in the ejection of milk (Fig. 3–27).

Hormones may control the release of other hormones. Exposure to painful injury, or the threat of injury, initiates a sequence of neural and endocrine events that prepares the body for a fight or flight. Stimuli transmitted to the brain are relayed to cells of the hypothalamus that secrete *adrenocorticotrophin-releasing hormone* (ACTH-RH) into the hypophyseoportal blood vessels. On reaching the pituitary, this

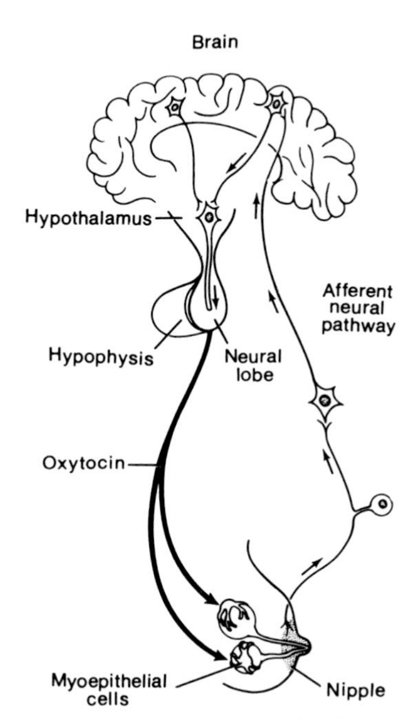

Figure 3–27. Diagram of neuroendocrine interrelationships involved in the suckling reflex. Stimulation of the nipples generates sensory impulses that pass to the central nervous system via the dorsal root ganglia. In the brain, these impulses are relayed to the hypothalamus, where they activate neurosecretory cells whose processes extend into the neural lobe of the hypophysis. Stimulation of cells there results in release of the hormone oxytocin which is carried in the blood to the breast where it causes contraction of myoepithelial cells around the acini of the gland, expelling milk. No feedback mechanism is involved.

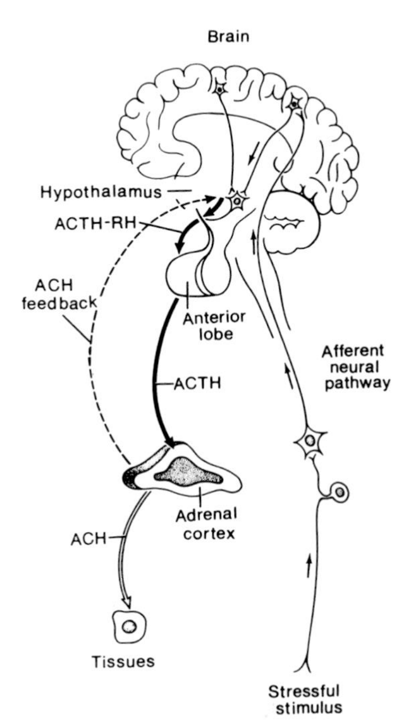

Figure 3–28. Diagram of the neuroendocrine relationships involved in response to stress. A painful peripheral stimulus reaching the brain is relayed to neurosecretory cells in hypothalamus. These liberate ACTH-releasing hormone (ACTH-RH) into vessels of the hypophyseoportal system. Carried downstream to the anterior lobe of the pituitary, this stimulates corticotrophs to release ACTH. Carried in the blood to the adrenal cortex, this hormone causes release of corticosteroids (ACH) which induce protective metabolic responses in cells throughout the body. The adrenocortical hormones act back on the hypothalamus to suppress liberation of ACTH-RH.

hormone stimulates cells of the anterior lobe to release a *adrenocorticotrophic hormone* (ACTH). Carried in the circulation to the adrenal cortex, this hormone induces release of steroid hormones (*glucocorticoids*) that are carried to a wide variety of tissues and organs, influencing their functions in ways that collectively enhance the body's ability to endure prolonged exertion, injury, and infection. The responses to this train of endocrine events are limited by negative feedback on the cells of the hypothalamus to reduce their secretion of ACTH-releasing hormone (Fig. 3–28).

Traditionally, the two major integrating systems of the body were considered to be quite distinct, with the nervous system providing rapid communication with effector cells using *neurotransmitters*, and the endocrine system, acting more slowly, and using *hormones* transported in the blood to distant target organs. The nature of the signaling molecules in the two systems was thought to be different, with neurotransmitters usually being monoamines or amino acids, whereas hormones were generally polypeptides, glycoproteins, or steroids. In the past 30 years, the distinction between nerve cells and endocrine cells on the basis of their mode of action and the chemical nature of their signaling molecules has gradually broken down, with the discovery that certain neurones in the brain secrete peptides that are carried in the blood to their target cells and that the classical neurotransmitter, norepinephrine, is also secreted by cells of the adrenal medulla and acts as a hormone. Conversely, vasopressin, a hormone secreted by the pituitary gland, has been found to serve as a neurotransmitter for certain cells of the hypothalamus. Clearly, an endocrine function is not confined to cells gathered together to form discrete glands.

DIFFUSE ENDOCRINE SYSTEM

In recent years, there has been intense interest in small granule-containing cells that occur individually or in small groups in the epithelium lining the gastrointestinal tract. Some of these have been found to release, into the capillaries of the lamina propria, hormones that are carried to target cells within the gut or its associated digestive glands. Fifteen or more morphologically similar, but functionally distinct, *enteroendocrine cells* have now been identified. Some secrete peptide hormones that influence the secretory activity of intestinal glands or the motility of the gut. Others seem to release diffusible substances that have local trophic effects on cells in their immediate vicinity. Still others secrete some of the same molecules that serve as neurotransmitters in the nervous system. Thus, endocrine cells occurring individually or in small groups in the brain and in the epithelia of the intestinal and respiratory tracts can be thought of as forming a *diffuse endocrine system* that controls and coordinates the activities of other cells in the same organ system.

Studies of the immune system have led to the discovery that individual lymphocytes which do not have secretory granules secrete signaling molecules that affect the differentiation and behavior of other cells in this system. These constitutively secreted soluble mediators are called *interleukins* or *lymphokines* (Fig.3–29). Some 20 years ago, antigen-stimulated T-lymphocytes were found to secrete a polypeptide, *interleukin-1* (Il-1) which induced proliferation and differentiation of B-lymphocytes. This was followed by the discovery of *interleukin-2* (Il-2), a growth factor for B-lymphocytes which also activates cytotoxic T-lymphocytes. *Interleukin-3* (Il-3), secreted by activated T-lymphocytes, is carried in the blood to the bone marrow where it induces proliferation of pluripotential stem cells. The number of identified interleukins has now grown to eight or more. The functions of some of these will be discussed in more appropriate context in the chapter on the immune system (Chapter 13).

In studies on blood formation, several other signaling molecules were discovered which act on stem cells in the bone marrow. Collectively these are called *colony-stimulating factors* (CSF) and there are separate factors specific for each blood cell type. For example, *granulocyte colony-stimulating factor* (G-CSF) induces develop-

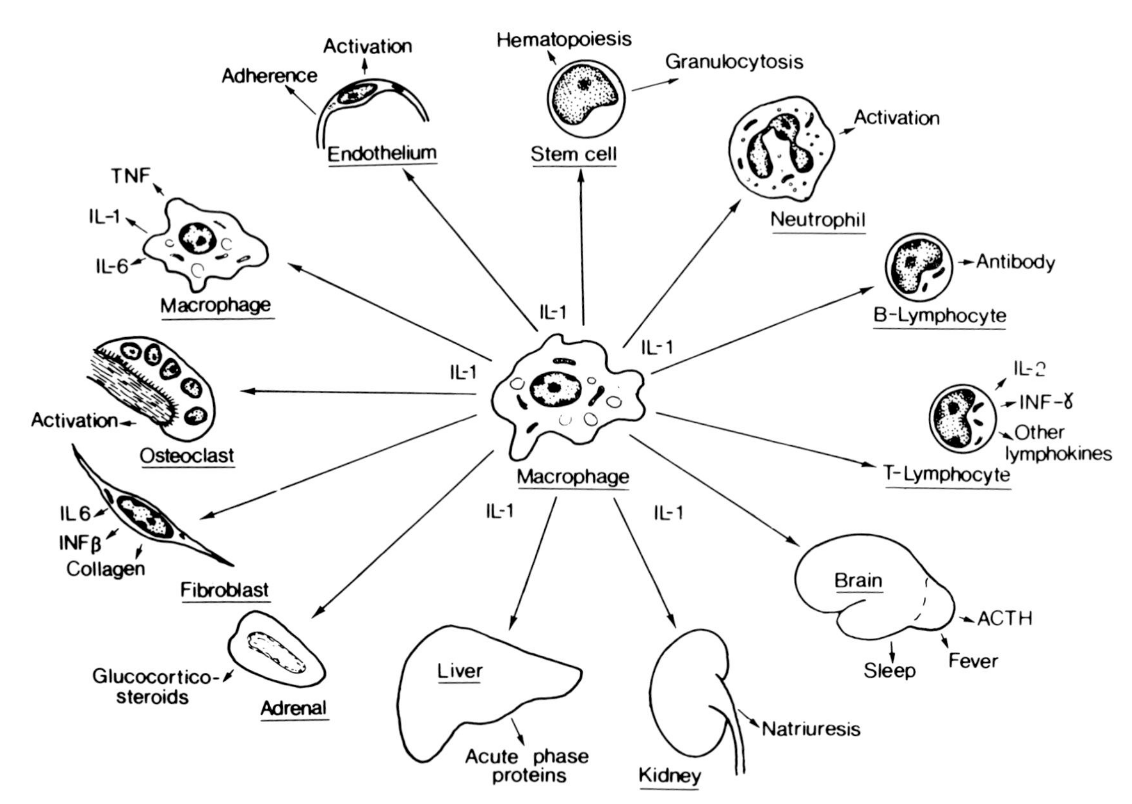

Figure 3–29. A diagram illustrating the multiplicity of targets that may be reached by cytokines of the diffuse endocrine system. Shown here are the cells activated by interleukin-1, secreted by macrophages, and the activities induced in those target cells.

ment of colonies of granulocytes. Another (M-CSF) stimulates production of monocytes, and yet another (GM-CSF) stimulates development of both granulocytes and monocytes. These will be discussed further in the chapter on blood (Chapter 4).

The proliferation of lymphokines, growth factors, and other signaling molecules continues and all of them are now grouped together under the general term *cytokines*, defined as soluble mediators released by individual cells and acting on target cells having appropriate receptors.

BIBLIOGRAPHY

PROTEIN SECRETION

Amsterdam, A., I. Ohad, and M. Schramm. 1969. Dynamic changes in the ultrastructure of the acinar cell of the rat parotid gland during the secretory cycle. J. Cell Biol. 41:753.

Blobel, G., P. Walter, C.N. Chang et al. 1979. Translocation of proteins across membranes. The signal hypothesis. *In* Secretory Mechanisms. Symp. Soc. Exp. Biol. Vol. 33. Cambridge, England, Cambridge University Press.

Burgess, T.L. and R.B. Kelly. 1987. Constitutive and regulated secretion of proteins. Annu. Rev. Cell Biol. 3:243.

Castle, J.D., J.D. Jamieson, and G.E. Palade. 1972. Radio autographic analysis of the secretory process in the parotid acinar cell of the rabbit. J. Cell Biol. 53:290.

Dunphy, W.G. and J.E. Rothman. 1985. Compartmental organization of the Golgi stack. Cell 42:13.

Farquhar, M.G. 1985. Progress in unraveling pathways in Golgi traffic. Annu. Rev. Cell Biol. 1:447.

Gilmore, R., G. Blobel, and P. Walter. 1982. Protein translocation across the endoplasmic reticulum. I. Detection in the microsomal membrane of a receptor for the signal recognition particle. J. Cell Biol. 95:463.

Kelly, R.B. . 1985. Pathways of protein secretion in eukaryotes. Science 230:25.

Neutra, M. and C.P. Leblond. 1966. Synthesis of the carbohydrate of mucus in the Golgi complex as shown by electron microscope radioautography of goblet cells from rats injected with glucose-H3. J. Cell Biol. 30:119.

Walter, P., I. Ibrahimi, and G. Blobel. 1981. Translocation of proteins across the endoplasmic reticulum. J. Cell Biol. 91:545.

Walter, P., R. Gilmore, and G. Blobel. 1984. Protein translocation across the endoplasmic reticulum. Cell 38:5.

CONTROL OF SECRETION

Berrage, M.J. 1985. Calcium: A universal second messenger. Triangle 24:79.

Rassmussen, H. 1970. Cell communication, calcium ion, and cyclic adenosine monophosphate. Science 170:404.

Sutherland, E.W. 1970. On the biological role of cyclic AMP. J. Am. Med. Assn. 214:1281.

ENDOCRINE SECRETION

Evans, R.E. 1988. The steroid and thyroid hormone receptor superfamily. Science 240:889.

Fawcett, D.W., J.A. Long, and A.L. Jones. 1969. The ultrastructure of the endocrine glands. Recent Progr. Hormone Res. 25:315.

O'Malley, B.W. and W.T. Schrader. 1976. The receptors of steroid hormones. Sci. Am. 234:32.

Schalley, A.U., A.J. Kastin, and A. Arimura. 1977. Hypothalamic hormones: the links between brain and body. Am. Scientist 65:712.

Smith, A.D. 1972. Storage and secretion of hormones. Sci. Basis Med. 74:102.

PARACRINE SECRETION

Fujita, T. 1977. The concept of paraneurons. Arch. Histol. Japan 40 (Suppl. 1) 1.

Fujita, T., T. Iwanaga, Y. Kusumato, and S. Yoshie. 1982. Paraneurons and neurosecretion. *In* Farner, D.S. and K. Lederis, eds. Neurosecretion: Molecules, Cells, Systems. New York, Plenum Publishing Co.

Pearse, A.G.E. 1977. The diffuse neuroendocrine system and the APUD concept: related endocrine peptides in brain, intestine, pituitary, placenta, and anuran cutaneous glands. Med. Biol. 55:115.

CYTOKINES

Akira, S., T. Hirano, T. Taga, and T. Kishimoto. 1990. Biology of multifunctional cytokines: Il-6 and related molecules (Il-1 and TNF). FASEB J. 4:2860.

Beutler, B. and A. Cerami. 1988. The common mediator of shock, cachexia, and tumor necrosis. Adv. Immunol. 43:213.

Durum, S.K., J.A. Schmidt, and J. Oppenheimer. 1985. Interleukin-1: an immunological perspective. Annu. Rev. Immunol. 3:263.

Fibbe, W.E., M.R. Schaafsma et al. 1989. The biological activities of interleukin-1. Blut 59:147.

Howard, M. and W.E. Paul. 1983. Regulation of B-cell growth and differentiation by soluble factors. Annu. Rev. Immunol. 1:307.

Kishimoto, T. 1985. Factors affecting B-cell growth and differentiation. Annu. Rev. Immunol. 7:145.

Kishimoto, T. 1989. The biology of interleukin-6. Blood 74:1.

Smith, K.A. 1984. Interleukin-2. Annu. Rev. Immunol. 2:283.

4

BLOOD

Blood is a tissue composed of *erythrocytes* (red blood cells), *leukocytes* (white blood cells), and *blood platelets* suspended in a fluid *blood plasma*. It circulates in the vascular system, transporting oxygen from the lungs and nutrients from the gastrointestinal tract to other tissues throughout the body. It also carries carbon dioxide from the tissues to the lungs and nitrogenous wastes to the kidneys for elimination from the body. It also plays an essential role in the integrative function of the endocrine glands by carrying hormones from their origin to their distant target cells.

A *tissue* is an aggregation of cells, predominantly of the same type, distributed in an abundant extracellular matrix. The *connective tissue*, which will be described in the next chapter, consists of fibroblasts in an extracellular matrix that is reinforced by numerous fibers. Similarly, cartilage is a connective tissue composed of cells in a gelatinous matrix, and bone is made up of cells in a highly organized matrix of calcified fibers. The early histologists considered blood to be a connective tissue with a fluid matrix. Unlike the others, it does not bind things together to preserve the integrity of the organism, but it is *connective* in the sense that it circulates to maintain logistical support and communication between all of the other tissues and organs of the body.

Blood cells were formerly thought to carry out their principal functions in the bloodstream, but when it became possible to radiolabel cells and trace their migrations, it was found that only the erythrocytes and blood platelets function within the confines of the vascular system. The several types of leukocytes are constantly migrating through the walls of capillaries and venules to become free cells in the connective tissues. It is there that they carry out their functions, complete their short life span, and degenerate. They are only transiently in the blood which simply serves as a vehicle for their transport and dissemination.

The volume of blood in the human is approximately 5 liters, accounting for 7% of the body weight. Erythrocytes make up about 45% of this volume, the leukocytes and platelets 1%, and the remainder is blood plasma, the transparent yellow fluid that constitutes the extracellular matrix of this tissue. When blood is drawn from a blood vessel, it rapidly clots into a deep red jelly-like mass, but if clotting is prevented by an anticoagulant, the cellular elements can be separated from it by centrifugation, and if it is centrifuged in a graduated tube, this procedure gives the clinician a useful measure of the percentage of the blood volume occupied by cells.

A thorough knowledge of the normal appearance of the blood cells is important in medical and veterinary practice because no tissue is examined more often for diagnostic purposes. The microscopic study of stained blood smears not only yields information about diseases that primarily affect the blood, it can also provide indirect evidence of viral, bacterial, and parasitic infections and may enable the physician to identify the disease, to follow its course, and to evaluate the effectiveness of his treatment.

ERYTHROCYTES

Erythrocytes are the minute corpuscles that impart a red color to the blood. They develop in the bone marrow as true cells, but before entering the blood, they extrude their nucleus, thereby losing the capacity for DNA-directed protein synthesis. Their mitochondria and other organelles are also lost and they are reduced to a membrane-bounded corpuscle containing cytoplasm that consists predominantly of the pigment *hemoglobin*. In this transformation, the erythrocytes are specialized for their primary function of transporting oxygen from the lungs to the tissues and carbon dioxide from the tissues to the lungs. Anucleate erythrocytes are characteristic of mammals. In birds, reptiles, fish, and

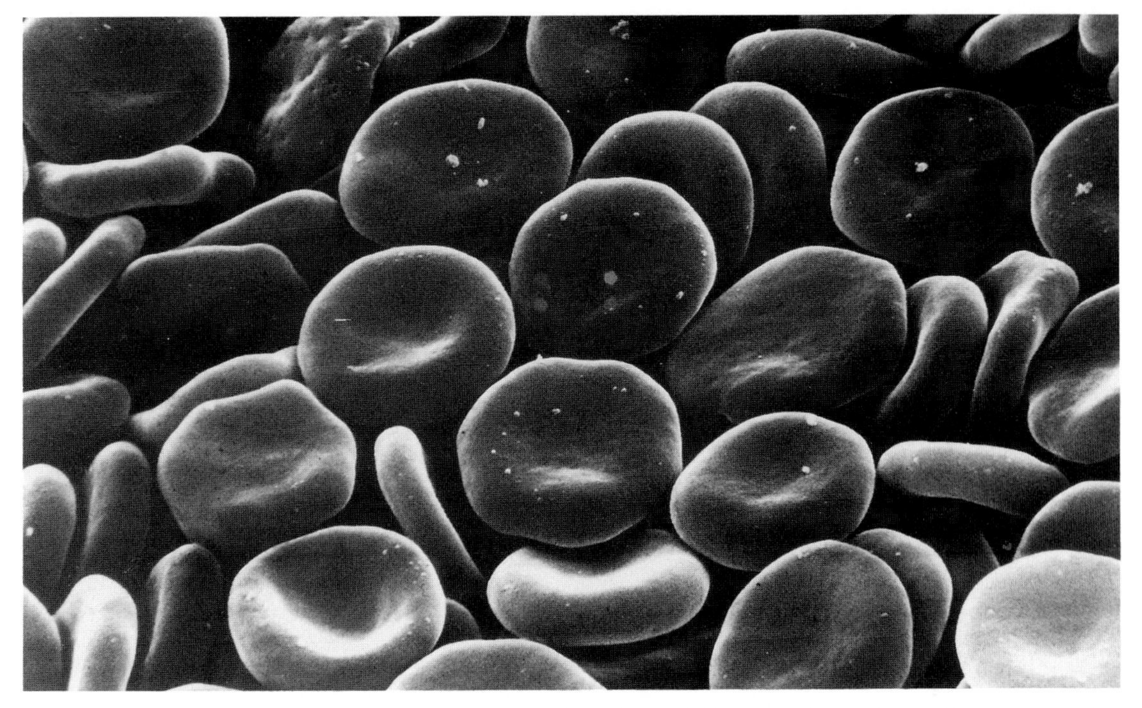

Figure 4–1. A scanning electron micrograph of erythrocytes illustrating their biconcave discoid shape. (Micrograph courtesy of D. Phillips.)

amphibia, the erythrocytes retain their nucleus, but its DNA is inert.

The normal number of erythrocytes is about 5.4 million per cubic millimeter of blood in men, and 4.8 million in women. These numbers are slightly increased by residence at high altitude. The erythrocyte has a very characteristic shape (Figs. 4–1 and 4–2). It is a biconcave disc about 7.5 μm in diameter, 1.9 μm in maximum thickness, and has a surface area of approximately 140 μm^2. The biconcave shape is well adapted to its function because, in this form, it presents a surface area 20–30% greater in relation to its volume than it would have if it were spherical. This increased surface area favors the immediate saturation of its hemoglobin with oxygen as the erythrocyte passes through the pulmonary capillaries. The total surface area of the erythrocytes in an average human is 3800 m^2. That is some 2,000 times the surface area of the body. This results in great efficiency in oxygen and carbon dioxide transport.

Erythrocytes are quite pliable and may be deformed to bell-like or paraboloid shapes when flowing through narrow capillaries. This deformation is the result of hydrodynamic forces and viscous drag and is dependent on the velocity of flow. Gas exchange is unimpaired by this shape change because it slightly increases the surface area. The shape of erythrocytes is also influenced by the osmolarity of the surrounding medium. In moderately hypotonic solutions, they swell and may become uniconcave or cup-shaped. In solutions that are more hypotonic, swelling stretches the membrane and it can become leaky, permitting the hemoglobin to escape and leaving behind the empty membrane, called an *erythrocyte ghost*. Hypotonic disruption of erythrocytes is called *hemolysis*.

Under certain conditions, erythrocytes round up with 10–30 short, conical projections radiating from their surface. In this form, they are called *echinocytes* and the adoption of this shape is called *crenation* (Fig. 4–3). The maintenance of their normal biconcave shape is dependent on ATP. When this falls below a critical level, erythrocytes are transformed to echinocytes. If they are then allowed time to regenerate ATP, the shape change is reversed. Crenation can also be induced, in vitro, by exposure of erythrocytes to anionic compounds, fatty acids, or lysolecithin. It is speculated that erythrocyte shape is, in part, a function of the relative areas of the outer and inner leaflets of the membrane. Amphipathic compounds that intercalate in

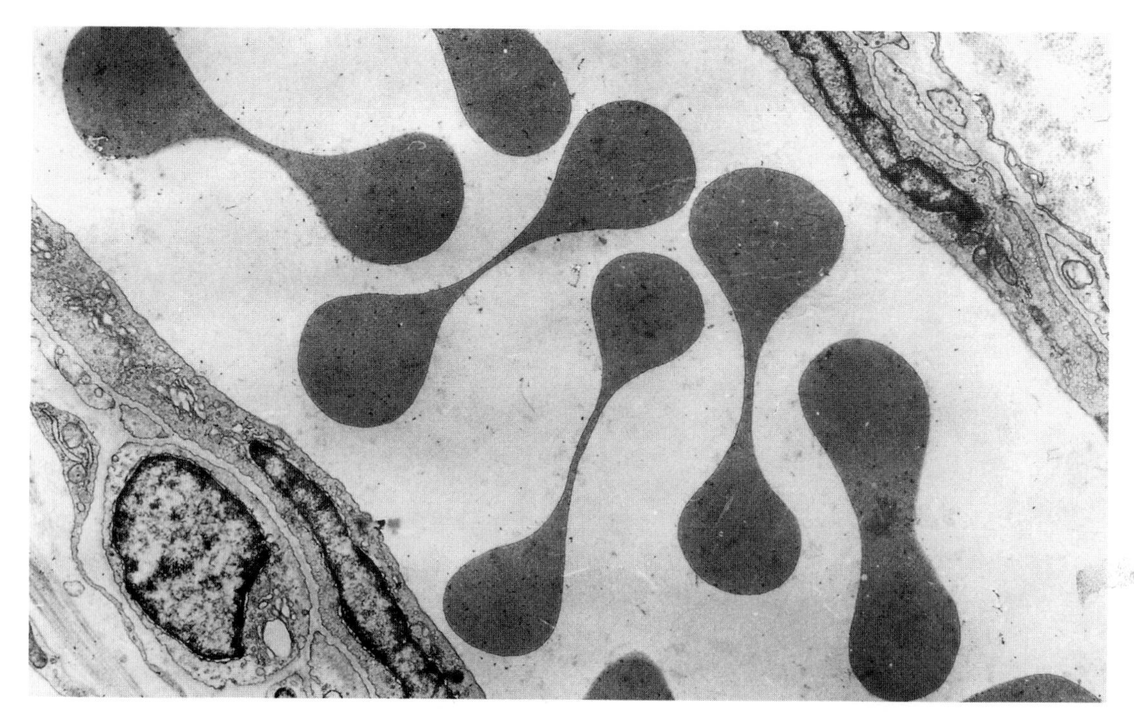

Figure 4–2. An electron micrograph of erythrocytes in a longitudinal section of a capuillary, illustrating their biconcave shape in cross section.

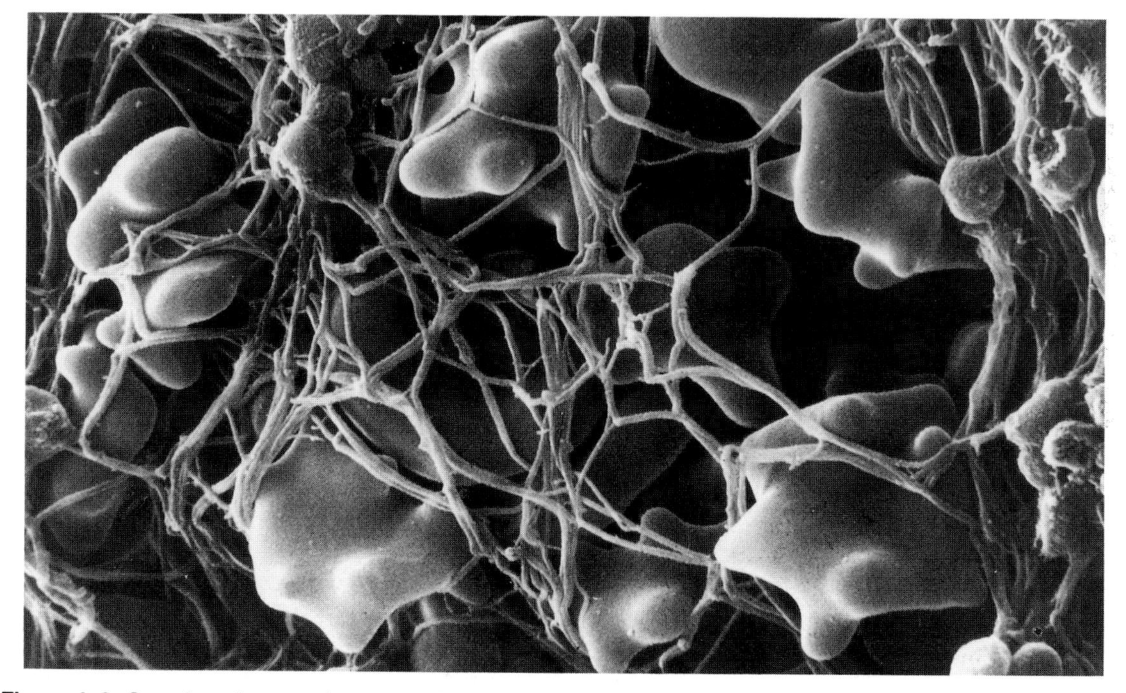

Figure 4–3. Scanning electron micrograph of a forming clot showing several crenated erythrocytes enmeshed in a meshwork of fibrin. (Micrograph courtesy of D. Phillips.)

the outer leaflet increases its area relative to the inner leaflet, resulting in the spiny projections on echinocytes.

When a thick smear of fresh blood is observed under the microscope, the discoid erythrocytes are often seen to form aggregates that resemble stacks of coins. These are called *rouleaux*. This happens only in stagnant blood, in vitro, and does not occur when blood is circulating. It is attributed by some to surface tension, but its basis is actually not understood.

Blood cells are usually studied in thin *blood smears* spread on a glass slide, dried, and stained with Wright's stain, which is a mixture of acid and basic dyes. In such preparations, the great majority of erythrocytes stain a deep pink (Fig. 4–4). A small number which have recently entered the circulation from the bone marrow have a bluish or greenish tint owing to the basophilic staining of residual ribosomes in their cytoplasm. These are called *polychromatophilic erythrocytes*. They may also be called *reticulocytes* because, when stained with brilliant cresyl blue, their residual ribonucleoprotein is precipitated by the dye as a delicate basophilic network in the otherwise acidophilic cytoplasm. Within 24 h after entering the circulation, the reticulocytes mature, losing their basophilia. In the adult human, the number of reticulocytes averages about 0.8% of the total number of erythrocytes. The *reticulocyte count* is used clinically as a rough index of the rate of erythrocyte production. In patients with anemia, an elevated reticulocyte count is an encouraging sign of response to treatment.

Unstained erythrocytes have a pale yellow or tan color due to their content of hemoglobin, the respiratory pigment that makes up about 33% of their mass. Hemoglobin is a protein with a molecular weight of 68,000, consisting of four polypeptide chains: two identical α-chains and two identical β-chains, with an iron-containing heme group bound to each chain of the tetramer. In the lung, oxygen combines loosely, and reversibly, with the heme portions of the hemoglobin molecule, and the oxygen is released in passage of the blood through the capillaries of the tissues. Concurrently, the enzyme carbonic anhydrase catalyzes the interaction of carbon dioxide with water in the erythrocytes to form carbonic acid which immediately dissociates into hydrogen and bicarbonate ions. Bicarbonate is the principal form in which carbon dioxide is carried to the lungs. This reaction is accelerated about 5000-fold by the carbonic anhydrases of the erythrocyte so that a large amount of bicarbonate ion is formed in a fraction of a second as the blood flows through the tissues. Carbon dioxide also reacts directly with hemoglobin, but this accounts for a relatively small fraction of the total uptake. Carbon dioxide dissociates from both bicarbonate and hemoglobin in the lungs and is exhaled.

Erythrocyte numbers are normally maintained at a nearly constant level. Patients who have a significant reduction in the oxygen-carrying capacity of the blood suffer from *anemia*. This may involve lower than normal numbers of erythrocytes or a reduction in their content of hemoglobin. Examination of stained blood smears can shed light on the nature of the underlying defect in blood formation (hemopoiesis). A number of terms are employed to describe the erythrocytes in various kinds of anemia. Abnormal variations in cell *size* is termed *anisocytosis*. Diversity in cell *shape* is called *poikilocytosis*. If the anemia is characterized by erythrocytes that are larger than normal, it is a *macrocytic* anemia; if they are of normal size, it is a *normocytic* anemia; and if they are small, it is *microcytic* anemia. Also needed is some judgment as to the concentration of hemoglobin as reflected in the depth of staining of the erythrocytes. Therefore, they are described as *hyperchromic, normochromic*, or *hypochromic*. For example, a dietary deficiency of iron needed for hemoglobin synthesis leads to a *hypochromic microcytic anemia*. Chronic inflammation or liver disease may lead to an anemia in which the cells are of normal size and color, and it is, therefore, a *normochromic normocytic* anemia, and so on. These terms are in common use in clinical medicine and may occasionally be encountered in the literature of basic science.

Human DNA contains the genes necessary for synthesis and incorporation into hemoglobin of four different polypeptide chains designated alpha (α), beta (β), gamma (γ), and delta (δ). Hemoglobin of the normal adult, called *hemoglobin A* (HbA), contains two α- and two β-chains. This form constitutes 96% of the hemoglobin, whereas 2% is of a second type, consisting of two α- and two δ-chains, and less than 2% is *fetal hemoglobin* (HbF), composed of two α- and two γ-chains. In fetal life, HbF greatly predominates over the other forms, but rapidly decreases in amount after birth. However, in one kind of anemia (*thalassemia*) there is a persistence of abnormally high levels of fetal hemoglobin. The structure of each

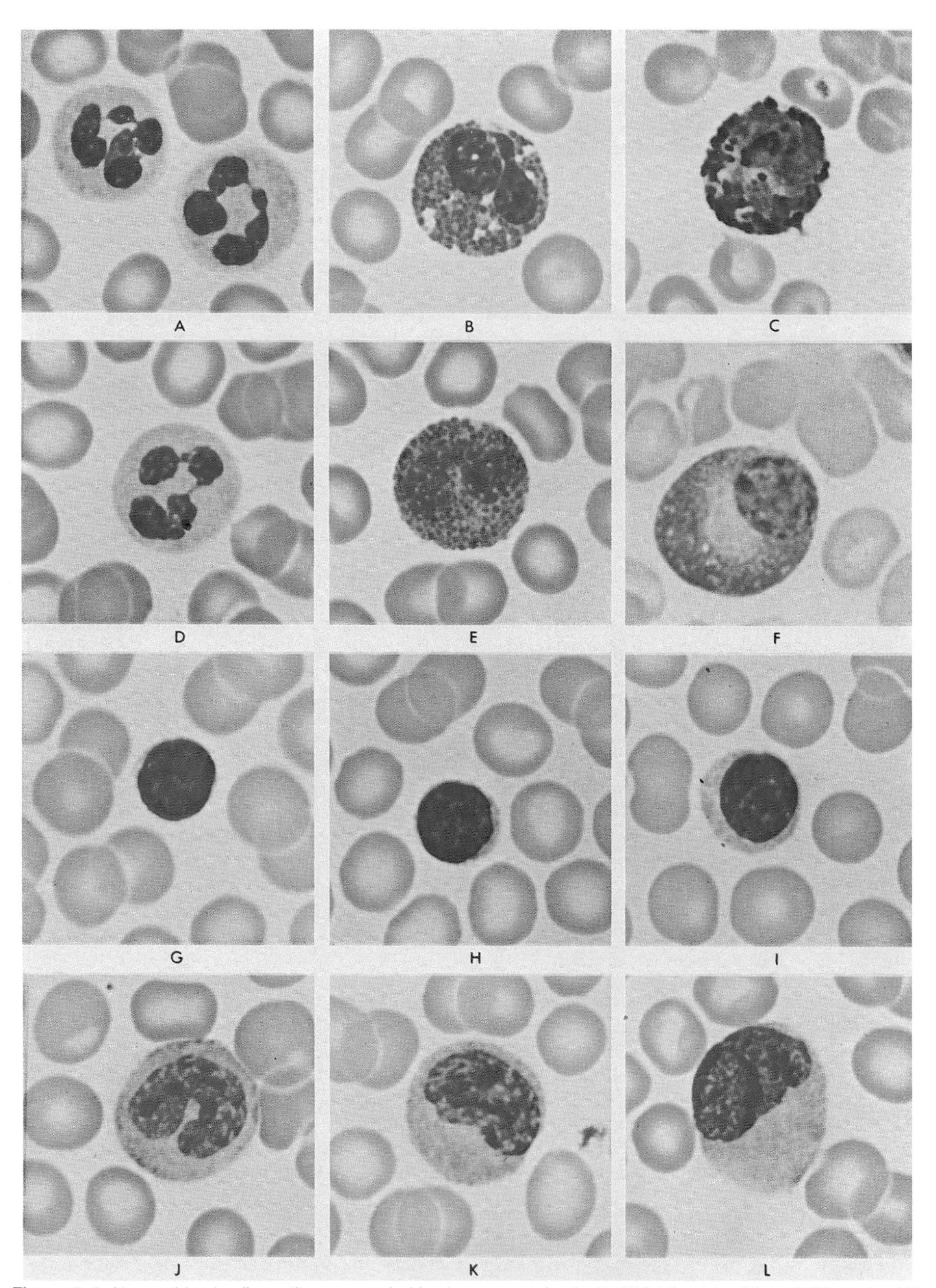

Figure 4–4. Human blood cells as they appear in blood smears stained with Wright's stain; (A) and (D) neutrophilic leukocytes; (B) and (E) eosinophilic leukocytes; (C) basophilic leukocyte; (F) plasma cell. This is not a normal constituent of the peripheral blood but is included here for comparison with the nongranular leukocytes; (G) and (H) small lymphocytes; (I) medium lymphocyte; (J)–(L) monocytes.

kind of globin chain is determined by a separate genetic locus. A great variety of inherited disorders of hemoglobin synthesis involve relatively minor amino-acid substitutions which, nevertheless, have profound physiological effects. For example, *hemoglobin S* (HbS), associated with *sickle cell anemia*, differs only in the substitution of valine for glutamine at one site on the β-chain, but this is enough to make this hemoglobin less soluble and it forms long tactoids that deform the erythrocytes into bizarre sickle shapes. These erythrocytes tend to block capillaries. They are also prone to hemolysis.

ULTRASTRUCTURE OF ERYTHROCYTES

The biconcave shape of the erythrocyte is clearly revealed in scanning electron micrographs (Fig. 4–1) and in thin sections (Fig. 4–2). The plasma membrane is a typical lipid bilayer containing various integral protein particles. In the interior, cell organelles are lacking, but there is a moderately dense homogeneous content which, at high magnification, has a granular texture, attributable to the molecules of hemoglobin. Immediately beneath the membrane, there is a two-dimensional network of short filaments. This *membrane skeleton* is composed of *spectrin, actin*, and two associated proteins designated only on the basis of their electrophoretic mobility in gels (band 4.1 and band 4.9 proteins). The major component of this flexible subplasmalemmal network is spectrin, a heterodimer of α- and β-polypeptide chains (100 nm) bound end-to-end to form double-stranded tetramers about 200 nm in length. These are bound at their ends to nodal structures consisting of actin and two other proteins (band 1 and band 4.9), forming a close-meshed network. Near the middle of each spectrin tetramer, there is a binding site for *ankyrin*, a phosphoprotein that serves to link the network to the cytoplasmic domain of a transmembrane protein (band 3). The actin of erythrocytes does not form visible filaments as it does in the cytoskeleton of other cell types, but forms short polymers 7 nm in length stabilized by *tropomyosin*. These are components of the nodal complexes that join the ends of the spectrin filaments to form a network.

These details of the molecular architecture of the membrane skeleton may seen beyond the scope of a textbook of histology, but they influence the form of the erythrocyte and recently have acquired clinical significance in helping to explain the abnormalities observed in certain anemias of humans, including *hereditary spherocytosis* and *hereditary ellipsocytosis*. These patients are found to have deficiencies of spectrin or defective binding of spectrin to the integral proteins of the membrane, resulting in varying degrees of instability of the erythrocyte membrane.

In their 120-day life span, erythrocytes must be able to withstand frequent deformations during thousands of passages through the vascular system. Their membrane skeleton provides the necessary stability and resilience. Because erythrocytes are readily available in quantity, and their membranes can easily be isolated after hemolysis, we know more about the components of their membrane skeleton than we do about the subplasmalemmal cytoskeleton of any other cell type. It is becoming apparent, however, that these findings have broader relevance because proteins closely related to spectrin, ankyrin, and band 4 are now being found in association with the membranes of other more complex cell types.

SURFACE ANTIGENS AND BLOOD GROUPS

The carbohydrate chains of the glycolipids and glycoproteins in the human erythrocyte membrane contain a number of antigenic determinants that can trigger severe immune reactions. Two of these are of clinical significance, in relation to blood transfusion, and are the basis of the *ABO blood-group system*. The erythrocytes of some individuals have antigen-A on their membrane, some have antigen-B, others have both A and B, and still others have neither of these antigens. Thus, there are four major blood-groups: A, B, AB, and O. For reasons that are not clear, nearly all individuals have, in their blood plasma, antibodies against certain of the antigens that do not occur on their own erythrocytes. Therefore, before giving a transfusion, it is necessary to determine what antigens occur on the erythrocytes of the blood donor and what antibodies are present in the plasma of the recipient. Failure to carry out this cross-matching may result in massive intravascular agglutination and lysis of erythrocytes in the recipient of the transfusion.

Another immunogen that may have undesirable effects is the *Rh-antigen*. Antibodies to Rh do not develop spontaneously, as they do for antigen of the ABO system, but if an Rh-negative individual receives a transfusion of Rh-positive blood, any subsequent transfusion of Rh-positive blood may have serious consequences. Moreover, if an Rh-negative woman is carrying an Rh-positive fetus, she may produce antibodies that can cross the placenta and cause hemolytic disease of the newborn.

BLOOD PLATELETS

The *blood platelets* or *thromboplastids* are minute, colorless, anucleate corpuscles found in the blood of all mammals. They function in the clotting of blood at sites of injury to blood vessels and serve to protect the organism against excessive blood loss. Their functional equivalents in lower vertebrates are nucleated cells called *thrombocytes*.

The platelets are thin biconvex discs, 2–3 μm in diameter, which are round or ovoid when viewed on the flat and fusiform when seen in profile (Fig. 4–5). In the human, their number ranges from 150,000 to 350,000 per cubic millimeter of blood. In stained blood smears, they exhibit two concentric zones: a thin pale-blue peripheral zone called the *hyalomere* and a thicker central region called the *granulomere*, which contains small azurophilic granules. In electron micrographs, the hyalomere is electron-lucent and contains no organelles. In equatorial sections, its most conspicuous structural element is a circumferential bundle of 10–15 microtubules near the plasma membrane (Fig. 4–6B). In transverse sections, the bundle of microtubules is seen as a cluster of small circular profiles at either end of the platelet (Fig. 4–6A). This ring of microtubules beneath the membrane serves to maintain the discoid form of the platelet.

Platelets arise in the bone marrow by fragmentation of the cytoplasm of very large nucleated cells called *megakaryocytes*. They are continuously formed and released into the blood, where they have a life span of 9 to 10 days. Despite their lack of a nucleus and inability to synthesize proteins, they are able to carry out many of the activities of complete cells. They consume oxygen and have an active metabolism that depends on the energy-generating enzymes of the one or two small mitochondria in their cytoplasm. Their azurophilic granules store substances that were synthesized in the megakaryocyte prior to their release.

Platelets have, in their hyaloplasm, a greater concentration of actin and myosin than any cell type, other than muscle. In circulating platelets, these are present mainly in monomeric form, but activation of platelets during the clotting process seems to initiate polymer-

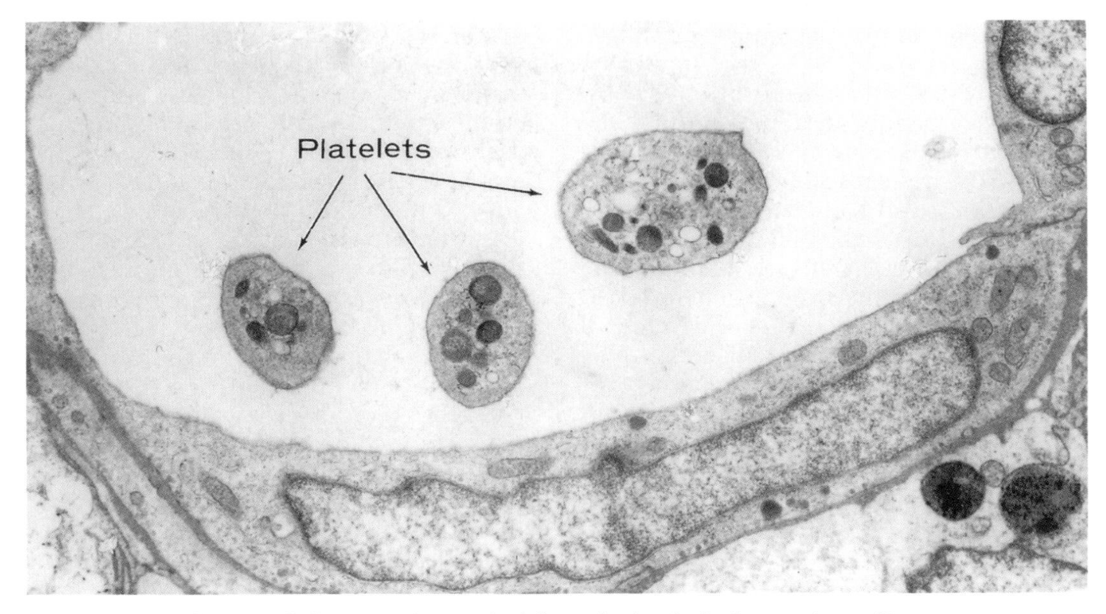

Figure 4–5. Electron micrograph of three platelets in the lumen of a capillary.

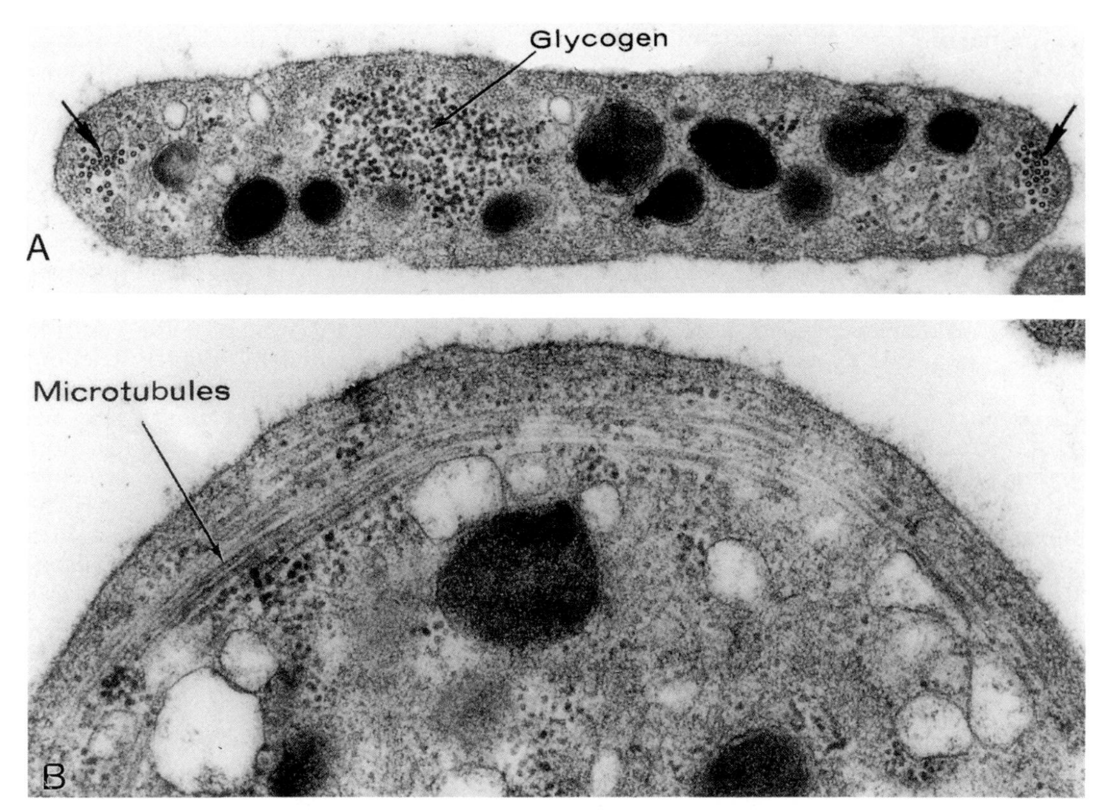

Figure 4–6. (A) Micrograph of a platelet sectioned transversely, showing its dense secretory granules and an aggregation of glycogen particles. At the arrows are cross sections of the circumferential bundle of microtubules. (B) A platelet sectioned parallel to its broad dimension. Here, the bundle of microtubules is seen in longitudinal section. (Micrograph courtesy of O. Behnke.)

ization of actin and myosin into the filamentous form necessary for contraction.

The granulomere of the platelet contains a few ribosomes and scattered particles of glycogen. There are also round or elongated membrane-bounded profiles that represent sections of small *canaliculi* that open at 10 or more sites on the surface. These are believed to be a major pathway for the uptake of solutes and discharge of secretory products upon activation of the platelets. In addition to the canaliculi, there may be a system of slender anastomosing tubules that have a content of moderate density. These are interpreted as residues of the endoplasmic reticulum of the megakaryocyte and are probably of no functional significance in the platelet.

Varying numbers of membrane-bounded granules, about 0.2 μm in diameter, are a conspicuous feature of the granulomere. These *alpha granules* contain several biologically active substances, including: (1) *platelet factor-IV*, which counteracts the anticoagulant heparin; (2) *von Willebrand factor*, a glycoprotein that facilitates adhesion of platelets to the vessel wall; (3) *platelet-derived growth factor* that stimulates fibroblast proliferation, thus contributing to repair after damage to blood vessels; and (4) *thrombospondin*, another glycoprotein involved in platelet aggregation in blood clotting. In some species other than man, there is a second category of granule, called *beta granules*. These contain *serotonin, adenosinetriphosphate* (ATP), and *adenosinediphosphate*, all potent promoters of platelet aggregation.

FUNCTION OF PLATELETS

Circulating platelets constantly patrol the vascular system. They normally exhibit no tendency to adhere to each other, to other blood cells, or to the vessel wall, but if any disruption of the endothelium is detected, they become sticky and rapidly adhere to one another and to the site of injury to initiate a blood clotting that limits blood loss and begins the process of repair. The magnitude of their defensive mission is evident from the reckoning that, during each minute of circulation time, approximately 10^{12} platelets pass over 1000 m^2 of capillary surface, lined by 7×10^{11} endothelial cells. Their adhesive property is expressed in vitro by their sticking to glass, plastic, and other solid substrates. In common usage, the term *platelet adhesion* is defined as the sticking of platelets to solid surfaces, and *platelet aggregation* is their sticking to each other.

Where the continuity of the endothelium is interrupted, exposing the underlying connective tissue, platelets quickly adhere to the collagen via a collagen-binding protein in their membrane. Adhesion *activates* the platelets resulting in breakdown of ATP and release of ADP and adhesive glycoproteins into their immediate environment. ADP is a potent inducer of platelet aggregation, inducing them to adhere, in increasing numbers, to those already adhering to collagen. These new platelets, in turn, are activated, contributing to continuing aggregation to form a coherent mass called a *platelet thrombus*.

Concurrent with these events, other complex reactions of clotting are set in motion. A substance called *tissue thromboplastin*, released by injured endothelial cells, initiates a series of reactions in the blood plasma that converts *prothrombin* to *thrombin*. Thrombin, in turn, catalyzes the conversion of *fibrinogen* to *fibrin* which polymerizes to form a meshwork of fine cross-striated fibrils. These bind to specific receptors on the membrane of the platelets, helping to bind them together and, at the same time, entrapping numerous erythrocytes in the fibrin meshwork to form a gelatinous *blood clot* (Fig. 4–7).

Clotting is a very complicated process. When platelets are activated, they undergo dramatic morphological changes, extending numerous slender processes, and releasing their α-granules. An adhesive protein called *thrombospondin*, released from their granules, binds to their membrane, promoting further platelet aggregation. Phospholipids released during degranulation reacts with plasma components to generate *platelet thromboplastin*, and platelet cyclo-oxygenase enzymes convert prostaglandin endoperoxides to *thromboxane*. The products of both of these reactions accelerate clotting. It has now been found that the platelet cyclo-oxygenase enzymes can be irreversibly inactivated by aspirin in low concentrations. This prevents the synthesis of thromboxane for the remainder of the life of the platelet. Clinicians now take advantage of this in certain cardiac patients to diminish the risk of coronary thrombosis.

Within an hour after formation of a clot, it shrinks to about half its original size. This is attributed to polymerization of actin and myosin monomers to form filaments that interact in contraction. The hemostasis achieved by occlusion of the lumen of the vessel by a clot is supplemented by vasoconstriction of the injured vessel. In nonhuman species, serotonin released from the beta granules of activated platelets also stimulates contraction of smooth muscle in the wall of the vessel. The complex process of blood coagulation involves the interaction of 12 or more plasma factors in addition to those produced by the platelets.

In recent years, there has been increasing interest in a group of growth-promoting factors that make an important contribution to tissue repair by stimulating cell migration and proliferation. One of the first of these to be identified was the *platelet-derived growth factor* (PDGF). The term is unfortunate because this factor has since been found to be secreted by monocytes, macrophages, and endothelial cells as well as platelets. It is a cationic protein of about 30,000 molecular weight and is a mitogen for cells of connective tissue origin. It is responsible for much of the mitogenic activity of blood serum on cells in tissue culture. It is synthesized in the megakaryocytes in the bone marrow and reaches the blood in the alpha granules of the platelets. When platelets are exposed to thrombin or ADP during blood clotting or to collagen at sites of injury, they release this growth factor. It induces a chemotactic response in fibroblasts and smooth muscle cells attracting them to the site of injury and stimulating their proliferation to initiate the repair process.

Inherited abnormalities of platelets or deficiencies of plasma factors are responsible for several human diseases. The best known is *hemophilia*, a serious bleeding disorder that occurs in about 1 in 10,000 males in the population. It is due to the absence of just one of the many plasma factors necessary for clotting. Defects attributable to platelets include a deficiency in their production *thrombocytopenia* or abnormalities in their structure and function *thrombocytopathia*. In one such inherited disease, *thrombocytopenic purpura*, a defect in platelet production is linked to abnormal fragility of the small blood vessels resulting in sponta-

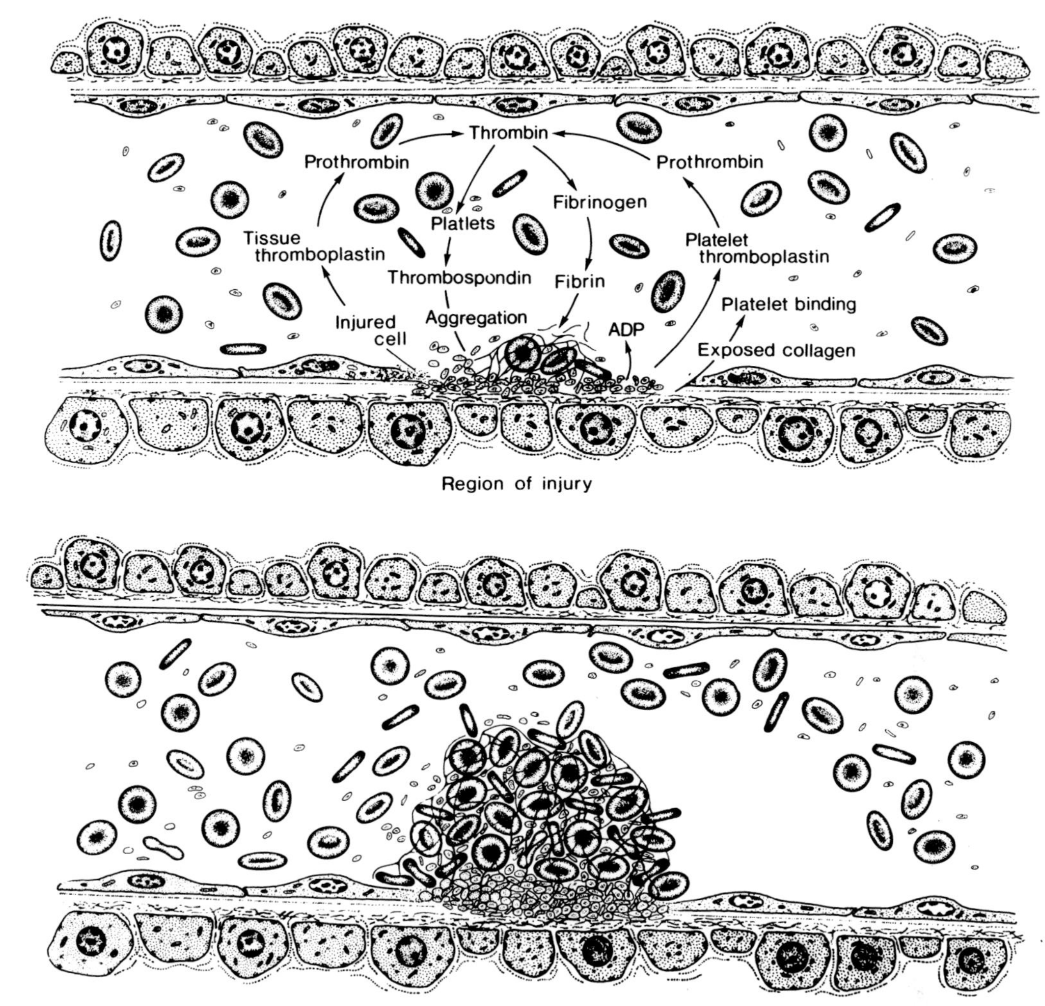

Figure 4–7. (A) Schematic representation of the events in formation of a blood clot in an injured vessel. Platelets adhere to the site of injury and release ADP and adhesive glycoproteins that accelerate platelet aggregation. Tissue thromboplastin released from injured cells induces conversion of plasma prothrombin to thrombin. This catalyzes conversion of fibrinogen to fibrin which polymerizes to form fibers enmeshing the platelets and impounding erythrocytes in a gelatinous clot. (B) A later stage in the process of clot formation.

neous capillary bleeding manifested by black-and-blue areas over the surface of the body.

LEUKOCYTES

The several kinds of white blood cells, collectively called *leukocytes*, have a nucleus and are colorless in the fresh state. They are spherical in the bloodstream but are pleomorphic amoeboid cells in the tissues, or on a solid substrate, in vitro. They are classified as *granular leukocytes* or *nongranular leukocytes*, depending on whether they do or do not have specific granules in their cytoplasm. The granular leukocytes are identified as *eosinophils, basophils*, and *neutrophils* on the basis of the affinity of their granules for the dyes in the Romanovsky stains commonly used for blood smears. The nongranular leukocytes include the *lymphocytes* and the *monocytes*. All leukocytes have a single nucleus, but in the clinical literature, the nongranular leukocytes are sometimes referred to as "mononuclear leukocytes," a regrettable contraction of the term monomorphonuclear leukocyte, which was intended to distinguish them from the polymorphonuclear cells (neutrophils) in which the single nucleus has a variable number of lobes.

The number of leukocytes in the circulation ranges from 5000 to 9000 per cubic millimeter of blood, but this number is subject to some variation with age, and even at different times of day. The number in the tissues and organs, where they carry out their functions, is very large but cannot be quantitated. Minor variations in the white cell count are of little clinical significance, but in the presence of an infection anywhere in the body, the blood leukocyte count may rise to 20,000 or even 40,000 per cubic millimeter. The relative numbers of the several types of leukocyte, called the *differential leukocyte count*, is normally fairly constant: neutrophils 55–60%; eosinophils 1–3%; basophils 0–0.7%; lymphocytes 25–33%; and monocytes 3–7%. Different disease processes affect the numbers of some cell types more than others and the differential count is often helpful in diagnosis.

NEUTROPHILIC LEUKOCYTES

Neutrophils are the most abundant of the granular leukocytes. In absolute numbers, there are 3000–6000 per milliliter, or 20–30 billion in the entire circulation at any one time. They remain in the blood for only about 8 h before migrating out of the vessels and into the tissues, where they carry out their mission and die. They are 7 μm in diameter in the blood, and 10–12 μm in diameter in dried blood smears. They are easily recognized by their characteristic nucleus, consisting of two or more lobules connected by narrow constrictions (Fig. 4–8). The number of nuclear lobes depends, in part, on their age. When first released from the bone marrow into the blood, their nucleus has a simple ovoid or elongated form. Such young cells are described as "band forms." A local constriction later develops, resulting in a bilobed nucleus. The process of nuclear elongation and constriction continues until, in older neutrophils, there may be five or more segments or lobes. The number of band forms in the differential count is a useful index of the rate of entry of new neutrophils into the blood. Their variability in nuclear form is the basis for the other name applied to this cell type—*polymorphonuclear leukocyte*. The chromatin of the nucleus is in deeply staining clumps at the periphery and a nucleolus usually cannot be identified. In the neutrophils of females, the chromatin representing the condensed X-chromosomes may form an additional minute lobule, often referred to as "the drumstick" owing to its characteristic shape (Fig. 4–8A). It is possible, in a blood smear, to determine the genetic sex of the individual by examining a large number of neutrophils for the presence of this nuclear appendage.

In a stained blood smear, the cytoplasm of the neutrophils is stippled with very fine *specific granules* that have little affinity for dyes and somewhat larger *azurophilic granules* that stain more deeply (Fig. 4–9). The granules are larger in neutrophils of the guinea pig and rabbit than they are in the human. Owing to the larger size of the granules in these species and their affinity for eosin, these cells are sometimes called *pseudoeosinophils* in the literature of hematology.

In electron micrographs, the neutrophil granules are widely distributed in the cytoplasm but tend to be excluded from the thin zone of ectoplasm that is rich in actin filaments involved in the amoeboid motility of these cells. The two types of granules are not easily distinguished in human neutrophils, but specific granules are slightly elongated, resembling rice grains, and the azurophil granules are slightly larger and more electron-dense. The two types can best be distinguished by cytochemical staining methods. The azurophil granules give a positive reaction for the enzymes *peroxidase, acid phosphatase*, and *β-glucuronidase* and are considered to correspond to the lysosomes of other cell types. The specific granules lack these lysosomal hydrolases but give a positive reaction for *alkaline-phosphatase, collagenase, lysozyme, lactoferritin*, and several poorly characterized basic proteins collectively called *phagocytins*. These latter are believed to have nonenzymatic antibacterial activity.

The neutrophils are the body's first line of defense against invasion by bacteria. A chemical mediator released at a site of infection is carried in the blood to the bone marrow, where it induces increased production and release of neutrophils into the blood. Many of these then adhere to the wall of postcapillary venules at the site of infection and migrate between endothelial cells into the surrounding connective tissue. Exposed there to low concentrations of bacteria products, their cytoskeletons reorganizes and become polarized for migration up the concentration gradient of the chemoattractant. This is called *chemotaxis*. When they reach the region of maximum concentration of the chemoattractant in the immediate vicinity of the bacteria, they cease to migrate and become avidly phagocytic (Fig. 4–10). Pseudopods are ex-

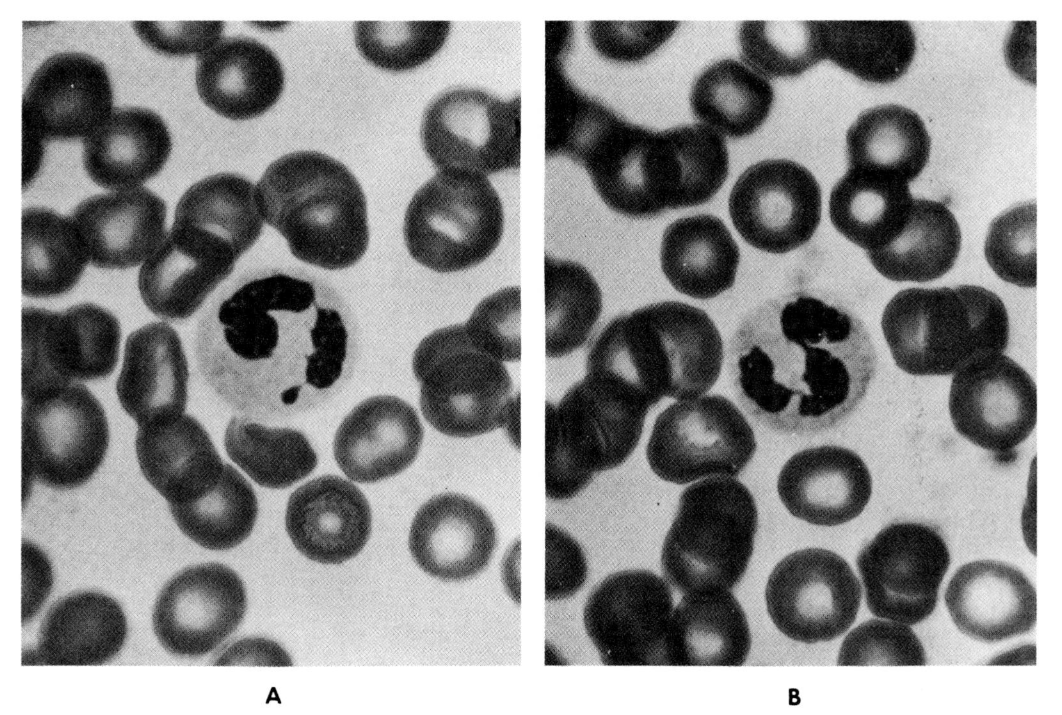

Figure 4–8. (A) Photomicrograph of a blood smear including a neutrophilic leukocyte from a female. Note the "drumstick" nuclear appendage characteristic of the female. (B) A comparable field of a blood smear from a male.

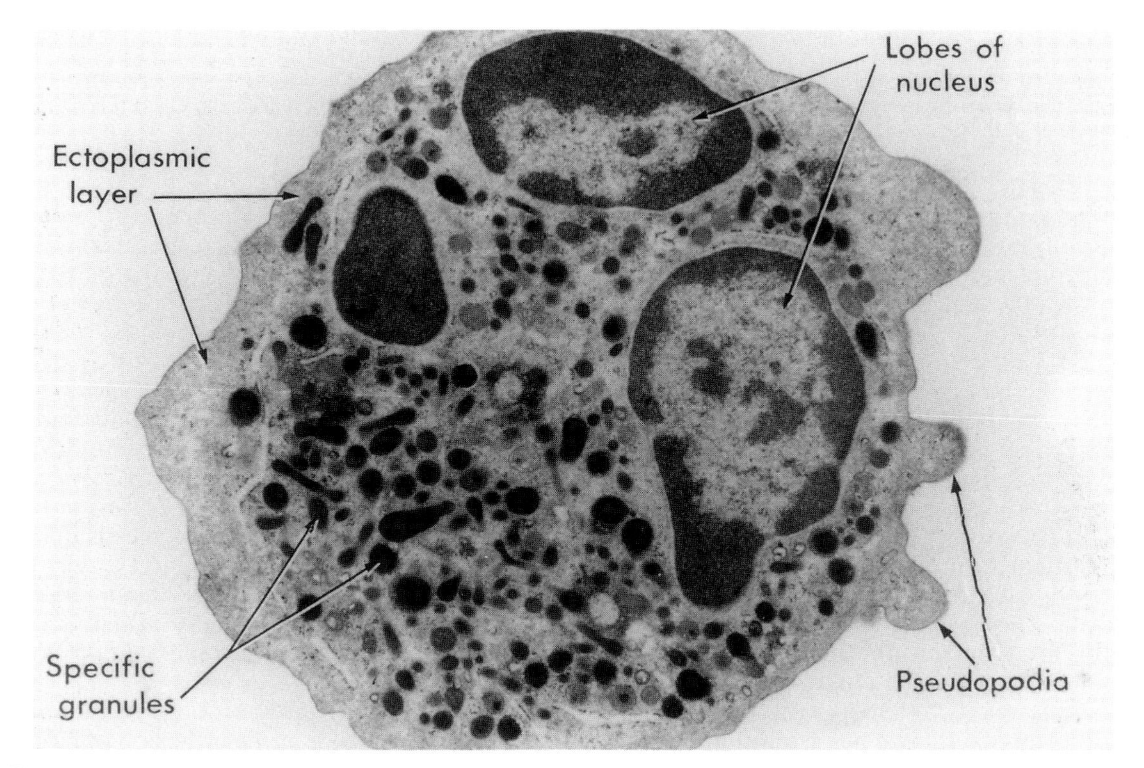

Figure 4–9. Electron micrograph of a guinea pig polymorphonuclear leukocyte. The three lobules of the nucleus appear separate in this plane of section but are, in fact, continuous. The cytoplasm contains specific granules of varying shape. There is a thin ectoplasmic zone of cytoplasm rich in actin which is important in pseudopod formation and in the amoeboid locomotion of the cell.

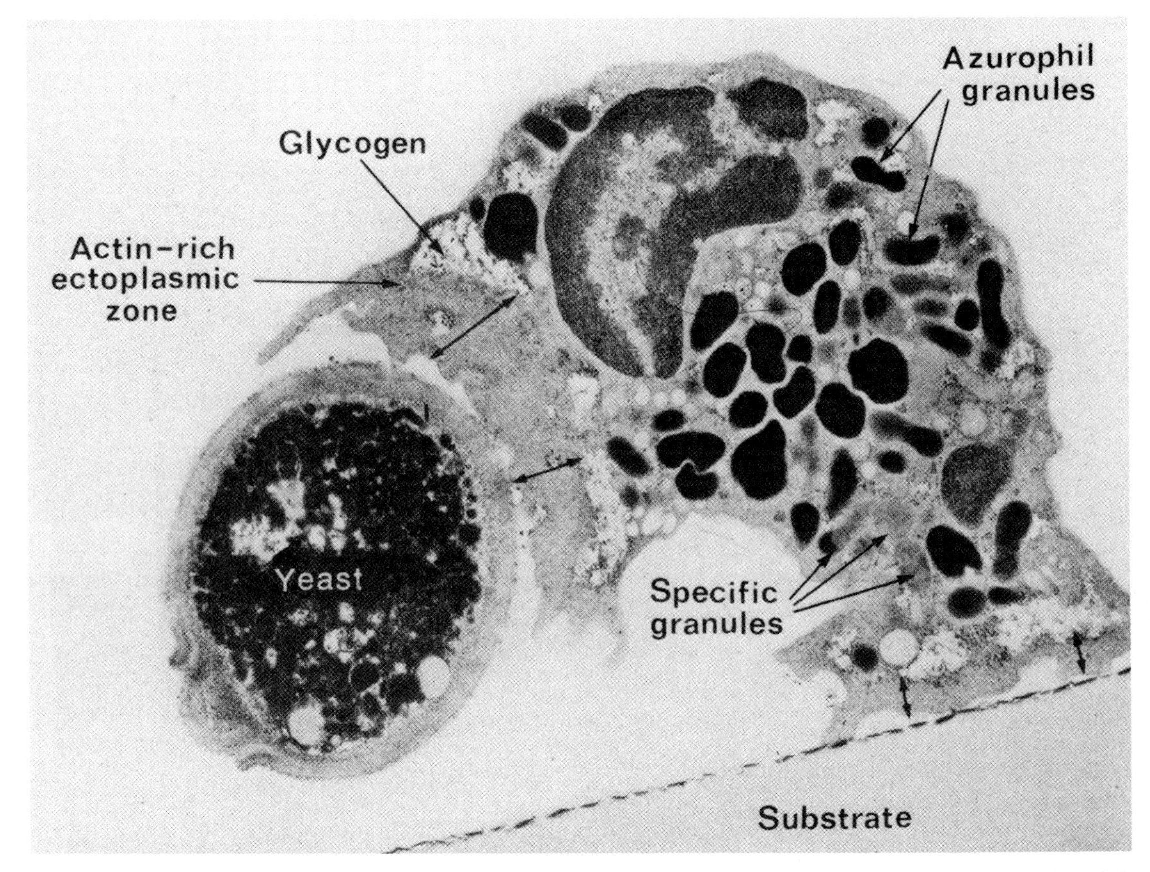

Figure 4–10. Electron micrograph of a neutrophil beginning to phagocytize a yeast in vitro. Note the thickening of the ectoplasmic zone (double arrows) and the extension of lamellipodia in the region of contact with the organism. (Micrograph courtesy of D. Bainton.)

tended around a bacterium and it is taken into the cytoplasm in a large vacuole (Fig. 4–11). Azurophil and specific granules then fuse with the vacuole, discharging their hydrolytic enzymes into it to destroy the bacterium (Fig. 4–12). The *pus* that accumulates at sites of infection consists of hundreds of thousands of dying and dead neutrophils and other leukocytes that have completed their mission.

The ingestion and destruction of bacteria by neutrophils is more efficient if the individual has previously been invaded by the same kind of bacterium and has developed specific antibodies to its surface antigens. In what is called *immune phagocytosis,* a blood-borne antibody (IgG) binds to the surface of the bacterium and a complement component of the blood plasma (C_3b) binds to the antigen–antibody complex. There are receptors for IgG and C_3b in the membrane of the neutrophil and these serve as ligands promoting adherence of the bacterium to its surface, thereby facilitating phagocytosis. Plasma components, such as IgG and C_3b, that coat bacteria and increase the efficiency of phagocytosis are referred to collectively as *opsonins.* When neutrophils phagocytize and digest cellular debris and particulate matter without the aid of opsonins, this is called *nonspecific phagocytosis.*

Adherence of neutrophils to capillary endothelium at sites of infection is attributed to a protein in their membrane called *leukocyte cell adhesion molecule-1* (LCAM-1), but this is not solely responsible. Other activated cells in the area release cytokines, such as interleukin-1β (IL-1β), and tumor necrosis factor alpha (TNF-α), that stimulate the endothelial cells to synthesize and insert into their membrane *endothelial leukocyte adhesion molecule-1* (ELAM-1). Thus, the neutrophils and the endothelial cells both participate in the adhesion of circulating cells so that they can leave the vessels to combat a bacterial invasion.

In addition to their assault on bacteria, neu-

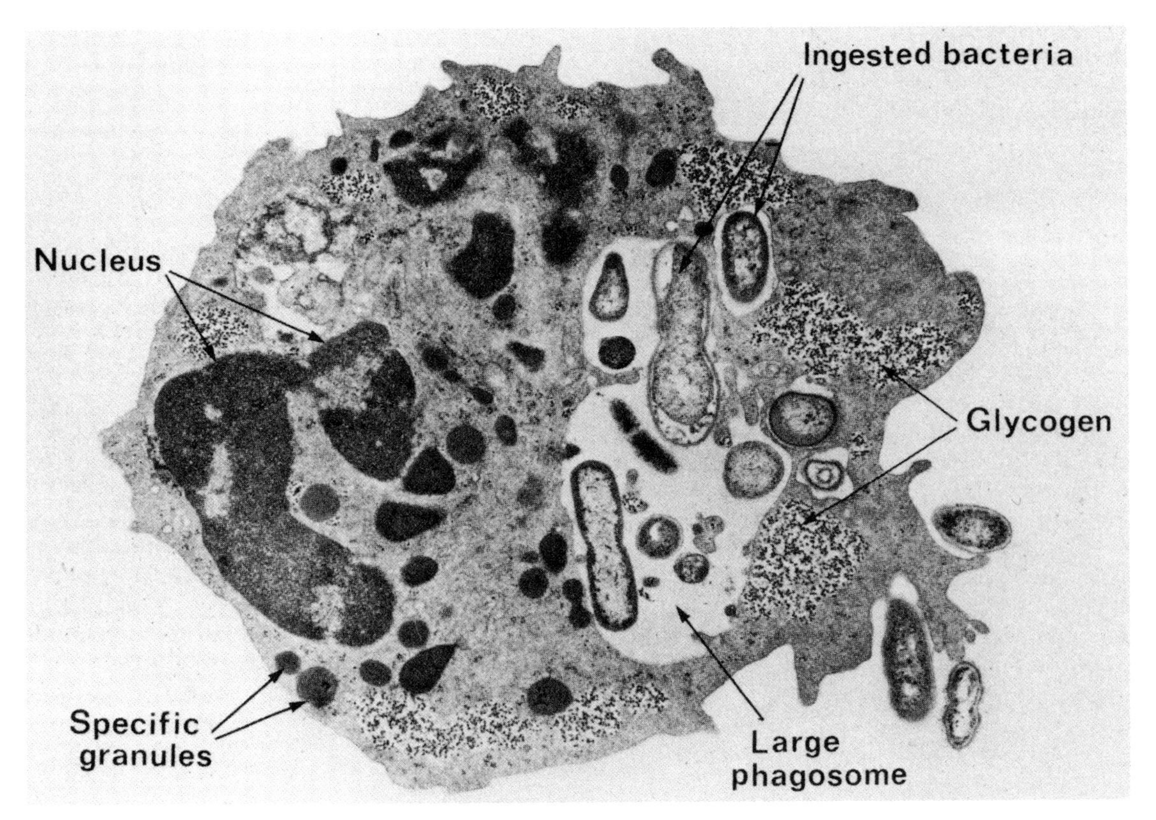

Figure 4–11. Micrograph of a neutrophil that has phagocytized several bacteria. The bacteria in the large vacuole show signs of incipient degeneration in this bacteriostatic and hydrolytic environment. (Micrograph courtesy of D. Bainton.)

trophils and certain other phagocytic cells generate compounds that contribute in other ways to the inflammatory process. From arachidonic acid in their plasma membrane, they synthesize a group of compounds called *leukotrienes* (LTs). Alphabetically, these are designated LTA_4, LTB_4, LTC_4, LTD_4, and LTE_4. Leukotriene B_4 promotes adhesion of neutrophils to endothelium and their emigration into the tissues. It is also a chemoattractant for eosinophils, monocytes, and other neutrophils and, thus, participates in the recruitment of such cells to sites of infection. The cysteine-containing leukotrienes LTC_4, LTD_4, and LTE_4 increase the permeability of postcapillary venules contributing to the edema and swelling at sites of inflammation. These leukotrienes are also potent vasoconstrictors that are responsible for much of the respiratory distress suffered by persons with asthma. Drugs blocking the synthesis of leukotrienes promise to be effective in preventing the constriction of bronchi and bronchioles that occurs when asthmatics are exposed to antigens to which they are hypersensitive.

EOSINOPHIL LEUKOCYTES

Eosinophils enter the blood from the bone marrow and circulate for only 6–10 h before migrating into the connective tissues, where they spend the rest of their 8–12-day life span. Eosinophils make up only 1–3% of the blood leukocytes and it is estimated that for every one in the blood there are 300 in the tissues. They are 9 μm in diameter in suspension, and about 12 μm in diameter in blood smears. They are easily distinguished from neutrophils by their large specific granules which stain pink with the eosin in Wright's blood stain (Fig. 4–4B and E). Their nucleus is less segmented and the chromatin less coarse than that of neutrophils. In the human, the nucleus is bilobed, and in the rat it is annular. A small Golgi complex and a few mitochondria are found around a granule-free cell center containing a pair of centrioles. There is very little endoplasmic reticulum. The specific granules are the most conspicuous feature of the cytoplasm. These exhibit a rather striking interspecific variation in their ultrastructure. In

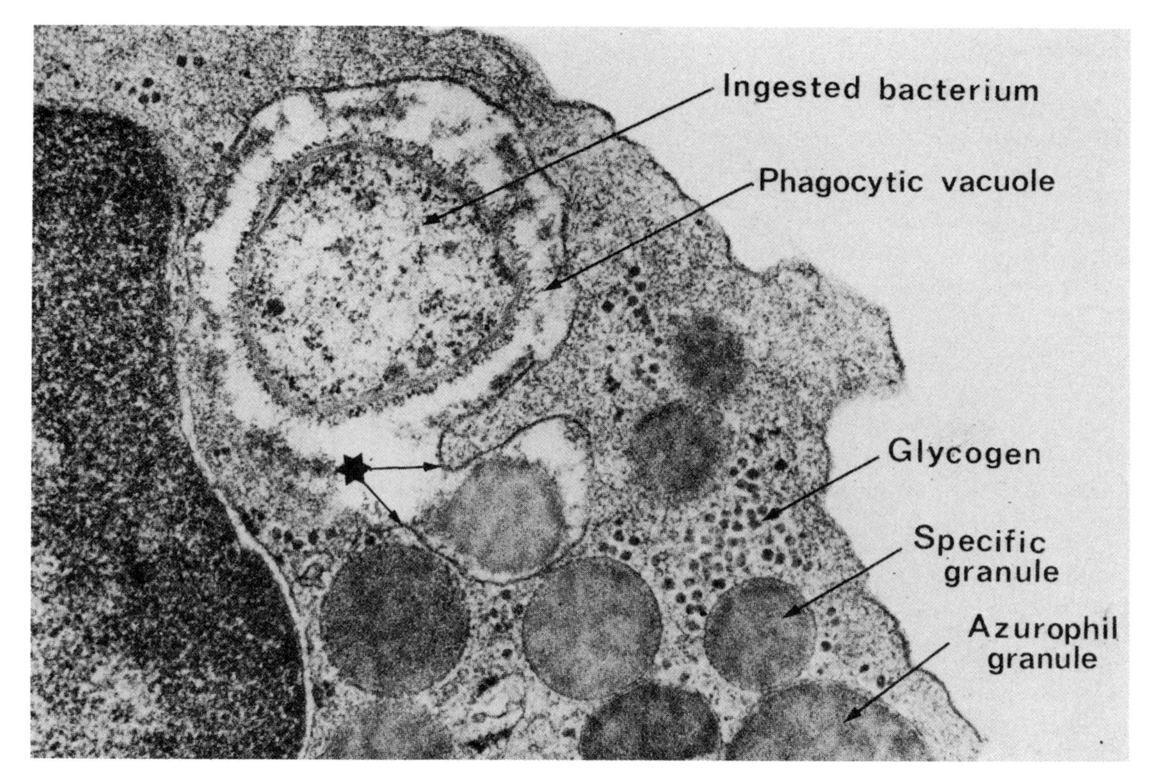

Figure 4–12. Micrograph of a portion of a neutrophil that has recently phagocytized a bacterium. Arrows from * indicate sites of continuity of the membrane of the phagosome with that of a granule about to discharge its contents into the phagosome. (Micrograph from D. Bainton. *In* R.C. Williams and H.H. Fudenberg, eds. Phagocytic Mechanisms in Health and Disease. New York, Intercontinental Medical Book Corp.)

the laboratory rodents, each granule contains a disc-like equatorial crystal (Fig. 4–13). In the cat, the granules have a single, dense, cylindrical inclusion that has a concentric lamellar substructure when viewed at high magnification. In humans, the granules contain single or multiple crystals of varying shape. In all species, these inclusions are embedded in an amorphous, or finely granular, matrix and enclosed in a membrane. The eosinophils also contain a few small azurophil granules.

Eosinophil granules contain several of the lysosomal hydrolases, including aryl sulfatase, β-glucuronidase, acid phosphatase, histaminase, and ribonuclease. In addition, they contain three cationic proteins not found in lysosomes of other cell types. These are *major basophilic protein* (MBP), *eosinophil cationic protein* (ECP), and *eosinophil-derived neurotoxin.* The significance of these proteins is still under investigation, but they are believed to be important in the role of eosinophils in allergic reactions and in defense against parasites. In both of these conditions, the number of circulating eosinophils is greatly increased. MBP and ECP are both quite damaging to the schistosomula of *Schistosoma mansoni*, to the larvae of *Trypanosoma cruzi*, and to many mammalian cells as well. Their cytotoxic effects appear to include the creation of transmembrane pores in the target cells and the release of superoxide ions and hydrogen peroxide that damage membranes by lipid peroxidation. Eosinophil-derived neurotoxin was so named because it induces a paralytic syndrome when injected into the cerebrospinal fluid of guinea pigs. Its role in the normal functioning of eosinophils is not understood.

Eosinophils do not phagocytose bacteria and destroy them intracellarly to any great extent. Although widely distributed in the connective tissue, they are especially numerous beneath the epithelia of the alimentary and respiratory tracts, where entry of foreign proteins is most likely to occur. Eosinophils are involved in damage control in allergic reactions. They are attracted to sites of histamine release and their enzymes are capable of degrading this and other mediators of allergic reactions. Repeated exposure to antigens is

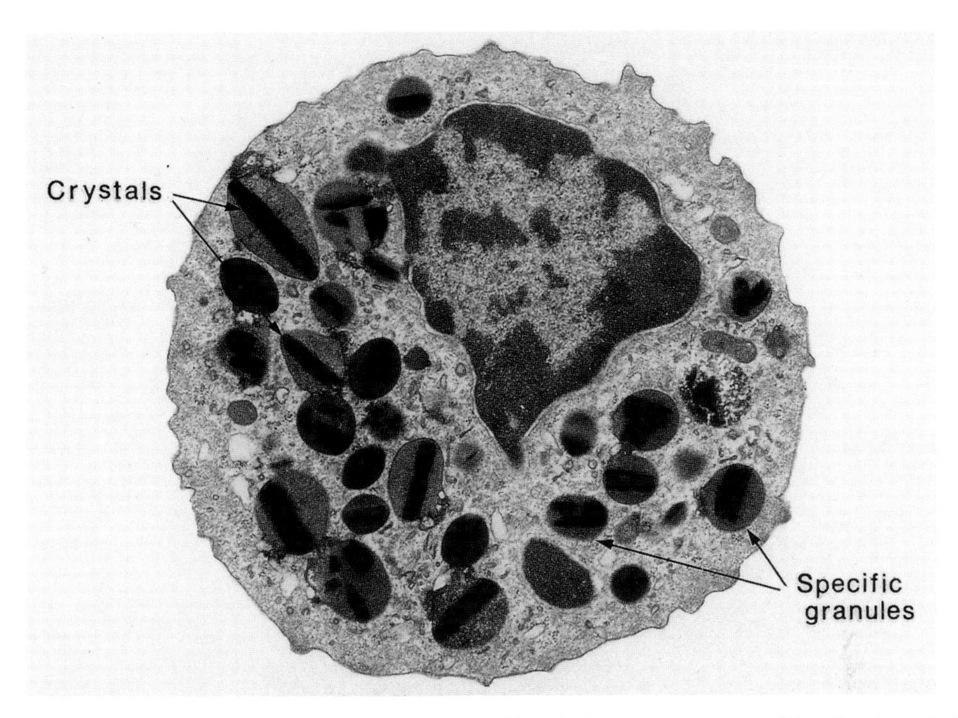

Figure 4–13. Electron micrograph of an eosinophilic leukocyte. Note the large granules containing rhombohedral crystals.

attended by an increase in eosinophils. The factors regulating their release from the bone marrow are poorly understood, but there is some evidence that interleukin-5 and other cytokines released at sites of antigen–antibody interaction stimulate proliferation of precursors and release of eosinophils into the blood. Injections of the hormones adrenocorticotrophin or hydrocortisone result in a marked reduction in circulating eosinophils.

BASOPHIL LEUKOCYTE

The *basophils* are the least numerous of the granular leukocytes, accounting for only 0.5% of the white blood cell count. They are slightly smaller than neutrophils, measuring about 10 μm in diameter in stained blood smears. The nucleus is often U- or J-shaped and may, therefore, appear bilobed in section. The specific granules are relatively few and larger than those of eosinophils (Fig. 4–14). They are metachromatic, staining purple with toluidine blue or alcoholic thionine. In the human, they are partially water-soluble and may be distorted or partially dissolved by aqueous stains, but in dried smears, they are usually preserved. The size, staining, and solubility properties of the granules vary from species to species. In the guinea pig, they are large and insoluble in water but stain only faintly. In the dog, they are small and closely aggregated. In the cat, rat, and mouse, basophils are not found in the blood.

In electron micrographs, the basophils have a small Golgi complex, a few mitochondria, and somewhat more endoplasmic reticulum than other leukocytes. Particles of glycogen may be found in their cytoplasm. The specific granules are round or oval and about 0.5 μm in diameter, with a substructure consisting of dense particles in a less-dense matrix (Fig. 4–14). In some mammalian species, the dense subunits of the granules are arranged in a highly ordered lattice. Basophil granules contain *histamine* and the sulfated mucopolysaccharide *heparin* which is responsible for their metachromatic staining. There is no evidence that they contain any of the common lysosomal hydrolases.

The basophil leukocytes share a number of properties with *mast cells* of the connective tissue. Both have large metachromatic granules containing histamine and heparin. The mast cells are larger and have round nuclei and many more granules. The basophils are short-lived and the mast cells are relatively long-lived. The mast cells are relatively sessile, whereas basophils can be rapidly mobilized

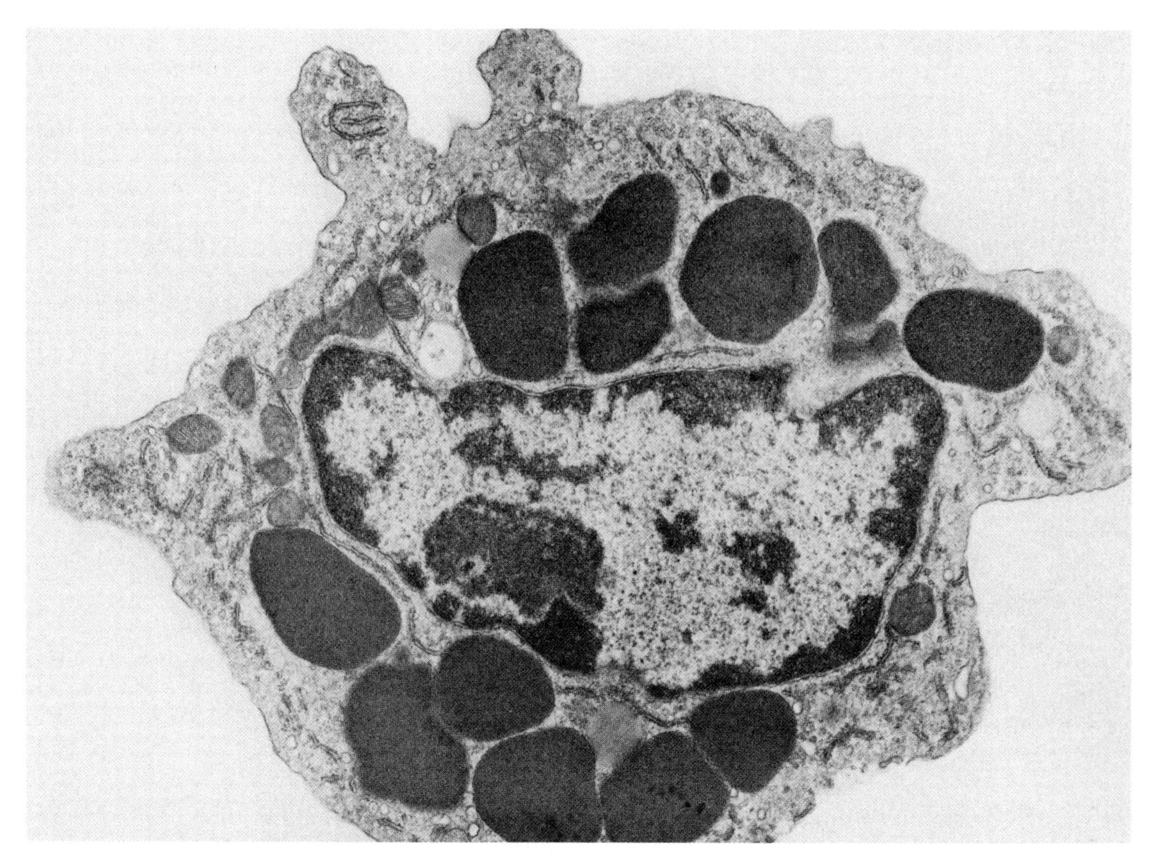

Figure 4–14. Electron micrograph of a basophil leukocyte. The large granules are somewhat irregular in outline and may vary in their electron density.

at sites where they are needed. Both release histamine when they degranulate and they evidently have very similar functions. It is speculated that both may arise from a common bipotential stem cell that gives rise to precursors, some of which enter the blood and become basophils, whereas others migrate into the connective tissue and differentiate into mast cells.

Because basophils make up such a small fraction of the leukocyte count, there is a tendency to consider them relatively unimportant, but the total number in the blood is of the order of 100 million and any condition that causes their rapid degranulation can have serious consequences. In some individuals, certain antigens induce the formation of a distinct class of immunoglobulins (antibodies), designated IgE. Blood basophils have receptors for IgE in their membrane. As such immunoglobulins are formed following exposure to antigen, they accumulate on the surface of the basophils and mast cells. Within minutes after reexposure of that individual to the same antigen, binding of the antigen to the IgE on basophils and mast cells may cause their rapid degranulation, with the release of histamine and other mediators. This may precipitate an asthma attack or urticaria and other cutaneous manifestations of hypersensitivity. Less commonly, massive systemic release of these mediators may result in *anaphylactic shock*, characterized by acute respiratory distress and generalized vascular collapse, culminating in death.

LYMPHOCYTES

Lymphocytes are the second most numerous class of the leukocytes, accounting for 20–35% of the circulating white blood cells. In blood smears, they are small round cells 7–12 μm in diameter, with a deeply staining, slightly, indented nucleus and a thin rim of clear blue cytoplasm (Fig. 4–4H). They contain no specific granules but may have a few small azurophil granules. Studied in electron micrographs, they have a very small Golgi complex, a pair of centrioles, and one or two mitochondria (Figs. 4–15–4–17). The endoplasmic reticulum is virtually absent, but there are many free ribosomes in the cytoplasm.

On the basis of their diameter and relative amount of cytoplasm, lymphocytes are described as *large, medium,* and *small.* These categories were originally believed to represent successive stages in their development from a larger precursor, the *lymphoblast,* located in the marrow. The small lymphocytes were considered to be end stages that survived for only a few days and then degenerated or were eliminated by migration into the lumen of the intestine. When methods were developed for radiolabeling cells to follow their migrations and determine their longevity, these assumptions proved to be erroneous. It was found that there are two major categories of small lymphocytes, *B-lymphocytes* and *T-lymphocytes* that differ in their developmental background, life span, and functions. They are not morphologically distinguishable, but they do have distinctive surface molecules that serve as type-specific markers identifiable by immunocytochemical methods. There is a third heterogeneous category of small lymphocytes that lack identifying surface markers and are referred to collectively as *null cells.*

LYMPHOCYTES AND IMMUNITY

Lymphocytes are the principal agents of the body's *immune responses* and, as such, they will be discussed at length in a later chapter on the *immune system* (Chapter 13). It will suffice here to define immunity and sketch the functions of lymphocytes in broad outline. The immune system provides mechanisms for recognizing invading microorganisms and other foreign matter entering the body and for neutralizing their potentially harmful effects. Any foreign substance capable of inducing an immune response is called an *antigen.* The surface of bacteria contains numerous proteins and polysaccharides that are antigenic. When presented to B-lymphocytes for the first time, an antigen induces the cell to synthesize and insert in its membrane *immunoglobulin* molecules that bear a *recognition site* specific for that antigen. Thereafter, the lymphocyte is irreversibly committed to producing immuno-

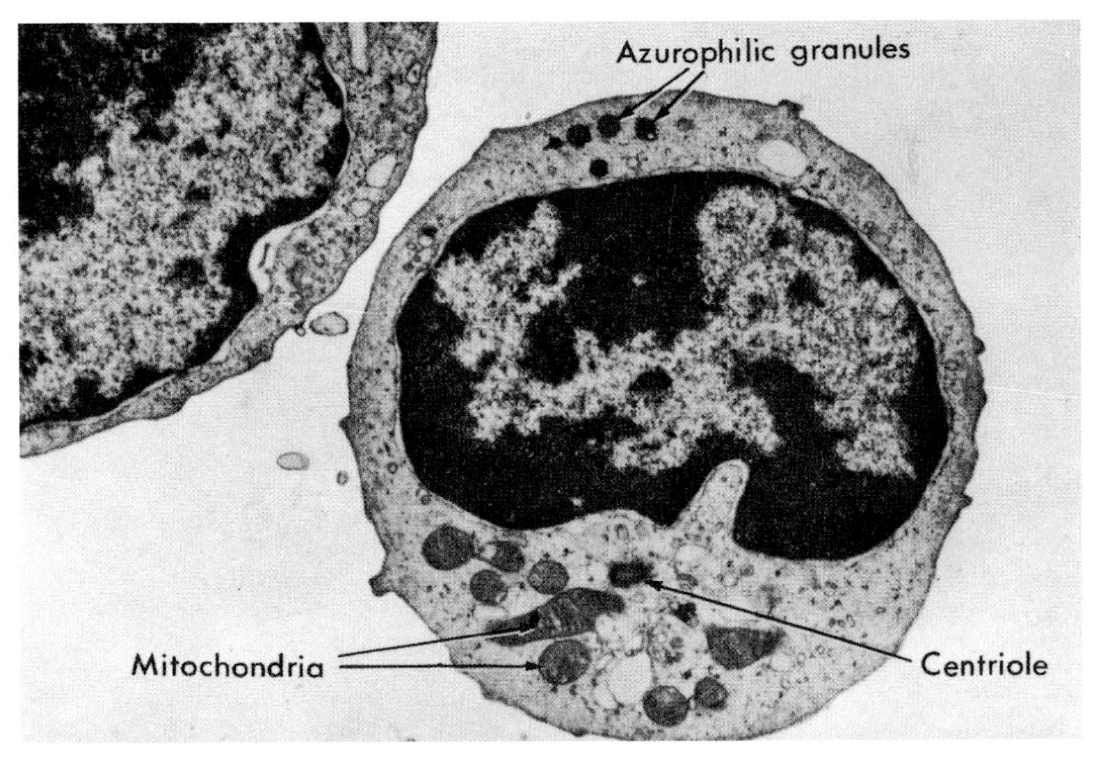

Figure 4–15. Micrograph of a guinea pig lymphocyte. The nucleus is indented and has a coarse pattern of heterochromatin. A centriole and several mitochondria are seen in the cytoplasm. Although it is classified as a nongranular leukocyte, the lymphocyte may contain a few small azurophilic granules.

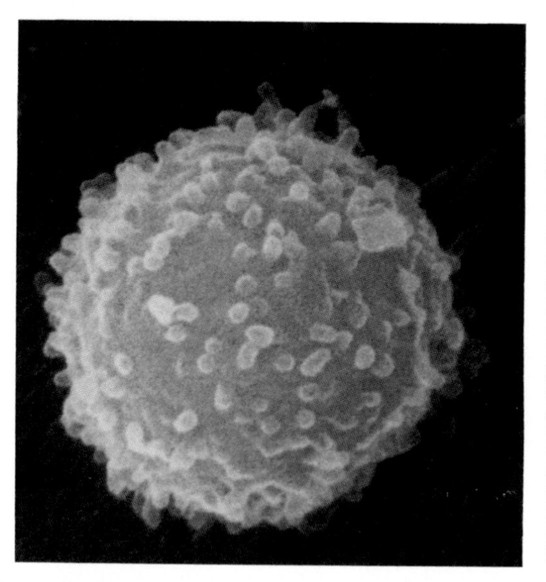

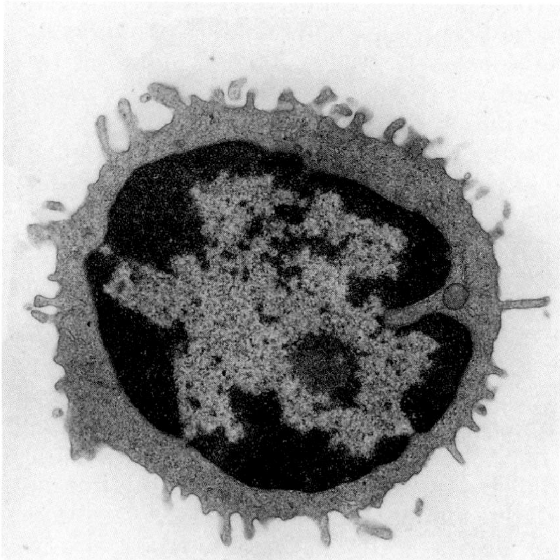

Figure 4–16. Scanning and transmission electron micrographs of a small lymphocyte, showing the numerous short microvilli on its surface.

globulin of the same antigenic specificity. In this *primary immune response,* B-lymphocytes are said to be *antigenically determined* or *programmed.* These cells produce low levels of circulating immunoglobulin (antibody). Because they retain, for a long time, the ability to recognize and respond to the inducing antigen, they are sometimes referred to as "memory cells." Although we consider B-cells to be a single class of lymphocytes, there are actually as many kinds of memory cells as the number of different antigens that have entered the body.

A second exposure to the same antigen, initiates a *secondary immune response* that is rapid in onset and soon raises the titer of circulating antibody to 10 to 100 times the previous level. Small lymphocytes in the circulation, or in the tissues, do not normally divide, but when lymphocytes bearing a specific surface immuno-

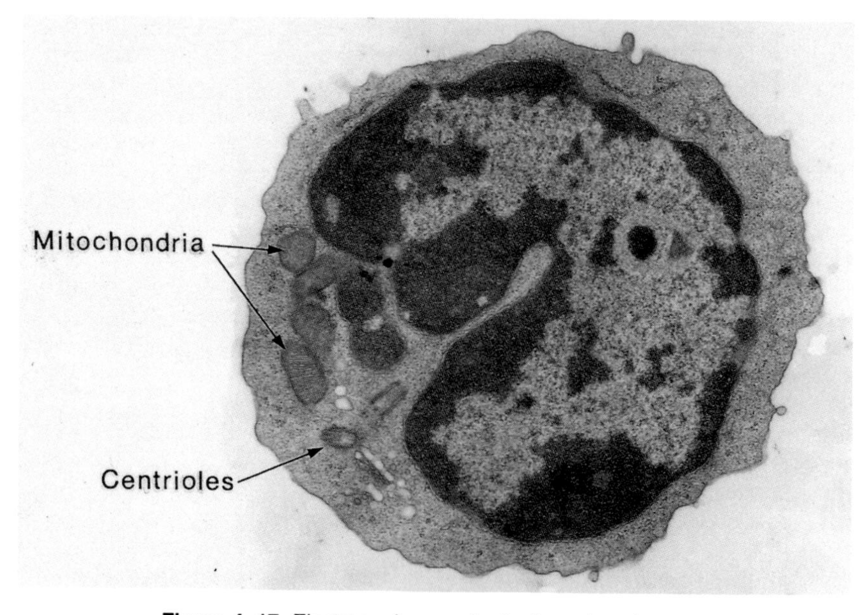

Figure 4–17. Electron micrograph of a large lymphocyte.

globulin are reexposed to the same antigen, they become transformed into lymphoblasts. In this process, they rapidly enlarge, their nucleus becomes euchromatic and acquires a large nucleolus, and they then undergo several divisions, giving rise to many lymphocytes of the same antigenic specificity. Some of these remain in lymphoid organs, amplifying the population of memory cells, whereas others migrate into other tissues and differentiate into *plasma cells* that produce large quantities of specific antibody. If there are multiple exposures to the same antigen, the elevated level of circulating antibody may be maintained for years. The morphological changes and ensuing proliferation that occur in antigen-stimulated lymphocytes during a secondary immune response in vivo can be reproduced in vitro by treatment of lymphocytes with the lectin concanavalin-A (Fig. 4–18).

T-lymphocytes participate in the immune response by regulating the activity of the B-lymphocytes. This regulation is mediated by the secretion of lymphokines that influence the behavior of B-lymphocytes. For many antigens, cells of a subpopulation of T-cells are required to provide an additional stimulus to the B-lymphocytes for antibody production. These are called *helper T-lymphocytes*. Under certain circumstances, another subpopulation of T-lymphocytes may depress production of antibody by B-cells; these are called *suppressor T-lymphocytes*. The exact mechanisms of T-cell regulation of the B-cell function are quite complex and can be deferred to a later chapter.

The defense mechanism described above, which depends on blood-borne antibodies, is called the *humoral immune response*. Another defensive reaction that requires cell-to-cell contact between the lymphocyte and its target is called *cell-mediated immunity*. The principal agents of this form of immunity are members of another subpopulation of T-cells called *cytotoxic T-lymphocytes*. These cells are the principal cause of graft rejection after tissue or organ transplantation. They can also destroy fungi, certain parasites, and virus-infected cells. Their mechanism of killing is revealed in electron micrographs that show, in the membranes of their target cells, numerous minute circular lesions with a central pore about 16 nm in diameter. Upon recognition of their target cell as foreign and attachment to it, the organelles of the killer cell are activated to synthesize a *pore-forming protein* (PFP), also called *perforin*. This is released between the two cells, where it polymerizes to form circular transmembrane channels in the membrane of the target cell. The creation of such pores results in leakage of water, salts, and proteins from the cytoplasm, leading to lysis of the cell. The pores also serve as avenues of entry of lytic toxins or enzymes that contribute to target cell destruction.

T-lymphocytes possess surface receptors for antigens, but these are not immunoglobulins. To activate T-cells, antigen must be presented together with a glycoprotein encoded by genes of the *major histocompatibility complex* (MHC) of the host. Macrophages play a major role in the humoral immune response by presenting antigen–MHC complexes to the T-cells. The antigen-dependent proliferation of T-cells is augmented in the presence of macrophages and, conversely, certain functions of macrophages are modified by T-lymphocytes. The communication between these cell types is mediated by the signaling molecules called lymphokines that were briefly discussed in the previous chapter.

ORIGIN AND RECIRCULATION OF LYMPHOCYTES

The lymph nodes, and other lymphoid organs, contain enormous numbers of lymphocytes. This led early histologists to conclude that lymphocytes arise in the lymphoid organs and reach the blood via the thoracic duct. This interpretation has proven to be wrong. The B-lymphocytes in mammals arise from stem cells in the bone marrow. When tritiated thymidine is infused into the efferent lymphatic vessel of a lymph node to label newly formed lymphocytes, it is found that fewer than 5% of the cells emerging in the efferent lymphatic are labeled. Thus, the vast majority of the lymphocytes in the node have arisen from precursors in the bone marrow and have been carried to the nodes in the blood. After a sojourn in the lymph node, they return to the blood via the efferent lymph that ultimately mingles with the blood at the opening of the thoracic duct into the subclavian or internal jugular vein. The B-lymphocytes have a life span of several months and during this time they circulate and recirculate through the blood, lymph nodes, spleen, and lymph many times. This extensive recirculation of lymphocytes increases the probability of their encountering and responding to any antigens that may have entered the body.

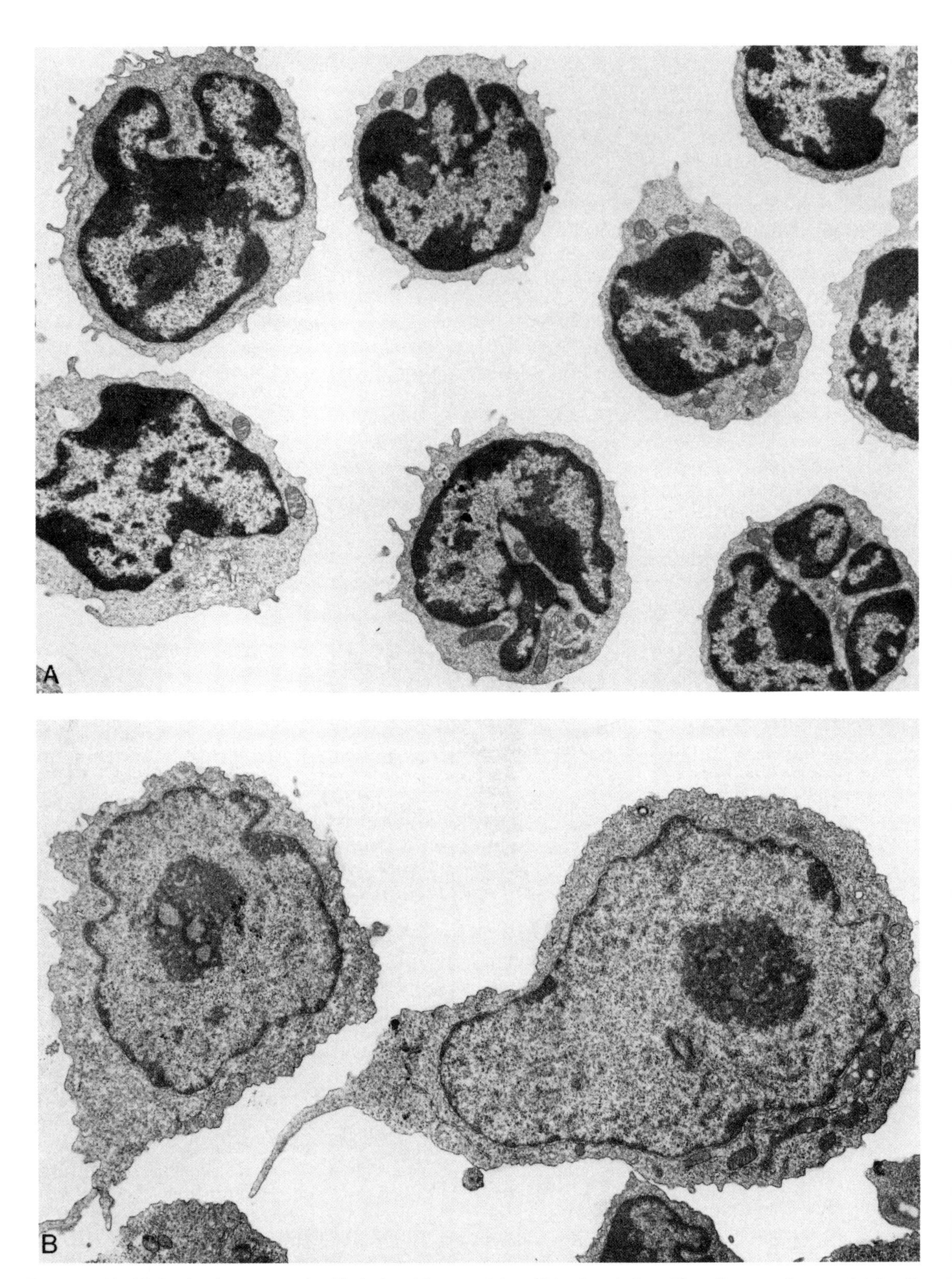

Figure 4–18. (A) Bovine lympocytes freshly isolated from peripheral blood and placed in culture medium containing the lectin concanavalin-A. (B) At the same magnification, after 72 h in culture, many of the lymphocytes have transformed into large lymphoblasts with prominent nucleoli and little heterochromatin. This in vitro transformation mimics that occurring in vivo in a secondary immune response.

T-lymphocytes have a different life history. Stem cells destined to give rise to T-lymphocytes originate in the bone marrow but soon enter the blood and then leave the circulation to settle in the *thymus* where they proliferate. As their progeny move through the cortex of this organ toward its medulla, they differentiate, acquiring the surface markers and receptors characteristic of T-lymphocytes. After entering the blood from the thymus, they may undergo some further differentiation in the spleen, but then they join the population of continuously recirculating lymphocytes. They constitute 70% or more of the small lymphocytes of the blood and have a life span, in humans, that may extend over several years.

MONOCYTES

Monocytes account for 3–8% of the circulating leukocytes. They are spherical cells 9–12 μm in diameter in suspension, but when flattened in dried blood smears, they may measure up to 17 μm in diameter. They might be confused with large lymphocytes, but are somewhat larger and have more cytoplasm. This does not stain a clear blue, but tends to have a pale blue-gray tint. The nucleus is eccentric and round or, more commonly, reniform. Its chromatin stains less intensely than that of lymphocytes, and there are one or two nucleoli, but these are not obvious in routine blood smears. The cytoplasm contains a few azurophil granules (Fig. 4–4J,K, and L).

In electron micrographs, the chromatin is less condensed than that of lymphocytes and the nucleoli are clearly seen. The cytoplasm contains a small Golgi complex, a few cisternae of endoplasmic reticulum, scattered particles of glycogen, and a moderate number of free ribosomes. There are also a number of moderately dense granules corresponding to the azurophil granules seen with the light microscope (Figs. 4–19 and 4–20). With cytochemical methods, these react positively for the acid hydrolases characteristic of lysosomes.

Monocytes originate in the bone marrow and circulate in the blood for a day or two and then migrate through the walls of post-capillary venules into the connective tissue of organs throughout the body. There, they differentiate into *tissue macrophages*. The monocytes in the blood perform no essential function and are simply a mobile reserve of cells capable of developing into voracious phagocytes that ingest senescent cells and cellular debris in the normal tissue and are active participants in the body's defense against invasion by bacteria. Moreover, as indicated above, they play an indispensable role in humoral immune responses by processing antigen and presenting it to the lymphocytes.

Monocytes take on a variety of shapes and staining characteristics in the tissues that may make it difficult to identify them with certainty in histological sections, but they possess specific surface markers that facilitate their identification by means of monoclonal antibodies to these integral membrane proteins. Connective tissue macrophages, alveolar macrophages in the lung, and Kupffer cells in the liver all share the same surface markers as monocytes and are assumed to originate from them. These cell types are now grouped together as the *mononuclear phagocyte system*, which will be discussed more fully in Chapter 5. There are antigen-presenting cells (Langerhans cells) in the skin and dendritic cells in T-lymphocyte-rich areas of the lymphoid organs that lack some of these surface markers, and their relationship to the monocytes remains uncertain.

OTHER BLOOD COMPONENTS

Blood plasma is the fluid matrix in which the blood cells are suspended and it contains a number of physiologically important proteins. When blood clots and the clot contracts, some of the larger plasma proteins are removed by incorporation in the clot. The fluid remaining is called *blood serum*. The major categories of plasma proteins include *albumin, globulins, fibrinogen*, and *complement*.

Albumin, with a molecular weight of about 50,000, is the smallest and the most abundant plasma protein. Synthesized in the liver and released more-or-less continuously into the blood, albumin is essential for maintaining the colloid osmotic pressure of the blood, thereby preventing excessive loss of fluid to the extracellular matrix of the tissues. It also binds some molecules that are not soluble in blood serum and because the bound form is soluble, albumin plays an important role in the transport of small molecules in the blood.

The *globulins* are proteins ranging in molecular weight from 80,000 to over a million. They are divided into three main categories, the *α-globulins*, the *β-globulins*, and the *γ-globulins*. The α- and β-globulins combine reversibly with various substances and serve as vehicles

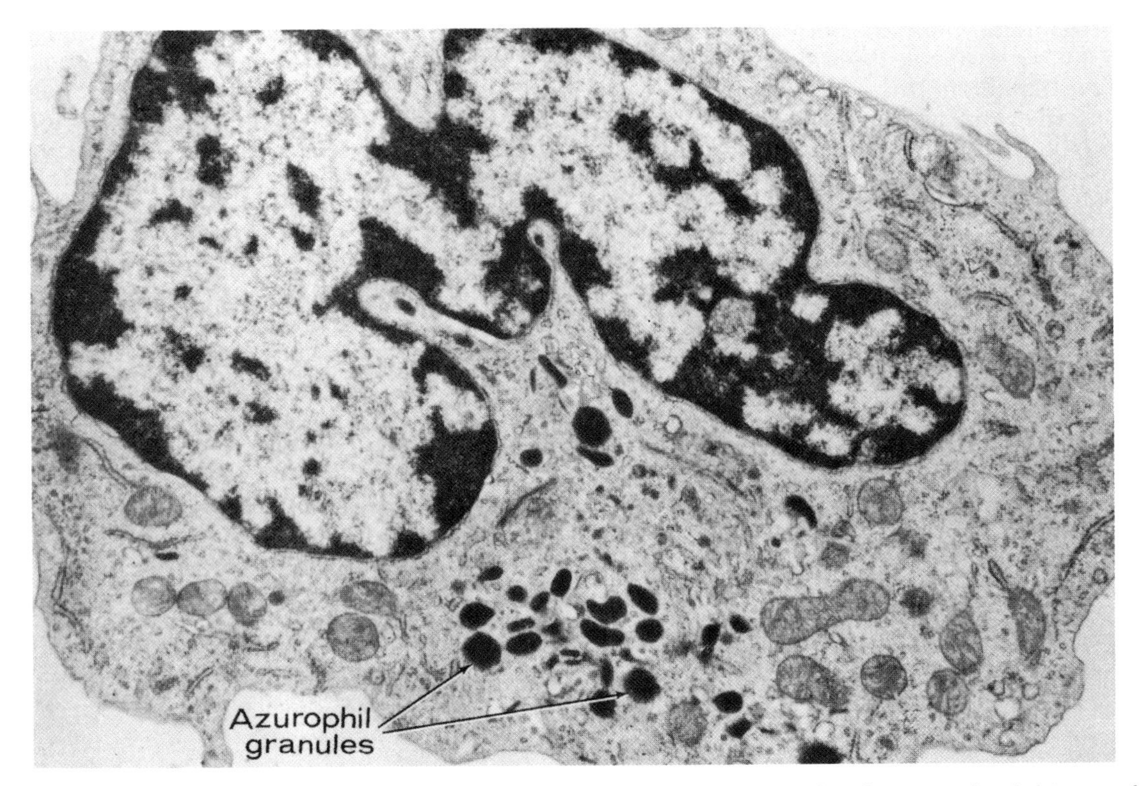

Figure 4–19. Electron micrograph of a rabbit monocyte showing its irregularly shaped nucleus, occasional cisternae of rough endoplasmic reticulum, and a small cluster of azurophil granules.

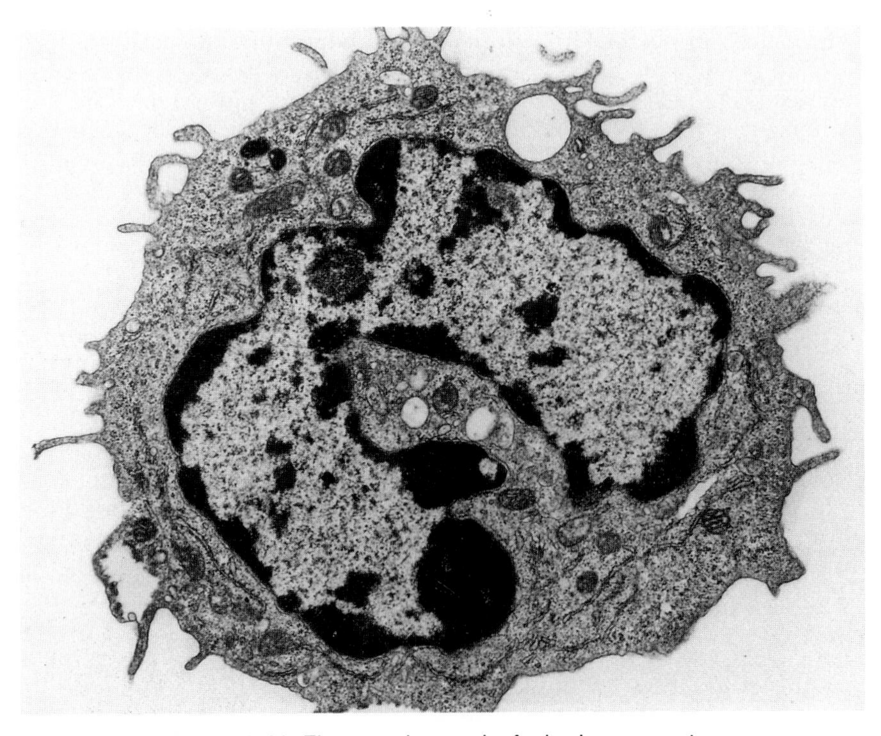

Figure 4–20. Electron micrograph of a bovine monocyte.

for their transport. For example, *transferrin*, a β-globulin, has as its major function the transport of iron, and *ceruloplasmin* transports copper. The γ-globulins include the immunoglobulins (antibodies) of the immune system.

The *complement system* is a group of 12 or more serum proteins that interact in a cascade of reactions whose products contribute to humoral immune responses, to initiation of inflammation, and to the lysis of invading microorganisms. At sites of tissue injury, complement in the extravasated plasma is activated to form components (C3a and C5a) that bind to mast cells, stimulating their release of histamine and chemoattractants that mobilize neutrophils and macrophages to assemble at the site. Phagocytic cells can ingest and destroy bacteria only if they recognize them as cells foreign to the body. The coating of bacteria with specific antibody, together with subunits of the complement system, ensures their recognition and binding to neutrophils and macrophages. In addition to facilitating phagocytosis of bacteria, other components of complement become incorporated in the surface of bacteria to form pores that result in their lysis by osmotic forces.

Plasma lipoproteins are involved in the transport of lipid from the intestine to the liver, and from the liver to the tissues. Three or more categories are identified on the basis of their size or their density which, in turn, depends on the amount of lipid each contains. *Chylomicra*, 100–500 μm in diameter are large enough to be visible by dark-field microscopy. *Very low-density lipoproteins* (VLDL), ranging in size from 25 to 70 nm, are visible in electron micrographs and are relatively rich in triglycerides. *Low-density lipoproteins* (LDL) are still smaller and are the principal vehicle for transport of cholesterol throughout the body. Many cell types have receptors for LDL and they take up these particles by receptor-mediated endocytosis to meet their need for fatty acids, as an energy source, and for cholesterol as a constituent of their membranes. This category of lipoproteins is of considerable clinical interest because inherited defects in LDL–receptor function may result in high blood levels of cholesterol and a predisposition to atherosclerosis.

BIBLIOGRAPHY

ERYTHROCYTES

Backman, L. 1986. Shape control in the human red cell. J. Cell Biol., 80:281.

Bennett, V. and D. Branton. 1977. Selective association of spectrin with the cytoplasmic surface of human erythrocyte plasma membranes. J. Biol. Chem. 252:2753.

Bennett, V. and P.J. Stenbuck. 1980. Human erythrocyte ankyrin. Purification and properties. J. Biol. Chem. 255:2540.

Bishop, C. and D.M. Surgenor, eds. 1964. The Red Blood Cells. New York, Academic Press.

Branton, D., C.M. Cohen, and J. Tyler. 1981. Interaction of cytoskeletal proteins on human erythrocyte membrane. Cell 24:24.

Cohen, C.M. 1983. The molecular organization of the red cell membrane skeleton. Sem. Hematol. 20:141.

Harrison, P.R. 1976. Analysis of erythropoiesis at the molecular level. Nature 262:253.

Ingram, V. 1963. The Hemoglobins in Genetics and Evolution. New York, Columbia Univ. Press.

Liu, S., L.H. Derick, and J. Palek. 1987. Visualization of the hexagonal lattice in the erythrocyte membrane skeleton. J. Cell Biol. 104:527.

Patek, J. and S.E. Lux. 1988. Red cell membrane skeleton defects in hereditary and acquired hemolytic anemias. Sem. Hematol. 20:189.

Perutz, M.F. 1978. Hemoglobin structure and respiratory transport. Sci. Am. 239:92.

PLATELETS

Biggs, R. and R.G. Macfarlane. 1962. Human Blood Coagulation and its Disorders, 3rd ed. Philadelphia, F.A. Davis Co.

Fox, J.E.B. and D.R. Phillips. 1983. Polymerization and organization of actin filaments within platelets. Sem. Hematol. 20:243.

George, J.N., A.T. Nurden, and D.R. Phillips. 1984. Molecular defects in the interaction of platelets with the vessel wall. N. Engl. J. Med. 311:1084.

Johnson, S.A., R.W. Monto, J.W. Rebeck, and R.C. Horn. eds. 1961. Blood Platelets. A Symposium. Boston, Little Brown & Co.

Lawler, J. 1986. The structural and functional properties of thrombospondin. J. Am. Soc. Hematol. 67:1197.

Marcus, A.J. and B.M. Zucker. 1965. The Physiology of Blood Platelets. New York, Grune & Stratton.

Oates, J.A., J. Hawiger, R. Ross, eds. 1985. Interaction of Platelets with the Vessel Wall. Baltimore, Williams and Wilkins.

Shattil, S.J. and J.S. Bennett. 1981. Platelets and their membranes in hemostasis: physiology and pathophysiology. Ann. Int. Med. 94:108.

Weiss, H.J. 1975. Platelet physiology and abnormalities of platelet function. N. Eng. J. Med. 203:531,580.

White, J.G. and C.C. Clausen. 1980. Overview article: Biostructure of blood platelets. Ultrastr. Pathol. 1:533.

Ross, R., C.W. Raines, and D.F. Bowen-Pope. 1986. The biology of platelet derived growth factor. Cell 46:155.

Ross, R., J. Glomset, B. Kariya, and L. Harker. 1974. A platelet-dependent serum factor that stimulates the proliferation of arterial smooth muscle cells, in vitro. Proc. Nat. Acad. Sci. USA 71:1207.

Xu, Z. and B. Afzelius. 1988. The substructure of the marginal bundle in human blood platelets. J. Ultrastr. Mol. Struct. Res. 99:244.

NEUTROPHILS

Anderson, D.R. 1966. Ultrastructure of normal and leukemic leukocytes in human peripheral blood. J. Ultrastr. Res. 16 (Suppl. 9):5.

Athens, J.W. 1969. Granulocyte kinetics in health and disease. Nat. Cancer Inst. Monogr. 30:135.

Bretz, U. and M. Baggiolini. 1974. Biochemical and morphological characterization of azurophil and specific granules of human neutrophilic leukocytes. J. Cell Biol. 63:251.

Cohn, Z.A. and S.I. Morse. 1965. Functional and metabolic properties of polymorphonuclear leukocytes. I. Observations on the requirements and consequences of particle ingestion. J. Exp. Med. 111:667.

Daems, W. 1968. On the fine structure of human neutrophilic leukocyte granules. J. Ultrastr. Res. 24:353.

Furie, M.B., B.L. Naprstek, and S.C. Silverstein. 1987. Migration of neutrophils across monolayers of microvascular endothelial cells. J. Cell Sci. 88:161.

Hirsch, J.G. and Z.A. Cohn. 1960. Degranulation of polymorphonuclear leukocytes following phagocytosis of microorganisms. J. Exp. Med. 118:1005.

Huber, A.R., S.L. Kunkel, R.E. Todd, and S. Weiss. 1991. Regulation of transendothelial neutrophil migration by endogenous interleukin-8. Science 254:99.

Klebanoff, S.J. 1975. Antimicrobial mechanisms in neutrophilic polymorphonuclear leukocytes. Sem. Hematol. 12:117.

Lisiewicz, J. 1980. Human Neutrophils. Bowie, MD, Charles Press Publishers.

Movat, H.Z. 1985. The Inflammatory Reaction. Amsterdam, Elsevier Press.

Spitznagel, J.K., F.G. Dalldorf, and M.S. Liffell. 1978. Characterization of azurophil and specific granules purified from human polymorphonuclear leukocytes. Lab. Invest. 30:774.

Wright, D.G., D.A. Bralove, and J.I. Gallin. 1977. The differential mobilization of human neutrophil granules. Am. J. Pathol. 87:273.

EOSINOPHILS

Ackerman, J.S., D.A. Loegering, P. Venge, I. Olsson et al. 1983. Distinctive cationic proteins of the human eosinophilic granule: major basic protein, eosinophilic cationic protein, and eosinophiul derived neurotoxin. J. Immunol. 131:2977.

Beeson, P.B. and D.A. Bass. 1977. The Eosinophil. Philadelphia, W.B. Saunders Co.

Henderson, W.R. and E.Y. Chi. 1985. Ultrastructural characterization and morphometric analysis of human eosinophil degranulation J. Cell Sci. 73:33.

Hudson, G. 1968. Quantitative study of eosinophil granulocytes. Sem. Hematol. 5:166.

Littg. M. 1964. Eosinophils and antigen–antibody reactions. Ann. N.Y. Acad. Sci. 116:964.

Young, J.D., C.G.B. Peterson, P. Venge, and Z.A. Cohn. 1986. Mechanism of membrane damage mediated by human eosinophil cationic protein. Nature 321:613.

BASOPHILS

Ackerman, G.A. 1963. Cytochemical properties of the blood basophilic granulocyte. Ann. N.Y. Acad. Sci. 103:376.

Askenase, P.W. 1977. Role of basophils, mast cells and vasoamines in hypersensitivity reactions with a delayed time course. Prog. Allergy 23:199.

Dvorak, H.F. and A.M. Dvorak. 1975. Basophilic leukocytes: structure, function, and role in disease. Clin. Hematol. 4:651.

Dvorak, H.F. and A.M. Dvorak. 1972. Basophils, mast cells and cellular immunity in animals and man. Human Pathol. 3:454.

Ishizaka, T. and K. Ishizaka. 1975. Biology of immunoglobulin E. Molecular basis of reaginic hypersensitivity. Prog. Allergy 19:60.

Terry, R.W., D.F. Bainton, and M.G. Farquhar. 1969. Formation and structure of specific granules in basophilic leukocytes of the guinea pig. Lab. Invest. 21:65.

Zucker-Franklin, D. 1967. Electron microscope study of human basophils, Blood 29:878.

Lymphocytes

See Bibliography, Chapter 7 and 13.

Monocytes

See Bibliography, Chapter 5.

5

CONNECTIVE TISSUE

The *connective tissues* are a diverse group of tissues that share a common origin from the mesenchyme of the embryo. Cartilage and bone are connective tissues with a firm extracellular matrix specialized for support of the body as a whole. Adipose tissue is specialized for storage of lipid as an energy source. These will be the subject of separate chapters. This chapter is concerned with the more generalized connective tissue that is found throughout the body and provides for cohesion of other structural elements and serves as the medium through which blood vessels are distributed to nourish the organs and to eliminate the waste products of their metabolism. Its cells are widely scattered in an abundant extracellular matrix consisting of fibrous and amorphous components.

The relative abundance of cells, fibers, and ground substance in this kind of connective tissue varies greatly from region to region. Different terms are used to facilitate description of some of these variations. *Loose connective tissue* and *dense connective tissue* differ according to whether the fibers are moderately abundant and loosely interwoven or very abundant and densely packed. Modifiers are added to these terms to indicate the organization of the fibers. Where fibers are closely interwoven in seemingly random orientation, the tissue is described as *dense irregular connective tissue*, and where the fibers are closely packed in parallel bundles, as in tendon, or in flat sheets, as in aponeuroses, the tissue is called *dense regular connective tissue*.

The several cell types of loose connective tissue are categorized as *fixed cells* or *free cells*. The fixed cells are a stable population of long-lived, relatively immobile *fibroblasts*, so named because they produce and maintain the surrounding fibers. They also secrete the amorphous *ground substance* of the extracellular matrix. The free cells are a heterogeneous population of motile cells of limited life span that emigrate from the blood and wander through the interstices among the fibers. These transients are concerned with the defense of the tissue and are normally present in limited numbers but may increase dramatically in mounting an inflammatory reaction against invading bacteria.

The principal function of loose connective tissue is to bind together and support the parenchyma of the organs in the body, but it has recently become apparent that it has other important roles. The polarity of epithelial cells, the stabilization of their basal surface, the organization of their cytoskeleton, and some of their metabolic functions are dependent on the interaction of the epithelial cells with matrix components of the underlying connective tissue. The nature of these interactions is now a subject of intensive investigation.

THE GROUND SUBSTANCE

The translucent material in which the cells and fibers of connective tissue are embedded is a highly hydrated gel commonly referred to as the *ground substance*. Its aqueous phase is the medium through which all nutrients and waste products must pass in transit between the blood and the parenchymal cells of the organs. The ground substance is poorly preserved in routine histological preparations, but its residues can be detected by use of certain dyes that undergo a change in color on binding to it, a staining property called metachromasia. The dye toluidine blue, for example, takes on a purple color when bound to the ground substance. It can also be stained with the periodic-acid–Schiff reaction, owing to the numerous polysaccharide chains on some of its molecules.

The stainable components of the ground substance were formerly classified as *acid mucopolysaccharides*, but as more has been learned about their chemical nature, this term has fallen into disuse. The major polysaccharides of the ground substance are now identified as

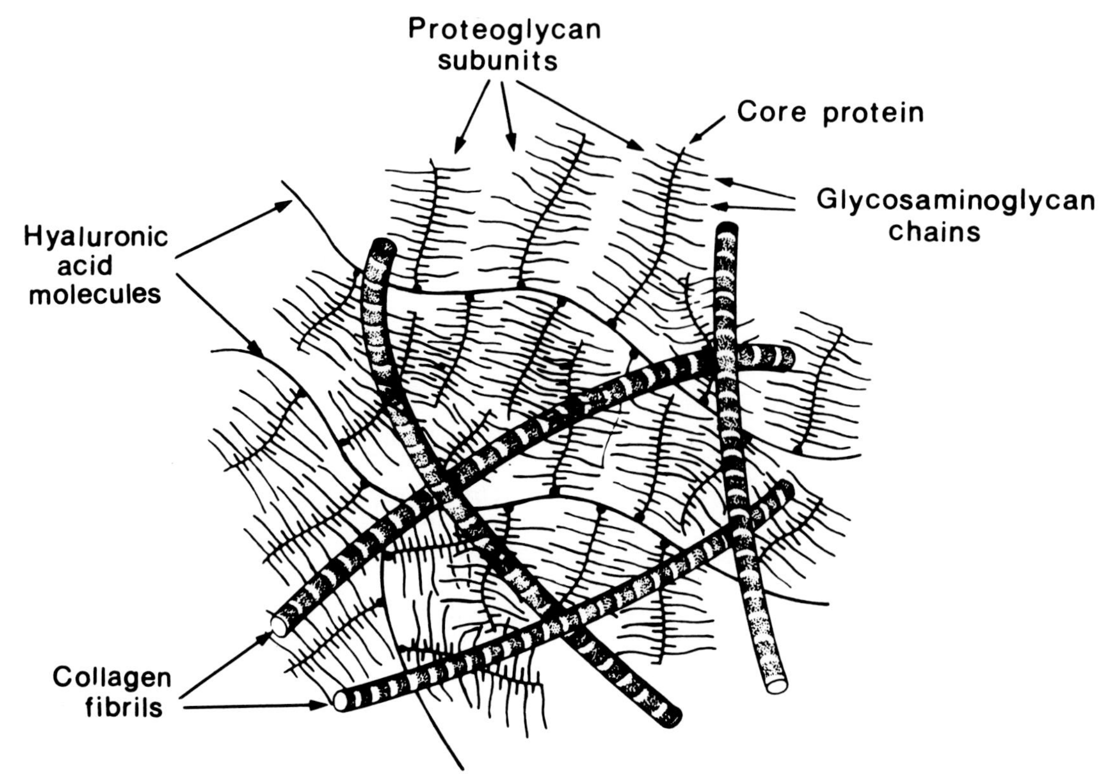

Figure 5–1. Drawing of the organization of the extracellular matrix of cartilage in which the interstices between collagen fibers are believed to be occupied by entwining long proteoglycan molecules with hundreds of polysaccharide side-chains.

glycosaminoglycans, a class of macromolecules that are long, linear polymers of disaccharide subunits. The major glycosaminoglycans of connective tissue are *chondroitin sulfate, keratan sulfate, heparan sulfate*, and *hyaluronic acid*. Hyaluronic acid, which is abundant in loose connective tissue in joint fluid and in the vitreous humor of the eye, is a very large molecule made up of some 5000 disaccharides in a chain that would be nearly 2.5 μm in length (Fig. 5–1). One of its important properties is its high viscosity in aqueous solution, which contributes to the gel-like consistency of the ground substance. This consistency is no barrier to diffusion of metabolites through its aqueous phase, but it is believed to be a significant barrier to the spread of bacteria that may enter the tissues. In this context, it is interesting that the most invasive species of bacteria are those that have acquired the ability to produce the enzyme *hyaluronidase* to depolymerize the hyaluronic acid of the ground substance.

There is no entirely satisfactory method for the microscopic study of the ground substance. Its extraction by the aqueous fixatives commonly used in specimen preparation can be partially avoided by fixation of frozen sections in ether-formaldehyde vapor. The proteoglycans, in such preparations, are polyanions due to the sulfate and hydroxyl groups on the disaccharide groups of the glycosaminoglycans, and they can be stained by cationic dyes such as Alcian-blue or by colloidal iron, which has a high affinity for anionic groups. For electron microscopy, incorporation of the polycationic dye ruthenium-red in the fixative appears to improve the preservation of the glycosaminoglycans by interaction with their anionic groups. However, the chains collapse onto the core protein during dehydration and the glycosaminoglycans appear as 10–20-nm granules in the interstices of the extracellular matrix. By high-pressure freezing, freeze-substitution, and low-temperature imbedding, the proteoglycans of cartilage matrix have been successfully preserved in a more extended state believed to resemble their true form. With this method of preparation, they appear as a network of very fine strands throughout the cartilage matrix, and those in loose connective tissue probably have a similar form.

Most of the tissue fluid is held by the hydrophilic glycosaminoglycans, but small molecules are able to diffuse through this bound water. A lesser amount of free fluid, carrying gases and nutrients in solution, also circulates through the ground substance. When the rate of exit of fluid from the arterial end of the capillaries exceeds the rate of its uptake at the venous ends, fluid accumulates in the extracellular matrix resulting a swelling of the tissue, called *edema*.

COLLAGEN FIBERS

Fibers of *collagen* are present in all kinds of connective tissue. In unstained preparations, they are colorless strands 0.5–10 μm in diameter and of indefinite length. In histological sections, they are acidophilic, staining pink with eosin, blue with Mallory's trichrome stain, and green with Masson's trichrome stain. They are unbranched and, in loose connective tissue, they appear to be randomly oriented (Fig. 5–2). When not under tension, they have an undulant course. In larger fibers, a faint longitudinal striation is evident, suggesting that these are bundles of smaller fibers. Under the polarizing microscope, even the smallest fibers exhibit birefringence, indicating that they are made up of submicroscopic subunits oriented parallel to the fiber axis.

With the electron microscope, collagen fibers are seen to consist of parallel fibrils 50–90 nm in diameter. These are the subunits responsible for the form of birefringence observed with polarization microscopy. In micrographs of lead-stained thin sections, these *unit fibrils* are cross-striated, with denser staining transverse bands repeating every 67 nm along their length (Fig. 5–3). The unit fibrils are polymers of collagen molecules, each 300 nm in length and 1.4 nm in diameter. They are made up of three polypeptide chains, called *α-chains*, each having a molecular weight of about 100,000. The chains have a left-handed helical configuration, and the three are entwined to form a right-handed triple helix, in which each turn spans a distance of 8 nm (Fig 5–4). The α-chains are held together within the triple helix by hydrogen bonds.

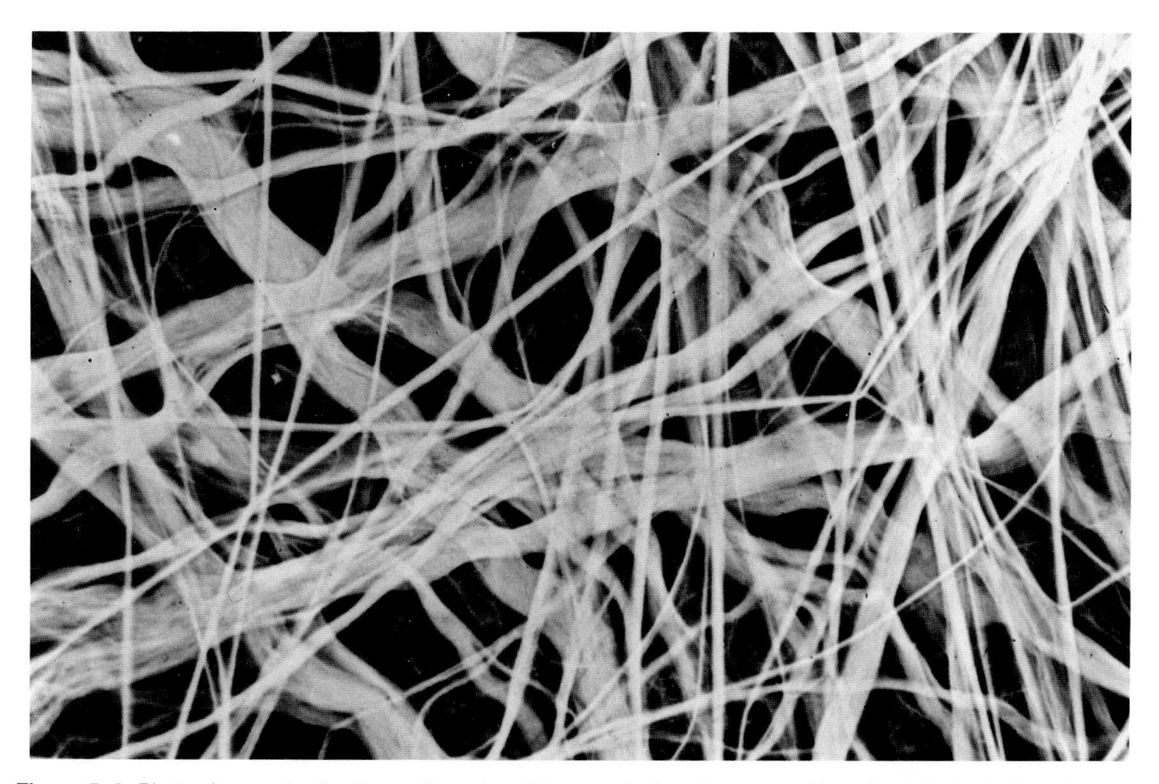

Figure 5–2. Photomicrograph of collagen fibers in a thin spread of rat mesentery. Note the variation in fiber diameter and the wavy course of the larger fibers. The preparation was stained by a silver method and the photograph printed as a negative to simulate more closely the appearance of the fibers in unfixed material. (From Fawcett, D.W. *In* Greep, R.O., ed. 1953. Histology, Blakiston Co. Reproduced by permission of McGraw-Hill Book Co.)

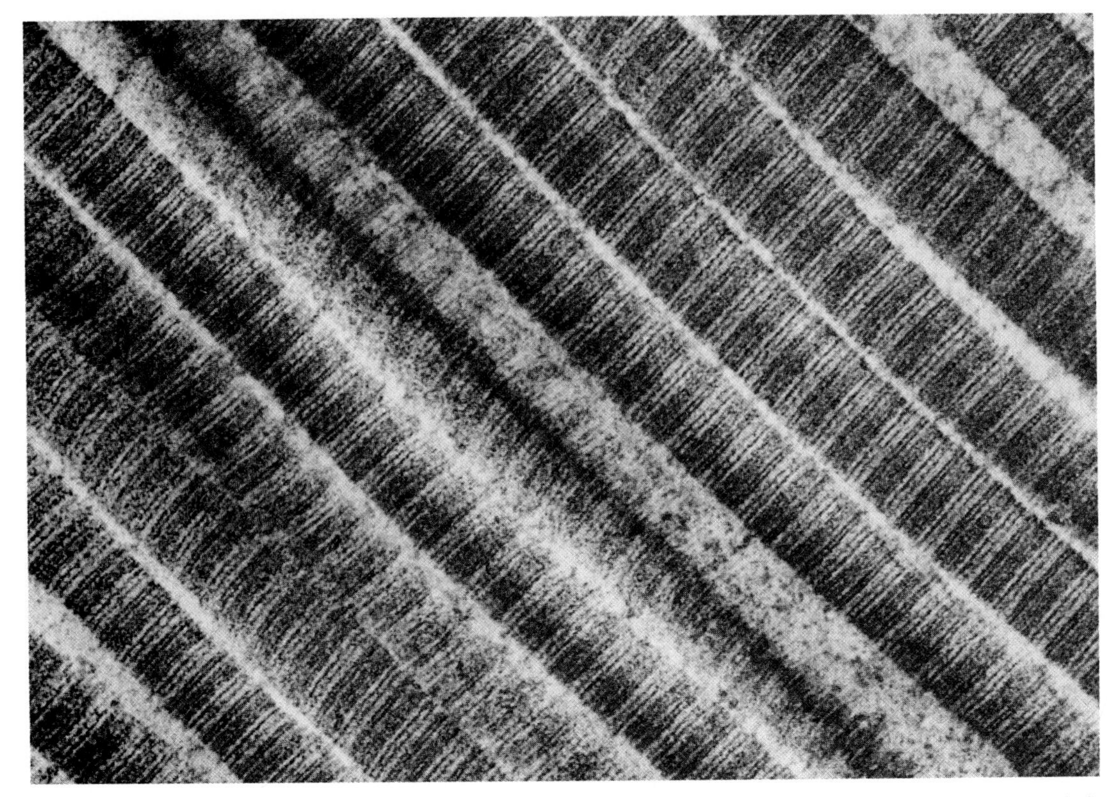

Figure 5–3. Electron micrograph of the unit fibrils of collagen, showing their characteristic pattern of cross-striations. (Micrograph courtesy of D. Friend.)

Molecular collagen can be extracted from developing or repairing connective tissue. When such extracts are warmed, in vitro, to body temperature, the collagen molecules spontaneously polymerize to form cross-striated fibrils with the 67-nm periodicity of native collagen. In this process, the molecules orient parallel, overlapping one another by a quarter of their length and leaving a short gap between the amino terminus of one molecule and the carboxy terminus of the next (Fig. 5–5). The gaps between molecules and their staggered arrangement are responsible for the cross-striation seen in negatively stained fibrils. The penetration of the contrast medium into the gaps results in the dark bands, and the light bands are regions in which molecular overlapping is complete and no stain penetrates.

Some banding patterns that do not occur in nature can be produced in vitro by varying the conditions under which polymerization takes place. If a solution of collagen and serum-glycoprotein is dialyzed against water, fibrils are formed that have a periodicity of 240 nm instead of 67 nm. This is called *fibrous long-spacing collagen* (FLS-collagen) (Fig. 5–6). Precipitation of collagen from acid solution

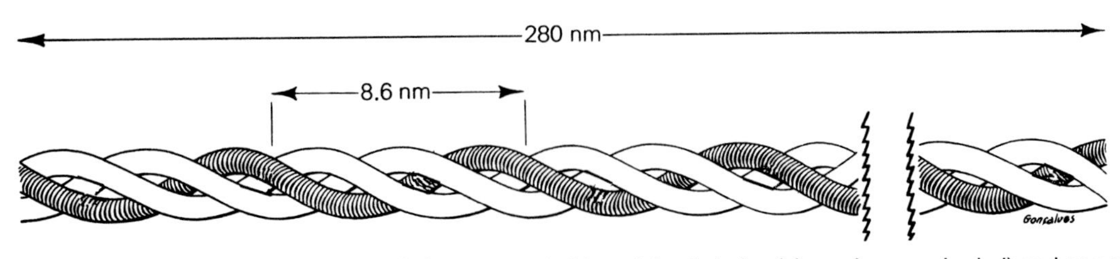

Figure 5–4. In type-I collagen, each molecule is composed of two alpha-1 chains (shown here unshaded) and one alpha-2 polypeptide chain (shaded), intertwined in a helical configuration. Each gyre of the helix spans a distance of 8.6 nm. (From Junquiera, L.C., and J. Carniero. 1980. Basic Histology, 3rd ed. Los Altos, CA, Lange Medical Publications.)

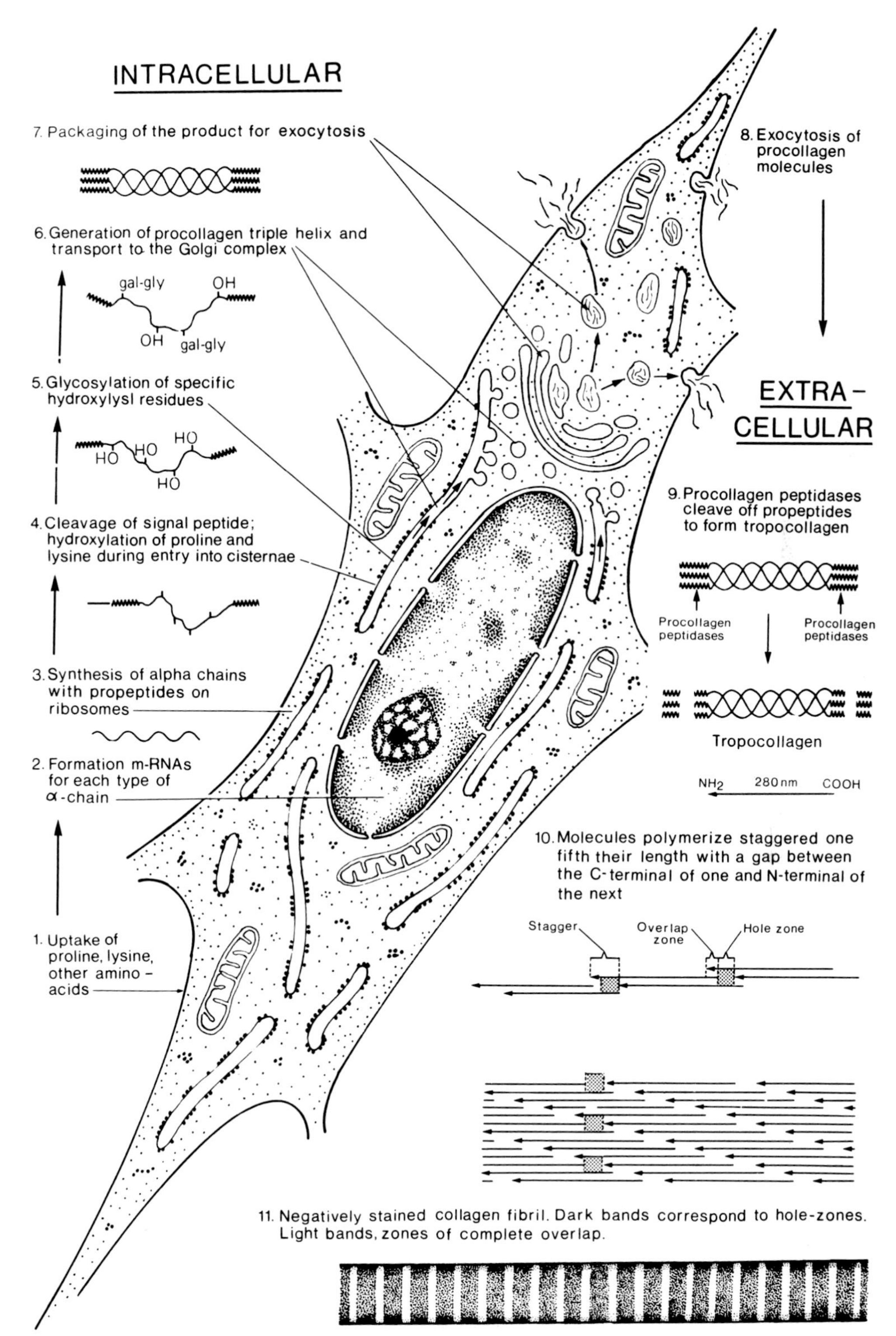

Figure 5–5. Schematic presentation of the biosynthetic events and organelle participation in the formation of collagen. On the left, successive intracellular events are defined; and on the right, the steps leading to extracellular assembly of cross-striated collagen fibrils. (Modified after Junquiera, L.C. and J. Carneiro. Basic Histology, 3rd ed. Los Altos, CA, Lange Medical Publications.)

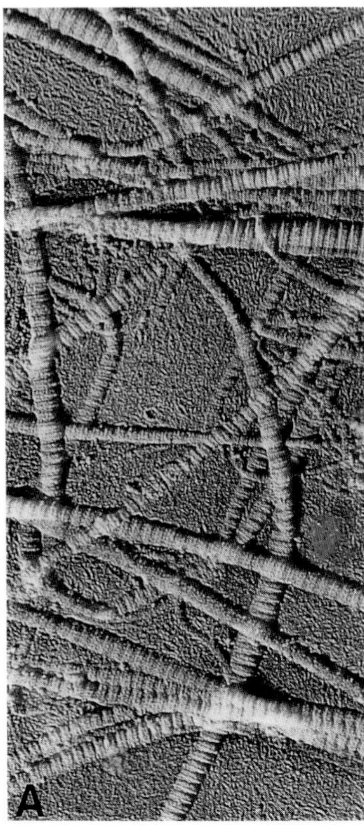

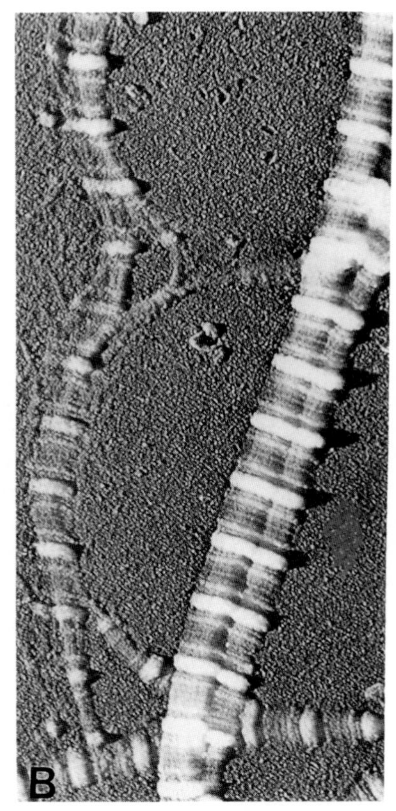

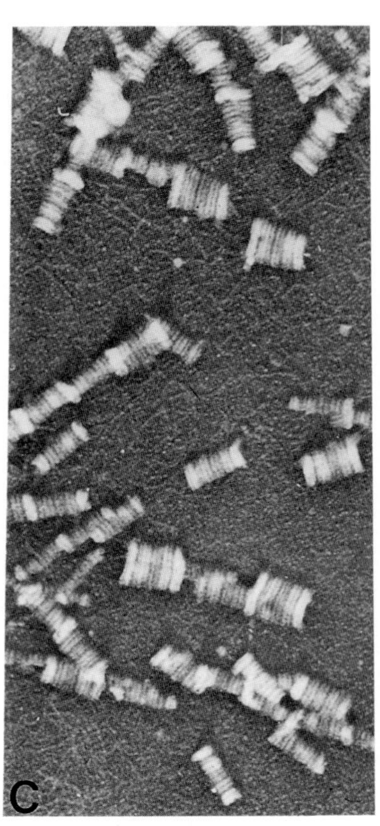

Figure 5–6 Electron micrographs of the different forms that can be produced on reconstitution of collagen in vitro. (A) Fibrils with 64-nm period of native collagen—precipitated from solution by dialysis against 1% NaCl. (B) Fibrous long-spacing collagen (FLS) produced from a mixture of acid glycoprotein of serum and collagen solution dialyzed against water. (C) Segment long-spacing collagen solution (SLS) precipitated from acid solution of collagen by addition of ATP. (Micrograph courtesy of J. Gross, F.O. Schmitt, and J.H. Highberger.)

by addition of adenosine triphosphate (ATP) does not result in fibrils but short segments about 300 nm long. This form is called *segment long-spacing collagen* (SLS-collagen). In both of these, the molecules come together side-to-side and in register with no overlap. The length of the segment is, thus, approximately the same length as the collagen molecule. Knowledge of these unnatural forms of collagen is of little use to the histologist or pathologist, but their study has contributed significantly to our understanding of the development and molecular organization of collagen fibers.

Collagen was formerly thought to be a single protein with an amino-acid composition that had been highly conserved in the course of evolution, but improved methods of analysis have led to the discovery of differences in the collagen extracted from various tissues in the body. Collagen is now regarded as a family of closely related, but genetically distinct, proteins that share certain features of molecular organization but have α-chains that differ in their amino-acid composition and sequence. Twelve types of collagen have been identified to date. Types I, II, III, V, and IX form quarter-staggered fibrils and can be localized by means of labeled antibody techniques. A standard terminology has been developed for specifying the α-chains in each type of collagen, but this is beyond the scope of this chapter. The interested reader is referred to texts of biochemistry for this information.

Type-I collagen is the most ubiquitous, occurring in the dermis, bone, tendon, fascia, and in the capsules of organs. Its cross-striated fibrils, 50–90 nm in diameter, aggregate to form collagen fibers and fiber bundles of a wide range of sizes (Fig 5–7) The fibers are flexible but offer great resistance to tension. The breaking force of the tendon, composed of this type of collagen, is reached at several hundred kilograms per square centimeter, and at this tension, the collagen fibers have elongated by only a few percent of their original length.

Type-II collagen is found in hyaline and elastic cartilage, in the nucleus pulposus of the intervertebral discs and in the vitreous body of the eye. It forms very thin fibrils that are embedded in an abundant ground substance. No larger fibers are formed. It is visible only with the polarizing microscope or after staining with picro-sirius.

Type-III collagen is abundant in loose connective tissue, in the walls of blood vessels, in the stroma of various glands, and in the spleen, kidney, and uterus. It forms the argyrophilic fibers traditionally called *reticular fibers* (see below). Collagens I, II, and III which form microscopically visible fibers are referred to as *interstitial collagens* to distinguish them form a larger group of collagens that are detectable in tissue sections only by means of fluorescein-labeled antibody.

Type-IV collagen is a specialized form largely restricted to the basal lamina of epithelia. Together with laminin and heparan sulfate proteoglycan, it forms a close meshwork of fine filaments that is the physical support of epithelia and a selective filtration barrier for macromolecules (Fig. 5–8).

Type-V collagen is of widespread occurrence but is present only in very small amounts. It is associated with the external lamina of smooth and striated muscle fibers and the basal lamina of epithelia but does not seem to be an integral component of those structures. It is also associated with the interstitial collagens where it may be involved in linkage within and between fibers.

Type-VI collagen is a short-chain molecule consisting of a triple helical segment about 100 nm in length with globular domains at either end. These molecules assemble laterally into tetramers, which, under certain circumstances, may polymerize end-to-end forming thin fibrils 5–10 nm in diameter having, along their length, prominent knobs or beads with a periodicity of 110 nm. This collagen is present, in small amounts, at most sites where types-I and -III are found. In the kidney, liver, and uterus, it constitutes less than 0.5% of the

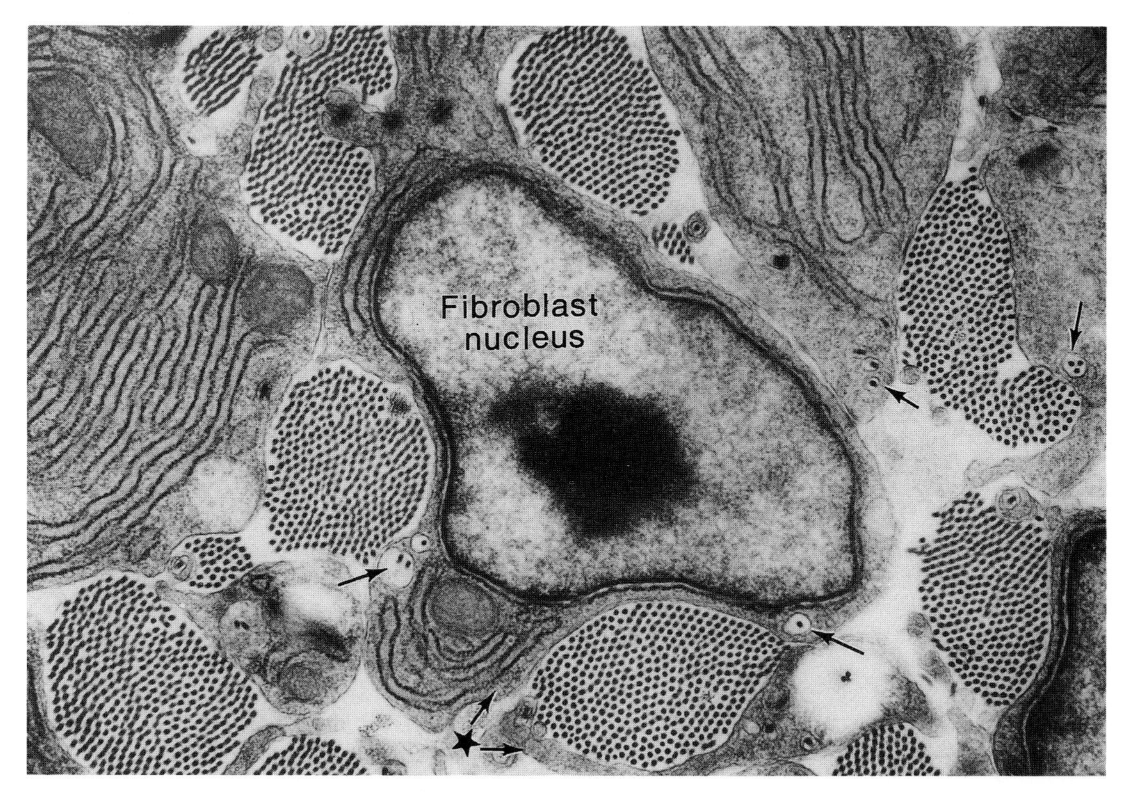

Figure 5–7. Micrograph of fibroblast and collagen bundles in a developing tendon. Small groups of fibrils can be seen within narrow recesses in the cell surface (at arrows). Larger bundles are partially or completely surrounded by fibroblast processes (at asterisk). (Micrograph courtesy of D. Birk and R.E. Trelstad [J. Cell. Biol. 103:231–240 (1986).])

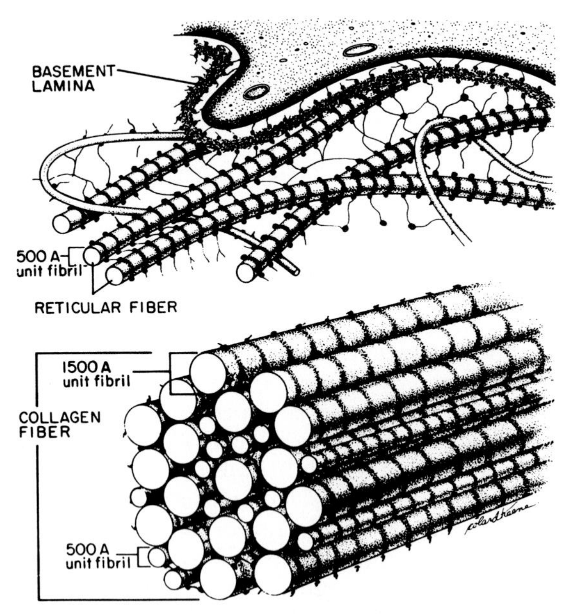

Figure 5–8. Drawing comparing type-IV collagen of basal lamina (top) with type-III collagen of the underlying reticular fibers and with type-I collagen of tendon (bottom). Fibers characteristic of tendons are a mixture of fibrils 30–150 nm in diameter, whereas reticular fibrils average 50–55 nm in diameter. (From Hay, E.D. et al. *In* H. Gastpar, K. Kuhn, and R. Marx, eds. Collagen Platelet Interactions. Stutttgart, Schattauer.)

total collagen, but in the cornea of the eye it makes up nearly 25% of the total collagen. Its precise structural role remains obscure.

Type-VII collagen is associated with the basal lamina of many epithelia, but it is most abundant at the dermo-epidermal junction of the skin. Its molecules are the largest of the collagen family, being some 800 nm in length. Aggregates of type-VII collagen form striated *anchoring fibrils* that originate and terminate in the basal lamina of the epithelium, forming loops around the underlying type-I and type-III collagen fibers of the dermis. Other fibrils, originating in the basal lamina, terminate in *anchoring plaques* of type-IV collagen in the connective tissue beneath the epithelium. They serve to stabilize and firmly anchor the epithelium to the dermis.

Type-VIII collagen was discovered as a secretory product of endothelial cells growing in vitro and is sometimes called *endothelial collagen.* It is very intimately associated with the surface of these cells, but the significance of this relationship is unknown. It is a major component of Descemet's membrane, the atypical basal lamina of the corneal epithelium.

Type-IX collagen is found mainly in cartilage. It differs markedly from the fibrillar collagens and apparently does not form supramolecular aggregates. In cartilage that has been digested with hyaluronidase to remove proteoglycans, a fluorescein-labeled antibody reveals that this collagen is coextensive with type-II collagen fibers of this connective tissue. It is believed to maintain the three-dimensional arrangement of the type-II collagen fibers in the matrix by serving as a coupler at their sites of intersection.

Type-X collagen is also confined to cartilage and is found in the matrix immediately surrounding hypertrophic chondrocytes involved in endochondral bone formation. It is speculated that it may play some role in initiating calcification of the matrix. *Type-XI collagen* is associated with type-II collagen in cartilage. Its function is not known. *Type-XII collagen* has recently been discovered in the screening of a cDNA library constructed from mRNA of tendon fibroblasts. It has some properties in common with type-IX collagen, but, as yet, little is known about its location in the tissues or its function.

The functional significance of the multiple types of collagen and their differing distributions is still not well understood. Those most commonly observed by the histologist or pathologist are the interstitial collagens, types I, II, and III that form fibers visible with the light microscope. The collagen of loose connective tissue is most easily studied in spreads of intact mesentery. These are thin enough to be studied without disturbing the arrangement of the fibers. In such preparations, the collagen is seen as randomly interwoven fibers of varying diameter and of indefinite length (Fig 5–1). The largest, up to 15 μm in diameter, are bundles of smaller fibers and they often have a wavy course if not under tension. Such fibers are predominately type-I collagen.

In addition to the relatively coarse type-I collagen fibers, loose connective tissue contains networks of very thin, 0.5–2.0-μm, fibers traditionally called *reticular fibers.* These are not ordinarily distinguishable in thin spreads of connective tissue, but they can be selectively stained with silver salts or with the periodic-acid–Schiff reaction for carbohydrates. Reticular fibers consist mainly of type-III collagen, and in electron micrographs, they are seen to be made up of small numbers of cross-striated unit fibrils of collagen. Their adsorption of silver salts and histochemical staining reaction for carbohydrates are probably attributable to a coating of bound proteoglycans. Reticular fibers are widespread in connective tissue

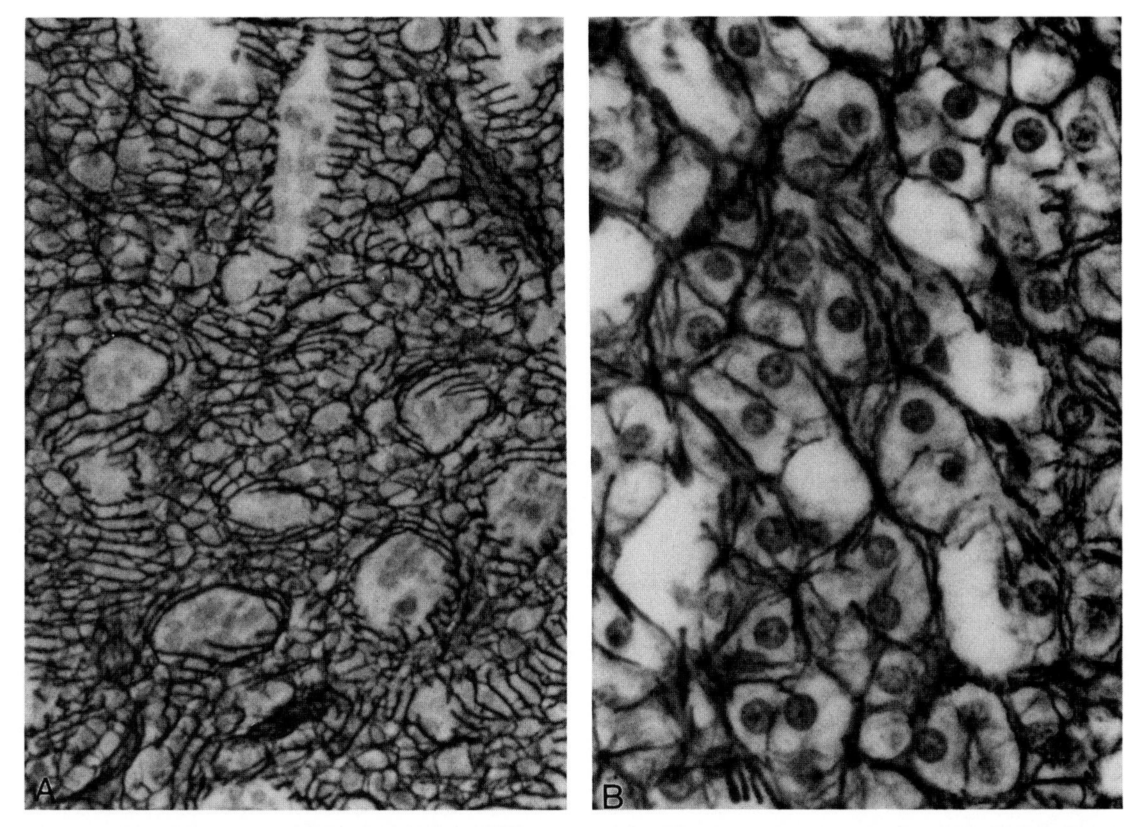

Figure 5–9. Reticular fibers are distinguished from other collagenous fibers by their smaller size, their reticular pattern, and by the fact that they blacken with silver stains. Two examples of the pattern of reticular fibers are presented: (A) reticulum of the spleen; (B) reticular fibers of the adrenal cortex.

throughout the body but are especially abundant in the intercellular clefts of smooth muscle, around the acini of glands, and beneath the epithelium of hollow organs that are subject to changes of volume, such as blood vessels, intestine, bladder, and uterus. They also make up most of the supporting framework of the spleen, lymph nodes, and bone marrow (Fig. 5–9).

Published tables giving the distribution of the several types of collagen are based largely on biochemical analyses. Although one type may predominate in a particular location, it should not be assumed that this is the only type present. The connective tissue, in most organs, includes more than one type of collagen. Identification of the predominant type by biochemical analysis does not provide information that may be desired on the range of fiber sizes, their arrangement, and their relation to other collagen types, or to the cells of the organ. Such information must be acquired by light microscopy, using polarization optics and selective stains, or by electron microscopy aided by immunohistochemical localization with type-specific antibodies.

When multiple types of collagen were first discovered, it was tempting to speculate that each type might polymerize into fibers of a characteristic size and that each type might be deployed in a characteristic pattern. This has not proven to be true. When examined with the electron microscope, fibril diameter is not closely correlated with collagen type. Tissues reported to be rich in type-I, type-II, or type-III collagen, by biochemical analysis, contain varying proportions of microfibrils (~4 nm in diameter), intermediate-sized fibrils (~10 nm), and larger striated fibrils (~25 nm). In the tendon, type-I collagen forms unusually large fibrils up to 190 nm in diameter, but in this tissue too, type-I collagen fibrils in the 50-nm range mingle with the larger fibrils. Thus, it is clear that the widely distributed 50-nm striated fibrils may be composed of type-I, type-II, or type-III collagen and fibrils of this size are not confined to reticular connective tissue, as has been commonly assumed. The size and pattern of collagen fibrils in different organs evidently does not depend on genetically determined differences in collagen molecules, but must be influenced by their posttranslational modification, by their relationship to matrix proteoglycans, and by other factors in their local microenvironment.

FIBRILLIN

Collagen and elastin are not the only fibrillar components of connective tissue. There are at least two other classes of microfibrils. The larger of these, 8–10 nm in diameter, consist of *fibrillin*, a nonsulfated 350 kD glycoprotein. These microfibrils appear as a beaded chain and, in cross-section, they have an electron-dense cortex around a lucid core. They are often closely associated with elastic fibers or with the basal lamina of epithelia. The smaller 3–5-nm microfibrils are associated with the granules of proteoglycan in the extracellular matrix. Their chemical nature and function remain unclear, but there is indirect evidence that they are essential for normal development.

Fibrillin is defective or deficient in *Marfan syndrome*, a heritable disorder of connective tissue, characterized by excessively long arms and legs and a progressive dilatation of the ascending aorta that may lead to fatal rupture. By molecular genetic analysis, the defect has been localized to a single gene on chromosome 15. It is speculated that President Lincoln may have had Marfan syndrome. Efforts are under way to verify this by searching for a mutant fibrillin gene in DNA from blood stains on garments preserved by the National Museum of Health and Medicine among other mementos of his assassination.

ELASTIC FIBERS

In selectively stained spreads of mesentery, very slender *elastic fibers* can be distinguished from the more abundant collagen fibers by their uniform small diameter and their tendency to branch and rejoin to form a loose

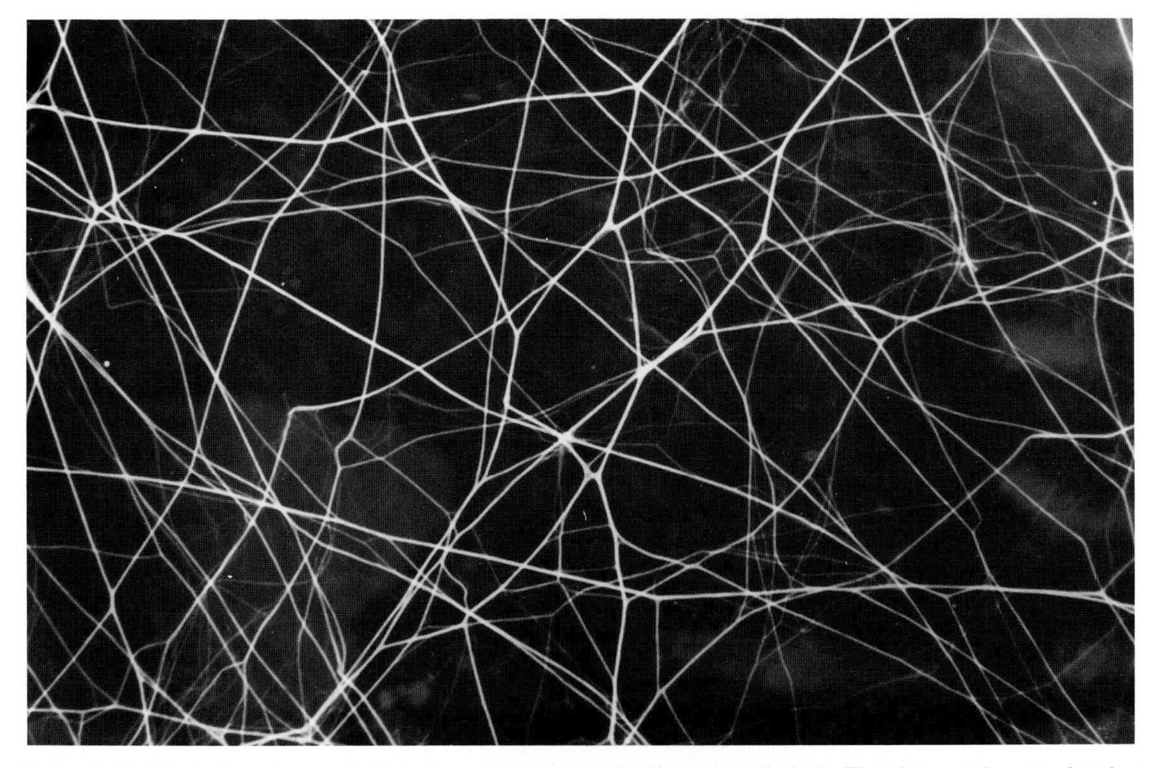

Figure 5–10. Elastic fibers in a spread of rat mesentery, stained with resorcin–fuchsin. The photograph was printed as a negative image. Note that the fibers are much more slender than the collagen fibers in Fig. 5–2, and they branch and anastomose to form a network. (From Fawcett, D.W. 1953. *In* R.O. Greep, ed. Histology, Philadelphia. Blakiston Co. Reproduced by permission of McGraw-Hill Book Co.)

network (Fig. 5–10). A branching pattern of fine elastic fibers is common in loose connective tissue but, in other tissues, elastin may take the form of fenestrated sheets or coarse parallel fibers. In the walls of large arteries, for example, there are multiple concentric fenestrated elastic laminae. Elastic ligaments, such as the ligamenta flava of the vertebral column, consist of coarse parallel fibers. In the ligamentum nuchae of ruminants, these fibers may be 4–5 μm in diameter. In sites where elastic fibers are abundant, they impart a yellow color to the tissue. Elastic fibers are difficult to identify in preparations stained with hematoxylin and eosin, but they can be selectively stained with Weigert's resorcin–fuchsin or Halmi's aldehyde–fuchsin method.

Elastic fibers consist of an amorphous core of *elastin* surrounded by the microfibrillar glycoprotein fibrillin. Elastin is composed of nonpolar amino acids and, in contrast to collagen, it contains little hydroxyproline and no hydroxylysine. It has an alanine content higher than that of any known protein and contains two unique amino acids, *desmosine* and *isodesmosine*. These unusual amino acids are thought to extensively cross-link the molecules into a three-dimensional network of randomly coiled chains that is responsible for its rubber-like properties. Elastic fibers can be stretched to one and a half times their original length by a force of 20–30 kg/cm and return to their original length when the tension is released. When a fiber breaks, its ends quickly retract and coil up like a broken rubber band. The fibrillar component is readily solubilized by chemical agents that break hydrogen bonds, but elastin is resistant to boiling and to hydrolysis by dilute acid or alkali, conditions that destroy collagen and other constituents of connective tissue. It can, however, be selectively digested by the pancreatic enzyme *elastase*.

The role of the microfibrils in the development of elastic fibers is not clear. Small bundles of microfibrils appear first in close proximity to fibroblasts or smooth muscle cells. Then, molecules of elastin, secreted by the cells, polymerize around and between the microfibrils. In the fully formed elastic fibers, the microfilaments are embedded in the periphery of the elastin. It is speculated that the microfibrils may serve to impose a fibrous form on the amorphous polymerizing elastin. Comparable studies of the formation of elastic laminae have not been carried out. During the extracellular polymerization of elastin, an enzyme, *lysyl oxidase*, catalyzes the formation and condensation of aldehydic groups on lysines to form the ring structure of the desmosines that cross-link elastin molecules. In the disease *lathyrism*, which occurs in domestic animals that eat the plant *Lathyrus odoratus*, the action of lysyl oxidase is inhibited and the polypeptide chains of both elastin and collagen are incompletely cross-linked.

Elastic fibers occur in connective tissues throughout the body but they are especially abundant in organs that must yield to externally or internally applied force, and then return to their original shape. The lungs, for example, are expanded during each inspiration but must have sufficient elasticity to return to their original volume during expiration. The connective tissue in the alveolar septa of the lung is rich in elastic fibers. The aorta, the large blood vessel conducting blood away from the heart, is distended by the outflow at each contraction of the ventricles. The elastic recoil of its wall is essential to maintain continuous flow from intermittent contractions of the heart. This expansion and recoil, after each heart beat, is made possible by multiple elastic laminae in the wall of the aorta

ADHESION GLYCOPROTEINS

In addition to the microscopically visible fibrous components of connective tissue, there are glycoproteins that are involved in the interaction of the cells with the extracellular matrix. Some cells have receptors in their membranes that can bind directly to collagen fibers, but the attachment of other cell types is mediated by adhesion glycoproteins such as *fibronectin, laminin*, and *thrombospondin* that have binding sites for cell membrane and for collagen or glycosaminoglycans of the extracellular matrix. These adhesive glycoproteins differ from proteoglycans in their higher proportion of protein and in characteristic differences in the nature of their polysaccharide side-chains. Their primary function is to maintain adhesion of cells to their substrate, but evidence is accumulating that they also influence the state of differentiation of the cells and the organization of their cytoskeleton.

FIBRONECTIN

Fibronectin is a large glycoprotein of 440,000 molecular weight (MW) that is a constituent of the extracellular matrix of connective tissue, the basal lamina of epithelia, and the external lamina that envelops smooth and striated muscle fibers. It is synthesized by connective tissue fibroblasts, by other mesenchymal derivatives, and by some epithelia. Because it is not directly visible by microscopy, what is known of its distribution is based on its immunocytochemical localization with fluorescent antibody.

The long flexible fibronectin molecule has cell-binding, collagen-binding, and glycosaminoglycan-binding domains along its length. These specific binding sites are the basis for its role in connecting the surface of the cells to the fibrous and amorphous components of the extracellular matrix. The receptor for fibronectin in the cell membrane is one member of a family of cell surface receptors, collectively called *integrins*, which interact with a variety of glycoproteins of the extracellular matrix. Some of these integral membrane proteins also have a cytoplasmic domain that binds to components of the cytoskeleton, thus linking structural proteins within the cell to proteins in the surrounding ground substance.

There is a fibronectin in blood plasma which is distinct from that of connective tissue but has a similar structure and function. *Plasma fibronectin* is synthesized by the liver cells and by endothelial cells. It binds to fibrin and may have a significant role in blood clotting.

LAMININ

Laminin is a large glycoprotein with a molecular weight of about one million. It is the most abundant constituent of the basal lamina of epithelia and of the corresponding layer investing muscle fibers. When isolated and rotary-shadowed, it can be resolved, with the electron microscope, as a cross-shaped molecule with rod-like and globular regions. It binds to the membrane of epithelial and muscle cells, to type-IV collagen, and to heparan sulfate proteglycans. The binding sites on the laminin molecule for each of these have been identified. The multiple interactions of laminin enable it to play a major role in the assembly of the basal lamina. It not only links epithelial cells to their basal lamina but also influences their phenotype. When epithelial cells devoid of a basal lamina are cultured in gels of type-I collagen, they change the nature of their intermediate filaments, cease to synthesize their normal products, and become transformed into cells resembling fibroblasts. However, if cultured in gels containing extracts of basal lamina, and therefore containing laminin, their normal differentiated state is retained. Thus, it is likely that laminin and other constituents of the basal lamina influence the form and function of epithelial cells.

THROMBOSPONDIN

Thrombospondin is an adhesive glycoprotein of 450,000 MW first identified as a product of activated platelets, secreted during blood clotting. It is the most abundant protein in the granules of blood platelets. It binds to fibrinogen, plasmalogen, and plasmalogen-activator and is an essential participant in blood clotting. Thrombospondin also binds to collagen, heparin, and fibronectin and has been localized by fluorescent antibodies in a number of tissues, including muscle, skin, and blood vessels. It is synthesized by the fibroblasts of connective tissue, by endothelial cells, and by smooth muscle cells. Upon secretion, it binds to the cell surface and to components of the extracellular matrix. Its exact function in the connective tissues is still poorly understood.

ORIGIN OF CONNECTIVE TISSUE FIBERS

The constant association of fusiform cells with collagen fibers led early histologists to conclude that these so-called *fibroblasts* produced the connective tissue fibers. This was later supported by the detection of collagen in the medium of tissue cultures of these cells. When radioisotopes became available, it was possible to trace the biosynthetic pathway of collagen within the fibroblast in autoradiographs. Radiolabeled proline was first localized in the endoplasmic reticulum, then in the Golgi complex, and later in the extracellular collagen fibers. These morphological observations were supplemented by biochemical studies showing that the α-chains of collagens are synthesized on ribosomes as a high-molecular-weight precursor called *preprocollagen α-chains* that have a short signal sequence at their amino-terminal end. This is removed as the precursor molecule traverses the membrane of the reticulum and *procollagen α-chains* accumulate in its lumen. There, they are modified by hydroxylation of certain proline and lysine subunits and by glycosylation of hydroxylysines. Disulfide bridges are formed as the chains associate in the triple helica configuration. The resulting *procollagen* is concentrated and packaged in the Golgi complex and then secreted. Procollagen molecules are unable to polymerize, but during, or immediately after, their release from the cell, amino- and carboxypropeptides are cleaved off by proteases, permitting the resulting *collagen* molecules to polymerize into cross-striated fibrils in the extracellular matrix (Fig. 5–5). Thus, in the fibroblast, the biosynthetic pathway for collagen is similar to that in other protein-secreting cells, but the final product is assembled extracellularly. Procollagen is secreted constitutively and, therefore, fibroblasts do not have the conspicuous secretory granules that are characteristic of cells involved in regulated secretion.

In developing connective tissue, delicate networks of argyrophilic reticular fibers (type-III collagen) are first to appear. Fibers formed somewhat later are not argyrophilic and are predominantly type-I collagen. This sequence of events suggests that the precursors of type-I and type-III collagen are secreted in amounts that change as development progresses. The relative amounts of these two collagens also vary from region to region and these differences have a major influence on the properties of the connective tissue. They are produced in ratios that provide the particular mechanical properties required in the various organs and tissues. In compliant organs, such as the lung and spleen, and in the lamina propria of the intestine, type-III collagen abounds, whereas in less-yielding structures, such as tendon or bone, type-I collagen greatly predominates. Little is known about the factors that modulate the secretory activity of the fibroblasts to produce these differences.

Equally obscure is the role of the fibroblasts, if any, in determining the arrangement of the fibers. It is generally assumed that they simply maintain, in the matrix, the appropriate physicochemical conditions to permit collagen fibers to polymerize and that the orientation of the fibers is determined by the direction of stresses in the tissue. However, some investigators contend that orthogonal patterns and other highly ordered arrangements of fibers, found at certain sites in the body, are hard to explain on the basis of mechanical forces within the tissue. Instead, they argue that the fibers only form in very close association with the cells and that these exercise some control over fiber orientation. Some support for this view has come from studies on the development of tendons, which consist of bundles of precisely parallel collagen fibers. Fibrils are reported to arise, a few at a time, in long grooves in the fibroblast surface that appear to be formed by alignment of procollagen-containing vacuoles within the cell and their subsequent fusion with each other and with the cell membrane (Fig. 5–7). Thus, although fiber formation is extracellular, it may take place in surface grooves or recesses wherein an environment favorable for polymerization is created by the fibroblast. It is suggested that this mode of fiber formation would enable the fibroblast to influence the orientation of the collagen fibers, but this remains speculative.

The principal producers of collagen and elastin of the connective tissues are the fibroblasts, but it is now known that these fibrous proteins can also be synthesized by smooth muscle cells and other cells of mesenchymal origin. Epithelia also secrete the type-IV collagen of their basal lamina and, in rare instances, may also produce fiber-forming collagens.

CELLS OF CONNECTIVE TISSUE

The cells of connective tissue are assigned to two categories, *fixed cells* and *free cells*. The fixed cells are a relatively stable population of long-lived cells that include the *fibroblasts* that secrete and maintain the extracellular components and *adipose cells* that store and release lipids to be used as an energy source in the metabolism of other cells throughout the body. The free cells are a changing population of motile cells that enter the connective tissue from the blood and wander through its ground substance. Most of these are short-lived and are continually replaced from the large pool of cells of the same type circulating in the blood. They include *eosinophils, monocytes, lymphocytes, macrophages, plasma cells* that differentiate from lymphocytes, and *mast cells* that are of uncertain provenance. Some of the free cells participate in short-term responses of the tissue to injury or bacterial invasion, whereas others participate in longer-term immunological defenses of the body.

MESENCHYMAL CELLS

The connective tissues develop from the embryonic tissue called *mesenchyme*. Its cells differentiate into the fibroblasts, the predominant sessile cell type of the connective tissues. The *mesenchymal cells* are small fusiform or stellate cells not easily distinguished from fibroblasts. In electron micrographs, they have a coarser chromatin pattern, fewer mitochondria and their sparse cytoplasm contains little or no endoplasmic reticulum.

A small population of these pluripotential cells is believed to persist into postnatal life, and to give rise to other cells types as the need arises. For example, when capillaries increase in diameter in response to altered hemodynamic conditions, and become transformed into arterioles, the smooth muscle cells of their wall are believed to arise by recruitment and differentiation of mesenchymal cells in the perivascular connective tissue. The adipose cells that accumulate in the connective tissue of overnourished individuals are believed, by some histologists, to arise by further differentiation of mesenchymal cells.

FIBROBLAST

As previously indicated, the *fibroblasts* are the cells that produce the extracellular components of developing connective tissue. When they become relatively inactive in fiber formation, some histologists prefer to call them *fibrocytes*. But because these cells have the potential for fibrogenesis in quiescent connective tissue of the adult, as well as during development, others prefer to use the term fibroblast in all circumstances. The shape of these cells depends, to some extent, on the nature of their substrate. They are usually deployed along bundles of collagen fibers and appear, in sections, as fusiform cells with long tapering ends (Figs. 5–12 and 5–13). In other situations, they may be flattened stellate cells with several slender processes (Fig. 5–14). Their elongated nucleus is always apparent, but the cell outline may be difficult to make out in histological sections because, when relatively inactive, their cytoplasm may be eosinophilic like the neighboring collagen fibers. Their shape is more clearly seen in sections stained with iron-hematoxylin.

Fibroblasts have been extensively studied in tissue cultures, where they can be observed in isolation from the interlacing fabric of fibers in which they reside in vivo. In this environment, the cells migrate out from the explant with their processes adhering to neighboring cells to form a cellular network (Fig. 5–12). It is likely that fibroblasts in the connective tissue also maintain contacts with one another but, for technical reasons, this is difficult to demonstrate.

In electron micrographs, the long elliptical fibroblast nucleus contains one or two nucleoli and small clumps of chromatin adjacent to the nuclear envelope. A pair of centrioles and a small Golgi complex are situated near the nucleus. Long slender mitochondria are found mainly in the perinuclear cytoplasm but may extend a short distance into the tapering cell processes. The rough endoplasmic reticulum is sparse in inactive fibroblasts but it is abundant in those of developing connective tissue (Fig 5–15). Immediately beneath the plasmalemma, there is an organelle-free cortex rich in microfilaments. Actin and α-actinin are localized in this peripheral zone by immunocytochemical staining methods. Myosin appears to be diffusely distributed in the cytoplasm. Numerous microtubules that radiate from the centrosome are believed to maintain the elongated shape of the cell.

Fibroblasts are able to move through collagen gels in vitro and through the extracellular matrix in vivo, at a rate of about 1 μm/min, while maintaining their bipolar form. How this is accomplished is unclear, but there is suggestive evidence that new membrane and new contacts with the matrix are continuously generated at the leading end of the cell, and endoplasm flows forward within the sleeve of the actin-rich cortex that remains fixed to components of the surrounding matrix via specific transmembrane receptors. As the bulk of the cell slowly moves forward, the trailing process disintegrates, breaking away from its attachments and often leaving behind bits of membrane and cytoplasm.

Dividing fibroblasts are rarely seen in normal connective tissue, but in response to injury, they proliferate and become more active in their synthesis of matrix components. In healing wounds, they are larger than normal and more basophilic. In electron micrographs, it is apparent that the Golgi complex has enlarged and the endoplasmic reticulum

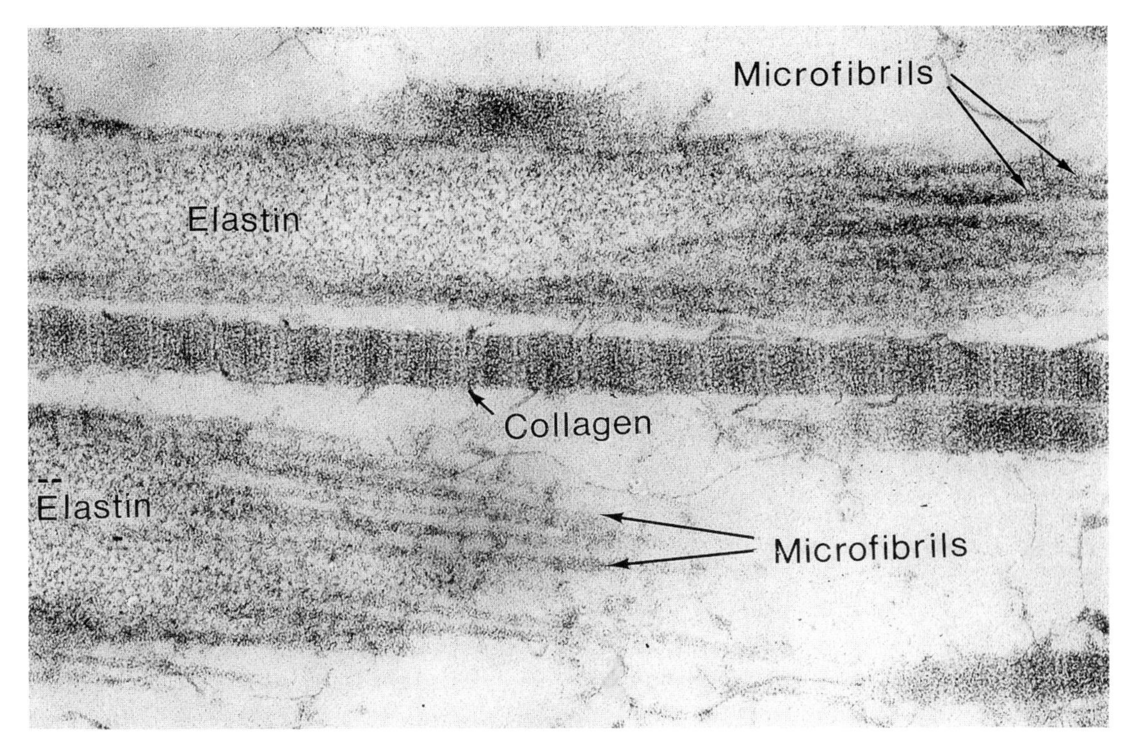

Figure 5–11 Electron micrograph of a portion of fetal calf nuchal membrane stretched to 150% of resting length and fixed under tension. The amorphous component, elastin, and associated microfibrils are clearly shown. (Micrograph courtesy of J.C. Fanning.)

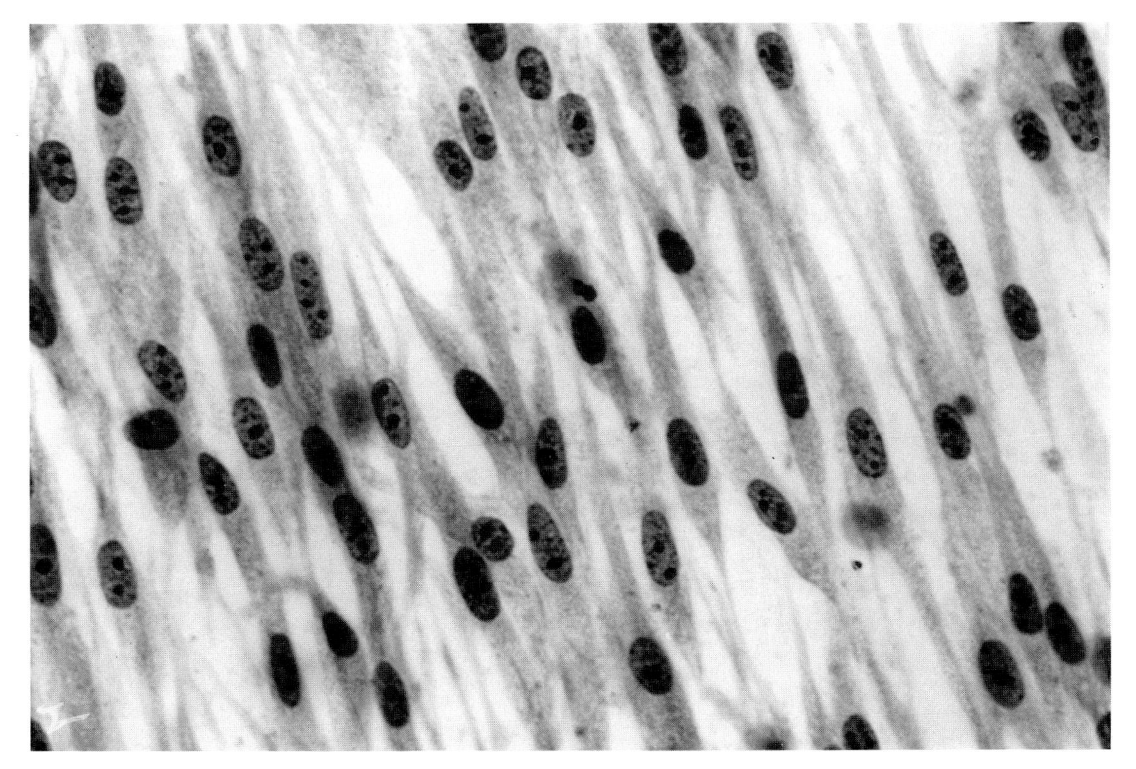

Figure 5–12. Photomicrograph of fibroblasts in tissue culture illustrating their long spindle shape. This shape is also common in the tissues, but there, the processes may be branched resulting in more stellate forms.

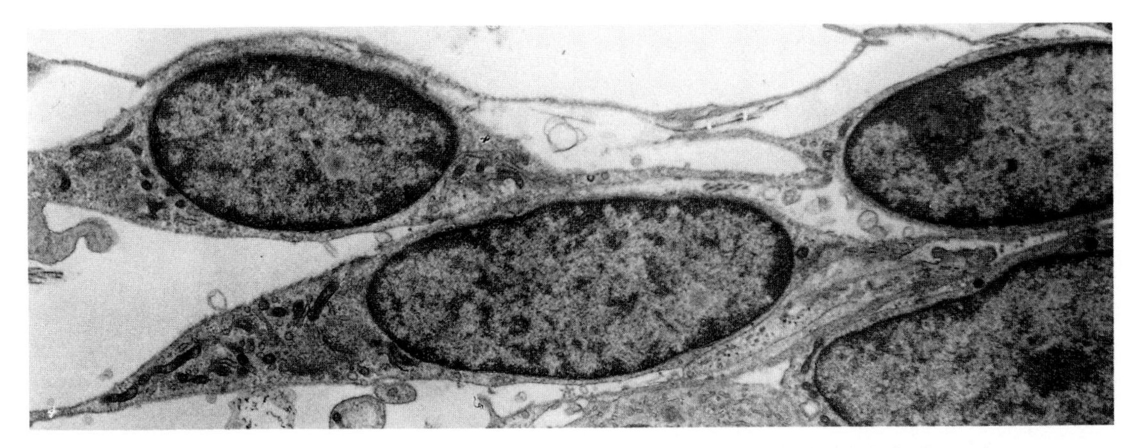

Figure 5–13. Electron micrograph of relatively inactive fibroblasts illustrating their fusiform shape.

has become more extensive. In histological sections, such stimulated fibroblasts contain numerous small periodic-acid–Schiff positive cytoplasmic granules that may represent intracellular precursors of collagen and glycosaminoglycans that are being secreted into the matrix in increased quantity.

Fibroblasts are commonly considered to be fully differentiated cells that do not give rise to other cell types, but this is debatable. Certainly, fibroblasts seem to accumulate lipid and become adipose cells, and in certain pathological conditions, they appear to transform into bone-forming cells, osteoblasts. However, in both of these examples, it is difficult to exclude the possibility that it is not the fibroblasts that have undergone these dramatic transformations, but pluripotential mesenchymal cells that persist in the connective tissue of adults. However, there is no doubt that fibroblasts can adopt a variety of shapes other than those they normally express in the connective tissues. With the increasing use of the scanning electron microscope, it has become apparent that the stromal cells, in some organs, have a form very different from the fusiform shape commonly attributed to connective tissue fibroblasts. In the intestinal villi, for example, the cells between the epithelium and the underlying capillaries appear fusiform in sections, but when viewed in three dimensions with the scanning microscope, they are found to form an elaborate cellular network of stellate cells having multiple radiating processes. Similarly, in the interstitium of the renal papilla, the interstitial cells form highly ordered arrays of elongated cells oriented perpendicular to the axis of the collect-

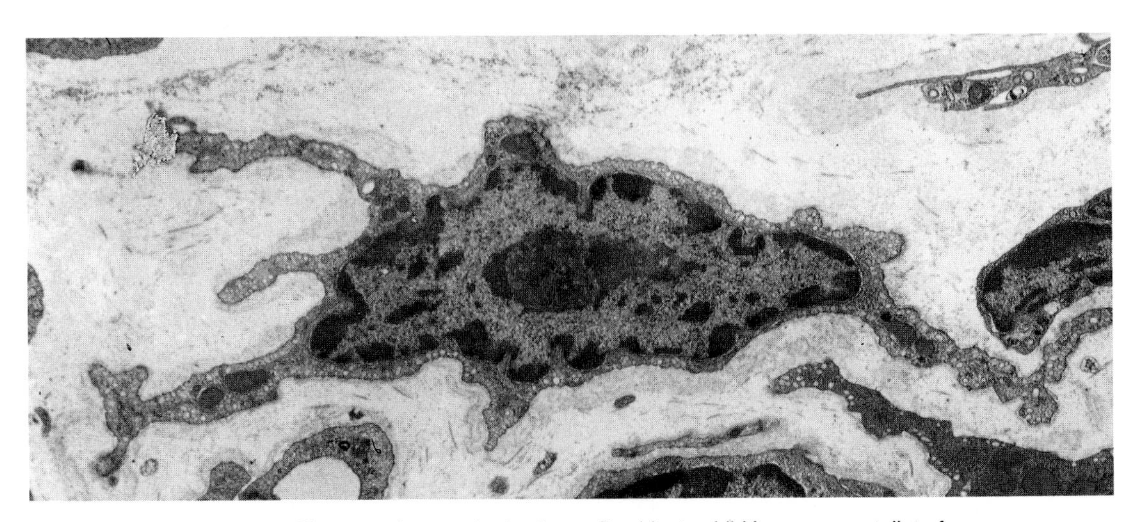

Figure 5–14. Electron micrograph of a tissue fibroblast exhibiting a more stellate form.

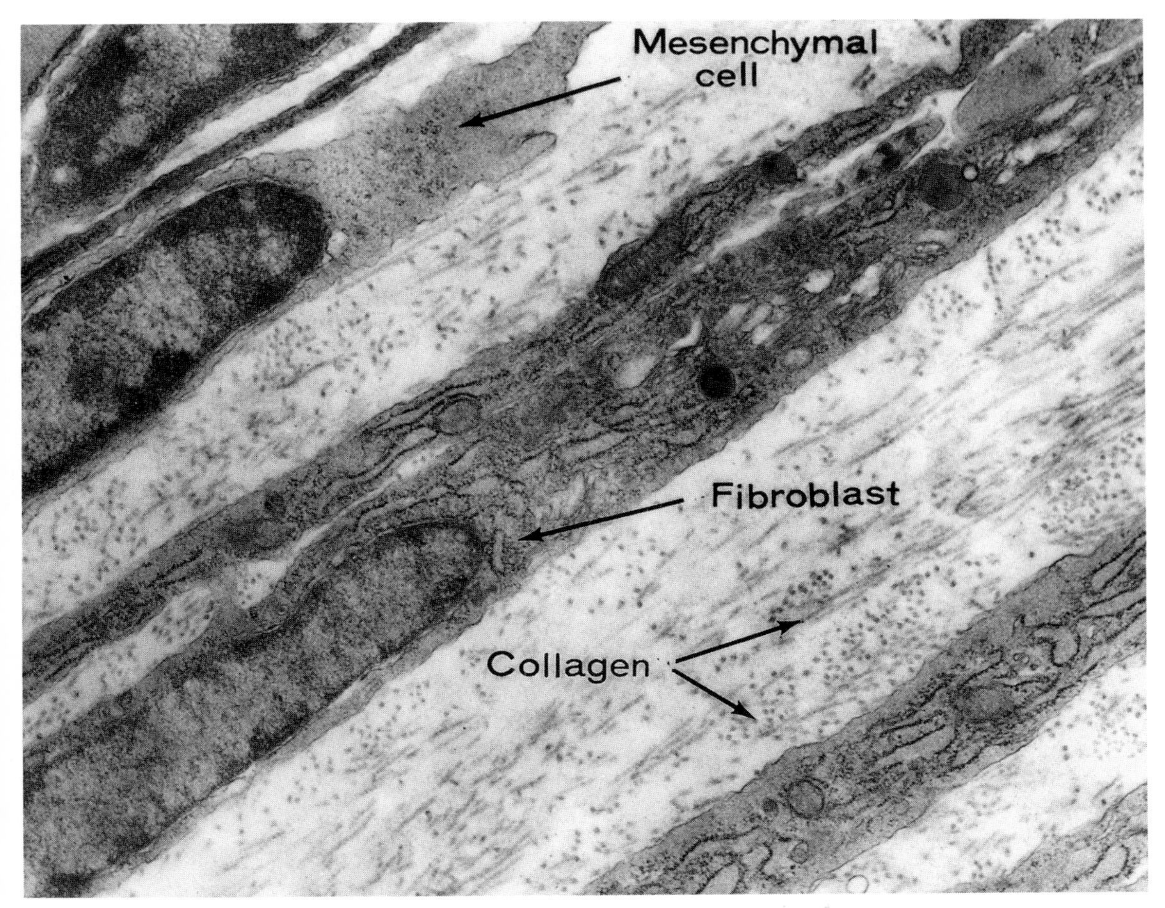

Figure 5–15. Electron micrograph of fibroblasts in developing connective tissue. Fibroblasts actively synthesizing collagen have a well-developed rough endoplasmic reticulum, often having distended cisternae. The relatively undifferentiated cell, at the upper upper left, having more heterochromatin and few cytoplasmic organelles is probably a mesenchymal cell.

ing ducts and joined to one another by zonulae adherentes and communicating through gap junctions. Although these cells have a supporting function, resemble fibroblasts, and secrete extracellular matrix, they have also been shown to have an endocrine function.

Experiments involving the labeling of fibroblasts to follow their participation in morphogenetic processes are revealing hitherto unsuspected versatility. The perineurium of peripheral nerves consists of one or more layers of cells joined together by tight junctions to form an epithelium-like barrier that serves to maintain a special endoneurial environment for the nerve axon. In ingenious reconstitution experiments using labeled fibroblasts, it has been shown that the perineurium that develops around axons, in vitro, is formed by fibroblasts that alter their shape to form a continuous layer of flattened cells joined by tight junctions. In the connective tissue, fibroblasts never form such junctions with neighboring cells. Thus, it has become apparent that although fibroblasts in the connective tissue are fully differentiated cells involved in maintenance of the extracellular matrix, they can take on a very different shape and acquire additional functions in other locations.

ADIPOSE CELLS

The *adipose cells* or *fat cells* are fixed cells of the connective tissue specialized for the synthesis and storage of lipid. These cells accumulate lipid to such an extent that their nucleus is flattened and displaced to one side and the cytoplasm is reduced to a thin film around a single very large droplet of lipid

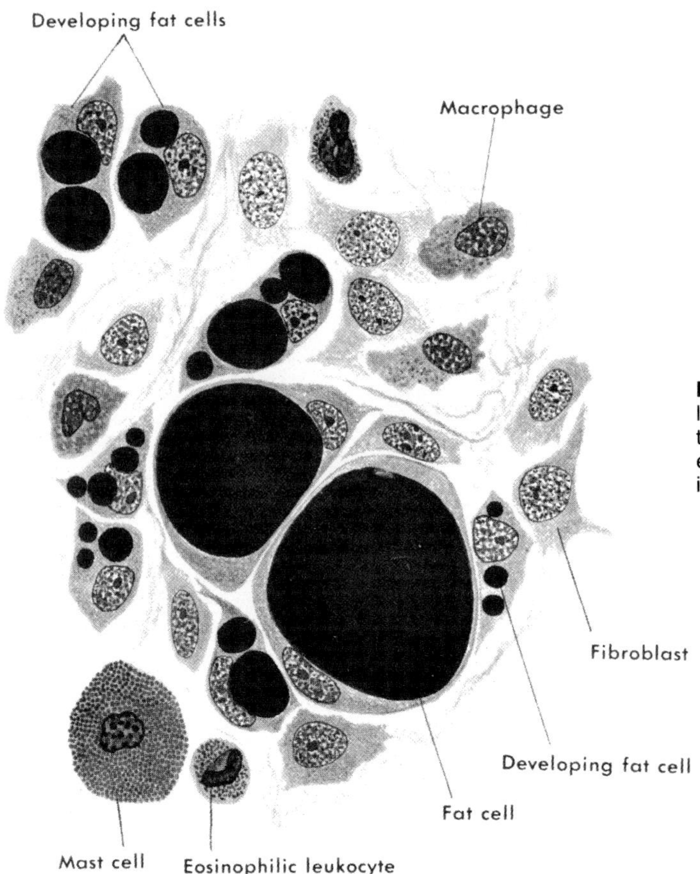

Figure 5–16. Drawing of cells in subcutaneous loose connective tissue of the rat. The osmium tetroxide of the fixative preserved and blackened the lipid droplets in several adipose cells in different stages of differentiation.

(Figs. 5–16 and 5–17). So inconspicuous are the nucleus and cytoplasm that the fat cells in unstained connective tissue have the appearance of large glistening drops of oil. They may occur singly in connective tissue but are often in groups of varying size. They tend to be concentrated along the course of small blood vessels. Where they accumulate in such large numbers that they become the predominant cellular component, they form *adipose tissue* which will be the subject of a separate chapter (Chapter 6).

MACROPHAGES

Connective tissue throughout the body contains a sparse population of mobile cells that have a remarkable capacity for phagocytosis. These *macrophages* (or *histiocytes*) play a role in the maintenance of normal tissues by ingesting dead cells and cellular debris and other particulate matter and breaking them down with their lysosomal enzymes (Figs. 5–19 and 5–20). They are also the first line of defense against infection, voraciously ingesting and destroying invading bacteria. They are also indispensable participants in the immunological defenses of the body by processing and presenting antigen to lymphocytes capable of producing protective antibodies.

When histologists had to rely exclusively on shape and staining properties of cells for their identification, two categories of macrophages were distinguished: *free macrophages*, motile cells of varying shape that wandered through the ground substance, and *fixed macrophages*, sessile cells that were stretched out along collagen fibers and had a shape not unlike that of fibroblasts. These two forms of macrophage were considered to be distinct in their origin and, to some extent, in their function. With the development of immunocytochemical methods for detecting specific surface molecules on cells and for tracing cell lineages by isotopic labeling, it became apparent that free and fixed macrophages are simply different phases in the life history of cells of the same lineage. All macrophages are now known to arise from monocytes that develop in the bone marrow, circulate in the blood for a day or two, and then migrate through the endothelium of postcapillary venules to take up residence in the connective tissue (Fig. 5–18). There they differentiate into macrophages that have a lifespan of about 2 months. Replacement of tissue macrophages goes on continuously at a slow basal rate, but the monocytes circulating in the blood constitute a very large reserve that can be rapidly mobilized at sites of injury or infection and there transform into macrophages.

The traditional terms free macrophages and fixed macrophages have now given way to more appropriate descriptive terms. Macrophages that are present at a given site, in the absence of an exogenous stimulus, are referred to as *resident macrophages*. Those mobilized at the site in response to a stimulus are *elicited macrophages* and those that have acquired enhanced phagocytic and antigen-processing activity in response to a local stimulus are called *activated macrophages*. These terms are useful in describing the sequence of events after local injury or in the development of an inflammatory reaction to bacterial invasion.

Unstimulated resident macrophages are fusiform or stellate cells widely distributed among the bundles of collagen fibers of connective tissue, but they tend to be more abundant in the vicinity of small blood vessels. They are distinguishable from fibroblasts by their slightly smaller, darker staining nucleus and a more heterogeneous cytoplasm, which often contains a number of vacuoles and small dense granules. The latter are identified in electron micrographs as primary and secondary lysosomes. Perhaps the most dependable method for identification of macrophages is by immunocytochemical detection of their distinctive surface markers. Their plasmalemma contains about 2×10^6 *Fc receptors* that bind immunoglobulins (antibodies). They also express surface receptors for the *C_3 component* of *complement*. Complement is a group of proteins synthesized in the liver and circulating in the blood plasma. Complement and immune globulins bind to the surface of bacteria, mak-

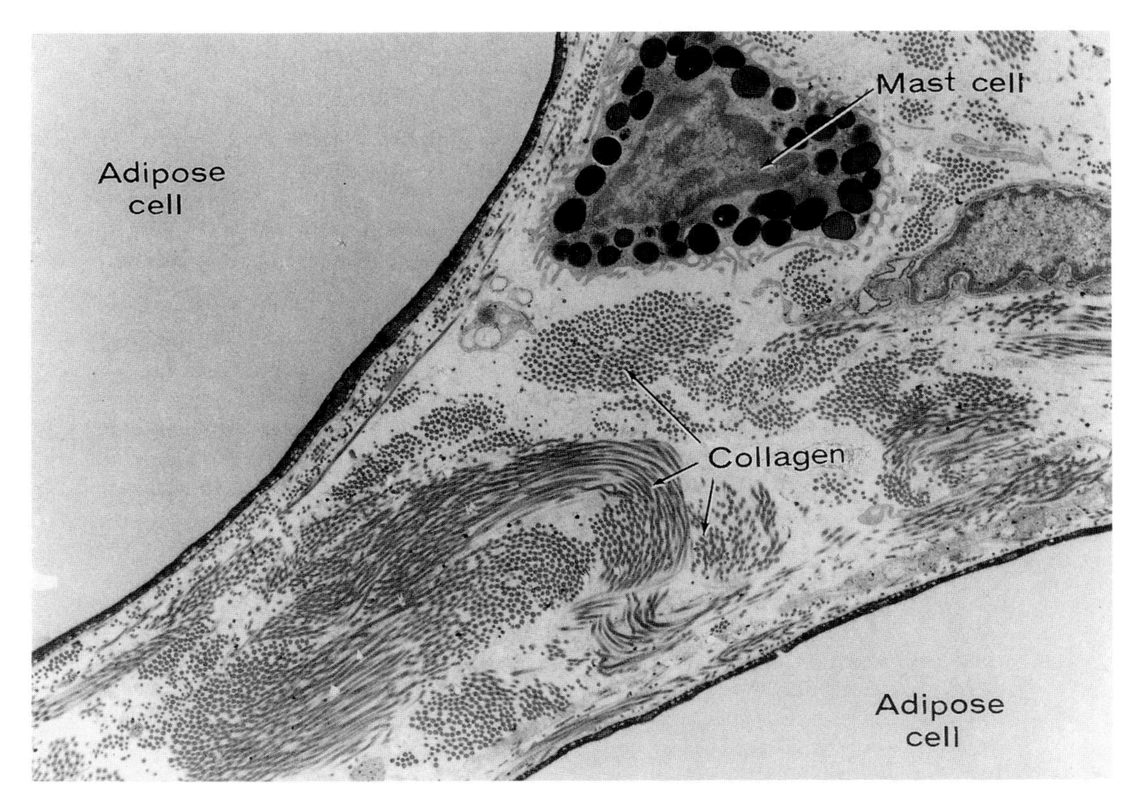

Figure 5–17. Electron micrograph of portions of two adipose cells and the intervening collagenous fibers. Relative to the mast cell and the fibroblast at the upper right, the adipose cells are enormous. Only a small portion of each is included in this field, but enough to show the thin peripheral layer of cytoplasm and the homogeneous lipid content, which usually is not stained black after primary glutaraldehyde fixation.

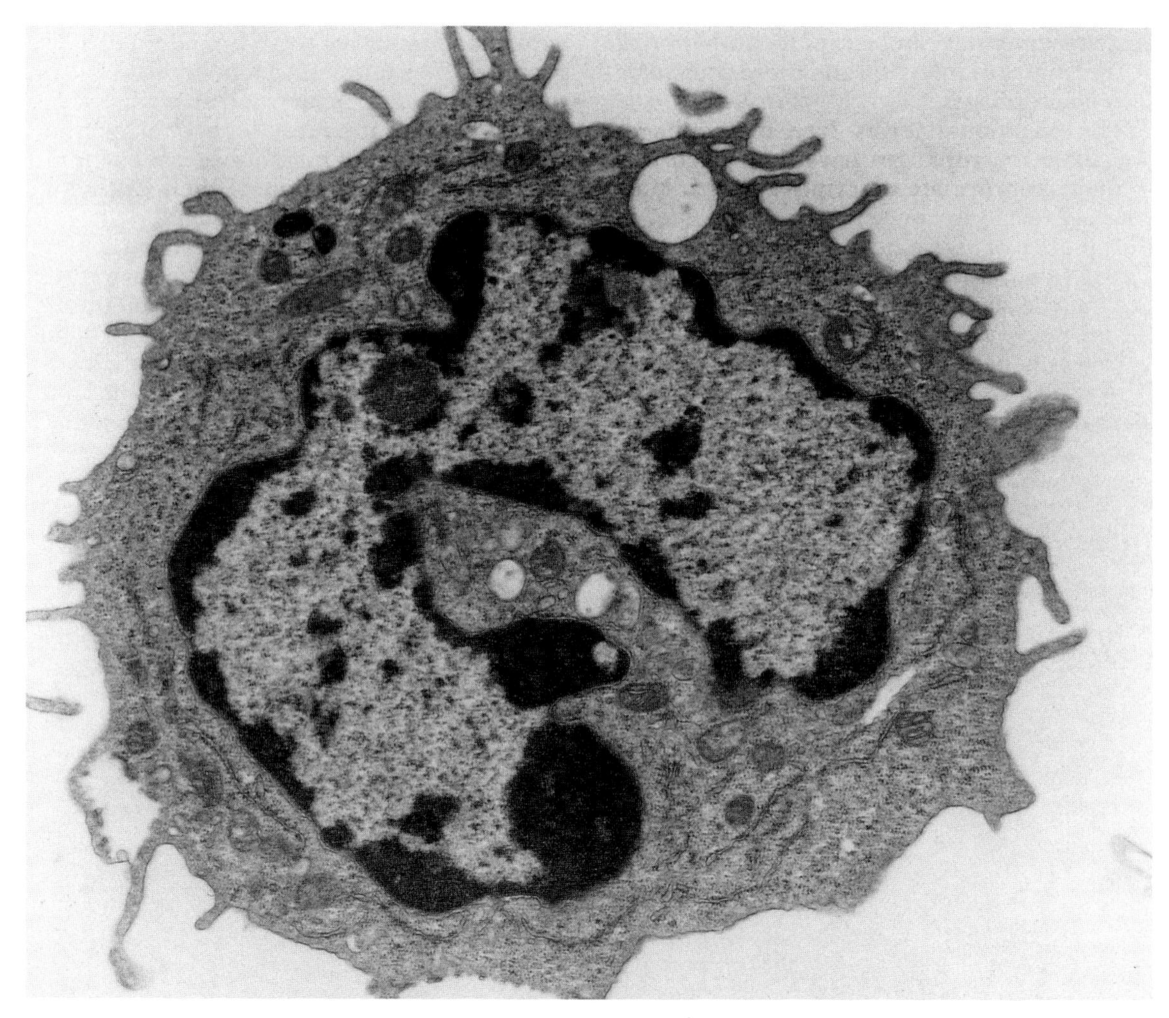

Figure 5–18. Electron micrograph of a monocyte, the precursor of the macrophage. Monocytes are not commonly found in the connective tissue because they transform into macrophages very soon after they leave the blood.

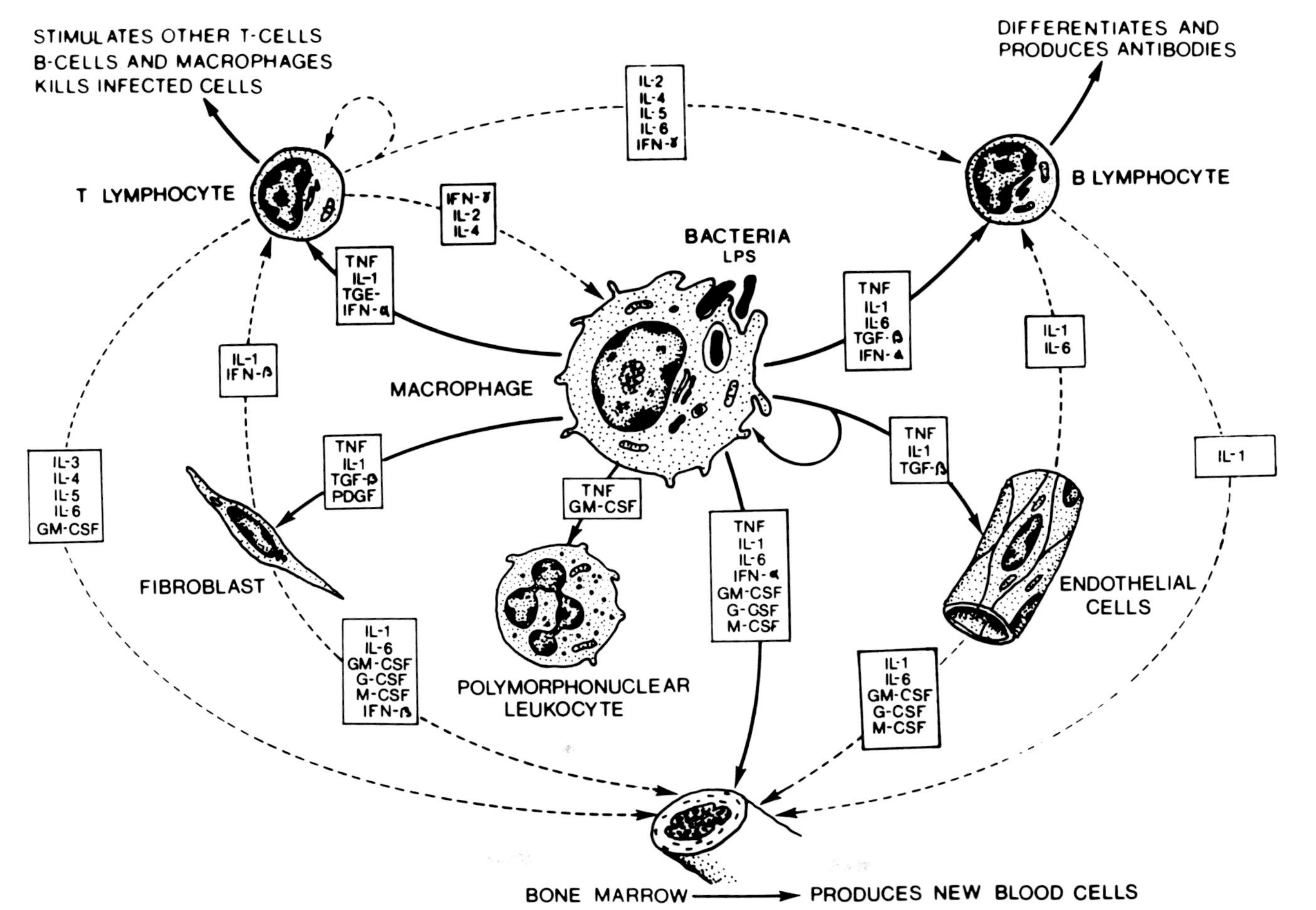

Figure 5–19. Diagram showing the activation of defenses against infection when macrophages are stimulated by bacterial lipopolysaccharide (LPS). Macrophage products influence polymorphonuclear leukocytes, T-lymphocytes, B-lymphocytes, fibroblasts, and endothelial cells (solid lines). These cells, in turn, secrete interferons, interleukins, and growth factors that act locally, as well as colony-stimulating factors that activate the hemopoietic cells of the bone marrow (dotted lines). (Redrawn after L.J. Old, *Scientific American*.)

ing them more vulnerable to phagocytosis, a process called *opsonization*. When an opsonized bacterium has bound to the surface of a macrophage, ingestion begins with a zipper-like progressive binding of Fc and C_3 receptors on its plasmalemma to the corresponding ligands on the surface of the bacterium until the latter is completely enveloped by folds of the macrophage surface. After membrane fusion at the leading edge of the encircling processes, the bacterium, now enclosed in a vacuole (phagosome), is drawn deeper into the cytoplasm. Lysosomes then fuse with the phagosome discharging into it microbicidal peptides and enzymes, including lysozyme that digests the bacterial cell wall and myeloperoxidase which generates oxygen, hydrogen peroxide (H_2O_2), and superoxide ions (O^{-2}). The actions of these and other lysosomal enzymes result in the complete destruction of the bacterium. It is interesting that certain strains of bacteria have developed a resistance to the microbicidal mechanisms of macrophages and have, therefore, become exceptionally virulent.

Macrophages do not act alone in combating infections. They interact with lymphocytes that also gather at sites of bacterial invasion. Macrophage activation depends on a *lipopolysaccharide* (LPS) that is a major component of the surface of gram-negative bacteria, and on *gamma interferon* (INF), a cytokine produced by antigen-stimulated T-lymphocytes. Macrophages, in turn, process antigen and present it to lymphocytes in a more immunogenic form. They also synthesize and release *interleukin-1* (IL-1), *tumor necrosis factor* (TNF), and *granulocyte-macrophage colony-stimulating factor* (GM-CSF), cytokines that have wide-ranging effects on the immune system (Figs. 5–19 and 5–20). Acting locally, interleukin-1 stimulates B-lymphocyte proliferation and antibody production. It is also chemotactic for neutrophils and mitogenic for fibroblasts. Carried in the blood, it acts on the bone marrow to increase the number of circulating neutrophils. The role of macrophages in immunity will be discussed in more appropriate context in Chapter 13.

In certain pathological conditions, macrophages may have unusual shapes. At sites of chronic inflammation, closely aggregated macrophages may take on a polygonal shape owing to their mutual deformation. In this configuration, they are described as *epitheloid cells*. Where macrophages gather around splinters or other foreign bodies that are too large to be engulfed, they may coalesce to form huge multinucleated masses that are called *foreign body giant cells*. This same transformation may be observed in vitro. Monocytes are the only leukocytes capable of surviving in cultures of blood leukocytes. They rapidly transform into macrophages that phagocytize dead and dying cells of other types and in a few days pure cultures of macrophages are obtained. The culture vessel acts as a foreign body and, after prolonged culture, the macrophages coalesce to form huge multinucleated giant cells.

Elicited and activated macrophages are highly variable in shape. In addition to the pseudopodia that they extend and retract in their locomotion, they have many short microvilli and thin undulating folds of their surface, called lamellipodia. Such macrophages are much more active in pinocytosis and phagocytosis than are resident macrophages. It is estimated that they may interiorize the equivalent of their total surface area every 30 min. They are selective in the kind of particles they ingest. They do not phagocytize viable cells, but they do recognize and ingest senescent, dead, or damaged cells of the connective tissue. The

Surface of Markers of Macrophages

Fc receptors
Il-2 receptors
Interferon receptors
Complement receptors
Adenosine triphosphatase
5-nucleotidase

Secretory Products of Marcrophages

Mediators

Interleukin-1 (Il-1)
Interleukin-6 (Il-6)
Tumor necrosis factor (TNF)
Interferon
Colony stimulating factors
(M-CSF, G-CSF, GM-CSF)
Erythropoietin
Platelet derived growth factor (PDGF)
Fibroblast growth factor (FGF)
Transforming growth factor (TGF)

Other products

Elastase
Collagenase
Lysozyme
Prostaglandins
Leukotrienes
Hydrogen peroxide

Figure 5–20. Table listing some of the secretory products and surface properties of macrophages.

scale of their waste disposal activities is not easily measured in the connective tissue but some indication of their voracity can be gained from the rate of disposal of erythrocytes by comparable sessile phagocytic cells that line the sinusoids of the liver and spleen. Every day about 10^{11} erythrocytes in the blood reach the end of their 120-day lifespan and are ingested by these sessile phagocytes.

FREE CELLS OF CONNECTIVE TISSUE

MONONUCLEAR PHAGOCYTE SYSTEM

Monocytes are rarely found in connective tissue for, on leaving the bloodstream, they rapidly differentiate into resident macrophages. These become rather uniformly distributed and either adhere to bundles of collagen fibers or wander through the tissue phagocytosing cellular debris. They respond to chemotactic metabolic products of bacteria by congregating at the site. Such actively phagocytic cells are not confined to connective tissue.

Phagocytic cells similar to macrophages were found, by early histologists, in other tissues and organs and were given different names. Metchnikoff (1892) recognized the desirability of including all such cells as members of a single diffuse cell system and proposed the term *macrophage system*. Relying on the uptake of the colloidal vital dye Trypan blue as a means of identifying such cells, Aschoff (1924) noted that the endothelial cells lining the sinusoids of the liver, spleen, and bone marrow also took up the dye and suggested the term *reticuloendothelial system* for all cells taking up this vital dye (Fig. 5–21). This more inclusive term is still widely used and strongly defended by its proponents. However, it has generated strong criticism on the ground that Trypan blue, when used in high concentration, is taken up by fluid-phase pinocytosis into cells that are not truely phagocytic, including endothelial cells, fibroblasts, and even adipose cells. Uptake of this dye is, therefore, a necessary, but not a sufficient, criterion for inclusion in the system of phagocytic cells. Later, the use of isotopic labeling to trace cell lineages and monoclonal antibodies for recognition of specific surface molecules made it possible to identify members of the system with greater certainty and Van Furth (1969) introduced the term *mononuclear phagocyte system* which is now widely accepted. It includes all highly phagocytic cell types and their monocyte precursor, but excludes the controversial sinuoidal endothelia and other cells that take up only small amounts of vital dye by pinocytosis, instead of by phagocytosis. As currently interpreted, the mononuclear phagocyte system includes: *monocytes* of the

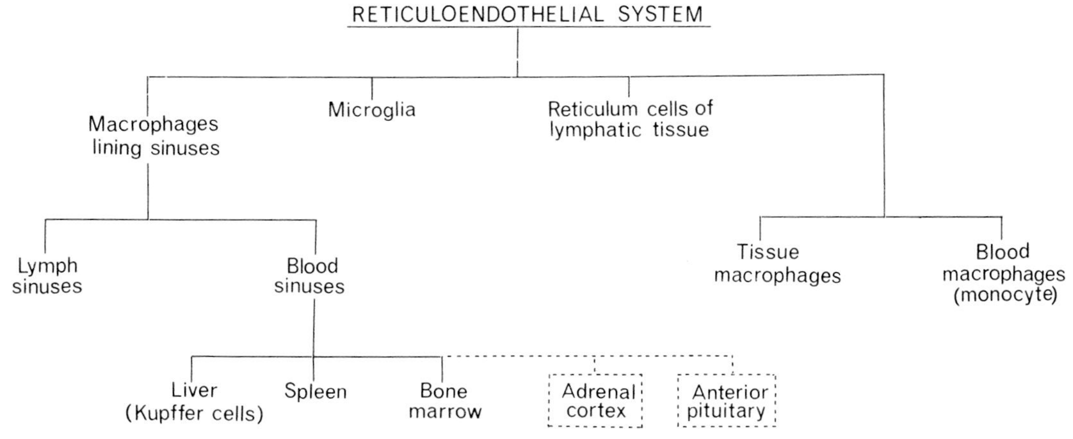

Figure 5–21. A chart of the reticuloendothelial system as traditionally defined—a diffuse system of macrophages and phagocytic endothelial cells that line blood sinuses in various organs. Although widely separated, these cells were grouped together because they shared phagocytic properties. The sinusoids of the adrenal and pituitary were originally included, but are shown here in interrupted lines grouped together because they shared phagocytic properties. The sinusoids of the adrenal and pituitary were originally included, but are shown here in interrupted lines because electron microscopy has revealed that it is not the endothelium, but perivascular macrophages, that are phagocytic in these organs. The alleged phagocytic activity of splenic sinusoids is now seriously questioned, and, in the liver, these properties reside in the Kupffer cells and not in the endothelium proper. Thus, the endothelial component of the system has been largely eliminated by application of modern research methods.

blood; *macrophages* of the connective tissue, lymphoid organs, and bone marrow; *alveolar phagocytes* of the lungs; *Kupffer cells* of the liver; and the *osteoclasts* of bone (Fig. 5–22). The appeal of this unifying concept is that labeling studies have shown that all of its members belong to the same lineage, originating from a comon precursor in the bone marrow and being transported in the blood to the various sites where they carry out their respective functions. They all take up vital dyes; react positively for peroxidase, esterase, and other lysosomal enzymes; and all have surface receptors for immunoglobulin (IgG) and complement.

NEUTROPHILIC LEUKOCYTES

Neutrophils are rarely found in normal connective tissue but they are included here, among its free cells, because they may gather in great numbers at sites of inflammation. Cleavage products of complement and cytokines liberated at sites of bacterial infection induce the endothelial cells of capillaries to synthesize and incorporate in their membrane, a glycoprotein called *endothelial cell adhesion molecule-1* (ELAM-1) that makes their lumenal surface sticky. Some of the same diffusible mediators of inflammation are believed to act on neutrophils to induce their synthesis of *leukocyte adhesion molecules* (LeuCAMs) that promote their adhesion to the sticky capillary endothelium. The adherent neutrophils then migrate through the wall of the capillary into the connective tissue, and up the concentration gradient of cytokines and other mediators diffusing from the site of inflammation. Neutrophils are very responsive to these factors which give direction to their movement (chemotaxis) and also increase its rate (chemokinesis). These mechanisms ensure rapid mobilization of large numbers of neutrophils to assist the resident macrophages in destruction of the invading bacteria.

EOSINOPHIL LEUKOCYTES

Eosinophils are normal constituents of the connective tissue. After leaving the bone marrow, they spend less than a day in the circulation before entering the connective tissues, where they survive for a few more days. They are more numerous in the connective tissue of the nasal cavity, lungs, skin, and lamina propria of the intestine than they are elsewhere. They have surface Fc and C3 receptors and their specific granules contain hydrolytic enzymes, but these cells are less efficient than neutrophils in destroying bacteria. Their functions are poorly understood. Their numbers are increased in persons suffering from allergies. They are attracted to sites of histamine release and their granules contain enzymes capable of degrading histamine and other mediators of inflammation. It is speculated that they may moderate the severity of allergic reactions.

Mononuclear Phagocyte System

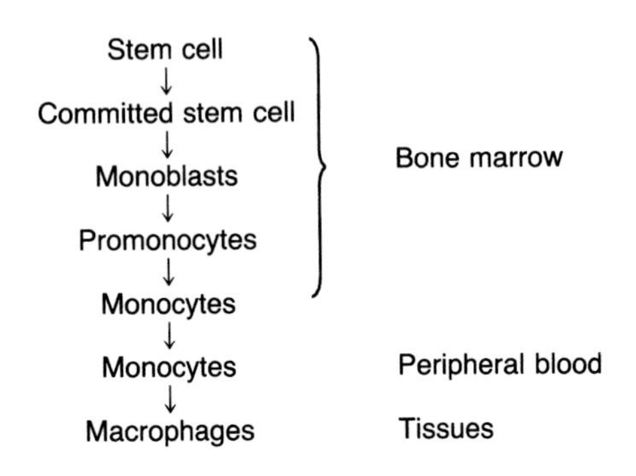

Normal State
connective tissue (histiocyte)
liver (Kupffer cell)
lung (alveolar macrophage)
lymph nodes (free and fixed macrophages; interdigitating cell?)
spleen (free and fixed macrophages)
bone marrow (fixed macrophage)
serous cavities (pleural and peritoneal macrophages)
bone (osteoclasts)
central nervous system (CSF macrophages; brain macrophages)
skin (histiocyte; Langerhans cell?)
synovia (type A cell)
other organs (tissue macrophage)

Inflammation
exudate macrophage
exudate-resident macrophage
epithelioid cell
multinucleated giant cell (Langhans type and foreign-body type)

Figure 5–22. The concept of a mononuclear phagocyte system has now largely replaced the reticuloendothelial system. This is a group of widely disseminated cell types that not only share similar morphology and phagocytic potential but also probably have a common origin from monocytes of the blood. Included in this system are all of the cell types in parentheses after the organ or tissue in which they are found. (After von Furth, R. 1982. Immunobiology 161:178.)

Eosinophils seem to be more responsive to parasitic infestations than they are to bacterial infections. In shistosomiasis, ascariasis, or trichinosis, eosinophils in the blood may increase to 90% of the leukocyte count, accompanied by an equally dramatic increase in their number in the connective tissues. In humans who have previously mounted an immune response to one of these parasites, a second invasion is rapidly followed by accumulation of eosinophils in great numbers around the parasites. There is recent evidence that proteins of the eosinophil granules participate in antibody-mediated, contact-dependent cytotoxicity. One of the proteins released, *eosinophil cationic protein* (ECP), appears to be incorporated in the membrane of the target parasite and to form there stable transmembrane pores that result in loss of ions and molecules from the cytoplasm, leading ultimately to death of the parasite. The *major basic protein* of eosinophil granules does not form pores but may damage the parasite membrane by other mechanisms yet to be defined. The enzyme *peroxidase* of eosinophil granules can also generate superoxide ions that cause membrane damage by lipid peroxidation. The eosinophils thus have multiple mechanisms that can be directed against invading parasites.

LYMPHOCYTES

Lymphocytes which are the principal agents of the immune system, are found in small numbers in the connective tissue throughout the body, but they are more abundant in the stroma of lymphoid organs and in the lamina propria of the intestinal tract. In the latter location, they function in protective immunosurveillance against the rich bacterial flora in the lumen of the gut. The selective accumulation of lymphocytes in certain organs depends on specific properties of the endothelium of venules in those sites. Tissue-specific *endothelial cell adhesion molecules* (also called *addressins* or *selectins*) serve as homing receptors binding lymphocytes as the blood passes through these vessels. The lymphocytes then migrate through the wall of the vessel into the surrounding connective tissue. The lymphocytes are of two kinds, T-lymphocytes and B-lymphocytes, which are identical in appearance but differ in their functions. This will be discussed in the chapter on the immune system (Chapter 13).

PLASMA CELLS

Plasma cells are widely distributed in the connective tissue. They arise by further differentiation of B lymphocytes and are major producers of humoral antibody. They are spherical or ovoid cells, with an eccentrically placed nucleus having a coarse pattern of heterochomatin. The cytoplasm is intensely basophilic. In electron micrographs, large radially arranged masses of chromatin give the nucleus a distinctive appearance. There is a small juxtanuclear Golgi complex and a pair of centrioles. Except for a few mitochondria, the surrounding cytoplasm is occupied by closely spaced cisternae of rough endoplasmic reticulum (Fig. 5–23). In a minority of the plasma cells, the reticulum is less ordered and the cisternae are distended with a flocculent material of low electron density that may be precipitated immunoglobulin. These differences in appearance of the plasma cells may reflect different degrees of secretory activity. No secretory granules are formed and their product is apparently secreted continuously in small vesicles shuttling between the Golgi complex and the cell surface.

Occasionally, plasma cells contain spherical inclusions 2–3 μm in diameter, called *Russell bodies*. These give a positive histochemical reaction for both protein and carbohydrate and are faintly reactive with fluorescin-conjugated antibody to immunoglobulin. They are located within distended cisternae of the endoplasmic reticulum. Their significance is unclear, but it is speculated that they may be accumulations of defective products of antibody synthesis.

MAST CELLS

The *mast cells* are the largest of the free cells of the connective tissue and are easily identified by the numerous basophilic granules in their cytoplasm, which may obscure the nucleus. The granules stain metachromatically with Toluidine blue. Their ability to change the color of this dye from blue to magenta is attributed to their content of the sulfated glycosaminoglycan *heparin*. They also contain *histamine*, neutral proteases *tryptase* and *chymase*, and an *eosinophil chemotactic factor*.

In electron micrographs, mast cells have a small round nucleus, several mitochondria, a few meandering cisternae of rough endoplas-

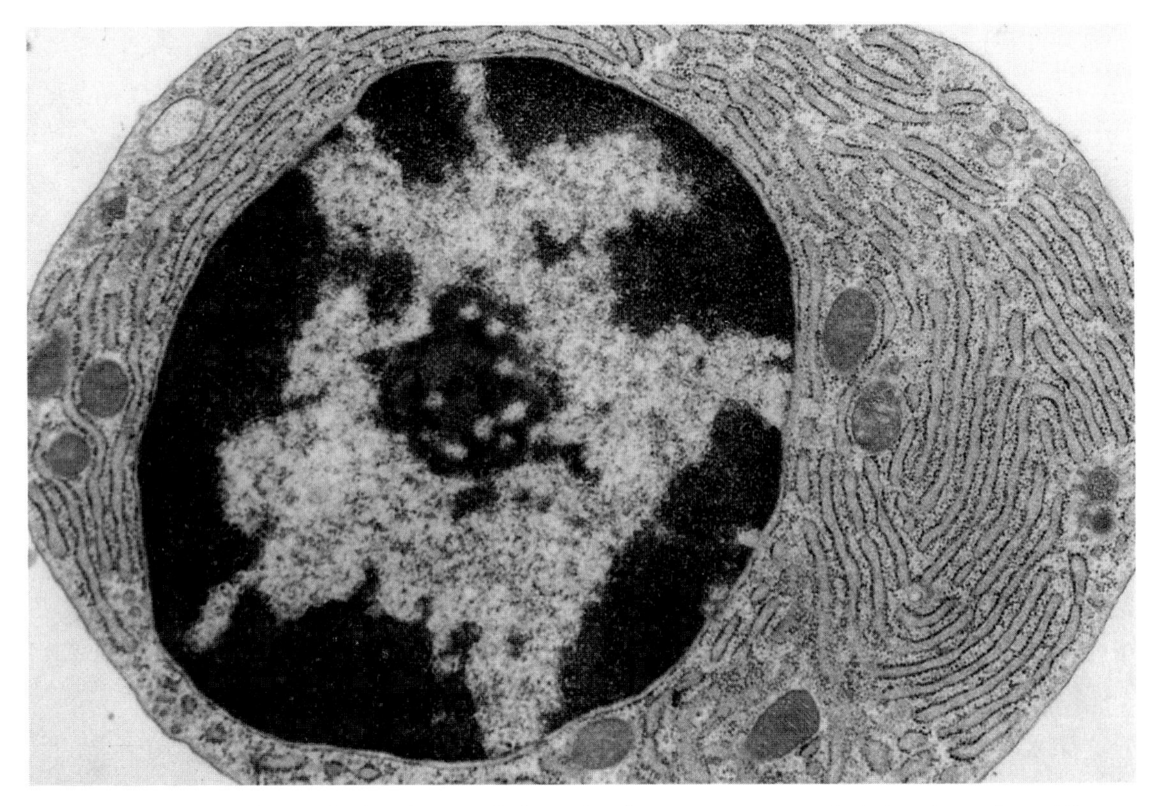

Figure 5–23. Electron micrograph of a plasma cell, illustrating the coarse pattern of its heterochromatin and the very extensive rough endoplasmic reticulum. The large Golgi complex is not included in this plane of section.

mic reticulum, and a small Golgi complex. The hundreds of specific granules are 0.3–0.8 μm in diameter and have a content of varying density (Fig. 5–24). There is considerable interspecific variation in the substructure of the granules. In the rat, they are homogeneous and electron dense. In the guinea pig, they have a crystal-like lattice with a 14-nm spacing that presents a honeycomb appearance in section. In the human, the granules are quite variable in size and more irregular in outline than those of rodents. At high magnification, differences in their ultrastructure can be observed from cell to cell and, indeed, within the same cell. Some contain short cylindrical scroll-like inclusions within a finely granular matrix. In cross section, these inclusions are made up of concentric lamellae having the dimensions of lipid bilayers. In other cells, the granules have a dense matrix surrounding a pale central region occupied by a lattice of parallel linear densities. The significance of these variations in the substructure of the mast cell granules is unknown.

Mast cells and the basophilic leukocytes of the blood both have conspicuous metachromatic granules that contain histamine and other mediators of inflammation. Both have surface receptors for immunoglobulin. These similarities prompted the speculation that the mast cells of connective tissue might arise from blood basophils; however, it is now generally accepted that they are separate cell types. Basophils are smaller and usually have a bilobed nucleus. They are found only in the blood and, like other granular leukocytes, they have a lifespan of only a few days and they are incapable of proliferation. Mast cells are found only in the tissues and have a lifespan of weeks or months, and under certain conditions they are able to divide. Both are thought to arise in the bone marrow. Basophils differentiate in the marrow and then enter the blood. Precursors of mast cells that are still unidentified are believed to circulate in the blood briefly and only acquire their granules during their subsequent differentiation in the connective tissues.

Mast cells are sparsely distributed throughout the connective tissue but are more numerous along the course of small blood vessels and beneath the epithelium of the respiratory and intestinal tracts, where antigens are likely to gain access to the underlying tissue. They are sensitive sentinels for the immune system, detecting the entry of foreign proteins and initiating a local inflammatory response. Their activation results in the prompt release of potent mediators stored in their granules, followed by a slower generation of cytokines that serve to recruit other cell types that participate in the body's defense. The content of mast cell granules is released by an unusual process that has been termed compound exocytosis. Instead of each granule fusing separately with the plasmalemma, a series of granules many fuse with one another and with one opening onto the surface, thus creating a membrane-limited channel that extends deep into the cytoplasm. The cells are able to survive this massive degranulation and recover to form new granules. The stimulus most commonly evoking degranulation is the presence of any foreign substance (antigen) to which the individual has been sensitized by an immune response to a previous exposure to the same antigen. Degranulation of mast cells can be induced, for experimental purposes, by a number of nonspecific agents including polymyxin-B, polylysine, compound 48/80, and certain snake venoms.

Among the several classes of immunoglobulin secreted by plasma cells, IgE is unique in not entering the circulation. Molecules of IgE, of varying antigenic specificity, bind to Fc receptors on mast cells. These cells are then primed to respond immediately when any of these antigens enter the tissues again (Fig. 5–25). The response is usually local and relatively mild, but the immune system of allergic individuals may overreact to a second exposure to one of these antigens, resulting in tissue damage and symptoms ranging from mild discomfort to serious anaphylaxis. Allergic individuals tend to produce antibodies of the IgE class against pollens and a host of other allergens. Upon reexposure, these antigens bind to, and cross-link, IgE molecules on the surface of mast cells, triggering their degranulation and liberation of *histamine* and *leukotrienes* which are responsible for the patient's unpleasant symptoms.

In *hay fever*, histamine released by mast cells in the connective tissue of the nasal mucosa results in increased permeability of the capillaries and consequent swelling of the mucosa, accompanied by sneezing and nasal discharge. In *asthma*, the immune response is mainly in the lungs, where histamine plays a less important role than the leukotrienes, which cause

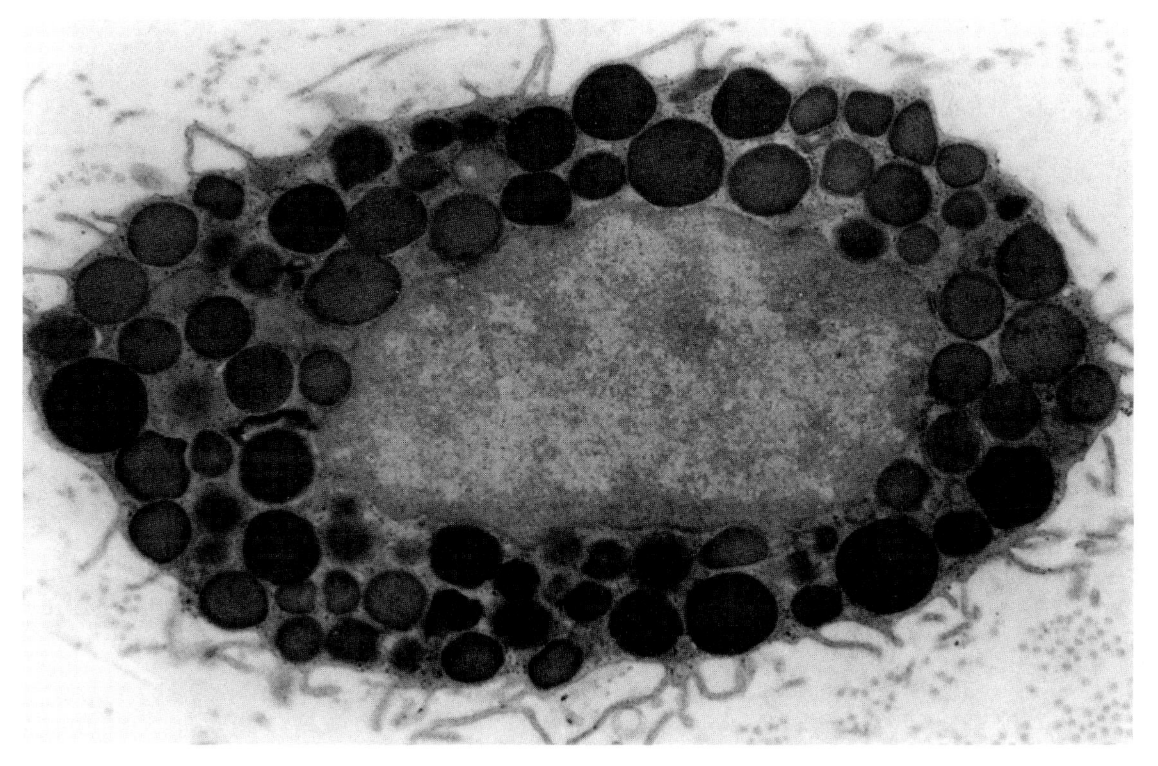

Figure 5–24. Electron micrograph of a mast cell from loose connective tissue of the rat.

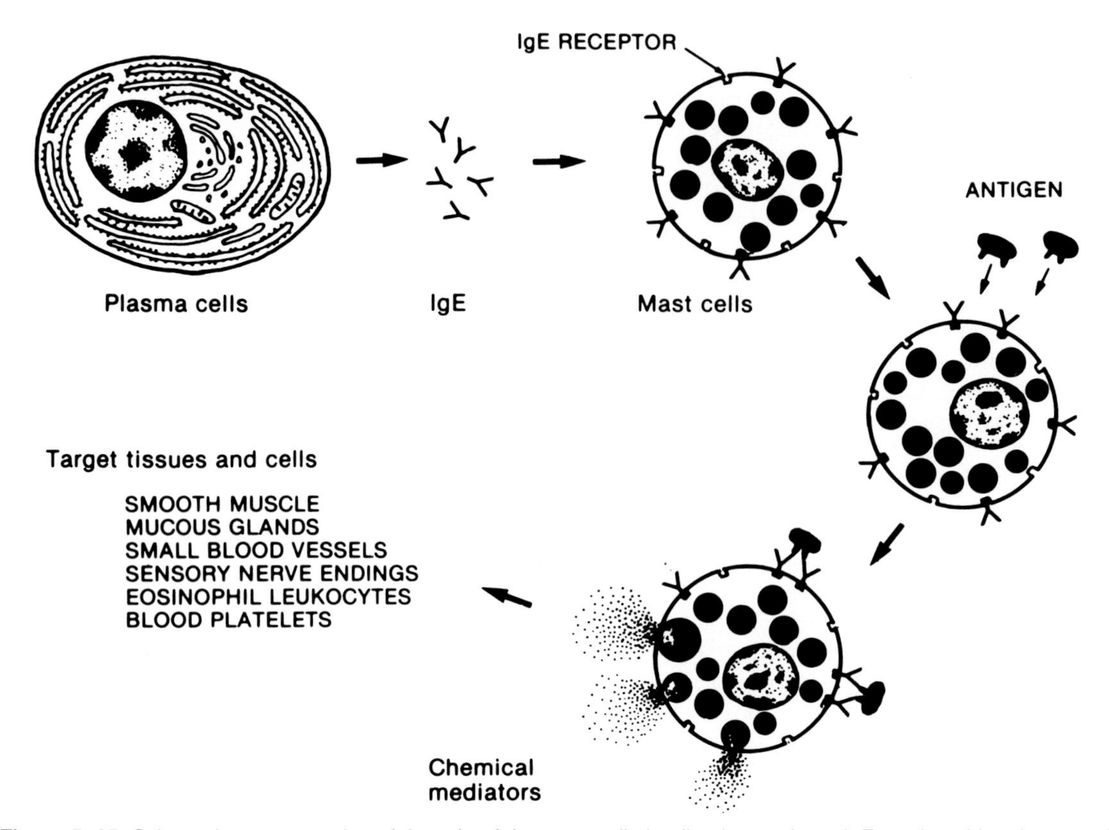

Figure 5–25. Schematic representation of the role of the mast cells in allergic reactions. IgE produced by plasma cells binds to IgE receptors in mast cell membranes. On a second exposure, antigen binds to this IgE and this event trigers mast cell degranulation with release of histamine and other mediators that affect various target tissues and organs.

spasms of the smooth muscle cells in the wall of the bronchioles, making breathing difficult. In *anaphylaxis*, the most serious of the IgE-mediated reactions, massive degranulation of mast cells along blood vessels releases histamine that is carried in the blood throughout the body, increasing capillary permeability with leakage of plasma into the tissues and a dramatic fall in blood pressure that may culminate in unconsciousness and, in rare instances, in death.

Although investigative attention has been focused mainly on the immunological role of mast cells, they may have other functions. In addition to histamine and neutral proteases, their granules contain β-glucuronidase, hexosaminidase, and aryl sulfatase. These enzymes would seem to have no role in the immune responses, but it is possible that they may degrade some of the glycosaminoglycans of the extracellular matrix. Therefore, it has been suggested that, under normal conditions, mast cells may have a low level of secretory activity that contributes to the continual turnover of the ground substance of connective tissue.

SEROUS MEMBRANES

The major cavities of the body are lined by *serous membranes*: the *peritoneum*, lining the abdominal cavity, and the *pleura*, lining the thoracic cavity. These consist of a thin layer of typical loose connective tissue covered by *mesothelium*, a squamous epithelium of mesodermal origin. Thin sheet-like extensions of the peritoneum extending from the posterior wall of the abdominal cavity form the *mesenteries* that support the intestines. These are very thin sheets of loose connective tissue covered on both sides by mesothelium. In small mammals, the mesenteries are so thin that they can be stretched over a glass slide to study the appearance of connective tissue, without sectioning or staining (Fig 5–26). Of greater clinical interest is the *omentum*, a large free fold of visceral peritoneum that hangs, like a curtain, from the greater curvature of the stomach and extends down over the anterior surface of the coiled intestines. In some areas, it has numerous large fenestrations that reduce it to a lace-like network of strands of loose connective tissue covered by mesothelium. Aggregations of adipose cells are found along its blood vessels. Scattered throughout its unfenestrated areas, there are small white patches, often referred to as *milky spots*. In stained preparations, these are found to be aggregations of macrophages, lymphocytes, and eosinophils. The omentum has an important role in limiting damage to abdominal viscera. It adheres to sites of inflammation, contributing the population of mobile phagocytic and cytotoxic cells in its milky spots to the inflammatory response and, at the same time, walling off the process so that a local abscess is formed instead of a generalized and potentially fatal peritonitis. When a patient with a recently perforated gastric ulcer is operated on, it is usually found that the omentum has already become adherent, partially closing the perforation.

VARIANT TYPES OF LOOSE CONNECTIVE TISSUE

Loose connective tissue, described in the foregoing pages, is the most widespread of the connective tissues, occurring in sites where relatively little resistance to stress is required. It supports the epithelial parenchyma of the major organs and is the tissue through which their blood vessels are distributed. It occupies the spaces around and between muscles. It

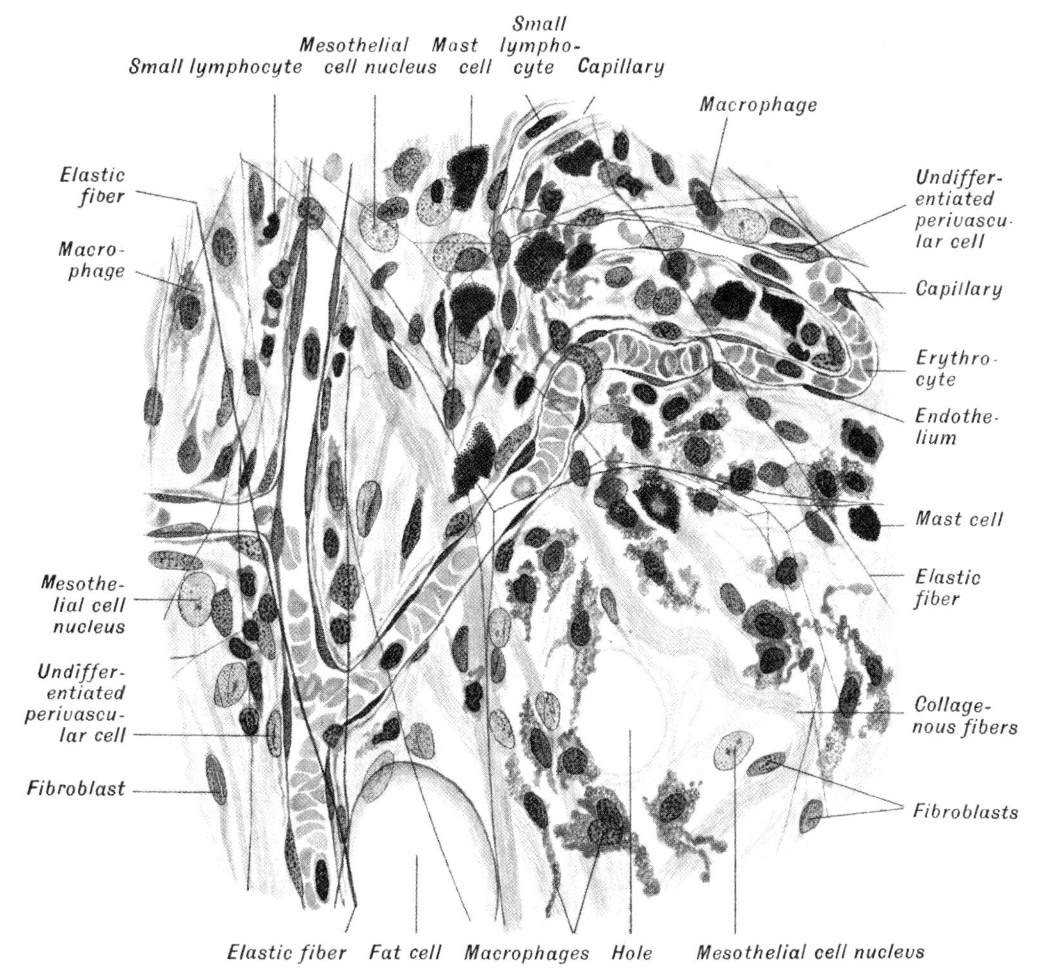

Figure 5–26. Drawing of a spread preparation of human omentum stained with hematoxylin and eosin, showing capillaries and the various cell types characteristic of loose connective tissue.

underlies the mesothelium lining the pleural and peritoneal cavities. There are, however, local differences in the relative proportions of its various fibrous and amorphous components and some of these have led to their designation as distinct types of connective tissue. These variants, of more limited distribution, will now be considered.

RETICULAR CONNECTIVE TISSUE

Reticular tissue is a form of loose connective tissue in which argyrophilic reticular fibers (type-III collagen) are the dominant fibrous component, forming a wide-meshed network. The cells tend to be stellate with slender radiating processes deployed along the intersecting strands of the reticulum. Their stellate form is probably a reflection of the three-dimensional configuration of the scaffold of fibers to which they adhere. They are not considered to be a distinct cell type, but merely fibroblasts which synthesize type-III collagen and little or no type-I collagen. In addition, there is a large population of resident macrophages adhering to the reticular fibers. Reticular connective tissue forms the stroma of the bone marrow and that of the spleen, lymph nodes, and thymus. In the lymphoid organs, the spaces in the loose reticulum are packed with lymphocytes, and in the marrow, with precursors of the blood cells.

MUCOUS CONNECTIVE TISSUE

The distinctive feature of mucous connective tissue is a very large amount of amorphous ground substance that is unusually rich in hyaluronic acid. Collagenous and reticular fibers make up a very small portion of its volume. Its widely spaced cellular elements are fusiform or stellate fibroblasts and very few macrophages. This kind of connective tissue is rare in adults, but common in the embryo. It is the principal component of the umbilical cord, where it was formerly called *Wharton's jelly.* Mucous connective tissue is also found in the pulp of developing teeth. Its occurrence in adult animals is largely limited to the cock's comb and the sexual skin over the ischium of baboons and other lower primates.

DENSE CONNECTIVE TISSUE

Dense connective tissue differs from loose connective tissue mainly in the great preponderance of its fibrous components and relatively few cells. Where the collagen fiber bundles are randomly oriented, the tissue is described as *dense irregular connective tissue.* Where the fibers are oriented parallel to one another or in some other ordered arrangement, it is called *dense regular connective tissue* (Fig. 5–27).

DENSE IRREGULAR CONNECTIVE TISSUE

Collagen fibers make up the greater part of the volume of this tissue. The fiber bundles are relatively coarse and interwoven in a compact meshwork with little space occupied by cells and ground substance. A network of elastic fibers is usually interspersed among the collagen fibers. Fibroblasts are lodged between the bundles of collagen, but generally only their elongated nuclei are visible in histological sections. Macrophages are present in small numbers but are recognizable as such, only after supravital staining with Trypan blue. Free cells are very few. Dense connective tissue is found in the dermis of the skin; the capsules of the spleen, liver, and lymph nodes; the tunica albuginea of the testis; the dura mater of the brain; and the sheaths of large nerves.

DENSE REGULAR CONNECTIVE TISSUE

This type of connective tissue occurs as robust cylindrical cords or flat sheets of closely approximated coarse collagen fibers that give the tissue a glistening white appearance in the fresh state. Its fibers are oriented in the direction best suited to resist the mechanical stresses to which they are subjected. *Tendons* that transmit the pull of muscles to the bones are typical examples of dense regular connective tissue. They are made up of parallel type-I collagen fibers, closely packed with very little intervening space for ground substance (Fig. 5–28). In cross sections of tendon viewed with the electron microscope, two size categories of collagen fibers are discernible, one averaging 60 nm in diameter and the other, 175 nm in diameter (Fig. 5–29A). The relative numbers of small and larger fibers vary from tendon to tendon and in different regions of the same tendon. The fibers appear to be con-

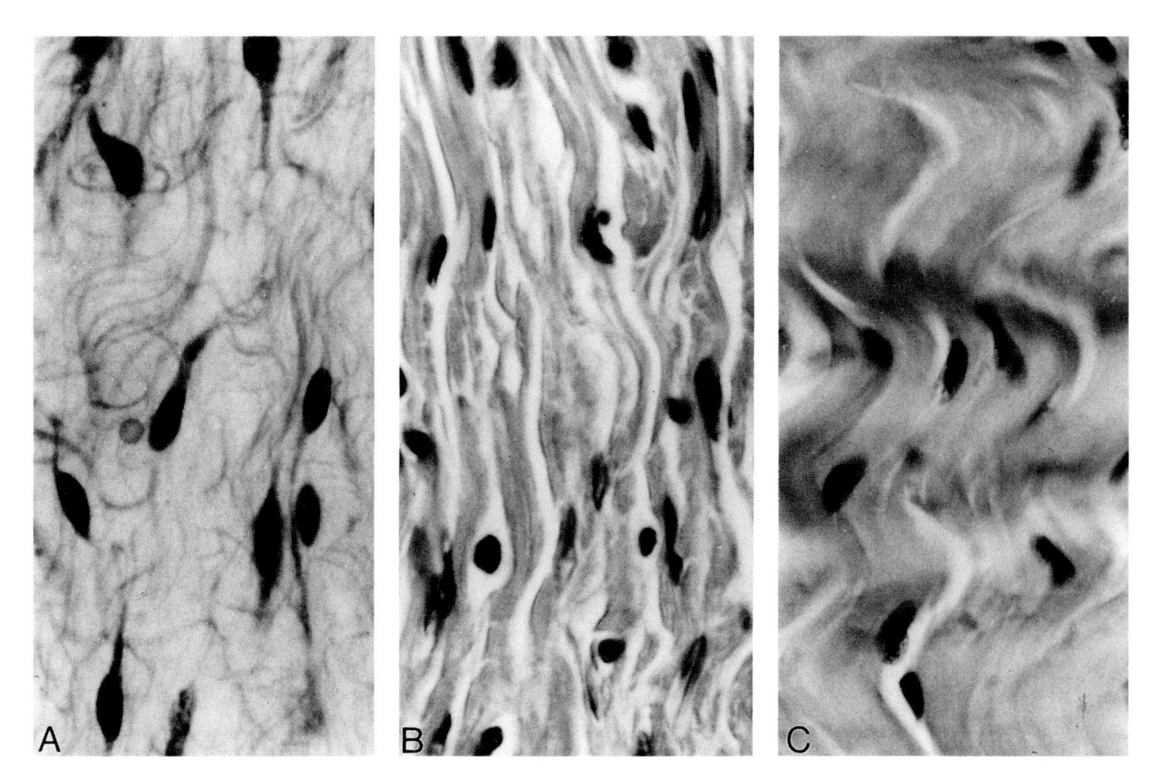

Figure 5–27. Photomicrographs illustrating connective tissues with different amounts of collagen. (A) Loose connective tissue from an 8-month-old fetus, showing relatively sparse, slender fibers. (B) Moderately dense irregular connective tissue with coarse, irregularly oriented bundles of collagen. (C) Dense connective tissue with very abundant collagen, in parallel wavy bundles.

nected laterally by delicate cross-bridges of unknown chemical nature (Fig. 5–29B).

The fibroblasts of tendons are aligned between fiber bundles and most of their cytoplasm is in thin fin-like processes that extend between, and partially surround, neighboring fiber bundles. Varying numbers of these primary bundles are assembled into larger secondary bundles that are surrounded by a very thin layer of loose connective tissue, through which run small blood vessels and nerves. At the periphery of the tendon, these thin septa are continuous with a layer of dense irregular connective tissue that forms the *tendon sheath.* In some long tendons, two layers can be distinguished in the sheath, an inner layer adjacent to the collagen and an outer layer that is loosely bound to the structures surrounding the tendon. Between these two layers is a narrow space lined by squamous cells and containing a viscous fluid similar in composition to the synovial fluid in joint cavities. This fluid serves as a lubricant permitting smooth sliding of the tendon within its sheath.

The parallel collagen fibers of tendons create a structure that is quite flexible but offers great resistance to a pulling force. In a runner, the tendons of the lower limb muscles are stretched when the ball of the foot strikes the ground, and they act like a spring, in that their recoil to their original length helps to push the foot off the ground at the beginning of the next stride. Unlike muscle contraction, the elastic energy of tendon recoil requires no energy input. Sprinters may derive as much as 50% of their locomotor energy from this source. Maximum use of this property of tendons is made by animals with a hopping or springing gait. In changing from a walking to a hopping gait, a kangaroo actually decreases its oxygen consumption and, at 30 miles an hour, uses no more oxygen that an animal half its size running at the same speed on all four legs. Thus, tendons can be an important source of "free energy" for locomotion.

Broad flat muscles do not have cylindrical tendons, but are attached to their insertions by thin sheets of dense regular connective tissue, called *aponeuroses.* These consist of multiple layers of coherent fascicles of collagen fibers. Within any one layer the fiber bundles are parallel, but their direction usually changes in

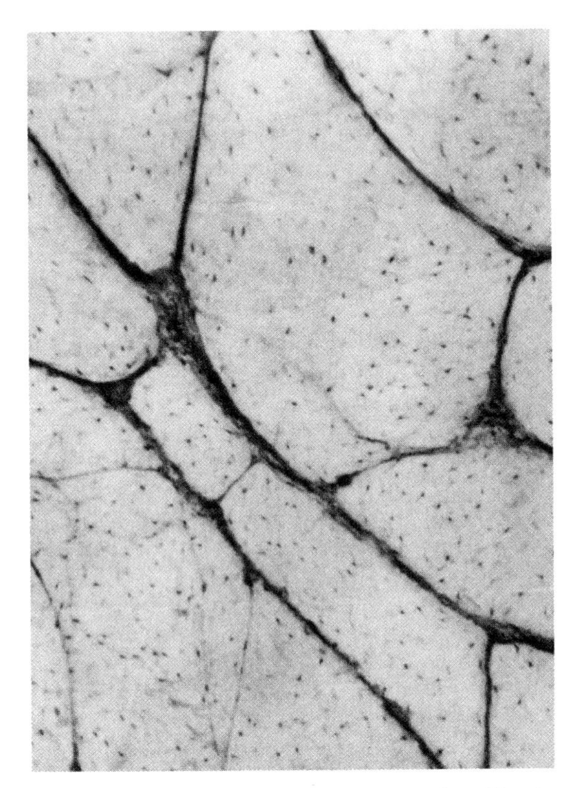

Figure 5–28. Cross section of human tendon. Massive bundles of collagen are separated by darker staining looser connective tissue. Dots in the pale areas of collagen are nuclei of fibroblasts in narrow clefts among the collagen fibers.

successive layers. Separation of the layers is prevented by some fibers that crossover between layers.

Dense irregular connective tissue forms the capsule around joints and this is often reinforced by *ligaments*, which are strong bands of parallel collagen bundles that serve to attach bone to bone and to limit the degree of movement at the joint. Ligaments may be independent structures or they may be incorporated within the capsule. There are usually few elastic fibers among the collagen bundles of ligaments. The *ligamenta flava* that connect successive vertebrae are exceptional in that elastic fibers outnumber collagen fibers. This is no doubt responsible for much of the flexibility of the vertebral column. The *ligamentum nuchae* associated with the cervical vertebrae of cattle and other grazers consists almost entirely of large parallel elastic fibers, and this has been the tissue of choice for biochemical studies of elastin (Fig. 5–11). The elastic recoil of this ligament reduces the energy needed for the cutting of grass with the lower incisor teeth of these animals.

The cornea of the eye is a unique form of dense regular connective tissue. It is composed of type-I collagen fibers in over 200 thin lamellae, each about 0.2 μm in thickness. Flattened fibroblasts are situated between the successive lamellae. The collagen fibers are of uniform diameter and consistent in orientation within any given lamella, but the direction of the fibers changes in each layer so that they are oriented at approximately 90° to those of the next layer (Fig. 5–30). The cells and fibers are embedded in a proteoglycan ground substance rich in keratan sulfate and containing lesser amounts of chondroitin-4 sulfate and condroitin-6 sulfate. The precise orientation of the fibers in the cornea is obviously not related to local mechanical stresses. Instead, it appears to be a specialization that contributes to the transparency of the cornea. Because of the alternation in orientation of fibers, the direction of light-scattering in one layer is reversed in the next.

HISTOPHYSIOLOGY OF CONNECTIVE TISSUE

NORMAL FUNCTIONS

Connective tissue functions in mechanical support; exchange of metabolites between the blood and the tissues; storage of energy reserves in adipose cells; protection against infection; and repair after injury. In the mechanical role of connective tissue, its fibrous components are the most important, and their abundance and orientation are adapted to local structural requirements. Delicate networks of reticular fibers support the basal lamina of epithelia, surround the capillaries and sinusoids, and envelope individual muscle fibers and the groups of parenchymal cells that form the functional units of organs. The elastic fibers give the tissue suppleness and the ability to spring back to its normal shape after deformation. They are especially abundant in the walls of hollow organs subject to periodic distension. Loose connective tissue is found in sites where a certain degree of mobility is advantageous. On the other hand, where strength is more important than mobility, dense connective tissue is formed and its bundles of coarse collagen fibers are so oriented that they resist the local mechanical stresses.

Loose connective tissue that surrounds and permeates the organs of the body plays an

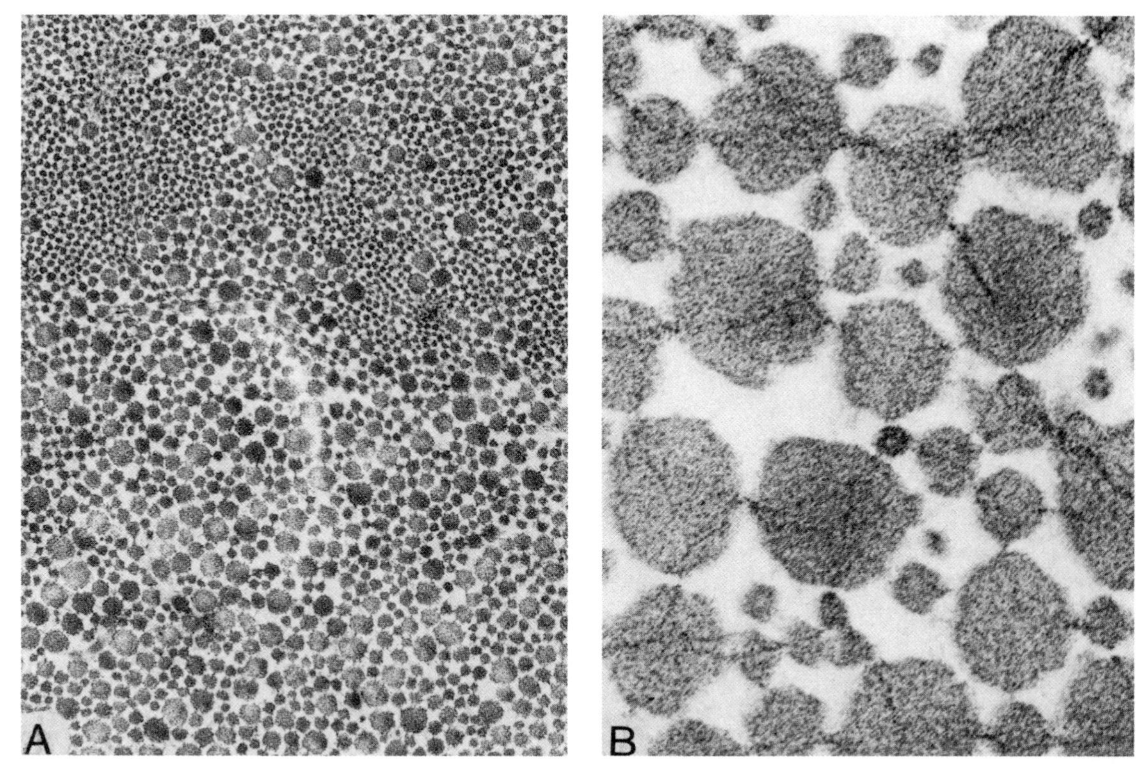

Figure 5–29. Electron micrographs of human tendon. (A) Transverse section of Achilles tendon showing variations in the distribution and ratio of larger, 175-nm, fibrils to smaller, 60-nm, fibrils. (B) Higher magnification of a small area of plantaris tendon illustrating linear densities extending from fibril to fibril. (Micrographs from Dyer, R.F. 1976. Cell Tissue Res. 168:247.

indispensable role in their nutrition. All nutrients reaching the cells of the organs from the blood and all of the waste products of their metabolism that are returned to the blood must pass through the connective tissue that surrounds the blood vessels. These substances diffuse through the aqueous phase of the gelatinous ground substance or along thin films of fluid that coat the fibers. The polyelectrolyte properties of the glycosaminoglycans of the ground substance help to maintain normal tissue hydration and electrolyte balance. In addition to its storage of lipid in adipose cells, connective tissue is a depot for protein. Approximately half of all the albumin, globulins, and other extracellular protein in the body is in the connective tissue.

INFLAMMATION

It may be helpful to review here the defensive role of the connective tissue. The invasion of tissues by microorganisms triggers a local response of the connective tissue called *acute inflammation*. A thorough study of this process falls within the scope of general pathology, but a superficial knowledge enables the student of histology to understand better the function of the free cells of the connective tissue.

At sites of infection, bacterial products that rapidly activate resident macrophages are released. These substances are also chemotactic for neutrophils and for monocytes that have recently migrated through the walls of postcapillary venules. These elicited phagocytes join the activated resident macrophages in ingesting and destroying bacteria. If the host has previously been invaded by microorganisms of the same kind and has developed antibodies, these bind to mast cells, inducing their release of histamine and other mediators that cause local dilatation and increased permeability of the blood vessels. These events are responsible for the *redness*, *swelling*, and *pain* that are the cardinal signs of inflammation.

The activated phagocytes release interleukin-1 which diffuses into the blood and is carried in the circulation throughout the body.

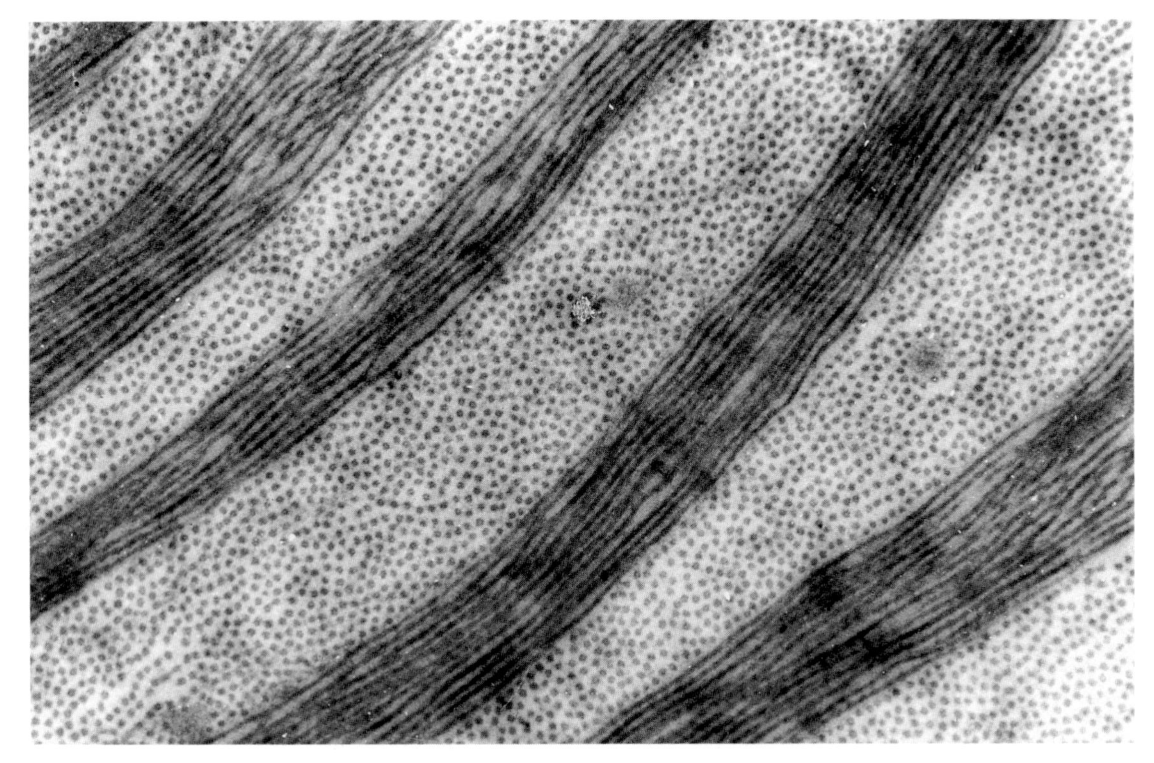

Figure 5–30. Electron micrograph of dense regular connective tissue of the cornea. The collagen is arranged in lamellae with the fibrils in alternate lamellae oriented at right angles to those in adjacent lamellae. (Micrograph courtesy of M. Jakus.)

In the brain, it acts on the thermoregulatory center in the hypothalamus, inducing the production of a prostaglandin that raises the thermostatic set-point, resulting in *fever*. On reaching the bone marrow, interleukin-1 stimulates the release of great numbers of neutrophils, resulting in the *elevated leukocyte count* that is invariably associated with an infection. Interleukin-1 also stimulates the liver to increase its synthesis of fibrinogen and complement. At the site of infection, coating of the bacteria with complement and with specific antibody greatly increases their susceptibility to phagocytosis. In addition to its systemic effects, interleukin-1 is chemotactic for neutrophils and lymphocytes and, thus, contributes to the accumulation of these cells at the site of infection.

Neutrophil leukocytes have in their cytoplasm lipoxygenases and dehydrases that are capable of transforming arachidonic acid, a constituent of biological membranes, into a number of biologically active compounds that act on the blood vessels and on the free cells of the connective tissue to contribute to the inflammatory reaction. Among these compounds are several leukotrienes (LTA, LTB, LTC, LTD, and LTE). LTB is the most potent chemotactic agent for human neutrophils yet discovered and is also chemotactic for monocytes. LTC and LTD, in nanogram concentrations, increase vascular permeability, contributing to the edema and local swelling. Release of these leukotrienes also stimulates the endothelial cells of local blood vessels to synthesize and insert into their membrane a factor that promotes the adherence of neutrophils to the vessels wall and their subsequent migration into the inflamed connective tissue. Clearly, inflammation is a very complex process involving several of the cell types of connective tissue that produce multiple cytokines. There is considerable redundancy in the process because mediators originating from different cells have similar effects.

If the invading bacteria are of a strain that is very resistant to elimination by phagocytosis, *chronic inflammation* ensues, with a gradual change in the population of infiltrating cells. The number of macrophages and neutrophils declines and the number of lymphocytes and plasma cells increases. Fibroblasts are stimulated to proliferate and increase their production of collagen fibers to form a dense wall of fibrous tissue around the site preventing the spread of the infection.

EFFECTS OF HORMONES

Some connective tissues appear to be influenced by sex hormones. In the human female, there is a slight increase in the degree of hydration of the tissues at certain phases of the menstrual cycle. More dramatic effects are observed in the mucous connective tissue of the cock's comb, and in that beneath the sex skin of lower primates, referred to earlier in the chapter. Testosterone stimulates the secretion of hyaluronic acid in the developing cock's comb, and estrogens cause a conspicuous swelling of the sex skin of baboons at midcycle, which subsides later in the cycle.

Normal levels of secretion of the glucocorticoid hormones of the adrenal cortex do not have any well-documented action on the connective tissues, but when given in excess, they have a marked effect on the inflammatory response to bacterial infection. Protein synthesis by fibroblasts is suppressed, decreasing fiber formation; permeability of capillaries is decreased, reducing swelling; lysosomal membranes of phagocytes are stabilized, reducing the escape of hydrolytic enzymes into the tissue; the synthesis of interleukin-1 and other cytokines is suppressed; and lymphocytes are destroyed, interrupting the immune response in the inflamed area. The hormone is often administered to protect the body against excesses of its own defense mechanisms and to reduce the associated pain, swelling, and redness.

REPAIR

After an injury anywhere in the body, the fibroblasts of the local connective tissue respond by proliferation and enhanced fibrogenesis, and they are the principal agents of the healing process. They not only heal defects in the connective tissue but also respond to injury to other tissues that have little capacity for repair. For example, after a heart attack, the degenerating cardiac muscle is replaced by a scar of dense connective tissue.

CONNECTIVE TISSUE DISEASE

Research on the intracellular events in the biosynthesis of collagen has led to a better understanding of the pathogenesis of certain inherited and acquired diseases. In the human, severe vitamin C deficiency leads to an acquired disorder of collagen formation, called *scurvy*. Vitamin C (ascorbic acid) is required for the enzymatic hydroxylation of prolyl and lysyl residues of collagen. In its absence, the procollagen molecules lack hydroxyproline residues and an unstable triple helix is formed. This results in abnormal bone growth, poor healing of fractures, and a bleeding tendency, owing to fragility of the capillaries and other small blood vessels.

A rare inherited disease of humans, *Ehlers-Danlos syndrome* is characterized by short stature, unusually stretchable skin, hypermobility of the joints, and poor wound healing. Recent evidence indicates that this mutant gene results in abnormal propeptide sequences in the region normally subject to cleavage by procollagen *N*-protease, and these patients also lack the lysyl hydroxylase and lysyl oxidase necessary for formation of stable cross-links in the assembly of collagen fibrils.

In another inheritable disease, *osteogenesis imperfecta*, there is unusually thin skin and multiple bone fractures and deformities. Type-I collagen is deficient in these individuals owing to a disorder in transcription of the gene for type-I procollagen and an altered structure of the α-chains which results in improper assembly of tripled helices.

Extensive skeletal deformities are also seen in an acquired disease of domestic ruminants called *lathyrism*. This disorder has been traced to ingestion of the sweet pea *Lathyrus odoratus* which contains a toxic compound that results in abnormal α-chains which are unable to cross-link to form stable collagen fibers.

BIBLIOGRAPHY

GENERAL

Hay, E.D., ed. 1981. Cell Biology of the Extracellular Matrix. New York, Plenum Press.

Hay, E.D. 1981. Extracellular matrix. J. Cell. Biol. (Suppl.) 91:205.

Ramachadran, G.N. and A.H. Reddi, eds. 1976. Biochemistry of Collagen. New York, Plenum Press.

Ross, R. 1975. Connective tissue cells, cell proliferation and synthesis of extracellular matrix—A review. Philos. Trans. Roy. Soc. London 271:247.

COLLAGEN

Bornstein, P. 1974. The biosynthesis of collagen. Annu. Rev. Biochem. 43:567.

Chapman, J.A. and D.J.S. Hulmes. 1984. Electron microscopy of the collagen fibril. *In* A. Ruggieri and P.M.

Motta, eds. Ultrastructure of the Connective Tissue Matrix. Boston, Martinius Nijhoff Publishers.

Dodson, J.W. and E.D. Hay. 1971. Synthesis of collagenous stroma by isolated epithelium grown in vitro. Exp. Cell Res. 65:215.

Junquiera, L.C.U., W. Cossermelli, and R.R. Brentani. 1978. Differential staining of collagens types I, II, and III by sirius red and polarization microscopy. Arch. Histol. Japan 41:267.

K. Kuhn. 1987. The classical collagen: types I, II, and III. *In* R. Mayne and R. Burgeson, eds. Structure and Function of Collagen Types. Orlando, FL, Academic Press.

LeRoy, E.C. 1975. Collagens and human disease. Bull. Rheum. Dis. 25:778.

Mimmi, M.E. 1974. Collagen: its structure and function in normal and pathological connective tissues. Semin. Arthritis Rheum. 4:95.

Montes, G.S. et al. 1984. Collagen distribution in the tissues. *In* A. Ruggieri and P.M. Motta, eds. Ultrastructure of the Connective Tissue Matrix. Boston, Martinius Nijhoff Publishers.

Prokop, D.J., K.I. Kivirikko, L. Tuderman, and N.A. Guzman. 1979. Biosynthesis of collagen and its disorders. N. Engl. J. Med. 301:77.

Sakai, L.Y., D.R. Keene, and E. Engvall. 1986. Fibrillin, a new 350 kD glycoprotein is a component of extracellular microfibrils. J. Cell. Biol. 103:2499.

ELASTIN

Cleary, E.G., and M.A. Gibson. 1983. Elastin-associated microfibrils and microfibrillar protein. Internat. Rev. Connective Tissue Res. 10:97.

Franzbau, C. and B. Faris. 1981. Elastin. *In* E.D. Hay, ed. 1981. Cell Biology of the Extracellular Matrix. New York, Plenum Press.

Gotte, L., M.G. Giro, D. Volpin, and R.W. Horne. 1974. The ultrastructural organization of elastin. J. Ultrastr. Res. 46:23.

Gray, W.R., L.B. Sandburg, and J.A. Foster. 1973. Molecular model for elastin structure and function. Nature 246:461.

Ross, R. 1973. The elastic fiber. A Review. J. Histochem. Cytochem. 21:199.

Sandberg, L. B., N.T. Soskel, and J.G. Leslie. 1981. Elastin, structure, biosynthesis and relation to disease states. N. Engl. J. Med. 304:506.

GROUND SUBSTANCE

Compar, W.D. and T.C. Laurent. 1978. Physiological function of connective tissue polysaccharides. Physiol. Rev. 58:255.

Hascall, V.C. and G.K. Hascall. 1981. Proteoglycans. *In* E.D. Hay, ed., 1981. Cell Biology of the Extracellular Matrix. New York, Plenum Press.

Hook, M.A., S. Woods, S. Johansson, L. Kjellen, and J.R. Couchman. 1986. Functions of proteoglycans at the cell surface. Ciba Found. Symp. 124:143–157.

Lindahl, U. and M. Hook. 1978. Glycosaminoglycans and their binding to biological macromolecules. Annu. Rev. Biochem. 17:385.

Stamatoglou, S.C. and J.M. Keller. 1982. Interactions of cellular glycosaminoglycans with plasma fibronectin and collagen. Biochim. Biophys. Acta 719:90–97.

ADHESIVE PROTEINS

Clegg, D.O., J.C. Helder, B.C. Hann, D.E. Hall, and L. Reichert. 1988. Amino-acid sequence and distribution of mRNa encoding a major skeletal muscle laminin-binding protein: An extracellular matrix associated protein. J. Cell. Biol. 107:699–705.

Galvin, N.J., P.M. Vance, V.M. Dexit, B. Fink, and W.A. Frazier. 1987. Interaction of human thrombospondin with types I–IV collagen: Direct binding and electron microscopy. J. Cell. Biol. 104:1413–1422.

Hall, D.A., K.A. Frazer, B.C. Hann, and L.F. Reichert. 1988. Isolation and characterization of a laminin-binding protein from rat and chicken muscle. J. Cell Biol. 107:687–697.

Hynes, R.O., and K.M. Yamada. 1982. Fibronectins: multifunctional modular glycoproteins. J. Cell Biol. 95:369–77.

Hynes, R.O. 1987. Integrins: A family of cell surface receptors. Cell 48: 549–554.

Kleinman, H.H., F.B. Cannon et al. 1985. Biological activities of laminin. J. Cell. Biochem. 27:317–325.

Mosher, D.F. 1984. Physiology of fibronectin. Annu. Rev. Med. 35:561–575.

Ruoslahti, E., E. Engvall, and E.G. Hayman. 1981. Fibronectin: Current concepts of its structure and function. Collagen Rel. Res. 1:95.

Ruoslahti, E., and M.D. Pierschbacher. 1987. New perspectives in cell adhesion: RGD and integrins. Science 238:491–497.

FIBROBLASTS

Bard, J.B.L. and E.D. Hay. 1975. The behavior of fibroblasts from the developing avian cornea: Morphology and movement in situ and in vitro. J. Cell Biol. 67:400–418.

Gabbiani, G. and E. Rungger-Brandle. 1981. The fibroblast. *In* L.E. Glynn, ed. Tissue repair and regeneration. Hundbook of Inflammation, Vol. 3 p. 1. Amsterdam, Elsevier/North Holland Biomedical Press.

Hay, E.D. 1985. Interaction of migrating embryonic cells with extracellular matrix. Exp. Biol. Med. 10:174–193.

Ross, R. 1975. Connective tissue cells, cell proliferation and synthesis of extracellular matrix—a review. Philos. Trans. Roy. Soc. London (Biol.) 271:247.

Tomasek, J.L., E.D. Hay, and K. Fujiwara. 1982. Collagen modulates cell shape and cytoskeleton of embryonic corneal and fibroma fibroblasts: Distribution of actin, a-actinin, and myosin. Devel. Biol. 92:107–122.

Willingham, M.C., G.S. Yamada et al. 1981. Intracellular localization of actin in cultured fibroblasts by electron microscopic immunocytochemistry. J. Histochem. Cytochem. 29:17–37.

MACROPHAGES

Cohn, Z.A. 1968. Structure and function of monocytes and macrophages. Adv. Immunol. 9:163.

Cohn, Z.A. and B. Benson. 1965. The differentiation of mononuclear phagocytes. Morphology, cytochemistry, and biochemistry. J. Exp. Med. 121:153.

Gordon, S. and Z.A. Cohn. 1973. The macrophage. Internat. Rev. Cytol. 36:171.

Griffin, F.M., C. Bianco, and S.C. Silverstein. 1975. Characterization of the macrophage receptor for complement and demonstration of its functional independence from the receptor for the Fc portion of immunoglobulin G. J. Exp. Med. 141:1269.

Griffin, F.M., J.A. Griffin, J.E. Leder, and S.C. Silverstein. 1975. Studies on the mechanism of phagocytosis. I. Requirements for circumferential attachment of particle-bound ligands to specific receptors on the plasma membrane. J. Exp. Med. 142:1263.

Page, R.C. 1978. The macrophage as a secretory cell. Internat. Rev. Cytol. 52:119.
Unanue, R.R. and J. Cerotti. 1970. The function of macrophages in the immune response. Semin. Hematol. 7:225.

MONONUCLEAR PHAGOCYTE SYSTEM

Aschoff, L. 1924. Das Reticulo-endotheliale System. Ergeb. Inn. Med. Kinderheilk. 26:1.
van Furth, R. 1982. Current view on the mononuclear phagocyte system. Immunobiol. 161:178.
van Furth, R., Z.A. Cohn, J.G. Hirsch, J.H. Humphrey, W.G. Spector, and H.L. Langevoort. 1972. The mononuclear phagocyte system. A new classification of macrophages, monocytes, and their precursor cells. Bull. W.H.O. 46:845.

MAST CELLS

Barrett, K.E. and D.D. Metcalf. 1984. Mast cell heterogeneity: Evidence and implications. J. Clin. Immunol. 4:253.
Crowle, P.K. and N.D. Reed. 1984. Bone marrow origin of mucosal mast cells. Internat. Arch. Allergy Appl. Immunol. 73:242–247.
Denberg, J.A., H. Messner, B. Kim et al. 1985. Clonal origin of human basophil/mast cells from circulating multipotential hemopoietic progenitors. Exp. Hematol. 13:185.
Dvorak, H.F. and A.M. Dvorak. 1972. Basophils, mast cells and cellular immunity in animals and man. Human Pathol. 3:454.
Fedorko, M.F. and J.G. Hirsch. 1965. Crystalloid structure in granules of guinea pig and human mast cells. J. Cell Biol. 26:973.
Froaese, A.S. 1984. Receptors of IgE on mast calls and basophils. Progr. Allergy 34:142–187.
Galli, S.J. 1990. New insights into the riddle of the mast cells Microenvironmental regulation of mast cell development and phenotypic heterogeneity. Lab. Invest. 62:5.
Ishizaka, T. and K. Ishizaka. 1984. Activation of mast cells for mediator release through IgE receptors. Progr. Allergy 34:188–235.
Lagunoff, O. 1978. Mast cell secretion: membrane events. J. Invest. Dermatol. 71:81.
Metzger, H. 1978. The IgE-mastcell system as a paradigm for the study of antibody mechanisms. Immunol. Res. 41:186.

EOSINOPHILS

Ackerman, S.J., D.A. Loegering, P. Venge et al. 1983. Distinctive cationic proteins of the human eosinophil granule: Major basic protein eosinophil cationic protein, and eosinophil-derived neurotoxin. J. Immunol. 131:2977.
Archer, R.K. 1965. On the functions of eosinophils in the antigen–antibody reaction. J. Br. Haemetol. 11:123.
Beeson, P.B. and D.A. Bass. The Eosinophil. Philadelphia, W.B. Saunders Co.
Hirsch, J.G. 1965. The eosinophil leukocyte. *In* B.W. Zweifach, L. Grant, and R.T. McCluskey, eds. The Inflammatory Process. New York, Academic Press.
Lewis, D.M., J.C. Lewis, D.A. Loegering, and J.I. Gleich. 1978. Localization of guinea pig eosinophil major basic protein to the core of the granule. J. Cell. Biol. 77:702.
Young, J.D., C.B. Peterson, P. Venge, and Z.A. Cohn. 1986. Mechanism of membrane damage mediated by human eosinophil cationic protein. Nature 321: 613.

INFLAMMATION

Dinarello, C.A. 1984. Interleukin-1 and the pathogenesis of the acute phase response. N. Engl. J. Med. 311:1413–1418.
Larsen, G.L. and P.M. Hensen. 1983. Mediators of inflammation. Annu. Rev. Immunol. 1:335–359.
Samuelsson, B. 1983. Leukotrienes: Mediators of immediate hypersensitivity reactions and inflammation. Science 220:568–575.

DENSE CONNECTIVE TISSUE

Cooper, R.R. and S. Misol., 1970. Tendon and ligament insertion—a light and electron microscopic study. J. Bone Joint Surg (Br.) 52:1.
Dyer, R.F. and C.D. Enna. 1976. Ultrastructural features of adult human tendon. Cell Tissue Res. 167:247.
Elliott, D.H. 1965. Structure and function of tendon. Biol. Rev. 40:392.
Field, P.L. 1971. Tendon fiber arrangement and blood supply. Australia New Zealand Journal of Surgery. 40:298.

6

ADIPOSE TISSUE

Most mammals, including man, feed intermittently but consume energy continuously. It is advantageous, therefore, to have a means of temporary storage of energy-rich material. Lipid is the most favorable substance for this purpose for it weighs less and occupies less volume per calorie of stored chemical energy than carbohydrate or protein. *Fat* or *adipose tissue* is a form of connective tissue specialized for storage of lipid. Although many cell types contain small reserves of carbohydrate and lipid, the adipose tissue is the body's most capacious reservoir of energy. In normal males, 12–14% of the body weight is fat, and in females, 25% or more, of their weight is fat, representing about a 2-month reserve of energy. By accumulating lipid in periods of excess food intake and releasing fatty acids in periods of fasting, adipose tissue is able to maintain a stable supply of energy-rich fuel. Although adipose tissue was long considered to be a relatively inert tissue, its *fat cells* or *adipocytes* are now known to actively synthesize lipid from carbohydrate as well as accumulating fat from the diet, and they are highly responsive to hormonal and nervous stimulation.

There are two distinct types of adipose tissue, which differ in distribution, color, vascularity, and metabolic activity. One is the familiar *white adipose tissue*, which is widespread and makes up the bulk of the body fat, and the other, called *brown adipose tissue*, which is less abundant and limited to certain specific areas. Although brown adipose tissue is present in all mammals, including man, it is most abundant in those species that hibernate.

WHITE ADIPOSE TISSUE (UNILOCULAR ADIPOSE TISSUE)

Adipose tissue of this kind varies in color from white to yellow, depending, in part, on the abundance of carotenoids in the diet. Carotenoids are fat-soluble plant pigments of carrots and other vegetables that may accumulate in the lipid droplets of adipose cells. The cells of white fat are very large, ranging up to 120 μm in diameter. They are typically spherical, but where closely packed together, they may take on polyhedral shapes due to mutual deformation (Fig. 6–1). Most of the volume of the cell is occupied by a single large droplet of lipid. The nucleus is displaced to one side of the cell and flattened by the accumulated lipid, and the cytoplasm is reduced to a thin rim around the lipid droplet, accounting for only about one-fortieth of the cell volume. Mature white adipose cells contain a single large lipid droplet and are described as *unilocular*, whereas cells of brown adipose tissue contain multiple small droplets and are designated as *multilocular*. However, this latter term does not apply exclusively to brown adipose cells because developing white fat cells contain multiple droplets of lipid for some time before these finally coalesce into a single large drop. They are, therefore, transiently multilocular.(Figs. 6–2 and 6–3).

In the preparation of histological sections of adipose tissue, the lipid droplet of each cell is extracted, leaving behind only the plasmalemma and the thin rim of cytoplasm containing the flattened nucleus. With silver stains, each fat cell is found to be surrounded by a network of reticular fibers. At low magnifications, well-preserved specimens of adipose tissue appear, in section, as a delicate three-dimensional network with large polygonal meshes (Figs. 6–1 and 6–4), but the thin cell rims often collapse to varying degrees during preparation, giving them very irregular outlines. Capillaries form a loose network throughout the tissue and are often found in cross-section in the angular spaces between the cells. Adipose tissue may be partitioned by connective tissue septa into lobules visible to the naked eye. This lobulation is most obvious in regions where adipose tissue is subject to pressure and has a cushioning or shock-absorbing effect. In other regions, the septa

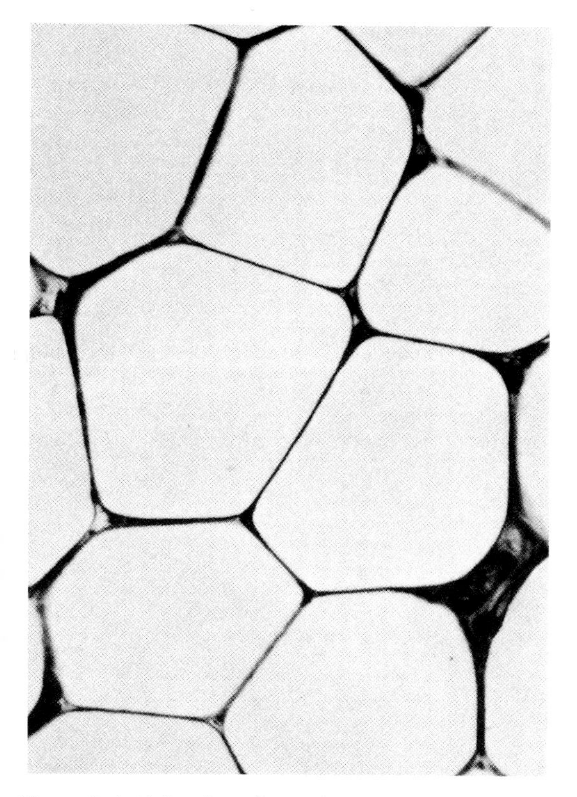

Figure 6–1. Unilocular adipose tissue prepared by routine methods. The large lipid droplet in each cell has been extracted during dehydration of the specimen and only the thin rim of cytoplasm remains.

are thinner and a lobular organization is less apparent.

In electron micrographs of unilocular adipose cells (Fig. 6–5), the lipid droplet is not bounded by a membrane but its interface with the cytoplasm stains more heavily and this may give the specious appearance of a limiting membrane. The cytoplasm contains a small juxtanuclear Golgi complex, a few filamentous mitochondria, occasional cisternae of endoplasmic reticulum, and a moderate number of free ribosomes. In immature fat cells, the lipid droplets that have not yet fused are often surrounded by a layer of 10-nm vimentin intermediate filaments (Fig. 6–6). Thin fenestrated cisternae of endoplasmic reticulum often partially envelope the lipid droplets, immediately peripheral to the monolayer of vimentin filaments. As development progresses and the droplets coalesce into a single lipid drop, the intermediate filaments become less obvious.

Each adipose cell has a glycoprotein envelope that bears a superficial resemblance to the basal lamina of epithelia. The plasma membrane has numerous minute invaginations of a kind that are usually interpreted as evidence of micropinocytosis. Their significance has been a subject of debate. Some have suggested that they may be involved in the uptake of materials used by the cell in lipid synthesis. However, their number is reported to increase greatly during prolonged starvation and after norepinephrine administration. This has led to the speculation that fatty acids and glycerol, formed during lipolysis, may be transported in small vesicles to the cell surface for release into the bloodstream. Because it is not easy to determine, from fixed images, the direction of vesicular transport, the role of these vesicles in the economy of the adipose cell remains unresolved.

In prolonged fasting or in the emaciation associated with chronic illness, adipose tissue gives up most of its stored lipid and reverts to a highly vascular tissue made up of small ovoid or polygonal cells with multiple small

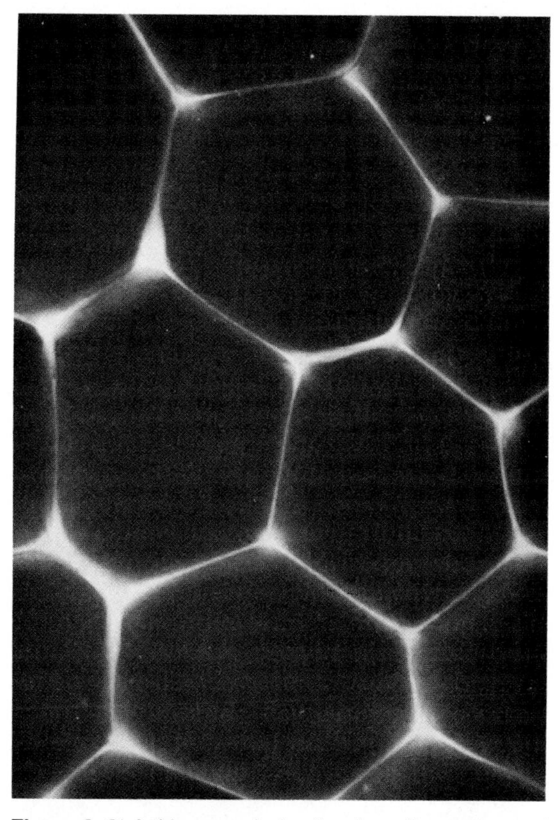

Figure 6–2. A thin spread of unilocular adipose tissue of the mesentery, stained with Sudan black without previous dehydration. The lipid droplet has been retained and is stained by the fat-soluble dye, whereas the surrounding rim of cytoplasm is unstained. (From Fawcett, D.W. 1953. *In* R.O. Greep, ed. Histology, Philadelphia, Blakiston Co. Reproduced by permission of McGraw-Hill Book Co.)

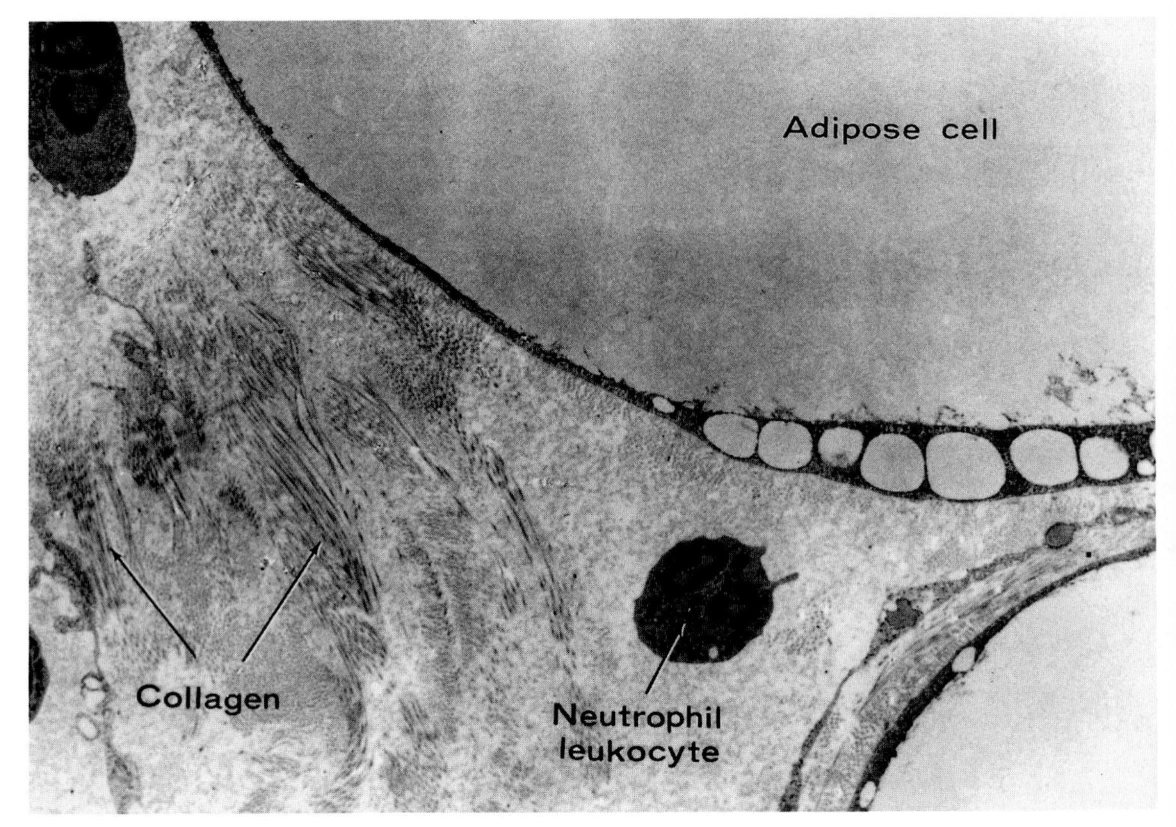

Figure 6–3. Electron micrograph of portions of two unilocular adipose cells from the epididymal fat pad of the rat. Note the relative sizes of the neutrophilic leukocyte and the very large fat cell. The cytoplasm of the fat cell at the upper right contains several small lipid droplets that have not yet coalesced with the main lipid drop.

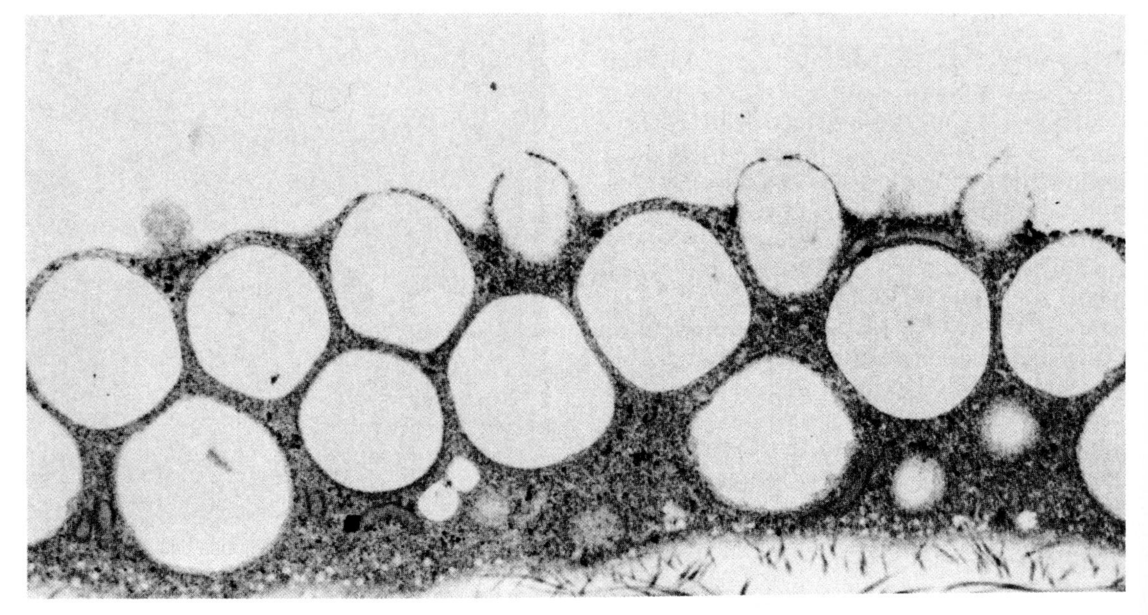

Figure 6–4. Micrograph of the rim of cytoplasm of a fat cell. A few of the numerous small lipid droplets appear to be discharging their contents into the main lipid drop at the top of the figure.

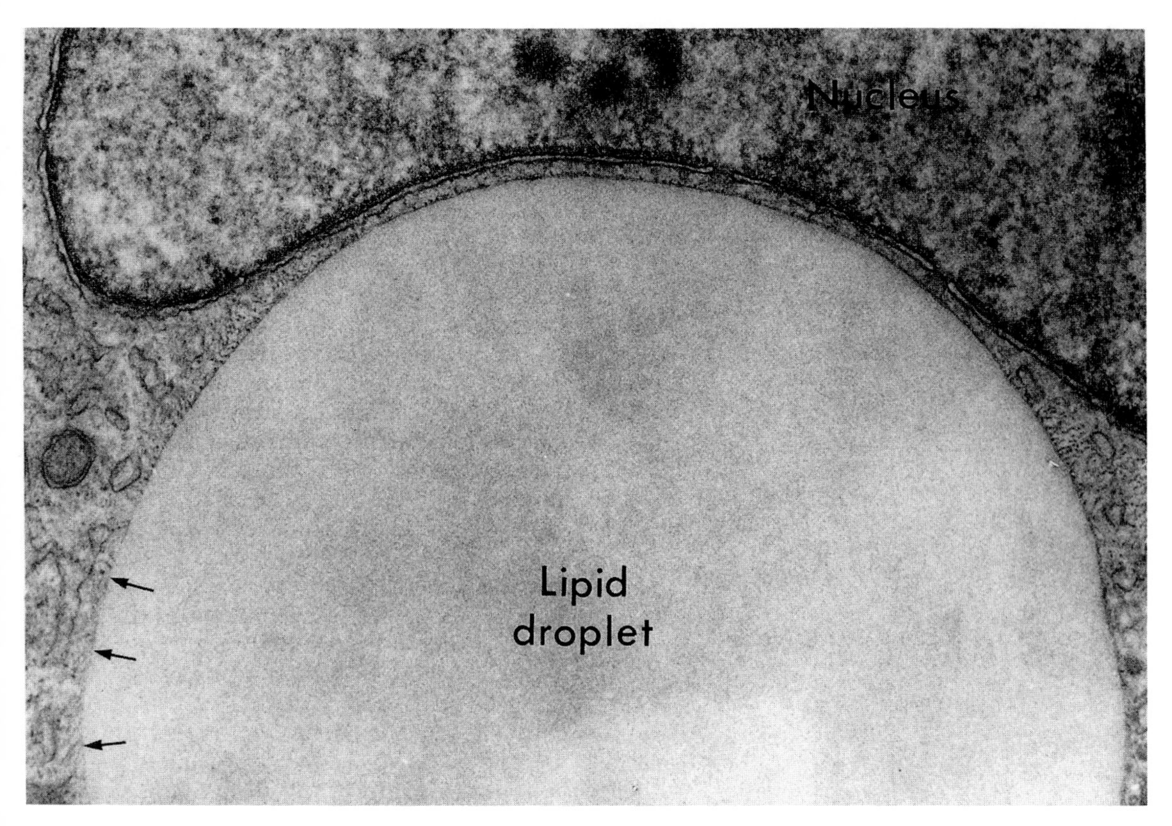

Figure 6–5. Electron micrograph of a portion of a developing adipose cell. After glutaraldehyde fixation, the lipid is often only slightly stained by osmium, and the interface between the lipid and the cytoplasm (at arrows) can be seen more clearly. Note the absence of a membrane around the lipid. (Micrograph courtesy of E. Wood.)

lipid droplets. In electron micrographs of fat cells decreasing in size during fasting, the cell surface becomes highly irregular in outline with multiple pseudopod-like processes. The redundant external lamina no longer conforms to the shape of the cell but becomes loosely folded around it. The adipose cells never revert to simple fusiform cells resembling preadipocytes or fibroblasts.

DISTRIBUTION OF WHITE ADIPOSE TISSUE

Unilocular fat is widely distributed in the subcutaneous tissue of the human but exhibits quantitative regional differences that are influenced by age and sex. In infants and young children, there is a continuous subcutaneous layer of fat, the *panniculus adiposus*, over the whole body. In adults, this layer thins out in some areas but persists and grows thicker in certain other regions. These sites of predilection differ in their distribution in the two sexes and are largely responsible for the characteristic differences in the body form of males and females. In the male, the principal regions are the nape of the neck, the subcutaneous area over the deltoid and triceps muscles, the lumbosacral region, and the buttocks. In the female, subcutaneous fat is most abundant in the breasts, the buttocks, the epitrochanteric region, and the anterior and lateral aspects of the thighs. In well-nourished individuals, the sex differences in fat distribution persist and become more obvious with advancing years, and the male tends to accumulate additional fat over the anterior abdominal wall.

In addition to these subcutaneous deposits, there are extensive accumulations of fat in the omentum, mesenteries, and the retroperitoneal area, in both sexes. All of these areas of white adipose tissue readily give up their stored lipid during fasting. However, there are other areas of adipose tissue that do not give up their stored lipid so readily. For example, the lipid in the adipose tissue of the orbit, in major joints, and on the palms and soles of the feet does not seem to be grist for the metabolic mill but contributes to the mechani-

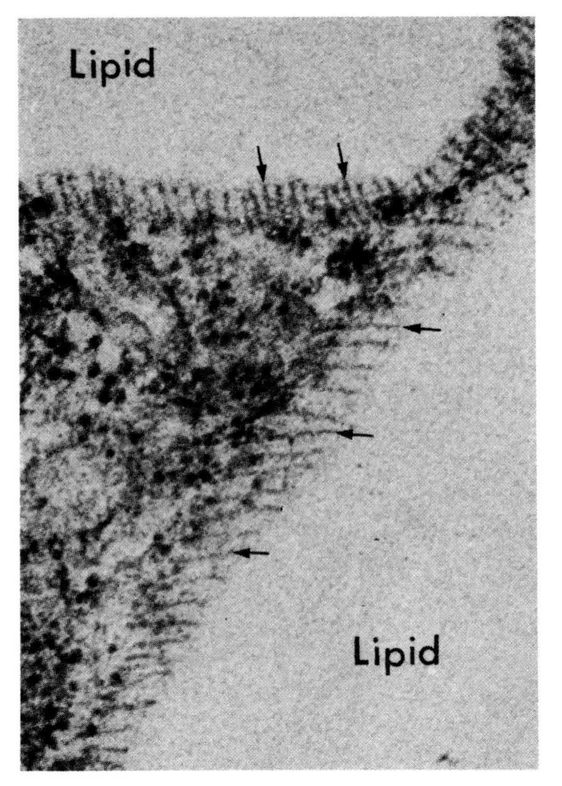

Figure 6–6. Micrograph of portions of two lipid droplets and the intervening cytoplasm of developing fat cells. The lipid-cytoplasm interface is sectioned obliquely, revealing (at arrows) an ordered array of 10-nm vimentin filaments at the boundary. (Micrograph courtesy of E. Wood.)

cal supportive role of fatpads in these locations. These areas of fat diminish in volume only after very long starvation.

HISTOGENESIS OF ADIPOSE TISSUE

In the 1800s, histologists considered adipose tissue to be merely loose connective tissue in which many of the fibroblasts had accumulated excess lipid. According to this interpretation, any connective tissue could become adipose tissue when dietary intake exceeded energy expenditure. Doubt was later cast on this view by the realization that, although connective tissue is ubiquitous, adipocytes do not become evenly distributed in obesity, but develop preferentially in some regions, whereas other remain devoid of fat cells. For example, the eyelids, nose, ears, scrotum, genitalia, and the back of the hands and feet rarely accumulate adipose tissue. This would be hard to explain if adipocytes could arise from fibroblasts wherever they occur.

It was later concluded that adipocytes differentiate from special precursor cells of mesenchymal origin, called *lipoblasts* or *preadipocytes,* but some histologists considered it unnecessary to postulate a separate category of committed precursors and prefered to regard *mesenchymal cells,* persisting in varying numbers in different regions, as the immediate precursors of the adipose cells. In either case, these stellate or fusiform precursor cells cannot, as yet, be distinguished from fibroblasts by cytological criteria. The view that adipocytes originate from specific precursors in particular locations, has derived support from studies in which it was shown that tissue cultures of the isolated stromal and vascular components of white fat yield cells that accumulate large amounts of lipid and exhibit adipocyte-specific enzyme activity, whereas the fibroblasts in cultures of the dermis from skin grown under the same conditions did not.

It is now the prevailing view that there are two processes of adipose tissue formation. In one taking place relatively early in the fetus and called *primary fat formation,* gland-like aggregations of *epitheloid* precursor cells are laid down in specific locations. These accumulate multiple lipid droplets and become brown adipose tissue. Later in fetal life and in the early postnatal period, other *fusiform* precursor cells differentiate in many areas of connective tissue and accumulate lipid that ultimately coalesces into a single large drop per cell. This so-called *secondary fat formation* results in the widely disseminated deposits of unilocular fat found in the adult human.

In affluent countries, obesity is a major health problem. Excess adipose tissue puts an added strain on the circulatory system, increasing the risk of hypertension and myocardial infarction. Obesity, developing in adult life, is commonly due to accumulation of excess lipid in a normal number of unilocular adipose cells (*hypertrophic obesity*). The fat cells in such individuals may be four times their normal size. In severe obesity, there may also be a greater than normal number of cells (*hypercellular obesity*). Fully differentiated adipocytes are unable to divide and their precursors, formed in the early postnatal period, are probably not able to proliferate later in life, but individuals vary in the number of their adipocyte precursor cells. There is now experimental and clinical evidence that overfeeding in the early weeks of life can result in the formation of greater than normal numbers of adipose cell precursors resulting in a greater danger of developing hypercellular obesity in adult life. Clinical data indicate that infants attaining a body weight above the 97th percentile are three times as likely as other infants to become obese adults. Conversely, infants who were born in a period of famine in Europe near the end of world War II had roughly one-third the incidence of adult obesity compared to a similar group born in a period of plenty in the first summer of peace. Thus, it seems clear that the level of nutrition in the early weeks of life can influence the number of adipose cell precursors. Whereas adult hypertrophic obesity may occur in anyone due to dietary excess, severe hypercellular obesity is more likely to occur in those who were overnourished as infants.

HISTOPHYSIOLOGY OF WHITE ADIPOSE TISSUE

After feeding, fats in the diet are degraded in the duodenum by the pancreatic enzyme *lipase* to yield fatty acids and glycerol. These are taken into the intestinal epithelial cells where they are recombined to form neutral fats (triglycerides). These are released at the basolateral membrane of the cells and carried via the lymph to the bloodstream in the form of minute droplets called *chylomicrons*. Reaching the capillaries of the adipose tissue, chylomicrons are exposed to the enzyme *lipoprotein lipase*, bound to the lumenal surface of their lining endothelium. This enzyme breaks down the chylomicrons, liberating fatty acids that are taken up by the fat cells and combined with endogenous glycerol to form triglycerides; these are added to the lipid droplet for storage. Triglycerides can also be synthesized by adipose cells from blood-borne glucose and amino acids resulting from digestion of carbohydrates and proteins of the diet (Fig. 6–7).

In fasting, the energy requirements of the body are met by drawing on the triglycerides stored in the adipose cells. Intracellular lipases are activated to break down triglycerides at the surface of the lipid droplet and the fatty

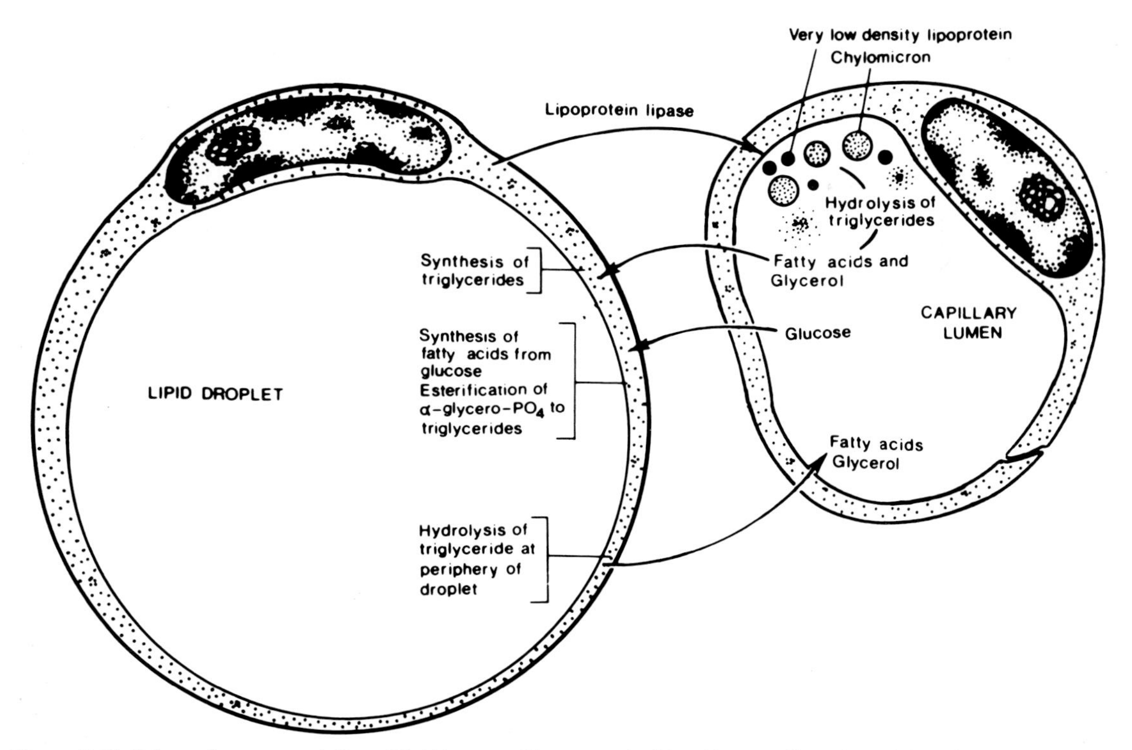

Figure 6–7. Schematic representation of lipid transport between the blood in a capillary (at right) and an adipose cell (at left). Lipid is carried in the bloodstream from the intestine to the adipose tissue in the form of chylomicrons and from the liver in the form of very low-density lipoprotein particles. In the capillaries, both of these are hydrolyzed by a lipoprotein lipase to fatty acids and glycerol, which diffuse from the capillary to the fat cell where they are reesterified to triglycerides that are added to the stored lipid. Blood glucose diffusing from the capillary to the adipose cells can also be used in the synthesis of triglycerides from carbohydrate. Upon neural or hormonal stimulation, elevated cyclic AMP activates a cytoplasmic lipase, which hydrolyzed triglyceride at the periphery of the droplet, and the resulting fatty acids and glycerol diffuse back to the capillaries and are carried in the blood to the tissues throughout the body.

acids so formed are released into the blood to be used as fuel for the other tissues of the body.

The changes occurring in adipose tissue can, thus, be compared to the deposits and withdrawals taking place in a checking account in a bank. Deposits are in the form of triglyceride synthesized from breakdown products of dietary fats or triglyceride formed from fatty acids synthesized from glucose in the liver or in the adipose cells themselves. Withdrawals are made by enzymatic hydrolysis of stored triglycerides. However, the lipid in adipose tissue is not an energy reserve drawn on *only* in times of fasting. Isotopic tracer studies have clearly shown that the lipid is continuously being mobilized and renewed even in an individual in caloric balance. The half-life of depot lipids in the rat is about 8 days, which means that almost 10% of the fatty acid stored in adipose tissue is replaced each day by new fatty acid. Continual renewal also occurs in man, but the quantity and rate of this process are not known with the same precision as they are in laboratory animals.

The plasma membrane of unilocular adipose cells contains receptors for certain hormones that influence their function. Secretion of *insulin* by the pancreatic islets accelerates the uptake of glucose and its conversion to triglycerides in the fat cells. It not only increases the rate of glucose transport into the cell and the deposition of glycogen (Fig. 6–8) but also activates the enzyme fatty-acid synthetase. Its effects can be detected microscopically in a transient increase in glycogen in the cytoplasm. *Epinephrine*, from the adrenal medulla, promotes the lipolysis of stored lipid and the release of fatty acids. The level of circulating *estrogens*, or the number of estrogen receptors expressed on preadipocytes, may influence the pattern of distribution of adipose tissue in the female. *Adrenocortical hormone*, in normal concentrations, has no known

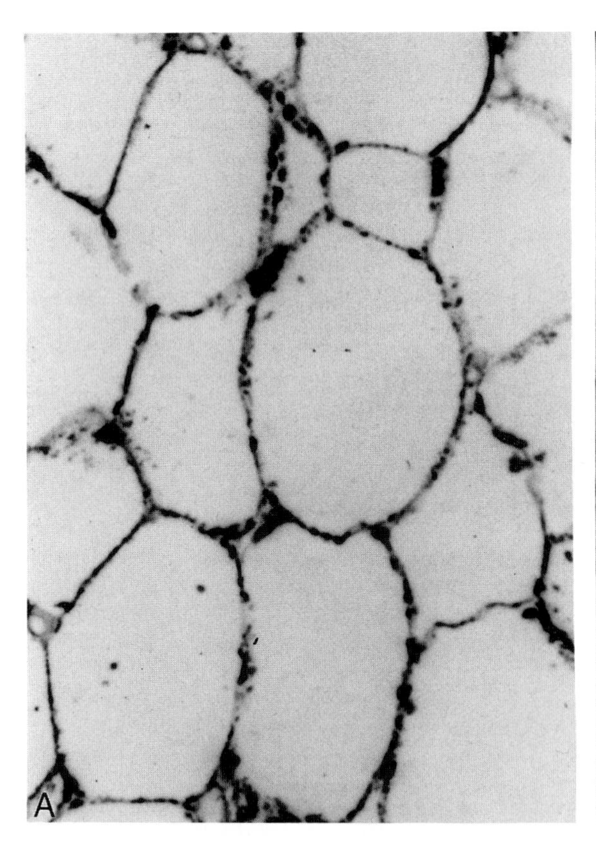

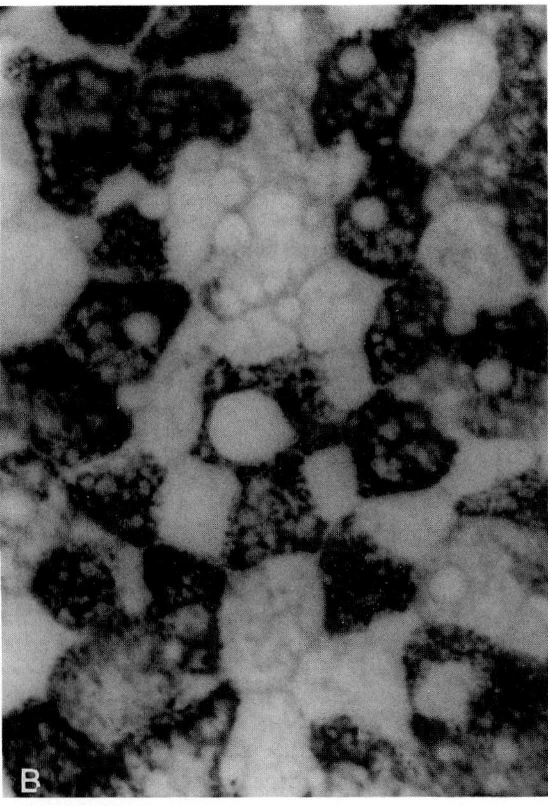

Figure 6–8. (A) White adipose tissue of a rat refeeding after a period of fasting. The dark granules around the periphery of each cell are deposits of glycogen which would later disappear as this carbohydrate was used in the synthesis of triglycerides. (B) Brown adipose tissue under the same experimental conditions. Considerably more glycogen has been deposited in these cells, but not all of the cells have accumulated glycogen to the same degree. Some, therefore, stain relatively little with the periodic-acid–Schiff reaction used here. A similar deposition of glycogen in fat cells can be induced by administration of insulin. (From Fawcett, D.W. 1952. J. Morphol. 90:363.)

physiological action on adipose tissue, but when present in excess, it results in a local hypertrophy of adipocytes over the lower cervical region resulting in a deformity referred to clinically as "buffalo hump."

BROWN ADIPOSE TISSUE (MULTILOCULAR ADIPOSE TISSUE)

Brown adipose tissue, in various species, ranges in color from tan to a rich reddish brown. Its color is due, in part, to its rich vascularity and, in part, to cytochromes in its extraordinarily abundant mitochondria. The cells are smaller than those of white fat and are polygonal in section. Their cytoplasm is relatively abundant and contains multiple lipid droplets of varying size (Fig. 6–9). The spherical nucleus is slightly eccentric in position but is never displaced to the periphery of the cell as in white fat. There is a small juxtanuclear Golgi complex and very numerous mitochondria. In electron micrographs, large spherical mitochondria occupy a large part of the cytoplasm. They have numerous cristae that often traverse the full width of the organelle (Fig. 6–10). Rough endoplasmic reticulum is generally lacking but a few profiles of smooth endoplasmic reticulum may be found. Small numbers of free ribosomes and variable amounts of glycogen are also present in the cytoplasm.

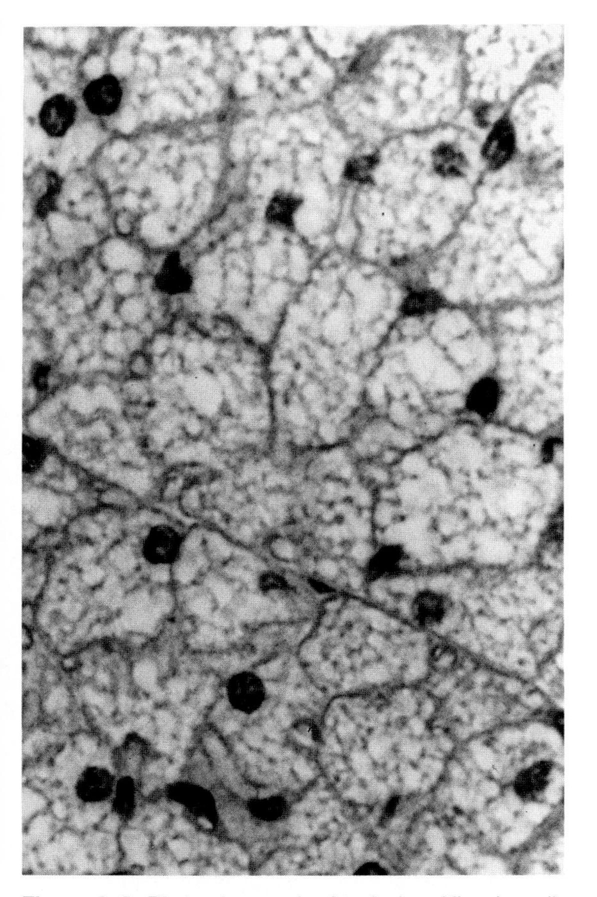

Figure 6–9. Photomicrograph of typical multilocular adipose tissue (brown fat). The polygonal cells contain more cytoplasm than those of unilocular adipose tissue and have multiple lipid droplets of varying size, instead of a single large globule.

Brown fat has a lobular organization and the pattern of distribution of blood vessels within the lobules is reminiscent of that of a gland (Fig. 6–11). In animals subjected to prolonged fasting, brown fat gradually loses lipid, becoming more deeply colored and reverting to a gland-like mass of epithelioid cells that bear no resemblance to cells of connective tissue (Fig. 6–12). Depletion of lipid is more rapid in animals exposed to a cold environment.

The connective tissue stroma of brown adipose tissue is very sparse and the blood supply exceedingly rich (Fig. 6–11). The cells are, therefore, in more intimate relation to one another, and to the capillaries, than in unilocular fat. Silver stains and electron micrographs reveal numerous small unmyelinated nerves in the brown adipose tissue. Axons are frequently found in close apposition to the surface of the cells. This contrasts with nerves in white adipose tissue which do not end on the fat cells but only innervate the blood vessels.

DISTRIBUTION OF BROWN ADIPOSE TISSUE

Brown adipose tissue has been found in representatives of at least seven orders of mammals. It is prominent in the newborn of all species in which it is found. In adults, it is most conspicuous in species that hibernate. In the common laboratory rodents, brown adipose tissue occurs in two symmetrical interscapular fat bodies, in thin lobules between muscles around the shoulder girdle, and in the axillae. It occupies the costovertebral angle and forms slender lobules along either side of the aorta and in the hilus of the kidneys. It has a similar distribution in young monkeys.

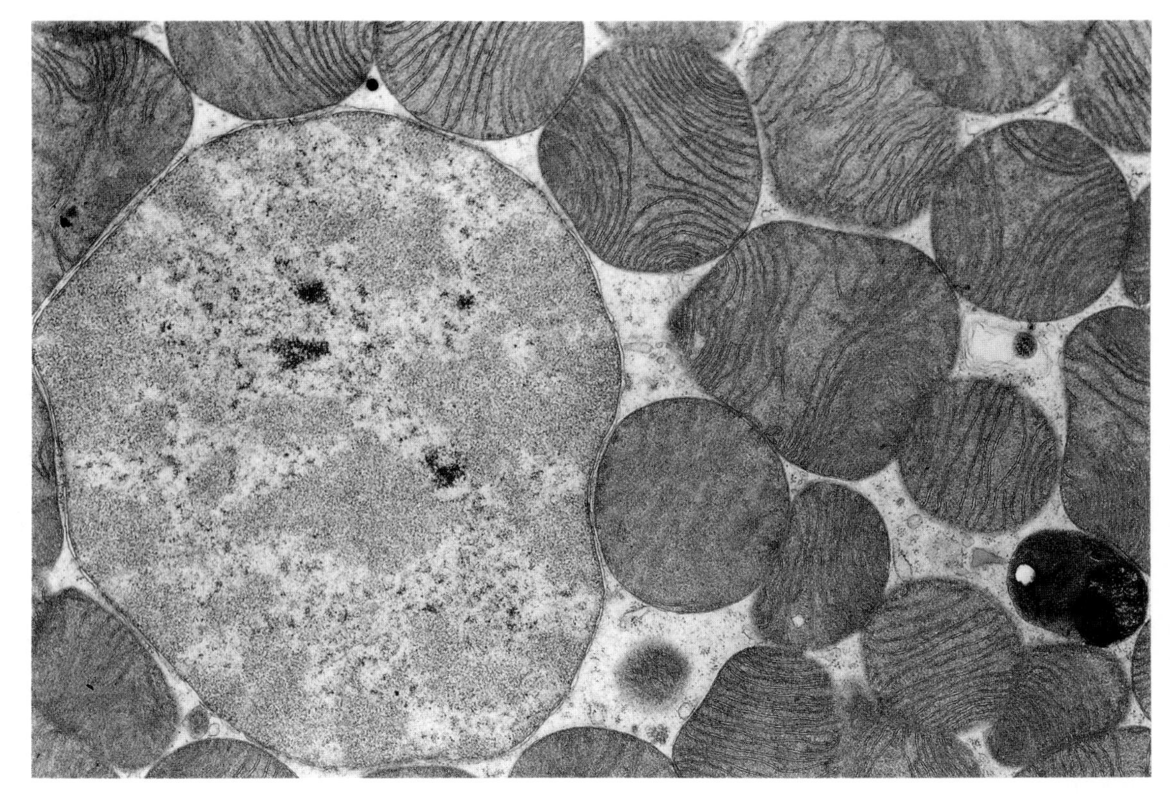

Figure 6–10. Electron micrograph of the nucleus and lipid-free surrounding cytoplasm of a brown adipose cell from a bat recently aroused from hibernation. Typical of this tissue is the great abundance of very large spheroidal mitochondria, with cristae traversing the entire width of the organelle.

In man, the multilocular condition of the lipid gradually diminishes by coalescence of the droplets and in adults, the cells gradually come to resemble those of white adipose tissue (Fig. 6–13). For this reason, there was formerly some debate as to whether or not two physiologically distinct types of adipose tissue occurred in humans. There is now compelling evidence that two types do exist, even though they may be difficult to distinguish in well-nourished adults. Brown fat is well developed in the neck and interscapular region of the human fetus by the 28th week and in the newborn it constitutes 2–5% of the body weight. All of the adipose tissue in the adult, may appear to be unilocular, but in the elderly with chronic wasting diseases and in starvation, masses of multilocular fat again become apparent in the same regions where it is found in the fetus and newborn. Further support for two types of fat in humans comes from the observation that there are two distinct types of *lipomas*, tumors of fatty tissue, occurring in man: one resembling unilocular adipose tissue and the other resembling brown fat. It is now the concensus that two kinds of adipose tissue are present in man throughout life.

HISTOPHYSIOLOGY OF BROWN ADIPOSE TISSUE

In addition to its storage of fuel, the subcutaneous white fat on most mammals has long been regarded as an insulating layer helping to conserve body heat. When this tissue was found to be metabolically active, it was realized that its chemical reactions might also generate a small amount of heat. It is now known that the brown fat is a tissue specialized for heat production. The very large number of its mitochondria give it an unusual capacity for generating heat through oxidation of fatty acids. The rate of oxidation of some substrates by brown adipose cells in vitro may be 20 times that of white fat. Each milliliter of oxygen consumed in the process contributes about 5 calories of body heat. In a cold environment, brown fat cells may treble their heat production.

Adult animals in a cold environment produce additional heat as a by-product of the muscular activity involved in shivering. Newborn and very young animals are unable to shiver and rely on their brown adipose tissue for *nonshivering thermogenesis*. On exposure to

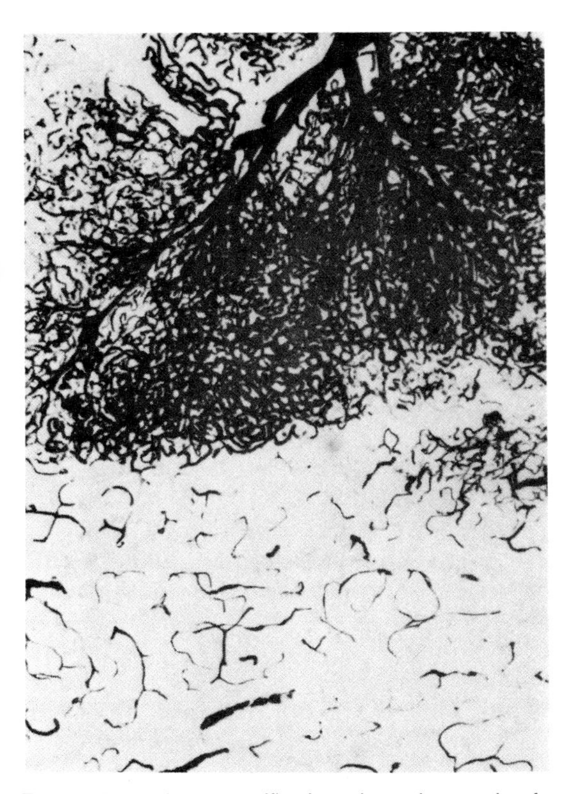

Figure 6–11. Low-magnification photomicrograph of a thick section of brown adipose tissue (top) and white adipose tissue (bottom). The blood vessels have been injected with India ink to show the relative vascularity of the two tissues. The vascular network of the brown adipose tissue is extraordinarily dense and has a gland-like pattern, whereas that of the white fat below is relatively sparse. (From Fawcett, D.W., 1952. J. Morphol. 90:363.)

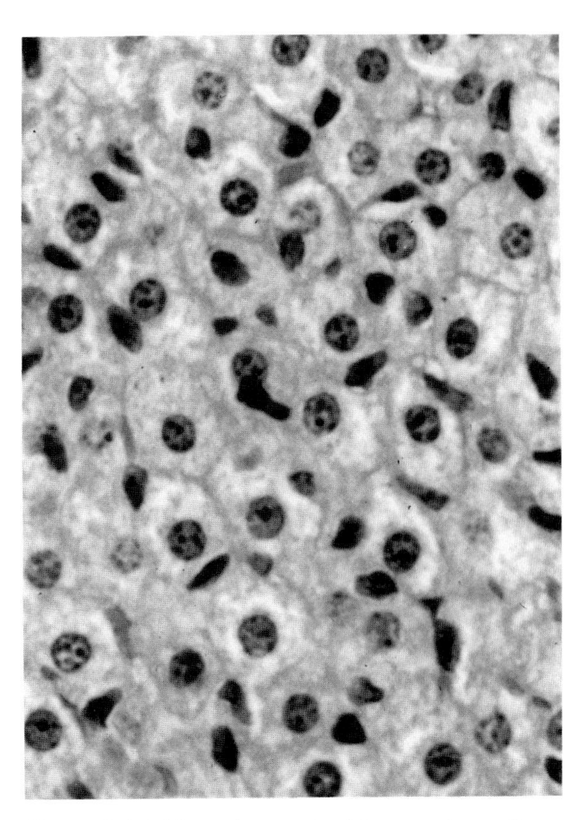

Figure 6–12. Photomicrograph of brown adipose tissue that has been depleted of lipid after prolonged fasting, or after hypophysectomy, takes on the appearance of a compact glandular epithelium. Its cells bear no resemblance to connective tissue fibroblasts.

cold, sensory receptors in the skin send nerve impulses to the temperature-regulating center in the brain. This relays impulses along sympathetic nerve pathways to the brown adipose tissue. Some nerves act on the blood vessels to increase blood flow; others, terminating on the adipose cells, release the neurotransmitter norepinephrine. This activates the enzyme that splits triglyceride molecules into fatty acid and glycerol, thereby triggering a heat-producing cycle of fatty-acid oxidation and regeneration of triglycerides that converts chemical-bond energy into heat energy. This is made possible by a unique *uncoupling protein* in brown fat mitochondria that results in its metabolism proceeding at a maximum rate under these conditions.

Hormones of the thyroid gland increase the metabolic activity of many tissues but they have an especially marked effect on adipose tissue. The action of thyroid hormones result from their binding to specific receptors in the nucleus. The principal hormone secreted by the thyroid is thyroxine (T4), but the affinity of nuclear receptors for triiodothyronine (T3) is 10 times higher than that for thyroxine. Therefore, T3 is physiologically the more important hormone, with T4 serving mainly as a prohormone. Deiodination of thyroxine to form triiodothyronine is generally carried out by an enzyme (thyroxine 5′ diiodinase) in the liver and kidneys and these organs are the principal sources of plasma triiodothyronine. However, brown adipose tissue has a similar enzyme that rises sharply on exposure to cold, reaching levels that may be 100 times those in this tissue of animals in the warm. The elevation of thermogenesis in response to cold may depend on activity of this enzyme.

Brown adipose tissue is abundant in species that hibernate and it is essential for their rapid warming during arousal from the torpid state. Heat generation by brown fat can be demonstrated visually by the technique of thermography (Fig. 6–14). The thermograph scans across the body, detecting the infrared radia-

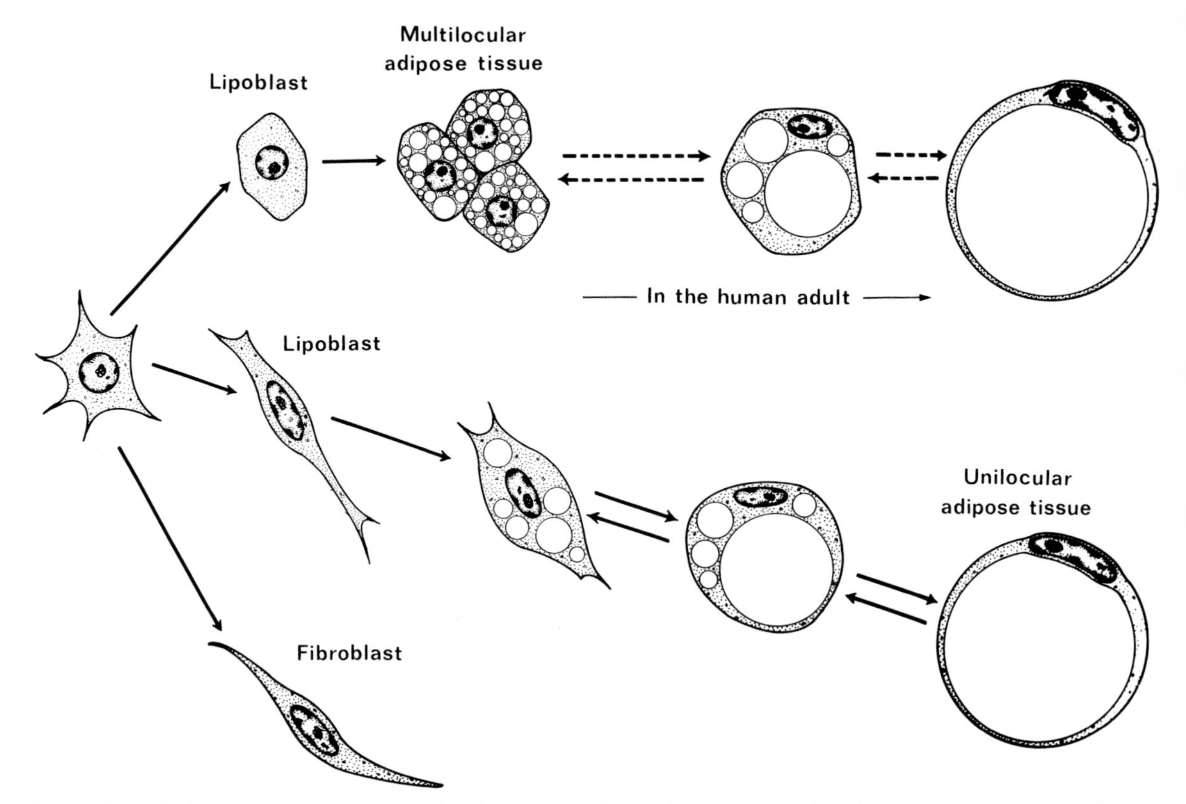

Figure 6–13. Schematic representation of the histogenesis of the adipose tissues. One forms gland-like aggregations of epithelioid lipoblasts, derived from mesenchymal cells. These accumulate multiple droplets of lipid, developing into multilocular brown adipose tissue. In primates, including man, the multiple lipid droplets coalesce to varying degrees in the adult, so that the tissue takes on an appearance similar to that of unilocular adipose tissue. Another kind of lipoblast, which is fusiform and more widely distributed in the embryonic connective tissues, accumulates lipid in a single large globule, giving rise to unilocular adipose tissue. When their lipid is depleted by prolonged fasting, the two types of fat revert to tissues of quite different appearance.

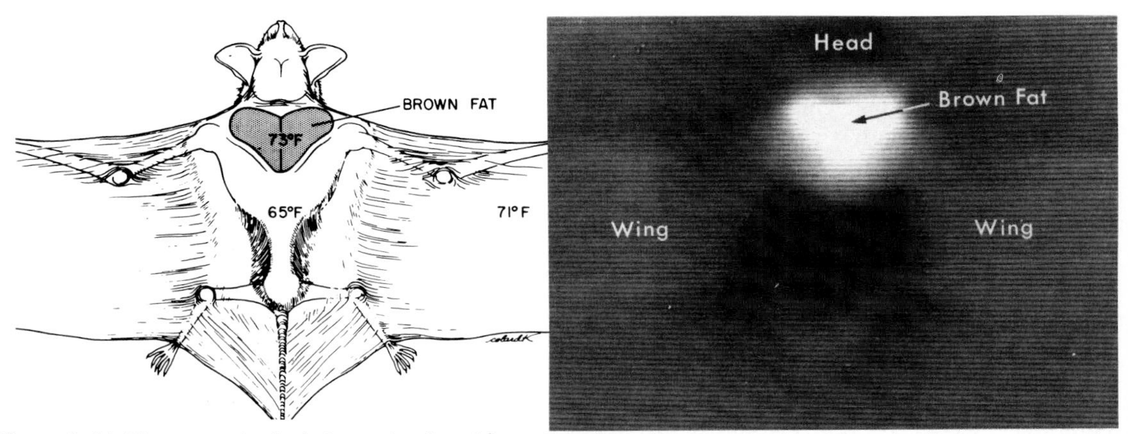

Figure 6–14. Thermograph of a bat arousing from hibernation. Scanning the animal for infrared radiation reveals a "hot spot" in the area corresponding to the interscapular brown adipose tissue. During arousal, this tissue serves as a chemical "furnace," producing heat that is carried in the bloodstream to warm the rest of the body. (Thermograph courtesy of J. Hayward.)

tion from the surface, and registers the temperature-dependent intensity of radiation on a photographic plate. When a bat, arousing from hibernation, is scanned, the thin wing membranes rapidly equilibrate with the ambient temperature and most of the body is still relatively cool. However, a sharply delineated "hot area" is found on the thermograph coinciding with the location of the interscapular brown fat.

It has been shown that the very young human infant uses this same mechanism for heat production. An infant placed in an environment at 23°C immediately after birth will have an increase in the level of glycerol in the blood resulting from lipolysis of triglycerides and will have approximately double the metabolic rate of an infant at 33°C. This will be accomplished without shivering. Thermography under these conditions reveal areas of elevated skin temperature over the sites of brown adipose tissue at the nape of the neck, interscapular region, and in the axillae.

BIBLIOGRAPHY

UNILOCULAR ADIPOSE TISSUE

Cushman, S.W. 1970. Structure–function relationships in the adipose cell. I. Ultrastructure of the isolated adipose cell. II. Pinocytosis and factors influencing its activity in the isolated adipose cell. J. Cell Biol. 46:326, 342.

Franke, W.W., M. Hergt, and C. Grund. 1987. Rearrangement of the vimentin cytoskeleton during adipose conversion: Formation of an intermediate filament cage around lipid globules. Cell 49:131.

Greenwood, M.R.C. and J. Hirsch. 1979. Prenatal development of adipose cellularity in the normal rat. J. Lipid Res. 15:474.

Heindel, J.J., L. Orci, and B. Jeanrenaud. 1975. Fat mobilization and its regulation by hormones and drugs in white adipose tissue. *In* C. Peters, ed. International Encyclopedia of Pharmacology and Therapy. Vol. I, p. 175. Oxford, Pergamon Press.

Hirsch, J. and B. Batchelor. 1976. Adipose tissue cellularity in human obesity. Clin. Endocrinol. Metabol. 5:299.

Jeanrenaud, B. 1961. Dynamic aspects of adipose tissue metabolism. A review. Metabol. Clin. Exp. 10:535.

Napolitano, L. 1963. The differentiation of white adipose cells: an electron microscope study. J. Cell. Biol. 18:663.

Napolitano, L. and H.T. Gagne. 1963. Lipid depleted white adipose cells. Anat. Rec. 147:273.

Renold, A.E. and G.F. Cahill, eds. 1965. Adipose Tissue. Handbook of Physiology, Section 5, Washington, D.C., American Physiological Society.

Sheldon, H. 1964. The Fine Structure of the Fat Cell. *In* K. Rodahl and B. Issekutz, eds. Fat as a Tissue. Baltimore, McGraw-Hill Book Co.

Slavin, B.G. 1972. The cytophysiology of mammalian adipose tissue. Internat. Rev. Cytol. 33:297.

MULTILOCULAR ADIPOSE TISSUE

Cannon, B. and B.W. Johansson. 1980. Non-shivering thermogenesis in the newborn. Mol. Aspects Med. 3:119.

Fawcett, D.W. 1952. A comparison of the histological organization and histochemical reactions of brown fat and ordinary fat. J. Morphol. 90:363.

Heaton, J.M. 1972. The distribution of brown adipose tissue in the human. J. Anat. 112:35.

Himms-Hagen, J. 1976. Cellular thermogenesis. Annu. Rev. Physiol. 38:315.

Lindberg, O., ed. Brown Adipose Tissue. New York, American Elsevier Publishing Co.

Lindberg, O., J. dePierre, E. Rylander et al. 1967. Studies of the mitochondrial energy-transfer system of brown adipose tissue. J. Cell Biol. 34:293.

Merklin, R.J. 1974. Growth and distribution of human fetal brown fat. Anat. Rec. 178:637.

Nedergaard, J. and O. Lindberg. 1982. The brown fat cell. Internat. Rev. Cytol. 74:310.

Nichols, D.G. and L. Locke. 1984. Thermogenic mechanisms in brown adipose tissue. Physiol. Rev. 64:1.

Nichols, D.G. 1979. Brown adipose tissue mitochondria. Biochim. Biophys. Acta 549:1.

Nnodim, J.O. and J.D. Lever. 1988. Neural and vascular provisions of rat interscapular brown adipose tissue. Am. J. Anat. 182:283.

Sidman, R.L. and D.W. Fawcett. 1954. The effect of peripheral nerve section on some metabolic responses of brown adipose tissue. Anat. Rec. 118:487.

Silva, J.E. 1986. Brown adipose tissue: an extrathyroid source of triiodothyronine. News Physiol. Sci. 1:119.

Smith, R.E. and B.A. Horwitz. 1969. Brown fat and thermogenesis. Physiol. Rev. 49:330.

7
CARTILAGE

Cartilage is a specialized form of connective tissue consisting of cells, called *chondrocytes*, sparsely distributed in a firm, gel-like extracellular matrix. This tissue is not penetrated by nerves or by blood vessels. Its cells, isolated in small cavities or lacunae, are nourished by diffusion through the aqueous phase of the matrix from capillaries in the tissues surrounding the cartilage. The viscoelastic properties of the extracellular matrix give cartilage unusual firmness and resilience. It is able to grow rapidly while maintaining a considerable degree of stiffness, a property which makes it an especially favorable skeletal material for the developing embryo. Most of the axial and appendicular skeleton is first formed of cartilage and later replaced by bone.

Cartilage is of more restricted occurrence in postnatal life, but it continues to play an important role in growth in length of the long bones of the extremities. When adult stature has been attained, the cartilage models of the bones have been entirely replaced by bone tissue except for a layer that persists throughout life on the surfaces that articulate with other bones.

Three kinds of cartilage, *hyaline, elastic,* and *fibrocartilage*, are distinguished on the basis of the amount of extracellular matrix and the relative abundance of collagen and elastic fibers encorporated in the matrix. Hyaline cartilage is the most common and archetypic form and the others can be regarded as variants of its basic structure.

HYALINE CARTILAGE

In the adult, hyaline cartilage is found in the tracheal rings, the nose and larynx, on the joint surfaces, and in the ventral ends of the ribs that connect them to the sternum. It is a semitranslucent tissue with a bluish-gray color. Its microscopic structure can be best understood by studying its development in the embryo.

HISTOGENESIS OF CARTILAGE

At sites of cartilage formation in the embryo, the mesenchymal cells withdraw their processes and become crowded together in dense aggregations recognizable as *centers of chondrification*. The cells are very close together and their boundaries are indistinct (Fig. 7–1B). As these precursor cells enlarge and differentiate, they secrete around themselves an amorphous metachomatic matrix (Figs. 7–1C and 7–2). Collagen is secreted concurrently, but the fibrils formed are masked by the hyaline matrix in which they are embedded. As the amount of this interstitial material increases, the cells become isolated in individual compartments or *lacunae* (Fig. 7–1D) and gradually take on the cytological characteristics of mature chondrocytes (Fig. 7–3).

In the expansion of centers of chondrification, growth occurs by two different mechanisms. The mesenchyme surrounding the developing cartilage condenses to form the *perichondrium*. The cells on its inner aspect, referred to as its *chondrogenic layer*, proliferate, differentiate into chondrocytes, and secrete matrix around themselves, thus becoming incorporated into the cartilage. This addition of new cells and matrix at the surface is called *appositional growth*. The ability of the perichondrium to form cartilage continues to be expressed in postnatal life and contributes to the growth in diameter of the cartilage models of the long bones.

In the interior of the developing cartilage, the cells retain, for a time, the ability to divide. After telophase, their secretion of matrix forms a partition of increasing thickness between the daughter cells so that they come to occupy separate lacunae. These cells, in turn, may later divide, resulting in a group of four chondrocytes in neighboring lacunae. The expansion of cartilage by formation of new cells and matrix in its interior is called *interstitial growth* and it accounts for the common

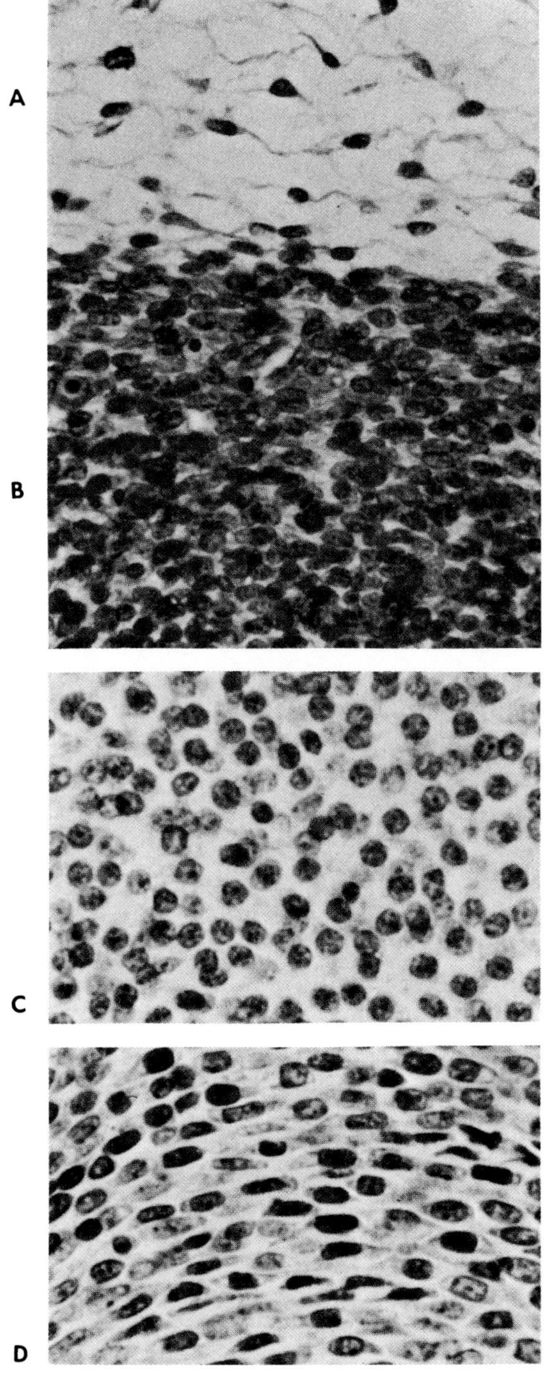

Figure 7–1. Stages in the histogenesis of cartilage. (A) Mesenchymal cells withdraw their processes and become crowded together to form (B) an area of precartilage. (C) The densely aggregated cells are moved apart by deposition of translucent hyaline matrix between them. (D) The cells become more fusiform, conforming to the shape of the lacunae in which they are isolated.

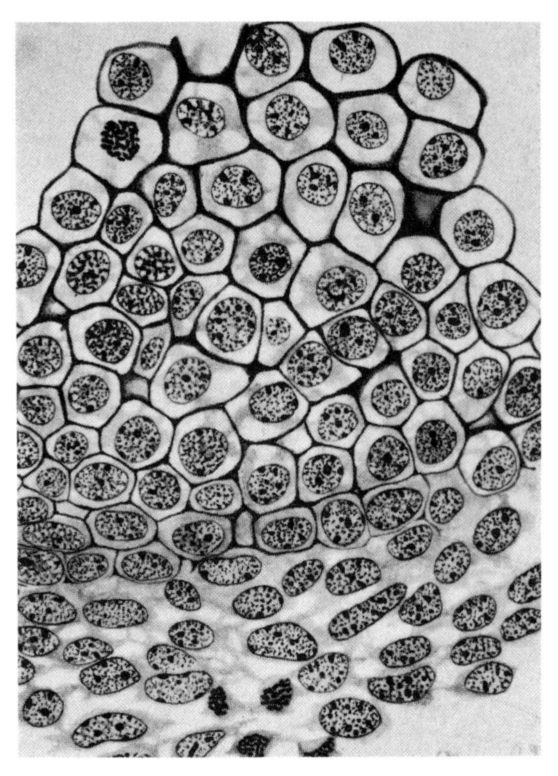

Figure 7–2. Drawing of procartilage (top) developing from mesenchyme (bottom) in a 15-mm guinea pig embryo. (After A.A. Maximov.)

occurrence of pairs and clusters of four or more lacunae in the cartilage of adults. Each cluster is said to be *isogenous* because it represents the progeny of a single chondrocyte that underwent a few divisions before becoming quiescent. The matrix immediately surrounding each group of isogenous cells stains more deeply than elsewhere (Fig 7–2). This more intensely basophilic halo is referred to as the *territorial matrix* and the less basophilic areas between cell groups are called *interterritorial matrix*.

In the epiphyseal cartilages of growing long bones, interstitial growth persists and cell divisions in a consistent orientation result in lacunae arranged in long columns parallel to the long axis of the bone (Figs. 7–4 and 7–5). The cells at the metaphyseal end of these columns degenerate and their lacunae are invaded by the advancing bone. The replacement of cartilage by bone will be described in Chapter 8.

THE CHONDROCYTES

Immediately beneath the perichondrium and under the free surface of articular carti-

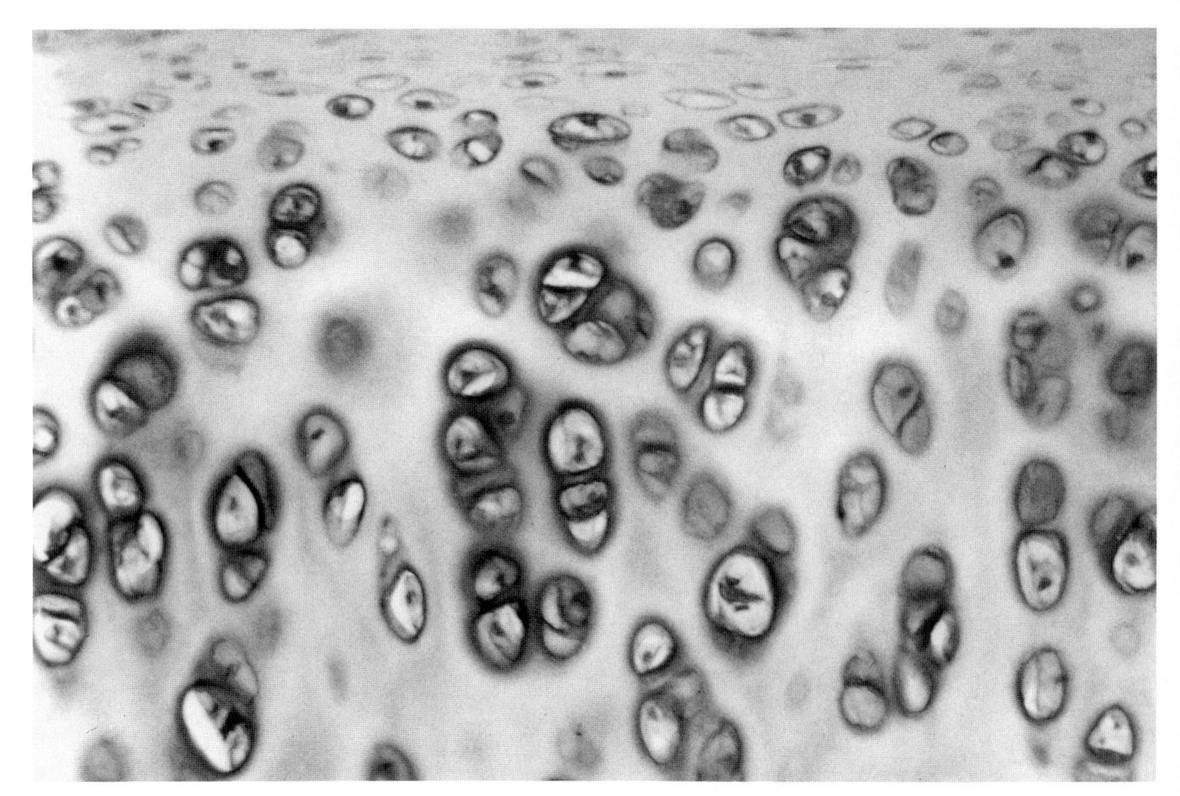

Figure 7–3. Hyaline cartilage from the trachea of a guinea pig. Note the more intense staining of the capsular, or territorial, matrix immediately surrounding the groups of isogenous cells. The cells immediately beneath the perichondrium (top) that have recently been added in appositional growth are single and fusiform. Their shape and that of their lacunae change as they move deeper into the cartilage.

lage, the lacunae are elliptical with their long axis parallel to the surface, whereas deeper in the cartilage, they are hemispherical or angular. In living cartilage, the cells conform to the shape of their lacunae, but in histological sections they often appear stellate owing to shrinkage and retraction of their surface from the wall of the lacuna. This is an artifact of specimen preparation which is less evident in specimens prepared for electron microscopy, but here too the quality of preservation is less than ideal. The cytoplasm is usually of low density and contains occasional lipid droplets and variable amounts of glycogen. The juxtanuclear Golgi complex is vacuolated and the cisternae of the endoplasmic reticulum often distended. The mitochondria may be distorted and have a matrix of low density. It is evident that the ultrastructure of chondrocytes is less well preserved by routine methods of specimen preparation than is that of other cell types. However, in electron micrographs of tissue prepared by high-pressure freezing and freeze-substitution followed by low-temperature embedding, their appearance is more representative of their state in vivo. There are few cytoplasmic vacuoles, the mitochondrial matrix is dense, and there is little or no distension of the cisternae of the Golgi or of the endoplasmic reticulum (Fig. 7–6).

When chondrocytes are actively engaged in synthesis of matrix components, their cytoplasm is more basophilic, and in electron micrographs, the Golgi complex is prominent and the endoplasmic reticulum more extensive.

CARTILAGE MATRIX

In the fresh condition, the matrix of hyaline cartilage has an opalescent blue-gray color and is semitranslucent. It appears homogeneous with the light microscope due in part to the fact that the ground substance and the collagen fibers within it have approximately the same refractive index. It stains deeply with the periodic-acid–Schiff reaction for carbohydrates, exhibits metachromasia with Toluidine blue, and has a strong affinity for other

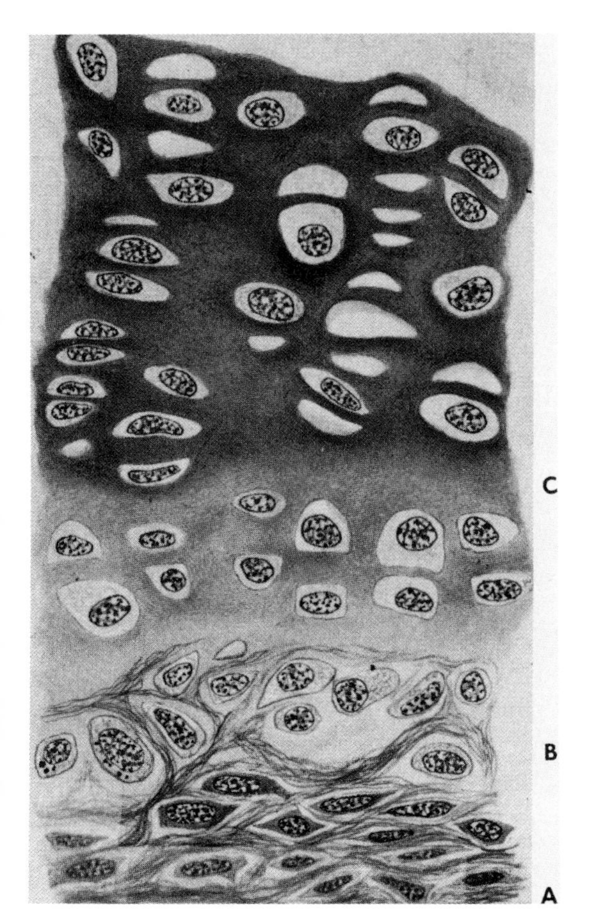

Figure 7–4. Drawing of hyaline cartilage from the xiphoid process of the rat. (A) Transitional layer adjacent to the perichondrium. (B) Collagen fibers can be seen continuing from the perichondrium into the matrix of the cartilage. (C) Columns of isogenous groups of chondrocytes, some of which have fallen out of their lacunae in processing. (After A.A. Maximov.)

basic dyes. These stains are of little use for studying the collagen that makes up 40% or more of the dry weight of cartilage. However, a solution of Sirius-red in picric acid applied to cartilage after digestion of its proteoglycans results in enhanced birefringence of collagen under polarization optics and, thus, permits analysis of fiber orientation in relation to local functional requirements.

The dominant collagen of cartilage matrix is type II. In contrast to the type-I fibers of other connective tissues, which average 75 nm in thickness, type-II collagen forms faint crossbanded fibers 15–45 nm in diameter that do not assemble into coarse bundles. The smaller fibers form a loose three-dimensional network throughout the matrix. There is a gradient of increasing fiber diameter from the lacunae outward into the interterritorial matrix. In articular cartilage, fiber diameter also increases from the surface inward. Studies employing the picro-Sirius stain and polarization microscopy reveal that, in addition to the small fibers forming a meshwork throughout the matrix, there are larger fibers that show a consistent preferential orientation. In articular cartilage, the fibers in a superficial zone are oriented parallel to the surface while deeper fibers curve inward to form vertical columns that extend down to the junction of the cartilage with bone. The trajectory of these fibers has been likened to a series of Gothic arches. Thin cartilages covered by perichondrium are traversed by similar transversely oriented columns of fibers joined by arches tangential to the perichondrium on both surfaces. Other cartilages have different patterns of collagen distribution suggesting that their fiber orientation is adapted to resist the stresses to which they are normally subjected.

Until recently, type-II was considered to be the only cartilage-specific collagen, but types-IX, -X, and -XI and three unclassified collagen chains have now been reported. Together, these three minor collagens amount to no more than 5–10% of the total collagen. There is no consensus on their organization or function. Type-IX and -XI are closely associated with the type-II fibers but what their exact relationship is remains unclear. Type-IX has been localized at the intersections of type-II fibers and it is speculated that it may contribute to stabilization of the fibrous network of the matrix. Type-X collagen has a very restricted distribution, limited to the matrix immediately surrounding cells in the zone of chondrocyte hypertrophy at sites of endochondrial ossification.

The territorial matrix varies in its extent in different cartilages but may be up to 50 μm wide. Its greater affinity for basic dyes is attributed to a higher local concentration of chondroitin sulfate. In recent years, another layer, the *pericellular capsule,* has been defined, immediately surrounding the lacunae. It is 1–3 μm thick and consists of a feltwork of very fine fibers and an amorphous material resembling that of basal laminae. Immunocytochemical studies suggest that some of the minor collagens may be localized in this layer. The pericellular capsule may play a significant role in protecting the chondrocytes in cartilages subjected to mechanical tension or compression.

Like the ground substance of other connective tissues, the cartilage matrix contains pro-

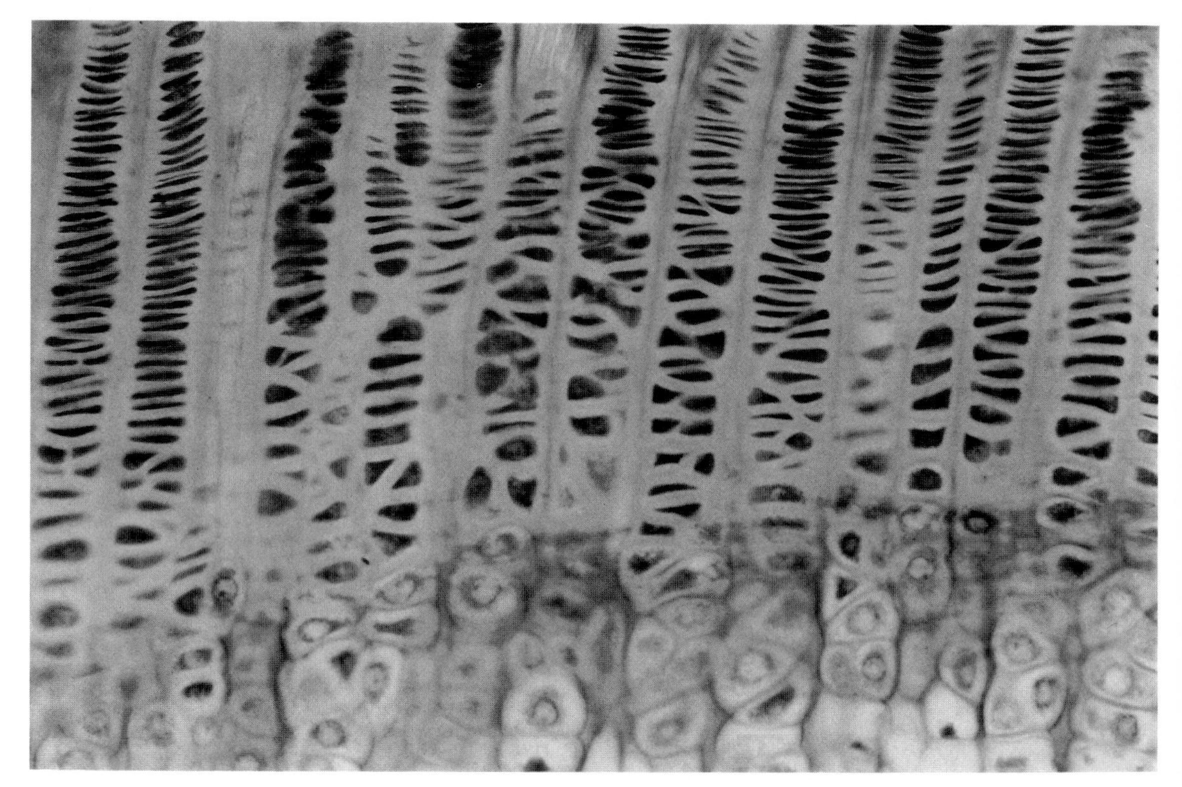

Figure 7–5. Hyaline cartilage of the epiphyseal plate of rabbit tibia. Here the cartilage cells are arranged in long parallel columns. From top downward, one can identify zones of chondrocyte proliferation, maturation, hypertrophy, and degeneration.

teoglycans, but here they are present in higher concentrations and form a very firm gel. The proteoglycans are among the largest molecules produced by cells, having molecular weights ranging up to 3.5×10^6 daltons. They are made up of a core protein, 200–300 nm in length, from which chains of disaccharides, called *glycosaminoglycans*, radiate in a bottle-brush configuration (see Fig. 6–1). The principal glycosaminoglycans of cartilage are *chondroitin sulfate* and *keratan sulfate*. A typical proteoglycan molecule may have as many as 100 chondroitin sulfate and 50 keratan sulfate chains radiating from its core protein. A convoluted polypeptide segment free of side-chains forms the globular end of the molecule which has binding sites for another large molecule, *hyaluronic acid*.

In the extracellular matrix, in vivo, the majority of the proteoglycan molecules are bound at their globular head to a long hyaluronic acid molecule via a *link-protein*, and spaced along its length at intervals of about 30 nm, forming *proteoglycan aggregates*. A single molecule of hyaluronic acid may have as many as 100 proteoglycan molecules linked to it. These aggregates are large enough to be immobilized by entanglement with the collagen fibers in the matrix. There is evidence that they may also interact specifically with particular sites in the cross-banding of the fibers.

These relationships cannot be directly visualized in routine electron micrographs because in fixation and dehydration of the tissue, the glycosaminoglycans collapse onto the core protein and in ruthenium-red-stained sections, the proteoglycan monomers then appear as dense granules dispersed in the meshes of the collagen meshwork. This collapse can be minimized and images that approach the normal state can be obtained from tissues prepared by high-pressure freezing, freeze-substitution, and low-temperature embedding. In micrographs of such preparations, the proteoglycan appears as a reticulum of delicate filaments. Two sizes can be discerned, slightly thicker, more intensely stained strands, and thinner ones that are very faintly stained. The former are interpreted as core proteins and the latter as the glycosaminoglycan side-chains (Fig. 7–7).

The molecular organization of cartilage ma-

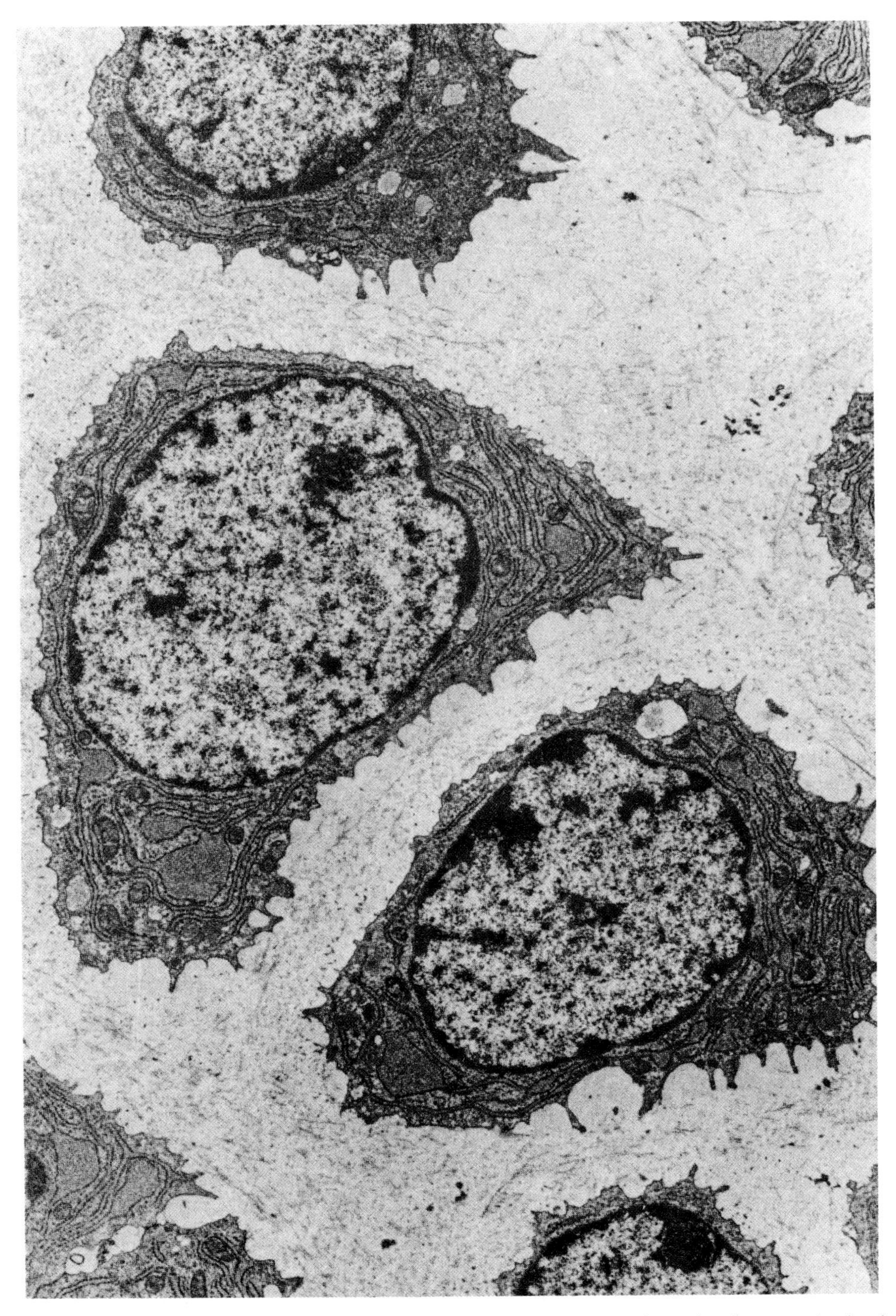

Figure 7–6. Electron micrograph of unusually well-preserved chondrocytes and matrix of mouse tracheal cartilage, illustrating the irregular outlines of the cells, their well-developed endoplasmic reticulum, and other organelles. (Micrograph from Seegmiller, R., C. Ferguson, and H. Sheldon. 1972. J. Ultrastr. Res. 38:288.)

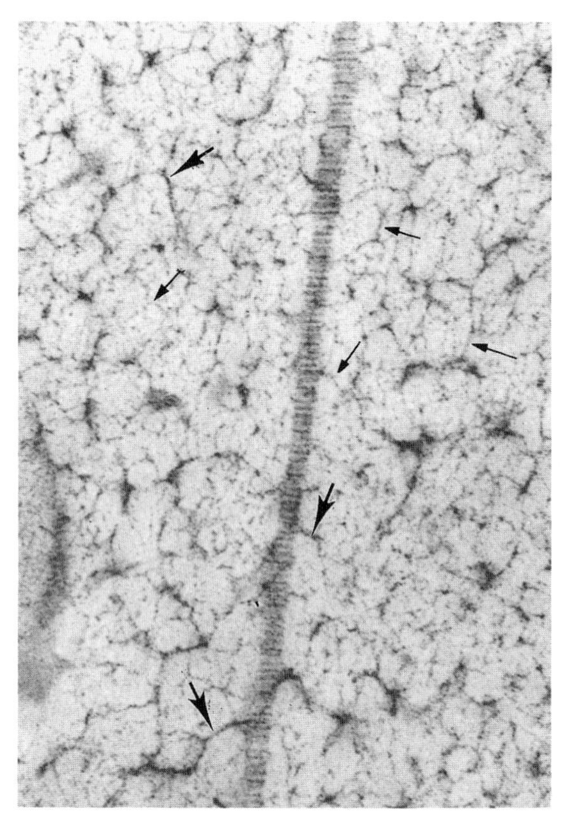

Figure 7–7. Electron micrograph of a small area of hyaline cartilage matrix, preserved by high-pressure freezing, freeze-substitution, and low-temperature embedding. A type-II collagen fiber crosses the field. Around it is a delicate reticulum of extended proteoglycans. The thicker, more heavily stained filaments (thick arrows) are probably the core proteins of proteoglycans, and the more slender filaments (small arrows) are the carbohydrate side-chains. 80,000×. (Micrograph courtesy of Hunziker, E.G., and R.K. Schenk. 1984. J. Cell Biol. 98:277.)

trix is ideally suited for its function on the weight-bearing articular surfaces of long bones. The fibrillar scaffolding of collagen maintains the shape of the tissue and resists tensile forces, whereas the proteoglycan aggregates occupying its interstices provide a firm hydrated gel that absorbs compressive forces. It also presents a virtually frictionless surface to the joint cavity. The numerous COO_- and $SO^4{}_{-2}$ groups on the carbohydrate chains of its glycosaminoglycans present a very large array of negative charges. Water becomes organized in multiple layers around such a focus of electric charge. The proteoglycans of the matrix thus trap and immobilize a large volume of water. More is simply sequestered in the interstices of the collagen framework so that water comes to constitute 70–80% of the wet weight of the tissue. The ability of cartilage to resist and recover from compression is said to be due, in large measure, to the structuring of water around its proteoglycans. When compressed, water is forced away from the charged domains of the proteoglycans. The negative charges of the carboxyl and sulfate groups then come into closer proximity and the repulsive force of like charges resists further compression. When the pressure is released, water returns to the charge domains of the proteoglycans restoring the normal organized hydrated state of the matrix.

SECRETION OF MATRIX COMPONENTS

Chondrocytes secrete the collagen and proteoglycans of the matrix. The intracellular biosynthetic pathway is much the same as that of other protein and glycoprotein secreting cells. If tritiated proline is injected into an animal actively forming cartilage, this amino-acid constituent of collagen can be localized by radioautography over the endoplasmic reticulum of the chondrocytes within 10 min; over the Golgi complex in 30 min; over secretory vacuoles in the peripheral cytoplasm in 2–3 h; and at longer time intervals, the label is found over the extracellular matrix (Fig. 7–8).

The same train of events can be followed with labeled precursors of the proteoglycans of the matrix. Synthesis of core protein and the initial steps of oligosaccharide addition appear to occur on the ribosomes of the endoplasmic reticulum. After transport of the initial products to the Golgi, chondroitin sulfate and other glycosaminoglycan chains are rapidly added to complete assembly of proteoglycans, which are packaged in secretory vesicles, moved to the cell surface, and released by exocytosis. In electron micrographs, both filamentous and granular material can be found within the same secretory vesicle, suggesting that collagen and proteoglycan are synthesized concurrently and packaged together for exocytosis. Synthesis of hyaluronic acid and link proteins no doubt follows a similar pathway. The proteoglycans are secreted as monomers and these are linked to hyaluronic acid extracellularly to form proteoglycan aggregates. In addition to these components of the matrix, chondrocytes synthesize and incorporate into their surface *chondronectin*, a fibronectin-like glycoprotein that binds specifically to type-II collagen and to glycosaminoglycans

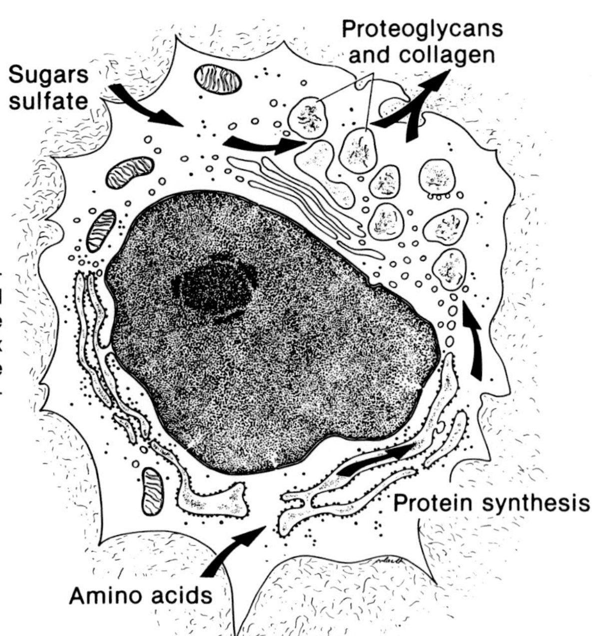

Figure 7–8. Diagram of the intracellular pathway for synthesis of matrix components. Amino acids are incorportated into proteins at the ribosomes. Sugars and sulfates are incorporated into polysaccharides in the Golgi complex and combined with protein from the reticulum to form the mucopolysaccharides released into the surrounding matrix. (Courtesy of E. Hay and J.P. Revel.)

and is believed to mediate attachment of these matrix components to the cell surface.

ROLE IN BONE GROWTH

In the embryo, the skeleton is first formed of hyaline cartilage. Later, centers of bone formation appear within the cartilage models and gradually expand, replacing the cartilage with bone. The establishment of a center of ossification appears to depend on precisely programmed intrinsic changes in the chondrocytes that set in motion a sequence of regressive changes in the matrix. In the center of the shaft of the cartilage model of a long bone, a group of chondrocytes hypertrophy, enlarging their lacunae at the expense of matrix (Fig. 7–9). Concurrent changes in the chemistry of the proteoglycans results in calcium deposition in the surrounding matrix and permits invasion of blood vessels and osteoprogenitor cells. After a period of increased activity, the hypertrophied chondrocytes die and bone-forming cells invade their lacunae and begin to deposit bone on residues of their walls of calcified cartilage. As this *primary center of ossification* expands, the proliferation of viable chondrocytes at either end of it results in a rearrangement of the cells into parallel columns. The same sequence of changes that took place in establishing the center of ossification is then repeated along the length of each column so that distinct transverse zones of cell *proliferation, maturation, hypertrophy*, and *degeneration* can be recognized. This provides for progression of the ossification process toward the ends of the shaft.

Secondary centers of ossification later appear near the ends of the cartilage model in a region designated the *epiphysis*, to distinguish it from the *diaphysis* or shaft. with continuing expansion of the primary and secondary centers of ossification, cartilage is reduced to two transverse discs at either end of the shaft called the *epiphyseal plates*. These contain the columns of cartilage cells whose proliferation will be responsible for the growth in length of the bone until adult stature is attained. Chondrocyte proliferation then ceases and the epiphyseal plates are replaced by bone.

In the formation of centers of ossification, mineralization of cartilage matrix is a prerequisite for vascular invasion of the cartilage and deposition of bone. What initiates the deposition of calcium salts is not entirely clear but much attention has been focused on *matrix vesicles*, small membrane-limited structures found in the extracellular matrix associated with hypertrophic chondrocytes. These vesicles arise by budding from the surface of cartilage cells. They have been isolated and their membrane is found to be rich in phosphatidylserine, which has a high binding affinity for

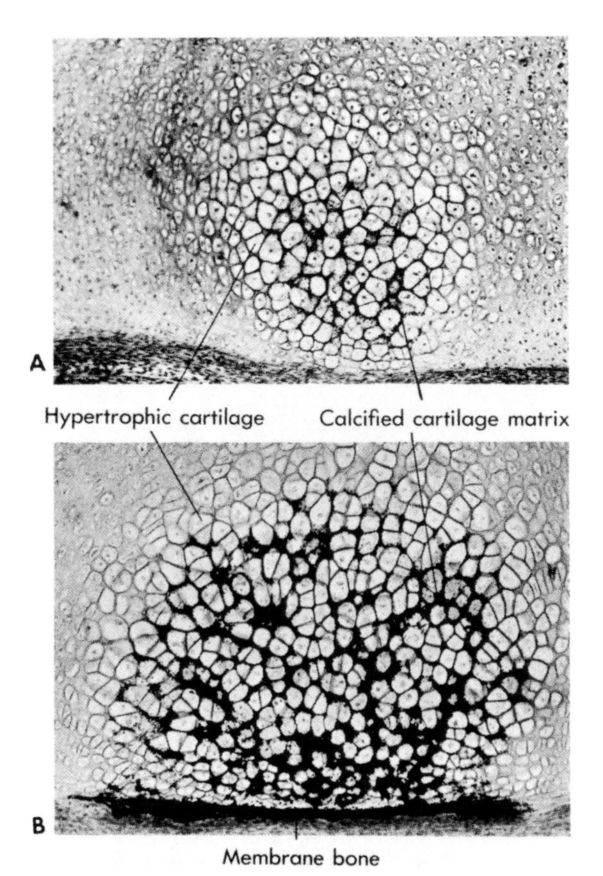

Figure 7–9. Photomicrographs of two stages in the calcification of the cartilage model of the calcaneus in the rat. (A) Two days after birth; (B) four days after birth. The calcium salts appear black due to the silver nitrate stain applied to the specimen (von Kossa's method). (After W. Bloom and M.A. Bloom.)

calcium, and alkaline phosphatase, a glycoprotein that makes phosphates available for mineralization. As calcium accumulates in the matrix vesicles, hydroxyapatite crystals are formed. The membrane subsequently breaks down and the mineral is released into the matrix. The alkaline phosphatase liberated is believed to bind firmly to matrix collagen and to contribute to the collagen-mediated calcification that follows the initial vesicle phase of mineralization. As hydroxyapatite deposition increases, the matrix becomes harder and more opaque. Owing to these changes in the matrix of epiphyseal cartilage, the zone of chondrocyte hypertrophy in developing long bones is also called the *zone of provisional calcification*. Calcification of cartilage is dependent on vitamin D and fails to occur in animals deficient in this vitamin. The relation of these early changes in cartilage to the process of bone growth will be discussed in greater detail in Chapter 8.

Deposition of bone in cartilage is not confined to the period of skeletal development and growth. In man, ossification of certain cartilages occurs as a normal age-change and may be seen in some parts of the larynx as early as age 25.

ELASTIC CARTILAGE

Elastic cartilage is found in the external ear, the walls of the auditory and eustachian canals, the epiglottis, and the corniculate and cuneiform cartilages of the larynx. It is distinguishable from hyaline cartilage by its greater opacity, yellowish color, and greater flexibility.

The chondrocytes are similar to those of hyaline cartilage and are housed in lacunae scattered singly or in isogenous groups of two or four. The matrix is somewhat less abundant and much of its substance consists of frequently branching elastic fibers (Fig. 7–10). In specimens stained for elastin, the fibers may be so closely packed that the amorphous proteoglycan component of the matrix is partially obscured. Near the periphery, the elastic network is looser and its fibers can be seen to continue into the perichondrium.

Elastic cartilage does not develop from highly cellular centers of chondrification but in areas of primitive connective tissue containing mesenchymal cells and bundles of fibers that do not have the characteristics of either collagen or elastin. These indifferent fibers later acquire the staining properties of elastin and the mesenchymal cells, withdraw their processes, and differentiate into chondrocytes, secreting matrix around themselves and the fibers. Condensation of connective tissue around the periphery forms a perichondrium.

Although the matrix is less abundant than in hyaline cartilage, it makes an equally important contribution to the mechanical properties of the tissue. This is dramatically demonstrated in the following simple experiment. When a crude preparation of papain is injected intravenously into a young rabbit, the proteoglycans of the matrix are partially degraded and the ears collapse. However, the chondrocytes quickly respond by secreting new matrix components and the ears are largely restored to their normal erect position within 48 h.

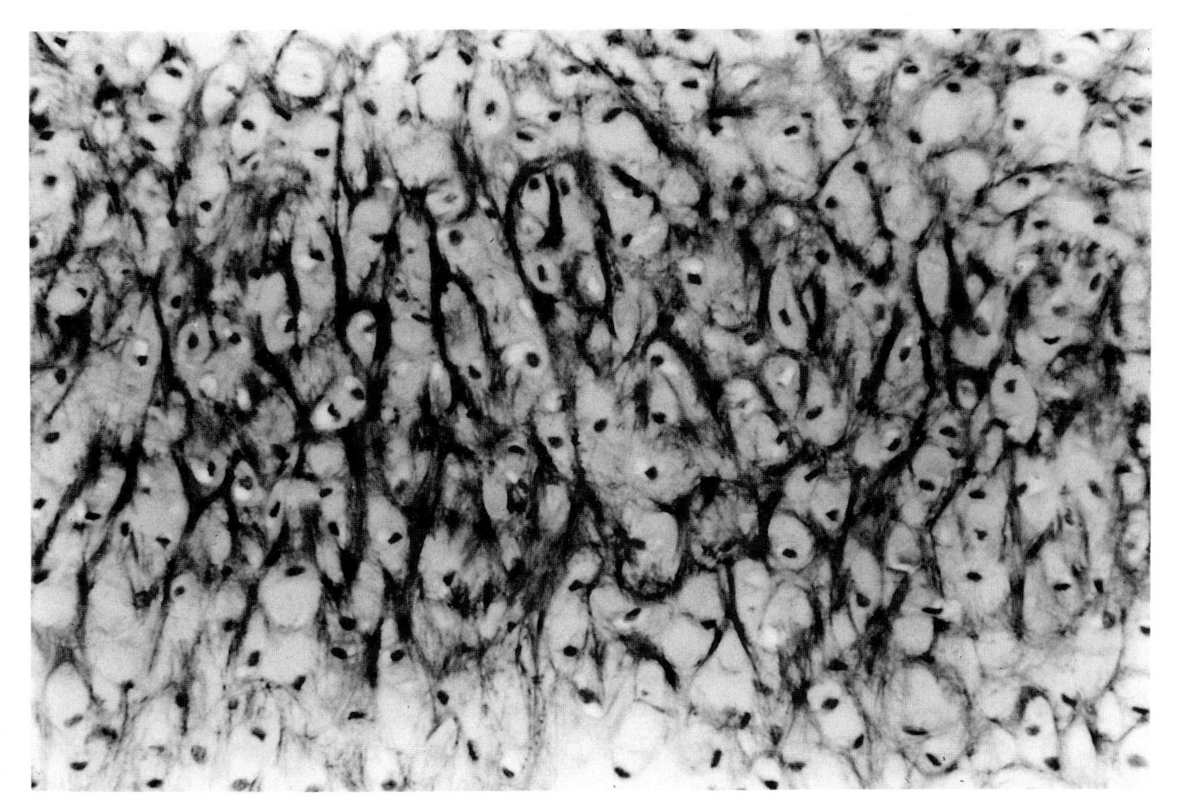

Figure 7–10. Photomicrograph of elastic cartilage from the epiglottis of a child. Note the dark-staining bundles of elastic fibers in the matrix between the groups of chondrocytes. (From Fawcett, D.W., *In* R.O. Greep, ed. Histology. Philadelphia, Blakiston Co. Reproduced by permission of McGraw-Hill Book Co.)

FIBROCARTILAGE

Fibrocartilage closely resembles dense regular connective tissue and the two are often continuous without any clear line of demarcation between them. Thus, fibrocartilage is found at sites of insertion of ligaments and tendons into bone. In place of fusiform fibroblasts, chondrocytes surrounded by a small amount of cartilage matrix are aligned in rows between coarse parallel bundles of type-I collagen fibers (Fig 7–11). A well-defined perichondrium is usually lacking. The cells are contained in lacunae with very thin capsules that may be basophilic but the tissue as a whole is usually acidophilic owing to the predominance of collagen. What little amorphous matrix is present is rich in chondroitin sulfate and dermatan sulfate. The greater part of the fibrocartilage in the body is found in the intervertebral discs which constitute about one-fifth of the length of the spine. The vertebrae have a thin layer of hyaline cartilage on their superior and inferior surfaces. Between the cartilage layers of successive vertebrae is an intervertebral disc consisting of a soft gelatinous material in its center, the *nucleus pulposus*, bounded peripherally by a tough ring of fibrocartilage, called the *annulus fibrosus*. The nucleus pulposus is a derivative of the notochord of the embryo. It consists of a small number of cells sparsely dispersed in a soft matrix rich in hyaluronic acid. The cells diminish in number with time, and after the age of 20, none may be found. The annulus fibrosus is made up of multiple concentric lamellae of type-I collagen fibers which run obliquely between the vertebrae, ending in the hyaline cartilage of the vertebrae it joins together. The fiber bundles in adjacent lamellae of the annulus are oriented at an angle, producing an arrangement that gives the fibrocartilage a great capacity to resist forces that would tend to displace the vertebrae with respect to one another. The nucleus pulposus, impounded between the vertebrae and restrained by the annulus fibrosus around its periphery, cushions compressive forces along the axis of the spine.

The annulus fibrosus may rupture, most

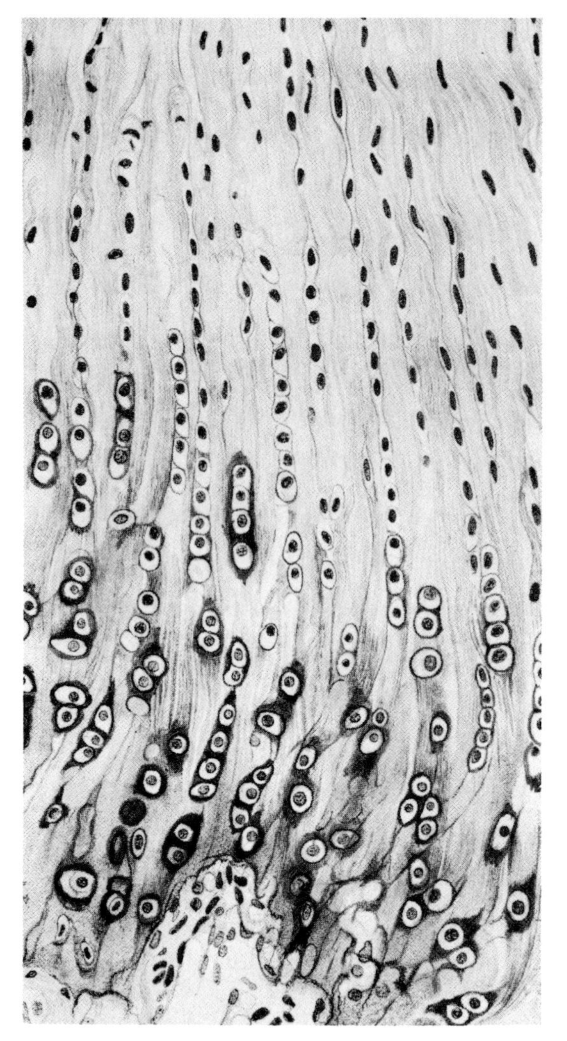

Figure 7–11. A drawing, at low magnification, of fibrocartilage at the insertion of a tendon into the tibia of a rat. Note the direct transformation of rows of tendon cells (top) into cartilage cells surrounded by deeply staining matrix (below).

commonly in the lumbar region. When the herniation is posterior, extrusion of the nucleus pulposus may cause pressure on the spinal nerves attended by severe pain and neurological disturbances in the region supplied by those nerves.

HISTOPHYSIOLOGY OF CARTILAGE

The specialized extracellular matrix of cartilage enables it to withstand great compressive forces at the articulations between weight-bearing bones, while at the same time permitting smooth frictionless joint movements. The ability of cartilage to grow interstitially makes possible the growth in length of the long bones of the extremities. It appears to be a relatively inert avascular structural material, but in its participation in bone growth, it is, in fact, a fairly sensitive indicator of nutritional deficiencies of protein, minerals, and vitamins. When a young animal is placed on a protein-deficient diet, or one lacking vitamin A, the thickness of the epiphyseal plates is rapidly diminished. When vitamin C is withheld from guinea pigs, resulting in *scurvy*, there is cessation of matrix production and distortion of the columnar arrangement of cells in the epiphyseal plate. Deficiency in absorption of calcium and phorphorus from the diet, due to the absence of vitamin D, leads to *rickets*, a condition in which the epiphyseal cartilage cells continue to proliferate but the matrix fails to calcify and the growing bones become deformed by weight-bearing.

The growth in length of bones is also influenced by hormones, of which, the most important is pituitary *growth hormone* (*somatotrophin*). Hypophysectomy in young rats results in thinning of the epiphyseal plates of long bones due to cessation of mitosis and decrease in size and number of chondrocytes. The cartilage fails to be eroded at the base of the cell columns and growth ceases. When growth hormone is injected into such animals, the epiphyseal cartilage is restored to normal and bone growth is resumed. Long continued administration of the hormone produces giant rats, due in part to the growth of cartilage beyond the time when the epiphyseal plates would normally have been obliterated.

In articular cartilage, the collagen seems to be quite enduring, but the proteoglycans are slowly turned over, being replaced by newly synthesized molecules. There is evidence that the chemistry of the proteoglycans produced changes with age. If chondrocytes that have been liberated from articular cartilage of old animals are placed in culture, they secrete smaller proteoglycans, with shorter chondroitin sulfate chains than those produced in vitro by chondrocytes of young individuals. It is possible that the prevalence of osteoarthritis in old people is related to such changes in the cartilage matrix. It is speculated that the smaller proteoglycans would structure less water and be less able to resist compressive forces. The matrix would then be more vulnerable to repeated small injuries in weight-bearing, and an associated inflammatory response to injury would result in the painful symptoms of arthritis.

Hyaline cartilage has a very limited capacity for repair. Its cells are dependent on diffusion of nutrients and oxygen over considerable distances through the matrix. If the blood flow to tissues around the cartilage is compromised, its cells may die. The cartilage is then invaded by blood vessels and phagocytes and the matrix is resorbed and replaced by a fibrous scar tissue. It is believed that the chondrocytes produce a factor that specifically inhibits the ingrowth of blood vessels. Extracts of cartilage have been shown to suppress vascularization of tissues commonly used in experimental studies of angiogenesis. This factor has not yet been isolated and characterized.

The unique properties of the extracellular matrix of cartilage have an interesting clinical significance for reconstructive surgery. As is well known, the transplantation of tissues from one individual to another is followed by rejection, unless measures are taken to suppress the host's immune system. Cartilage is exceptional in that it can be taken from the victim of a fatal accident and used in cosmetic or reconstructive surgery of another individual without immunosuppression. This is attributed to the avascularity of cartilage and its impermeability to molecules as large as immunoglobulins. The matrix also constitutes an impenetrable physical barrier to cytotoxic lymphocytes, preventing them from contacting and lysing the foreign chondrocytes of the donor. If the grafted cartilage is placed in a highly vascular bed, the cells will receive, by diffusion, sufficient oxygen and nutrients to survive.

BIBLIOGRAPHY

Ali, S.Y., S.W. Sajdera, and H.C. Anderson. 1970. Isolation and characterization of calcifying matrix vesicles from epiphyseal cartilage. Proc. Natl. Acad. Sci. USA 67:1531.

Anderson, H.S. 1969. Vesicles associated with calcification of the matrix of epiphyseal cartilage. J. Cell Biol. 41:59.

Anderson, D.R. 1964. The ultrastructure of elastic and hyaline cartilage in the rat. Am. J. Anat. 114:403.

Anderson, H.C. and S.W. Sajdera. 1971. The fine structure of bovine nasal cartilage. Extraction as a technique to study proteoglycans and collagen in cartilage matrix. J. Cell Biol. 49:650.

Benjamin, M. and E.J. Evans. 1990. Fibrocartilage. A review. J. Anat. 171:1.

Bonucci, E. 1967. Fine structure of early cartilage calcification. J. Ultrastr. Res. 20:35.

Bonucci, E. 1970. Fine structure and biochemistry of calcifying globules in epiphyseal cartilage. Zeitschr. Mikroskop. Anat. 103:192.

Carney, S.L. and H. Muir. 1988. The structure and function of cartilage proteoglycans. Physiol. Rev. 68:858.

Comper, W.D. and T.C. Laurent. 1978. Physiological function of connective tissue polysaccharides. Physiol. Rev. 58:255.

Gibson, B.J. and M.H. Flint. 1985. Type X collagen synthesis by chick sternal cartilage and its relationship to endochondral ossification. J. Cell. Biol. 101:277.

Goldman, G.C. and K.R. Porter. 1960. Chondrogenesis, studies with the electron microscope. J. Biophys. Biochem. Cytol. 8:719.

Hascall, G.K. 1980. Cartilage proteoglycans; comparison of sectioned and spread whole molecules. J. Ultrastr. Res. 70:369.

Hascall, V.C. 1977. Interaction of cartilage proteoglycans with hyaluronic acid. J Supramol. Struct. 7:101.

Hunziker, E.B., W. Herrmann, R.S. Schenk, M. Muller, and H. Moor. 1984. Cartilage ultrastructure after high-pressure freezing, freeze-substitution, and low temperature embedding. I. Chondrocyte ultrastructure. J. Cell Biol. 98:267.

Hunziker, E.B. and R.K. Schenk. 1984. Cartilage ultrastructure after high-pressure freezing, freeze-substitution, and low temperature embedding. II. Intracellular matrix ultrastructure. Preservation of proteoglycans in their native state. J. Cell Biol. 98:277.

Lane, J.M. and C. Weiss. 1975. Review of articular cartilage collagen research. Arthritis Rheum. 18:553.

Mecham, R.P. and J. Heuser. 1990. Three dimensional organization of extracellular matrix in elastic cartilage as viewed by quick-freeze, deep-etch electron microscopy. Connective Tissue Res. 24:83.

Minns, R.J. and F.S. Stevens. 1977. The collagen fibril organization in human articular cartilage. J. Anat. 123:437.

Poole, C.A., M.H. Flint, and B.W. Beaumont. 1984. Morphological and functional interrelationships of articular cartilage matrices. J. Anat. 138:113.

Revel, J.P. and E.D. Hay. 1963. An autoradiographic and electron microscopic study of collagen synthesis in differentiating cartilage. Zeitschr. Zellforsch. 61:110.

Schmid, T.M. and T. Linsenmeyer. 1985. Developmental acquisition of type X collagen in the embryonic chick tibiotarsus. Dev. Embryol. 107:373.

Sheldon, H. and F.B. Kimball. 1962. Studies on cartilage. III. The occurrence of collagen within vacuoles of the Golgi apparatus. J. Cell Biol. 12:599.

Sheldon, H. and R.A. Robinson. 1958. Studies on collagen. I. Electron microscope observations on normal rabbit ear cartilage. J. Biophys. Biochem. Cytol. 4:401.

Sheldon, H. and R.A. Robinson. 1960. II. Electron microscopic observations on rabbit ear cartilage following the administration of papain. J. Biophys. Biochem. 8:151.

Silverberg, R., M. Silverberg, and D. Feir. 1964. Life cycle of articular cartilage cells: an electron microscope study of the hip joint of the mouse. Am. J. Anat. 114:17.

Thomas, L. 1956. Reversible collapse of rabbit ears after intravenous papain and prevention of recovery by cortisone. J. Exp. Med. 104:245.

Wolbach, S.B. and C.L. Maddock. 1952. Vitamin-A acceleration of bone growth sequences in hypophysectomized rats. Arch. Pathol. 52:273.

Zambrano, N.Z., G.S. Montes, G.S. Shigihara, K.M. Sanchez, and L.C. Junqueira. 1982. Collagen arrangement in cartilages. Acta Anat. (Basel) 113:26.

8
BONE

Bone, like other connective tissues, consists of cells, fibers, and ground substance, but unlike the others, its extracellular components are calcified, making it a hard, unyielding substance ideally suited for its supportive and protective functions in the skeleton. It provides for the internal support of the body and for the attachment of the muscles and tendons essential for locomotion. It protects the vital organs of the cranial and abdominal cavities, and it encloses the blood-forming elements of the bone marrow. In addition to these mechanical functions, it plays an important metabolic role as a mobilizable store of calcium, which can be drawn on as needed in the homeostatic regulation of the concentration of this important ion in the blood and other body fluids.

Bone possesses a remarkable combination of physical properties—high tensile and compressive strength and some elasticity while, at the same time, being a relatively lightweight material. At all levels of the organization of bones, from their gross form to their submicroscopic structure, their construction ensures great strength with great economy of material and minimal weight. But, with all its strength and hardness, bone is a dynamic living material, constantly being renewed and reconstructed throughout the lifetime of the individual. Owing to its continual internal reorganization and its responsiveness to external mechanical forces, it can be modified by the surgical procedures and appliances of the orthopedic surgeon or orthodontist. Disuse leads to atrophy with some loss of substance, and increased use is accompanied by hypertrophy, with a slight increase in bone mass. Bone is also quite responsive to metabolic, nutritional, and endocrine influences.

MACROSCOPIC STRUCTURE OF BONES

Upon inspection with the naked eye or with a hand lens, two forms of bone are distinguishable, *compact* (*substantia compacta*) and *spongy* or *cancellous bone* (*substantia spongiosa*). The latter consists of a three-dimensional lattice of branching bony spicules, or trabeculae, delimiting a labyrinthine system of interspaces that are occupied by *bone marrow*. The compact bone, as the name implies, appears as a solid continuous mass in which spaces can be seen only with the aid of a microscope. The two forms of bone grade into one another without a sharp boundary (Figs. 8–1 and 8–2).

In typical long bones, such as the femur or humerus, the shaft (*diaphysis*) consists of a thick-walled hollow cylinder of compact bone with a voluminous central marrow cavity (*medullary cavity*) occupied by the bone marrow. The ends of long bones consist mainly of spongy bone covered by a thin *cortex* of compact bone (Figs. 8–1 and 8–2). The intercommunicating spaces among the trabeculae of this spongy bone, in the adult, are directly continuous with the marrow cavity of the shaft. In the growing animal, the ends of the long bones, called the *epiphyses*, arise from separate centers of ossification and are separated from the shaft (*diaphysis*) by a cartilaginous *epiphyseal plate* (Fig. 8–3), which is united to the diaphysis by columns of spongy bone in a transitional region called the *metaphysis*. The epiphyseal cartilage and the adjacent spongy bone of the metaphysis constitute a growth zone in which all increment in length of the growing bone occurs. On the articular surfaces, at the ends of the long bones, the thin cortical layer of compact bone is covered by a layer of hyaline cartilage, the *articular cartilage*.

With few exceptions, bones are invested by *periosteum*, a layer of specialized connective tissues, which is endowed with *osteogenic potency*. That is to say, it has the ability to form bone. A covering of periosteum is lacking on those areas on the ends of long bones that are covered by articular cartilage. It is also absent where tendons and ligaments insert into the bone and on the surface of the patella (kneecap) and other *sesamoid bones* that are formed

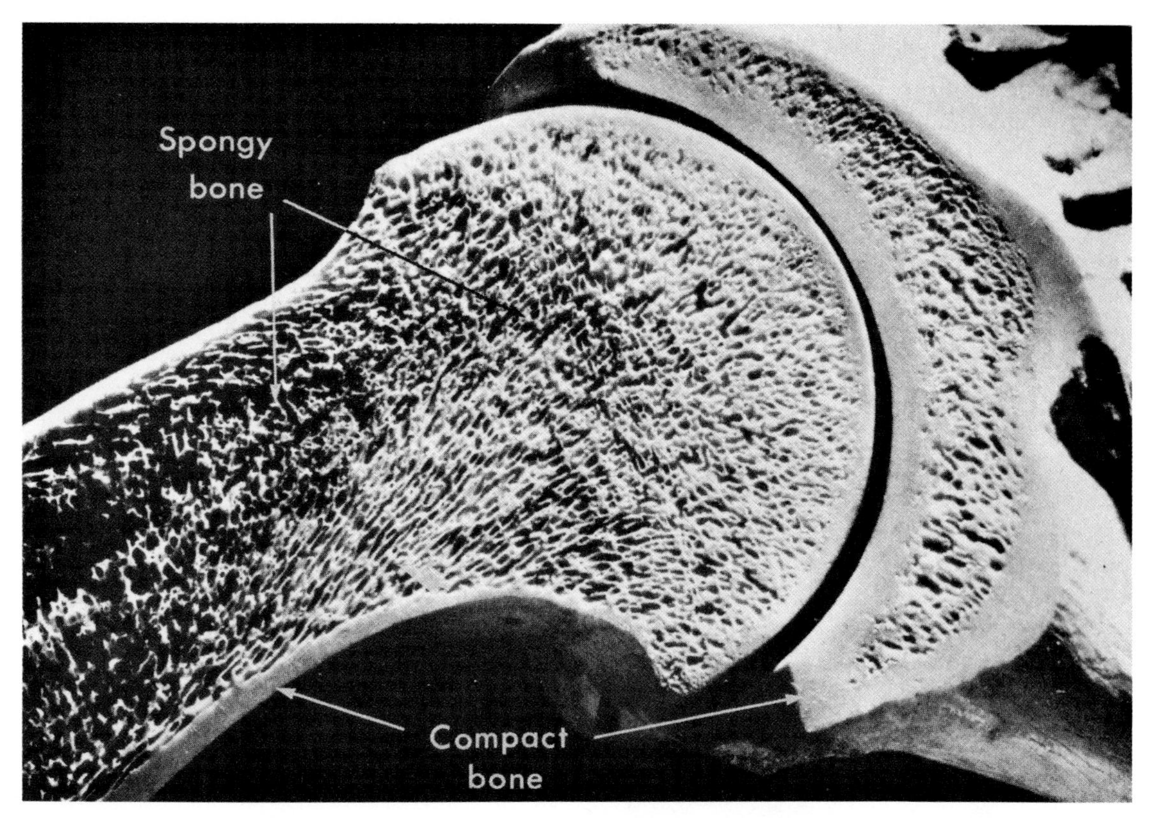

Figure 8–1. Photomicrograph of a saggital section of the proximal end of the humerus in relation to the glenoid fossa of the scapula at the shoulder joint. These are dry bones and the cartilaginous articular surfaces of the joint are not present. The figure is presented here to illustrate the appearance and distribution of spongy and compact bone. (After A. Feininger. 1956 Anatomy of Nature. New York, Crown Publishers. With permission of Time, Inc.)

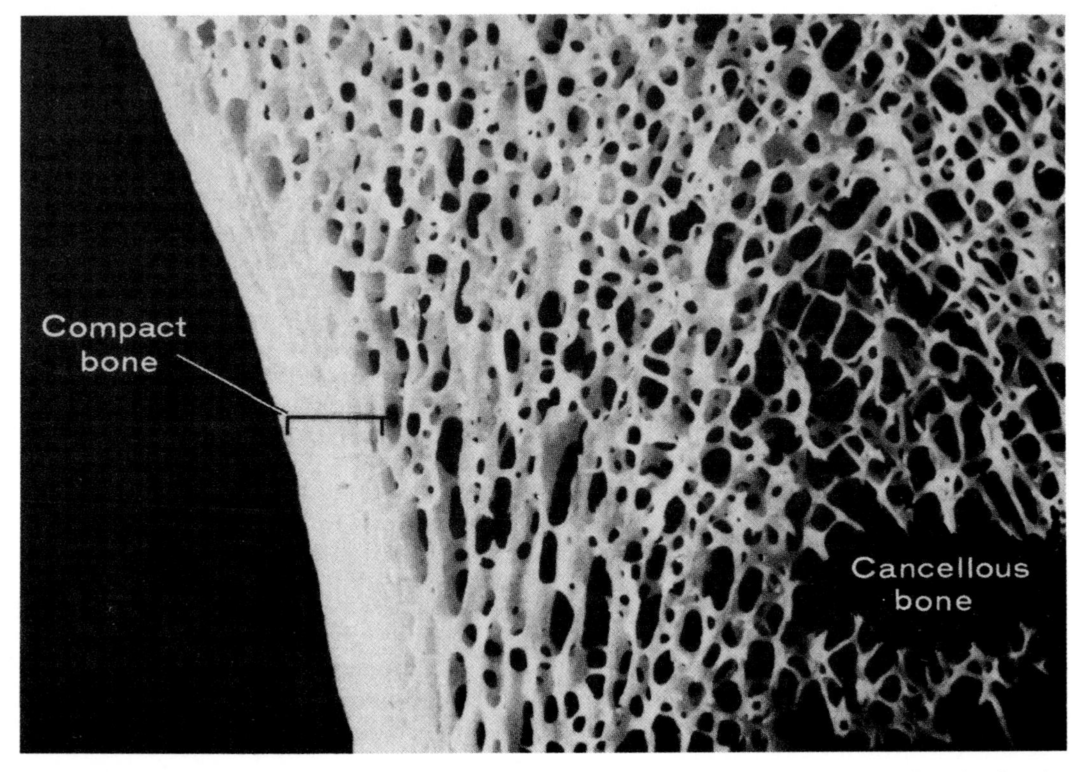

Figure 8–2. A thick ground section of the tibia, illustrating the cortical compact bone and the lattice of trabeculae of cancellous bone.

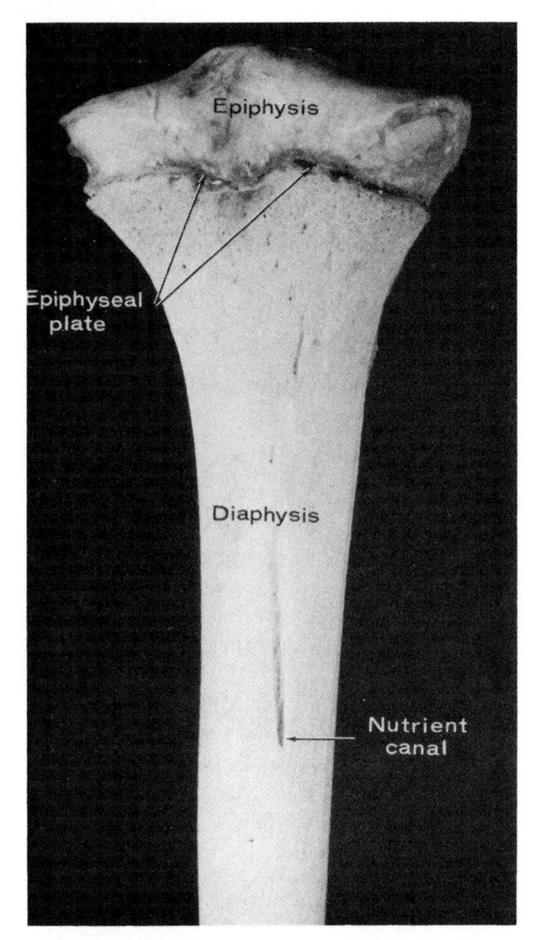

Figure 8–3. Photograph of the upper half of the tibia of a young girl showing the proximal bony epiphysis, the cartilaginous epiphyseal plate, and the diaphysis.

within tendons. It is also absent in the subcapsular areas of the neck of the femur and of the astragulus. Where functional periosteum is absent, the connective tissue in contact with the surfaces of bone lacks osteogenic potential and, therefore, does not contribute to the healing of fractures at these sites. The marrow cavity of the diaphysis and the cavities within spongy bone are lined by *endosteum,* a thin cellular layer that also possesses osteogenic properties.

In the flat bones of the skull, the substantia compacta forms, on both outer and inner surfaces, relatively thick layers that are often referred to as their *outer* and *inner tables.* Between them is a thin layer of spongy bone called the *diploe.* The periosteum on the outer surface of the skull is called the *pericranium,* whereas that on the inner surface is the *dura mater.* Although these connective tissue coverings of the flat bones are designated by different terms, they do not differ significantly in their structure or osteogenic potency from the periosteum and endosteum of long bones. However, defects in the skull vault (*calvarium*) resulting from injury often do not heal completely in adults.

MICROSCOPIC STRUCTURE OF BONES

If a thin ground section of the shaft of a long bone is examined with the microscope, it is apparent that the contribution of the cellular elements of bone to its total mass is small. It is largely composed of *bone matrix,* a mineralized interstitial substance deposited in layers or lamellae 3–7 μm thick (Figs. 8–4 and 8–5). Rather uniformly spaced throughout the interstitial substance of bone are lenticular cavities, called *lacunae,* each occupied by a bone cell, or *osteocyte.* Radiating in all directions from each lacuna are very slender, branching *canaliculi* that penetrate the lamellae of the interstitial substance and anastomose with the canaliculi of neighboring lacunae (Figs. 8–6 and 8–7). Thus, although the lacunae of bone are spaced some distance apart, they form a continuous system of cavities interconnected by an extensive network of minute canals. These slender passages are essential to the nutrition of the bone cells. In cartilage, the cells can be sustained by diffusion through the aqueous phase of the gel-like matrix; the deposition of calcium salts in the matrix of bone reduces its permeability to solutes. However, the system of intercommunicating canaliculi between lacunae provides avenues for exchange of metabolites between the cells and the nearest perivascular space.

The lamellae of compact bone are disposed in three common patterns: (1) The great majority are arranged concentrically around longitudinal vascular channels, forming cylindrical units called *haversian systems* or *osteons.* These vary in diameter, being made up of 4–20 lamellae. In cross section, the haversian systems appear as concentric rings around a circular opening (Fig. 8–8). In longitudinal section, they are seen as closely-spaced layers parallel to the vascular channels (Figs. 8–8 and 8–9). (2) Between the haversian systems are angular pieces of lamellar bone of varying size and irregular shape. These are the *interstitial systems* (Fig. 8–9). The limits of the haversian systems and the interstitial systems are

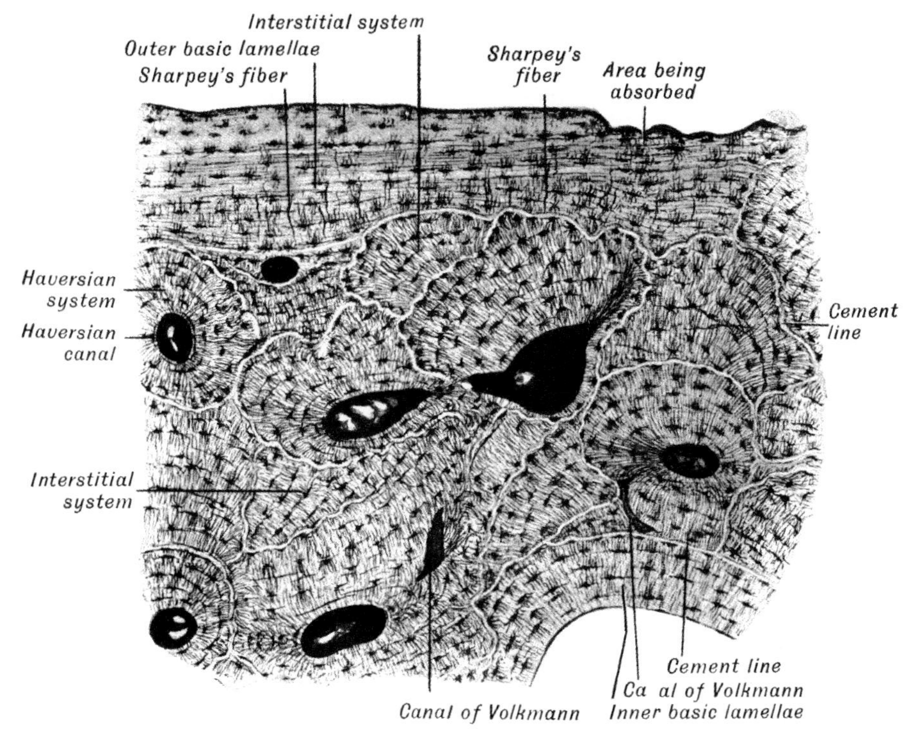

Figure 8–4. Photomicrograph of a ground section of a portion of a human metacarpal bone, stained with fuchsin and mounted in Canada balsam. (After Schaffer.)

sharply demarcated by thin refractile layers called *cement lines.* In cross section, compact bone thus appears as a mosaic of round and angular pieces cemented together (Fig. 8–9). (3) At the external surface of cortical bone, immediately beneath the periosteum, and on the internal surface, subjacent to the end-osteum, there may be several lamellae that extend uninterruptedly around much of the circumference of the shaft. These are called the *outer* and *inner circumferential lamellae* (Fig. 8–8).

Two categories of vascular channels are distinguished in compact bone on the basis of their orientation and their relation to the lamellar structure of the surrounding bone. The longitudinal channels in the centers of the osteons are called *haversian canals.* They are 22–110 μm in diameter and contain one or two small blood vessels ensheathed in loose connective tissue. The vessels are, for the most part, capillaries and postcapillary venules, but occasional arterioles may be found. The haversian canals are connected with one another and with the free surface and marrow cavity, via transverse or oblique channels, called *Volkman's canals.* These can be distinguished from haversian canals by the fact that they are not surrounded by concentrically arranged lamellae. Instead, they traverse the bone in a direction perpendicular or oblique to the osseous lamellae. Blood vessels from the marrow, and to a lesser extent from the periosteum, communicate with those of the haversian systems via Volkman's canals. These vessels are often larger than those of the osteons.

Although generally true, the traditional description of haversian canals as being longitudinal and Volkman's canals as being oblique or transverse is an over simplification. Reconstruction of osteons from serial sections has shown that they are not always simple cylindrical units, but that they may branch and anastomose and have a rather complex three-dimensional configuration. Thus, obliquely oriented vascular channels surrounded by concentric lamellae may be encountered. These are lateral branches of longitudinally oriented haversian systems.

The relatively slender trabeculae of cancellous bone are also composed of lamellae but they are not penetrated by blood vessels and, therefore, do not have haversian systems. They consist of a mosaic of angular pieces of lamellar bone. Their bone cells are nourished by diffusion along the intercommuni-

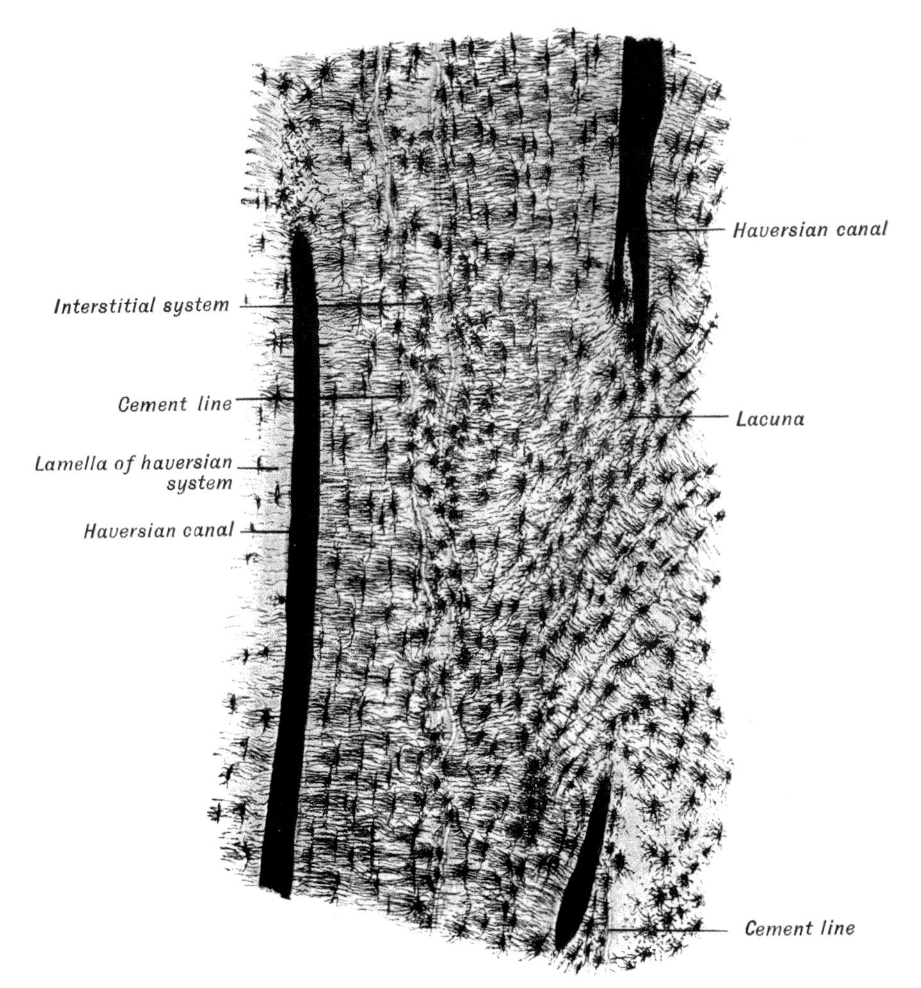

Figure 8–5. A portion of a longitudinal ground section of the ulna, stained with fuchsin. (After Schaffer, J. 1922. Lehrbuch der Histologie und Histogenese. Verlag von W. Engelmann, Leipzig.)

cating canaliculi that connect the lacunae and extend to the endosteal surface of the trabeculae.

The periosteum varies in its microscopic appearance depending on its functional state. During embryonic and postnatal growth, it has an inner layer of bone-forming cells, *osteoblasts,* that are in direct contact with the bone. After growth of the bone has ceased, the osteoblasts revert to inactive bone-lining cells, indistinguishable from other fusiform connective tissue cells. However, they retain their osteogenic potential, and if the bone is injured, they are reactivated and take on, once again, the appearance of osteoblasts while they participate in new bone formation to repair the damage.

The outer layer of the periosteum is a relatively acellular connective tissue containing many blood vessels. Branches of these vessels penetrate the inner layer of the periosteum to enter *Volkmann's canals,* through which they communicate with the vessels in the haversian canals. The numerous small vessels entering Volkmann's canals from the periosteum may contribute to maintaining its attachment to the underlying bone. In addition, coarse bundles of collagen fibers from the outer layer of the periosteum turn inward, penetrating the outer circumferential lamellae and extending between the interstitial lamellae deeper in the bone. These are called *Sharpey's fibers* (Fig. 8–10). They arise during the growth of the bone, when thick bundles of periosteal collagen fibers become incarcerated in bone matrix in the subperiosteal deposition of new lamellae. When these perforating fibers are uncalcified, they occupy irregular channels extending into the compact bone from the periosteum in a direction perpendicular or oblique to the cir-

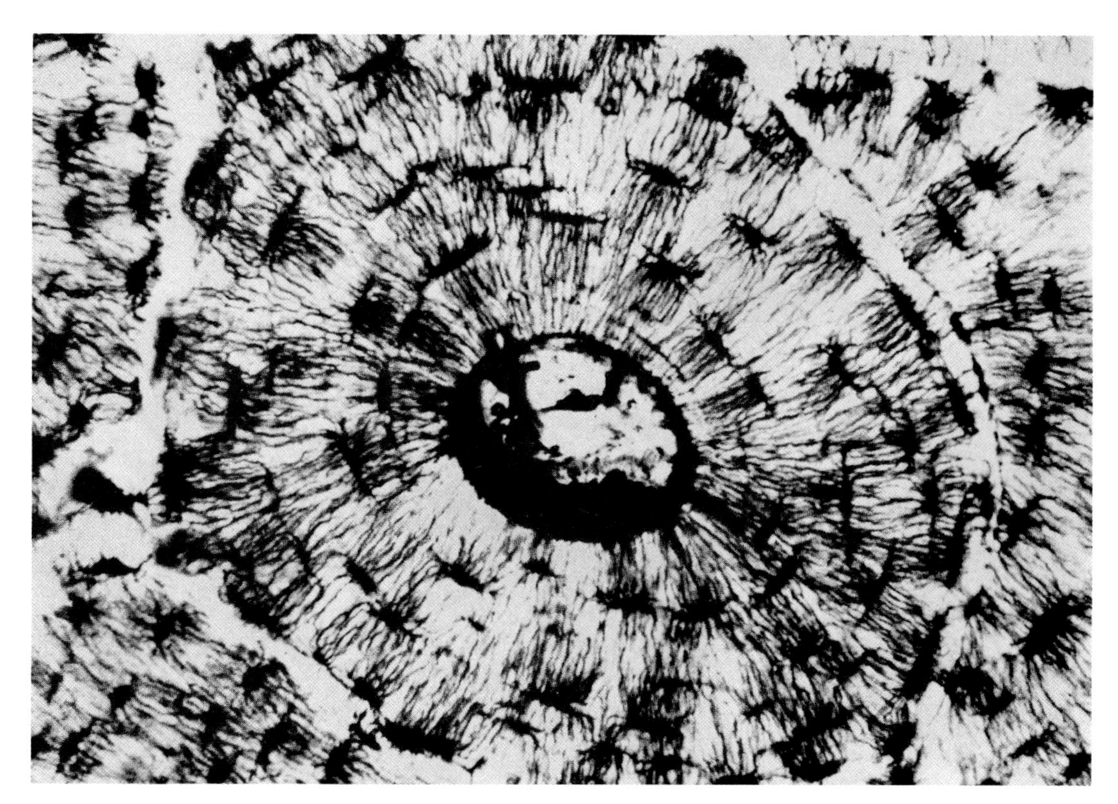

Figure 8–6. Photomicrograph of a ground section of a typical haversian system, showing the lacunae and canaliculi in black. (After Facett, D.W. 1953. *In* R.O. Greep, ed. Histology. Philadelphia, Blakiston Co. Reproduced by permission of McGraw-Hill Book Co.)

cumferential lamellae. When they are calcified, they are distinguishable in histological sections, only as faint streaks in the outer portion of the cortical bone. They serve to anchor the periosteum firmly to the underlying bone. They vary greatly in number in different regions, being especially numerous in some bones of the skull and near the sites of attachment of tendons to the long bones. In addition to Sharpey's fibers, some elastic fibers penetrate cortical bone from the periosteum, either together with, or independent of, the bundles of collagen fibers.

The *endosteum* is a thin layer of squamous cells lining the walls of those cavities in the bone that house the bone marrow. Endosteum is the peripheral layer of the stroma of the marrow, where it is in contact with bone. It resembles the periosteum in its osteogenic potencies, but is much thinner—usually a single layer of flat cells and associated connective tissue fibers. All the cavities of bone, including the haversian canals and the marrow spaces within spongy bone, are lined by endosteum.

BONE MATRIX

The interstitial substance of bone is composed of two major components, an organic matrix comprising 35%, and inorganic salts, comprising 65% of its dry weight. The organic matrix consists of collagen fibers embedded in a ground substance rich in proteoglycans.

GROUND SUBSTANCE

The amorphous ground substance of bone has been less thoroughly studied than that of cartilage due, in part, to the fact that it constitutes only a small fraction of the extracellular matrix. A positive periodic-acid–Schiff reaction, faint metachromasia, and incorporation of ^{25}S by the ground substance provided indirect histochemical evidence for the presence of glycosaminoglycans. This was verified by identification of *chondroitin sulfate,*

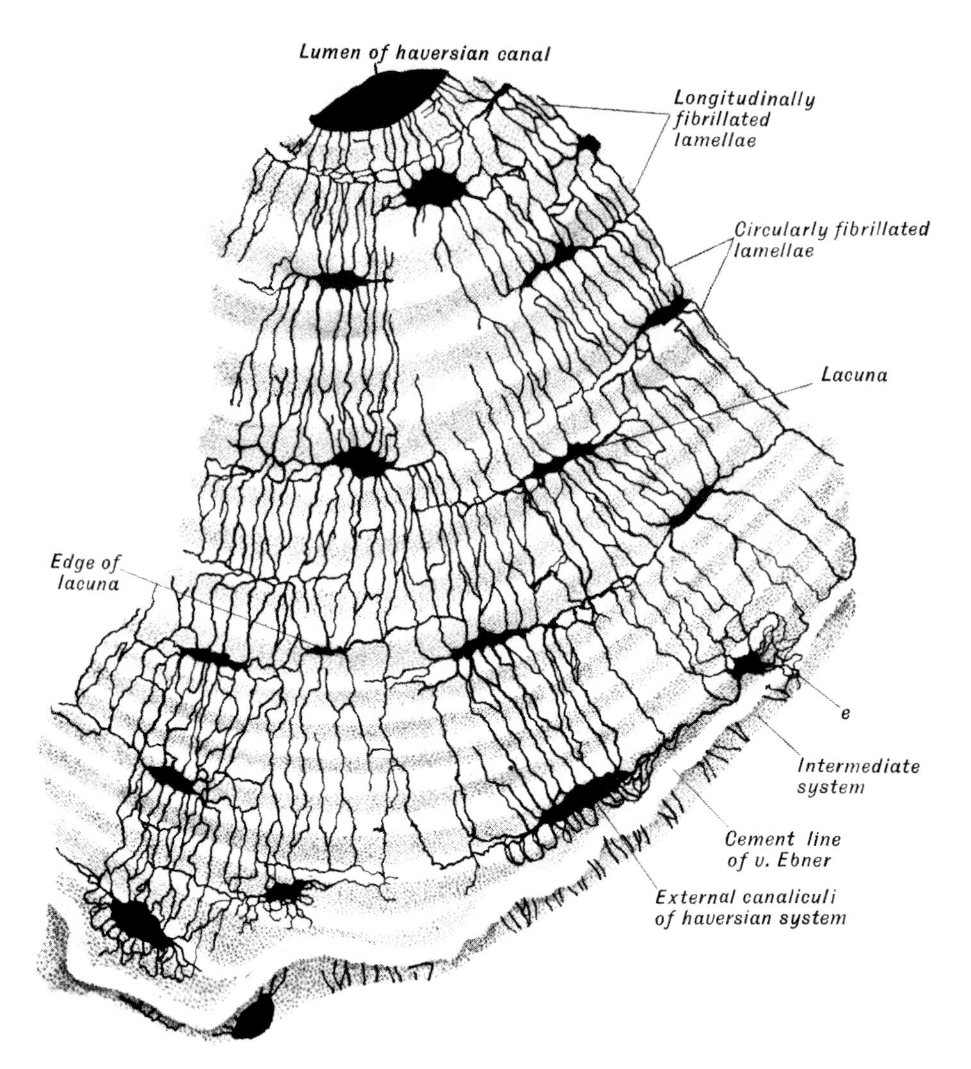

Figure 8–7. Drawing of a sector from a cross section of an haversian system in a macerated human hip bone. The cavities and canaliculi are filled with a dye.

keratan sulfate, and *hyaluronic acid* in extracts of bone. Despite the presence of sulfated glycosaminoglycans, bone matrix is acidophilic in histological sections, owing to its content of abundant closely packed collagen. In contrast to the proteoglycans of cartilage matrix which are very large, those of bone consist of short core proteins with relatively few glycosaminoglycan side-chains.

In addition to the noncollagen matrix proteins common to connective tissues, there are several that are found only in bone. Among these are two small, vitamin-K-dependent proteins. *Osteocalcin,* a 5.8 kD protein, constituting 2% of the total matrix protein, has three γ-carboxyglutamic acid residues per molecule and is found in the extracellular matrix, bound to hydroxyapatite. Its function is not known. *Osteopontin* is a 63 kD sialoprotein that binds tightly to hydroxyapatite and contains a cell-binding sequence similar to that of fibronectin. It is speculated that it may be involved in binding of osteoblasts or osteoclasts to bone. Both osteocalcin and osteopontin are products of osteoblasts and their synthesis is stimulated by 1,25-dihydroxycholecalciferol, the active metabolite of vitamin D. A third matrix component, *bone sialoprotein* (BSP), is a 78kD protein that also has a cell-binding sequence. Its synthesis is stimulated by 1,25-OH_2D_3 and its function is unclear.

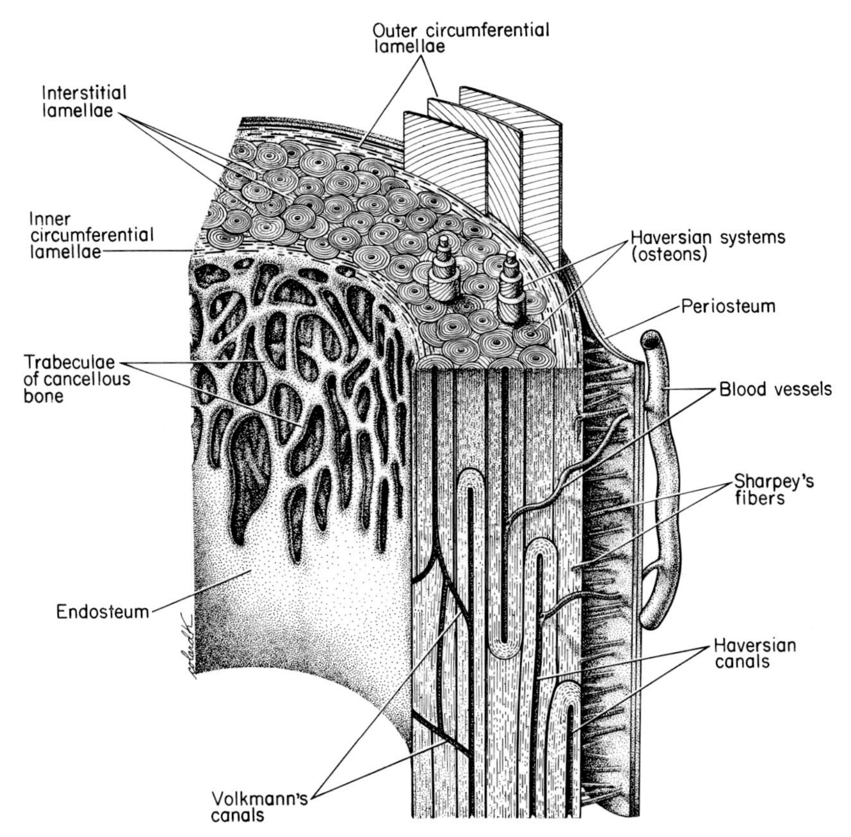

Figure 8–8. Diagram of a sector of the shaft of a long bone, showing the disposition of the lamellae in the osteons, the interstitial lamellae, and the outer and inner circumferential lamellae. (Redrawn after Benninghoff A., Lehrbuch der Anatomie des Menschen. Berlin, Urban and Schwarzenberg.)

COLLAGEN

Collagen, which constitutes 90% of the organic portion of bone matrix, is predominantly type-I. The fibers are 50–70 nm in diameter and have the typical 67-nm cross-banding. Bone collagen differs slightly from soft-tissue collagen of the same type in having a greater number of intermolecular cross-links, which accounts for its failure to swell in dilute acid and its insolubility in some solvents that are used successfully to extract collagen from other tissues. The lysines of bone collagen are also more highly hydroxylated. Minute amounts of some minor collagens have been reported, but it is likely that these are contaminants from traces of cartilage in the samples analyzed.

In mature lamellar bone, the collagen fibers have a highly ordered arrangement. Those within each lamella of an osteon are parallel in their orientation, but the direction of the fibers changes in successive concentric lamellae. This change in orientation of the fibers is responsible for the alternation of bright and darker layers in haversian systems viewed with polarization optics (Fig. 8–9B). Some disagreement persists as to the arrangement of the fibers. In decalcified preparations, viewed at high magnification, refractile lamellae with a fine circumferential striation alternate with less refractile layers having a stippled or punctuate appearance. This observation was originally interpreted as indicating a regular alternation of lamellae with circularly, and with longitudinally, oriented fibrils. This proved to be an oversimplification. Some investigators have insisted that collagen-rich lamellae alternate with collagen-poor lamellae and that this quantitative difference is as important as the direction of the fibers in accounting for the microscopic appearance of the haversian systems. Others have suggested that the fibrils within a given collagen-rich lamella are not parallel but form two sets intersecting in a lattice-like pattern. However, it is now the opinion of the majority, that the fibrils in all lamellae run helically with respect to the axis

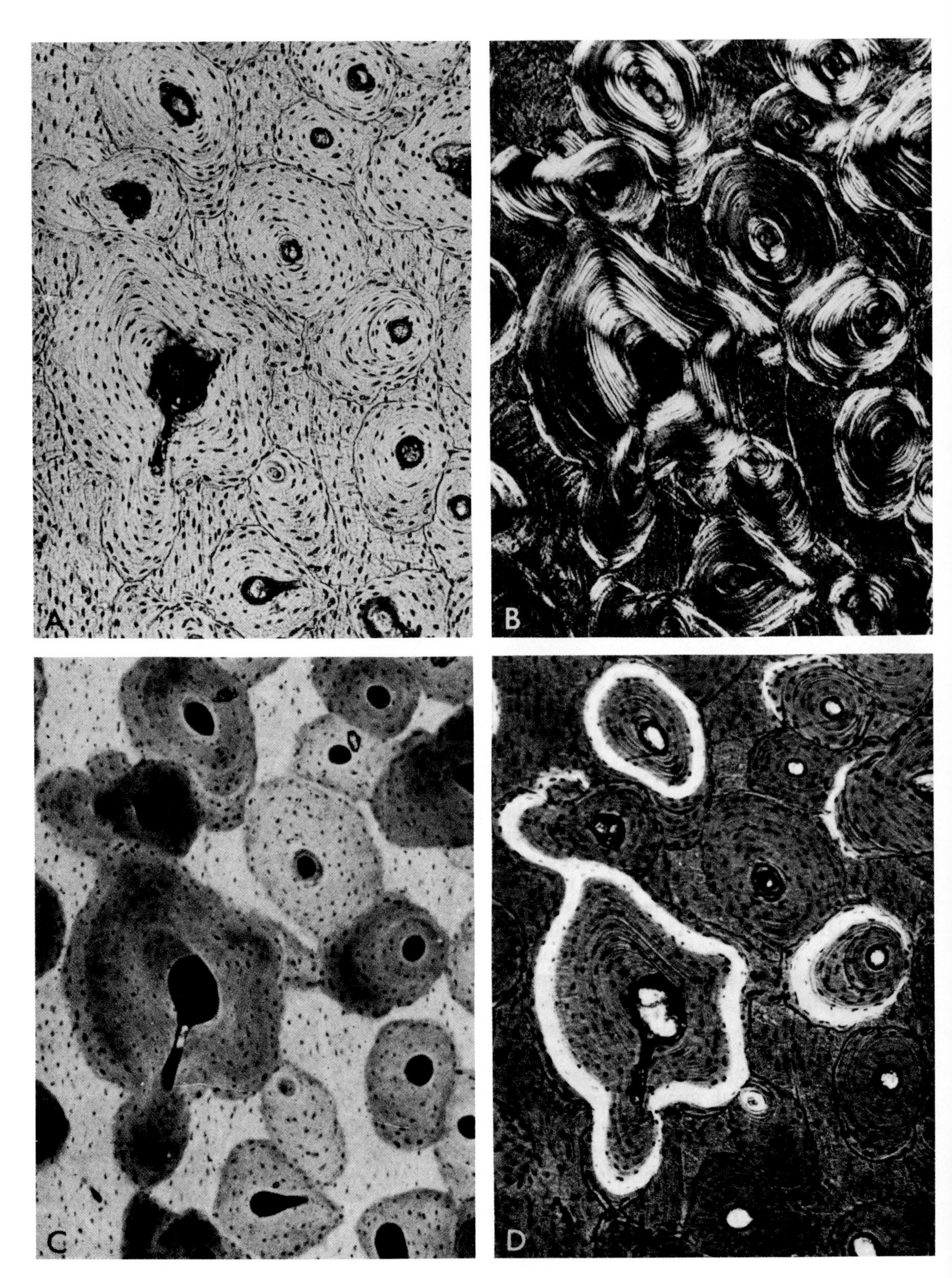

Figure 8–9. *See opposite page for legend.*

of the haversian canal, but that the pitch of the helix changes sufficiently from one lamella to the next to account for the differences observed under bright-field and polarization microscopes.

BONE MINERAL

The inorganic matter of bone consists of submicroscopic deposits of a form of calcium phosphate very similar, but not identical, to the mineral hydroxyapatite ($Ca_{10}[PO_4]_6[OH]_2$). Opinion varies as to whether bone mineral is deposited initially as amorphous calcium phosphate and is subsequently reordered to form crystalline hydroxyapatite or whether it is crystalline from the outset. It is clear, however, that in mature bone the mineral is in the form of slender rod-like crystals about 40 nm in length and 1.5–3 nm in thickness. The crystals are not randomly distributed but recur at regular intervals of 60–70 nm along the length of the collagen fibers. This disposition of mineral reflects the underlying geometry of the molecular lattice in collagen. In type-I collagen, the molecules are parallel, with nearest neighbors staggered by 67 nm. This arrangement results in an ordered array of gaps roughly 40 nm long and 2.5 nm wide within the substance of the fiber. The crystals of hydroxyapatite reside mainly in these gaps, but in heavily mineralized bone they may extend longitudinally a short distance into the regions of overlap of the collagen molecules.

Bone mineral contains significant amounts of the citrate ion $C_6H_5O_7^{\equiv}$ and the carbonate ion $CO_3^{=}$. Citrate is considered to be a separate phase, located on the surfaces of the crystals. The site of carbonate is still a matter of debate; it may be located on the surface of the crystals or it may substitute for $PO_4^{\equiv}$ in the crystal structure, or both. Substitution of the fluoride ion F^- for OH^- in the apatite crystal is common. Its amount depends mainly on the fluoride content of the drinking water. Magnesium and sodium, which are normal constituents of the body fluids, are also present in bone mineral, which, to some extent, serves as a storage depot for these elements. The isotopes ^{45}Ca and ^{32}P can, of course, substitute for the stable ^{40}Ca and ^{31}P in the hydroxyapatite crystal. Foreign cations such as Pb^{++}, Sr^{++}, and Ra^{++} (^{226}Ra), if ingested, may also substitute for Ca^{++}. In the fission of uranium in nuclear reactors, or of uranium and plutonium in the detonation of nuclear weapons, a large number of radioactive elements are liberated. On gaining access to the body, some of these are incorporated in bone. The most hazardous of these *bone-seeking isotopes* is ^{90}Sr. As a result of their radioactivity, these isotopes may cause severe damage to bone and to the blood-forming cells in the bone marrow. A few of these bone-seeking isotopes, including ^{239}Pu, do not enter the bone mineral but instead have a special affinity for the organic constituents of bone. Studies of the rate of turnover of the inorganic substances in bone have been greatly aided by the use of bone-seeking isotopes.

During growth, the amount of organic material per unit volume of bone remains relatively constant, but the amount of water decreases and the proportion of bone mineral increases, attaining, in adults, a maximum of about 65% of the fat-free dry weight. In the poorly calcified bone of individuals suffering from *rickets* or *osteomalacia,* the mineral content may be as low as 35%.

If bone is exposed to a weak acid or a chelating agent, the inorganic salts are removed. Thus demineralized, the bone loses most of its hardness but is very tough and flexible. It retains its gross form and a nearly normal

Figure 8–9. Section of bone from the midshaft of the human fibula as revealed by four different optical methods. (A) Ground section photographed through the light microscope. Lacunae, haversian systems, and interstitial lamellae are clearly shown. (B) The same section photographed through the polarizing microscope shows the alternating light and dark concentric layers in the haversian systems that result from the differing orientation of collagen fibers in the successive lamellae. (C) A historadiogram of the same section. The differing shades of gray from nearly white to nearly black, reflect the differing concentrations of calcium. The most recently deposited haversian systems are incompletely calcified and appear dark gray, whereas older ones containing higher concentrations of calcium are lighter. The old intersitial lamellae, being fully calcified, are the most highly absorptive and, therefore, appear white. (D) The 14-year-old girl from whom this specimen was taken had been given a daily dose of the antibiotic Achromycin (tetracycline) for 15 consecutive days at one period of her illness. Amputation of the leg was carried out 230 days later. Achromycin was incorporated in bone matrix being deposited at the time of its administration, and it imparted a fluorescence to the bone deposited in that period. In the section shown here, transilluminated with ultraviolet light in a fluorescence microscope, the white areas represent the new bone deposited during the 15-day Achromycin treatment. The nonfluorescent central areas of the same haversian systems represent bone deposited after cessation of the treatment. (Micrographs courtesy of R. Amprino.)

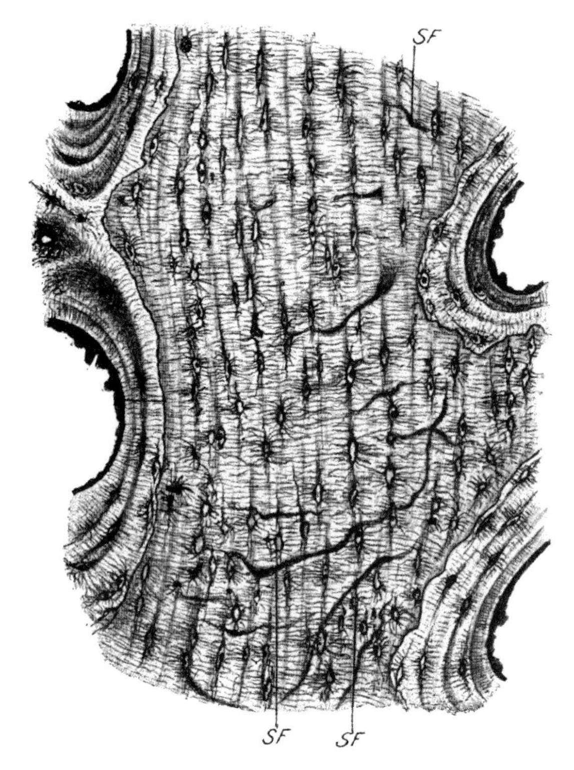

Figure 8–10. A portion of a cross section of a human fibula, showing Sharpey's fibers (SF). (After Schaffer, J. 1922 Lehrbuch der Histologie und Histogenese Verlag von W. Englemann, Leipzig.)

microscopic appearance. On the other hand, if the organic components are extracted from a bone, the remaining inorganic constituents retain the gross form of the bone and, to a certain extent, its microscopic topography, but the bone has lost its tensile strength and is as brittle as porcelain. Thus, it is apparent that the hardness of bone depends on its inorganic constituents, whereas its great toughness and resilience reside in its organic matrix, particularly in its abundant collagen fibers. Without either one, bone would be a poor skeletal material, but, with both, it is a highly ordered, remarkably resistant tissue, superbly adapted, at all levels of its organization, for its mechanical and metabolic functions.

THE CELLS OF BONE

In actively growing bone, four kinds of cells are distinguishable: *osteoprogenitor cells, osteoblasts, osteocytes,* and *osteoclasts.* Although the first three are usually described as distinct cell types, there is clear evidence for transformation from one to the other, and it is probably more reasonable to regard them as different functional phases of the same cell type. Reversible changes in microscopic appearance of this kind are examples of *cell modulation,* not to be confused with *cell differentiation,* which is a term reserved for progressive and apparently irreversible specialization in the structure and function of cells. The osteoclasts have a separate origin coming from precursors of bone-marrow origin.

OSTEOPROGENITOR CELLS

Like other connective tissues, bone develops originally from embryonic mesenchymal cells that have a very broad range of development potentialities, giving rise to fibroblasts, adipose cells, muscle, and so on. Along the pathway of their differentiation into bone-forming cells, a population of cells is formed that have more limited potential, being able to proliferate and differentiate only into chondroblasts or osteoblasts. These *osteoprogenitor cells* persist throughout postnatal life and are found on or near all of the free surfaces of bones: in the endosteum, in the inner layer of the periosteum, and on the trabeculae of calcifying cartilage at the metaphysis of growing bones. Their nuclei are pale-staining and oval or elongated and their scant cytoplasm is acidophic or faintly basophilic.

Osteoprogenitor cells are most active during the growth of bones but are reactivated in adult life in the repair of bone fractures and other forms of injury. Osteoblasts and osteocytes are thought to be incapable of division. After administration of tritiated thymidine, the osteoprogenitor cells are the only cells found to be labeled in autoradiographs at early time intervals. At later times, silver grains can also be found over the nuclei of osteoblasts. Thus, it is evident that as the population of osteoblasts is depleted in the continual internal remodeling of bone, they are replaced by proliferation and differentiation of the osteoprogenitor cells.

In bone remodeling, osteoblasts are transiently active at sites of reformation of bone. When they cease to form bone matrix, they lose their basophilia and revert to a quiescent state, forming a layer of flat cells on the bone surface. They are not morphologically distinguishable from osteoprogenitor cells. In this resting phase, they are referred to as *bone-lining cells.* It is assumed that they are simply the resting phase in the functional modulations of osteoblasts and that they differ from osteoprogenitor cells in not being capable of division or of alternative pathways of differentiation. There is, however, some ambivalence on this point in the literature.

OSTEOBLASTS

Osteoblasts are the bone-forming cells of developing and mature bones. During active deposition of new matrix, they are arranged as an epithelioid layer of cuboidal or columnar cells on the bone surface. The nucleus is usually located at the end of the cell farthest away from the bone surface. The cytoplasm is intensely basophilic and a prominent Golgi complex appears as a paler staining area between the nucleus and the cell base. Osteoblasts give a strong histochemical reaction for acid phosphatase. With the periodic-acid-Schiff reaction, a number of small cytoplasmic vacuoles are found to contain pink-staining material believed to represent precursors of bone matrix. When formation of new bone ceases, these vacuoles are no longer seen, the phosphatase reaction of the cytoplasm diminishes, and the osteoblasts revert to relatively inactive squamous cells covering the surface of the bone.

In electron micrographs, osteoblasts have the structure expected of cells actively engaged in protein synthesis (Fig. 8–11). The extensive endoplasmic reticulum is studded with ribosomes and many free ribosomes are found in the cytoplasm. Numerous small vacuoles associated with the Golgi complex contain an amorphous or flocculent material of appreciable density that corresponds to the PAS-staining material observed with the light microscope. Occasional small lipid droplets are present in some cells. Neighboring osteoblasts on advancing bone surfaces are usually less closely apposed to one another than in typical epithelia, but they are connected by gap junctions.

Although osteoblasts are polarized toward the underlying bone, the release of their products is apparently not confined to the basal pole because some cells among them gradually become enveloped by their own secretions and are transformed into *osteocytes,* imprisoned in lacunae within the newly formed bone matrix.

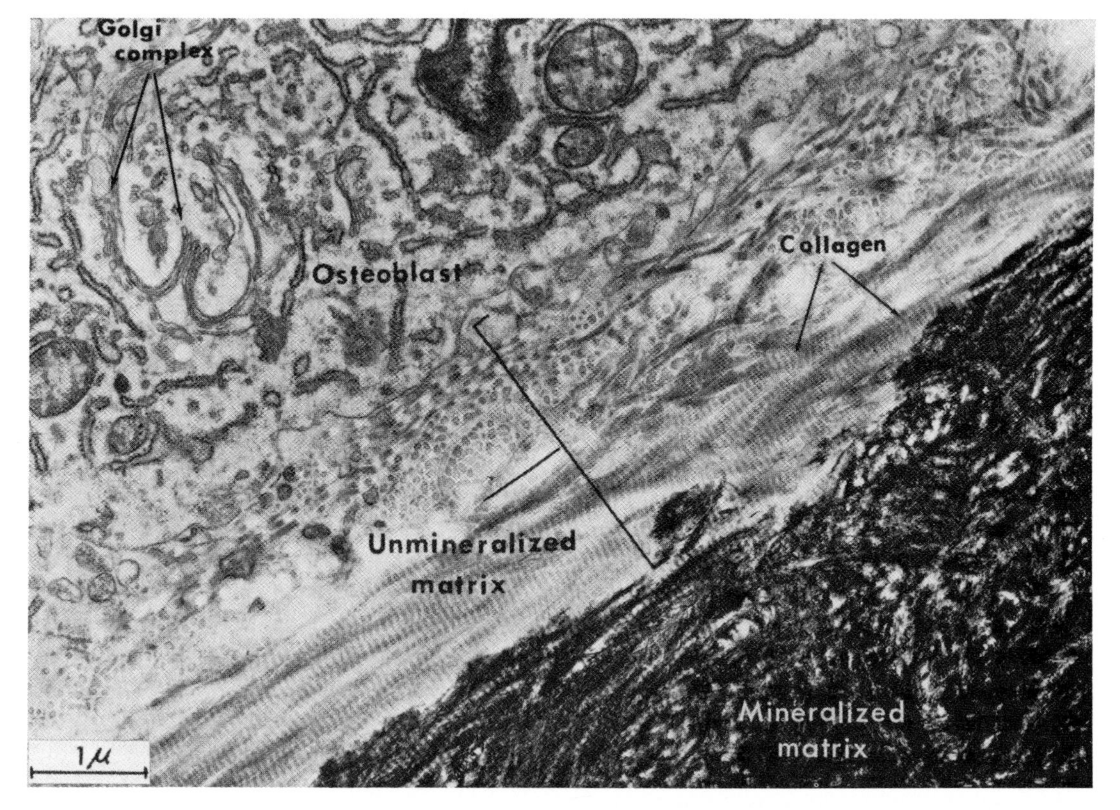

Figure 8–11. Electron micrograph of the edge of a resorption canal being filled in by lamellar bone. At the upper left is a portion of an osteoblast containing a prominent Golgi zone and abundant rough endoplasmic reticulum. Below it, one can see the collagen fibrils of two unmineralized lamellae; at the lower right are the older, dense, mineralized lamellae. (From Cooper D. et al. 1966. J. Bone Joint Surgery 48A:1239.)

In addition to secreting several matrix components including type-I collagen, proteoglycans, osteocalcin, osteonectin, and osteopontin, osteoblasts also produce growth factors that probably have important autocrine and paracrine effects on bone growth. They also have surface receptors for a variety of hormones, vitamins, and cytokines which influence their activity.

The traditional view that bone is deposited by osteoblasts and removed by large multinucleate osteoclasts has proven to be too simplistic. In vitro experiments have now shown that osteoblasts also have an essential role in bone resorption. Osteoclasts are effective only when in direct contact with mineralized bone matrix. Bone normally has a thin layer of unmineralized matrix called *osteoid.* Osteoblasts are believed to participate in bone resorption by secreting enzymes that remove this superficial layer of osteoid, thereby exposing mineralized matrix that can be attacked by osteoclasts. If bone is stripped of its layer of osteoblasts and exposed to isolated osteoclasts in vitro, no resorption pits are formed beneath the osteoclasts. But, if osteoblasts are added to the cultures, bone resorption does occur.

Parathyroid hormone administration, in vivo, results in increased bone resorption. Receptors for parathyroid hormone have not been found on osteoclasts, but they are present on osteoblasts which are believed to respond to the hormone by secretion of an *osteoclast-stimulating factor* that induces activation of quiescent osteoclasts in their vicinity. They also secrete the enzymes *procollagenase* and *plasminogen activator.* Plasminogen activator catalyzes the conversion of serum plasminogen to the neutral protease *plasmin.* This in turn, releases *collagenase* from its proenzyme procollagenase. These enzymes then depolymerize the layer of osteoid, making the underlying mineralized matrix accessible to the activated osteoclasts. The effect of parathyroid hormone on bone resorption by osteoclasts, thus, appears to be indirect, depending on osteoblast release of osteoid-destroying enzymes and an osteoclast-stimulating factor.

OSTEOCYTES

The principal cells of mature bone are the *osteocytes,* which reside in lacunae within the calcified matrix. Their cell body is flattened, conforming to the shape of the lenticular cavity that it occupies, but there are numerous slender cell processes that extend for some distance into canaliculi that radiate from the lacuna into the surrounding matrix (Fig. 8–15). How far the processes extend into the canaliculi of adult mammalian bone could not be ascertained by light microscopy, but studies with the electron microscope have shown that processes of neighboring osteocytes are in contact at their ends. Moreover, their apposed membranes are specialized to form gap junctions at their sites of contact (Fig. 8–12). Thus, these cells are not completely isolated in their lacunae but are in communication with one another, and ultimately with cells at the surface via a series of junctions of low electrical resistance, permitting flow of ions and possibly of small molecules from cell to cell. This finding helps to explain how cells deep within the calcified matrix can be nourished and possibly can respond to hormones that would seem to have access only to cells in the vicinity of small blood vessels outside of the matrix.

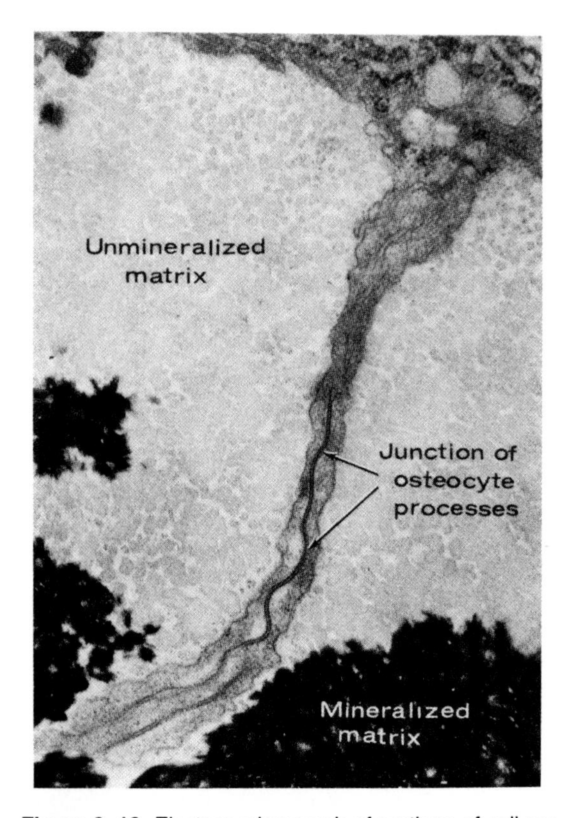

Figure 8–12. Electron micrograph of portions of cell processes from two neighboring osteocytes traversing the zone of unmineralized matrix lining a lacuna. Note the gap junction where the two processes overlap. (From Holtrop, M.E. and M.J. Wenger. 1971. Proc. 4th Parathyroid Conference, International Congress Series No. 243. Amsterdam, Excerpta Medica.)

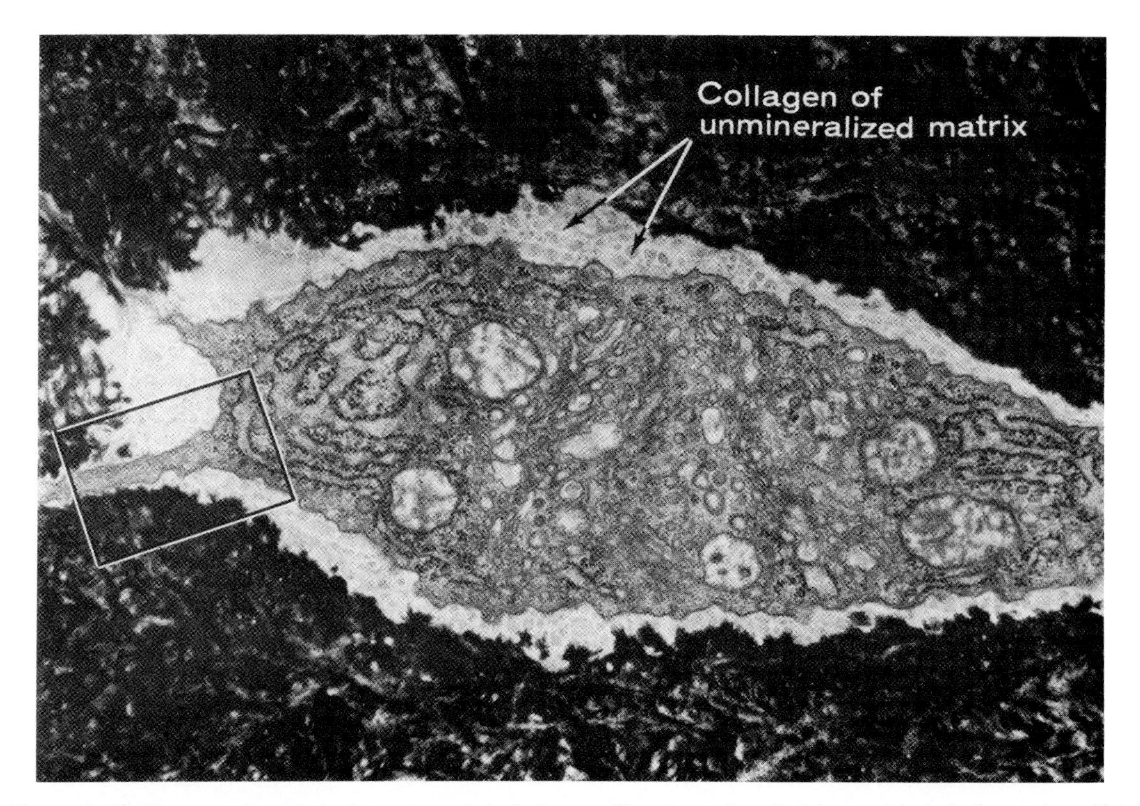

Figure 8–13. Electron micrograph of an osteocyte in its lacuna. The plane of section does not include the nucleus. Note that there is a prominent Golgi complex and numerous cisternal profiles of the endoplasmic reticulum. At the left, a cell process is seen extending into a canaliculus. An area similar to that in the rectangle is seen at higher magnification in Fig. 8–15. (Micrograph courtesy of M. Holtrop.)

The nuclear and cytoplasmic characteristics of osteocytes, as observed with the light microscope, are similar to those of osteoblasts, except that the Golgi area is less conspicuous and the surrounding cytoplasm exhibits less affinity for basic dyes. In electron micrographs of osteocytes that have only recently been incorporated into bone, the Golgi complex may still be rather large and the endoplasmic reticulum quite extensive (Fig. 8–13). In osteocytes situated deeper in the matrix, these organelles have undergone some regression (Fig. 8–14) and the cells are obviously relatively inactive in protein synthesis. But, it is possible that they may continue to produce components needed to maintain the surrounding matrix.

It was formerly believed that osteocytes were responsive to parathyroid hormone and could withdraw calcium ions from bone mineral and transfer them to the tissue fluid, thus contributing to maintenance of normal levels of blood calcium. This process, called *osteocytic osteolysis,* is no longer widely accepted. The retrieval of calcium from bone matrix which is stimulated by parathyroid hormone is now believed to depend on the interaction of osteoblasts and osteoclasts described earlier. When osteocytes are liberated from their lacunae by osteoclastic bone resorption, they revert to quiescent bone-lining cells. Whether they can subsequently undergo modulation to active osteoblasts is debated.

OSTEOCLASTS

Throughout life, bone undergoes a continuous process of internal remodeling and renewal that involves removal of bone matrix at multiple sites, followed by its replacement by newly deposited bone. In this process, the agents of bone resorption are the *osteoclasts,* huge cells up to 150 μm in diameter and containing as many as 50 nuclei. These cells occupy shallow concavities, called Howships lacunae, produced by the erosive action of the osteoclast on the underlying bone.

Osteoclasts exhibit an obvious polarity, having their nuclei congregated near their

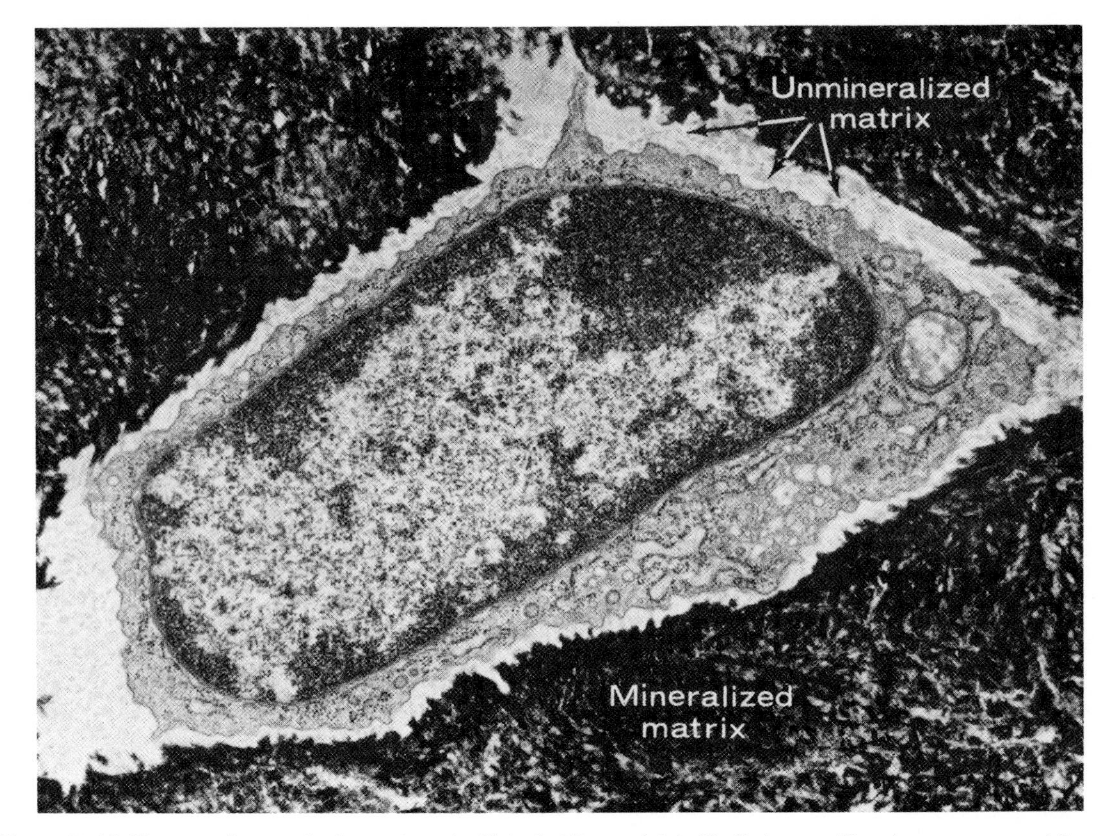

Figure 8–14. Electron micrograph of an osteocyte. Note that it completely fills its lacuna. The clear area around the cell is not a space but is occupied by unmineralized matrix in which collagen fibers are faintly visible. This osteocyte is less active than that in Fig. 8–13, as evidenced by its lesser amount of rough endoplasmic reticulum. The mineralized matrix is black owing to the electron scattering of the apatite crystals. (Micrograph courtesy of M. Holtrop.)

smooth-contoured free surface, whereas the surface adjacent to the bone shows a radial striation that was formerly interpreted as a brush border. However, electron micrographs have revealed that it is less ordered than a typical brush border and consists of deep infoldings of the membrane that delimit a large number of clavate and foliate processes, separated by narrow clefts. Unlike a brush border, which is a very stable surface specialization, the border of the osteoclast is highly active and continually changing its configuration. Cinematographic studies document frequent extension and retraction of border processes and changes in their shape. The descriptive term *ruffled border* is now commonly used to distinguish this specialization at the base of osteoclasts from the brush border found on the lumenal surface of absorptive epithelia (Fig. 8–16).

In electron micrographs, the nuclei are unusual only in their number. Associated with each is a Golgi complex and a pair of centrioles. The multiple diplosomes may gather together in a single large centrosomal region. In the surrounding cytoplasm, the endoplasmic reticulum is sparsely represented and there are many mitochondria of varying length that tend to congregate near the ruffled border. In this region of the cytoplasm, there are also numerous electron-dense lysosomes, about 0.5 μm in diameter, and larger vesicles, up to 3 μm in diameter. Some of the latter also react positively for acid phosphatase. The plasmalemma of the border bears, on its cytoplasmic face, a nap of exceedingly fine bristle-like appendages, 15–20-nm long and spaced about 20 nm apart. This bristle coat makes the elaborately infolded membrane of the border appear thicker than the rest of the plasma membrane. Around the circumference of the ruffled border, the membrane is very closely applied to the bone and the subjacent cytoplasm is unusually rich in actin filaments. This annular specialization, termed the *sealing zone,* bounds a closed *subosteoclastic compartment* between the border and the bone that is undergoing resorption (Fig. 8–17).

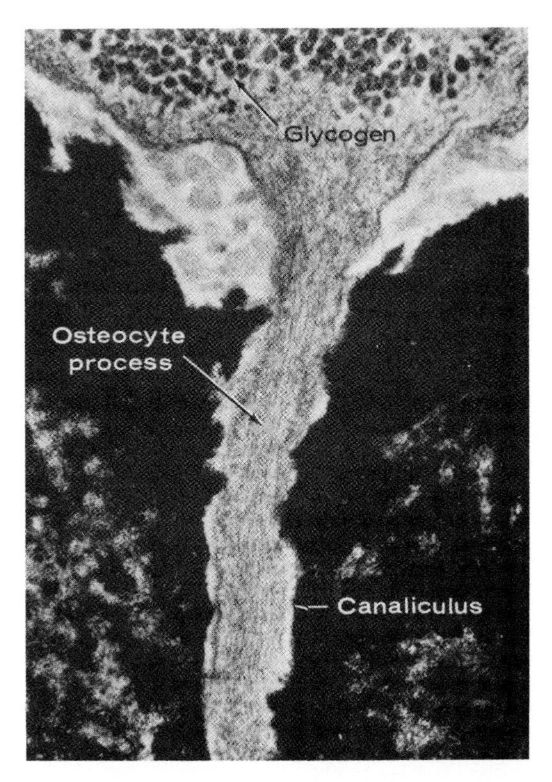

Figure 8–15. Micrograph of an osteocyte process extending from the cell body (top) into a canaliculus (bottom). Note the cytoplasmic filaments in the cell process. (Micrograph courtesy of M. Holtrop.)

How osteoclasts could erode mineralized bone matrix was long puzzling to histologists. It was known, however, that bone can be decalcified by acid and it was logical to expect that acidification of the subosteoclastic compartment might be involved. For a cell to lower the pH in an intracellular vacuole or an external compartment, it must pump H^+ ions across the limiting membrane. In the familiar case of the gastric parietal cells that acidify the content of the stomach, the action of the enzyme carbonic anhydrase on water and CO_2 results in the formation of bicarbonate and H^+ ions, and the H^+ ions are actively transported into the lumen by an ATP-dependent proton pump in the plasma membrane. The same mechanism is employed by cells, in general, to create an acid pH in secondary lysosomes. In osteoclasts, carbonic anhydrase has been localized on the inner aspect of the ruffled border and a 100 kD protein, present in the membrane, has been found to be similar, or identical, to the ATP-dependent proton pump in lysosomal membranes. The fact that the subperiosteal compartment is sealed off enables the cell to pump H^+ ions into it and create an acidic microenvironment capable of solubilizing bone mineral. Thus, this extracellular compartment can be considered functionally equivalent to a secondary lysosome. The acid environment of the compartment also favors the action of secreted acid hydrolases that digest the organic components of bone matrix. The lysosomal enzymes, β-glycerophosphatase, aryl sulfatase, and the cysteine proteases cathepsin-B and cathepsin-L can be localized in osteoclasts along the entire biosynthetic pathway from the endoplasmic reticulum, through the Golgi complex, to vesicles that discharge their contents at the ruffled border. Thus, the osteoclast must be regarded as a secretory cell releasing acid hydrolases and pumping H^+ ions into the subosteoclastic compartment to remove calcium salts and to digest collagen and other organic components of bone matrix.

For over a century, it has been generally accepted that the multinucleate osteoclasts arise by coalescence of uninucleate cells, but there has been little agreement until recently as to the identity of the precursor. Over the years, the osteoprogenitor cell, osteoblast, osteocyte, monocyte, and macrophage have all had their advocates. When the technique of radiolabeling cells became available, it was observed that some osteoclasts contained labeled nuclei. Because the nuclei of osteoclasts do not divide and would, therefore, not incorporate tritiated thymidine during DNA replication, it was concluded that the labeled nuclei had been incorporated through cell fusion and that the uninucleate precursor probably originated in the bone marrow. More compelling evidence for the origin of osteoclasts from cells transported in the blood came from ingenious experiments with a mutant strain of mice in which some individuals exhibit *osteopetrosis,* an excessive accumulation of spongiosa in their long bones, due to impaired ostoclastic resorption of bone during development. When an osteopetrotic mouse was joined, in parabiosis, with a normal littermate, the excess spongiosa disappeared from its bones within 6 weeks, and it remained cured even after separation from the normal parabiont. The inescapable conclusion from this experiment was that the osteoclasts that removed the excess bone originated from blood-borne uninucleate precursors from the blood of the normal mouse while their circulatory systems were joined. For a time, thereafter, monocytes were considered the most likely

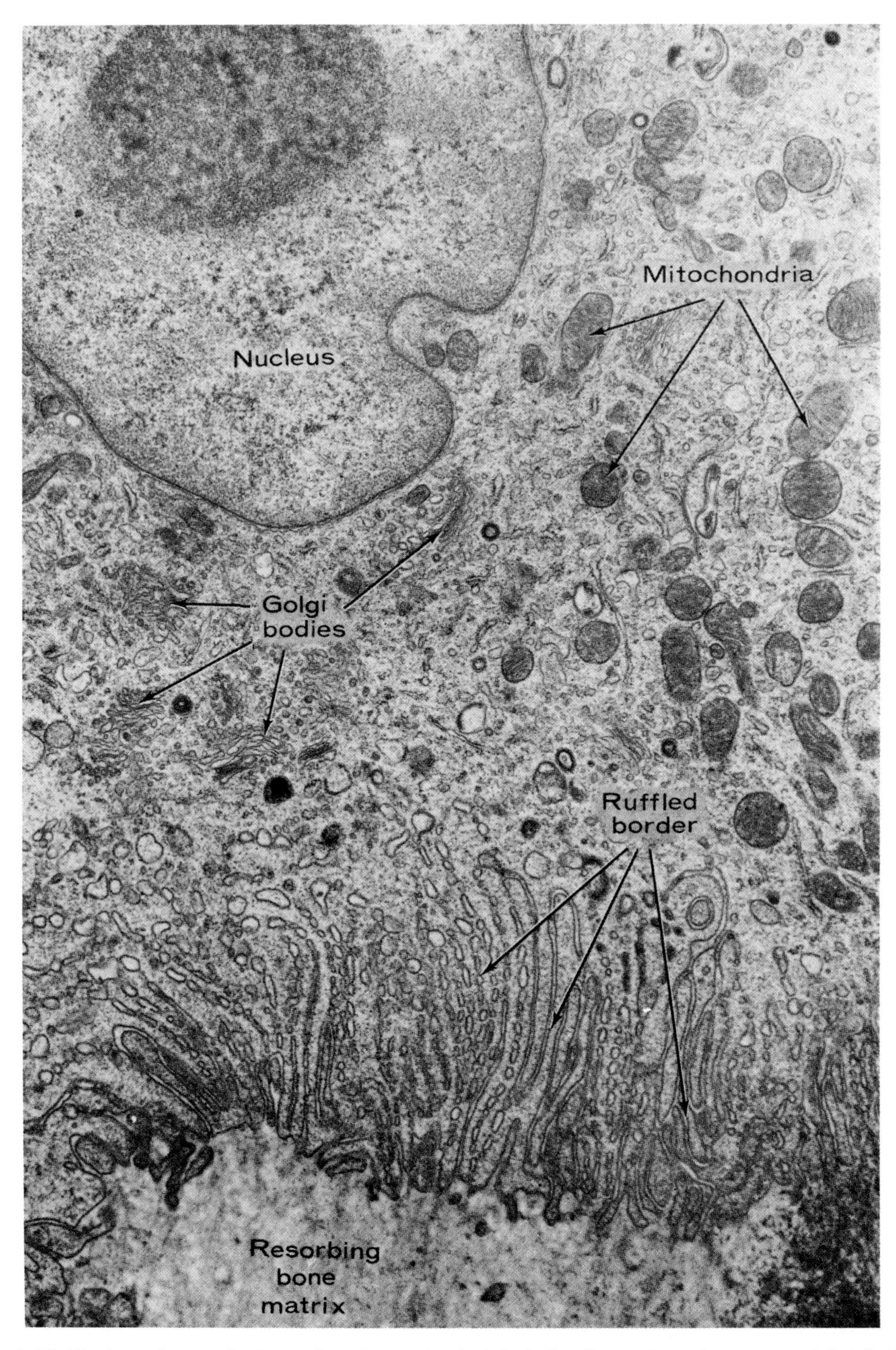

Figure 8–16. Electron micrograph of a portion of an osteoclast, including the nucleus above, several Golgi elements, and the ruffled border closely applied to an area of resorbing bone matrix, at the bottom of the figure. (Micrograph courtesy of P. Garrant.)

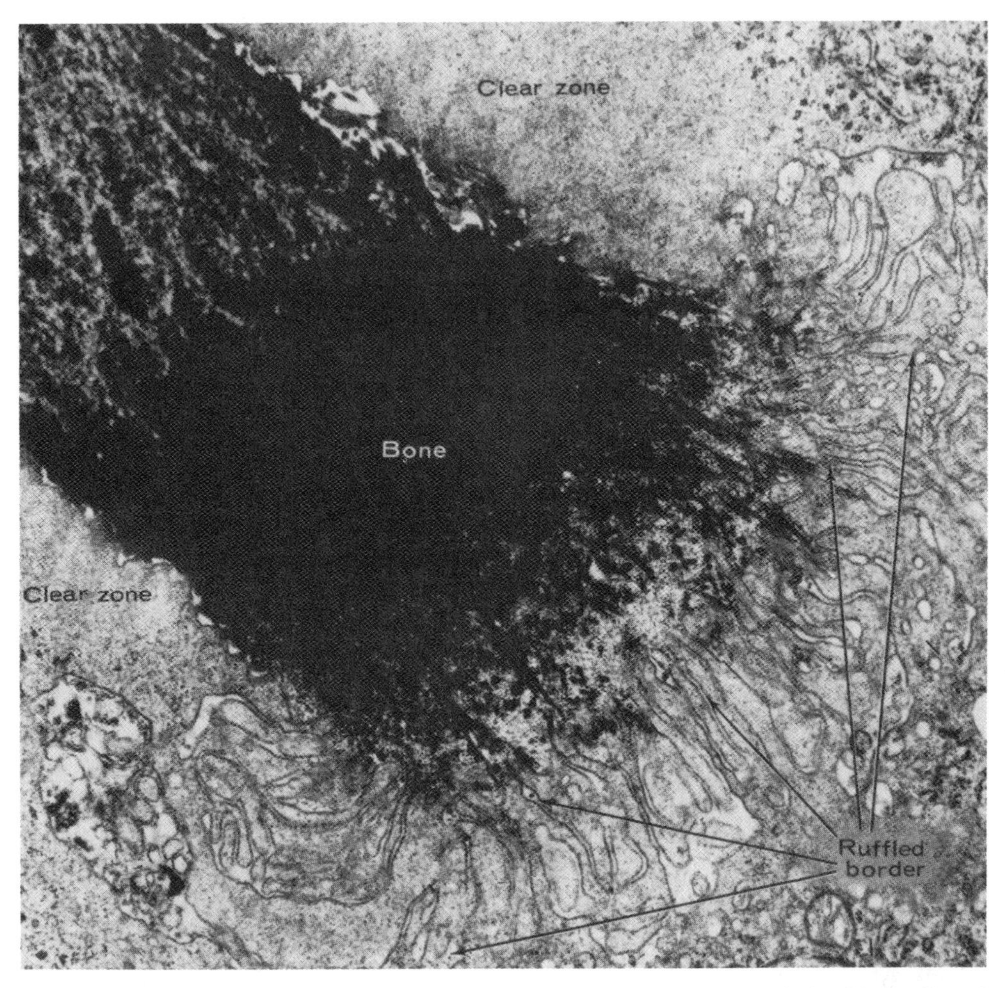

Figure 8–17. Electron micrograph of a portion of an osteoclast around the end of a spicule of bone. Note the ruffled border at the end of the bone where it is undergoing resorption. A smooth-contoured portion of the osteoclast surface, with a subjacent clear zone of ectoplasm, is closely adherent to the bone around the periphery of the ruffled border. This zone is believed to seal the space into which the osteoclast is releasing hydrogen ions and lysosomal enzymes. (Micrograph courtesy of M. Holtrop.)

precursors. However, monocytes and macrophages are not able to resorb bone, even after they have fused to form multinucleate giant cells that resemble osteoclasts. It is now believed that monocytes, macrophages, and osteoclasts share a common precursor in the bone marrow, the *granulocyte–macrophage progenitor cell* (GM-CSF), but that, at some stage in its development, an osteoclast progenitor is generated that follows a diverging path of differentiation and is distributed in the blood to the bones. Although these so-called preosteoclasts resemble monocytes, they contain lysosomes that are rich in a tartrate-resistant acid phosphatase which is thought to be specific to lysosomes of osteoclasts. These precursor cells can be found, in limited numbers, in other tissues but they fuse to form osteoclasts, only in bone. It is postulated that this final step in osteoclast differentiation is dependent on an unidentified soluble factor, or factors, produced by osteoblasts or osteocytes.

Osteoclasts are long lived but they are not continuously active. A response to an unusual metabolic demand for mobilization of calcium from bone does not depend on the generation of additional osteoclasts but on the activation of quiescent members of the total population. When the demand for calcium has been met, the ruffled border of many of the osteoclasts disappears and they revert to a resting phase. These modulations of osteoclast activity are controlled by hormones and cytokines. Osteoclasts have receptors for *calcitonin,* a hormone that suppresses bone resorption. They do not appear to have receptors for *parathyroid hormone,* which increases bone resorption. As indicated earlier, their activation by this hormone is indirect, being mediated by an *osteoclast-stimulating factor* produced by osteoblasts.

HISTOGENESIS OF BONE

Bone always develops by replacement of a preexisting connective tissue. In the embryo, two different modes of osteogenesis are observed. Where bone is formed directly in primitive connective tissue, it is called *intramembranous ossification.* Where bone formation takes place in preexisting cartilage, it is called *endochondral ossification.* The actual deposition of bone matrix is essentially the same in the two modes of bone formation, but in endochondral ossification the bulk of the cartilage must be removed before bone deposition begins. In both, bone is first laid down as a network of trabeculae, called the *primary spongiosa,* and this is then transformed into more compact bone by a filling-in of the interstices between trabeculae.

INTRAMEMBRANOUS OSSIFICATION

Certain flat bones of the skull—the frontal, parietal, occipital, and temporal bones—develop by intramembranous ossification and are, therefore, referred to as *membrane bones.* The embryonic mesenchyme first condenses into a richly vascularized layer of connective tissue in which the cells are in contact with one another via long tapering processes, and the intercellular spaces are occupied by delicate, randomly oriented bundles of collagen in a thin gel-like extracellular matrix. The first sign of bone formation is the appearance of thin strands, or trabeculae, of eosinophilic *bone matrix* (Fig. 8–18). These tend to be deposited equidistant from neighboring blood vessels, and because the vessels form a network, the earliest trabeculae of bone matrix also develop in a branching and anastomosing pattern (Fig. 8–19). Concurrent with the appearance of trabeculae in the connective tissue, there are changes in the cells. They enlarge, become intensely basophilic, and gather on the surface of the trabeculae, where they assume a cuboidal or columnar form while still remaining in contact with one another via short processes. Thenceforth, they are called *osteoblasts* and through their secretion of additional bone matrix, the trabeculae become longer and thicker.

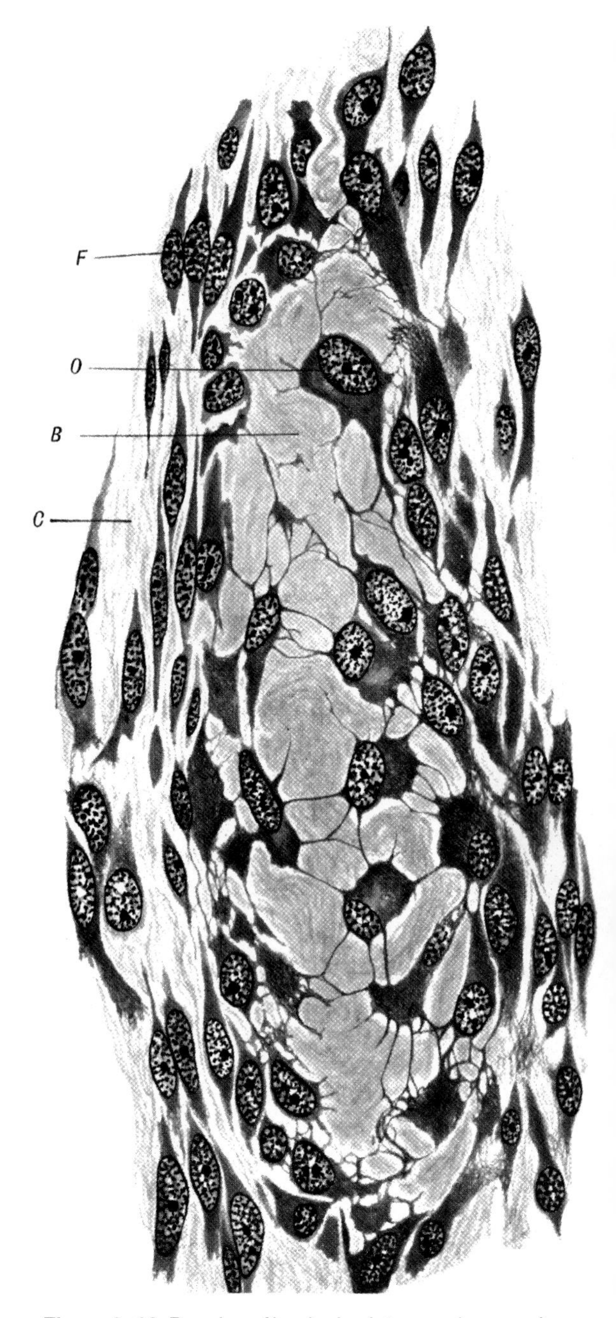

Figure 8–18. Drawing of beginning intramembranous bone formation in the skull of a 5.5-cm cat embryo. (B) Homogeneous appearing collagen fibers and newly deposited extracellular matrix. (C) Collagen fibers of the surrounding connective tissue. (F) Fibroblasts. (O) Cells with multiple processes in transition to osteoblasts, and later into osteocytes.

Collagen molecules secreted by the osteo-

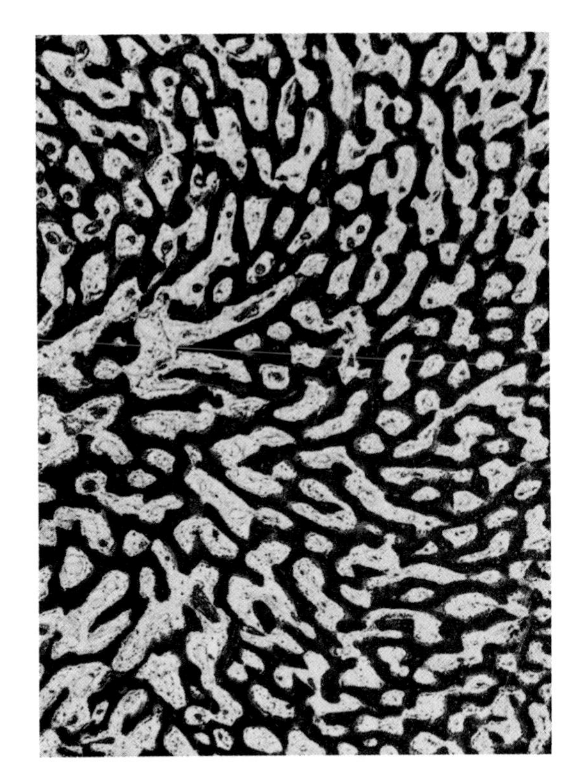

Figure 8–19. Photomicrograph of the pattern of trabeculae in the primary spongiosa of intramembranous bone formation.

blasts during embryonic bone deposition polymerize extracellularly to form numerous randomly oriented fibrils throughout the trabeculae. The early intramembranous bone, in which the collagen fibers run in all directions, is often described as *woven bone* to distinguish it from the *lamellar bone* formed during subsequent bone remodeling, which has highly-ordered parallel collagen fibers that change direction in alternate layers. The woven bone initially formed in intramembranous ossification is permeated by relatively large tortuous channels occupied by blood vessels and connective tissue. The lacunae containing its osteocytes are uniformly distributed but random in their orientation. In lamellar bone, on the other hand, the osteocytes are consistent in their orientation and are arranged concentrically around relatively straight vessels within slender haversian canals (Fig. 8–20).

The trabeculae of bone matrix laid down in primitive connective tissue soon become a site of deposition of calcium phosphate and all of the matrix added by the osteoblasts calcifies after a short lag period. Thus, only a thin layer of osteoid is found between the bases of the osteoblasts and the heavily mineralized matrix of the underlying trabeculae (Figs. 8–13 and 8–14). As the trabeculae thicken by accretion, individual osteoblasts at their surface are incarcerated in the newly deposited matrix, and, one by one, they become isolated in lacunae to join the ranks of the osteocytes within the trabeculae. Although sequestered in newly deposited matrix, they remain connected to osteoblasts at the surface by slender cell processes. The canaliculi of bone are formed by deposition of matrix around these cell processes. As rapidly as the osteoblasts on the surface of the trabeculae are depleted by their incorporation in bone, their numbers are restored by proliferation and differentiation of new osteoblasts from osteoprogenitor cells in the perivascular connective tissue. Mitotic division is not observed in osteoblasts but is frequent in osteoprogenitor cells.

In areas of the primary spongiosa that are destined to become compact bone, the trabeculae continue to thicken at the expense of the connective tissue until the spaces around the blood vessels are largely obliterated. In this progressive encroachment on the perivascular spaces, bone is deposited in irregularly concentric layers that bear some resemblance to haversian systems but it is not true lamellar bone because its collagen fibers are randomly oriented.

In those areas where spongy bone will persist in postnatal life, the thickening of the trabeculae does not progress and the vascular connective tissue between them is gradually transformed into hemopoietic tissue. The connective tissue investment of the bone condenses to form the *periosteum*. As growth ceases, the osteoblasts on the external and internal surfaces of the bone take on a fibroblast-like form and persist as quiescent bone–lining cells of the periosteum and *endosteum,* respectively. If they are subsequently called on to form bone in the repair of fractures, their osteogenic potentialities are reactivated and they again become osteoblasts.

ENDOCHONDRAL OSSIFICATION

Bones of the vertebral column, pelvis, and the extremities are first formed of hyaline cartilage, and the cartilage model is then replaced by bone in the process called *endochondral ossification*. These bones are, therefore, referred to as *cartilage bones* in contradistinction to the *membrane bones* of the skull. In the develop-

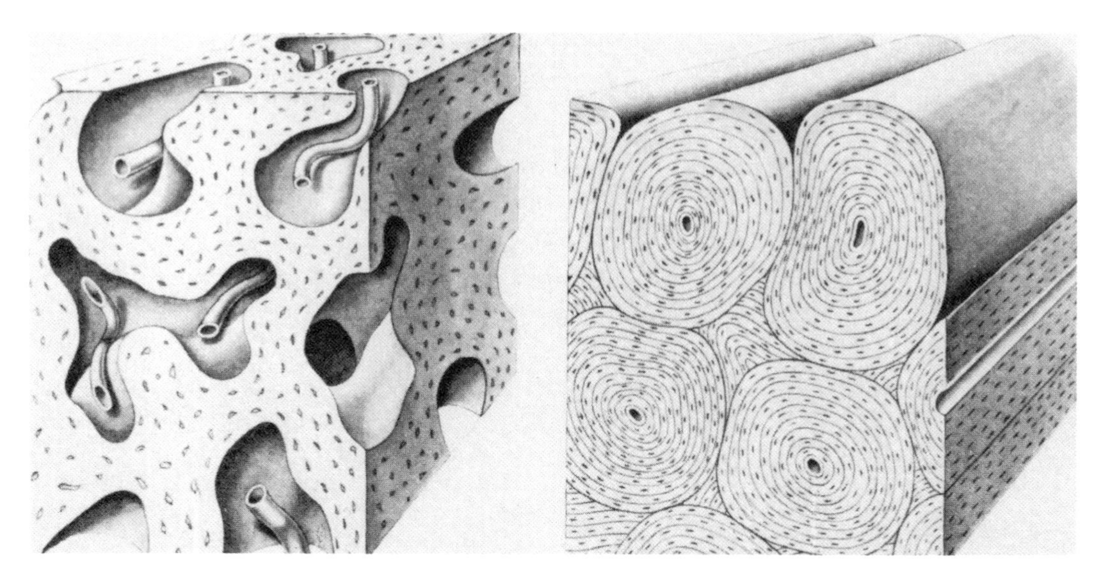

Figure 8–20. Three-dimensional diagramatic representation of the differences in architecture of woven bone (A) and lamellar bone (B). (From Hancox, N.M. 1972. Biology of Bone. Cambridge, England, Cambridge University Press.)

ment of a long bone, the first indication of the formation of a *center of ossification* is a local enlargement of the chondrocytes in the middle of the shaft of its cartilage model (Fig. 8–21). Glycogen accumulates in the hypertrophied chondrocytes and their cytoplasm becomes vacuolated. As their lacunae enlarge, the intervening cartilage matrix is gradually reduced to thin fenestrated septa or irregularly shaped spicules. These become calcifi-

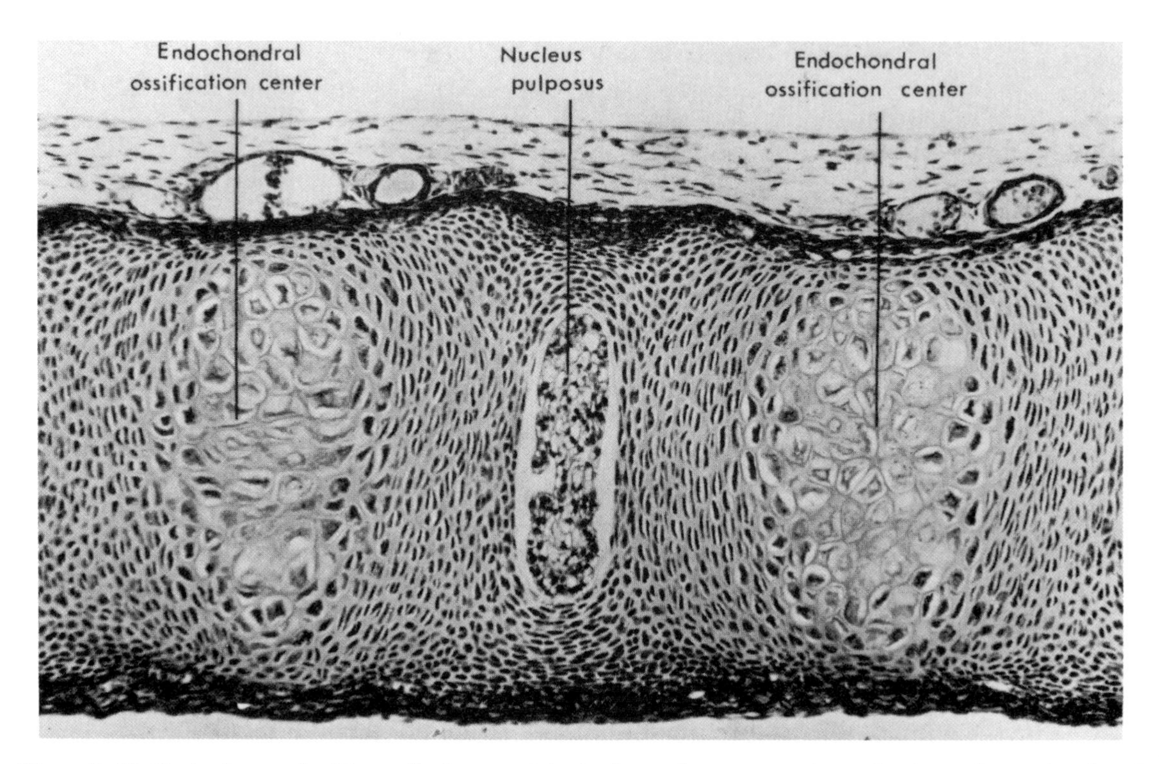

Figure 8–21. Photomicrograph of the cartilaginous vertebral column of a mouse embryo, showing in the center of each vertebra, an area of hypertrophied cartilage cells which represent an early stage in the establishment of a center of endochondral ossification.

able and small aggregations of calcium phosphate crystals are deposited within them. Hypertrophy of the chondrocytes is followed by regressive changes leading to their death and degeneration.

Concurrent with these changes in the interior of the cartilage model, the osteogenic potentialities of cells in the perichondrium are activated and a thin *periosteal collar* of bone is deposited around the midportion of the shaft, now called the diaphysis (Fig. 8–22B, C). At the same time, blood vessels invade the irregular cavities in the cartilage created by the confluence of the enlarged lacunae formerly occupied by the hypertrophied chondrocytes (Figs. 8–22D, 8–23, and 8–24). The vessels branch and grow toward either end of the center of ossification, forming capillary loops that extend into the blind ends of the cavities created in the calcified cartilage. Osteoprogenitor cells and hemopoietic stem cells are carried into the interior of the cartilage with the perivascular connective tissue of the invading blood vessels. Osteoprogenitor cells differentiate into osteoblasts that congregate on the irregular surfaces of the spicules of calcified cartilage and begin to deposit bone matrix on them. The earliest bony trabeculae formed in the interior of the cartilage model, thus, have a core of calcified cartilage and an outer layer of bone of varying thickness. Owing to the different staining affinities of calcified cartilage and bone, these trabeculae have a mottled appearance that distinguishes them from the trabeculae of woven bone that are formed under the periosteum by intramembranous ossification.

At this stage of development, a long bone consists of epiphyses of hyaline cartilage at either end, and a diaphysis consisting of an hour-glass shaped region of endochondral ossification surrounded by a collar of bone of periosteal origin. In common usage, the term *primary center of ossification* embraces all of the developmental events described above, whether they occur in the interior of the cartilage model or under the perichondrium. It is intended to distinguish the diaphyseal center of ossification, which appears first, from secondary centers of ossification that develop much later in the epiphyses. Some investigators, however, reserve the term primary center for the periosteal collar on the grounds that it is the first true bone formed, even though its formation is heralded by earlier changes in the chondrocytes in the interior of the model.

GROWTH IN LENGTH OF LONG BONES

While cartilage is being replaced by bone in the diaphyseal center of ossification, interstitial growth of the hyaline cartilage of the epiphyses continues. The chondrocytes near the diaphysis become arranged in longitudinal columns, within which the cells are separated by thin septa, whereas adjacent columns are separated by wider longitudinally oriented septa of cartilage matrix (Figs. 8–25 and 8–26). As endochondral ossification progresses from the diaphysis into the epiphyses, the chondrocytes in the longitudinal columns undergo changes similar to those described in the primary center of ossification. Four zones representing successive stages in the cytomorphosis of the cartilage cells are recognizable along the length of the columns. At their epiphyseal ends, there is a *zone of proliferation* where frequent division of the flattened chondrocytes provides for continuing elongation of the cartilage model. Next, toward the diaphysis, is a *zone of maturation* in which the cells undergo significant enlargement which reaches its peak in the *zone of hypertrophy,* where the cells are very large and highly vacuolated. Because the matrix in this zone is a site of deposition of calcium salts, it is also referred to as the *zone of provisional calcification.* Finally, at the diaphyseal end of the columns is the *zone of degeneration,* where the hypertrophied chondrocytes are dying and the open ends of their vacated lacunae are being invaded by capillary loops and associated osteoprogenitor cells from the marrow-filled spaces of the diaphysis. The osteoprogenitor cells congregate on the irregularly shaped spicules of calcified cartilage that remain between the columns and deposit on them a thin layer of bone matrix, which begins to calcify nearly as rapidly as it is formed. However, electron microscopy has shown that a thin superficial layer of uncalcified osteoid, 1 μm or less in thickness, is always present. The distribution of calcified cartilage and bone matrix is best demonstrated in undecalcified sections in which the bone mineral has been stained black by the von Kossa method (Fig. 8–26A).

In growing children with a dietary deficiency of vitamin D or of calcium and phosphate, calcification of newly deposited matrix at the junction of diaphysis and epiphysis of long bones may be seriously impaired, resulting in excessive accumulation of osteoid. In this condition, called *rickets,* the poorly

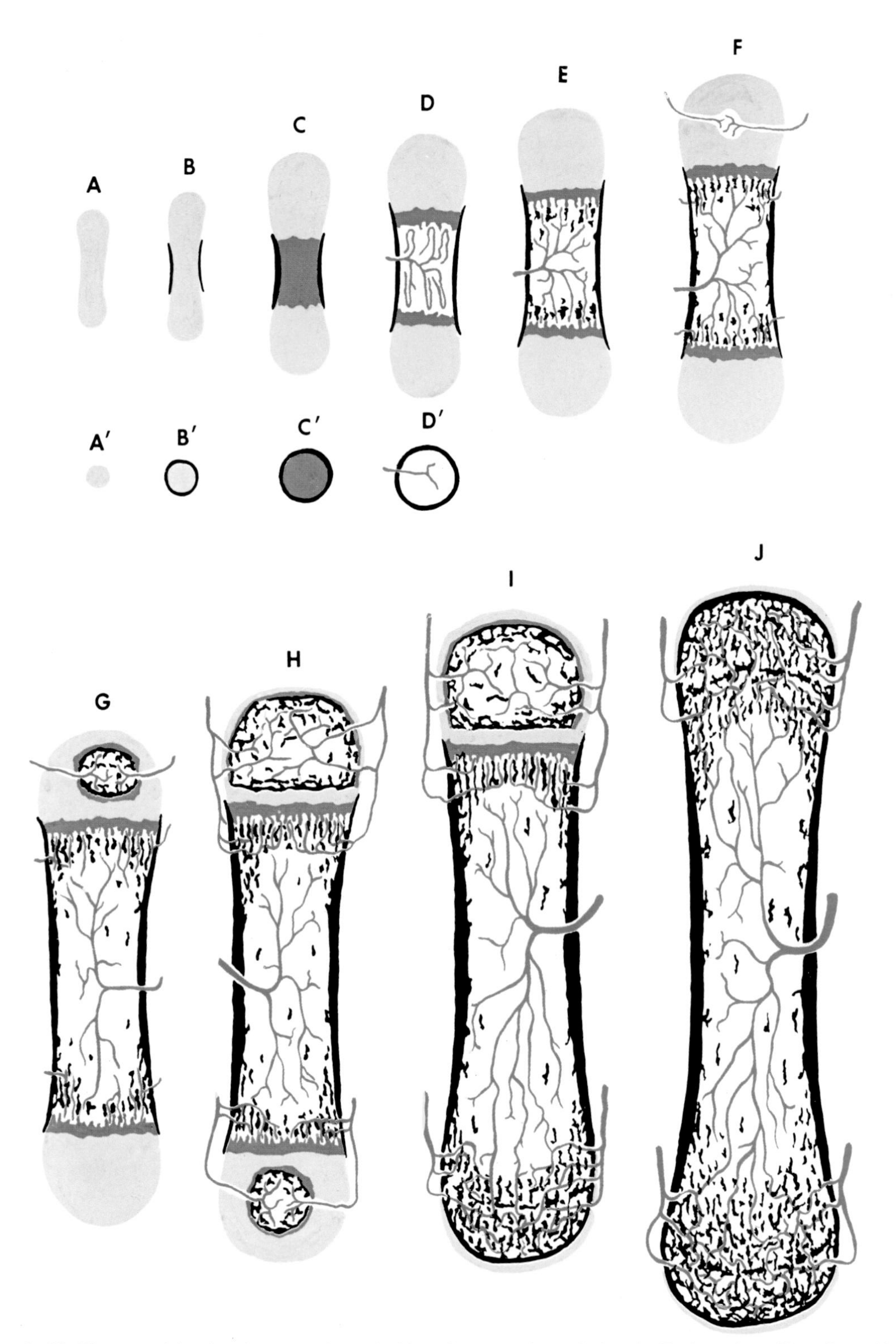

Figure 8–22. Diagram of the development of a typical long bone as shown in longitudinal sections (A to J), and in cross sections A′, B′, C′ and D′, through the centers of A, B, C, and D. Pale blue is cartilage; purple, calcified cartilage; black, bone; red, arteries. (A) The original cartilage model of the bone; (B) a periosteal collar of bone appears before any calcification of cartilage occurs; (C) cartilage begins to calcify; (D) vascular mesenchyme enters the calcified cartilage and divides it into two zones of ossification (E) and (F); blood vessels and mesenchyme penetrate the epiphyseal cartilage and the epiphyseal ossification center develops within it (G); a similar ossification center develops in the lower epiphyseal cartilage (H); as the bone ceases to grow in length, the lower epiphyseal plate disappears first (I) and then the upper epiphyseal plate (J). The marrow cavity then becomes continuous throughout the length of the bone, and the blood vessels of the diaphysis, metaphyses, and epiphyses intercommunicate.

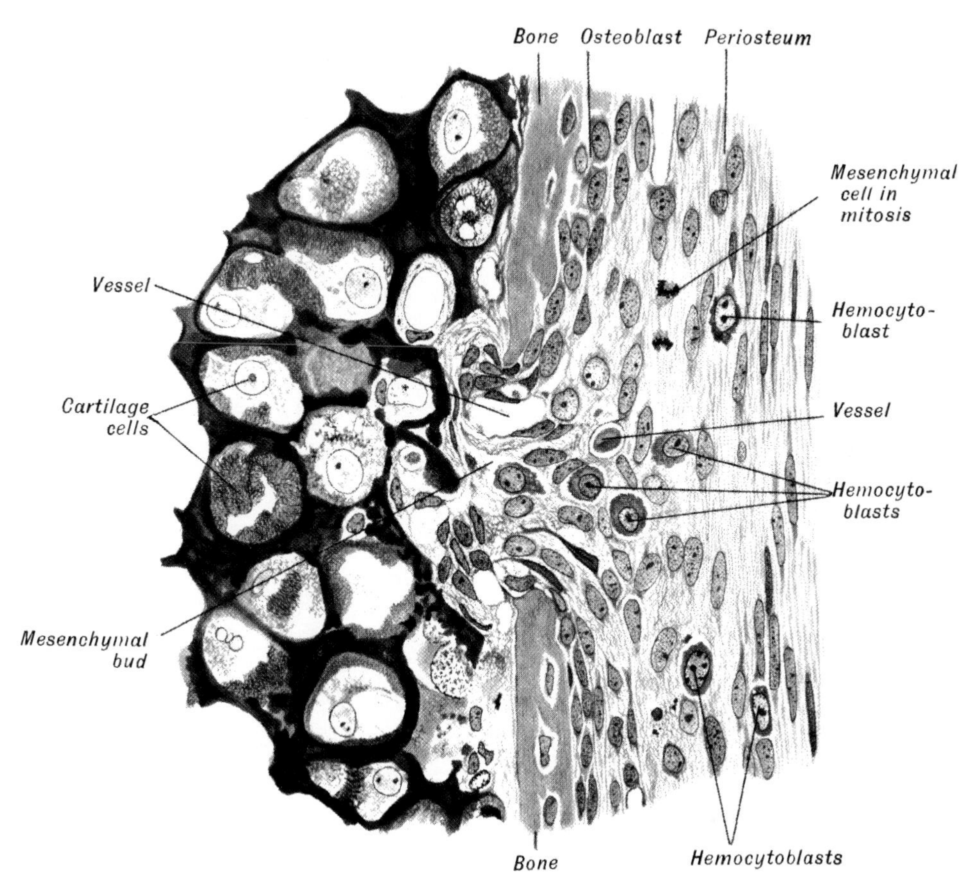

Figure 8–23. Drawing from a longitudinal section through the middle of the diaphysis of the femur of a 25-mm human embryo. Mesenchyme and vessels are beginning to enter calcified cartilage through an opening in the periosteal bone collar. (After A.A. Maximov.)

calcified bones are often deformed under the strain of weight-bearing, resulting in the permanent skeletal deformities commonly described as bowlegs and knock-knees.

In the transitional zone, called the *metaphysis,* where the cartilage of the epiphyses is being invaded and replaced by bone, the trabeculae are continually eroded by osteoclasts at their diaphyseal ends at about the same rate that they are being added to at the epiphyseal end. As a result, the primary spongiosa of the metaphysis remains relatively constant in length, while the marrow cavity elongates.

Primary centers of ossification have developed in the diaphysis of each of the principal long bones by the third month of fetal life. Much later, usually after birth, the chondrocytes in the interior of the epiphyses begin to hypertrophy, heralding the onset of ossification. The spaces vacated by their subsequent degeneration are invaded by blood vessels and osteoprogenitor cells from the perichondrium, establishing *secondary centers of ossification* in the epiphyses at either end of the developing bones (Fig. 8–22G). These differ from the primary center in that there is no associated subperichondrial deposition of bone. In their subsequent expansion, all of the epiphysial cartilage is ultimately replaced by bone, except for a layer that persists as the *articular cartilage* and a thin transverse disc, called the *epiphyseal plate,* between the epiphyses and the diaphysis. All subsequent growth in length of the bone is attributable to proliferation of chondrocytes in the epiphyseal plate and their replacement by bone. In normal growth, the rate of cell division in the proliferative zone of the epiphyseal plate is in balance with the rate of chondrocyte degeneration and replacement by bone at the diaphyseal ends of the cell columns. The net effect is a progressive increase in the length of the diaphysis with little or no change in the thickness of

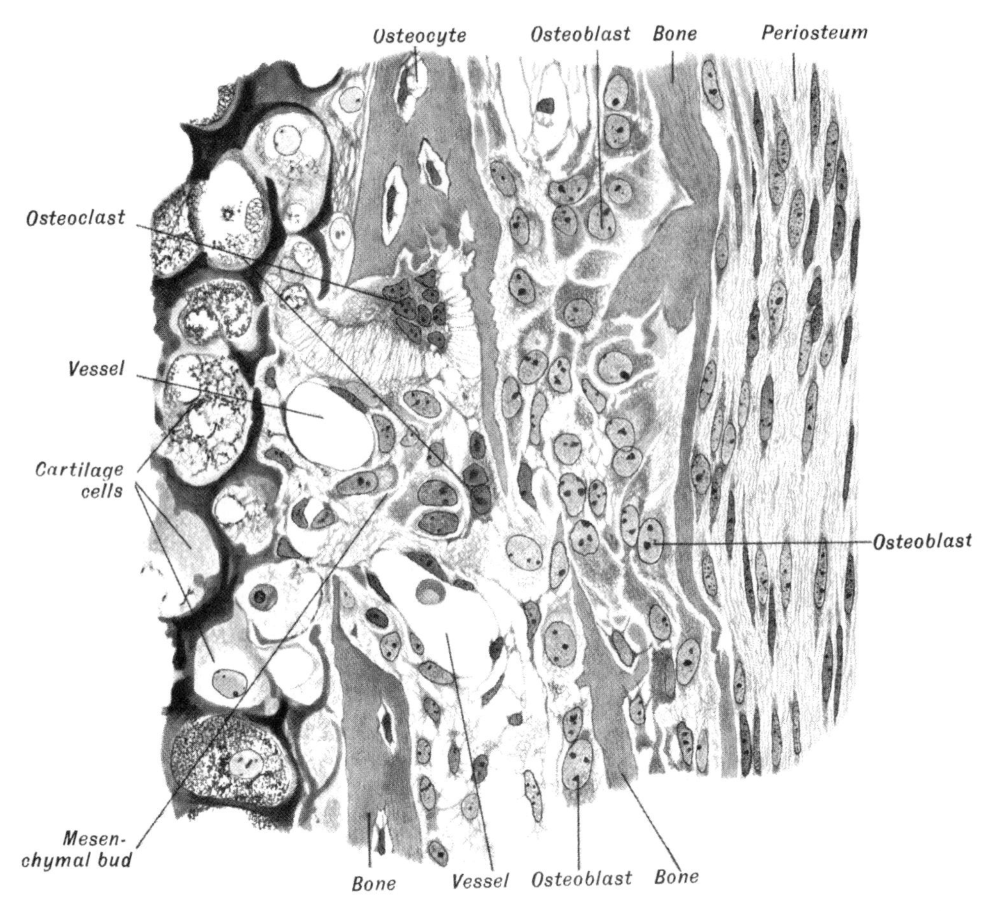

Figure 8–24. Drawing of a longitudinal section through the middle of the diaphysis of the humerous of a human embryo of 8 weeks. The process of ossification has advanced slightly farther than in Fig. 8–23 with vessels clearly penetrating into lacunae of the degenerating chondrocytes. (After A.A. Maximov.)

the epiphyseal plate throughout the period of growth.

At the end of the growing period, proliferation of the cartilage cells slows and finally ceases. Continued replacement of cartilage by bone at the diaphyseal ends of the cell columns then results in obliteration of the epiphyseal plate. The bony trabeculae of the diaphysis are then continuous with the spongiosa of the bony epiphyses. The elimination of the plates is referred to as *closure of the epiphyses.* When this is completed, no further longitudinal growth of the bone is possible. The times of closure and the relative contribution of each of the two epiphyseal plates of a long bone to its overall growth may differ markedly. Growth of the femur takes place mainly at the distal plate and growth of the tibia mainly at the proximal epiphyseal plate. This has clinical relevance in orthopedic surgery. For example, a child may have retarded growth of one leg following poliomyelitis. In such a case, the orthopedic surgeon can take advantage of existing knowledge of the rates of growth at the respective epiphyseal plates and the times of their normal closure to select the time and site for surgical obliteration of an epiphysis in the normal leg. If appropriately timed, such a procedure can retard the growth of the normal leg just enough to permit the slower-growing leg to catch up, and thus ensure an equalization of leg length by the time growth in stature of the child ceases. A seriously disabling distortion of gait can, thus, be avoided.

MECHANISM OF CALCIFICATION

In endochondral ossification, calcification of cartilage matrix is a critical step, upon which a number of subsequent events de-

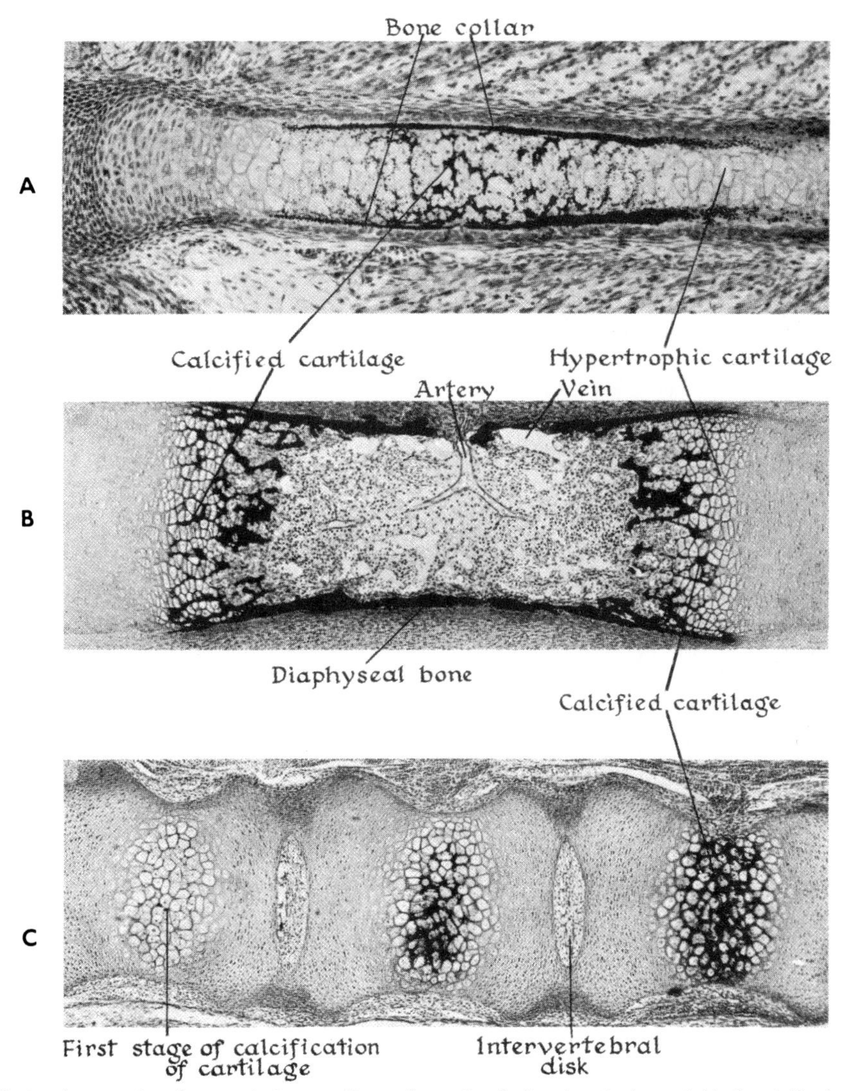

Figure 8–25. Photomicrographs of several stages of bone formation in the developing rat. Undecalcified sections stained with silver nitrate. Bone salts appear black. (A) Longitudinal section through the second rib of an 18-day-old rat embryo; calcification of the periosteal bone collar is evident. (B) Section of a metatarsal of a 4-day-old rat in which calcification is proceeding toward both epiphyses; the hypertrophied cartilage is not completely calcified. (C) Three stages in the calcification of vertebrae in a 20-day-old rat embryo. (Courtesy of W. Bloom and M.A. Bloom.)

pends. The mechanism of mineral deposition has been a subject of much debate and remains unsettled. A widely accepted hypothesis holds that it is analogous to induction of crystallization from metastable solutions by adding a crystal or scratching the wall of the beaker—a process called *heterogeneous nucleation.* The foreign matter disturbs the equilibrium of the solution causing a clustering of molecules that form "nuclei" that are capable of growing to form crystals. It is suggested that collagen fibers of the matrix act as nucleation sites for transformation of calcium and phosphate in solution, into solid phase mineral deposits. In support of this theory, it has been shown that reconstituted collagen fibers induce the formation of apatite crystals when introduced into metastable solutions of calcium and phosphate. Only native collagen, having a 67-nm periodicity, is effective, leading to the speculation that nucleation of bone mineral is dependent on the arrangement of molecules within the fiber. This is consistent with electron microscopic observations indicating that the earliest deposits of mineral are localized in the holes between the ends of the quarter-staggered collagen molecules (Fig. 8–27).

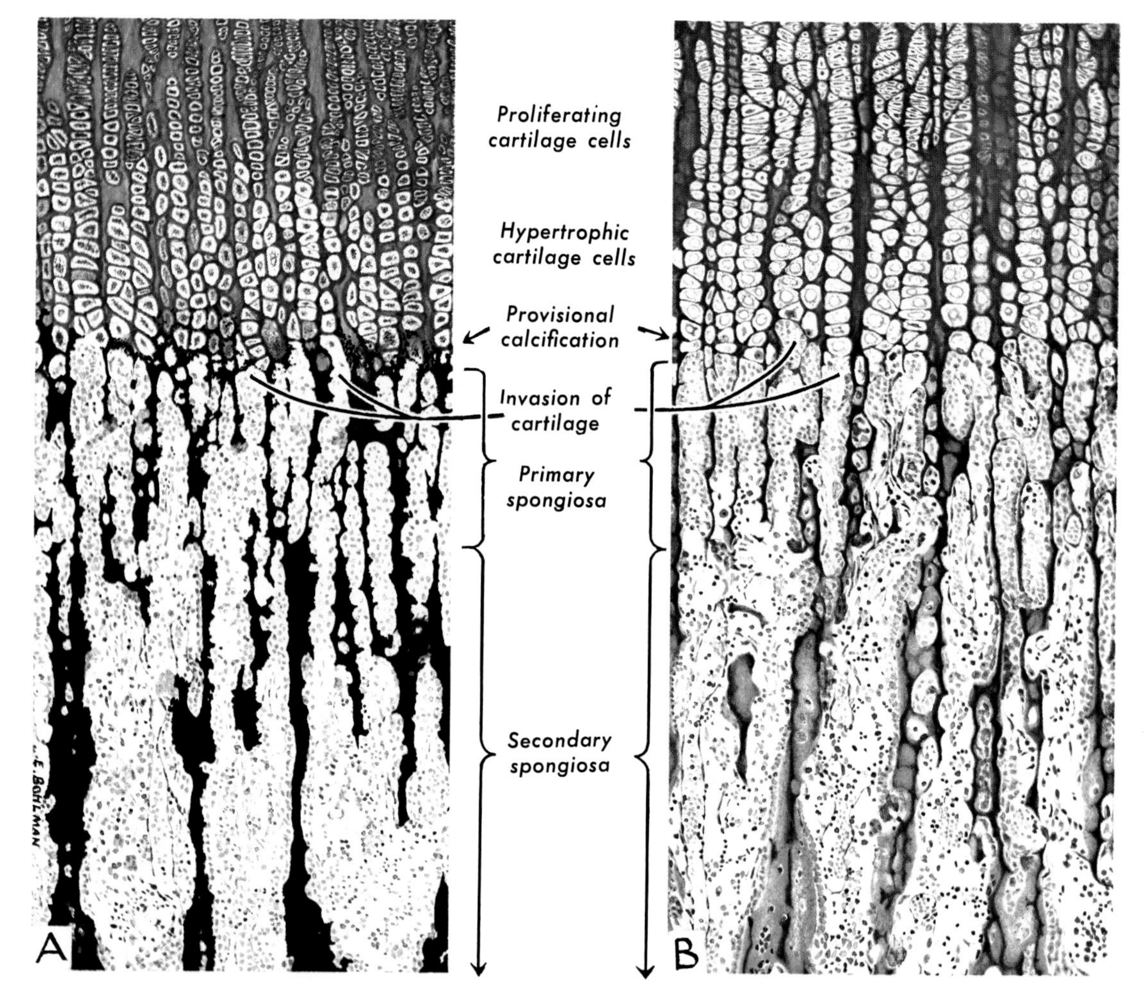

Figure 8–26. Endochondral ossification in longitudinal sections of the zone of epiphyseal growth of the distal end of the radius in a puppy. (A) Neutral formalin fixation, no decalcification, von Kossa and hematoxylin-eosin stains. All deposits of bone salt are stained black; thus, bone and calcified cartilage matrix stain alike. (B) Zenker-formol fixation, specimen decalcified, and stained with hematoxylin-eosin-azure II. Persisting cores of cartilage matrix in the trabeculae of bone take a deep blue or purple stain, whereas the bone matrix stains red. It is not possible with this method to see where calcium has been deposited.

As persuasive as the evidence is for this hypothesis, it does not explain the absence of calcification in many other collagen-rich tissues. Moreover, the heavily mineralized matrix of tooth enamel contains a very different protein, so it is evident that collagen cannot be the only initiator of calcification.

As detailed in Chapter 7, much attention has been devoted in recent years to *matrix vesicles* as possible initiators of calcification. These vesicles bud off from the hypertrophied cartilage cells and are rich in an alkaline phosphatase that is responsive to vitamin D, a vitamin essential for bone mineralization. Hydroxyapatite crystals are said to be deposited in these matrix vesicles, which then break down liberating mineral into the matrix. In the zone of proliferation where the matrix does not calcify, the chondrocytes also produce matrix vesicles but these differ from those in the zone of hypertrophy, in their enzymatic activity and responsiveness to vitamin D. This proposed mechanism of calcification now has many advocates, but how the vesicles move some distance from the cells in a matrix that is a barrier, even for some macromolecules, remains to be explained. Moreover, no such vesicles have been reported, to date, in the calcification of dentine or enamel.

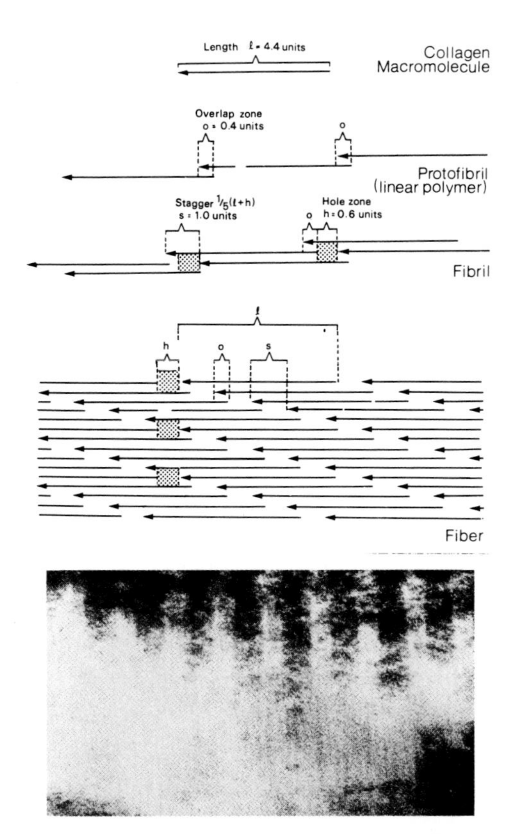

Figure 8–27. Diagram of the overlapping staggered arrangement of molecules in a collagen fiber showing the small discontinuities or holes that are thought to be the sites of nucleation of apatite crystals in the mineralization of bone. Bottom: a collagen fiber stained for bone salts suggests such a localization of the sites of initial mineralization. (Modified from Glimcher, M.J. and S.M. Crane. 1968. *In* B.S. Gould and G.N. Ramachandran, eds. A Treatise on Collagen. Vol. II. New York, Academic Press.

GROWTH IN DIAMETER OF LONG BONES

As indicated in the foregoing section, growth in length of long bones is dependent on proliferation of cartilage cells. However, growth in diameter of the diaphysis is the result of appositional deposition of membrane bone beneath the periosteum. The diaphysis of the original cartilage model is later removed in the progressive enlargement of the marrow cavity, and the bone constituting the shaft of a fully developed long bone is entirely the product of subperiosteal intramembranous ossification.

After establishment of the primary ossification center, the ends of the cartilage model continue to elongate and broaden by interstitial proliferation of chondrocytes and elaboration of new matrix. Such interstitial growth is not possible in the diaphysis where the cartilage has been replaced by bone. To keep pace with the interstitial growth of the cartilaginous epiphyses and maintain the shape of the developing bone, there is a progressive thickening of the periosteal collar that was formed around the middle of the diaphysis at the onset of endochondral ossification. This results in deposition of a lattice of trabeculae of woven bone around the diaphysis.

In skeletal development, resorption of bone is as important as bone deposition. The laying down of new bone on the outside of the shaft is accompanied by the appearance of osteoclasts on its inner aspect to resorb bone and enlarge the marrow cavity. The rates of external apposition of new bone and of internal resorption are such that the diameter of the cylindrical diaphysis expands rapidly with a relatively slow increase in thickness of its wall.

The extent of the contribution of subperiosteal bone deposition to bone development is seldom fully appreciated because evidence of the original topographical distribution of endochondral and intramembranous ossification is erased by the continual internal resorption and reorganization that takes place in later stages of development. It is informative, therefore, to examine developing long bones of the manatee, an aquatic mammal in which resorption of bone to form a marrow cavity does not take place. In fetal bones of this species (Figs. 8–28 and 8–29), the primary spongiosa of endochondral bone has a characteristic hour-glass distribution. The two conical regions with their apices meeting at the site of the original ossification center, result from the interstitial growth in length and breadth of the epiphyseal ends of the cartilage model. The area between the diverging sides of the two cones is filled by a thick collar of trabeculae of periosteal origin. Manatee bones, lacking the capacity for bone resorption, that forms the marrow cavity in other species, provide an instructive view of the basic topography of the endochondral and intramembranous components of mammalian long bones, in general (Fig. 8–29).

SURFACE REMODELING OF BONES

Although growing bones are continuously changing their internal organization, they retain approximately the same external form

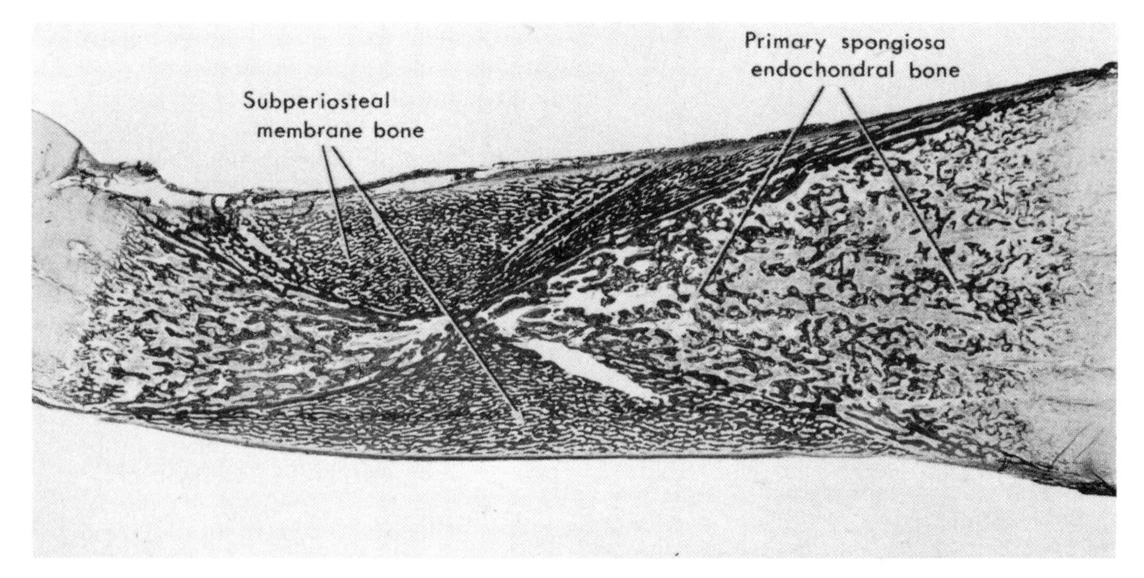

Figure 8–28. Photomicrograph of the humerus of a fetal manatee in longitudinal section. In this species, long bones lack a marrow cavity, and the respective contributions of subperiosteal and endochondral bone to the formation of the shaft are more evident than in the bones of other species where these topographical relationships are obscured by bone resorption to create a marrow cavity. (After Fawcett, D.W. 1942. Am. J. Anat. 71:271.)

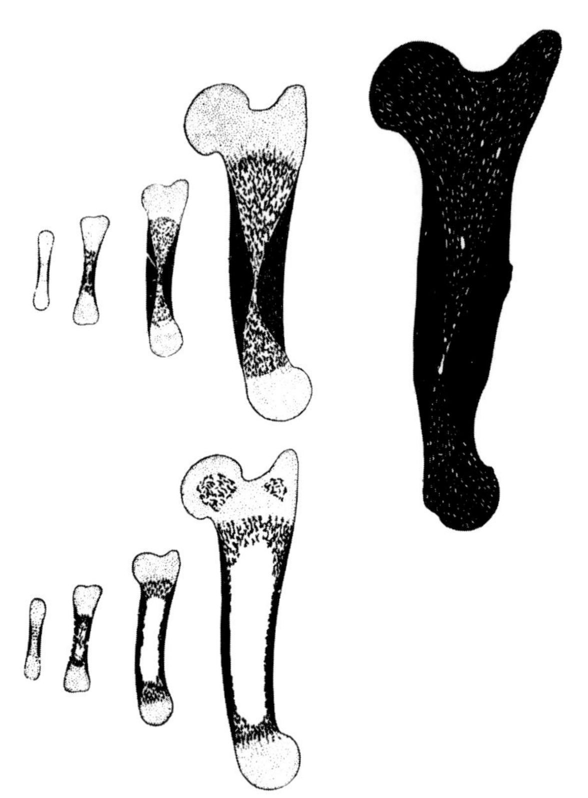

Figure 8–29. Diagrammatic representation of the development of a manatee humerus (top) compared to that of a typical mammal (bottom). (After Fawcett, D.W. 1942. Am. J. Anat. 71:271.)

from an early fetal stage into adult life. It is obvious this would not be so if new bone were deposited at a uniform rate at all points beneath the periosteum. Instead, the shape of a bone is maintained during growth by a continual remodeling or sculpturing of its surface, which involves bone deposition under some areas of the periosteum and bone absorption in other areas. That this is true was demonstrated in the middle of the eighteenth century by experiments in which animals were fed on madder-root. Bone deposited during the period of madder feeding was stained red, whereas areas that were stable or undergoing resorption remained unstained. It was clear that some areas of the surface of long bones were stained, whereas others were not. The findings of these early experiments in vital staining of bone have since been confirmed and extended with newer techniques employing bone-seeking isotopes or the fluorescent antibiotic tetracycline, both of which are deposited preferentially in newly deposited bone.

Typical of such experiments are those localizing the sites of osteogenesis in the growing rat tibia (Fig. 8–30). This bone supports a large articular surface and the epiphysis is considerably broader than the shaft. Thus, it is possible to recognize a cylindrical region in the middle of the shaft and conical regions toward the ends where it expands to the width

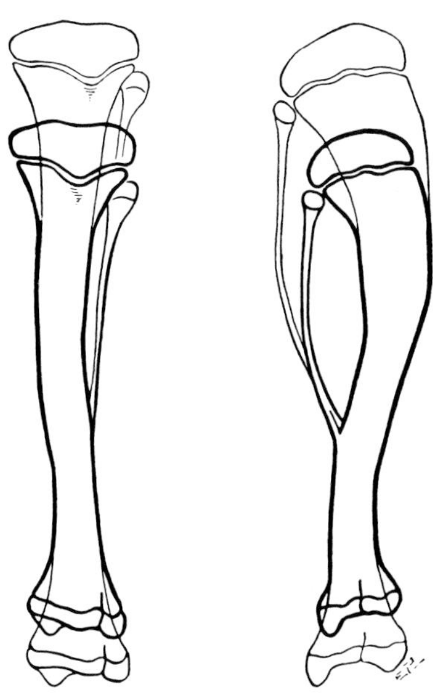

Figure 8–30. Diagram to illustrate the remodeling occurring during the growth of the tibia and fibula of the rat, viewed from anterior and in lateral profile. (After Wolbach.)

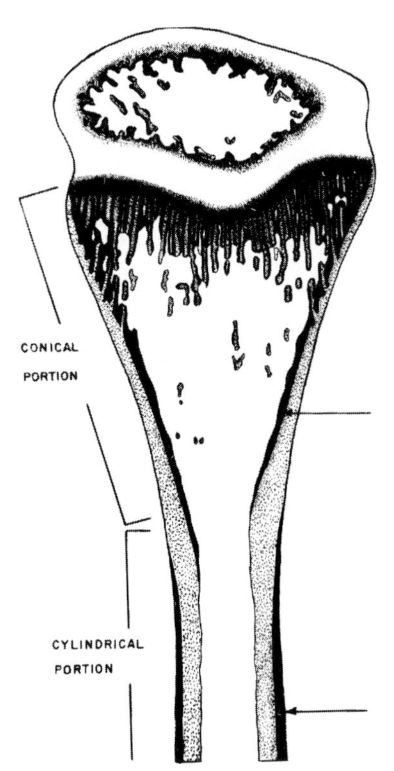

Figure 8–31. Diagram based on an autoradiograph of the head of the tibia of a growing rat killed a few hours after receiving an injection of ^{32}P. The localization of high concentrations of silver grains in the autoradiograph is shown here in black. In addition to the new bone in the epiphysis and at the metaphysis, bone is being deposited under the endosteum in the conical portion of the bone, and beneath the periosteum in the cylindrical portion of the shaft (at arrows). (Drawing based on studies of Leblond, C.P. et al. 1950. Am. J. Anat. 86:289. After Fawcett, D.W. 1954. *In* R.O. Greep, ed. Histology. Philadelphia, Blakiston Co. Reproduced by permission of McGraw-Hill Book Co.)

of the epiphysis. If a bone-seeking isotope is given to a growing rat and autoradiographs are then made of longitudinal sections of the tibia, the sites of new bone formation are disclosed by the distribution of silver grains in the overlying photographic emulsion. In the conical region of the bone, the silver grains are aligned immediately subjacent to the *endosteum,* whereas in the cylindrical portion of the shaft, they are found beneath the *periosteum* (Fig. 8–31). Study of parallel histological sections reveals numerous osteoclasts beneath the periosteum of the conical region and beneath the endosteum of the cylindrical shaft. Thus, it is clear that in the surface remodeling of this bone the periosteum plays opposite roles in neighboring regions of the same bone. Subperiosteal bone deposition is occurring in the cylindrical shaft while subperiosteal bone resorption is taking place in the conical region. Similarly, bone is being formed at the endosteal surface of the conical region and absorbed on the inner aspect of the cylinder. As a result of these activities, the midportion of the shaft is expanding radially and its marrow cavity is being enlarged. As the bone, as a whole, is elongating by growth at the epiphyseal plate, the diverging walls of the conical region of the shaft is being straightened by bone deposition on its inner surface and absorption on its outer surface. It is, thus, contributing, at its lower end, to the lengthening of the cylindrical portion of the shaft while maintaining the same general shape of the bone.

In the skull vault, the assumption that growth of the flat bones at the sutures alone could account for the enlargement of the cranial cavity to accommodate the growing brain is flawed because as the radius of curvature of the growing skull vault increases, the bones become less convex. Therefore, not only must bone resorption take place on the inside of the calvarium concurrently with bone deposition on its outer surface, but the rates of deposition and absorption must differ from the center to the periphery of each cranial bone to account for its flattening as the radius of curvature of the skull vault increases. How these local variations in the function of the endosteum and periosteum are controlled in space and time so as to mold and shape the bone constantly during its growth is a fascinating unsolved problem in morphogenesis.

INTERNAL REORGANIZATION OF BONE

The conversion from the primary lattice of trabeculae produced by intramembranous ossification into compact bone is attributable to thickening of the trabeculae and the progressive encroachment of bone on the perivascular spaces. As this process advances, bone is deposited in ill-defined layers containing randomly oriented collagen fibers, but because these layers are disposed more-or-less concentrically around the vascular channels, they bear a superficial resemblance to haversian systems. They are sometimes called *primitive haversian systems,* but they should be clearly distinguished from the more precisely ordered lamellar systems comprising the *definitive haversian systems* of adult bone. The latter are first formed only during the internal reorganization of primary compact bone that is referred to as *secondary bone formation.*

In this process, cavities appear in the primary compact bone as a result of local osteoclast activity. Such *absorption cavities* are enlarged by continuing osteoclastic activity to form long cylindrical cavities which are invaded by blood vessels growing out from the embryonic bone marrow. When the cavities reach considerable length, bone absorption ceases and the osteoclasts are replaced by osteoblasts that begin to deposit concentric lamellae of bone on the wall of the cylindrical cavity until it is filled in to form a typical haversian system. The lamellae of this and subsequent generations of haversian systems have the ordered arrangement of collagen fibers, with changing orientation in successive layers, that is characteristic of the osteons of adult bone. In the human, from the age of one year onward, only lamellar bone of this character is deposited within the shafts of long bones, and this secondary bone eventually replaces all of the primitive haversian systems (Fig. 8–32).

The outer limits of secondary haversian systems are defined by distinct *cement lines,* which are a layer of uncalcified matrix laid down whenever a period of resorption is followed by new bone formation. Cement lines are collagen-poor, have staining properties differing from other layers of matrix, and they are not traversed by canaliculi.

Internal bone resorption and reconstruction do not end with the replacement of primary by secondary bone, but continue actively throughout life. Resorption cavities continue to appear and to be filled in by third, fourth, and higher orders of haversian systems (Fig. 8–32). The *interstitial lamellae* of adult bone represent persisting fragments of earlier generations of haversian systems that have been largely removed in the course of the continuing internal reorganization. Thus, in crosssections of adult bone, one may see (1) mature osteons in which rebuilding activity has come to an end; (2) actively forming new osteons; and (3) absorption cavities being hollowed out in preparation for formation of new osteons.

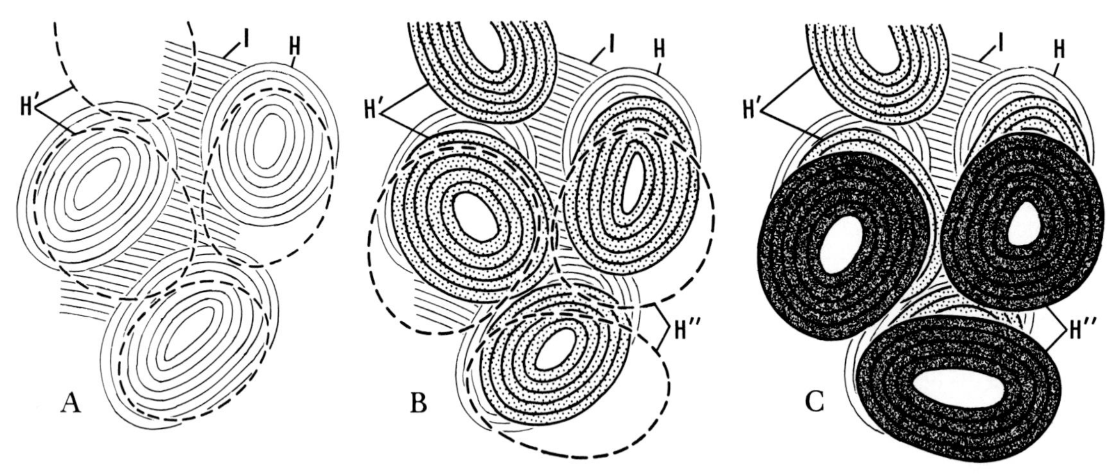

Figure 8–32. Diagram of stages in formation of three successive generations of haversian systems. The areas outlined by dotted lines in (A) are removed by osteoclasts, and replaced by deposition of new haversian systems (B) (stippled). Portions of these, outlined by dotted lines are, in turn, absorbed and the cylindrical cavities so formed are filled in to form a third generation of haversian systems (C) (heavily stippled). H, H′, and H″ successive generations of haversian systems, I, interstitial lamellae.

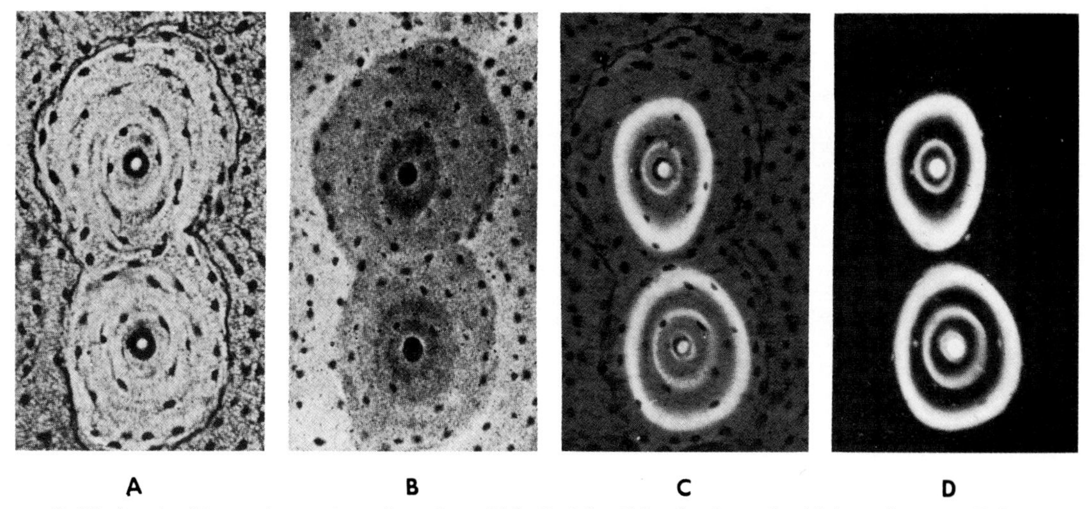

Figure 8–33. A pair of haversian systems from the midshaft of the tibia of a 9-month-old dog, given two 5-day courses of treatment with a tetracycline, separated by an interval of 19 days. (A) Ordinary microscopy; (B) historadiogram; (C) and (D) fluorescence microscopy. The bone deposited during the treatments fluoresces and the design of this experiment permits one to visualize the amount of bone deposited in each 5-day period. Of particular interest is the fact that the inner fluorescent band, corresponding to the second period of administration, is narrower than the first, demonstrating that there is a slowing down of the rate of concentric bone deposition as the formation of the haversian system progresses. (Courtesy of R. Amprino.)

The rate of new bone formation can be determined by administration of tetracycline at two different times and measurement of the thickness between the two labeled bands of bone (Fig. 8–33). Such studies show that about 1 μm per day is a fair average for the human. For any given haversian system, the rate of deposition slows as the osteon nears completion. The formation time of an haversian system in the adult is 4–5 weeks. Different values are obtained in young growing bone and in pathological states. The newly deposited lamellar bone continues to calcify over a considerable period of time after the osteon is completed. A historadiogram of the bone, therefore, reveals a mixture of haversian systems of varying age, displaying all degrees of mineralization (Fig. 8–34). With this continuous turnover, the organism is assured a continuing supply of new bone to meet its skeletal and metabolic requirements. It also provides the plasticity that enables bone to alter its internal architecture to adapt to new mechanical stresses.

REPAIR OF BONE

In the formation of intramembranous bone in the embryo, mesenchymal cells in primitive connective tissue are transformed into osteoprogenitor cells and ultimately into osteoblasts. The osteogenic potential of these cells, having been expressed in embryonic life, can be evoked again even after the cells have been quiescent for an indefinite period. After a bone fracture in postnatal life, the blood clot formed at the site is soon organized by formation of granulation tissue which condenses into connective tissue and later into a *fibrocartilaginous callus* between the bone fragments. At the same time, previously quiescent cells in the periosteum are reactivated by the trauma and begin to deposit new bone that contributes to formation of the *bony callus,* a meshwork of trabeculae of woven bone that will ultimately bridge the gap between the fragments. A similar activation of cells of the endosteum results in deposition of bone around the fibrocartilaginous callus which is slowly eroded and replaced by bone. The spongy bone, then uniting the fragments, is transformed over the next few weeks into compact bone by continuing osteoblastic deposition of bone which gradually obliterates the interstices among the trabeculae. Subsequent resorption of excess bone reestablishes continuity of the marrow cavity and restores normal surface contours to the bone.

Many attempts have been made to utilize the osteogenic potentialities of periosteum and bone by transplantation of these tissues to sites where bone formation is desired. The fruit of these efforts is the modern "bone bank" which supplies fragments of bone, preserved by freezing or other means, for use in orthopedic procedures. Transplants of bone from the same individual (autografts) are usu-

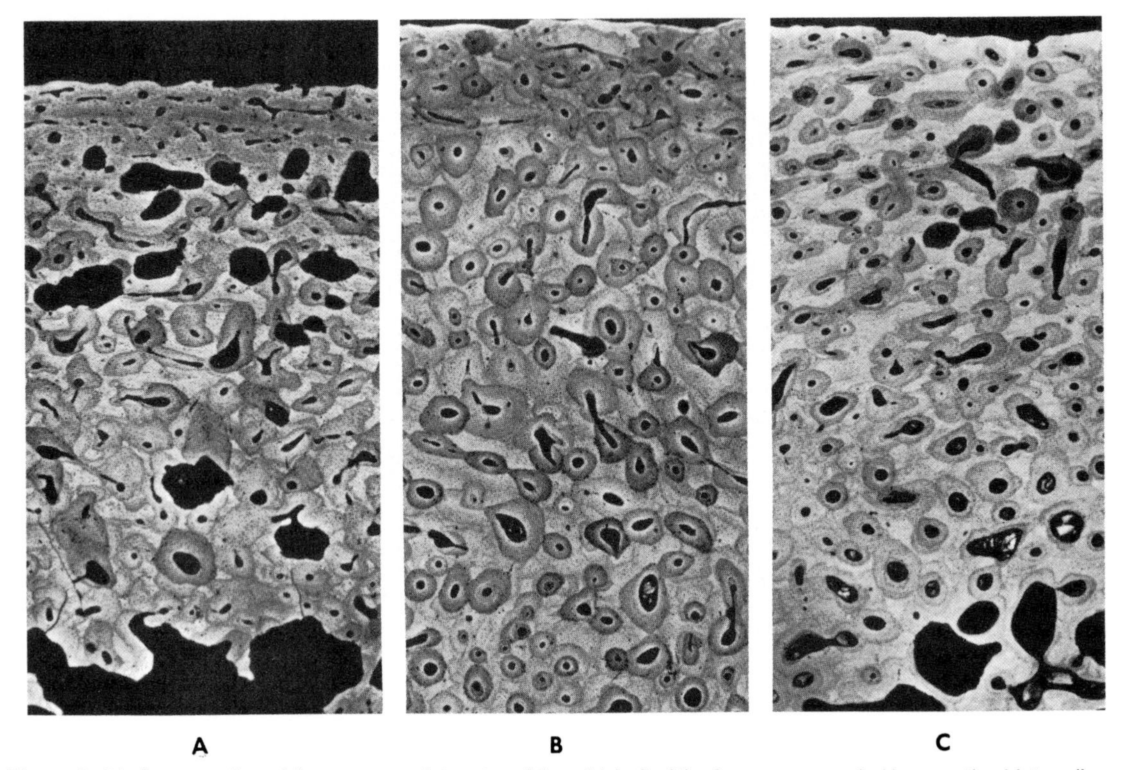

Figure 8–34. Cross section of the anteromedial sector of the midshaft of the femur, as revealed by negative historadiography: (A) at age 7; (B) at age 20; (C) at age 65. Note that in the child (A), there are large resorption cavities (black) and large irregularly shaped haversian systems. Large remanents of periosteal primary bone are found in the interstices between the secondary osteons, in the middle zone of the compacta. These remanents are fewer and smaller in the older perimedullary zone at the bottom of the figure. In the 20-year-old man (B), the compacta is much thicker. Secondary haversian systems and remanents of primary bone persist in the subperiosteal zone. Elsewhere, the osteons are fairly regular in outline and are separated by remanents of preexisting osteons. (Courtesy of R. Amprino.)

ally quite successful. Transplants of bone from another individual of the same species (homografts) often induce an immune response that leads to their rejection. Transplants of bone from another species (heterografts) do not survive. However, if calf bone is refrigerated and stored for some time, it seems to lose some of its antigenicity and may be suitable for use by bone banks. Even if such grafts do not survive, they seem to have a favorable influence on activation of bone formation by the cells of the host. These observations suggest that bone itself may contain a substance capable of inducing osteogenesis, but until very recently, attempts to isolate it have been unsuccessful.

ECTOPIC BONE FORMATION

Under certain conditions, bone is formed in connective tissue that is not associated with bone. This *ectopic ossification* has been reported in such diverse locations as the pelvis of the kidney, the walls of arteries, and in muscles and tendons. In the long tendons in the legs of chickens and turkeys, bone formation is a common occurrence. It has been inferred from this that connective tissue in some sites contains cells with latent osteogenic potentialities that are not normally expressed. This can be verified by experiment.

It has long been known, for example, that bone can be induced by implanting demineralized bone matrix or bladder epithelium into connective tissue. Chemotaxis of cells to the site is followed by their proliferation and differentiation. Cartilage is first formed and then replaced by bone, as in normal ossification. Within 2 weeks, a small ossicle is formed that contains hemopoietic bone marrow. Repeated attempts to isolate an osteoinductive component from bone matrix have recently met with some success. In one procedure, extraction of 40 kg of bovine bone powder yields about 40 μg of a highly purified fraction designated *bone morphogenetic proteins* (BMP). Further reduction yields several polypeptides, BMP-1,

BMP-2A, BMP-2B, and BMP-3. Of these, BMP-2A and BMP-2B induce endochondral bone formation in rats. Another extraction procedure has isolated *osteogenin,* a glycoprotein in the size range 28–43 kD that is capable of initiating ectopic bone formation. The exact structure and mechanism of action of these factors are subjects of current research.

It is increasingly apparent that bone formation involves the interaction of multiple regulatory substances. After induction of osteogenesis, the process is promoted and maintained by several *growth factors* that are not confined to bone. Among these is the *transforming growth factor-β,* (TGF-β), an ubiquitous 25 kD peptide originally described as a mitogen for fibroblasts, but later found to be present in highest concentration in bone and in blood platelets. After injury to soft tissues, release of this peptide from platelets stimulates the formation of granulation tissue and accelerates the healing process. It seems to have a similar role in the healing of bone fractures, inducing proliferation and further differentiation of periosteal and endosteal osteoprogenitor cells. This growth factor has been localized immunocytochemically in chondrocytes and osteoblasts and has been shown to stimulate synthesis of matrix components by these cells. Because these cell types both produce and are stimulated by TGF-β, it is considered to be an important *autocrine* growth factor in bone formation.

HISTOPHYSIOLOGY OF BONE

As the principal component of the skeletal system, bone supports the soft tissues of the body; it carries the articulations and provides attachment for the muscles involved in locomotion; and it forms a rigid covering for protection of the nervous system and the hemopoietic tissue. In addition to these mechanical functions, it has an important role as a very large reservoir of calcium and phosphate that can be drawn on to maintain the normal levels of these elements in the blood and to provide for the mineral requirements of other tissues.

BONE AS A STORE OF MOBILIZABLE CALCIUM

The importance of calcium cannot be overemphasized. Calcium ions are essential for the activity of many enzymes and for many other intracellular functions. It is required for maintenance of cell cohesion and in the regulation of membrane permeability. It is required in coagulation of the blood, contraction of smooth and striated muscle, and numerous other vital functions in the body. It is not surprising, therefore, that homeostatic mechanisms have evolved to maintain the plasma calcium concentration, with remarkable constancy, in a range of 9–11 mg/100 ml.

Most of the calcium in the body (99%) is stored in bone as hydroxyapatite crystals, but as much as 1% of the calcium of bone is in the form of more readily mobilizable salts and there is a constant exchange of calcium ions between the blood and bone. Diffusion and simple equilibrium between blood and the labile fraction of bone mineral is adequate to maintain a low calcium level (~7 mg/100 ml) in the plasma. Not all of the bone contributes to this exchange. The most labile calcium is located in the recently formed and incompletely mineralized osteons. It is these that are most sensitive to ionic variations in the body fluids. The continual remodeling of the adult skeleton provides a pool of young osteons that can respond to homeostatic regulation, releasing or taking up calcium. As these osteons mature and become more heavily mineralized, their calcium becomes less available to the interstitial fluids and blood plasma. These older osteons contribute more to the mechanical function of bone than to its metabolic function.

The principal mechanism for maintaining the blood calcium level involves the resorption of bone by osteoclasts. The cells of the parathyroid gland are sensitive to changes in the level of blood calcium. When it falls significantly below normal, their secretion of parathyroid hormone is increased. The hormone acts on osteoblasts to suppress their deposition of bone and induce their secretion of the *osteoclast-stimulating factor.* The activated osteoclasts then resorb bone, releasing calcium to restore the normal blood level. Conversely, if the blood calcium concentration becomes too high, secretion of parathyroid hormone is suppressed and the continuing deposition of bone by the osteoblasts soon brings the calcium level down to normal.

It has been argued that parathyroid hormone-stimulated osteoclastic activity could not account for the rapidity of the response to a metabolic need for calcium, and other explanations have been sought. The early response was formerly attributed to retrieval of calcium from bone by the process of osteocytic osteolysis, referred to previously, but this has now fallen into disfavor for lack of compelling evidence. A satisfactory explanation of the rapid mobilization of calcium has not been forthcoming. Possibly involved are other functions of parathyroid hormone, such as its action on the kidney, promoting enhanced resorption of calcium from the glomerular filtrate or its stimulation of increased production of a vitamin-D metabolite, *1,25-dihydrocholecalciferol,* which accelerates calcium absorption by the intestine. There is no doubt, however, that quantitatively, the most important mechanism is activation of bone resorption by osteoclasts.

The response of the parathyroid and of the bones to the body's need for circulating calcium is most dramatic in those species that have periodic unusual demands for calcium. The most familiar example is the laying cycle of birds, during which large amounts of calcium are required in the oviduct for deposition of the egg shell. To meet this need, many trabeculae of cancellous bone in the marrow cavities are resorbed, only to be reformed after that egg is laid, and again removed to provide shell for the next egg in the clutch. Less dramatic examples of mobilization of calcium from the skeleton are also observed in mammals. During the growth of deer antlers, there is a slight rarification of bone throughout the skeleton, and in dairy cows producing large volumes of milk there may be a detectable osteoporosis. In the human, there is no doubt some withdrawal of calcium from the maternal skeleton during pregnancy and lactation to provide for calcification of the bones of the baby, but in normal females, this does not result in radiologically demonstrable changes. However, superimposition of pregnancy and prolonged lactation on nutritional deficiency or impaired intestinal absorption of calcium may lead to decalcification so severe as to result in pathological fractures.

In addition to the direct effect of parathyroid hormone on bone, the hormone acts on the kidney, increasing the rate of reabsorption of calcium ions in the proximal tubules and concurrently decreasing the reabsorption of phosphate ions. These renal effects of parathyroid hormone prevent a continual loss of calcium in the urine that would ultimately result in depletion of the calcium content of bone.

The polypeptide hormone *calcitonin* has an effect opposite to that of parathyroid hormone. A *rise* in the plasma concentration of calcium stimulates release of calcitonin just as a *fall* in plasma calcium induces increased secretion of parathyroid hormone. Calcitonin is produced by the parafollicular cells of the thyroid gland and acts directly on the osteoclasts to inhibit bone resorption. These multinucleated cells have numerous receptors for the hormone on their surface. The presence of surface receptors for calcitonin is a useful marker for the mononuclear precursors of osteoclasts which are difficult to identify by morphological criteria alone.

EFFECTS OF OTHER HORMONES ON BONE

Although parathyroid hormone is principally concerned with calcium homeostasis, other hormones have significant effects on skeletal growth and bone remodeling. The growth hormone of the pituitary gland, *somatotrophin,* has a major influence on skeletal development. A deficiency of the hormone in children results in dwarfism. An excess of the hormone prior to epiphyseal closure results in gigantism. In adults, excessive secretion of somatrophin leads to the unsightly deformities characteristic of the condition called *acromegaly.* Remodeling of adult bone normally involves a controlled coupling of new bone formation to bone resorption with little or no net change in bone mass. In acromegaly, the rate of bone deposition exceeds that of bone resorption, resulting in local thickening of some bones, particularly those of the face. There is an accompanying soft tissue enlargement that contributes to the cosmetic disfigurement.

The gonadal hormones, *estrogens* and *androgens,* influence the rate of skeletal maturation. The time of fusion of the epiphyses with the diaphysis of long bones is normally remarkably constant. The progress of these events at any given time is closely related to the developmental state of the reproductive system. Thus, in cases of precocious sexual development, skeletal maturation is accelerated and growth is stunted owing to premature epiphyseal closure. On the other hand, in individuals with testicular hypoplasia, epiphyseal union is delayed and the arms and legs become disproportionately long. The basis of the linkage between gonadal development and skeletal maturation is still not well understood.

The influence of ovarian hormones, *estrogens,* is of clinical interest because of the prevalence of *osteoporosis* in aging women. After age

40, some loss of bone mass begins in both sexes at a rate of 0.3–0.5% a year. This becomes a more serious problem in women when the production of estrogen declines in the years immediately following menopause. The rate of bone loss may then increase to 2–3% a year. Nearly one-third of women who live into their late 80s will have had fractures of the hip or of vertebrae due, in part, to the fragility of their osteoporotic bones. This age-dependent loss of bone mass is attributed to continuing osteoclastic activity combined with a failure of osteoblasts to completely fill the resorption cavities. Evidence for estrogen receptors on osteoblasts has been elusive but it has recently been shown that 17β-estradiol stimulates osteoblast proliferation in vitro and increases the steady-state level of mRNA encoding the α1-chain of type-I collagen. Thus, it appears that estrogen stimulates bone formation by direct action on osteoblasts. Postmenopausal osteoporosis is no doubt due to decline in the anabolic functions of osteoblasts. Administration of exogenous estrogens slows or arrests bone loss.

NUTRITIONAL EFFECTS ON BONE

Growth of the skeleton is dependent on several nutritional factors. Deficiencies of dietary mineral or essential vitamins are often more easily detectable in the structure of the bones than in other tissues. A gross dietary deficiency of calcium or phosphorus leads to a rarification of the bones and increased risk of fractures. Even when the intake of these minerals is adequate, a deficiency of *vitamin D* in children may lead to *rickets.* In this condition, ossification of epiphyseal cartilages is disturbed, the regular columnar arrangement of cartilage cells in the epiphyseal plate disappears, and the metaphysis becomes a disordered mixture of uncalcified cartilage and poorly calcified bone matrix. Such bones become deformed by weight-bearing. A prolonged deficiency of calcium and vitamin D in adults leads to accumulation of an excessive proportion of uncalcified osteoid. This condition called osteomalacia or *adult rickets* is aggravated by pregnancy. The diminished calcium content of the bones is due to the failure of newly deposited bone to calcify in the course of bone remodeling.

Endogenous vitamin D (cholecalciferol) is formed by ultraviolet irradiation of a precursor in the synthesis of cholesterol in the skin. More than a dozen metabolites of the vitamin have been identified, but the majority of its biological effects are attributed to a single metabolite, 1,25-$(OH)_2$D3 (calcitriol), a steroid hormone. Its principal site of action is in the intestinal mucosa, where it stimulates synthesis of a calcium-binding protein in the brush border that is involved in the transport of calcium across the epithelium. This protein is essential to the uptake of sufficient calcium to sustain bone growth. 1,25-$(OH)_2$D3 also has direct effects on bone, binding to receptors on osteoclasts. It is believed to complement the action of parathyroid hormone on bone resorption. The effects of this steroid are more widespread than previously realized. Studies using radiolabeled hormone have disclosed the presence of receptors for it on B-cells of the pancreatic islets, the somato-mammotrophs of the pituitary, C-cells of the thyroid, cells of the parathyroid, and smooth and cardiac muscle fibers.

Deficiency of vitamin C leads to profound changes in tissues of mesenchymal origin, resulting in the condition known as *scurvy* or *scorbutus* in which the primary defect is an inability to produce and maintain the intercellular substance of connective tissues. In the case of bone, it results in deficient production of collagen and bone matrix, with consequent retardation of growth and delayed healing of fractures.

Deficiency of vitamin A results in a slowing in the rate of growth of the skeleton. This vitamin controls the activity, distribution, and coordination of osteoblasts and osteoclasts during development. Among other effects, resorption and remodeling fail to enlarge the cranial cavity and spinal canal at a rate sufficient to accommodate growth of the brain and spinal cord. Serious damage to the central nervous system, therefore, results. In hypervitamin A, on the other hand, erosion of the cartilage columns accelerates without a compensatory increase in the rate of multiplication of the cells in the proliferative zone. The epiphyseal plates may, therefore, be completely obliterated, and growth may cease prematurely.

JOINTS AND SYNOVIAL MEMBRANES

Bones are joined together at *joints* or *articulations* of several kinds. The bones of the skull interdigitate and are connected by the *sutural ligament,* a thin intervening layer of dense connective tissue that permits no movement. In the vertebral articulations, the successive vertebrae are joined by *intervertebral discs* of dense connective tissue and cartilage that permit slight movement. In joints in the limbs, the ends of the bones are covered by cartilage and surrounded by a *joint capsule* that permits a rather wide range of movement. Joints in which there is little or no motion are called *synarthroses.* Within this category, those in which bone connects directly with bone are called *synostoses.* Those in which the bones are connected by cartilage are *synchondroses.* Those in which the connection is connective tissue are *syndesmoses.* Joints that permit free movement of the bones are called *diarthroses* (Fig. 8–35).

In diarthroses, the articular surfaces of the bones are covered with hyaline cartilage and enclosed in a *joint capsule.* The capsule is composed of an outer *fibrous layer* of dense connective tissue that is continuous with the periosteum of the bones and an inner *synovial layer* (*synovium*) about 25 μm thick, which is more cellular (Fig. 8–36). The latter is sometimes referred to as the *synovial membrane,* but this term is misleading in that it suggests an epithelial lining such as that found in other body cavities. There is no continuous cellular lining. Over most of its surface, connective tissue of the synovium is directly exposed to the synovial fluid in the joint cavity (Figs. 8–37 and 8–38). Two kinds of cells are found on or near the surface: fibroblast-like cells that secrete the collagen, protoglycans, and other components of the interstitium, and macrophages that clear any debris from wear-and-tear within the joint. Lymphocytes are present, in limited numbers, deeper in the synovium.

Where the synovium covers intraarticular ligaments and tendons or lines parts of the joint subject to considerable strain, it rests directly on the fibrous layer. Elsewhere, it is separated from it by loose connective tissue or adipose tissue. In these areas, folds or broad-based villi of synovium project into the joint cavity. These villi increase in size and number

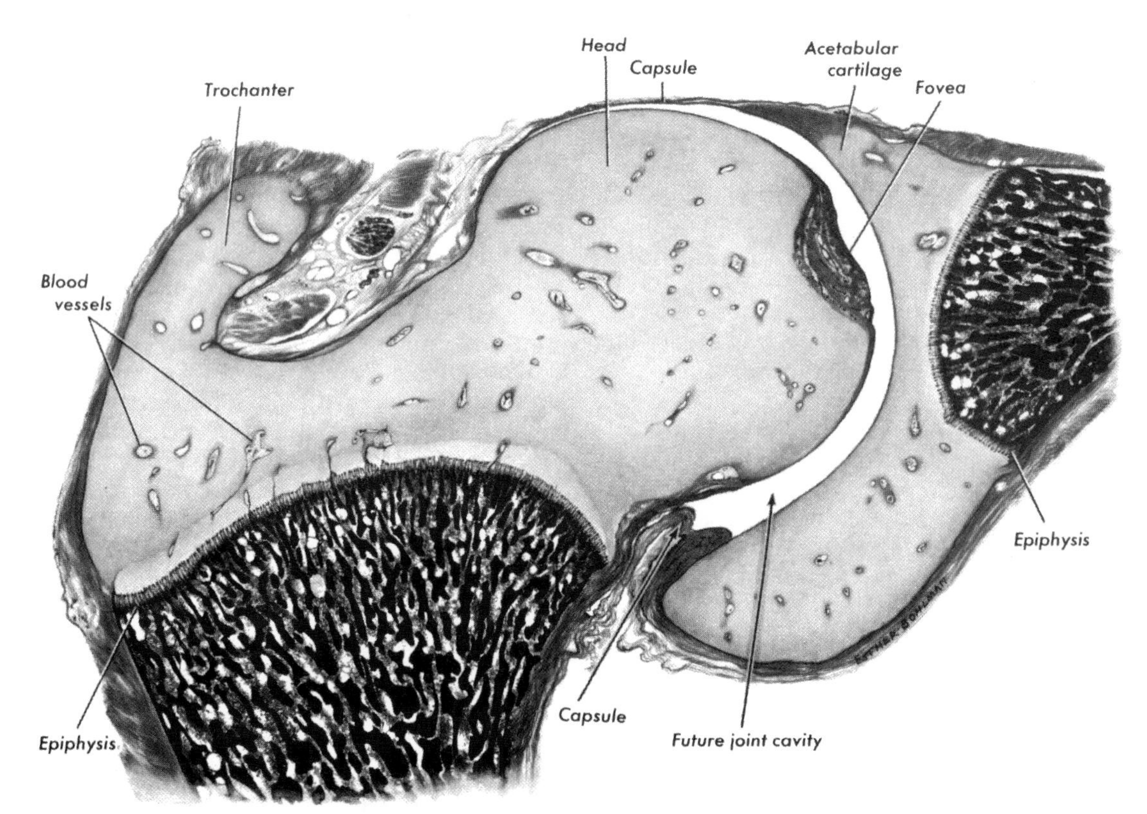

Figure 8–35. Section through the head of the femur and the conforming acetabulum of a human fetus (26 weeks). Both consist of hyaline cartilage at this stage but, in subsequent development, bone replaces the cartilage except for thin layers of cartilage that persist over the head and lining the acetabulum, forming the articular surfaces of the diarthrosis in postnatal life. (Preparation of H. Hatcher.)

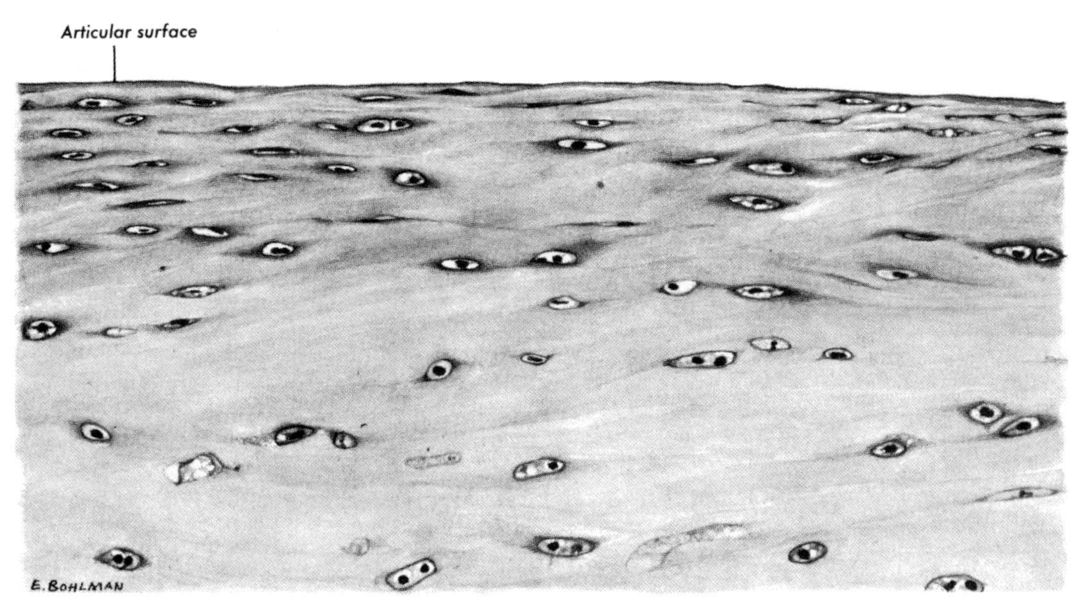

Figure 8–36. Histological section of articular cartilage of the femur, illustrating the flattening of the chondrocytes in planes parallel to the articular surface. (Preparation of H. Hatcher.)

with age, and islets of cartilage may form within them.

The synovium is highly vascular with a rich network of capillaries about 10 μm below the surface. About half of the capillaries have fenestrations, usually on the side toward the joint cavity. The synovial fluid is a transudate of water and solutes from the blood and, therefore, has a composition similar to that of the interstitial fluid of tissues in general. To this fluid are added *hyaluronate* and a glycoprotein, *lubricin,* both of which are molecules with lubricating properties. These are believed to be secreted by the fibroblast-like cells of the synovium. Also present in small amount are other glycoproteins that are normally found in cartilage where they stabilize the binding of proteoglycan monomers to hyaluronic acid

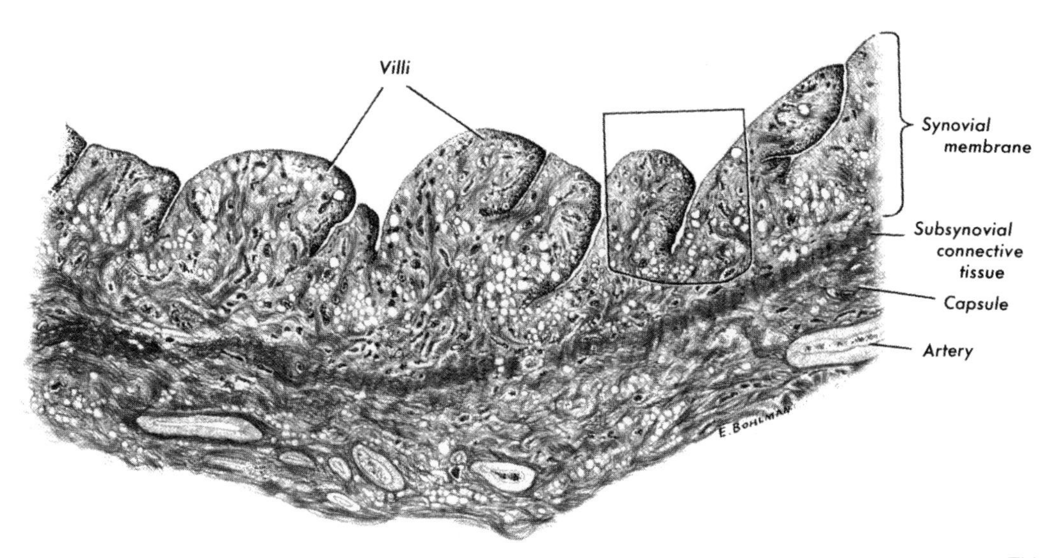

Figure 8–37. Section through the capsule of a knee joint, showing the villi and connective tissue components. This area outlined is shown at higher magnification in Fig. 8–38. (From a preparation by H. Hatcher.)

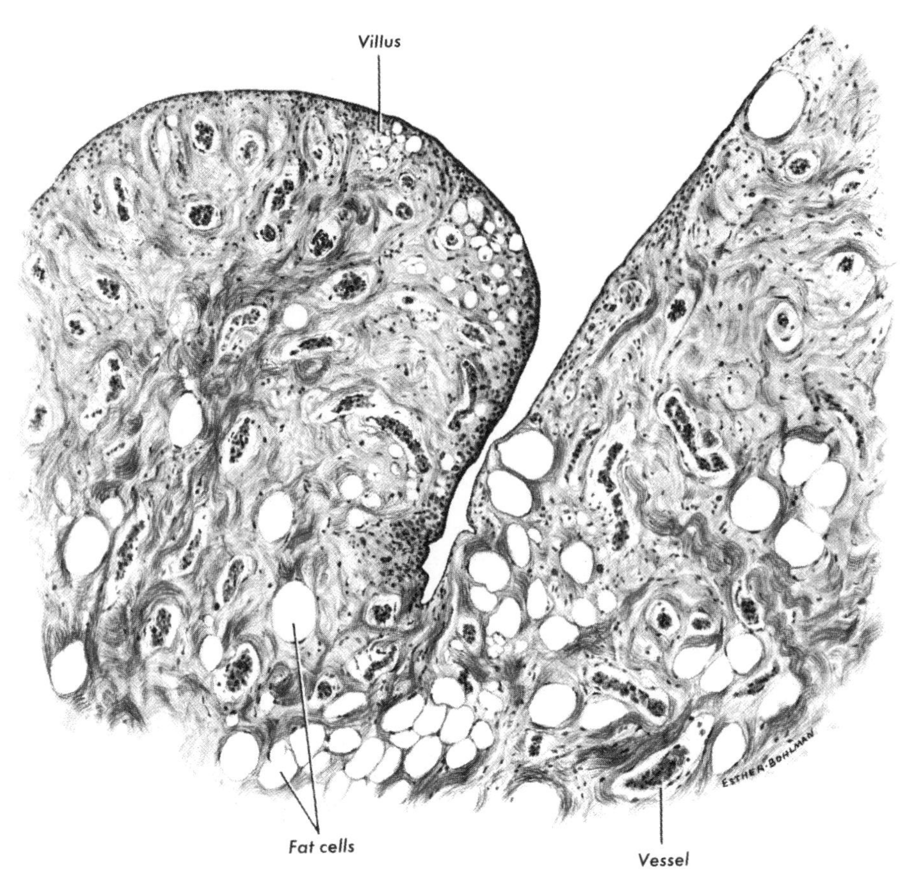

Figure 8–38. Synovial membrane of a young adult. Note the irregularity in concentration of cells toward the free surface of the villus and the irregular distribution of fat cells. (From a preparation by H. Hatcher.)

to form aggregates. These link proteins are synthesized by synovial cells in culture but their function, if any, in the synovial fluid is not known. A few lymphocytes and monocytes are found in the synovial fluid.

Exchange of fluid in diarthrodial joints depends on its continual renewal by transudation from the blood capillaries into the joint cavity and by its escape via transsynoveal movement of fluid and macromolecules to lymphatic capillaries, promoted by transient increases in pressure produced by intermittent flexion at the joint.

BIBLIOGRAPHY

GENERAL

Cohen, J. and W.H. Harris. 1958. The three dimensional anatomy of the haversian systems. J. Bone Joint Surg. 40A:419.

Cooper, R.R., J.W. Milgram, and R.A. Robertson. 1966. Morphology of the osteon. An electron microscopic study. J. Bone Joint Surg. 48A:1239.

Curtis, T.A., S.H. Ashrafi, and D. Weber. 1985. Canalicular communication in the cortices of human long bones. Anat. Rec. 212:336.

Holtrop, M.E. 1975. The ultrastructure of bone. Am. Clin. Lab. Sci. 5:264.

Jowsey, J. 1966. Studies of the haversian systems in man and some animals. J. Anat. 100:857.

Miller, E.J. and G.R. Martin. 1968. The collagen of bone. Clin. Orthop. 59:195.

HISTOGENESIS

Bernard, G.W. and D.C. Pease. 1969. An electron microscopic study of initial intramembranous osteogenesis. Am. J. Anat. 125:271.

Fawcett, D.W. 1942. The amedullary bones of the Florida manatee. Am. J. Anat. 71:271.

Glimcher, M.J. and S.M. Krane. 1968. The organization and structure of bone and the mechanism of calcification. *In* G.N. Ramachandran and B.S. Gould, eds. Treatise on Collagen II B: Biology of Collagen. London, Academic Press.

Glimcher, M.A., A.J. Hodge, and F.O. Schmitt. 1957. Macromolecular aggregation states in relation to mineralization: The collagen-hydroxyapatite system as studied in vitro. Proc. Nat. Acad. Sci. USA 43:860.

Leblond, C.P., G.W. Wilkinson, L.F. Belanger, and J. Robichon. 1950. Radioautographic visualization of bone formation in the rat. Am. J. Anat. 86:289.

McLean, F.C. and W. Bloom. 1940. Calcification and ossification: calcification in normal growing bone. Anat. Rec. 78:333.
Owen, M. 1978. Histogenesis of bone cells. Calcif. Tissue. Res. 25:205.
Scott, B.L. 1967. Thymidine-H electron microscopic radioautography of osteogenic cells in the fetal rat. J. Cell Biol. 35:115.
Whitson, S.W. 1972. Tight junction formation in the osteon. Clin. Orthoped. 86:206.
Young, R.W. 1962. Cell proliferation and specialization during endochondral osteogenesis in young rats. J. Cell Biol. 14:357.

REMODELING

Baron, R., L. Neff, D. Louvard, and P.J. Coutoy. 1985. Cell-mediated extracellular acidification and bone resorption: Evidence for a low pH in resorbing lacunae and localization of a 100 kD lysosomal membrane protein at the osteoclast ruffled border. J. Cell. Biol. 101:2210.
Belanger, L.F. 1969. Osteocytic osteolysis. Calcif. Tissue. Res. 4:1.
Bloom, W., M.A. Bloom, and F.C. McLean. 1941. Calcification and ossification: Medullary bone changes in the reproductive cycle of female pigeons. Anat. Rec. 81:443.
Fishman, D.A. and E.D. Hay. 1962. Origin of osteoclasts from mononuclear leukocytes in regenerating new limbs. Anat. Rec. 143:329.
Hancox, N.M. and B. Boothroyd: 1963. The osteoclast in resorption. *In* R.F. Sognnaes, ed. Mechanisms of Hard Tissue Destruction. Washington, D.C., American Association for the Advancement of the Sciences, 1963.
Harris, W.H. and R.P. Heaney. 1969. Skeletal renewal and metabolic diseases of bone. N. Engl. J. Med. 28:253.
Jones, S.J. and A. Boyde. 1977. Some morphologic observations on osteoclasts. Cell Tissue Res. 185:387.
Kallio, D.M., P.R. Garant, and C. Minkin. 1971. Evidence of coated membranes in the ruffled border of the osteoclast. J. Ultraster. Res. 37:169.
McLean, F.C. and R.E. Rowland. 1963. Internal remodeling of compact bone. *In* R.F. Sognnaes, ed. Mechanisms of Hard Tissue Destruction. American Association for the Advancement of the Sciences. Washington, D.C., 1963.
Schenk, R.K., D. Spiro, and J. Wiener. 1967. Cartilage resorption in the tibial epiphyseal plate of growing rats. J. Cell Biol. 34:275.
Scheven, B.A., J.W. Visser, and P.J. Nijweide. 1986. In vitro osteoclast generation from different bone marrow fractions, including a highly enriched hemopoietic stem cell population. Nature 321:79.
Vaes, G. 1988. Cellular biology and biochemical mechanism of bone resorption. Clin. Orthoped. Related Res. 231:239.
Walker, D.G. 1973. Osteopetrosis cured by temporary parabiosis. Science 180:875.

HISTOPHYSIOLOGY

Canalis, E., T.L. McCarthy, and M. Centrella. 1988. Growth factors and the regulation of bone remodeling. J. Clin. Investig. 81:277.
Centrella, M., T.L. McCarthy, and E. Canalis. 1988. Skeletal tissue and transforming growth factor-B. (review). FASEB J. 2:3066.
Ernst, M., C. Schmidt, and E.R. Froesch. 1988. Enhanced osteoblast proliferation and collagen gene expression by estradiol. Proc. Nat. Acad. Sci. 85:2307.
Gaillard, P.J. 1959. Parathyroid gland and bone in vitro. VI. Dev. Biol. 1:152.
Heller, M., F.C. McLean, and W. Bloom. 1950. Cellular transformations in mammalian bones induced by parathyroid extract. Am. J. Anat. 87:315.
Henry, H.L. and A.W. Norman. 1984. Vitamin-D metabolism and biological activities. Ann. Rev. Nutrition 4:493.
Marks, S.C. and S.N. Popoff. 1988. Bone cell biology: Regulation of development, structure and function in the skeleton. Am. J. Anat. 183:1.
Mears, D.C. 1971. Effects of parathyroid hormone and thyrocalcitonin on the membrane potential of osteoclasts. Endocrinology 88:1021.
Norman, A.W., J. Roth, and L. Orci. 1982. The vitamin-D endocrine system: steroid metabolism, hormone receptors, and biological response (calcium binding protein). Endocrin. Res. 3:331.
Raisz, L.G. and B.E. Kream. 1981. Hormonal control of skeletal growth. Annu. Rev. Physiol. 43:225.
Raisz, L.G. and B.E. Kream. 1983. Regulation of bone formation. N. Engl. J. Med. 309:29, 83.
Rasmussen, C.D. and A.R. Means. 1987. Calmodulin is involved in regulation of cell proliferation. EMBO J. 6:3961.
Sampath, T.K., N. Muthukumaran, and A.H. Reddi. 1987. Isolation of osteogenin, an extracellular matrix associated bone inductive protein, by heparin affinity chromatography. Proc. Nat. Acad. Sci. USA 84:7109.
Tam, C.S., J.N. Heersche, T.M. Murray, and J.A. Parsons. 1982. Parathyroid hormone stimulates the bone apposition rate independently of its resorptive action. Differential effects of intermittent and continuous administration. Endocrinology 110:506.
Urist, M.R., R.J. Delange and G.A. Finerman. 1983. Bone cell differentiation and growth factors. Science 220:680.
Vincent, J. 1963. Microscopic aspects of mineral metabolism in bone tissue with special reference to calcium, lead and zinc. Clin. Orthoped. 26:161.
Walker, D.G. 1975. Control of bone resorption by hemopoietic tissue. J. Exp. Med. 142:651.
Wakefield, L.M., D.M. Smith, T. Masui, C.C. Harris, and M.B. Sporn. 1987. Distribution and modulation of the cellular receptor for transforming growth factor beta. J. Cell Biol. 105:965.
Wozney, J.M., V. Rosen, A.L. Celeste et al. 1988. Regulators of bone formation: molecular clones and activities. Science 242:1528.
Zichner, D. 1971. The effects of calcitonin on bone cells in young rats: an electron microscopic study. Israel J. Med. Sci. 7:359.

9

BONE MARROW AND BLOOD CELL FORMATION

The relatively short life span of mature blood cells, ranging from a few days to a few months, requires their continual replacement throughout life. In the adult human, it is estimated that some 200 billion erythrocytes and 10 billion neutrophilic leukocytes are formed each day. Erythrocytes, monocytes, neutrophils, eosinophils, and platelets are produced in the marrow and their formation is called *hemopoiesis*. Precursors of the lymphocytes arise in the marrow but migrate in the bloodstream to the thymus, where T-lymphocytes proliferate and differentiate, and to the spleen and lymph nodes, where B-lymphocytes develop and multiply. The generation of lymphocytes outside of the marrow is called *lymphopoiesis* and will be discussed in Chapter 13.

Marrow occupies the cylindrical cavities of the long bones and the interstices of the spongiosa in the vertebrae, ribs, sternum, and the flat bones of the cranium and pelvis. It accounts for 4–6% of the body weight and has a total volume nearly equal to that of the liver. It is a soft, highly cellular tissue consisting of the precursors of the blood cells, macrophages, adipose cells, fibroblast-like reticular cells, and reticular fibers. The relative proportions of the several cell types vary in different regions of the skeleton and change with age. At birth, all of the bones contain deep red hemopoietically active marrow. At 4–5 years of age, the number of blood–forming cells begins to decline and the number of adipose cells increases. With the progressive increase in the abundance of adipose cells, relative to blood-forming cells, there is a change in the color of the marrow from deep red to yellow. The gradual transformation of red marrow to relatively inactive yellow marrow begins earlier and progresses further in the distal portions of the long bones. In adults, red marrow persists only in the proximal ends of the humerus and femur, and in the vertebrae, ribs, sternum, and ilia of the pelvis. The fatty transformation of the marrow in the distal segments of the appendicular skeleton may be related to a slightly lower temperature in these parts. Yellow marrow can revert to red marrow in response to elevated temperature or unusual demands for blood cells.

PRENATAL HEMOPOIESIS

During prenatal life, the principal site of hemopoiesis shifts from one region of the embryo to another in three successive stages. In the first of these, called the *mesoblastic phase of hemopoiesis*, during the second week of gestation when the embryo is only a few millimeters long, blood formation is detectable in the mesenchyme of the body stalk and neighboring areas of the yolk sac. Some of the mesenchymal cells in these areas withdraw their processes and differentiate into *primitive erythroblasts* (*hemocytoblasts*), large, spherical, basophilic cells that gather to form aggregations called *blood islands*. There they proliferate, synthesize hemoglobin, and develop into *polychromatophilic erythroblasts* that gradually lose basophilia in their cytoplasm to become *primitive erythrocytes* (Figs. 9–1 and 9–2). These differ from erythrocytes of postnatal life in that they retain their nucleus. At about 6 weeks of gestation, round basophilic cells also appear in the primordium of the liver, initiating the *hepatic phase of hemopoiesis*. These *definitive erythroblasts* more closely resemble the erythroblasts of postnatal life and they go on to form typical anucleate erythrocytes. By the second month of gestation, a small number of granular leukocytes and megakaryocytes also appear in the sinusoids of the liver. Somewhat later, the spleen also becomes a site of hemopoiesis.

In the early embryo, the entire skeleton consists of hyaline cartilage. In the fourth month,

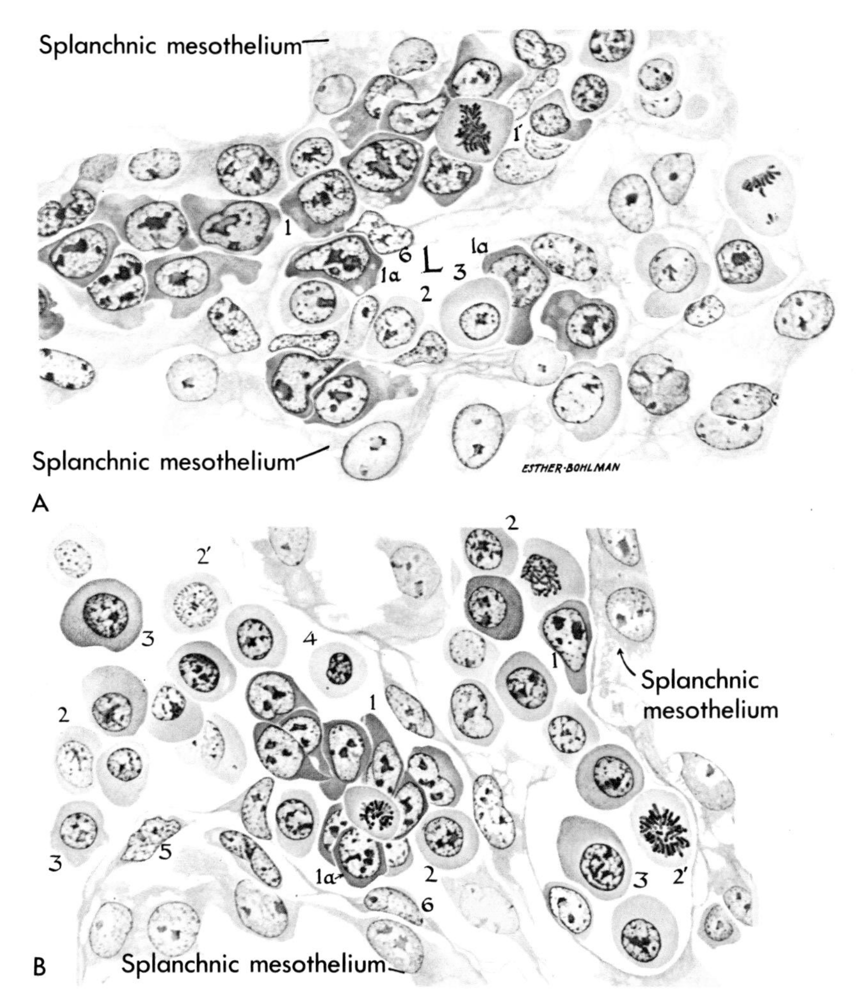

Figure 9–1. Two sections through folds in the wall of the yolk sac of a 24-day old human embryo. (A) Early stage of hemopoiesis, consisting of proliferating extravascular stem cells (hemocytoblasts) 1, 1′; L, lumen of a small vessel containing a few early polychromatophilic erythroblasts. (B) Later stage of hemopoiesis, showing transformation of hemocytoblasts 1, into early basophilic erythroblasts, 1a; polychromatophilic erythroblasts, 2, 3; primative erythrocytes 4; mesenchymal cells, 5; and endothelium, 6. Hematoxylin-eosin-axure II stain. (From Bloom, W. and F.W. Bartelmez. 1940. Am. J. Anat. 67:21.)

blood vessels and associated mesenchymal cells penetrate into cavities created in certain cartilages by the programmed degeneration of chondrocytes that precedes the establishment of centers of ossification. The mesenchymal cells accompanying the vessels differentiate into osteoblasts and into *reticular cells* that are destined to form the stroma of the bone marrow. With the establishment of ossification centers in the cartilaginous skeleton, blood formation begins within the primitive bone marrow, establishing the *myeloid phase of hemopoiesis.* Blood cell formation in the liver and spleen then declines and, thenceforth, the bone marrow is the predominant site of hemopoiesis. Although the liver and spleen do not normally participate in blood formation in the adult, extramedullary hemopoiesis may be reestablished in those organs in diseases attended by extensive damage to the bone marrow.

It was the traditional view that in the transition of hemopoiesis from yolk sac, to liver, and then to bone marrow, mesenchymal cells in each of these sites gave rise to blood-forming cells independently. It is now the prevailing view that the successive sites of hemopoiesis are seeded by stem cells that are carried in the bloodstream from the previous site of blood formation.

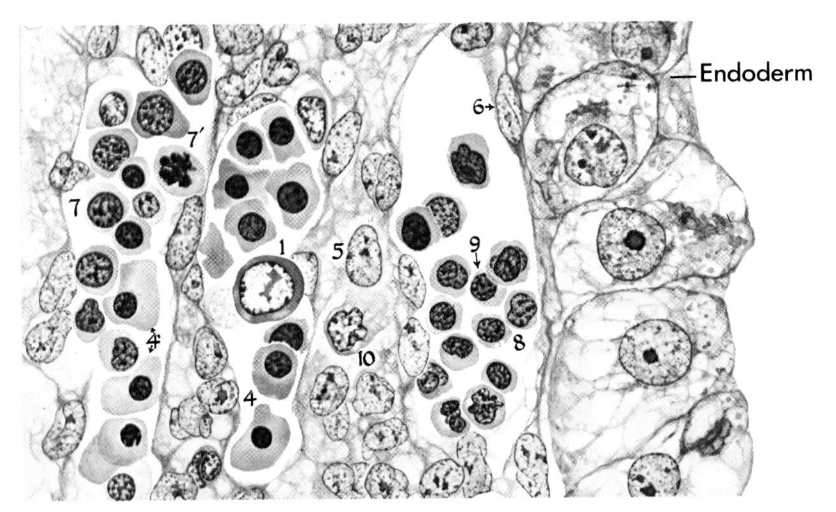

Figure 9-2. Section through the yolk sac of a 20-mm human embryo. In addition to circulating primitive erythrocytes, there are two foci of developing polychromatophilic definitive erythroblasts. Hemocytoblast, 1; primitive erythrocytes, 4; mesenchymal cells, 5; endothelium, 6; early and late definitive polychromatophilic erythroblasts, 7, 8, with one in mitosis at 7′; normoblast, 9; lymphoid wandering cell, 10. Hematoxylin-eosin-azure II stain (From Bloom, W. and F.W. Bartelmez. 1940. Am. J. Anat. 67:21.)

STRUCTURAL ORGANIZATION OF BONE MARROW

Most of the *marrow,* or myeloid tissue, occupies the *marrow cavity* (medulla) of the long bones of the skeleton. There, it is surrounded by the compact osseous tissue of the cortex or the trabeculae of the spongiosa. It does not have an independent blood supply, but receives blood that has first circulated through the osseous tissue of the bone. A major nutrient artery enters the bone through a nutrient canal in the diaphysis and bifurcates into ascending and descending branches that course along the axis of the marrow cavity giving off lateral branches. Very few of the finer ramifications of these vessels communicate with the vascular bed of the marrow. The great majority enter the osseous tissue, which is also supplied from the outside by branches of a network of blood vessels in the periosteum. At the corticomedullary interface of the bone, some of the capillaries of the cortex are continuous with a system of thin-walled anastomosing *sinuses* within the marrow. These, in turn, converge on larger *collecting sinuses* arranged radially around a longitudinally oriented *central sinus.* Thus, most of the blood reaching the sinuses of the marrow has first entered the osseous tissue, either from the periosteal vessels or from endosteal branches of the nutrient artery, and has secondarily entered the medullary sinuses. The significance of this indirect transosteal routing of the blood supply to the marrow is not known, but it is speculated that this may be necessary to maintain an optimal physicochemical environment for hemopoiesis.

The vascular sinuses of the marrow are 50–75 μm in diameter and have a very thin endothelium. It was long believed that the endothelium was discontinuous to allow passage of newly formed blood cells into the circulation. This view seemed to be sustained by early electron microscopic studies, but it is now agreed that the openings described in the wall of the sinuses were artifacts. In more recent scanning and transmission electron microscopic studies in which care was taken to preserve the marrow in situ and avoid mechanical damage, the sinuses have been shown to have no permanent apertures that would permit passage of blood cells. The endothelium is composed of very flat cells joined together by junctional complexes as in other endothelia. Clusters of transendothelial pores 80–100 nm in diameter are often found in the extremely attenuated peripheral portions of the cells. A continuous basal lamina is absent, but there may be scattered deposits of material of similar nature.

The stroma of the marrow consists of *reticular cells,* reticular fibers, macrophages, and adipose cells. The reticular cells are of mesenchymal origin but differ somewhat from connective tissue fibroblasts in their appearance and functions. They are pale-staining cells that are difficult to study in histological sections because their outlines are obscured by the closely packed hemopoietic cells. They synthesize and maintain the delicate framework of reticular fibers found throughout the marrow, but there is evidence that their role is not limited to mechanical support. They are essential for maintenance of hemopoiesis in long-term marrow cultures and are believed to produce growth factors required for proliferation and maturation of blood-cell precursors.

Adventitial reticular cells, in normal marrow, are estimated to cover 40–60% of the ablumenal surface of the sinuses, leaving the remainder accessible to mature blood cells for transmural migration into the bloodstream. In response to hemopoietic stimulation, the reticular cells may change their shape, exposing more endothelial surface for the egress of newly formed blood cells. When transmural cell migration is enhanced experimentally, the adventitial cover may be reduced to less than 20% of the sinus surface.

The passage of mature blood cells into the lumen of the sinuses does not take place by separating endothelial cells at their junctions, but is transcellular. The migrating cell appears to press the ablumenal membrane of the endothelial cell into contact with the adlumenal membrane and the two fuse to form a transient *migration pore* (Fig. 9–3). The opening, so formed, may be somewhat enlarged by the cell in transit but does not exceed 4 μm in diameter, and continuity of the endothelium is rapidly restored after the blood cell has become free in the lumen of the sinus. The endothelium appears to be actively involved in the process and there is suggestive evidence that it may exercise some selectivity in control of the transcellular traffic.

Reticular cells are capable of accumulating lipid and developing into cells that are morphologically indistinguishable from the adipose cells of connective tissue. Because they develop from adventitial reticular cells, they tend to be located near the sinuses. Despite the

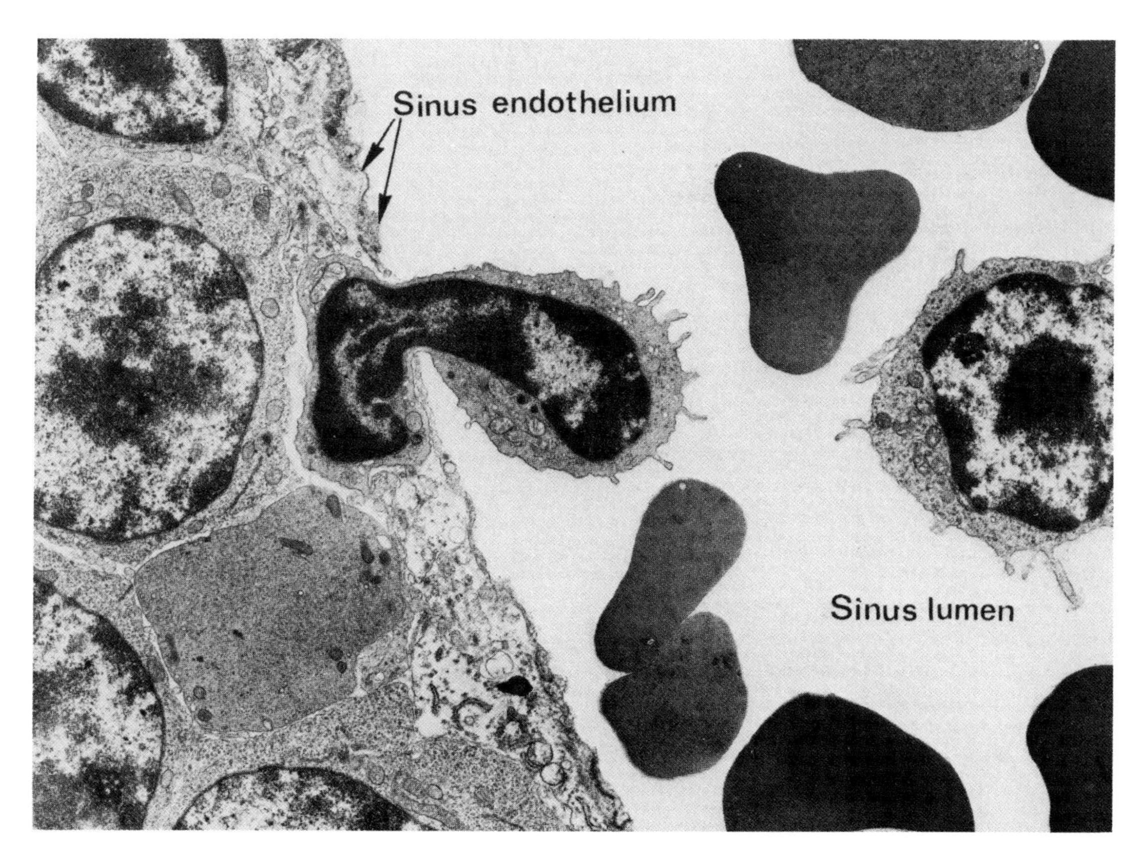

Figure 9–3. Electron micrograph showing the transmural migration of a lymphocyte through the very thin endothelium into the lumen of a sinus.

resemblance of adipose cells of the marrow to extramedullary fat cells, there is compelling biochemical and experimental evidence that they differ significantly in their functions. They are somewhat smaller and more active in their metabolism, having a fivefold greater rate of palmitate turnover than ordinary fat cells. Whereas lipogenesis in extramedullary fat cells is stimulated by insulin, lipogenesis in adipose cells of the marrow is stimulated by glucocorticoids. Acute starvation induces release of fatty acids from the lipid stores in the peripheral adipose tissues of the body, but does not induce lipolysis in adipose cells of the marrow. An interesting reciprocal relationship exists between the partial volume of the marrow occupied by adipose cells and the volume occupied by hemopoietic cells. When hemopoiesis is stimulated by experimentally induced hemolysis, the volume of marrow adipose cells is reduced by lipolysis of their lipid stores, and conversely, an experimentally induced reduction in the volume of hemopoietic tissue is attended by increased lipogenesis in the adiopose cells of the marrow, whereas extramedullary fat cells are unaffected by these experimental conditions. The significance of the differences in the two kinds of adipose cells is not entirely clear, but it is apparent that those in the peripheral fat depots are primarily responsive to the nutritional state of the organism, whereas those of the marrow are somehow related to its hemopoietic function.

In histological sections, the hemopoietic tissue of the marrow generally appears as an

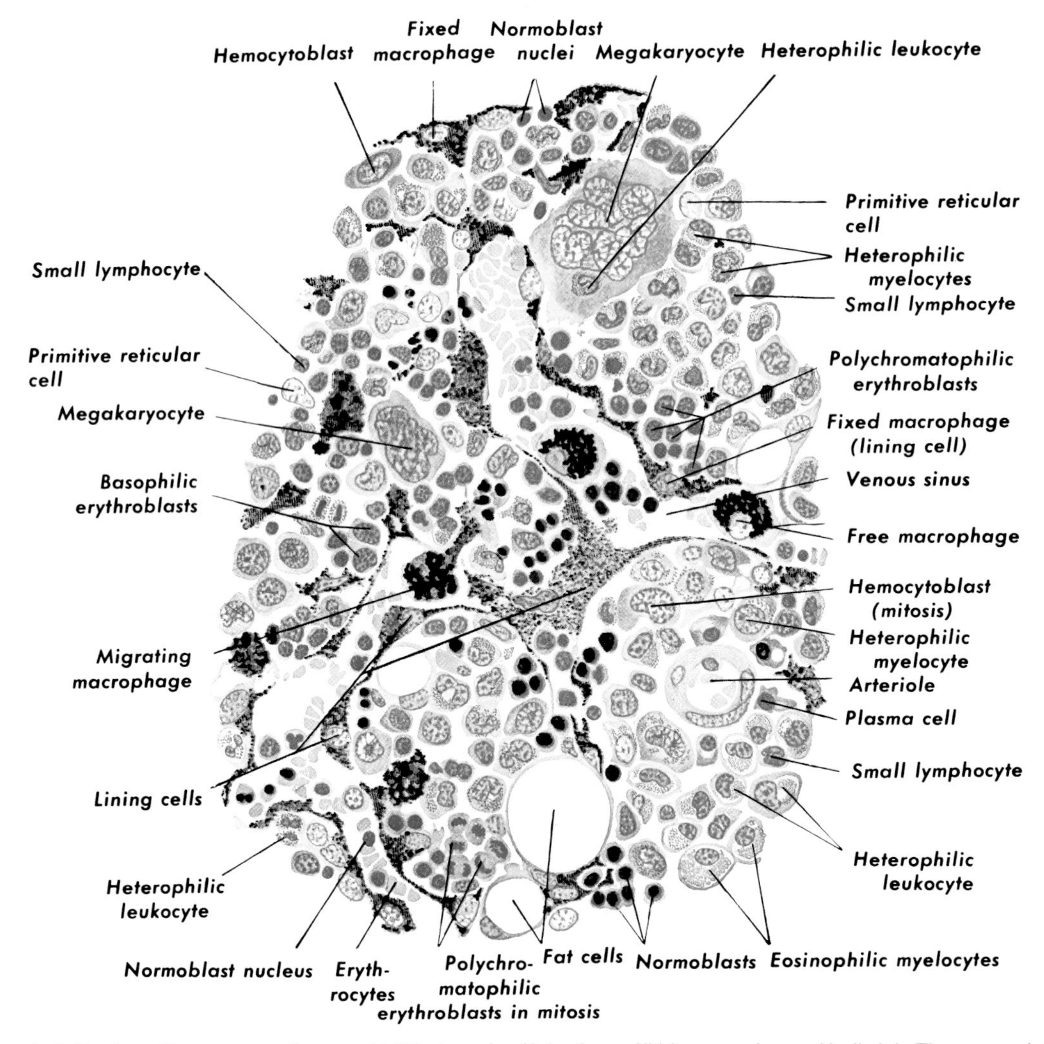

Figure 9–4. Section of bone marrow from a rabbit that received injections of lithium carmine and India ink. The macrophages and some of the cells lining the sinuses contain phagocytosed particulate tracer. Hematoxylin-eosin-ezure II stain.

unorganized mixture of closely packed cells of different lineages in various stages of differentiation (Fig. 9–4). However, on careful study, preferential localization of certain lineages is detectable. Erythroid cells tend to be localized very near the adventitial reticular cells, and megakaryocytes are typically situated adjacent to a sinus wall with platelet-shedding processes projecting into the lumen. Granulocyte precursors are reported to be concentrated near the centers of the intervascular spaces. Macrophages are widely distributed in the marrow but they are commonly found in the center of clusters of erythroid cells and the maturation of granulocytes appears to take place in intimate contact with macrophage cell processes. The finding that macrophages and reticulum cells produce a number of cytokines and growth factors suggests that the close association of hemopoietic cells with these stromal cells may be significant.

HEMOPOIETIC STEM CELLS

Blood-cell formation depends on the presence in the marrow, of *pluripotential hemopoietic stem cells,* cells whose proliferation and differentiation can generate all of the blood-cell types. These stem cells constitute less than 0.2% of the total population of nucleated cells in the marrow. The majority of them are dormant and only resume division after varying time intervals, or in response to unusual demands for new blood cells. Cycling stem cells may either undergo *self-renewing divisions* to maintain the pool of pluripotential cells or they may undergo *differentiating divisions* that give rise to *progenitor cells*—cells that have a more limited potential for development along alternative pathways. Progenitor cells have little or no capacity for self-renewal and are irreversibly committed to differentiation into a single blood-cell type. The stem cells and the lineage-specific progenitor cells that arise from them are morphologically and cytochemically indistinguishable. All are small round cells with a thin rim of basophilic cytoplasm around a nucleus with inconspicuous chromatin and two or more nucleoli. In their differentiation, the progeny of the progenitor cells of the several cell lineages progress through a series of intermediate stages that are morphologically distinguishable on the basis of size, nuclear configuration, staining properties, and the presence or absence of specific cytoplasmic granules. The identifying characteristics of these developmental stages will be described later.

A microenvironment that will permit the proliferation and development of hemopoietic cells is not confined to the bone marrow. The stromal cells of the spleen share a number of properties with those of the marrow and much of our knowledge of the hemopoietic potential of stem cells and their immediate progeny is based on a *spleen assay* developed in the 1960s. In this procedure, a suspension of hemopoietic cells from the bone marrow is injected into a syngeneic mouse that has been X-irradiated with a dosage sufficient to destroy the proliferative capacity of its own cells. The injected cells, carried in the blood, "home" into the favorable microenvironment of the spleen and bone marrow of the irradiated host and begin to proliferate. The spleen is more accessible to observation, and after several days it contains grossly visible small colonies, each having developed by proliferation of a single stem cell and differentiation of its progeny. This assay detects a broad class of stem cells that have been designated *colony-forming units spleen* (CFU-S). The developmental potentialities of individual colony-forming cells can be more narrowly defined by microscopic identification of the kind of mature blood cells present in the colony. If all blood-cell lineages are represented, the cell of origin was a pluripotential hemopoietic stem cell (PHSC). If both granulocytes and monocytes are found, their bipotential progenitor is designated a *colony-forming unit granulocyte monocyte* (CFU-GM). If only granulocytes are found, the colony originated from a *colony-forming unit-granulocyte* (CFU-G), and if only monocytes are present the cell of origin was a *colony-forming unit monocyte* (CFU-M). Unipotential progenitor cells giving rise exclusively to each of the other cell types, namely, erythrocytes, eosinophils, and megakaryocytes, are similarly designated CFU-E, CFU-Eo, CFU-Meg, and so on (Fig. 9–5).

Although our understanding of the kinetics of stem cells has been based on spleen colony assays in irradiated mice, there was reason to believe that the same principles would hold for hemopoiesis in other mammals including man. This has been borne out in more recent studies using an in vitro culture system in which pluripotential cells from human marrow are stimulated to form colonies in a semisolid matrix of agar or methyl cellulose. This system now permits studies of the kinetics and

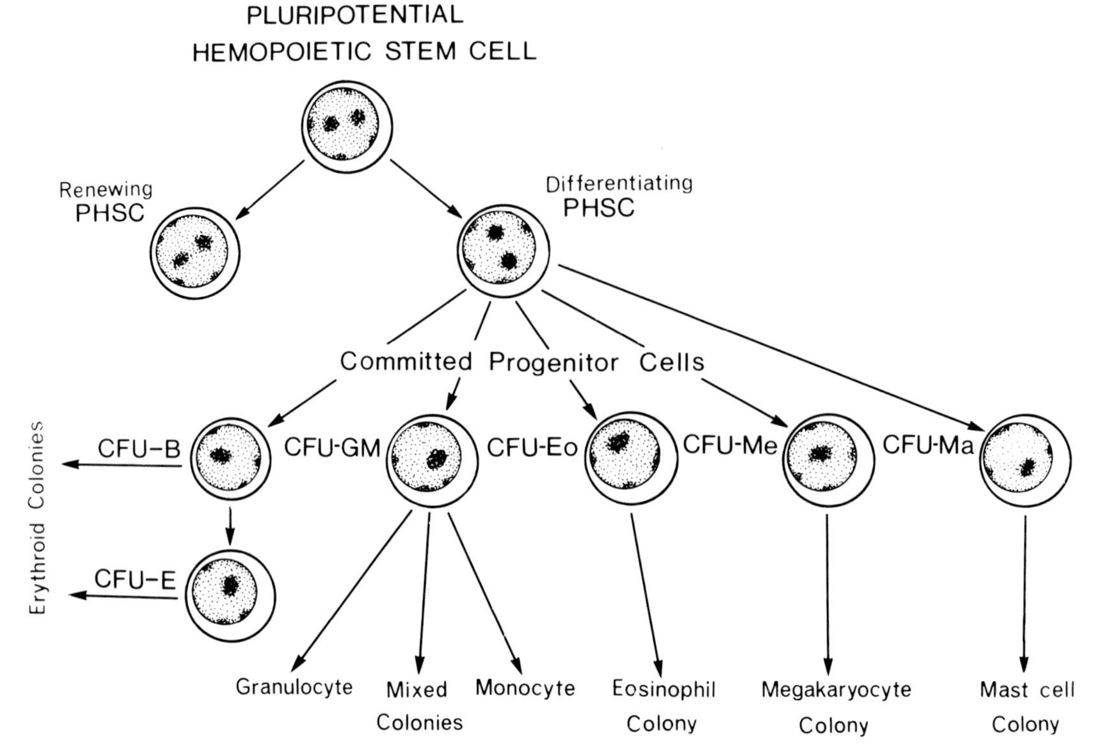

Figure 9–5. Stem cells and successive stages of differentiation up through the committed precursors of the several blood-cell lines are very similar in their morphology. Since the development of spleen assays and in vitro methods for studying hemopoiesis, progenitor cell types have been designated colony-forming units (CFU) and have been further identified by the initial letter of the cell type, or types, found in the colony resulting from their cultivation in vitro. Thus, CFU-E is the committed precursor of erythrocytes and CFU-GM is the progenitor of granulocytes and monocytes, and so on.

regulation of hemopoiesis comparable to those carried out with spleen assays in mice.

By taking advantage of lineage-specific surface antigens to identify committed progenitors and more differentiated cells, it has been possible to eliminate them, leaving behind a population of cells believed to be the long-sought hemopoietic stem cells. Injection of as few as 30 of these into lethally irradiated mice is sufficient to save half of the animals and to completely repopulate the marrow of those surviving. If human stem cells could be isolated by a comparable procedure, it might be possible to inject these instead of transplanting bone marrow to patients receiving heavy X-ray therapy for cancer.

ERYTHROPOIESIS

Erythrocytes have a life span of about 120 days. The effete erythrocytes are removed from the blood in its passage through the spleen and are destroyed there. The maintenance of normal numbers in the circulation requires continuous formation in the bone marrow. Some 2.5×10^{11} new erythrocytes enter the circulation each day.

Development in all myelopoietic cell lineages progresses from the pluripotential *stem cell* to a unipotential *progenitor* and then through a sequence of microscopically identifiable *maturation stages* leading to functional blood cells. It is customary to refer to the first recognizable cells of the maturational sequence as *precursor cells* of that lineage in contradistinction to the earlier *progenitor* cells which usually cannot be distinguished microscopically from stem cells or from the corresponding stage of other lineages.

In erythropoiesis, two categories of progenitors are distinguished on the basis of their colony generation in cultures. One called the *erythroid burst-forming unit* (BFU-E) has a high rate of proliferation when stimulated by an incompletely characterized regulatory factor called *burst-promoting activity* (BPA). Its proliferation produces a large number of the second type of progenitor, called the *erythroid colony–forming unit* (CFU-E). This is a larger and more slowly proliferating cell that is responsive to low concentrations of *erythropoietin,* the principal humoral regulator of erythrocyte production.

CFU-Es have now been isolated from mouse spleen colonies by elutriation and density-gradient centrifugation. They are distinctly larger than CFU-B. Their rim of cytoplasm is wider and contains a greater number of mitochondria. There is a small amount of marginated chromatin and a large nucleolus (Fig. 9–5). The progeny of the CFU-E become the morphologically identifiable *proerythroblasts.* In smears, these are round cells up to 16 μm in diameter with a rim of moderately basophilic cytoplasm around a large nucleus that often has two nucleoli. As they differentiate, their cytoplasm becomes more basophilic and, in electron micrographs, is found to contain an increasing number of polyribosomes.

Division of the proerythroblasts produces slightly smaller *basophilic erythroblasts* that have intensely basophilic cytoplasm and a somewhat smaller nucleus with more heterochromatin. In electron micrographs, their cytoplasm contains a profusion of polyribosomes but no profiles of endoplasmic reticulum. The synthesis of hemoglobin is occurring in the cytoplasm and it can be recognized in micrographs as particles of very small size and low electron density. In preparations stained for light microscopy, its presence is obscured by the intense basophilia of the ribosome-rich cytoplasm.

The progeny of basophilic erythroblasts are smaller cells called *polychromatophilic erythroblasts.* They are readily identifiable by their greater degree of chromatin condensation and by the color of the cytoplasm which ranges from blue-gray to a dull olive green (Fig. 9–6). A nucleolus is no longer present and a cessation of ribosome production is associated with its loss. Characteristic variations in the color of the cytoplasm reflect progressive changes in the relative abundance of ribosomes (which bind the blue component of the dye mixture) and of hemoglobin (which has an affinity for the pink dye, eosin). Polychromatophilic erythroblasts are the last cells of the erythroid lineage that are capable of division. The concentration of ribosomes is reduced by cytokinesis while continuing accumulation of hemoglobin in the cytoplasm of the daughter cells results in increasing eosinophilia.

As a result of these changes, cells of the next stage of erythropoiesis, called *orthochromatic erythroblasts* (or *normoblasts*) have a pinker cytoplasm with only a faint tinge of blue. Chromatin condensation has progressed and the nucleus is now quite small, eccentric in position, and intensely stained. In electron micrographs, the dense heterochromatin is in large clumps with little or no intervening euchromatin. The cytoplasm, rich in hemoglobin, has a finely granular appearance and is devoid of organelles other than an occasional mitochondrion (Figs. 9–8 and 9–9). Widely scattered small clusters of ribosomes can still be found (Fig. 9–9C).

The eccentric nucleus of the orthochromatic erythroblast is ultimately extruded, enclosed in a thin film of cytoplasm and a portion of the cell membrane (Fig. 9–8), leaving behind an anucleate *erythrocyte.* The extruded nucleus is ingested and destroyed by macrophages in the stroma of the bone marrow. When the newly formed erythrocytes are released into the circulation, they do not yet have the clear salmon-pink color of mature erythrocytes but have a faint greenish tint attributable to the presence of small numbers of ribosomes. If fresh blood smears are stained with cresyl blue the residual ribosomes in these *polychromatophilic erythrocytes* form aggregates that appear as a bluish network in an otherwise pink cytoplasm. The newly formed erythrocytes are, therefore, described as *reticulocytes.* This staining method is clinically useful in assessing the rate of erythropoiesis in patients suffering from anemia or recovering from blood loss. Normally there is a reserve of reticulocytes in the marrow somewhat greater than the number in the circulation.

In their further differentiation, reticulocytes divest themselves of cytoplasmic organelles and membrane constituents that would serve no purpose in the erythrocyte which is little more than a membrane-bounded solution of hemoglobin. Although these late modifications go unobserved with the microscope, they can be detected biochemically. The clumped ribosomes that are responsible for the distinctive staining of reticulocytes are believed to be degraded intracellarly. A number of functions associated with the surface membrane are lost, including those involved in the transport of glucose and amino acids. The receptors for the iron-transporting protein, transferrin, are also lost in the transition from reticulocyte to erythrocyte. These integral membrane proteins aggregate and are taken into the cytoplasm where they are processed and subsequently extruded in vesicles, about

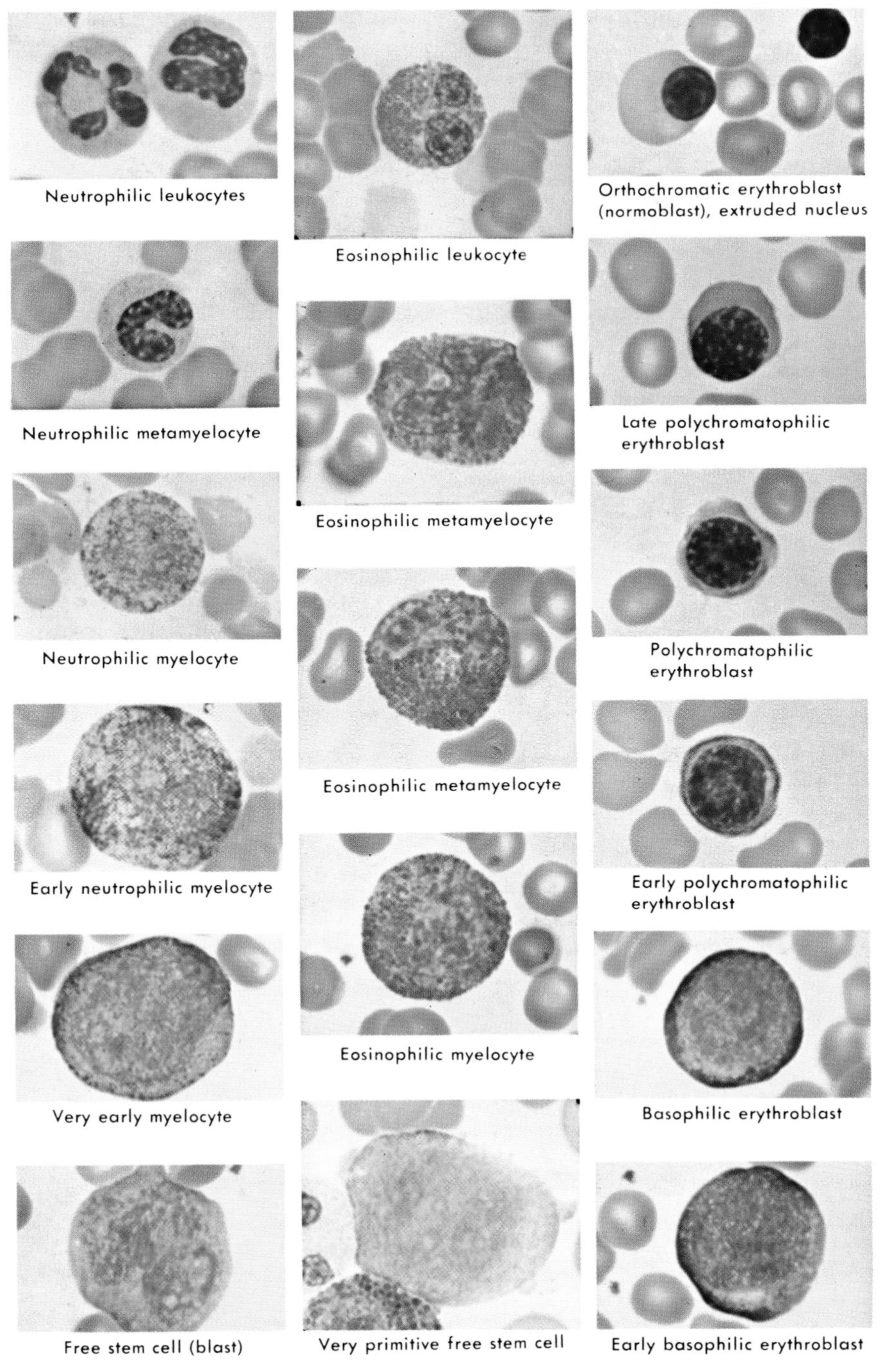

Figure 9–6. Photomicrographs of the morphologically identifiable stages in the development of erythrocytes, eosinophils, and neutrophils, as seen in dry smears stained with Wright's blood stain.

50 nm in diameter, that can be recovered from culture medium or plasma by very high-speed centrifugation.

In the continual turnover of erythrocytes in the blood, the number released into the circulation from the marrow each day is about the same as the number of aged and damaged erythrocytes removed and destroyed in the spleen. The iron released in the degradation of hemoglobin by macrophages in the spleen is returned to the marrow by the transport protein *transferrin* and reutilized in hemoglo-

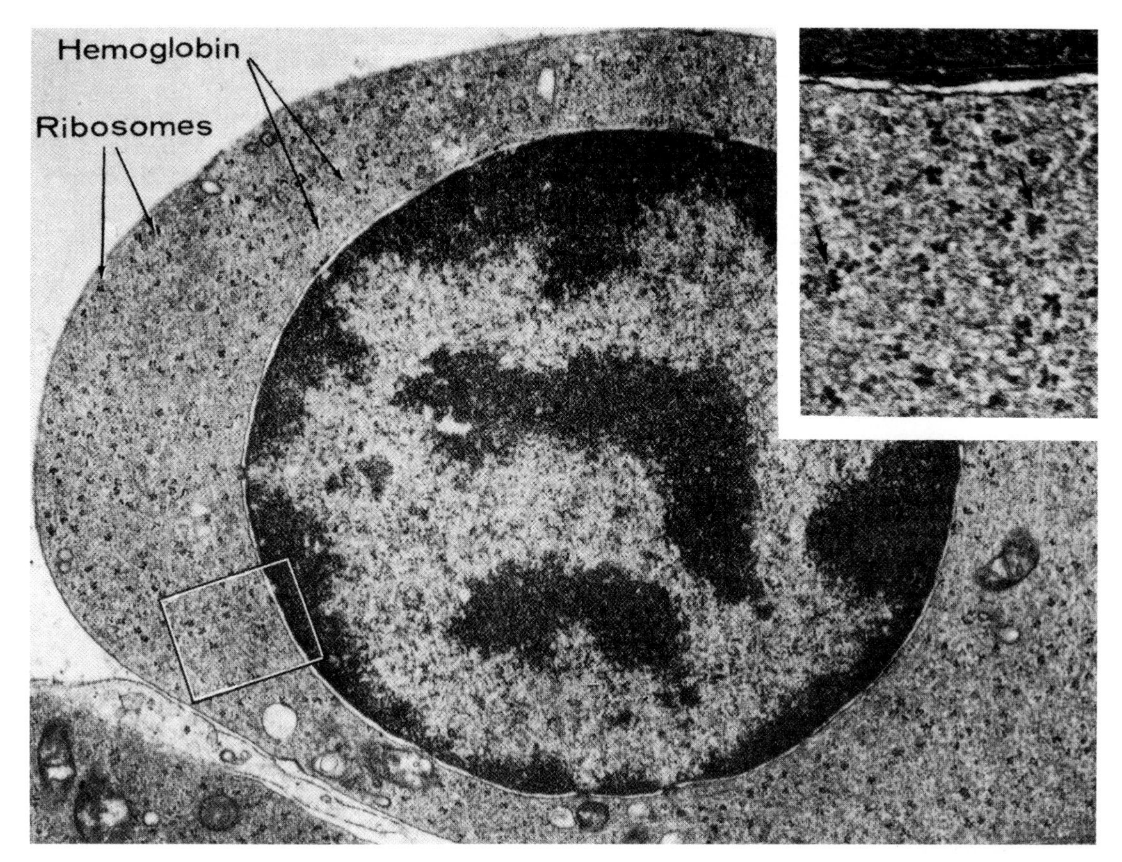

Figure 9–7. Electron micrograph of a polychromatophilic erythroblast from guinea pig bone marrow, showing the coarse blocks of heterochromatin in the nucleus and a cytoplasm consisting mainly of hemoglobin and polyribosomes. In the inset, polyribosomes (at arrows) can be distinguished from the smaller, less dense background of hemoglobin.

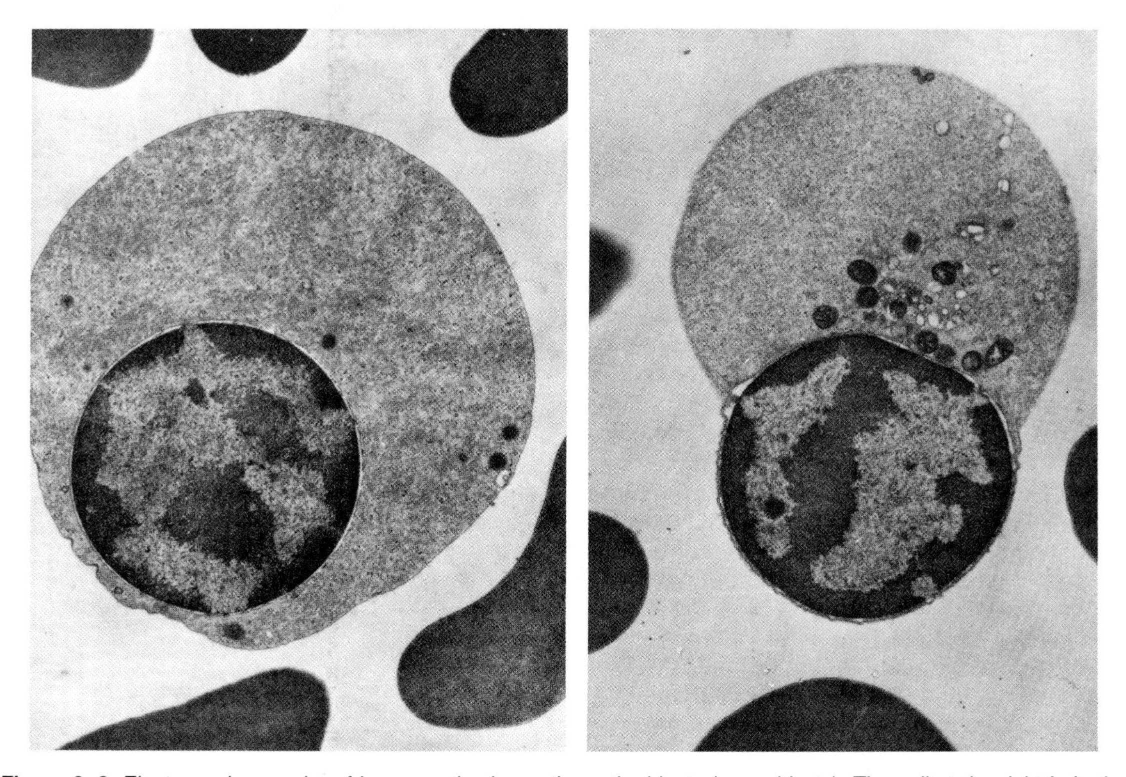

Figure 9–8. Electron micrographs of human orthochromatin erythroblasts (normoblasts). The cell at the right is in the process of extruding its nucleus. The nucleus is pinched off enclosed in a thin layer of cytoplasm. It does not pass out through a break in the membrane, as previously believed.

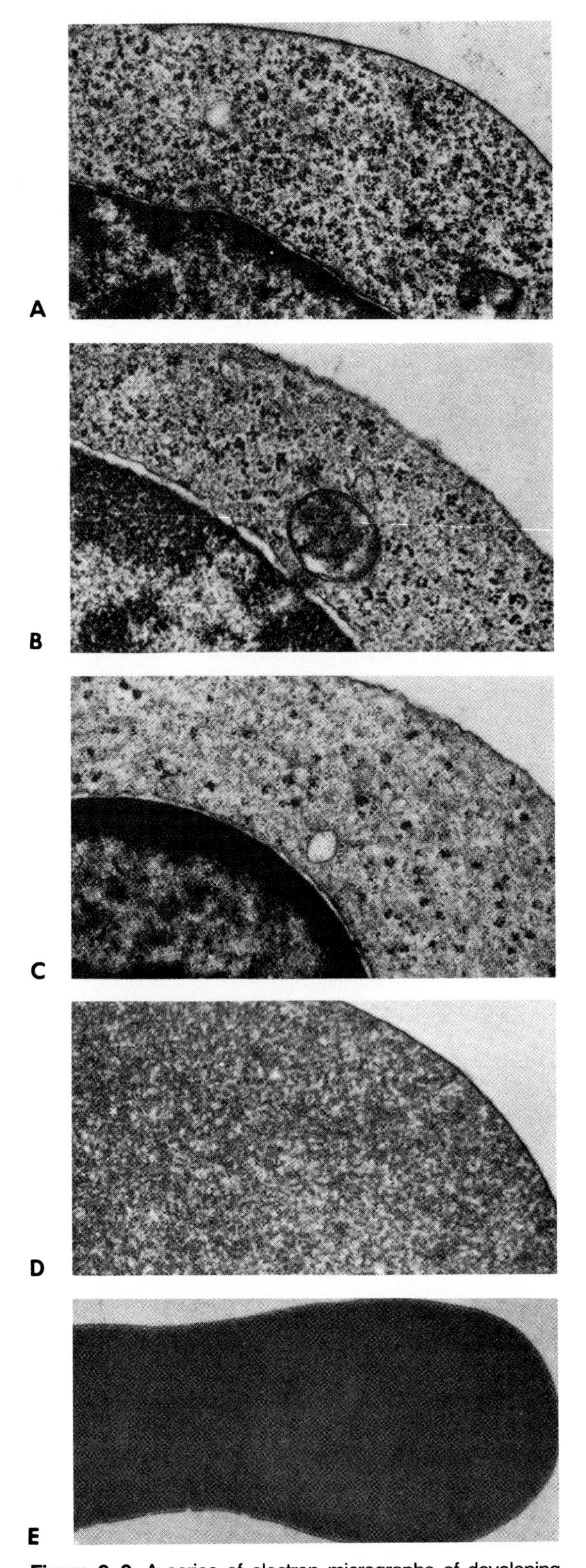

Figure 9–9. A series of electron micrographs of developing erythrocytes illustrating the decline in the number of ribosomes and the progressive increase in the concentration of hemoglobin in the cytoplasm. (A) Basophilic erythroblast; (B) polychromatophilic erythroblast; (C) orthochromatic erythroblast (normoblast); (D) reticulocyte; (E) nature erythrocyte.

bin synthesis by the erythropoietic cells. Other residues of the degraded hemoglobin are transformed by the liver and excreted as the bile pigment *bilirubin.*

GRANULOPOIESIS

The neutrophil and monocyte (macrophage) cell lineages arise from the bipotential progenitor CFU-GM which subsequently gives rise to the unipotential progenitors CFU-G and CFU-M. The progenitors of eosinophils and basophils appear to arise from the pluripotential stem cell separately (Fig. 9–5). The first morphologically identifiable precursors of the granulocytes are the *myeloblasts.* These are round cells about 16 μm in diameter that have a large nucleus with dispersed chromatin and multiple nucleoli. The cytoplasm is moderately basophilic and devoid of granules. They are capable of division, producing daughter cells that increase in size (24 μm) and acquire metachromatic *azurophilic granules* in their cytoplasm. With these changes, they become recognizable as early *promyelocytes.* Their nucleus is indented and contains more marginated heterochromatin than that of myeloblasts. The cytoplasm is deeply basophilic and, in electron micrographs, contains numerous mitochondria and meandering cysternae of endoplasmic reticulum. The azurophil granules are electron-dense, membrane-bounded, and slightly irregular in outline (Fig. 9–10). Initially, they are clustered around the small juxtanuclear Golgi complex but become dispersed throughout the cytoplasm as they become more numerous (Fig. 9–12). Promyelocytes are the largest cells of the granulocyte lineages but after one or more divisions, late promyelocytes are considerably smaller, their chromatin is more condensed, and nucleoli are no longer conspicuous (Fig. 9–11). Although azurophil granules still occupy much of the cytoplasm, the peak period of their formation has passed and there is a notable decrease in the size of the Golgi complex and in the extent of the endoplasmic reticulum.

From the stem cell to the late promyelocytes, the precursors of neutrophils, eosinophils, and basophils are morphologically indistinguishable. Their separate paths of differentiation first become detectable with appearance of *specific granules* in the cytoplasm that differ in their staining properties and in their ultrastructure. This divergence takes

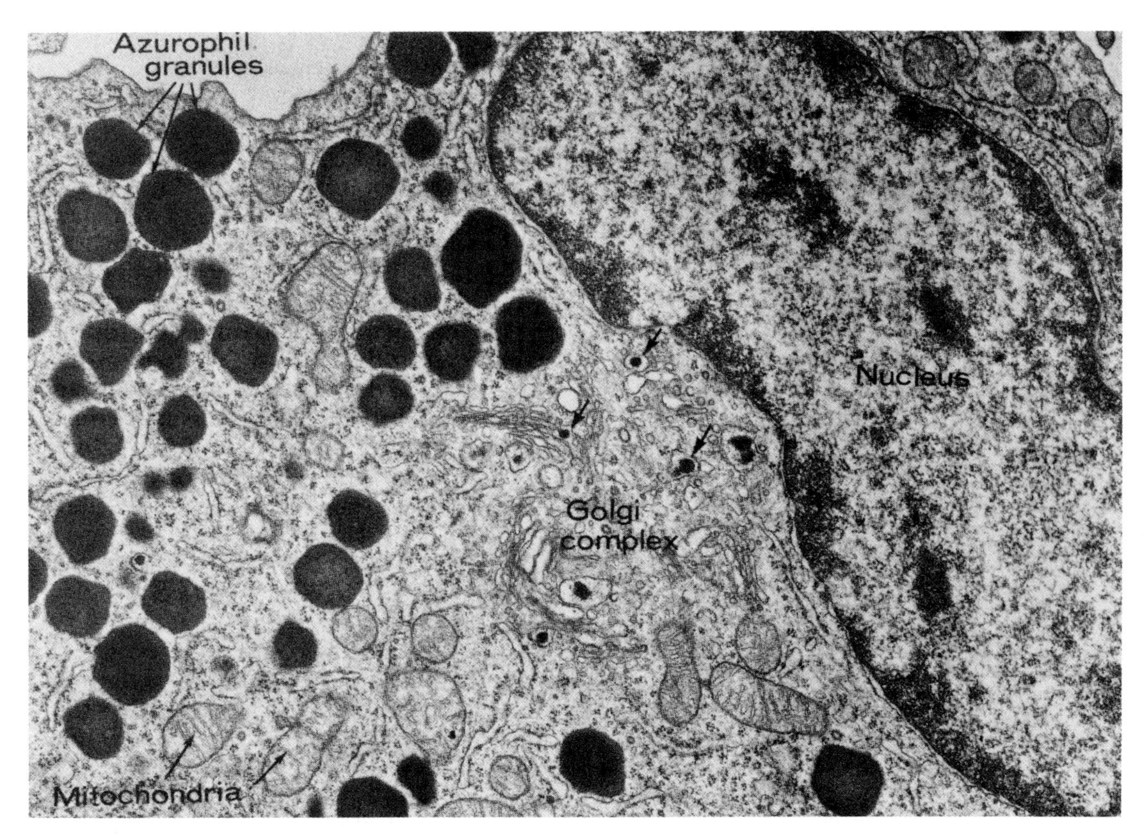

Figure 9–10. Electron micrograph of a promyelocyte from rabbit marrow. Dense-cored vacuoles associated with the Golgi complex represent formative stages of the azurophil granules. Enlargement and coalescence of these give rise to the large dense granules seen at the upper left. (Micrograph from Bainton, D. and M. Farquhar. 1966. J. Cell. Biol. 28:277.)

place at the *myelocyte* stage of their development.

NEUTROPHILIC MYELOCYTES

The *neutrophilic myelocyte* is distinguishable from the promyelocyte by its smaller size, by the more variable shape of the nucleus and greater condensation of its chromatin, by its smaller Golgi complex, and especially by the presence in its cytoplasm of a second type of granule that has little affinity for the stains used for routine marrow smears. In electron micrographs, these *specific granules* are less dense than the azurophil granules and are often elongated, resembling rice grains (Fig. 9–13). Thus, two populations of granules are formed at different times in the development of neutrophils. The azurophil granules arise in the promyelocyte stage and the specific granules are formed in the myelocyte stage. The azurophil granules contain histochemically demonstrable peroxidase, acid phosphatase, β-galactosidase, β-glucuronidase, esterase, and 5′-nucleotidase and, therefore, correspond to the primary lysosomes of other cell types (Fig. 9–13). The specific granules contain alkaline phosphatase, collagenase, lysozyme, and basic proteins collectively called phagocytins.

From the progenitor cell through the myelocyte stage, four to seven mitotic divisions occur. Cell division then ceases and subsequent differentiation involves changes in nuclear form, a decrease in number of mitochondria and other organelles, and the appearance of small amounts of glycogen in the cytoplasm.

The next stage, called the *metamyelocyte,* is distinguishable from the myelocyte mainly by the shape of its nucleus, which is deeply indented. Two types of granules are still present, but the specific granules now make up over 80% of the granule population. Nuclear modeling continues resulting in a cell with a straight or slightly curved elongated nucleus. Such cells are often referred to as *band-forms.* During the final stage of neutrophil matura-

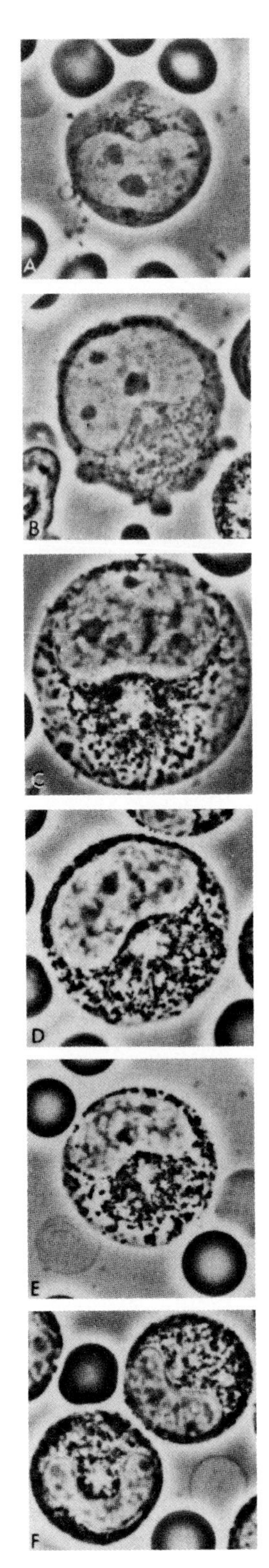

Figure 9–11. Phase contrast photomicrographs of promyelocytes (A, B, C). Neutrophilic myelocytes (D, E) and metamyelocytes (F) from human bone marrow. (Photomicrograph from Ackerman, A. 1972. Zeitschr. Zellforsch. 121:153.)

tion, local constrictions appearing in the nucleus result in its division into multiple small lobules joined by very thin segments (Fig. 9–14).

The entire transit time from stem cell to mature granulocyte is about 10 days. The rate of production of granulocytes of all types, in the human, is estimated to be about 1.6×10^4/kg/day, of which the great majority are neutrophils. A large reserve of metamyelocytes, band forms, and mature neutrophils is maintained in the marrow, perhaps as many as 10 times the daily production. These can be rapidly mobilized to meet unusual demands. Mature neutrophils are preferentially released, but in infections, band forms and even metamyelocytes may enter the circulation.

EOSINOPHILIC MYELOCYTES

The first morphologically recognizable stage of eosinophil development is the *eosinophilic myelocyte.* The nucleus has a rather coarse pattern of peripheral clumps of chromatin. The cytoplasm is slightly basophilic and the specific granules are eosinophilic and distinctly larger than those of neutrophilic myelocytes. In electron micrographs, there are numerous cisternae of rough endoplasmic reticulum and moderately abundant free ribosomes (Fig. 9–15). As in neutrophilic myelocytes, two types of granules are recognizable. The specific granules are somewhat less electron-dense than the azurophil granules. They are rich in peroxidase, and cytochemical reactions for this enzyme are useful in tracing their development. In early myelocytes, peroxidase is demonstrable in the perinuclear cistern, and throughout the endoplasmic reticulum, in the Golgi saccules, and in the forming granules (Fig. 9–16). A similar distribution is reported for acid phosphatase and aryl sulfatase. Thus, the eosinophilic myelocyte is capable of synthesizing and concentrating several enzymes simultaneously. In later stages of differentiation, after granule formation has ceased, these enzymes are detectable only in the granules.

Band forms do not occur in eosinophilic metamyelocytes and the nucleus never acquires the degree of lobulation seen in neutrophils. The nucleus is slightly indented in metamyelocytes and usually bilobed in mature eosinophils. In electron micrographs of metamyelocytes, the ultrastructure of the specific granules varies. Some are still moderately

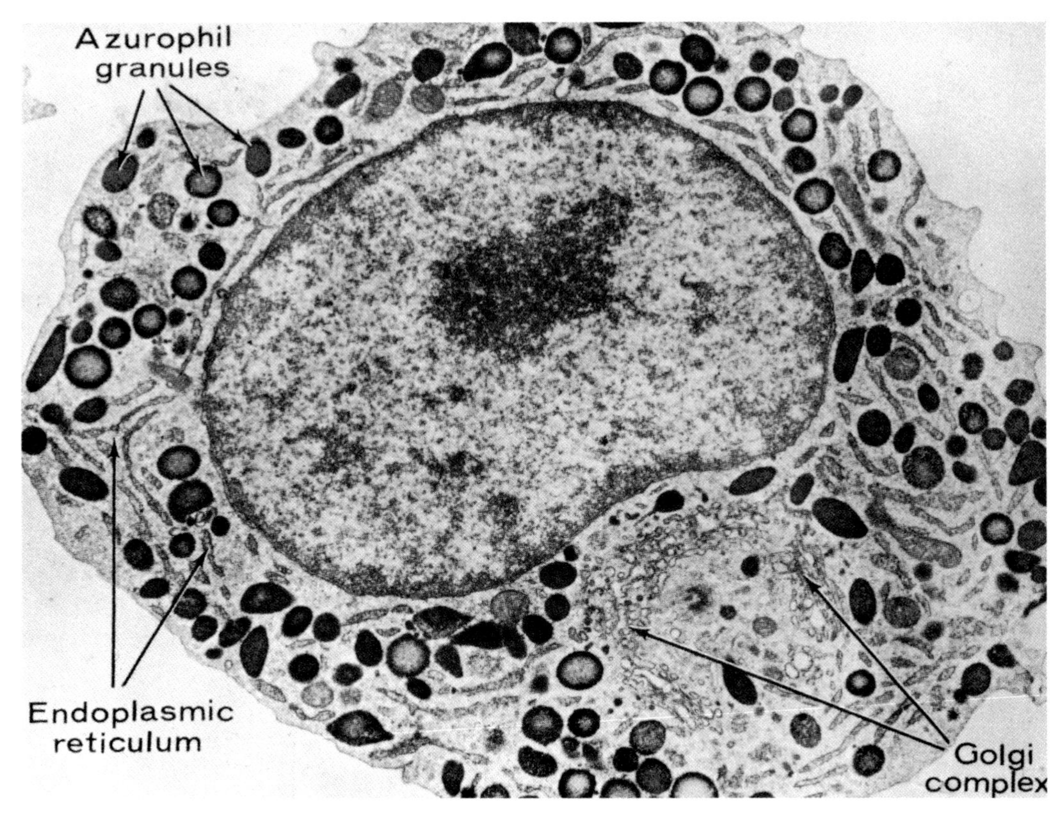

Figure 9–12. Electron micrograph of a polymorphonuclear promyelocyte, the largest cell of the neutrophil series, stained for peroxidase. The cytoplasm is packed with peroxidase-positive azurophil granules, and a positive reaction is seen throughout the endoplasmic reticulum. Specific granules have not yet formed. (From Bainton, D., J. Ullyot, and M. Farquhar. 1971. J. Exp. Med. 134:907.)

dense and homogeneous, whereas others show varying degrees of crystallization of the granule content. In mature eosinophils, the granules all contain one to three protein crystals of varying shape surrounded by a matrix of lower density (Fig. 9–17).

BASOPHILIC MYELOCYTES

Basophilic myelocytes are rarely observed in preparations of human marrow owing to their small number and the difficulty of preserving their granules, which are water soluble and are partially or completely extracted during fixation and staining. The nucleus contains little condensed chromatin and is paler-staining than that of other myelocytes. In mature basophils, the nucleus is deeply indented or bilobed. The slightly basophilic cytoplasm contains few specific granules. When successfully preserved, the granules vary in size and stain intensely with basic dyes. Like the granules of mast cells, they are metachromatic with Toluidine blue or thionine.

MONOPOIESIS

As previously stated, the pluripotential stem cell (PHSC) gives rise to several kinds of stem cells of more restricted potential. Among these is the bipotential granulocyte/macrophage colony-forming unit (CFU-GM). The progeny of this cell differentiate either into precursors of granulocytes or into *monoblasts.* These are difficult to identify in marrow, but have been studied in colonies formed in tissue culture. The division of monoblasts give rise to *promonocytes.* Some of the promonocytes proliferate rapidly and give rise to *monocytes* that enter the circulation. Others form a reserve of very slowly renewing precursor cells in the marrow that can be activated to meet unusual demands for macrophages elsewhere in the body. The transit time from stem cell

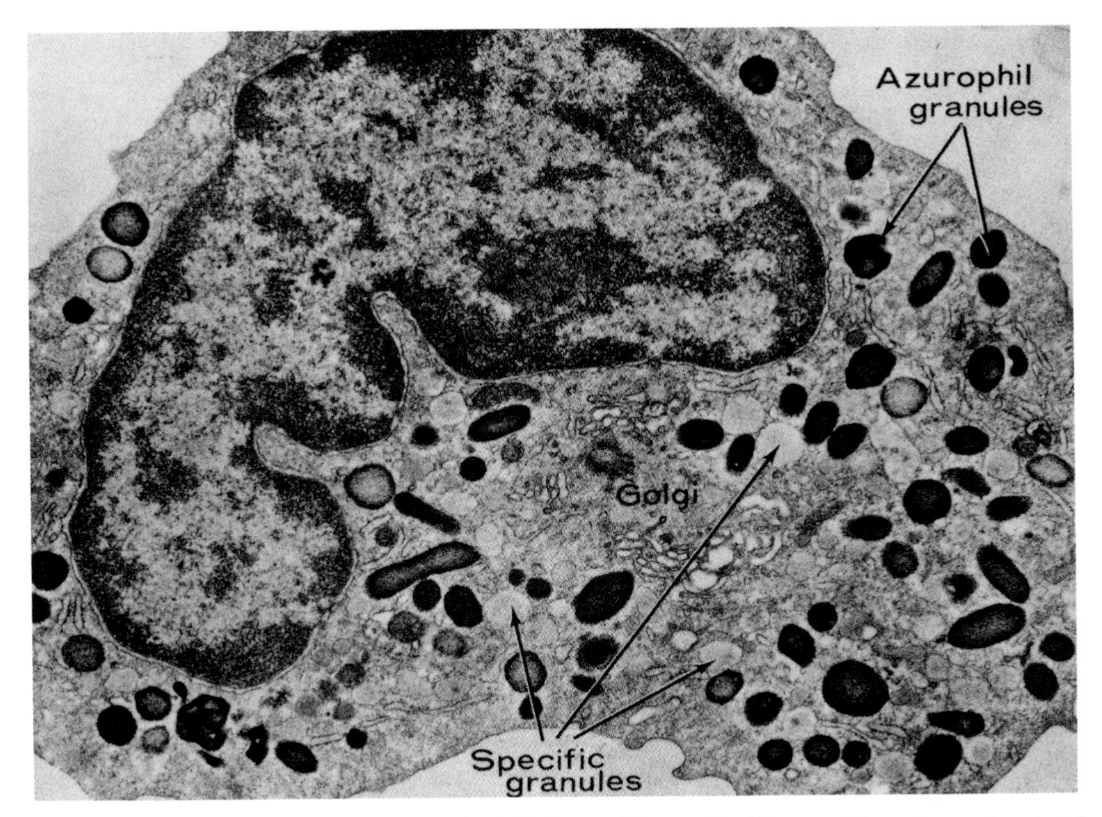

Figure 9–13. Micrograph of a neutrophilic myelocyte stained with the peroxidase reaction. The azurophil granules are strongly stained, but the specific granules are unstained. (From Bainton, D., J. Ullyot, and M. Farquhar. 1971. J. Exp. Med. 134:907.)

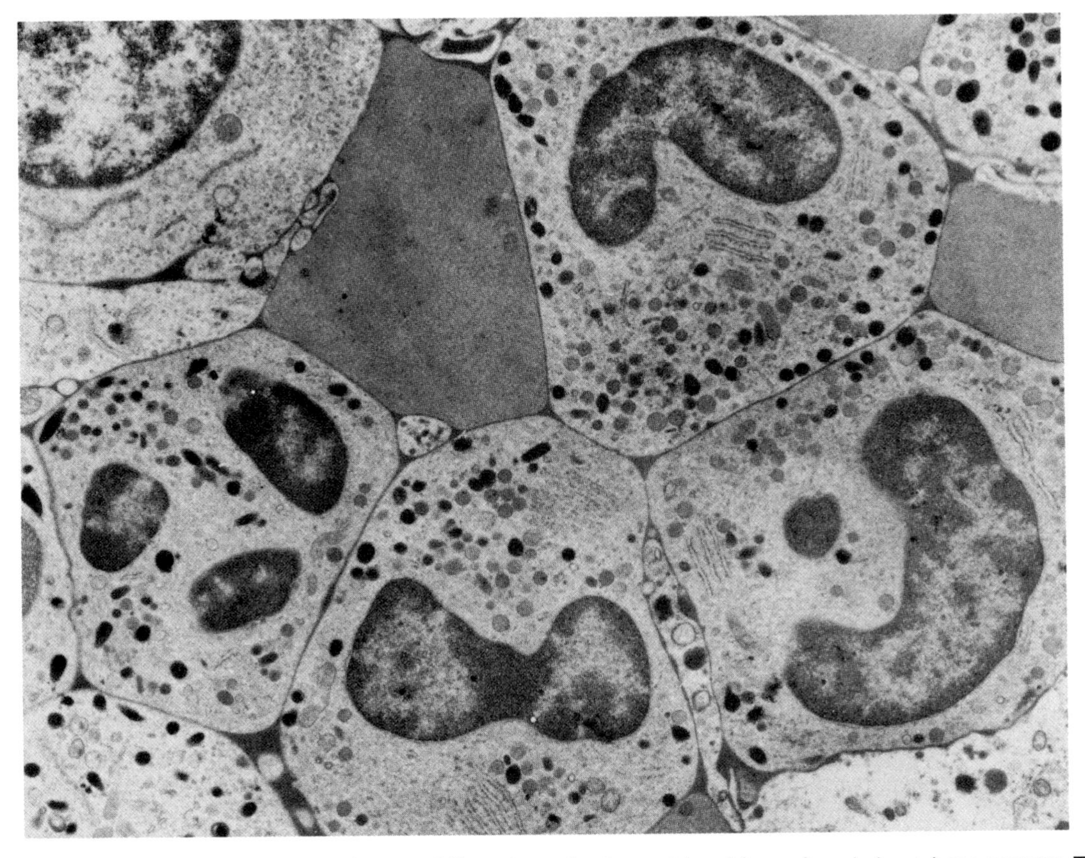

Figure 9–14. Micrograph of a group of neutrophilic metamyelocytes and band forms from baboon bone marrow. The dense azurophil granules are few in number relative to the less dense specific granules.

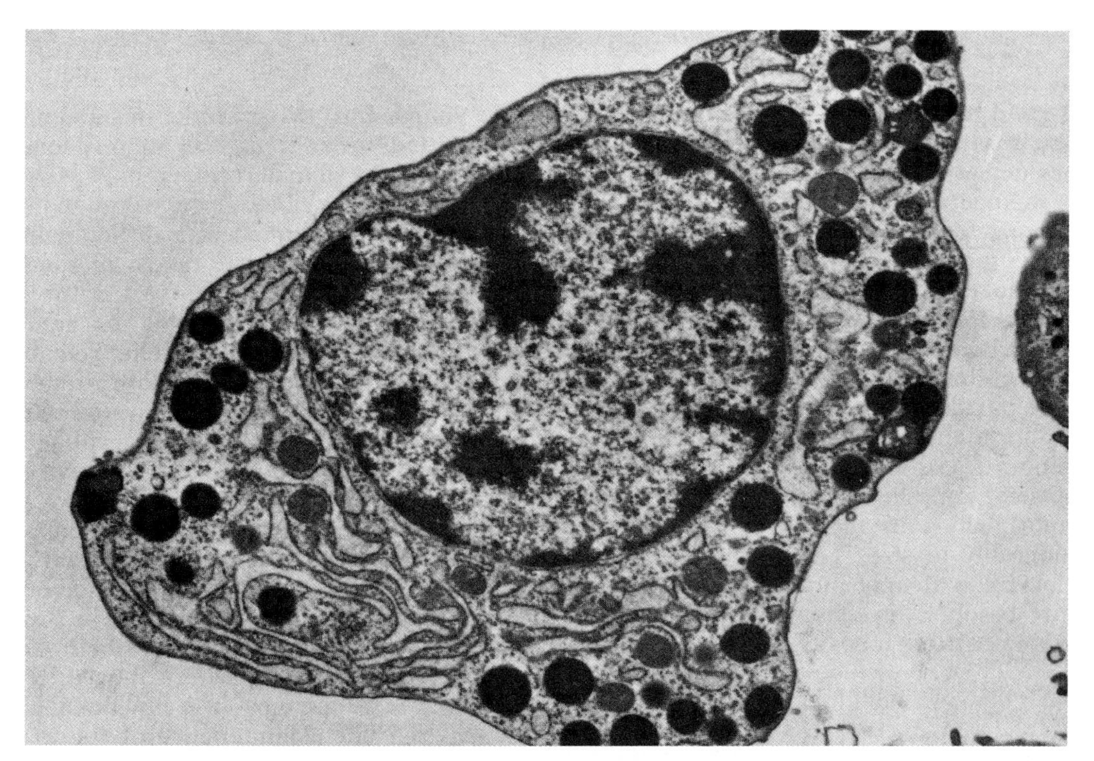

Figure 9–15. Micrograph of an eosinophilic myelocyte from guinea pig bone marrow. There is a well-developed endoplasmic reticulum and the specific granules are distinctly larger than those of the neutrophilic myelocyte. The crystals present in the granules of the mature eosinophil of this species have not developed as yet.

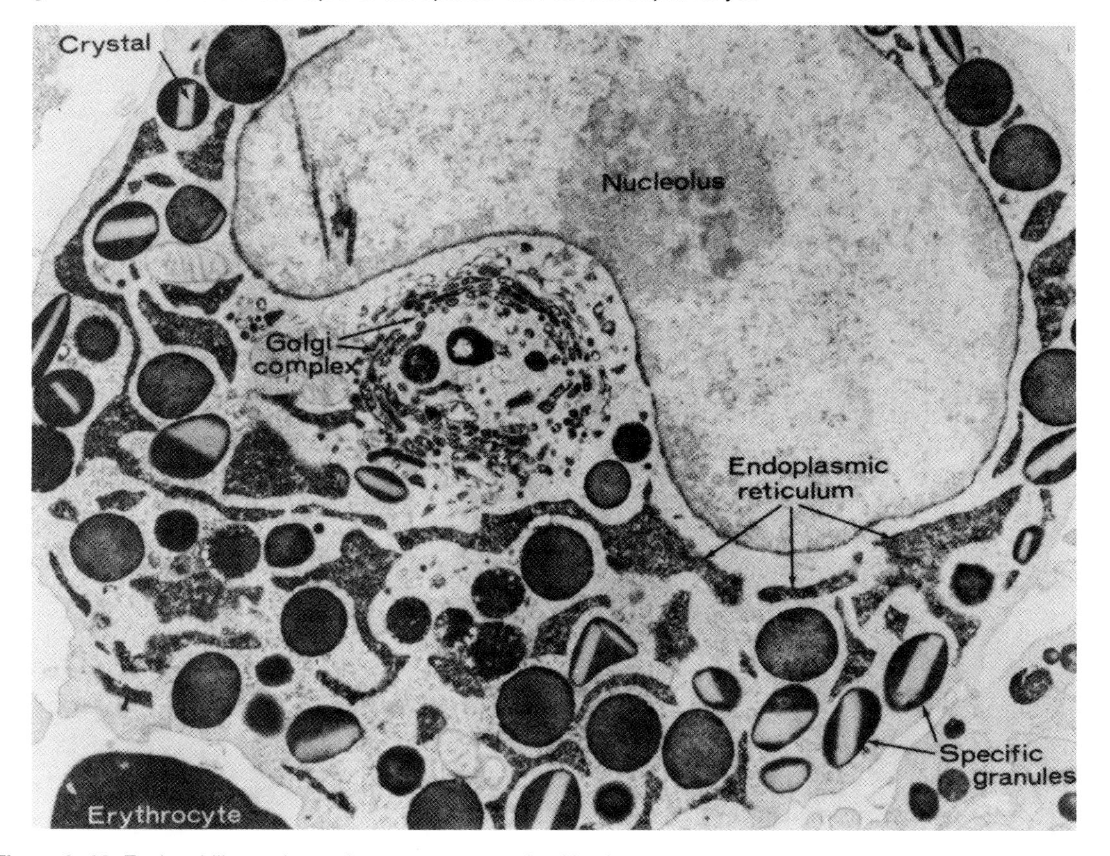

Figure 9–16. Eosinophilic myelocyte from rat marrow stained by the cytochemical reaction for peroxidase. The formation of specific granules is continuing in the Golgi complex and reaction product is found in the perinuclear cisterna and throughout the endoplasmic reticulum. Negative images of crystals are clearly visible in the granules. (From Bainton, D., and M. Farquhar. 1970. J. Cell Biol. 45:54.)

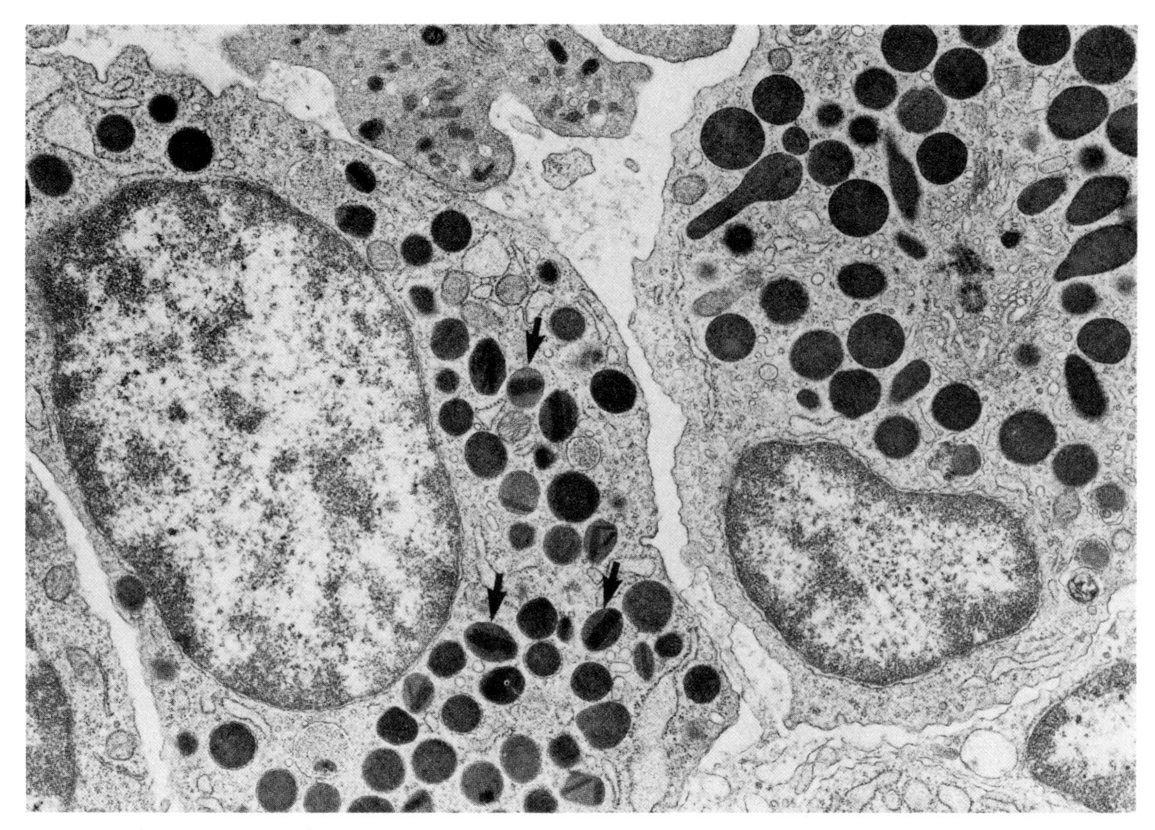

Figure 9–17. Micrograph of a pair of late eosinophilic myelocytes from rat bone marrow. Endoplasmic reticulum is now less extensive and crystals are forming in the specific granules (at arrows) but are difficult to see owing to the density of the background.

to monocyte is about 55 h. The pool of promonocytes in the human marrow is estimated to be about 6×10^8/kg body weight.

Monocytes are not retained in the marrow in great numbers, but migrate into the sinuses soon after they are formed. They probably remain in the circulation for no more than 36 h before migrating into the connective tissues, where they increase in size, acquire multiple lysosomes, and become active in phagocytosis. They are then recognizable as tissue *macrophages.* They are capable of division, but their proliferation does not contribute significantly to renewal of the population in the tissues. This depends mainly on continuous emigration of monocytes from the circulation. The life span of macrophages varies in different tissues but may be as long as several months.

THROMBOPOIESIS

The blood of vertebrates contains cells that provide protection against blood loss by promoting the clotting of blood at the site of injury to blood vessels. In lower vertebrates, these are nucleated cells called *thrombocytes.* In mammals, the functional equivalent of thrombocytes are the *blood platelets.* The term *thrombopoiesis* refers to the development of either thrombocytes or platelets. We are concerned here only with the genesis of blood platelets. These are small anucleate, membrane-limited bits of cytoplasm cast off by large polymorphonuclear cells called *megakaryocytes,* situated adjacent to the marrow sinuses. They extend cell processes between the endothelial cells and into the lumen, where the processes break up into platelets that are swept away in the slow flow of blood.

The very large size of the megakaryocytes, 50–70 μm, makes them the most conspicuous blood-forming cell in the marrow. The cell body is roughly spherical but may have a few short blunt processes (Fig. 9–18) other than the one extending into a sinus. The nucleus is remarkably pleiomorphic, with multiple lobes of varying size interconnected by narrower segments. The nucleoplasm has a moderately

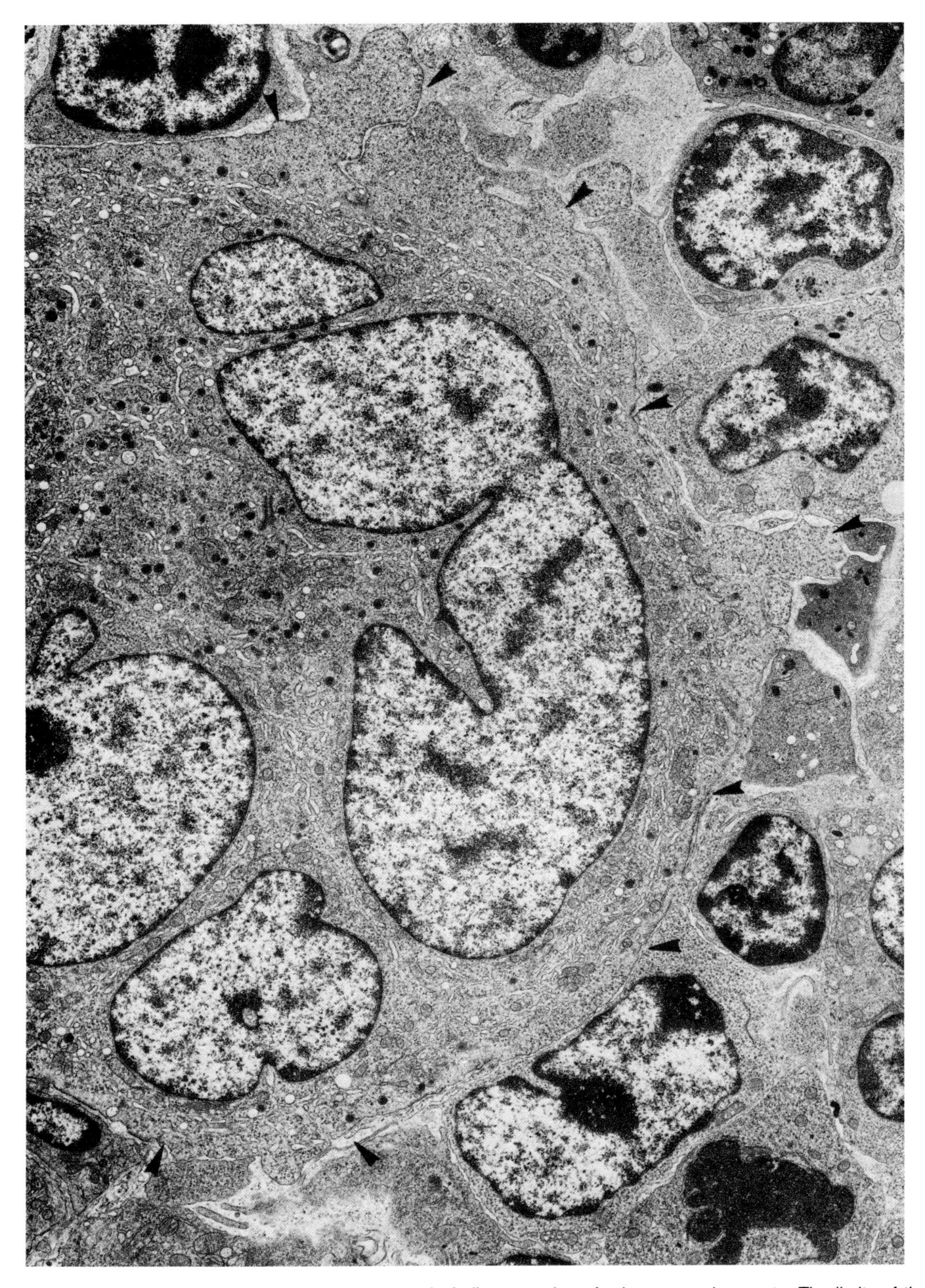

Figure 9–18. Electron micrograph of rat bone marrow including a portion of a large megakaryocyte. The limits of the cell are outlined by the arrow heads. Its very large size and multilobulate nucleus can be contrasted with the smaller hemopoietic cells at the right of the figure.

coarse chromatin pattern and contains multiple indistinct nucleoli. The cytoplasm appears rather homogeneous in routine marrow preparations, but after appropriate fixation and special staining methods, a concentric zonation is apparent. A narrow perinuclear zone, devoid of granules, is surrounded by a broad region that is stippled with many fine azurophilic granules which may be either uniformly distributed or gathered in small clusters, depending on the stage of development of the megakaryocyte. Groups of centrioles can be found in bays between the lobules of the nucleus. Small mitochondria are numerous and dispersed throughout the cytoplasm. In early megakaryocytes, there is a single Golgi complex, but in mature forms, multiple small complexes are found widely dispersed in the cytoplasm. At the periphery of the cell, there is a rim of clear cytoplasm of irregular outline and varying width which is devoid of azurophil granules.

The nucleus of these giant polyploid cells commonly contains from 8 to 16 sets of chromosomes, and occasionally as many as 64. Thus, if platelets arose by nuclear and cytoplasmic division, as do thrombocytes of lower vertebrates, 64 cells would be formed, at most. Megakaryocytes may produce from 4000 to 8000 platelets. Therefore, in mammals, a significant increase in productivity has been gained by the unique device of casting off membrane-limited fragments of cytoplasm endowed with procoagulant properties.

MEGAKARYOCYTE DEVELOPMENT

The committed precursor cell of mammalian thrombopoiesis, called the *colony-forming unit megakaryocyte* (CFU-Meg) gives rise to the *megakaryoblast,* the earliest morphologically identifiable cell of this lineage. It is a large cell with a round or indented nucleus, a loose chromatin pattern and inconspicuous nucleoli. The cytoplasm is basophilic and devoid of specific granules. In electron micrographs, it contains a juxtanuclear Golgi complex, a few cisternae of rough endoplasmic reticulum, and large mitochondria. In subsequent development, these cells increase greatly in size and become polyploid in a series of atypical nuclear divisions that are not followed by cytoplasmic division, a process called *endomitosis.* In each of these endomitotic events, the centrioles replicate and a complex multipolar spindle is formed. At metaphase, the chromosomes become arranged in several planes and, at anaphase, form several distinct groups. Instead of forming several nuclei, these are incorporated in a single lobulated nucleus of larger size. After a brief interval, another episode of endomitosis occurs with daughter groups of chromosomes again reconstituting a single larger nucleus at telophase. Thus, cells with $4n$, $8n$, $16n$, $32n$, and even higher orders of polyploidy are formed without division of the cytoplasm which continues to increase in volume. The repeated doubling of DNA content has been verified by microspectrophotometric analysis and the frequencies of the various degrees of ploidy were found to be $4n$ (1.6%), $8n$ (10%), $16n$ (71.2%), $32n$ (17.1%), and $64n$ (0.1%).

Although the volume of the cell increases progressively during this period, there is little detectable differentiation of the cytoplasm until the cell has acquired all of the DNA it will possess. Because megakaryocytes represent different degrees of polypoidy, they vary considerably in size and in the number of platelets they can produce in their life span.

The *promegakaryocyte,* formed in the process described above, is a cell 30–50 μm in diameter with a prominent cytocentrum containing a number of pairs of centrioles corresponding to the degree of polyploidy. In its further differentiation, numerous small azurophilic granules appear in the cytoplasm. The fully formed *reserve megakaryocyte,* not yet active in platelet formation, is a cell 50–70 μm in diameter with a very large multilobular nucleus. Azurophil granules are uniformly distributed throughout the central region of the cytoplasm but are usually absent from a narrow ectoplasmic zone at the periphery. In mature *platelet-forming megakaryocytes,* the azurophil granules are clustered in small groups, separated by aisles of granule-free cytoplasm. The pale blue ectoplasmic zone is now less conspicuous.

ULTRASTRUCTURAL BASIS OF PLATELET FORMATION

Fragmentation of the megakaryocyte cytoplasm to form platelets was first reported by Wright in 1906, but a more detailed description of the process had to await the development of the electron microscope. In megakaryocytes in which the azurophilic granules had formed small discrete aggregations, early electron micrographs revealed small vesicles

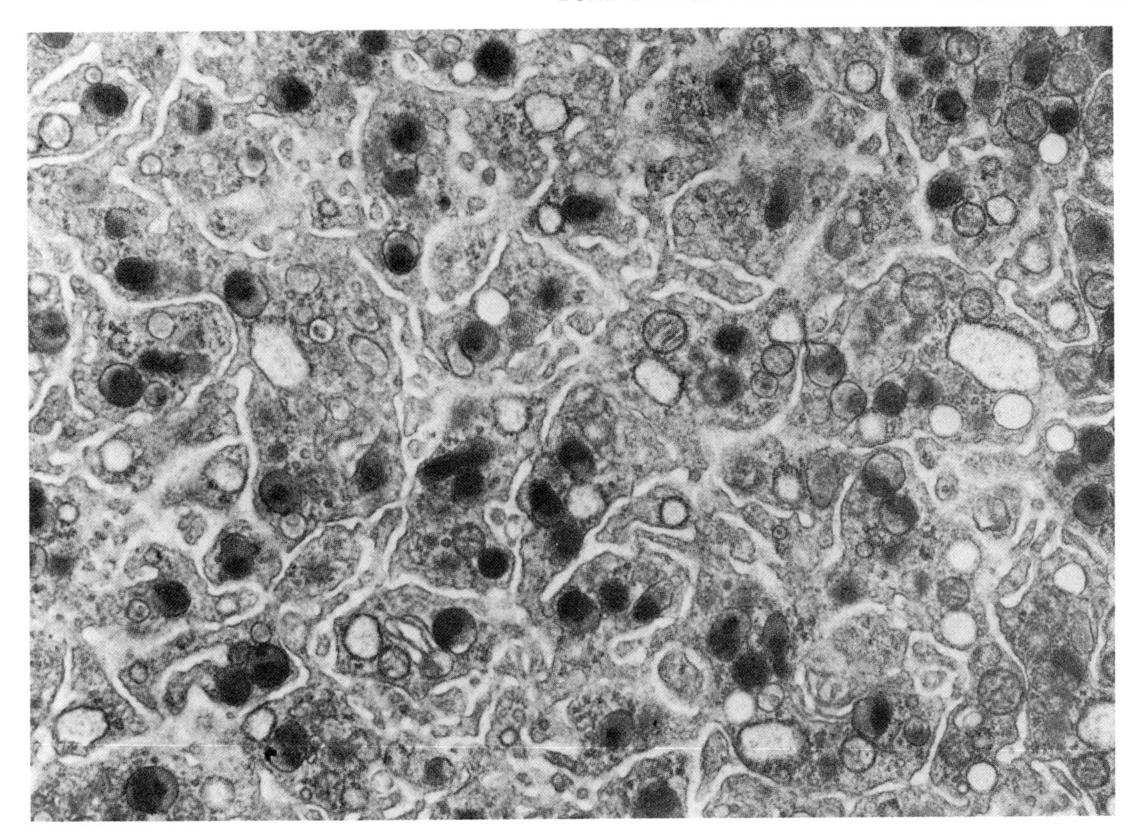

Figure 9–19. Micrograph of a small area of megakaryocyte crytoplasm, showing the platelet demarcation channels outlining future platelets.

aligned in rows between neighboring clumps of granules. This later proved to be a fixation artifact. With improved specimen preparation, what were previously been described as rows of vesicles are found to be membrane-limited, tubules or flattened saccules, oriented in intersecting planes so that they partition the cytoplasm into units 1–3 μm in diameter, each unit containing a cluster of azurophil granules. In maturing megakaryocytes, the limiting membranes of these membrane-limited elements coalesce, resulting in a three-dimensional lattice of paired *platelet demarcation membranes* that bound a continuous system of narrow clefts outlining the nascent platelets (Fig. 9–19).

When first described, the platelet demarcation system was variously interpreted as (1) an unusual form of smooth endoplasmic reticulum; (2) a derivative of the Golgi complex; or (3) a product of deep invasion of the cytoplasm by invaginations of the cell membrane. Its communication with the extracellular space was soon demonstrated by exposing megakaryocytes to suspensions of large molecules that do not cross biomembranes, such as ferritin or horseradish peroxidase. In electron micrographs, these probes were found within the demarcation channels throughout the cytoplasm. It is now widely accepted that the system of platelet demarcation membranes arises from invaginations of the plasmalemma that ramify throughout the cytoplasm and subsequently coalesce into a labyrinth of fenestrated cisternae bounding small areas of cytoplasm destined to become platelets.

RELEASE OF PLATELETS

From their position along the marrow sinuses, mature megakaryocytes extend large processes through the endothelium into the lumen. These processes, sometimes called *proplatelets,* may contain as many as 1200 platelet subunits and it is estimated that a single megakaryocyte may form up to six such processes in its life span. The discharge of platelets from these processes ultimately leaves only a thin layer of cytoplasm bounded by an intact cell membrane. The possibility that these *residual megakaryocytes* may reconstitute their cytoplasm and produce another set of platelets has not been excluded. However, it is generally assumed that they degenerate and are replaced by newly formed megakaryocytes. About 10% of megakaryocytes observed in bone marrow appear to be degenerating cells that have lost nearly all of their cytoplasm through the formation of platelets.

Fragmentation of proplatelets into individual platelets generally takes place in the lumen of the marrow sinuses, but entire proplatelets may occasionally be carried in the bloodstream to the lungs, where they lodge in small vessels and break up into platelets. That entire megakaryocytes may also enter the circulation, has been abundantly documented. They can be found occasionally in the spleen or liver, but are more commonly observed in the small vessels in the lung. Indeed, thousands of megakaryocytes are believed to reach the lung. The observation that the platelet count in blood drawn from the pulmonary vein is higher than in blood taken from the pulmonary artery verifies that these ectopic megakaryocytes continue to make a significant contribution to platelet production.

A considerable body of information has accumulated on the kinetics of thrombokinesis. The generation time from stem cell to mature platelet-producing megakaryocyte is estimated to be about 10 days in humans. A humoral regulatory mechanism seems to ensure that their rate of development is responsive to the need for circulating platelets. Bleeding or an exchange transfusion that results in low levels of platelets (*thrombocytopenia*) is followed, in several days, by a three-to fourfold increase in the number of megakaryoces in the marrow and a rebound of circulating platelets to 150–200% of the initial level. This positive feedback control of platelet production is attributed to a humoral agent, *thrombopoietin*. The source of this hypothetical stimulating factor is unknown and, to date, efforts to purify and characterize it have not been successful.

LYMPHOPOIESIS

Histologists of the nineteenth century and the early part of the present century divided the blood cells into two categories according to their presumed sites of origin. Erythrocytes, platelets, and granular leukocytes developing in the bone marrow were called the *myeloid* elements of the blood, and their collective development was termed *myelopoiesis*. Lymphocytes and monocytes were believed to originate in the lymph nodes, spleen, and thymus and were referred to as the lymphoid elements of the blood. Their development was termed *lymphopoiesis*. This terminology has persisted although the assumption of a dualistic origin of the blood cells, on which it was based, is no longer valid. The existence, in the marrow, of pluripotential stem cells capable of giving rise to blood cells of all kinds is now widely accepted. The monocyte, formerly believed to arise by further differentiation of large lymphocytes, is now known to develop in the marrow from a bipotential progenitor cell (CFU-GM) that also gives rise to granular leukocytes. The monocyte is now assigned to the myeloid rather than the lymphoid category.

Lymphopoiesis has continued to be a subject of debate but much has been learned in recent years from techniques for labeling lymphocytes to follow their migrations and from immunological methods for distinguishing different types by detecting specific molecules on their surface. It is now clear that the lymphopoietic stem cells originate in the bone marrow. The unipotential stem cells destined to form T-lymphocytes leave the marrow and are carried in the blood to the cortex of the thymus. There they proliferate and differentiate as they move from the cortex to the medulla. During their differentiation, they acquire a surface marker (Thy-1) characteristic of all T-cells, and different subsets of T-cells acquire their own distinctive surface markers. For reasons that remain obscure, a high percentage of T-lymphocytes degenerate during their transit from the cortex to the medulla. Mature T-lymphocytes leave the medulla via blood vessels and lymphatics and many home to the spleen for a short period before joining the recirculating pool of lymphocytes.

The genesis of B-lymphocytes in birds has been established beyond doubt. Stem cells migrate from the marrow to an appendage of the avian cloaca, called the *bursa of Fabricius*, in much the same way that T-cell precursors populate the thymus. In the bursa, they differentiate into mature B-lymphocytes and then enter the recirculating pool of small lymphocytes. The functional equivalent of the bursa of Fabricius in mammals has been a subject of controversy, but it seems that the genesis of B-lymphocytes may take place in multiple sites, including bone marrow, spleen, and possibly the submucosal lymphoid tissue of the intestine. However, the bone marrow appears to be the primary site of lymphopoiesis in mammals. In laboratory rodents in which lymphocyte development can be studied with radiolabelled tracers, the marrow has a high rate of lymphocyte production throughout fetal and postnatal life. Lymphocytes constitute 30% of all nucleated marrow cells and exceed the number of erythroblasts at all ages.

The proliferating precursors of small lymphocytes are somewhat larger cells with a pale-staining nucleus, a very thin rim of cytoplasm, and few organelles. These so-called *transitional cells* are actively proliferating and constitute about one-fifth of all marrow lymphocytes. In the mouse, the rate of lymphocyte production is estimated to be about 10^8 per day. For ethical reasons, quantitation of lymphocyte production by similar methods cannot be carried out in humans, but a proportionally high rate of lymphocyte production is assumed. The cells acquire surface markers characteristic of B-lymphocytes and enter the circulation. They then continuously recirculate through the spleen, lymph nodes, and peripheral blood. The origin and functions of the T- and B-lymphocytes will be discussed in more appropriate context in the chapter on the Immune System.

REGULATION OF HEMOPOIESIS

Much remains to be discovered about the factors that determine which path of differentiation will be taken by the progeny of pluripotential stem cells and about the mechanisms that enable the body to respond to unusual demands for specific blood-cell types needed to recover from blood loss or to combat infection. However, it is apparent that multiple factors are involved. Some of these reside in the stromal cells and extracellular elements that create the local *microenvironment* for hemopoiesis. Others are regulatory *humoral agents* that originate elsewhere in the body and are carried in the blood to the bone marrow where they stimulate proliferation and differentiation of particular cell lineages.

HEMOPOIETIC MICROENVIRONMENT

Although stem cells may enter the circulation and be carried throughout the body, hemopoiesis occurs in only a few sites that provide an environment capable of sustaining their proliferation. That the appropriate local conditions can be acquired by an organ and can subsequently be lost is evident from the changing location of the principal site of blood formation in the embryo, from the yolk sac, to liver and spleen, and finally to the bone marrow. It is assumed that the successful colonization of these organs is due to distinctive properties of the cells and extracellular components of their stroma. This is strongly supported by animal experiments in which ectopic hemopoiesis can be established only by first transplanting to the site, stroma from the bone marrow. Further evidence of the dependence on this specific microenvironment has come from efforts to grow hemopoietic cells in vitro. Long-term proliferation of stem cells and progenitor cells was achieved only if the floor of the culture vessel was first covered with an adherent layer of cells derived from the stroma of bone marrow. A feeder layer of fibroblasts from other organs was ineffective. The hemopoietic cells in vitro, or in vivo, maintain an intimate relationship to the stromal cells, but whether the beneficial effects are mediated by cell contact or by diffusable products of the stromal cells is not known.

The stroma of different hemopoietic organs, or indeed of separate regions in the same organ, may favor the development of different cell lineages. Stem cells lodging in the spleen of irradiated mice give rise to colonies that are predominantely erythroid, whereas those settling in depleted bone marrow produce a preponderance of granulocyte/monocyte colonies. Stem cells rarely form lymphoid colonies in the spleen or marrow, but those lodging in the thymus or lymph nodes do so regularly. It has been speculated that these differences may be attributable to organotypic variations in the relative numbers of reticular cells, fibroblasts, and macrophages because it has been noted that erythroid cells cluster around macrophages, forming assemblages called erythroblastic islets, whereas the precursors of granulocytes appear to be related to the dendritic processes of reticular cells. Confidence in such judgments is compromised, however, by the difficulty of analyzing three-dimensional relationships from thin sections of the closely packed cells in these complex organs.

There is suggestive evidence that extracellular components of the stroma may be involved. Extracellular matrix extracted from bone marrow has been shown to stimulate proliferation and differentiation when used as a substrate for cultures of hemopoietic cells. The growth-stimulating factor GM-CSF is reported to bind to glycosaminoglycans of the marrow. Granulocyte precursors have also been shown to bind preferentially to *hemonectin,* an adhesion protein found only in the marrow, whereas mature neutrophils are not bound. It is proposed that the presence of such an organ-specific, lineage-specific component in the extracellular matrix may help to explain the predominance of granulocytopoiesis in the marrow compared to the spleen. Although our understanding of the mechanisms is fragmentary, there is no doubt that the induction and maintenance of hemopoiesis are decisively dependent on the stromal microenvironment.

HUMORAL REGULATION OF HEMOPOIESIS

In the continuous renewal of circulating blood cells, the relative numbers of the several cell types remain remarkably constant. This led to the assumption that there must be some mechanism for monitoring their numbers in the circulation and type-specific humoral growth regulators that act back on the hemopoietic tissue to control the rate of formation and release of new cells of each type. The means of sensing changes in the numbers of cells in the circulation remain obscure, but some progress has been made in detecting and characterizing the molecules involved in the humoral regulation of specific cell lineages.

The control of erythropoeisis was the first to be studied and is best understood. Blood loss stimulates the marrow to increase its production and release of erythrocytes. Transfusion of excess erythrocytes is followed by suppression of erythropoiesis. An enhanced need for oxygen also stimulates the marrow. In the physiological adaptation to residence at high altitude, the body responds to hypoxia by increasing the number of circulating erythrocytes. When this was first observed, it was assumed that the marrow was *directly* responsive to the oxygen content of the blood. However, this reasonable conclusion was later shown to be incorrect. In ingenious experiments on parabiotic rats that share a common circulation, it was found that when only one member of the conjoined pair was exposed to hypoxia in a hypobaric chamber, *both* members showed enhanced erythropoiesis. This, and other experiments, clearly demonstrated that the hypoxic stimulus to the marrow was mediated by a blood-borne humoral agent. This hypothetical substance was originally referred to as the *erythropoiesis-stimulating factor.* It has since been isolated and named *erythropoietin.* It is a glycoprotein of about 34,000 MW. It can be detected in the plasma and urine of hypoxic animals and of humans with blood or respiratory diseases that are attended by oxygen deficiency. Erythropoietin synthesis is inversely related to the oxygen tension prevailing in the tissues. The monitor for tissue oxygenation and site of synthesis of erythropoietin is located mainly in the juxtaglomerular apparatus of the kidney.

Maintenance of normal numbers of circulating erythrocytes depends on (1) continuing stimulation of the marrow by erythropoietin, (2) a marrow capable of responding, and (3) an adequate supply of iron to meet the needs of the differentiating cells of the erythroid lineage for hemoglobin synthesis. A normal marrow not only provides for slow continuous replacement of aging erythrocytes, but is also capable of a rapid increase in output to four or five times the basal rate. Such rapid increases in erythrocyte production may tax the stores of iron. The body contains only limited reserves of iron in the form of *ferritin,* a large protein capable of accumulating 2000 or more atoms of iron. It is found in many cell types throughout the body but is especially abundant in the liver. Iron is transported in the blood plasma by an iron-binding globulin, *transferrin,* which binds to specific receptors on the surface of erythropoietic cells in the marrow and is internalized in coated vesicles. Within the cells, acidification of the vesicles results in dissociation of iron from transferrin and its transfer to the intracellular iron carrier *ferritin.* Iron is made available from this store for hemoglobin synthesis. An inadequate supply of iron may limit the response of the marrow to erythropoietin stimulation, resulting in *iron-deficiency anemia.*

It was long believed that leukocyte production would prove to be regulated by humoral factors comparable to erythroietin, but validation of this assumption was delayed because some of the variations observed in leucocyte numbers can be explained by mechanisms other than formation of new cells. In the presence of bacterial invasion, there is a very rapid increase in circulating neutrophils. The rapidity of this response suggests that it results from mobilization of reserves, rather than production of new cells. The population of neutrophils is envisioned in two categories: (1) those that move with the flow of blood, the so-called *circulating pool of leucocytes* and (2) those that are temporarily adherent to the endothelium in various parts of the vascular system, the *marginated pool of leucocytes*. Normally, the leucocyte population is about equally divided between these two, but in response to exercise, epinephrine injection, or bacterial toxins, there is a massive movement of the marginated cells into the bloodstream, doubling the number in the circulating pool without increased granulocytopoiesis. In addition, there are large reserves of bandforms and mature neutrophils in the marrow and these can be released on demand. Indeed, it is estimated that there may be 10 times as many in the marrow as there are in the circulation. Therefore, dramatic increases in circulating neutrophils can be achieved early in an infection by their release from the marginated pool and from the marrow without an immediate change in the rate of production of new cells.

As infection continues, however, there is a marked increase in granulocytopoiesis. The capacity for leucocyte production under these conditions is enormous. In a prolonged infection, the leukocyte count may progress from a normal level of about $5000/ml^3$ to 50,000 or more. This represents both mobilization of reserves and formation of astounding numbers of leukocytes over the course of several days or weeks. Humoral agents carried in the blood from the site of infection to the marrow are now known to be responsible for the increased granulocytopoiesis.

Identification of the humoral agents has been facilitated by the development of methods for the cultivation of hemopoietic cells in vitro. The stem cells and committed precursors of the various types of blood cells were found to be incapable of self-renewal or differentiation into more mature cell types in the absence of specific stimulating factors. However, the addition of one of these to the culture medium stimulated clonal development of the target progenitor, resulting in the formation of a mixed colony or a pure colony of a single cell type. As previously stated, the various stem cells and committed precursors all look alike and, as in the spleen-colony assay, the developmental potential of the cell of origin, called a colony-forming unit (CFU), is determined by identifying the end-cell type, or types, present in the resulting colony. Hemopoietic cell cultures have verified that there are some progenitor cells that are multipotential (CFU-GMMMe), others are bipotential (CFU-GM), and still others are unipotential, that is, they are committed to a single cell lineage (CFU-G, CFU-M, CFU-Eo, CFU-Me), as depicted in Fig. 9–5.

To date, four *colony-stimulating factors* (CSFs) have been isolated and characterized. Two of these stimulate early progenitor cells that are still capable of differentiating into more than one cell type:—*granulocyte-monocyte colony stimulating factor* (GM-CFS), which stimulates CFU-GM to form mixed colonies of neutrophils and monocytes; and *multi-CSF,* also called *interleukin-3* which stimulates the multipotential progenitor cell CFU-GEMMe to form colonies containing neutrophils, erythrocytes, monocytes, and megakaryocytes. Two other CSFs stimulate the differentiation of more advanced progenitors that are committed to a single cell lineage:—*granulocyte-colony stimulating factor* (G-CSF), which acts upon the unipotential CFU-G resulting in colonies containing only meutrophils; and *monocyte-colony stimulating factor* (M-CSF) producing pure colonies of monocytes. There is however, some redundancy in the effects of the stimulating factors. The development of several cell lineages is stimulated, to some extent, by interleukin-3, as well as by their specific CSF, and erythropoietin, which is required for erythrocyte development, also weakly promotes the differentiation of the megakaryocyte progenitor.

The colony-stimulating factors are glycoproteins ranging in molecular weight from 18,000 to 90,000. They are effective in extremely low concentrations, and are believed to be synthesized by a variety of cell types both within and outside of the bone marrow. They are detectable in the blood and in most organs that have been assayed.

The maintenance of normal levels of circulating leucocytes is believed to depend upon the production of CSFs by cells in the stroma of the bone marrow. This basal rate of leucocyte production controlled within the marrow is sometimes referred to as *constitutive hemopoiesis* to distinguish it from *induced hemopoiesis* that results from stimulating factors produced by cells remote from the marrow that are activated by products of invading bacteria. Injection of bacterial endotoxin into experimental animals results in a thousand-fold increase in circulating CSFs. The genes for CSFs are evidently not expressed in cells outside of the marrow until they are activated by reception of signals from T-lymphocytes and macrophages which serve as sentinels detecting microbial invasion. In infections, these cells produce CSFs themselves and also release cytokines that induce other cells to synthesize them. T-lymphocytes, reacting to a specific bacterial antigen, produce GM-CSF and also release lymphokines that activate the macrophages mobilized at the site. Similarly, macrophages exposed to bacterial products respond by producing GM-CSF, G-CSF and M-CSF which are transported in the blood to the marrow where they stimulate leucocyte production. Activated macrophages also release the cytokines *interleukin-1* (Il-1) and *tumor necrosis factor* (TNF) which act locally upon fibroblasts and endothelial cells triggering their synthesis of CSFs that contribute to the stimulation of myelopoiesis in the marrow.

All four colony-stimulating factors have been purified and characterized. The chromosomal location of their genes has been determined, and the sequences encoding each factor have been cloned. This raises the hope that sufficient quantities may be produced by DNA technology to be used clinically in the treatment of humans with leukopenias resulting from therapeutic radiation for cancer or from viral diseases such as AIDS.

There is, as yet, no convincing evidence for a feedback control of B-lymphocyte production comparable to the colony-stimulating factors or hemopoietins that regulate the circulating levels of other blood cells. By analogy with the effects of bleeding or induced hemolysis on erythropoiesis, one might expect a marrow response to depletion of blood lymphocytes. However, immunological suppression of circulating lymphocytes is reported to have no significant effect on lymphocyte production. It is concluded that the normal basal rate of lymphopoiesis is regulated mainly by local conditions in the lymphoid organs and to a lesser extent in the marrow. As will be discussed in a later chapter on the immune system, the majority of B-lymphocytes are programmed to respond specifically to foreign protein or bacteria that have previously entered the body. When B-lymphocytes encounter such an antigen again, they are activated to proliferate, producing more lymphocytes of the same antigenic specificity. Their proliferation is further stimulated by lymphokines released by T-lymphocytes responding to the same antigens.

BIBLIOGRAPHY

GENERAL

Tavassoli, M. and J.M. Yoffey. 1983. Bone Marrow Structure and Function. New York, Alan Liss.

Wickramasinghe, S.N. 1975. Human Bone Marrow. Oxford, Blackwell Scientific Publications.

PRENATAL HEMOPOIESIS

Bloom, W. and F.W. Bartelmez. 1940. Hemopoiesis in young human embryos. Am. J. Anat. 67:21.

Johnson, F.R. and M.A.G. Moore. 1975. Role of stem cell migration in initiation of mouse fetal liver hemopoiesis. Nature (London) 258:726.

Moore, M.A.G. and D. Metcalf. 1970. Ontogeny of the hemopoietic system: yolk sac origin of in vivo and in vitro colony forming cells in developing mouse embryos. Br. J. Hematol 18:279.

ORGANIZATION OF THE BONE MARROW

Becher, R.P. and P.P. DeBruyn. 1976. The transmural passage of blood cells into myeloid sinuses and the entry of platelets into the sinusoidal circulation. A scanning electron microscopic investigation. Am. J. Anat. 145:183.

Campbell, A.D. and M.S. Wicha. 1988. Extracellular matrix and the hematopoietic microenvironment. J. Lab. Clin. Med. 112:140.

DeBruyn, P.P., P.C. Breen, and T.B. Thomas. 1970. The microcirculation of the bone marrow. Anat. Rec. 168:55.

Dexter, T.M. 1982. Stromal cell associated hemopoiesis. J. Cell Physiol. 110 (Suppl. 1):87.

Weiss, L. 1976. The hemopoietic microenvironment of the bone marrow: an ultrastructural study of the stroma in rats. Anat. Rec. 186:161.

Weiss, L. and L.T. Chen. 1975. The organization of hemopoietic cords and vascular sinuses in bone marrow. Blood Cells 1:617.

Wolf, N.S. 1979. The hemopoietic microenvironment. Clin. Hematol. 8:469.

HEMOPOIETIC STEM CELLS

Deldar, A., H. Lewis, and L. Weiss. 1985. Bone living cells and hematopoiesis: An electron microscopic study of canine bone marrow. Anat. Rec. 213:187.

Dexter, T.M. 1979. Hemopoiesis in long-term bone marrow cultures. A review. Acta. Haematol. 62:299.

Lajtha, L.G. 1979. Haemopoietic stem cells. Concepts and definitions. Blood Cells 5:447.

Quesenberry, P. and L. Levitt. 1979. Haematopoietic stem cells. N. Engl. J. Med. 30:755, 819.

Spangrude, G.J., S. Heimfeld, and I.L. Weissman. 1988. Purification and characterization of mouse hematopoietic stem cells. Science 241:58.

Till, T.E. and E.A. McCulloch. 1980. Hemopoietic stem cell differentiation. Biochim. Biophys. Acta. 605:431.

ERYTHROPOIESIS

Campbell, F.R. 1968. Nuclear elimination from the normoblast of fetal guinea pig liver as studied with electron microscopy and serial section techniques. Anat. Rec. 160:539.

Harrison, P.R. 1976. Analysis of erythropoiesis at the molecular level. Review article. Nature (London) 262:353.

Hillman, R.S. and C.A. Finch. 1967. Erythropoiesis normal and abnormal. Semin. Hematol. 4:427.

Nijhof, W. and P.K. Wierenga. 1983. Isolation and characterization of the erythroid progenitor cell: CFU-E. J. Cell Biol. 96:386.

GRANULOPOIESIS

Ackerman, G.A. 1971. The human neutrophil myelocyte. A correlated phase and electron microscopic study. Z. Zellforsch. Mikrosk. Anat. 121:153.

Bainton, D.F. and M.G. Farquhar. 1966. Origin of granules in the polymorphonuclear leukocytes. Two types derived from opposite faces of the Golgi complex in development. J. Cell Biol. 28:277.

Bainton, D.F. and M. Farquhar. 1968. Differences in enzyme content of azurophil and specific granules of polymorphonuclear leukocytes. II. Cytochemistry and electron microscopy of bone marrow cells. J. Cell Biol. 39:299.

Bainton, C.F. and M. Farquhar. 1970. Segregation and packaging of granule enzymes in eosinophilic leukocytes. J. Cell Biol. 45:54.

Boggs, D.R. 1967. The kinetics of neutrophilic leukocytes in health and disease. Semin. Hematol. 4:1.

Cannistra, S.A. and J.D. Griffin. 1988. Regulation of production and function of granulocytes and monocytes. Semin. Hematol. 25:173.

Scott, R.E. and R.G. Horn. 1970. Ultrastructural aspects of neutrophil granulocyte development in humans. Lab. Invest. 23:202.

MONOPOIESIS

Meuret, G. 1976. Origin, ontogeny, and kinetics of mononuclear phagocytes. Adv. Exp. Med. Biol. 73, Pt.A:71.

Nichols, B.A., D.F. Bainton, and M. Farquhar. 1971. Differentiation of monocytes: origin nature and fate of their azurophil granules. J. Cell Biol. 50:498.

van Furth, R. and Z. Cohn. 1968. The origin and kinetics of mononuclear phagocytes. J. Exp. Med. 128:415.

Whitlaw, D.M., M.F. Bell, and H.F. Batho. 1968. Monocyte kinetics. Observations after pulse labelling. J. Cell Physiol. 72:65.

THROMBOPOIESIS

Becher, R.P. and P.P. DeBruyn. 1976. The transmural passage of blood cells and entry of platelets into the sinusoidal circulation: a scanning microscope investigation. Am. J. Anat. 145:183.

Behnke, O. 1968. An electron microscope study of the megakaryocyte of rat bone marrow. I. The development of the demarcation membrane system and the platelet surface coat. J. Ultrastr. Res. 24:412.

Metcalf, D., H.R. MacDonald, N. Odartchenki, and B. Sordat. 1975. Growth of mouse megakaryocyte colonies in vitro. Proc. Nat. Acad. Sci. USA, 72:1744.

Pedersen, N.T. 1978. Occurrence of megakaryocytes in various vessels and their retention in the pulmonary capillaries in man. Scand. J. Hematol. 21:369.

Radley, J.M. and G. Scofield. 1980. The mechanism of platelet release. Blood 56:996.

Shaklai, M. and M. Tavassoli. 1978. Demarcation membrane system in rat megakaryocyte and the mechanism of platelet formation. J. Ultrastr. Res. 62:270.

Tavassoli, M. 1980. Megakaryocyte–platelet axis and the process of platelet formation and release. Blood 55:537.

Williams, N. and R.F. Levine. 1982. The origin, development, and regulation of megakaryocytes. Br. J. Hematol. 52:173.

Zucker-Franklin, D. and S. Peterson. 1984. Thrombocytopoiesis: Analysis by membrane tracer and freeze-fracture studies on fresh human and cultured megakaryocytes. J. Cell Biol. 99:390.

LYMPHOPOIESIS

Osmond, D.G. 1975. Formation and maturation of bone marrow lymphocytes. J. Reticuloendo. Soc. 17:99.

Osmond, D.G., M.T. Fahlman, G.M. Fulop,and D.M. Rahal. 1981. Regulation and localization of lymphocyte production in the bone marrow. *In* Microenvironment in Hemopoietic and Lymphoid Differentiation. Ciba Found. Symposium 84. London, Pitman Medical.

Rosse, C. 1976. Small lymphocyte and transitional cell populations of the bone marrow. Their role in the mediation of immune and hemopoietic progenitor cell function. Internat. Rev. Cytol. 62:311.

REGULATION OF HEMOPOIESIS

Campbell, A.D. and M.S. Wicha. 1988. Extracellular matrix and the haemopoietic microenvironment. J. Lab. Clin. Med. 112:140.

Cannistra, S.A. and J.D. Griffin. 1988. Regulation of production and function of granulocytes and monocytes. Semin. Hematol. 25:173.

Clark, S.C. and R. Kamen. 1987. The hemopoietic colony stimulating factors. Science 236:1229.

Dexter, T.M. 1987. Growth factors involved in hemopoiesis. J. Cell Sci. 88:1.

Golde, D.W. and M.J. Cline. 1974. Regulation of granulopoiesis. N. Engl. J. Med. 231:1388.

Gordon, M.Y., G.P. Riley, S.M. Watt, and M.F. Greaves. 1987. Compartmentalization of a hemopoietic growth factor (GM-CSF) by glycosaminoglycans in the bone marrow microenvironment. Nature 326:403.

Metcalf, D. 1985. The granulocyte-macrophage colony stimulating factors. Science 229:16.

Reissman, K.R. 1960. Studies on the mechanism of erythropoietic stimulation in parabiotic rate during hypoxia. Blood 5:372; 16: 1411.

Rifkin, R.A. and P.A. Marks. 1975. The regulation of erythropoiesis. Blood Cells 1:417.

Robinson, W.A. and A. Magalik, 1975. The kinetics and regulation of granulopoiesis. Semin. Hematol. 12:7.

10 MUSCULAR TISSUE

Contractility is a fundamental property of protoplasm exhibited, in varying degree, by nearly all cells. In cells of muscular tissue, the ability to convert chemical energy into mechanical work has become highly developed. Locomotion of multicellular animals, the beating of their hearts, and the movements of their internal organs depend on muscle of different types, each specialized for the kind of force or motion required.

Three categories of muscle are distinguished in vertebrates: *smooth muscle, striated muscle,* and *cardiac muscle.* Smooth muscle is composed of fusiform, uninucleate cells that are not subject to voluntary control but respond to stimulation by the autonomic nervous system. Striated muscle, associated with the skeleton, is innervated by the cerebrospinal nervous system and is responsible for locomotion and other voluntary movements. Its long cylindrical subunits, called *muscle fibers,* are multinucleate syncytia containing closely packed *myofibrils,* exhibiting along their length alternating dark and light bands that are in register across the width of the fiber. This highly ordered arrangement results in a distinctive pattern of repeating cross-striations that are the basis for the term *striated muscle.* This type of muscle is also frequently called *skeletal muscle* to distinguish it from *cardiac muscle* which is also cross-striated but differs in that its fibers are not syncytial but are made up of uninucleate cellular units joined end-to-end. Cardiac muscle is not under voluntary control. It is endowed with an intrinsic system for generating rhythmic contractions but receives input from the central nervous system influencing its rate.

SMOOTH MUSCLE

Smooth muscle forms the contractile portion of the wall of the digestive tract from the middle of the esophagus to the internal sphincter of the anus. It provides the motive power for mixing the ingested food with digestive juices and for its propulsion through the tract. Smooth muscle is also found in the walls of the ducts in the glands that are associated with the alimentary tract and in the walls of the respiratory passages from the trachea to the alveolar ducts. Blood vessels also have smooth muscle in their wall that controls their caliber.

SMOOTH MUSCLE FIBERS

In the histological literature, the organizational subunits of all types of muscle have traditionally been called *fibers.* Those of smooth muscle are fusiform or spindle-shaped with their elongated nucleus situated in their wider central portion (Fig. 10–1). They vary greatly in their length in different organs. In the gravid human uterus, smooth muscle fibers may reach a length of 0.5 mm. In the wall of the intestine, their average length is about 0.2 mm, and in the walls of blood vessels, the smallest smooth muscle fibers may be only 20 μm long. Where smooth muscle is organized in bundles, or extensive layers, the individual fibers are offset such that the wide portion of the cells are adjacent to the thin tapering ends of neighboring cells. Therefore, in transverse sections, smooth muscle appears as a mosaic of rounded or polygonal profiles, varying from one to several microns in diameter, with nuclei found only in the larger profiles (Fig. 10–2). The nucleus contains one or two nucleoli and its chromatin is distributed in small clumps along the inner aspect of the nuclear envelope. The major cell organelles are confined to conical regions of cytoplasm extending in either direction from the poles of the elongate nucleus. The peripheral cytoplasm, containing the contractile components, generally appears rather homogeneous under the light microscope, but in favorable preparations studied at high magnification, longitudinally oriented bundles of filaments can be

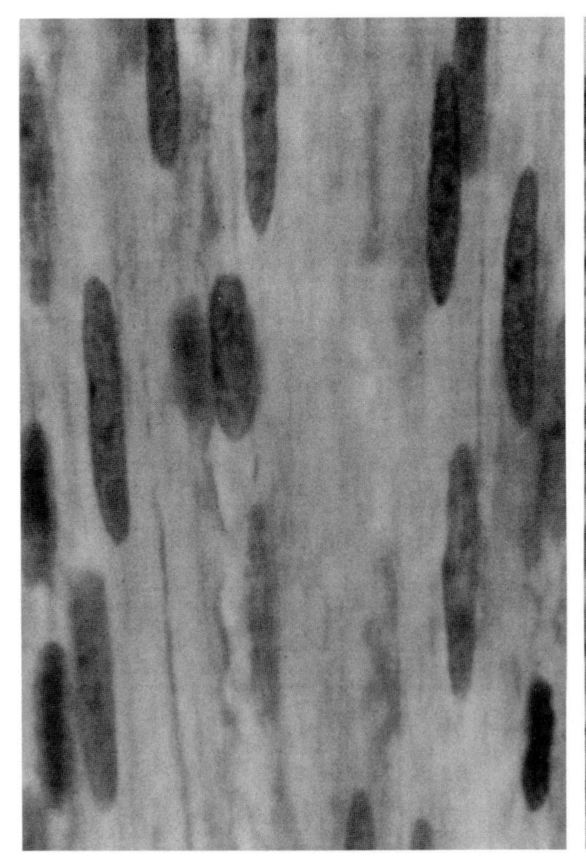

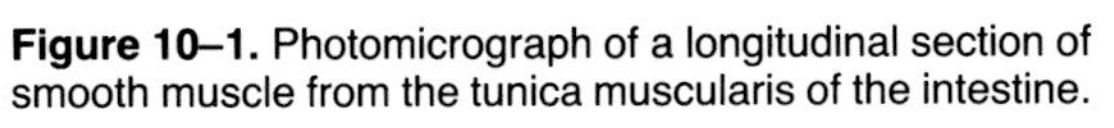

Figure 10–1. Photomicrograph of a longitudinal section of smooth muscle from the tunica muscularis of the intestine.

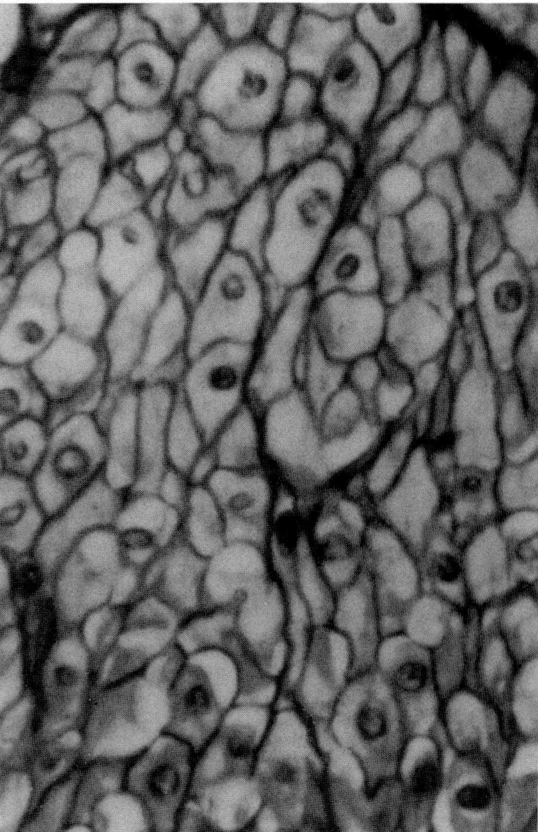

Figure 10–2. Photomicrograph of a transverse section of smooth muscle from the tunica muscularis of the human stomach. The section was stained with the periodic-acid–Schiff reaction which stains the glycoprotein of the lamina externa of the muscle cells, accentuating their outline.

resolved. These can be revealed more clearly by their distinct birefringence, when examined with the polarizing microscope.

In sections stained with the periodic-acid–Schiff reaction, the cytoplasm of the smooth muscle cells in some organs may contain pink-staining deposits of glycogen. In preparations stained by this method, the individual smooth muscle fibers are also outlined by a carbohydrate-rich *external lamina,* comparable to the basal lamina of epithelia (Fig. 10–2). Silver impregnation methods reveal a delicate network of reticular fibers closely associated with the external lamina enveloping each muscle cell.

ORGANIZATIONAL DIVERSITY

Smooth muscle fibers are organized in different patterns to meet local requirements. They may occur singly in loose connective tissue, or gathered together in slender fascicles, as in the tiny arrector pili muscle associated with each hair bulb, or in an annular band, as in the constrictor pupillae muscle of the iris. In precapillary arterioles, single circumferentially oriented fibers are spaced at intervals along the vessel. Their contraction narrows the lumen, decreasing blood flow through the capillary bed. In the wall of larger arteries, flow is controlled by a continuous layer of circular smooth muscle. In the wall of the intestine, smooth muscle fibers form two concentric layers with the fibers of the inner layer oriented circumferentially and those of the outer layer longitudinally. Contraction of the inner layer constricts, and the outer layer tends to shorten the intestine. Their coordinated action produces peristaltic waves of contraction that are propagated along the intestine to propel its contents. In other hollow organs, such as the urinary bladder, smooth muscle is not organized in distinct layers but in interwoven coarse bundles oriented in various directions. The force generated by contraction of the fibers is transmitted through their investment of reticular fibers to the interstitial connective tissue, and thus spreads throughout the muscle mass, diminishing the size of the organ to void its contents.

VARIATIONS IN FORM

Although smooth muscle is usually made up of fusiform cells of varying length, scanning microscopy, combined with methods for digesting the surrounding connective tissue, has revealed examples of morphological diversity that were hitherto unsuspected. The fibers in the urinary bladder and ductus deferens are often branched. In other organs, the fibers may have short lateral processes that contact neighboring cells. Where muscle fibers attach to the central tendon in the gizzard of birds, they have multiple finger-like processes at their ends resembling those seen on skeletal muscle fibers at myotendinous junctions.

There are other cell types, of limited distribution, that differ from smooth muscle fibers in form but share some of their characteristics. In the mammary gland, *myoepithelial cells* of putative ectodermal origin have several long radiating processes that contain myofibril-like bundles of actin and myosin filaments. The cell processes embrace the acini of the gland and their hormonally induced contraction serves to expel the milk. Similar myoepithelial cells are associated with the secretory portions of the tubular sweat glands in the skin. Cells, called *pericytes,* are found at intervals on the surface of certain capillaries and postcapillary venules. They have a rounded cell body and several tapering processes that extend around the vessel. They have been little studied but are assumed to be capable of contracting to influence blood flow.

ULTRASTRUCTURE OF SMOOTH MUSCLE

In electron micrographs of low magnification, the juxtanuclear cytoplasm of smooth muscle fibers contains a small Golgi complex, a cluster of elongate mitochondria, a few short profiles of endoplasmic reticulum and many free ribosomes (Fig. 10–3). The bulk of the contractile cytoplasm presents a homogeneous appearance, save for widely spaced,

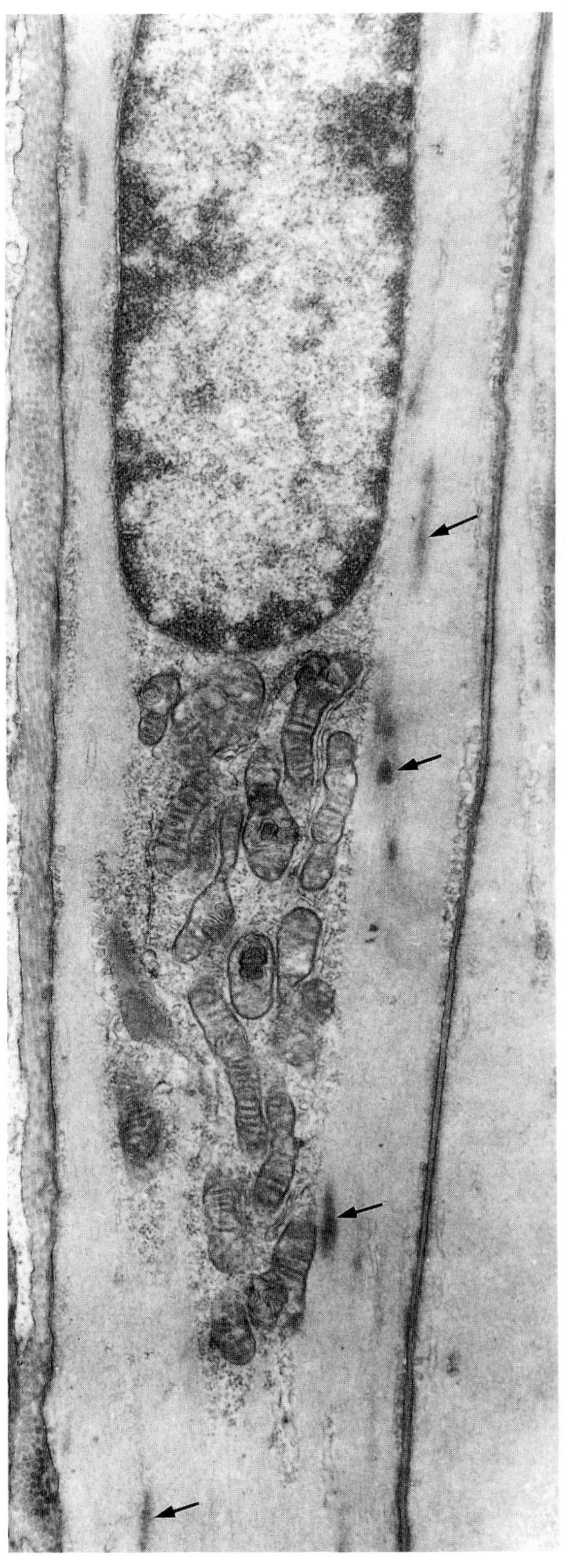

Figure 10–3. Micrograph of a smooth muscle cell in longitudinal section. The uniform gray region at the periphery is occupied by myofilaments that are not resolved at this magnification. A conical region of cytoplasm extending downward from the pole of the elongate nucleus contains numerous mitochondria and a few profiles of endoplasmic reticulum.

rather ill-defined fusiform densities termed *cytoplasmic dense bodies* (Figs. 10–3 and 10–4). Similar densities, uniformly spaced along the inner aspect of the cell membrane, are called *subplasmalemmal dense plaques*. The cytoplasmic dense bodies can be selectively stained with fluorescent antibodies to the actin-binding protein *α-actinin* (Fig. 10–5) and the dense plaques, at the cell surface are reactive with antibodies to *vinculin* and *talin*.

In micrographs of high magnification, three kinds of filaments can be resolved: thin *actin* filaments 4–8 nm in diameter; thicker *myosin* filaments, about 15 nm in diameter; and 10-nm *intermediate filaments*. The latter generally consist of *desmin*, a cytoskeletal protein characteristic of muscle, but they may be *vimentin* in vascular smooth muscle. These filaments occur in longitudinal or oblique bundles that converge on, and attach to, the cytoplasmic dense bodies and subplasmalemmal dense plaques to form a robust cytoskeletal network. Microtubules are rarely found in smooth muscle.

The contractile units of smooth muscle are identified with difficulty. Short myosin filaments (1.5–2.2 μm) seem to be intercalated within bundles of relatively long actin filaments (~4.5 μm) that probably correspond to the myofibrils described with the light microscope. The ratio of actin filaments to myosin filaments is 12 to 1 to 14 to 1 in smooth muscle (Fig. 10–6, inset) compared to 2 to 1 or 4 to 1 in skeletal muscle. The orientation of the bundles of filaments is longitudinal or oblique and there is no hint of lateral register of the myosin filaments such as that responsible for the cross-banding of skeletal muscle. The myofibrils terminate in the cytoplasmic dense bodies and the actin filaments on the two sides of a dense body are of opposite polarity. This suggests that the dense bodies of smooth muscle are the functional equivalent of the Z-lines of skeletal muscle. There is a different molecular organization of the thick filaments in smooth muscle. In isolated thick filaments, the projecting heads of the myosin molecules, which form cross-bridges to the surrounding

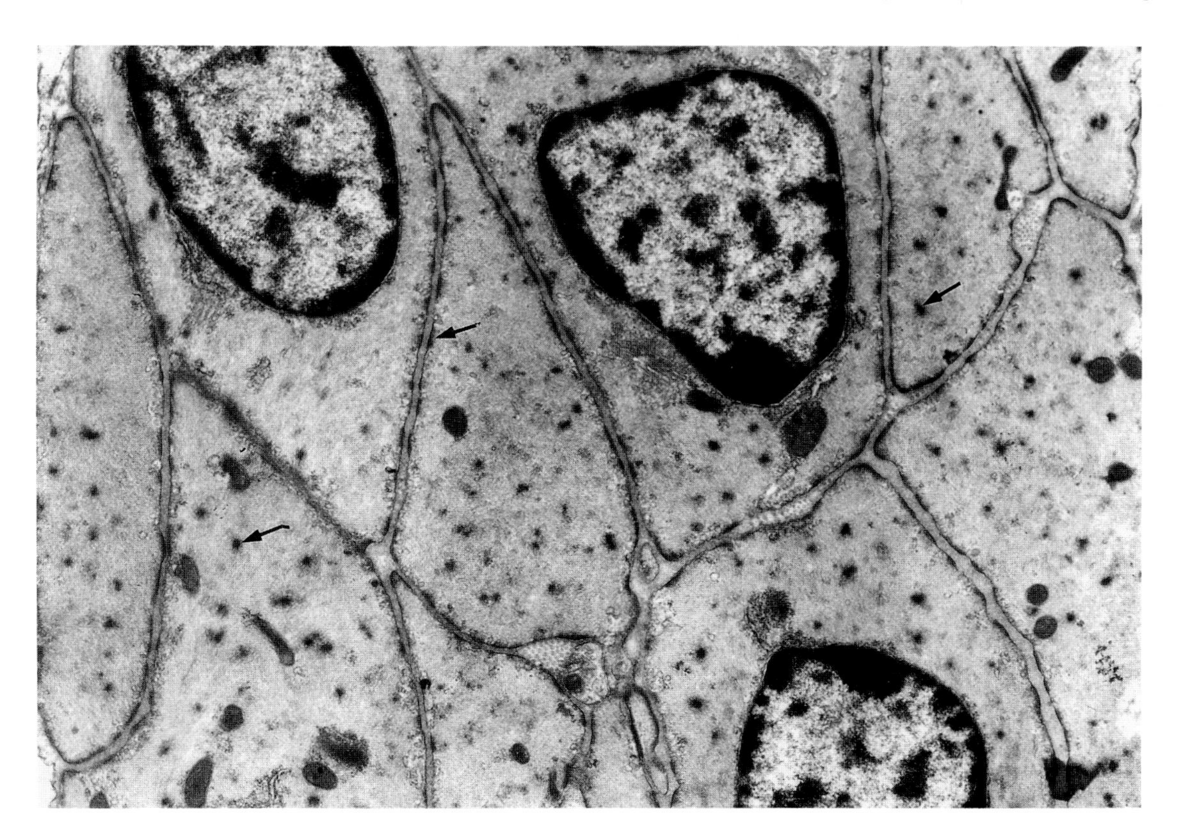

Figure 10–4. Electron micrograph of smooth muscle in cross section. The cells are separated by wide intercellular spaces occupied by glycoprotein cell coats and small bundles of collagen fibers. Scattered through the cytoplasm are densities (at arrows) that are sites of lateral bonding of filaments of the cytoskeleton and of actin filaments. Those at the periphery of the cells are sites of attachments of filaments to the cell membrane. Fusiform densities, indicated by arrows, are sites of lateral bonding of bundles of myofilaments.

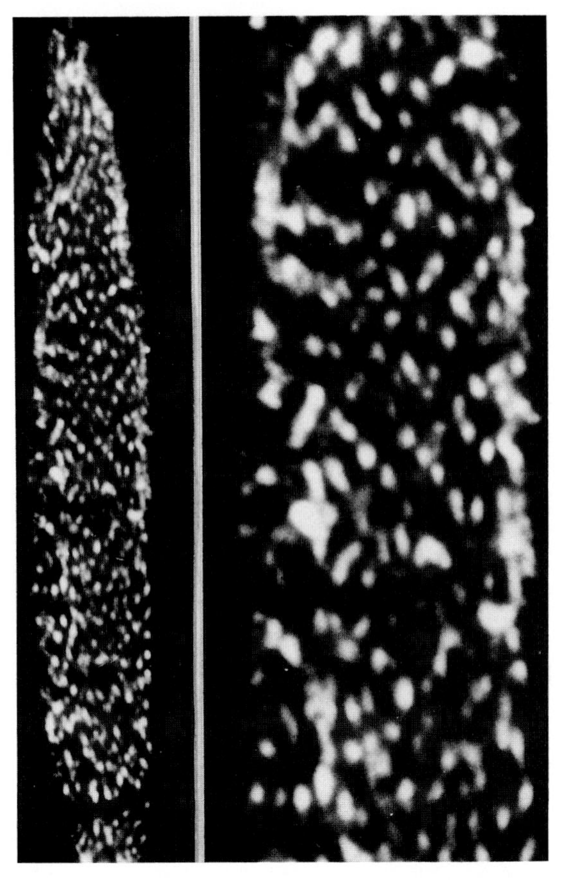

Figure 10–5. Confocal images of contracted, isolated smooth muscle cells labeled with fluorescent antibody to α actinin, showing the number and distribution of the cytoplasmic dense bodies. (A) ×1600, (B) ×4400. (Micrographs courtesy of Draeger, A. et al., 1990. J. Cell Biol. 11:2463.)

actin filaments are found along their entire length, whereas thick filaments of skeletal muscle have a bare central segment that is devoid of cross-bridges.

A distinctive feature of the ultrastructure of smooth muscle fibers is the presence of a great number of vesicular invaginations of the plasmalemma (caveolae), associated with all areas of the membrane between the subsurface dense plaques. These resemble vesicles involved in pinocytosis in other cell types, but in smooth muscle, there is no evidence that they detach and move into the cytoplasm. Their functional significance is puzzling. In skeletal muscle, the coupling of excitation to contraction is dependent on release of free calcium from stores in a network of endoplasmic reticulum (sarcoplasmic reticulum) that surrounds the individual myofibrils. Calcium release is triggered by impulses conducted along tubular invaginations of the plasma membrane (T-tubules) to the reticulum in the interior of the muscle fiber. No comparable tubular invaginations of the membrane are found in smooth muscle fibers. However, a close relationship exists between the caveolae and elements of smooth endoplasmic reticulum that course among them, parallel to the surface. This has led to the suggestion that they may function in electromechanical coupling in a manner comparable to the interaction of T-tubules with the sarcoplasmic reticulum in skeletal muscle. This speculation is in need of further validation, because other investigators contend that in such small fibers inward diffusion of extracellular calcium, accompanying depolarization of the membrane, would be adequate to trigger contraction of smooth muscle.

The argyrophilic reticulum observed around smooth muscle fibers, with the light microscope, is represented in electron micrographs by small bundles of slender collagen fibrils in the intercellular clefts. The cells are thus held apart over most of their surface by their external laminae and the intervening collagen fibers. However, in visceral smooth muscle these extracellular components are lacking at certain sites, permitting the membranes of adjacent cells to come into contact and form gap junctions. In certain other smooth muscles, such low-resistance junctions appear to be absent.

PHYSIOLOGY OF SMOOTH MUSCLE

Smooth muscle differs considerably from skeletal muscle in its physiology. Its contraction is slow but it can be sustained for long periods. It can shorten to one-quarter of its resting length and can generate a force, per cross-section area, comparable to that of striated muscle, while consuming far less energy. How this economy of energy is achieved is not entirely clear. The mechanism of contraction is less well understood than that of skeletal muscle due, in part, to the difficulty of defining a contractile unit comparable to the sarcomere. It is generally assumed, however, that shortening is produced by a similar sliding of actin filaments with respect to the myosin filaments. Its relatively slow speed and broad range of shortening may be attributable to the fact that the actin filaments are considerably longer (4.6 μm) than those of skeletal muscle (1.6 μm). The force generated is believed to

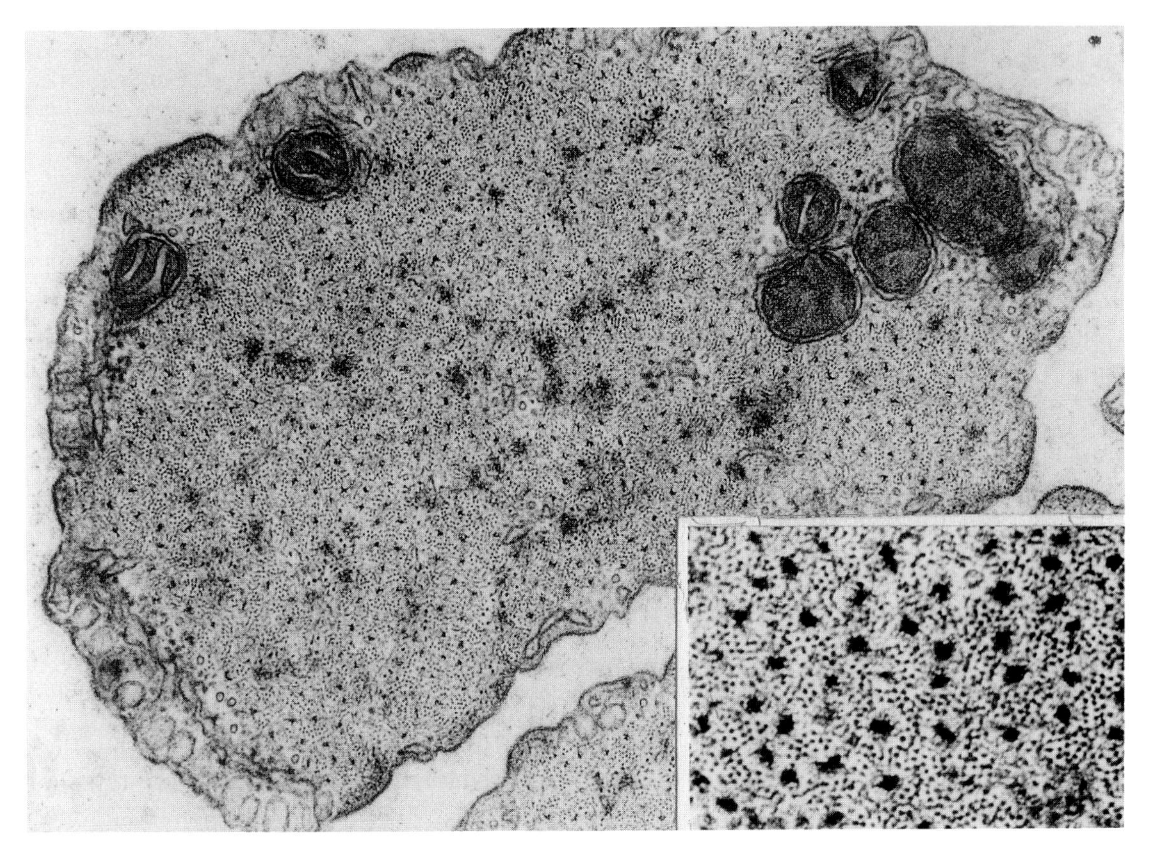

Figure 10–6. Electron micrograph of a vascular smooth muscle cell in cross section, clearly showing thick and thin filaments. The inset shows a portion of cytoplasm at higher magnification. (Micrograph from Somlyo, A.P., E. Devine, and A.V. Somlyo. 1972. *In* Vascular Smooth Muscle. Heidelberg, Springer-Verlag.)

be transmitted to the cell surface via the attachment of the contractile units to the cytoplasmic dense bodies at nodal points in the cytoskeleton.

The mechanism of triggering contraction is also different. The tropomyosin complex that is activated by calcium ions to initiate contraction of skeletal muscle is absent in smooth muscle. Instead, calcium diffusing into the cell with depolarization of the membrane, or calcium released from the subplasmalemmal reticulum, binds to a protein *calmodulin.* The complex, so formed, activates ATPase in the heads of the myosin molecules, and cleavage of ATP induces a conformational change in the myosin heads that results in translocation of the adjacent actin filaments.

Smooth muscles in various tissues and organs differ in their mode of activation. Visceral smooth muscle, also called *unitary smooth muscle,* exhibits an autorhythmicity. Intrinsically generated stimuli are conducted, via gap junctions, from cell to cell throughout a large area of muscle that contracts in unison. This type of smooth muscle is responsible for the waves of peristalsis that sweep along the intestine to advance its contents. Similar spontaneous waves of contraction are observed in the ureters and bile ducts. The mechanism of intrinsic excitation of the unitary smooth muscle in the viscera is still poorly understood. However, its ability to perform slow, synchronized contractions is attributable to the electrical coupling of adjacent fibers by gap junctions that permit the spread of excitation from fiber to fiber. Skeletal muscle fibers, on the other hand, are electrically isolated from one another, with each requiring stimulation by its own neuromuscular junction.

The smooth muscle in the walls of large arteries, in the ciliary body and iris of the eye, and in the wall of the ductus deferens of the male reproductive tract is described as *multiunit smooth muscle.* In this kind of muscle, there is little evidence of impulse conduction from fiber to fiber via gap junctions. Instead, each fiber is innervated and contraction is relatively rapid. Postganglionic autonomic nerve fibers pass over the muscle surface or penetrate into it, synapsing with fibers *en passant.*

Smooth muscle in the walls of blood vessels normally maintains a state of partial contraction called *muscle tonus,* but this is subject to modulation by blood-borne hormones. The cells have receptors for norepinephrine, angiotensin, and vasopressin which stimulate their contraction, resulting in *vasoconstriction,* a decrease in the caliber of the vessel. Other substances, such as brandykinin and, prostaglandins produced locally in the tissues irrigated, may result in loss of smooth muscle tone and consequent *vasodilatation.* Response to hormones is not confined to vascular smooth muscle. Changes in circulating levels of estrogens during the menstrual cycle are reflected in variations in the actin and myosin content of uterine smooth muscle, and during pregnancy, the fibers undergo a remarkably hypertrophy.

Smooth muscle fibers were formerly thought to be highly specialized cells incapable of proliferation, or of protein synthesis, other than that required to maintain their contractile components. It is now known that they synthesize laminin, collagen, elastin, and other components of the external lamina and extracellular matrix. An abnormal proliferation of smooth muscle cells and their production of excess collagen contribute to the formation of atherosclerotic plaques in the aorta and coronary arteries of aging humans.

STRIATED MUSCLE

The units of organization of skeletal muscle are the muscle *fibers,* long cylindrical multinucleated cells. They are much larger than smooth muscle fibers, ranging from 10 to 30 cm in length and from 0.1 to 0.5 mm in diameter. Parallel fibers are aggregated in bundles or *fascicles* large enough to be visible to the naked eye. The individual fibers, the fascicles, and the muscle as a whole are invested by connective tissue that forms a continuous supporting framework. However, to facilitate description, its different portions are designated by separate terms. The dense connective tissue surrounding the whole muscle is called the *epimysium.* Thin septa that extend inward from it to surround each of the fascicles constitute the *perimysium* and the delicate reticulum investing the individual fibers is the *endomysium* (Figs. 10–7 and 10–8). Although the con-

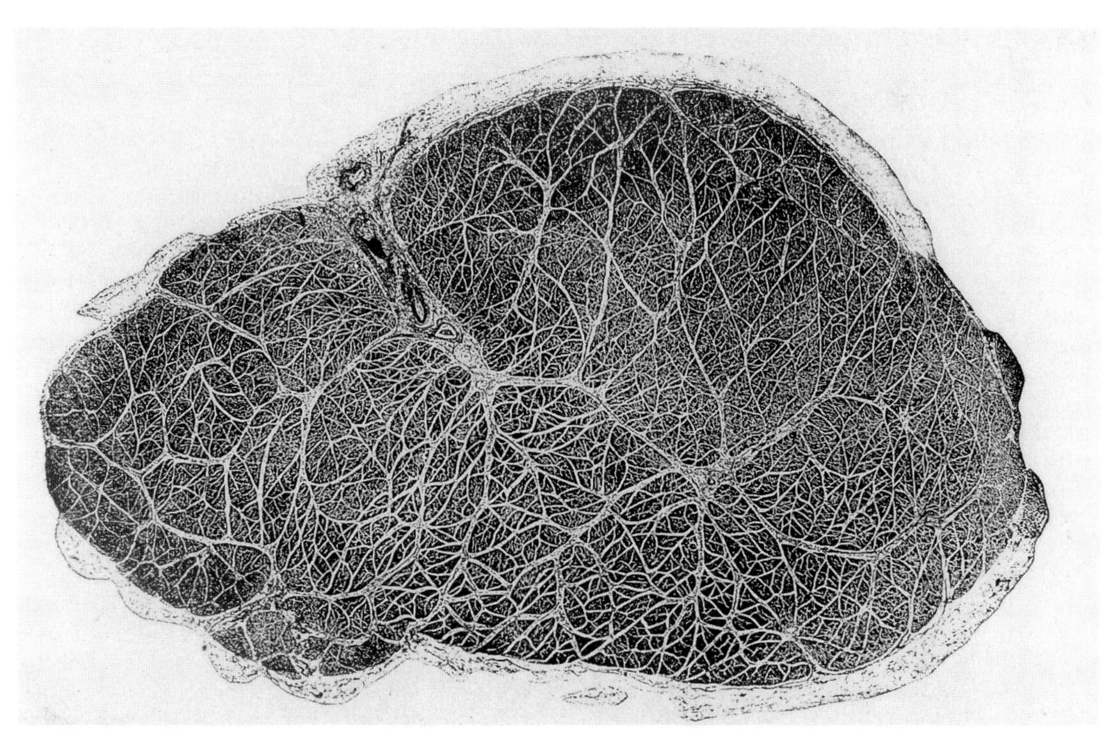

Figure 10–7. Photograph of a cross section of a human sartorius muscle showing the connective tissue of the epimysium around the entire muscle and the perimysium enclosing muscle fiber bundles of varying size. (From Heidenhain, 1911. Plasma und Zella 2 Leif. Jena.)

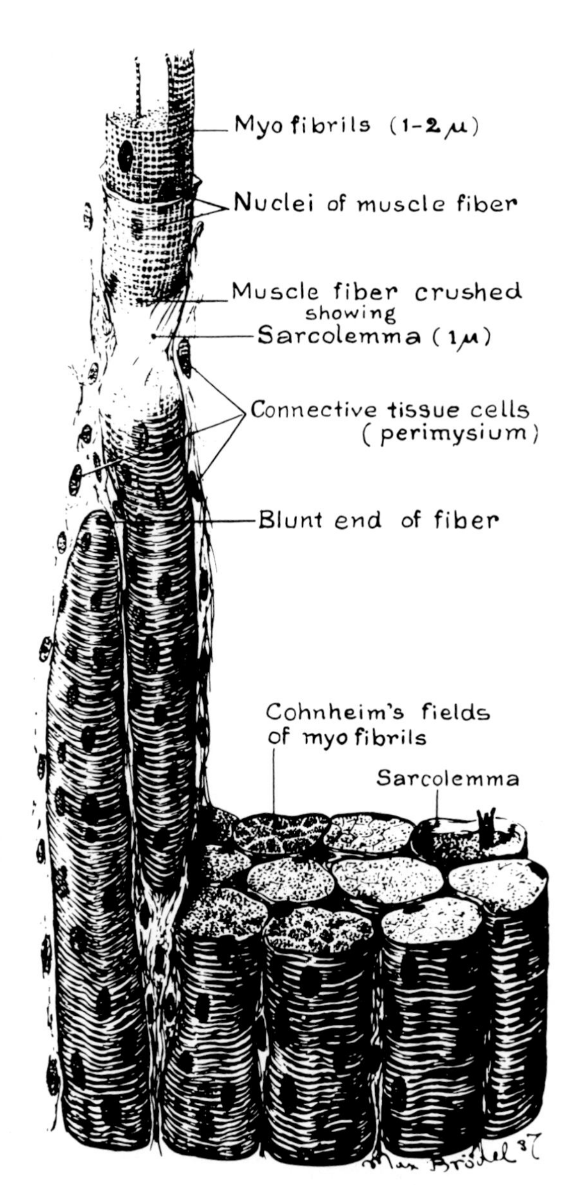

Figure 10–8. Drawing of the relationships of skeletal muscle fibers and the surrounding connective tissue forming the endomysium. (From Brödel, M. 1937. Bull. Johns Hopkins Hosp. 61:295.)

nective tissue serves to bind together the subunits of the muscle, it permits a certain degree of freedom of motion between them. Some longitudinal movement of fascicles with respect to one another is possible and each muscle fiber can move independently of neighboring fibers.

The blood vessels supplying skeletal muscle ramify in the epimysium and penetrate via the septa of the perimysium to form, in the endomysium, a rich capillary network around the individual muscle fibers (Fig. 10–9). The capillaries are sufficiently tortuous to accommodate changes in fiber length by straightening somewhat during relaxation and becoming more contorted during contraction.

The arrangement of the fascicles varies from muscle to muscle. In some relatively short muscles, they are oriented parallel to the direction of pull and may continue without interruption throughout its length. In very long muscles, fibers are usually shorter than the muscle as a whole and are connected to one or more transverse bands of connective tissue spaced at intervals along the length of the muscle. In other muscles, described as *unipinnate,* the fasciculi are oriented obliquely with respect to a longitudinal band of connective tissue along one side of the muscle. Others are *bipinnate,* having oblique fascicles that radiate from a connective tissue core in the muscle, resulting in a pattern resembling that of the barbs extending obliquely from the axial core of a feather. A few muscles are *multipinnate,* with oblique fascicles radiating from several longitudinal connective tissue strands within the muscle. These strands converge on the tendon. Some loss of efficiency associated with oblique fascicular architecture is offset by the very large number of fibers that can be accommodated in this arrangement. It is generally found in muscles where considerable power and a short range of motion are required.

DEVELOPMENT AND REPAIR

In the embryo, skeletal muscle develops from uninucleate precursors called *myoblasts.* These proliferate and fuse to form long multinuclear cells that are often referred to as *myotubes,* an unfortunate term that erroneously implies that they have a hollow structure. These elongated syncytia then develop, in their cytoplasm, *myofibrils,* the contractile elements of differentiated muscle fibers. During postnatal growth, the muscle fibers increase in length and thickness, reaching a diameter of 10–70 μm, depending on the muscle and the species. Fibers in the same muscle may vary considerably in their thickness. In adults, they may undergo further increase in diameter in response to prolonged and intense muscular activity—a phenomenon called *hypertrophy of use.* Conversely, the fibers may become thinner in muscle immobilized for a long period by a cast applied in treatment of a fractured bone—a change called *atrophy of disuse.*

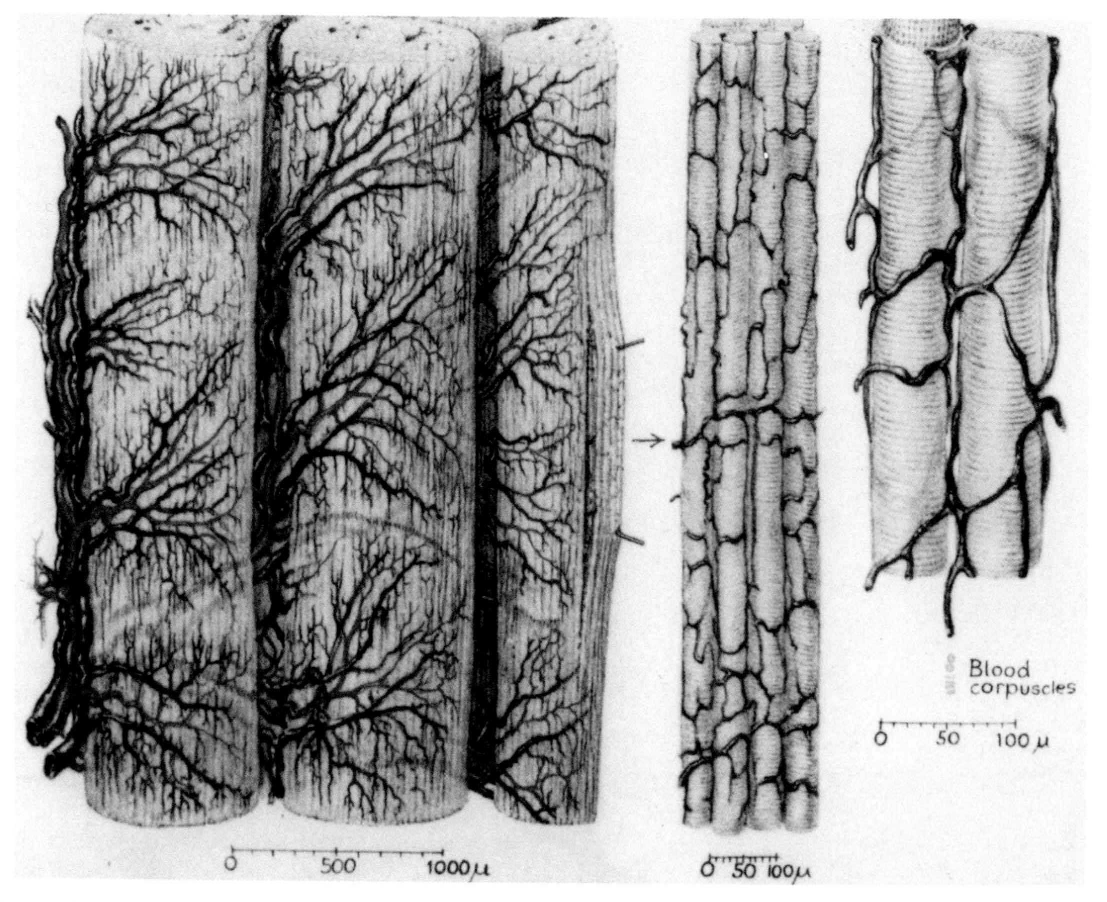

Figure 10–9. Drawing of the blood supply of muscle fiber bundles from the human rectus abdominis muscle (left) and the capillary network around the individual muscle fibers (right). (From Brödel, M. 1937. Bull. Johns Hopkins Hosp. 61:295.)

In muscle of adults, occasional small cells with an elongate nucleus and a relatively coarse chromatin pattern can be found occupying shallow depressions in the surface of muscle fibers. These so-called *satellite cells* are situated within the external lamina that surrounds the individual muscle fibers. They are believed to be a residual population of myoblast-like stem cells that persist in fully differentiated muscle and participate in muscle repair after injury. However, skeletal muscle has only limited capacity for repair in adults. After minor injury, satellite cells, within an intact endomysium may divide and fuse to restore damaged fibers. If the injury is more extensive, disrupting the endomysium, regeneration of muscle fibers does not occur. Instead, the damaged area is invaded by fibroblasts that deposit collagen, resulting in a fibrous scar. Restoration of muscle function after such an injury depends mainly on hypertrophy of the remaining undamaged fibers.

THE STRUCTURE OF MUSCLE FIBERS

Fresh muscle can be teased apart, under a dissecting microscope, into its individual fibers. At higher magnification, these show a closely spaced transverse striation that is characteristic of skeletal and cardiac muscle and is the basis for the term *striated muscle* used to distinguish them from smooth muscle (Fig. 10–10). A fine longitudinal striation is also detectable. Its structural basis becomes apparent if samples of muscle are macerated in dilute nitric acid. This treatment destroys cell membranes, extracts organelles, and cytoplasmic matrix. The contractile components left behind separate into thousands of thin cross-striated *myofibrils* that appear to be made up of alternating short segments of differing refractive index. It is evident that the cross-striation of the intact muscle fiber is due to the fact that corresponding segments of the closely packed myofibrils are in register across the entire width of the fiber.

In the literature of histology, the plasma membrane of muscle fibers has traditionally been called the *sarcolemma* and the cytoplasm, the *sarcoplasm*. These terms persist but no fundamental difference from the corresponding structures in other cells is implied by their use. The sarcolemma of the long cylindrical fibers is reinforced by an external lamina comparable to the basal lamina of epithelia. Numerous nuclei, spaced along the length of the fiber, are displaced to the periphery by the column of myofibrils that occupies the bulk of the sarcoplasm (Fig. 10–11). They are flattened against the sarcolemma and, thus, present a long profile in section. Their number cannot be specified because it varies from muscle to muscle, but in a fiber several centimeters in length, the nuclei would number in the hundreds. The peripheral location of the nuclei is useful in distinguishing skeletal muscle from cardiac muscle in which the nuclei are central.

The cytoplasmic surface of the sarcolemma in skeletal muscle is coated with the 400 kD protein *dystrophin* which appears to provide mechanical reinforcement to the membrane, thereby protecting it against stresses developed during muscular contraction. In the X-linked heritary myopathy *Duchenne muscular dystrophy* this protein is lacking resulting in structural weakness of the sarcolemma. Onset of the disease is apparent by age 5, and there is a progressive replacement of damaged muscle fibers by connective tissue and adipose tissue. By age 12 these individuals are usually unable to walk.

All of the common cell organelles are represented in the sarcoplasm. A small Golgi complex is associated with one pole of most of the nuclei. Mitochondria (*sarcosomes*) congregate in the juxtanuclear sarcoplasm and are also deployed in longitudinal rows between the myofibrils where they provide energy for muscle contraction. Lipid droplets are found in small numbers between the myofibrils or among the mitochondria at the poles of the nuclei. After staining with the periodic-acid–Schiff reaction, glycogen can be demonstrated throughout the sarcoplasm. In addition to these microscopically demonstrable components, the sarcoplasm contains, in solution,

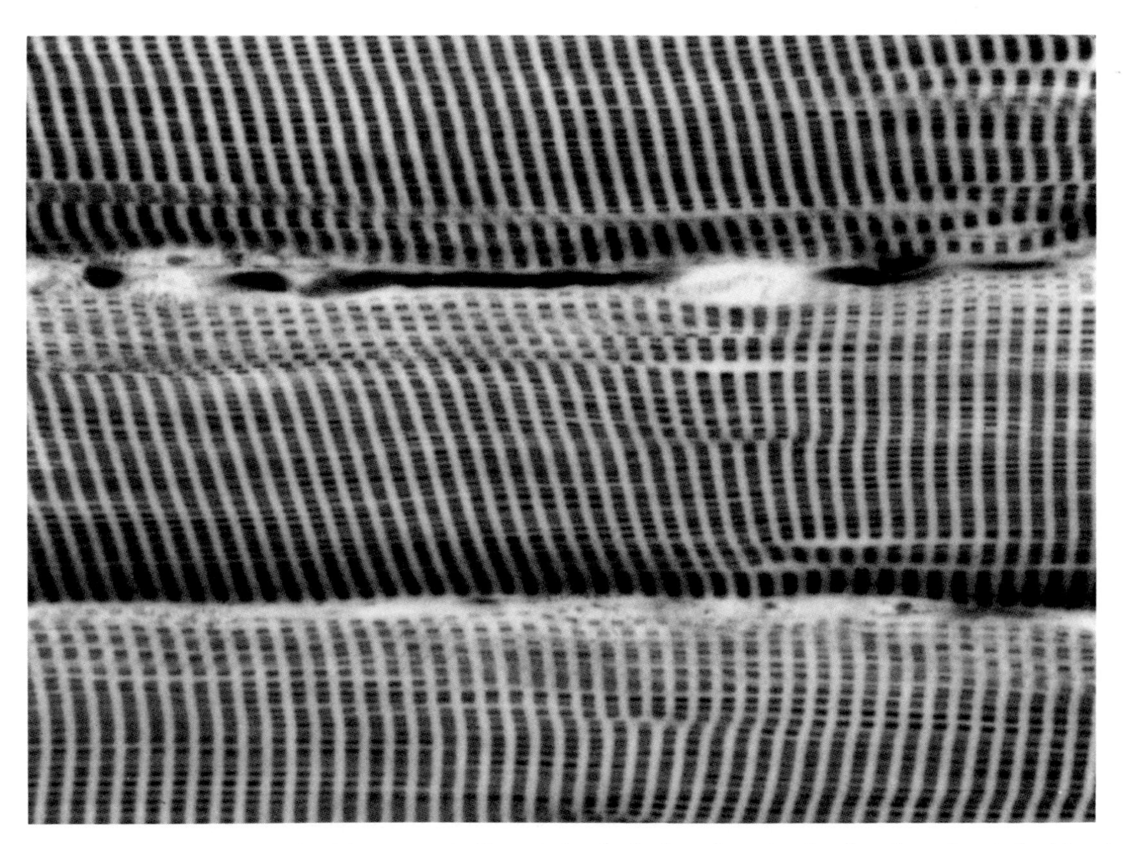

Figure 10–10. Photomicrograph of three muscle fibers in longitudinal section, showing the alternating dark, A-bands, and light I-bands. Preparation stained with iron hematoxylin.

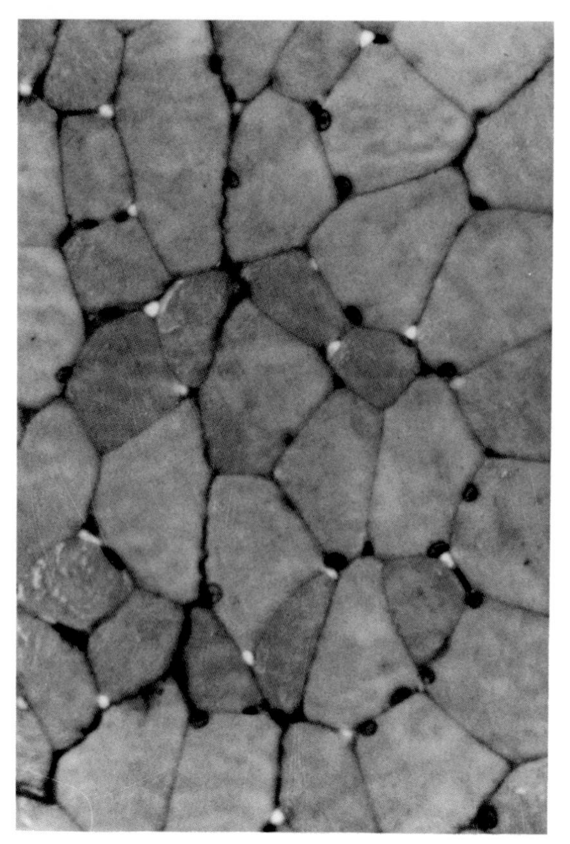

Figure 10–11. Photomicrograph of skeletal muscle fibers in cross section, illustrating their polygonal outline, due to mutual deformation, and the peripheral location of their nuclei.

myoglobin, an oxygen-binding protein which is largely responsible for the slightly brown color of muscle. As required, oxygen dissociates from myoglobin and becomes available for oxidations. Myoglobin is present in low concentration and is possibly of little functional significance in the relatively pale muscles of humans, but in the deeply colored muscle of diving birds and mammals, it is abundant and probably of greater physiological significance.

In transverse sections, myofibrils occupy most of the interior of the fiber and are resolved as fine dots either uniformly distributed or in polygonal areas formerly referred to as the *fields of Cohnheim.* Whether the latter represent the true distribution of myofibrils or are a result of shrinkage during specimen preparation was long debated. The weight of evidence now favors their interpretation as a shrinkage artifact.

In longitudinal sections, stained with iron haematoxylin, the cross-striations that are barely detectable in fresh muscle are greatly accentuated, with heavily stained bands alternating with relatively pale bands (Fig. 10–12). The bands that appear dark in stained preparations are *anisotropic* (birefringent) when examined with the polarizing microscope and are, therefore, designated *A-bands,* whereas the lighter-staining bands are *isotropic* and are called the *I-bands.* The relative lengths of the bands depends on the state of contraction of the muscle. The I-bands are very short during contraction, longer during relaxation, and longest in muscle that has been passively stretched. The length of the A-bands remains constant in all phases of the cycle of contraction and relaxation.

Each I-band is bisected by a transverse line, the *Z-line* or *Z-disc.* The segments of myofibrils between successive Z-lines are called *sarcomeres* and all of the morphological changes during the contractile cycle are described with reference to this structural unit. The sarcomere includes an A-band and half of the two contiguous I-bands. The A-bands, I-bands, and the Z-discs are usually the only cross-striations visible with the light microscope, but in exceptional preparations a slightly paler zone, called the *H-band,* may be seen traversing the center of each A-band. The structural basis of the cross-striations of skeletal muscle becomes apparent in electron micrographs and will be discussed below.

HETEROGENEITY OF SKELETAL MUSCLE FIBERS

The myofibers that make up a given muscle are not all identical. They vary in diameter and in their cytochemical and physiological properties. The relative proportions of the different fiber types vary from muscle to muscle. Two major categories of muscle fibers are distinguished by physiologists: *twitch fibers* (fast fibers) which propagate an action potential and respond with all-or-none contraction, and *tonic fibers* (slow fibers), which are unable to propagate an action potential and require a series of nerve impulses. Their contraction is more prolonged than that of twitch fibers. By these criteria, slow fibers are common in amphibian and reptilian muscle but rare in mammals. The discussion that follows will refer to heterogeneity among twitch fibers, which are the dominant physiological type in mammalian skeletal muscle.

Mammalian muscle fibers vary in diameter over a narrow range, but other differences are

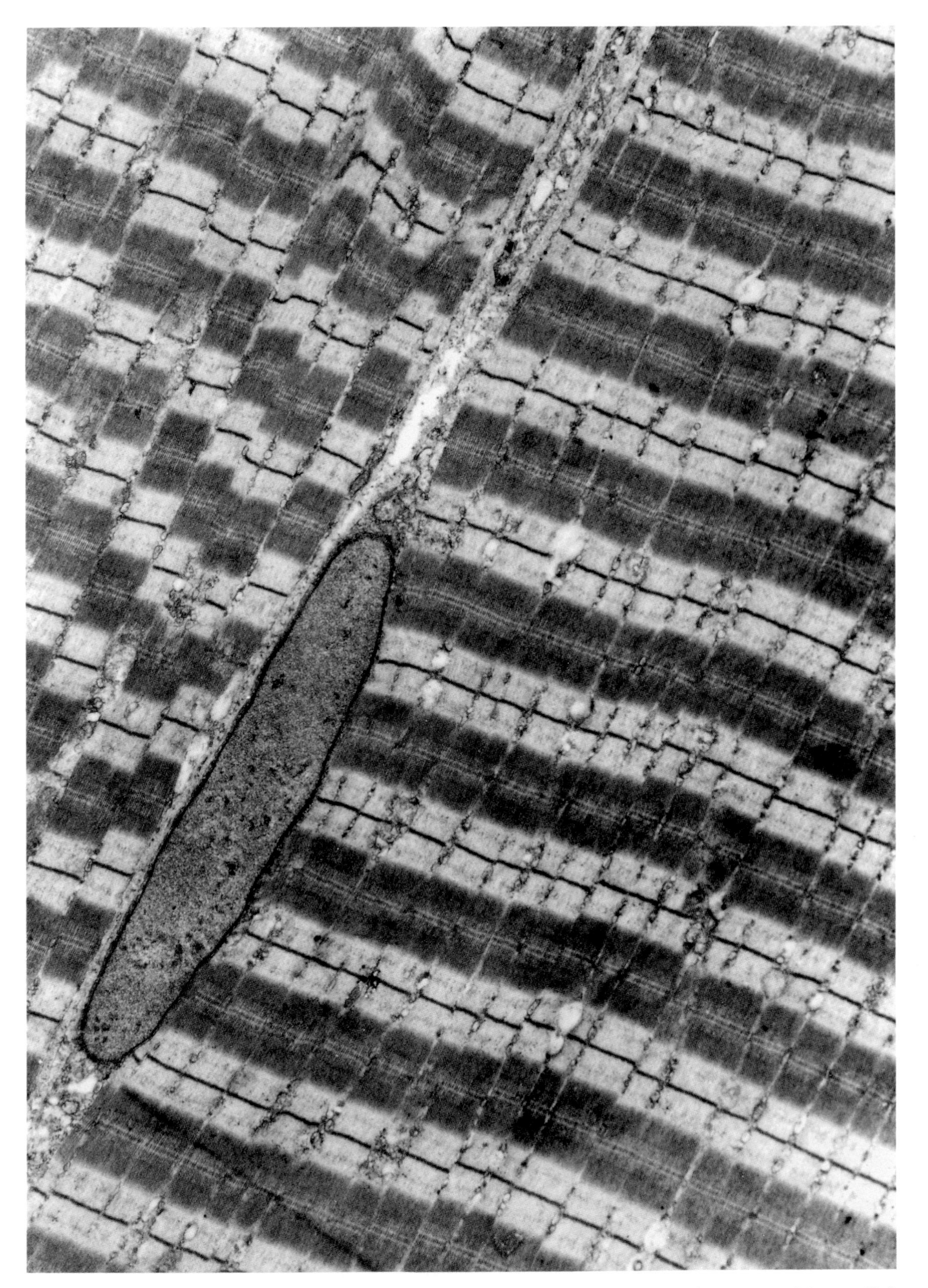

Figure 10–12. Electron micrograph of skeletal muscle, extracted with glycerin to improve the contrast of the myofibrils. Observe the uniform diameter of the myofibrils and the location of the nucleus immediately beneath the sarcolemma. Corresponding bands of the myofibrils are usually in register across the muscle fiber. Where they are out of register, as at the upper left, this is thought to be an artifact of specimen preparation.

Structural and Functional Characteristics of Muscle Fiber Types

Fiber Type	**White** Fast twitch glycolytic (FC)	**Red** Slow-twitch Oxidative (SO)	**Intermediate** Fast-twitch oxidative, glycolytic (FOG)
Structural Characteristics			
Color	White	Red	Pink
Fiber diameter	Large	Small	Medium to small
Mitochondria	Few	Many	Many
Capillary density	Sparse	Rich	Rich
Metabolic Characteristics			
Twitch rate	Fast	Slow	Fast
Rate of Fatigue	Fast	Slow	Intermediate
Primary pathway for ATP synthesis	Anaerobic	Aerobic	Aerobic
Myosin ATPase activity	Fast	Slow	Fast
Myoglobin content	Low	High	High
Histochemistry			
Glycogen content	High	Low	Intermediate
Neutral fat content	Low	High	Intermediate
ATPase, pH 9.4	High	Low	High
ATPase, pH 4.3	Low	High	Low
Succinic dehydrogenase	Low	High	Medium to high
NADH dehydrogenase	Low	High	Medium to high

Figure 10–13. Table presenting the structural, metabolic, and histochemical characteristics of the three types of skeletal muscle fibers. At the top of the columns are the traditional terms (red, white, and intermediate) and the corresponding terms employed by physiologists. (Modified after Burke, R.E. 1981. *In* Handbook of Physiology, The Nervous System II, pp. 345–422. American Physiology Society, Bethesda and Table 9-2, from Morieb, E.N. 19xx. *In* B. Cummins, ed. Human Anatomy and Physiology.

not apparent in routine histological sections. However, with cytochemical staining methods, three fiber types are easily distinguished. These have traditionally been designated *red fibers, white fibers,* and *intermediate fibers.* Regrettably, some terminological confusion has resulted from recognition of four types by physiologists and by their use of descriptive terms based on different criteria from those used by histologists. The divergences in terminology are set forth in the table in Fig. 10–13.

Red fibers (slow twitch, oxidative fibers) are relatively small in diameter and have a darker color, attributable to their greater content of myoglobin and rich supply of capillaries. They have numerous large mitochondria beneath the sarcolemma and between the myofibrils. Lipid droplets are common in the sarcoplasm of these fibers and, owing to the abundance of their mitochondria, they stain intensely with the cytochemical reaction for the enzyme succinic dehydrogenase (Fig. 10–14). The Z-bands tend to be wider than those of other fiber types. They are innervated by small axons with small and relatively simple motor end plates. Motor units consisting of red fibers contract more slowly than other types and are very resistant to fatigue because of their ability for oxidative regeneration of ATP, the high-energy compound needed to recycle the contractile process. These proper-

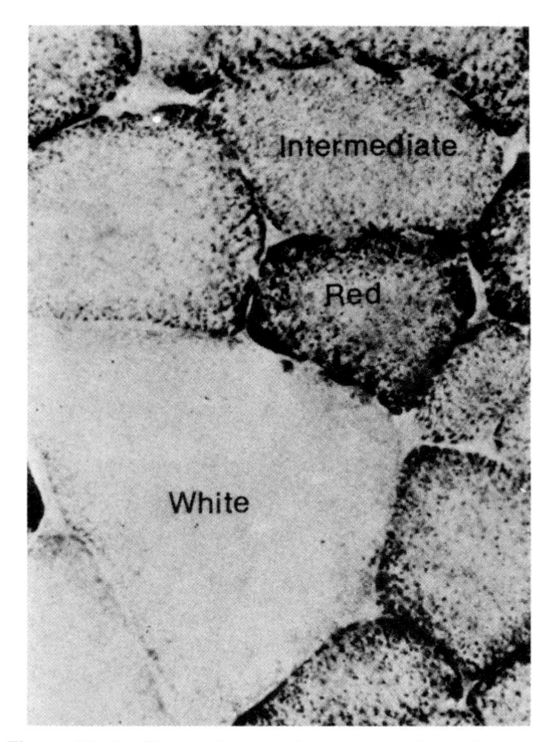

Figure 10–14. Photomicrograph of several skeletal muscle fibers in cross section, stained for the mitochondrial enzyme succinic dehydrogenase. Three categories of fibers are distinguished: small red fibers rich in peripheral mitochondria; large white fibers, with relatively few mitochondria; and fibers with intermediate characteristics. (Photomicrograph courtesy of G. Gautier.)

ties make them particularly effective in postural maintenance.

The *white fibers* (fast-twitch fibers) are the largest of the fiber types. Their subplasmalemmal mitochondria are smaller and less numerous than those of red fibers and interfibrillar mitochondria are relatively few. Their cytochemical reaction for succinic dehydrogenase is correspondingly weak (Fig. 10–14). Their generation of ATP depends on anaerobic glycolysis of glucose derived from abundant deposits of glycogen in the sarcoplasm. White fibers are innervated by larger axons that form motor end plates about twice the size of those of red fibers. They contract rapidly and generate a large force but they fatigue rapidly. They are best suited for brief bursts of intense muscle activity.

The form and disposition of mitochondria in the three types of muscle fibers has been studied by field emission scanning electron microscopy, after removal of the cytoplasmic matrix (Fig. 10–16). In red fibers, spherical subsarcolemmal mitochondria are large and abundant. Slender, paired mitochondria are transversely oriented on either side of the Z-lines. In the interfibrillar spaces, mitochondria, one sarcomere in length, form longitudinal columns. These may be thick, consisting of multiple mitochondria, or thin, consisting of rows of single mitochondria (Fig. 10–16A). In white fibers, subsarcolemmal mitochondria are fewer and longitudinal columns are rare and often interrupted (Fig. 10–16B). Mitochondrial disposition in intermediate fibers is similar to that of red fibers, but thick mitochondrial columns are rarely found.

A subclass of fast-twitch fibers, recognized by physiologists, are relatively rich in myoglobin and have a capacity for aerobic glycolysis, but also have considerable capacity for anaerobic metabolism and are relatively resistant to fatigue. Such fibers are classified by some authors as *fast-twitch fatigue resistant fibers* (FR) and by others as *fast-twitch oxidative glycolytic fibers* (FOG). A fourth class intermediate between these and fast fatiguable twitch-fibers has also been described. It is not entirely clear how many of these subclasses fall within the histologist's category of intermediate fibers, which are simply defined as those that are intermediate between red and white fibers in diameter, mitochondrial volume, and cytochemical staining intensity.

Muscle fibers do not contract individually, but in *motor units,* groups of fibers of the same type innervated by branches of the same nerve axon. The number of fibers innervated by a single motor neuron varies from 100 to 300, in the small muscles of the hand, to 600–1700, in large muscles of the arm and leg. The muscle fibers in any one motor unit are not grouped together but are scattered over a considerable area which may be shared by 20 or more other motor units. The intermingling of the fibers of many different motor units explains the differences in staining reactions of neighboring fibers (Fig. 10–15).

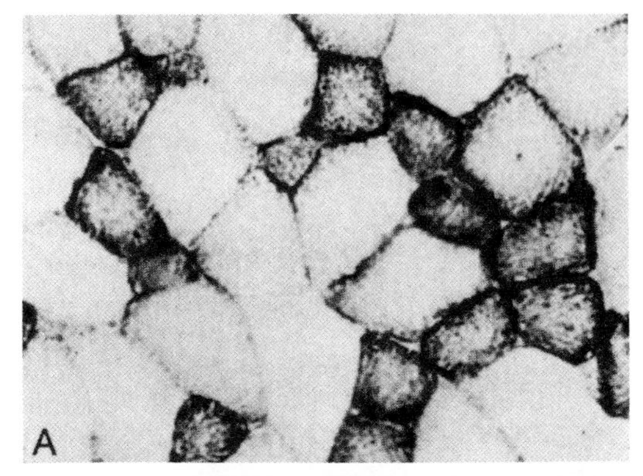

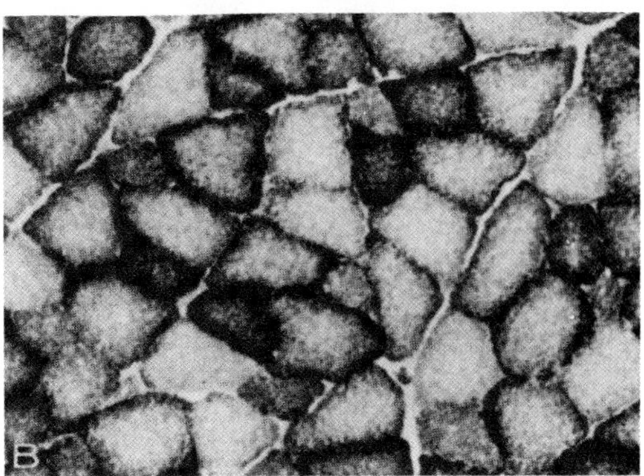

Figure 10–15. Succinic dehydrogenase reaction in skeletal muscle. (A) Plantaris muscle of a control guinea pig. (B) Same muscle of an animal after 8 weeks of running on a treadmill. The fiber population of the exercised muscle is more homogeneous—nearly all fibers are small and rich in mitochondria. (Photomicrograph from Faulkner. J.A. 1944. *In* Podolsky, R.J., ed. Contractility of Muscle Cells and Related Processes. Englewood Cliffs, NJ, Prentice-Hall.)

When muscles are examined with the naked eye, they vary somewhat in color. The difference between the white and dark meat of a chicken is a striking example. In mammalian muscles, slight differences in color are also detectable. These variations are a reflection of differences in vascularity and differing proportions of the fiber types. The ratio of fiber types in any given muscle is fairly constant,

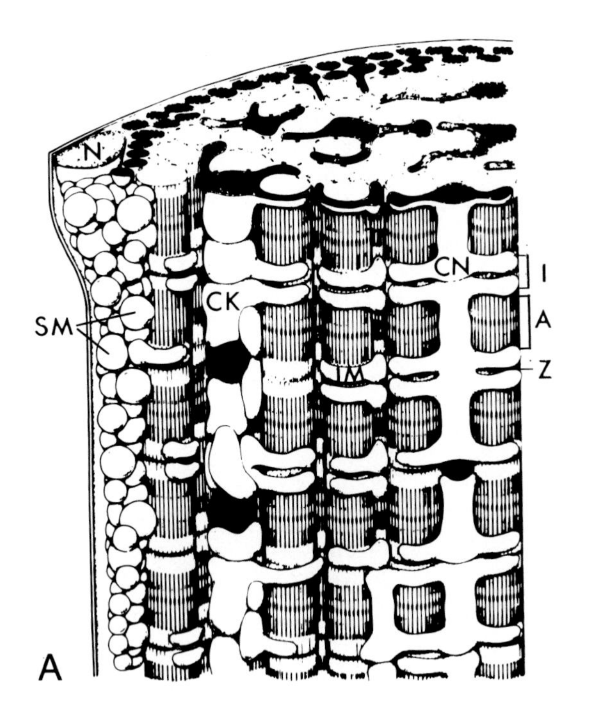

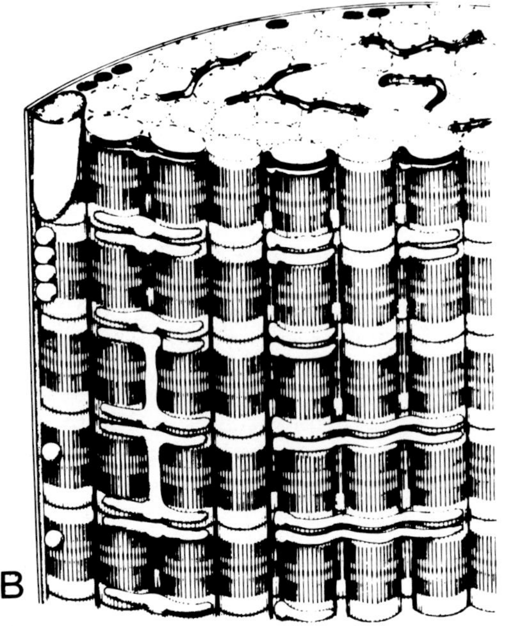

Figure 10–16. The three-dimensional organization of the mitochondria in red muscle fibers (A) and white fibers (B). N: nucleus; SM: subplasmalemmal mitochondria; CK: thick mitochondrial column; CN: thin mitochondrial column; IM: I-band-limited mitochondria. (Drawings from Ogata, T. and Y. Yamasaki. 1985. Cell Tissue Res. 241:251.)

but it is not immutable. It has now been shown that fast-switch fibers can be transformed to slow twitch fibers, and vice versa. If the nerves to a slow postural muscle and a fast locomotor muscle are exchanged, there is gradual change in the structural and physiological characteristics of both muscles to those of the other type.

ULTRASTRUCTURE OF STRIATED MUSCLE FIBERS

Our understanding of the mechanism of shortening and the generation of force by skeletal muscle has been greatly advanced by examination of the fibers with the electron microscope. The structure of the common organelles is not fundamentally different from that in other cells. However, consistant with the high-energy requirement for contraction, the mitochondria have numerous closely spaced cristae and their distribution, in intimate relation to the myofibrils, brings the source of energy (ATP) close to its site of utilization. The endoplasmic reticulum is highly organized and has acquired physiological properties not typical of this organelle in other cell types.

In the latter part of the nineteenth century, a cytologist examining muscle that had been impregnated with a heavy metal described a lace-like network of blackened strands that appeared to surround each of the myofibrils. This he called the *sarcoplasmic reticulum.* Efforts of others to demonstrate it were only partially successful and its validity remained in doubt until it was rediscovered with the electron microscope in 1954. It consists of membrane-bounded tubules that form a continuous network occupying the narrow spaces between the myofibrils throughout the muscle fiber. Although it corresponds to the endoplasmic reticulum of other cells, it is largely devoid of associated ribosomes and is specialized for a different function. It is the site of sequestration of calcium during muscle relaxation and for release, into the sarcoplasm, of the free calcium ions that trigger contraction in response to a nerve impulse. It is, therefore, essential for the termination and initiation of muscle contraction. The reticulum around each myofibril exhibits a repeating pattern of local differentiations, related to specific regions of the sarcomeres. The prevailing orientation of the sarcotubules is longitudinal, but anastomosing lateral branches form a denser network encircling the myofibril at the level of the H-zone of each A-band. At the junction of the A-band with the I-band, the longitudinal sarcotubules are confluent with a transversely oriented tubule of larger caliber, called the *terminal cisterna*. The longitudinal tubules that span successive I-bands and the intervening Z-line also terminate in a separate terminal cisterna at the A–I junction. Thus, a pair of parallel terminal cisternae is associated with each A–I junction along the length of the myofibril, two pairs to each sarcomere. Between each pair of terminal cisternae, there is a slender *transverse tubule* (T-tubule) that is not an integral part of the sarcoplasmic reticulum but is a long tubule extending inward from the sarcolemma (Fig. 10–17). At the surface of the muscle fiber, its limiting membrane is continuous with the sarcolemma and its lumen opens onto the extracellular space. Thus, the T-tubules are slender invaginations of the sarcolemma that penetrate deep into the interior of the muscle fiber crossing many myofibrils. The two parallel terminal cisternae and the intervening T-tubule form a complex referred to as the *triad*. Like the sarcomeres, the triads are in register across the entire width of the muscle fiber. The above description applies to skeletal muscle of all mammals. In amphibia, the triads are located at the Z-line instead of at the A–I junction (Fig. 10–18).

The sarcoplasmic reticulum is continuous throughout the muscle fiber, but two functionally distinct regions are now distinguished. The expanded transverse cisternae that are associated with the T-tubules to form triads, are designated the *junctional reticulum*. It has properties that enable it to respond to an action potential, spreading inward along the adjacent T-tubule, by releasing calcium into the sarcoplasm. The tubules making up the remainder of the reticulum are commonly referred to as *longitudinal sarcotubules*, even though they have lateral branches that form a network around the A-bands of the myofibrils. In freeze–fracture preparations, the membrane of these tubules is rich in intramembrane particles that are thought to con-

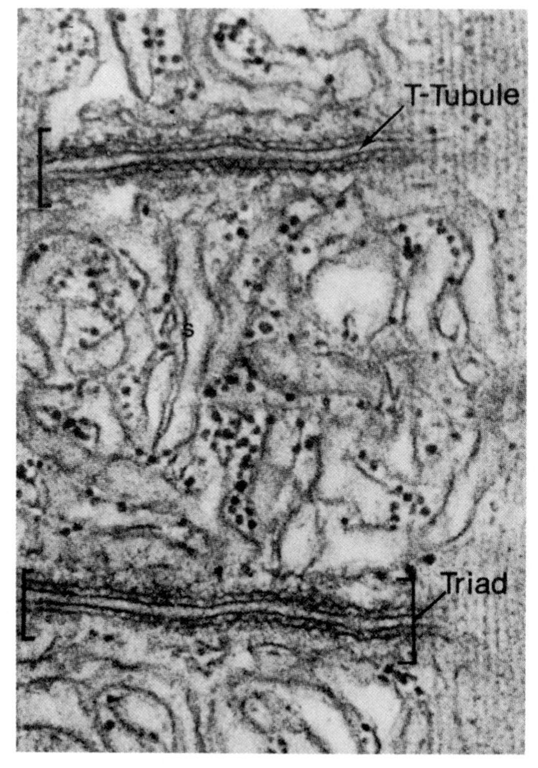

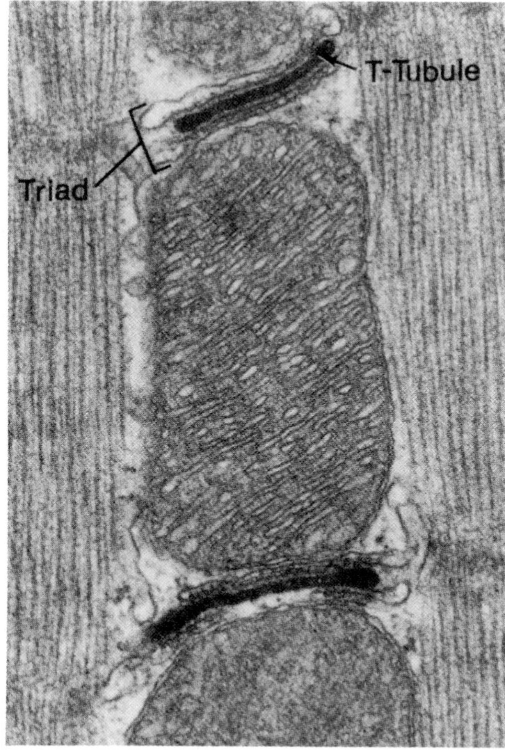

Figure 10–17. (A) Micrograph of a small area from a longitudinal section of skeletal muscle, passing tangenital to a myofibril. Observe the longitudinal tubules of the sarcoplasmic reticulum and two transversely oriented triads at the level of the A–I junctions. Glycogen particles are present among the sarcotubules. (B) Longitudinal section of muscle that has been immersed in peroxidase. The dense reaction product of the peroxidase is present in the lumen of the two T-tubules, verifying the continuity of their lumen with the extracellular space. (Micrograph courtesy of D. Friend.)

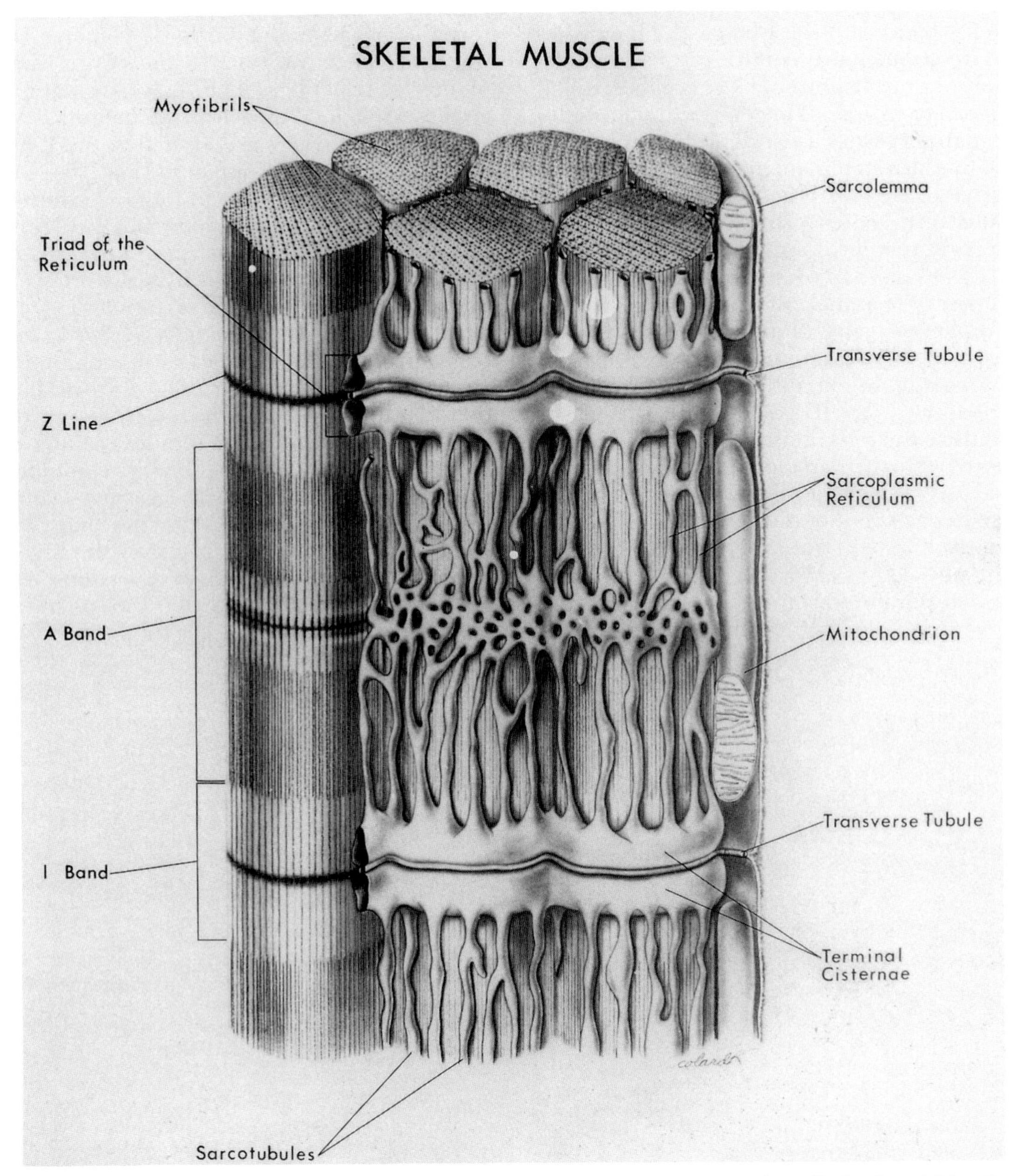

Figure 10–18. Schematic drawing of the distribution of the sarcoplasmic reticulum around myofibrils of amphibian skeletal muscle. The longitudinal sarcotubules are confluent with transverse terminal cisternae. A slender transverse T-tubule extending inward from the sarcolemma is flanked by two terminal cisternae to form the "triads" of the reticulum. In amphibian muscle, depicted here, the triads are at the Z-lines. In mammalian muscle, there are two to each sarcomere, located at the A–I junction. (From McNutt, S. and D.W. Fawcett. 1969. J. Cell Biol. 42:46; modified from Peachey, L. 1965. J. Cell Biol. 25:209.)

tain the Ca^{++}–Mg^{++}-ATPase responsible for transporting calcium from the sarcoplasm back into the lumen of the reticulum during muscle relaxation. The contents of the longitudinal sarcotubules is extracted in specimen preparation and their lumen generally appears empty. The lumen of cisternae of the junctional reticulum, on the other hand, contains an amorphous material of low density that consists mainly of *calciquestrin.* This 55 kD protein can bind 300 nM of calcium per milligram and is believed to serve as a sequestering agent for the storage of calcium within the reticulum.

EXCITATION–CONTRACTION COUPLING

The term excitation–contraction coupling refers to the sequence of electrical and chemical events leading to the activation of muscle contraction. Some of these have already been alluded to, but a brief overview of the process may facilitate understanding of additional detail to follow. In brief, it begins at the myoneural junction with the generation of an action potential that spreads over the sarcolemma and along the membrane of the T-tubules into the interior of the muscle fiber. This activates events at the interface between the T-tubules and the terminal cisternae of the triads that result in the rapid release of calcium from the sarcoplasmic reticulum. The calcium set free in the sarcoplasm binds to the myofibrils and triggers their shortening. When depolarization of the sarcolemma by nerve impulses ceases, calcium is actively transported back into the lumen of the terminal cisternae. The consequent lowering of the calcium concentration around the myofibrils brings about muscle relaxation.

In recent years, the structural and chemical components of the triad involved in excitation–contraction coupling have been pursued down to the molecular level. In electron micrographs of high resolution, the T-tubules and adjoining cisternae are seen to be joined by small regularly-spaced electron-dense structures that bridge the 15-nm gap between their membranes. These so-called *junctional feet* (also called *spanning proteins* or *junctional channel complexes*) are arranged on the surface of the cisterna in two or three rows, parallel to the long axis of the T-tubule. In sections tangential to the junctional face of the cisterna, each foot appears to be made up of four subunits about 14 nm in diameter arranged in a quadrifoil configuration. In freeze–fracture preparations, the intramembranous domain of these complexes is represented by groups of four rounded profiles projecting from the inner surface of cleaved junctional membrane. Images of cleaved T-tubule membrane reveal groups of four particles that have the same center-to-center spacing as the subunits of the junctional feet. These are also arranged in longitudinal rows and are believed to be in contact with the subunits of foot proteins that span the gap between the junctional membranes of the triads.(Fig. 10–19)

These ultrastructural observations have been supplemented by biochemical studies on isolated T-tubules and junctional reticulum. Two proteins have been isolated that are believed to be involved in signal transduction at the junction. An 1800 kD protein composed of four identical subunits has been extracted from terminal cisternae. It binds *ryanodine,* a plant alkaloid known to release calcium from the sarcoplasmic reticulum. In electron micrographs, this protein has an appearance identical to that of the junctional feet in situ. A second protein of 212 kD, extracted from T-tubules, binds *1,4,dihydroxypyridine,* a known voltage dependent blocker of Ca^{++} channels. In electron micrographs, this protein matches the tetrads seen in freeze–fracture preparations of T-tubules. It is believed to sense the voltage change associated with depolarization of the T-tubule membrane and to activate opening of the Ca^{++} channels in the junctional feet.

SUBSTRUCTURE OF THE MYOFIBRILS

The smallest units of the contractile material of muscle that are visible with the light microscope are the myofibrils (Fig. 10–20D), but in electron micrographs, these are found to be composed of even smaller units, the *myofilaments* (Fig. 10–20E). These are of two kinds, thin *actin filaments* and thicker *myosin filaments.* The cross-banded pattern of striated muscle is due to a highly ordered arrangement of interdigitating sets of these filaments. Myosin filaments, 1.5 μm in length and 15 nm in diameter, are oriented longitudinally in parallel array and spaced about 45 nm apart. They are the principal constituent of the A-bands of the sarcomeres. Each is slightly thicker in the middle and tapers toward its ends. They are held in lateral register by slender cross-links in the middle of the A-band. The transverse alignment of these links creates a thin linear density called the *M-line* that bisects the paler *H-band* at the middle of each A-band (Fig. 10–20F). Actin filaments are the dominant component of the I-bands, but at their ends, they interdigitate with myosin filaments in the neighboring A-bands to varying degrees depending on the state of muscle contraction. It follows that in cross sections at the level of the I-band, only punctate profiles of thin actin filaments are found (Fig. 10–20G), whereas in cross sections near the middle of the A-band, only larger punctate profiles of myosin filaments are found (Fig. 10–20H). However, in cross sections through the region

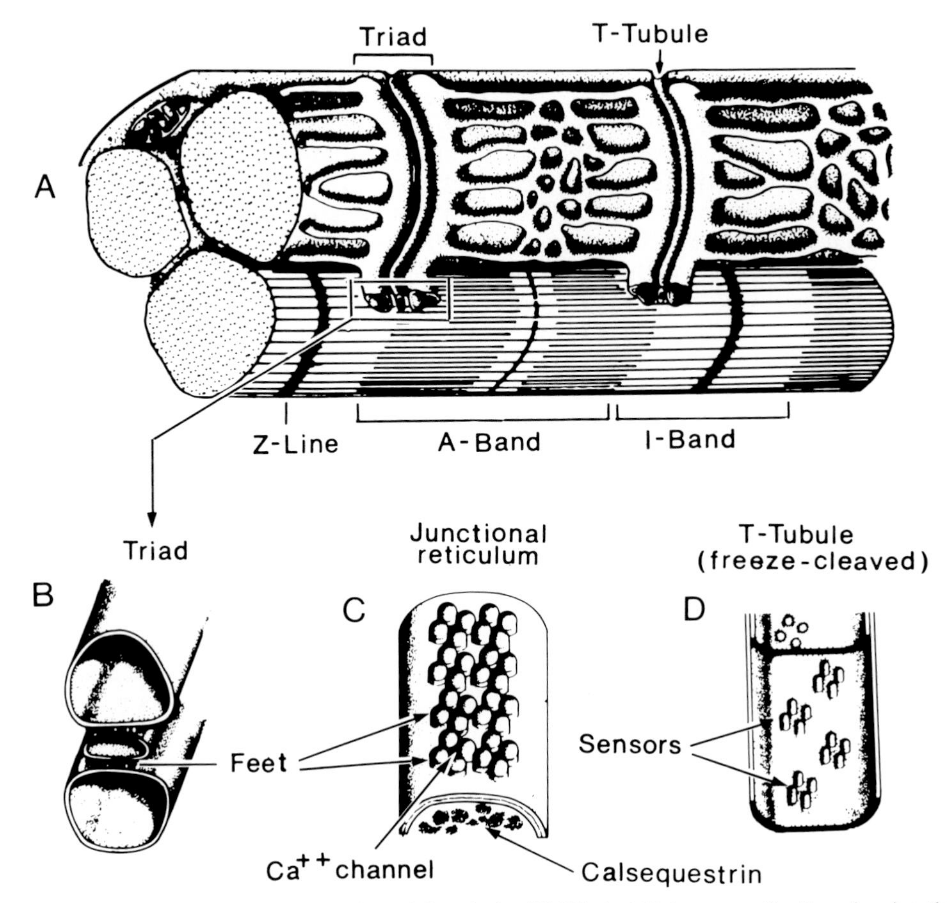

Figure 10–19. (A) Diagram showing the location of the triads. (B) Triad at higher magnification showing the so-called feet connecting the cisternae to the T-tubule. (C) Drawing of the freeze–fracture appearance of the junctional surface of a terminal cisterna, showing the groups of four subunits of the feet. The lipophilic intramembrane portions of these subunits surround the calcium-release channel. (D) Appearance of freeze–fracture image of the T-tubule, showing diamond-shaped clusters of particles that correspond in their distribution to that of the protein subunits of the feet. These presumably detect the depolarization of the membrane and transmit a signal to the foot processes that results in opening of the calcium channels. (Figure based on diagrams in Block, B.A. et al. 1988. J. Cell Biol. 107:2587.)

of filament interdigation, near the ends of the A-band, both kinds of filaments are found, with thin filaments in hexagonal array around each myosin filament (Fig. 10–20I, 20–21). In longitudinal sections, the 10–20-nm interval between thick and thin filaments is traversed by regularly-spaced cross-bridges radiating from each myosin filament toward the neighboring actin filaments (Figs. 10–20F, 10–23 and 10–24). Little additional detail can be seen in routine electron micrographs of thin sections, but analysis of the myofilaments has been carried further by their isolation and examination at high magnification after shadowing with heavy metals and with negative-staining procedures.

Isolated thick filaments have a smooth central segment, but toward either end, they bear short lateral projections 14 nm apart. These correspond to the cross-bridges seen between thick and thin filaments in intact myofibrils. Further dissociation of a thick filament yields about 350 *myosin molecules,* each 300 nm long and 2–3 nm in diameter. These, in turn, consist of two α-helical polypeptide chains with a globular region at one end. The two chains are entwined to form the straight, rod-like "tail" of the molecule, whereas the globular regions diverge to form two "heads," corresponding to one of the cross-bridges of an intact myosin filament. The junction of the head and tail of the molecule is flexible, permitting a change in configuration which, as will be shown later, results in movement of the adjacent actin filament (Fig. 10–25). Enzymatic proteolysis of the myosin molecule cleaves it into two fragments, a straight portion called *light meromyosin* (LMM), representing the

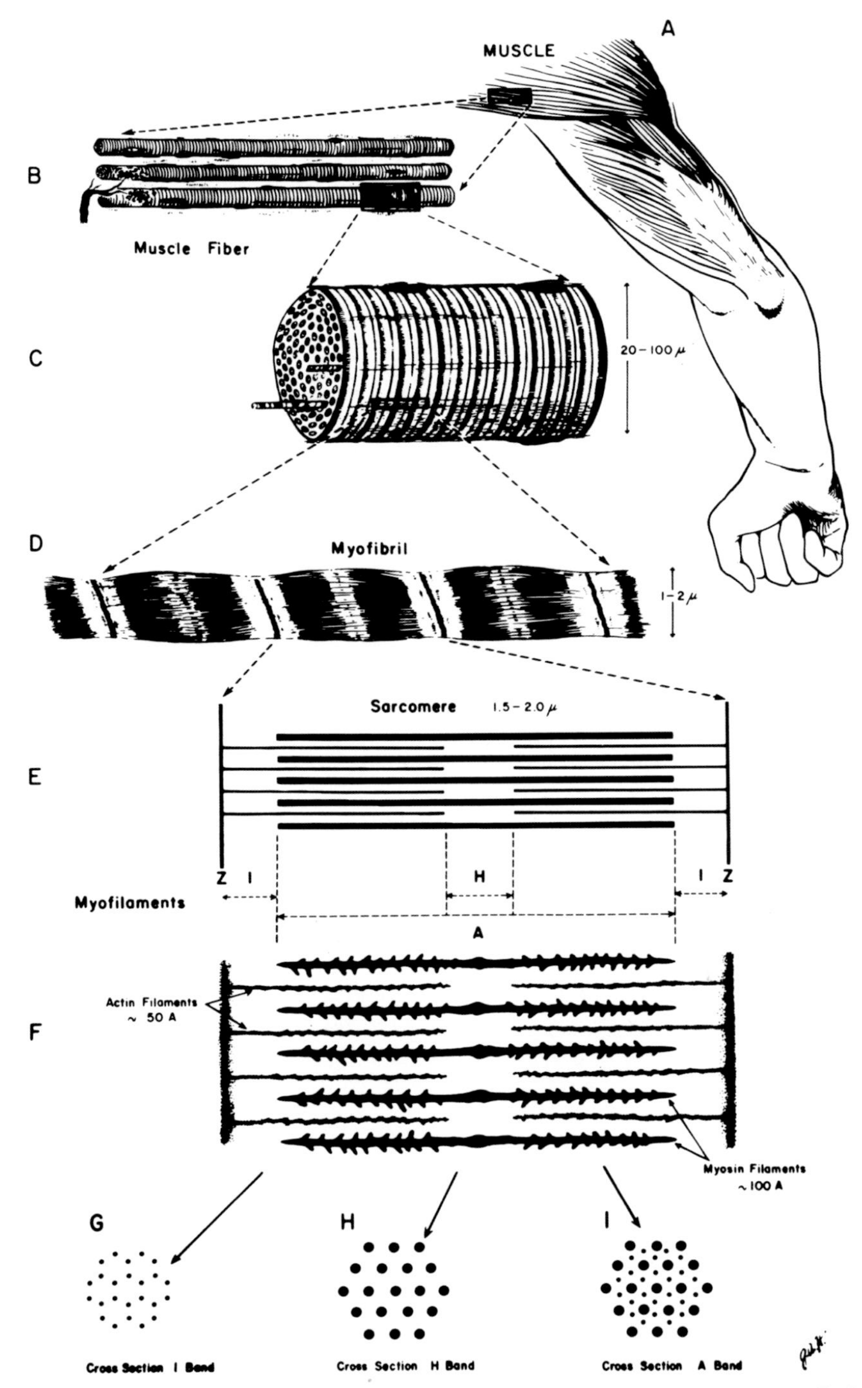

Figure 10–20. Diagram of the organization of skeletal muscle from the gross to the molecular level. F, G, H, and I show the arrangement of filaments in cross section at the levels indicated in E. (Drawing by Sylvia Colard Keene.)

greater part of the tail, and a shorter segment called *heavy meromyosin* (HMM), which includes the heads and a short portion of the backbone of the molecule. When a heavy meromyosin fraction is added to isolated actin filaments, large numbers of these HMM fragments attach to the filaments decorating them in a distinctive arrow-head pattern. This clearly demonstrates, in vitro, the actin-binding property of the heads of the myosin molecules that is essential for muscle contraction.

Under appropriate physicochemical condi-

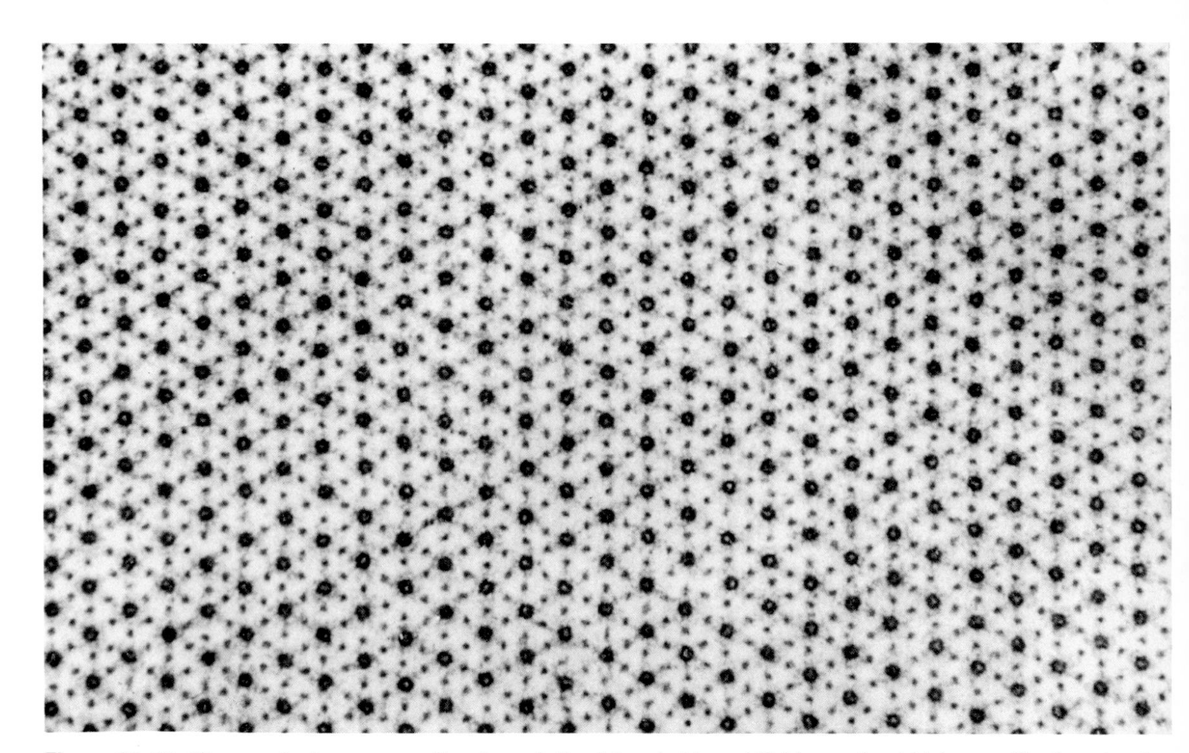

Figure 10–21. Micrograph of a cross section through the A-band of insect flight muscle at high magnification showing the orderly arrangement of actin filaments around the larger myosin filaments, as in Fig. 10–20, I. The pattern is similar in vertebrate muscle but it usually does not exhibit such a highly ordered "crystalline" lattice, and the myosin filaments do not appear hollow in cross section in mammalian muscle. (Micrograph courtesy of H. Ris.)

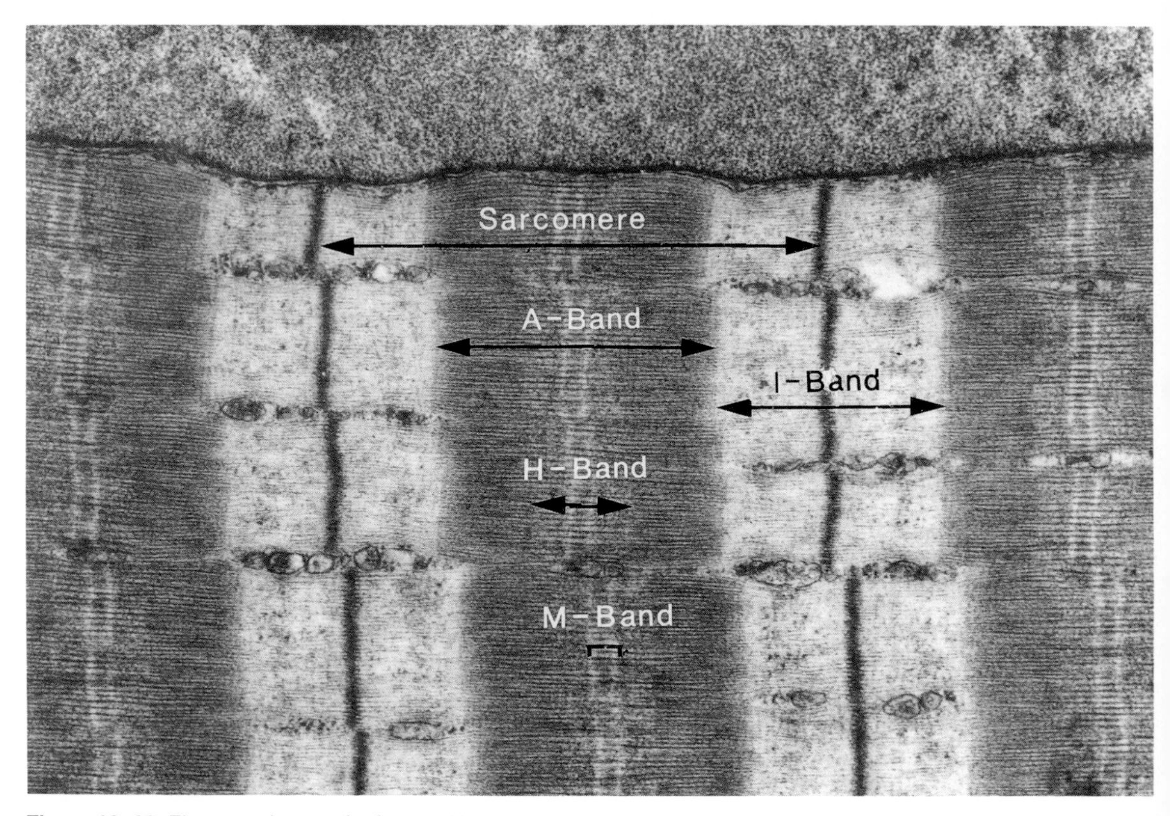

Figure 10–22. Electron micrograph of several juxtanuclear myofibrils labeled to indicate the various bands in the normal pattern of cross-striations in a relaxed mammalian muscle.

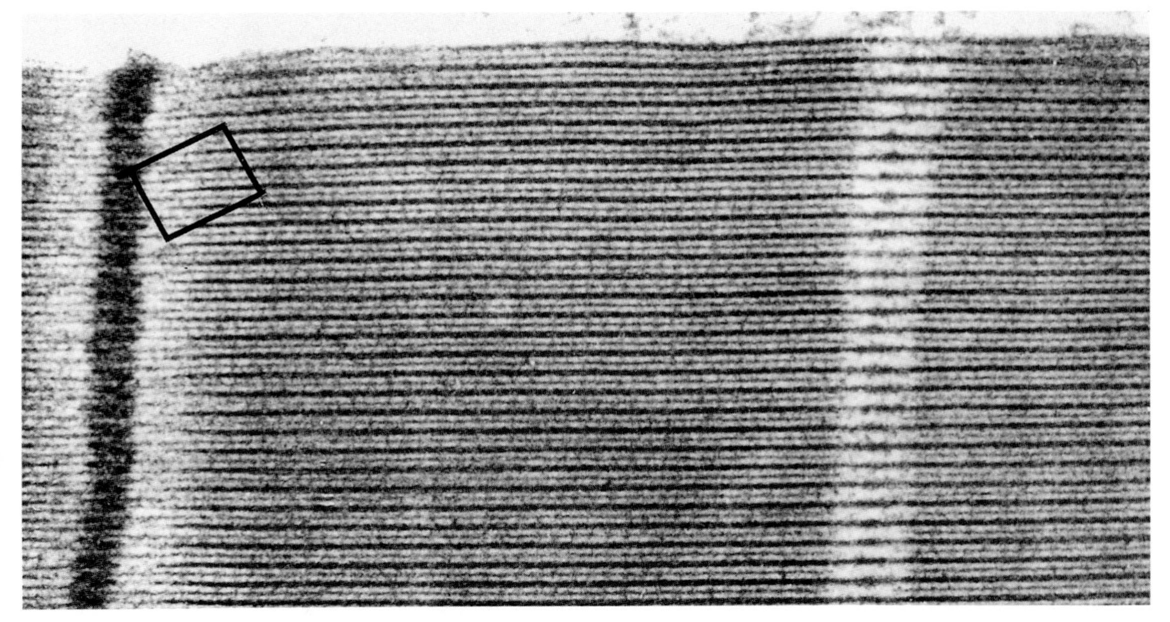

Figure 10–23. Micrograph of the major portion of one sarcomere of insect flight muscle. Cross-bridges between the think and thin filaments are just detectable. These are more apparent in the Fig. 10–24, an area comparable to that outlined in the square on this figure. (High-voltage micrograph courtesy of H. Ris.)

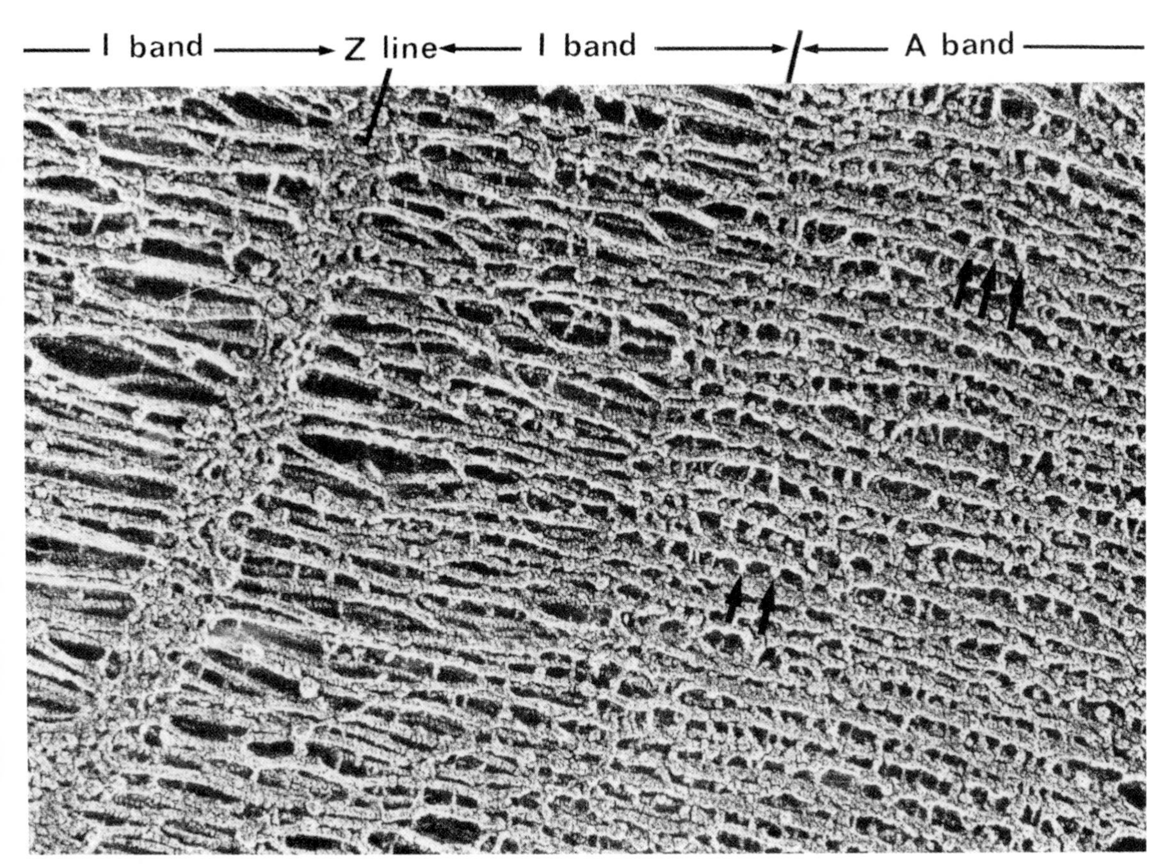

Figure 10–24. Micrograph of an area of skeletal muscle prepared by rapid freezing in liquid helium, deep etching, and rotary-shadowing. The cross-bridges between the myosin and actin filaments are clearly visible (at arrows). (Micrograph courtesy of N. Hirokawa and J. Heuser.)

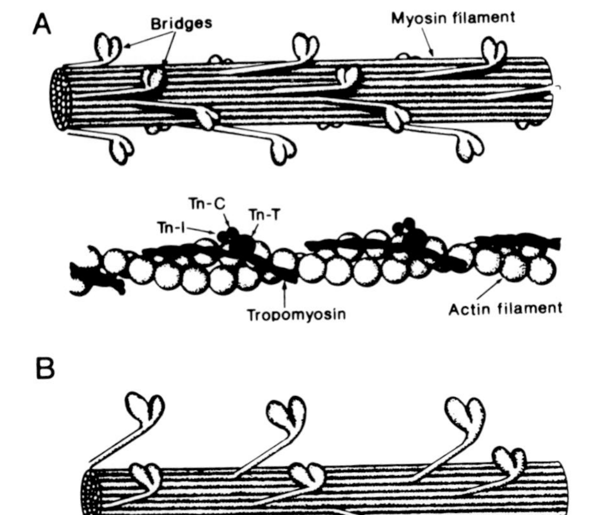

Figure 10–25. (A) Schematic representation of the arrangement of myosin molecules in a segment of a thick filament, and the double helical configuration of the actin filament with its periodic associated tropomyosin and troponin complexes. (B) In the current interpretation of the mechanism of movement of the actin filaments, calcium binding causes a change in the configuration of the tropomyosin–troponin complexes, exposing the myosin-binding sites on the actin filament. The myosin heads, energized by ATP, then change their angle to bind and move the actin filament.

tions, myosin molecules will self-assemble in vitro to form myosin filaments. In so doing, they assume an antiparallel arrangement with the rod portions toward the center of the nascent filament and the heads toward its ends. The overlapping molecules are staggered so that the projecting heads recur at intervals of 14 nm and each is rotated 120° with respect to its neighbors. This results in a spiral disposition of the heads along much of the filament toward either end. A central segment consisting only of the overlapping antiparallel rod portion of the molecules is devoid of bridges. In intact myofibrils, the lateral register of these smooth segments of the myosin filaments results in the paler H-band in the center of the A-bands (Fig. 10–22).

Thin filaments isolated by dissociation of myofibrils are about 1 μm in length and consist predominantly of filamentous actin (F-actin). At very high magnification, they have a slightly beaded appearance because they are formed by polymerization of globular monomers (G-actin), 5.6 nm in diameter, into two strands helically entwined, with each gyre about 36 nm in length. Study of polymerization of G-actin, in vitro, has shown that the monomers are consistently oriented, giving the resulting filaments a definite polarity. Within the myofibrils, in vivo, the actin filaments on either side of the Z-discs are of opposite polarity. Associated with the actin filaments are molecules of *tropomyosin,* a protein about 40 nm in length consisting of two polypeptide chains in α-helical configuration. These long molecules are arranged end-to-end in the grooves between the helically entwined actin chains (Fig. 10–25). Bound to each molecule of tropomyosin, at regular intervals of about 40 nm, is a complex of three *troponin* peptides (Tn-T, Tn-I, and Tn-C) that have distinct functions. Tn-T binds the complex to tropomyosin, Tn-C has a binding site for calcium, and Tn-I inhibits binding of myosin heads to actin in resting muscle. These submicroscopic components of the thin filaments have key roles in the sliding filament mechanism of muscle contraction that will be discussed later in this chapter.

Muscle exhibits a resistance to stretch that is independent of the interaction of actin and myosin filaments and a third type of filament, responsible for this passive elasticity, was postulated. This has now been verified by the discovery of very thin filaments that extend from the A-band to the Z-line. They are seldom resolved in routine electron micrographs, but when muscle is greatly stretched, they can be seen in the gap created between the ends of the thick and thin filaments. In addition, if the actin filaments are selectively depolymerized with gelsolin, delicate strands can be seen extending the full length of the I-band. These extremely thin strands (~ 4 nm) consist of *titin,* an exceptionally large protein having a molecular weight of about 3×10^6 D. The molecules are approximately 1 μm long, spanning the distance from the M-line of the A-band to the Z-disc (Fig. 10–26). The portion of the molecule that extends into the A-band may be an integral part of the thick filaments. There are probably six per filament. The I-band region of the molecules forms an elastic connection between the thick filaments and the Z-line. Titin is the main structural basis for myofibrillar elasticity. In addition, it is believed to maintain the central position of the thick filaments in the sarcomere. This is supported by the observation that, after radiation damage to titin, the central position of the A-band is lost.

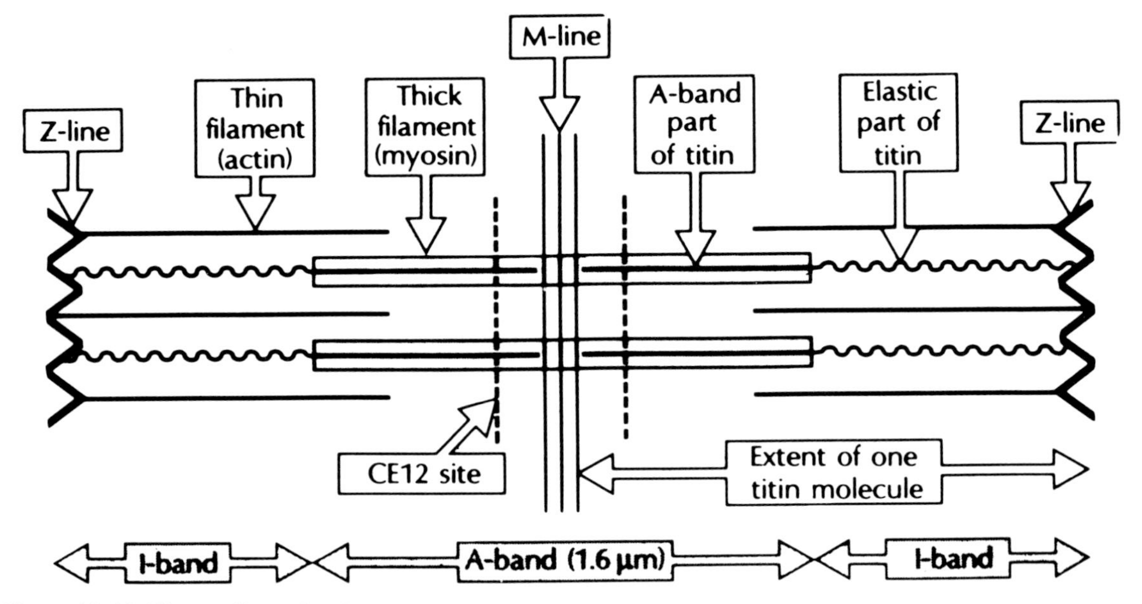

Figure 10–26. Diagram illustrating the probable arrangement of titin molecules within the sarcomere. The elastic part of the molecule is shown only in the I-band. (From Trinnick, J. 1991. Current Opinion Cell Biol. 6:112.)

The myofilaments of successive sarcomeres are linked end-to-end by the Z-disc. The structural basis for this linkage is still a matter of debate because, in electron micrographs, the density of the disc and the superimposition of its components in sections of normal thickness makes its substructure difficult to analyze. In very thin sections of muscle from a species with a relatively simple disc, the actin filaments appear to terminate at the edge of the disc. There, each filament is attached to four thin diverging *Z-filaments.* These course obliquely across the disc to attach to four actin filaments of the next sarcomere. In transverse sections passing through the disc, the ends of the actin filaments, and the Z-filaments connecting them project a square lattice (Fig. 10–27). The filaments of one sarcomere are slightly offset with respect to those approaching the disc from the other side. Therefore, in longitudinal sections, the connecting Z-filaments form a zigzag pattern across the myofibril. The chemical nature of the Z-filaments has yet to be established, but other important components of the disc have been identified. Much of its electron density is attributed to *α-actinin,* a 100 kD actin-binding protein which is also involved in the end-to-end linkage of actin filaments in the cytoplasmic dense bodies of smooth muscle. A 200 kD protein, *zeugmatin,* can be localized in two parallel lines along the boundaries of the disc. Another actin-binding protein, *filamin,* originally isolated from

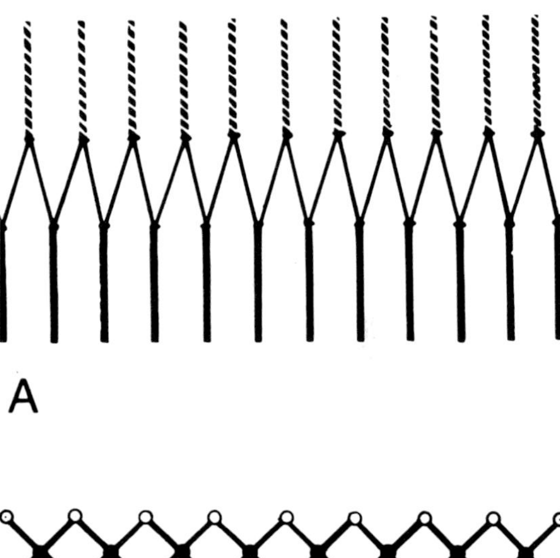

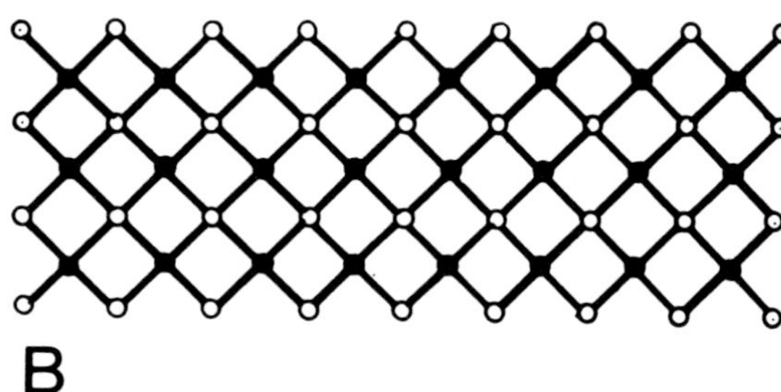

Figure 10–27. Diagram illustrating one interpretation of the structure of the Z-disc. At (A) the actin filaments terminate at the edge of the Z-disc, where each is attached to four diverging Z-filaments, coursing across the disc to attach to four actin filaments of the next sarcomere. (B) In transverse sections through the disc, the ends of the actin filaments and the Z-filaments, project a square lattice. (After Kelly, D.E. and M.A. Cahill. 1972. Anat. Rec. 172:623.)

smooth muscle, is also found in the Z-discs of skeletal muscle. The respective roles of these proteins in maintaining the structural integrity of the disc has yet to be worked out.

A complex cytoskeleton of sarcoplasmic intermediate filaments supports the myofibrils and maintains the transverse alignment of sarcomeres that results in the characteristic cross-striated appearance of skeletal and cardiac muscle. A ring of interwoven filaments encircles the myofibrils at each Z-line and the rings around the Z-lines of successive sarcomeres are connected by longitudinal filaments in the intermyofibrillar spaces. Thus, each myofibril is enclosed in a delicate sleeve of 10-nm filaments and the collars around the Z-lines of neighboring myofibrils are interconnected by short transverse filaments. Beneath the sarcolemma, there are inconspicuous rib-like bands, called *costameres,* seen in longitudinal sections as small densities that repeat along the fiber in register with the Z-lines of the peripheral myofibrils. These appear to be sites where the myofibrils are loosely connected to the sarcolemma by filaments of the cytoskeleton. In contracted or swollen muscle fibers, indentations occur along the length of the fiber at these subsarcolemmal densities which can be shown to contain the anchoring protein, *vinculin.* The contribution of this elaborate cytoskeleton to the active tension and passive elasticity of muscle has yet to be explored.

SLIDING FILAMENT MECHANISM OF CONTRACTION

Histologists using the light microscope observed the changes in relative length of the sarcomeres during contraction but could offer no satisfactory explanation of the mechanism of contraction. In the past three decades, detailed analysis of muscle by electron microscopy and X-ray diffraction has revealed the structural basis for its periodic cross-striations and has led to a widely accepted explanation of the mechanism of myofibril shortening.

Any acceptable theory had to account for the observation that, during contraction, the length of the A-band remains constant while the length of the I-band and H-band both decrease. An explanation became apparent when the electron microscope revealed two sets of interdigitating filaments. In the *sliding filament theory,* it is proposed that when muscle contracts, the thick and thin filaments maintain the same length as in resting muscle, but the thin filaments are moved relative to the thick filaments, sliding more deeply into the A-bands, thus shortening the sarcomeres along the entire length of the myofibrils (Fig. 10–28). Consistent with this interpretation are the changes in length of the H-band in different phases of the contractile cycle. Its dimensions are determined by the distance between the ends of the actin filaments that extend into the A-band from opposite ends. Therefore, it is widest in resting muscle and becomes narrower in contracted muscle, owing to the deeper penetration of the actin filaments into the A-band.

The only visible structures that could produce the observed displacement of the actin filaments are the heads of the myosin molecules that form cross-bridges between the two sets of filaments. It is assumed that it is these that develop the force necessary for actin filament sliding. During contraction, the displacement of the actin filaments may be as much as 300 nm in each half-sarcomere, whereas the movement of the distal ends of the bridges could be no more than 10 nm. Therefore, hundreds of bridge-forming and bridge-breaking cycles must take place to produce the observed displacement of the actin filaments.

The observation that the distance between filaments, in some phases of contraction, appeared to be greater than the length of the myosin heads, initially cast some doubt on their involvement in translocation of the actin filaments. Reluctance to accept this explanation was dispelled by the subsequent discovery of two flexible regions in the myosin molecule, one at the base of the heads and one at the junction of the heavy and the light meromysin subunits. The existence of these two flexible regions permits the heads to attach over a range of interfilament distances and still maintain the same orientation of the heads relative to the actin filaments (Fig. 10–25). What part of the myosin molecule develops the force that results in filament movement is still not entirely clear, but it is believed that a force-generating change occurs in the angle of attachment of the heads to the actin filaments.

For the conversion of chemical energy to mechanical work, actin filaments are a necessary cofactor in the release of energy by the ATPase in the heads of the myosin molecules. If *purified* actin is added to myosin filaments, in vitro, there is rapid hydrolysis of ATP. However, in resting muscle, the binding sites for myosin on the thin filaments are blocked

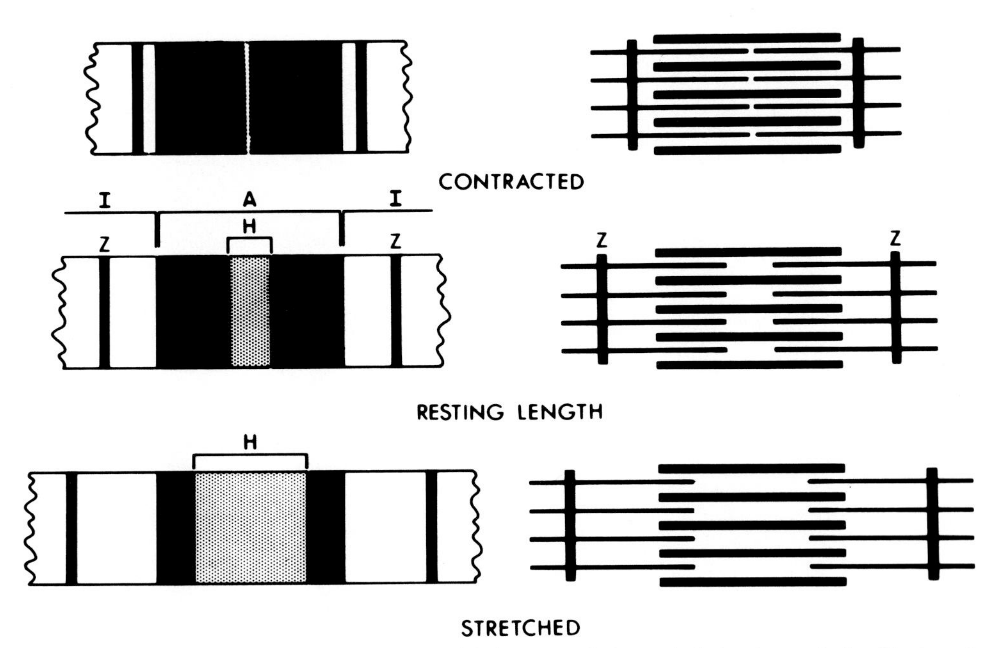

Figure 10–28. Diagram of the changing appearance of the cross-striations of skeletal muscle in different phases of contraction (on left) and the corresponding differences in the degree of interdigitation of the thick and thin filaments (on right).

by the tropomyosin–troponin complexes, preventing myosin-actin interaction. Release of calcium into the sarcoplasm, in response to a nerve impulse, is followed by binding of calcium to troponin C in each of the subunits along the length of the actin filaments (Fig. 10–25). This is believed to cause a conformational change that moves the tropomyosin chains deeper into the groove of the actin helix, exposing the myosin-binding sites. Binding then activates the myosin ATPase and the resulting release of energy induces a flexion of the myosin heads that displaces the thin filaments a short distance toward the center of the A-band of the sarcomeres. The heads then detach and realign with the next set of actin subunits for a new cycle of bridge-making and bridge-breaking. The progressive translocation of the actin filaments toward the center of the A-bands shortens the sarcomeres along the entire length of the myofibrils, resulting in a contraction that continues until calcium ions are taken up and sequestered in the terminal cisternae. The tropomyosin–troponin complexes then cover the binding sites on the actin filaments, restoring the resting state.

INNERVATION OF SKELETAL MUSCLE

Muscle is innervated by nerves containing the axons of many motor neurons in the spinal cord. At the muscle, the nerve divides into branches that penetrate into its interior via the perimysial septa. Individual axons then ramify in the endomysium to form endings, from a few to several hundred, on individual muscle fibers. A single motor neuron, its axon, and the muscle fibers it innervates together constitute a *motor unit.* Activity of a motor unit is all-or-none; that is, the fibers of the unit either contract fully in response to a nerve impulse or not at all. The largest motor units may generate a tension 200 times that of the smallest motor units. In the graded response that is possible in whole muscles, the strength of contraction depends on the number of motor units activated. Small muscle tensions are generated by selective recruitment of varying numbers of small motor units. When greater tension is required, the larger motor units are activated.

In addition to differences in size of the units, there are different kinds, corresponding to the different fiber types. *Slow-twitch motor units* (red fibers) generate little tension but can remain active for long periods with little fatigue. *Fast-twitch motor units* (white fibers) generate high peak tension but fatigue rapidly. Muscles generally consist of a mixture of the two types. Thus, muscle tension can be regulated in two ways: (1) control of the number and kind of motor units recruited and (2) control of the firing frequency of the units that have been activated.

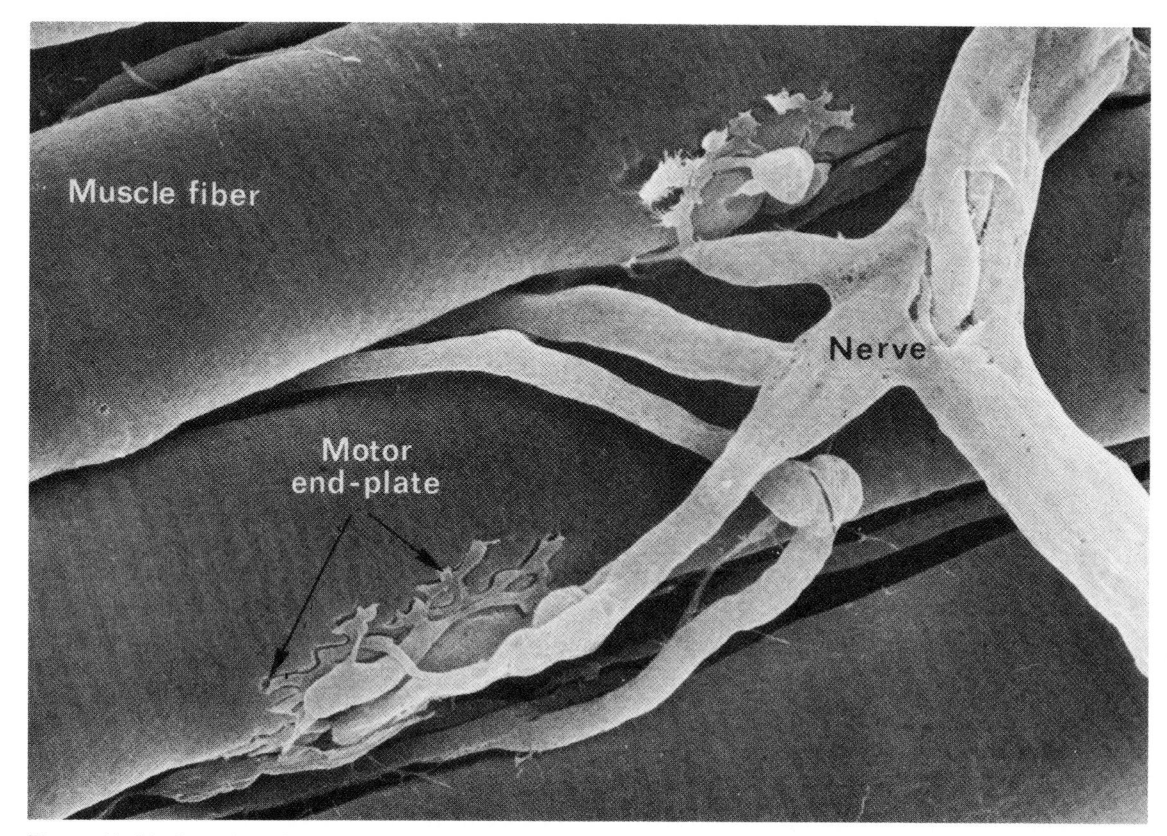

Figure 10–29. Scanning micrograph of a motor nerve and two end plates on adjacent muscle fibers. (Micrograph from Desaki, J. and Y. Uehara. 1981. J. Neurocytol. 10:101.)

At the site of contact with the muscle fiber, the axon loses its myelin sheath and it branches to form several short *axon terminals* that occupy a shallow depression in the fiber surface, called the *primary synaptic cleft.* The sarcolemma underlying the axon terminals is infolded to form numerous narrow *secondary synaptic clefts* (Figs. 10–29 and 10–30). These evidently serve to increase the area of sarcolemma exposed to neurotransmitter. At the margins of the junction, the basal or external lamina of the axon fuses with that covering the sarcolemma to form a single layer that lines the primary and secondary synaptic clefts. The specialized region of the muscle fiber underlying the nerve terminal is called the *motor end plate.* Several nuclei and numerous mitochondria are clustered in the sarcoplasm in this area (Fig. 10–31). The axoplasm of the nerve terminals contains a few mitochondria and a very large number of 40–60-nm vesicles, identical to the *synaptic vesicles* seen at axodendritic synapses in the central nervous system (Fig. 10–32). These vesicles are the sites of storage of the neurotransmitter *acetylocholine.* It is estimated that each vesicle may contain 10,000 molecules of acetylcholine. In neural transmission, the content of these vesicles is released by exocytosis. This takes place at specialized sites in the presynaptic membrane, referred to as *active zones* (Fig. 10–33). In freeze–fracture preparations, the active zones are recognized as linear specializations of the membrane that run parallel to the subneural ridges and furrows in the motor end plate. The synaptic vesicles cluster in the axoplasm near these active zones, and in preparations of nerve endings frozen with liquid helium within milliseconds of nerve stimulation, linear arrays of discharging synaptic vesicles can be seen along the active zones.

In rapidly frozen, deep-etched, and rotary-shadowed preparations of the sarcolemma covering the ridges and folds of the muscle fiber, one can see a high concentration of closely packed intramembrane particles believed to be the *acetylcholine receptors* (Fig. 10–34). The acetylcholine receptors have been isolated and their structure analyzed in some detail. They consist of five similar subunits

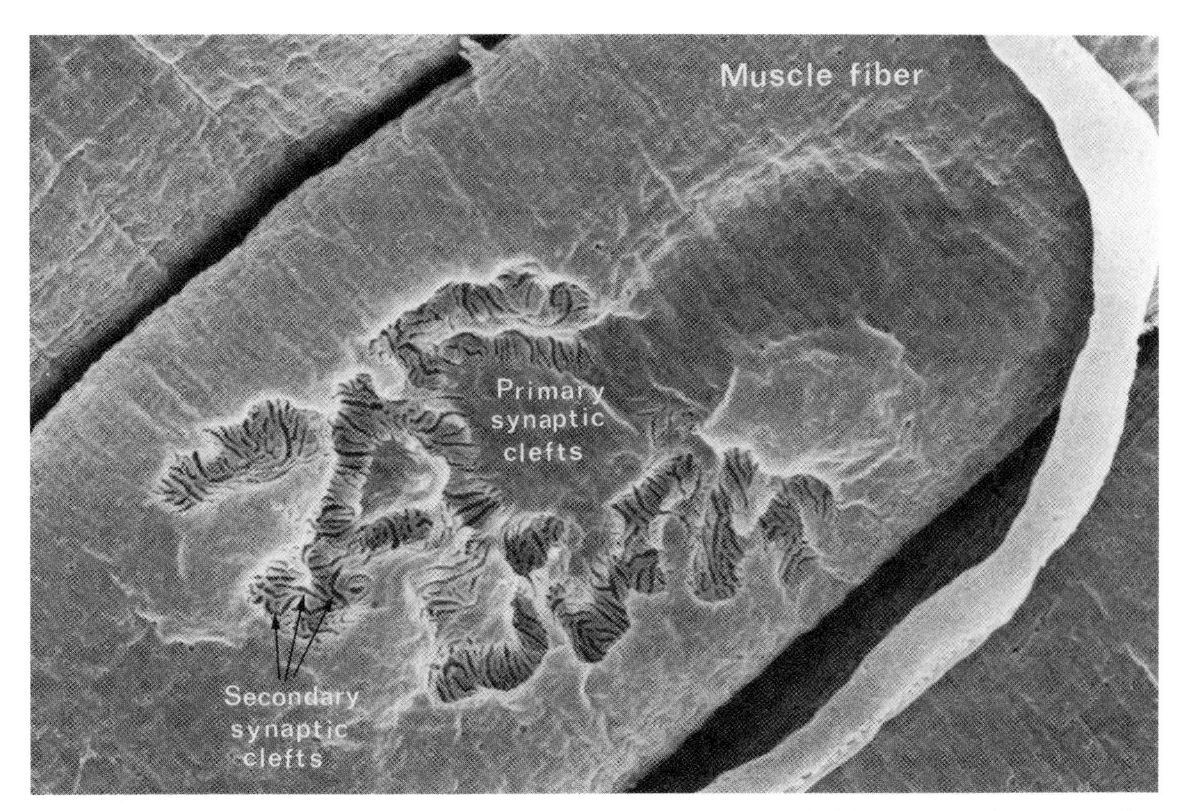

Figure 10–30. Scanning micrograph of a muscle fiber from which the nerve terminal has been pulled away, revealing the underlying primary and secondary synaptic clefts. (Micrograph from Desaki, J. and Y. Uehara. 1981. Dev. Biol. 119: 390, 1987.)

forming a funnel-shaped complex around a central ion channel. The receptor complex extends through the membrane and has a cytoplasmic domain, a membrane domain, and an extracellular domain that projects about 6 nm into the synaptic cleft.

According to current interpretations of the initiation of a neural impulse, a wave of depolarization traveling down the nerve axon opens channels that permit influx of Ca^{++} into the nerve ending. This causes synaptic vesicles to release acetylcholine into the synaptic cleft. Its binding to receptors results in a transient change in the conformation of their subunits, opening ion-conducting channels. The channel in each receptor remains open for a few milliseconds permitting entry of thousands of sodium ions per millisecond. Influx of sodium depolarizes the postsynaptic membrane, generating an action-potential that is propagated over the sarcolemma and into the T-tubules, activating the intracellular release of calcium from the terminal cisternae of the sarcoplasmic reticulum to trigger muscle contraction. Acetylcholine, diffusing laterally in the synaptic cleft, is hydrolyzed by acetylcholine esterase located in the basal lamina lining the clefts, thereby limiting the duration of the response to the transmitter.

A reduction in the number of available acetylcholine receptors in the myoneural junctions is the basic defect in the human disease *myasthenia gravis,* which is characterized by weakness and fatigability of skeletal muscle. There are normally 30 million or more receptors per neuromuscular junction. In myasthenia gravis, there is a 70–90% reduction in their number.

NEUROMUSCULAR SPINDLES

For muscles to be used in a coordinated manner for locomotion and other voluntary movements, the central nervous system continuously needs information about the position of the limbs and the state contraction of the various muscles. Such sensory inputs are collectively called *proprioception.* To meet this need, muscles contain complex sensors called

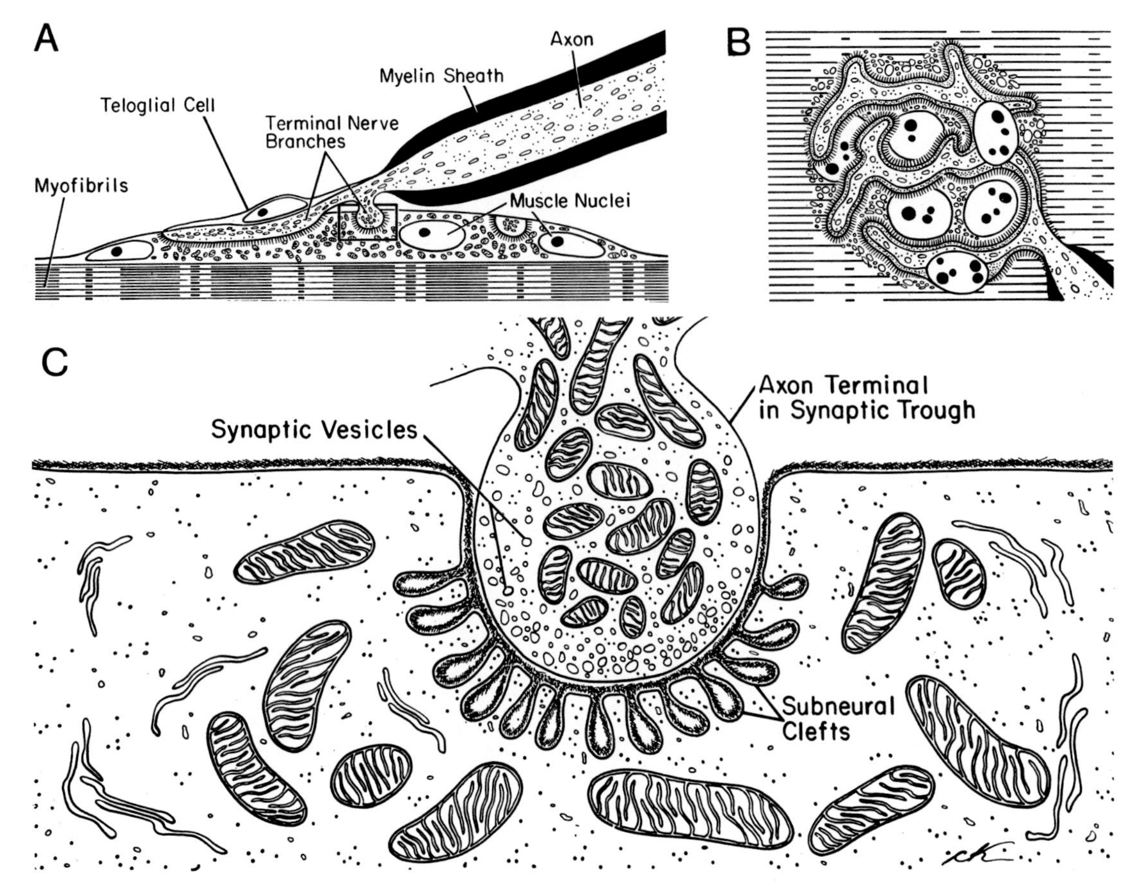

Figure 10–31. Schematic representation of the motor end plate. (A) End plate as seen in a longitudinal histological section of a muscle fiber; (B) as seen in surface view with the light microscope; (C) as seen in an electron micrograph of an area such as that in the rectangle in (A). (Modified after Couteaux, R. 1960. In Structure and Function of Muscle. J.H. Bourne, ed. Academic Press, New York, Vol. 1, p. 337.

neuromuscular spindles and *Golgi tendon organs.* The muscle spindles consist of several modified striated muscle fibers enclosed in a fusiform sheath or capsule. They are 5–10 mm long and therefore much shorter than the surrounding muscle fibers. The number of spindles varies greatly from muscle to muscle. Fifty have been counted in a limb muscle of moderate size in the cat. Comparable figures for human muscles are not available, but it is likely that the number would be several times greater.

The specialized muscle fibers in the interior of the spindle are referred to as *intrafusal fibers* to distinguish them from the unspecialized *extrafusal fibers* that make up the bulk of the muscle (Fig. 10–35). They number from 6 to as many as 12. They are of two kinds, *nuclear bag fibers (2–4)* and *nuclear chain fibers (4–8).* In a central region occupying about half the length of the nuclear bag fibers, the intrafusal fibers are enclosed in a connective tissue capsule which is expanded in its central 2–3 mm to limit a fusiform cavity filled with a gelatinous substance comparable to that of the vitreous body of the eye (Fig. 10–36). This material is usually extracted in specimen preparation, leaving the intrafusal fibers surrounded by an empty-appearing *periaxial space.* The nuclear bag fibers extend for some distance in either direction beyond the ends of the capsule and are attached at their ends to the connective tissue septa that form the endomysium of the muscle. The relatively short nuclear chain fibers are largely confined to the capsule. Cross-striations are lacking in the midportion of the intracapsular segment of both fiber types. This region of the nuclear bag fibers contains 50 or more spherical nuclei that completely fill, and slightly distend, the fiber. From this central *nuclear bag* region to either end of the capsule, the fiber contains oval nuclei aligned in a single row in its core, surrounded by a layer of cross-striated myofibrils. The nuclei

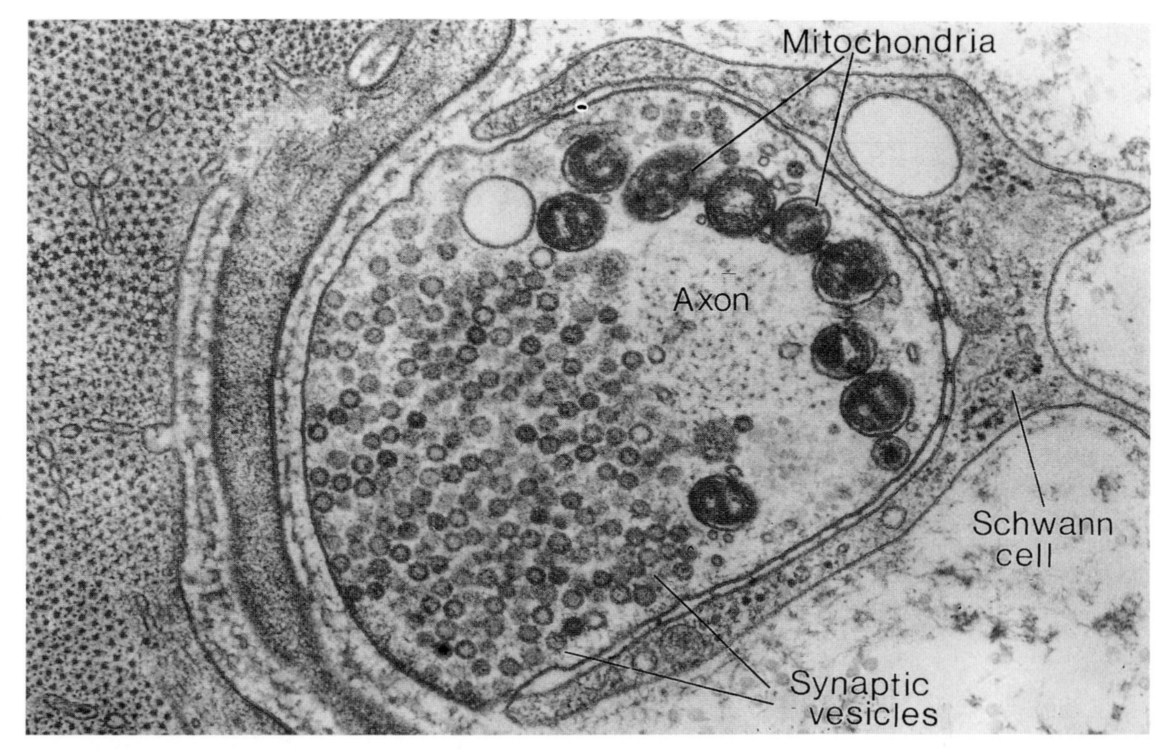

Figure 10–32. Electron micrograph of the nerve ending at the myoneural junction, showing an accumulation of mitochondria in the axoplasm and a large number of synaptic vesicles. (Micrograph courtesy of T. Reese.)

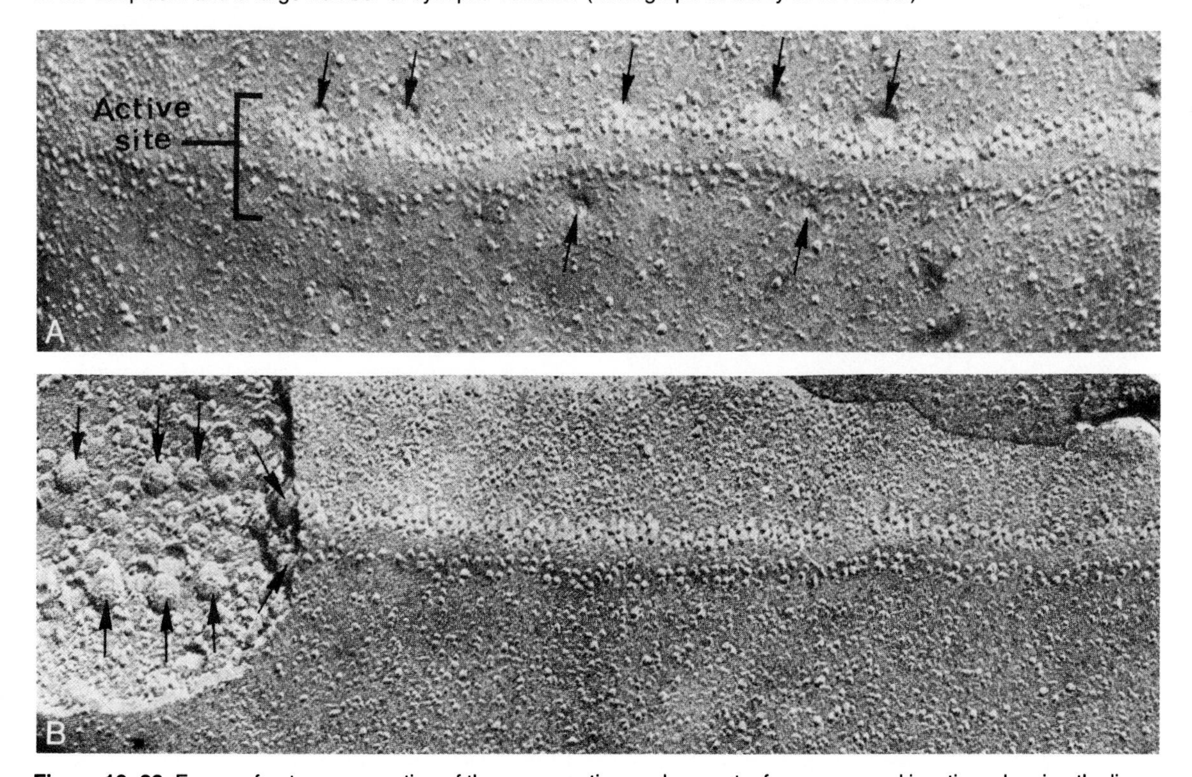

Figure 10–33. Freeze–fracture preparation of the persynaptic membrane at a frog myoneural junction, showing the linear active site. (A) The nerve was electrically stimulated and the junction frozen within milliseconds. Exocytosis of several synaptic vesicles can be seen along the active site (at arrows). (B) Similar preparation of the presynaptic membrane of an unstimulated nerve ending. No exocytosis of vesicles is seen. The fracture plane has broken into the axoplasm, at the left, showing synaptic vesicles (arrows) clustered near the active site. (Micrograph courtesy of T. Reese.)

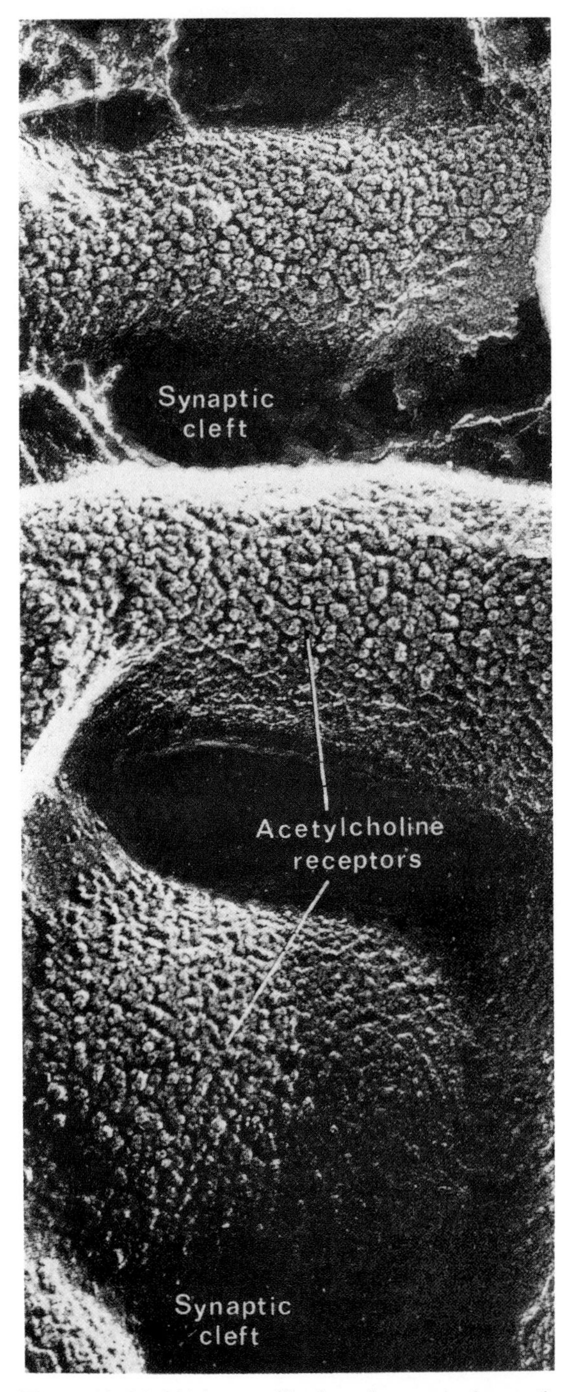

Figure 10–34. A high-magnification micrograph of synaptic ridges and clefts of a motor end plate prepared by rapid freezing, deep etching, and rotary-shadowing. The etching exposes large intramembranous particles in the postsynaptic membrane that are believed to be the acetylcholine receptors. (Micrograph courtesy of N. Hirokawa and J. Heuser.)

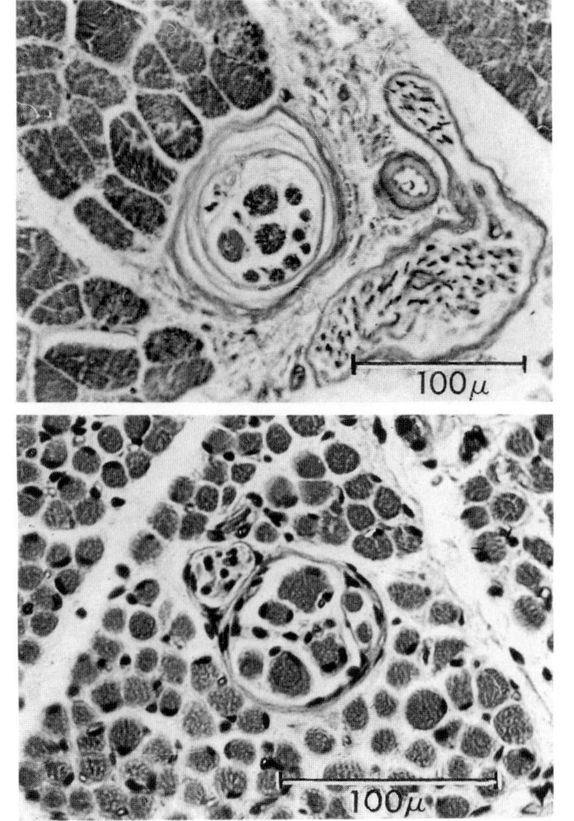

Figure 10–35. (A) Photograph of a muscle spindle in the lumbrical muscle of a human hand. The equatorial region of the spindle is seen with its laminated capsule and large periaxial space, containing cross sections of nine intrafusal muscle fibers, of which three are nuclear bag fibers. The other six smaller ones are nuclear chain fibers. (B) Muscle spindle in human extrinsic eye muscle. Seven of the fibers are surrounded by a thin capsule and there is a small nerve trunk attached. Spindles in eye muscles are usually smaller than those in the limb muscles and have no nuclear bag fibers in man. (Photographs courtesy of S. Cooper.)

in the polar regions of the fiber, and beyond, are spaced at longer intervals and gradually assume a position under the sarcolemma at the periphery of the fiber. The several nuclear chain fibers are only about half the diameter of the nuclear bag fibers and have an axial row of nuclei in their nonstriated central segment.

The muscle spindles have a complex innervation. In the anterior horn of the gray matter of the spinal cord, there are cell bodies of *anterior motor neurons* of two types. Larger *alpha motor neurons* give rise to motor nerve fibers, 9–20 μm in diameter, that innervate the extrafusal fibers of muscles. Smaller *gamma motor neurons* give rise to gamma motor fibers that innervate the contractile portions of the intrafusal fibers in the spindles. The nuclear bag fibers are of two types, *dynamic*

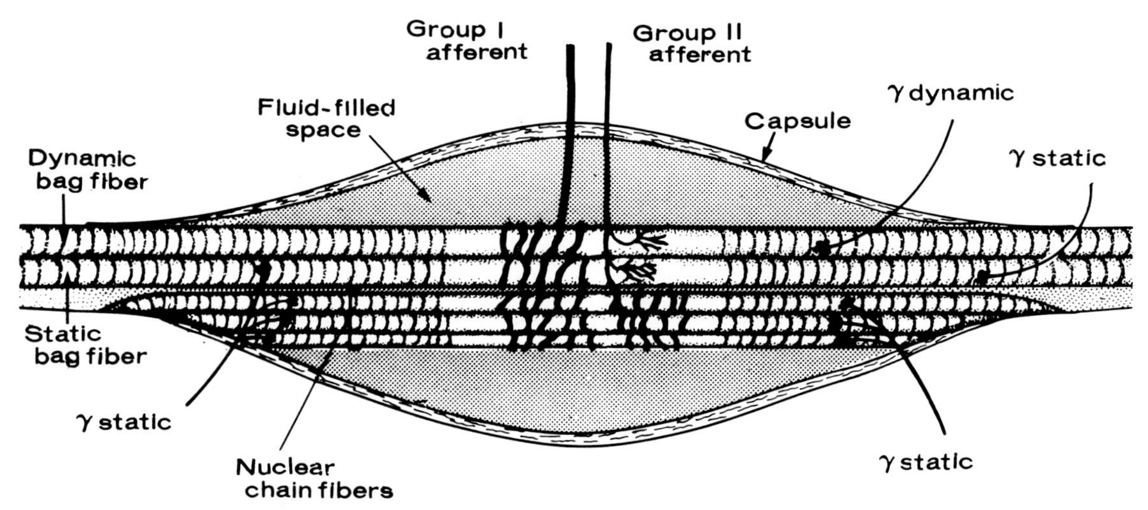

Figure 10–36. Diagram of the central portion of a cat muscle spindle. Three types of intrafusal fibers are distinguished: dynamic nuclear bag fibers, static nuclear bag fibers, and nuclear chain fibers. Also shown, are group-I primary sensory endings, group-II secondary sensory endings, and the fusimotor dynamic and static efferent nerve fibers. (Based on Boyd, I.A. 1985. *In* Motor Systems in Neurobiology. New York, Elsevier Biomedical Press.)

nuclear bag fibers and *static nuclear bag fibers*. These are similar in appearance in histological sections but differ in histochemical and functional properties. They are innervated by distinct axon types. Dynamic bag fibers are innervated by *dynamic gamma axons*, whereas the static nuclear bag fibers and chain fibers are both innervated by *static gamma axons*. Activity of these motor nerves to the intrafusal fibers is believed to stretch their noncontractile portion to maintain its sensitivity near threshold, so that they respond more readily when the muscle as a whole contracts.

The primary sensory nerve endings of the spindle are elaborate *annulospiral endings* that envelope the noncontractile central portion of each of the intrafusal fibers (Fig. 10–37). The afferent fibers from these endings course from the spindles to cell bodies in the posterior horn of the spinal cord. The axons are of relatively large diameter and have a high conduction velocity. The primary afferent nerve from the spindle is accompanied by a smaller nerve containing axons that have spiral secondary nerve endings on each nuclear chain fiber and a spray ending on the nuclear bag fibers near their primary sensory nerve ending.

Spindles respond to changes in length of the muscle in two different ways depending on the rate of change. When the central receptor segment of the intrafusal fibers is stretched *slowly*, impulses are transmitted from the sensory endings on the static nuclear bag fibers

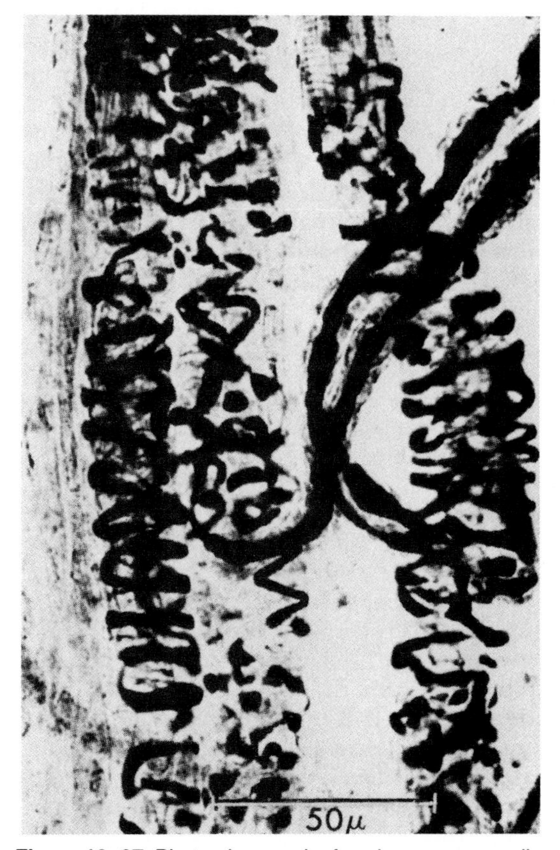

Figure 10–37. Photomicrograph of a primary nerve ending in a muscle spindle of a cat's plantaris muscle. Two branches of an afferent nerve fiber supply the ending which consists of two large spirals around the nuclear bag regions of the muscle fibers. (Courtesy of S. Cooper.)

and nuclear chain fibers at a rate proportional to the degree of stretch for as long as the stretch endures. This is called the *static response* of the spindle. If the length of the primary receptor on the dynamic nuclear bag fibers is increased *suddenly*, a very large number of afferent impulses are transmitted. This is called the *dynamic response.* It lasts only during the period that the length of the fiber is increasing and the rate of impulse discharge then returns to the level that the spindle emits more or less continuously. A familiar example of the dynamic response is seen in the stretch reflex induced in the clinically useful "knee-jerk test." When the doctor taps the patellar tendon, spindles in the extensor muscles are quickly stretched. Their afferent impulses activate alpha motor neurons in the spinal cord and the muscles on the front of the thigh contract, extending the lower leg.

To summarize, spindles scattered through skeletal muscles appear to function like miniature strain gauges, sensing the degree of tension in the muscle. Stimulation of motor nerves to the contractile portions of the intrafusal fibers exerts sufficient tension on the noncontractile sensory portion to maintain its stretch receptor ending near its threshold. A further stretch of the equatorial region of the fibers results in discharge of the spindle afferent fibers, and the frequency of their discharge is proportional to the tension exerted on the intrafusal fibers.

SENSORY NERVE ENDINGS IN TENDONS

There appear to be more than one kind of nerve ending in tendons. In the simplest, unmyelinated nerve fibers ramify over and between collagen fibers of the tendon. It is speculated that these may give rise to pain upon excessive stretching of the tendon. Of greater interest are the *encapsulated tendon organs* also called *Golgi tendon organs.* These occur near the junction of muscle and tendon. They are smaller than muscle spindles, being only about 1 mm long. They consist of a small fascicle of collagen fibers of the tendon, enclosed in a connective tissue capsule. The myelinated sensory nerve to the organ, on traversing the capsule, gives rise to multiple unmyelinated branches that are insinuated among those collagen fibers of the tendon that pass through the organ. It is believed that when the muscle is relaxed, the spaces between the bundles of collagen fibers of the tendon spread open, slightly reducing pressure on the nerve endings, but during muscle contraction, the collagen bundles under tension draw closer together, compressing the nerve endings. The electrochemical events generated in the axons then results in transmission, to the spinal cord, of information about the degree of tension.

Tendon organs detect changes in muscle tension, whereas spindles detect changes in muscle length. The tendon organs normally have a rather steady rate of impulse transmission to the spinal cord, one that is proportional to the degree of muscle tension. However, if the tension is suddenly increased, an intense response of the tendon organ results in a reflex inhibitory effect on the muscle that presumably prevents the development of potentially destructive excessive tension.

MUSCLE–TENDON JUNCTION

The force generated by contraction of a muscle is transmitted to its insertion through a tendon. The specialized region of attachment at the interface between muscle cells and the bundles of collagen fibrils comprising the tendon is called the *myotendinous junction.* Muscle fibers are bounded by a plasmalemma like that of other cells and it seems unlikely that the delicate lipid bilayer of this membrane alone would be capable of withstanding and transmitting the considerable tension produced by myofibrillar contraction. Indeed, extraction of the myotendinous junction with lipid solvents has been shown to have little effect on tension transmission. Interest in this problem in recent years has focused on the ultrastructure of the ends of muscle fibers and a search for possible transmembrane linkages between the intracellular actin filaments and the extracellular collagen of the tendon.

The three-dimensional configuration of the ends of muscles was difficult to analyze with the light microscope. Now with the aid of scanning and transmission electron microscopy, it has been shown that at the ends of muscle fibers there are very large numbers of anastomosing folds and cylindrical processes that interdigitate with the collagen fiber bundles of the tendon (Figs. 10–38 and 10–39). This local elaboration of the cell surface greatly increases the area of the muscle–tendon interface and its complex geometry ensures that most of the tension generated is applied to

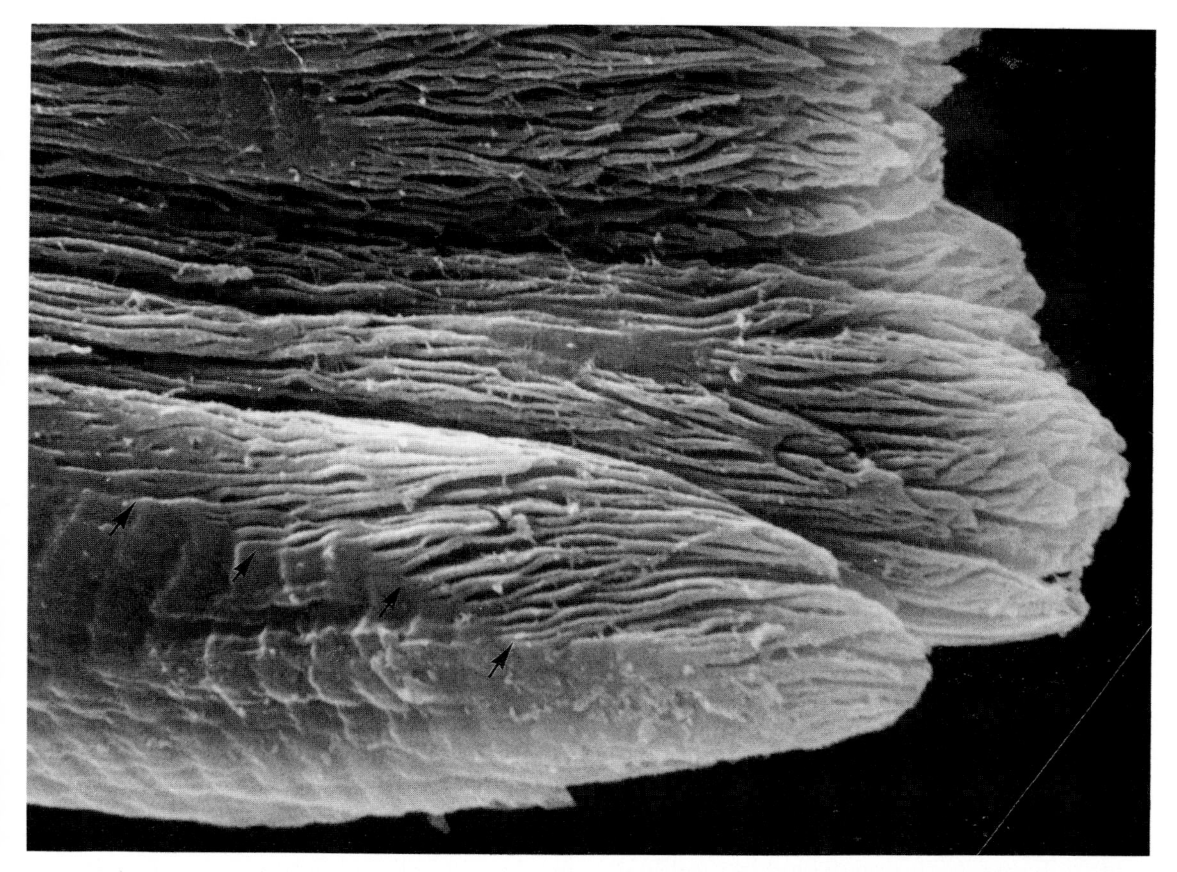

Figure 10–38. Scanning micrograph of a portion of the end of a single muscle fiber after extraction of the tendon collagen. The area of the junctional surface, at the right, is greatly amplified by innumerable branching and anastomosing processes. The transition from the nonjunctional to the junctional portion of the fiber is indicated by arrows. (Micrograph courtesy of Trotter, J. et al. 1985. Anat. Rec. 213:16).

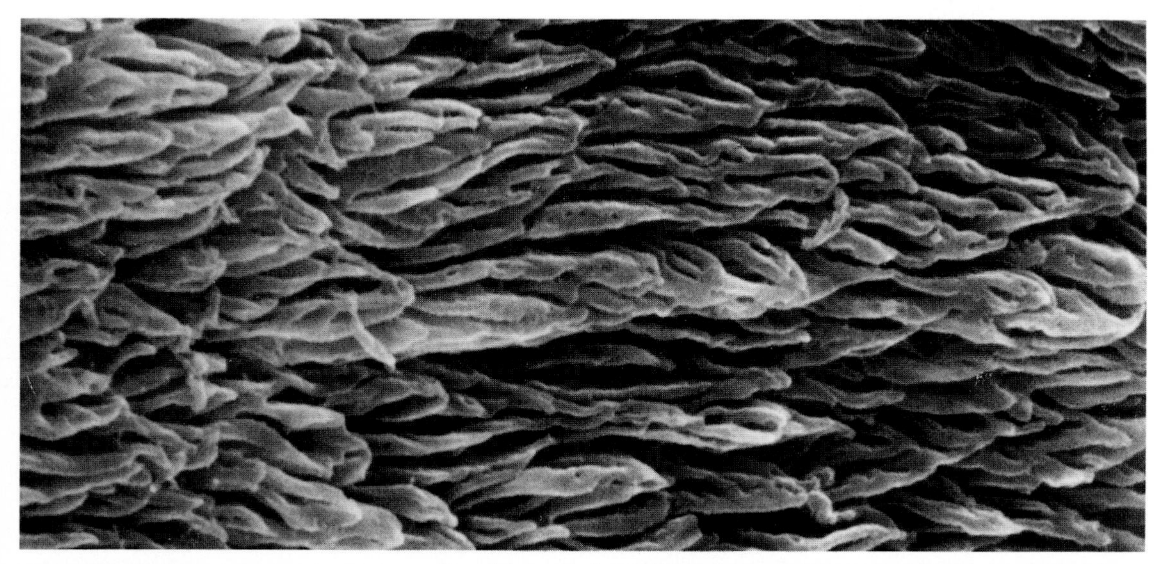

Figure 10–39. Scanning micrograph of a portion of the end of an individual muscle fiber from which the tendon has been removed. The area of sarcolemma across which the force of contraction is transmitted is greatly increased by the very numerous folds and tapering processes. (Micrograph courtesy of Trotter, J. et al. 1987. Anat. Rec. 218:288.)

the membrane of the longitudinally oriented processes as shear stresses. Moreover, the considerable amplification of the area of the membrane across which force is transmitted results in a reduction of stress that is proportional to the ratio between the force-transmitting area of sarcolemma and the total force-generating cross-sectional area of the myofibrils. This ratio varies from 10 : 1 to 14 : 1 in muscles that have been studied.

In transmission electron micrographs of high magnification, the external lamina investing the sarcolemma at the end of the muscle fiber consists of a 20-nm-thick lamina lucida and a 30-nm-thick lamina densa. The lamina lucida is traversed by fine 2–7-nm filaments which appear to cross the membrane and mingle with the meshwork of filaments that form the subsarcolemmal dense layer in which the actin filaments of the myofibrils terminate. It seems likely that these transmembrane thin filaments bind the muscle to the type-IV collagen in the lamina densa and to the type-II collagen bundles of the tendon. The chemical nature of these filaments has not been established. However, *α-actinin, talin,* and *vinculin* have been localized immunocytochemically in this region. Inasmuch as these proteins have been found to bind intracellular filaments to desmosomes and other focal contacts between cells, it is not unreasonable to speculate that they are also involved in attachment of muscle fibers to tendon.

CARDIAC MUSCLE

Unlike skeletal muscle, cardiac muscle consists of separate cellular units about 80 μm in length and 15 μm in diameter. These *cardiac myocytes* are joined end-to-end at junctional specializations called *intercalated discs* (Figs. 10–40 and 10–41). Although the strands so-formed are predominantly parallel, the individual myocytes branch and form oblique interconnections with neighboring strands, resulting in a complex three-dimensional organization that is quite different from the parallel arrangement of discrete cylindrical fibers of skeletal muscle. Prior to the discovery that the intercalated discs are intercellular junctions, the structural units of cardiac muscle were called "fibers," as in skeletal muscle. Although it is questionable whether this term is appropriate for cardiac muscle, it continues to be used in the contemporary literature.

The human heart beats at a rate of 60 to 100 times a minute throughout life. Its contraction is *myogenic,* i.e., it is independent of nervous stimulation. All cardiac myocytes are capable of spontaneous rhythmic depolarization and repolarization of their membrane. However, a group of myocytes in the atrium constitute the *pacemaker* and excitation spreads from there throughout the myocardium via gap junctions between myocytes. Thus, although made up of separate cellular units, cardiac muscle behaves as though it were a syncytium.

HISTOLOGY OF CARDIAC MUSCLE

Under the light microscope, cardiac muscle has a pattern of cross-striations similar to that of skeletal muscle but branching and interconnection of neighboring fibers is evident. The sarcoplasm is more abundant and a longitudinal striation is more apparent owing to the separation of bundles of myofibrils by rows of mitochondria. The myofibrils diverge around a centrally placed nucleus, outlining a fusiform axial region of sarcoplasm rich in organelles and inclusions. A small Golgi complex is located near one pole of each elongate nucleus. Lipid droplets are common in this region and, in older animals, granular deposits of lipochrome pigment may be abundant. In aged humans, such pigment may constitute up to 20% of the dry weight of the myocardium. In smaller animal species, occasional lipid droplets are found throughout the intermyofibrillar sarcoplasm.

A unique feature of cardiac muscle is the occurrence of transverse *intercalated discs* at regular intervals along the length of the fibers. They are relatively inconspicuous in routine preparations but are heavily stained by iron haematoxylin. A disc may extend straight across the fiber, but, more commonly, segments of it are slightly offset longitudinally giving it a step-like configuration in section. In the pattern of cross-striations, the intercalated discs invariable occur at the I-bands.

ULTRASTRUCTURE OF CARDIAC MUSCLE

Under the electron microscope a distinctive feature of cardiac muscle in cross section is the absence of separate myofibrils (Fig. 10–42). It will be recalled that, in similar sections of skeletal muscle, the myofilaments are as-

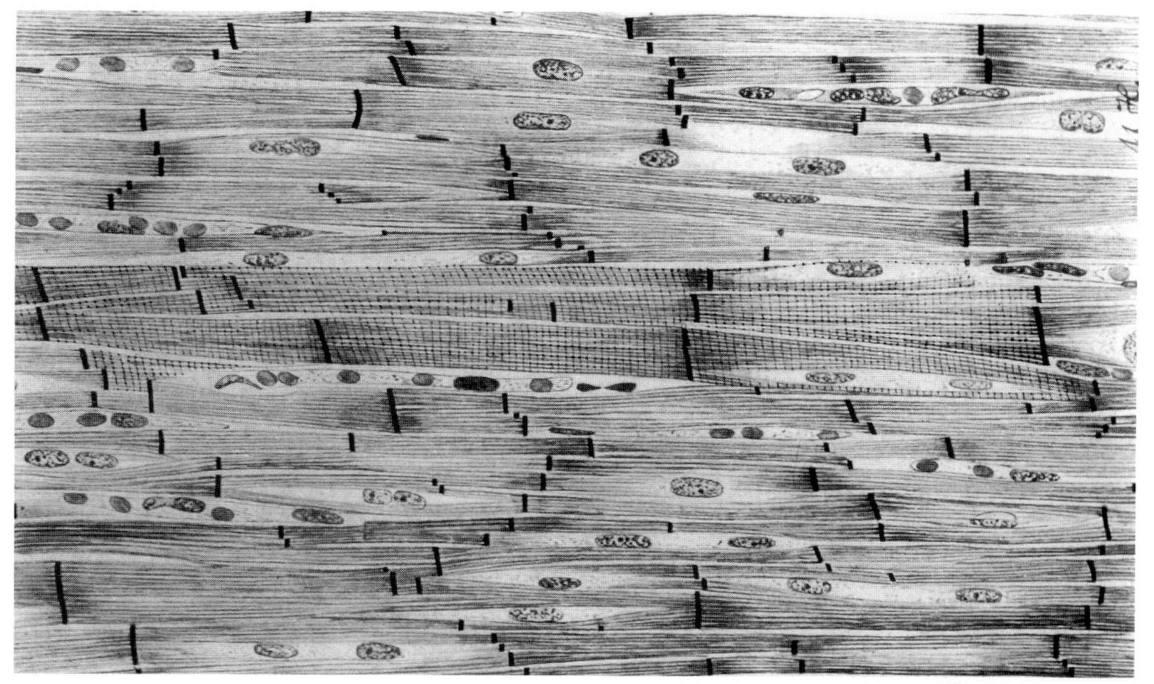

Figure 10–40. Drawing of a histological section of human cardiac muscle that was stained with thiazin red and toluidine blue to show the intercalated discs, a characteristic feature of this type of striated muscle. (From H. Heidenhein. 1901, Anat. Anz. 20,1.)

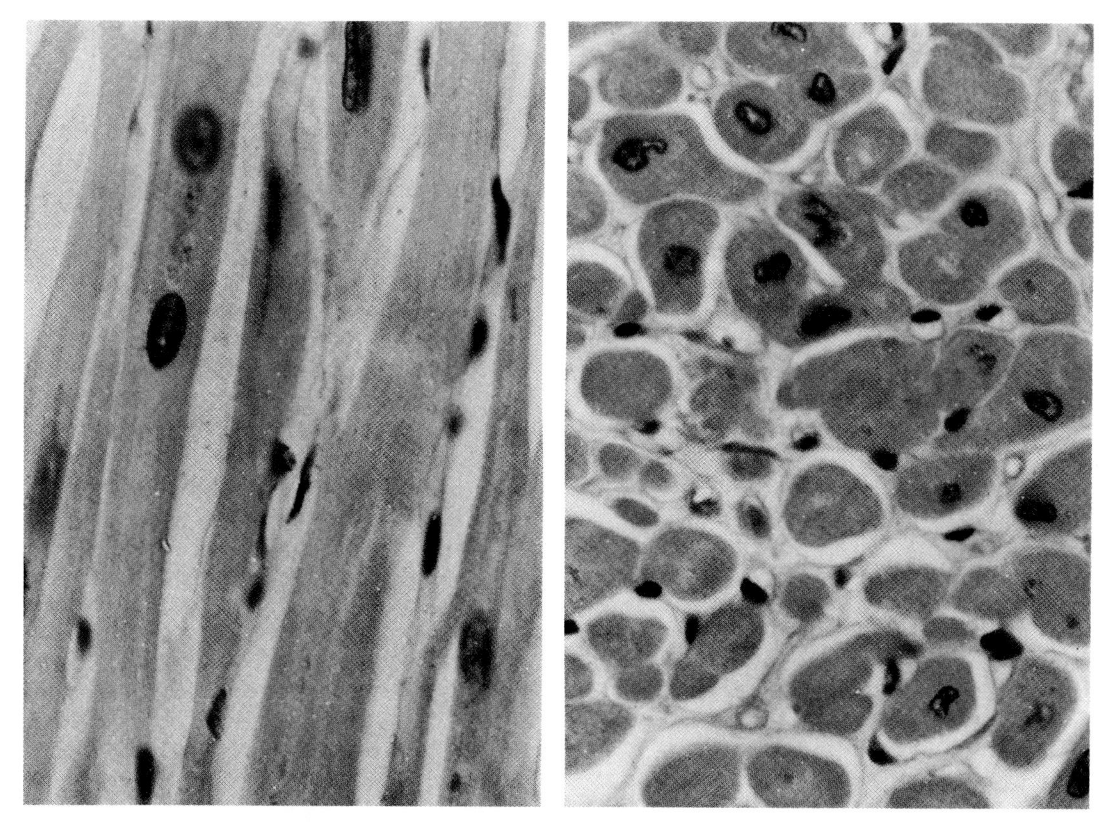

Figure 10–41. Photomicrograph of a longitudinal section of cardiac muscle (left) illustrating the variable diameter of the fibers and the central position of their nuclei. In routinely stained preparations, the intercalated discs are not evident. At the right, a cross section of human cardiac muscle.

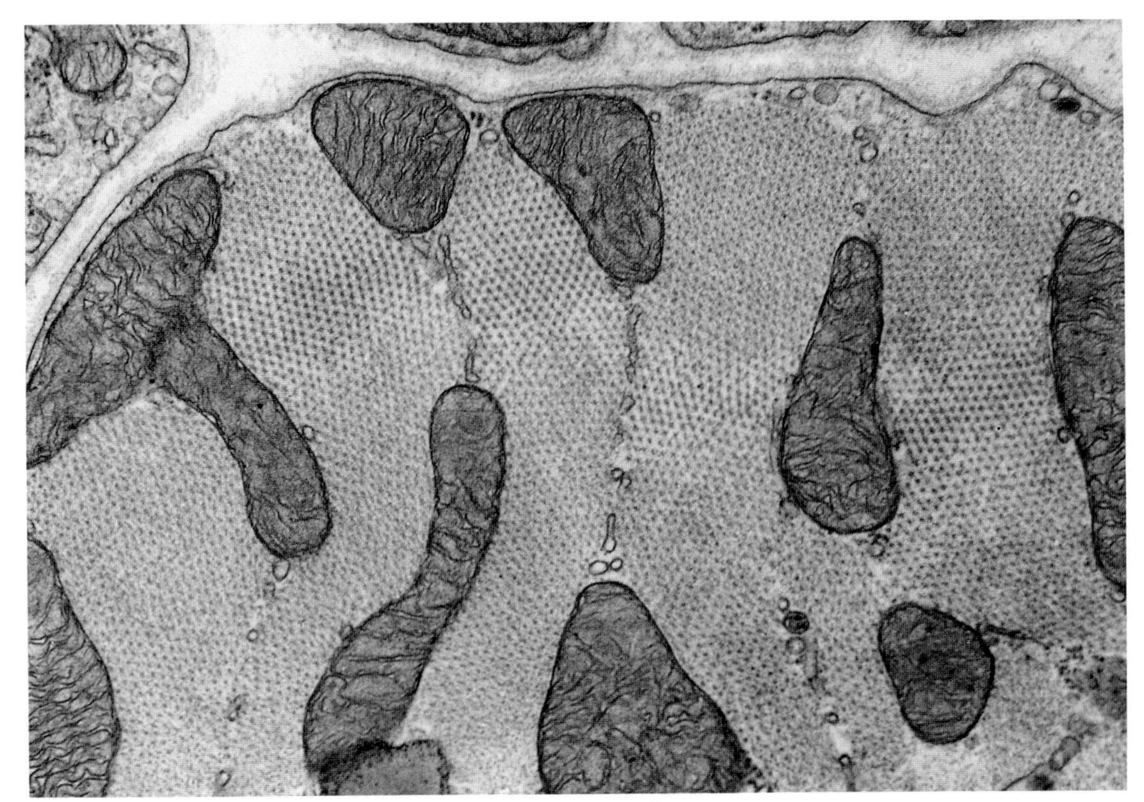

Figure 10–42. Electron micrograph of a small peripheral area of a cardiac muscle cell in cross section. Observe that the myofilaments are not associated in discrete myofibrils with clearly defined limits, as in skeletal muscle, but form a more-or-less continuous mass interrupted by mitochondria and elements of the sarcoplasmic reticulum.

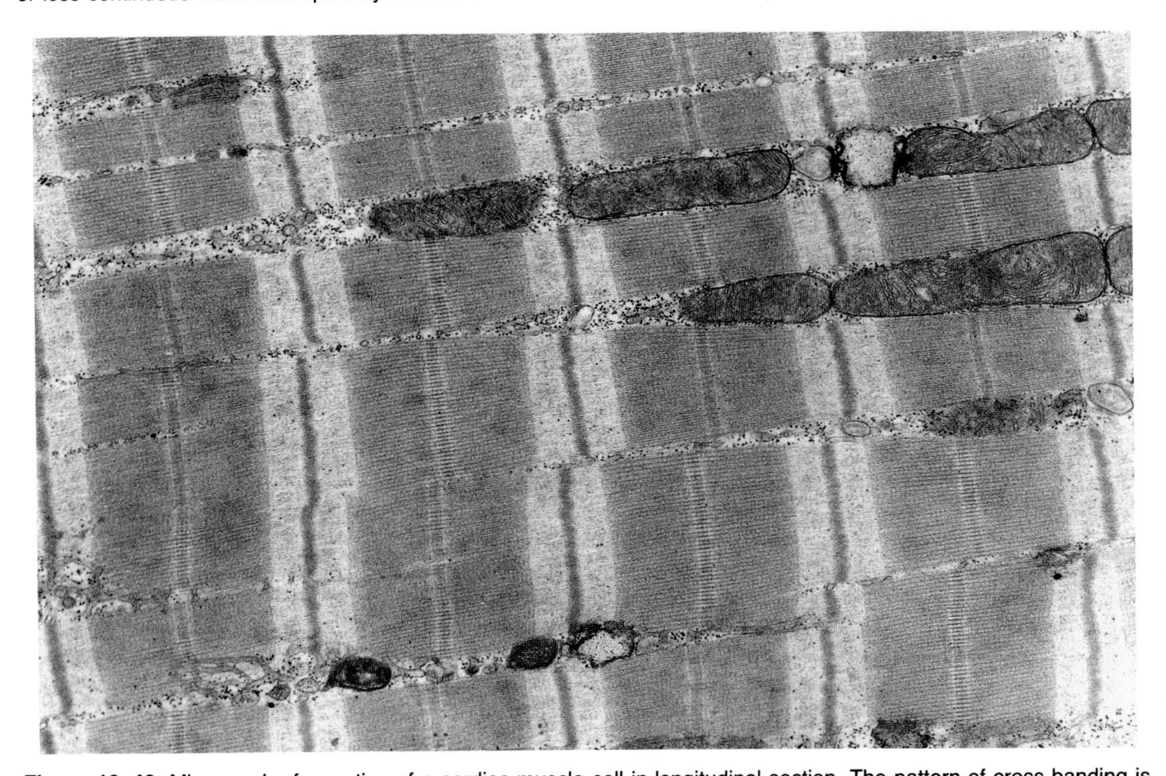

Figure 10–43. Micrograph of a portion of a cardiac muscle cell in longitudinal section. The pattern of cross-banding is similar to that of skeletal muscle. Mitochondria occupy fusiform spaces that may appear to subdivide the mass of myofilaments into myofibril-like units of varying width for short distances.

sembled into discrete myofibrils of uniform diameter, each outlined by a thin layer of sarcoplasm containing longitudinal elements of the sarcoplasmic reticulum and occasional mitochondria. In cardiac muscle, separate myofibrils are not distinguishable. Instead, the cross section of a myocyte is occupied by a continuum of myofilaments, interrupted here and there by mitochondria and profiles of sarcoplasmic reticulum that penetrate into the cylindrical mass of myofilaments from its periphery. In longitudinal sections, these incursions appear as slender fusiform areas of sarcoplasm containing mitochondria and circular profiles of sarcotubules (Fig. 10–43). Locally, these may appear to define the lateral limits of myofibrils of varying width, but this is misleading because they are of limited longitudinal extent and, at their ends, lateral continuity of the mass of myofilaments is again evident. Absence of distinct myofibrils is also reported in certain slow-acting tonic skeletal muscles found mainly in amphibians.

The mitochondria of cardiac muscle have numerous cristae that often show a periodic angulation that gives them a zig–zag form. As a rule, the mitochondria are about the length of a sarcomere (2.5 μm), but they may be as long as 7–8 μm. Glycogen tends to be more abundant in cardiac than in skeletal muscle. It occurs in the form of 30–40-nm dense particles located in the areas of intermyofilament sarcoplasm that contain mitochondria, but particles may also be found aligned in rows between myofilaments (Fig. 10–44). These are more numerous in the I-bands than in the A-bands. Glycogen and lipid are both important energy sources for the contractile activity of the myocardium.

The T-tubules of cardiac muscle differ significantly from those of skeletal muscle. They are located at the level of the Z-discs instead of at the A–I junctions and there is, therefore, only one per sarcomere. They are of greater diameter and penetrate deep into the cell where they communicate with occasional tubules of slightly smaller diameter that course parallel with the long axis of the cell. Thus,

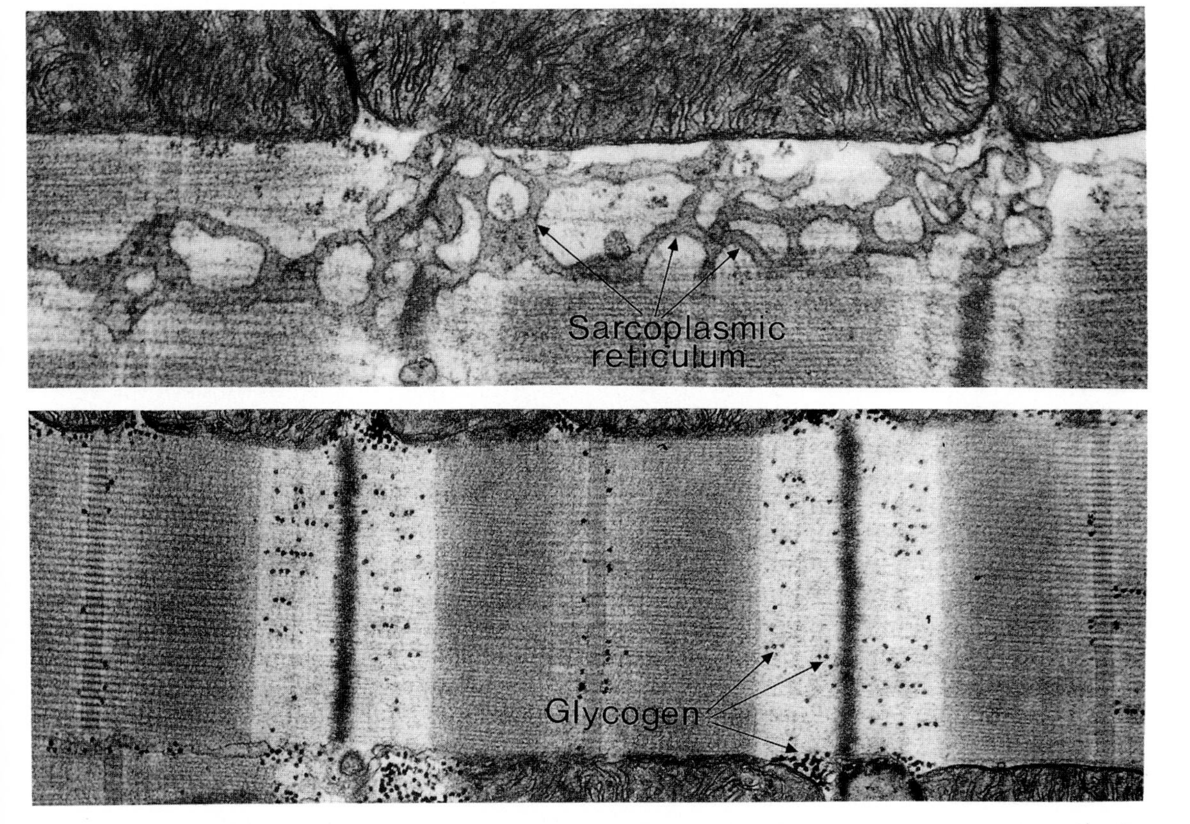

Figure 10–44. (A) Longitudinal section of a small area of cardiac muscle showing a loose network of tubular elements of the sarcoplasmic reticulum. (B) Particles of glycogen are abundant around the mitochondria and may be found between the myofilaments in the I- and H-bands. The muscle in the two figures was fixed in slightly different degrees of relaxation. Note the difference in length of the I-band (indicated by brackets), the A-band is of constant length.

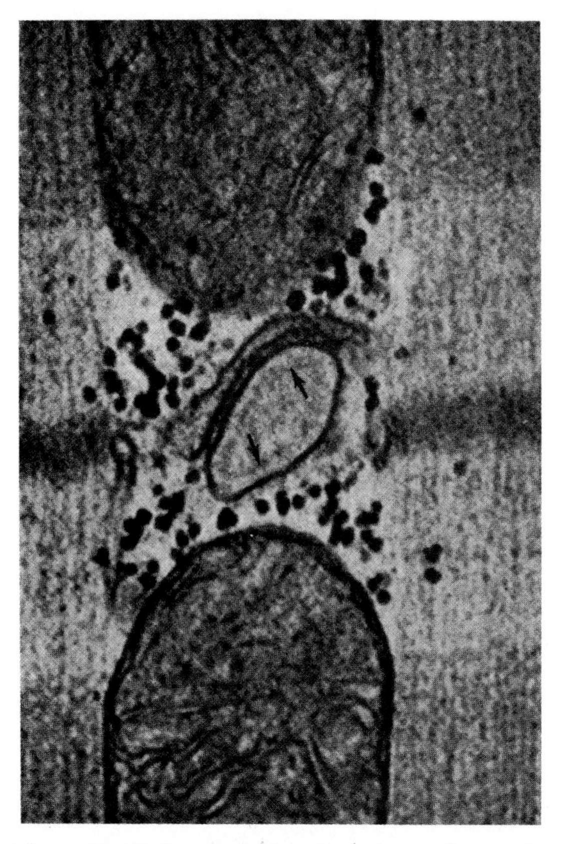

Figure 10–45. Longitudinal section of a small area of a cardiac muscle cell including a cross section of a T-tubule and an adjacent tubule of the sarcoplasmic reticulum. The larger T-tubule is lined with a layer of glycoprotein (at arrows) like that coating the sarcolemma at the surface of the cell. The dense granules in the surrounding sarcoplasm are glycogen.

channels with a lumen that opens to the extracellular space ramify throughout the myocyte. The transverse tubules are lined by a layer continuous with the external lamina of the sarcolemma (Fig. 10–45). This system of branching tubules is called the *transverse-axial-tubular system* (TATS) to distinguish it from the T-system of skeletal muscle.

The longitudinal sarcoplasmic reticulum is less elaborate than that of skeletal muscle. It consists of a subsarcolemmal network of tubules 20–35 nm in diameter that extends into deep clefts within the column of myofilaments. Its pattern varies at different levels in the sarcomere, being close-meshed adjacent to A-bands and more loosely organized at I-bands. Terminal cisternae and triads are not found in cardiac muscle. Their functional counterparts are relatively small flattened saccules that establish junctional contacts with the transverse-axial system of tubules at the level of the Z-discs (Figs. 10–46 and 10–47). The total area of junctional contact of these saccules is considerably less than that of the terminal cisternae with the T-tubules of skeletal muscle. In both, transduction of excitation from the sarcolemma to the reticulum takes place at rows of intramembrane particles called *feet* or *spanning proteins* bridging the gap between the apposed membranes. In addition, there are small saccules or cisternae of the superficial reticulum that are connected directly to the sarcolemma by junctional feet. These are sometimes referred to as the *corbular sarcoplasmic reticulum.* The calcium-binding protein calsequestrin is localized in the junctional saccules and in the corbular reticulum.

As in skeletal muscle, contraction is dependent on free calcium ions in the sarcoplasm. But cardiac muscle, with relatively small saccules in place of terminal cisternae, has more limited intracellular reserves of calcium. During depolarization of the sarcolemma and its invaginations, there is an influx of extracellular calcium. This is followed and supplemented by release of intracellular calcium stored in the reticulum. Calcium from these two sources activates sliding of the filaments and consequent contraction.

The structure of cardiac muscle in the atria and ventricles of the heart is similar, but the atrial myocytes have a smaller average diameter and the transverse-axial tubule system is poorly developed. Such tubules are seen only in the largest of the atrial myocytes. It is possible that in the more slender myocytes there is less need for transverse tubules for inward conduction of excitation. The spread of the action potential is reported to be more rapid in atrial myocytes than in those of the ventricles. The contractile elements are identical in their ultrastructure, but minor differences have been discovered at the molecular level. The heavy chains of myosin molecules occur in two isoforms, α-HMC and β-HMC. In the atrium, α-HMC is more abundant, whereas in the ventricle, β-HMC is the predominant isoform. Myocytes in the sinoatrial and atrioventricular nodes (vide infra) show specific immunoreactivity for a third isoform. The significance of these regional differences in the myosin molecules remains obscure.

THE INTERCALATED DISC

At the intercalated discs, the conjoined myocytes have a highly irregular surface with

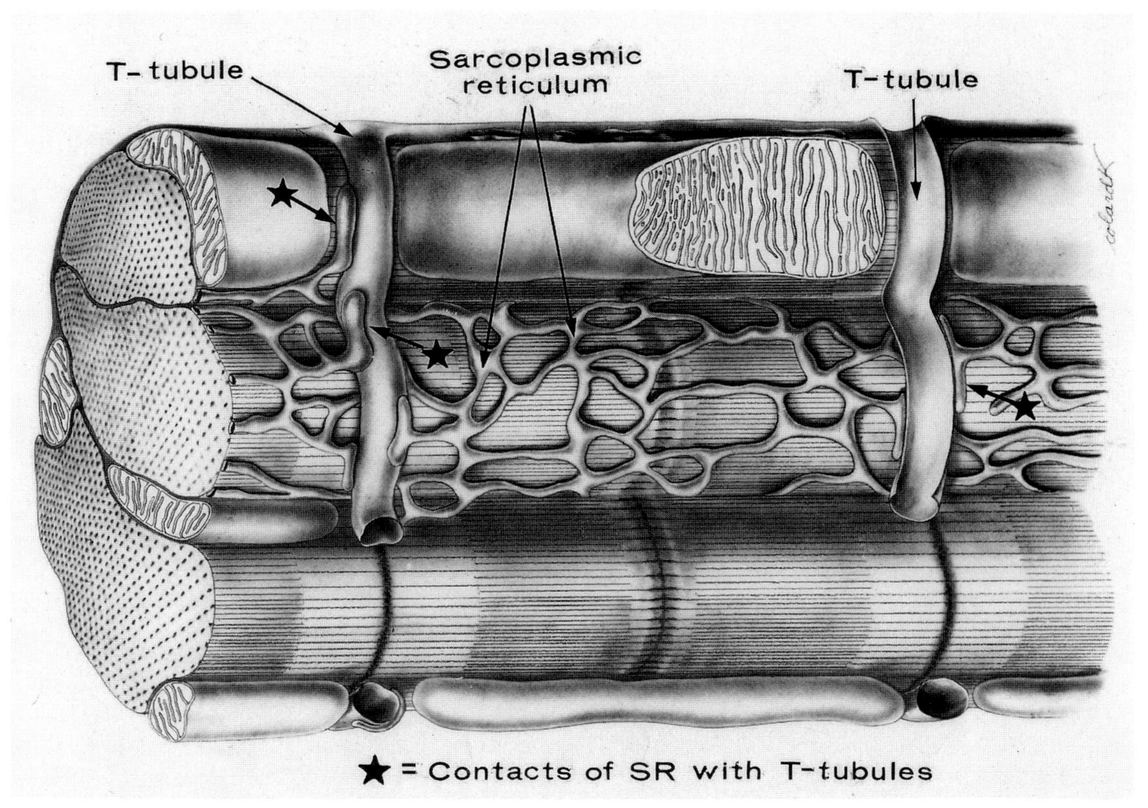

Figure 10–46. Schematic drawing of the disposition of the T-system and sarcoplasmic reticulum of cardiac muscle. The transverse tubules are much larger than those of skeletal muscle. The relatively simple reticulum has no terminal cisternae and, therefore, there are no triads. Instead, small expansions of some of its tubules end in close apposition to the sarcolemma, either at the surface of the fiber or at its inward extension in the T-tubules. (From Fawcett, D.W. and N.S. McNutt. 1969. J. Cell Biol. 42:1.)

multiple ridges and papillary projections on the end of one cell fitting into complementary grooves and pits on the other (Fig. 10–48). On this interface, one can distinguish areas identical to desmosomes, other areas that appear to be gap junctions, and large areas that resemble the zonula adherens of epithelia. In this mosaic of junctional specializations, only the desmosomes are typical in respect to their shape. The areas having a fine structure resembling that of zonulae adherentes are not circumferential, as the term zonula implies, but are more-or-less continuous areas of specialization extending over much of the contact surface of the cells. The term *fascia adherens* has been suggested as a more appropriate designation for this component of the intercalated disc. In longitudinal thin sections, the opposing cell membranes can be identified as two parallel dense lines that follow a sinuous course, separated by a 15–20-nm intercellular cleft (Fig. 10–49). The myofilaments of the conjoined cells terminate in a very dense layer of sarcoplasm of varying width on the inner aspects of the apposed membranes. A high concentration of the actin-binding proteins *α-actinin* and *vinculin* can be demonstrated in this dense layer. These proteins are often found in other cell types at sites of anchorage of actin or intermediate filaments to the membrane. In the intercalated disc, they evidently serve to bind the ends of the myofilaments to the sarcolemma. The 83 kD polypeptide, *plakoglobin,* and another adhesive glycoprotein (A-CAM) are localized in the narrow cleft between the membranes.

The fascia adherens, comprising the greater part of the disc, is interrupted in certain areas by typical desmosomes. The myofilaments diverge at these sites and do not terminate in the dense plaque of the desmosomes, but intermediate filaments of the cytoskeleton may attach there. In other small areas in the transverse portion of the intercalated disc, the opposing membranes come into close contact to form small gap junctions.

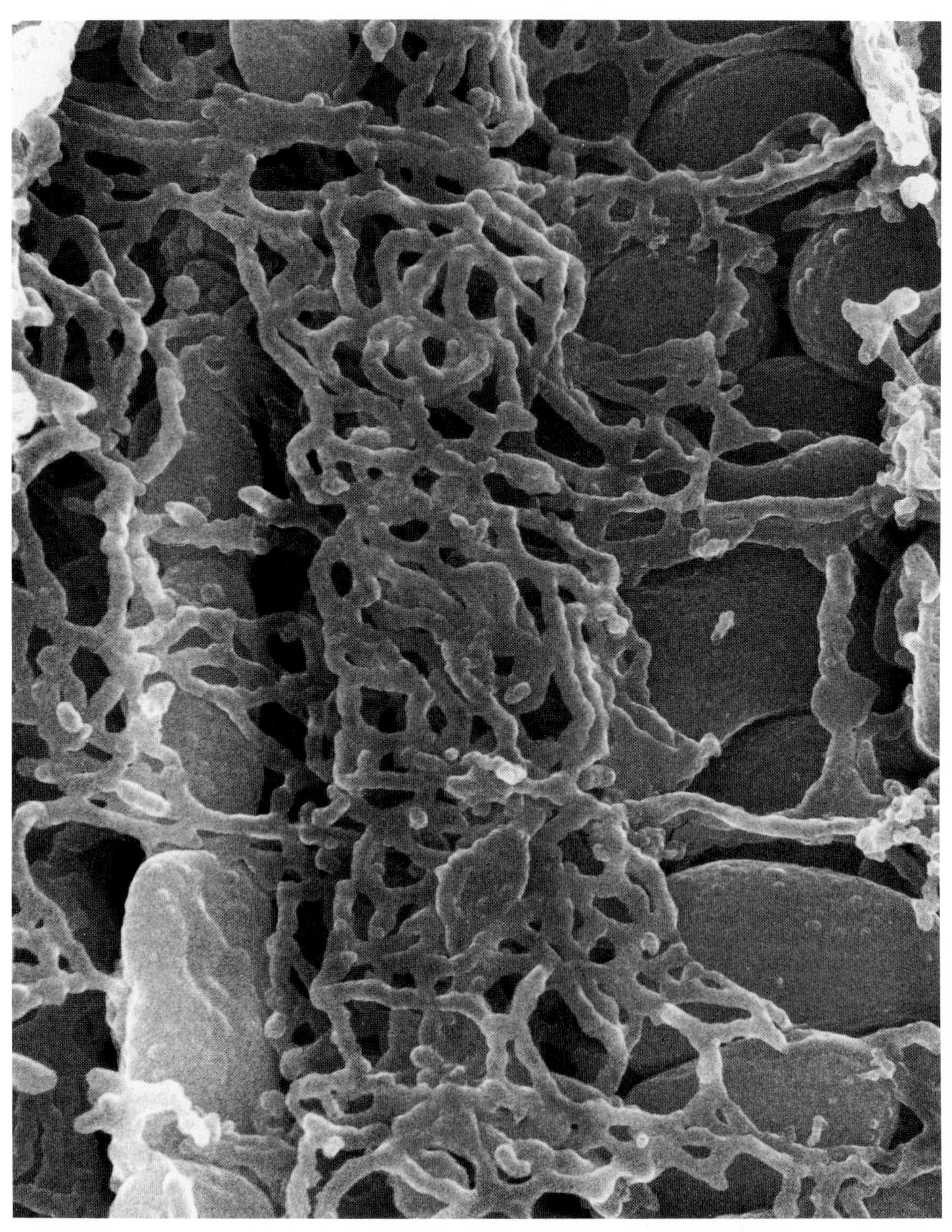

Figure 10–47. Scanning micrograph of the sarcoplasmic reticulum of rat cardiac muscle, showing a dense network of tubules associated with the A- and I-bands of a myofibril. Transverse tubules are also identifiable at the level of the Z-discs. The round profiles between myofibrils are mitochondria. (Micrograph courtesy of Ogata, T. and Y. Yamasaka. 1990. Anat. Rec. 228:227.)

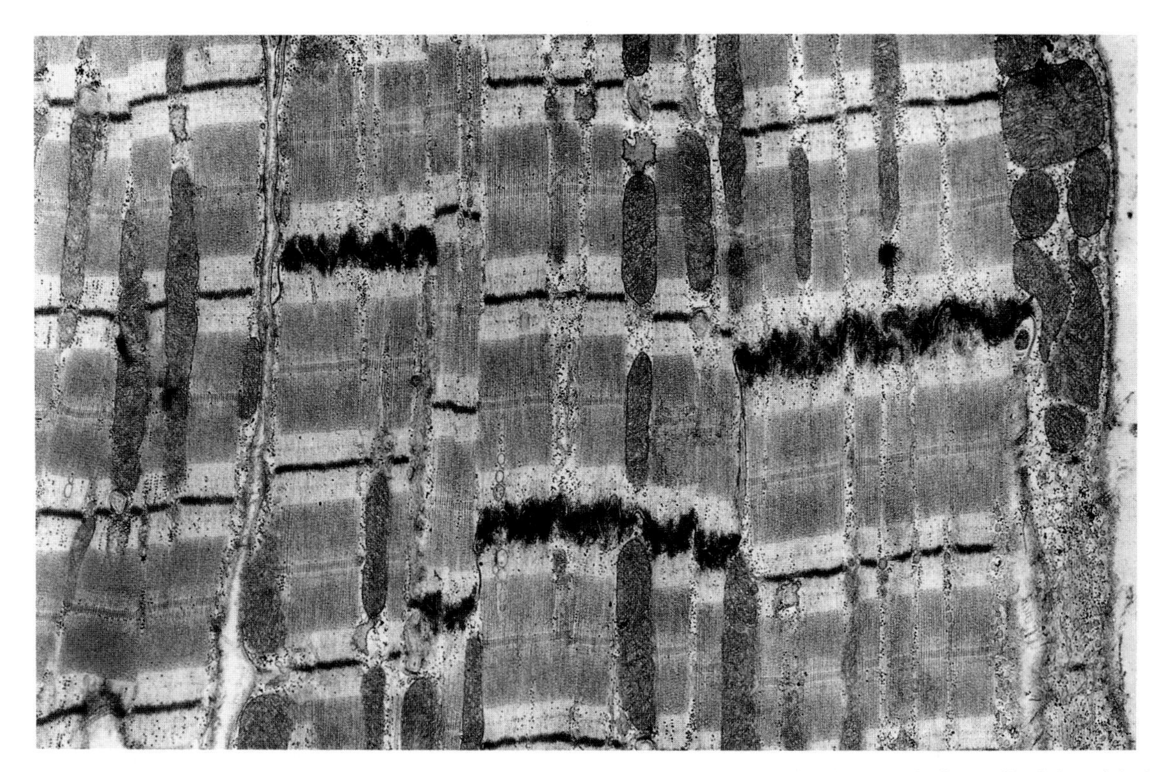

Figure 10–48. A low-power micrograph of cardiac muscle in longitudinal section showing a typical step-like intercalated disc. The transverse portions are highly interdigitated and there is an abundance of dense material at the attachment of the myofilaments to the end of the cell. The longitudinal segments of the disc are smooth, devoid of dense material, and difficult to see at this magnification.

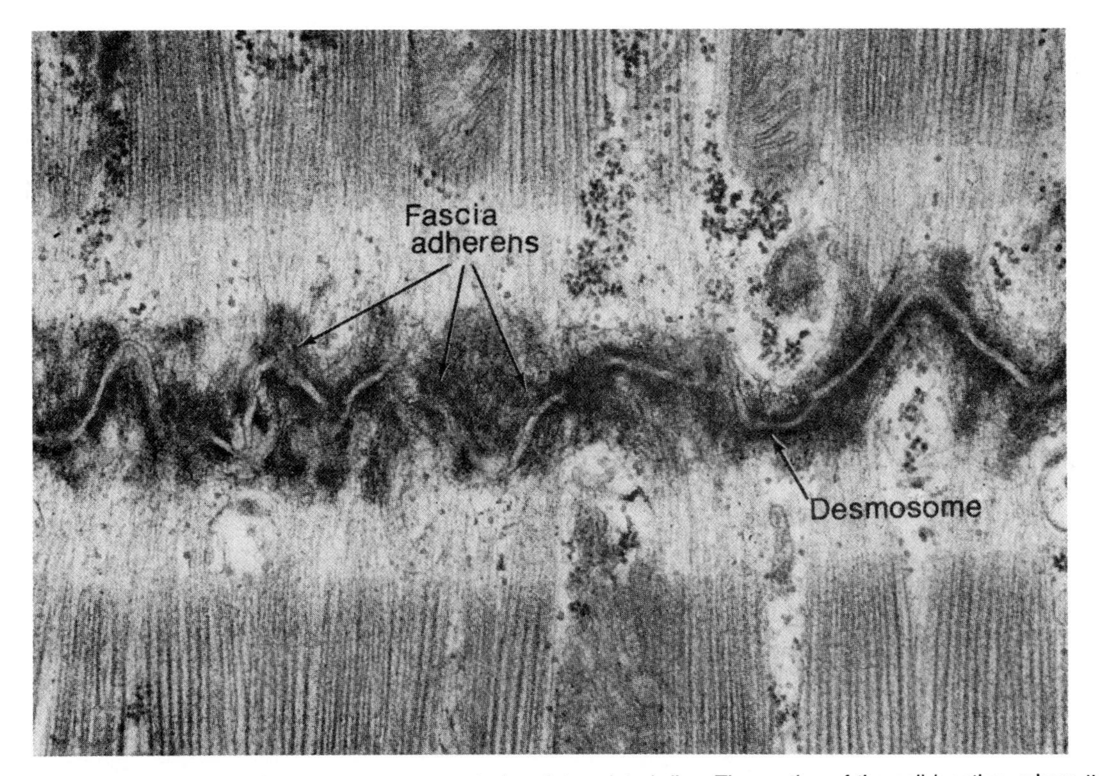

Figure 10–49. Micrograph of a transverse segment of an intercalated disc. The portion of the cell junction, where the myofilaments terminate, resembles the zonula adherens of epithelia but is here called the fascia adherens. Between sites of myofilament attachment are typical desmosomes. (From Fawcett, D.W. and N.S. McNutt. 1969. J. Cell Biol. 42:1.)

More extensive junctions of this kind are found on the longitudinal segments of the step-like intercalated discs. These are of great physiological importance because diffusion of ions through the pores in such junctions permits coordination of the activities of the myocytes. Measurements of current across intercalated discs, in atrial and ventricular muscle, have shown that all parts of the heart are electrically coupled. Thus, although made up of separate cells, cardiac muscle behaves physiologically as though it were a syncytium. The very firm attachment of myocytes at the intercalated discs ensures transmission of the traction generated by the individual cells throughout the myocardium.

MYOCARDIAL ENDOCRINE CELLS

The functions of the cells in the myocardium were formerly believed to be limited to contraction or excitation and conduction, but in the past two decades, morphological and biochemical studies have identified myocytes in the atrium that synthesize and secrete peptide hormones involved in the regulation of blood volume and the electrolyte composition of the extracellular fluid.

The *myoendocrine cells* are specialized myocytes localized mainly in the right and left atrial appendages, but they are also found scattered within other areas of the atria and along the conductive system in the ventricular septum. They resemble the working myocytes in having longitudinally oriented myofilaments that diverge around a centrally placed nucleus and insert into intercalated discs at either end of the cell. The numerous mitochondria and the sarcoplasmic reticulum do not differ significantly from those of nonendocrine myocytes. The Golgi complex is commonly located at one pole of the nucleus but may be paranuclear and, rarely, isolated dictyosomes may be found near the sarcolemma.

The most conspicuous feature distinguishing myoendocrine cells from other atrial myocytes is the presence of membrane-bounded dense secretory granules 0.3–0.4 μm in diameter (Fig. 10–50). These are concentrated in the core of sarcoplasm that extends in either direction from the poles of the nucleus, but

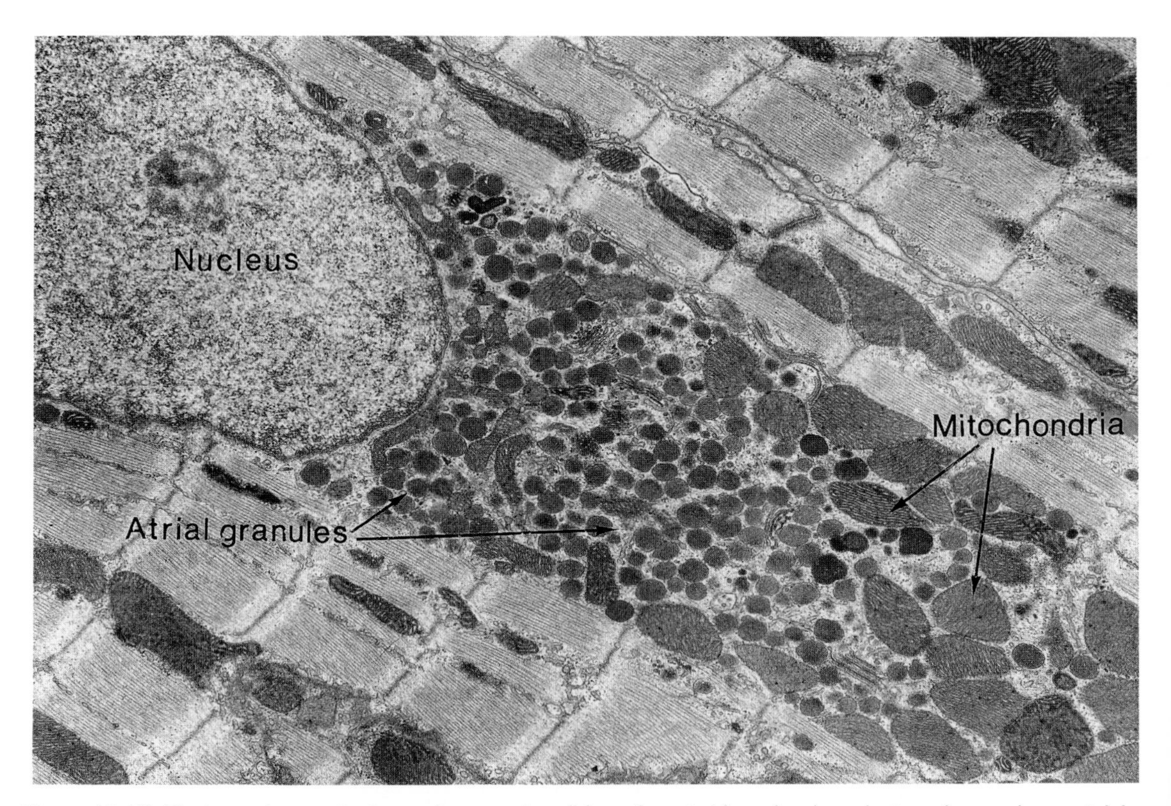

Figure 10–50. Electron micrograph of a cardiac muscle cell from the rat atrium showing a juxtanuclear region containing mitochondria and numerous spherical secretory granules. These granules contain the precursor of the peptide hormone, cardiodilatin, also called atrial natriuretic factor. (Micrograph courtesy of J. Hansen.)

they can also be found among the myofilaments and occasionally near the sarcolemma. The granules contain the precursor of a family of biologically active polypeptides collectively called *cardiodilatins* (CDD) or *atrial natriuretic polypeptides* (ANP).

As in other peptide–hormone-secreting cells, the product is synthesized as a large precursor molecule and reduced to the active form by an endopeptidase. The prohormone, a polypeptide of 126 amino acids (CDD 1–126) is cleaved during or immediately after exocytosis to peptides of lower molecular weight, including a peptide of 28 amino acids (CDD 99–126) which is the only product that circulates in the blood.

The hormone causes vasodilatation, lowering of blood pressure and decreased blood volume. Some of its effects are mediated by its inhibition of arginine–vasopressin secretion by the posterior pituitary and of aldosterone production by the adrenal cortex. It causes constriction of the efferent arteriole of the renal glomeruli resulting in diuresis and increased excretion of sodium. It is the most potent endogenous natriuretic agent discovered to date. Injection of an extract of cardiac atria into an experimental animal may result in a 30-fold increase in sodium excretion. The regulation of fluid balance in the central nervous system is regulated by the epithelium of the choroid plexus that secretes the cerebrospinal fluid; by the arachnoid villi of the dural sinuses that are the outflow system for this fluid, and by the cerebral capillary endothelium that constitutes the blood-brain barrier. All of these structures have been shown to possess receptors for atriopeptides. It is likely, therefore, that the atriopeptides also have a role in maintenance of fluid balance in the brain.

CONDUCTION SYSTEM OF THE HEART

The heart does not contract synchronously throughout the myocardium. To function effectively as a pump, the contraction of the atria must be completed slightly before the onset of ventricular contraction. The precise timing and coordination of events in the cardiac cycle depends on myocytes that are specialized for initiation of excitation and its conduction to different regions of the myocardium at a rate that will ensure their activation in the correct sequence. These specialized myocytes are located in the *sinoatrial node,* at the junction of the superior vena cava with the right atrium; in the *atrioventricular node* situated in the lower part of the interatrial septum; in *internodal tracts* connecting the sinoatrial and atrioventricular nodes; and in the *atrioventricular bundle* (bundle of His) which originates in the atrioventricular node and enters the fibrous portion of the interventricular septum where it divides into *right* and *left bundle branches* that ramify beneath the endocardium of the right and left ventricles, establishing communicating junctions with the unspecialized working myocytes.

All myocytes are autonomously excitable cells that undergo rhythmic depolarization and repolarization independent of nervous influences, but the inherent rate of this activity in myocytes of the atria is greater than that of the ventricles. The rhythm of cells of the sinoatrial node is still more rapid and their depolarization, propagated over tracts of myocytes specialized for conduction, overrides the slower rhythm of the working myocardium. The sinoatrial node is, therefore, the site of initiation of excitation and the "pacemaker" of the heart.

The sinoatrial node is 10 to 20 mm long, 3 mm wide, and about 1 mm in thickness. It is made up of pale-staining branched cells enmeshed in a framework of collagen. These *nodal myocytes* contain relatively few myofilaments, aggregated into inconsistently oriented myofibrils of varying diameter in sarcoplasm rich in mitochondria. They are joined to like cells and to other myocytes by conspicuous gap junctions. The nature of the cellular constituents of the internodal tracts is disputed. They are identified by some as *transitional myocytes* and are described as being more slender than ordinary atrial myocytes and having more myofibrils than nodal myocytes. Little is known about their conduction velocity. Interposed between the nodal myocytes and the rapidly conducting distal portions of the conduction system, it is speculated that they may be relatively slow and, thus, contribute to the atrioventricular delay essential for optimal filling of the ventricles. Transitional myocytes are also the principal cellular elements of the atrioventricular node which contains a relatively small population of nodal myocytes in its center. At its periphery, there are many *Purkinje myocytes.* These uninucleate cylindrical cells, associated end-to-end in long rows, continue from the node into the atrioventricular bundle. The long strands or tracts that they form were traditionally called "Pur-

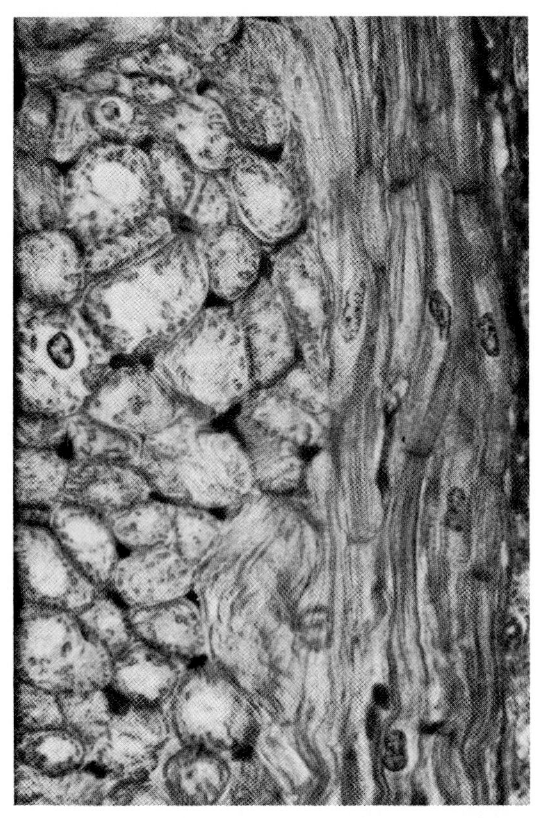

Figure 10–51. Photomicrograph of the specialized conduction tissue of the human atrioventricular bundle. The large Purkinje fibers seen in cross section, at the left of the figure, can be compared with the smaller unspecialized heart muscle cut longitudinally at the right.

kinje fibers" before their multicellular nature was revealed by the electron microscope. Purkinje myocytes are relatively short (~50 μm) compared to ordinary myocytes (~80 μm) but are nearly twice their diameter (30 μm)(Figs. 10–51 and 10–52). In cross section, they are often quite irregular in outline with one cell partially surrounding another or extending large processes into conforming concavities in the neighboring cell (Figs. 10–53 and 10–54). Their irregular shape increases the area of cell-to-cell contact. Intercalated discs are not found but there are large gap junctions both at the ends and sides of the cells. Their ultrastructure and membrane properties favor rapid impulse conduction. In the "Purkinje fibers" of the bovine heart, which are exceptionally large and have been well studied, the conduction velocity is said to be 2–3 m/s compared to 0.6 m/s in the unspecialized myocardium.

The atrioventricular bundle contains an admixture of cellular elements. Transitional myocytes extend from the node into its initial portion, but more distally, Purkinje myocytes predominate. The common bundle and its right and left bundle branches are ensheathed by a layer of connective tissue that appears to insulate the conducting tissue from the surrounding cardiac muscle, but where the conduction system terminates in profuse subendocardial plexuses, functional contacts between Purkinje cells and the ventricular myocardium are common.

Lesions of the conduction system may cause asynchrony in the beating of the ventricles or disorders in the timing of atrial and ventricular contraction that result in impaired efficiency of the heart.

INNERVATION OF THE MYOCARDIUM

Although the initiation of each heartbeat is myogenic, the heart is innervated and its rate is modulated by the autonomic nervous system. Parasympathetic nerve fibers from the vagus and fibers from the sympathetic trunk form extensive plexuses at the base of the heart. Ganglion cells and numerous nerve axons are found in the wall of the right atrium, especially in the regions of the sinoatrial and atrioventricular nodes. The heart rate is slowed by stimulation of the vagus and accelerated by sympathetic nerve stimulation. The autonomic nervous system acts on the myocardium indirectly by modifying the inherent rhythm of the pacemaker.

Light and electron microscopic observations confirm the presence of many unmyelinated axons among the specialized myocytes of the nodes and conduction pathways (Fig. 10–53). The nerves do not form specialized endings comparable to the myoneural junctions of skeletal muscle but merely pass close to the specialized myocytes. They are identifiable as functional endings only by the presence of local aggregations of small vesicles identical to those found in synapses elsewhere in the body. Dense-cored vesicles, found in some of these axons, identify them as sympathetic nerve endings. Similar endings occasionally observed in close relation to ordinary working myocytes suggest that there may also be a direct action of the nerves on the myocardium, but this has yet to be convincingly established in physiological studies.

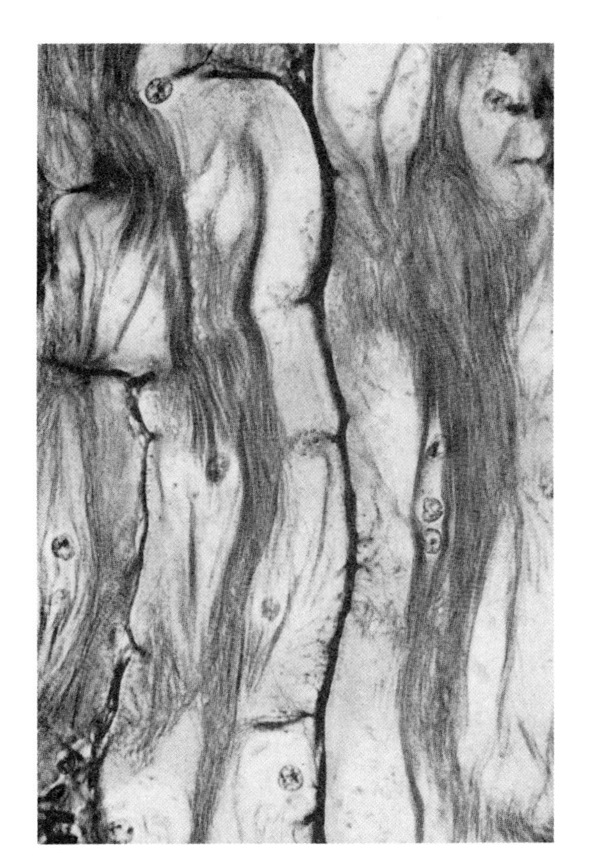

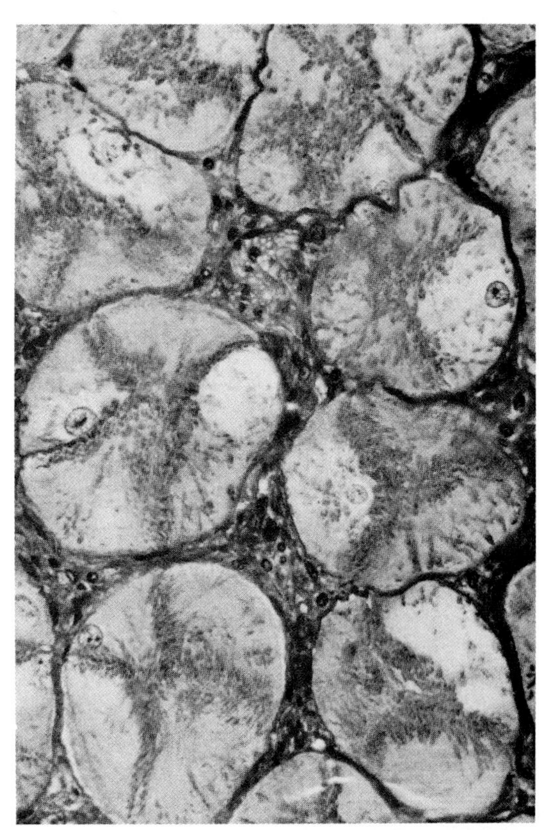

Figure 10–52. Photomicrographs of the very large Purkinje fibers in the moderator band of the bovine heart. In the figure at the left, the fibers are cut longitudinally and in the figure at the right they are cut transversely. In both, it is evident that the myofilaments occupy only a small part of the sarcoplasm. The large clear areas are rich in glycogen, not stained here.

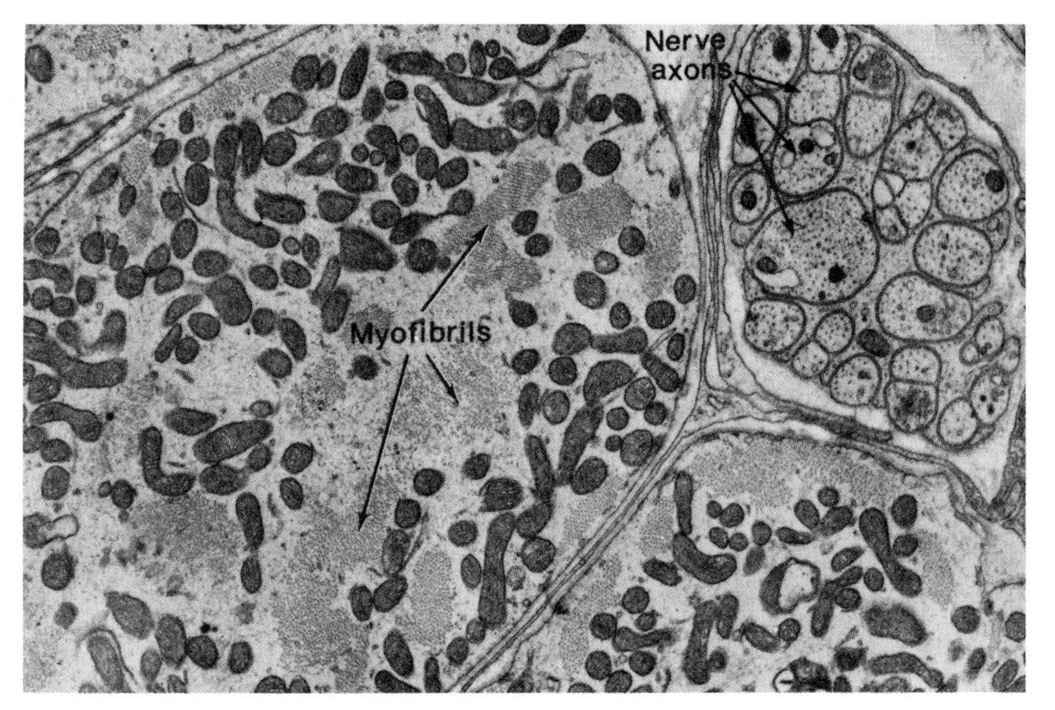

Figure 10–53. Micrograph of portions of two adjacent Purkinje fibers and an accompanying nerve from the atrioventricular bundle of the cat heart. Mitochondria are abundant and myofilaments occur only in scattered bundles.

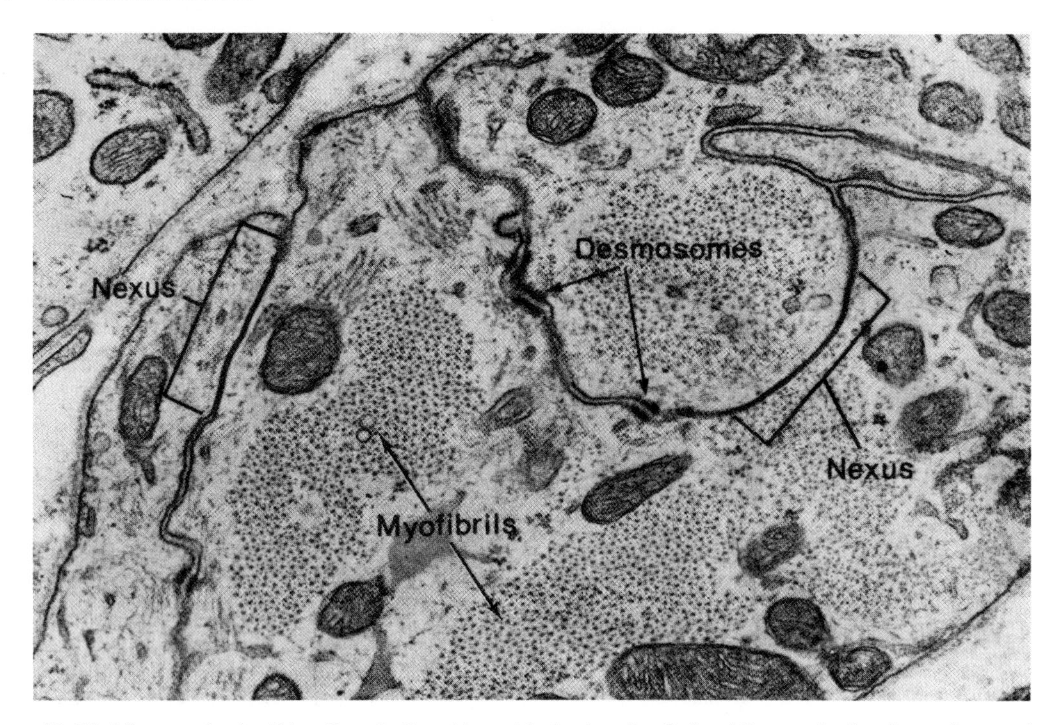

Figure 10–54. Micrograph of cell junctions in the atrioventricular bundle. Cells of the conduction tissue have extensive areas of cell-to-cell apposition forming large gap junctions or nexuses.

BIBLIOGRAPHY

SMOOTH MUSCLE

Bagby, R. 1986. Toward a comprehensive three-dimensional model of the contractile system of vertebrate smooth muscle cells. Internat. Rev. Cytol. 105:67.

Bond, M. and A.V. Somlyo. 1982. Dense bodies and actin polarity in vertebrate smooth muscle cells. J. Cell Biol. 95:403.

Cooke, P. 1976. A filamentous cytoskeleton in vertebrae smooth muscle fibers. J. Ce. . Biol. 68:539.

Devine, C.E., A.V. Somlyo, and A.P. Somlyo. 1972. Sarcoplasmic reticulum and excitation–contraction coupling in mammalian smooth muscle. J. Cell Biol. 52:690.

Devine, C.E. and A.P. Somlyo. 1971. Thick filaments in vascular smooth muscle. J. Cell. Biol. 49:636.

Dewey, M.M. and L. Barr. 1962. Intercellular connection between smooth muscle cells: the nexus. Science 137:670.

Draeger, A., W.B. Amos, M. Ikebe, and J.V. Small. 1990. The cytoskeleton and contractile apparatus of smooth muscle. J. Cell Biol. 111:2463.

Fay, F.S., K. Fujiwara, D.D. Rees, and K.E. Fogarty. 1983. Distribution of alpha actinin in single isolated smooth muscle cells. J. Cell Biol. 96:783.

Gabella, G. and D. Blundell. 1979. Nexuses between smooth muscle cells of guinea pig ileum. J. Cell Biol. 82:239.

Jones, P.A., T. Scott-Burden, and W. Gevers. 1979. Glycoprotein, elastin and collagen secretion by rat smooth muscle cells. Proc. Nat. Acad. Sci. USA 76:353.

Murphy, R.A. 1979. Filament organization and contractile function in vertebrate smooth muscle. Am. Rev. Physiol. 41:737.

Nonomura, Y. and S. Ebashi. 1980. Calcium regulatory mechanismin vertebrate smooth muscle. Biomed. Res. 1:1.

Rhodin, J.A.G. 1962. Fine structure of vascular walls in mammals with special reference to smooth muscle component. Physiol. Rev. 42:49.

Ross, R. and S.J. Klebanoff. 1971. The smooth muscle cell I. In vivo synthesis of connective tissue proteins. J. Cell Biol. 50:172.

Somlyo, A.P. 1985. Excitation–contraction coupling and the ultrastructure of smooth muscle. Circulat. Res. 57:497.

Small, J.V. 1977. Studies on isolated smooth muscle cells: The contractile apparatus. J. Cell Sci. 24:317.

Small, J.V., M. Herzog, M. Barth, and A. Draeger. 1990. Supercontracted state of vertebrate smooth muscle fragments reveals myofilament lengths. J. Cell Biol. 111:2541.

Small, J.V. 1985. Geometry of actin-membrane attachments in the smooth muscle cell: localization of vinculin and alpha actinin. EMBO J. 4:45.

Stromer, M.H. and M. Bendayan. 1988. Arrangement of desmin intermediate filaments in smooth muscle cells as shown by high-resolution immunocytochemistry. Cell Motil. Cytoskel. 11:117.

Warsaw, D.M., J.M. Derosiers et al. 1990. Smooth muscle myosin cross-bridge interactions modulate actin filament sliding velocity in vitro. J. Cell Biol. 11:453.

SKELETAL MUSCLE

Allbrook, D. 1981. Skeletal muscle regeneration. Muscle Nerve 4:234.

Block, B.B., T. Imagawa, K.P. Campbell, and C. Franzini-Armstrong. 1988. Structural evidence for direct interaction between molecular components of the transverse tubule-sarcoplasmic reticulum junction in skeletal muscle. J. Cell Biol. 107:2587.

Burke, R.E. 1981. Motor units: anatomy, physiology and functional organization. *In* Handbook of Physiology, The Nervous System II. pp. 345–352. American Physiology Society, Bethesda, MD.

Caswell, A.H. and J.P. Brunschweig. 1984. Identification and extraction of proteins that compose the triad junction of skeletal muscle. J. Cell Biol. 99:929.

Cooper, S. and P.M. Daniel. 1963. Muscle spindles in man: their morphology in lumbricals and the deep muscles of the neck. Brain 86:563.

Ebashi, S. 1974. Regulatory mechanism of muscle contraction with special reference to the Ca-troponin-tropomyosin system. Essays Biochem. 10:1.

Ferguson, D.G., H.W. Schwartz, and C. Franzini-Armstrong. 1984. Subunit structure of junctional feet in triads of skeletal muscle: a freeze-drying rotary-shadowing study. J. Cell Biol. 99:1735.

Franzini-Armstron, C. and L.D. Peachey, 1981. Striated muscle: contractile and control mechanisms. J. Cell Biol. 88:166.

Fanatsu, K., H. Higuchi, and S. Tshiwata. 1990. Elastic filaments of skeletal muscle revealed by selective removal of thin filaments with plasma gelsolin. J. Cell Biol. 110:53.

Gautier, G.F. 1971. The structural and cytochemical heterogeneity of mammalian skeletal muscle fibers. *In* R.J. Podolsky, ed. Contractility of Muscle Cells and Related Processes. New York, Prentice-Hall.

Hanson, J. and L. Lowy. 1964. The structure of actin filaments and the origin of the axial periodicity in the I-substance of vertebrate skeletal muscle. Proc. Roy. Soc. London B 160:449.

Hanson, J. and L. Lowy. 1965. Molecular basis of contractility in muscle. Br. Med. Bull. 21:264.

Horowitz, R., E.S. Kempner, M.E. Bisher, and R.J. Podolsky. 1986. A physiological role for titin and nebulin in skeletal muscle. Nature 323:160.

Huxley, H.E. 1964. Evidence for continuity between the central elements of the triads and extracellular space in frog sartorius muscle. Nature 202:1067.

Huxley, H.E. 1969. The mechanism of muscle contraction. Science 164:1356.

Jorgenssen, A.O., A.C. Shen, K.P. Campbell, and D.H. MacLennon. 1983. Ultrastructural localization of calsequestrin in rat skeletal muscle by immunoferritin labelling of ultrathin frozen sections. J. Cell Biol. 97:1573.

Kawamoto, R.M., J.P. Brunschweig, K.C. Kim, and A.H. Caswell. 1986. Isolation, characterization, and localization of the spanning protein of skeletal muscle triads. J. Cell Biol. 103:1405.

Kelly, D.E. and M.A. Cahill. 1972. Filamentous and matrix components of skeletal muscle Z-discs. Anat. Rec. 172:623.

Merrillees, N.C.R. 1960. The fine structure of muscle spindles in the lumbrical muscles of the rat. J. Biophys. Biochem. Cytol. 7:725.

MacLennon, D.H. and P.T.S. Wong. 1971. Isolation of a calcium sequestering protein from the sarcoplasmic reticulum. Proc. Nat. Acad. Sci. USA 68:1231.

Maruyama, K. 1986. Connectin, and elastic filamentous protein of striated muscle. Internat. Rev. Cytol. 104:81.

Ogata, T. 1988. Morphological and cytochemical features of the fiber types in vertebrate skeletal muscle. CRC Crit. Rev. Anat. Cell Biol. 1:229.

Page, S. 1968. Structure of the sarcoplasmic reticulum in vertebrate muscle. Br. Med. Bull. 24:170.

Pardo, J.V., J.D.F. Siciliano, and S.W. Craig. 1983. A vinculin containing cortical lattice in skeletal muscle: Transverse lattice elements (costomeres) mark sites of attachment between myofibrils and sarcolemma. Proc. Nat. Acad. Sci. USA. 80:1008.

Patten, R.M. and W.E. Ovalle. 1991. Muscle spindle ultrastructure revealed by conventional and high-resolution scanning microscopy. Anat. Rec. 230:183.

Peachey, L.D. 1965. The sarcoplasmic reticulum and transverse tubules of the frog's sartorius. J. Cell Biol. 15:209.

Pierbon-Bormoli, S., R. Betto, and G. Salviati. 1989. The organization of titin (connectin) and nebulin in the sarcomeres: an immunocytolocation study. J. Muscle Res. Cell Motil. 10:446.

Porter, K.R. 1961. The sarcoplasmic reticulum, its recent history and present status. J. Biophys. Biochem. Cytol. 10 (Suppl.):219.

Porter, K.R. and G.E. Palade. 1957. Studies on the endoplasmic reticulum. III. Its form and distribution in striated muscle cells. J. Biophys. Biochem. Cytol. 3:269.

Somlyo, A.V. 1979. Bridging structures spanning the junctional gap at the triad of skeletal muscle. J. Cell Biol. 80:743.

Trinnick, J. 1991. Elastic filaments and giant proteins in muscle. Current Opinion Cell Biol. 3:112.

Trotter, J.A., A. Samora, and J. Baca. 1985. Three dimensional structure of the murine muscle–tendon junction. Anat. Rec. 213:16.

Uehara, Y., and K. Hama. 1965. Some observations on the frog muscle spindle. I. On the sensory terminals and motor endings of the muscle spindle. J. Electron Microsc. 14:34.

Wang, K. and R. Ramirez-Mitchell. 1983. A network of transverse and longitudinal intermediate filaments is associated with the sarcomeres of vertebrate skeletal muscle. J. Cell Biol. 96:562.

INNERVATION OF MUSCLE

Desaki, J. and Y. Uehara. 1981. The overall morphology of neuromuscular junctions as revealed scanning electron microscopy. J. Neurocytol. 10:101.

Heuser, J.E. 1976. Morphology of synaptic vesicle discharge and reformation at frog neuromuscular junction. *In* S. Thesleff ed. The Motor Innervation of Muscle. London, Academic Press.

Heuser, J.E., T.S. Reese, M.J. Dennis, J.L. Jan, and L. Evans. 1979. Synaptic vesicle exocytosis by quick-freezing and correlated with quantal transmitter release. J. Cell Biol. 81:275.

Zacks, S.I. 1964. The Motor End Plate. Philadelphia, W.B. Saunders Co.

CARDIAC MUSCLE

Fawcett, D.W. and N.S. McNutt. 1969. The ultrastructure of the cat myocardium. I. Ventricular papillary muscle. J. Cell Biol. 42:1.

Forbes, M. and N. Sperelakis. 1985. Intercalated discs of mammalian heart: A review of structure and function. Tissue Cell 17:605.

Forssmann, W.G., D. Hock, F. Lottspeich et al. 1983. The right auricle of the heart is an endocrine organ. Cardiodilatin as a peptide hormone candidate. Anat. Embryol. 168:307.

Forssmann, W.G. 1986. Cardiac hormones I. Review on morphology, biochemistry, and molecular biology of the endocrine heart. Eur. J. Clin. Investig. 16:439.

Gorza, L.J., J. Mercadier, K. Schwartz, L.E. Thornell, S. Sartore, and J. Schiaffino. 1984. Myosin types in the human heart. An immunofluorescent study of normal and hypertrophied atrial and ventricular myocardium. Circ. Res. 54:694.

Gorza, L., S. Sartore, L.E. Thornell, and S. Schiaffino. 1986. Myosin types and fiber types in cardiac muscle, III. Nodal conduction tissue. J. Cell Biol. 102:1758.

Jamieson, J.D. and G.E. Palade. 1964. Specific granules in atrial muscle cells. J. Cell Biol. 23:151.

McNutt, N.S. and D.W. Fawcett. 1969. The ultrastructure of the cat myocardium. II. Atrial muscle. J. Cell Biol. 42:46.

McNutt, N.S. and D.W. Fawcett. 1974. Myocardial ultrastructure. *In* Mammalian Mycardium. New York, John Wiley and Sons.

Metz, J., V. Mutt, and G. Forssmann. 1984. Immunochemical localization of cardiodilatin in myoendocrine cells of cardiac atria. Anat. Embryol. 170:123.

Muir, A.R. 1975. Electron microscope study of the embryology of the intercalated discs in the heart of the rabbit. J. Biophys. Biochem. Cytol. 3:193.

Rhodin, J.A., P. Missier, and L.C. Reid. 1961. The structure of the specialized impulse-conducting system of the steer heart. Circulation 24:349.

Simpson, F.O. and S.J. Oertelis. 1961. Relationship of the sarcoplasmic reticulum to the sarcolemma in sheep cardiac muscle. Nature 189:758.

11

THE NERVOUS TISSUE

Jay B. Angevine

The nervous system comprises the entire mass of nervous tissue in the body. A basic function of the nervous system, from which others derive, is *communication;* it depends on special chemical and electrical properties of the nerve cells and their long cell processes. These properties reflect two fundamental attributes of protoplasm: *irritability,* the capacity to react in a graded manner to physical or chemical stimuli, and *conductivity,* the ability to transmit excitation rapidly from one place to another.

On reception of a stimulus from outside or inside the body, the form and flux of stimulus energy (mechanical, thermal, chemical, etc.) is transduced by specialized structures, *receptors,* into electrical potentials that, in turn, generate *nerve impulses.* Trains of these impulses are then rapidly transmitted to nerve centers, where they evoke in other nerve cells additional patterns of activity that result in sensations or motor responses. By such means, the organism reacts to events around or within it and coordinates the functions of its organs. Moreover, the nervous system generates impulses within itself. Thus, it has endogenous activity as well as its ability to respond to stimuli. These attributes constitute the structural and chemical basis of conscious experience, provide mechanisms for behavior and its regulation, and maintain those qualities that collectively define the personality.

The *central nervous system* (CNS) consists of the brain and spinal cord and contains the nerve cells, or *neurons,* and a host of supporting cells called the *neuroglia.* Nerve impulses pass to and from the CNS over long neuronal processes called axons (see below). The *peripheral nervous system* (PNS) comprises all of these processes which travel in cranial and spinal *nerves* and related clusters of outlying neurons known as *ganglia.* The functions of all parts of the body are integrated by this system. Although exceptions are seen in certain locally generated neural responses (as in the skin and viscera), *centralization* is the paramount principle of neural organization.

The communicative functions of neurons depend not only on their irritability and conductivity but also on their structure, integrative properties, and connections, as well as on chemical compounds that they synthesize and deliver to other neurons, to muscle, or to glands. These *neuroactive substances* are of three types: *neurotransmitters,* which act rapidly and locally to alter the activity of the target cells; *neuromodulators,* which regulate, but generally do not directly effect neurotransmission; and *neurohormones,* which exert slow and widespread influences, usually through the extracellular fluid or the blood. Neurons elaborating neurohormones are, thus, similar to cells of the endocrine system: Their secretory products are released from axon terminals into the perivascular space, transported into the lumen of blood vessels, and carried by the blood to distant tissues and organs. Indeed, studies of the interplay of the nervous and endocrine systems have been combined in the field of neuroendocrinology. And as other interactions of the brain and body have been explored, a field of neuroimmunology has emerged.

In the evolution of the nervous system, it is believed that certain cells of primitive Metazoa developed the properties of irritability and conductivity to a high degree, and as a result, a rudimentary nervous system evolved. By further specialization, some nerve cells developed the capacity to react to various exogenous and endogenous stimuli, and these cells, together with accessory cells in some cases, gave rise to three systems of sensory receptors: *exteroceptors* near the body surface; *interoceptors* in the internal organs; and *proprioceptors* in the muscles, tendons, and joints. Other neurons became connected with muscles, forming *neuromotor systems.* Still others collected in a large mass, the central nervous system, and as-

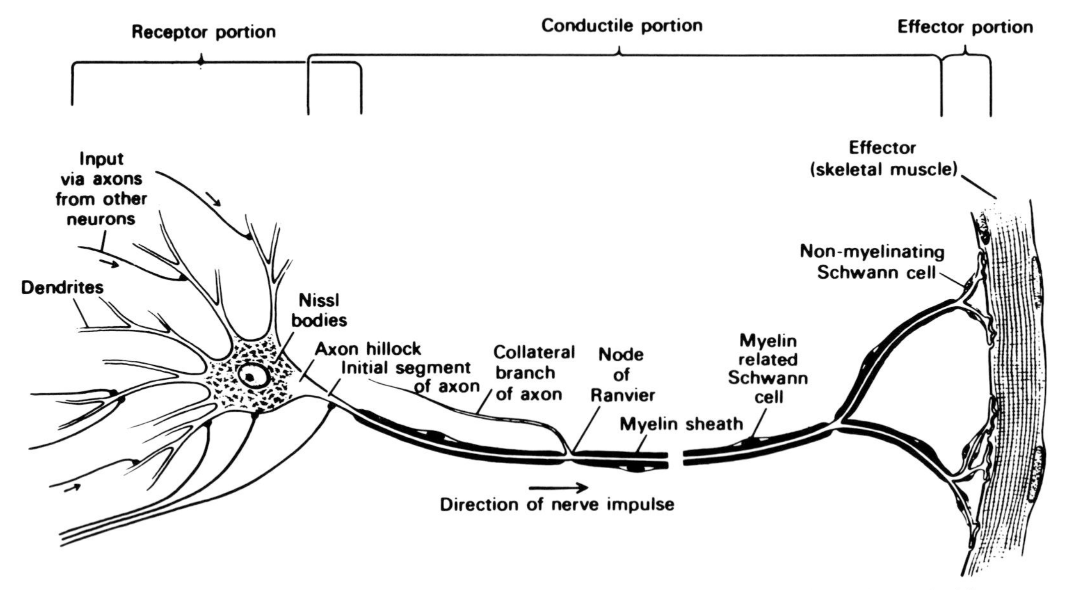

Figure 11–1. Diagrammatic representation of the effector, conductile, and receptor portions of a typical large neuron. The effector endings on skeletal muscle identify this as a somatic motor neuron. The effector endings of many neurons may terminate on the receptor portions of a single neuron. The myelin sheath on the conductile portion acts as "insulation" and serves to increase its conduction velocity. The discontinuity in the axon indicates that it is much longer than can be illustrated; a motor neuron to a limb may be 2–3 feet long. (Drawing after Bunge, in *Bailey's Textbook of Histology,* 16th ed. Williams and Wilkins Co. Baltimore, 1971.)

sumed the functions of integration of stimuli and initiation of appropriate responses.

Neurons exhibit an astonishing variety of forms, but each has a cell body, or *soma,* consisting of a nucleus and its surrounding cytoplasm, the *perikaryon.* The body usually has several radiating processes called *dendrites* and a single long slender process, the *axon* (Fig. 11–1). An axon may attain great length, emit branches, or *axon collaterals,* along its course, and undergo additional finer ramification into so-called *preterminal branches* near its end, or *axon terminal.* In rare instances, there may be no axon, only dendrites, which have complex relationships to other neurons.

The size and shape of the cell body and the mode of branching of its processes are highly variable, resulting in a great diversity of morphologically distinguishable kinds of nerve cells (Fig. 11–2). They range from simple bipolar neurons with only two processes, found in some invertebrates, to huge multipolar neurons in the mammalian cerebellum that have a single axon and hundreds of spiny dendrites. Neurons in the CNS are functionally interrelated at specialized sites of contact called *synapses,* where chemical or electrical signals pass from cell to cell. Transmission between two neurons via a chemical synapse is unidirectional, whereas in electrical synapses, it is bidirectional. Mixed modes of transmission also occur, neurons may have multiple contacts and reciprocal synapses, and there are examples of synaptic complexes that involve the processes of many neurons. The number of synapses on a neuron is partially dependent on the number and length of its dendrites, which is subject to great variation: Small local-circuit neurons with few dendrites receive few synapses, larger spinal motor neurons with moderately large dendritic arborizations may have 10,000, and cerebellar Purkinje cells, with their huge elaborately branched dendritic tree, may have in excess of 250,000. These variables make for the extraordinary complexity of cellular interactions within the CNS and permit a considerable range of adaptive changes referred to as *neural plasticity.*

Although functionally interrelated by synapses, the countless neurons in the CNS are morphologically and trophically independent. This is the basic concept of the *neuron doctrine,* enunciated in the late 1800s as a restatement of the cell theory for the nervous system. It held, among other things, that the nervous system was entirely cellular and that its cells did not have protoplasmic continuity, but were juxtaposed, with only a very narrow extracellular space intervening. The electron microscope confirmed these basic tenets and

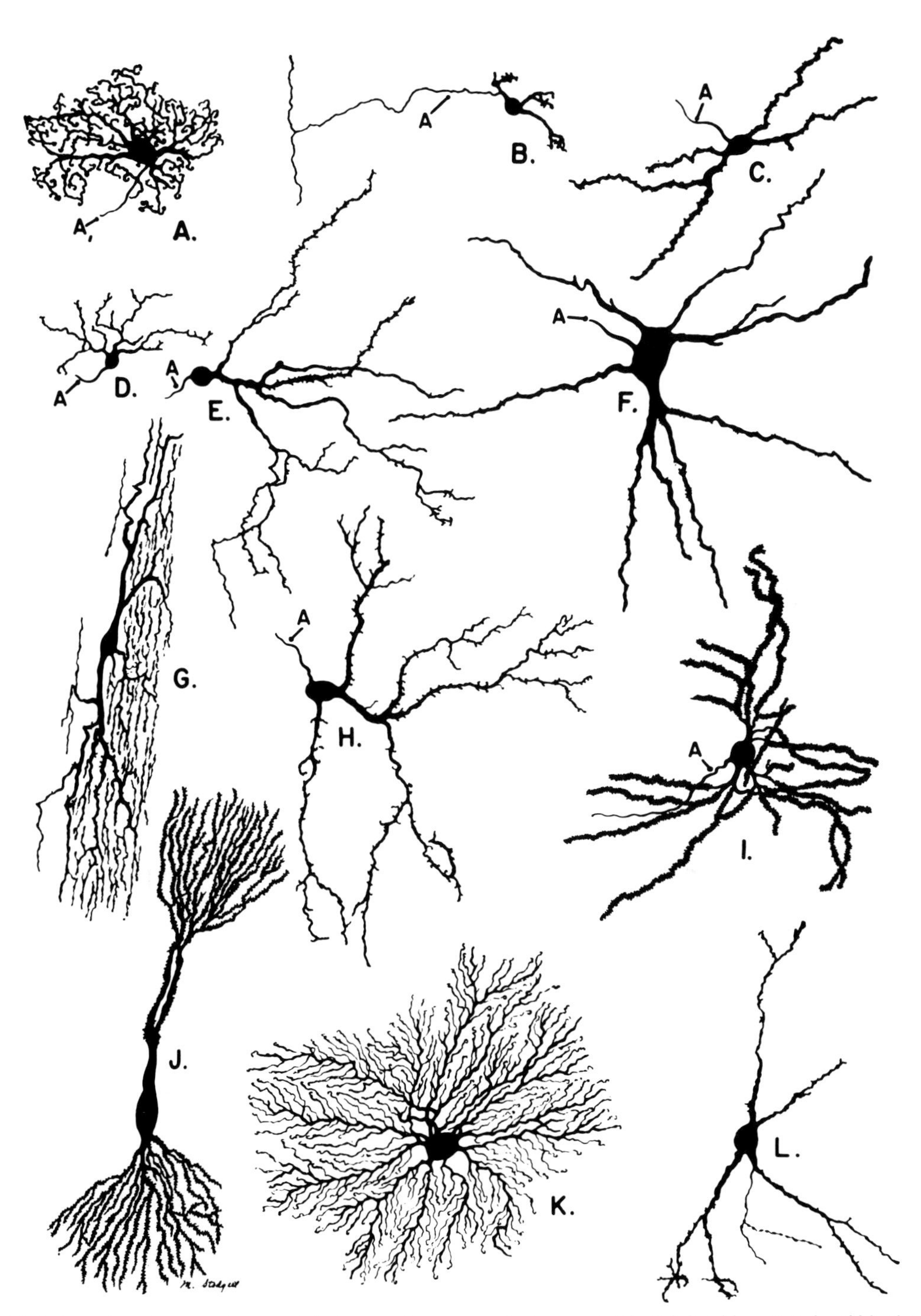

Figure 11–2. Drawing of some characteristic types of neurons whose axons (a) and dendrites remain within the central nervous system, illustrating some of the remarkable diversity of cell form exhibited by neurons. (A) Neuron of the inferior olivary nucleus; (B) granule cell of the cerebellar cortex; (C) small cell of the reticular formation; (D) small gelatinosa cell of the spinal trigeminal nucleus; (E) ovoid cell, nucleus of the tractus solitarius; (F) large cell of the reticular formation; (G) spindle-shaped cell, substantia gelatinosa of spinal cord; (H) large cell of spinal trigeminal nucleus; (I) neuron of putamen of lenticular nucleus; (J) double pyramidal cell, Ammon's horn of hippocampal cortex; (K) cell from thalamic nucleus; (L) cell from globus pallidus of lenticular nucleus. Golgi preparations, monkey brain. (Courtesy of Clement Fox, from Truex, R. and M.B. Carpenter. 1969. Human Neuroanatomy, 6th ed. Baltimore, MD, Williams and Wilkins.)

showed that nervous tissue is a highly specialized epithelium in which the myriad cellular constituents have extremely varied and complex shapes. Interpretation of the nervous system as a highly modified epithelium is consistent with its phylogeny and its origin from the embryonic ectoderm.

Like other epithelia, nervous tissue exhibits various types of junctional complexes: the *gap junction,* at electrotonic synapses; the *zonula occludens* between cells of the choroid plexus; and the *zonula adherens,* at chemical synapses and elsewhere. Of these, the latter is often of punctuate form and called a punctum adherens. *Puncta adherentia* appear to be important in stabilizing the spatial relationships of the cells and cell processes on which interneuronal communication depends. However, unlike other epithelia, in which the cells are all rather similar in form, those that make up the nervous tissue are extraordinarily heterogeneous.

THE NEURON

The neuron generally has several cell processes which collectively contain the bulk of its cytoplasm. In the CNS, the perikaryon is typically angular or polygonal with slightly concave surfaces between the processes (Figs. 11–3 and 11–4); motor neurons (Fig. 11–7) and pyramidal cells on the cerebral cortex (Fig. 11–5) are examples. Cell bodies in the dorsal root ganglia, on the other hand, are rounded and only one process projects from the perikaryon (Fig. 11–6).

Nucleus

The nucleus is usually large and spherical or ovoid, with a conspicuous nucleolus and relatively little heterochromatin. In primates, the *sex chromatin* representing the condensed, inactive X-chromosome of the female lies adjacent to the nuclear envelope, but in some species (cat, rat, mouse), it appears as a small satellite mass of heterochromatin (Barr body) associated with the nucleolus. In very large, synthetically active neurons, the chromatin is largely dispersed as euchromatin, making much of the genome available for transcription. Therefore, owing to the lack of stainable material, the nucleus appears pale when stained with basic dyes and is often described as "vesiculate." However, this description does not hold for the much more numerous small neurons, which have more condensed chromatin. In tiny neurons, such as the cerebellar granule cells, there are numerous coarse clumps of heterochromatin, like those seen in lymphocytes or plasma cells. In electron micrographs, the fine structure of the karyoplasm and the nuclear envelope is much like those of cells elsewhere in the body. In some neurons, the nucleus may be irregular in shape with deep infoldings of the nuclear envelope.

Perikaryon

The cytoplasm of the neuron is crowded with organelles, inclusions, and filamentous elements of the cytoskeleton arranged more or less concentrically around the centrally placed nucleus. In nervous tissue stained with basic aniline dyes and viewed with the light microscope, the most conspicuous of these components are clumps of intensely chromophilic material, traditionally called *Nissl bodies* (Fig. 11–7. In living neurons, these are visible with the phase contrast microscope. In electron micrographs, they are found to consist of cisternae of granular endoplasmic reticulum in ordered parallel array (Figs. 11–8 and 11–9). As in other cells engaged in active protein synthesis, ribosomes are arranged in rows, loops, and spirals on the outer surface of the cisternae, and polyribosomes are also found free in the cytoplasm. Rough endoplasmic reticulum is present in the dendrites, but there it takes the form of branching and anastomosing tubules and short cisternae, except at sites of branching, where small groups of parallel cisternae may be found. Endoplasmic reticulum is usually absent from the area of the perikaryon from which the axon arises, the *axon hillock* (Fig. 11–7). It is also lacking in the axon, which contains only agranular reticulum.

The form, size, and distribution of the Nissl bodies vary greatly in different types of neurons, with each type seeming to have a characteristic pattern. Small neurons always have many very small Nissl bodies, but among larger neurons, there is no clear correlation between cell size and the size of the Nissl bodies. Some large nerve cells (motor neurons and the giant Betz cells of the cerebral cortex) have large Nissl bodies, whereas in other large neurons (Purkinje cells of the cerebellar cortex) they are relatively small. Although the ganglion cells of the dorsal roots may attain a large size, they typically contain uniformly

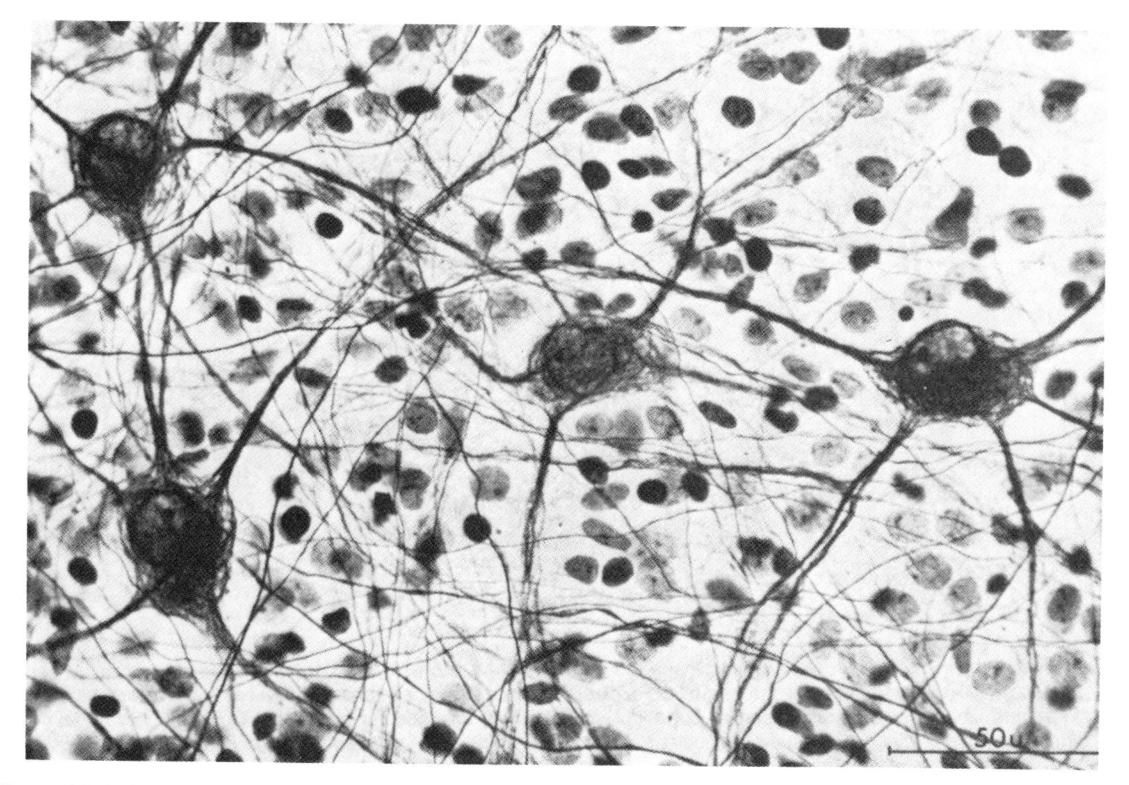

Figure 11–3. In tissue cultures of the nervous system, the three-dimensional configuration of the intact neuron can be seen to better advantage than in sections. Shown here are multipolar neurons from the deep nuclei of the rat cerebellum in a 12-day culture. Note the neurofibrils in the cell bodies. (From Hild, W. 1966. Zeitschr. Zellforsch. 69:155.)

distributed very small Nissl bodies. The appearance of the Nissl bodies may change in different physiological and pathological conditions (axonal fatigue or injury), and these changes can be quite striking in large neurons.

The *smooth endoplasmic reticulum* of neurons is less obvious and has attracted less investigative attention than the rough endoplasmic reticulum, but it is abundant and widely distributed. A network of smooth reticulum pervades the perikaryon and extends into the axon and dendrites. It often forms a broad, flat, fenestrated hypolemmal cisterna immediately beneath and parallel to the plasmalemma of the cell body. The smooth reticulum is in continuity with the rough reticulum and may occupy much of the space between Nissl bodies. Its functional role in neurons remains unclear. It is known to sequester calcium and to contain proteins and may provide a pathway for their distribution throughout the cell. It is speculated that transport vesicles, and possibly synaptic vesicles, may bud off from it, as they do from the trans-Golgi network, but this has not been firmly established. The significance of the hypolemmal cisternae of smooth reticulum that are characteristic of some neurons is still unknown.

As expected of cells active in protein synthesis, the Golgi apparatus is prominent in all neurons. When impregnated with osmium or silver methods for light microscopy, it appears as a juxtanuclear loose network of wavy strands. In electron micrographs, these are resolved as several arciform stacks of closely apposed flat cisternae, often slightly dilated at their ends (Fig. 11–8). These are surrounded by many small vesicles. These stacks of Golgi membranes correspond to the *dictyosomes* of classical cytology. In the current literature, the several stacks of Golgi cisternae are collectively referred to as the *Golgi complex* rather than the Golgi apparatus. The tubules linking the stacks of cisternae together are usually not evident in thin sections, but they have been reconstructed in serial sections. At the concave surface of each stack, the innermost cisterna is fenestrated and is continuous with branching and anastomosing tubules forming the *trans-Golgi network* (See Chapter 1).

In general, the function of the Golgi com-

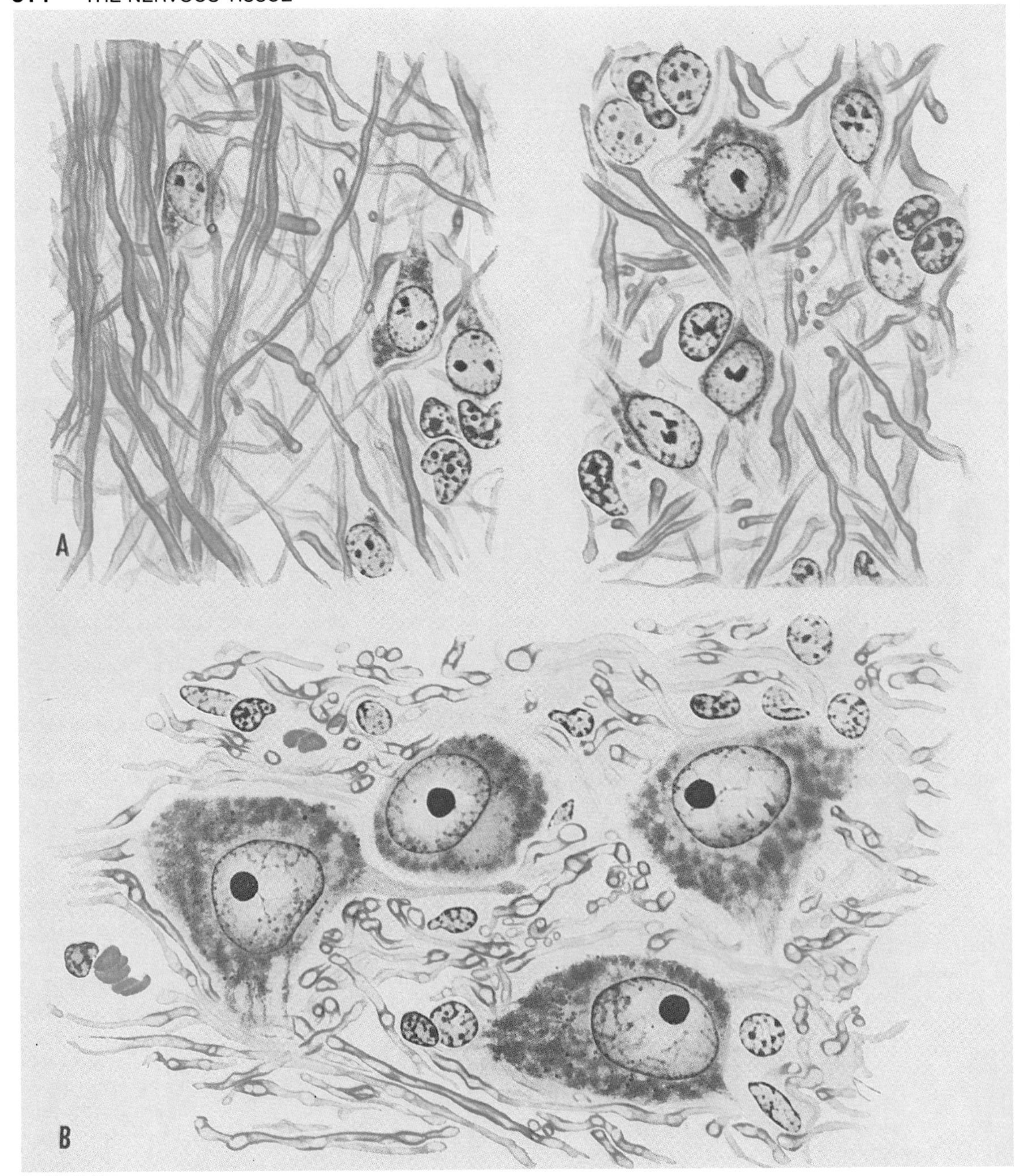

Figure 11–4. (A) Two areas of a section through the optic tectum of a leopard frog showing blue-stained myelin sheaths and the nerve cell bodies. The small dark nuclei are supporting cells. (B) Section from pons of man, showing myelin sheaths, nerve cell bodies, and glial cells. (A) is from a frozen section fixed in formalin; (B) Paraffin section after postmortem formalin fixation, Kluver and Barrera staining method for cells and myelin sheaths. (Drawn by Esther Bohlman.)

plex in neurons is similar to that in other cells, but it may have additional specialized functions not yet elucidated. It concentrates and slightly modifies proteins synthesized in the granular endoplasmic reticulum. It is also involved in production of components of the cell membrane and the formation of lysosomes. These functions are most apparent in neurosecretory cells and more subtle in cells that synthesize neurotransmitters. In these, it is thought that the Golgi either produces transmitter molecules or the enzymes necessary for their production in the axon terminals. It also produces constituents of the mem-

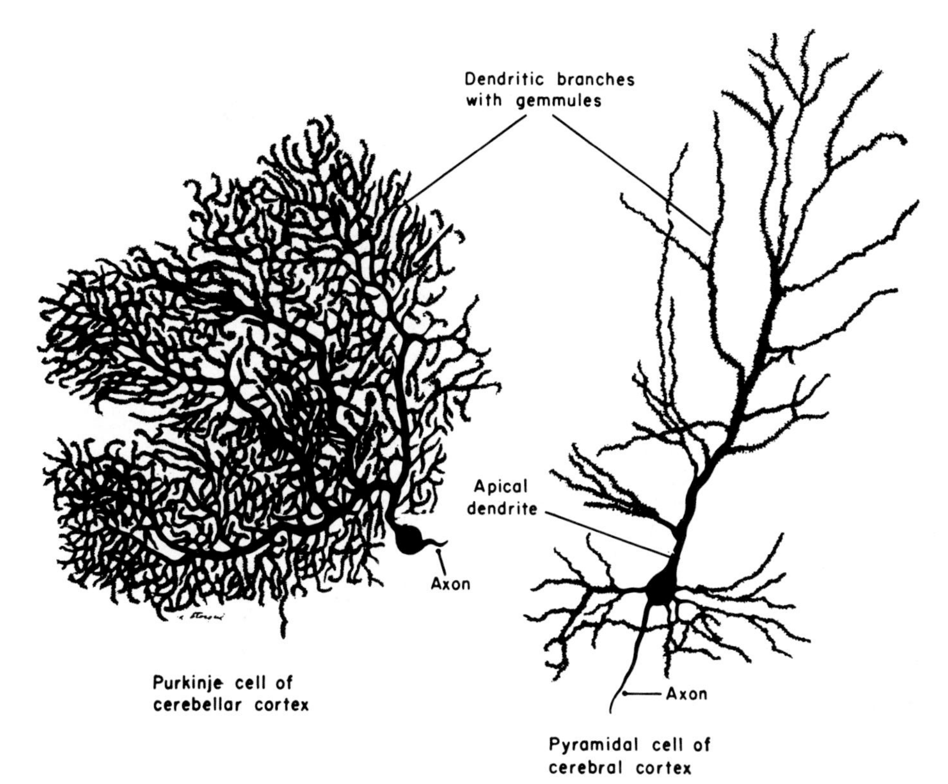

Figure 11–5. Drawing of two principal cell types in cerebellar and cerebral cortex. Dendritic branches may provide a very extensive area for attachment of synaptic terminals of many other cortical and subcortical neurons. Golgi preparations, monkey brains. (Courtesy of Clement Fox, from Truex, R.C. and M.B. Carpenter. 1966. Human Neuroanatomy, 5th ed. Baltimore, MD. Williams and Wilkins.)

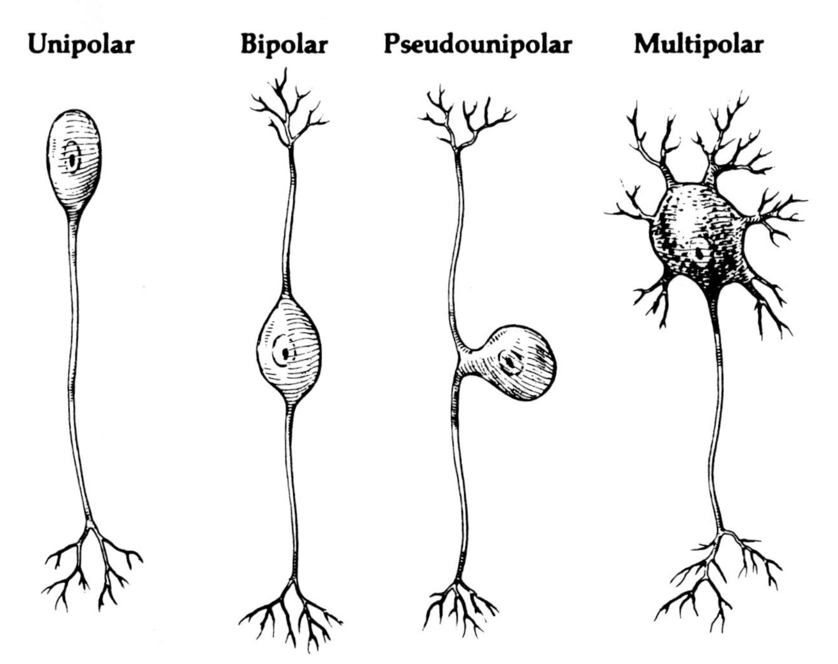

Figure 11–6. Types of neurons according to their polarity. (Adapted from Ham, A.W. 1969. Histology, 6th ed. Philadelphia, J.P. Lippincott Co.

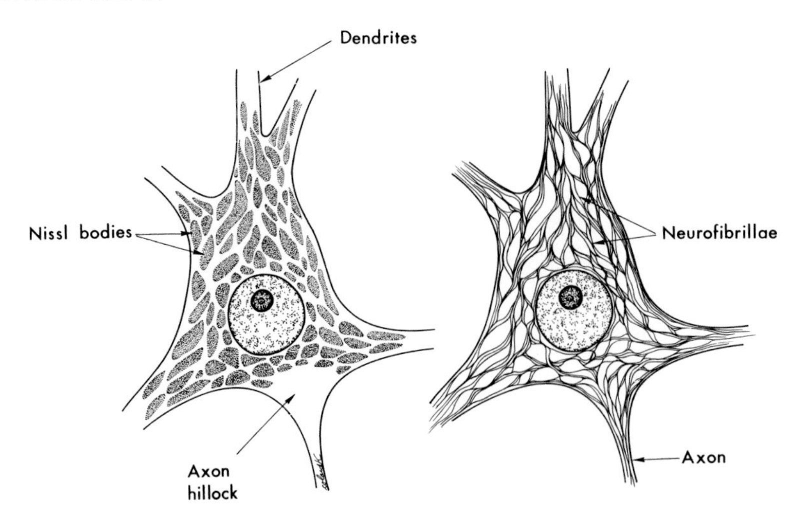

Figure 11–7. Drawings of a motor neuron from the gray matter of the ventral horn of the cat spinal cord stained for Nissl substance (A) and stained by the silver method for demonstrating neurofibrillae (B). The two images are complimentary, the network of neurofibrillae running between the areas occupied by Nissl bodies and continuing into the processes. The Nissl bodies are largely confined to the perikaryon but may extend into the dendrites. They usually are not found in the axon hillock.

brane of synaptic vesicles and components of the plasma membrane that are essential to the signaling properties of neurons. After severance of the axon, neurotransmitter production ceases and the Golgi complex regresses to such an extent that it may no longer be detectable with the light microscope.

Neurons have low energy reserves and a great need for glucose and oxygen. Accordingly, numerous mitochondria are widely distributed in the cell. They are rod-like or filamentous and may be closely associated with the Nissl bodies. They are often more slender than those in cells of non-nervous tissues, ranging from 0.1 to 0.8 μm in diameter, but more plump, rounded mitochondria are occasionally encountered. Mitochondria also occur in the dendrites (Figs. 11–10 and 11–11). They are scattered at intervals along the axon and are especially numerous in axon terminals. Their cristae are not always oriented transversely but may run parallel to their long axis, so that in cross section the membranes appear as concentric light and dark rings. Another peculiarity is the paucity of the electron-dense granules normally found in the mitochondrial matrix. Microcinematography of neurons in culture reveals that the mitochondria are constantly moving, at varying rates, throughout the cytoplasm and between the perikaryon and its processes. Their movement appears to be along microtubules in open tracts between the other organelles.

In neurons of the adult, two centrioles are found only occasionally. A single centriole associated with the basal body of a cilium is more common. At its origin, the cilium has a 9+0 complement of longitudinal elements in place of the usual 9+2 found in active cilia. More distally, one of the peripheral doublets often is displaced inward, resulting in an 8+1 pattern in cross section. Although sensory and other roles have been suggested for these abnormal cilia, they are generally considered to be nonmotile vestigial structures.

All neurons have the organelles described above, but the great majority contain relatively few inclusions other than pigment granules. Coarse dark-brown or black granules of *melanin* are found in neurons of the substantia nigra of the midbrain, in the locus coeruleus of the upper pons, in the dorsal motor nucleus of the vagus nerve in the medulla oblongata, and in the spinal cord and sympathetic ganglia. Its physiological significance in these sites is unknown. Of more widespread occurrence are the golden brown granules of *lipofuscin.* These are irregular in shape and are believed to be accumulations of end products of lysosomal enzyme activity. A gradual increase in the amount of lipofuscin occurs with aging and may even displace the nucleus and organelles to one side of the perikaryon, possibly affecting cell function in advanced stages. Deposits of iron-containing pigment are found in the neurons of the substantia nigra, globus pallidus, and a few other centers. Their number also increases with aging. Occasional lipid

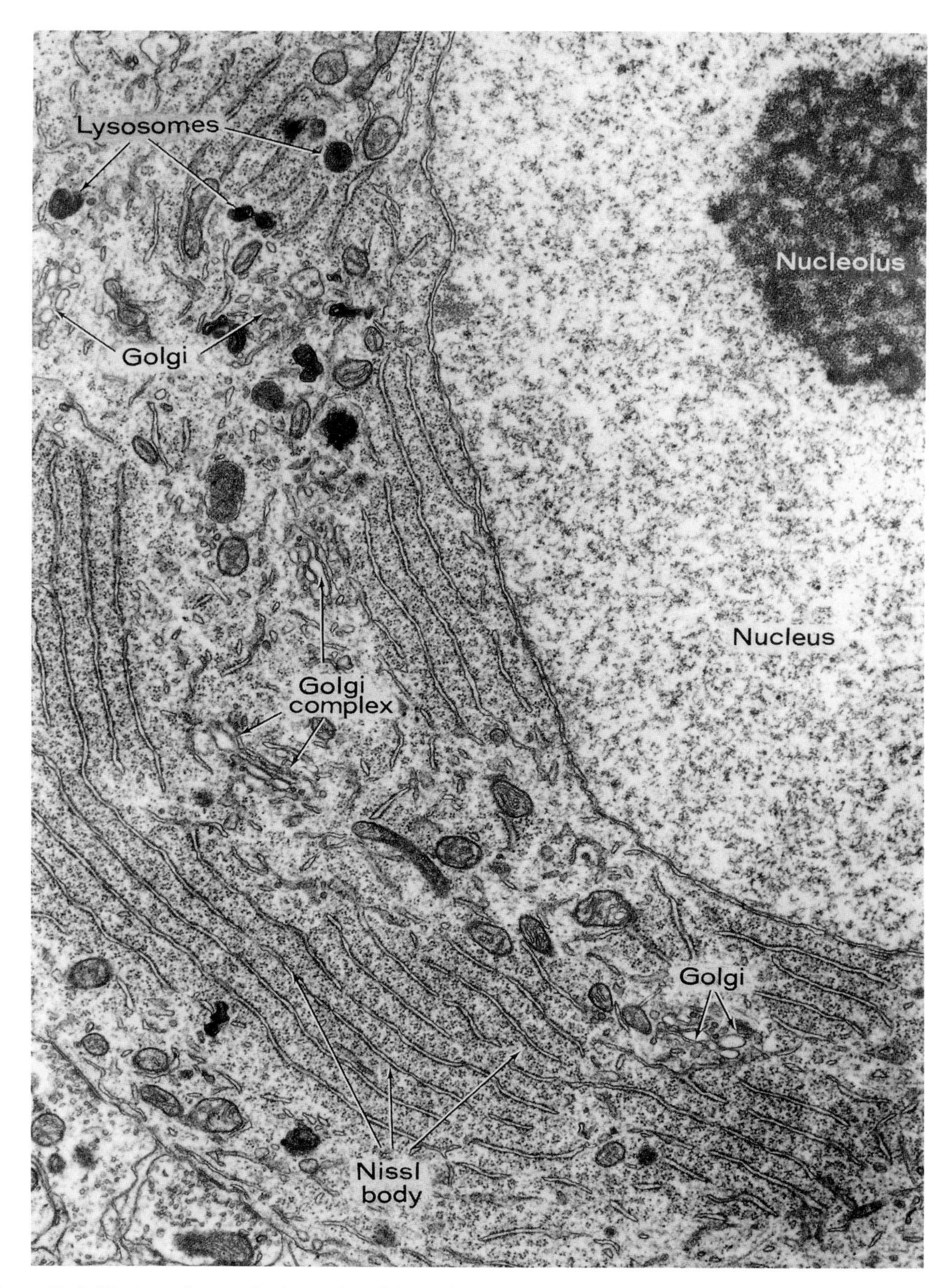

Figure 11–8. Electron micrograph of a portion of the perikaryon of a typical neuron illustrating the principal organelles. The Golgi complex of the neurons is highly developed and forms a continuous network in the perinuclear cytoplasm; therefore, in thin sections such as this, it is transected at multiple sites. (Micrograph courtesy of Sanford Palay.)

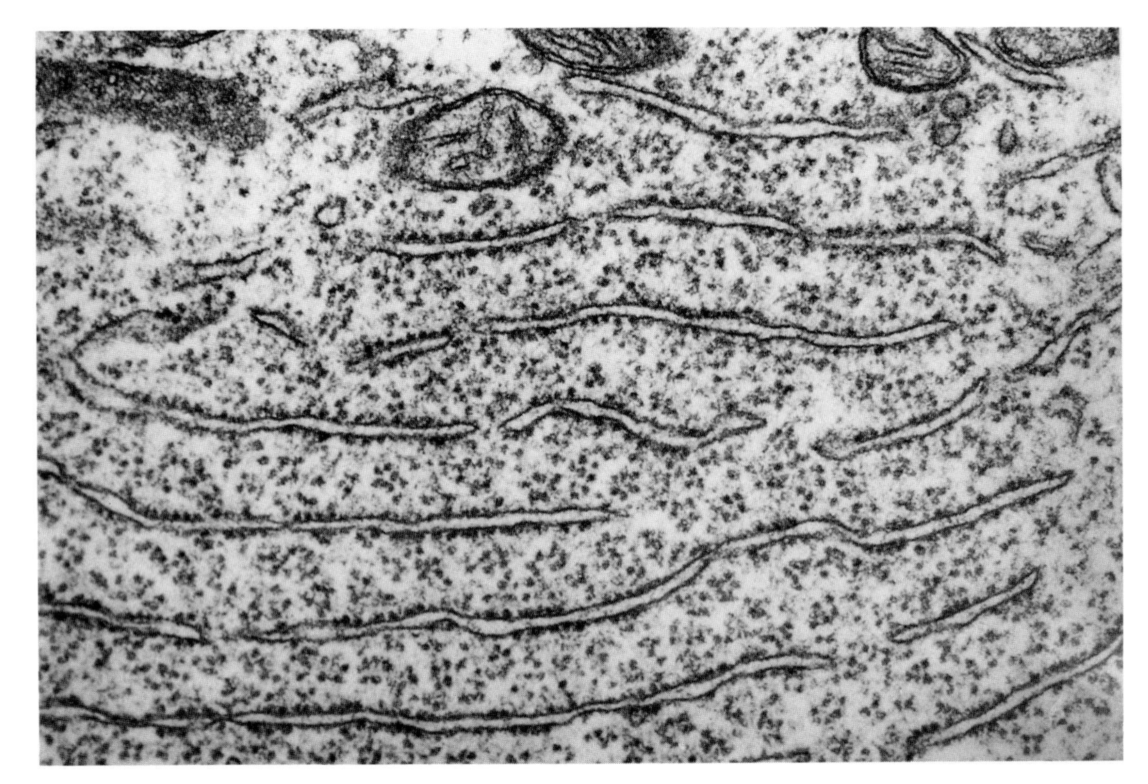

Figure 11–9. Electron micrograph of a Nissl body at higher magnification. It consists of flattened cisternae of the endoplasmic reticulum oriented parallel to each other. In addition to the ribosomes associated with the membranes, there are many clusters of ribosomes in the cytoplasmic matrix between cisternae.

droplets in the cytoplasm may represent normal energy reserves or may be a product of abnormal metabolism. Glycogen, a common energy source for cells outside the nervous system, is not present in histochemically demonstrable quantity in the cytoplasm of neurons.

Neurosecretory cells contain small membrane-limited secretory granules. Those secreting catecholamines contain dense-cored vesicles 80 to 120 nm in diameter. The neurosecretory cells of the hypothalamus contain granules 10–30 nm in diameter containing the hormones vasopressin and oxytocin and their carrier peptides, neurophysins. These granules are transported along the axon to the neurohypophysis where their hormones are discharged and diffuse into the bloodstream. In recent years, isolated granule-containing cells of several kinds have been found widely dispersed in the CNS. Their granules are immunoreactive for a number of peptides that are also found in endocrine cells of the gastrointestinal tract (vasoactive intestinal peptide, cholecystokinin, and others). The functional significance of these cells and their peptides is now a subject of intensive study, especially as to actions they may, or may not, have on the signaling activities of neurons.

Cytoskeleton of Neurons

In specimens prepared for light microscopy by silver-impregnation methods, a network of *neurofibrils* up to 2 μm in diameter can be seen in the perikaryon, weaving among the organelles and extending into the dendrites and the axon (Fig. 11–7). With the electron microscope, three kinds of filamentous structures are found in the neuron; *microtubules,* 20–28 nm in diameter (Figs. 11–12 and 11–14); *neurofilaments,* 10 nm in diameter (Figs. 11–12 and 11–14); and *microfilaments,* 3–5 nm in diameter. The relationship of these to the neurofibrils of classical cytology has been subject to varying interpretations. According to some, the neurofibrils are aggregates of both microtubules and neurofilaments, whereas others consider them to consist only of bundles of neurofilaments. The latter interpretation is more likely because the neurofilaments are the principal elements that retain silver ni-

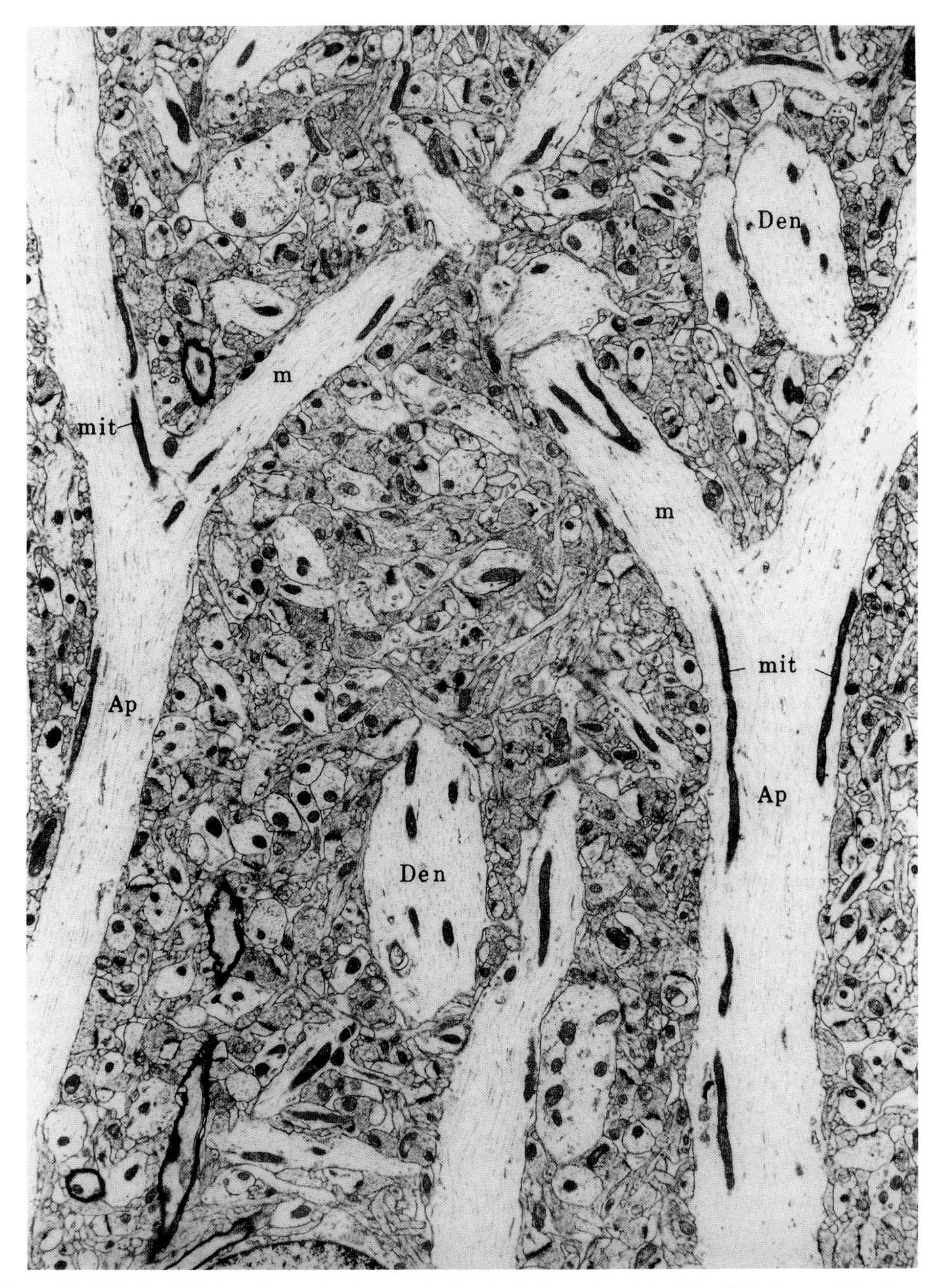

Figure 11–10. In this field, from the rat visual cortex, two longitudinally sectioned dendrites (Ap) of pyramidal cells, can be seen, both of which are branching as they begin to form their apical tufts. The cytoplasm of the dendrites contains microtubules (m) and long thin mitochondria (mit). Portions of other dendrites are also visible (Den). Note the absence of neuroglia covering the outside of these dendrites. (Micrograph from Peter, A. S.L. Palay, and H. deF. Webster. 1991. The Fine Structure of the Nervous System. New York, Oxford University Press.)

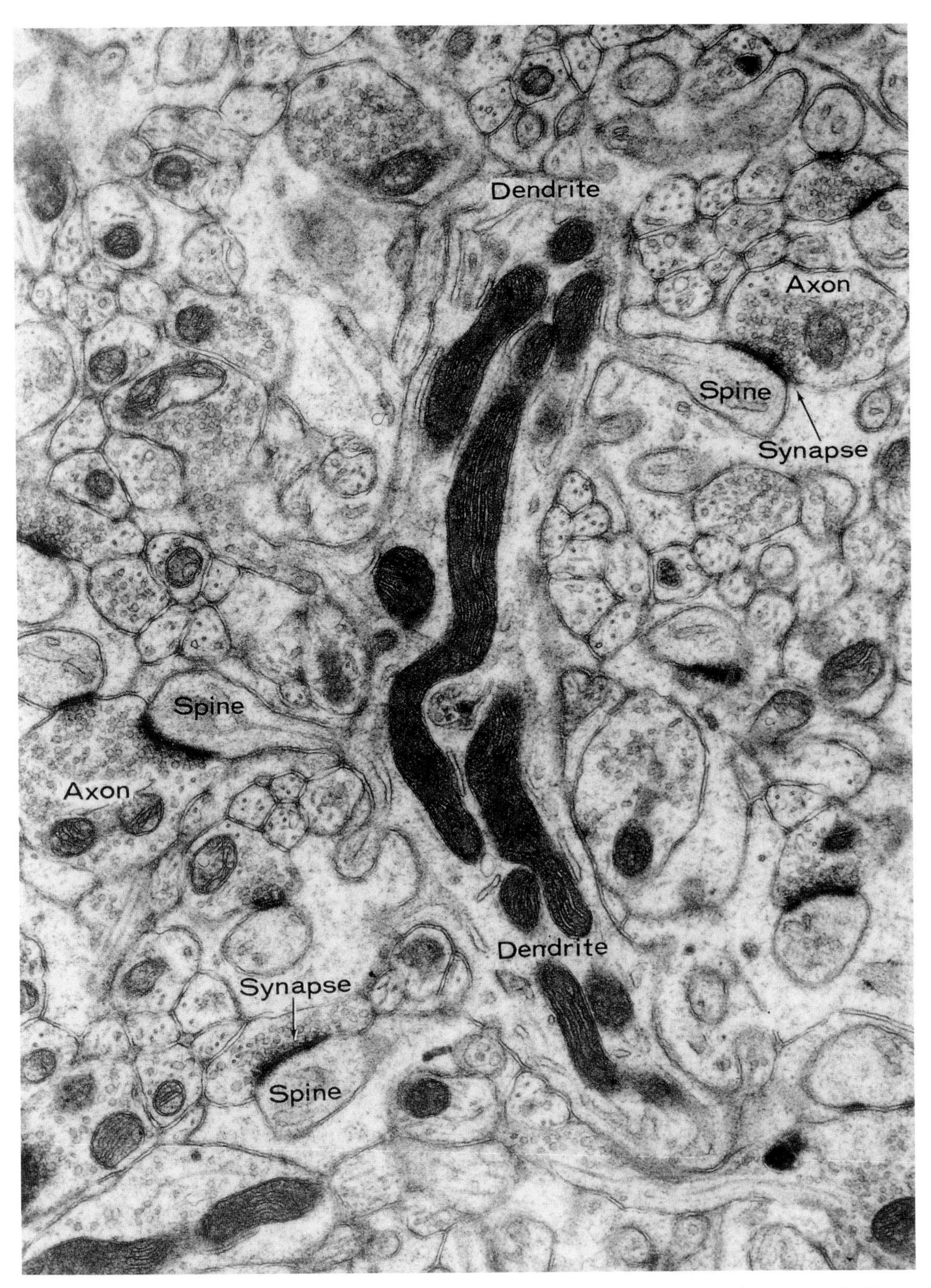

Figure 11–11. Electron micrograph of a small area of cerebellum. A small branch of the dendritic tree of a Purkinje cell running vertically through the field contains several conspicuous mitochondria. Projecting laterally from the dendrite are "spines" or "thorns" with bulbous tips and narrow stalks. Axons of granule cells form synapses with the Purkinje cell dendrite. (From Palay, S.L. and V.C. Palay. 1974. Cerebellar Cortex. Berlin. Springer-Verlag.)

trate. The neurofilaments are related to the intermediate filaments of other cell types that all belong to a family of proteins called cytokeratins. *Neurofilaments* are made up of minute filaments, of molecular dimensions, that twist around each other in a helical fashion to form heterodimers. Four of the dimers form a protofilament, and two of these form a protofibril. Two protofibrils, in turn, coil around one another to form a neurofilament. The subunits are so arranged that the neurofilaments appear, in cross section, to be minute tubules with a thick wall and a clear center about 2–3 nm in diameter.

The *microfilaments* of neurons are composed of two strands of polymerized G-actin arranged in a helix, and they are not significantly different from the actin filaments of other cells. Most of the actin is associated with the plasma membrane and bound to it by an anchoring protein called fodrin. The actin in cortical dendrites is especially concentrated in the dendritic spines.

The *microtubules* are identical to those of other cells, but there are slight differences in the *microtubule-associated proteins* (MAP-1, MAP-2, MAP-3) that regulate the stability of the microtubules and promote their assembly. MAP-2 is abundant in the perikaryon and dendrites but absent in the axon. MAP-3 is present only in the axon.

The cytoskeleton of the neuron is important in supporting the organelles and in changes in shape of the cell as a whole. The microtubules also have an essential role in transport of vesicles and organelles that move along their surface within the cell body and along the length of the axon (see below). They are constantly turning over, and their influence on cell shape is not expressed by contraction but in changes of their length by polymerization or depolymerization or by self-assembly of new microtubules of different orientation. The neurofilaments are less dynamic. In certain degenerative diseases, including Alzheimer's disease, their protein seems to be modified, resulting in the formation of characteristic lesions called neurofibrillary tangles.

PROCESSES OF NEURONS

The cell processes of neurons are perhaps their most remarkable features. Long or short, thick or thin, smooth or spiny, simply or elaborately branched—on them depends most of the capacity of nerve cells to transmit, receive, and integrate messages. Although their length and complexity have been obstacles to visualizing the entire nerve cell in all but the smallest of neurons, their infinitely varied patterns of ramification and distribution are of great interest to neurobiologists, as well as examples of beauty in nature. In almost all neurons there are two kinds of processes: the *dendrites* and the *axon.*

Dendrites

Neurons usually have multiple dendrites arising directly from the cell body, and these branches provide most of the surface for receiving signals from other neurons. However, the cell body and the initial segment of the axon may also receive afferent synapses. Where the dendrites emerge from the perikaryon they are relatively thick but they taper gradually along their length. Dendrites of most neurons are fairly short and confined to the immediate vicinity of the soma. They bifurcate, typically at acute angles, into primary, secondary, tertiary, and higher orders of branches that form patterns ranging from simple to highly complex (Figs. 11–10 and 11–12). The number and length of the dendrites bears little relation to the size of the soma, but the pattern of branching is typical for each kind of neuron. Dendrites may appear thorny owing to the presence of numerous minute projections, *spines,* from their surfaces (Fig. 11–11). While the role of the spines is debated, they are clearly specialized sites of synaptic contact that could provide some selectivity and control of input. Spines decrease in number after neuronal deafferentation or nutritional deprivation and exhibit structural changes in aged persons and in individuals with certain chromosomal abnormalities (trisomies 13 and 21).

At their base, the fine structure of the dendrites is similar to that of the perikaryon. They may contain extensions of the Golgi apparatus, small Nissl bodies, mitochondria, agranular endoplasmic reticulum, microtubules, and neurofilaments (Fig. 11–12). With increasing distance from the soma, longitudinal microtubules become prominent and the organelles are usually aligned parallel to them. Neurofilaments diminish in number away from the cell body and are reduced to single filaments or small bundles, with delicate cross-links between the filaments and between them and the microtubules. Spinal motor neurons and

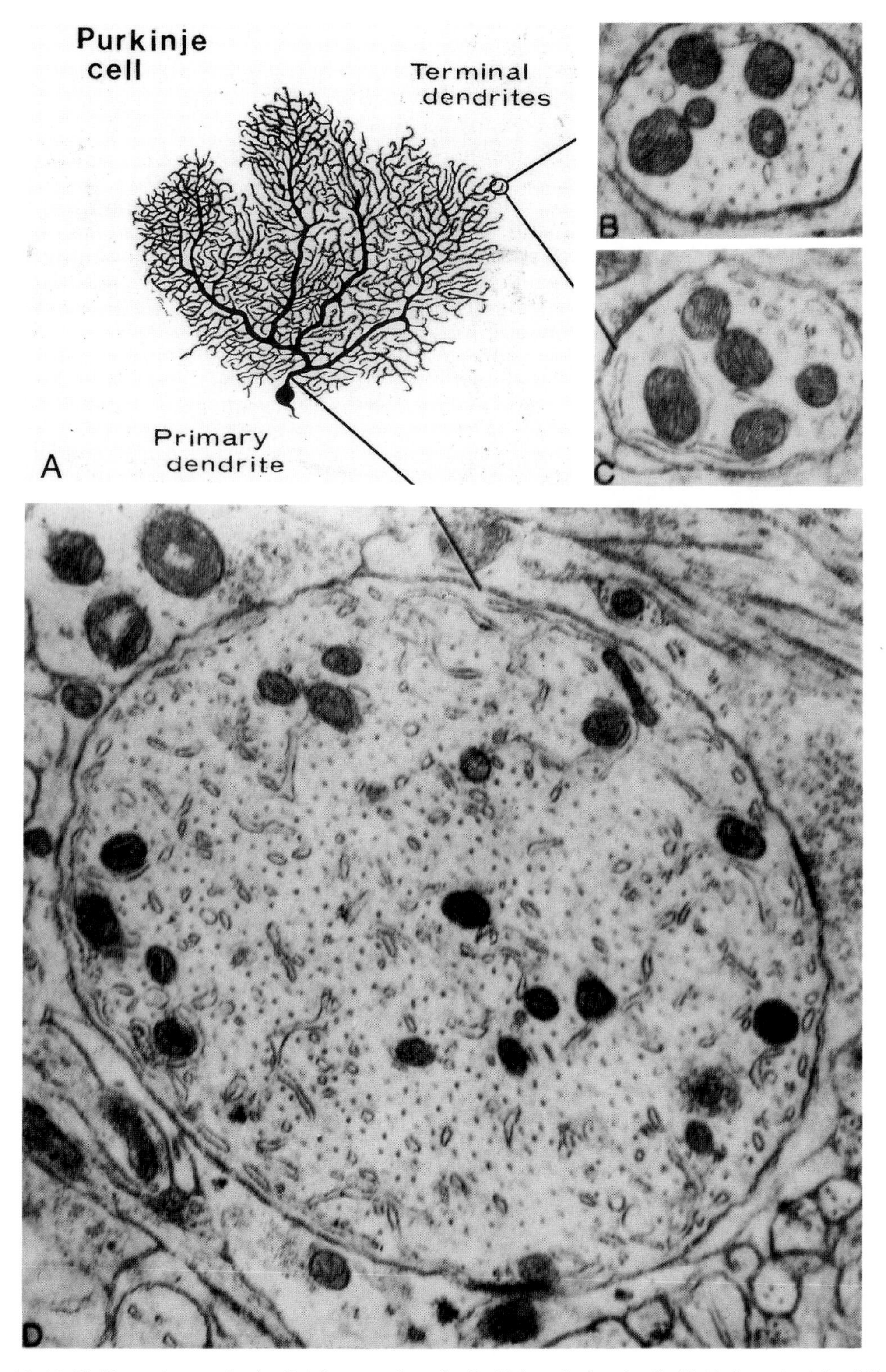

Figure 11–12 (A) Photomicrograph of a Golgi preparation of a Purkinje cell, showing its highly branched dendritic tree. (B) and (C) Electron micrographs of small terminal dendrites of the Purkinje cell located in the molecular layer of the cerebellum. (D) Cross section of the primary dendrite of a Purkinje cell. Mitochondria, tubular elements of the endoplasmic reticulum, and punctate profiles of microtubules are found throughout the dendritic tree. (Micrograph from Wuerker and Kirkpatrick, 1972. *In* G.H. Bourne, and J.F. Danielli, eds. International Review of Cytology, Vol. 33. New York, Academic Press.)

Betz cells are exceptional in having very large numbers of dendritic neurofilaments. Tubules of endoplasmic reticulum and free ribosomes diminish, whereas mitochondria become more numerous and are concentrated in the finer ramifications of the dendrites.

Dendrites receive impulses from other neurons via their synapses with axon terminals. The number of such inputs may be very large. As stated earlier, the terminals on the dendritic tree of the large Purkinje cells may number in the hundreds of thousands. The degree of branching of the dendrites and the number of their spines are directly related to the capacity of a neuron to integrate inputs from many different sources. Arriving nerve impulses excite, or inhibit, electrical activity in local regions of the dendritic membrane and, thus, continually shift the neuron toward, or away from, its threshold for generating nerve impulses of its own. The impulse carried over an axon is "all-or-none," but the integrative capacity of the dendrites depends on graded local changes in electrical potential. In rare instances, dendrites may transmit as well as receive and may, therefore, influence adjacent dendrites at special dendrodendritic synapses. They may also rapidly propagate summated signals along dendrites that attain great length, acting somewhat like axons. These varied attributes of the dendrites illustrate the ability of the neuron to adapt to special requirements.

THE AXON

The axon arises from a conical extension of the cell body called the *axon hillock* (Fig. 11–13). Occasionally, it may arise from the base of a principal dendrite. In certain very small local-circuit neurons (e.g., amacrine cells of the retina) there may be no axon, but this is quite uncommon. The axon is usually thinner and very much longer than the dendrites of the same cell. The axoplasm does not contain Nissl bodies but does contain short tubular profiles of agranular endoplasmic reticulum, long and extremely slender mitochondria, microtubules, and neurofilaments.

The part of the axon between the hillock and the beginning of the myelin sheath is called the *initial segment.* Here, the plasmalemma is underlain by a thin layer of moderately electron-dense material of unknown nature. A similar layer occurs at the nodes of Ranvier, but not elsewhere along the length of the myelinated axon. The microtubules in the axon hillock and initial segment may occur in small bundles. More distally, they are numerous, but the individual microtubules are uniformly spaced a short distance apart, with neurofilaments in the interspaces between them. The neurofilaments greatly outnumber the microtubules (Fig. 11–14).

The axon carries the response of the neuron, the nerve impulse, in the form of a propagated *action potential.* The axon hillock and initial segment give rise to this potential and constitute the so-called "spike trigger zone." These two regions also provide a receptive zone for inhibitory afferents. Impulse conduction is only one function of the axon. *Signal transmission* at its ending and *trophic relationships* with target neurons, muscles, and glands are others. Basic to these is the function of *axonal transport,* the movement of substances up and down the axon. This commerce with the cell body is essential because the axon lacks the synthetic machinery present in the dendrites. Two forms of axonal transport exist: *anterograde transport* from the perikaryon to the axon terminal and *retrograde transport* in the opposite direction. In the anterograde transport, two components have been identified, fast and slow. Subcellular organelles are moved down the axon by fast transport, whereas the cytosol is transported by slow axoplasmic flow.

The velocity of fast transport varies from 20 to 400 mm per day. The bulk of the materials transported at this rate are membrane-bounded organelles, such as short tubules of reticulum, mitochondria, small vesicles, actin, myosin, and the clathrin used in recycling of synaptic vesicle membrane. Rapid retrograde transport also occurs from the nerve terminals to the cell body, returning materials for degradation or reuse. The velocity of fast retrograde transport is one-half to two-thirds that of fast anterograde transport. Slow transport proceeds at a rate of 0.2–0.4 mm per day and carries protein subunits of neurofilaments, tubulins of the microtubules, and soluble enzymes. In addition, proteins and small molecules picked up by the axon terminal are conveyed upward in vesicles or multivesicular bodies that fuse with lysosomes when they reach the cell body.

An important role of axon transport is the delivery to the axon ending of synaptic vesicles and enzymes involved in transmitter synthesis. Although neurotransmitters can also be transported along the axon, the quantity

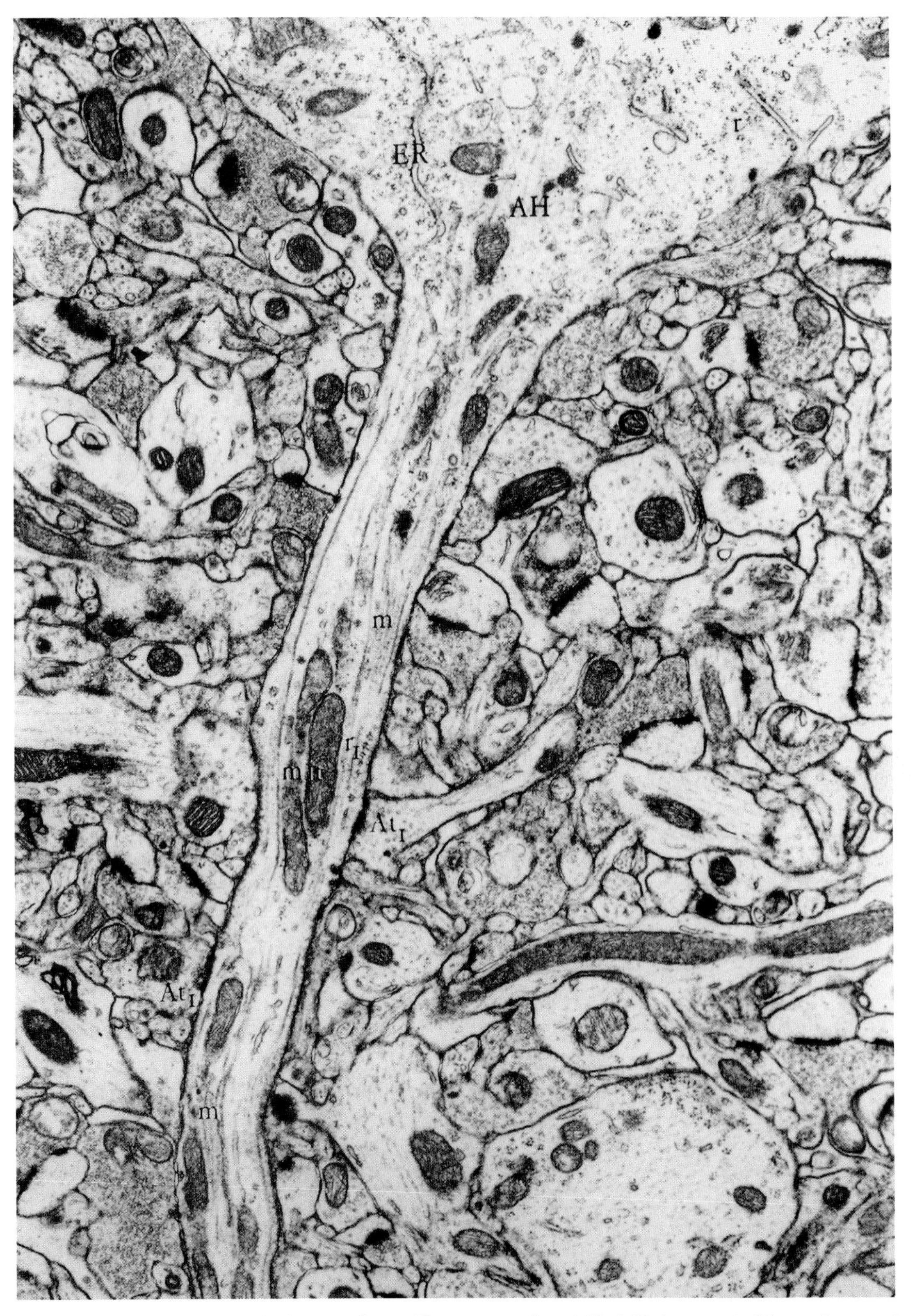

Figure 11–13. An area of the cerebral cortex of a rat. The upper portion of this field shows part of the perikaryon of a pyramidal neuron. The axon leaves the perikaryon at the axon hillock (AH) and courses downward. Note the axon terminal (AT1) synapsing with the initial segment of the axon. (Micrograph from Peters, A., S.L. Palay, and H. DeF Webster. 1991. The Fine Structure of the Nervous System, 3rd ed. New York, Oxford University Press.)

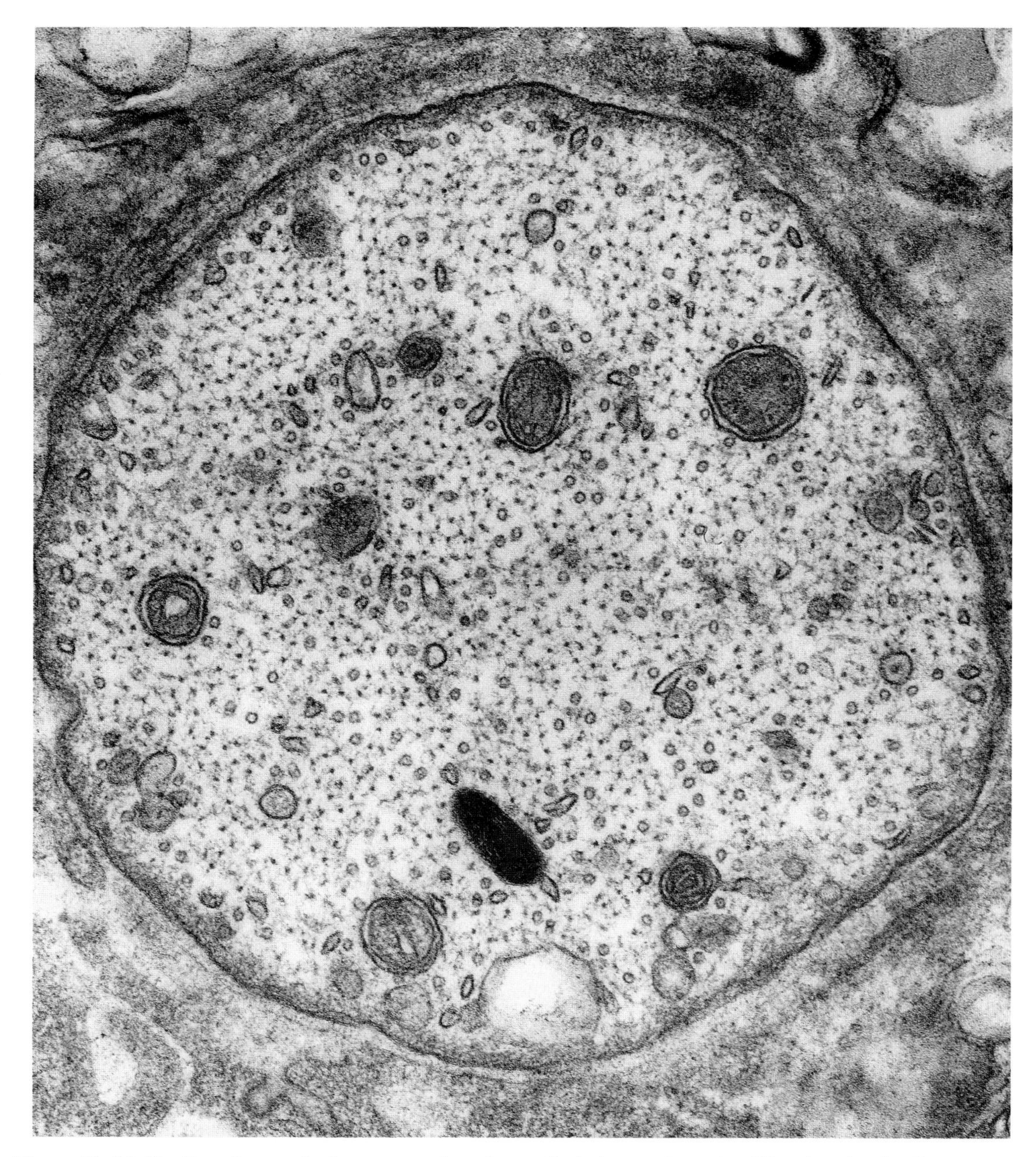

Figure 11–14. Electron micrograph of a cross section of a myelinated axon at a node of Ranvier, showing the very even distribution of neurofilaments and of microtubules that are essential for axonal transport. (Micrograph by Price, R.L. 1989. Proc. 47th Annual Meeting, Electron Microscope Society of America, p. 948.)

reaching the ending by this mechanism is probably small compared to the amount synthesized at the endings. Exceptions to this include the neuropeptides and neurosecretory granules that are definitely produced in the cell body. In neurons that use biogenic amines as transmitters, large dense-cored vesicles can be seen in the cell body and traveling along the axon.

Axoplasmic transport is vital to nerve cell functions. It provides for replacement of catabolized proteins in the axon and its endings, transport of enzymes for transmitter synthesis at the endings, movement of macromolecular precursors of cytoskeletal elements, and feedback from the periphery, contributing to regulation of the synthetic activity of the cell body. Unfortunately, however, retrograde transport can be a liability because it may carry tetanus toxin and neurotropic viruses such as those of herpes simplex and rabies directly to cell bodies in the CNS.

Traditionally, the complex interconnections within the CNS could only be studied by cutting nerve axons, waiting for them to degenerate, and then searching for the affected cell bodies—a laborious and uncertain method. In the past two decades, it has been possible for the neuroanatomist to take advantage of retrograde transport in axons to establish the location of the cell of origin. Particles of the enzyme horseradish peroxidase injected in the periphery are taken up by nerve endings and transported to the cell bodies, where they can be detected by a histochemical reaction for the enzyme. Conversely, a tracer, such as a radiolabeled amino acid, injected near neuron cell bodies will be taken up and carried by anterograde transport to the endings of the axons where the radioactivity can be detected by autoradiography. The distribution of axons from nerve centers can, thus, be studied and the "wiring diagram" deduced with considerable accuracy.

The mechanisms of axonal transport have recently been under intensive study and it has become apparent that the microtubules play an important role in the fast component. Axonal microtubules have a fixed polarity with their "plus end" toward the axon ending and their "minus end" toward the cell body. They are constantly turning over with tubulin dimers being added at their plus end and depolymerized at their minus end at about the same rate. In the absence of rough endoplasmic reticulum in the axoplasm and protein synthesis confined to the perikaryon, its products are conveyed down the axon in small vesicles. A microtubule associated protein, *kinesin,* is the motor responsible for anterograde transport. One end of this molecule attaches to a vesicle, and the binding site on the other end undergoes cyclic interaction with the wall of a microtubule, resulting in movement of the vesicle toward the plus end at about 3 μm/s. The retrograde transport depends on another protein, *dynein,* which moves vesicles along microtubules toward the perikaryon. The mechanism of slow axonal transport is less clear. One hypothesis holds that the cytoskeleton of the axoplasm moves as a whole due to the continual polymerization at the distal end and depolymerization at the proximal end, and the axoplasmic matrix moves with it. Other explanations will no doubt be forthcoming.

In developing neurons, microtubules are believed to have an important role in elongation of the axon toward its target cell. In the growth cone, at the distal end of the axon, the microtubules occur in bundles and are connected by regularly spaced cross-bridges consisting of another protein, *dynamin.* It is proposed that, in the presence of ATP and a co-factor, dynamin acts as a motor, causing some microtubules to slide relative to others in the bundle. The resulting elongation of the bundle of overlapping microtubules is believed to contribute to the advance of the growth cone.

Axons of motor neurons may be up to 1 m in length. On reaching their targets, a second phase of growth begins in which the axon thickens. Concurrently, neurofilaments become the most abundant cytoskeletal elements of the axoplasm and there is suggestive evidence that they are involved in determining the diameter of the axon. This dimension is important because axon caliber is the principal determinant of its conduction velocity. Under experimental conditions in which neurofilament mRNA in the cell body is diminished, fewer neurofilaments are formed and the axon diameter is decreased.

The axons of many neurons have a prominent sheath of *myelin,* a sleeve of material that is highly refractile in the fresh condition and appears black in tissues fixed in osmium tetroxide. The myelin sheath of the axon is not a part of the neuron but an enveloping layer produced by ensheathing glial cells, called Schwann cells (see below). The presence or absence of a myelin sheath exerts a major influence on the conduction velocity of the nerve axon. Because myelin is associated only with axons, myelin provides a convenient criterion for their recognition. There are, however, numerous *unmyelinated axons.* In electron micrographs of the CNS, these may appear quite similar to dendrites but can usually be distinguished by their greater number of neurofilaments.

Along its course, an axon may give rise to lateral branches, *axon collaterals.* Unlike dendritic branches, which diverge at acute angles, these generally depart at right angles. In some instances, axons may display an extensive system of collaterals which individually ramify into even finer branches. In such cases, the total length of axon may approach, or even exceed, that of the dendrites and can extend the sphere of influence of the neuron to a great number of other neurons—a key principle of neural organization known as *divergence.* On the other hand, axon collaterals and axon terminals may combine to form a plexus of great complexity, enveloping the cell bodies of other neurons and exemplifying an equally fundamental principle, *convergence.* In the simplest case, the tips of one or two twigs make very localized contacts with the dendrites or soma of another neuron. At the other extreme, the terminal arborizations of axons may exhibit several orders of branching, varying greatly in number, shape, and distribution. These branches often assemble into compact networks that surround the body of the postsynaptic cell in the form of a basket or twist around its dendrites like a clinging vine. In all of these specialized endings, the axon transmits signals across synapses to other neurons, or to muscle or glandular cells.

DISTRIBUTION AND DIVERSITY OF NEURONS

The core of the CNS, the *gray matter* (Fig. 11–15), contains the cell bodies of the neurons, their dendrites, and the proximal parts of their axons, along with the terminal reaches of axons arriving from other regions. Clusters of functionally related cell bodies in the gray matter are referred to as *nuclei* (not to be confused with cell nuclei). Surrounding the gray matter is a zone devoid of nerve cell bodies but containing axons from perikarya in the gray matter or in ganglia of the PNS. This zone is *white matter,* so named because the axons are invested by myelin, which is glistening white in the fresh state. Bundles of myelinated axons in the white matter, called *tracts,* are cable-like functional groupings of nerve fibers. In the cerebral hemispheres, cerebellum, and roof of the midbrain, additional gray matter with neuronal perikarya arranged in distinct layers forms a *cortex* outside the white matter.

As indicated earlier, a great variety of neurons can be distinguished in the CNS on the basis of shape, size, position of the cell body, and the number, length, and mode of branching of their processes (Fig. 11–2). Neurons may have long axons that leave the gray matter, traverse the white matter, and terminate at some distance in another part of the gray matter. Or, axons may leave the CNS and end elsewhere in the body. Traditionally, such large cells with long axons have been called *Golgi type-I neurons;* they include the neurons contributing axons to the peripheral nerves and to the tracts of the brain and spinal cord.

In other neurons, the axon is relatively short and does not stray far from the perikaryon; such *Golgi type-II neurons* are usually small and are especially numerous in the cerebral and cerebellar cortices and in the retina. A recent and more useful scheme of classification recognizes *projection neurons* and *local-circuit neurons;* here, the classification rests on whether the cell is involved in long-distance or local communication, rather than on cell size and the length of the axon.

The shape of the perikaryon may be spherical, ovoid, pyriform, fusiform, or polyhedral and its size may also vary from 4 μm (smaller than an erythrocyte) in certain dwarf neurons to 150 μm in some giants. The pyramidal cells of Betz in the mammalian cerebral cortex and the paired Mauthner cells in the medulla oblongata of certain fishes and amphibia are large enough to be seen with the naked eye.

A clear manifestation of the position and function of a neuron in the overall circuitry of the nervous system is its *polarity,* i.e., the number of poles or processes stemming from its cell body (Fig. 11–6). True *unipolar neurons* are rare in vertebrates except in early embryonic stages. They are, however, the preeminent population in invertebrates, displaying a single process, or neurite, that has both dendritic and axonal properties. In *bipolar neurons,* a process projects from each end of a fusiform cell body. Cells of this type are found in the vestibular and cochlear ganglia and in the nasal olfactory epithelium. During early development, neurons of the other craniospinal ganglia are also bipolar, but in time the two processes shift around the perikaryon and combine into one. Such neurons are, therefore, *pseudounipolar.* As this single process lengthens, it may tangle about the globular cell body and travel some distance to the region of fusion where it divides, like the letter T. One branch (usually slightly thicker than the other) leads distally in a peripheral nerve, the other proximally to the CNS in a posterior nerve root. Such cells serve as primary sensory neurons. Except for the smallest examples, the stem process and both branches of pseudounipolar neurons are myelinated. All these processes are axonal, displaying the structural features of axons and propagating nerve impulses. There may be short dendritic processes of some sort, but these are found far out in the periphery at the end of the distal

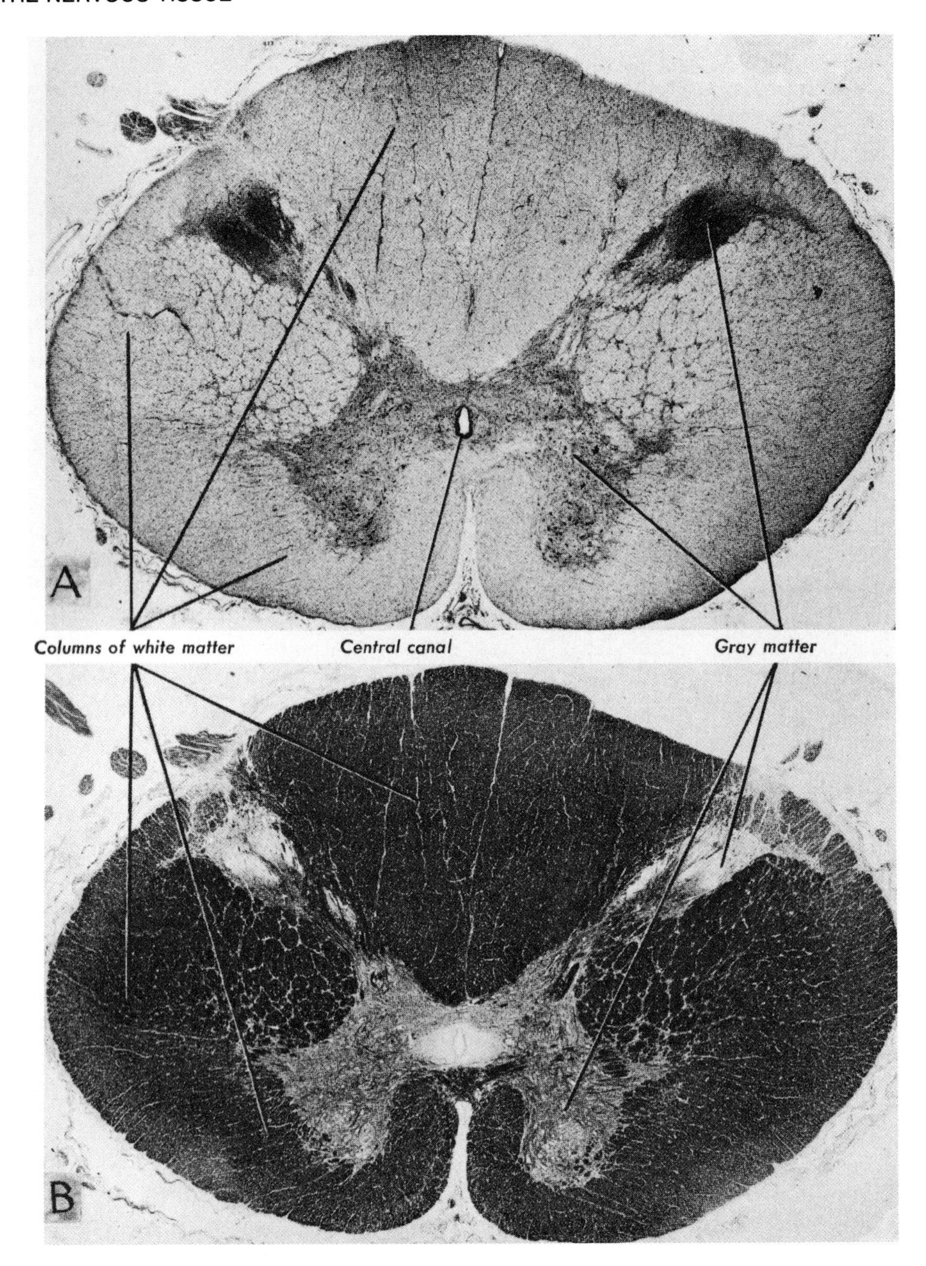

Figure 11–15. Sections through human upper cervical spinal cord stained with thionine (A) to show cells and with the Weigert–Weil method (B) to show myelinated fibers. Note the external arrangement of the fibers (white matter) and the central, cruciate area containing the cell bodies (gray matter). The ventral surface is below. (Courtesy of P. Bailey.)

branch, often in association with some kind of receptor structure.

Dorsal root ganglion cells are atypical, occurring in fairly small numbers (a few million), but they exemplify the variety and versatility of neurons. They receive no inputs from other neurons, except for presynaptic axoaxonic endings that regulate transmission by their central branches as they enter the central gray matter. What integrative capacity they have resides in a remote dendritic shrub in some sensory region of the body, with the intervening length of the axon serving to speed sensory messages inward to the CNS. The perikaryon has only trophic significance, and the sensory impulse passes it by at the axonal branch point, only secondarily backfiring the cell body by way of the stem process.

Most vertebrate neurons are *multipolar*. This type of nerve cell is the hallmark of the CNS and the kind most commonly studied in neuroanatomy. The integrative power of the nervous system is rooted in such cells and communications within the CNS and with the effector organs depends on them. Their variety is so great that it has been said that there are more kinds of cells in the brain of a mammal than in all the rest of the body. In multipolar neurons the shape of the cell body is largely determined by the number and arrangement of the dendrites, but the configuration of the dendritic tree depends more on the number, direction of approach, mode of arrival, and diversity of afferent axons.

Stellate, or star-shaped, neurons include the motor neurons of the spinal cord and brain stem, whereas pyramidal cells are characteristic of the cerebral cortex. The Purkinje cells of the cerebellar cortex have the most specialized form known (Figs. 11–5 and 11–12). One to four thick dendrites with stubby spines, arising from a flask-shaped body, branch profusely to form a dense arborization in which the branchlets bear tens of thousands of finer thorns with a delicate thread-like stem and a knobby end. The dendritic tree has a very orderly appearance, like a well-trimmed hedge. It is relatively flat, being 300–400 μm wide but only 15–20 μm deep, and shaped like a fan turned at a right angle to the axis of the cerebellar convolution in which it lies. This cell type has enormous integrative capacity, for hundreds of thousands of afferents terminate in various ways on specific parts of its widespread dendritic tree. The Purkinje cell is a good example of a Golgi type-I cell, or a projection neuron, because it has a long axon that descends into the white matter and runs to distant target cells deep in the cerebellum or in the brain stem.

Many other types of cells are found in the cerebral and cerebellar cortices. Among these are diminutive *granule cells* that have a few short dendrites radiating in all directions, whereas the axon and its collaterals remain in the vicinity of the cell or at least within the cortical gray matter. These cells would be classified as Golgi type-II cells, or as local-circuit neurons (LCNs). Perhaps the most interesting neurons are the archaic and deceptively simple-looking cells found in the reticular formation of the brain stem. These come in many sizes, but most have an angular perikaryon and long sparsely branched dendrites with few thorns. Their form, like that of the Purkinje cell, suggests great integrative capacity and an even larger sphere of influence, but this is achieved in a different way. The dendrites reach out at right angles to the long axis of the brain stem toward various ascending and descending tracts, intermingling with axons and axon collaterals of these tracts. The axon typically has long ascending and descending branches with a profusion of collaterals, at many different levels, infiltrating numerous centers. At first inspection, these sprawling neurons convey an impression of great disorder, yet they are found in the core of the brain in areas involved in the delicate control of homeostasis. Apparently their patterns of dendritic and axonal branching permit the widest possible range of inputs and outputs and are, thus, ideally suited for control of sleep and wakeful states, arousal, attention, emotion, mood, and regulation of sensory and motor activity.

A more complete description of the wealth of different kinds of neurons would be beyond the scope of a text of histology, but the few examples presented above may give some appreciation of the complexity of the CNS and the relation of cell form to cell function. From studies in which electron microscopy has been combined with classical chrome-silver-staining methods, it has become apparent that each ganglion, nucleus, or cortical area is made up of a characteristic variety of neurons and a highly ordered meshwork of dendritic, axonal, and neuroglial processes having the relationships and fine structure necessary for a particular type of organized activity. The term used to describe the feltwork of interwoven cell processes is the *neuropil.* The neuropil is of great importance in communication within the CNS, providing an enormous area for synaptic contact and functional interaction between cell processes. However, details of its dense, but purposeful, entanglements cannot be resolved in silver preparations, and the two-dimensional images in electron micrographs offer little insight into the three-dimensional relationships of the processes.

The number of cells in the entire human nervous system is astronomical, being estimated by some at one trillion. The tremendous increase in this number in the course of evolution has been mainly in the integrator cells or *interneurons* of the central nervous system. The number of *sensory neurons* and associated receptors has also increased, but to a far lesser extent. The number of *motor neurons* has remained relatively small and probably does not exceed two million. These cells, which collect influences from many central and peripheral sources before activating muscles, are often referred to as the *final common path.*

THE NERVE FIBER

A *nerve fiber* consists of an axon enveloped in a sheath of Schwann cells from near its origin to near its termination. Many peripheral axons also have a *myelin sheath* interposed between the Schwann cells and the axon. The myelin sheath is derived from the Schwann cell. Other axons lack a myelin sheath and simply lie in deep grooves in the surface of the Schwann cells, with multiple axons often enveloped by the same cell (Figs. 11–16 and 11–17). Therefore, it is customary to designate axons as *myelinated* or *unmyelinated.*

In the living, unfixed state, myelinated fibers appear as glistening tubes, and this refractile property of myelin is responsible for the white color of many peripheral nerves and fiber tracts in the CNS. In histological preparations, the appearance of nerve fibers depends on the technique used. After routine preparative procedures and hematoxylin and eosin staining, the lipid constituents of the myelin have been extracted during dehydration, leaving behind a loose network of *neurokeratin* around each faintly stained axon (Figs. 11–18 and 11–24). After supravital staining with methylene blue, the axon is stained blue and the intact myelin is unstained. The Weigert method darkens myelin, leaving the axon colorless or pale gray, whereas the Kluver–Barrera method stains myelin a blue-green. With fixation by glutaraldehyde and osmium tetroxide, the lipid of the myelin sheath is preserved and appears in cross sections as a nearly black ring around each faintly stained axon. Thus, although nerve fibers may be difficult to identify by routine histological methods, they can be clearly revealed by these special staining techniques.

THE SHEATH OF SCHWANN

The sheath of Schwann (formerly called the neurilemmal sheath) consists of flattened cells that form a thin sleeve around the myelin of a nerve fiber. Their nuclei are flattened and their attenuated cytoplasm contains a small Golgi apparatus and a few mitochondria. With the light microscope, the myelin and the Schwann sheath appear to be separate structures, but the electron microscope has revealed that the myelin is actually part of the Schwann cell, consisting of redundant cell membrane wrapped spirally around the axon (see below).

The Schwann sheath and its myelin are interrupted at regular intervals along the length of the nerve fiber by *nodes of Ranvier* (Fig. 11–18), which are sites of discontinuity between successive Schwann cells along the axon. There, the axon is partially uncovered, being only incompletely enclosed by small interdigitating processes at the margins of the two adjoining Schwann cells. The sheath of myelinated axons is, thus, divided into segments delimited by successive nodes of Ranvier and called *internodal segments.* Each consists of a single Schwann cell and its concentric lamellae of myelin around the axon. The internodal segments tend to be shorter near the terminal region of the fiber. Their length also varies from species to species and in different nerves within the same species, ranging from 200 μm to over 1000 μm. The longer and thicker the nerve fiber, the longer the internodal segments. If an axon emits collaterals, they emerge at a node of Ranvier.

In peripheral nerves fixed in osmium tetroxide, the myelin in each segment appears interrupted by cone-shaped discontinuities, the *incisures of Schmidt–Lantermann* (Figs. 11–16 and 11–22). There are several such incisures in each segment, having the specious appearance of oblique clefts on either side of the axon. In electron micrographs, it is apparent that these are not discontinuities, but are aligned sites of local separation of the myelin lamellae. The lamellae are continuous across these sites, but separated by residues of cytoplasm trapped in the spiral and presumably continuous with the cytoplasm of the cell body. Incisures are always present but may become more numerous with aging.

The exact relationship of the Schwann sheath to unmyelinated axons cannot be made out with the light microscope, but electron micrographs show that several axons occupy deep recesses in the surface of the Schwann cell (Figs. 11–17 and 11–18). The Schwann cell membrane is very closely applied to each of the axons around their circumference, but turns away from it to form a *mesaxon* consisting of two parallel membranes extending from the axon to the surface of the Schwann cell. Because a myelin sheath consists of multiple layers of Schwann cell membrane, it is perhaps misleading to describe axons surrounded by a single layer of Schwann cell membrane as

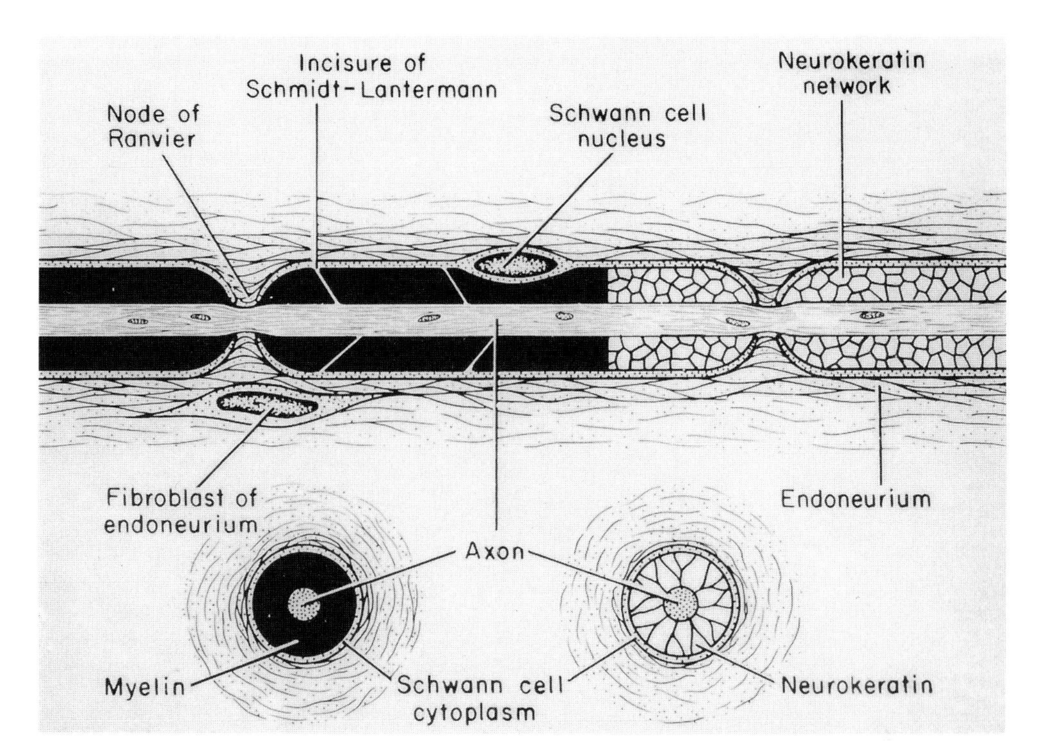

Figure 11–16. Diagrammatic representation of a longitudinal section of a single myelinated nerve and its endoneurial sheath. The left half of the drawing represents what would be seen after fixation with osmium tetroxide, which preserves the lipid of the myelin. Right half represents the appearance after ordinary methods of preparation, which extract the myelin and leave behind an artifactitious network of residual protein described as "neurokeratin." (Redrawn from Ham, A.W. 1965. Histology, 5th ed. Philadelphia, J.B. Lippincott Co.)

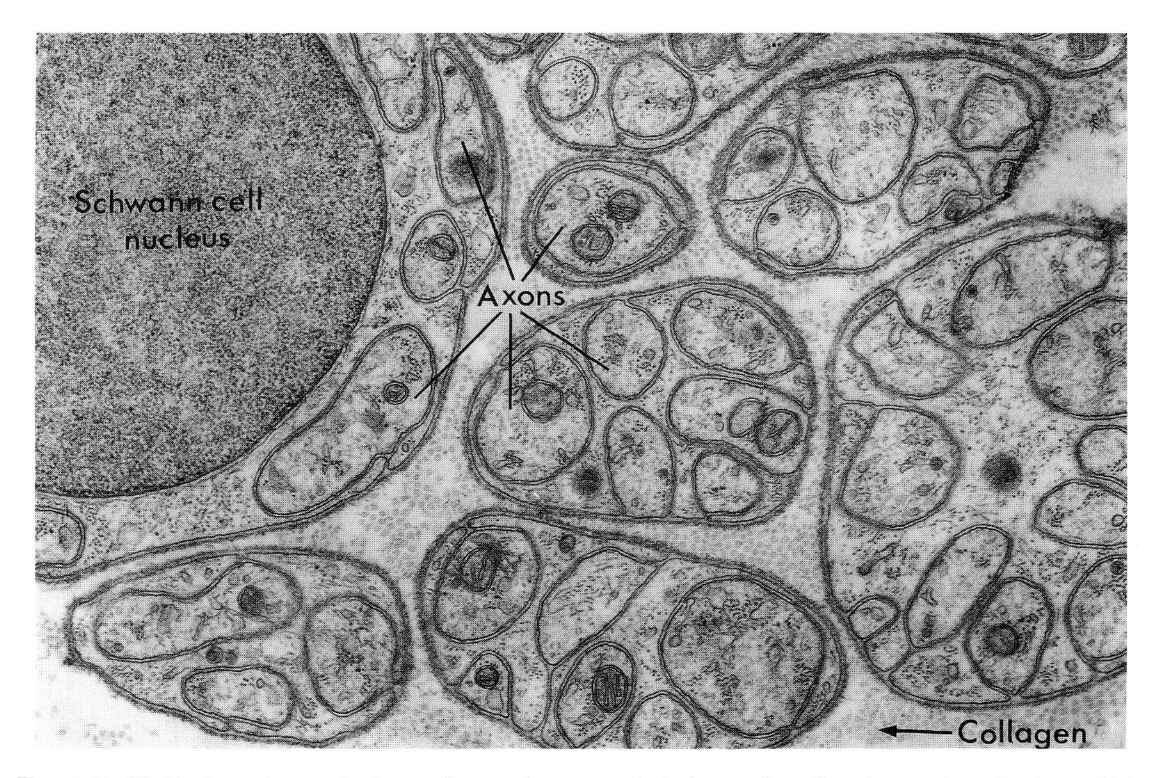

Figure 11–17. Electron micrograph of a small area of an unmyelinated nerve from the rat mesentery showing multiple axons associated with the cross-sectional profile of each Schwann cell. Between these fasciles of unmyelinated axons are unit fibrils of collagen of the endoneurium.

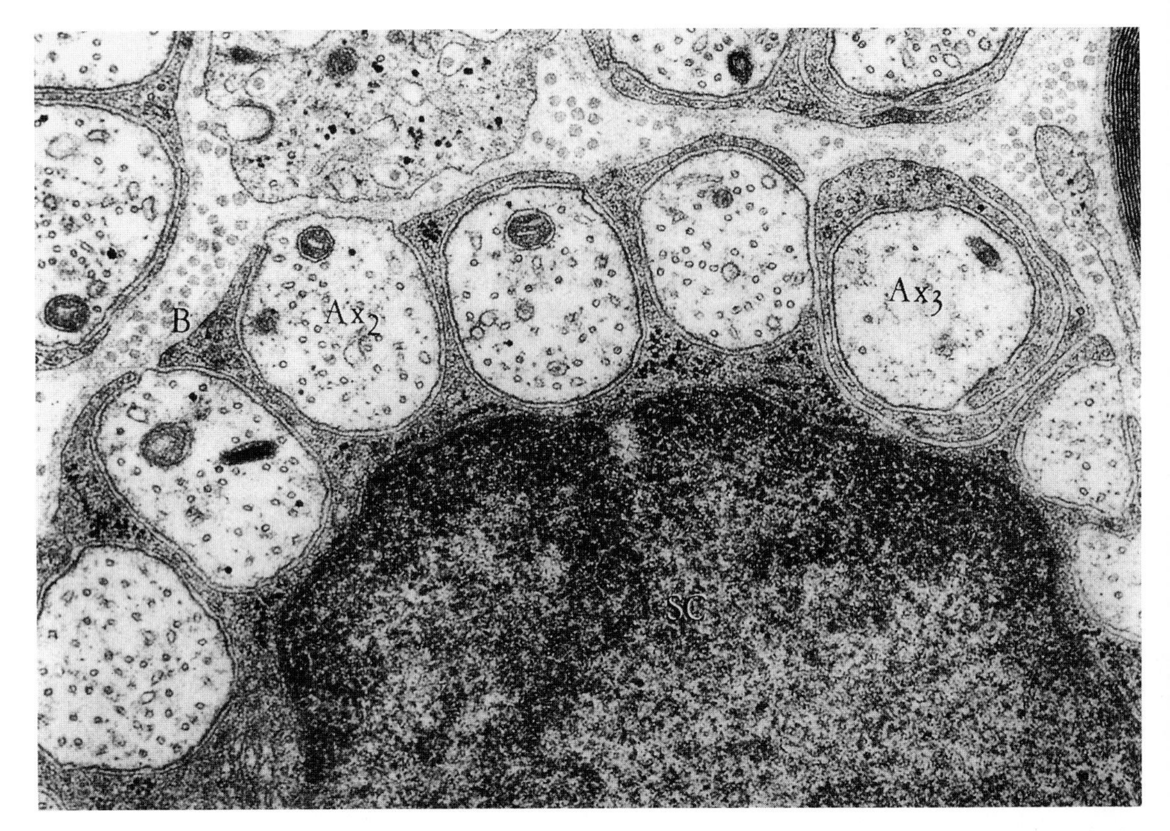

Figure 11–18. Electron micrograph of a Schwann cell in a peripheral nerve showing several unmyelinated axons occupying deep recesses in its surface. Most are completely surrounded by Schwann cell cytoplasm, but one (Ax 2) is only partially enclosed. In such cases, the axon is covered only by the basal lamina (B). Another unmyelinated axon (AS 3) appears to be embedded in this Schwann cell, but is actually surounded by a completely separate process which is probably an extension of the next Schwann cell in the row. (Micrograph from Peters, A., S.L. Palay, and H. deF. Webster. 1991. The Fine Structure of the Nervous System, 3rd ed. New York, Oxford University Press.)

"unmyelinated," implying that they are uncovered. They are covered by a single layer of membrane and the cytoplasm of the enveloping Schwann cell.

Schwann cells are essential to the viability and normal functioning of the axons of peripheral nerves. In regeneration following nerve transection or other injury, an axon grows from the proximal stump along the path formed by the Schwann cells, and these undergo a number of changes essential to the establishment of appropriate connections and resumption of normal function.

THE MYELIN SHEATH

There has long been great interest in the organization of the myelin sheath. Before the advent of the electron microscope, X-ray diffraction analysis suggested that it was composed of concentric layers of mixed lipids alternating with thin layers of the protein neurokeratin. Within the layers, the lipid molecules were thought to be oriented with their hydrocarbon chains extending radially and their polar groups aligned at the aqueous interface and loosely bonded to the proteins. In general, this interpretation of the molecular organization of myelin has been confirmed by electron microscopy, which has shown that the alternating layers of mixed lipid and proteins are, in fact, successive layers of Schwann cell membrane wrapped spirally around the axon.

In electron micrographs of high magnification, compact myelin appears as a series of alternating light and dark lines with a 12-nm repeat (Fig. 11–19). Bounding each repeating unit is the dark *major dense line,* about 3 nm thick, representing the apposition of the cytoplasmic surfaces of the Schwann cell membrane. Between major dense lines is the less dense *intraperiod line,* which has been interpreted as representing the apposition of the outer leaflets of the Schwann cell membrane. How-

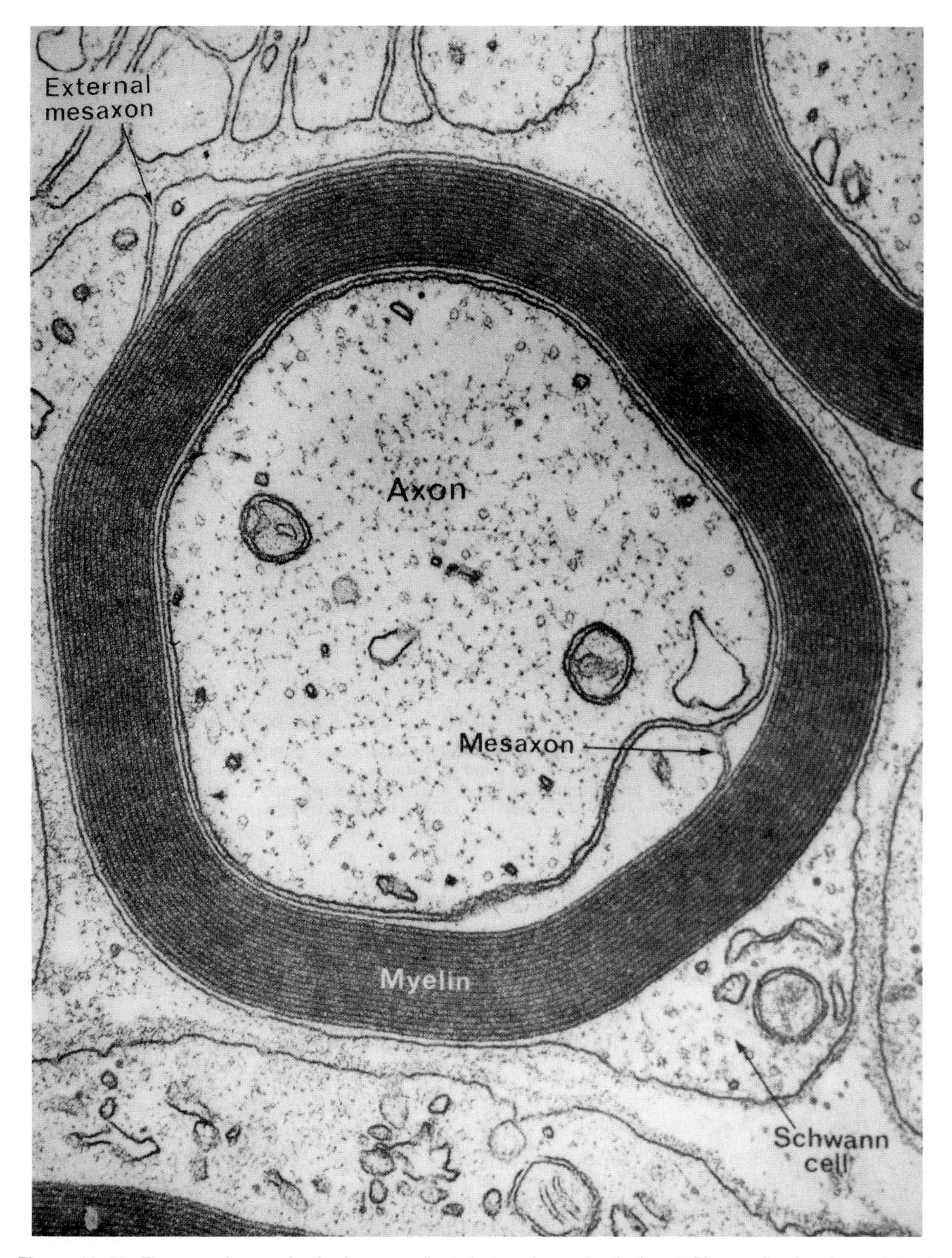

Figure 11–19. Electron micrograph of a large myelinated nerve in a rat spinal root. The myelin sheath consists of a multilayered spiral wrapping of Schwann cell membrane. Two apposed portions of Schwann cell membrane from the internal mesaxon extend from the periaxonal space to the innermost layer of myelin. Similarly the two membranes extending from the outermost turn of myelin to the endoneurial space are called the external mesaxon. (Micrograph from Coggeshall, R. 1979. Anat. Rec. 194:201.)

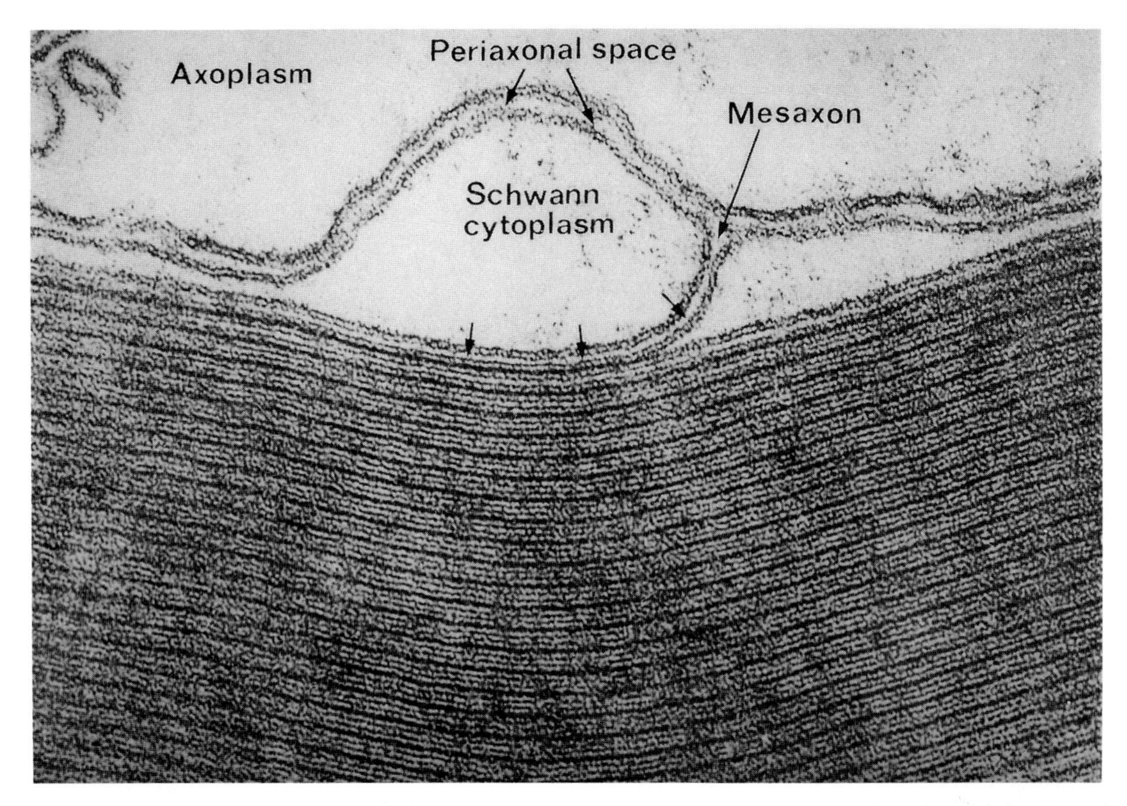

Figure 11–20. At high magnification, it can be seen that the periaxonal space continues into the cleft between the opposing external leaflets of the membranes forming the mesaxon. This cleft, in turn, is continuous with a narrow intraperiod gap in the innermost turn of the myelin sheath (at arrows). (Micrograph from Coggeshall, R. 1979. Anat. Rec. 194:201).

ever, in recent studies based on high-resolution micrographs of optimally fixed myelin in spinal roots, a narrow cleft (2 nm) is evident between the membranes (Fig. 11–20). This *intraperiod gap* is continuous through the myelin spiral from the periaxonal to the endoneurial extracellular space. Very small tracer molecules such as lanthanum can enter it, but rows of tight junctions block passage of larger molecules.

Externally, the Schwann cell is covered by a basal lamina and it, in turn, by endoneurium. Where the myelin sheath is interrupted at a nodes of Ranvier, the basal lamina turns inward covering the minute finger-like processes (paranodal loops) of the adjoining Schwann cells. On reaching the axon, the basal lamina continues over its surface to the paranodal loops of the next Schwann cell, where it turns outward again. Successive Schwann cells and the axonal surface at the nodes are, thus, surrounded by a thin continuous sleeve of basal lamina. Persistence of such sleeves after injury to the nerve serves to guide the regenerating axons along the right path.

The gap between the Schwann cells (Fig. 11–21) has physiological significance in that it permits current flow between the axoplasm and its surround during propagation of the action potential. Almost no current flows through the axonal membrane in the internodal segments owing to its insulation by the surrounding myelin. Because current can only flow outward at the nodes of Ranvier, only the nodal regions undergo depolarization. Conduction of the nerve impulse, therefore, does not proceed continuously along the axonal membrane, but each depolarized node initiates depolarization in the succeeding node by flow of current through the axoplasm and the extracellular fluid. This regenerative propagation of the nerve impulse is called *saltatory conduction.* It is more rapid and requires less energy than continuous conduction along the axonal membrane, as occurs in unmyelinated fibers.

The above interpretation of the significance of the nodes of Ranvier for conduction is widely accepted, but some investigators consider the gaps between successive Schwann cells to be artifacts. The gaps cannot be seen in fresh nerves with phase contrast microscopy, and it is claimed that, in vivo, the ends of the Schwann cells are closely interdigitated with no intervening intercellular space and that the images seen with light and electron microscopy are caused by shrinkage during fixation and dehydration of the specimen. This possibility may deserve more consideration than it has received, but the majority of investigators are convinced that the electron microscopic images are valid and that the relationships of the Schwann cell processes do not preclude nodal current flow.

The stages of myelinization can be observed in developing nerves. It begins with a single turn of a pair of Schwann cell membranes around the axon, progressing to many turns followed by compaction of the myelin by elimination of the intervening cytoplasm (Fig. 11–22). The mechanism of formation of the spiral, consisting of a few to more than 50 turns, is still poorly understood. It has been suggested that the spiral disposition of the lamellae is established during myelinization by rotation of the sheath cell with respect to the axon. It is difficult, however, to imagine how such movements could be initiated or controlled to produce the uniformly lamellated structure observed. It is even more unlikely that the myelin spiral results from rotation of the axon during its growth. If this were the mechanism, the direction of the spiral would be uniform throughout all of the internodal segments, and such is not the case. It is possible that early turns are produced by Schwann cell movement, and later turns result from amplification of total membrane area by continuous insertion of membrane constituents into it wherever it overlies the cytoplasm. The mechanism of generation of the myelin spiral remains a mystery.

Myelin also occurs in the CNS, in an amount varying with the caliber of the axons. In general, axons of major tracts, which represent long-distance connections, have thick myelin sheaths and, hence, high conduction velocity. Similarities to peripheral myelin include the presence of nodes of Ranvier and incisures in the sheaths of the larger fibers, but there are also important differences. Central myelin is not made by Schwann cells which are found only in the PNS. It is made by a type of *neuroglial cell* called the *oligodendrocyte,* which will be discussed in more detail later. In contrast to the Schwann cell, which forms a myelin sheath around a single axon, the oligodendrocyte can somehow produce helical turns of plasma membrane at the tips of its processes that can myelinate a number of axons, perhaps 10–60. Other peculiarities of central myelin include a paucity of associated cytoplasm, periodic thickenings of the axonal membrane at its point of contact with paranodal loops, presence of a longitudinal ridge of cytoplasm on the outside of the spiral, instead of a continuous enveloping layer of cytoplasm, and absence of the basal lamina around the ensheathing cell. There are also no connective tissue investments around the myelin sheaths in the CNS, as there are in the peripheral nerves.

During human development, peripheral

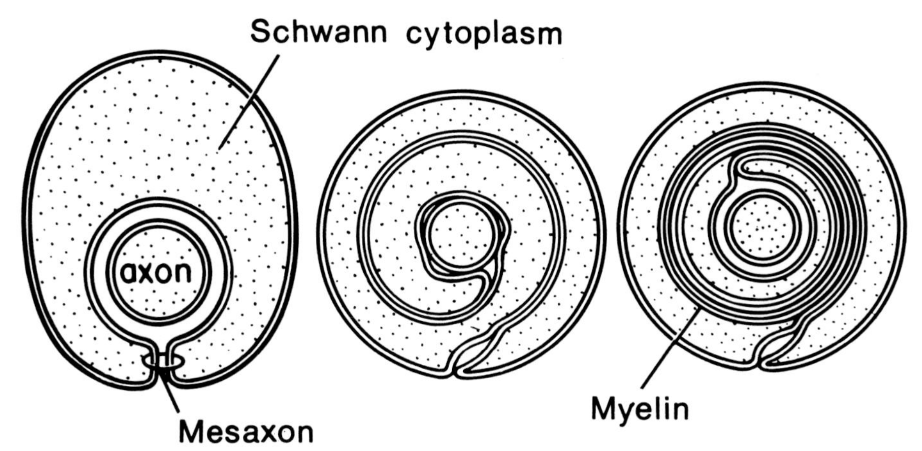

Figure 11–21. Diagrams illustrating the development of nerve myelin. (A) Earliest stage: axon enveloped by a relatively large Schwann cell. (B) Intermediate stage: unit membranes of the mesaxon and, to some extent, of the axon have come together, the line of contact representing the future intraperiod line of the myelin. (C) Later stage: a few layers of compact myelin have formed by contact of cytoplasmic surfaces of mesaxon loops to make the major dense line of myelin. (Redrawn from Robertson, J.D. 1960. Progr. Biophys. 10:349.)

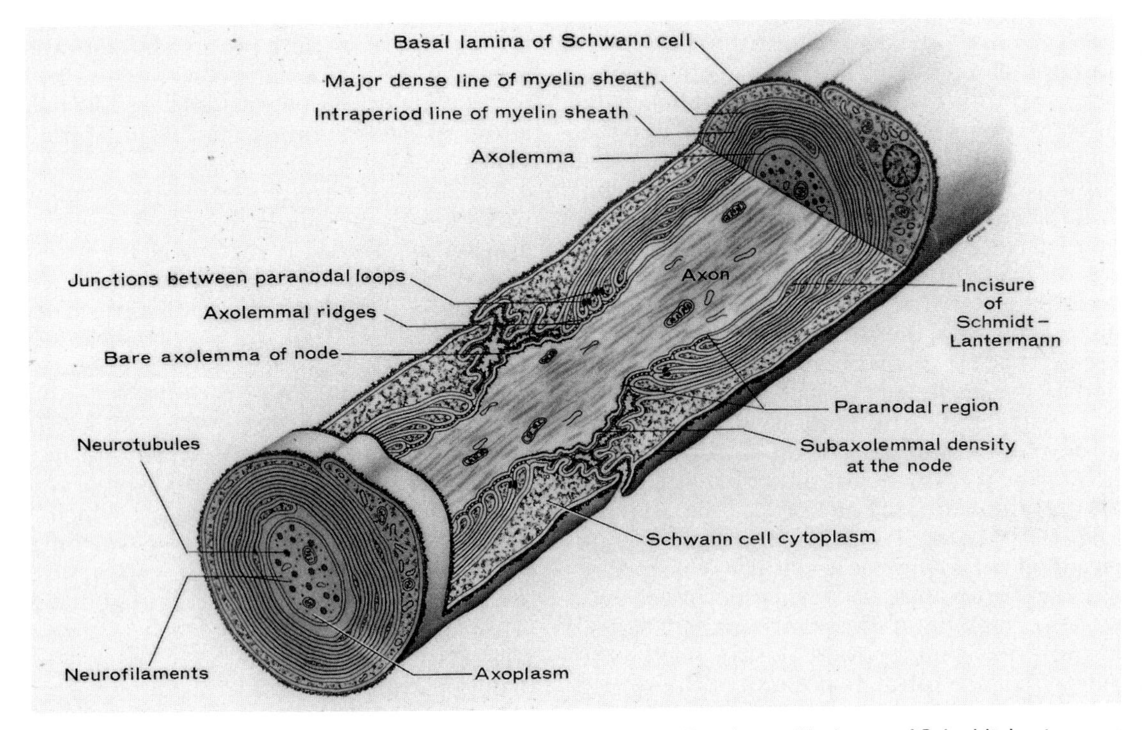

Figure 11–22. Diagrammatic representation of the myelin shealth, node of Ranvier, and incisures of Schmidt–Lantermann in a peripheral nerve. (Courtesy of Kent Morest.)

nerves and central tracts become myelinated at different times. Motor nerve roots are largely myelinated at birth, but the optic nerve and sensory roots lag behind by 3 or 4 months. The corticospinal tracts require a year for full myelinization, and commissural axons of the cerebral hemispheres, 7 years or more. In this protracted progressive process, the onset of many functions is correlated with the degree of myelinization, for example when the baby can see, begin to walk, perform directed movements, and so on.

The function of the myelin sheath is generally believed to be that of increasing the speed of conduction: from 1 m/s in slender unmyelinated axons, to nearly 120 m/s in heavily myelinate axons of large caliber. As indicated above, myelin serves as a high-resistance low-capacitance insulator. It confines the ionic current set up within the axon by the action potential generated at a node of Ranvier and forces it onward to the next node where membrane depolarization regenerates the potential. But in many neural pathways in both the central and peripheral nervous systems, speed of communication may be neither necessary nor desirable. Slower, but more persistent, delivery of impulses may better suit the function of the structure innervated. Thus, grouping of axons by Schwann cells, or oligodendrocytes, so as to provide a range of conduction velocities may be advantageous. It has been postulated that myelin may have a role in nutrition of the axon, based on the observations that tracers pass from the outer collar of Schwann cell cytoplasm inward along the cytoplasm in the incisures and that the tracer may later be found in vesicles and elements of the agranular reticulum in the axoplasm. However, it is not known whether metabolites follow this same pathway. Lastly, myelin may have a protective role assuring continuing conductivity: In demyelinating diseases, such as multiple sclerosis, axons denuded of myelin can still conduct impulses, albeit less rapidly and efficiently. The improvement in neural function seen during remissions is greater than would be expected from the degree of remyelinization that occurs.

PERIPHERAL NERVES

SHEATHS

The larger peripheral nerves are enclosed in three layers of tissue of differing character. From outside inward these are the *epineurium,* the *perineurium*, and the *endoneurium* (Figs. 11–23 and 11–24). The endoneurium is a delicate, loose connective tissue consisting of small fibrils of collagen, fibroblasts, fixed macrophages, capillaries, perivascular mast cells, and extracellular fluid. It is bounded internally by the basal lamina around the Schwann cells and externally by the relatively impermeable inner layer of the perineurium. Its collagen fibers tend to be randomly oriented and more concentrated near the nerve fibers and around the capillaries. Near the perineurium they are longitudinally oriented, somewhat thicker, and more closely packed. The extracellular fluid of the endoneurium is isolated from the general extracellular space of the body by the perineurium and epineurium and from the circulation by tight junctions between the endothelial cells of the capillaries. This isolation of the endoneurium is believed to be important for maintaining the appropriate physicochemical environment for the axons and for protecting them from harmful agents. Unfortunately, if it chances to be invaded by bacteria or neurotropic viruses, the sleeve of endoneurism can provide a route through which they can spread and ultimately enter the CNS.

The *perineurium* is more dense and consists of a few to several layers of flattened fibroblast-like cells bounded both internally and externally by a basal lamina. In larger nerves, layers of longitudinally oriented collagen fibers and a few elastic fibers are found between the layers of cells. The squamous cells within each layer often interdigitate along their margins and may have tight junctions. These epithelium-like layers of tightly adherent cells present a significant barrier to passage of particulate tracers, dye molecules, or toxins into the endoneurium, thus protecting the *perineurial compartment*, the controlled environment within the endoneurium.

The outermost sheath, the *epineurium*, envelops the nerve and sends extensions into it to surround the separate nerve fascicles within it, if such exist. It is a relatively thick and strong investment composed of dense irregular connective tissue in which longitudinally oriented collagen fibers predominate. Unusually thick fibers of elastin are also present, as well as fibroblasts, occasional fat cells, and perivascular mast cells associated with the walls of arterioles and venules. The collagen fibers are so deployed as to limit the extent to which the nerve can be stretched, either by movements of the body or by externally applied forces. Without this layer, the fragile

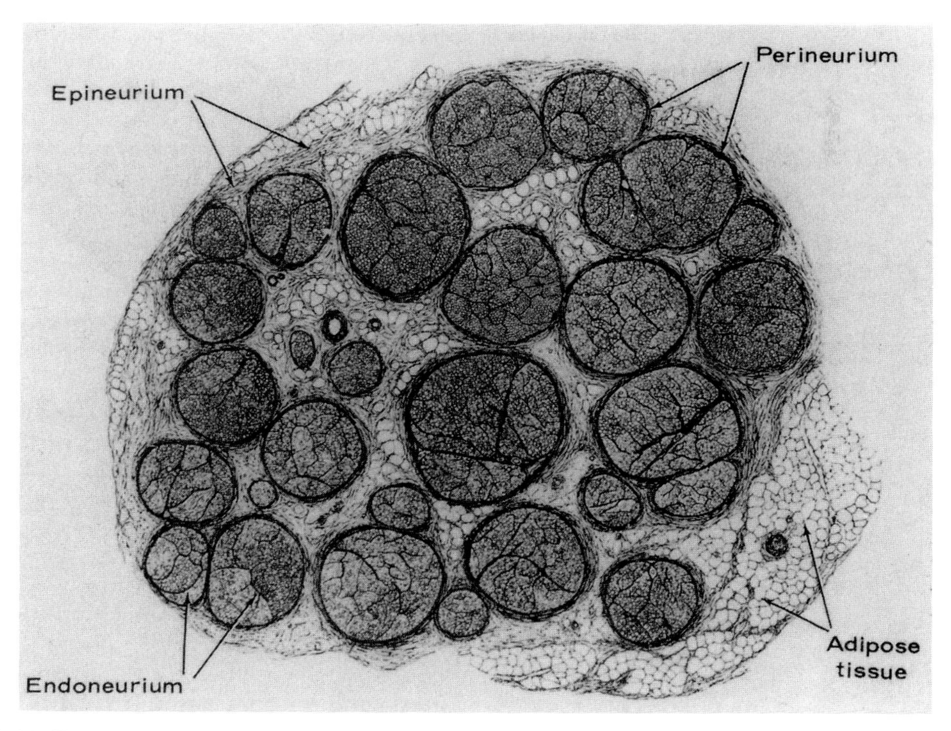

Figure 11–23. Drawing of a histological cross section of a human ulnar nerve at very low magnification illustrating the perineurial adipose tissue, epineurium, perineurium, and endoneurium. (From Bargmann, W. 1959. Histologie und mikroschopische Anatomie des Menschen. Stuttgart, Georg Thieme.)

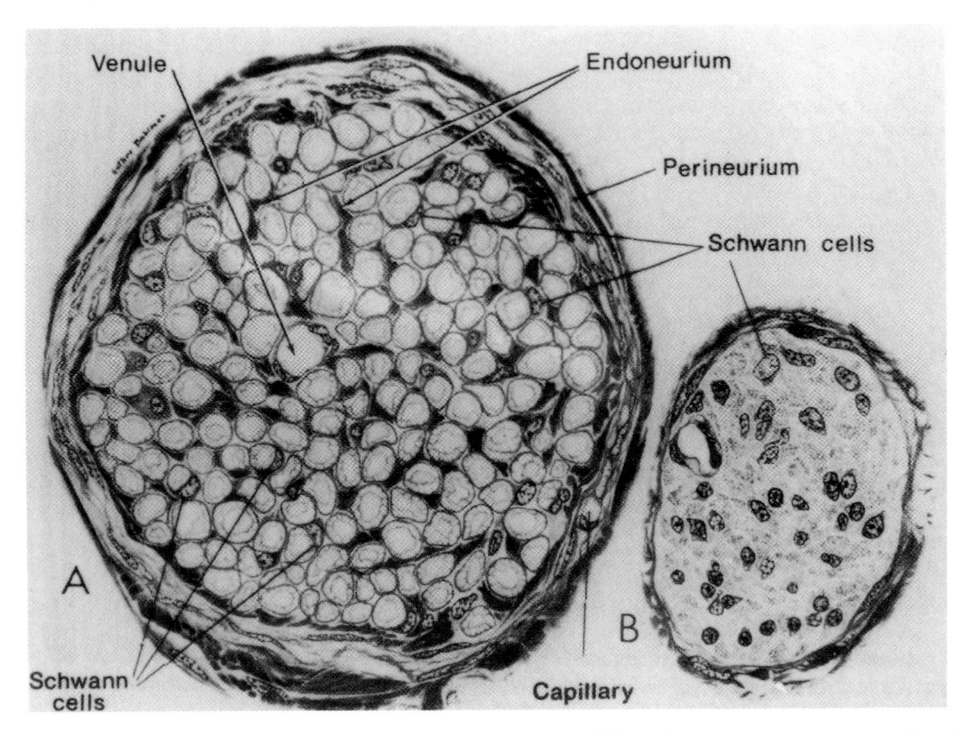

Figure 11–24. Drawing of a myelinated (A) and unmyelinated nerve (B) as they appear in cross section in routine histological preparations. The lipid of the myelin sheaths in (A) has been extracted in specimen preparation.

axons within the nerve might be injured or stretched to the breaking point. At the proximal end of the spinal and cranial nerves, the epineurium is continuous with the dura mater, the tough outer envelope of the central nervous system.

As large nerves branch in their course to the periphery, the epineurium is progressively reduced in thickness, and in small nerves it is usually absent, its residues having been incorporated into the perineurium. That sheath, in turn, diminishes in thickness and eventually is reduced to a single sleeve of flattened cells that ends near the termination of enclosed axons. There, the endoneurium is reduced to a network of delicate reticular fibers around the Schwann cells and their enclosed axons.

Turning now to the nerve fibers in the core of peripheral nerves, it is customary to classify them according to diameter because speed of conduction varies with the diameter of the fiber. They range from 0.3 μm to 20 μm and, in one system of classification, letter prefixes (A, B, C) are used to designate three size categories. Large type-A fibers conduct at from 15 to 120 m/s (270 miles per hour). These include the skeletomotor fibers and most of the somatosensory fibers. The latter, in order of increasing velocity, conduct fast pain, temperature, tactile sensation, and afferent impulses from muscle. Type-B fibers, which include many autonomic and visceral afferents, conduct at 3 to 15 m/s. Type-C are small unmyelinated fibers that conduct at 0.5 to 2 m/s and carry visceromotor and some sensory impulses (slow pain). Over two-thirds of the fibers in nerves are type-C. Unfortunately, there is another system of classification that was developed for somatosensory nerves only, and it uses Roman numerals (I, II, III, IV). Its fastest conducting fibers, group-Ia, originate in muscle spindles and are among the largest fibers in type-A of the other system of classification. Its slowest, group-IV, conduct pain, corresponding to the C-fibers of the other system and are found in the dorsal roots. All fibers between these extremes (groups-Ib, -II, and -III) fall into type-A of the other system.

There is a clear segregation of functionally distinct nerve fibers in the *spinal roots* emerging from the spinal cord. The anterior root contains motor fibers: large, heavily myelinated fibers innervating extrafusal skeletal muscle fibers; smaller myelinated fibers to the intrafusal muscle fibers; and fine, thinly myelinated autonomic fibers. On the other hand, the posterior roots contain sensory fibers from the skin, muscles, tendons, joints, and viscera. More than half of the dorsal root fibers are very thin fibers distributed via the cutaneous rami. The relative numbers of myelinated and unmyelinated fibers vary widely in different spinal segments. In the mixed nerve trunks, distal to the spinal ganglia, the fibers of the anterior and posterior roots mingle, together with sympathetic fibers from the communicating rami.

THE NERVE IMPULSE

As previously stated, a major function of the axon is to carry electrical signals from the cell body of a neuron to a nerve ending on another cell. Having described the structure of nerves in some detail, it may be appropriate to review here the mechanism of the axon's signaling function. The *nerve impulse* that travels along the axon is a wave of transient membrane depolarization. In an unstimulated nerve, the concentration of positively and negatively charged ions in the cytoplasm and in the extracellular fluid are unequal, with a higher concentration of positive ions outside the cell and a higher concentration of negatively charged ions inside. This difference in charge across the membrane (about −70 mv) is the *resting potential.* It is maintained by an ion pump that enables the cell to move Na^+ ions out and K^+ ions in against their concentration gradients. This is achieved by controlling membrane permeability to those and other ions, by opening or closing specific ion channels in the plasmalemma, and by large intracellular anions to which the membrane is impermeable. Both sodium and potassium are positively charged, and the total concentration of positive ions is greater outside of the cell. Therefore, in a resting neuron, the inner aspect of the membrane is negative relative to its outer aspect, and is, thus, said to be *polarized.*

A stimulus applied to a nerve opens sodium channels, permitting influx of Na^+ ions down their concentration gradient into the cytoplasm, reducing the total positive charge outside the cell and increasing it inside. As the Na^+ ion concentration inside the axon equilibrates with that of the extracellular fluid, the membrane becomes *depolarized* and the resting potential at the site of stimulation disappears. The movement of ions across the membrane constitutes a current that generates an electrical signal called the *action potential.* The initial flux of Na^+ ions renders the axoplasm at that site positively charged, and a local circuit is established that enables current to flow, via the axoplasm and extracellular fluid, between the depolarized site and the surrounding polarized regions of the axolemma. This current triggers depolarization of the neighboring regions of the membrane.

The action potential, thus, spreads along the axon from the site of initial stimulation. As the influx of Na^+ ions reaches its peak, potassium channels in the axolemma open and a net outward flux of K^+ ions restores the membrane potential. The spread of the potential is unidirectional; on closure of the sodium channels in the repolarized site, the channels become refractory to further activation, thus preventing retrograde propagation of the wave of depolarization. The net effect of these events is propagation of the nerve impulse from the *spike trigger zone* (axon hillock plus initial segment) to the axon terminal. The changes described take place in milliseconds and the impulse travels along the axon, depending on its caliber and its degree of myelinization, at speeds up to 120 m/s.

When the axon terminal lies in skeletal muscle and is, therefore, a *neuromuscular synapse,* it releases its neurotransmitter, acetylcholine, from synaptic vesicles. Acetylcholine was the first transmitter identified and is the major transmitter of the PNS. It binds transiently to specific receptor channels in the postsynaptic membrane. These open, causing current to flow across the membrane and initiate an action potential in the sarcolemma. Unbinding of acetylcholine then causes the channels to close. In synapses of the CNS, a host of substances serve as neurotransmitters, including acetylcholine and a number of monoamines, peptides, and amino acids.

In recent years, ingenious methods have been developed to study the ion channels that mediate transmission between neurons. Artificial membranes of pure lipid are impermeable to ions, so it is the pore-like channels formed by the proteins in natural membranes that permit the transmembrane passage of charged ions that is necessary for conductivity. Some of these proteins have been isolated and characterized, and the DNA encoding their subunits has been cloned and sequenced. This has made it possible to change critical sequences of amino acids in the channel proteins and to observe the effects on their function. Functional artificial ion channels have even been synthesized by attaching long polyethylene chains around annular macrocyclic rings and incorporating these complexes into artificial lipid membranes. Such studies are contributing to our understanding of ion channels. There is reason to believe that a number of clinical disorders will be found to be due to defects in channel function.

NERVE ENDINGS

Peripheral nerve fibers—sensory, motor, or secretory—end in one or more terminal arborizations. Sensory endings which serve as sensory receptors are, in effect, dendrites lying far from the neuronal cell body (see unipolar neurons), whereas motor and secretory endings are axonal terminations. In general, the morphology of the ending is adapted to increase the surface of contact between the neuron and the structure innervated. Three groups of nerve terminations are distinguished: endings in muscle, endings in epithelium, and endings in connective tissue.

MOTOR NERVE ENDINGS IN SKELETAL MUSCLE

The ending of *somatic motor nerves* has been described in the previous chapter and need only be reviewed here. The motor neuron, together with the muscle fibers it innervates, is called a *motor unit.* Each motor nerve fiber branches to supply many muscle fibers. The myelin sheath around each branch of the nerve ends as it nears the muscle fibers, but the Schwann sheath continues to cover the axon terminal (Fig. 11–25). Muscle nuclei and mitochondria accumulate in the sarcoplasm beneath the *motor end plate,* and the terminal branches of the axon occupy grooves in the surface of the muscle fiber. Their axoplasm contains mitochondria and numerous synaptic vesicles (40–60 μm), but microtubules and neurofilaments usually terminate proximal to the end plate. The axolemma and sarcolemma are separated by a glycoprotein boundary layer that is continuous with the external lamina of the Schwann cell and that of the muscle fiber. The gap between the axon and the muscle fiber varies but may be as wide as 50 nm.

ENDINGS IN SMOOTH AND CARDIAC MUSCLE

In these tissues, thin unmyelinated nerve fibers emerge from nerve plexuses and approach the surface of muscle fibers. *Visceral motor axons* give rise to many slender terminal branches with small dilatations closely spaced along their length. These expansions contain synaptic vesicles and are referred to as *boutons en passant.* Such endings remain a short distance from the smooth or cardiac muscle cells and do not form specialized junctions with them. The *visceral sensory fibers,* on the other hand, ramify in the connective tissue between bundles of muscle fibers and may contact their surface. In cardiac muscle, the afferents permeate the myocardium as a multitude of thin fibers passing between the muscle trabeculae and ending, again without specialized contact, near the surface of the muscle fibers.

SOMATIC SENSORY RECEPTORS IN GENERAL

Acoustic, visual, or olfactory stimuli reach us from our environment, often from considerable distances, and are detected by specialized receptors in the ear, eye, or nose, highly complex organs of the special senses. However, the nervous system must also receive information about forces acting directly on the surface of the body and about other forces generated within the body. This is accomplished by highly diverse receptors in the tissues and organs that convert various forms of energy into action potentials in sensory nerves that carry this information to the CNS. The *transduction* of stimuli within the body to nerve impulses is carried out by various kinds of somatic sensory or *somesthetic receptors,* some of which will be described below. Such receptors always include the peripheral terminations of a primary sensory neuron, and, in some instances, also contain cells so arranged that they encapsulate the nerve ending. These associated cells are not neurons and are not themselves excitable, but they serve to modulate, amplify, or otherwise influence the threshold, speed, or duration of the transduction function of the receptor.

SENSORY NERVE ENDINGS IN SKELETAL MUSCLE

Sensory nerve endings of varying degrees of complexity are found in skeletal muscle. *Interstitial endings* are in the connective tissue between muscle fibers. They may be simple naked branches of axons or elaborate encapsulated structures. *Epilemmal endings* contact

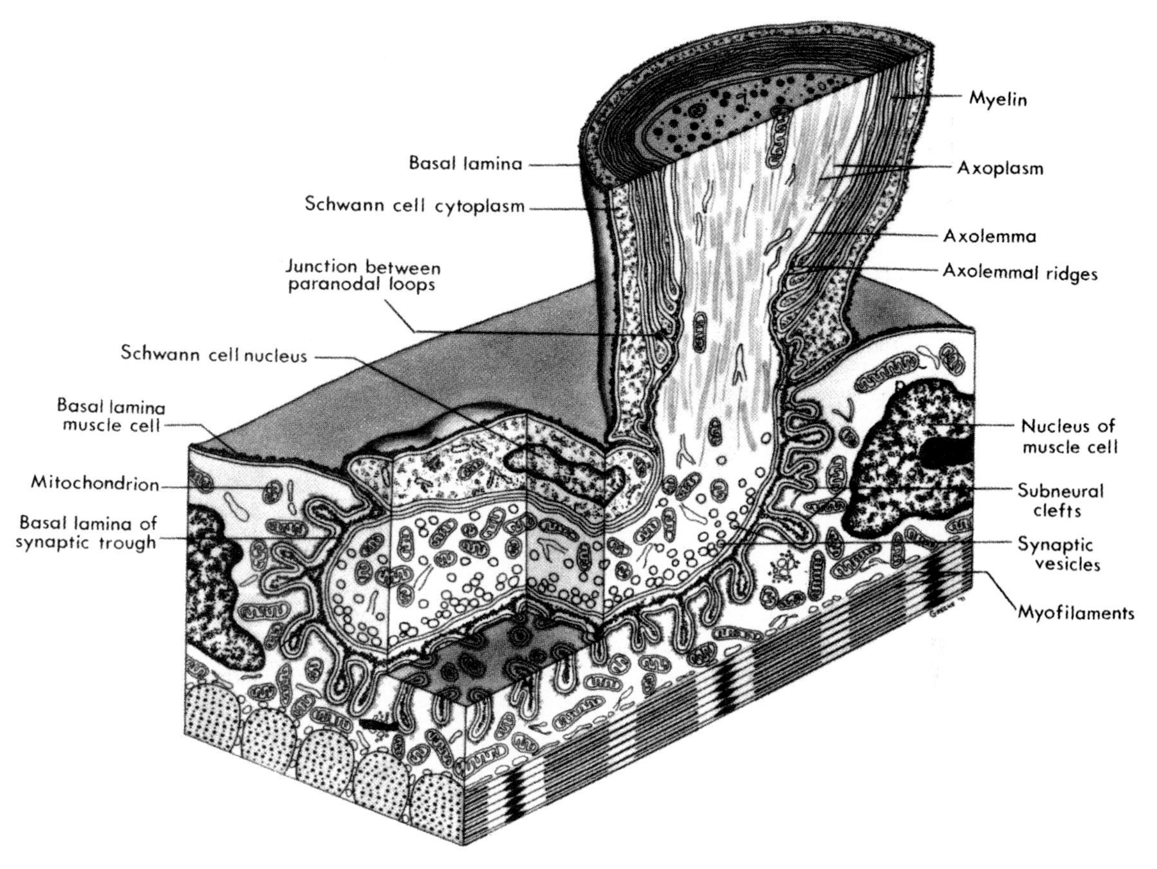

Figure 11–25. Diagrammatic representation of a myoneural junction (motor and plate) illustrating a typical chemical synapse in the peripheral nervous system. Synapses in the central nervous system have some features in common with this, but they occur between neurons and have no basal lamina or postjunctional folds. (Courtesy of D. Kent Morest.)

the muscle fibers. They may be simply tortuous axons spiraling around the muscle fiber, with varicose branches terminating in nodular expansions. In addition to these relatively simple endings, mammals have complex *neuromuscular spindles* in most of their muscles. These are 1–5-mm-long, narrow fusiform structures arranged between the muscle fascicles or near myotendinous junctions. Each spindle consists of a connective tissue capsule containing a gelatinous material through which 2 to 12 longitudinally oriented *intrafusal muscle fibers* run from one end of the spindle to the other. These fibers are shorter and more slender than the surrounding extrafusal muscle fibers. In their midportion, their cross-striated contractile filaments are replaced by an aggregation of nuclei. Two types of intrafusal fiber are distinguished on the basis of the arrangement of their nuclei. When the nuclei are aligned in a single row, it is called a *nuclear chain fiber*, and when they are closely clustered, with little or no order, it is a *nuclear bag fiber*. The bag fibers are few in number but longer (8–10 mm) than chain fibers, extending well beyond the ends of the capsule, and their rate of contraction is slower. The chain fibers are more numerous, shorter (4–5 mm), and are capable of fast (twitch) contractions. The spindles are situated within the interfascicular connective tissue of the muscle, but their intrafusal fibers are attached to the endomysium around the neighboring fascicles of extrafusal muscle fibers. As a result, they are stretched whenever the muscle as a whole is stretched.

Each neuromuscular spindle is supplied by myelinated sensory nerve fibers of two sizes. The thicker axons (group-1a) make *primary endings*, formerly described as annulospiral endings, on the nuclear region of all of the intrafusal fibers of the spindle, regardless of type. These axons signal irregular rate changes and, to some degree, the extent of muscle lengthening. Thinner axons (group-II) make *secondary endings* (formerly called flower-spray endings) near the nuclear region of chain fibers and provide a relatively faithful signal of the extent of muscle lengthening. Thus, these two types of nerve endings serve as *stretch afferents.* Both report static (steady-state) stretch to the CNS, but the primary endings are sensitive to the dynamic phases of stretch, especially to irregular changes in rate of stretch.

Neuromuscular spindles are also supplied by thin efferent axons called *gamma motor fibers,* to distinguish them from the large axons of the *alpha motor neurons* innervating the extrafusal muscle fibers. The gamma fibers come from small *gamma motor neurons* in the CNS and end on intrafusal muscle fibers in typical motor end-plates, stimulating contraction of their polar regions. This contraction does not contribute significantly to the tension produced by the muscle as a whole, but it does serve to stretch the non-contractile central region of the intrafusal fibers, where the primary endings are located, and this results in the stretch receptor firing more rapidly. In this way, the gamma efferent or *fusimotor system* acts constantly to regulate the sensitivity of the spindle to stretch over the normal range of muscle length. Spindle efferent discharge is, thus, maintained in an optimal midrange between extremes in either direction. This normal range varies, of course, for different types of movement.

The foregoing description of muscle spindles and their innervation has been considerably simplified. Their structure and function are highly complex and remain a challenging area in the study of motor control. *Beta motor fibers,* first described in muscles of nonmammals have now been identified in mammals. They innervate combinations of intrafusal and extrafusal fibers. Fusimotor regulation is now known to apply to both parameters of stretch. *Gamma dynamic fibers* end on bag fibers and, thus, enhance the primary afferent response in dynamic phases of stretch. *Gamma static fibers* supply chain fibers and, thus, enhance group-Ia discharge to static stretch. Spindle group-II afferents are regulated only by gamma static axons because secondary endings are mainly restricted to chain fibers. However, these details are of greater interest to the specialist than to students of histology, for whom the simplified explanation offered above is more than enough.

SENSORY NERVE ENDINGS IN TENDONS AND MYOTENDINOUS JUNCTIONS

In these structures, several kinds of nerve endings are observed. In the simplest of these, naked axons simply arborize over the surface of a tendon, and probably sense high tension and pain. More complex endings, called *Golgi tendon organs,* are found at the junction of the tendon with the intramuscular connective tissue, rarely within the tendon itself. The slender tendon organ, about 1 mm in length, has a thin capsule surrounding braided bundles of collagen fibers. At one end, 5 to 25 muscle fibers enter through a narrow orifice and end on the bundles of collagen fibers within the tendon organ. Intertwined with the bundles of collagen fibers are branches of a large, thickly myelinated axon that enters the capsule near its midpoint. Such axons comprise the group-Ib sensory fibers of peripheral nerves. In this designation, the "I" signifies their large diameter and high conduction velocity, and the "b" distinguishes them from the Ia axons that innervate the muscle spindles.

In contrast to muscle spindles, which lie *in parallel* with the muscle fibers, a Golgi tendon organ is *in series* with a relatively small set of muscle fibers and operates like a strain-gauge, responding to local intramuscular tension, not to change in muscle length. As the entering muscle fibers contract, the undulant collagen fibers, to which they attach, straighten, compressing the many branches of the axon that weave in and out among them. This compression depolarizes (excites) their mechanosensitive terminations. The local depolarizations are summed at a spike trigger zone within the capsule of the tendon organ, where they initiate action potentials that are propagated to the CNS.

Tendon organs are exquisitely sensitive and can respond to the contraction of even one muscle fiber. Their intrinsic muscle fibers belong to different motor units so that the discharge of each tendon organ signals the amount of force developed in different regions of the muscle. Thus, a tendon organ acts not only as an accurate stimulus transducer but also to sample local forces generated within the muscle. This integrative role is no doubt enhanced when input from all the tendon organs comes together centrally.

Complex connections in the CNS relate the activity of receptors in muscle and tendon to that of the alpha, gamma, and beta motor neurons, so that they participate in postural and phasic adjustments of the skeletal musculature. These CNS connections and the roles they play in motor control are a major field of investigation in modern neuroscience, but beyond the scope of this chapter. It will suffice to state that the activity of the muscle spindles, of mechanoreceptors in joints, of the vestibular apparatus of the inner ear all contribute to *proprioception* or "position sense." Awareness of the position of the body in space, of the position of the limbs, and of limb movements appears to depend, at least in part, on the muscle spindles, because our sense of joint angle seems to be derived from information about muscle length. The receptors of the joints themselves are thought to report only extremes of joint angle and pressure changes within the joint.

NERVES IN EPITHELIAL TISSUE

Endings in the epithelial layers of the skin and mucous membranes are probably only sensory, whereas in glandular epithelia some are secretory and others sensory, but there are no dependable morphological criteria for distinguishing the receptors from effectors in histological sections. Endings in the lacrimal and salivary glands, the kidney, and other epithelial organs are all unmyelinated sympathetic fibers forming networks just outside of the basal lamina of the epithelium. From there, branches penetrate the lamina, often forming a second network on its inner surface, and end between the bases of the glandular cells.

Free sensory endings in epithelia are abundant in particularly sensitive areas of the body, such as the cornea, skin, and mucous membranes of the oral cavity and respiratory tract. Free nerve endings in the hair follicles are important tactile organs. In these, there are two sets of endings—one arranged circularly in the middle layer of the dermal sheath and the other consisting of fibers running parallel to the hair shaft and terminating in the outer root sheath. These endings are classified as mechanoreceptors (see below) and are extremely sensitive. Even the slightest bending of any hair is sufficient to stimulate the nerve entwined around its base. Thus, each hair is a tactile receptor. It is rapidly adapting because as soon as displacement of the hair ends, the tactile sensation ceases.

FREE, EXPANDED-TIP, AND ENCAPSULATED ENDINGS

Many sensory nerve fibers terminate as so-called *free nerve endings*. These slender, unmyelinated axonal branches with a tapering tip are the most widely distributed somesthetic receptors in the body. They are extremely important in cutaneous sensation, mediating pain (*nociceptors*), heat and cold sensations (*thermoreceptors*), as well as the input from tactile hairs (*mechanoreceptors*). They are found throughout the dermis and in the epidermis, where they penetrate nearly to the stratum corneum. The cornea of the eye is richly supplied with free nerve endings in the stroma, and some of these penetrate Bowman's membrane to ramify among all but the outer two layers of epithelial cells. They are often enfolded by epithelial cell membranes and, unlike free endings elsewhere, these axons become beaded near their termination.

In other sensory endings, the branches of the axons have specializations in the form of minute terminal expansions. These *endings with expanded tips* include the Merkel receptors (Merkel's discs) and Ruffini endings (Ruffini corpuscles). Unlike the rapidly adapting tactile hairs, these endings are slowly adapting mechanoreceptors. Merkel receptors are found in the papillary layer of the dermis, closely associated with certain distinctive cells of the stratum germinativum in the epidermis, notably on the lips and skin of the distal regions of the limbs. Leaf-like expansions of the axon terminals establish intimate contact with these tactile cells. These complexes appear to signal prolonged touch or pressure on the skin.

Ruffini endings are more widely distributed in the dermis and consist of numerous axonal branches terminating in tiny bulb-like expansions located among collagen fibers that run through a thin uniform capsule and are in continuity with those of the surrounding dermis. Tension exerted along the axis of the capsule is the most effective stimulus for a Ruffini corpuscle. Tension on the capsule is presumed to tighten the collagen fibers within and so compress and depolarize the axonal endings entwined among them. Thus, Ruffini corpuscles appear to serve as low-threshold stretch receptors of the skin, signaling the direction and magnitude of the forces acting on them.

In still other endings, a special connective tissue capsule of varying thickness surrounds the actual nerve ending. A good example is the *Pacinian corpuscle*, the largest of the sensory receptors, often being visible with the naked eye. It is a white ovoid structure up to 1 mm in length. Each Pacinian corpuscle receives one or more thickly myelinated axons which lose their myelin sheath on entering the corpuscle. Flattened Schwann cells surround the axon terminals, and these, in turn, are surrounded by numerous concentric lamellae forming the thick capsule. The lamellae consist of thin flat cells, and successive lamellae are separated by a thin semisold layer of a gel-like material. This gives the corpuscle an organization that is often compared to that of an onion. Pacinian corpuscles are found in the reticular layer of the dermis, especially that under the skin of the finger tips. They are also common in the subcutaneous connective tissue, in the stroma of the pancreas, in the mesenteries, and in the external genitalia.

The Pacinian corpuscles are illustrated in the chapter on the skin (Fig. 22–31). It is instructive to note here the role played by the capsule in its signaling function. The structure of the capsule endows the corpuscle with the property of *rapid-adaptation.* Steady force applied on the outer region of the capsule results in deformation of the axons deep inside, but slippage of the lamellae, lubricated by the intervening gel, redistributes the force and diminishes the effectiveness of the stimulus within milliseconds. Owing to the rapid accommodation of its capsule, the Pacinian corpuscle responds only to rapid changes in pressure, and not to sustained pressure, and hence serves as a high-frequency sinusoidal mechanoreceptor, that is, a *vibration receptor.* It is interesting that removal of its capsule transforms the Pacinian corpuscle into a slowly adapting receptor.

The *Meissner corpuscle* is also an encapsulated receptor. This pear-shaped or elliptical structure is smaller and is encountered more superficially than the Pacinian corpuscle. It occurs in certain dermal papillae in regions of the skin that are especially sensitive—palms, soles, tips of fingers and toes, lips, and external genitalia. Like the other corpuscle, it contains lamellae and flattened cells that may be modified Schwann cells. Their orientation, however, is not concentric, but across the corpuscle, which usually has its long axis perpendicular to the skin surface. The axon enters the corpuscle at its lower pole, loses its myelin sheath, and spirals upward between the cell layers until it ends at the upper pole immediately beneath the epidermis. The Meissner corpuscle is also a fast-adapting mechanoreceptor but is tuned by its capsule to low-frequency sinusoidal mechanical stimuli. Therefore, although the sensitivity of sensory fibers to particular stimuli is considered an intrinsic property of the fiber, the capsule sets the threshold of response to certain temporal parameters and the speed of accommodation. The Meissner corpuscle is illustrated in Chapter 22 (Fig. 22–34).

SYNAPSES OF NEURONS

Neurons differ from other cells in their greater capacity to communicate rapidly with one another. Two signaling mechanisms are involved, namely, axonal conduction of nerve impulses and synaptic transmission. The extremely large number of neurons in the nervous system are arranged so as to permit transmission of nerve impulses from cell to cell. Thus, all parts of the system are physically coherent and functionally linked so that each part can communicate with many other parts. Each neuron receives inputs from other neurons, integrates them, and transmits signals to still other neurons or to peripheral effector cells. The site of transmission is the *synapse* (Greek: "to fasten together"). Two distinct modes of transmission are recognized: *electrical* and *chemical.*

Electrical synapses are uncommon in the mammalian CNS, but have been described in a few places in the brain stem, retina, and cerebral cortex. They have been noted more frequently in nonmammalian nervous systems. Such cell-to-cell contacts for communication are not confined to the nervous system. Examples are the familiar *gap junctions* that provide electrotonic cell coupling in epithelia and in smooth and cardiac muscle. In these, particles bridging opposing plasma membranes form channels permitting the movement of ions from one cell to the other. Where such junctions connect neurons, they permit direct flow of ionic current between the two cells—possibly in either direction, but usually in a direction determined by the position of the cells in the circuit or pathway. Because the cells are so closely apposed and no chemical transmitter is involved, transmission is much more rapid than in chemical synapses. Gap junctions are also common between CNS cells other than neurons, for example, astrocytes.

At chemical synapses, the axonal terminal or other presynaptic component secretes a *neurotransmitter* that diffuses across a *synaptic cleft* (12–20 nm wide) and binds to specific *receptors* on the postsynaptic membrane. These receptors undergo immediate conformational change that leads to opening of channels so as to alter permeability of the membrane to certain ions, thus changing the membrane potential. Such effects are brief (2–20 ms) and depend entirely on the events in the postsynaptic cell triggered by the receptor, not on any intrinsic property of the neurotransmitter. If these events depolarize the postsynaptic neuron (i.e., shift its membrane potential in a positive direction toward the threshold for generation of an action potential), the result is an *excitatory postsynaptic potential* (EPSP). On the other hand, if the events act to maintain membrane potential at a given level or hyperpolarize the cell (i.e., shift its membrane potential toward greater negativity, thus lessening the probability of cell firing), the result is an *inhibitory postsynaptic potential* (IPSP).

Although they vary greatly in the nature of their neurotransmitters, chemical synapses are by far the most common type and are referred to hereafter simply as synapses. Their number in the human CNS is astronomical: 10^{14} (one hundred quadrillion) is the current estimate. The number of established neurotransmitters continues to grow (some 30–50 to date) and shows remarkable diversity, including six different classes of compounds, among which are acetylcholine, amino acids, monoamines, peptides, purines, and even gases.

At a synapse, the presynaptic and postsynaptic membranes run a parallel, and often gently curving course convex toward the presynaptic cytoplasm (Fig. 11–26). The cleft between the membranes contains a moderately dense material that may contribute to cohesion of the opposing membranes, but it does not form a discrete layer comparable to the basal lamina of epithelia. The cytoplasm of the presynaptic component typically contains several mitochondria and one or two tubules of smooth endoplasmic reticulum. Its most distinctive constituents are the numerous *synaptic vesicles* aggregated near the presynaptic membrane. These small organelles (40–60 nm in diameter), unique to neurons, are spherical packets all containing the same quanta of neurotransmitter. The transmitter is usually synthesized and packaged in the nerve terminal, but in some cases (e.g., peptide neurotransmitters), it may be produced in the cell body. Transmitter stored in the synaptic vesicles is protected from degradation by axoplasmic enzymes.

The inner aspect of the presynaptic membrane is decorated with a dense material in the form of conical densities extending a short distance into the cytoplasm. Many of the synaptic vesicles are closely associated with this material, and some lie very close to the membrane between these densities. A less prominent discontinuous layer of dense material is found on the cytoplasmic side of the postsynaptic membrane. The region of the presynaptic membrane bearing the densities and associated synaptic vesicles is referred to as the *active zone* of the synapse.

In electron micrographs, vesicles are rarely seen fusing with the presynaptic membrane. However, in a stimulated neuron, many vesicles fuse with the membrane and release their contents into the synaptic cleft. The constituents of the limiting membrane of the vesicles added to the membrane in this process are believed to diffuse outward from the release site and are retrieved at the periphery of the active zone by endocytosis in coated vesicles. The clathrin coat of these vesicles is then lost, and the vesicles fuse with elements of the smooth endoplasmic reticulum. New vesicles are formed and charged with transmitter by this organelle. Membrane is, thus, recycled repeatedly. The neuronal soma may also contribute new vesicles that are transported to the nerve ending along microtubules of the axoplasm. Few vesicles are observed in transit in the axoplasm and the soma is, therefore, considered to be a less important source of synaptic vesicles than the reticulum in the axon terminal.

The relative thickness of the densities on the cytoplasmic surface of the presynaptic and postsynaptic membranes is the basis for a useful classification of synapses. In many synapses, the postsynaptic density is relatively thicker and the synaptic cleft is about 30 nm wide. Such synapses are called *asymmetric.* They are generally, but not always, characteristic of terminals associated with excitatory responses on the part of the postsynaptic neuron. In contrast, other synapses show a relatively thin postsynaptic density, no thicker than the presynaptic density, and they have a narrower synaptic cleft of about 20 nm. These so-called *symmetric* synapses are almost always associated with inhibitory postsynaptic responses. Differences in the appearance of the synaptic vesicles are also reported. They are said to be somewhat flattened in the inhibitory synapses, in contrast to their spherical form in the excitatory synapses. Although the flattening of the vesicles may be an artifact attributable to the use of hypertonic fixatives, their pleomorphic appearance no doubt reflects some difference in the properties of the vesi-

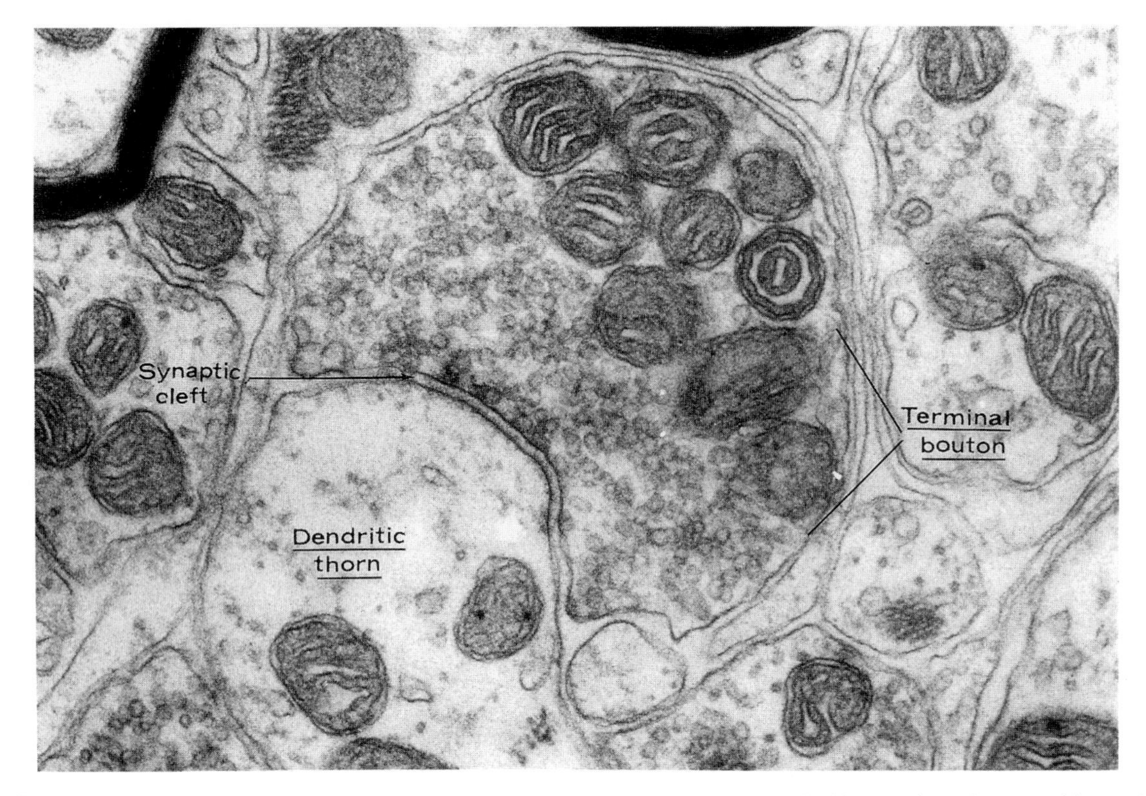

Figure 11–26. Electron micrograph of the tip of a dendritic spine capped by a terminal bouton from the ventral horn of the spinal cord in a rat. The typical features of synapses—mitochondria, clustered synaptic vesicles, and the cleft—are well shown. The terminal is enclosed within a thin astrocytic process. (Micrograph courtesy of S.L. Palay.)

cle membrane and can, thus, be used as a provisional basis for distinguishing the two types of synapses.

Freeze–fracture preparations of the presynaptic membrane reveal a population of randomly distributed large particles and crater-like deformations, where the fracture plane has broken through the necks of synaptic vesicles (Fig. 11–27). The large particles may represent the transmembrane proteins that form ion channels for entry of calcium ions. In the cleaved postsynaptic membrane of synapses associated with excitation of the target neuron, a cluster of large intramembranous particles are often found (Fig. 11–27). These may be the membrane proteins that recognize and bind the transmitter released by the synaptic vesicles.

The physiological events taking place at a synapse can be summarized as follows. Arrival of the action potential causes opening of voltage-gated ion channels that permit Ca^{++} ions to enter the terminal. This influx triggers quantal release of the neurotransmitter by exocytosis (Fig. 11–28). This process is much more rapid than exocytosis elsewhere. It is, in

Figure 11–27. Freeze–fracture preparations of the synaptic membrane. (A) Active zone in the presynaptic membrane of a myoneural junction. The pits indicated by arrows are the cross-fractured necks of synaptic vesicles discharging their transmitter. (Courtesy of T. Reese). (B) Synaptic junction from the inner plexiform layer of the macaque retina. The presynaptic active zone is characterized by an aggregation of large intramembrane particles (arrow heads). A synaptic vesicle in exocytosis is indicated by an arrow with asterisk (Courtesy of E. Raviola and G. Raviola.) (C) Specialization of the P-face of the presynaptic membrane in a synapse in the inner plexiform layer of the retina. The fracture plane has passed through the cluster of synaptic vesicles and then cleaved the presynaptic membrane, exposing its P-face at the active zone (arrow heads). The aggregation of large particles is in register with the underlying cluster of synaptic vesicles. (Courtesy Raviola, E, and G. Raviola. 1982. J. Comp. Neurol. 209:233. (D) In one type of synapse in the CNS the postsynaptic membrane is characterized by an aggregation of large particles that remain associated with the E-face (arrows). In this synapse, from the inner plexiform layer of the retina, two postsynaptic processes occur side by side, each with its aggregation of particles (From Raviola, E. and G. Raviola. 1982. J. Comp. Neurol. 209:233.)

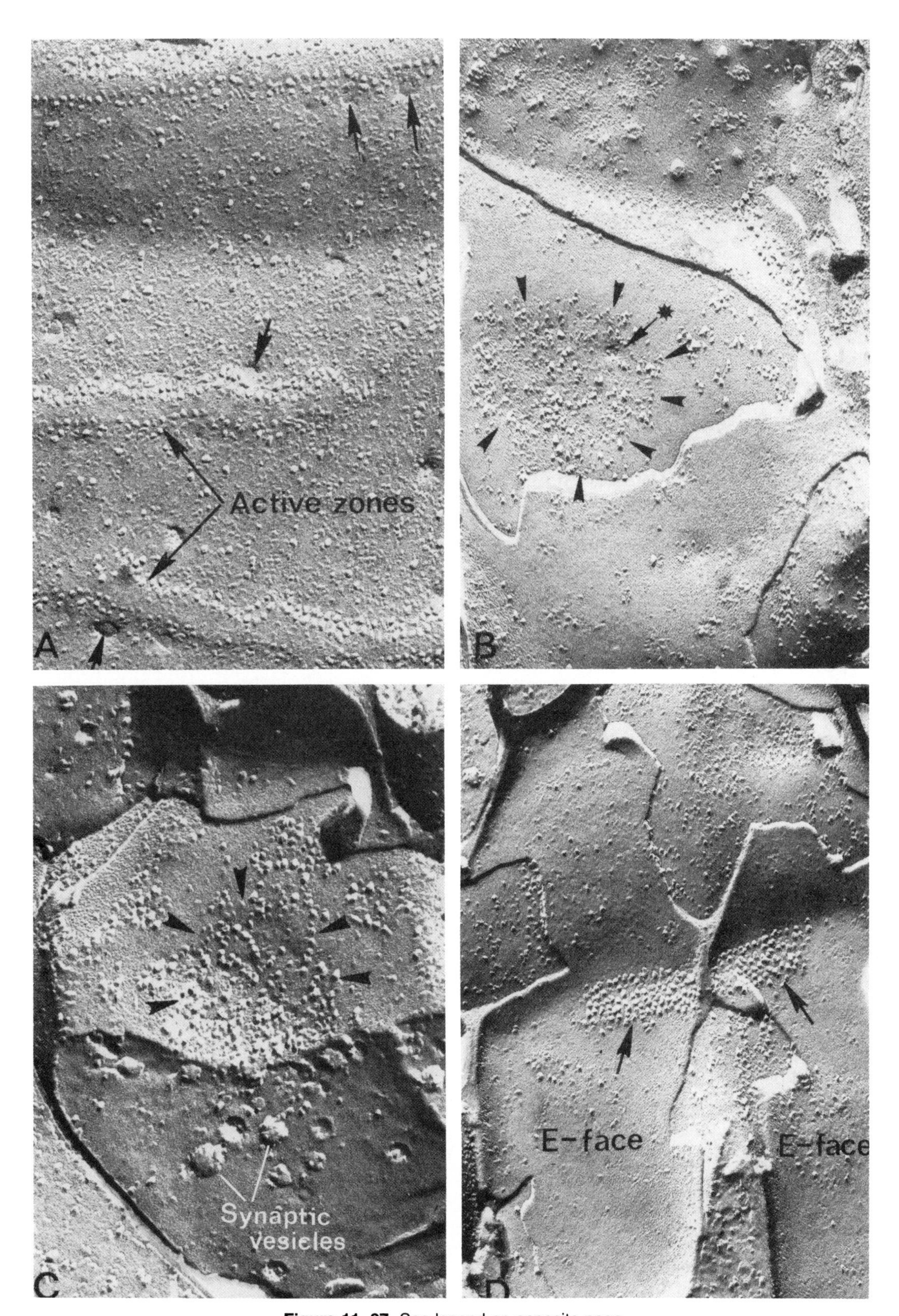

Figure 11–27. See legend on opposite page.

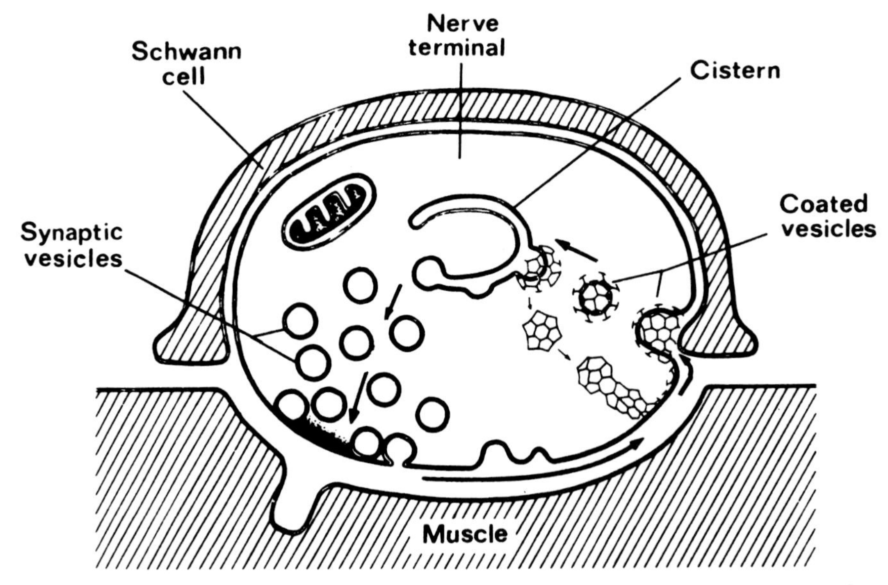

Figure 11–28. The pathway for synaptic vesicle membrane recycling at the neuromuscular junction. Synaptic vesicles coalesce with the plasma membrane in discharging their transmitter. Equal amounts of membrane are retrieved by formation of clathrin-coated vesicles in regions of membrane adjacent to the Schwann sheath. The coated vesicles coalesce with each other and with cisternae within which transmitter accumulates, and new synaptic vesicles are budded off to return to the active zone, as needed. (After Heuser, J.E. and T.S. Reese. Reproduced from J. Cell Biol. 57:315, 1973, by copyright permission of Rockefeller Institute Press).

fact, almost instantaneous, apparently owing to the fact that a subset of vesicles are already docked at the active zone. The transmitter diffuses across the synaptic cleft and binds to specific receptors in the postsynaptic membrane. These cause ion channels to open, thereby changing the permeability of the membrane and resulting, as explained earlier, in its depolarization and consequent excitation of the target neuron, or in its hyperpolarization and resultant inhibition.

Within the axon terminal, there are two functional pools of synaptic vesicles: a relatively small releasable pool, some members of which fuse with the presynaptic membrane when the nerve impulse arrives, and a larger pool of vesicles tethered to the actin cytoskeleton and mobilized to the other pool as required. Following transmitter release, membrane is taken up by endocytosis and vesicles are reloaded with locally synthesized transmitter. Details of how the content of new vesicles are synthesized from precursors transported to the terminal by kinesin-mediated axonal transport are currently receiving investigative attention.

Mechanisms for modulating transmitter release and reception are also under study and these appear to play important roles in regulating synaptic transmission. In general, neuromodulation does not depend on the action of *ion-channel-coupled receptors* as in the case of neurotransmission, that is, it does not involve direct binding of a chemical messenger to an ion-channel protein. Instead, the neuromodulator binds to *second-messenger-coupled receptors.* These activate one or more second-messenger systems, usually via signal-transducing guanyl-nucleotide-binding proteins (G-proteins). A neurotransmitter itself, once released, may act as its own modulator by binding to *autoreceptors* on the presynaptic membrane. These receptors then act in various ways to inhibit (or sometimes facilitate) further transmitter release.

In second-messenger systems, a cascade of events (e.g., generation of cyclic AMP from ATP, activation of cAMP-dependent protein kinases, and phosphorylation of proteins within the cell) leads indirectly to changes in conductance of ion channels. Such influences have long latencies (100–250 ms) and may last from milliseconds or minutes up to days or weeks. They usually act to regulate postsynaptic sensitivity to the fast synaptic events described earlier, rather than to rapidly alter membrane potential.

Neuromodulation may also occur presynaptically. One mechanism is by regulation of the relative numbers of synaptic vesicles in the reserve and releasable pools. Several proteins are associated with the cytoplasmic surface of the vesicle membrane. Some of these are phosphoproteins, and second-messenger systems that activate protein kinases result in their phosphorylation. One such protein, *synapsin-I,* appears to form a complex with the vesicle surface and with actin. Such complexes are believed to be responsible for the clustering of reserve vesicles near the active zone. Phosphorylation of synapsin-I seems to cause dissociation of the complex, resulting in detachment of vesicles from the cytoskeleton and an increase in free synapsin-I in the cytosol. Vesicles are, thus, liberated to join the releasable pool. Recent studies indicate that the process is reversible, with dephosphorylation of synapsin-I favoring its interaction with actin of the cytoskeleton and recapture of synaptic vesicles within its meshwork.

Another phosphorprotein, *synapsin-II,* together with a peripheral membrane protein, *rab3a,* is also thought to mediate synaptic vesicle interactions with the cytoskeleton. Still other proteins, *synaptotagmin* and *synaptophysin,* are candidate controllers of the docking and fusion of vesicles at the presynaptic membrane. In overview, synthesis of neurotransmitter, transport and packaging in vesicles, clustering, cytoskeletal anchoring, dissociation, docking, fusion, release of contents, membrane reuptake, and recycling are simply stages in a continuous, extremely rapid process which we are just beginning to understand at the submicroscopic level. Although much work remains to be done, the application of the techniques of molecular biology to the synapse have revealed important details of the submicroscopic organization of the axon terminal and have greatly clarified some of the mechanisms of synaptic transmission.

Synapses have been found to exhibit great diversity in their form and ultrastructure, in their number and location on target neurons, in their functional effects, in type and number of chemical messengers, and in their relationships to neuroglia. This great variability has strained traditional concepts of the synapse and stimulated a reappraisal of neuronal communication that mandates greater precision in describing the actions of neuroactive substances. Among these new developments, three are singled out for mention here: (1) *Multiple transmitters* now seem to be the rule for neurons; (2) a given transmitter may have *different actions* in different situations; and (3) the effect of a neuroactive substance on its target cell is determined *exclusively* by the postsynaptic receptors to which it binds. As an example, the well-established neurotransmitter dopamine may (1) coexist in the terminals of certain brainstem neurons with two neuropeptides, cholecystokinin (CCK), and neurotensin, (2) function as a *neurotransmitter* when secreted by axonal endings of neurons in the substantia nigra, but may act as a neurohormone in the adenohypophysis after release into the hypophyseoportal circulation by neurons of the hypothalamus, and (3) excite, inhibit, or merely modulate the activity of the target cell, depending on the nature of the receptor molecule in the postsynaptic membrane. In view of the latter, terms such as "excitatory neurotransmitter" are imprecise and may be incorrect. Although widely used, and possibly useful in discussing specific circuits, they are misleading and should be used with care.

The list of neuroactive substances continues to grow. The neurotransmitters identified to date include acetylcholine, monoamines (three catecholamines—adrenaline, dopamine, and noradrenaline; two indolamines—serotonin and tryptamine gamma-amino butyric acid, or GABA, aspartate, glutamate, glycine, histamine, taurine and certain amino acids). These last appear to be the major transmitters of the mammalian CNS; the others mediate transmission at only a small percentage of central synapses.

In recent years, it has been found that 30 or more small peptides are synthesized by neurons and released at nerve endings, often along with one of the above neurotransmitters. They are relatively slow acting, but can affect the discharge rate of the target neurons and are generally regarded as neuromodulators rather than transmitters. These peptides include cholecystokinin (CCK), endorphins, methionine- and leucine-encephalins, neuropeptide Y, neurotensin, substance-P, and vasoactive intestinal peptide (VIP). Several of these also occur, and were first found, in the gastrointestinal tract where they exert paracrine effects on neighboring cells and, in a few instances, may be released into the blood as hormones. Other peptides appear to serve importantly, although not exclusively, as neurohormones: luteinizing hormone-releasing hormone (LHRH), oxytocin, somatostatin, thyroid hormone-releasing hormone (THRH), and vasopressin. The list also includes purines: Adenosine and its phosphates AMP, ADP, and ATP play crucial roles in second messenger systems and discharge other modulatory functions. Recently a novel class of transmitters has been discovered, namely, gases. Nitric oxide (NO) has been shown to mediate the neural aspects of penile erection, and carbon monoxide (CO) is also receiving attention as a possible transmitter.

Demonstration by electron microscopy, in the 1950s, of the synaptic cleft between the presynaptic and postsynaptic membranes provided definitive proof of the "neuron doctrine" postulating the structural independence of nerve cells, a subject that had been vehemently debated for nearly a century. The cells which confront each other across this cleft may be two neurons, a neuron and a skeletal or smooth muscle, or a neuron and a gland. When the two synaptic elements are both parts of neurons (i.e., dendrites, somata, or axons), numerous combinations have been found and given compound designations indicating the parts in synaptic contact, for example, *axodendritic, axosomatic,* and *axoaxonic* synapses (Fig. 11–29). These are ubiquitous in the mammalian CNS and, having been recognized for years, they are referred to as "conventional." However, other combinations that have been recognized only since the advent of the electron microscope are inappropriately termed "unconventional." Their discovery has strained the traditional concepts of information processing at the neuronal level to no small degree and led to radical changes in modeling the operation of neural networks.

Of these conceptually novel couplings, *dendrodendritic* synapses were the first to be found. They are now well known, having been encountered in many regions of the CNS, including the olfactory bulb, retina, and thalamus. At the time of their discovery, they aroused great interest. They shattered the idea that dendrites cannot hold presynaptic positions, and they were the first example of a synapse between homologous neuronal components. They were highly unusual in that, reciprocal synapses with opposite polarities occurred in juxtaposition at the same interface, and they exhibited both asymmetric

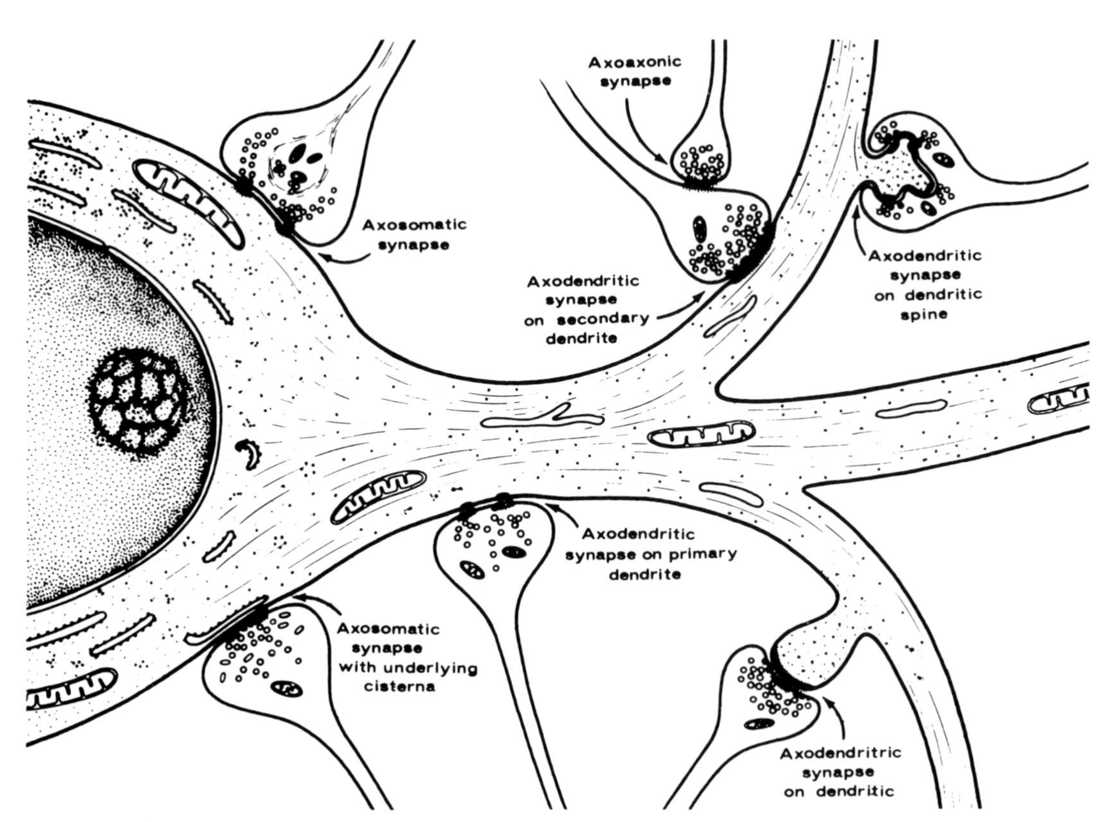

Figure 11–29. Illustration of the types and terminology of synapses occurring on various portions of the neuron (Drawn after Bunge, R. 1971. *In* Copenhaver, W.M. and R. Bunge, eds. Baileys Textbook of Histology, 16th ed. Baltimore, MD, Williams and Wilkins.)

and symmetric membrane densities, respectively, in the two adjacent junctions.

Since then, *somatodendritic, dendrosomatic, somatosomatic, somatoaxonic, dendroaxonic,* and *axoaxodendritic* (serial) junctions have been described. Thus, it appears that any part of a neuron can participate in the formation of a synapse. Even more intriguing are nests of synapses, called *synaptic glomeruli.* These more-or-less discrete globular tangles of neuronal processes are so named for their resemblance to the capillary knots in renal corpuscles. They are usually partially enclosed and separated from the surrounding neuropil by veil-like astrocytic processes. Within this glial capsule, various neuronal components articulate in an intricate fashion around a central component—usually an axon, but sometimes a dendrite or a dendritic thorn. These complexes are found in many regions of the brain and spinal cord and have attracted much study. Although varying greatly in details, they all seem to display a triadic arrangement of components—axonal elements containing synaptic vesicles and forming asymmetric synapses with dendritic elements, and a third set of elements, either dendritic or axonal in origin, containing pleomorphic vesicles and thought to be associated with inhibition of one of the other two groups. In at least one example, this complexity is compounded by the presence of gap junctions between the dendritic elements.

Axons commonly terminate in fine branches that have small expansions along their course (*boutons en passant*) or at their ends (*boutons terminaux*). These knobs are applied to the surface of the postsynaptic neuron. In some cases, the terminal branches form loose basket-like networks adhering to the soma or dendrites of other nerve cells. In rare instances, the axon gives rise to a single large ending that occupies an extensive area of the surface of the target cell; these endings are called *end bulbs* or *calyces,* depending on their size and shape. As mentioned earlier, the number of synapses on a neuron in the CNS varies within wide limits—from a dozen to one-quarter of a million.

As explained earlier, chemical synapses are by far the standard mode of communication between nerve cells in mammals. They mediate transfer of neuronal activity by release of a neurotransmitter and, in some instances, two or three different transmitters. They also regulate the activity of both presynaptic and postsynaptic cellular components of a synapse in various ways, including the actions of neuromodulators and neurohormones—sometimes at a great distance and over a life span. But over and above these considerations, such synapses, unlike the less common electrical synapses, establish the polarization of the nervous system. With the important qualification that neuromodulation can occur in both anterograde and orthograde manner, they are one-way gates or "turnstiles" that allow most messages to pass from neuron to neuron in only one direction. So-called "two-way synapses" have been described, but rather inaccurately. These dendrodendritic, or other comparable homologous synapses, are, in fact, a pair of reciprocally polarized synapses side-by-side. The unidirectional feature of the synapse is of cardinal importance because the other parts of a neuron—the axon, cell body, and dendrites—can, and in certain instances do, conduct in both directions. Thus, the polarity of the synapse determines the one-way traffic flow that takes place in most pathways and in most regions of the CNS.

Before leaving the synapse, it is appropriate to return to two of the junctional complexes found between the cells of the specialized epithelium that forms the nervous system: the *zonula adherens* and its smaller counterpart, the *punctum adherens.* The puncta adherentia are widely distributed in the nervous system. Although most conspicuous between astrocytes, they have also been found between virtually every other combination of CNS components; between dendrites, dendrites and axons, dendrites and cell bodies, adjacent cell bodies, axon terminals and axon initial segments, axon membranes and their sheaths, and neuronal processes and astrocytes. Although these specialized regions of contact are believed to play a purely adhesive role, binding cells tightly to one another as in other epithelia, their importance cannot be overstated. They hold the neurons together and stabilize their areas of synaptic contact, somewhat as soldered connections stabilize electrical circuits. Although not sites of synaptic transmission in themselves, they are frequently found in close association with chemical synapses, as well as at many other nonspecific sites. Indeed, the active zone of a synapse is believed, by some, to represent a greatly modified zonula adherens. Thus, it seems that within the central nervous system both the site of chemical transmission and its stability derive from simple adhesive junctions found universally in epithelial tissues.

AUTONOMIC NERVOUS SYSTEM

As classically defined, the autonomic nervous system (ANS) is a largely involuntary effector system concerned with maintaining the constancy of the body's internal environment. Closely related to it, however, is a visceral sensory or *interoceptive system,* the neurons and fibers of which form the afferent side of visceral reflex arcs. The ANS has three subdivisions: *sympathetic* (thoracolumbar), *parasympathetic* (craniosacral), and *enteric.* In all three, it acts via two motor neurons in series: the first located in a nucleus in the brain stem or spinal gray matter; the second in a ganglion outside of the CNS. In contrast, in the voluntary part of the peripheral nervous system, a motor neuron acts directly on the effector organ.

The sympathetic division includes a chain of interconnected ganglia on either side of the vertebral column. The cell bodies of its preganglionic neurons are situated in the gray matter of the spinal cord. Their axons exit the cord through the ventral roots joining the spinal nerves, but soon leave them to pass through the communicating rami and enter one of the paravertebral ganglia (Fig. 11–30). Each preganglionic neuron synapses with multiple postganglionic neurons in the ganglia of the same segment, or of neighboring segments of the chain. Their axons, in turn, return to peripheral nerves and travel to virtually all parts of the body: to blood vessels (*vasomotor fibers*), sweat glands (*sudomotor fibers*), hair follicles (*pilomotor fibers*), the dilator pupillae muscle of the iris, and to the salivary glands, heart, and lungs.

Some preganglionic fibers of this system pass through the paravertebral ganglia without synapsing and travel in the splanchnic nerves to synapse on neurons in the prevertebral ganglia (celiac ganglion, superior and inferior mesenteric ganglia) in the abdominal cavity. Postganglionic fibers from these ganglia innervate the gastrointestinal tract, kidneys, pancreas, and liver and provide the sympathetic innervation of the bladder and external genitalia. Thus, the sympathetic trunks and their ganglia, as well as the prevertebral ganglia, are the avenues of communication for the thoracolumbar outflow between the CNS and the viscera.

In the parasympathetic division of the ANS, the preganglionic cell bodies are located in the brain stem and in several sacral segments of the spinal cord. Their axons do not synapse in paravertebral ganglia, but extend for long distances to postganglionic neurons in ganglia near or within the visceral targets. Axons of the cranial component emerge in the oculomotor, facial, glossopharyngeal, and vagus nerves and synapse with postganglionic neurons in the ciliary, pterygopalatine, submandibular, and otic ganglia. Those of the spinal component derive from the second, third, and fourth sacral segments, depart via ventral roots and sacred nerves, and project to postganglionic neurons in ganglia associated with the pelvic viscera.

The enteric division controls the gastrointestinal tract, pancreas, and gallbladder. Its neurons are arranged in complex networks of ganglia and interconnecting nerve fibers within the wall of the target organs. The two major networks are the *myenteric plexus* located between the longitudinal and circular muscle of the gut, and the *submucosal plexus,* between the mucosa and the circular muscle layer. This division can function autonomously but is also regulated by extrinsic parasympathetic preganglionic fibers of the vagus and splanchnic nerves and by postganglionic sympathetic fibers from the prevertebral ganglia.

AUTONOMIC NERVE CELLS

The preganglionic visceral efferent neurons are small, spindle-shaped cells in the intermediolateral gray column of the spinal cord. They receive a number of axodendritic endings that is small compared to the numerous terminals found on the cell bodies and dendrites of somatic motor neurons. Because the preganglionic neurons of the craniosacral division are close to the viscera innervated, the preganglionic fibers are relatively long and the postganglionic fibers are short. In the thoracolumbar region, on the other hand, the synapses are in the paravertebral sympathetic chain, and so it is the postganglionic fibers that are long.

In both divisions of the ANS, preganglionic fibers are usually myelinated and of variable but small diameter, whereas postganglionic fibers as a rule are unmyelinated and thin. Another generalization is that *acetylcholine* is the principal neurotransmitter of pregangli-

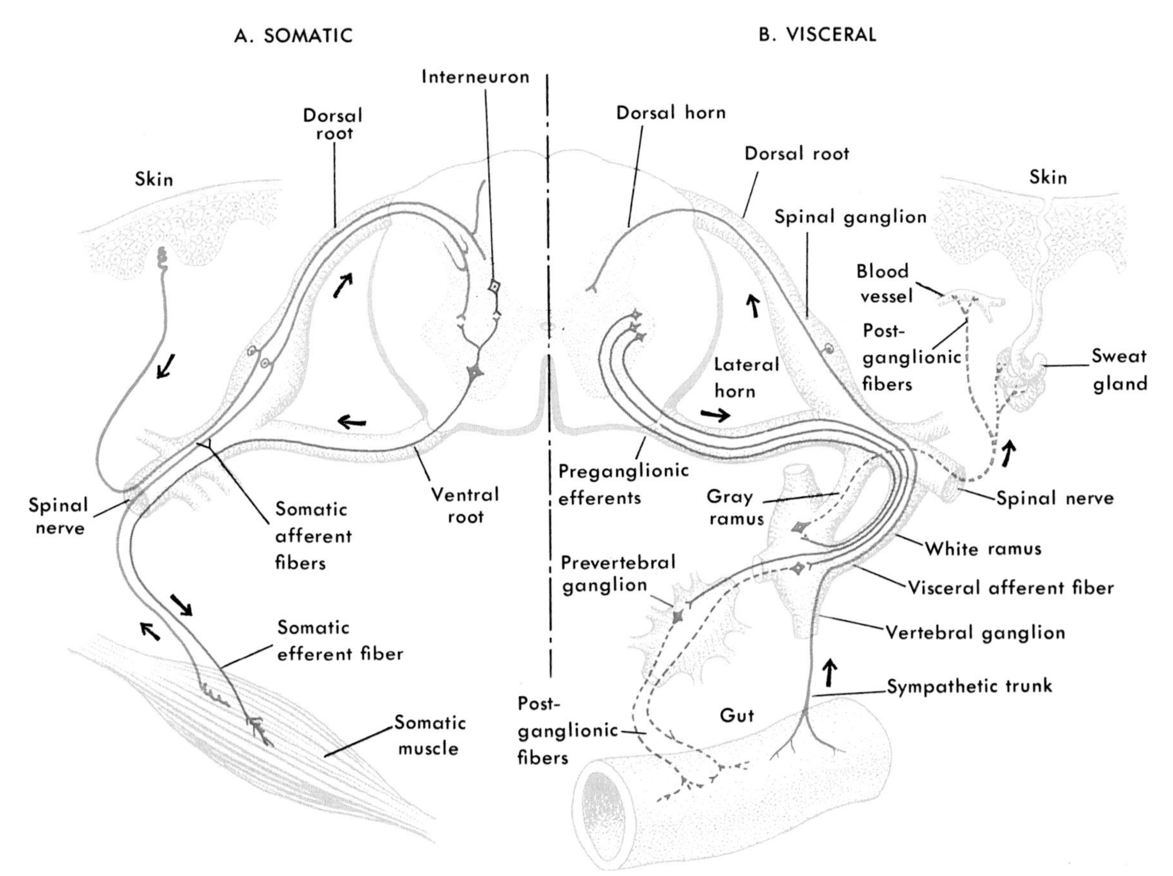

Figure 11–30. In this drawing of the spinal cord and dorsal and ventral roots, the left half (A) shows the somatic nerves and (B) shows the visceral nerves. The pattern of afferent and efferent nerve fibers in both the somatic and the visceral system can be directly compared. (From Copenhaver, W. and R. Bunge, eds. 1971. Bailey's Textbook of Histology, 16th ed. Baltimore, MD, Williams and Wilkins.)

onic neurons and of postganglionic parasympathetic neurons, whereas *norepinephrine* is the neurotransmitter of most postganglionic sympathetic neurons.

An important difference between autonomic and somatic modes of innervation is that postganglionic fibers usually do not form typical synapses with their effector organs, but instead break up into multiple branches bearing varicosities in which neurotransmitter is contained within vesicles. On release, the transmitter diffuses, often over some distance, before reaching the target cells. In many cases, this makes for widespread effects, long latencies of response, and prolonged action. Moreover, when the effectors are smooth muscle cells, the activity evoked within those cells that are within the range of the neurotransmitter, is then transmitted electrotonically to other smooth muscles in the target organ via gap junctions. As these cells may also be activated hormonally, or by stretching of the organ, the role of their autonomic innervation is generally contributory or modulatory rather than definitive. Nevertheless, an interesting similarity to somatic patterns of innervation is the varying degree of precision of these patterns: The ratio between the number of efferent nerve fibers and the number of effector cells varies greatly in both systems, depending on the accuracy and delicacy of control required.

The cells of the sympathetic ganglia are generally small and quite diverse in shape. They are usually multipolar with little detectable difference between dendrites and axon. Preganglionic fibers often synapse with the dendrites of the ganglion cell in elaborate glomeruli. The cell body may be encapsulated by satellite cells of ectodermal origin that are similar to Schwann cells of peripheral nerve sheaths. Such cells may be absent in the outlying sympathetic ganglia, but Schwann cells accompany the peripheral sympathetic fibers everywhere.

INTERRELATIONSHIPS OF NEURONS

Nearly every neuron is connected to from several to many other neurons. Many different types of relationship have been shown with the Golgi impregnation technique, by electron microscopy, and with newer methods involving observation of the distribution within living cells of substances injected or applied iontophoretically. For example, attached to the soma and dendrites of large motor neurons in the spinal cord are hundreds of synaptic boutons of axons coming from neurons in the cerebral cortex, nuclei of the brain stem, neurons in the overlying layers of the spinal gray matter, monosynaptic group-Ia afferents from muscle spindles, and from elsewhere. Thus, motor neurons serve as the *final common pathway* by which activity from many sources is transmitted to effector organs. Their responses are determined by the net effect of excitatory, inhibitory, and modulatory inputs from many neurons. Therefore, in a spinal reflex arc, the excitation of peripheral sensory elements is only one of the determinants of motor neuron response.

Details of the organization of the CNS are beyond the scope of this book and must be sought in textbooks of neuroanatomy, but some concept of its complexity can be derived from the enormous number of cells involved, which is estimated to be 9×10^9 neurons in the cerebral cortex alone. It may be useful, nonetheless, to present an overview of some of the regions where these cellular interactions take place.

A photomicrograph of the spinal cord (Fig. 11–15) illustrates the gray matter containing the nerve cell bodies, surrounded by the white matter, consisting of masses of myelinated nerve fibers. In the cerebral hemisphere and cerebellum, there is an additional layer of gray matter, the cortex, located outside of the white matter. The myelinated and unmyelinated fibers of the white matter serve to transmit patterns of nerve impulses from the body to the CNS, from the CNS to the body, and from one region of the CNS to another.

In the gray matter of the CNS, the nerve cell bodies are arranged in some order, in clusters called *nuclei* or in *cortical layers.* Innumerable reciprocal contacts between types of neurons permit a variety of mutual influences. The spaces between neurons are packed with axons, neuroglial elements, and blood vessels. In these areas, the axons usually lack myelin sheaths, which accounts for their gray color in the unfixed condition. When stained by routine methods, the regions between nerve cell bodies have a stippled appearance characteristic of the *neuropil.* In the cerebellar and cerebral cortices and in the retina, certain layers consist almost exclusively of neuroglial and naked neuronal processes. Huge numbers of synaptic contacts are made in such synaptic fields.

The pattern of cells and fibers, the *cytoarchitecture,* varies from place to place in the gray matter. Every peripheral ganglion, subcortical nucleus, and locality of the cerebral cortex has cytoarchitectural features of its own. For example, the *motor area* in the precentral gyrus of the cerebral hemisphere differs noticeably from the postcentral gyrus, where *somatosensory function* is represented, and indeed from all other parts of the cerebral cortex. Another important cortical region having a distinctive cytoarchitecture is the visual area in the occipital lobe. Generally, however, efforts to correlate cytoarchitectonic and functional parameters have largely failed.

Anatomical and physiological studies provide compelling evidence that the nervous system is not a random tangle of neurons and neuroglial cells and their processes. Neurons in most regions, including the seemingly chaotic mass of cells and fibers of the brain-stem reticular formation, display remarkable structural and functional individuality, as expressed in the connections between particular cells, and in the number, type, and location of synaptic endings on different regions of the same cell. Particular neurons among the astronomical numbers making up the visual cortex may respond to specific modes of activation—in this instance, to the specific orientation of a straight line or edge, or to other parameters of visual stimuli to the retina, such as direction of movement.

NEUROGLIA

Although the numbers of neurons in the CNS are astronomical, they are exceeded 5–10-fold by the supporting cells collectively called the *neuroglia.* These are not merely mechanically supportive cells but are metabolically active elements that assist nerve cells in performing their integrative and communicative functions. The term neuroglia, meaning "nerve-glue" was coined by the German pathologist Rudolf Virchow in 1846 and it includes *astrocytes, oligodendroglia,* and the *microglia.* The Schwann cells of peripheral nerves and the satellite cells of peripheral ganglia may be considered the peripheral neuroglia. Also included in this category is the *ependyma,* a cuboidal epithelium lining the ventricular system of the brain and the central canal of the spinal cord. In modified form, the ependyma also provides the epithelial lining of the choroid plexus (see p. 361).

With notable exceptions, the neuroglia has been relatively neglected by anatomists and physiologists because their study seemed less promising than that of the neurons, which were obviously the major elements involved in the functions of the brain. Unlike neurons, glial cells do not seem to play a direct role in neural communications. They respond passively to electrical currents and do not generate or propagate impulses even though they are linked by gap junctions. Other factors contributing to the neglect of the glial cells have been their small size and the general assumption that they have only a trophic function.

NEUROGLIAL CELLS

The star-shaped glial cells called astrocytes occur in many specialized varieties, but there are two major kinds (Fig. 11–31). *Protoplasmic astrocytes* are found mainly in the gray matter of the CNS. In silver-impregnated preparations, they have a stellate form with multiple highly branched processes. Some of these end on blood vessels in expanded "sucker feet" or pedicels. Other astrocytes have their cell body directly apposed to the wall of a blood vessel. Some, near the surface of the brain or spinal cord, extend processes with pedicels that contact the pia mater and collectively form the *pia glial membrane.* Protoplasmic astrocytes have abundant cytoplasm and a nucleus that is larger and paler-staining than that of other neuroglial cells. Smaller cells of this type lie close to the bodies of neurons and represent another form of satellite cell. *Velate astrocytes* have thin veil-like processes that extend as sheets between neurons and their processes. A striking example of the partitioning of the inputs to a neuron by such thin processes is seen in the astrocytic envelopment of groups of axons terminating on dendrites of Purkinje cells. Other protoplasmic astrocytes have very distinctive modes of ramification, as exemplified by the so-called subpial candelabra cells and similar, but smaller, feather cells of Fananas.

Astrocytes have an important role in homeostasis in the CNS. K^+ ions, glutamate, and α-aminobutyric accumulate in the extracellular spaces as a result of increased neuronal activity. The extracellular spaces are believed to be cleared of these substances by the astrocytes. They are also the principal cell type in which glycogen is stored as an energy reserve, and certain neurotransmitters (norepinephrine and VIP) induce glycogenolysis and release of glucose. Therefore, astrocytes make a significant contribution to energy metabolism in the cerebral cortex.

Fibrous astrocytes are found mainly in the white matter but also in some regions of the periventricular gray matter. They have long thin processes that branch infrequently and, like those of protoplasmic astrocytes, often attach to the pia mater or to blood vessels but are separated from these structures by a distinct basal lamina. Protoplasmic and fibrous astrocytes may be a single cell type that varies in form in different locales. Their shape cannot be made out in routine histological preparations but only with classical metallic-impregnation techniques. In such preparations, it was possible to detect *fibrils* in their cytoplasm. In electron micrographs, these have been resolved as bundles of slender intermediate filaments. They are unlike the neurofibrils of neurons, being more closely packed and having a diameter of only 8 nm. They are also chemically distinct, consisting of *glial fibrillar acidic protein* of 51,000 D molecular weight. The cell nucleus is euchromatic and the cytoplasm contains relatively few organelles, including scant, rough endoplasmic reticulum, few free ribosomes, and glycogen particles.

Oligodendrocytes resemble astrocytes to some degree, but as their name implies, they have fewer processes and these seldom branch (Fig. 11–31D). The cell body is small and the nucleus smaller than that of astrocytes and is rounded, heterochromatic, and deeply staining. The cytoplasm is relatively dense, rich in endoplasmic reticulum and free ribosomes, and contains a conspicuous Golgi complex and many mitochondria. The overall density of the cytoplasm is perhaps the most characteristic feature of these cells. Although a few less dense types have been described, oligodendrocytes are usually among the darkest cells

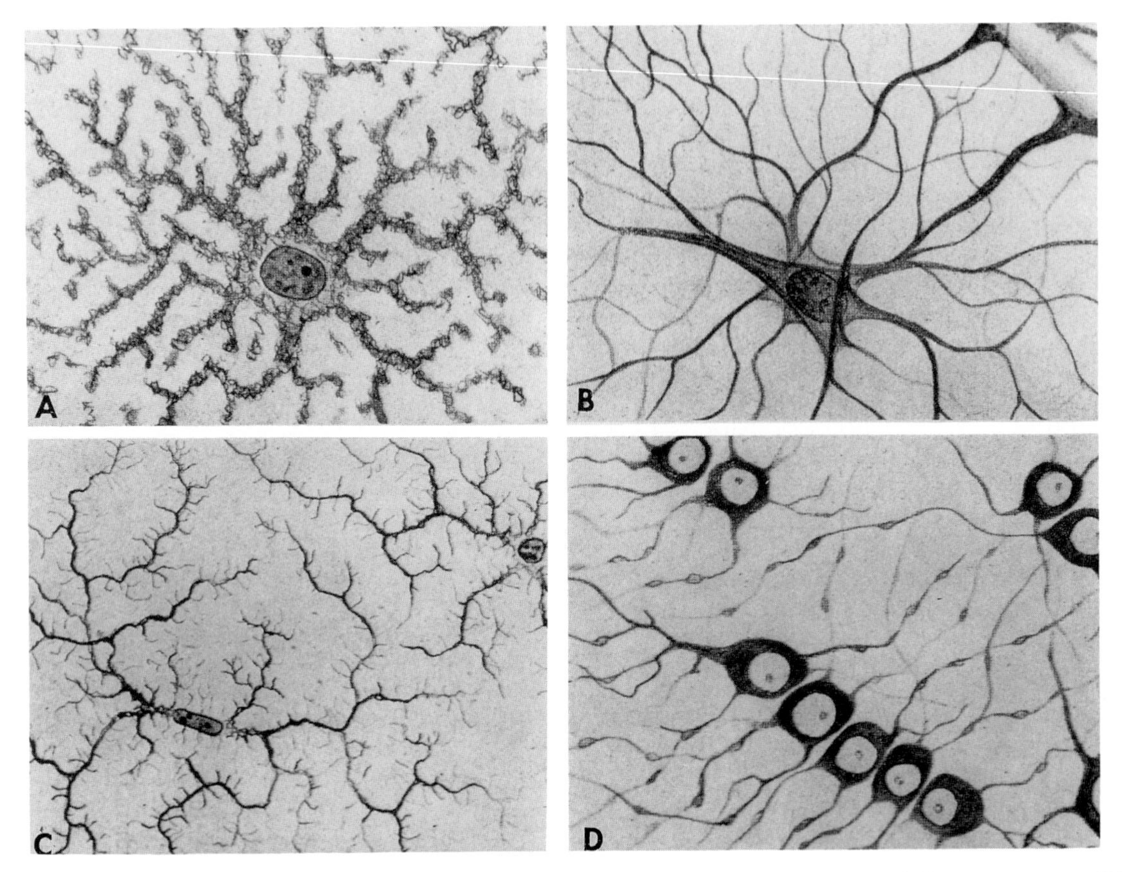

Figure 11–31. Neuroglial cells of the central nervous system. (A) Protoplasmic astrocyte; (B) fibrous astrocyte; (C) microglia. (D) oligodendroglia.

seen in electron micrographs of the CNS. Microtubules are prominent, both in their perinuclear cytoplasm and in the processes.

One type of oligodendrocyte makes and maintains central myelin. These cells, found in rows or columns between bundles of axons in the white matter, are called *interfasicular oligodendrocytes.* Each internodal segment of the myelin sheath of CNS axons is formed by apposed membranes of such a cell wrapped spirally about the axon, so this cell is the homologue of the Schwann cell of the peripheral nervous system. Unlike the latter, however, one oligodendrocyte may form myelin segments on several adjacent axons. At the nodes of Ranvier, the sheaths are interrupted, as in the PNS, to permit current flow.

In the gray matter, another type, *satellite oligodendrocytes,* is closely associated with the somata of nerve cells. Their exact relationship with the neurons is unclear. Electron micrographs show only a smooth, unspecialized zone of apposition between neuron and glial cell and do not suggest what may transpire between them. In tissue culture, such cells exhibit shallow rhythmic pulsations. The significance of this activity in relation to their function is not known.

The *microglia* is composed of small cells scattered throughout the CNS. They bear some resemblance to oligodendrocytes, but are even smaller and darker. They have a dense oval, elongated or roughly triangular nucleus, scant cytoplasm, and short tortuous processes. The cell body and processes are decorated with minute pointed spines. The embryological origin of the microglia is disputed. Some believe it is of mesodermal origin, possibly invading the developing CNS with the blood vessels. Others favor other possible origins, including blood-borne cells derived from the bone marrow. In areas of injury, microglial cells proliferate, enlarge, and become phagocytic, clearing up cellular debris and ingesting damaged myelin.

In the developing nervous system, astrocytes provide scaffoldings for the inward migration of young neurocytes into final position. In the adult, they form an elaborate framework in which the neurons are deployed. In this glial labyrinth, neurons and their processes are often individually encapsulated and, thus, isolated from one another. In electron micrographs, wherever a neuron or neuronal process is not in synaptic contact with another neuron, it is enveloped by the cell body or the processes of glial cells. The distribution of these glial processes appears neither random nor merely arranged to fulfill the requirements of mechanical support and nutrition of the neurons. Early on, the great neuroanatomist Ramon y Cajal proposed that they are always so disposed as to prevent contact of neuronal processes at sites other than those appropriate to their specific signaling function. This hypothesis has been revived by electron microscopists. Each neuron has a characteristic pattern of glial investment complimentary to the pattern of its synaptic connections. Only at synapses are these barriers interrupted to permit contact with other neurons. Therefore, by isolating the many pathways that converge on a neuron, the neuroglia may play a key role in the communication functions of the nervous system.

Through their processes and foot plates on the walls of blood vessels, the neuroglia is thought to influence the formation of tight junctions between the endothelial cells that make up the blood-brain barrier (see p. 364). The intimate relationship of the glial processes to the blood vessels also suggests that they may have some role in the nutrition of the neurons, but as yet there is little firm evidence for this. However, there is evidence that glial cells buffer the potassium ions that accumulate in the intercellular space following neuronal activity. They also appear to take up and degrade excess neurotransmitter released during chemical transmission. Whenever neurons are affected by local or distant pathological processes, the surrounding glial elements react in some way. They are also actively involved in the degeneration and regeneration of nerve fibers, in vascular disorders, and in various infectious diseases. Unfortunately, they are also the commonest source of tumors of the CNS.

EPENDYMA

The ventricles of the brain and the central canal of the spinal cord are lined by the *ependyma,* a layer of cuboidal or columnar epithelium. It arises indirectly from the pseudostratified embryonic neuroepithelium from which the neurons and glial cells develop. That epithelium is ciliated in places and some cilia persist on the mature ependyma. Ependymal cells often have an accumulation of mitochondria in their apical cytoplasm and they contain conspicuous bundles of intermediate filaments. The bases of some cells taper into long, slender processes. In the embryo, these reach to the surface of the brain, but in the adult they are less extensive and disappear, apparently ending among other cellular components. Where the wall of neural tissue is thin, some of these processes span the entire distance between the central canal and the pia, as in the embryo. In these cases, the ependymal cells form a dense *internal limiting membrane* at the ventricular surface. Beneath the pia, the thin ependymal processes expand into pedicels that fuse into a thin, smooth *external limiting membrane.* In the ventricles of the brain, ependymal cells are modified, in one region, to form the secretory epithelium of the *choroid plexus.* Other modified ependymal cells, the *tanycytes,* have processes extending into the hypothalamus to terminate near blood vessels and neurons. It is suggested that tanycytes transport cerebrospinal fluid to neurosecretory cells there. In general, ependymocytes are thought to play various roles in relation to that fluid.

MENINGES, VENTRICLES, AND CHOROID PLEXUS

The neurons and macroglia are of ectodermal origin, but the blood vessels of the CNS are derived from the mesenchyme, and the three layers enveloping the brain and spinal cord are composed of connective tissue. The outermost, the *dura mater* or *pachymeninx,* is dense connective tissue, whereas the innermost, the *pia mater,* and the intermediate layer, the *arachnoid,* are of looser connective tissue. The latter two together constitute the *leptomeninges.*

DURA MATER

The spinal dura and that of the brain differ in their relationship to the surrounding bony tissue. The inner surface of the vertebral canal is lined by its own periosteal layer of connective tissue, and a separate cylindrical dural membrane loosely encloses the spinal cord. The wide *epidural space,* between the periosteum and the dura, contains loose connective tissue, adipose cells, and the epidural venous plexus. The inner surface of the dura is lined by squamous cells and firmly connected to the spinal cord along each side by a series of denticulate ligaments. Generally, the dural collagenous fibers are oriented longitudinally and it contains fewer elastic fibers than the cerebral dura.

The dura mater of the brain initially has two layers, but in the adult these are closely joined. Both consist of collagenous fibers and elongated fibroblasts. There is no distinct border between the two, but there are some differences in their organization. The outer layer, or *periosteal dura,* adheres rather loosely to the inner aspect of the skull except at the cranial sutures, and at the base of the skull, where it is more firmly adherent. It functions as a periosteum, is richer in cells than the inner layer, and contains many blood vessels. Its collagen fibers are organized in distinct bundles.

The inner layer, the *meningeal dura,* is made up of fine fibers forming an almost continuous sheet. Its fibers coursing upward and backward from the frontal region are oriented at an angle to those of the outer layer. Its fibroblasts have a slightly darker cytoplasm, elongated processes, and ovoid nuclei with more condensed chromatin than those of the outer layer. Small blood vessels are present in both layers of the dura.

Internal to the inner dura is a *border cell layer* of modified, flattened fibroblasts with long sinuous processes that intermingle with those of neighboring cells (Fig. 11–32). The cells have the usual organelles. Their processes are attached at occasional desmosomes and gap junctions that are lacking on the cells of the meningeal dura. The intercellular

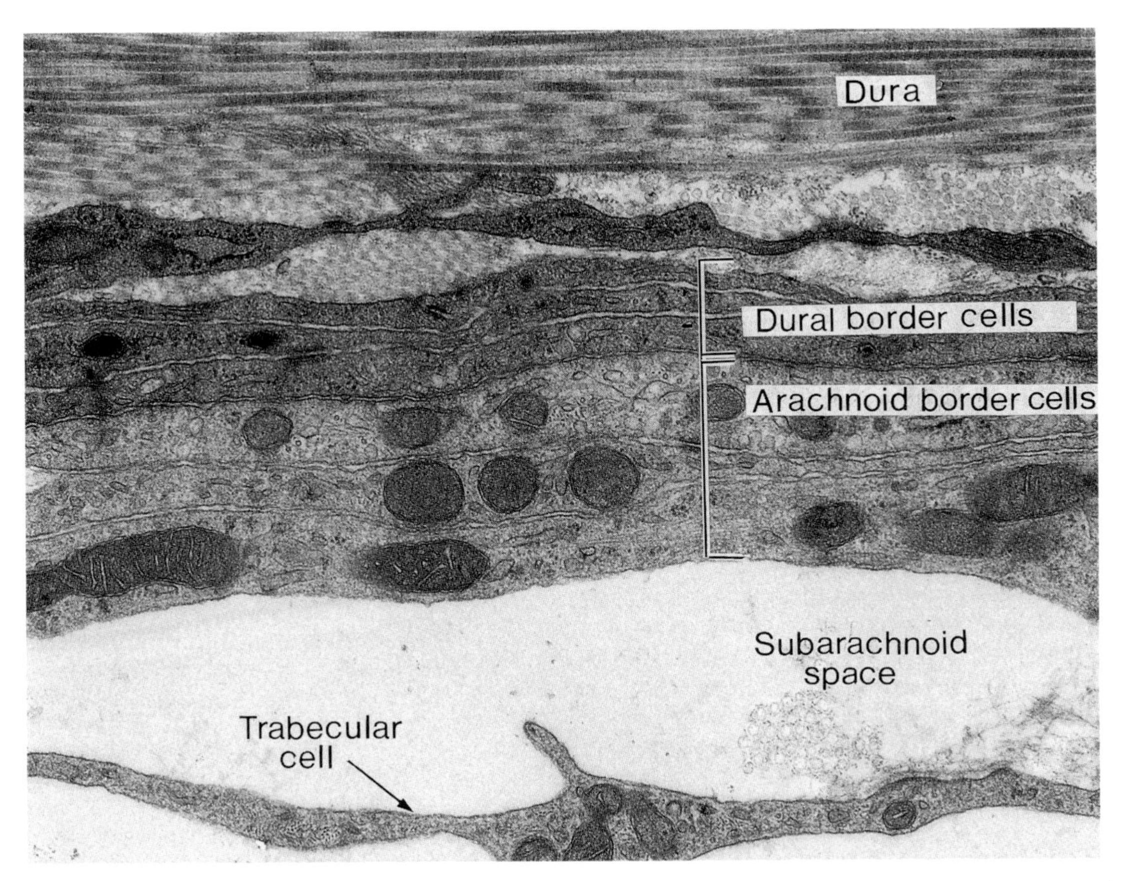

Figure 11–32. Electron micrograph of the inner dura (D), the cells comprising the dura border cell layer (DBC), and the arachnoid barrier cell layer (ABC) in the guinea pig. The DBC and ABC layers are continuous and there is no evidence of a subdural space. (Courtesy of Haines, D.E. 1991. Anat. Rec. 230:3.)

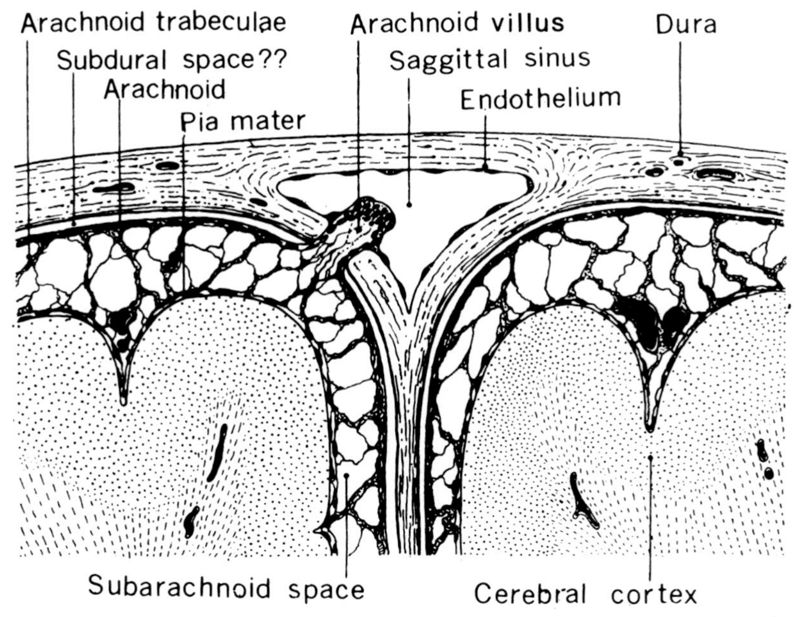

Figure 11–33. Diagram of the organization of the connective tissue sheaths of the brain. Cerebrospinal fluid formed in the choroid plexus circulates in the subarachnoid space and is absorbed into the venous sinuses through the arachnoid villi, of which one is shown here projecting into the saggittal sinus. The subdural space shown here is now thought to be an artifact. (From Weed, L.H. 1922. Am. J. Anat. 31:191.

spaces are not occupied by collagenous fibers but by a flocculent material, possibly mucopolysaccharide in nature. The dark, highly branched fibroblasts, amorphous intercellular material, and absence of connective tissue fibers are distinctive features of this layer. In the transitional zone between the border cell layer and the meningeal dura, flocculent intercellular material is found, together with small collagen fibers.

ARACHNOID

The arachnoidal component of the leptomeninges consists of a layer of closely apposed cells, the *arachnoid barrier layer,* and an inner region of very loosely associated cells oriented, for the most part, perpendicular to that layer and traversing the *subarachnoid space* between it and the pia mater (Figs. 11–33 and 11–34). These *arachnoid trabecular cells* are modified fibroblasts. With long processes attached to each other and to the cells of the barrier layer by desmosomes and gap junctions. A few collagen fibers are associated with the trabecular cells. The cells of the barrier layer are separated by little or no extracellular space and are attached to one another by many desmosomes and tight junctions. A thin basal lamina is present on the inner aspect of this layer.

PIA MATER

This layer, closely adherent to the brain and spinal cord, is composed of flattened, modified fibroblasts that closely conform to the contours of the underlying nervous tissue. They may form a thin, single layer or, in some areas, they may overlap one another. They closely resemble the cells of the arachnoid trabeculae. Numerous blood vessels are associated with this layer, but owing to its thinness, these are often partially surrounded by trabecular cells. The pia mater and arachnoid are so intimately related that they are often treated as a single layer, the *pia arachnoid.* Fine collagenous and elastic fibers are interposed between the pial cells and the underlying neural tissue. Macrophages are also found between the pial cells and the glial basement membrane around the pial blood vessels. In humans, they often contain large amounts of a yellow pigment that reacts positively for iron. Scattered mast cells and small groups of lymphocytes may be found along the pial vessels. In certain pathological conditions, these may greatly increase

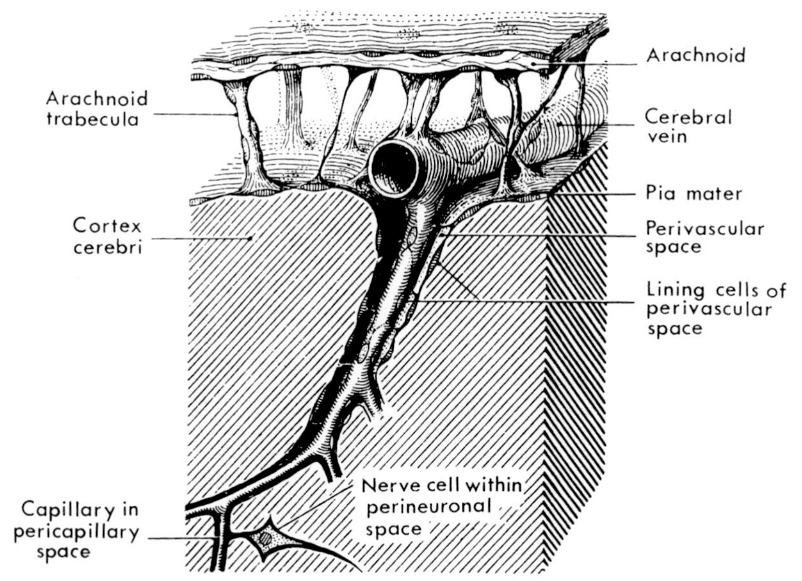

Figure 11–34. Diagram of the cerebral pia arachnoid showing the relations of the subarachnoid space and perivascular channels with the brain. (From Weed, L.H. 1922. Am. J. Anat. 31.)

in number. In the pia covering the ventral surface of the medulla oblongata, a variable number of melanocytes may be found.

MENINGEAL SPACES

In the anatomical and clinical literature, frequent reference is made to a "subdural space," and such a space is included in the Nomina Anatomica. But, it is clear from the foregoing description of the histology of the meninges that there is normally no such space between the dura and the arachnoid. When such a space appears to be present, it is now considered to be an artifact of specimen preparation. The dural border cell layer, with its abundant intercellular spaces, is evidently a relatively weak plane within the meninges, and extravasation of blood, or other fluids, enlarges its spaces, disrupts cell junctions, or tears off cell processes and so creates a larger space where none normally exists. Therefore, the "subdural hematoma" that commonly follows head injuries is not beneath the dura as the name implies but is an accumulation of blood within the dural border cell layer and, thus, intradural.

Between the arachnoid barrier cell layer and the pia mater, there is a true *subarachnoid space,* traversed by arachnoid trabeculae and normally containing a large amount of fluid (Figs. 11–32 and 11–33). Over the convolutions of the brain, it is narrow, but in the sulci between the cerebral hemispheres, it is wide and deep. The subarachnoid space is especially wide throughout the length of the spinal cord. In the brain, it is greatly enlarged in a few places where the arachnoid barrier layer is widely separated from the pia, and trabeculae are few or absent. Such areas are referred to as *cisternae.* The largest, the *cisterna magna,* lies above the medulla oglongata and below the posterior border of the cerebellum. The fourth ventricle communicates with it through three openings in the tela choroidea: a medial *foramen of Magendie* and two lateral *foramina of Luschke.*

NERVES OF THE MENINGES

The dura and pia mater are richly supplied with nerves. All vessels of the pia, and of the choroid plexus, are surrounded by extensive nerve plexuses in their adventitia. The axons, belonging to the sympathetic system, originate in certain cranial nerves and in the carotid and vertebral plexuses. Nonencapsulated sensory nerve terminations, and even single nerve cells, are also present in the adventitia of the blood vessels.

In addition to the nerves to the vessels, the cerebral dura contains many sensory nerve endings. The pia also contains extensive nerve plexuses, most abundant in the tela choroidea of the third ventricle. The axons end either in large pear-shaped or bulbous expansions or in spiral convolutions like those of Meissner's corpuscles. In the spinal pia, the vessels receive their nerves from the plexuses following the larger spinal blood vessels. Afferent nerve endings are also present, but these are unevenly distributed.

Both myelinated and unmyelinated nerve fibers accompany the blood vessels into the substance of the spinal cord and the brain, ending on the smooth muscle cells of the vessel walls. These come from similar nerves of the pial vessels.

VENTRICLES

The CNS develops from the embryonic neural tube and remains a hollow organ in the adult. The ventricular cavities of the brain form a continuous channel for the flow of the cerebrospinal fluid (CSF). If part of this channel is occluded by disease preventing free circulation of fluid, intracerebral pressure increases, with resulting hydrocephalus and other serious consequences. The central canal of the spinal cord is minute in the adult and may be completely obliterated.

The ventricular cavity is normally dilated in four regions: the two *lateral ventricles* in the medial wall of the cerebral hemispheres; the *third ventricle* in the roof of the diencephalon between the two thalami; and caudad to the nondilated cerebral aqueduct traversing the midbrain, the *fourth ventricle* in the roof of the pons and rostral medulla oblongata. Choroid plexuses develop in all four regions and most of the fluid in the ventricles is derived from the blood vessels of these plexuses.

CHOROID PLEXUSES

The entire CNS is bathed in the cerebrospinal fluid secreted by the *choroid plexuses.* In these plexuses, there is no nervous tissue in the wall, and the highly vascular pia mater, therefore, comes into direct contact with the ependymal epithelium lining the ventricle. In forming each choroid plexus, these two layers give rise to elaborate folds that project into the lumen (Fig. 11–35). The folds, in turn, bear numerous villi, each covered by epithelium and containing afferent and efferent pial vessels and an intervening capillary network. The choroid plexuses, thus, present a very large surface area, estimated to be in excess of 200 cm^2.

The cells of these specialized regions of the ependymal epithelium are cuboidal, with a single spherical nucleus, numerous rod-shaped mitochondria, and a moderately extensive endoplasmic reticulum. The free surface has an atypical brush border consisting of irregularly oriented microvilli that often have bulbous expansions at their tips (Fig. 11–36). Although it is possible that these expansions are artifacts of fixation, microvilli of other cell types, prepared similarly, do not have this appearance.

The choroid plexuses serve as a selective barrier, maintaining constancy of the fluid environment of the CNS. They produce CSF at a mean rate of 14–36 ml/h, replacing the total volume of about 150 ml, four or five times per day. This is accomplished by creation of an ion gradient. At the basal and basolateral surfaces of the cells, H^+ ions are exchanged for Na^+ ions in the plasma and these are pumped out at the cell apex. Cl^- and HCO^- ions move from the cytoplasm across the apical membrane to neutralize the excess Na^+ ions. The osmotic gradient so produced results in diffusion of water into the ventricle. Although water makes up 90% of the CSF, its ionic composition is actively regulated.

Movement of substances across the choroid epithelium takes place in both directions. Molecules such as glucose and amino acids required by the brain in large amounts move by facilitated diffusion down a concentration gradient, whereas substances required in small amounts such as vitamin C, vitamin B, and foliates move by active transport. Proteins are generally excluded from the CSF, but very small amounts present are believed to be secreted by the choroid plexuses, which also excrete metabolic by-products and certain drugs into the blood for degradation in the liver or elimination by the kidneys. The capillary endothelium of a choroid plexus is very thin and has many pores closed by thin diaphragms. If vital dyes, such as trypan blue, are repeatedly injected intravenously, they are taken up and stored in the choroid epithelium, or ingested by macrophages found in the perivascular connective tissue. When horseradish peroxidase is injected into the blood, the protein can be shown to cross the

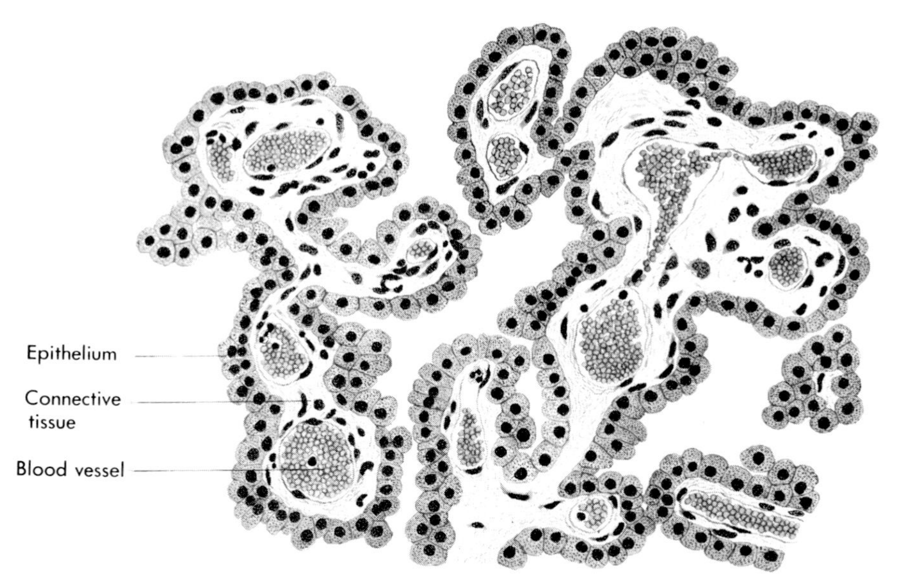

Figure 11–35. Drawing of the choroid plexus of the fourth ventricle of man.

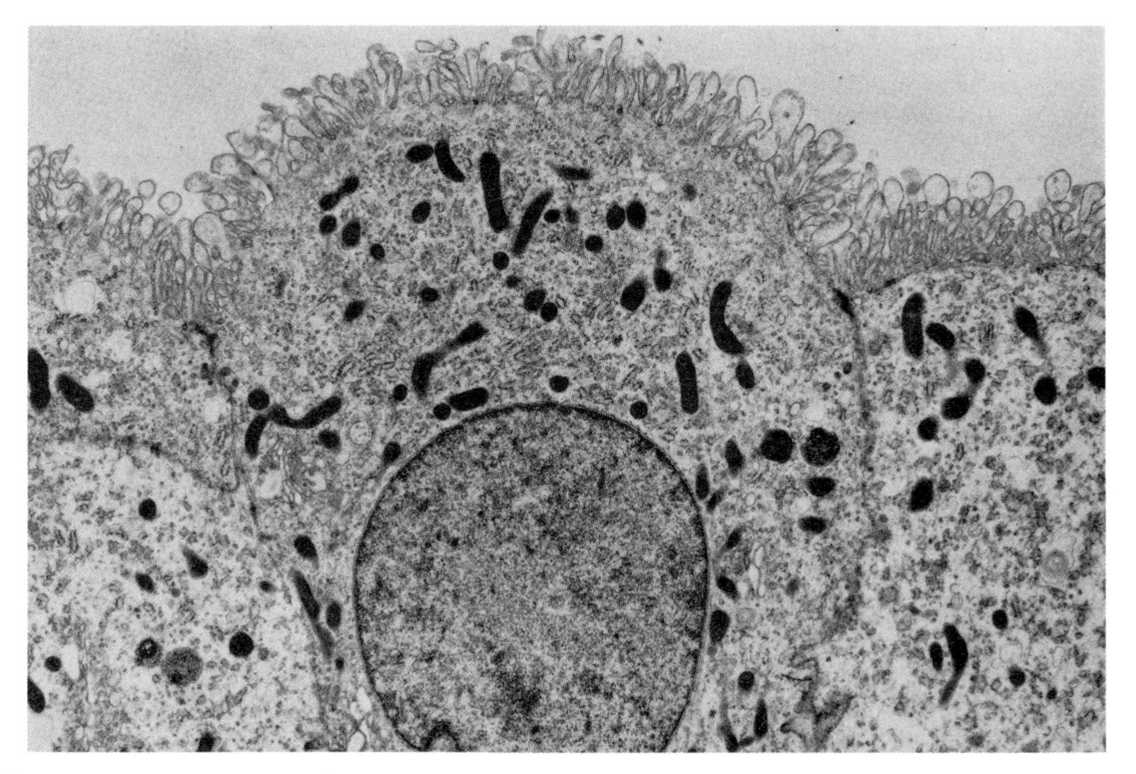

Figure 11–36. Electron micrograph of the epithelium of the choroid plexus at high magnification illustrating its unusual free border consisting of bulbous or clavate microvilli.

capillary endothelium and accumulate in the extracellular spaces. It also moves between the epithelial cells but is denied entry to the CSF by the occluding junctions between the cell apices.

CEREBROSPINAL FLUID

The CSF produced by the choroid plexuses in the lateral ventricles flows to the third ventricle, where more fluid is produced, and from there, via the cerebral aqueduct, into the fourth ventricle, where still more fluid is added. It then escapes through the foramina of Magendie and Luschka into the subarachnoid space, within which it flows upward over the surface of the brain and downward around the spinal cord. Metabolites from the brain diffuse freely from the extracellular spaces, across the ependyma, and into the CSF in the subarachnoid space.

In addition to its role in maintaining the appropriate fluid environment for the brain, the CSF provides some protection against mild concussions and other mechanical injuries. It is formed at a rate of 350 μl/min or about 500 ml per day. Of this, perhaps 30 ml is contained within the ventricles, with the rest occupying the subarachnoid space and cisterns. Although the bulk of the CSF (probably well over half) is formed in the choroid plexus, substantial amounts appear to arise elsewhere, from the parenchyma of the brain, with the fluid then moving across the ependyma into the ventricle. An additional contribution may be made in the area postrema at the caudal margin of the fourth ventricle. In the constant loss of fluid that counterbalances continued CSF production, a small amount may enter extracranial lymphatics through perineural spaces around cranial and spinal nerve roots, and some may diffuse into small superficial veins. Most of it, however, passes through local specializations of the arachnoid where it is returned to the venous blood.

ARACHNOID VILLI

The large endocranial venous sinuses are surrounded over most of their surface by thick dura. However, in certain places, chiefly in the sagittal sinus of the falx cerebri, the dura is penetrated by many small protrusions of the arachnoid (Fig. 11–33). Through each of these openings, a small projection of the arachnoid, called an *arachnoid villus,* extends a short distance into the lumen of the sinus. At its base, the interior of the villus communicates freely with the subarachnoid space. Thus, at a villus, CSF in that space is separated from the blood in the sinus only by a thin cap of epithelium and the overlying endothelium (Fig. 11–37).

Arachnoid villi provide the main pathway for outflow of cerebrospinal fluid. The low hydrostatic pressure and relatively high colloid osmotic pressure of the blood favor diffusion of fluid across the thin layers of cells intervening, but even if the pressure gradient is reversed, the outward flow continues. Thus, the arachnoid villi act like one-way valves. How the flow is maintained is debated. Some believe that open channels between the endothelial cells capping the villus allow fluid to pass, whereas others fail to find such openings (Fig. 11–37). A recent suggestion proposes that giant vacuoles form on the subarachnoid side of the endothelial cells and are then trans-

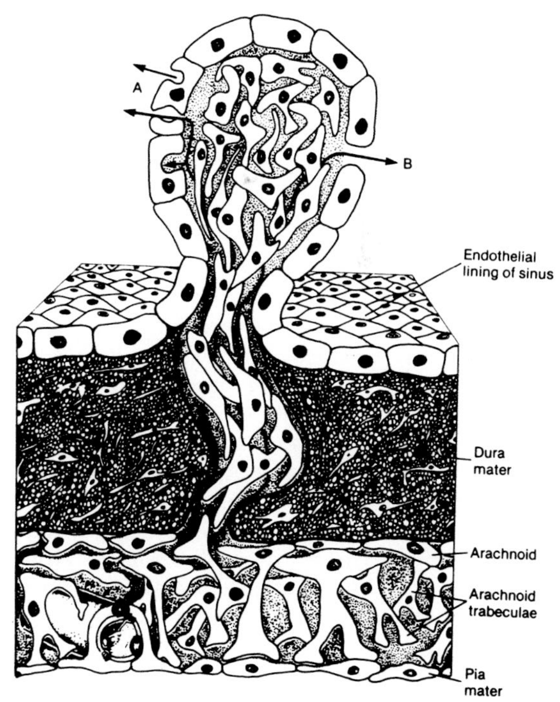

Figure 11–37. Diagram of an arachnoid villus showing the passage of cerebrospinal fluid from the subarachnoid space into a dural venous sinus. (A) Cerebrospinal fluid movement through large vacuoles in the endothelial cells as described by some workers. (B) Movement through channels between cells, as described by other workers. (From Nolte, J. 1988. The Human Brain, 2nd ed. St. Louis, MO, C.V. Mosby Co.; modified after Shabo, A.L. and D.S. Maxwell. 1968. J. Neurosurg. 29:451.)

ported to the venous side, with these vacuoles sometimes opening briefly on both sides at the same time. However accomplished, the outflow is quite rapid. Dyes injected into the subarachnoid space can be detected in the bloodstream in from 10 to 30 s, and after 30 min they can be found in the lymphatics.

Arachnoid villi have been found in dogs, cats, monkeys, and man and are presumed to be present in other mammalian species. In humans, they enlarge with advancing age and become corpuscles or granulations readily visible with the naked eye, and they may become a site of calcium deposition.

BLOOD-BRAIN BARRIER

When dyes such as trypan blue or Evans blue are injected into the blood, they rapidly diffuse through capillary walls and stain most of the tissues of the body, but the brain remains colorless, save for the choroid plexus and a few subependymal areas. Thus, between the blood and the brain, there is an effective *blood-brain barrier.* Although this is the term used universally, it is important to recognize that it applies equally to the spinal cord. It is not an absolute barrier, except to some vital dyes and other large molecules, but is a highly selective interface between the blood and the entire CNS (Fig. 11–38). Many substances can pass through it in both directions and under some degree of neural control, thus acting to preserve the homeostasis of the CNS.

Electron micrographs show that the barrier depends on special properties of the capillary endothelium. Whereas capillaries elsewhere are often fenestrated, or have intercellular junctions of low resistance, the endothelial junctions in the CNS have tight junctions that are highly resistant to passage of ions or small molecules. Moreover, unlike peripheral capillaries, those of the brain do not exhibit transendothelial transport in small vesicles. How is it that these endothelial cells differentiate differently than those elsewhere is not clear, but it is speculated that the astrocyte foot-processes that normally surround brain capillaries may somehow influence the endothelium to acquire its unique properties when blood vessels invade the CNS during development.

The blood-brain barrier serves to protect the CNS from abrupt changes in the concentration of ions in the extracellular fluid and from molecules in the general circulation that might interfere with normal neural function. The need for nutrients and for exchanging hormones and other compounds with the rest of the body is met by facilitated diffusion, as in the case of glucose, or by specific active transport systems within the capillary endothelial cells. Such systems for amino acids, transferrin, and insulin ensure that the CNS continuously receives the compounds it needs.

The advantages of the barrier are somewhat offset by the fact that it excludes antibiotics, certain neurotransmitters (e.g., dopamine), and other potentially beneficial drugs. Some success has been achieved in transiently breaching the barrier by perfusion of a hypertonic solution of mannitol, which transiently opens the tight junctions and permits entry of therapeutic drugs. Another ingenious approach to this problem is to take advantage of an existing transport system of the endothelium by binding a drug to antibodies against transferrin receptors. After binding, these receptors then actively shuttle the antibody and drug molecules across the blood-brain barrier.

RESPONSE OF NEURONS TO INJURY

This topic may seem more appropriate to pathology than to histology, but it is included here because much of our knowledge of the origin, course, and connections of nerve tracts was gained by tracing the visible degenerative changes in neuronal cell bodies and their axons after localized lesions. When an axon is crushed or severed, degeneration extends only a short distance proximally and repair soon begins with the appearance of new axonal sprouts. Distally, however, the axon, its myelin sheath, and its terminal arborization completely degenerate. This process is commonly called *Wallerian degeneration* after Augustus Waller, the nineteenth century British physician who first described it in 1850. In peripheral nerves, these changes usually proceed simultaneously along the nerve fibers distal to the point of injury. Within 24–48 h, axonal mitochondria swell and aggregate, neurofilaments break up, and the axon takes on a beaded appearance. At the same time, the myelin sheath breaks down, first into concentric lamellated columns, then into lipid droplets around the axon. Macrophages then move in to remove the debris.

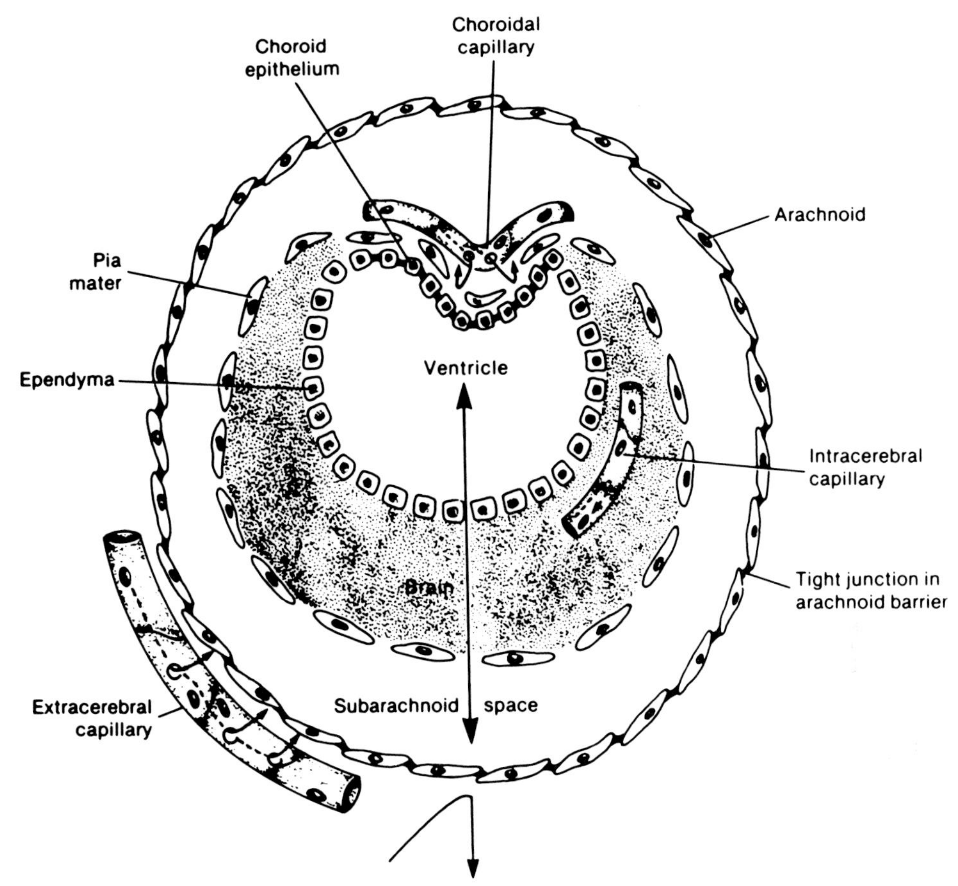

Figure 11–38. Barrier systems in and around the brain. Substances can leave extracerebral capillaries but are then blocked by the arachnoid barrier. They can also leave choroidal capillaries but are then blocked by the choroidal epithelium. They cannot leave any other capillaries that are inside the arachnoid barrier. The ventricular and subarachnoid spaces are in free communication with each other and both communicate with the extracellular space of the brain. (From Nolte, J. 1988. The Human Brain, 2nd ed. St. Louis, MO, C.V. Mosby.)

The Schwann cells remain intact during axonal degeneration, but, shortly thereafter, they hypertrophy and also divide, aligning themselves along the nerve as a long train of cells each separated from the next, but with extensively overlapping ends, so as to form a tube containing fluid and the residues of the axon. As the wall of the tube thickens, its lumen is reduced in diameter and ultimately is obliterated, forming a solid band (band of Bungner) recognizable by the alignment of Schwann cell nuclei along its length. Concurrently with these changes, the plasmalemma of the Schwann cells and adjacent basal lamina separate and additional basal laminae may be formed concentrically around the band. This serves to create multiple tubular compartments between the Schwann cells and the endoneurium, through which axonal sprouts grow from undamaged regions of the axon proximal to the injury or from neighboring undamaged axons. Such bands remain for months awaiting the slow growth of axons toward their peripheral targets. If axon regeneration does not occur, the bands are gradually reduced by encroaching endoneurial connective tissue.

The brief and limited degeneration of the proximal stump of a severed peripheral nerve is usually followed by axonal regeneration. Fine growth cones and filopodia appear at the tip of the viable proximal end of the axon and these slowly advance along the outer surface of the columns of Schwann cells and are progressively enveloped by them. The rate of axon elongation is 3–4 mm per day, but the distance to be traversed may be 1 m or more, depending on the site of the original injury. The abundance of the regenerative sprouts from the axons involved, and the capacity of the columns to accommodate and direct hundreds of axons, favor successful reinnervation. Functional recovery depends on successful reestablishment of appropriate sensory or motor connections at the periphery. In the case of a denervated muscle, it will have undergone some degree of atrophy, and full recovery must await its recovery as well, along with return of effective neuromuscular transmission. Also required is deletion of maladaptive endings and central remodeling of reflex arcs. Intensive physical therapy to maintain and strengthen those muscle fibers that remain innervated also appear to play an important role in the recovery process, which may take 2 years or longer.

Nerve fibers in the central nervous system undergo a slower Wallerian degeneration. Loss of myelin in a tract may not be evident in routine Weigert-stained preparations for 2 months, but the special selective silver method of Nauta, in which impregnation of normal axons is suppressed, may reveal degenerative changes in the myelin sooner, and this is useful in tracing connections after experimental ablation of nuclei and tracts in neuroanatomical research.

The changes in the nerve cell body after severance of the axon were described by Nissl in 1892. Chief among these is *retrograde chromatolysis,* the apparent disappearance of the cytoplasmic basophilic bodies which have long been referred to as the Nissl substance. This is now known to consist of parallel arrays of cisternae of rough endolasmic reticulum. Under the light microscope, the break up of this material is first seen near the axon hillock. It then spreads from around the nucleus to other parts of the cell body. In addition, the perikaryon takes up water and swells and the nucleus shifts from its normal central position to one at the periphery, away from the axon hillock. Electron micrographs show disperson of the arrays of cisternae of endoplasmic reticulum, diminution in number of ribosomes, and the appearance of many neurofilaments. This process begins about a day after axonal injury and reaches its peak in about 2 weeks. It is most obvious in motor neurons but also occur to varying degrees in other nerve cells. Neuroanatomists familiar with the normal pattern of Nissl substance in the cells of various regions of the CNS can cut a nerve or tract and locate its origin by looking for neurons exhibiting chromatolysis. Until the advent of techniques exploiting orthograde and retrograde axonal transport, such a time-consuming search for chromatolysis and tracing Wallerian degeneration were the only methods available for working out the organization of the CNS.

In general, the more axoplasm that is detached from the cell body, the greater is the retrograde chromatolysis. Cutting an axon near its distal termination may elicit no detectable response. Conversely, if the damage to the axon has been near the cell body, the cell may die, with the chromatolytic reaction progressing to complete lysis of the neuron. If regeneration of the axon takes place, the changes in the cell body are slowly reversed, with reconstitution of the Nissl substance, sometimes to such a degree that it becomes superabundant. Return to normal may take several months because an enormous metabolic effort is required to synthesize an amount of axoplasm that may be 100–200 times the volume of the cell body. Not surprisingly, even after apparent recovery, the neuron may later die.

Chromatolysis may occur in neuronal perikarya for reasons other than axonal section. Such a loss of stainable Nissl substance may differ in the direction of its disappearance within the cell body, fading away from the cell periphery inward toward the nucleus, rather than outward from the nucleus, as in the case in retrograde or *central chromatolysis.* In some instances, this *peripheral chromatolysis* has been considered to reflect either an advanced stage of neuronal degeneration or a neuron's fight for life. It is seen in certain infectious or degenerative diseases of the nervous system, such as poliomyelitis and progressive muscular atrophy. Another interpretation is that peripheral chromatolysis of early onset after neuronal damage is a step toward cell death, whereas a late reaction is a sign of recovery in progress. The validity of such interpretations is questionable.

BIBLIOGRAPHY

Bray, D. and D. Gilbert. 1981. Cytoskeletan elements in neurons. Annu. Rev. Neurosci. 4:505.

Bray, G.M., M. Rasminsky, and A.J. Aguayo. 1981. Interactions between axons and their sheath cells. Annu. Rev. Neurosci. 4:127.

Bunge, R.P. 1968. Glial cells and the central myelin sheath. Physiol. Rev. 41:197.

Cleveland, D.W. and P.N. Hoffman. 1991. Neuronal and glial cytoskeletons. Current Opinion Neurobiol. 1:346.

Coggeshall, R.E. 1979. A fine structural analysis of the myelin sheath in rat spinal roots. Anat. Rec. 194:201.

Davis, H. 1961. Some principles of censory receptor action. Physiol. Rev. 41:391.
Davison, P.F. and E.W. Taylor. 1960. Physical-chemical studies of proteins of squid nerve axoplasm, with special reference to the axon fibrous protein. J. Gen. Physiol. 43:801.
Eccles, J.C. 1957. The Physiology of Nerve Cells. Baltimore, MD. Johns Hopkins Press.
Fox, C.A. and J.W. Barnard. 1957. A quantitative study of the Purkinje cell dendritic branchlets and their relation to afferent fibers. J. Anat. 91:299.
Furshpan, E.J. 1964. "Electrical transmission" at an excitatory synapse in a vertebrate brain. Science 144:878.
Geren, B.B. 1956. Structural studies of the formation of the myelin sheath in peripheral nerve fibers. *In* D. Rudnick ed. Cellular Mechanisms in Differentiation and Growth. Princeton, NJ, Princeton University Press.
Gershon, M.D. 1981. The enteric nervous system. Annu. Rev. Neurosci. 4:227.
Glees, P. 1955. Neuroglia: Morphology and Function. Springfield, IL, Charles C. Thomas.
Grafstein, B. and D.S. Forman. 1980. Intracellular transport in neurons. Physiol. Rev. 60:1167.
Gray, E.G. and R.W. Guillery. 1962. Synaptic morphology in the normal and degenerating nervous system. Internat. Rev. Cytol. 19:41.
Guth, L. 1956. Regeneration in the mammalian peripheral nervous system. Physiol. Rev. 36:441.
Haines, D.E. 1991. On the question of a subdural space. Anat. Rec. 230:3.
Harrison, R.G. 1910. The outgrowth of the nerve fiber as a mode of protoplasmic movement. J. Exp. Zool. 9:787.
Heuser, J.E. and T.S. Reese. 1977. Structure of the synapse. *In* Handbook of Physiology, Section I: The Nervous System, Vol. I, Cellular Biology of Nurons, Part I, p. 261. Bethesda, MD, American Physiological Society.
Heuser, J.E. and T.S. Reese. 1979. Changes in structure of presynaptic membranes during transmitter secretion. *In* Neurobiology. New York, John Wiley & Sons.
Heuser, J.E., T.S. Reese, M.J. Dennis, Y. Yan, L. Jam, and L. Evans. 1979. Synaptic vesicle exocytosis captured by quick freezing and correlated with quantal transmitter release. J. Cell Biol. 81:275.
Katz, B. 1959. Mechanism of synaptic transmission, and nature of the nerve impulse. *In* J.L. Oncley et al. eds. Biophysical Science—A Study Program. New York, John Wiley & Sons.
Kelly, R.B. 1988. The cell biology of the nerve terminal. Neuron 1:431.
Kunz, A. 1953. The Autonomic Nervous System, 4th ed. Philadelphia, Lea & Febiger.
Landis, D.M., T.S. Reese, and E. Raviola. 1974. Differences in membrane structure between excitatory and inhibitory components of the reciprocal synapse in olefactory bulb. J. Comp. Neurol. 155:67.
Maycox, P.R., E. Link, A. Reetz, S. Morris, and R. Jahn. 1992. Clathrin-coated vesicles in nervous tissue are involved primarily in synaptic vesicle recycling. J. Cell Biol. 118:1379.
Morris, J.F. and D.V. Pow. 1991. Widespread release of peptides in the central nervous system: Quantitation of tannic acid-captured exocytoses. Anat. Rec. 231:437.
Ortiz-Picón, J.M. 1955. The neuroglia of the sensory ganglia. Anat. Rec. 121:513.
Palay, S.L. 1963. The structural basis for nerve action. *In* M.A.B. Brazier, ed. Brain Function, Vol. II. Berkeley, University of California Press.
Palay, S.L. and V. Chan-Palay, 1974. Cerebellar Cortex. Cytology and Organization. New York, Springer-Verlag.
Palay, S.L. and G.E. Palade. 1955. The fine structure of neurons. J. Biophys. Biochem. Cytol. 1:69.
Peters, A.S., S.L. Palay, and H. deF. Webster. 1991. The Fine Structure of the Nervous System, 3rd ed. Philadelphia, W.B. Saunders Co.
Polyak, S. 1957. Vertebrate Visual System. Chicago, IL, University of Chicago Press.
Ramón y Cajal, S. 1909. Histologie du Systeme Nerveux de l'Homme et des Vertébrés. Paris, A. Maloine.
Ramón y Cajal, S. 1929. Degeneration and Regeneration of the Nervous System. London, Oxford University Press.
Raviola, E. and G. Raviola. 1982. Structure of the synaptic membranes in the inner plexiform layer of the retina. A freeze-fracture study in monkeys and rabbits. J. Comp. Neurol. 209:233.
Revel. J.P. and J. Hamilton. 1969. The double nature of the intermediate dense line in peripheral nerve myelin. Anat. Rec. 163:7.
Robertson, J.D. 1955. The ultrastructure of adult vertebrate myelinated nerve fibers in relation to myelinogenesis. J. Biophys. Biochem. Cytol. 1:271.
Robertson, J.D. 1958. The ultrastructure of Schmidt–Lantermann clefts and related shearing defects of the myelin sheath. J. Biophys. Biochem. Cytol. 4:39.
Scharrer, E. and B. Scharrer. 1954. Neurosekretion. *In* W. Von Mollendorff and W. Bargmann, eds. Handbuch der Mikroschopischen Anatomie des Menschen. Vol. 6., Part 5. Berlin, Springer-Verlag.
Schwartz, J.H. 1979. Axonal transport. Components, mechanisms, and specificity. Annu. Rev. Neurosci. 2:467.
Snyder, S.H. 1992. Nitric oxide: First of a new class of neurotransmitters. Science 257:494.
Trimble, W.S., M. Linial, and R.H. Scheller. 1991. Cellular and molecular biology of the presynaptic nerve terminal. Annu. Rev. Neurosci. 14:93.
Vallee, R.B. and G.S. Bloom. 1991. Mechanism of fast and slow axonal transport. Annu. Rev. Neurosci. 14:59.

12

BLOOD AND LYMPH VASCULAR SYSTEMS

Multicellular animals require a mechanism for distribution of oxygen, nutritive materials, hormones, and other signaling molecules to the tissues, and for collecting from them carbon dioxide and other metabolic waste products to be transported to the excretory organs for elimination. In vertebrates, these essential functions are carried out by the *blood vascular system* which consists of a muscular pump, the *heart,* and two systems of *blood vessels.* One of these, the *pulmonary circulation,* carries blood to and from the lungs; the other, the *systemic circulation* (peripheral circulation), distributes blood to all the other tissues and organs of the body. In both, the blood pumped from the heart passes successively through *arteries* of diminishing diameter, to networks of minute *capillaries,* and then back to the heart through *veins* of increasing caliber.

At each beat, the heart ejects into two large vessels, the *pulmonary artery* and the *aorta,* about 80 ml of blood, resulting in an outflow of about 6 L/min. The initial velocity of blood flow is about 33 cm/s, but the rate gradually decreases as the total cross-sectional area of the vascular system is increased by the repeated branching of the arteries. A further expansion of the cross-sectional area of the system occurs quite abruptly at the level of the *capillaries,* resulting in a decrease in rate of flow to about 0.3 cm/s. The extensive capillary networks of the body have a total surface area of 700 m^2, available for exchange of metabolites with the tissues. It is only in the capillaries and small venules that the vessel walls are thin enough and permeable enough to permit diffusion of substances to and from the surrounding tissues. The larger vessels are concerned with distribution of blood to the capillaries. At any given moment, only about 5% of the total blood volume is in the capillaries and 95% is on its way to or from them. The structure and functional properties of the capillaries are of great physiological importance because it is this part of the circulation that carries out the primary function of the vascular system.

ARTERIES

Blood is carried from the heart to the capillary networks in the tissues by *arteries.* These constitute an extensive system of vessels beginning with the aorta and pulmonary artery, which emerge from the left and right ventricles of the heart, respectively. As they course away from the heart, these vessels branch repeatedly and, thus, give rise to large numbers of arteries of progressively diminishing caliber.

The basic organization of the wall of all arteries is similar in that three concentric layers can be distinguished: (1) an inner layer, the *tunica intima,* consisting of an endothelial tube whose squamous cells generally have their long axis oriented longitudinally; (2) an intermediate layer, the *tunica media,* composed mainly of smooth muscle cells oriented circumferentially; and (3) an outer coat, the *tunica adventitia,* made up of fibroblasts and associated collagen fibers oriented, for the most part, longitudinally (Fig. 12–1 and 12–2A). This outer layer gradually merges with the loose connective tissue around the vessel. The boundary between the tunica intima and tunica media is marked by the *internal elastic lamina* (*elastica interna*), which is especially well developed in arteries of medium caliber. Between the tunica media and the tunica adventitia, a more delicate *external elastic lamina* (*elastica externa*) is also distinguishable in many arteries.

There is a continuous gradation in diameter and in the character of the vessel wall, from the largest arteries down to the capillaries, but arteries are usually classified as (1) *elastic*

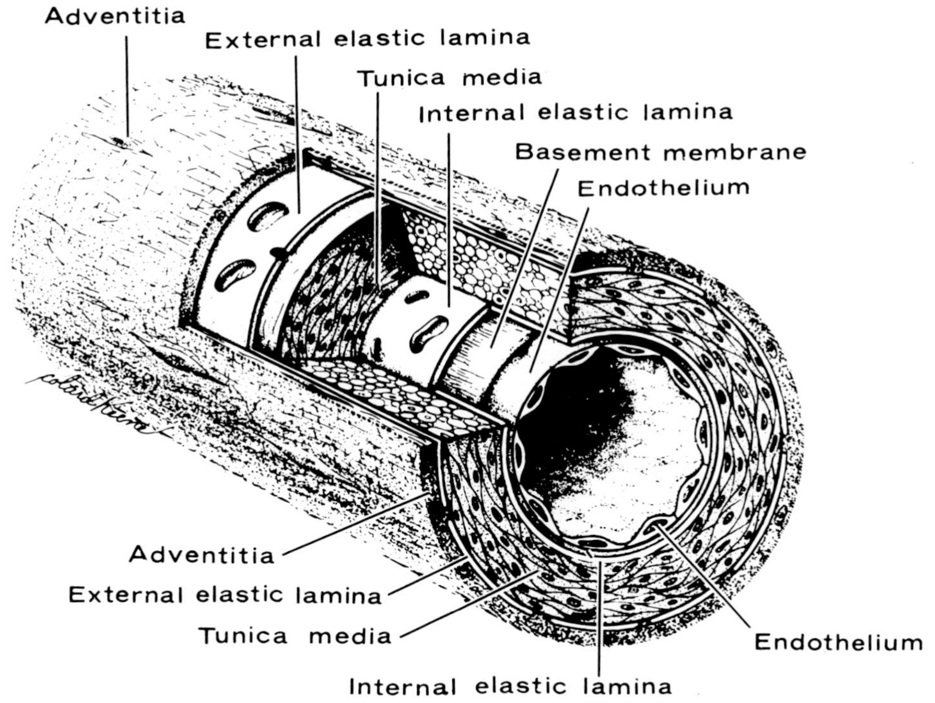

Figure 12–1. Schematic representation of the principal structural components of a medium-sized artery. (Redrawn after Williams and Warwick. 1980. *In* Gray's Anatomy, 38th British ed. Philadelphia, W.B. Saunders Co.

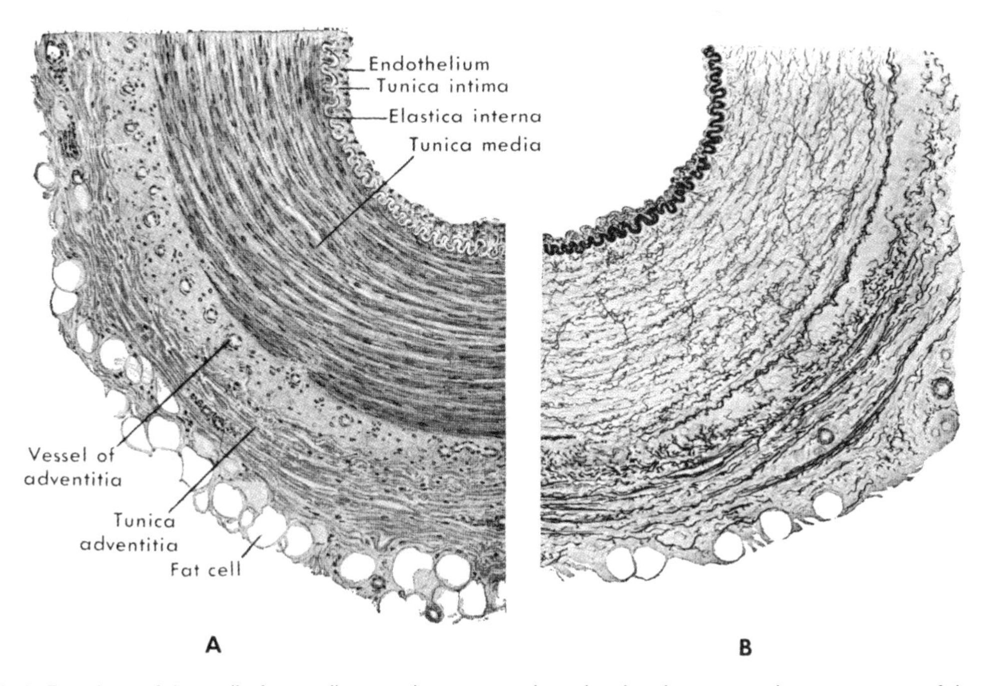

Figure 12–2. Drawings of the wall of a small artery, in cross section, showing the concentric arrangement of the tunica intima, media, and adventitia. (A) Stained with hematoxylin and eosin; (B) stained with orcein to reveal the elastic tissue component.

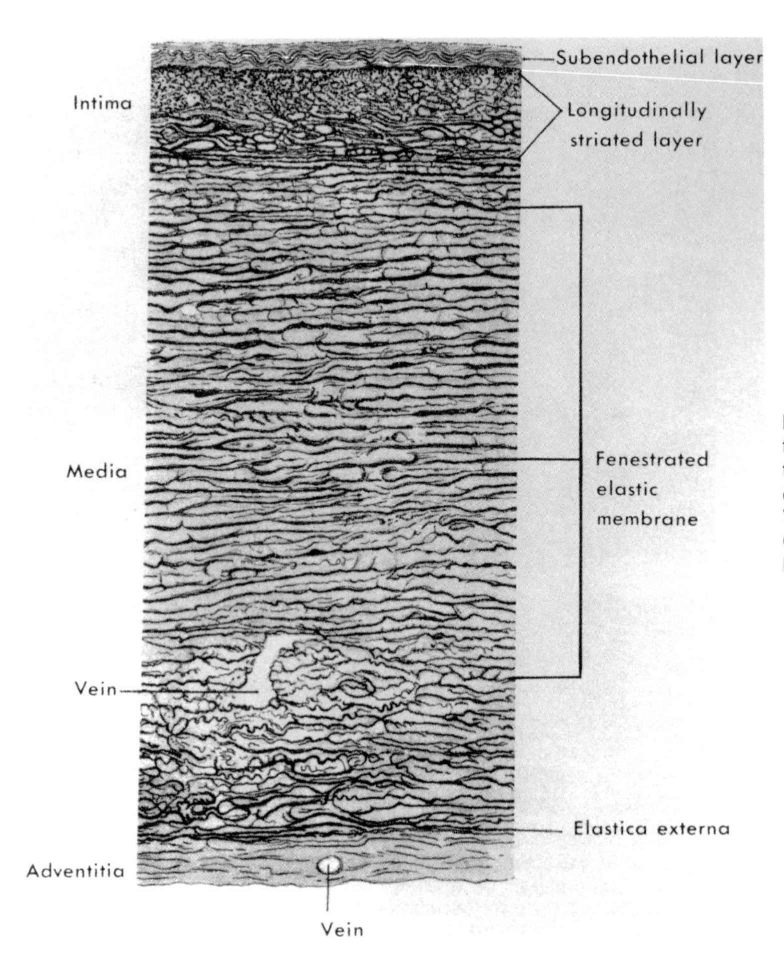

Figure 12–3. Section through the posterior wall of the human aorta. Elastic tissue is black, other components are essentially unstained (after von Ebner, V. 1902 in Kolliker, A., Handbuck der Gewebelehre, Vol. 3, Leipzig.) [Publisher not available]

arteries (conducting arteries), (2) *muscular arteries* (distributing arteries) and *arterioles,* on the basis of their size, the predominant component of their tunica media, and their principal function.

ELASTIC ARTERIES

The large elastic arteries, such as the pulmonary and aorta, brachiocephalic, subclavian, common carotid, and common iliac have walls containing many fenestrated layers of elastin in their tunica media (Fig. 12–3). Their walls may be distinctly yellow in the fresh state due to the abundance of elastin. These major conducting vessels are distended during contraction of the heart (systole), and the subsequent elastic recoil of their walls during diastole serves as a subsidiary pump maintaining continuous flow despite the intermittency of the heart beat.

The tunica intima of these arteries consists of the *endothelium,* a thin squamous epithelium, separated from the elastica interna by loose connective tissue containing a few fibroblasts, occasional smooth muscle cells, and thin collagen fibers. The endothelium provides a smooth lining layer for the vessel and a partially selective diffusion barrier between the blood and the outer tunics of the vessel wall. Its cells are polygonal in outline, 10–15 μm wide and 25–50 μm long, with their long axis oriented longitudinally. Adjacent endothelial cells are attached by simple occluding junctions and occasional gap junctions. The cells contain all of the common organelles, usually located in the thicker region of cytoplasm around the centrally placed and flattened nucleus. The endothelium is a very slowly renewing population of cells that are rarely found in division. Their adluminal and abluminal membranes have numerous associated small vesicles that are believed to be involved in transendothelial transport of water, electrolytes, and certain macromolecules. Short blunt processes occasionally extend from the base of the endothelial cells through fenestrae in the elastica interna and establish junctions with smooth muscle cells in the media.

Rod-like cytoplasmic inclusions are observed in electron micrographs of arterial endothelium. These are named *Weibel–Palade bodies* after the cytologists who first described them. They are membrane-bounded structures about 0.1 μm in diameter and up to 3 μm long and they contain tubular elements of unknown composition in a moderately dense matrix. They are sites of storeage of *von Willebrand factor,* a very large glycoprotein synthesized by endothelial cells throughout the vascular system but stored in Weibel–Palade bodies only in arteries. This factor is believed to be secreted continuously into the blood plasma. It is a major participant in blood platelet aggregation and adhesion to form a clot at sites of injury to the vessel wall. Its congenital absence results in *von Willebrand disease,* characterized by prolonged blood coagulation time and excessive bleeding after injury.

The tunica media of elastic arteries is made up of multiple concentric, fenestrated lamellae of elastin alternating with thin layers consisting of circularly oriented smooth muscle cells, and fibers of collagen and elastin in a proteoglycan extracellular matrix. The elastic lamellae and other extracellular components are apparently secreted by the smooth muscle cells. The elastica interna is less prominent than it is in muscular arteries. It is merely the innermost of the many elastic laminae in the wall. In the adult, these may number 50 or more in the thoracic aorta and about 30 in the abdominal aorta. The three-dimensional configuration of the elastic components of the vessel wall are difficult to visualize in histological sections, but it is possible to remove all other components with hot formic acid and to examine the unextracted elastin with the scanning electron microscope. In such preparations, it is apparent that the elastic lamellae have relatively large fenestrations of varying size and shape and the successive lamellae are joined by slender interconnecting strands of elastin (Figs. 12–4 and 12–5). Owing to the abundance of elastin in the large elastic

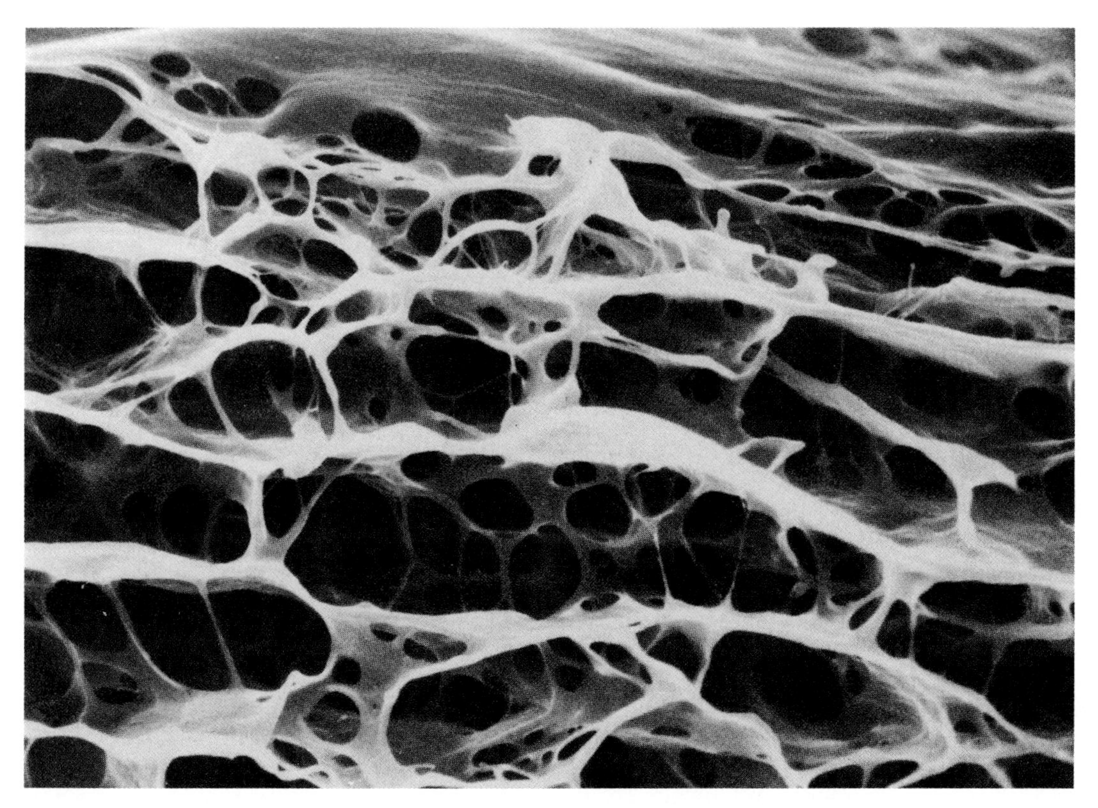

Figure 12–4. Scanning electron micrograph of the three-dimensional architecture of the elastin in the wall of rat aorta extracted with hot formic acid to remove all other tissue components. The elastic tissue consists of multiple concentric sheets or laminae interconnected by radially oriented strands and fenestrated septa. In the intact aorta, smooth muscle cells occupied the spaces demarcated by these elastic elements. (Micrograph courtesy of Wasano, K. 1983. J. Electron Microsc. 33:32.)

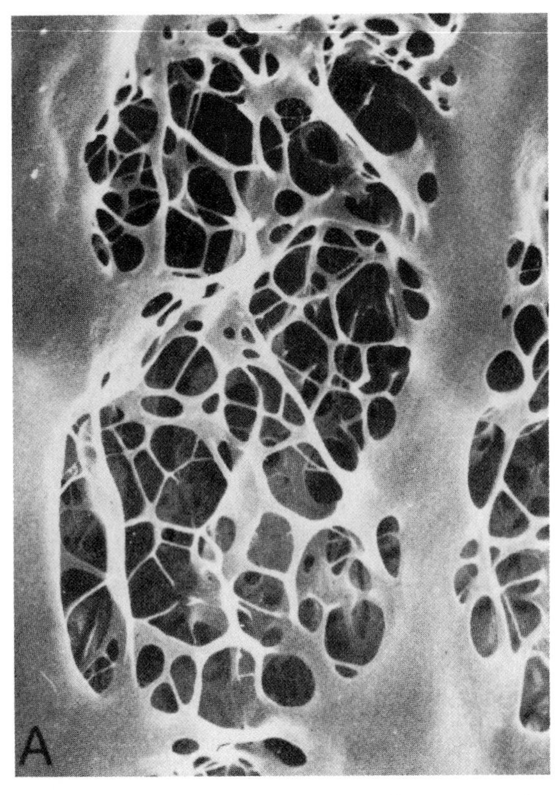

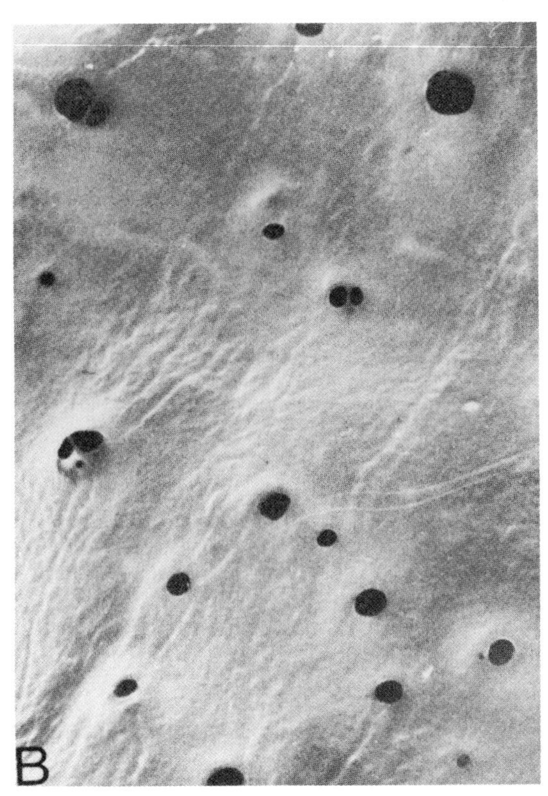

Figure 12–5. (A) Scanning micrograph showing a surface view of the aortic internal elastic lamina of the rat. It is characterized by large fenestrations traversed by an irregular meshwork of thin strands of elastin. (B) In contrast, the internal elastic lamina of the femoral artery shows relatively small round fenestrations. (Micrograph courtesy of Wasano, K. 1983. J. Electron Microsc. 32:33.)

arteries, smooth muscle makes up a relatively small fraction of the media. In the aorta of the rabbit, smooth muscle constitutes only 35% of the volume of the wall, compared to 74% in the tibial artery, a distributing artery.

The tunica adventitia of elastic arteries is relatively thin and consists of fibroblasts, longitudinal bundles of collagen fibers, and a loose network of thin elastic fibers. The walls of the large elastic arteries are too thick to be nourished by diffusion from the lumen of the vessel. Such arteries have a microvasculature of their own. Small blood vessels called *vasa vasorum* ramify over the surface of the vessel to form a network in the adventitia from which capillaries penetrate into the media. How far inward they extend is debated, but it is likely that at least the outer half and possibly more of the wall receives nutrients and oxygen from the vasa vasorum. This still leaves a considerable thickness of the wall dependent on diffusion from the lumen. Fenestration of the elastic lamellae is thought to facilitate diffusion of nutrients. Blood is returned via small veins that are confluent with nearby larger veins.

MUSCULAR OR DISTRIBUTING ARTERIES

As the elastic arteries gradually diminish in diameter and in the thickness of their wall, they give off lateral branches with walls containing less elastin and more smooth muscle. These *muscular* or *distributing arteries* include the branchial, femoral, radial, and popliteal arteries and their branches. This category includes the majority of vessels in the arterial system, spanning a wide range of sizes down to 0.5 mm in diameter.

The intima is thinner than that of the elastic arteries but otherwise similar in its organization. Peripheral to the intima, in cross sections, there is a conspicuous elastica interna which often has an undulating contour, owing to agonal contraction of the media of the vessel (Figs. 12–6 and 12–7). The endothelium closely conforms to the undulations of the elastica interna and extends processes through its fenestrations to establish junctions with the innermost smooth muscle cells of the media. The fenestrations in the elastica interna are also believed to be essential for nutrition of the avascular media, permitting diffusion of small molecules from the lumen. The gap junctions formed by the cell processes that traverse the fenestrae serve to maintain metabolic coupling of the endothelium to the smooth muscle of the media.

The thickness of the media varies from three or four layers of smooth muscle cells in small arteries to as many as 40 in large arteries. The size and arrangement of the cells are best observed in scanning electron micrographs of vessels, after extraction of perivascular and intramural connective tissue. The myocytes are circumferentially oriented and closely packed in parallel array. A few slender bundles of longitudinally oriented smooth muscle cells may be found at the interface between the intima and media and between the media and adventitia. Vascular smooth muscle cells are much smaller than those in the walls of the hollow viscera. In laboratory rodents, the vascular smooth muscle cells are about 40 μm in length in arterioles and 130 μm in large arteries, compared to 400–500 μm in smooth muscle cells in the wall of the intestine.

The individual cells of the media are enveloped by a typical basal lamina (Fig. 12–8). Short processes extend through discontinuities in this layer to form gap junctions with neighboring cells. These low-resistance junctions are essential for coordination of muscle contraction throughout the tunica media. With traditional silver-staining methods, the cells were also seen to be surrounded by a network of reticular fibers. In electron micrographs, these are identified as bundles of thin collagen fibrils in the narrow intercellular spaces. The collagen fibrils of the media and those of the intima are of small diameter (30 nm) and chondroitin sulfate is the predominant glycosaminoglycan of the surrounding matrix. The collagen fibrils of the adventitia are distinctly larger (60–100 nm) and the associated matrix is rich in dermatan sulfate and

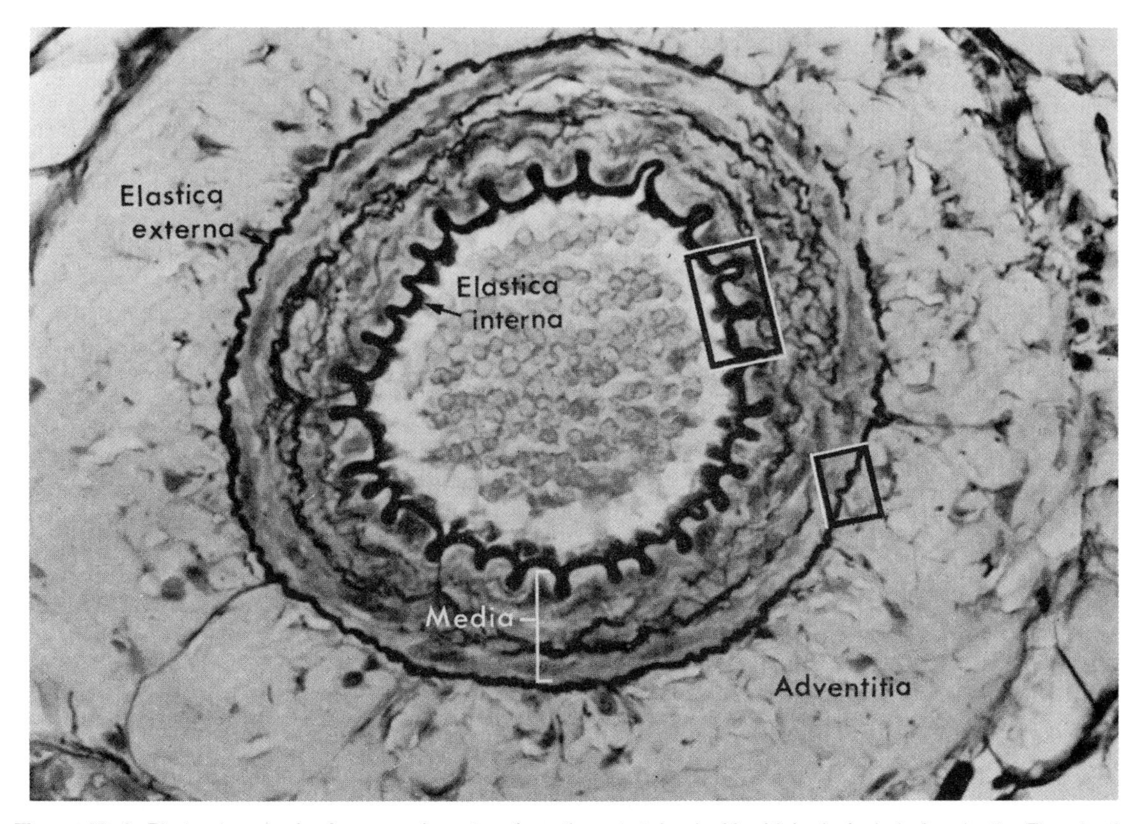

Figure 12–6. Photomicrograph of a muscular artery from the rat stained with aldehyde fuchsin for elastin. The elastica interna, elastica externa, the media, and the thick adventitia are clearly shown. An area comparable to that enclosed in the larger rectangle is illustrated in an electron micrographs in Fig. 12–7.

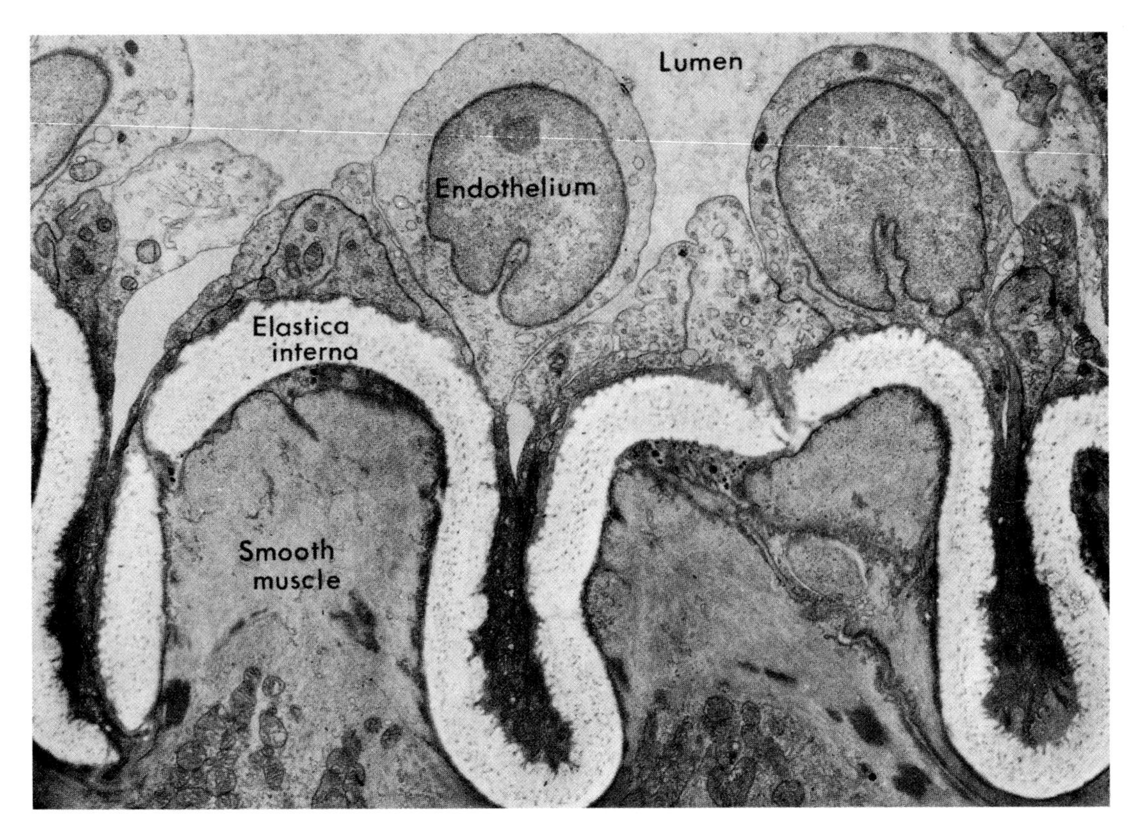

Figure 12–7. Transmission electron micrograph of a section through the wall of a small muscular artery (for orientation, see the rectangle in Fig. 12–6). The elastica interna has a wavy outline owing to agonal contraction of the vessel wall. It is traversed at intervals by small fenestrations through which processes of endothelial cells pass to contact smooth muscle cells in the tunica media.

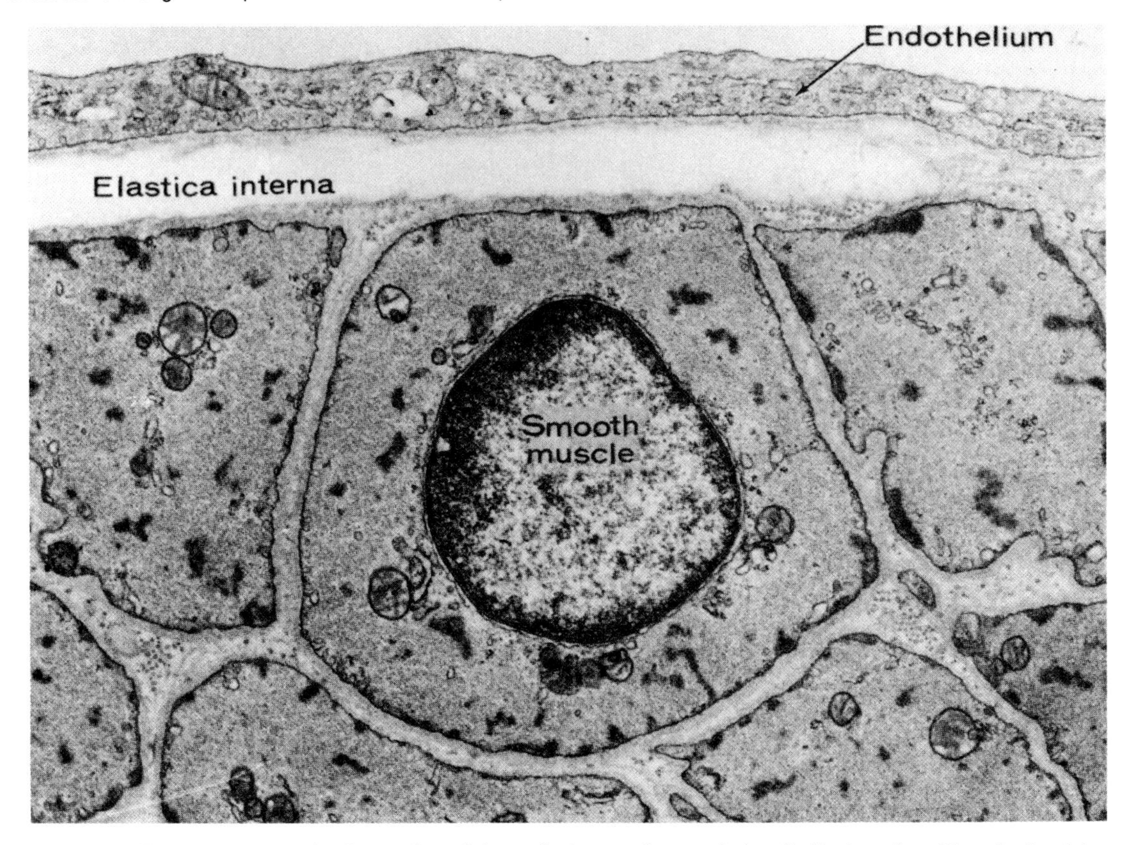

Figure 12–8. Electron micrograph of a portion of the wall of a small artery in longitudinal section. The elastica interna is not stained and, therefore, appears as a clear area between the endothelium and the smooth muscle of the media.

heparan sulfate. The smaller fibrils in the media are a product of the smooth muscle cells whereas the larger ones, in the adventitia, are formed by fibroblasts. It is not clear whether this difference in fiber diameter is directly related to the cell of origin or whether the chondroitin sulfate glycosaminoglycan in the extracellular matrix of the media limits fiber diameter by influencing collagen assembly.

The media also contains slender elastic fibers with a prevailing circumferential orientation. In preparations stained with aldhyde-fuchsin or resorcin-fuchsin, they appear as dark wavy lines among the smooth muscle cells (Fig. 12–2B). In electron micrographs, they are recognizable as irregular linear profiles that are unstained by osmium or the uranyl acetate commonly used.

In histological sections, the elastica externa often appears as a continuous lamina at the junction of the media and adventitia (Fig. 12–9), but in electron micrographs, it is a discontinuous layer of elastin, considerably thinner than the elastica interna. Closely applied to its outer surface are occasional small fascicles of unmyelinated nerve axons, some containing local accumulations of mitochondria and numerous synaptic vesicles (Fig. 12–10). The

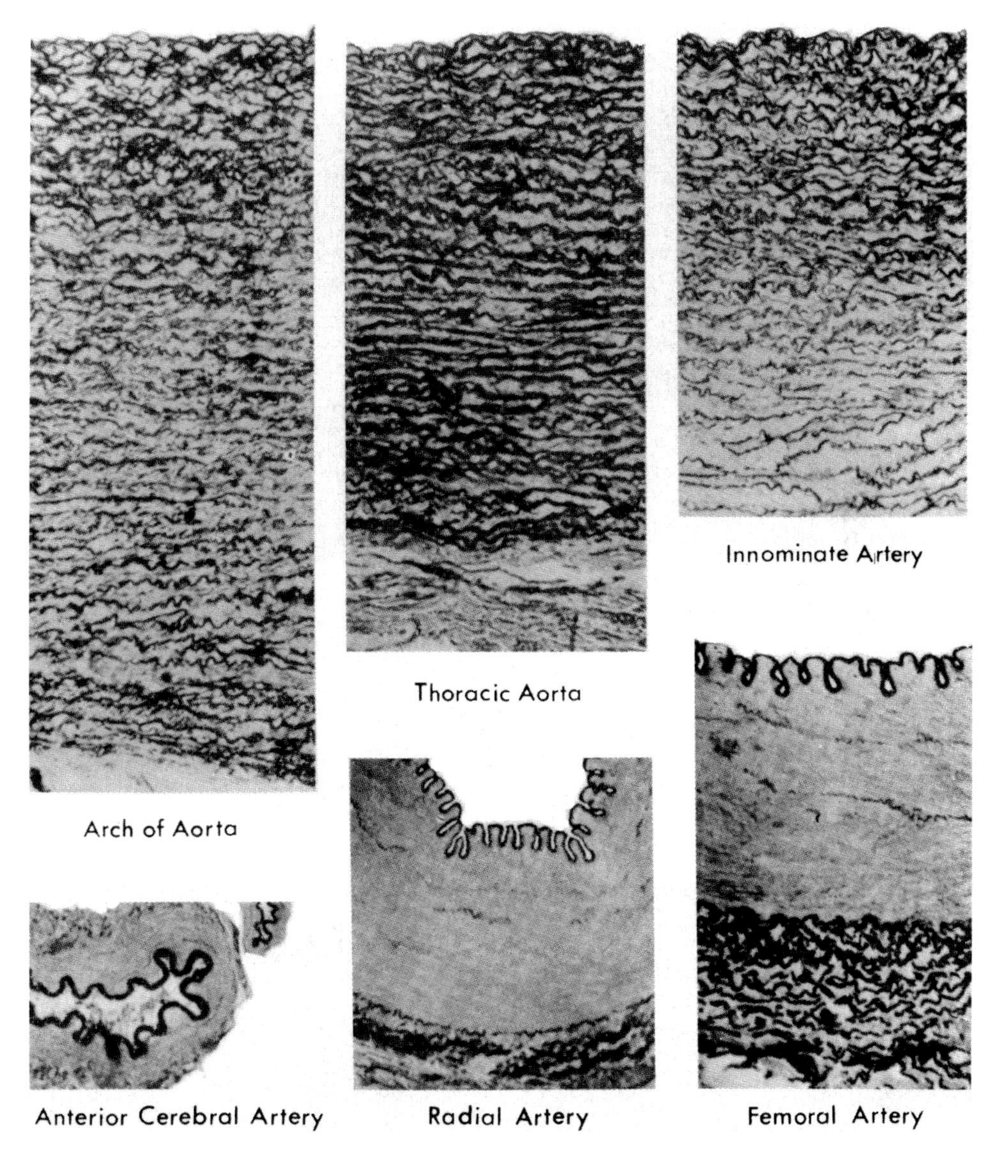

Figure 12–9. Photomicrographs of the wall of elastic and muscular arteries of a macaque, illustrating variations in relative thickness and the differing amounts and distribution of the elastic tissue, which has been stained with resorcin-fuchsin. (From Cowdry, E.V. 1950. Textbook of Histology. Philadelphia, Lea and Febiger.)

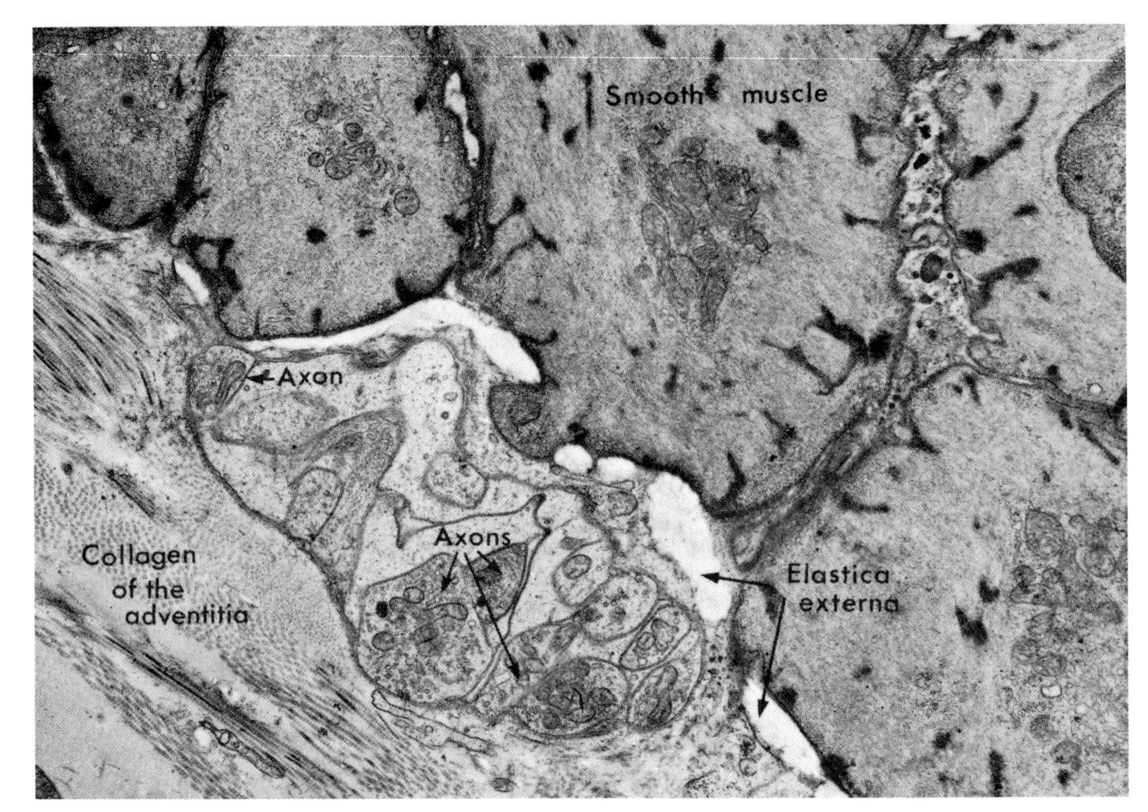

Figure 12–10. Electron micrograph of the junctional zone between the media and adventitia of a small muscular artery. (For orientation, see lower box in Fig. 12–6). The media is limited, on its outer aspect, by a discontinuous elastica externa. Closely applied to this are small nerves, some of whose axons contain numerous synaptic vesicles.

nerves do not penetrate into the media but appear to terminate at the elastica externa. The neural stimulation of the smooth muscle cells evidently depends on diffusion of the neurotransmitter through fenestrations in this layer of elastin. The resulting depolarization of the peripheral smooth muscle cells is propagated throughout the media via the gap junctions between cells.

The tunica adventitia of muscular arteries may be thicker than the media (Figs. 12–2, 12–6). It consists of fibroblasts, elastic and collagen fibers, oriented, for the most part, longitudinally. These grade into the surrounding connective tissue without a clearly defined boundary. The loose organization and prevailing longitudinal orientation of its components imposes little restraint on changes in diameter of the vessel in vasoconstriction and vasodilatation.

TRANSITIONAL AND SPECIALIZED ARTERIES

In the gradual structural changes from one type of artery to another, it is often difficult to classify vessels in the transitional region. Some arteries of intermediate caliber (e.g., popliteal and tibial arteries) have walls that resemble those of larger arteries, whereas some large arteries (e.g., external iliac) have walls not unlike those of medium-sized arteries. The transitional regions between elastic and muscular arteries are often designated *arteries of mixed type*. Examples are the external carotid, axillary, and common iliac arteries. Their walls contain islands of smooth muscle in the tunica media that either separate the elastic laminae or interrupt their continuity. The visceral arteries that arise from the abdominal aorta are also of mixed type. In the transitional region, the tunica media may consist of two distinct zones—an inner muscular zone and an outer zone of elastic laminae.

The thickness of the tunica media of arteries varies according to the internal pressure to which it is subjected. The coronary arteries of the heart are subjected to relatively high internal pressure and have a wall that is thicker than that of other muscular arteries of comparable size. Similarly, in the arteries of the lower limbs, the media is thicker than in corresponding arteries of the upper limbs.

Blood pressure in the pulmonary circulation is considerably lower than in the systemic circulation. Accordingly, the blood vessels in the lung are relatively thin-walled. A unique feature of the pulmonary circulation is the presence of cardiac muscle extending from the heart, for a short distance, into the initial portion of the large pulmonary artery.

Within the cranial cavity, where vessels are protected from external pressure and tension, the dural and cerebral arteries have relatively thin walls. The elastica interna is well developed but the tunica media is thin and virtually devoid of elastic fibers (Fig. 12–9).

In other sites, where vessels are subject to frequent bending and traction, as in the popliteal artery behind the knee joint and in the axillary artery in the axilla, longitudinal bundles of smooth muscle are more prevalent in the tunica intima than they are in comparable vessels elsewhere in the body.

ARTERIOLES

The small arteries and *arterioles* are a physiologically important segment of the circulation because they constitute the principal component of the peripheral resistance to flow that regulates the blood pressure. Arterioles range in diameter from 200 μm down to about 40 μm. Their tunica intima consists of a continuous endothelium and a very thin subendothelial layer consisting of reticular and elastic fibers. A very thin and fenestrated elastica interna is present in the larger arterioles but absent in terminal arterioles. In the larger arterioles, the tunica media consists of two layers of smooth muscle cells, but in the smallest arterioles, there is a single layer and the individual cells completely encircle the endothelium (Figs. 12–11, 12–12, and 12–13). Collagen fibers and occasional fibroblasts form a very thin tunica adventitia. In the vessels of the short transitional region between arterioles and capillaries, sometimes called *metarterioles,* smooth muscle does not form a continuous layer, but individual smooth muscle cells, completely encircling the endothelial tube, are spaced a short distance apart. Their contraction is believed to give this region a sphincter-like function, controlling the inflow of blood into the capillary bed.

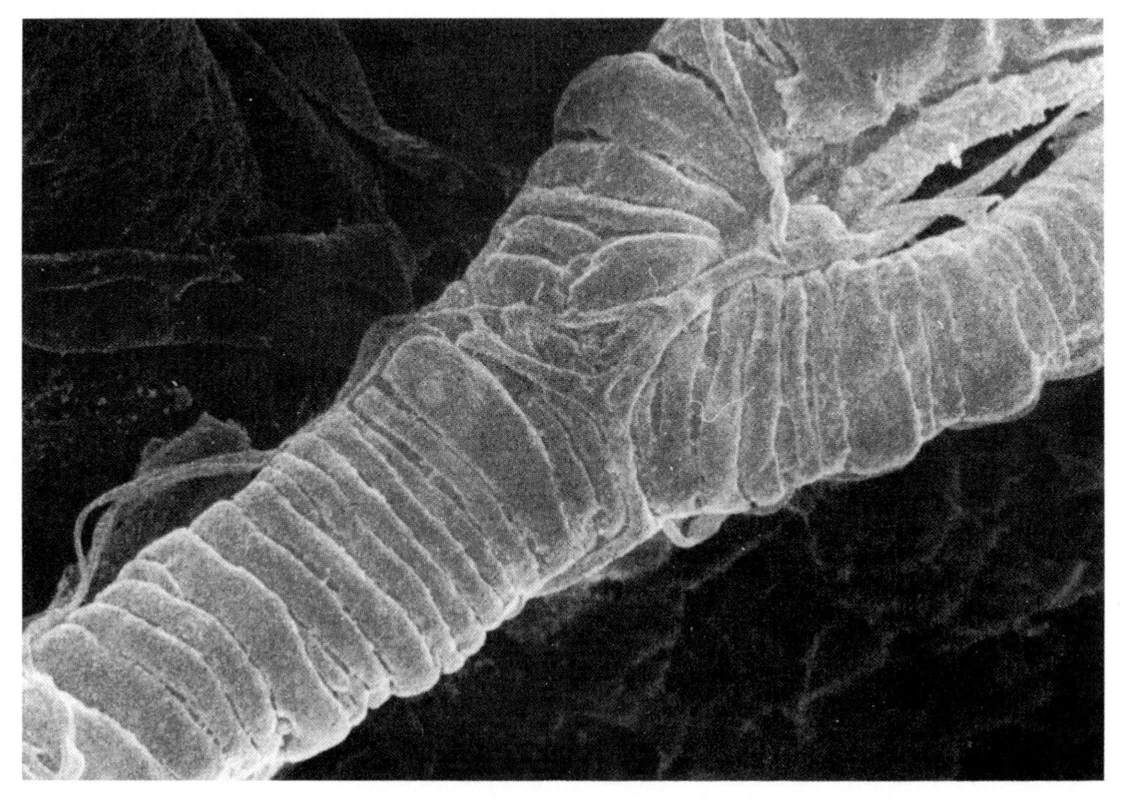

Figure 12–11. Scanning electron micrograph of a branching arteriole showing the circumferential arrangement of the single layer of smooth muscle cells. (Micrograph courtesy of J. Desaki and Y. Uehara.)

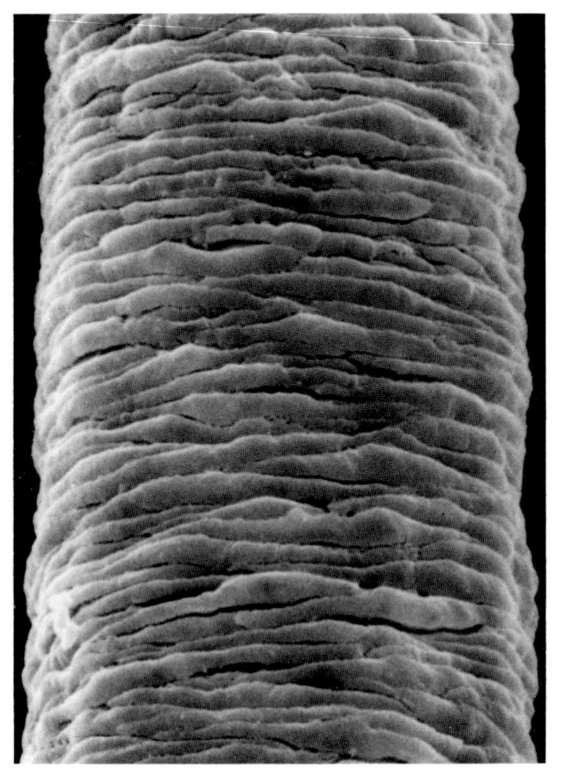

Figure 12–12. Scanning micrograph of the wall of a subarachnoid muscular arteriole, showing the closely apposed, circumferentially oriented smooth muscle cells. (Micrograph from Uehara, Y. T. Fujiwara, and K. Kaidoh. 1990. *In* D.M. Motta, ed. Ultrastructure of Smooth Muscle. Boston, Kluwer Academic Publishers.)

ARTERIOVENOUS ANASTOMOSES

In many parts of the body, the terminal ramifications of arteries are connected to the veins not only through an intervening network of capillaries, but also by direct *arteriovenous anastomoses* (AVA) of larger caliber. These arise as side branches of small arteries and directly join small veins. Three morphologically distinct segments are recognizable along their course. The initial segment is similar in structure to the small artery of which it is a branch. The terminal segment resembles the small vein with which it is confluent. Between these is a contractile intermediate segment with a wall that is unusually thick for a vessel of this size. In addition to a media, it has a subendothelial layer of plump cells that are polygonal in cross sections viewed with the light microscope. These were traditionally described as "epithelioid," but ultrastructural studies have now shown that they are longitudinally oriented modified smooth muscle cells.

Arteriovenous anastomoses provide a path for shunting arterial blood directly into the venous system. When they are contracted, all of the blood passes through the network of capillaries; when they are relaxed, opening their lumen, a considerable volume of blood passes directly into the veins. Arteriovenous anastomoses, therefore, play an important role in regulating blood flow to the region. This regulatory function is perhaps best exemplified in the skin where arteriovenous anastomoses are an important component of the physiological mechanism for thermoregulation. When they are open, blood at deep body temperature can flow through the hypodermal venous plexus at an increased rate, resulting in a much greater loss of heat to the environment. In various mammalian species, the number and distribution of cutaneous arteriovenous anastomoses is adapted to their special requirements for thermoregulation. For example, in sheep in which the insulating fleece limits evaporative heat loss from much of the body surface, the bare nose, ears, and lower legs are of greatest importance in heat regulation. The number of arteriovenous anastomoses per square centimeter of skin on the lower leg (72) is about five times the number on the trunk (15). Even more impressive examples are to be found in seals and other aquatic mammals continuously exposed to arctic seawater. In addition to an external insulation of thick fur, they have a subcutaneous insulating layer of blubber to minimize heat loss. But on land, excess heat is dissipated through the fore and hind flippers which lack this insulation. The arteriovenous anastomoses in the skin of the flippers number up to 1200 per square centimeter compared to about 100 in the skin of the trunk. Comparable studies of the AVAs of human skin have not been made. They are much less numerous than in the above species and the regional differences in their abundance are less marked.

Arteriovenous anastomoses are richly innervated with both adrenergic and cholinergic periadventitial nerves. The nerves are most abundant around the thick intermediate segment with the majority being adrenergic. The contractions of arteriovenous anastomoses are described as being rapid, forceful, and relatively independent of the vasomotor activity of neighboring arteries. There is evidence that they are under control of the thermoregulatory centers in the brain, whereas other peripheral arteries are more responsive to locally generated stimuli.

In addition to these relatively simple shunts

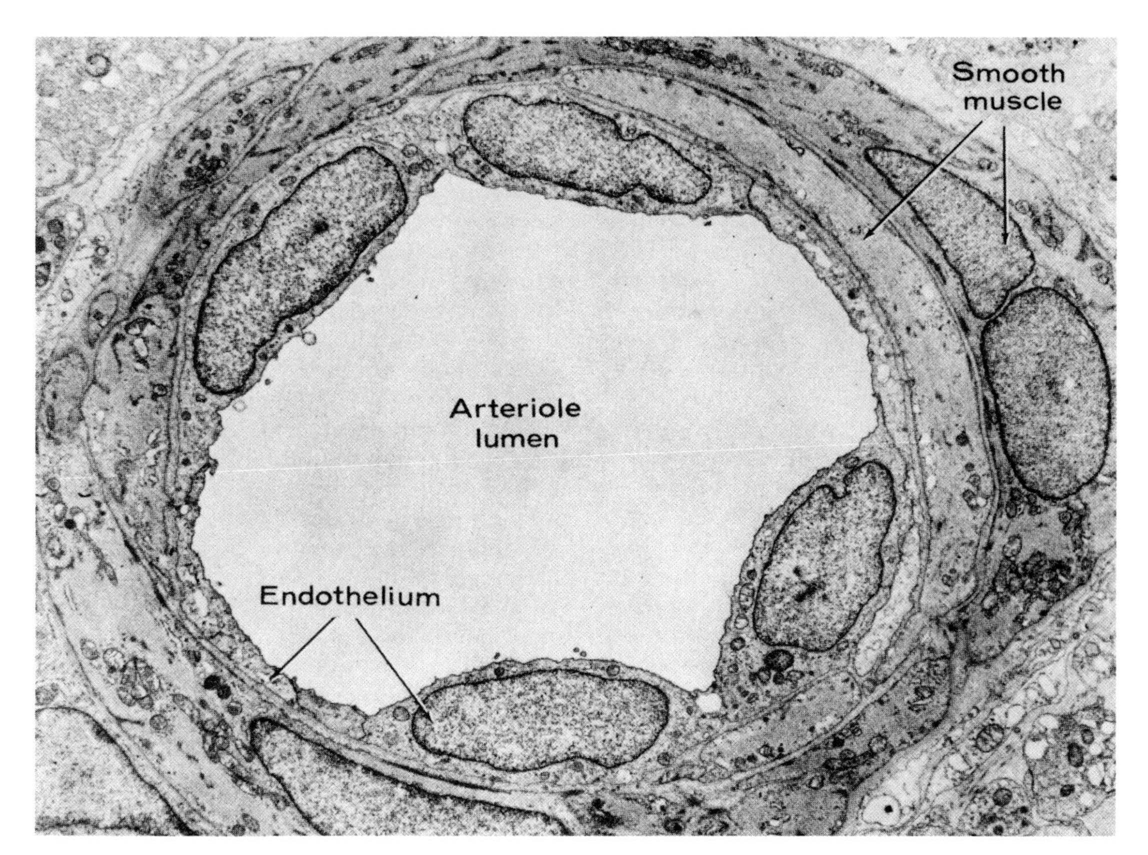

Figure 12–13. Electron micrograph of a typical small arteriole with a single layer of smooth muscle cells around the endothelium.

between small arteries and veins, there are more complex communications through small organs called *glomera* located mainly in the nailbeds, the pads of the fingers and toes, and in the ears. An afferent arteriole traverses the connective tissue capsule of the *glomus*, loses its internal elastic lamina, and acquires a subendothelial layer of epithelioid smooth muscle cells. The vessel may branch or become highly convoluted within the glomus before continuing as a short, thin-walled vein that emerges from the glomus and joins the hypodermal venous plexus. The glomera are very richly innervated. They seem to be far more complex than is required for simple shunting of blood from arteries to veins and are suspected by some investigators to have an additional function that is yet to be discovered.

PHYSIOLOGICAL IMPLICATIONS OF THE STRUCTURE OF ARTERIES

The intermittent contraction of the heart results in a pulsatile flow of blood in the large arteries. If the walls of the arteries were rigid, flow of blood through the capillaries would be intermittent, but, in fact, it is continuous. Because the wall of the large elastic arteries is distensible, only a portion of the force generated by contraction of the heart is dissipated in advancing the column of blood in their lumen. The rest of the force goes to expanding the walls of the large arteries. The potential energy accumulated in the stretching of their walls during contraction of the heart (systole) is dissipated in the elastic recoil of their walls during relaxation of the heart (diastole). The release of tension in the wall of the elastic arteries serves as an auxiliary pump, forcing the blood onward during diastole when no force is being exerted by the heart. Thus, although the flow is pulsatile throughout the initial portion of the system, the elasticity of the wall of the large arteries ensures a continuous flow through the capillaries.

A *vasomotor center* in the brain continuously generates impulses that travel via nerves in the spinal cord to the sympathetic chain, and then over *vasomotor nerves* to all of the blood vessels except the capillaries. As a result of these impulses, the smooth muscle in the media of the distributing arteries is maintained in a state of partial contraction referred to as *vasomotor tone*. The nerves to the blood vessels include both *vasoconstrictor* and *vasodilator fibers,* permitting modulation of the caliber of the vessels to change the pressure in the system as a whole or to increase or decrease blood flow to particular areas.

In histological sections, the smooth muscle of the majority of the arteries has undergone some degree of contraction after death or in response to immersion in a chemical fixative. One, therefore, gets an erroneous impression of the thickness of the arterial wall in relation to the diameter of the lumen. The remarkable capacity of arteries to change their caliber is best observed in the living, anaesthetized animal. If a droplet of the neurotransmitter, *norepinephrine,* is applied to an artery, the underlying portion of the vessel will undergo a marked local vasoconstriction. The vessel can then be rapidly fixed in situ and prepared for histological study. In sections through the open and the constricted segments of the vessel, one can observe the striking differences in the caliber of the lumen and in the character of the vessel wall, that are associated with vasoconstriction (Fig. 12–14). Because the arteries provide the principal resistance to flow in the system, a generalized vasoconstriction results in a marked increase in the blood pressure.

Smooth muscle cells of the arteries have receptors for a number of humoral agents other than the sympathetic neurotransmitter norepinephrine. A fall in blood pressure causes the kidneys to secrete *renin,* an acid protease that cleaves angiotensinogen in the circulating blood, to yield *angiotensin,* a potent vasoconstrictor. The resulting generalized vasoconstriction raises the blood pressure. A fall in blood pressure, associated with severe hemorrhage, also causes the posterior lobe of the pituitary gland to release a peptide hormone, *vasopressin,* which is another very potent vasoconstrictor.

Local constriction of arteries may also be induced by products of tissue injury, an effect

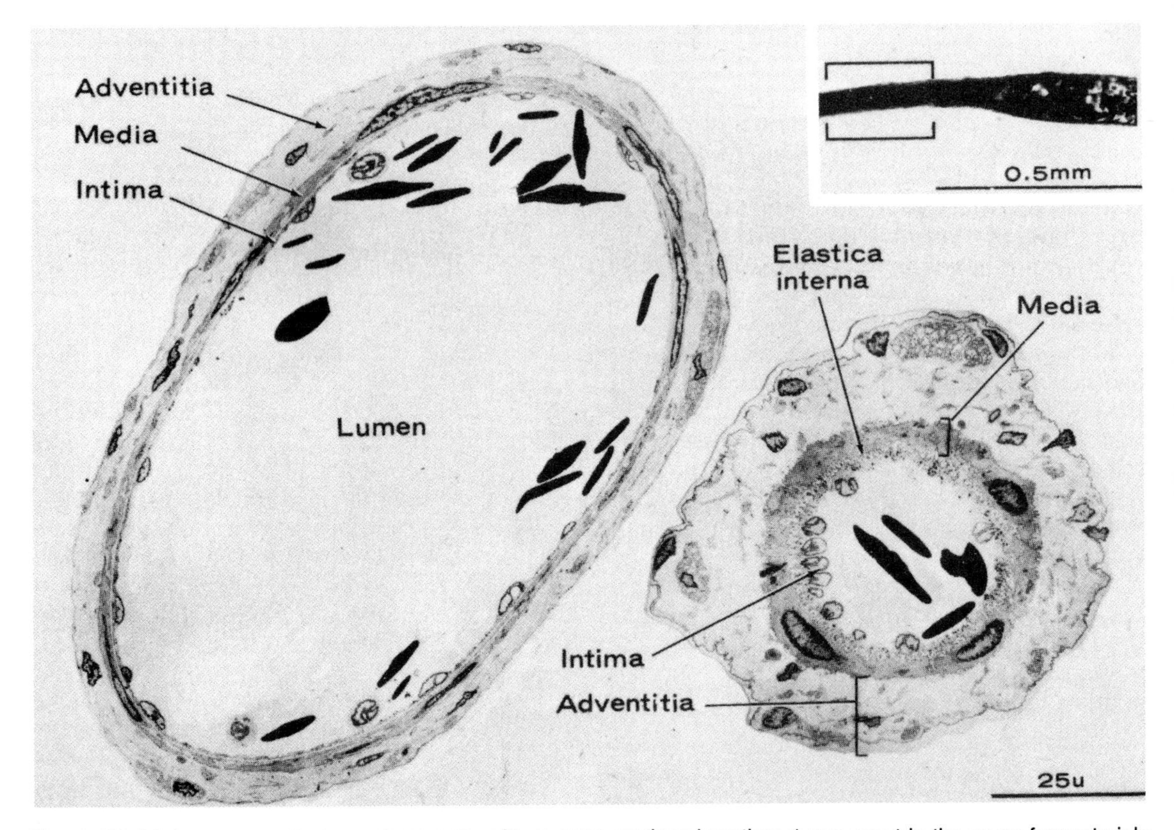

Figure 12–14. Low-power electron micrographs of two cross sections less than 1 mm apart in the same frog arteriole. A microdroplet of norepinephrin was applied to the living vessel, causing local vasoconstriction in the area indicated by brackets (inset). The vessel was then fixed, in situ, and sectioned. These two sections provide a dramatic demonstration of the structural correlates of vasoconstriction. (From Phelps, P.C. and J.H. Luft. 1969. Am. J. Anat. 125:3999.)

that is important in limiting blood loss. There are other local factors acting at the level of small arteries and arterioles that influence blood flow. If flow is briefly interrupted, oxygen deprivation and accumulation of carbon dioxide and lactic acid in the tissues cause relaxation of smooth muscle in the walls of these small vessels so that when circulation is restored the rate of flow may be two to six times greater than it was before. This *reactive hyperaemia,* tending to correct a local deficit of metabolites, is independent of the nervous system.

SENSORY ORGANS OF ARTERIES

Sensory nerves are associated with arteries throughout the vascular system, but at certain sites, there are specialized neural organs whose function is to monitor the pressure and composition of the blood. Chief among these are the *carotid bodies, aortic bodies,* and *carotid sinus.* These sensory organs are of great importance in regulating respiration, heart beat, and the vasomotor activities controlling blood pressure.

The *carotid bodies* are inconspicuous organs about 3 mm wide and 5 mm long located in the connective tissue associated with the vessel walls at the bifurcation of the common carotid artery to form the external and internal carotid arteries. They are richly innervated, have a large blood flow in relation to their size, and contain *chemoreceptors* responsive to changes in the oxygen, carbon-dioxide, and hydrogen ion concentrations of the blood. Afferent nerves from these organs transmit signals to a *respiratory center* in the brain that controls respiration.

The carotid body consists of multiple clusters of pale-staining cells embedded in a highly vascular connective tissue stroma. The parenchymal cells are of two types identifiable with the light microscope on the basis of their nuclear form and staining properties. They are more easily distinguished in electron micrographs. The *glomus cells* (*type-I cells*) usually appear round or oval in section but they may have a few processes of varying length that contact other glomus cells or capillaries. They occur in clusters that are surrounded by *sheath cells* (*type-II cells*).

The glomus cells have a large nucleus, a prominent juxtanuclear Golgi complex, numerous mitochondria, and ribosome-studded cisternae of endoplasmic reticulum that are often stacked in parallel array. The most distinctive feature of these cells is the presence in their cytoplasm of dense-cored vesicles (60–200 nm) which resemble those in cells of the adrenal medulla. The cell processes contain longitudinally oriented microtubules, a few dense-cored vesicles and numerous small vesicles with an electron-lucent interior. In some species, two categories of glomus cells (types A and B) are distinguishable on the basis of the size and number of their dense-cored vesicles. In type A, these are about 30% larger and twice as numerous as those in type B. Nerve endings are closely associated with type-A cells, but are seldom seen in contact with cells of type B.

Sheath cells have a more complex three-dimensional configuration, including long tapering or lamelliform processes that envelope from two to six glomus cells, covering nearly all of their surfaces, that are not in contact with nerve endings or other glomus cells. The nuclei of the sheath cells are more irregular in shape and contain more heterochromatin than those of the glomus cells. Their cytoplasm contains no dense-cored vesicles. Sheath cells are quite similar to sustentacular cells in other sensory organs and to the glial cells of the nervous system. Where nerves enter groups of glomus cells they lose their investment of Schwann cells and their terminal portion is surrounded by sheath cells. These cells do not form a complete diffusion barrier around the glomus cells because when probes such as horseradish peroxidase are injected intravascularly, they permeate the intercellular clefts throughout the carotid body.

Certain cells of the carotid body exhibit a brown color of the cytoplasm when exposed to a solution of potassium dichromate. This staining, referred to as the *chromaffin reaction,* is believed to detect the presence of catecholamines. It is characteristic of the cells of the adrenal medulla and of *paraganglia,* small clusters of epithelioid cells that are widely scattered in the retroperitoneal tissues. Owing to its chromaffinity, the carotid body was included in the system of paraganglia. This has been questioned by some histologists who found marked species differences in the chromaffinity of the glomus cells and a variable, and marginal, reaction among cells in the same glomus. However, it is now widely accepted that cells of the carotid body exhibit some degree of chromaffinity and that they contain catecholamines demonstrable by other histochemical procedures. Whether some of the cells also contain peptide hormones remains unsettled, but the presence of two size categories of dense-cored vesicles in their cytoplasm suggests this possibility.

The carotid bodies are richly innervated by branches of the glossopharyngeal nerve that are made up of axons whose cell bodies are located in the petrosal ganglion. The axon terminals associated with the glomus cells are quite pleomorphic, some being calyceal and others simple boutons. An enduring controversy as to whether these nerves are afferent (conducting toward the brain) or efferent (conducting away from the brain) has been resolved in favor of the view that they are afferent sensory nerves. In the great majority of the synapses, the glomus cells are presynaptic. Aggregations of dense-cores vesicles and of small lucent-cored vesicles are found in the cell body near the synaptic cleft, whereas relatively few vesicles are found in the axoplasm of the nerve ending. In the great majority of synapses, the glomus cell is presynaptic, but, rarely, two synapses may be found in close proximity with the aggregation of vesicles in one, being presynaptic, and in the other, postsynaptic, thus constituting a *reciprocal synapse*. The significance of these is unclear.

The localization of the chemoreceptor function of the carotid body has not been definitely established, but it is assumed that it resides in the glomus cells and that these release signals carried over afferent sensory neurons. An alternative interpretation postulates that the receptor function is in the nerve endings, with the glomus cells acting as interneurons modulating the chemoreceptive sensitivity of the nerve endings.

Other chemoreceptor organs, the *aortic bodies,* are situated on the arch of the aorta between the origins of the subclavian and common carotid arteries on the right, and medial to the origin of the subclavian on the left. The structure and function of these bodies appear to be identical to those of the carotid bodies.

In the internal carotid artery immediately above the bifurcation of the common carotid, there is a slight dilatation called the *carotid sinus.* In this local specialization of the vessel wall, the tunica media is thinner than elsewhere, whereas the adventitia is thicker and contains numerous sensory nerve endings of the carotid sinus branch of the glossopharyngeal nerve. The thinning of the media makes this region of the vessel wall more distensible. The nerve endings in the adventitia are stimulated by stretch. The carotid sinus, therefore, serves as a *baroreceptor* reacting to changes in blood pressure and initiating afferent impulses that trigger appropriate vasomotor adjustments to maintain a pressure within normal limits. A few baroreceptors are also present in the wall of the aorta and other large arteries in the thorax and neck, but these are not visually identifiable.

CHANGES IN ARTERIES WITH AGE

The walls of large arteries undergo a gradual process of further growth and development from birth to age 25. In elastic arteries, there is a progressive thickening of the wall and development of increasing numbers of elastic laminae. In muscular arteries, the thickness of the tunica media increases with little or no addition of elastin. From middle age onward, there is a relative increase in collagen and proteoglycans and the walls of the larger arteries consequently become less pliant. More significant age-related changes are found in the intima. Extracellular matrix components slowly accumulate and intimal smooth muscle cells become more numerous.

The late stages of development of the arterial wall cannot be clearly differentiated from the early regressive changes associated with aging and the onset of *arteriosclerosis* ("hardening of the arteries"). Arteries are constantly subjected to mechanical stresses due to the oscillations of intralumenal pressure associated with intermittent contractions of the heart and they seem to be more susceptible to wear-and-tear than other tissues. The larger arteries, particularly the aorta, iliac, femoral, coronary, and cerebral arteries, are especially prone to develop *atherosclerosis,* a disease that is the principal basis of heart attack (*myocardial infarction*) and stroke (*cerebral thrombosis*).

Atherosclerosis is characterized by patchy thickenings of the intima that contain intracellular and extracellular deposits of lipid. By the age of 15, small focal accumulations of lipid-laden smooth muscle cells, surrounded by deposits of cholesterol-rich lipid, form yellow "fatty streaks" visible to the naked eye in the intima of the aorta. These gradually increase until they occupy 30% or more of the intimal surface by the age of 25. Whether these early-appearing fatty streaks are physiological or are precursors of the more advanced lesions of atherosclerosis is debated. More patently pathological are the *fibrous plaques* that appear in older individuals. These are white in color and thicker, so that they project slightly into the lumen. These arise by local proliferation of the smooth muscle cells of the intima and by migration of smooth muscle cells of the tunica media through fenestrations in the internal elastic lamina to join those in the intima. Normally, smooth muscle cells of the arterial wall are a very slowly renewing population, but where there is damage to the endothelium and aggregation of blood platelets, as there is in the earliest stages of atherosclerosis, there is a local release of *platelet-derived growth factor* (PDGF), which stimulates proliferation of smooth muscle cells. Lipid accumulates in and around these cells and they are stimulated to produce more collagen and proteoglycans that contribute to the local thickening of the tunica intima. As the disease progresses, there is cell necrosis, erosion of the endothelium, and aggregation of blood platelets to form a mural thrombus (blood clot) that may occlude the lumen.

The principal processes involved in arteriosclerosis, thus, seem to be local proliferation of smooth muscle cells, their production of excess extracellular matrix, and the intracellular and extracellular accumulation of lipid. Research on the pathogenesis of the disease is now concentrating on the role of cholesterol, various plasma lipoproteins, and mitogens released at the site by activated blood platelets.

CAPILLARIES

The terminal branches of the arterioles have a short transitional region in which occasional smooth muscle cells persist around the endothelial tube. Where these adventitial cells end, the vessels continue as small, thin-walled, endothelium-lined tubes of uniform diameter that branch and anastomose frequently to form extensive capillary networks in the tissues throughout the body (Figs. 12–15 and 12–16). The capillary wall consists of extremely attenuated endothelial cells, with their basal lamina supported by a sparse network of reticular fibers. Scattered along the outside of the capillaries are cells called *pericytes*. Unlike the fusiform, circumferentially oriented smooth muscle cells associated with arterioles, the pericytes usually have long primary processes deployed longitudinally along the capillary wall and secondary processes extending from the primary processes, circumferentially around the vessel (Figs. 12–17 and 12–18). Pericytes are enclosed in a thin external lamina that is continuous with the basal lamina of the endothelium, except at focal gap junctions between their processes and the underlying endothelial cells. Pericytes have the usual complement of cytoplasmic organelles, including a small Golgi complex, mitochondria, and a few meandering tubules and cisternae of the endoplasmic reticulum. Lysosomes are common in the pericytes of brain capillaries but are relatively few in the pericytes of capillaries elsewhere. Microtubules, originating at the centrosome, extend along the axis of the primary cell processes, and bundles of filaments in the peripheral cytoplasm terminate in densities on the inner aspect of the plasma membrane.

It has long been speculated that the pericytes might be contractile. This has now been verified by the demonstration that pericytes, in large capillaries and postcapillary venules, contain tropomyosin, isomyosin of the smooth muscle type, and a protein kinase that is involved in the control of contraction in muscle. Thus, pericytes appear to be contractile cells involved in the control of blood flow through the microvasculature. There is suggestive evidence that, in the revascularization following tissue injury, pericytes may undergo further differentiation to become smooth muscle cells in the walls of arterioles and venules.

The caliber of the capillaries in different regions of the body varies within relatively narrow limits, averaging from 9 to 12 μm in diameter, which is just large enough to permit unimpeded passage of the cellular elements of the blood. In organs that are in a state of minimal functional activity, many of the capillaries are narrowed so that little or no blood circulates through them. Normally, only about 25% of the total capillary bed of the body is patent, but with increased physiological activity, the narrowed vessels open, and flow through them is restored to meet an increased need for exchange of metabolites.

In cross sections of small capillaries, the lumen may be encircled by a single endothelial cell (Fig. 12–19). In larger capillaries, the wall may be made up of portions of two or three cells. The cell nucleus is greatly flattened and, thus, appears elliptical in section. The thicker nuclear region of the cell bulges into the lumen, whereas the attenuated peripheral portion of the cell is extremely thin, with the adlumenal and ablumenal membranes separated by a layer of cytoplasm 0.2 to 0.4 μm thick. A small Golgi complex and a few mitochondria are found in the juxtanuclear cytoplasm.

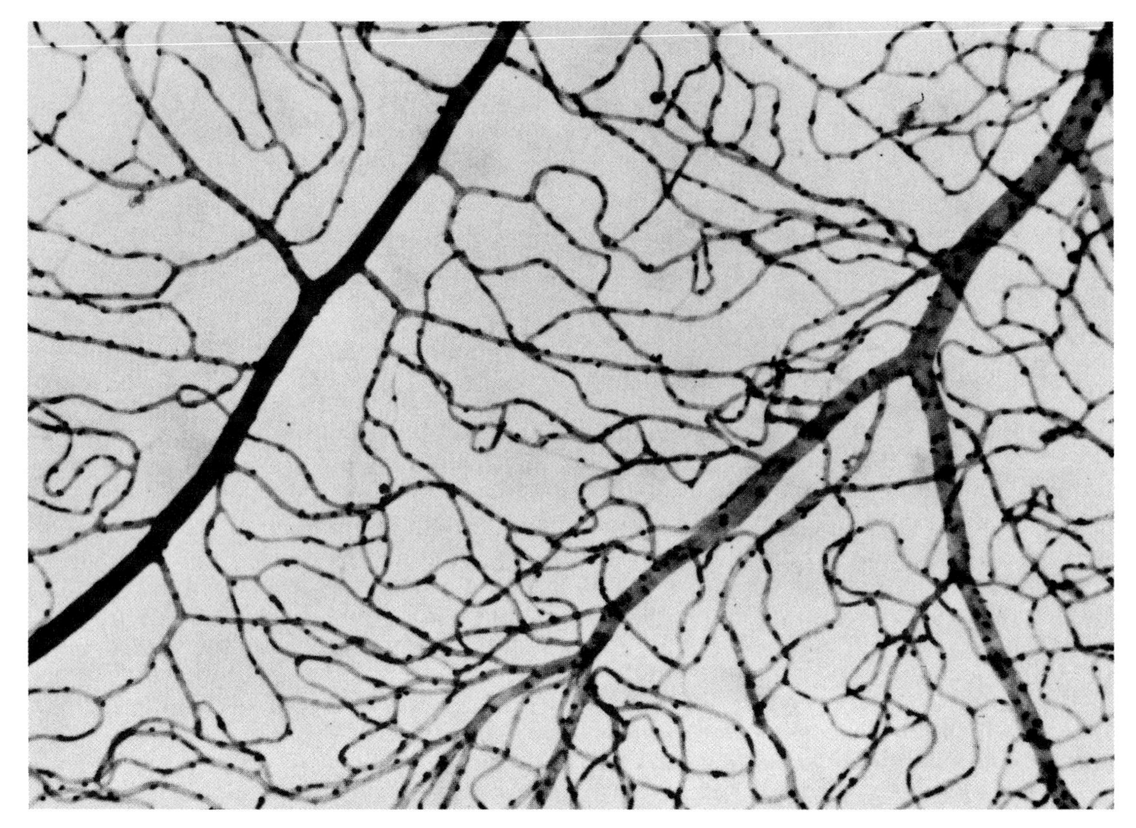

Figure 12–15. Photomicrograph of normal human retinal blood vessels. These were isolated by tryptic digestion of the neural and receptor elements, leaving behind only the vessels. At the left is an arteriole, and at the right, a venule; between them is a network of capillaries of very uniform caliber. (Photomicrograph courtesy of T. Kuwabara.)

Tubular elements of the endoplasmic reticulum extend into the thinner peripheral portions of the cell. A conspicuous feature of endothelial cells is the presence of a large number of vesicles associated with the plasmalemma at both surfaces of the cell (Figs. 12–20, 12–24).

Although endothelial cells are similar in appearance throughout most of the vascular system, they have been shown to have regional differences in the types of intermediate filaments that make up their cytoskeleton. Some contain desmin filaments only, others vimentin filaments only, and still others have both. Whether these variations reflect different functional properties or different embryological origins of the cells is not clear. The lumenal surface of the endothelium is generally smooth contoured, but the thin margins of the adjacent cells may overlap slightly and a thin marginal ridge, or flap, may project a short distance into the lumen (Fig. 12–21). Zonulae adherentes and desmosomes are not found between adjoining cells, but two or three narrow sites of closer membrane approximation can be detected (Fig. 12–22). At these sites, in freeze–fracture preparations, one finds, on the E-face, parallel intramembranous strands comparable to those occurring in the zonulae occludentes of other epithelia.

At the resolution afforded by the light microscope, capillaries, in most tissues and organs, appear quite similar, but with the electron microscope, two distinct types can be distinguished (Figs. 12–23 and 12–24). In muscle, nervous tissue, and the connective tissues, the endothelium forms an uninterrupted layer around the lumen of the capillary. Such vessels are designated *continuous capillaries* (or muscle-type capillaries). In the pancreas, intestinal tract, kidney cortex, and endocrine glands, the peripheral portions of the endothelial cells are interrupted by circular fenestrations or *pores,* 60–70 nm in diameter, each closed by a very thin *pore diaphragm* (Figs. 12–24B and 12–25). When examined in tissues that have been prepared by quick freezing, deep-etching, and replication by

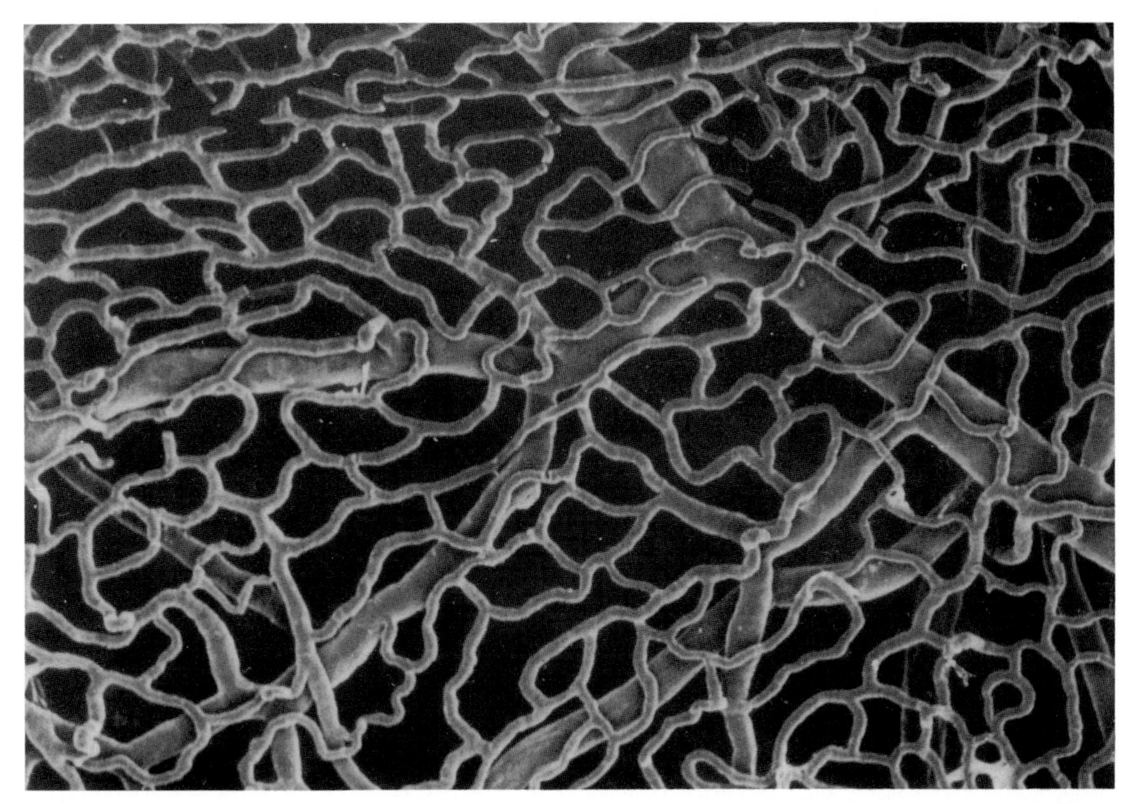

Figure 12–16. Scanning electron micrograph of a corrosion cast of a typical capillary network from the submucosa of the hamster forestomach. (Micrograph from Imada, M., H. Tatsumi, and H. Fujita. 1987. Cell Tissue Res. 250:287.)

platinum-carbon shadowing, the structure of the diaphragm is more clearly revealed. It is made up of about eight fibrils that radiate, like spokes, from a central meshwork. The geometry of these fibrils create wedge-shaped channels with their bases at the periphery of the pore. The maximum width of the broad end of each wedge-shaped opening is about 5.5 nm. The dimensions of these channels are, therefore, consistent with physiological studies showing that the particulate tracer, *horseradish peroxidase* (4.5 nm in diameter) readily escapes from such capillaries, whereas *ferritin* (11 nm in diameter) does not. In such *fenestrated capillaries* (visceral capillaries), seen in surface view under the scanning microscope or in freeze–fracture preparations, the pores are very uniformly distributed with a center-to-center spacing of about 130 nm (Fig. 12–25). However, the areas exhibiting pores make up only a fraction of the vessel wall, with the remainder resembling the uninterrupted endothelium of muscle capillaries. In the resulting mosaic, the relative proportions of fenestrated and unfenestrated areas vary in capillaries of different organs. Among the fenestrated capillaries of the body, those of the renal glomerulus appear to be exceptional in that the pores do not have pore diaphragms and their basal lamina is as much as three times thicker than that of other capillaries. This may account for the fact that fluid traverses the wall of glomerular capillaries as much as 100 times more rapidly than in muscle capillaries.

TRANSENDOTHELIAL EXCHANGE

Physiologists have long speculated about the mechanism of exchange across the capillary wall. The observed rates of passage of water-soluble molecules could be accounted for by postulating two fluid-filled systems of pores traversing the endothelium: one of "small pores" about 9 nm in diameter and of relatively high frequency, and the other of "large pores" up to 70 nm in diameter and of lower frequency. These pores were not seen in electron micrographs of muscle capillaries and the structural equivalent of the postulated two sets of pores was a subject of lively debate. To clarify this issue, electron-dense molecules

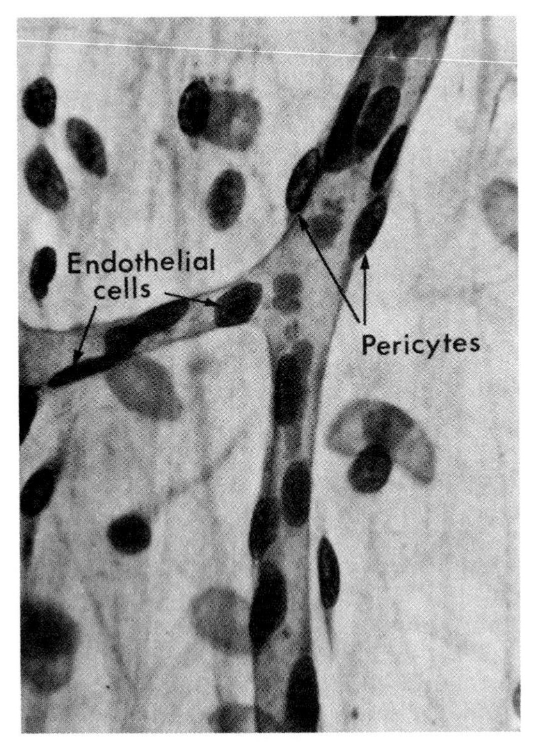

Figure 12–17. Photomicrograph of an intact capillary in a whole-mount of rat mesentery. The nuclei of the flattened endothelial cells lining the capillary can be distinguished from those of the pericytes, which bulge outward from the wall.

of known dimensions greater than 10 nm have been introduced into the circulation and their fate followed in electron micrographs. In muscle capillaries, these particles are rapidly taken up in vesicles opening onto the adlumenal surface of the continuous endothelium, then ferried across the cytoplasm, and discharged into the extravascular space by fusion of the vesicles with the ablumenal plasmalemma (Fig. 12–26).

The uptake of materials in small vesicles is a form of endocytosis common to many cell types and is generally referred to as *micropinocytosis.* In cells other than endothelium, the micropinocytosis vesicles moving into the cytoplasm from the plasmalemma usually fuse with lysosomes or become incorporated in multivesicular bodies. The use of vesicles to ferry fluid and solutes across the cell is largely confined to endothelial cells and is an expression of their specialization for transport. The term *transcytosis* has been suggested to distinguish this process from pinocytosis. In addition to the translocation of vesicles from one surface of the endothelium to the other, serial sections have revealed that transient transendothelial channels may be formed by fusion of several vesicles, or in extremely thin areas, a single vesicle may open at both surfaces of the cell Fig. 12–26). Because the capillaries are the principal site of exchange of substances between the blood plasma and the tissue fluid, it is not surprising that there are more vesicles in capillary endothelium (~$1000/\mu m^2$) than in the endothelium of arterioles (~$190/\mu m^2$) or postcapillary venules (~$645/\mu m^2$).

Albumin is largely responsible for the colloid osmotic pressure of the blood plasma and interstitial fluid and there is abundant physiological evidence for continuous movement of albumin from blood to the extra-vascular fluid. In addition to its oncotic properties, albumin serves as an important carrier of various kinds of molecules including fatty acids, steroid hormones, and thyroid hormone from the blood to their target tissues. Electron micrographs of capillaries perfused with gold-labeled albumin and fixed within 3 min reveal the dense gold particles selectively bound to the membranes of pits and vesicles open on the lumenal surface of the endothelium. After 5 min, the vesicles carrying the tracer are located on the ablumenal side of the endothelium discharging their contents into the extravascular space. The endothelium of continuous capillaries in lung, heart, diaphragm, and various other organs evidently has albumin-receptors in its membrane that aggregate in uncoated pits and vesicles that provide a mechanism for selective transport of albumin and any molecules bound to it.

The process of transcytosis was originally envisioned as involving continuous formation of vesicles at the adlumenal plasmalemma, their detachment and movement across the cytoplasm, and fusion with the opposite membrane. To account for the measured rate of albumin clearance, there would have to be a continuous massive translocation of membrane from the lumenal to the ablumenal surface of the endothelium. Recent evidence suggests that, instead, the transport vesicles are not all newly formed at the expense of the plasma membrane but may be a separate and relatively stable population arising from the Golgi complex and simply shuttling back and forth, undergoing alternate fusion and fission without intermixing of membrane constituents at the plasmalemma (Fig. 12–26B). This model would be consistent with the images observed in electron micrographs and would not involve translocation of very large

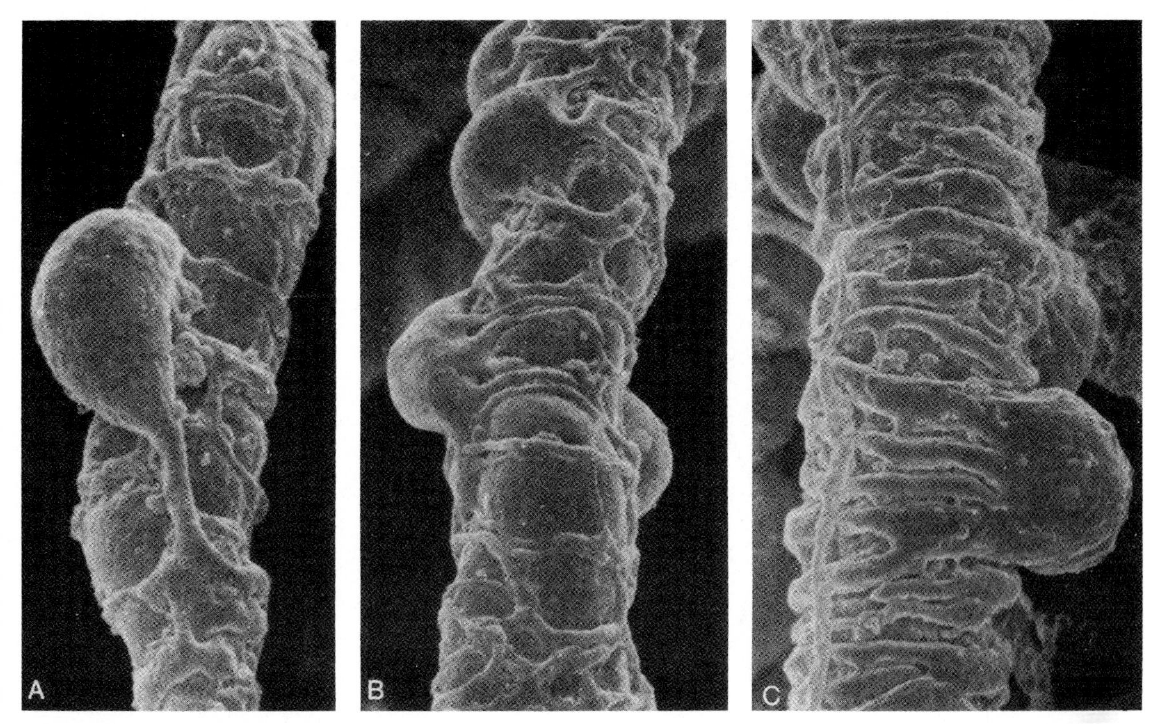

Figure 12–18. Scanning micrographs of small blood vessels showing pericyte processes encircling the vessel wall. (A) Pericyte of a capillary with primary processes directed longitudinally and secondary processes deployed circumferentially. (B) Capillary with numerous associated pericytes. (C) Terminal arteriole showing a mixture of pericytes and circular smooth muscle cells. (Micrographs from Fujinara, T., and Y. Uehara. Amer. J. Anat. 170:39, 1984.)

amounts of the plasmalemma from one side of the cell to the other.

There is general agreement that the vesicles in muscle capillaries and the pores of fenestrated capillaries are the structural equivalents of the "large pores" postulated by physiologists, but there is still disagreement as to the location of the "small pores" permitting passage of molecules smaller than 9 nm. It is possible that molecules of this size may pass through discontinuities in the intercellular junctions.

Transendothelial transport is influenced by factors other than molecular size, namely, by the chemical nature of the molecules, their net charge, and the charge in the pathways involved. In general, the surface of the endothelium is negatively charged. When tracers of opposite charge, such as cationized ferritin, are perfused, they bind randomly on the plasmalemma and tenaciously to the diaphragms of fenestrated capillaries, but not to the vesicles involved in transcytosis, which appear to be neutral. Thus, the endothelial surface presents to the blood a mosaic of microdomains of varying charge. It is speculated that these may be able to sort macromolecules according to their differing charge. Cationic tracers are taken up mainly by adsorptive endocytosis in clathrin coated vesicles, whereas anionic or neutral tracers are shuttled across the endothelium in noncoated transport vesicles.

SPECIALIZED CAPILLARIES

Capillaries with the same morphological appearance may exhibit marked differences in their permeability properties. Some 70 years ago it was observed that intravenously injected dyes that readily escape from the capillaries of most tissues are retained in brain capillaries. This gave rise to the concept of a special *blood-brain barrier.* Its structural basis remained conjectural until these capillaries could be studied with the electron microscope. Their endothelial lining was found to be continuous and devoid of fenestrations, transendothelial channels, and transcellular vesicular transport. The cells are joined by continuous tight junctions that prevent passage of molecules through the intercellular clefts. In this and other respects, the endothelium of brain capillaries is similar to epithelia. It has a low permeability to many polar solutes and a high

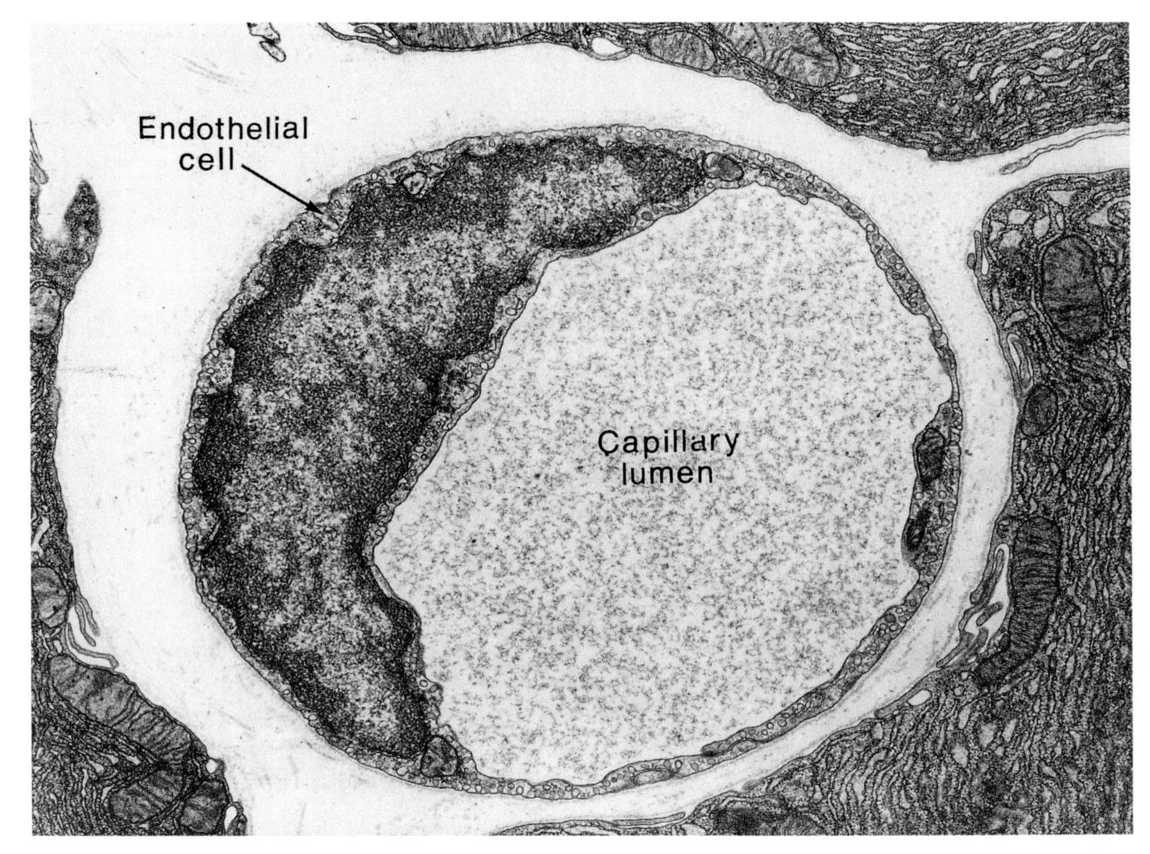

Figure 12–19. Electron micrograph of a typical capillary from guinea pig pancreas. The entire circumference is made up of a single endothelial cell. There is a thin basal lamina and a few associated collagen fibers. No pericyte is present in this plane of section. (Micrograph from Bolender, R.J. 1974. J. Cell Biol. 61:269.)

transcellular gradient for proteins, ions, and amino acids.

The barrier obviously cannot be absolute because the brain, like other tissues, is dependent on the blood to supply its metabolic substrates and to remove its wastes. The transendothelial movement of glucose, amino acids, nucleosides, and purines have been extensively studied and appears to depend on specific carrier-mediated transport. The cells exhibit a polarity with different transport systems in the lumenal and basal membranes. For example, Na^+, K^+–ATPase is found in the basal and not in the apical plasma membrane of endothelial cells in brain capillaries.

There is now evidence that the barrier properties of brain capillaries are not intrinsically determined but are induced by a product of astrocytes, a type of glial cell that is closely associated with the capillaries of the brain. If clumps of astrocytes are implanted in the anterior chamber of the eye, the capillaries growing from the iris into the transplant develop tight junctions between the endothelial cells. Capillaries invading transplants of other cell types do not.

A blood-ocular barrier and a blood-thymus barrier have been shown to depend on properties similar to those of the brain. In the thymus, segments of the microvasculature only a few millimeters apart have very different permeability properties. The endothelium prevents access of circulating macromolecules to the lymphocytes in the cortex, whereas the endothelium of capillaries in the medulla are freely permeable to the same electron-opaque probes that are excluded from the cortex.

SECRETORY FUNCTIONS OF THE ENDOTHELIUM

The endothelium of blood vessels was long believed to have a rather passive role, simply providing a smooth nonthrombogenic lining to facilitate the flow of blood. It is now known to secrete several components of the underlying extracellular matrix, including fibronec-

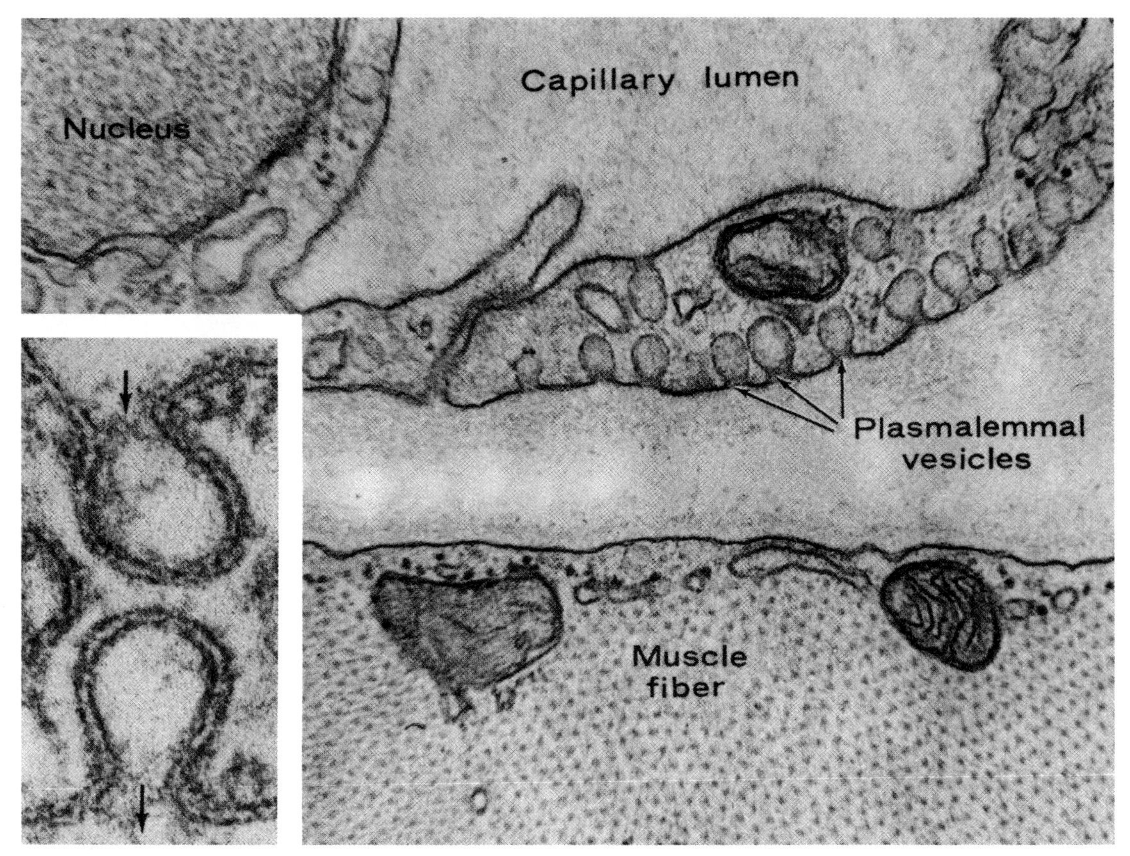

Figure 12–20. Electron micrograph of capillary endothelium, illustrating the small vesicular invaginations of the luminal and basal membranes that are characteristic of capillaries in muscle. (From Fawcett, D.W. 1965. J. Histochem. Cytochem. 13:75.). The inset shows two such vesicles on opposite surfaces of the endothelium at high magnification. (From Bruns, R. and G.E. Palade. 1968. J. Cell Biol. 37:244.)

tin, laminin, collagens, II, IV, and V. Other products of the endothelium are involved in blood clotting, emigration of neutrophils, recirculation of lymphocytes, and maintenance of vascular tone.

The functional versatility of the endothelium long went unsuspected because the cells lack the degree of development of the endoplasmic reticulum and Golgi complex that is expected of secretory cells, and they usually have no secretory granules in their cytoplasm. The majority of their products are secreted constitutively. An exception is the von Willebrand factor, already referred to in describing the ultrastructure of arteries. Small amounts of this large glycoprotein may be secreted constitutively, but it also follows the regulated secretory pathway, being stored in atypical secretory granules, called Weibel–Palade bodies. These are believed to discharge their contents into the blood by exocytosis in response to cytokines such as interleukin-1 and tumor necrosis factor that are liberated at sites of injury to blood vessels. The von Willebrand factor facilitates the binding of platelets to the endothelium to form a hemostatic plug and, thus, plays an important role in limiting blood loss from damaged vessels.

Small arteries respond to the shear stress associated with an increased rate of blood flow by vasodilatation. This response was formerly attributed to local release of a diffusable substance acting on the smooth muscle of the vessel wall to decrease vascular tone. Pending its isolation and characterization, this hypothetical mediator was called the *endothelium-derived relaxing factor* (EDRF). It has now been discovered that endothelial cells synthesize *nitric oxide* (NO) from L-arginine and this activates an enzyme that causes relaxation of smooth muscle. The postulated endothelium-derived relaxing factor is now considered to be nitric oxide.

Endothelium responds to anoxia by release of vasoconstrictor substances. The most potent of these is *endothelin-I,* a peptide that binds

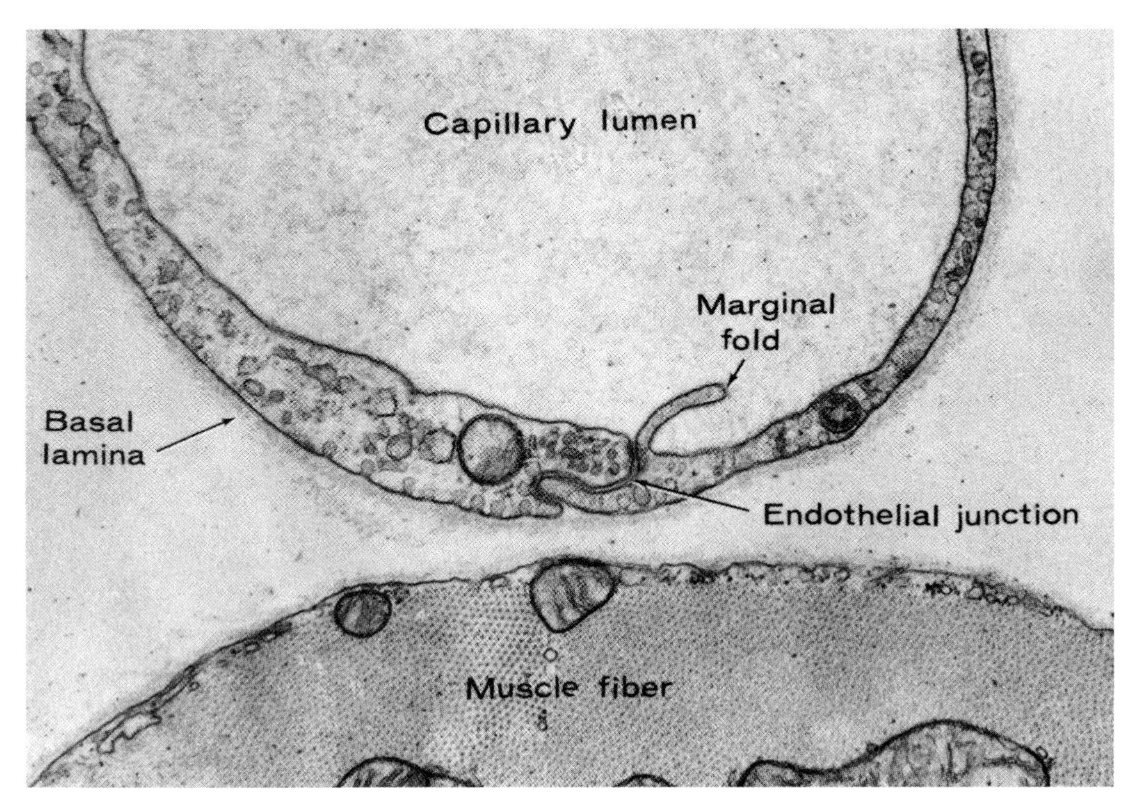

Figure 12–21. Electron micrograph of a capillary from cardiac muscle, illustrating the interdigitating cell junction and a marginal fold.

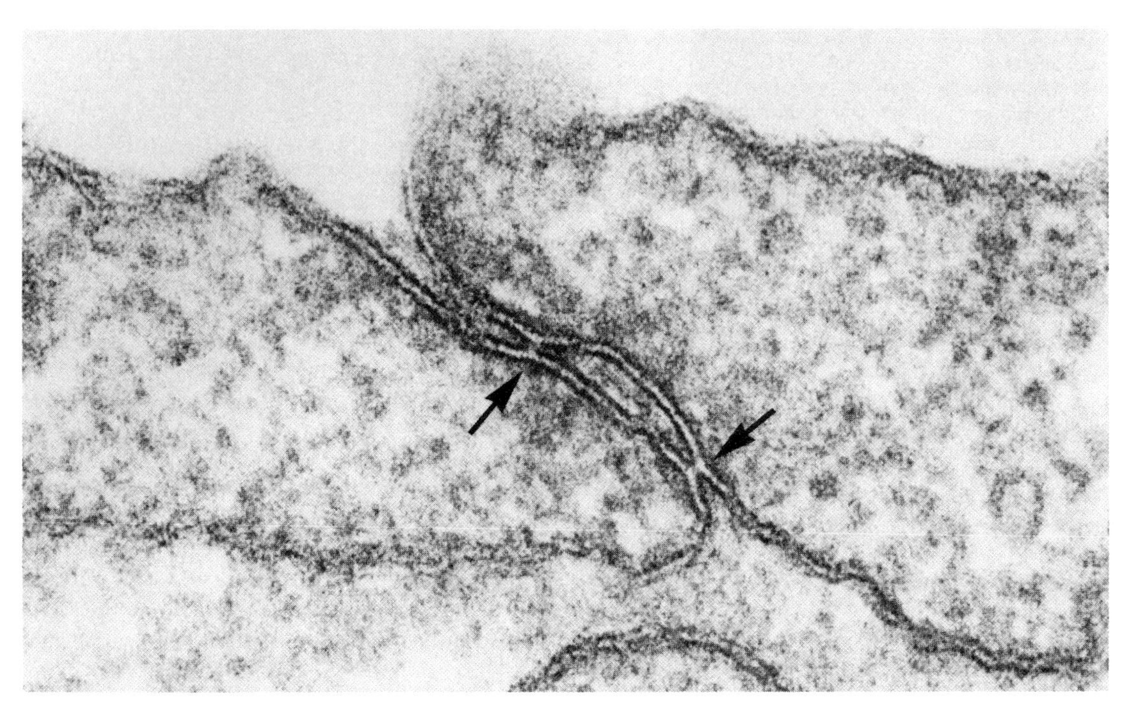

Figure 12–22. Micrograph of the junction between two endothelial cells in a muscle capillary. At the arrows, the opposing membranes are joined to form an occluding junction. (Micrograph courtesy of E. Weihe.)

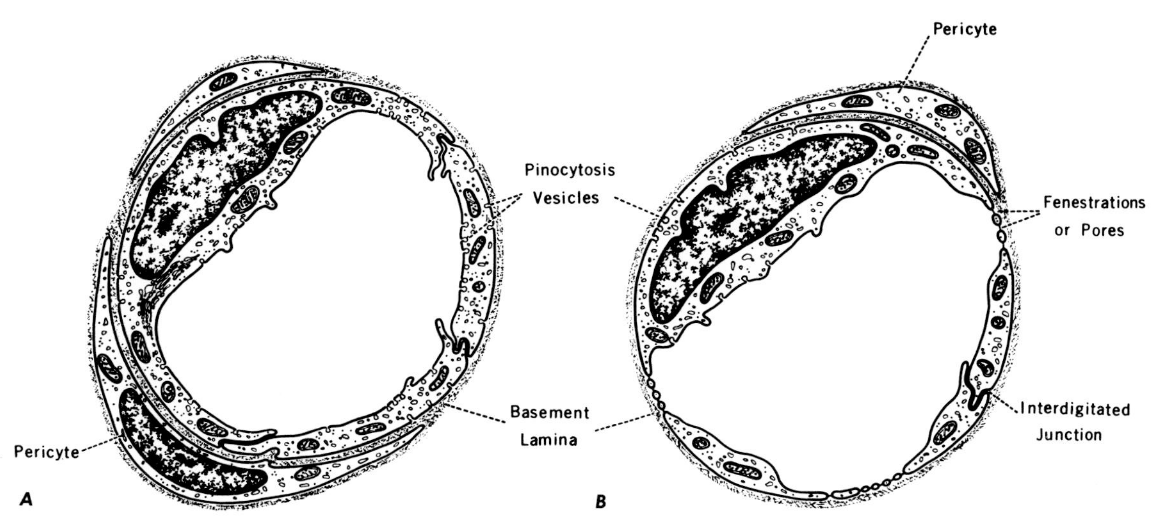

Figure 12–23. Schematic representation of the two most common types of capillaries. (A) The continuous or muscle type with an uninterrupted endothelium. (B) The fenestrated type in which the endothelium varies in thickness and the thinnest areas have multiple small pores closed by an exceeding thin diaphragm. (After Fawcett, D.W. 1962. *In* J.L. Orbison and D. Smith, eds. Peripheral Blood Vessels. Baltimore, Williams and Wilkins.)

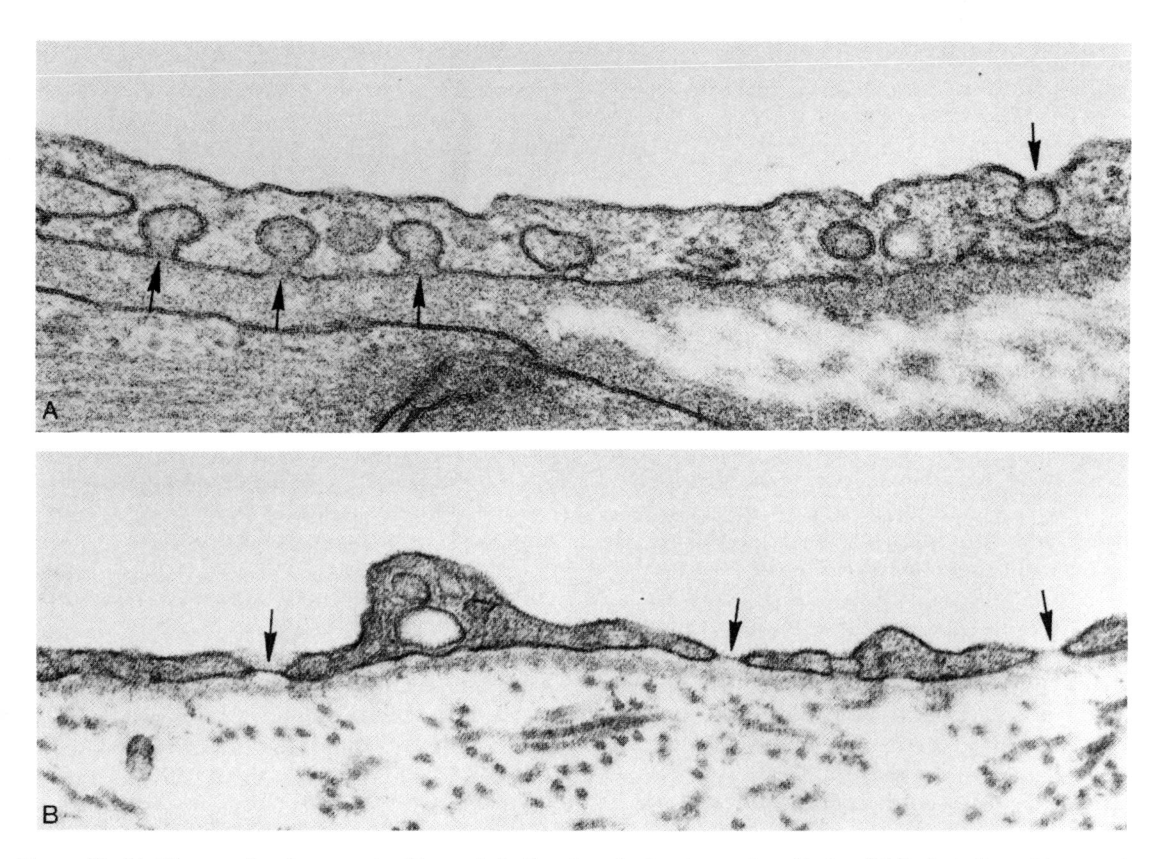

Figure 12–24. Micrographs of segments of the endothelium from the two types of capillaries. (A) Endothelium of the muscle-type capillary has vesicular invaginations of both adluminal and abluminal plasma membranes (arrows). (B) Endothelium of a fenestrated capillary from the lamina propria of the colon is very thin and has pores closed by a thin diaphragm. (Micrographs courtesy of E. Weihe.)

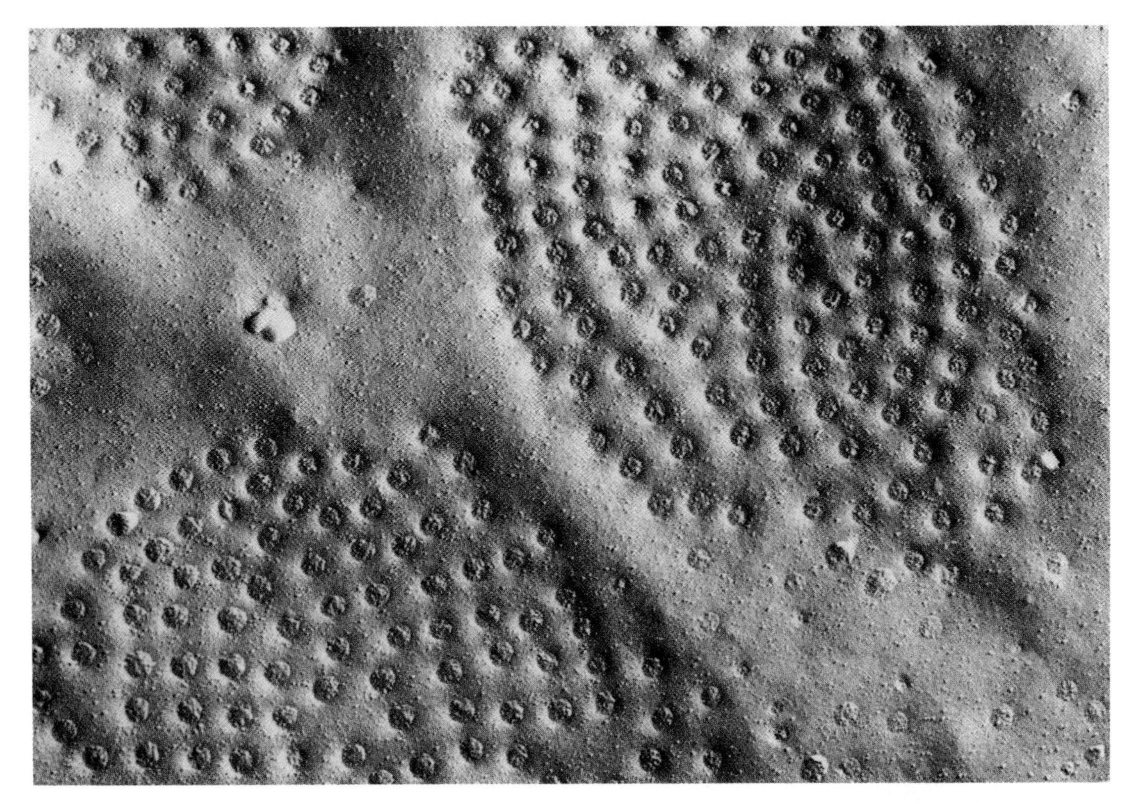

Figure 12–25. Replica of a freeze–fracture preparation of a fenestrated capillary. The extensive surface view of the cleaved membrane of an endothelial cell shows fenestrated areas separated by nonfenestrated areas. Note the uniform size and spacing of the pores. (Micrograph courtesy of S. McNutt.)

to smooth muscle of arteries and is several times as effective in the elevation of blood pressure as angiotensin-II, the systemic regulator of vascular tone. Endothelin-I has a hypertensive action of relatively long duration. It is not yet clear whether it is involved in regulation of the cardiovascular system as a whole or is produced locally in defensive events such as haemostasis after injury.

The leukocytes are transported in the blood but carry out their functions in the tissues. To reach their ultimate destinations, they must first adhere to the endothelium and then migrate between its cells. The interactions of leukocytes with the endothelium of postcapillary venules are early and essential events in inflammation. Circulating polymorphonuclear leukocytes normally express on their plasma membrane-adhesion molecules called *L-selectin* and *B_2-integrins* (CH11a–CH18 and CH11b–CH18). These lectins are capable of binding to receptors on the surface of endothelial cells at sites of inflammation. Bacterial lipopolysaccharide, histamine, and cytokines (TNF, Il-1) activate endothelial cells to synthesize and incorporate in their membrane, *intercellular-adhesion molecules* (ICAM-1, ICAM-2), and *platelet-activating factor* (PAF). Concurrently with the synthesis of PAF, *P-selectin* is released from granules in the endothelial cytoplasm and inserted in the membrane. The initial arrest of circulating leukocytes at sites of inflammation is mediated by their binding to P-selectin on the endothelium and binding of L-selectin on their surface to endothelial receptors, causing the leukocytes to roll slowly over the surface. PAF on the endothelial cells also serves as a signal inducing a structural change in the integrins on the leukocytes that increases their binding affinity for the ICAMs on the endothelium, resulting in tighter binding and cessation of their rolling. PAF also enhances the responsiveness of leukocytes to chemotactic factors emanating from the site of bacterial invasion. After adhering to the endothelium, they become polarized and migrate through the endothelium to ingest and destroy the bacteria.

VESICULATION OF THE PLASMALEMMA

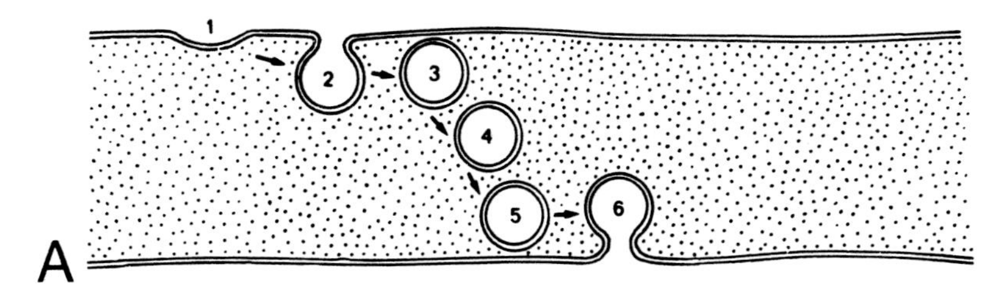

FUSION-FISSION WITHOUT MIXING OF VESICLE AND PLASMA MEMBRANES

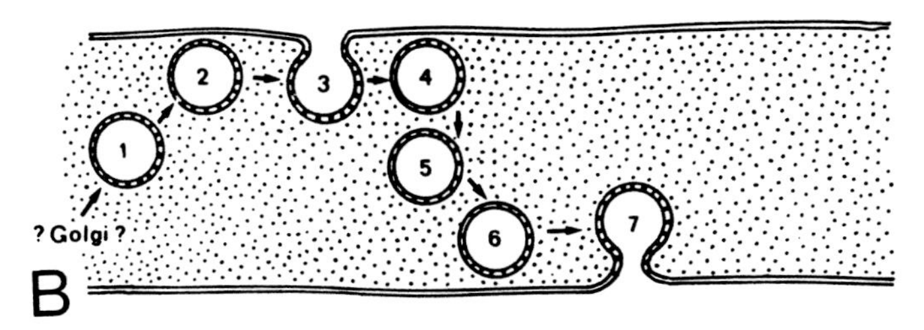

FORMATION OF CHANNELS AND FENESTRAE

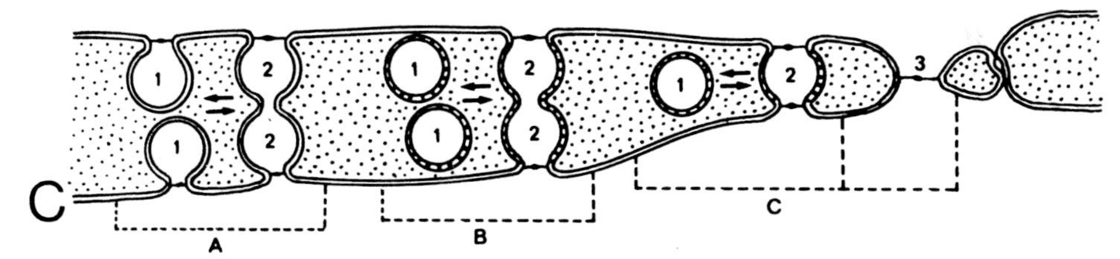

Figure 12–26. Alternate models for transport of water-soluble molecules across the endothelium. (A) Continuous formation of plasmalemmal vesicles followed by detachment, transit, and fusion with the membrane on the other side of the endothelium. (B) Transport mediated by a separate cytoplasmic population of vesicles, possibly of Golgi origin, which undergo transient fusion and fission first at one surface and then at the other, without mixing their membrane with the plasmalemma. This would not require massive movement of membrane from one surface to the other. (C) Transcellular passage involving fusion of vesicles to form channels or formation of fenestrate in thin areas of the endothelium. Current opinion favors (A) and/or (C). (Redrawn after Simionescu, N. and M. Simionescu. 1981. *In* H.H. Ussing, N.B. Bindslev, and O. Sten-Knudsen, eds. Water Transport Across Epithelia. Copenhagen, Munksgaard.)

SINUSOIDS

The vascular channels in the liver, bone marrow, certain endocrine glands, and lymphoid organs are *sinusoids* of relatively large caliber and irregular cross-sectional outline. Unlike capillaries that are cylindrical in form, sinusoids vary in shape and usually conform to the spaces between the epithelial sheets and cords of the organ that they supply. Their form is a consequence of their mode of development. Capillaries develop as branching cellular cords that secondarily acquire a lumen and then grow by addition of vasoformative cells at their ends. In liver and other epithelial organs, sinusoids develop during organogenesis by ingrowth of cords of epithelium into preexisting large, thin-walled embryonic vessels. The walls of the resulting vascular channels, therefore, conform to the irregular spaces between the epithelial components of the organ. Macrophages may be incorporated in the sinusoidal endothelium. Because of their active endocytosis and phagocytosis, sinusoids have traditionally been grouped together with the monocyte-derived macrophages of the body as components of the so-called *reticulo-endothelial system.*

In some lymphoid organs, the sinusoidal endothelium is extremely thin but continuous. In endocrine glands, its cells present a mosaic of fenestrated and unfenestrated areas. The hepatic sinuoids are unique in having larger fenestrations of varying size and shape through which the blood plasma has direct access to the liver cells with no interposed permeability barrier.

VEINS

From the capillaries, blood is carried back to the heart in the veins. These normally accompany the corresponding arteries (Fig. 12–27, and as they progress toward the heart they increase in diameter and their walls become thicker. Because veins are more numerous than arteries and have a larger lumen, the venous system has a much greater capacity than the arterial system. The walls of veins are thinner, more supple, and less elastic than those of arteries. Thus, in histological sections, veins are usually collapsed and have a slit-like lumen, unless a special effort has been made to fix them in distension.

For descriptive purposes, it is customary to distinguish three categories: small, medium, and large veins. However, this subdivision is not entirely satisfactory because the structure of the wall is not always closely correlated with the diameter of the vessel. Veins in the same category show greater variation in their structure than do arteries, and the same vein may vary in the structure of its wall in different segments along its length.

Most authors distinguish three layers in the wall of veins: tunica intima, tunica media, and tunica adventitia, as in arteries. However, the boundaries of the layers are often quite indistinct. The muscular and elastic components are not nearly as well developed in veins as they are in arteries, and connective tissue components are more prominent. In certain veins, a tunica media cannot be identified.

VENULES AND SMALL VEINS

Capillaries converge to form postcapillary venules of slightly larger size (15–20 μm) (Fig. 12–28). The ultrastructure of the wall of these vessels is not significantly different from that of capillaries (Fig. 12–29). It consists of very thin endothelium surrounded by reticular fibers and pericytes. Although it is not evident in histological sections, the pericytes differs somewhat from those of capillaries in their shape and interrelationships. In scanning electron micrographs, their multiple branching processes form a rather elaborate loose network around the vessel (Fig. 12–30). In larger venules, these give way to smooth muscle cells. In venules about 50 μm in diameter, circumferentially oriented smooth muscle cells are spaced some distance apart, but they become more closely spaced in vessels of larger size. In larger venules and small veins, smooth muscle forms a more-or-less continuous layer, but the cells are more irregular in shape and are spaced farther apart than those of arterioles (Fig. 12–31).

Not all of the exchange between the blood and the tissues takes place in the capillaries. The postcapillary venules also participate in this function. Indeed, their wall seems to be

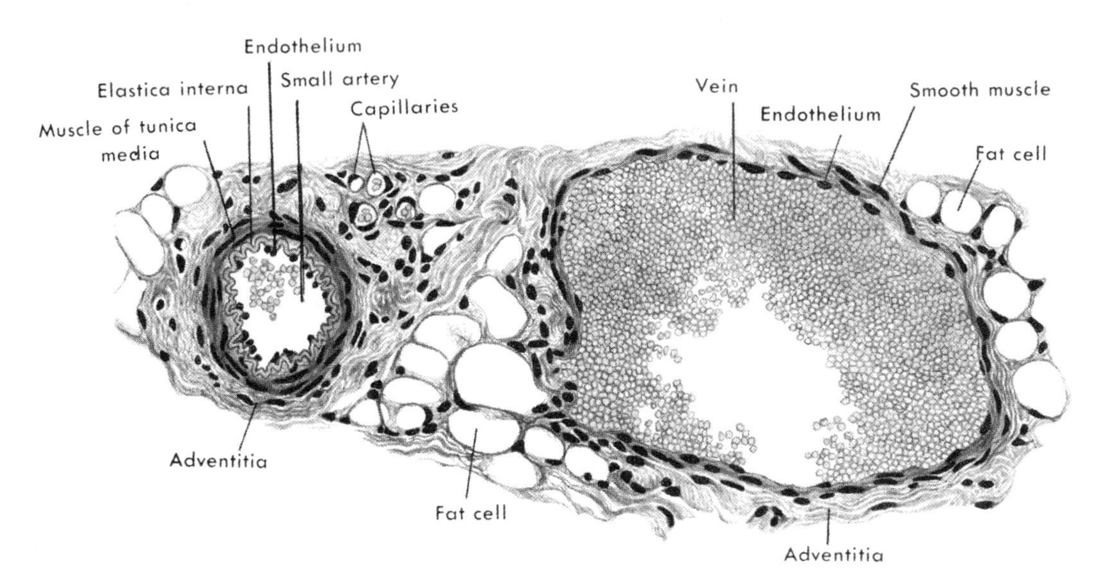

Figure 12–27. Cross section through a small artery and its accompanying vein from the submucosa of the human intestine.

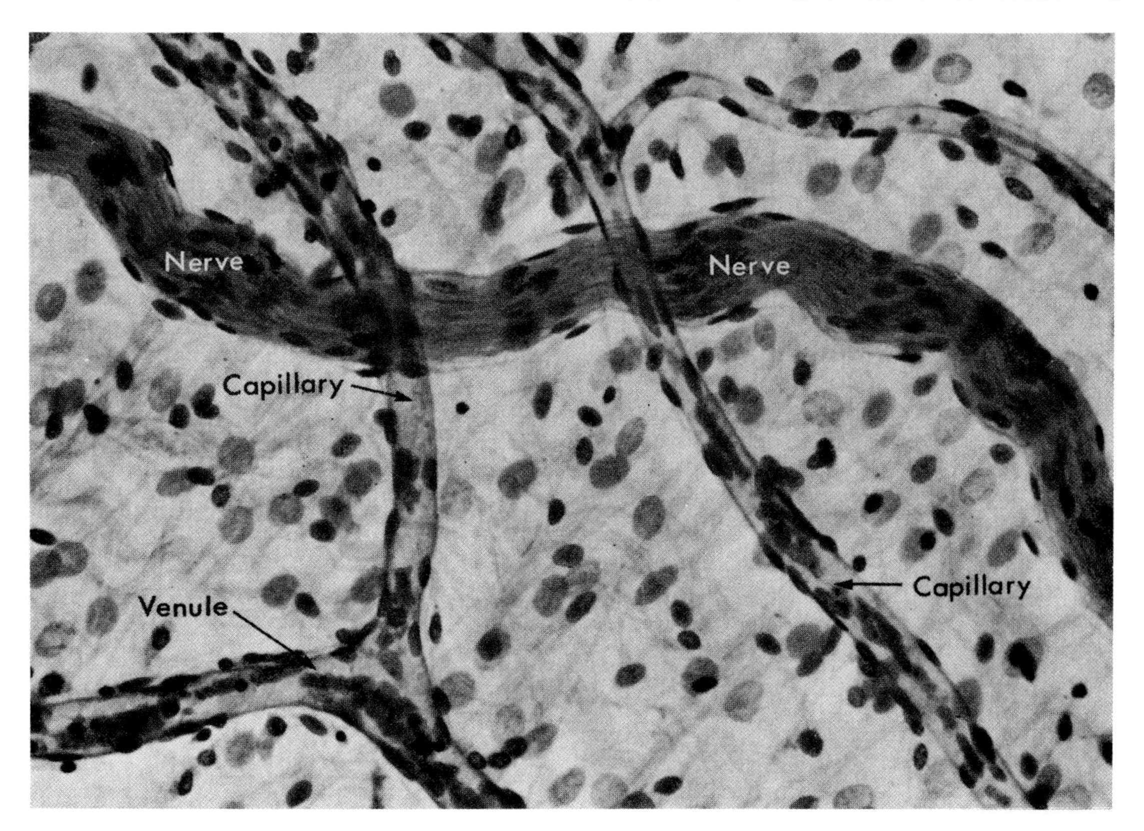

Figure 12–28. Photomicrograph of a thin-spread intact mesentery showing a nerve, venule, and capillaries.

even more permeable. When particulate tracers are injected intravascularly, the first particles found outside of the vessels are not at the capillaries, but are along slightly larger vessels interpreted as venules. This segment of the vascular system is also the preferential site for emigration of leukocytes from the blood into the tissues. These vessels are also especially susceptible to the effects of histamine, serotonin, and other substances known to increase vascular permeability. If one of these substances is injected locally into an animal that has previously received an intravascular injection of an electron-opaque particulate tracer, the particles accumulate in small gaps formed by retraction of endothial cells of the venules, thus marking the sites of increased permeability (Fig. 12–32). Such leaks can occasionally be found in typical capillaries but much less often than in venules. There is some evidence of a gradient in permeability from the arterial to the venous side of the capillary bed which extends into the postcapillary venules.

In lymph nodes and submucosal lymphoid accumulations called Peyer's patches, the postcapillary venules have a unique structure. Their endothelial cells are not squamous but cuboidal. Such vessels are called *high-endothelial venules*. This local specialization of the vessels is an important component of the mechanisms that ensure localization of specific categories of lymphocytes in the lymphoid tissues. For example, T-lymphocytes predominate in lymph nodes, whereas B-lymphocytes are most abundant in Peyer's patches. This selective distribution depends on the fact that lymphocytes possess type-specific molecules (homing receptors) on their surface. As blood circulates, lymphocytes destined to home into the submucosal lymphoid tissue bind to type-specific molecules on the luminal surface of the high-endothelial cells that recognize the ligand on the surface of the lymphocytes. Having adhered to the high-endothelial cells, the lymphocytes then migrate through the wall of the vessels into the surrounding lymphoid tissue. A protein molecule of 58–60 kD that is responsible for lymphocyte homing to mucosal lymphoid tissue has been isolated and partially characterized. Recognition molecules which are specific for lymphocytes bearing "addresses" to other tissues having high-endothelial cells, such as peripheral lymph nodes, and the synovium of inflamed joints, will no doubt be identified in the future.

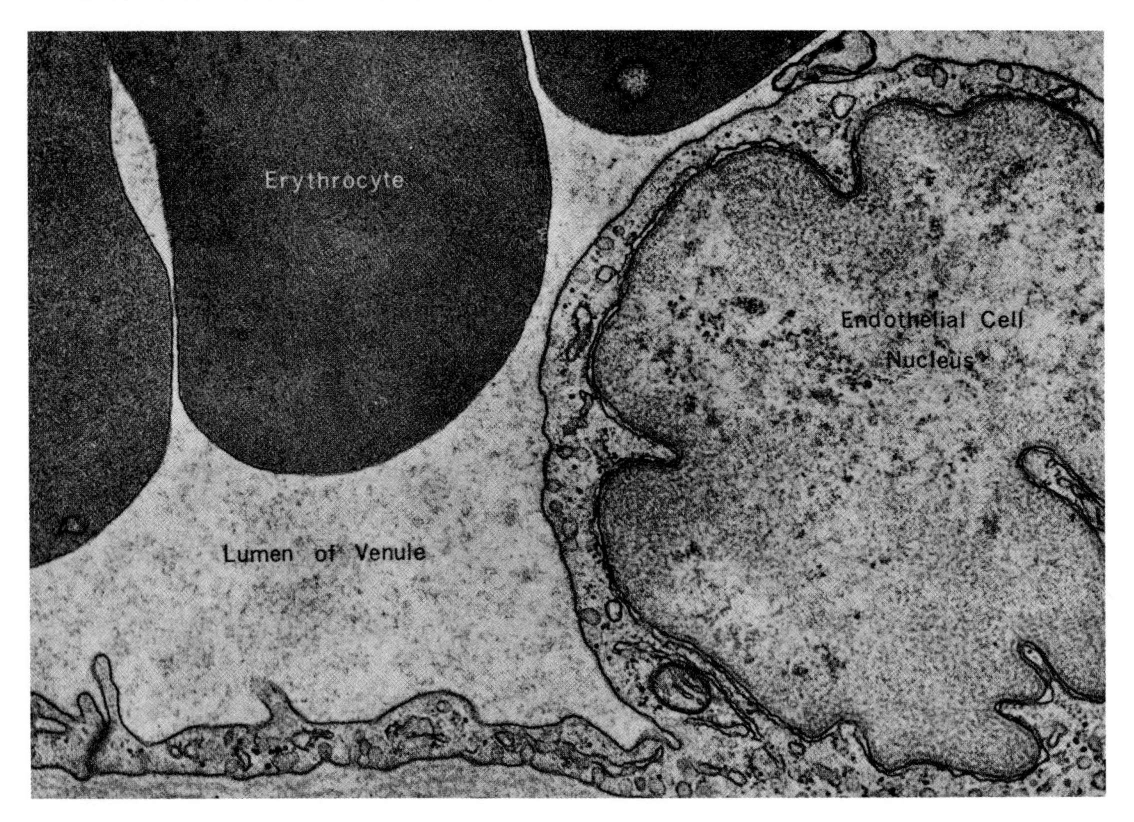

Figure 12–29. Electron micrograph of a portion of the wall of a small venule from the myocardium. The appearance of the thin continuous endothelium is essentially the same as that of a capillary. The nuclear region of the endothelial cell bulges into the lumen.

VEINS OF MEDIUM SIZE

Veins in the size range 2–9 mm include the cutaneous and deeper veins of the extremities distal to the brachial and popliteal, the veins of the head, and many of those of the viscera. Their tunica intima consists of endothelium, its basal lamina, and associated reticular fibers. It is sometimes bounded externally by a moderately dense network of elastic fibers, but there is no true elastica interna. In surface view, the endothelial cells tend to have elaborate interdigitating outlines. The media consists of a layer of circular smooth muscle but this is thinner and more loosely organized than in arteries. Numerous longitudinal collagen fibers and a few fibroblasts intermingle with, and tend to separate, the smooth muscle cells. The tunica adventitia of medium-sized veins is usually their thickest layer and consists of bundles of collagen and networks of elastic fibers. A few longitudinally oriented smooth muscle cells may found between the adventitia and the media.

LARGE VEINS

The large veins include the inferior vena cava, the portal, splenic, superior mesenteric, external iliac, renal, and azygos veins. Their tunica intima has much the same structure as in medium-sized veins, but in these larger trunks, the subendothelial connective tissue may be considerably thicker. It contains scattered fibroblasts and is bounded externally by a network of elastic fibers. The amount of smooth muscle in the wall of veins is highly variable. Smooth muscle is a prominent component of the veins in the gravid uterus, and the pulmonary veins have a well-developed media containing circular smooth muscle, but in the great majority of large veins, a media is lacking and a thick adventitia makes up the greater part of the thickness of the wall. Smooth muscle is entirely absent in veins of the meninges, retina, placenta, corpora cavernosa, and spongiosa of the penis. Where vessels are shielded from pressure of surrounding structures, there is very little smooth

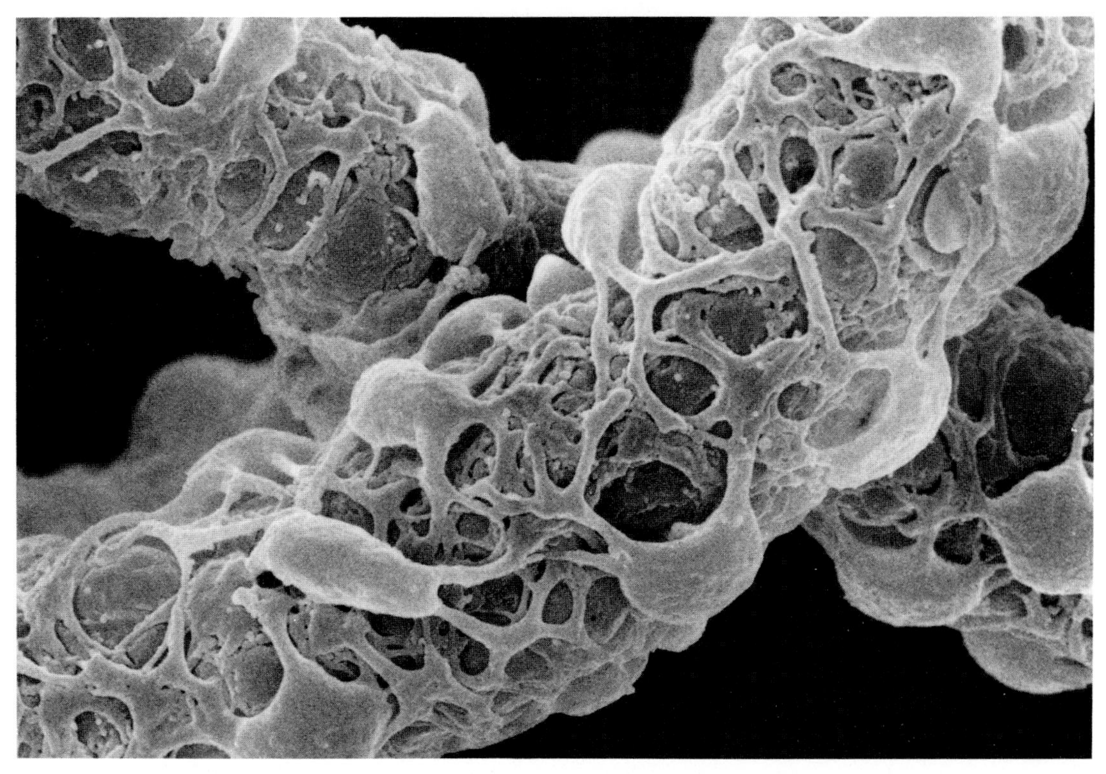

Figure 12–30. The pericytes differ in their form along the length of the microvasculature, from the arterial to the venous end. Here in a postcapillary venule of a cat mammary gland, the highly branched pericyte processes form a lace-like network over the surface of the vessel. (Micrograph from Fujiwara, T. and Y. Uehara. 1984. Am. J. Anat. 170:39.)

muscle in their wall. On the other hand, the superficial veins of the legs have a rather well-developed media. This may possibly be an adaptation to resist distension due to the resistance to flow that is attributable to the force of gravity. The great saphenous vein of the lower extremity has circular smooth muscle in its media and may also have an inner layer of longitudinal fibers.

The thick adventitia of larger veins is rich in elastic fibers and bundles of collagen that are oriented, for the most part, longitudinally. In the inferior vena cava, the collagen fibers are reported to have a spiral course that is believed to facilitate the slight lengthening and shortening that the vessel undergoes in the ascent and descent of the diaphragm. The inferior vena cava is also exceptional in that its adventitia contains scattered longitudinal bundles of smooth muscle. Where the pulmonary veins and the vena cava enter the heart, cardiac muscle extends a short distance into their adventitia.

Minute vessels, called *vasa vasorum,* penetrate the wall of both large arteries and veins to supply oxygen to their tissues. These are more numerous and extend more deeply into the wall of veins than they do in arteries.

VALVES OF VEINS

Many medium-sized veins have valves that prevent flow of blood away from the heart. Each of the two opposing semilunar valve leaflets is a thin fold of the intima, internally reinforced by a thin layer of collagen and a network of elastic fibers that are continuous with those in the intima of the vessel wall (Fig. 12–33). On the side toward the vessel wall, the endothelial cells are elongated transversely, whereas on the other side, the long axis of the cells is longitudinal. The space between the valve and the vessel wall is called the *sinus of the valve.* Just above the arc of attachment of each valve cusp, the wall of the vein is thinner and slightly expanded. In distended veins, this thin region of the wall bulges slightly, making it possible to detect the location of valves in intact vessels with the naked eye.

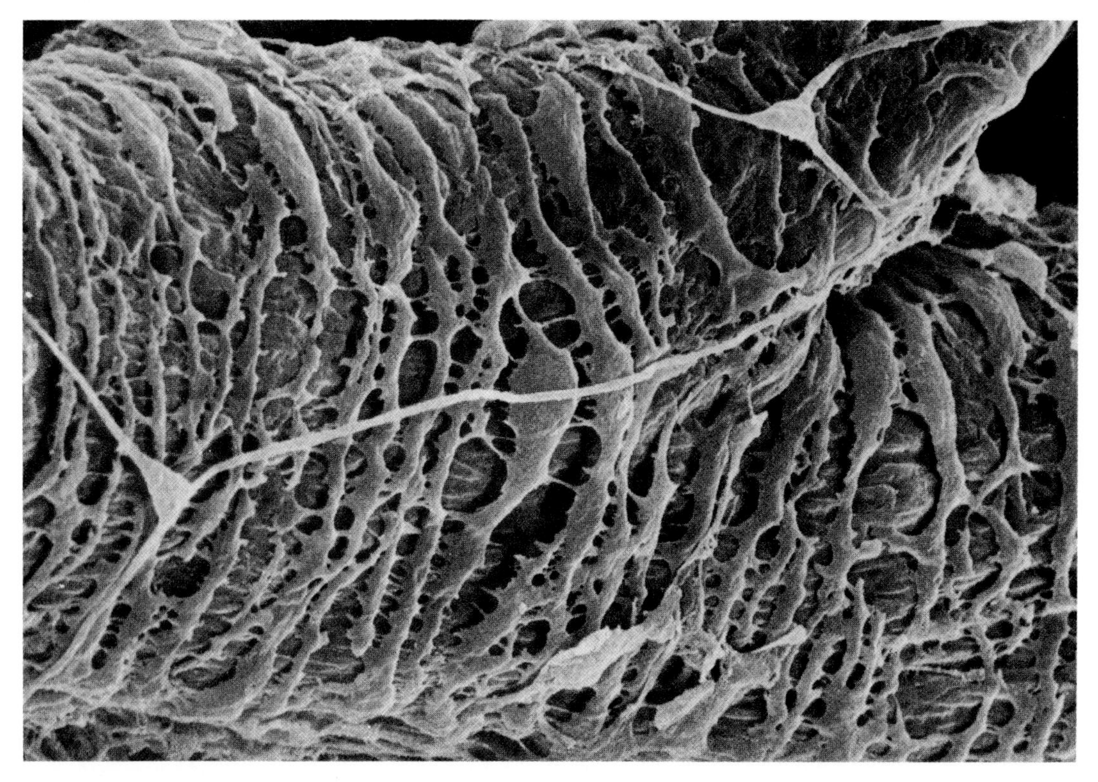

Figure 12–31. Scanning micrograph of a large venule joined at the upper right by a smaller tributary. The smooth muscle cells are more irregular in shape and are spaced further apart than in arterioles. Elements of the perivascular nerve net can be seen branching over the vessel. The fibrous and amorphous connective tissue components have been removed, in this preparation, by enzymatic digestion to reveal the underlying structures. (Micrograph from Uehara, Y., J. Desaki, and T. Fujiwara. 1981. Biomed. Res. 2 (Suppl.): 139.)

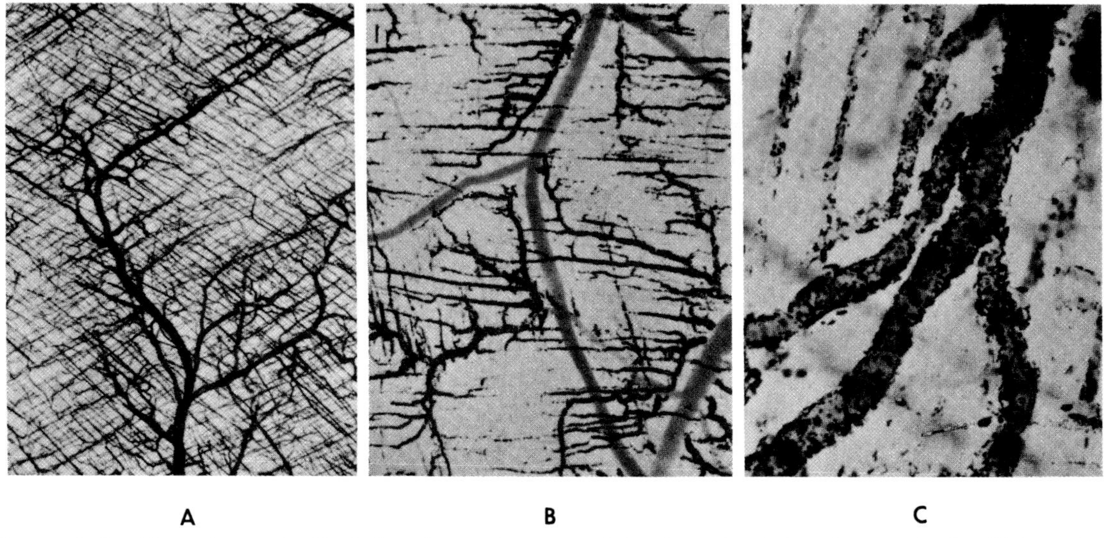

Figure 12–32. Photomicrographs illustrating the greater permeability of venules, induced by serotontin. (A) Vessels of the cremaster in the normal rat injected with carbon to demonstrate the blood vessels. (B) Vascular labeling resulting from leakage of opaque particles from the vessels after local application of serotonin. The blackened vessels are venules. The permeability of many of the capillaries, visible in (A), has not been affected by this treatment. (C) Higher magnification of a venule after 7 days, showing intracellular masses of particulate matter in the vascular wall. (From Majno, G., G.E. Palade, and G.I. Schoefl. 1961. J. Biophys. Biochem. Cytol. 11:607.)

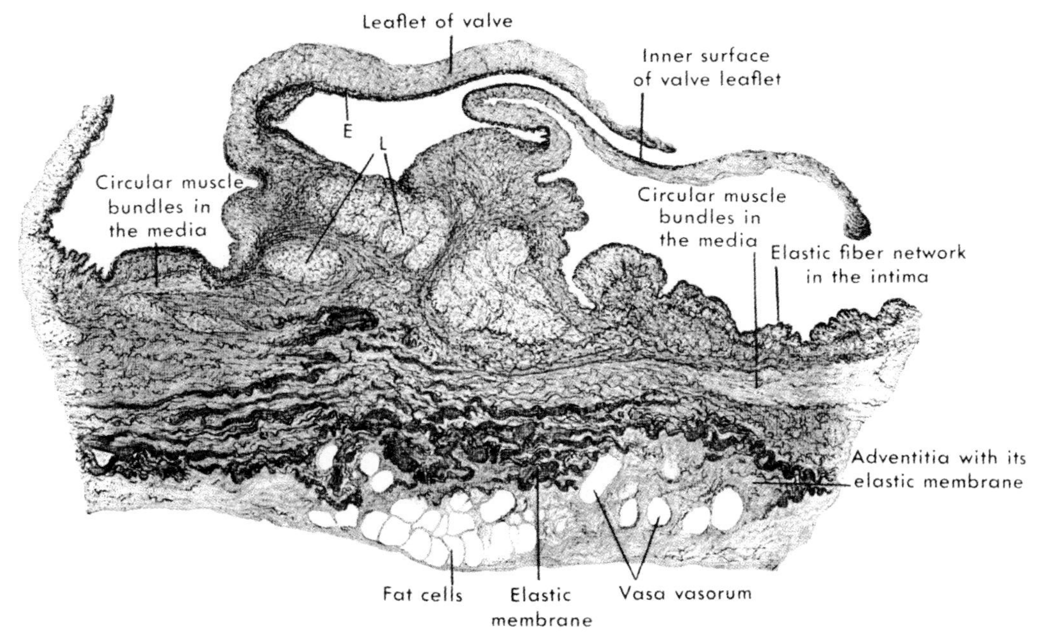

Figure 12–33. From a cross section of a human femoral vein. The section passes through the origin of a valve, seen projecting upward into the lumen. (E) Elastic fiber network in the intima on the inner surface of the valve leaflet. (L) Bundle of longitudinal muscle fibers at the base of the valve.

The free margins of valves project in the direction of blood flow. When blood is flowing toward the heart, the cusps of the valves are flattened against the vessel wall, but if the contraction of surrounding muscles exerts pressure on the vein, the edges of the valve leaflets come into close apposition, preventing backflow. Valves are numerous in the veins of the lower extremity where they facilitate venous return by helping to resist the force of gravity on the column of blood. Valves are not found in small veins or in the very largest veins.

PORTAL SYSTEMS

As a rule, networks of capillaries are interposed between the terminal ramifications of the arterial system and those of the venous system. This arrangement is modified in several places in the body to meet special functional requirements. In one physiologically important modification of the general plan, the blood from one capillary bed flows into a larger vessel, having the histological characteristics of a vein, and this vessel later ramifies into capillaries so that the blood flows through a second capillary network before returning to the heart. The vessel or vessels interposed between two capillary beds constitute a *portal system.*

In the hepatic portal system, the capillary networks of the intestine and of certain other abdominal organs are drained via the *portal vein* to the liver. There, the portal vein ramifies into an extensive network of sinusoids between cords of liver cells. Blood then flows from the sinusoids through a converging system of vessels of increasing caliber to the hepatic vein and then back to the heart via the inferior vena cava. This arrangement permits nutrients absorbed in the intestines to be exposed to, and processed by, the liver cells before being distributed throughout the body in the general circulation.

In another example, the capillaries in the median eminance of the hypothalamus are continuous with the *hypophyseoportal system,* a plexus of small veins that course along the hypophyseal stalk and then ramify into the sinusoids of the anterior lobe of the hypophysis. This arrangement permits releasing factors liberated by neurosecretory axons in the hypothalamus to be carried downstream to activate the endocrine cells of the hypophysis (see Chapter 19).

In the kidney, we have a unique example of a vessel with the structure of an artery interposed between two capillary beds. Afferent arterioles break up into a spherical mass of contorted capillaries, called a *glomerulus*. These capillaries coalesce to form an efferent arteriole, which goes on to ramify into another set of capillaries that surround the tubules of the kidney. In this case, the efferent arteriole conforms to the definition of a portal vessel (see Chapter 30).

ANGIOGENESIS

In the mammalian embryo, the first blood vessels are formed in the area vasculosa of the yolk sac, where mesenchymal cells aggregate and differentiate into a layer of flattened cells lining a system of discontinuous spaces. These spaces later coalesce to form thin-walled vessels within which blood cells formation begins. In the embryo proper, the primordia of the heart and great vessels also arise from mesenchymal cells that form a squamous epithelium lining fluid-filled spaces between the ectoderm and endoderm. These discontinuous spaces later unite with each other and with those of the area vasculosa to form a closed system of vessels through which blood cells soon begin to circulate. As the tissues and organs of the embryo develop, new capillaries are formed by budding from preexisting vessels. Endothelial cells first proliferate and migrate to form a solid strand of cells that extends laterally from the parent vessel. Rearrangement of the cells creates a lumen, permitting blood cells to enter. The growing ends of these blind-ending tubes contact and fuse with sprouts from neighboring vessels. In this way, an expanding three-dimensional network of capillaries is formed to nourish the growing tissues. Small and medium-sized arteries and veins are first formed as capillaries. They then expand by proliferation of endothelial cells and their walls are thickened by addition of smooth muscle cells and various extracellular components. The smooth muscle cells are added by recruitment and differentiation of mesenchymal cells.

The factors that cause the larger arteries to develop in a consistent pattern are not well understood. It is probable that the pattern of major vessels is genetically determined in the early embryo, but the pattern of small vessels that develop later may depend, at least in part, upon local hemodynamic forces.

In postnatal life, the vascular system retains the capacity to develop new capillaries in the repair of tissues that have been injured. Moreover, in tissues such as the endometrium of the uterus, which is normally subject to cyclic degeneration and renewal, new capillaries are rapidly formed to ensure that the regenerating tissue will have an adequate supply of oxygen. The number of capillaries needed is very large because diffusion of oxygen is limited to about 2.5 nm. Thus, the growth of normal or tumorous tissue depends on *angiogenesis*, the formation of new capillaries. This involves a sequence of events not unlike that occurring in the embryo: (1) There is a local degradation of the basal lamina in persisting capillaries and small venules; (2) migration of endothelial cells toward the site of new growth; (3) their proliferation and alignment to form capillary sprouts; (4) rearrangement of the endothelial cells to form a lumen; (5) anastomosis of neighboring sprouts to form loops or networks; and (6) the establishment of blood flow through the new vessels. If this process fails, the growth of the tissue ceases or its center degenerates due to local anoxia.

The factors responsible for the initiation of capillary growth have recently been the subject of intensive research. A substance has been extracted from tumors which, at extremely low concentrations, will stimulate endothelial proliferation and formation of capillaries. This cationic polypeptide of 18,000 MW is called *tumor angiogenesis factor* (TAF). A convenient system for its study has been the proliferation of capillaries induced by small implants of tumor on the chorioallantoic membrane of the chick embryo. One of the early changes observed at the site of the implant is a 20- to 40-fold increase in the concentration of mast cells. Heparin, one of the products of mast cells, potentiates the action of TAF. This factor binds to heparin and heparin-affinity has been used to purify it and other endothelial growth factors. Because heparin-sulfate is a major glycosaminoglycan on the endothelial cell surface and in the basal lamina, it is speculated that it may bind and concentrate endothelial growth factors that stimulate locomotion and proliferation of endothelial cells during angiogenesis. In recent years, five unrelated polypeptides secreted by various cell types have been shown to be angiogenic. One of these, *tumor necrosis factor* (TNF.) is secreted by activated macrophages that accumulate in wounds. It may, therefore, be involved in the generation of capillaries in wound healing. Why there are multiple angiogenic factors and which are the most important in vivo remains unclear.

HEART

The heart is a muscular, rhythmically contracting portion of the vascular system that provides the motive force for circulation of the blood. Its myocardium is analogous to the media of other blood vessels, but instead of smooth muscle, it consists of striated cardiac muscle, which has been described in Chapter 10. The heart is about 12 cm long, 9 cm wide, and 6 cm in antero-posterior diameter. It consists of four chambers: right and left *atria* and right and left *ventricles*. Blood returning to the heart in the superior and inferior venae cavae enters the right atrium and passes from it to the right ventricle. From there, it is pumped, via the pulmonary artery, to the lungs, where it is aerated and then returned to the left atrium via the pulmonary vein. Contraction of the left atrium expels blood into the left ventricle, from where it is pumped into the aorta and through its branches throughout the body.

The orifice between the right atrium and right ventricle is closed by the *tricuspid valve* and that between the left atrium and ventricle by the *mitral valve*. *Aortic* and *pulmonary semilunar valves* prevent reflux of blood from these vessels during relaxation of the heart. The mitral and tricuspid valves remain open while the heart is filling between beats and during contraction of the atria, but when the ventricles contract, both valves are closed by the pressure developed within these chambers. At the same time, the rising pressure opens the aortic and semilumar valves, permitting outflow of blood into the pulmonary and systemic circulations.

The wall of the heart consists of three layers *endocardium, myocardium,* and *epicardium* which are homologues of the tunica intima, tunica media, and tunica adventitia, of the blood vessels.

ENDOCARDIUM

The *endocardium* is lined by an endothelium of polygonal squamous cells that is continuous with the endothelium of the vessels entering and leaving the heart. Directly underlying the endothelium is a thin layer of collagenous and elastic fibers containing occasional fibroblasts (Fig. 12–34). External to this, there is a layer of denser connective tissue that makes up the bulk of the thickness of the endocardium. This layer is rich in elastic fibers and contains varying numbers of smooth muscle cells, especially in the region of the ventricular septum. A *subendocardial layer* of loose connective tissue binds the endocardium to the myocardium and is continuous with its endomysium. This layer contains small blood vessels, nerves, and bundles of fibers of the conduction system of the heart. In the thin wall of the atria, the connective tissue of the endocardium may extend through narrow spaces between muscle-fiber bundles to become continuous with that of the epicardium. A subendocardial layer is absent on the papillary muscles and chordae tendineae that tether the free edges of the mitral and tricupid valves.

MYOCARDIUM

The myocardium consists mainly of working cardiac muscle fibers that are responsible for pumping blood through the circulation. Their structure and mechanism of contraction have been described in Chapter 10. Some cardiac myocytes also have an endocrine secretory function. Some are specialized for initiation of the impulses that control the rhythmic contraction of heart, and others are specialized for conduction of those impulses from the atria to the ventricles.

The heart normally beats about 70 times a minute. This rate is largely determined by *pacemaker cells* in the *sinoatrial node,* a small area about 10 mm in length and 3 to 5 mm in width, located at the junction of the superior vena cava with the right atrium. The nodal myocytes are much more slender than those of the rest of the atrium and are endowed with the special property of undergoing spontaneous depolarization at a frequency of about 70 times a minute, resulting in the generation of impulses that spread to the surrounding atrial myocardium and over special bundles of myocytes, called the *anterior, middle,* and *posterior internodal pathways,* to the *atrioventricular node,* which is located beneath the endocardium of the interatrial septum, just above the attachment of the septal leaf of the tricuspid valve.

The atrioventricular node is about 6 mm long and 2–3 mm wide and consists of a complex meshwork of specialized myocytes embedded in connective tissue. The terminals of the internodal conduction path are in contact with special impulse-conducting Purkinje fibers which continue from the node as compo-

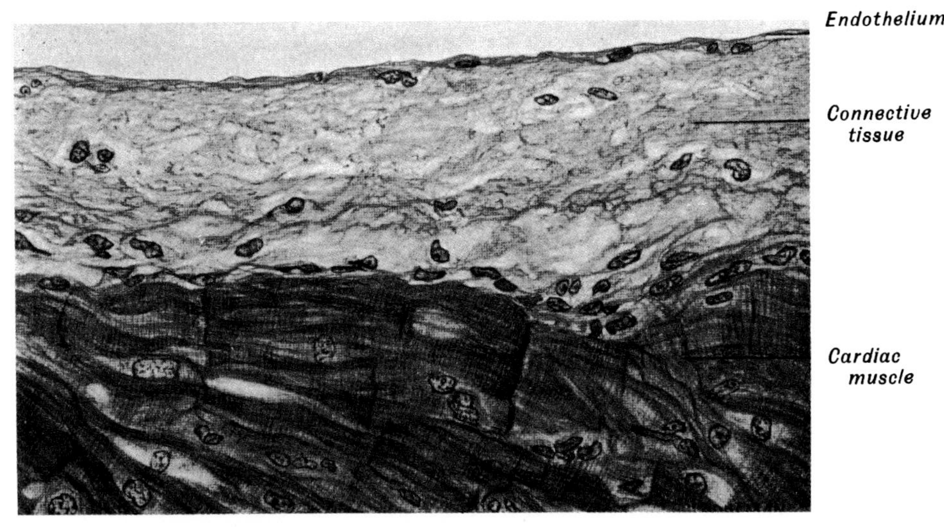

Figure 12–34. Section of the endocardium from the human ventricle.

nents of the *atrioventricular bundle* (bundle of His). The bundle penetrates the annulus of dense connective tissue that separates the atrial and ventricular myocardium and courses down the interventricular septum for about 1 cm and then divides into right and left branches. The right branch, a cylindrical bundle 1–2 mm thick, courses down the septum beneath the endocardium and gives rise to many branches that fan out to the papillary muscles and all parts of the right ventricle. The left bundle branch is a flat band that proceeds down the left side of the septum and breaks up into branches that radiate throughout the wall of the left ventricle. The conduction system of the heart enables impulses generated in the pacemaker cells of the sinoatrial node to activate the atrium and to travel rapidly to the atrioventricular node and then to spread from there over both ventricles.

Myoendocrine cells of the myocardium are located mainly in the atrial appendages and ventricular septum. Their ultrastructure has been described in Chapter 10. Their most conspicuous feature is an accumulation of small secretory granules in the central column of sarcoplasm that contains the nucleus and Golgi complex. Smaller numbers of granules are found between the myofibrils throughout the cell. These cells synthesize a prohormone of 126 amino acids which is broken down to a family of smaller peptides that have been variously designated *cardionatrin, cardiodilatin, atriopeptin,* and *atrial natriuretic polypeptide.* These are believed to be released by exocytosis and to enter the blood flowing in the capillaries of the myocardium. Distributed in the circulation, they act on cells in the kidney, adrenal, hypophysis, and brain. Collectively, they have a potent diuretic action and increase sodium excretion. They suppress aldosterone secretion by the adrenal and induce relaxation of vascular smooth muscle. Therefore, these peptides have an important role in the regulation of fluid and electrolyte balance, blood volume, and blood pressure.

EPICARDIUM

The *epicardium* consists of an inner layer of fibroelastic connective tissue and an outer layer of squamous mesothelial cells. The connective tissue of the inner layer is continuous with the endomysium of the underlying myocardium. The major coronary blood vessels course through the connective tissue layer of the epicardium, enveloped by varying amounts of adipose tissue. The epicardium also forms the visceral layer of the *pericardium,* a serous cavity that surrounds the heart. Around the roots of the aorta and pulmonary artery, the epicardium is continuous with the parietal layer of the pericardium, a similar mesothelium-coated layer of fibroelastic tissue. The visceral and parietal layers of the pericardium bound a narrow space, called the *pericardial cavity.* This contains a small amount of fluid that permits the smooth mesothelial surfaces of the epicardium and parietal pericardium to glide freely over one another during contraction and relaxation of the heart. If the pericardial cavity becomes infected (*pericarditis*), these layers may become adherent, obliterating the space between them. They then impose considerable restraint on the beating of the heart.

CARDIAC SKELETON

The heart has a continuous framework of dense connective tissue components that are referred to collectively as the *cardiac skeleton* because they provide attachment for many of the working muscle fibers. Its principal components are the *annuli fibrosi,* encircling the base of the aorta, pulmonary artery, and the atrioventricular orifices. The annuli associated with the great vessels are not planar but consist of three scallops conforming to the bases of the valve cusps. The scallop associated with the left posterior cusp of the aortic valve has a roughly triangular thickening called the *trigonum fibrosum* which is continuous with the mitral valve annulus and provides attachment for the anterior leaf of this valve. A comparable thickening of the scallop associated with the posterior cusp of the aortic valve provides attachment for the septal leaf of the tricuspid valve and continues downward as the *septum membranaceum,* the thin upper portion of the interventricular septum.

In addition to providing attachment for myocytes and for the valve leaflets, the annuli around the atrioventricular orifices ensure discontinuity between the myocardium of the atria and ventricles so that the only electrophysiological connection between them is via the specialized conduction tissue of the atrioventricular bundle. This is necessary to maintain the orderly sequence of events in the cardiac cycle. In man, these annuli contain some elastic fibers but are mainly dense collagenous tissue. The trigona fibrosa contains small islets of chondroid, a cartilage-like tissue consisting of globular cells in an amorphous matrix that stains deeply with hematoxylin and basic aniline dyes. In old age, the cardiac skeleton may undergo calcification, and, in rare instances, true bone may be found within it. In bovine species, bone is normally found in the trigona fibrosa.

BLOOD SUPPLY OF THE HEART

The blood supply to the heart is carried by the *coronary arteries* which arise from the anterior and left posterior aortic sinuses just above the valve cusps. The right coronary artery descends between the right atrial appendage and the pulmonary trunk, then along the atrioventricular sulcus to supply the right atrium and ventricle. The larger left coronary artery courses downward between the pulmonary trunk and the left atrial appendage and turns to the left in the atrioventricular sulcus. It gives rise to two or three branches running toward the apex of the heart. Anastomoses have been described between the branches of the right and left coronary arteries.

The coronary arteries and their main branches are located in the epicardium and send small branches into the underlying myocardium. Compared to other arteries of similar size, the coronaries are somewhat atypical in their structure. The intima is not in direct contact with the internal elastic lamina, but in some segments of the vessel, is separated from it by a layer of longitudinally oriented smooth muscle and associated reticulum and elastic fibers. Some histologists interpret this layer as a thickening of the intima; others consider the media to have two layers separated by a fenestrated elastic lamina. The significance of this unusual configuration is unknown.

The main coronary arteries and their epicardial branches normally undergo little change in caliber, but the small intramyocardial arterioles have a great capacity for dilatation and constriction to regulate the supply of blood and oxygen under varying physiological conditions. Because the vessels are somewhat compressed by contraction of the myocardium during systole, most of the flow is believed to take place during diastole.

In older individuals, the coronary arteries are especially vulnerable to *atherosclerosis.* Subintimal collections of cells and lipid lead to the formation of *atherosclerotic plaques* that reduce the cross-sectional area of the epicardial coronary arteries. When this process progresses to the point that flow is insufficient to enable their small branches to respond to increased demands for oxygen, the patient may experience attacks of angina. Further narrowing may result in ischemia of a large area of the ventricular myocardium and a fatal heart attack.

LYMPHATIC VESSELS

Most tissues and organs contain another system of endothelium-lined vessels in addition to the blood vessels. These constitute the *lymph vascular system.* The blood vessels form a closed "circulatory system" with a central pump (the heart), an outflow pathway (the arteries and capillaries), and a return pathway (the veins). The lymph vascular system, on the other hand, is a "drainage system." Its terminal branches, the *lymphatic capillaries,* end blindly and transport a clear fluid, called *lymph,* from the extracellular spaces, through successively larger *lymphatic vessels* that ultimately converge to form two *lymphatic ducts* that are confluent with the great veins at the base of the neck. Lymphatics are found in all tissues with the exceptions of the central nervous system, cartilage, bone and bone marrow, thymus, teeth, and placenta. Along the course of lymphatic vessels, there are encapsulated aggregations of lymphoid tissue called *lymph nodes* (see Chapter 15). Within these, the *afferent lymphatic vessel* breaks up into a labyrinthine system of minute channels lined by endothelium and macrophages. The lymph then emerges from the node in *efferent lymphatic vessels.* Exposed to a very large number of phagocytic cells during its passage through the lymph node, the lymph is cleared of any particulate matter. The only cellular elements in the lymph are lymphocytes that are added to the efferent lymph and carried back to the bloodstream.

In its composition, lymph is essentially an ultrafiltrate of the blood plasma formed by continual seepage of fluid constituents of the blood across the capillary walls and into the surrounding interstitial spaces. It consists of water, electrolytes, and 2–4% protein, depending on the site and conditions of its formation. The walls of blood capillaries are less permeable to plasma proteins than they are to water and electrolytes. Plasma proteins, therefore, maintain a significant colloid osmotic pressure in the blood. At the arterial end of the capillaries, where the hydrostatic pressure exceeds the colloid osmotic pressure of the blood, water, solutes, and some protein move across the wall of the capillaries. At the venous end, the hydrostatic pressure is lower and the colloid osmotic pressure tends to draw water, electrolytes, and products of tissue catabolism back into the blood. However, some of the fluid and much of the plasma protein that have left the blood do not return to it directly, but are drained off in the lymph and returned to the blood via the lymph vascular system. A delicate balance is thus maintained, which keeps the volume of extracellular fluid reasonably constant and conserves the small amount of plasma protein that continually escapes through the walls of the blood capillaries.

It follows from this mechanism of lymph formation that the flow of lymph will be increased by (1) an increase in blood capillary permeability, (2) an increase in hydrostatic pressure, or (3) a decrease in colloid osmotic pressure of the blood plasma. If fluid accumulates in the tissues in excess of the capacity of the lymphatic vessels to drain it away, the resulting swelling of the tissues is referred to as *edema.* The increased resistance to venous return in congestive heart failure may raise pressure in the blood capillaries, resulting in edema of the ankles. Similarly, obstruction of major lymphatic vessels of an extremity by parasites or by radical surgery may result in persistent edema.

The principal functions of the lymph vascular system are (1) to return to the blood, fluid, and plasma protein that escape from the circulation, (2) to return lymphocytes of the recirculating pool to the blood, and (3) to add to the blood immune globulins (antibodies) produced in the lymph nodes. We are concerned here only with the structure of the lymph vessels. The organization of the associated lymphoid tissue will be discussed with the immune system in Chapter 15.

LYMPHATIC CAPILLARIES

The lymphatic capillaries are far more variable in form and cross-sectional area than blood capillaries (Figs. 12–35 and 12–36). The endothelium is very thin and the edges of the cells often overlap for some distance. Throughout most of the region of overlap, there is a distinct intercellular cleft, but one or two small areas of closer adherence can usually be found along the boundary. A continuous basal lamina is usually lacking (Fig. 12–37). Extracellular bundles of 5–10-nm filaments terminate on the abluminal plasma membrane. These filaments appear to end in patches of amorphous material of low electron density resembling that which forms the basal lamina of blood capillaries. The chemical nature of these *lymphatic anchoring filaments* has not been clearly established, but they are probably very thin filaments of collagen. They extend outward to mingle with collagen bundles

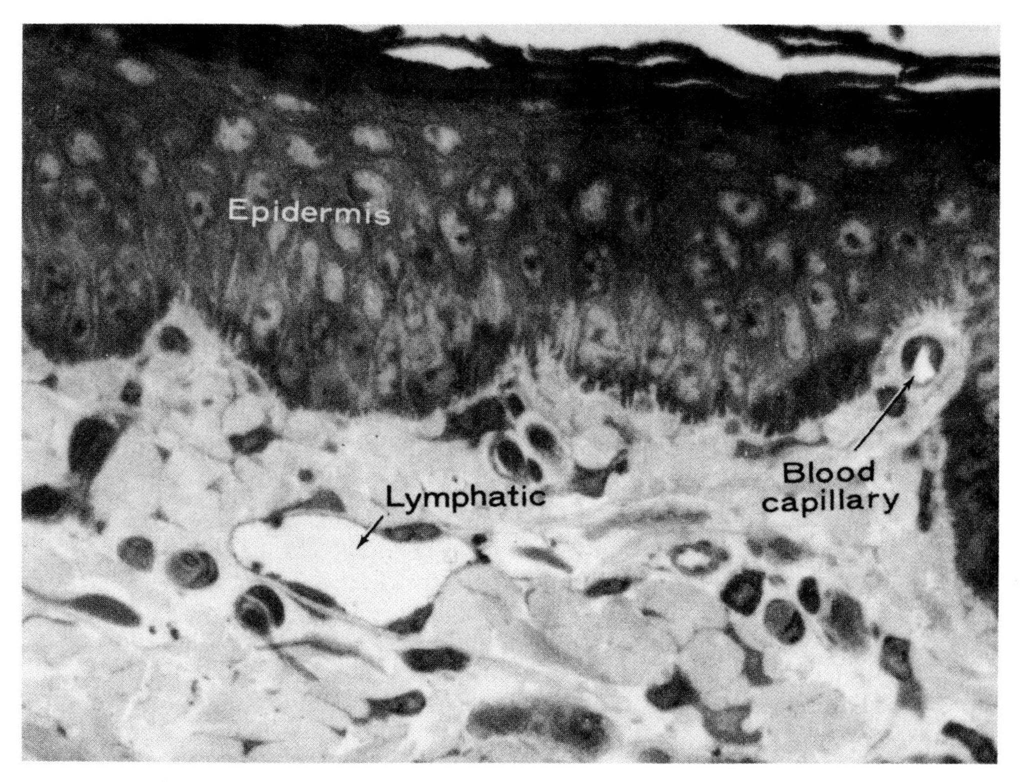

Figure 12–35. Photomicrograph of a section of guinea pig skin, showing a typical lymphatic capillary in the dermis. This can be compared to the blood capillary at the upper right. (Photomicrograph courtesy of L.V. Leak.)

in the surrounding areolar tissue. It is believed that they have a mechanical role in maintaining the patency of these very thin vessels.

The shape and arrangement of lymphatic capillaries vary greatly from region to region. In the skin and mucous membranes, lymphatics form a plexus of more-or-less cylindrical vessels that are generally parallel to the network of blood capillaries but tend to be more deeply situated. In the lamina propria of the intestine, a single lymphatic capillary extends from the submucous plexus into the core of each intestinal villus and ends blindly near its tip. In the lining of the oviduct, terminal lymphatics are flattened sinusoids extending into each fold of mucous membrane. In the testis of rodents, lymphatics form labyrinthine peritubular sinusoids that have no consistent geometry, but conform to the shapes of the intertubular spaces which they occupy and to the contours of the perivascular clusters of Leydig cells which they surround. In larger species, including man, testicular lymphatics are not sinusoidal but occur as one or two cylindrical vessels in each intertubular space. They are usually of considerably greater diameter than the neighboring blood capillaries.

Larger lymphatics are distinguishable from blood vessels by the large size of their lumen relative to the thickness of their wall. In lymphatics with a diameter greater than 0.2 mm, some histologists describe layers corresponding to the intima, media, and adventitia of blood vessels, but the boundaries between them are indistinct and designation of these layers seems rather contrived. Outside of the endothelium, there is a thin layer of elastic fibers, then a layer of smooth muscle one or two cells thick, followed by a typical adventitia of elastic and collagenous fibers that blend with those of the surrounding connective tissue.

A characteristic feature of small and medium-sized lymphatics is the presence of valves, at rather close intervals along their length. As in veins, the valves have two leaflets on opposite sides of the lumen with their free edges pointing in the direction of lymph flow. The valve leaflets are folds of the intima consisting of back-to-back layers of endothelium with an intervening thin layer of connective

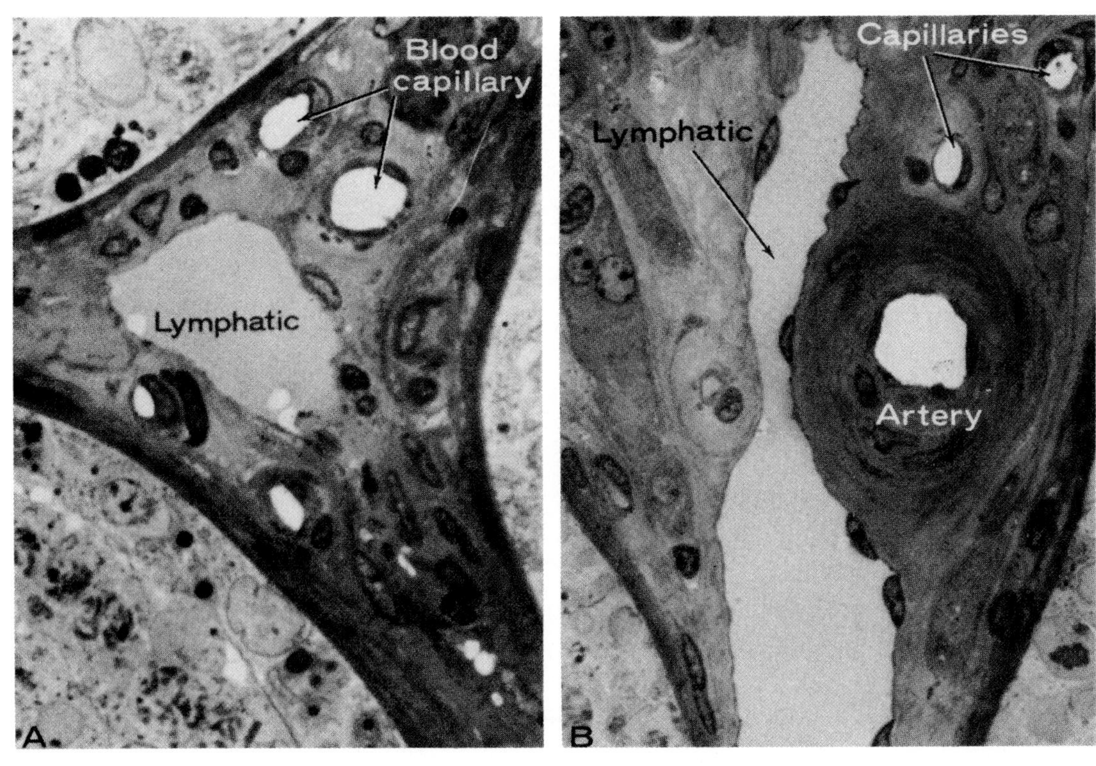

Figure 12–36. Photomicrographs of a lymphatic in the interstitial tissue of the ram testis. (A) and lymphatic in the interstitium of the bull testis (B) Both preparations were fixed by vascular perfusion. Therefore, the blood vessels are empty, whereas the lymphatics have a light gray content representing precipitated protein of the lymph. (From Fawcett, D.W., W.B. Neaves, and M.N. Flores. 1973. Biol. Reprod. 9:500.)

tissue near their base. Although not found elsewhere, a tenuous basal lamina may be found supporting the endothelium of the vessel wall at the site of valves. The wall is often slightly dilated distal to each valve. This gives intact lymphatics a distinctive beaded appearance.

Valves are essential to the function of the lymph vascular system, which has no pump comparable to the heart. The flow of lymph in the extremities is believed to depend, in large measure, on the massaging effect of movement of the surrounding tissues that results from muscle contraction. The pressure thus applied to the thin wall of lymphatics expels lymph from the segments between valves, while the valves ensure unidirectional flow. This interpretation is supported by the observation that there is little or no flow of lymph from an immobile limb of an anaesthetized animal, but if passive movements of the limb are initiated, a slow flow of lymph is reestablished.

This does not adequately explain lymph flow in organs where there is no muscle-generated movement. However, larger lymphatics are innervated and there is visual and cinematographic evidence of contraction of smooth muscle in the vessel wall. This contractile activity seems to depend on the volume of lymph produced. If this is small, the vessel walls are quiescent, but slight distension initiates rhythmic contractions at a rate of 2–3 per minute. This pulsatile activity was formerly believed to be limited to small animals in which it was first observed but it has now been demonstrated in sheep and it probably occurs in other large animals as well. Thus, there is a growing awareness that intrinsic rhythmic contraction of larger lymphatics may be a significant factor in maintenance of normal lymph flow.

LYMPHATIC DUCTS

By their confluence, the lymphatics form progressively larger vessels and these converge to form two main trunks: (1) the *right lymphatic duct,* which is relatively short and

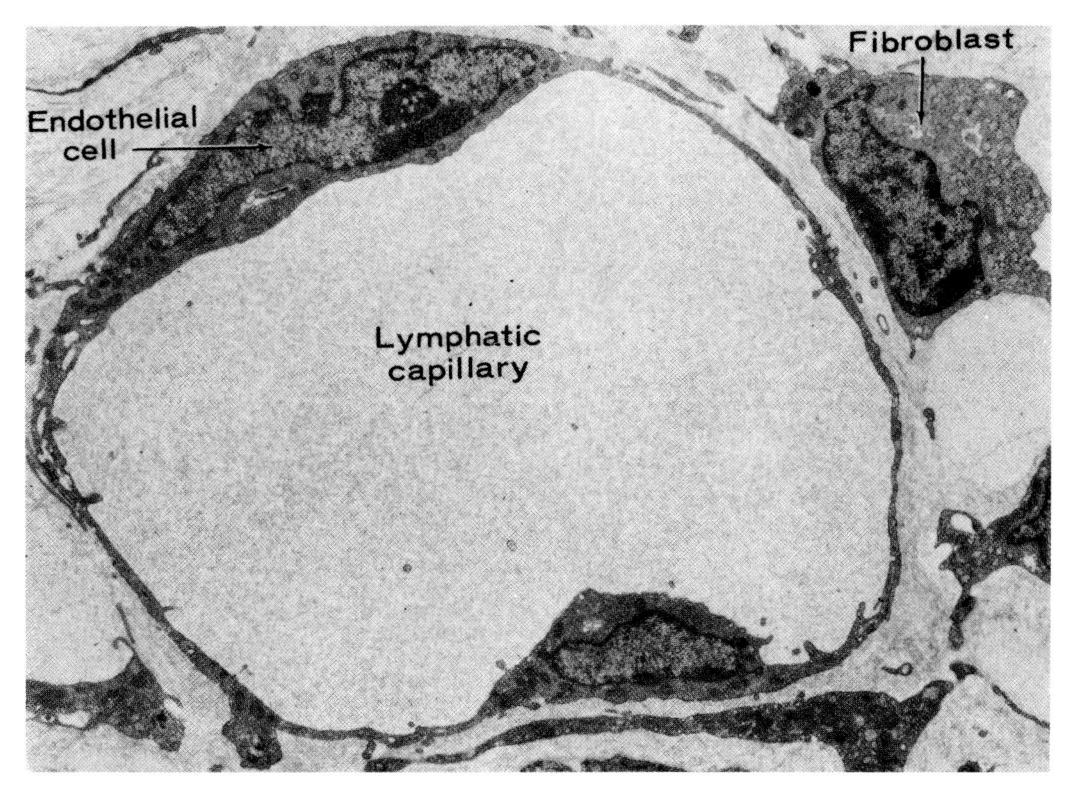

Figure 12–37. Electron micrograph of a subcutaneous lymphatic capillary from guinea pig. Note its irregular outline, thin wall, and the slight variations in thickness of the endothelium. The absence of a basal lamina cannot be verified at this magnification. (Micrograph courtesy of L.V. Leak.)

opens into the right brachiocephalic vein at the junction of the internal jugular and subclavian veins. It carries lymph drainage from the right upper portion of the body; and (2) the *thoracic duct* which arises in the abdomen and courses upward along the anterior aspect of the vertebral column, through the thorax and into the base of the neck, where it joins the venous system at the junction of the left jugular and subclavian veins.

The wall of the lymphatic ducts differs from that of veins in less distinct demarcations of the three layers and a somewhat greater development of smooth muscle in a tunica media. The tunica intima consists of the endothelium and several thin layers of elastic and collagenous fibers. Near the junction of the intima and media, the elastic fibers condense into a layer similar to the internal elastic lamina of blood vessels. Elastic fibers extend outward among the smooth muscle cells of the media. The tunica adventitia contains longitudinally oriented smooth muscle and collagenous fibers that gradually merge with the surrounding loose connective tissue. The wall of the thoracic duct is provided with small blood vessels in the adventitia that extend inward to the outer portion of the tunica media. These vessels correspond to the vase vasorum of large blood vessels.

BIBLIOGRAPHY

BLOOD VESSELS, GENERAL

Brightman, M.W. and T.S. Reese. 1969. Junctions between intimately apposed membranes in the vertebrate brain. J. Cell Biol. 40:648.

Burton, A.D. 1954. Relation of structure to function of the tissues of the wall of blood vessels. Physiol. Rev. 34:619.

Rhodin, J.A.G. 1962. Fine structure of the vascular wall in mammals. Physiol. Rev. 42 (Supp. 5):48.

Rhodin, J.A.G. 1980. Architecture of the vessel wall. 1962. *In* D.F. Bohr et al., eds. Handbook of Physiology. The Cardiovascular System, p. 1. Bethesda, MD, American Physiology Society.

ARTERIES AND ARTERIOLES

Fujiwara, T. and T. Uehara. 1982. Scanning electron microscopical study of vascular smooth muscle cells in mesenteric vessels of the monkey. Biomed. Res. 3:649.

Movat, H.Z. and N.V.P. Fernando. 1963. The fine structure of the terminal vascular bed. I. Small arteries with an internal elastic lamina. Exp. Mol. Pathol. 2:549.

Palmer, R.M., D.S. Ashton, and S. Moncada. 1988. Vascular endothelial cells synthesize nitric oxide from L-arginine. Nature 333:664.

Rhodin, J.A.G. 1967. The ultrastructure of mammalian arterioles and precapillary sphincters. J. Ultrastr. Res. 18:181.

Ross, R. and J.A. Glomset. 1976. The pathogenesis of atherosclerosis. Parts I and II. N. Engl. J. Med. 259:369, 420.

Simionescu, M., N. Simionescu, and G.E. Palade. 1976. Segmental differentiations of cell junctions in the vascular endothelium. Arteries and Veins. J. Cell Biol. 68:705.

Somlyo, A.P. and A.V. Somlyo. 1968. Vascular smooth muscle, I. Normal structure, pathology, biochemistry, and biophysics. Pharmacol. Rev. 20:197.

Uehara, Y., T. Fujiwara, and T. Kaidoh. 1990. Morphology of vascular smooth muscle fibers and pericytes: Scanning electron microscopic studies. P.M. Motta, ed. *In* Ultrastructure of Smooth Muscle. Boston, Kluwer Academic Publishers.

Vanhoutte, P.M., G.M. Rubanyi, V.M. Miller, and D.S. Houston. 1986. Modulation of vascular smooth muscle contraction by the endothelium. Annu. Rev. Physiol. 48:307.

Weibel, E.R. and G.E. Palade. 1964. New cytoplasmic components in arterial endothelia. J. Cell Biol. 23:101.

CAROTID BODY

Adamsa, W.E. 1958. The Comparative Morphology of the Carotid Body and Carotid Sinus. Springfield, IL, Charles C Thomas.

Biscoe, T.J. 1971. Carotid body: Structure and function. Physiol. Rev. 51:437.

Boyd, J.D. 1939. The development of the human carotid body. Carnegie Contrib. Embryol. 152:1.

Chen, I.L. and R. Yates. 1969. Electron microscopic radioautographic studies of the carotid body following injections of labeled biogenic amine precursors. J. Cell Biol. 42:794.

De Kock, L.L. 1959. The carotid body system of the higher vertebrates. Acta Anat. 37:265.

Duncen, D. and R. Yates. 1967. Ultrastructure of the carotid body of the cat as revealed by various fixatives and the use of reserpine. Anat. Rec. 157:667.

Eyzaguirre, C. and S.J. Fidone. 1980. Transduction mechanisms in the carotid body: glomus cells, putative neurotransmitters, and nerve endings. Am. J. Physiol. (Cell Physiol.) 8:C135.

McDonald, D.M. 1981. Peripheral chemoreceptors: structure–function relationships of the carotid body. *In* Regulation of Breathing. Part I. T.F. Hornbein ed. New York, Marcel Dekker, Inc.

Verna, A. 1979. Ultrastructure of the carotid body in mammals. Internat. Rev. Cytol. 60:271.

Yates, R.D., I. Li-Chen, and D. Duncen. 1970. Effects of sinus nerve stimulation on carotid body glomus cells. J. Cell Biol. 46:544.

ARTERIOVENOUS ANASTOMOSES

Bryden, M.M. and G.S. Molyneux. 1978. Arteriovenous ansastomoses in the skin of seals II. California sealion and the northern fur seal. Anat. Rec. 191:253.

Cauna, N. 1970. The fine structure of the arteriovenous anastomosis and its nerve supply in the human nasal respiratory mucosa. Anat. Rec. 168:9.

Hales, J.R., A. Fawcett, J.W. Bennett, and A.D. Needham. 1978. Thermal control of blood flow through capillaries and arteriovenous anastomoses in the skin of sheep. Pfluger's Arch. 378:55.

CAPILLARIES AND PERICYTES

Bearer, E.L. and L. Orci. 1985. Endothelial fenestral diaphragms: A quick-freeze, deep etch study. J. Cell Biol. 100:418.

Bennett, H.S., J.G.H. Luft, and J.C. Hampton. 1959. Morphological classification of vertebrate capillaries. Am. J. Physiol. 196:381.

Bruno, R.R. and G.E. Palade. 1968. Studies on blood capillaries I. General organization of muscle capillaries. J. Cell Biol. 37:244.

Bundegaard, M. 1984. The three dimensional organization of tight junctions in a capillary endothelium, revealed by serial section electron microscopy. J. Ultrastr. Res. 88:1.

Ghitescu, L.A., M. Fixman, M. Simionescu, and N. Simionescu. 1986. Specific binding sites for albumen restricted to plasmalemmal vesicles of continuous capillary endothelium: Receptor mediated transcytosis. J. Cell Biol. 102:1304.

Herman, I.M. and P.A. D'Amore. 1985. Microvascular pericytes contain muscle and non-muscle actins. J. Cell Biol. 101:43.

Joyce, N.C., M.F. Haire, and G.E. Palade. 1985. Contractile proteins in pericytes. I. Immunolocalization of tropomyosin. J. Cell Biol. 100:1376.

Joyce, N.C., M.F. Haire, and G.E. Palade. 1985. Contractile proteins of pericytes. II. Immunocytochemical evidence of two isomyosins in graded concentrations. J. Cell Biol. 100:1387.

Maul, G.G. 1971. Structure and formation of pores in fenestrated capillaries. J. Ultrastr. Res. 36:768.

Palade, G.E. 1960. Transport in quanta across the endothelium of blood capillaries. Anat. Rec. 136:254.

Palade, G.E., M. Simionescu, and N. Simionescu. 1979. Structural aspects of the permeability of the microvascular ensdothelium. Acta Physiol. Scand. (Suppl.) 463:11.

Simionescu, N. 1983. Cellular aspects of transcapillary exchange. Physiol. Rev. 63:1536.

Simms, D.E. 1986. The pericyte—a review. Tissue Cell 18:153.

Wagner, D.D., J.B. Olmsted, and V.J. Marder. 1982. Immunolocalization of von Willebrand protein in Weibel–Palade bodies of human endothelial cells. J. Cell Biol. 95:355.

Zimmerman, G.A., S.M. Prescott, and T.M. McIntyre. 1992. Endotheliel cell interactions with granulocytes: tethering and signaling molecules. Immunology Today 13:93.

BLOOD-BRAIN, BLOOD-OCULAR, AND BLOOD-THYMUS BARRIERS

Betz, A.L. 1985. Epithelial properties of brain capillary endothelium. Fed. Proc. 44:2614.

Brightman, M.W. 1977. Morphology of blood-brain interfaces. Exp. Eye Res. 25 (Suppl.): 1.

Crerr, H.F. 1971. Physiology of the choroid plexus. Physiol. Rev. 51:273.

Dobbing, J. 1961. The blood-brain barrier. Physiol. Rev. 41:130.

Rapoport, S.I. 1976. Blood-brain Barrier in Physiology and Medicine. New York, Raven Press.

Raviola, E. and M.J. Karnovsky. 1972. Evidence for a blood–thymus barrier using electron-opaque tracers. J. Exp. Med. 136:466.
Reese, T.G. and M.J. Karnovsky. 1967. Fine structural localization of the blood-brain barrier for exogenous peroxidase. J. Cell Biol. 34:207.

VENULES AND VEINS

Majno, G., G.E. Palade, and G. Schoeffl. 1961. Studies on inflammation. II. The site of action of histamine and serotonin along the vascular tree. J. Biophys. Biochem. Cytol. 11:607.
Movat, H.C. and N.V.P. Pernando. 1964. Fine structure of the terminal vascular bed. IV. Venules and their perivascular cells. Exp. Mol. Pathol. 3:98.
Rhodin, J.A.G. 1968. Ultrastructure of mammalian venous capillaries, venules and small collecting venules. J. Ultrastr. Res. 25:452.
Simionescu, N., M. Simionescu, and G.E. Palade. 1978. Open junctions in the endothelium of post-capillary venules of the diaphragm. J. Cell Biol. 79:27.

HEART

Cantin, M. and G. Genest. 1985. The heart and the atrial natriuretic factor. Endocr. Rev. 6:107.
Forssmann, W.G. 1986. Cardiac hormones I: Review on morphology, biochemistry, and molecular biology of the endocrine heart. Eur. J. Clin. Invest. 16:1.

LYMPHATIC VESSELS

Drinker, C.K. and J.M. Yoffey. 1941. Lymphatics, Lymph, and Lymphoid Tissue. Cambridge, MA, Harvard University Press.
Leak, L.V. 1972. Normal anatomy of the lymphatic vascular system. *In* H. Messen ed. Handbuch der Algemeine Pathologie. Berlin, Springer-Verlag.
Leak, L.V. 1970. Electron microscopic observations on lymphatic capillaries and structural components of the connective tissue interface. Microvasc. Res. 2:361.

ANGIOGENESIS

Fett, J.W., D.J. Strydom, R.R. Lobb, E.M. Alderman, J.L. Bethune, J.F. Riordan, and B.L. Vallee. 1985. Isolation and characterization of angiogenin, an angiogenic protein from human carcinoma cells. Biochemistry 24:5480.
Folkman, J. 1985. Toward an understanding of angiogenesis: search and discovery. Perspectives Biol. Med. 29:10.

13
THE IMMUNE SYSTEM

Elio Raviola

The *immune system* includes the bone marrow, thymus, spleen, and lymph nodes; aggregations of lymphocytes found in the lungs and the mucosa of the intestinal tract; lymphocytes in the blood and lymph; and lymphocytes and plasma cells that are widely distributed in the connective tissues throughout the body. The collective function of this heterogeneous group of cells and organs is to protect the organism against the potentially harmful effects of invasion by exogenous macromolecules, whether these enter the body as such, or as components of viruses, bacteria, or protozoa. This is accomplished by cellular and humoral defense mechanisms that together constitute an *immune response.*

The molecular constituents of organisms of different species, and of members of the same species, differ sufficiently to give each individual a unique biochemical identity. Fundamental to the ability to mount an immune response is the ability to distinguish *self* from *non-self.* The cellular elements of the immune system that possess this ability are two kinds of lymphocytes. Some lymphocytes have immunoglobulin molecules on their surface that serve as receptors binding *antigen,* which is any substance recognized as foreign. Antigen binding stimulates proliferation of this kind of lymphocyte and their synthesis and release of *antibodies,* immunoglobulin molecules identical to those on their surface. These combine with antigenic surface components of pathogenic microorganisms, initiating their destruction. This train of events, involving the production of specific antibodies, is called a *humoral immune response.* Other lymphocytes do not produce antibodies but have on their surface immunoglobulin-like receptors that enable them to bind directly to virus-infected cells or other foreign cells and to kill them by secreting cytotoxic agents. They also secrete signaling molecules (*interleukins*) that regulate the immune response or mobilize and activate macrophages and granulocytes to help in elimination of the invader. To distinguish it from the humoral response, this direct cell-to-cell mechanism for destruction of antigen-bearing cells is called a *cell-mediated immune response.*

How lymphocytes recognize foreign molecules long puzzled immunologists. The answer was found in studies of their surface immunoglobulins that serve as receptors. There are several classes, designated *immunoglobulin-M* (IgM), *immunoglobulin-D* (IgD), *immunoglobulin-G* (IgG), *immunoglobulin-A* (IgA), and *immunoglobulin-E* (IgE). Of these, IgG is the most abundant form in the globulin fraction of blood plasma. It has a high affinity for *antigen determinants,* the part of the molecule recognized by antibody, and it is very effective in establishing humoral immunity. It has a molecular weight of about 150,000 and consists of four polypeptide chains so arranged that each half of the molecule is made up of one long heavy chain (*H-chain*) and one shorter light chain (*L-chain*), bound together by disulfide bonds. The longer chains have a flexible hinge-region near their middle and the upper halves of the two H-chains and their associated L-chains diverge, giving the molecule a Y-shape. The enzyme papain cleaves the molecule into three parts: two *Fab fragments,* corresponding to the arms of the Y, with each consisting of an L-chain and half of an H-chain; and one *Fc fragment,* representing the stem of the Y, and consisting of two half H-chains (Fig. 13–1). The binding sites for antigen are confined to the Fab fragments, whereas the Fc fragment has a binding site for *complement,* a group of plasma proteins that can produce a cascade of enzymatic reactions leading to lysis of foreign cells. Immunoglobulin molecules are not all the same in the sequence of amino acids within the H- and L-chains of their Fab fragments. There are constant and variable regions within these chains. The variable regions of H- and L-chains are bound

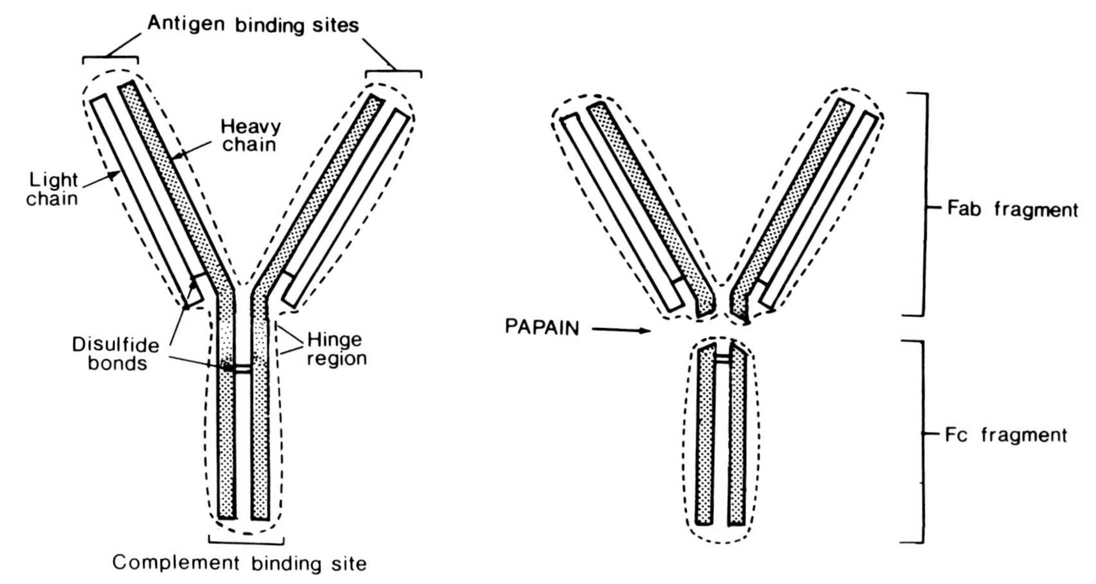

Figure 13–1. (A) Diagram of the structure of a monomeric immunoglobulin molecule. It is made up of two longer heavy chains and two shorter light chains in a Y-shaped configuration, with a complement binding region at the stem end and antigen-binding regions at the ends of the arms. (B) Treatment with papain cleaves the molecule into two Fab fragments that bind antibody and one fragment that binds complement.

together to form an *antigen-binding site.* On any given lymphocyte, the IgG molecules are all identical but will differ from those on another lymphocyte in the amino-acid sequence of the variable regions. Advances in molecular biology have revealed that the constant regions of the H- and L-chains are products of a single gene, but the variable regions are coded by multiple gene segments. A relatively small number of gene segments can be recombined in hundreds of thousands of different ways. This accounts for the great diversity of antigen-binding specificities within the lymphocyte population. The ability of the body to mount an immune response to an antigen, to which it has not previously been exposed, is due to the fact that one or more of its myriad lymphocytes is likely to have an amino-acid sequence complementary to a determinant on that antigen.

Immunoglobulin-M is produced transiently by lymphocytes early in their response to antigenic challenge and it makes up only 10% of serum immunoglobulin. It is a large molecule with a molecular weight of 900,000. It is a pentamer of radially arranged monomeric immunoglobulin units joined together by disulfide bonds, and a J-protein that evidently serves to hold the circle of monomers together. IgM is the immunoglobulin first expressed in the embryo and is present with IgD on the surface of resting lymphocytes in postnatal life. It serves as receptor for antigen and transduces the signal for proliferation and secretion of antibody early in an immune response, but it is soon replaced by IgG. It is also very effective in activating *complement.* Complement is a group of blood proteins, which, when activated, cause a cascade of enzymatic reactions that result in chemotaxis, phagocytosis, and lysis of foreign cells and bacteria.

Immunoglobulin-A (IgA) constitutes about 20% of the serum immunoglobulin. It has a molecular weight of about 160,000 and occurs either as a monomer or as a dimer joined by J-protein. In addition to its presence in blood, IgA occurs in glandular secretions such as milk, tears, saliva, and mucus. In these fluids, it is a dimer with an additional *secretory component* that is added as the molecule passes through the epithelial cells of glands and those lining the intestinal tract. It is believed to play a role in protecting the intestinal epithelium from the bacterial flora in the lumen. Although found in relatively low concentration in the blood, its presence in these extravascular sites make it the most abundant immunoglobulin in the body.

Immunoglobulin-D is present in very low concentration in the serum and has a molecular weight of about 180,000. It occurs with IgM on the surface of mature resting lymphocytes that have not yet been challenged by antigen. It has been difficult to study owing to its low concentration in blood. Its function in the immune response is not well understood.

Immunoglobulin-E (IgE) has a molecular weight of 72,000 and occurs in the serum in only trace amounts. It does not play a significant role in the response to invasion of the body by pathogenic microorganisms, but it is involved in some forms of *allergic reactions.* Its Fc portion binds firmly to mast cells of the connective tissue. Subsequent interaction of the bound IgE with an allergen causes the mast cells to degranulate, liberating histamine and other active molecules that are responsible for the clinical symptoms associated with allergy.

Lymphocytes arise from stem cells in the bone marrow that divide to give rise to an expanding population of uncommitted *lymphocyte precursors.* In birds, some of these are carried in the blood to an appendix-like diverticulum of the cloaca, called the *bursa of Fabricius.* There they proliferate and differentiate into cells capable of responding to antigen and producing antibodies. These cells are designated *bursa-dependent lymphocytes* or *B-lymphocytes.* In mammals, which have no bursa of Fabricius, lymphocyte precursors do not seem to require a special extramedullary environment to continue their development into B-lymphocytes. They are believed to complete their differentiation in the bone marrow. In both mammals and birds, other lymphocyte precursors are carried in the blood from the bone marrow to the thymus, where soluble factors produced by stromal cells induce their differentiation into *T-lymphocytes,* which are capable of binding antigen and causing lysis of foreign cells. There are several kinds of T-lymphocytes, but the principal categories are *cytotoxic T-lymphocytes,* which are the effector cells of cell-mediated immune responses, and *helper T-lymphocytes,* which participate in both humoral and cell-mediated responses. The various kinds of T-lymphocytes cannot be distinguished under the microscope, but they can be identified by monoclonal antibodies to specific surface molecules.

Because lymphocytes, programmed to participate in cell-mediated immune responses, originate in the bone marrow and thymus, these are called *primary lymphoid organs.* From there, they are carried in the blood to *secondary lymphoid organs* such as the spleen, lymph nodes, and tonsils, where the B- and T-lymphocytes tend to be segregated in discrete areas. There they proliferate and interact with antigen, macrophages, and dendritic cells, and subsequently enter the blood and lymph to be disseminated throughout the connective tissues of the body.

CYTOLOGY OF THE CELLS OF THE IMMUNE SYSTEM

LYMPHOCYTES

Lymphocytes have already been considered as cellular elements of the blood (Chapter 4) and of the connective tissues (Chapter 5), but those descriptions need review and amplification in the context of the immune system. As previously stated, the lymphocytes are not a uniform population of cells, but a family of cell types generally characterized by a round, centrally placed nucleus, a cytoplasm usually lacking specific granules and displaying varying degrees of basophilia (Figs. 13–2 and 13–3A). Although they are morphologically similar, lymphocytes are physiologically heterogeneous. Within the two major classes, B- and T-lymphocytes, individual lymphocytes have the ability to recognize different antigens and they may vary considerably in their function, life span, sensitivity to ionic radiation, and to hormones. In addition to those circulating in the blood and residing in the connective tissues, lymphocytes make up the bulk of the thymus, lymph nodes, and spleen and of localized masses of lymphoid tissue associated with the mucosa of the digestive, respiratory, and urinary tracts.

When suspended in a fluid medium, lymphocytes are round, but when crowded together in lymphoid tissues, they may be mutually deformed into polyhedral shapes. In the tissues, motile lymphocytes exhibit a slow amoeboid progression and may conform to the shape of the interstices through which they are advancing. When moving on a solid flat substrate in vitro, they take on a characteristic hand-mirror shape with their nucleus ahead, followed by a short tail consisting of the bulk of the cytoplasm and its organelles.

Lymphocytes vary in size in different organs and in different phases of their functional activity. Those in the blood usually have a diameter of 4–8 μm, but when spread on a slide in dried blood smears, their diameter increases to 7–10 μm. In lymphoid organs and tissues not involved in an acute inflammatory

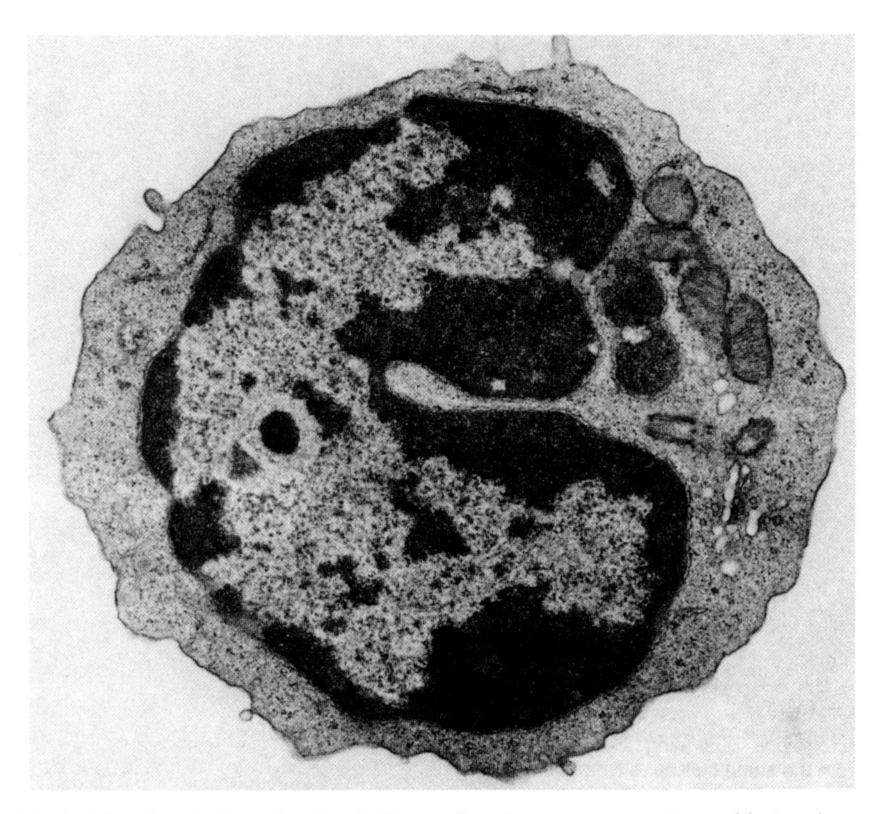

Figure 13–2. A typical lymphocyte from the blood. The nucleus has a coarse pattern of heterochromatin. A pair of centrioles and a small Golgi complex are located in or near a slight concavity in the nucleus.

reaction, lymphocytes range from 4 to 11 μm in diameter, but the larger ones are relatively few. For descriptive purposes, histologists commonly divide them into *small* (4–7 μm), *medium* (7–11 μm), and *large lymphocytes* (11–15 μm) on the basis of their size, nuclear characteristics, and the intensity of their cytoplasmic basophilia, but such a subdivision is quite arbitrary because these features vary without discernible discontinuity. In this classification, the lymphocytes of the blood are exclusively small and medium-sized. Those of the lymph include a variable proportion of large lymphocytes. The lymphoid organs contain the whole range of cell sizes. Upon stimulation by antigen, cells arise in these sites that are 25 μm or more in diameter (Fig. 13-B). These are called *lymphoblasts* and there is good evidence that these very large cells arise by transformation of small lymphocytes and that they can, in turn, divide to generate greater numbers of small and medium-sized lymphocytes.

Small lymphocytes have a densely staining nucleus surrounded by a thin rim of cytoplasm. The nucleus is central and round or slightly indented on the side toward the cytoplasm and has coarse peripheral clumps of heterochromatin and a barely discernible nucleolus. The cytoplasm is basophilic and when stained by the Giemsa method, it contains a few small azurophilic granules. In electron micrographs, a diplosome is located adjacent to the nuclear indentation where it is surrounded by a small Golgi complex and a few mitochondria. Free ribosomes are scattered throughout the cytoplasm as single units. Cisternae of endoplasmic reticulum are lacking. There are usually a few small dense lysosomes that correspond to the azurophilic granules seen with the light microscope. Medium-sized lymphocytes have a somewhat larger nucleus with more abundant euchromatin, a prominent nucleolus, and a more basophilic cytoplasm. In large lymphocytes and lymphoblasts, the large relatively pale nucleus is largely euchromatic and contains one or two prominent, loosely organized nucleoli (Fig. 13–3B). The cytoplasm is relatively abundant and intensely basophilic owing to the presence of numerous free polyribosomes. The Golgi complex is larger and the mitochondria and lysosomes somewhat more numerous than in

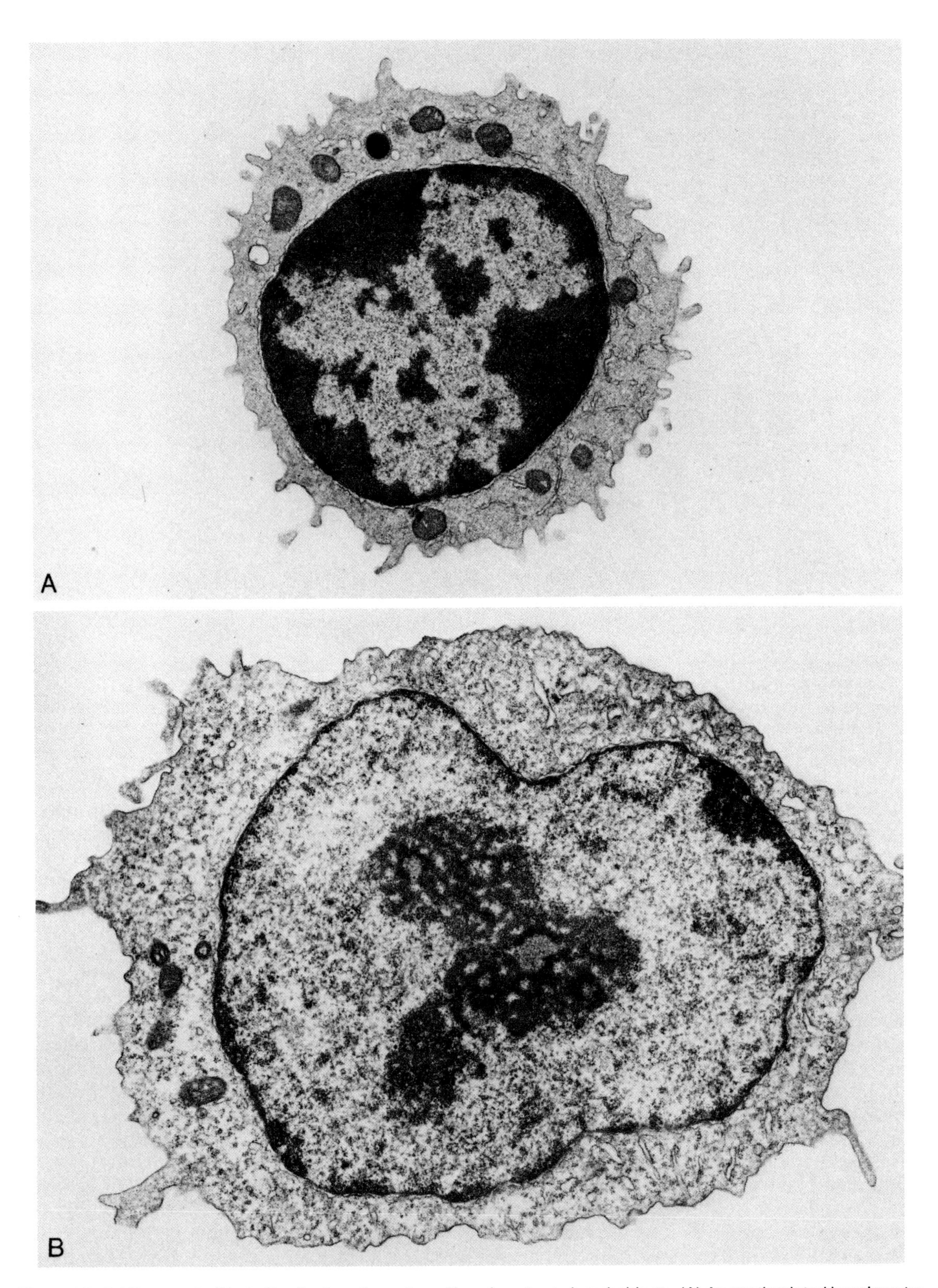

Figure 13–3. Micrographs illustrating the transformation of lymphocytes to lymphoblasts. (A) An unstimulated lymphocyte; (B) a lymphoblast from the same culture, 36 h after transformation induced by treatment with the lectin concanavalin-A. The micrographs are at the same magnification and show the great increase in cell volume and the development of a euchromatic nucleus with a very prominent nucleolus. Lectin-induced transformation is similar to that which occurs in response to antigenic stimulation.

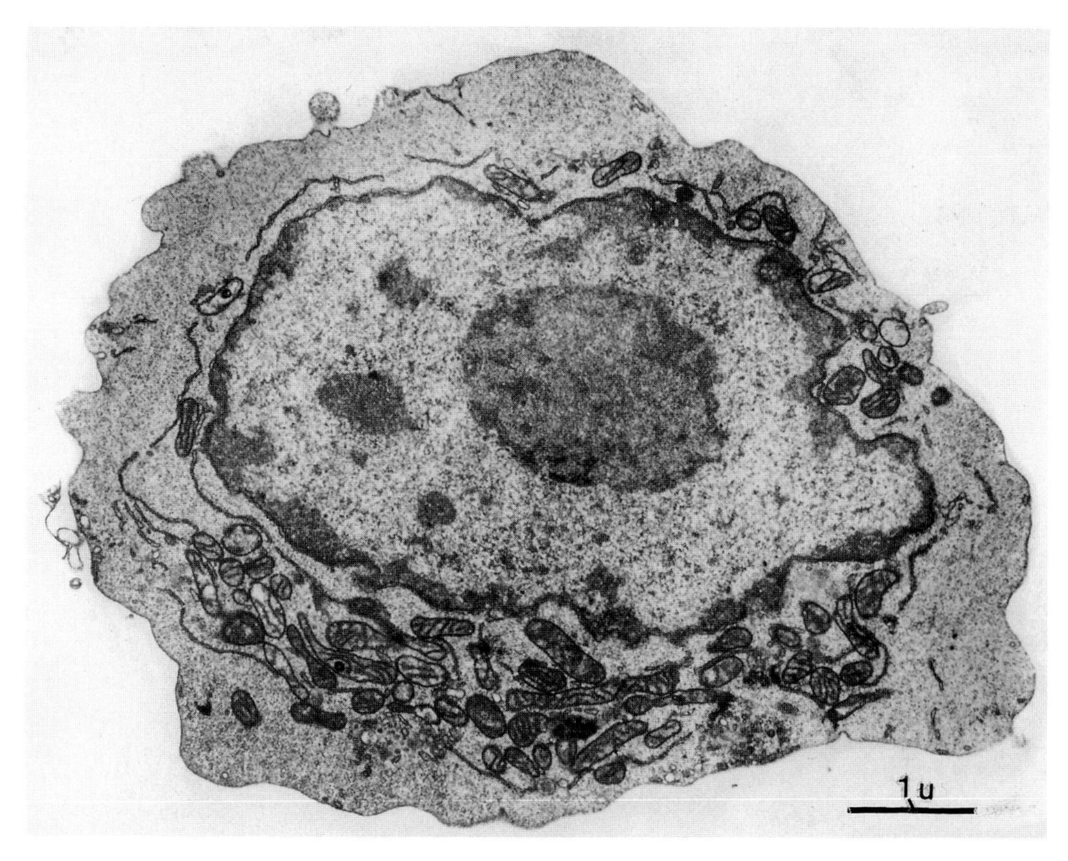

Figure 13–4. Electron micrograph of a lymphoblast showing the large nucleolus, numerous mitochondria, and a few short profiles of endoplasmic reticulum.

smaller lymphocytes. Cisternae of rough endoplasmic reticulum are uncommon in large lymphocytes but may occasionally be observed in lymphoblasts (Fig. 13–4).

PLASMA CELLS

Plasma cells represent a late stage in the differentiation of B-lymphocytes. Their function is to synthesize and release antibody. They are found in the medullary cords of the lymph nodes, in the marginal zone and cords of the spleen, and scattered through the connective tissues of the body. They are also especially numerous in the lamina propria of the intestinal mucosa where most of them secrete IgA instead of IgG. During the acute phase of a humoral immune response, large numbers of relatively small immature plasma cells appear in the deep portion of the cortex of lymph nodes and at the boundary between the white and red pulp of the spleen. Mature plasma cells are sessile elements that apparently never enter the blood and lymph. However, after an antigenic challenge, immature forms do appear in the lymph. Moreover, under these conditions, a limited number of cells may be found in the blood that appear with the light microscope, to be lymphocytes but which, in electron micrographs, display the extensive rough endoplasmic reticulum typical of plasma cells (Fig. 13–5). These are evidently cells in transition from B-lymphocytes to plasma cells.

Fully differentiated plasma cells are 8–20 μm in diameter and have a round or ovoid shape. They have a spherical, eccentrically placed nucleus with a small nucleolus and coarse masses of heterochromatin arranged radially in a cartwheel-like configuration. The cytoplasm is much more abundant than in lymphocytes and is strongly basophilic except for a conspicuous juxtanuclear pale area that contains the diplosome and surrounding Golgi complex. In electron micrographs, it is evident that the intense basophilia of plasma cells is due to their content of many parallel cisternae of rough endoplasmic reticulum. With immunocytochemical methods, the con-

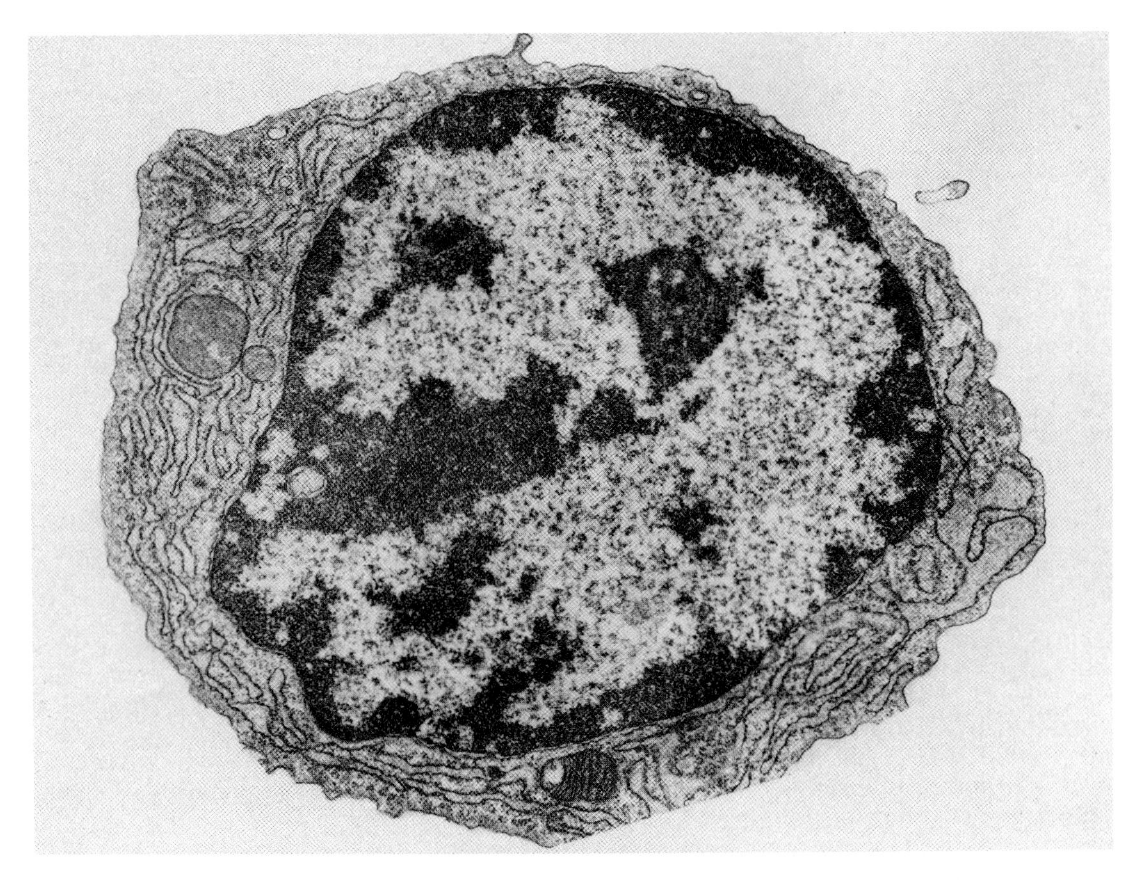

Figure 13–5. A rare immature plasma cell from peripheral blood. The cell has developed an extensive rough endoplasmic reticulum. At its destination in the tissues, its pattern of chromatin would become coarser, the cytoplasm would increase in volume, and the reticulum would become ordered into closely spaced parallel arrays of cisternae. For an illustration of a mature plasma cell, see Fig. 5–25.

tent of these cisternae can be shown to consist largely of antibody. Synthesis of the light and heavy chains of the immunoglobulin molecules takes place on polyribosomes associated with the cisternae and the chains undergo covalent interchain linkage in the lumen. Glycosylation begins in the reticulum and is completed in the Golgi. The antibody so formed is transported to the cell surface in small vesicles. With the light microscope, dense bodies 2–3 μm in diameter were occasionally observed in the cytoplasm of plasma cells and were called *Russell bodies*. These have been shown to be accumulations of incomplete immunoglobulin molecules within one or more cisternae of the reticulum. It is now speculated that these may be indicative of abnormal synthesis or faulty intracellular transport of antibody, but the evidence for this interpretation is inconclusive.

Antibody secreted by plasma cells into the interstitial spaces of the surrounding connective tissue ultimately reaches the blood via the lymphatics. The product of plasma cells in the spleen can be released into the blood more directly.

MACROPHAGES

Macrophages are important participants in the immune response. They have been described in some detail in Chapter 5 (Connective Tissue) and the reader is referred to that chapter to review the general features of their structure and function.

HISTOPHYSIOLOGY

SURFACE PROPERTIES OF T- AND B-LYMPHOCYTES

Owing to the fact that B- and T-lymphocytes are identical in appearance, studies of their distribution and their respective roles in the immune response have depended on ingenious immunocytochemical methods for their identification that are based on differences in the molecules expressed on their surface. In these methods, the immune response is used to make reagents that detect type-specific surface markers. Immunoglobulin from one animal species is injected into another and the anti-immunoglobulin antibodies produced in the resulting immune response are isolated and conjugated with molecules that render them visible. When conjugated with the fluorescent dye fluorescein, anti-Ig antibody complexes can be localized in tissues by using the fluorescence microscope (Fig. 13–6); or, the anti-Ig antibody can be conjugated with hemocyanin molecules which are large enough to be visible with the electron microscope (Fig. 13–7). A third alternative is to label the anti-Ig antibody with radioactive iodine. This makes it feasible to localize the bound antibody by autoradiography. Any of these methods make it possible to identify B-lymphocytes by the binding of labeled antibody to the IgM and IgD molecules on their surface. One can also use antibody and complement to demonstrate that the B-lymphocyte is the effector cell of humoral immune responses. Anti-Ig antibody injected into an animal will bind to its B-lymphocytes. A subsequent injection of complement will bind to the Fc fragment of the bound antibody and induce lysis of the B-cells. An animal deprived of its B-lymphocytes by this device is no longer able to mount a humoral immune response but can still reject a graft with a cell-mediated immune response.

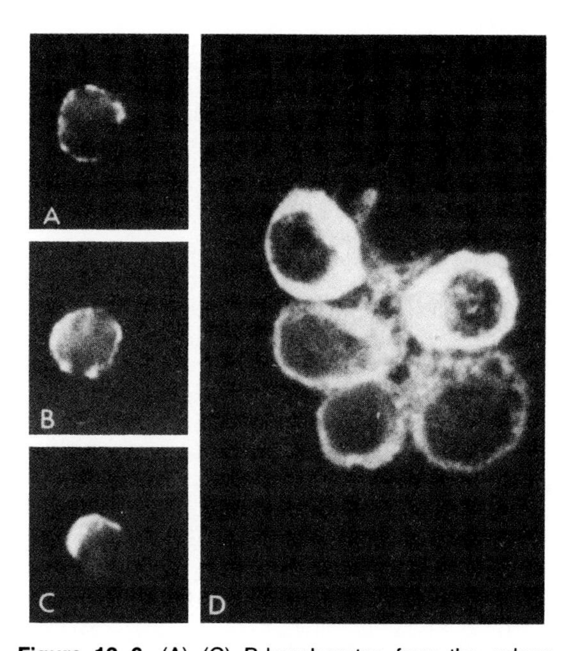

Figure 13–6. (A)–(C) B-lymphocytes from the spleen, stained with anti-immunoglobulin antibody conjugated to fluorescein isothiocyanate and photographed with the fluorescence microscope. In (A), the lymphocyte was reacted with labeled antibody at 4°C. The anti-immunoglobulin is dispersed over the entire surface. (B) and (C) Upon warming at 37°C, the fluorescent antibody becomes concentrated over one pole of the cell (capping). For comparison, (D) illustrates the intense staining of the antibody in the cytoplasm of splenic plasma cells treated with fluorescent anti-immunoglobulin. (Courtesy of E.R. Unanue.)

T-lymphocytes do not possess immunoglobulins as integral membrane proteins, but they do have *antigen-receptors* that consist of two polypeptide chains with constant and variable regions similar to those of the immunoglobulin molecules on the surface of B-lymphocytes. Some T-lymphocytes of mice also have a surface antigenic determinant, called Thy-1, which is lacking on B-cells. If such T-lymphocytes are transferred from one mouse to another that is genetically different (an *allogeneic* recipient), they elicit formation of antibodies that bind to T-cells but not to B-lymphocytes. These antibodies, appropriately labeled, can then be used to identify T-lymphocytes in tissue sections. When injected into a mouse whose T-cells bear this antigen, the antibodies will cause a specific complement-mediated lysis of its T-lymphocytes, making it possible to study the immunological impairment resulting from their elimination. As in animals lacking T-lymphocytes as a result of neonatal thymectomy, these animals are unable to respond to antigen with an immune response. If they are subsequently given an infusion of T-lymphocytes, this ability is restored. These experiments clearly demonstrate that an animal must have T-lymphocytes to mount an immunological response to antigenic challenge.

Certain properties of B-lymphocytes make it possible to separate them from mixed populations of lymphocytes. They have a lower electrophoretic mobility than T-cells and they adhere preferentially to nylon wool at 37°C in the presence of serum. They can also be passed through a column coated with monoclonal antibody to which they adhere; or, after selectively staining with a fluorochrome, they can be separated with a fluorescent-cell sorter. Differences in the reactivity of B- and T-lymphocytes to various mitogens, to X-ray irradiation, and to cortisone administration, and their differing distribution and patterns of recirculation will be discussed on later pages.

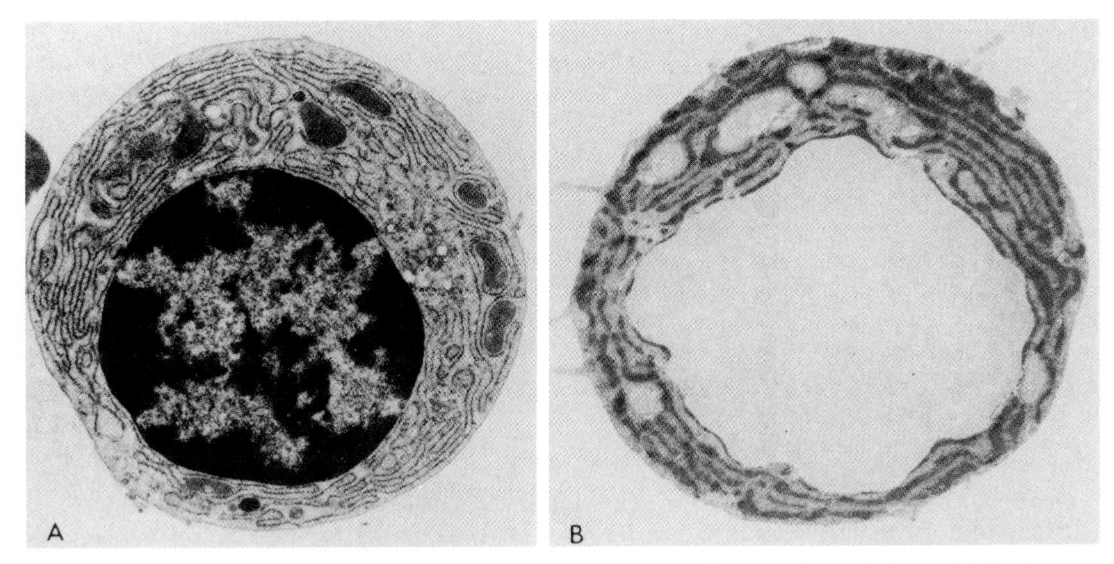

Figure 13–7. (A) Electron micrograph of a plasma cell from the rat spleen. The cytoplasm displays a highly developed rough endoplasmic reticulum. (B) Plasma cell from the spleen of a rabbit, which was injected with horseradish peroxidase, used as an antigen. (B) The spleen cells were subsequently exposed to the peroxidase antigen and stained by the histochemical reaction for demonstrating peroxidase activity. The dense reaction product is seen in the cisternae of endoplasmic reticulum, indicating the presence of anti-peroxidase antibody. (Micrograph courtesy of E.D. Leduc and S. Avrameas.)

RESPONSE OF B-LYMPHOCYTES TO ANTIGEN

Before discussing in more detail the role of B-lymphocytes in a humoral immune response, it may be useful to consider what constitutes an antigen and to define more narrowly some terms we have used heretofore rather loosely. We have stated that the function of the surface immunoglobulins on lymphocytes is *recognition* of the antigen. That portion of a large antigen molecule that is recognized by an antibody, or by a T-cell receptor, is called an *antigenic determinant.* The property of a molecule that enable it to *react* with an antibody is called its *antigenicity,* whereas the ability of the molecule to induce an immune response is called its *immunogenicity.* Most molecules are able both to bind to antibody and to induce an immune response. However, some small molecules can react with antibody but are not able to induce production of antibody. Such small molecules are called *haptens.* But when a hapten is conjugated with a larger carrier molecule and an animal is injected with the *hapten-carrier complex,* it responds by producing antibodies to both the hapten and the carrier portions of the complex. These antibodies are then able to react with the hapten alone. The hapten acts as an additional determinant on a carrier molecule that was already immunogenic.

Prior to their first encounter with an antigen, B-cells synthesize IgM and IgD immunoglobulin molecules that are incorporated in the plasma membrane to serve as antigen receptors. These may number 50,000 to 100,000 per cell and all are specific for a single antigenic determinant. In an immune response, all of the progeny of any given lymphocyte produce antibody of the same specificity, termed *monoclonal antibody.* However, because most immunogenic molecules have multiple determinants, multiple lymphocytes of differing specificities are activated by the same molecule and their proliferation of a number of clones, each reacting to a single determinant, results in the production of *polyclonal antibody.* Normal antibody producing B-lymphocytes cannot be grown in tissue cultures. To obtain monoclonal antibodies in bulk, it is necessary to fuse them with malignant myeloma cells that can proliferate indefinitely in vitro. Such *hybridomas,* combining the antibody synthesis of the B-lymphocytes and the proliferative capacity of the myeloma cells, are used in the production of monoclonal antibodies as valuable reagents for immunological research.

In addition to the stimulus provided by antigen-binding, the activation and proliferation of B-lymphocytes in an immune response requires the participation of *helper T-lymphocytes* whose receptors are believed to bind to a different determinant on the same immunogen. Their activation turns on a gene for the synthesis of the lymphokine *interleukin-2* (Il-2), which is released to stimulate the proliferation of the activated B-lymphocytes. At the same time, the helper T-lymphocytes express I1-2 receptors on their surface and respond to their own interleukin production by proliferating. Thus, the paracrine and autocrine effects of interleukin greatly amplify the immune response. The activated B-lymphocytes are initially stimulated to synthesize more IgM molecules. Some of these lack the hydrophobic region of the molecule necessary for insertion into the membrane and have, instead, a *signal sequence* that results in their release as antibody. Under the influence of helper T-cells, IgM production declines as the immune response progresses and synthesis of the more efficient IgG antibody accelerates.

Thus, under the influence of helper T-cells, small B-lymphocytes, activated by antigen, become transformed to large lymphocytes. During this process, antibody of the same specificity as the immunoglobulin deployed on the cell surface is synthesized in increasing amount and is released as a secretory product, instead of being inserted in the plasma membrane. Some of these actively secreting and proliferating large B-cells develop a larger Golgi complex and a few cisternae of endoplasmic reticulum, becoming transitional elements in the differentiation of plasma cells. Some of these cells may enter the lymph of the node draining the site of antigen entry and colonize other lymph nodes in the same path of lymph drainage. Others may enter the blood for distribution throughout the body. As their differentiation progresses in their new locations, they become immotile, increase in size, and lose their surface immunoglobulins, while continuing to produce antibody. Compared to the plasma cells, the amount of antibody produced by lymphocytes is relatively small, but it is released at an earlier stage of the immune response at the site of antigen invasion, where it can be more effective than antibody circulating, in relatively low concentration, within the vascular system.

Some of the lymphocytes activated in the primary response engage only transiently in antibody production and revert to long-lived small *memory-cells* that retain surface immunoglobulins of the same specificity. On subsequent exposure to the same antigen, these cells initiate a secondary immune response resulting in an exponential increase in high-affinity IgG antibody, and with a shorter lag phase than in the primary response. Although it is widely believed that the memory cells arise from some of the progeny of the B-cells involved in the primary response, there is some evidence suggesting that they arise from a separate precursor population that did not participate in the primary response. This matter remains unsettled.

RESPONSE OF T-LYMPHOCYTES TO ANTIGEN

To be activated, T-lymphocytes must interact with certain *histocompatibility molecules.* These are a group of glycoproteins occurring on the surface of all cells in the body. They are encoded by a set of genes known as the *major histocompatibility complex* (MHC). These genes and their products are grouped in three classes. Class-I genes encode molecules found on *all* cells, class-II genes encode molecules expressed exclusively on cells of the immune system, and class-III encode serum proteins and components of complement. The histocompatibility molecules that are expressed on all cells differ from individual to individual and their diversity is the basis for the uniqueness of every member of the population. They constitute the antigen that is recognized by the T-lymphocytes in rejection of grafts between individuals.

The T-lymphocyte receptor consists of two chains (α and β) containing constant and variable regions. The receptor is unusual in that it must recognize both antigen and the associated histocompatibility molecules. In the differentiation of T-cells in the thymus, the gene segments for the variable region of the receptors are thought to be randomly rearranged in many different ways, resulting in a population of T-cells that express receptors with a host of different specificities. Those cells that express receptors which recognize the histocompatability molecules of that individual (self-MHC) die during their sojourn in the thymus. This elimination of the self-reactive cells results in a remaining population of mature T-cells that are able to react only with non-self, in cell-mediated immune responses.

During their differentiation, T-lymphocytes not only acquire receptors of differing specificity but they also express surface molecules that serve as markers, enabling immunologists to distinguish subpopulations that have different functions. As monoclonal antibodies were raised against differentiation markers, investigators often assigned different names to the same marker. To eliminate the resulting terminological confusion, an international conference examined over 100 monoclonal antibodies. All known antibodies that reacted with the same marker were grouped on the basis of immunofluorescence tests into what was termed a "cluster of differentiation" (CD). Previous designations were abandoned in favor of simpler designations CD-1, CD-2, CD-3, CD-4, and so on and these terms are now in general use. Two of the several subsets of lymphocytes are of special interest. Those bearing the CD-4 marker function as helper T-cells in antibody production and are, thus, involved in class-II MHC-restricted responses. Lymphocytes bearing the CD-8 marker are the cytotoxic T-cells that are the effector cells in cell-mediated responses and can only lyse foreign cells expressing class-I MHC molecules on their surface (a class-I-restricted response).

In the humoral immune response, B-lymphocytes are the effector cells, and CD-4 T-lymphocytes are helper cells. These T-cells can apparently be activated to carry out their function only by antigen presented together with class-II MHC molecules. The macrophage, which also bears class-II MHC on its surface, is the commonest *antigen-presenting cell.* Immunologists speculate that the antigen is processed intracellularly by macrophages which then incorporate an *antigen–MHC complex* in their surface, where it is recognized by CD-4 lymphocytes, leading to their activation and antibody production.

The cytotoxic T-lymphocytes contain cytoplasmic granules not observed in other subsets of lymphocytes. They recognize foreign cells as targets on the basis their class-I MHC molecules and closely bind to their membrane. The opposing membranes may even interdigitate in the area of adhesion. The Golgi complex of the lymphocyte becomes oriented toward the target cell and its cytoplasmic granules move to the surface, discharging a protein called *perforin.* Molecules of this protein become inserted in the membrane of the target cell where they form polymers that create circular pores in the membrane, permitting influx of water and ions that result in osmotic lysis of the cell. The granules also contain *lymphotoxin* and proteases that may participate in the destruction of the cell. After discharging its granules, the cytotoxic lymphocyte disengages and moves on to another target cell.

LYMPHOKINES IN THE IMMUNE RESPONSE

In recent years, we have become increasingly aware of the importance of communication between cells of the immune system accomplished by secretion of diffusable signalling molecules. In the 1970s, it was discovered that antigen-presenting macrophages also release a soluble factor, *interleukin-1* (Il-1), that activates T-lymphocytes and induces their production of a second factor, *interleukin-2* (Il-2), which stimulates proliferation and immunoglobulin production by B-lymphocytes. Release of these factors serves to amplify and sustain an immune response. More recently, interleukin-3 (Il-3), produced by T-lymphocytes, has been found to stimulate differentiation of neutrophils, macrophages, and mast cells. Three other lymphokines, distinct from Il-1 and Il-2, have been implicated in regulating B-cell growth and differentiation (Il-4, Il-5, and IL-6). These also have a wide variety of biological effects on other tissues. For example, Il-6 released by T-cells, monocytes, fibroblasts, and endothelial cells acts on the temperature-regulating center, causing the fever associated with infections; it induces the liver to produce certain proteins that bind to invading microorganisms and promote their destruction by phagocytosis; in cooperation with Il-3, it acts on the stem cells in the bone marrow to stimulate their division, increasing the output of leukocytes; and it promotes the maturation of megakaryocytes, increasing the production of platelets; Il-8, produced by monocytes and endothelial cells at sites of inflammation, enhance chemotaxis of neutrophils to combat the infecting microorganisms.

The interactions of the nine or more interleukins are quite complex and still not completely understood. There is considerable redundancy in their actions, with more than one having the same effect. One lymphokine may have diverse effects by acting on different cells and tissues. A lymphokine may induce, in its target cell, expression of receptors for a second lymphokine. A lymphokine may also have an autocrine effect acting back on the cell, producing it to increase its surface receptors for its own product. Much of what we know of the actions of these molecules has been based on assays in vitro and it is assumed that they have similar functions in vivo. In some instances, the validity of this assumption may be questionable.

Regrettably, the terminology in this field is inconsistent. Initially, when these soluble factors were thought to be produced by lymphocytes and to act on lymphocytes, the terms *interleukin,* or *lymphokine,* seemed appropriate. Later, when some of them were found to be produced also by other cell types and to have a broader range of target cells, the more general term *cytokine* was suggested. However, the term interleukin is still widely used and seems likely to persist.

ROLE OF MACROPHAGES IN THE IMMUNE RESPONSE

Macrophages are versatile participants in the body's immunological defenses. They actively eliminate antigens by phagocytosis and intracellular digestion. Their prey includes bacteria and other foreign cells whose viability has been impaired by the action of cytotoxic lymphocytes, and cells that have been lysed by binding of antibody and complement. Their efficiency increases as an immune response progresses. As the level of circulating antibody rises, invading microorganisms become coated with immunoglobulin molecules that bind to them by their Fab portion, leaving their Fc portion exposed. The antibody thus serves as an *opsonin,* that is, a molecule that binds both to a particle and to a receptor on a phagocyte, thus promoting phagocytosis. Fc receptors are normally present on the surface of macrophages and the binding of antibody-coated bacteria to them greatly increases the rate of phagocytosis. Granulocytes are also more efficient in disposing of bacteria that have been opsonized.

The role of macrophages is not limited to disposal of the invaders by phagocytosis. As mentioned earlier in this chapter, they also interact with lymphocytes in the inductive phase of the immune response. The evidence for this has come from a variety of experiments, all showing that antigens that are avidly taken up by macrophages are good immunogens, whereas those that are not phagocytosed are poor immunogens. Blockade of the body's macrophages by injection of large amounts of inert particulate matter significantly depresses a subsequently induced immune response. Moreover, if an animal is injected with an antigen that is feebly immunogenic and its macrophages are later transferred to a syngeneic recipient, the latter responds with a vigorous immune response. This clearly indicates that a small amount of an antigen, bound to the surface of a macrophage, is a much stronger immunogen than the antigen in its original free form. Perhaps the strongest evidence for an indispensible role for the macrophage has come from efforts to induce an immune response in vitro. In those experiments, mixing B-lymphocytes and helper T-lymphocytes failed to result in antibody formation, but on addition of macropages, production of antibody could be demonstrated.

The role of the macrophages in induction of an immune response has been a subject of intensive research which has led to the conclusion that they present, to T-lymphocytes, a processed fragment of the antigen, bound to class-II MHC. Recognition of this complex by receptors on the T-cells results in their activation and secretion of lymphokines that enhance antibody production by the B-lymphocytes. If this interpretation is valid, one would expect to find a very close spatial relationship between macrophages and lymphocytes at sites of antibody production. This is borne out in electron micrographs that show a close clustering of lymphocytes around macrophages both in vivo and in immune reactions induced in vitro (Fig. 13–8).

There is general agreement among immunologists that to carry out its role in helper T-lymphocyte activation, a macrophage must first bind, ingest, and process the antigen, then return a peptide fragment of it to the cell surface for presentation together with class-II MHC molecules. The evidence for this is quite compelling, but some cell biologists are puzzled by what the immunologist means by "processing" of the antigen. In phagocytosis, material is taken into the cell in a membrane-bounded endocytic vacuole. Lysosomes then fuse with the vacuole and lysosomal hydrolases completely degrade the contents to amino acids. In this process, it seems unlikely that a peptide bearing a specific antigenic determinant could be spared, conjugated with MHC molecules in the vacuole, and returned to the surface. Moreover, there is little morphological evidence for macrophages releasing partially digested material by exocytosis. Immunologists concede that they do not know just what antigen processing entails in a biochemical sense, but they believe it takes place in an acidic endocytic vacuole without the participation of lysosomes. They assume that there is another intracellular pathway for handling interiorized material that is yet to be discovered.

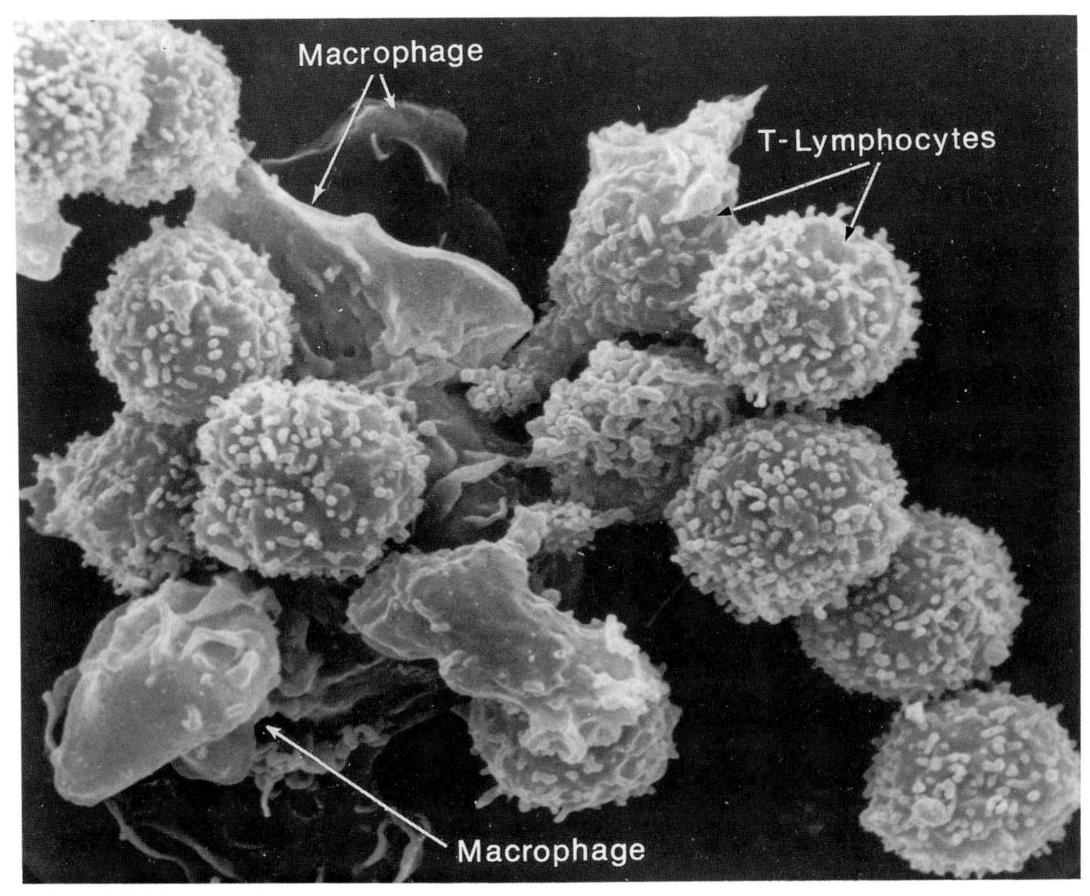

Figure 13–8. Scanning electron micrograph of T-lymphocytes closely associated with the surface of a macrophage for antigen presentation. (Micrograph courtesy of M.H. Nielsen and O. Werdelin.)

The possible existence of an alternate pathway is further suggested by the fact that cell types, other than macrophages, appear to be efficient in MHC-restricted antigen presentation, even though they are incapable of taking up particulates by phagocytosis. Among these are the *dendritic cells* that can be isolated from cell suspensions of thymus, lymph nodes, and spleen. These cells have numerous processes that may take the form of blunt pseudopodia or thin undulant veils. Their nucleus is irregular in outline, with a thin rim of heterochromatin and prominent nucleoli. The cytoplasm contains many mitochondria but few lysosomes. They possess class-II MHC on their surface and are believed to develop from bone-marrow precursors. The *follicular dendritic cells* in the germinal centers of lymph nodes and the *interdigitating cells* in thymus-dependent areas of lymph nodes and spleen have similar characteristics. The highly branched *Langerhans cells* of the epidermis are also capable of antigen presentation. They bind the Fc fragment of immunoglobulins and have some of the same surface markers as macrophages but do not appear to be active phagocytes. It is not clear whether all of these cells are a subpopulation of macrophages in some special state of differentiation, or are separate cell populations with different origins and distinctive biological properties. All seem to have a significant role in induction of immune responses.

NONSPECIFIC STIMULATION OF LYMPHOCYTES

Certain substances, other than antigen, have been found to stimulate lymphocytes, inducing their transformation into actively proliferating large lymphocytes. Whereas antigens react only with individual lymphocytes that bear receptors specific for their determinants, these agents, called *mitogens,* are effective on whole classes of lymphocytes. The mitogens include a variety of substances extracted from plants or their seeds and constituents or metabolic products of bacteria. All mitogens have the capacity to bind to chemical groupings on the plasma membrane of lymphocytes. Although some of them also bind to other cells, only lymphocytes respond by transformation and proliferation. There are other agents that bind to lymphocytes without stimulating them. Mitogens can, therefore, be regarded as belonging to a larger class of substances that share an affinity for certain chemical groups on the surface of cells. Such substances are referred to collectively as *ligands.* Mitogenic ligands have been of special interest because their mechanism of action, although nonspecific, appears to be identical to that of antigens. They have, therefore, been useful tools in studies aimed at understanding lymphocyte stimulation. Especially well studied have been certain extracts of plants that have long been known to cause agglutination of erythrocytes and lymphocytes. Agglutination by these substances, collectively called *lectins,* depends on the fact that they are multivalent ligands and, thus, form bridges between neighboring cells, resulting in the formation of cell clumps. The plant lectins are proteins or glycoproteins that have a strong affinity for oligosaccharides on the plasma membrane of mammalian cells. They can be conjugated to an electron-opaque marker, such as ferritin or hemocyanin. Using such conjugates, the distribution of the lectin-binding oligosaccharides on the cell surface can be visualized with the electron microscope.

In immunological research on experimental animals, advantage can be taken of the fact that these lectins do not stimulate all lymphocytes indiscriminately. *Phytohemagglutinin* (PHA), extracted from the red kidney bean, and *concanavalin-A* (Con-A) extracted from the jackbean, stimulate T-lymphocytes. *Pokeweed nitrogen* (PWM), extracted from the root of pokeweed, stimulates both T- and B-cells whereas a *lipopolysaccharide* (LPS), extracted from colon bacillus, is specific for B-lymphocytes. T-lymphocyte stimulation by PHA has been widely used as a means of mimicking the morphological and biochemical changes that follow the binding of antigen. The earliest event after addition of PHA to a culture of small lymphocytes (15 min) is enhanced endocytic activity (demonstrated by the uptake of the dye neutral red) and increased synthesis of RNA (15–30 min). Soon thereafter, the nucleus begins to enlarge (4 h). At 12–36 h, the nucleus becomes more euchromatic, the nucleolus becomes more loosely organized, and the cell volume increases. The cell begins DNA synthesis, entering the S-phase of the cell cycle, which lasts for 6–10 h. It then enters the G2 phase, characterized by active RNA and protein synthesis. Concomitantly, there is a striking increase in cytoplasmic polyribosomes with little increase in cisternae of rough endoplasmic reticulum. At the end of G2, which lasts for 2–4 h, the lymphocyte has undergone a fourfold increase in volume and it enters mitosis. DNA synthesis in cultures of PHA-stimulated lymphocytes reaches a peak at 72–120 h, and then slowly declines over a period of 5–7 days. Beginning at about 24 h after PHA exposure, the T-lymphocytes develop the capacity to promote the proliferation, and affect the behavior, of other cells by the secretion of lymphokines. This sequence of events, in vitro, closely parallels that occurring in T-lymphocytes after antigen-binding in vivo. The effects of lectins on B-lymphocytes is less well understood but there is some evidence that PWM stimulates their differentiation into plasma cells.

Studies employing ligands conjugated to a microscopically visible marker have cast some light on the events that immediately follow ligand-binding to the lymphocyte membrane. When anti-immunoglobulin antibody conjugated to ferritin is reacted at 4°C with a B-lymphocyte bearing that immunoglobulin, the label initially appears uniformly distributed over the cell surface. With the passage of time the marker becomes aggregated in patches. The *patching* depends on the fact that the surface immunoglobulins move randomly in the fluid domain of the membrane, and when they approach sufficiently close to one another, they are cross-linked by the multivalent anti-immunoglobulin antibody. However, if the cell suspension is warmed to 37°C, the marker molecules form a continuous cap localized in the region of the cell surface overlying the Golgi complex, a behavior called *capping* (Fig. 13–9). That portion of the membrane bearing the marker subsequently becomes interiorized by endocytosis, or the label is shed from the surface. This process leaves the B-cell de-

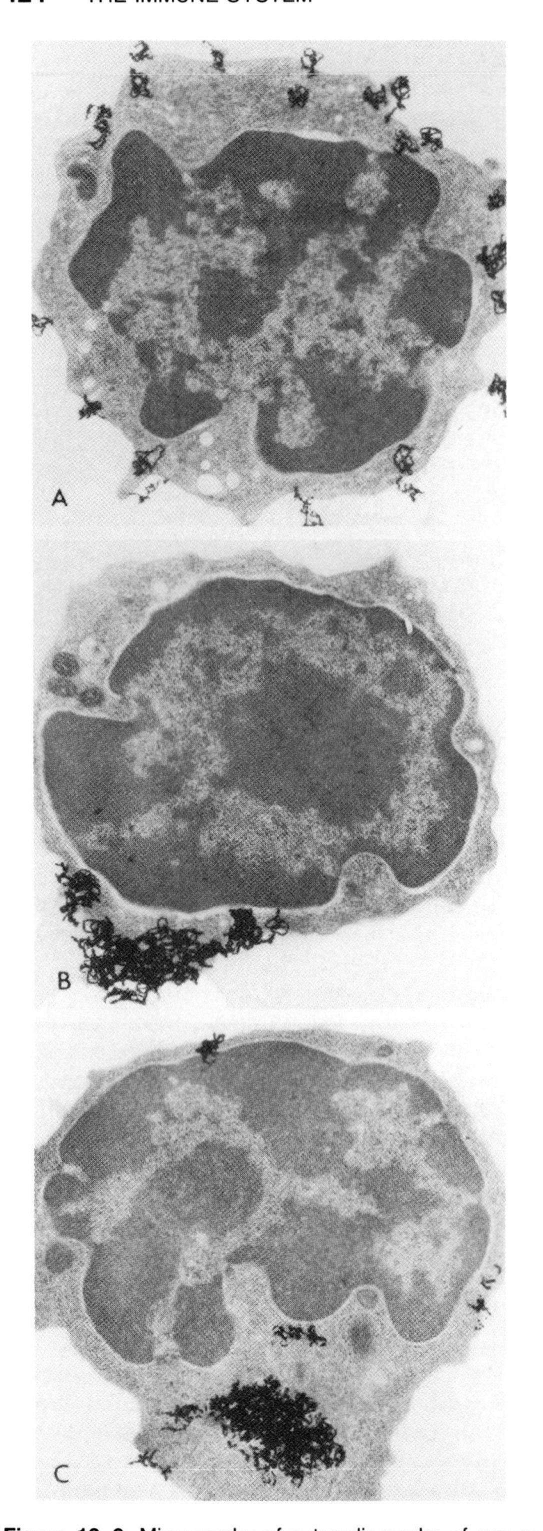

Figure 13–9. Micrographs of autoradiographs of mouse spleen B-lymphocytes treated with ^{125}I-labeled rabbit anti-immunoglobulin antibody. (A) At 4°C, the grains are randomly distributed over the entire cell membrane. (B) When the lymphocytes are incubated at 37°C, the label becomes concentrated at one pole of the cell, forming a "cap." (C) Finally, the label is interiorized by endocytosis. (From Unanue, E.R. et al. 1972. J. Exp. Med. 136:885.)

nuded of its surface immunoglobulin for several hours. It is thought that capping probably occurs on binding of antigen to the surface of B-lymphocytes, in vivo.

OTHER FUNCTIONAL PROPERTIES OF LYMPHOCYTES

Lymphocyte heterogeneity is not limited to the two classes B- and T-lymphocytes. Within each class, lymphocytes may differ considerably in functional properties, such as immunocompetence, life span, and sensitivity to ionizing radiation or to adrenal steroids. In T-lymphocytes which have been most thoroughly studied, these functional differences are related to their degree of differentiation. Most of the lymphocytes in the thymus, which represent precursors of T-cells, are not immunocompetent, that is, they lack the capacity to respond to antigen or to lectins, such as PHA, by transformation and proliferation. They are also more readily destroyed by X-ray irradiation or administration of cortisone. Furthermore, some of the thymic lymphocytes have a very short life span (see Chapter 14). On leaving the thymus, T-lymphocytes become immunocompetent and more resistant to ionizing radiation and cortisone. Their life span is unknown, but on interaction with antigen, they can give rise to memory cells that have the appearance of small lymphocytes and a life span, in man, of several years.

The changes in functional properties of the B-lymphocytes during their development are still poorly understood. There is evidence, however, that their bone-marrow precursors are resistant to corticosteroids, whereas peripheral B-lymphocytes are sensitive to both ionizing irradiation and adrenal steroids. Memory cells of the B-type also have a long life span.

An important property of lymphocytes is their motility, which enables them to cross the walls of postcapillary venules to enter, or leave, the bloodstream. They also move about in the parenchyma of lymph nodes and can leave the nodes by migrating through the walls of lymphatic vessels to enter the lymph. They also insinuate themselves between the cells of epithelia and freely wander through the connective tissues of the body. Their differentiation into plasma cells is accompanied by a loss of motility.

LYMPHOID TISSUE

Lymphocytes occur individually in the blood, in lymph, and in the connective tissues and epithelia of the body. They also occur, together with plasma cells, in densely packed masses in the loose connective tissue of the lamina propria in the digestive and respiratory tracts. The thymus, lymph nodes, tonsils, and white pulp of the spleen also consist mainly of enormous numbers of closely aggregated small lymphocytes. The terms "lymphoid" or "lymphatic tissue" are commonly used to include all of these aggregations of lymphocytes and the lymphocyte-rich organs. Although, in the past, these terms were often used with quite different connotations, advances in immunology have rendered those distinctions obsolete. However, our knowledge of the cell interactions at the tissue and organ level is still quite incomplete and a solid basis for classification of the various lymphocyte aggregations in the body is still lacking. In this book, the terms "lymphoid tissue" and "lymphoid organ" will be used to specify sites in which lymphocytes, with or without associated plasma cells, are the principal cellular component. It is emphasized, however, that this definition is purely descriptive and includes lymphocyte aggregations that may have very different functions.

A type of lymphoid tissue that is recognized as morphologically and functionally distinct from others is found in the thymus and in the avian bursa of Fabricius. It consists of lymphocytes and a few macrophages, contained within the meshes of a tridimensional network of stellate cells that are held together by desmosomes. These stellate stromal cells have traditionally been called *reticular cells,* simply because they form a network. They are not to be confused with the reticular cells of other organs that are of mesenchymal origin. The reticular cells of thymus arise from an epithelial outgrowth of the embryonic endoderm which is subsequently invaded by lymphopoietic stem cells. Reticular fibers which are commonly associated with reticular cells of mesenchymal origin are rare in the lymphoid tissue of the thymus and bursa of Fabricius.

A much more common type of lymphoid tissue is that making up the bulk of the mass of lymph nodes, the white pulp of the spleen, and the tonsils, and forming more-or-less discrete masses scattered sporadically in the loose connective tissues of other organs. For descriptive purposes, *diffuse* and *nodular* subvarieties of this type of lymphoid tissue can be distinguished (Fig. 13–10).

DIFFUSE LYMPHOID TISSUE

Lymphoid tissue of this description is typically found in the internodal, deep cortical, and medullary regions of lymph nodes; in the periarterial lymphoid sheaths of the spleen; in the internodal regions of the tonsils; and in Peyer's patches of the ileum. It consists of a sponge-like stroma with lymphocytes filling its meshes. The stroma is made up of reticular fibers and reticular cells of mesenchymal origin (Fig. 13–11). The reticular fibers, best revealed by silver impregnation methods, are intimately associated with the reticular cells, often occupying deep recesses in their surface. The reticular cells appear as elongate or stellate elements with an ovoid euchromatic nucleus and scant acidophilic cytoplasm. In animals injected with vital dyes, some of the cells take up the colloidal dye avidly, whereas others do not. This indicates that some of the cells are phagocytic and can be regarded as macrophages. Viewed with the electron microscope, reticular cells contain a few cisternae of rough endoplasmic reticulum and a moderately well-developed Golgi complex, but other organelles are rather inconspicuous. The peripheral cytoplasm is devoid of organelles and inclusions but contains bundles of fine filaments. Thus, some of the stromal cells of diffuse lymphoid tissue are regarded as fixed macrophages, whereas others are rather like the fibroblasts of connective tissue elsewhere in the body.

Experiments, involving the use of H^3-thymidine, have shown that the reticular cells in lymph nodes have a slow turnover rate. Moreover, during the regeneration of a lymph node following X-irradiation, no transformation of labeled reticular cells into free cells of the lymphoid parenchyma is observed. There appears, therefore, to be no evidence to support the traditional view that reticular cells are primitive undifferentiated cells capable of giving rise to lymphocytes or other cellular components of the connective tissue. It is now believed that reticular cells, other than those of the thymus, are simply fibroblasts involved in the synthesis and maintenance of the framework of reticular fibers. Scattered among them are occasional fixed macrophages. The free cells of diffuse lymphoid

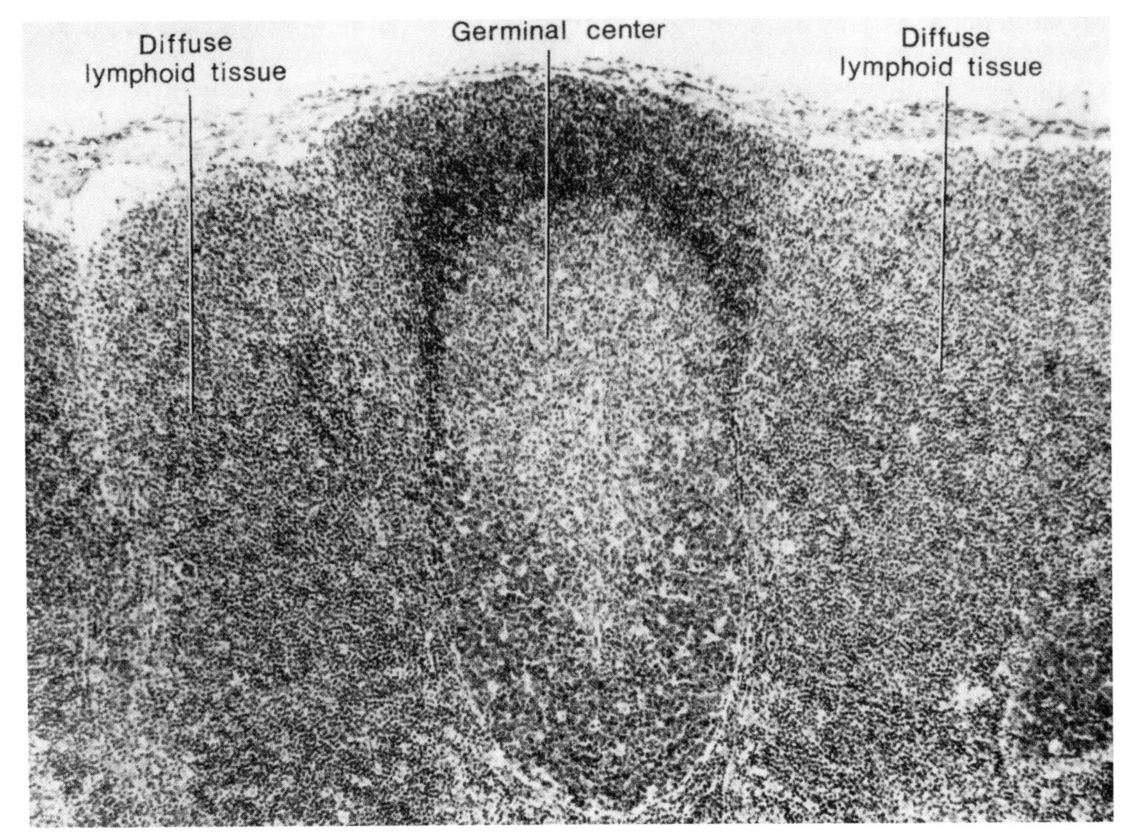

Figure 13–10. Photomicrograph of diffuse lymphoid tissue and a single germinal center in the outer cortex of a mesenteric lymph node from a dog.

tissue are lymphocytes, free macrophages, and a variable number of plasma cells.

LYMPHOID NODULES

Lymphoid nodules or *lymphoid follicles* are circumscribed closely packed collections of lymphocytes within areas of diffuse lymphoid tissue. They are found in the cortex of lymph nodes, at the periphery of the white pulp of the spleen, and in the lamina propria of the digestive and respiratory tracts. They are especially numerous in the tonsils, Peyer's patches, and the appendix. Some terminological confusion may be found in the literature in the application of the terms "primary nodule," "secondary nodule," and "germinal center" to different entities. *Primary lymphoid nodule* is commonly used to designate any rounded aggregation of closely packed small lymphocytes, whereas *secondary nodule* (also called *germinal center*) is applied to ovoid areas consisting of larger pale-staining cells covered by a "cap" of small lymphocytes. The precise functional significance of primary nodules is not known. Moreover, there is no convincing evidence that secondary nodules, with their cap of small lymphocytes, arise from preexisting primary nodules, as the word secondary would imply. Therefore, the term "secondary nodule" does not seem to be justified and should be discarded in favor of "germinal center."

A *germinal center* is a highly organized component of lymphoid tissues, other than that of the normal thymus (Fig. 13–12). When fully developed, it appears as a spherical or ovoid mass of cells with a darker, densely populated pole and a paler, less densely populated pole. It is surrounded by slender elongated cells in a thin layer, which, in turn, is invested at one pole by a crescentic cap of small lymphocytes. Germinal centers display an obvious polarity in that the cap of small lymphocytes is quite thick over its light region and gradually becomes thinner toward its darker pole (Fig. 13–10). In lymph nodes, the light region and lym-

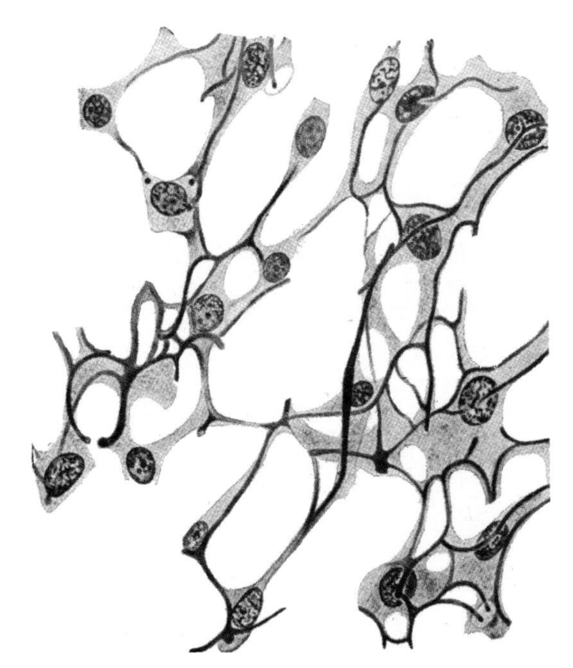

Figure 13–11. Section of a small area of a lymph node after the lymphocytes have been removed. The three-dimensional network of reticular cells is shown and their intimate relation to the reticular fibers.

phocyte cap of the germinal centers are directed toward the marginal sinus. In the spleen, they are directed toward the red pulp. In the digestive and respiratory tracts, they are directed toward the overlying epithelium. When the plane of a histological section passes through a germinal center perpendicular to its axis of symmetry, the polarity just described is not seen because the cap of lymphocytes appears as an encircling rim of uniform width around the center. For this reason, the cap has sometimes been erroneously described as a "mantle" or "corona."

The darker region of the germinal center (Fig. 13–12) results from staining of the nuclei and basophilic cytoplasm of numerous closely packed lymphoblasts, large, medium, and small lymphocytes, and cells in transition to plasma cells. All of these cells are actively proliferating, and antibody can be demonstrated in their occasional cisternae of endoplasmic reticulum. Macrophages loaded with residues of phagocytized degenerating lymphocytes are consistently found in the dark zone. The cells of the germinal center are contained within the meshes of a cellular framework of stellate cells whose processes are joined by desmosomes. These cells, which show little cytoplasmic specialization, are stained by silver methods and were called *dendritic cells* because of their numerous radiating processes. At the equator of the germinal center, the transition from the light to the dark region is gradual. The basophilic lymphoblasts and large lymphocytes progressively give way to small lymphocytes, mitotic figures disappear, and macrophage numbers decrease. The dendritic cells acquire more cytoplasm and extend great numbers of interdigitating peripheral processes.

The outer boundary of the germinal center consists of a few layers of flattened reticular cells joined by desmosomes. This layer is more disorganized over the light pole owing to its infiltration by many highly pleiomorphic small lymphocytes fixed in the process of migrating to, or from, the overlying lymphocyte cap. Plasma cells are scarce in germinal centers, except in those of the tonsils.

Germinal centers are believed to pass through a sequence of developmental changes and subsequently undergo involution and disappear. Their life span and the precise sequence of events leading to their disappearance are largely unknown. They seem to arise from small clusters of large lymphocytes or lymphoblasts which proliferate to form aggregations of increasing size and complexity up to 1 mm in diameter. In large germinal centers, phagocytosis of degenerating lymphocytes is very active and macrophages loaded with residual bodies form lighter areas on a background of darkly staining and closely spaced nuclei.

Until recently, little was known about the function of germinal centers. They are now known to be sites where B-lymphocytes are undergoing active proliferation following an initial, or a secondary, exposure to antigen. Consistent with this interpretation is the fact that they are not present in the lymph nodes at birth, and they do not appear in animals reared in a germ-free environment. In the germinal centers of lymph nodes and spleen, the lymphocytes of the cap are probably members of a long-lived class, whereas those arising in the germinal center probably move into the medulla, where a few may develop into plasma cells and others may enter the lymph and return to the circulation.

The function of the dendritic cells has been a subject of debate. They do not seem to be capable of phagocytosis. Therefore, the term "dendritic macrophage," formerly applied to

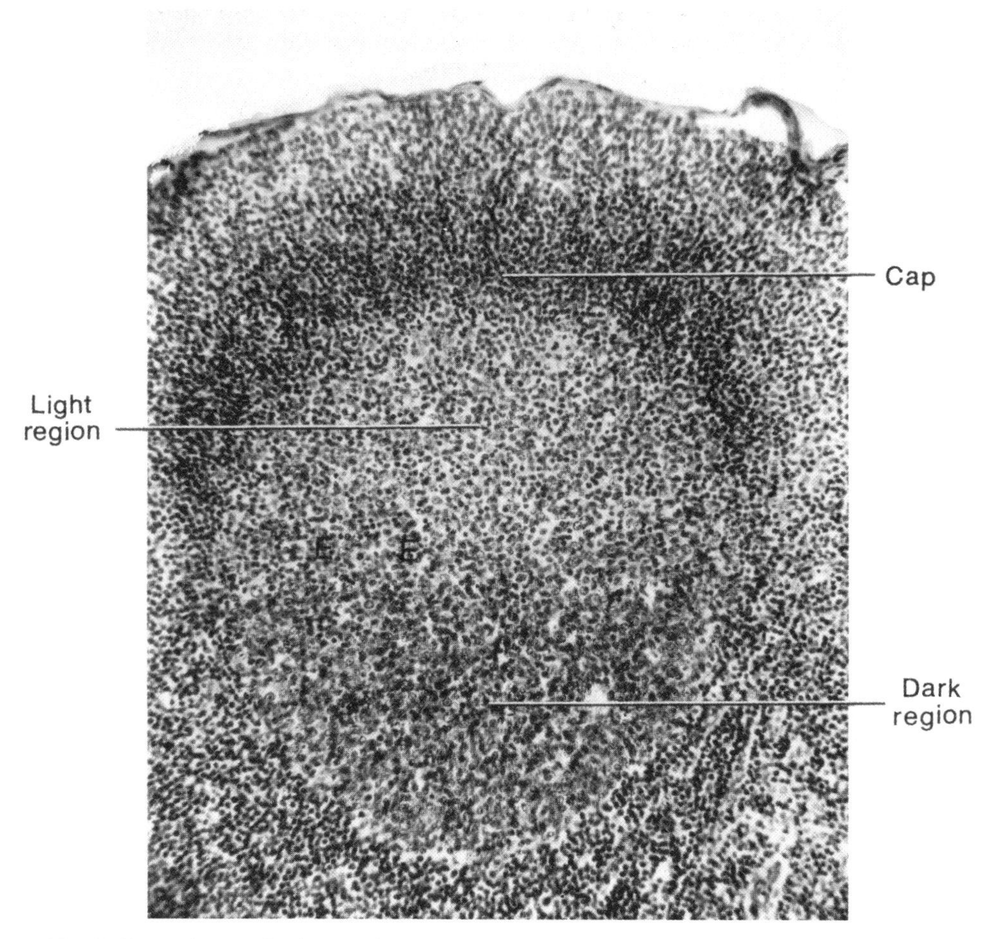

Figure 13–12. Photomicrograph of a germinal center in the outer cortex of an inguinal lymph node from a dog.

them, is no longer appropriate. However, they can bind and retain antigens on their surface for long periods and, like macrophages, they can present antigen, together with their own MHC molecules, to activate T-lymphocytes and may, therefore, participate in induction of an immune response.

Germinal centers are believed to be involved in the functional differentiation of B-lymphocytes. Their appearance is closely correlated with the evolution of humoral immune responses. They are formed de novo during the primary response to antigen, and increase very rapidly during a secondary response. Their cells secrete the IgG form of immunoglobulin, although relatively few develop into plasma cells. Each germinal center seems to produce monospecific antibody and it has been suggested that the whole lymphocyte population of an individual germinal center may represent a clone of cells all responding to the same antigen. Although there is a good correlation between the appearance of germinal centers and the humoral response to antigen, they are not indispensable for antibody production. In the human fetus, there is antibody secretion before germinal centers develop, and in the course of the primary response to antigen, plasma cells develop and antibody appears in the blood in small quantity before antibody-producing germinal centers can be demonstrated. In a secondary response to antigen, however, it is reported that germinal center formation does precede the rise in circulating antibody. On the basis of these and other observations, it is suggested that germinal centers develop following repeated contact with an antigen and that they may be involved in long-term memory of previous IgG responses. However, in the present state of our knowledge, it must be admitted that much remains to be learned about the precise function of the germinal centers of lymphoid tissue.

LYMPHOCYTE CIRCULATION

To recapitulate, the immune system consists of (1) specific lymphoid organs, (2) masses of lymphoid tissue embedded in other organs, (3) isolated lymphoid cells infiltrating the connective and epithelial tissues of the body, and (4) lymphocytes circulating in the blood and lymph. Among the organs of the immune system, the thymus and lymph nodes are made up exclusively of lymphoid tissue, whereas the spleen also possesses the red pulp which has nonimmune functions. Aggregations of lymphoid cells can be found anywhere in the body, with the exception of the central nervous system. The bone marrow, although not ordinarily considered a part of the immune system, is the source of the precursors of the lymphocytes in late fetal and in postnatal life and is regarded by many as the mammalian equivalent of the avian bursa of Fabricius and the site of differentiation of precursors into B-lymphocytes.

The various regions of the immune system have important functional interrelationships that depend on their communication via an orderly traffic of lymphocytes carried in the blood and lymph. Lymphocyte precursors are carried to the thymus, and in that special microenvironment, they proliferate and undergo differentiation into immunocompetent T-lymphocytes. In the bone marrow, lymphocyte precursors undergo antigen-independent differentiation into immunocompetent B-lymphocytes. From these sites of origin, the cells enter the bloodstream and populate the lymph notes, spleen, and connective tissues. On encountering an appropriate antigen, T- and B-lymphocytes are stimulated to proliferate and undergo further differentiation into activated T-lymphocytes, antibody-secreting B-lymphocytes, and plasma cells. Antigen stimulation results in the production of lymphocytes that propagate the response throughout the immune system. Some of these carry "memory" of a primary immune response and are capable of mounting a more rapid and vigorous response on exposure to the same antigen.

Efficient immunological surveillance is possible only if lymphocytes, each capable of responding to a single antigen, are able to move freely throughout the body, thereby increasing the chance of encountering their specific antigen, wherever it may enter. That such a scouting and patrolling of the body exists has been verified in a number of elegant experiments that have disclosed a continuous traffic of lymphocytes between the various lymphoid organs, via the blood and lymph. There are slow and fast modes of lymphocyte migration. The time course of lymphocytes moving to and through the thymus, and the subsequent seeding of lymphocytes, from the thymus and bone marrow to the peripheral lymphoid organs, is measured in weeks. Superimposed on this slow traffic is a second kind of migratory behavior in which long-lived small lymphocytes move rapidly to the lymphoid organs and tissues and then back into the blood for another circuit. This latter process, which does not involve lymphocyte proliferation or transformation, is called *recirculation* and is measured in hours. There are hints of a third pattern of cell migration in the course of an acute immune response. In this, effector lymphocytes and plasma cell precursors are seeded via the blood and lymph throughout the immune system and connective tissues, thus widely disseminating the immune response.

Recirculation was first demonstrated by experiments involving collection of lymphocytes from a chronic fistula of the thoracic duct, the large lymph channel that collects most of the lymph of the body and returns it to the bloodstream where the duct empties into the confluence of the left subclavian and internal jugular veins. The thoracic duct lymph contains varying numbers of cells in different animal species, but in man, the number ranges from 2,000 to 30,000 per cubic millimeter, of which 90–95% are small lymphocytes. The remaining cells are large lymphocytes, possibly precursors of plasma cells en route to the connective tissues. The outflow of small lymphocytes from the thoracic duct would be sufficient to replace all blood lymphocytes several times daily. Because the number of blood lymphocytes remains unchanged, it is reasoned that they must be continuously leaving the blood at the same rate that they enter it from the thoracic duct. Consistent with this idea is the finding that prolonged drainage through a thoracic duct fistula results in a marked leukopenia and extreme depletion of the lymphocyte population of the spleen, lymph nodes, and the gut-associated lymphoid tissue. The bone marrow is not obviously affected. The thymus shows some decrease in weight, but this does not seem to be a direct effect.

If lymphocytes recovered from the thoracic duct are radioactively labeled, in vitro, and then injected intravenously into a syngeneic recipient, it can be shown that they rapidly leave the bloodstream and localize in the peripheral lymphoid organs, but they do not enter the thymus or the bone marrow. These experiments gave rise to the concept that a population of small lymphocytes continuously migrate from the blood into the peripheral lymphoid organs, but soon leave them again to reenter the blood either directly or via the lymphatics. If this is true, it should be possible to delete the recirculating pool by destroying lymphocytes at any point along their migratory route. This has been verified by irradiation of the hilus of the spleen.

Recirculation is rapid, with an average transit time of small lymphocytes through the blood being 0.6 h; transit time through the spleen, 5–6 h; and through lymph nodes, 15–20 h. The recirculating lymphocytes represent a substantial fraction of the body's total small lymphocyte population. Most, if not all, of these are long-lived. Because the blood contains a much higher proportion of short-lived small lymphocytes (30–50% in the rat), than the thoracic duct lymph, only a portion of the blood lymphocytes must belong to the recirculating pool. The origin and fate of these short-lived lymphocytes are poorly understood. The vast majority of recirculating lymphocytes (85% in mice) are T-cells, and the remainder are B-lymphocytes. B-cells seem to recirculate at a slower rate than T-cells and are mobilized with difficulty by prolonged drainage of the thoracic duct lymph. It is not clear whether this is because they are inherently more sluggish or because they are somewhat segregated from the main recirculatory path.

Drainage of thoracic duct lymph causes a selective depletion in specific regions of the lymphoid organs. Early in such an experiment, lymphocytes disappear first from the deep portion of the cortex of lymph nodes, from the periarterial lymphoid sheaths of the spleen, and from the internodal regions of Peyer's patches. These are the same sites that appear devoid of lymphocytes in neonatally thymectomized rodents and which were, therefore, designated *thymus-dependent* regions. This is attributable to the fact that the T-lymphocytes are the main component of the recirculating pool and are rapidly mobilized from peripheral lymphoid organs. After more prolonged drainage of thoracic duct lymph, there is lymphocyte depletion in the *thymus-independent* regions of the peripheral lymphoid organs, namely, the superficial cortex and medullary cords of lymph nodes and the peripheral areas of the white pulp of the spleen. This finding probably reflects a relatively late mobilization of the recirculating B-lymphocytes. Recirculating T- and B-lymphocytes, labeled in vitro, and injected into a syngeneic recipient localize, respectively, in the thymus-dependent and thymus-independent regions of the peripheral lymphoid organs. The mechanism by which recirculating small lymphocytes leave and subsequently reenter the bloodstream in the spleen, or leave the blood and enter the lymph in lymph nodes will be discussed in later chapters devoted to these organs (Chapters 15 and 16).

Despite the continuous exchange of lymphocytes between the various regions of the immune system, a steady state is reached that ensures a consistent proportion of T- and B-lymphocytes in the blood, lymph, and lymphoid organs. In the mouse, 65–85% of the small lymphocytes in the lymph nodes and thoracic duct lymph, and 30–50% of those in the spleen, are T-lymphocytes. In human blood, 69–82% of the lymphocyte population are T-cells and the remaining 20–30% are B-lymphocytes. The significance of the recirculation of small lymphocytes is still open to investigation, but it is widely assumed that these cells represent, at least in part, "memory cells" patrolling the immune system, ready to quickly set up an immune response on encountering the appropriate antigen.

BIBLIOGRAPHY

GENERAL

Barrett, J.T. 1983. Textbook of Immunology. An Introduction to Immunochemistry and Immunobiology, 4th ed. St. Louis, MO, C.V. Mosby.

Benacerraf, B. and E.R. Unanue. 1979. Textbook of Immunology. Baltimore, MD, Williams and Wilkins.

Golub, E.S. and D.R. Green. 1991. Immunology. A Synthesis, 2nd ed., Sunderland, MA, Sinauer Associates, Inc.

Roitt, I.M. 1980. Essential Immunology. Oxford, Blackwell.

Weiss, L. 1972. The Cells and Tissues of the Immune System: Structure, Function, Interactions. Englewood Cliffs, NJ, Prentice-Hall.

IMMUNOGLOBULINS AND COMPLEMENT

Davies, D.R. and H. Metzger. 1983. Structural basis of antibody function. Annu. Rev. Immunol. 1:87.

Rabellino, E.S., S. Colo, H.M. Grey, and E.R. Unanue. 1971. Immunoglobulins on the surface of lymphocytes. I. Distribution and quantitation. J. Exp. Med. 133:156.

Tonegawa, S. 1985. The molecules of the immune system. Sci. Am. 253 (4):122.

van Bleek, G.M. and S.G. Nathanson. 1991. Structure of

the antigen-binding groove of major histocompatibility complex Class I molecules determines specific selection of self-peptides. Proc. Acad. Sci. USA 88:11032.

Wall, R. and M. Kuehl. 1983. Biosynthesis and regulation of immunoglobulins. Annu. Rev. Immunol. 1:393.

LYMPHOCYTES AND PLASMA CELLS

Everett, N.B. and R.W. Tyler. 1967. Lymphopoiesis in the thymus and other tissues: Functional implications. Internat. Rev. Cytol. 22:205.

Feldmann, M. and G.V.V. Nossal. 1972. Cellular basis of antibody production. Quart. Rev. Biol. 47:269.

Harris, T.N., E. Grimm, E. Mertens, and W.E. Ehrlich. 1945. The role of the lymphocyte in antibody formation. J. Exp. Med. 81:73.

Harris, T.N. and S. Harris. 1956. The genesis of antibodies. Am. J. Med. 123:114.

Henkart, P.A. 1985. The mechanism of lymphocyte-mediated cytotoxicity. Annu. Rev. Immunol. 3:31.

Hummeler, K., T.N. Harris, N. Tamassini, M. Hechtel, and M.B. Farber. 1966. Electron microscopic observation on antibody producing cells in lymph and blood. J. Exp. Med. 124:255.

Karnovsky, M.J., E.R. Unanue, and M. Leventhal. 1972. Ligand-induced movement of lymphocyte membrane macromolecules. II. Mapping of surface moieties. J. Exp. Med. 136:907.

Katz, B.H. and B. Benacerraf. 1962. The regulatory influence of activated T cells on B cell responses to antigen. Adv. Immunol. 15:1.

Leduc, E.H., S. Avrameas, and M. Bouteille. 1968. Ultrastructural localization of antibody in differentiating plasma cells. J. Exp. Med. 127:109.

Leduc, E.H., A.H. Coons, and J.M. Connolly. 1955. Studies on antibody production. II. The primary and secondary responses in the popliteal lymph node of the rabbit. J. Exp. Med. 102:61.

Murphy, M.J., J.B. Hay, B. Morris, and M.C. Bessis. 1972. Ultrastructural analysis of antibody synthesis in cells from lymph and lymph nodes. Am. J. Pathol. 66:25.

Perkins, W.D., M.J. Karnovsky, and E.R. Unanue. 1972. An ultrastructural study of lymphocytes with surface-bound immunoglobulin. J. Exp. Med. 135:267.

Persechini, P.M., J.D.E. Young, and W. Almers. 1990. Membrane channel formation by the lymphocyte pore-forming protein: Comparison between susceptible and resistent target cells. J. Cell. Biol. 110:2109.

Raff, M.C. 1973. T and B lymphocytes and immune responses. Nature 242:19.

Reinherz, E.L. and S.F. Schlossman. 1980. The differentiation and function of human T lymphocytes. Cell 19:821.

Sprent, J. 1973. Circulating B and T lymphocytes of the mouse. I. Migratory properties. Cell Immunol. 7:10.

Sprent, J. and A. Basten. 1973. Circulating B and T lymphocytes of the mouse. II. Lifespan. Cell Immunol. 7:40.

MACROPHAGES AND DENDRITIC CELLS

Berkovsky, J.A., S.J. Brett, H.Z. Streicher, and H. Takahashi. 1988. Antigen processing for presentation to T-lymphocytes. Immunol. Rev. 106:5.

Brodsky, F.M. and L.E. Guagliardi. 1991. The cell biology of antigen processing and presentation. Annu. Rev. Immunol. 9:707.

Cohn, Z.A. 1968. The structure and function of monocytes and macrophages. Adv. Immunol. 9:163.

Steinman, R.M. 1981. Dendritic cells. Transplantation 31:151.

Steinman, R.M. and M.C. Nussenzweig. 1980. Dendritic cells: features and functions. Immunol. Rev. 53:127.

LYMPHOID TISSUES

Belisle, C. and G. Saint-Marie. 1981. Tridimensional study of the deep cortex of the rat lymph node. III. Morphology of the deep cortex units. Anat. Rec. 199:213.

Coons, A.H. 1957–58. Some reactions of lymphoid tissues to stimulation by antigens. Harvey Lecture Series 53:113.

Doe, W.F. 1989. The intestinal immune system. Gut 30:1679.

Gutman, G.A. and I.L. Weissman. 1972. Lymphoid tissue architecture: Experimental analysis of the origin and distribution of T-cells and B-cells. Immunology 23:465.

Millikin, P. 1966. Anatomy of germinal centers in human lymphoid tissue. Arch. Pathol. 82:499.

Movat, H.Z. and N.V.P. Fernando. 1964. The fine structure of lymphoid tissue. Exp. Mol. Pathol. 3:546.

Movat, H.Z. and N.V.P. Fernando. 1965. The fine structure of the lymphoid tissue during antibody formation. Exp. Mol. Pathol. 4:155.

Saint-Marie, G., F.S. Peng, and C. Belisle. 1982. Overall architecture and pattern of lymph flow in the rat lymph node. Am. J. Anat. 64:275.

von Gaudecker, B. 1991. Functional histology of the human thymus. Anat. Embryol. 183:1.

LYMPHOCYTE RECIRCULATION

Gowans, J.L. 1959. The recirculation of lymphocytes from blood to lymph in the rat. J. Physiol. 146:54.

Gowans, J.L. and E.J. Knight. 1964. The route of recirculation of lymphocytes in the rat. Proc. Roy. Soc. London B. 159:257.

McGregor, D.D. and J.L. Gowans. 1963. The antibody response of rats depleted of lymphocytes by chronic drainage from the thoracic duct. J. Exp. Med. 117:303.

Sasou, S. and T. Sugai. 1992. Periarterial lymphoid sheath in the rat spleen: A light, transmission, and scanning electron microscopic study. Anat. Rec. 232:15.

14

THYMUS

Elio Raviola

The thymus is an organ situated in the superior mediastinum anterior to the great vessels where they emerge from the heart. It extends from the root of the neck, cranially, to the pericardial sac, caudally. It consists of two lobes, arising in the embryo as separate primordia on either side of the midline, but they later become closely joined by connective tissue (Fig. 14–1). The thymus attains its greatest relative weight at the end of the fetal life, but its absolute weight continues to increase, reaching 30–40 g at the time of puberty. It then begins to undergo involution that progresses until, in the adult, the organ is largely replaced by adipose tissue. However, the lymphoid tissue that remains retains some function.

The thymus is the only primary lymphoid organ that has been clearly identified, as such, in the mammal. The bone marrow is widely believed to constitute a second primary lymphoid organ which corresponds to the bursa of Fabricius in birds, but this has been difficult to verify, owing to its inaccessibility and its other hemopoietic functions. The thymus is the first organ to become lymphoid during embryonic life, being seeded with blood-borne lymphoblasts from the yolk sac, and later from the liver. These differentiate into T-lymphocytes within the special microenvironment of the thymus. These undergo intensive proliferation within the thymus, independent of antigenic stimulation, and, after differentiation, populate the peripheral lymphoid organs. These T-lymphocytes are capable of carrying out various functions in cell-mediated immune responses and cooperate with B-lymphocytes in humoral immune responses. Germinal centers are lacking in the thymus and no antibody production occurs there. Removal of the organ, before the immune system has completed its development, results in very serious impairment of immunological defenses.

HISTOLOGICAL ORGANIZATION

Each thymic lobule is invested by a thin capsule of loose connective tissue and is subdivided into a number of parenchymal lobules that appear roughly polyhedral in shape and are 0.5–2 mm in diameter (Fig. 14–1). However, the thymic lobules are not completely independent of one another. In serial sections, one can demonstrate continuity from lobule to lobule via slender connecting strands of lymphoid tissue. Thus, the thymus can be thought of as a convoluted strand of parenchyma with irregularly shaped expansions corresponding to the lobules.

The principal cellular constituents of the thymus are lymphocytes (thymocytes); epithelial cells of unusual form, traditionally called *reticular cells;* and a moderate number of macrophages. At the periphery of the lobules, the lymphocytes are numerous and densely packed, contributing to the intense basophilia of this region (Fig. 14–2). At the center of the lobules, the lymphocytes are somewhat fewer and epithelial cells with abundant eosinophilic cytoplasm are more prominent. Thus, each lobule has a dark-staining peripheral portion, the *cortex,* and a lighter-staining central portion, the *medulla.*

The thymic parenchyma consists of a tridimensional network of stellate, reticular cells bounding small, irregularly shaped compartments filled with lymphocytes that are in direct contact with one another. The thymic lymphocytes within the meshes of the reticulum are morphologically indistinguishable from the lymphocytes of the blood, lymph, and peripheral lymphoid organs. Thin secondary septa extend inward from the primary connective tissue septa of the organ, penetrating the lobules, as far as the corticomedullary boundary. These carry with them small blood vessels. Despite the paucity of intercellular space, small vessels, with a minimal amount of

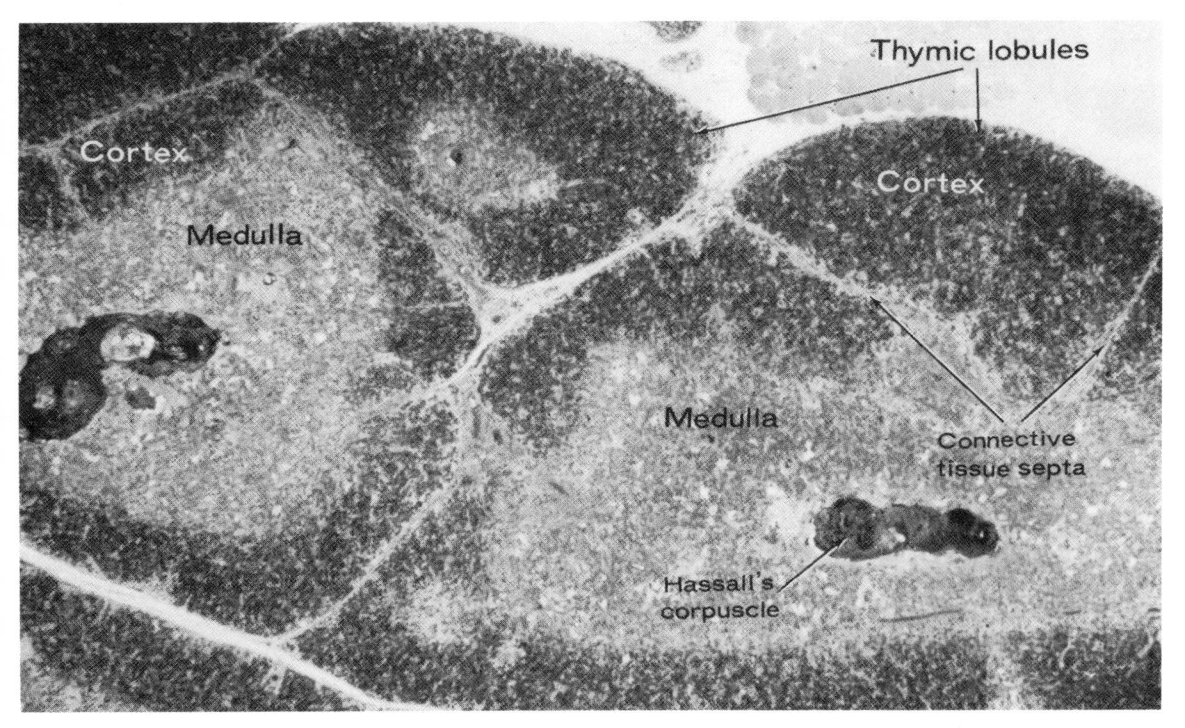

Figure 14–1. A section through the thymus of the guinea pig. The thymic lobes are made up of roughly polygonal lobules, separated from one another by connective tissue septa. Each lobe is comprised of a densely staining peripheral zone, the cortex, and a lighter staining central region, the medulla. The dark structures shown here in the medulla are Hassall's corpuscles. (Courtesy of G.B. Schneider and S. Clark, Jr.)

connective tissue in their adventitia, do thread their way through the thymic parenchyma.

Reference is often made to the stroma of the thymus as a *cytoreticulum* to emphasize the cellular nature of the framework of the parenchyma. Its cells, like those of the lymph nodes and spleen, are stellate in shape, but their embryological origin is from one or the other of the epithelial germ layers and not from mesenchyme. These cells exhibit considerable heterogeneity and their origin has been a subject of controversy. Some believe that they arise from both endoderm and ectoderm. Others conclude from immunocytochemical studies that they arise from a common stem cell, but they have not been able to assign that cell to either ectoderm or endoderm. Six morphologically distinct types of epithelial cells have been described, four in the cortex and two in the medulla. The epithelial nature of those in the medulla is more evident in that they may form cysts lined by cuboidal cells or concentric arrays of squamous cells comprising *Hassall's corpuscles* (Fig. 14–6).

The thymic lobule is a highly dynamic structure. Lymphocytes are continuously produced in the cortex, and although some undergo apoptosis and are disposed of by macrophages, many migrate toward the medulla and enter the bloodstream through the walls of postcapillary venules.

CORTEX

Beneath the capsule of the human thymus, the parenchyma is invested by an almost continuous layer of epithelial cells. These have an irregularly shaped nucleus and a prominent nucleolus. The cytoplasm contains a well-developed Golgi complex, mitochondria, a few cisternae of endoplasmic reticulum, and occasional electron-dense granules. Cells of the same type also ensheath the connective tissue septa and line the perivascular spaces of the cortex. These are called *type-1 epithelial cells* and are referred to collectively as the *subcapsular–perivascular epithelium.* Within this bounding layer, the three-dimensional supporting framework or cytoreticulum of the cortex consists of stellate reticular cells with their processes adhering to one another by small desmosomes (Figs. 14–3, 14–4, 14–5). Lymphocytes completely fill the interstices of

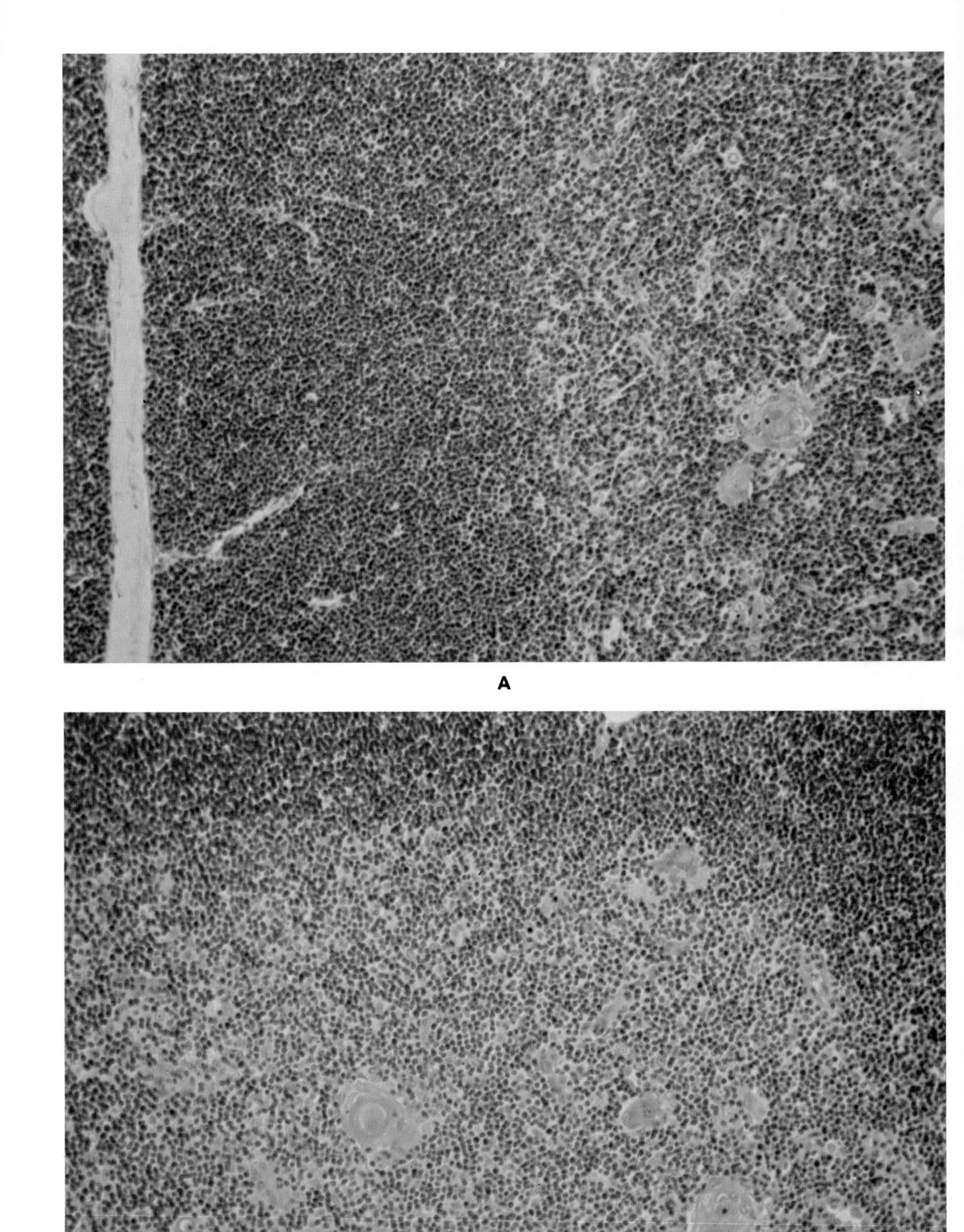

Figure 14–2. *See* legend on opposite page.

the reticulum. The outer and midregion of the cytoreticulum consists of *type-2 cells,* with a large pale nucleus 10–12 μm in diameter and a prominent nucleolus. The pale-staining cytoplasm contains bundles of tonofilaments, short profiles of endoplasmic reticulum, a sizable Golgi complex, surrounded by coated vesicles and a few small dense granules. A few lysosomes and multivesicular bodies may also be present.

Somewhat deeper in the cortex are *type-3 epithelial cells,* in which both nucleus and cytoplasm exhibit a wide range of electron densities. The irregularly shaped nucleus has some peripheral heterochromatin and its perinuclear cistern is often expanded. The cytoplasm contains numerous filaments, dilated cisternae of the endoplasmic reticulum, and a moderate number of cytoplasmic vacuoles. These two cell types, making up the greater part of the cytoreticulum, are considered to be the in vivo counterparts of the *thymic nurse cells* that have been isolated and extensively studied in vitro. In culture, they form large complexes, each encorporating 30 or more lymphocytes. They have been shown to have molecules of the major histocompatibility complex (HMC) on their surface, and it is speculated that the acquisition of self-tolerance and the MHC-restricted T-cell-mediated immune response are dependent on close contact of the lymphocytes with these cells during their differentiation in the thymus.

MEDULLA

Lymphocytes are much less abundant in the medulla of the thymus than in the cortex and they are predominantly small lymphocytes. They differ slightly from those of the cortex in having a more irregular shape and containing fewer ribosomes in their cytoplasm. Macrophages are rarely found in the medulla. Granulocytes, especially eosinophils, may be found in small numbers. Plasma cells are absent.

In the medulla, as in the cortex, there are multiple types of epithelial cells. Scattered *type-4 epithelial cells* are found in the deeper portion of the cortex but are more abundant in the medulla. They stain more deeply than the other epithelial cells described above and have an irregularly shaped nucleus with coarse clumps of heterochromatin and long slender processes rich in tonofilaments. Cisternae of endoplasmic reticulum, when present, are dilated, the mitochondria appear swollen, and a Golgi complex is identified with difficulty. There are numerous cytoplasmic vacuoles, some containing material of moderate electron density. These darkly staining stellate cells form the cytoreticulum of the medulla. *Type-5 epithelial cells* occur in small groups at the corticomedullary junction and scattered singly in the medulla. They have an irregularly shaped or elongate nucleus with peripheral condensations of heterochromatin and a prominent nucleolus. They have less cytoplasm than other reticular cells and it is rich in polyribosomes. They are believed to be relatively undifferentiated cells. Larger pale-staining *type-6 epithelial cells* are confined to the medulla. They have a euchromatic nucleus with a prominent nucleolus. Their cytoplasm contains endoplasmic reticulum which may take the form of long parallel cisternae with a moderately dense granular content. The cytoplasm also contains curious tubular structures 20 nm in diameter with a linear density in the middle which may appear as a dense dot in the circular cross sections of this organelle. Some of the type-6 cells are rounded, whereas others are flattened and tend to wrap around one another. These are the cells involved in the formation of *Hassall's corpuscles,* which are characteristic of the medulla of the thymus. These structures may reach a diameter of 100 μm and consist of a concentric mass of squamous cells joined together by many desmosomes and containing conspicuous bundles of intermediate filaments. The cells in the central portion of the corpuscle may lose their nucleus and come to resemble the superficial cells of the epidermis. They may also degenerate or become calcified. The close resemblance of the cells of Hassall's corpuscles to those of the epidermis has been interpreted as evidence for the origin of at least some of the epithelial cells of the thymus from ectoderm. This is supported by the finding that these cells react positively when exposed to antibody raised

Figure 14–2. Histological sections through the thymus of a monkey. (A) The cortex of a lobule, seen here on the left, consists mainly of densely packed lymphocytes. (B) In the medulla, seen here in the lower two-thirds of the figure, lymphocytes are fewer in number and the reticular cells have more abundant acidophilic cytoplasm than those of the cortex.

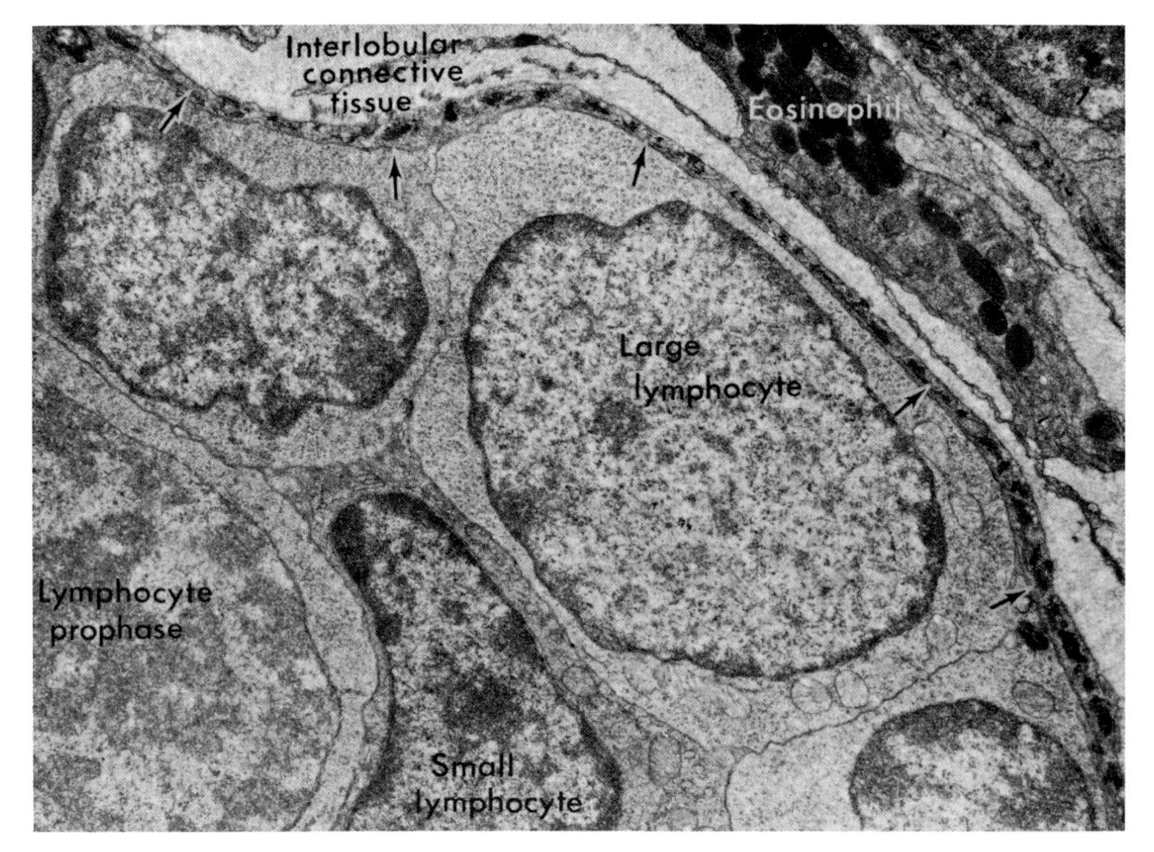

Figure 14–3. An electron micrograph of a small area of the peripheral portion of a rat thymic lobule. Large and small lymphocytes of the cortex are separated from the connective tissue of an interlobular septum (at the upper right) by a continuous layer of attenuated processes of reticular cells, indicated here by arrows. (Courtesy of E. Raviola.)

against epidermal cells or skin keratins. It is not entirely clear whether the six epithelial cell types that have been described are indeed distinct cell types or whether some of this number are different functional states of a smaller number of distinct cells types. Some properties are shared by all, but medullary and subcapsular epithelial cells have histochemical reactions not shared by those of the inner cortex. Type-6 epithelial cells of Hassall's corpuscles react with anti-epidermal antibodies, whereas the other epithelial cell types do not. In the thymus of reptiles and birds, and rarely in mammals, the medulla may contain other seemingly extraneous components, including muscle cells (Hammar's myoid cells); cysts lined with epithelium having a brush border; and even mucus-secreting cells. These are generally believed to be embryonic rests or errors of differentiation having no functional significance.

The significance of the pleomorphism of the epithelial cells (reticular cells) of the thymus is not well understood. There has been some reluctance to accept the existence of as many as six different types. Some contend that regional differences in their form are due to variations in the degree of packing of the lymphocytes and that other cytological differences simply reflect local differences in the physiological activity of a single cell type. Proponents of multiple cells types cite studies showing that medullary and subcapsular epithelial cells have histochemical properties distinct from those of the cytoreticulum of the inner cortex. These cells are also reported to share the same cytokeratin and to have thin filaments reactive with antibodies to smooth muscle actin and myosin whereas other reticular cells of the thymus are unreactive. Moreover, antibodies to certain thymic hormones stain subcapsular and medullary epithelial cells but not those of the inner cortex. The question as to the exact number of distinct reticular cell types and their respective functions remains unsettled. They are difficult to study in situ, owing to their intermingling with great numbers of lymphocytes, and when explanted to cell cultures, there is no assurance that their properties have not been altered in the in vitro microenvironment.

The vast majority of the cell population of the cortex is made up of lymphocytes. These include large, medium, and small forms. The largest lymphocytes have a round or oval nucleus, 9 μm in diameter, rich in euchromatin and containing one or two prominent nucleoli. The cytoplasm is relatively abundant and strongly basophilic. In electron micrographs, the most prominent feature of the cytoplasm is the abundance of free polyribosomes, whereas cisternae of rough endoplasmic reticulum are exceedingly rare. A diplosome, surrounded by a small Golgi complex, is located near a slight indentation of the nuclear envelope. Mitochondria are few. Multivesicular bodies, small dense granules, and lipid droplets are seen only exceptionally. The small lymphocytes have a round, deeply staining heterochromatic nucleus 4–5 μm in diameter with a single small nucleolus. The rim of cytoplasm is very thin and contains a few free ribosomes, mostly dispersed as single units. The cytocentrum and associated minute Golgi complex slightly indent the nucleus. Mitochondria and granular endoplasmic reticulum are encountered even less often than in large lymphocytes and multivesicular bodies and small dense granules are uncommon. The large and small lymphocytes are at the extremes of a continuous spectrum of cells displaying intermediate gradations of nuclear and cytoplasmic organization. Prominent features of cortical lymphocytes are their smooth surface contour and their polyhedral shape, due to mutual deformation.

Large lymphocytes make up only a small portion of the lymphoid population of the lobule and tend to be concentrated at the periphery of the cortex. There is a gradient of progressively smaller forms at deeper levels, and the inner cortex consists mainly of tightly packed small lymphocytes. Dividing cells are frequent at the periphery of the lobule and cells with pycnotic nuclei, undergoing

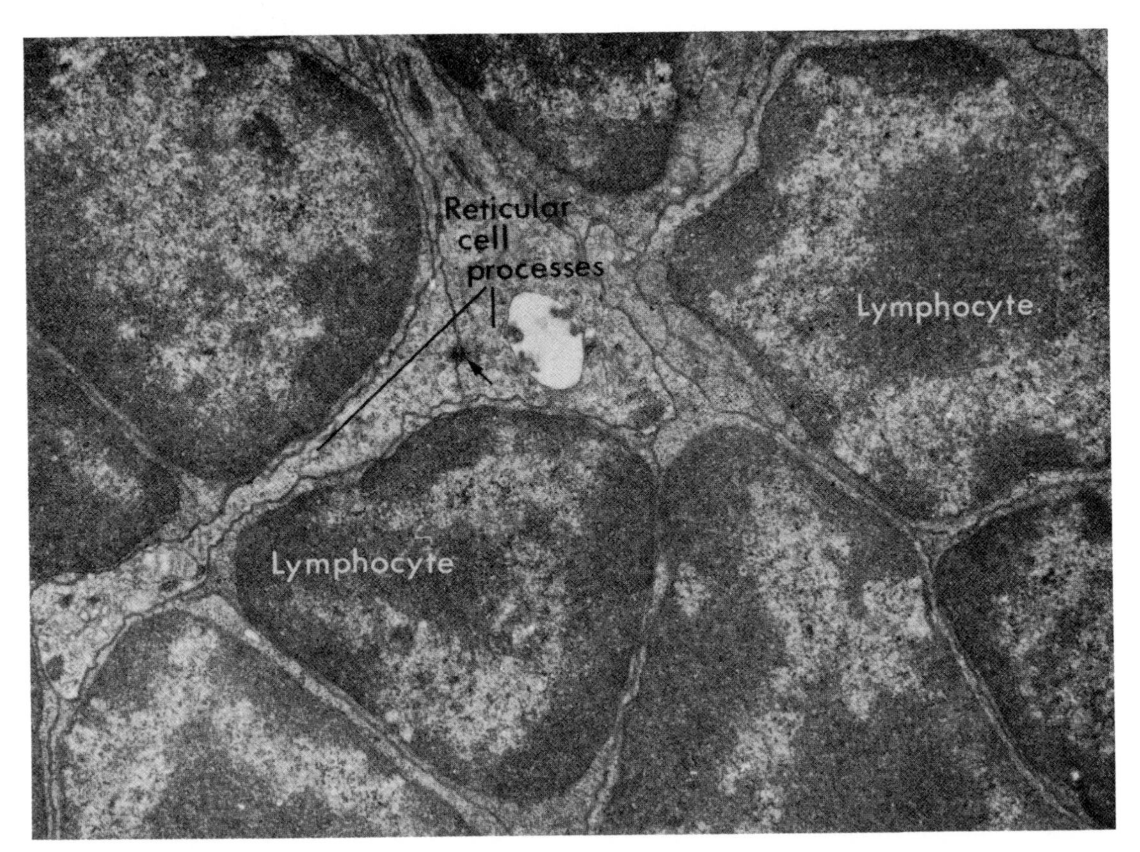

Figure 14–4. Electron micrograph from the deeper portion of the cortex of a rat thymic lobule. Among the crowded small lymphocytes, two reticular cell processes, are joined by a desmosome (at arrow). (Courtesy of E. Raviola.)

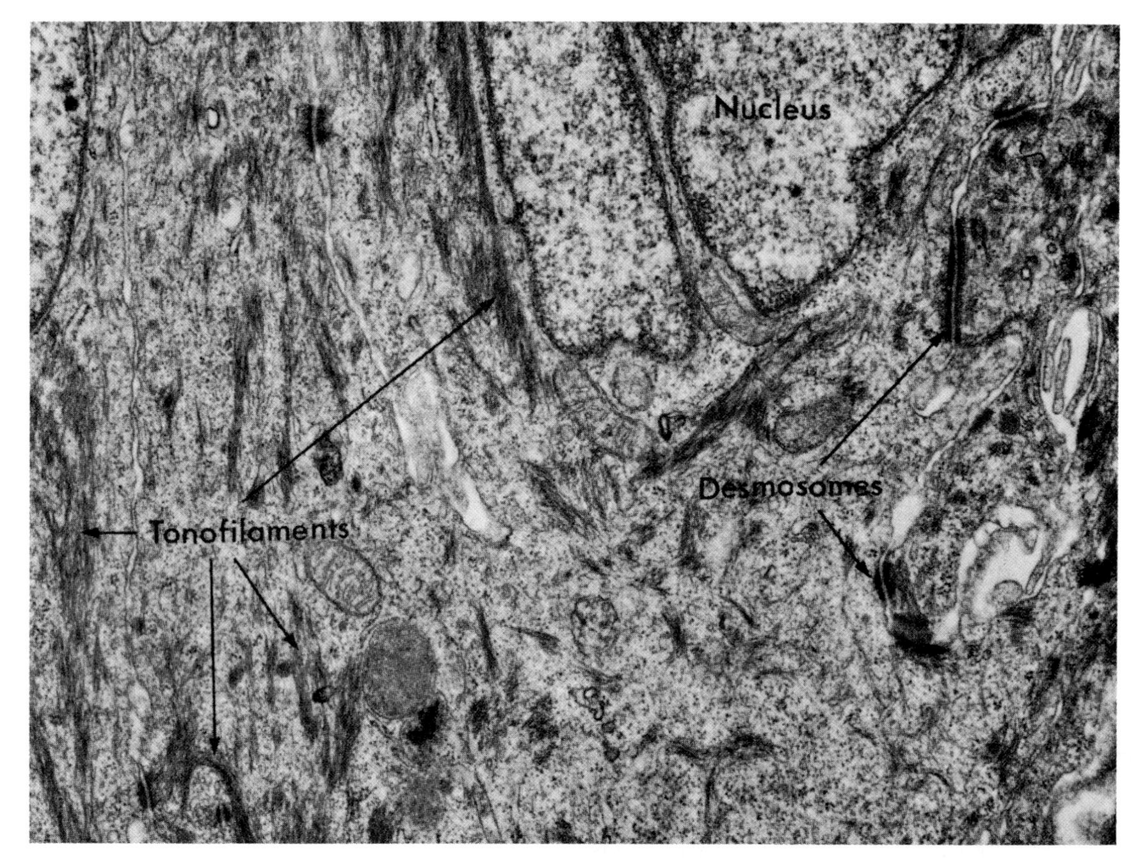

Figure 14–5. Electron micrographs from the medulla of rat thymus, showing portions of several reticular cells, joined by desmosomes and containing conspicuous bundles of tonofilaments. (Courtesy of E. Raviola.)

apoptosis, are abundant in the deep portion of the cortex.

Macrophages are a minor component of the cell population of the thymus; they are scattered throughout the cortex but, in most mammals, increasing in number near the boundary between the cortex and medulla. With the light microscope, they are distinguished from reticular cells with some difficulty, but with the electron microscope, they are easily recognized by their lack of desmosomes and by the presence, within the cytoplasm, of degenerating lymphocytes or residues of their digestion.

A few plasma cells are present in the interstitial connective tissue of the involuting thymus in adults. They also occur in the parenchyma at the extreme periphery of the cortex and along the blood vessels. Mast cells may also be found, but they are mainly outside of the lobules.

The reticular cells of the medulla are also quite pleomorphic. Some of the dark cells (type-4) described earlier as occurring deep in the cortex, are also scattered within the medulla. In addition, there are also groups of cells (type-5) with an irregular or elongated nucleus, having peripheral condensations of heterochromatin and a prominent nucleolus. They have relatively less cytoplasm than other reticular cells. The organelles are similar, but the cytoplasm is rich in polyribosomes. Larger paler cells (type-6), confined to the medulla, have a euchromatic nucleus about 15 nm in diameter with a prominent nucleolus. The endoplasmic reticulum is always present and may take the form of long parallel cisternae with a moderately dense granular content. The cytoplasm also contains the curious tubular structures 20 nm in diameter described above. Some of these cells are rounded, whereas others are flattened and tend to wrap around one another. These are the principal cells involved in formation of Hassall's corpuscles. Lymphocytes are much less abundant in the medulla than in the cortex and are predominantly small lymphocytes. These differ from those of the cortex in having a somewhat

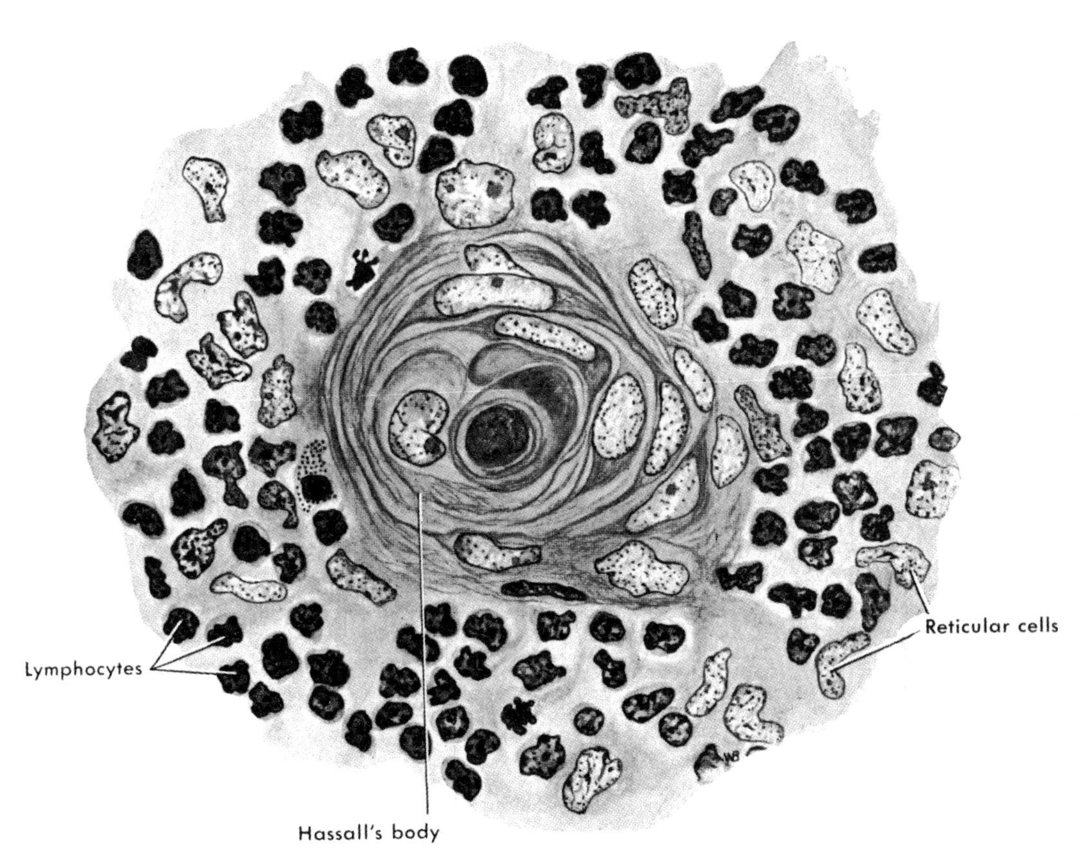

Figure 14–6. Drawing of a Hassall's corpuscle in the medulla of the thymus of an 8-year-old boy. It consists of a concentric array of modified reticular cells.

irregular shape and fewer ribosomes in their cytoplasm. Macrophages are rarely found in the medulla and plasma cells are absent. Granulocytes, especially eosinophils, may be found in small numbers.

VESSELS AND NERVES

The arteries supplying the thymus arise from the internal thoracic arteries and their mediastinal and pericardiacophrenic branches. They ramify in the interlobular connective tissue, and their ultimate subdivisions follow the secondary connective tissue septa that extend inward from the surface of the lobules. Thus, they penetrate the lobule at the corticomedullary boundary without coursing through the parenchyma of the cortex. The arterioles following the boundary between cortex and medulla give off capillaries that ascend into the cortex and these are connected to each other by collateral anastomoses. At the periphery of the cortex, but still within the parenchyma, the capillaries form a network of branching and anastomosing arcades turning back toward the interior of the lobule. In their recurrent course through the cortex, the capillaries join to form somewhat larger vessels that can still be classified as capillaries on the basis of their fine structure. These vessels are confluent with postcapillary venules at the corticomedullary boundary and in the medulla. As an exception to this basic pattern, capillaries may leave the periphery of the cortex and join superficial veins coursing within the interlobular connective tissue. The postcapillary venules of the corticomedullary boundary and the medulla leave the thymic parenchyma via the secondary connective tissue septa and join to form interlobular veins. The majority of these are ultimately drained by a single thymic vein, a tributary of the left brachiocephalic vein.

Because of the peculiar arrangement of the parenchymal blood vessels, the various segments of the vascular tree appear to be spatially segregated within the lobules, the cortex being supplied exclusively by capillaries, whereas the corticomedullary boundary and the medulla also contain arterioles and venules. Studies with electron-opaque tracers show that there is very little movement of macromolecules from blood to thymic parenchyma across the capillary walls in the cortex (Fig. 14–7), whereas the larger medullary vessels are highly permeable to substances in the plasma. Thus, only the lymphoid population of the cortex appears to be protected from circulating macromolecules. This finding gave rise to the concept that interendothelial cell junctions of the capillaries and the layer of epithelial cells lining the perivascular spaces constitute a *blood-thymus barrier* to antigens, comparable to the blood-brain barrier protecting the cells of the central nervous system. For nearly two decades, it was believed that the lymphocytes mature in an antigen-free environment. This has now been challenged by the finding that antigens injected peritoneally or into the mediastinum can enter the periphery of the cortex. In more recent studies, monoclonal antibodies, directed at MHC class-II antigen, injected intraperitoneally or intravenously were found to enter the subcapsular parenchyma and to spread with the flux of interstitial fluid toward the corticomedullary boundary. Thus, although a blood-thymus barrier certainly exists, the traditional view that the thymic microenvironment is free from exposure to antigens is no longer tenable. It is now thought that circulating self-antigens can enter the cortex via a transcapsular route and may contribute to induction of self-tolerance by clonal deletion.

Great numbers of lymphocytes enter the bloodstream from the thymus by traversing the walls of the postcapillary venules of the corticomedullary junction and medulla. The height of the endothelium in these venules is low, in contrast to the cuboidal epithelium of the postcapillary venules of lymph nodes. It is noteworthy, however, that in lymph nodes the lymphocytes are migrating in the opposite direction, from the blood to the parenchyma.

Small lymphatics are found in the connective tissue septa of the thymus, but they seem to be absent from the parenchyma of the lobules. Lymph is drained from these vessels to the sternal, tracheobronchial, and mediastinal lymph nodes.

The thymus receives branches from the vagus and sympathetic nerves. The sympathetic fibers are distributed to the blood vessels. The distribution of the branches of the vagus is not well known. The medulla does appear to contain acetylcholinesterase positive nerve fibers and cells, but the presence of cholinergic innervation is still unproven. A noradrenergic network of nerves has been reported in the subcapsular cortex and at the corticomedullary boundary, with varicose fibers penetrating into the cortex. Various neuropeptides have also been demonstrated in the thymus,

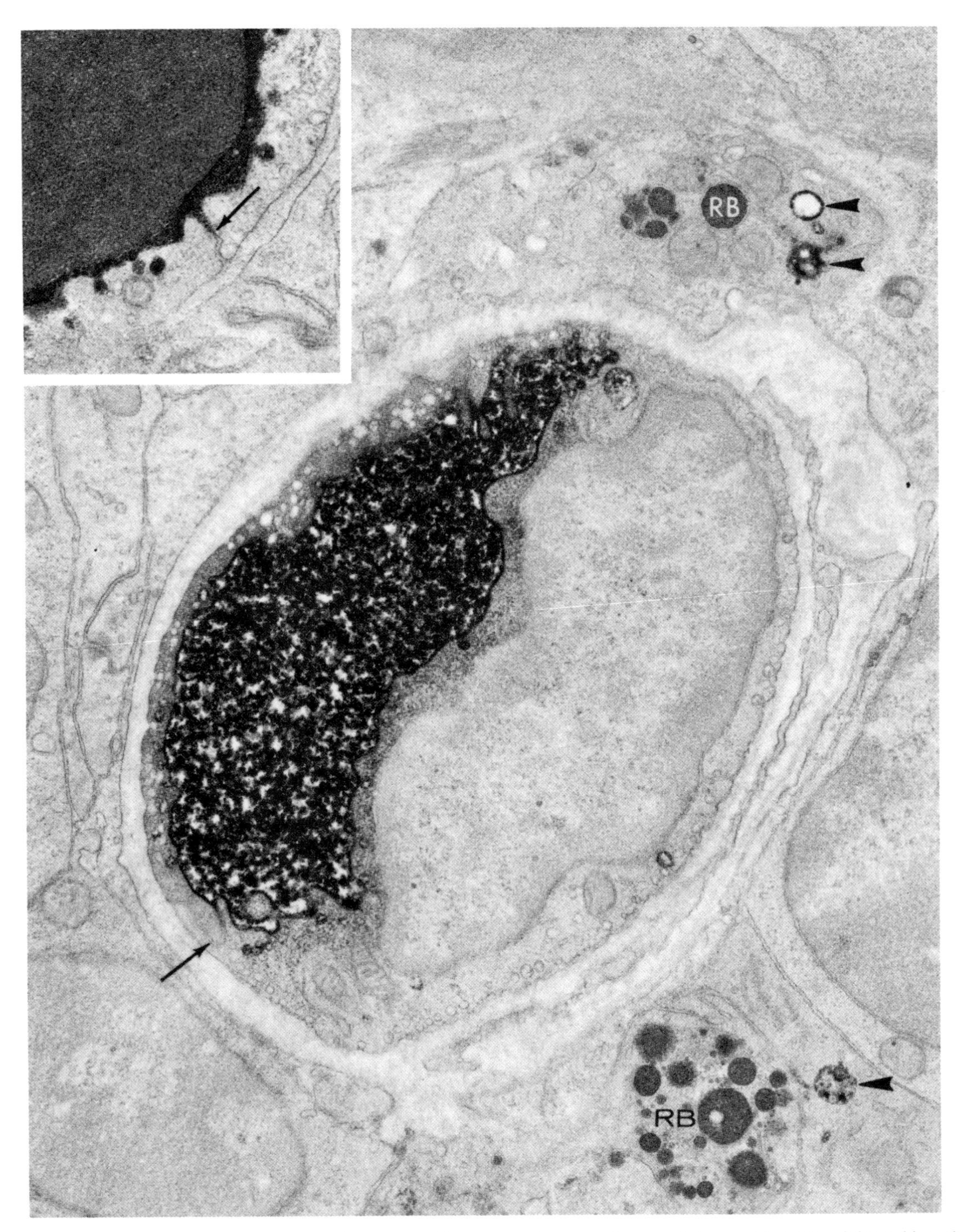

Figure 14–7. Micrograph of a capillary in the cortex of the mouse thymus. Horseradish peroxidase was injected into the bloodstream of the animal, as a large-molecular-weight tracer. It can be seen, at the arrow, that its progression along the intercellular clefts of the endothelium has been blocked by an impermeable tight junction. A little of the tracer has been transported across the endothelium by pinocytotic vesicles, and this was rapidly sequestered in perivascular macrophages. RB residual bodies. *Inset:* A much smaller tracer, cytochrome oxidase, is also arrested by interendothelial junctions (arrow). (From Raviola, E. and M. Karnovsky. J. Exp. Med. 136:466.)

but their physiological significance has yet to be ascertained.

HISTOGENESIS

In man, the thymus arises bilaterally as an outgrowth from the endoderm lining the third branchial pouch, and there may be a small contribution from the fourth. The primordia initially have a slit-like lumen continuous with that of the embryonic pharynx, but they soon become solid outgrowths with a peripheral layer of columnar epithelial cells surrounding a central region of similar cells of varying orientation. After considerable elongation ventrally and medially the separate primordia meet and fuse in the midline, in embryos of 8 weeks, and they acquire a common mesenchymal investment. The cells in the central region have intermingling processes connected by small desmosomes. At this stage, large lymphocyte precursors appear among the epithelial cells. These originate from stem cells in the yolk sac and migrate into the thymic primordium, where they proliferate and differentiate into lymphocytes.

By the 12th week, large pale-staining lymphocytes predominate in the outer portion of the organ and small lymphocytes are more abundant in its interior. At this stage, septa of mesenchyme begin to invade the organ. Among the mesenchymal cells of the septa and among the epithelial cells in the region of the organ destined to become the medulla, there are large pale-staining cells with irregularly shaped nuclei. The identity of these cells is uncertain, but it is suggested that they are precursors of interdigitating cells like those found in peripheral lymphoid organs.

By the 14th week, differentiation of the cortex and medulla is essentially complete. The epithelial cells of the cortex have formed a meshwork of stellate cells with a dense population of small lymphocytes occupying its interstices. This makes the cortex appear darker than the medulla which is dominated by fusiform epithelial cells and contains a smaller population of lymphocytes. By this time, the septa and their blood vessels have advanced to the corticomedullary boundary and have formed there the perivascular spaces which will be the principal avenues for exit of mature lymphocytes from the thymus.

Occasional myoid cells and small Hassall's corpuscles are found in the thymic parenchyma as early as the 8th week of gestation. The finding that cells of the thymic corpuscles contain keratin filaments of the same type as those in squamous cells of the epidermis has lent credence to the claim that ectoderm, as well as endoderm, contributes to formation of the thymus.

The thymus is the first organ of the immune system in which lymphocytes appear, and it continues to be the most active lymphopoietic tissue of the body throughout embryonic life.

INVOLUTION OF THE THYMUS

With advancing age, the thymus undergoes a physiological process of involution in which production of lymphocytes declines, the cortex becomes thinner, and the parenchyma becomes largely replaced by adipose tissue. This normal process of *age involution* was formerly thought to begin in humans at puberty, but it is now known that a decline in the relative volume of parenchyma actually begins in early childhood. In adults, the thymus has been transformed into a mass of adipose tissue containing scattered islands of parenchyma that include some lymphocytes but consist mainly of epithelial cells. In experiments on rodents involving destruction of most of their lymphocyte population, it has been shown that the thymus retains functional competence throughout life and can reacquire full lymphocytopoietic capacity. The same may be true of humans but it has not been demonstrated.

The gradual process of age involution can be acutely accelerated by so-called *accidental involution,* which may occur in response to disease, severe stress, ionizing radiation, bacterial endotoxins, and administration of adrenocorticotrophic hormone or adrenal and gonadal steroids. Under any of these conditions, the thymus rapidly diminishes in size due to massive death of cortical small lymphocytes and their elimination by macrophages. Medullary lymphocytes are more resistant. Therefore, the usual tinctorial pattern of the lobule, with a densely staining cortex and a pale medulla may be reversed. Acute involution, induced in experimental animals, is followed by intensive regeneration, and the thymus rapidly returns to its former size.

HISTOPHYSIOLOGY

Until recently, much of our knowledge of the function of the thymus was based on animal experiments involving thymectomy at a critical stage in development of the immune system, followed by examination of the deficiencies that resulted from removal of this organ. Thymectomy in adult rodents had little effect on the peripheral lymphocyte population or on immune responsiveness. However, thymectomy in the newborn caused lymphocytopenia, severe impairment of cellular immune responses, and depression of antibody production in response to injected antigen. It was concluded from these and other experiments that the thymus is a primary lymphoid organ that is essential for the development of T-lymphocytes, which are helper cells in humoral immune reactions and the effector cells in cell-mediated immune responses such as delayed cutaneous reactions to protein antigens; homograft rejection; and the immune response to fungi, facultative intracellular bacteria, and some viruses. All of these functions are carried out by lymphocytes circulating in the blood and lymph or residing in lymph nodes, spleen, and the connective tissues of the body. The vast majority of the lymphocytes in the thymus are still immature and incapable of participating in immune reactions, but they become functionally competent by the time they leave this organ.

In the past decade, a great deal has been learned about maturation of T-lymphocytes in the thymus. Their stem cells are carried in the blood from the yolk sac or embryonic liver and are induced to emigrate into the parenchyma of the thymus by a chemotactic peptide, *thymotaxin,* secreted by subcapsular reticular cells. Early in their differentiation, in the outer cortex, lymphocytes express different surface molecules that make it possible to identify several subsets by using specific antibodies to those surface markers. The fate of two of these, designated CD-4 and CD-8, has been most thoroughly worked out. The cells also acquire surface molecules of the major histocompatibility complex (MHC) that are involved in cell interaction in immune responses. Lymphocytes of the CD-8 phenotype bear class-I MHC molecules which are present on all cells throughout the body. T-lymphocytes of the CD-4 phenotype bear MHC class-II molecules that are found primarily on cells of the immune system. They serve as helper cells in immune responses. It is of current interest that it is these cells that are the targets of HIV type-I virus. The glycoprotein of the viral envelope binds to the cell surface protein CD-4. The resulting loss of this population of helper cells is largely responsible for the subsequent development of *acquired immune deficiency syndrome* (AIDS).

In addition to acquiring these surface marker molecules in the course of their differentiation in the thymus, the T-cells synthesize receptors for recognition of foreign antigens. These consist of two chains (α and β) that determine both the antigen- and the MHC-specificity of the receptor. In preparation for synthesis of receptors, the genes for the α- and β-chains undergo extensive rearrangement that results in the expression of a great variety of sequences in the receptor chains of the lymphocyte population. Those cells which, by chance, have chains that recognize and react to self-MHC, undergo apoptosis. This results in self-tolerance and leaves in the thymus only those T-cells capable of responding to antigen in association with non-self MHC. This so-called *negative selection* explains the very large numbers of immature lymphocytes (>90%) that die in the cortex of the thymus. A *positive selection* is achieved by the clonal expansion of those cells bearing receptors for non-self and it is these that are released into the bloodstream as mature CD-8 T-lymphocytes.

To recapitulate, maturation of thymocytes takes place in an orderly sequence of steps: (1) migration of T-cell precursors into the cortex of the thymus; (2) acquisition of distinctive surface markers and MHC class specificity; (3) gene segment rearrangement to create diversity in the chains of the receptor; (4) synthesis of T-cell receptors and insertion into the membrane; (5) negative selection involving elimination of self-reactive cells; (6) positive selection by clonal expansion of cells capable of reacting to non-self; (7) release of immunocompetent T-lymphocytes. This succession of events in T-cell differentiation is dependent on a special microenvironment within the thymus created by the resident nonlymphoid cell types. The respective contributions of these several cell types has been difficult to study, owing to the complex architecture of the thymus but it is known that stromal epithelial cells secrete cytokines (Il-1 and Il-4) that influence differentiation of the lymphocytes. The macrophages are also capable of secreting a variety of cytokines (Il-1, Il-2, Il-4, TNF) that may influence T-cell maturation and clonal proliferation.

The epithelial cells also secrete several peptides that have been interpreted as "thymic hormones." The function of these peptides is still poorly understood and earlier claims that they are hormones released into the bloodstream has not been substantiated. It seems more likely that they mediate short-range interactions within the thymus. One of these, *thymulin*, is reported to bind avidly to receptors on immature lymphocytes and to induce synthesis of T-cell surface markers in vitro. It may, therefore, have a similar role in the development of the different subsets of immature lymphocytes in vivo. *Thymic humoral factor* is said to be essential for differentiation and clonal expansion of T-lymphocytes.

Thymopoietin is also believed to promote thymocyte differentiation, but it may have other functions not directly related to the immune system. It has been found to bind with high affinity to acetylcholine receptors and is suspected of being involved in the pathogenesis of myasthenia gravis, a neuromuscular disorder characterized by extreme muscular weakness. This condition has long been attributed to an autoimmune response resulting in antibodies to acetylcholine receptors thereby reducing the number available for muscle excitation. An alternative hypothesis, now in favor, suggests that the benign tumor of the thymus (thymoma) and the thymic hyperplasia, often associated with this disorder, result in hypersecretion of thymopoietin which binds to ACh-receptors, impairing ACh-mediated transmission at the neuromuscular junctions. If this is confirmed, it would indicate that this thymic hormone is released into the circulation.

Another thymic peptide, *thymosin-1*, has been localized by immunocytochemical methods in subcapsular epithelial cells and in cells around Hassall's corpuscles in the medulla. Various immunomodulatory effects have been attributed to it on the basis of in vitro experiments. Doubt has now been cast on the functions assigned to it by a recent study showing that it occurs in vivo as a larger molecule *prothymosin* which appears to serve as a signaling peptide targeted at the nucleus. It is not confined to the thymus and, although it may have a role in DNA replication, there is no evidence that it is released from the cell and, therefore, probably has no paracrine effect in the thymus.

Although there is little evidence for distant effects of thymic hormones, the secretions of other endocrine glands do have an influence on the thymus. Adrenal and gonadal steroids administered in excess cause a significant diminution in the population of thymocytes in the cortex and adrenalectomy or gonadectomy are followed by an increase in the weight of the thymus. Thyroxin administration results in hypertrophy of epithelial cells and an increase in thymulin secretion. Somatostatin (somatotrophin release inhibiting hormone) was originally isolated from the hypothalamus and, until recently, was believed to be limited in its function to regulation of growth hormone secretion by the pituitary. It has now been shown to influence cells of the immune system. Receptors for the hormone have been found on lymphocytes and monocytes and it has been detected in low concentration in the spleen, thymus, and bursa of Fabricius. In the thymus, it has been localized, by immunostaining, to clusters of cells at the corticomedullary junction and in the medulla. Its physiological significance in this and other lymphoid organs is not known.

BIBLIOGRAPHY

Abe, K. and T. Ito. 1970. Fine structure of small lymphocytes in the thymus of the mouse: qualitative and quantitative analysis by electron microscopy. Z. Zellforsch. 110:321.

Aquila, M.C., W.L. Dees, W.E. Haensly, and S.M. McCann. 1991. Evidence that somatostain is localized and synthesized in lymphoid organs. Proc. Nat. Acad. Sci. USA 88:11485.

Bach, J.F. and M. Dardeene. 1973. Studies on thymus products. II. Demonstration and characterization of a circulating thymic hormone. Immunology 25:353.

Bennaceraf, B. and M.I. Greene. 1982. The thymus, transplantation and immunity. *In* B. Bennaceraf, ed. Immunogenetics and Immune Regulation. Milano, Masson.

van Bleek, G.M. and S.G. Nathanson. 1991. Structure of the antigen-binding groove of major histocompatability complex class I molecules determines specific selection of self-peptides. Proc. Soc. Nat. Acad. Sci. USA 88:11032.

Blomgren, H. and B. Anderson. 1969. Evidence for a small pool of immunocompetent cells in the mouse thymus. Exp. Cell Res. 57:185.

Cantor, H. and E. Boyse. 1977. Lymphocytes as models for the study of mammalian cellular differentiation. Immunol. Rev. 33:105.

Cantor, H., M.A. Mandel, and R. Asofsky. 1970. Studies of thoracic duct lymphocytes of mice. II. A quantitative comparison of the capacity of thoracic duct lymphocytes and other lymphoid cells to induce graft-versus-host reactions. J. Immunol. 104:409.

Claman, H.N. and F.H. Brunstetter. 1968. The response of cultured human thymus cells to phytohemagglutinin. J. Immunol. 104:409.

Claman, H.N. and F.H. Brunstetter. 1968. Effects of antilymphocyte serum and phytohemmaglutinin upon cultures of human thymus and peripheral blood lymphoid cells. I. Morphologic and biochemical studies of the thymus and blood lymphoid cells. Lab. Investig. 18:757.

Clark, S.L. Jr. 1963. The thymus in mice of strain 129/J studied with the electron microscope. Am. J. Anat. 112:1.

Clark, S.J. 1968. Incorporation of sulfate by the mouse thymus: its relation to secretion by medullary epithelial cells and to thymic lymphopoiesis. J. Exp. Med. 128:927.

Cohen, M.W., G.J. Thorbecke, G.M. Hochwald, and E.B. Jacobson. 1963. Induction of graft-versus-host reaction in newborn mice by injection of adult or newborn homologous thymus cells. Proc. Soc. Exp. Biol. Med. 114:242.

Colley, D.G., A. Malakian, and B.H. Waxman. 1970. Cellular differentiation in the thymus. II. Thymus specific antigens in rat thymus and peripheral lymphoid cells. J. Immunol. 104:585.

Colley, D.G., A.Y. Shih Wu, and B.H. Wazman. 1970. Cellular differentiation in the thymus. III. Surface properties of rat thymus and lymph node cells separated on density gradients. J. Exp. Med. 132:1107.

Dandenne, M. and J.F. Bach. 1973. Studies on thymus products. I. Modification of rosette-forming cells by thymic extracts. Determination of the target RFC subpopulation. Immunol. 25:343.

Davies, A.J., E. Leuchars, V. Wallis, R. Marchant, and E.V. Elliott. 1967. The failure of thymus-derived cells to produce antibody. Transplantation 5:222.

Defendi, V. and D. Metcalf. 1964. The Thymus. Wistar Institute Symposium, Monograph 2. Philadelphia, Wistar Institute Press.

Ernstrom, U. and B. Larsen. 1969. Thymic export of lymphocytes 3 days after labelling with tritiated thymidine. Nature 222:279.

Ford, W.L. and J.L. Gowans. 1969. The traffic of lymphocytes. Semin. Hematol. 6:67.

Goldschneider, I. and D.D. McGregor. 1968. Migration of lymphocytes and thymocytes in the rat. I. The route of migration from blood to spleen and lymph nodes. J. Exp. Med. 127:155.

von Gaudecker, B. and H.K. Muller-Hermekinck. 1980. Ontogeny and organization of the stationary nonlymphoid cells in the human thymus. Cell. Tissue Res. 207:287.

von Gaudecker, B. 1991. Functional histology of the human thymus. Anat. Embryol. 183:1.

Good, R.A. and A.E. Gabrielson, eds. 1964. The Thymus in Immunobiology. New York, Harper and Row.

Haelst, U. van. 1967. Light and electron microscopic study of the normal and pathological thymus of the rat. I. The normal thymus. Z. Zellforsch. 77:534.

Haynes, B.F. 1984. The human thymic microenvironment. Adv. Immunol. 36:87.

Henkart, P.A. 1985. Mechanism of lymphocyte cytotoxicity. Annu. Rev. Immunol. 3:31.

Imhof, B.A., M.A. Daegnier, B. Bauvois, D. Dunon, and J. Thiery. 1989. Properties of pre-T cells and their chemotactic migration to the thymus. Thymus Update 2:3.

Ishidate, M. and D. Metcalf. 1963. The pattern of lymphopoiesis in the mouse thymus after cortisone administration or adrenalectomy. Austr. J. Exp. Biol. Med. Sci. 4:637.

Izard, J. 1966. Ultrastructure of the thymic reticulum in guinea pig. Cytological aspects of the problem of thymic secretion. Anat. Rec. 155:117.

Kendall, M.D. 1991. Functional anatomy of the thymic microenvironment. J. Anat. 177:1.

Leckband, E. and E.A. Boyse. 1971. Immunocompetent cells among mouse thymocytes: a minor population. Science 172:1258.

Lundin, P.M. and U. Schelin. 1965. Ultrastructure of the rat thymus. Acta Pathol. Microbiol. Scand. 65:379.

Mandel, T. 1968. The development and structure of Hassall's corpuscles in the guinea pig. Z. Zellforsch. 89:180.

Mandel, T. 1968. Ultrastructure of epithelial cells in the cortex of guinea pig thymus. Z. Zellforsch. 92:159.

Miller, H.C., S.K. Schmiege, and A. Rule. 1973. Production of functional T cells after treatment of bone marrow with thymic factor. J. Immunol. 11:1005.

Miller, J.F. and D. Osoba. 1967. Current concepts of the immunological function of the thymus. Physiol. Rev. 47:437.

Mitchell, G.F. and J.F. Miller. 1968. Immunological activity of thymus and thoracic duct lymphocytes. Proc. Nat. Acad. Sci. USA 59:296.

Moore, M.A.S. and J.J.T. Owen. 1967. Experimental studies on the development of the thymus. J. Exp. Med. 126:715.

Murray, R.G., A. Murray, and A. Pizzo. 1965. The fine structure of the thymocytes of young rats. Anat. Rec. 151:17.

Order, S.E. and B.H. Waxman. 1969. Cellular differentiation in the thymus. Changes in size, antigenic character, and stem cell function of thymocytes during thymus repopulation following radiation. Transplantation 8:783.

Owen, J.J.T. and M.C. Raff. 1970. Studies on the differentiation of thymus-derived lymphocytes. J. Exp. Med. 132:1216.

Owen, J.J.T. and M.A. Ritter. 1969. Tissue interactions in the development of thymus lymphocytes. J. Exp. Med. 129:431.

Persechini, P.M., J.D.E. Young, and W. Almers. 1990. Membrane channel formation by the lymphocyte pore-forming protein: Comparison between susceptible and resistant target cells. J. Cell Biol. 110:2109.

Raviola, E. and M.J. Karnovsky. 1972. Evidence for a blood-thymus barrier using electron opaque tracers. J. Exp. Med. 136:466.

Raviola, E. and G. Raviola. 1967. Striated muscle cells in the thymus of reptiles and birds: an electron microscope study. Am. J. Anat. 121:623.

Ritter, M.A., C.A. Sauvage, and S.F. Cotmore. 1981. The human thymus microenvironment. In vitro identification of thymic nurse cells and other antigenically-distinct subpopulations of epithelial cells. Immunology 44:439.

Sainte-Marie, G. and F.S. Peng. 1971. Emigration of thymocytes from the thymus; a review and study of the problem. Rev. Can. Biol. 30:51.

Sanel, F.T. 1967. Ultrastructure of differentiating cells during thymus histogenesis. Z. Zellforsch. 83:8.

Small, M. and N. Trainin. 1971. Contributions of a thymic humoral factor to the development of an immunologically competent population from cells of mouse bone marrow. J. Exp. Med. 134:786.

Warner, N.L. 1964. The immunological role of different lymphoid organs in the chicken. II. Immunological competence of thymic cell suspensions. Austr. J. Exp. Biol. Med. Sci. 42:401.

Weber, W.T. 1966. Difference between medullary and cortical thymic lymphocytes of the pig in their response to phytohemagglutinins. J. Cell Physiol. 68:117.

Wijngaert, Van de, P., M.D. Kendall, H.J. Schuurman, L.H. Rademakers, and L. Kater. 1984. Heterogeneity of epithelial cells in the human thymus: An ultrastructure study. Cell Tissue Res. 237:227.

Weissman, I.L. 1967. Thymus cell migration. J. Exp. Med. 126:291.

Williams, R.N., A.D. Chanana, E.P. Cronkite, and B.H.

Waxman. 1971. Antigenic markers on cells leaving the calf thymus by way of the efferent lymph and venous blood. J. Immunol. 106:1143.
Winkelstein, A. and C.G. Craddock. 1967. Comparative response of normal human thymus and lymph node cells to phytohemagglutinins in culture. Blood 29:594.
Wolstenholme, G.E.W. and R. Porter, eds. 1966. The Thymus, Experimental and Clinical Studies. Ciba Foundation Symposium. Boston, Little and Brown, Co.

15
LYMPH NODES

ELIO RAVIOLA

Lymph nodes are small organs occurring in series along the course of lymphatic vessels. Their parenchyma consists of a highly organized accumulation of lymphoid tissue, which recognizes antigenic materials in the lymph that percolates through the node and initiates a specific immune reaction against them. Lymph nodes also contain many macrophages which clear the lymph of invading microorganisms and other particulate matter.

Large numbers of lymph nodes occur in groups scattered throughout the prevertebral region, along large blood vessels in the thoracic and abdominal cavities, between the leaves of the mesentery, and in the loose connective tissue of the neck, axilla, and groin. They are commonly ovoid or reniform in shape and 3–25 mm in diameter with a slight indentation, the *hilus*, where blood vessels enter and leave the organ. In most mammals, as the *afferent lymphatic vessels* approach the node, they give rise to a number of small branches that enter the node at multiple sites on its convex surface (Fig. 15–1). A smaller number of *efferent lymphatic vessels* leave the node at the hilus. The afferent vessels are provided with valves with the free edge of the cusps toward the node, whereas the valve cusps of the efferent lymphatics point away from the hilus. This arrangement of valves ensures unidirectional flow through the node.

The general organization of lymph nodes is much the same from species to species. Within the same species, there is considerable variation in the appearance of lymph nodes depending on their state of activity. In a healthy subject, the histological organization and cell population of each lymph node reflect both the background activity of the immune system as a whole and the local response of the node to small amounts of antigen reaching it from the region of the body drained by its afferent lymphatics. Lymph nodes, therefore, exhibit marked differences depending on their location in the body. A small unstimulated node in an extremity will have an appearance quite different from that of a large mesenteric lymph node which is continuously receiving a variety of antigens from the contents of the intestines. If bacteria, or a high dose of any other foreign substance, is injected subcutaneously, the lymphoid tissue of the nodes draining the site of injection undergo profound changes typical of an acute primary or secondary immune response.

HISTOLOGICAL ORGANIZATION

A lymph node consists of an encapsulated mass of lymphoid tissue traversed by specialized lymph vessels called *lymphatic sinuses* (Figs. 15–1 and 15–2). Its connective tissue framework consists of a *capsule* which invests the whole organ but which is greatly thickened at the hilus. A variable number of branching connective tissue *trabeculae* extend inward from the capsule into the parenchyma of the node. Between the trabeculae, the lymphoid tissue is supported by a tridimensional network of reticular fibers and associated reticular cells. The meshes of this network are filled with lymphocytes, plasma cells, and macrophages. The afferent lymphatics are continuous with a *subcapsular sinus,* a narrow lymph-filled space immediately beneath the capsule. From there, the lymph flows inward through narrow *cortical sinuses* and then to *medullary sinuses* that carry the lymph to the *efferent lymphatics* draining the node.

Viewed under low magnification, the sectioned lymph node is seen to have an outer, densely staining *cortex* and an inner paler *medulla.* The difference in appearance of these two regions is due, in part, to differences in the number, diameter, and arrangement of the lymph sinuses, but is also due to a somewhat higher concentration of lymphocytes in

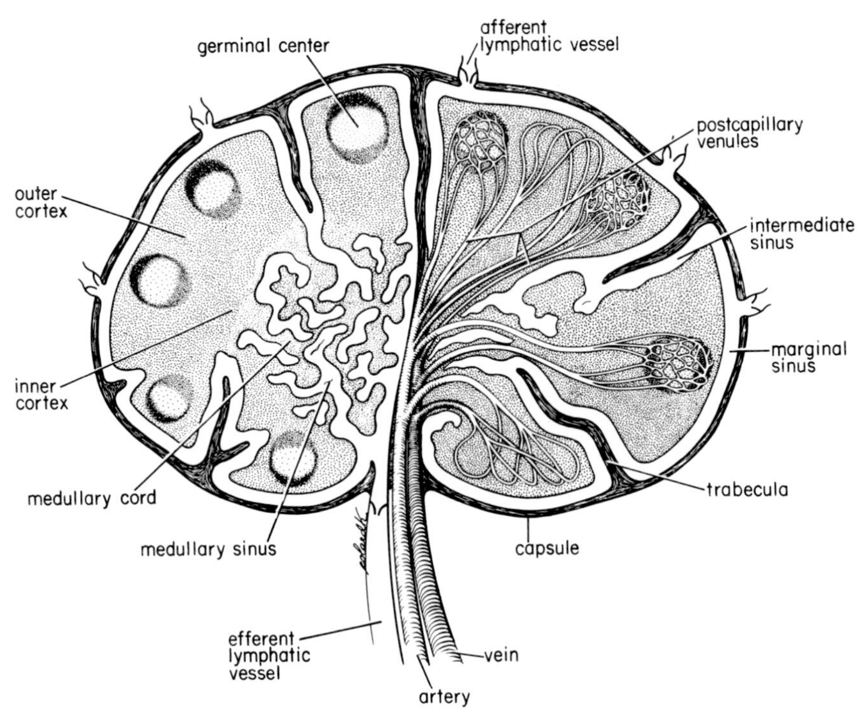

Figure 15–1. Diagram of the organization of a lymph node, with the parenchyma depicted on the left, and the blood supply on the right.

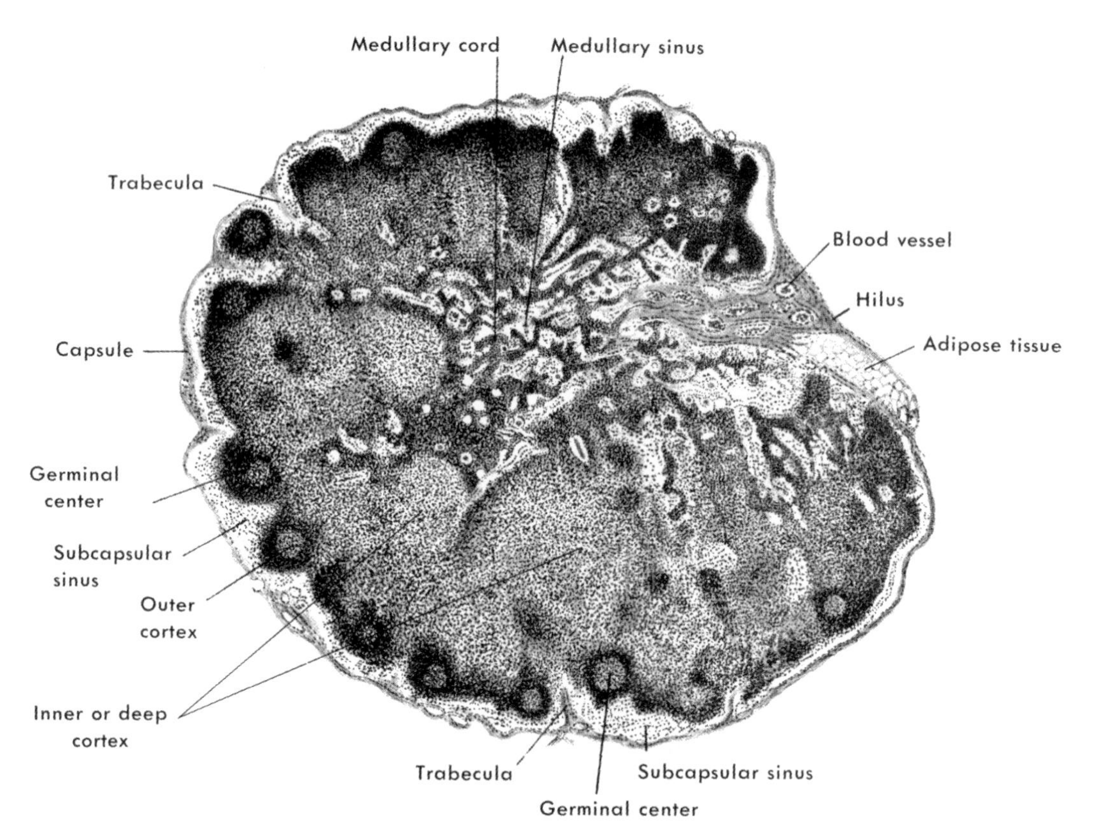

Figure 15–2. Drawing of a section through a small human lymph node. (Redrawn and slightly modified from Sobotta. Sobotta, J. Atlas of Human Anatomy Vol. II. G.E. Stechert & Co., New York, 1936.)

the cortex. Lymphocytes occupy all of the spaces within a *reticulum* of reticular fibers and reticular cells that make up the stroma of the organ. The medulla consists of many lymphatic vessels and medullary sinuses occupied by lymphocytes, macrophages, and plasma cells. The relative amounts of cortical and medullary tissue and their distribution vary considerably. The nodes in the abdominal cavity are especially rich in medullary substance. The cortex in some nodes may surround the medulla completely, but in others, the medullary tissue may border directly on the capsule for long distances. In large peripheral lymph nodes, trabeculae extending inward from the cortex are prominent, but in small nodes they are thin and often interrupted. Nodes deeper in the body, as in the abdominal cavity, have a relatively poor development of trabeculae and the cortex appears as a continuous mass of closely packed lymphoid cells.

LYMPH SINUSES

The afferent lymphatic vessels approach the convex surface of the node, traverse its capsule obliquely, and open into the *marginal* or *subcapsular sinus*. This is not a cylindrical vessel but an inverted bowl-shaped cavity which separates the capsule from the cortical parenchyma. It is traversed by many slender strands of collagen fibers of varying orientation. At the hilus, the subcapsular sinus communicates with the efferent lymph vessels. Arising from the marginal sinus are radially oriented *intermediate* or *cortical sinuses* which penetrate the cortical parenchyma, usually following along the similarly oriented trabeculae. These continue into the medulla as *medullary sinuses*—large, tortuous, irregular channels that branch and anastomose repeatedly, thus subdividing the lymphoid parenchyma into an number of *medullary cords* (Figs. 15–2 and 15–3B). The si-

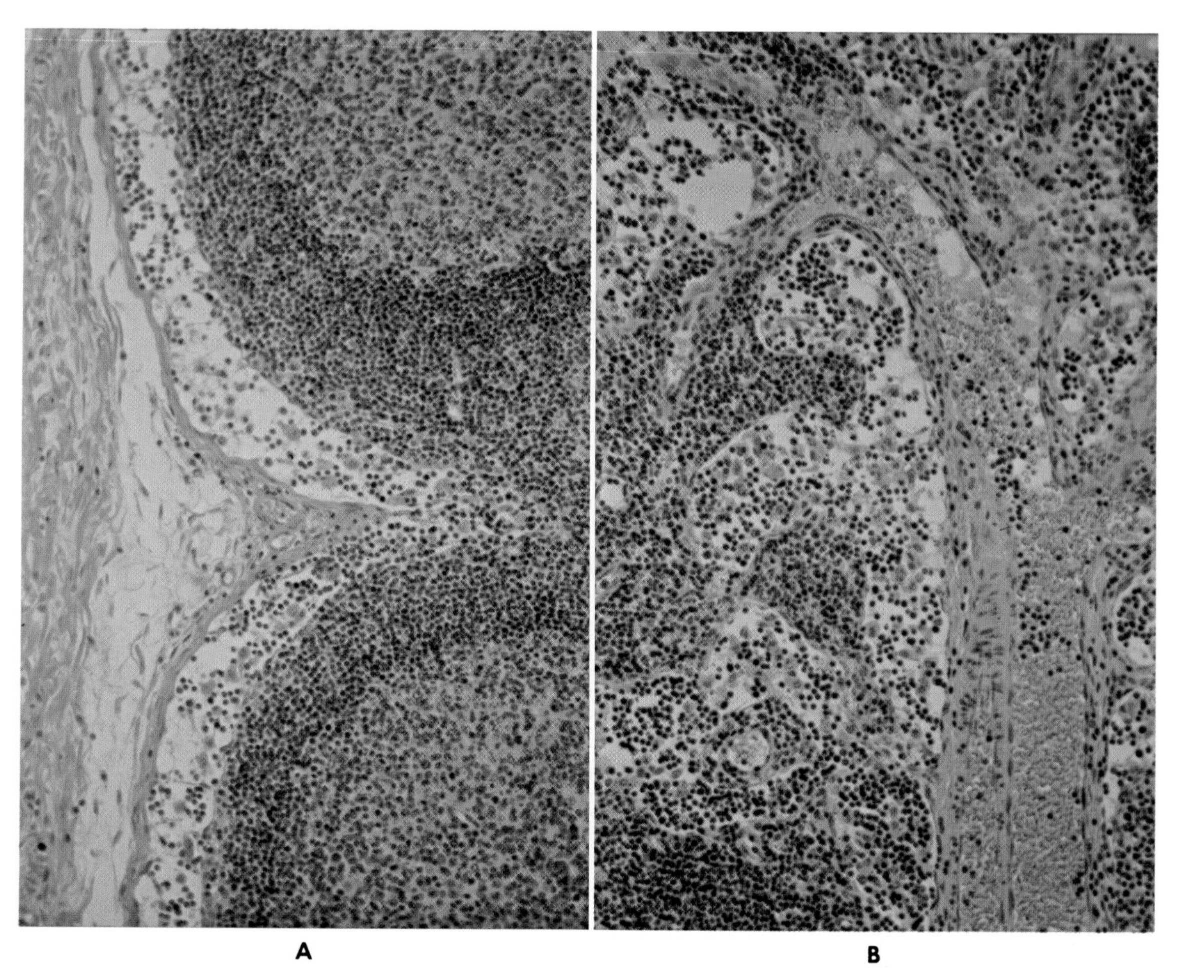

Figure 15–3. Histological sections of a mesenteric lymph node of the dog. (A) Capsule, marginal sinus, and part of two germinal centers; (B) medullary cords and sinuses. At the right is a trabecula containing a small artery and vein. The vein receives tributaries from neighboring medullary cords.

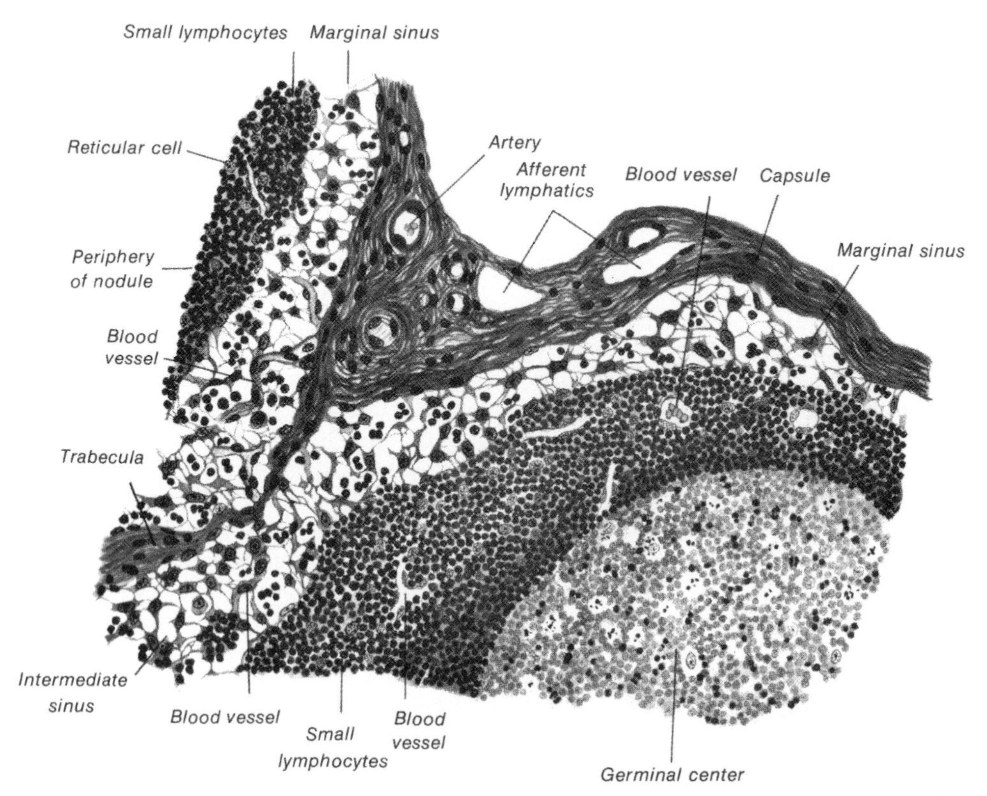

Figure 15–4. Diagram of the marginal sinus of a lymph node, showing the branching interconnected cells that cross the lumen. (After A.A. Maximov.) Sobotta, J. Atlas of Human Anatomy Vol. II. G.E. Stechert & Co., New York, 1936.

nuses of the medulla are confluent with the marginal sinus at the hilus near where it penetrates the capsule to join the efferent lymphatics.

Examined with the scanning electron microscope, the sinuses appear as channels lined by a layer of attenuated squamous cells, with the lumen bridged by a meshwork of stellate reticular cells connected to each other and to the walls of the sinus via slender cell processes (Figs. 15–4 and 15–5). Projecting into the lumen from the wall of the sinus and from the network of stellate cells are rounded macrophages that are covered with microvilli and thin undulant cell processes. Also present are lymphocytes, free in the lumen. The supporting framework of the sinuses is a layer of reticular fibers continuous with the parenchymal reticulum. No basal lamina intervenes between these reticular fibers and the cells lining the sinuses. The reticular fibers that traverse the lumen are not directly exposed to the lymph but are completely invested by the intraluminal stellate cells, and occupy deep invaginations of their plasmalemma.

The wall of the sinuses is freely permeable to the constituents of the lymph and is frequently crossed by wandering cells which move freely to-and-fro between the lymph and the lymphoid parenchyma. The nature and properties of the lining cells of the sinuses and those traversing their lumen have long been a subject of dispute. These cells were traditionally thought to be the same as the reticular cells of the lymphoid parenchyma and were assumed to be capable of phagocytosis. At present, it is widely believed that there are two distinct categories of cells lining the sinuses: (1) macrophages and (2) flattened or stellate cells similar to endothelial cells. The latter, like the endothelial cells of blood and lymph vessels, have inconspicuous organelles and they take up only small amounts of particulate matter by endocytosis. The macrophages are incorporated in the lining of the sinuses or adherent to the surface of the translumenal stellate cells. They lack specialized intercellular junctions and contain a complement of pleomorphic organelles and residual bodies typical of phagocytic cells. It is not clear whether the macrophages have migrated into the sinuses from the parenchyma and are permanently associated with the endothelium, or they are lymph-borne elements that take up residence in the sinus walls and acquire phagocytic properties.

The relative proportions of macrophages and endothelial cells vary in different regions of the node. The capsular wall of the marginal sinus and the wall of the intermediate sinuses that is adjacent to the collagenous trabeculae are composed exclusively of flattened endothelial cells. Their outlines are easily stained with silver nitrate. Macrophages, on the other hand, are especially numerous in the medullary sinuses, and, there, the outlines of the endothelial cells cannot be demonstrated by silver nitrate, suggesting that the membranes of adjacent cells may not be closely adherent.

The organization of the walls of the lymph sinuses is well suited to the filtering function of the lymph node. Lymph entering the node through the afferent vessels percolates through the intermediate and medullary sinuses, freely exchanging with the lymphoid parenchyma, substances in solution, particulate matter, and cells. The system of sinuses functions as a "trap" with the intraluminal strands serving as a multitude of microscopic baffles that increase the surface exposed to the lymph and facilitate the function of the macrophages deployed along the sinus walls.

CORTEX

The cortical parenchyma appears, with the light microscope, as a dense mass of lymphoid cells, traversed in places by the collagenous trabeculae and intermediate sinuses. Certain regional differentiations within the cortical parenchyma have traditionally been classified as *primary lymphoid nodules, secondary nodules,* and *diffuse lymphoid tissues.* Primary lymphoid nodules are spherical or ovoid areas of tightly packed small lymphocytes that are discernible within the continuum of lymphoid tissue comprising the cortex. Secondary nodules have a paler central zone, called the *germinal center,*

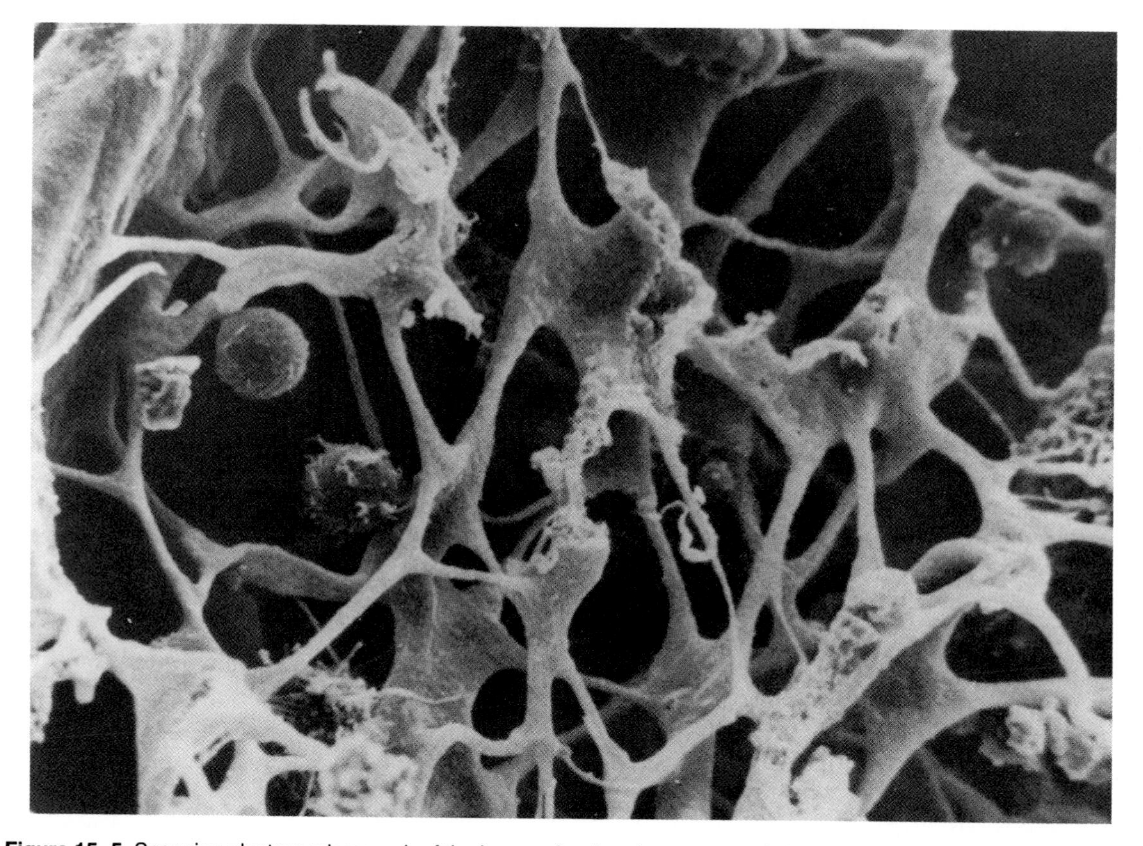

Figure 15–5. Scanning electron micrograph of the lumen of a sinus in a mesenteric lymph node of the dog. Many stellate cells form a network that serves to create turbulence in the lymph flow and provides a large surface for attachment of macrophages. On the left, there are two rounded cells in the lumen of the sinus that are probably lymphocytes. (From Fujita, T. et al. 1972. Z. Zellforsch. 133:147.)

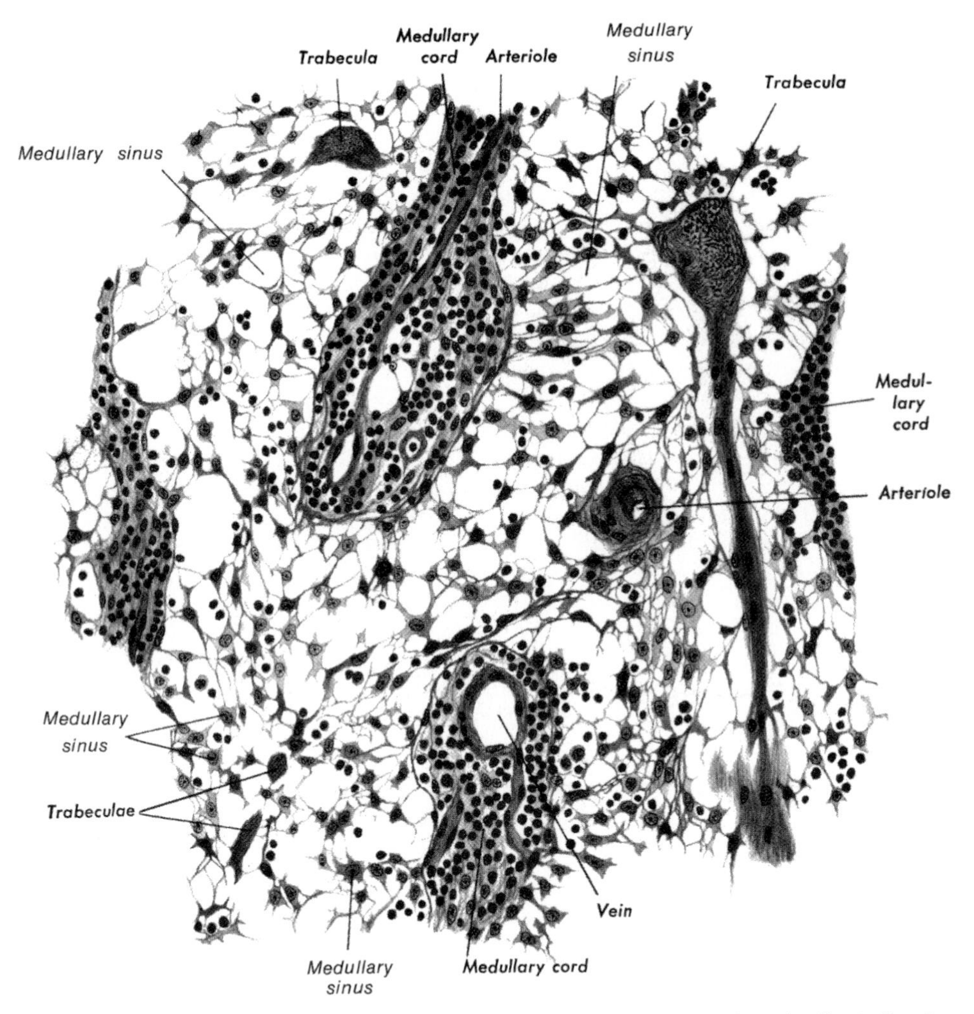

Figure 15–6. Diagrammatic representation of an area of the medulla of a dog lymph node, illustrating the medullary cords and medullary sinuses.

made up of large lymphocytes and macrophages. The paler staining of the germinal centers is due to the fact that the large lymphocytes and macrophages have more cytoplasm than small lymphocytes, and their nuclei are more euchromatic. The zone of small lymphocytes surrounding the germinal center is referred to as the *mantle* or the *crescent* if it forms a cap on the side toward the capsule. The primary and secondary nodules are usually located at the periphery of the node and together make up the bulk of the *outer cortex.* The *internodular cortex* and the *inner* or *deep cortex* consist of diffuse lymphoid tissue devoid of germinal centers (Fig. 15–7). There is no distinct boundary between the outer and inner cortices and the latter continues into the medullary cords without any discernible demarcation. The relative proportions of outer and inner cortices vary considerably in different nodes and in different functional states. Despite the absence of clear boundaries between these various zones, the distinctions are useful because the composition of the lymphocyte population differs from region to region. B-lymphocytes are concentrated in the primary nodules and T-lymphocytes are abundant in the diffuse lymphoid tissue. The germinal centers are sites of B-cell differentiation and antibody production, but they also contain some T-lymphocytes. Only the deep cortex is populated by lymphocytes of the recirculating pool and it contains specialized postcapillary venules with high endothelial cells. These vessels are the portal of entry of blood-borne lymphocytes into the lymph node.

In man and laboratory rodents, the primary

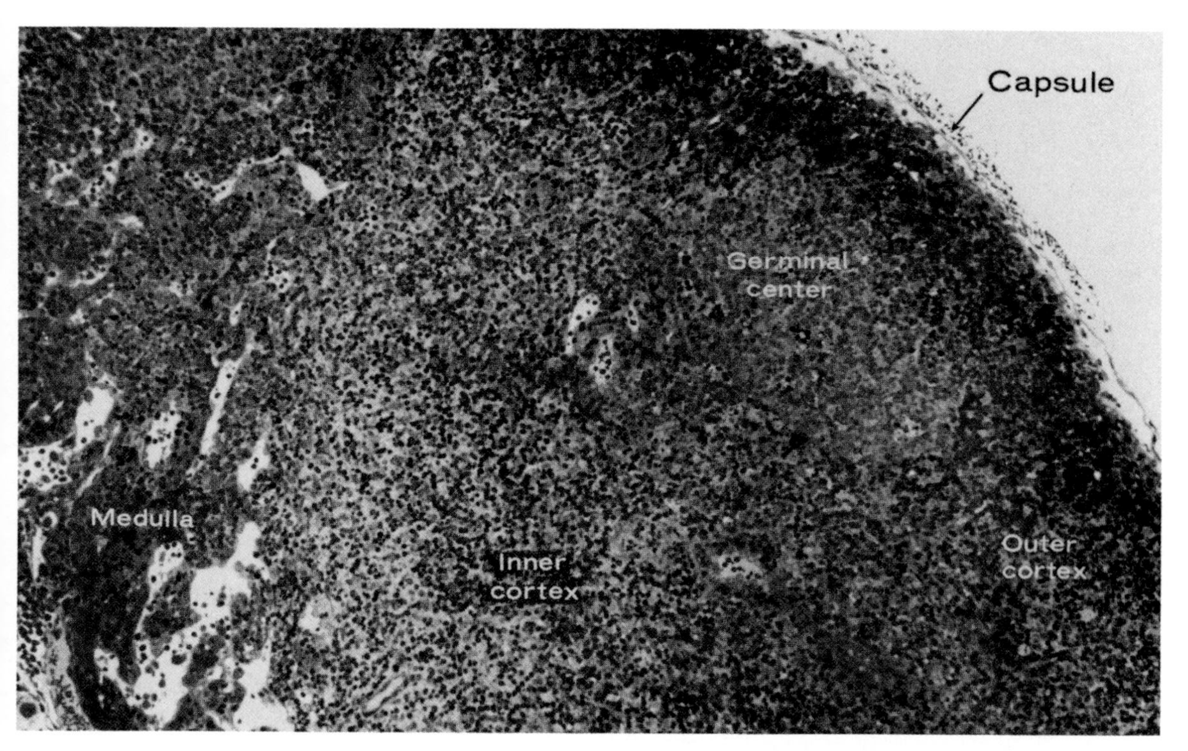

Figure 15–7. Histological section of a portion of an auricular lymph node of the mouse. Note the differing appearance of the outer and inner cortex and the medullary cords on the left. (Courtesy of G.B. Schneider.)

nodules are not clearly defined morphological entities. They consist merely of the lymphoid tissue intervening between the secondary nodules of the outer cortex. In other species, notably the ox, they appear as discrete rounded aggregates that may project slightly above the surface of the node. Germinal centers occur in variable numbers in the outer cortex, but are seldom found in the inner cortex. They are only very rarely found in the medulla. Those located in the outer cortex are polarized in such a way that their light region and cap or crescent of small lymphocytes are directed toward the marginal sinus that receives the incoming lymph (Fig. 15–8). In lymph nodes of the pig, these relationships are reversed, with the germinal centers polarized toward a central sinus which receives the incoming lymph in this species.

In the deep cortex, the cells are more loosely packed than in the outer cortex. Small lymphocytes predominate, whereas large lymphocytes, macrophages, and plasma cells are found only occasionally. Considerable interest has been directed, in recent years, to a cell type which is characterized by a euchromatic nucleus, pale cytoplasm, few organelles, and numerous surface processes that interdigitate among the surrounding lymphocytes. These are called *interdigitating cells* and are localized mainly in the deep cortex. They may contain cytoplasmic granules similar to Birbeck's granules found in the Langerhans cells of the epidermis. Cells with numerous surface ruffles, so-called *veil cells,* have been isolated from the afferent lymph. These occur in the lumen of the sinuses and may migrate across the endothelium of the marginal sinus. These cells also contain Langerhans-type cytoplasmic granules. It is speculated that these cells may arise in the bone marrow, but this remains controversial. The interdigitating cells, veil cells, and the Langerhans cells of the epidermis all bear molecules of the class-II MHC complex on their surface. T-lymphocytes cluster around them, and it is believed that they may be involved in presentation of antigen to lymphocytes.

MEDULLA

The *medullary cords* consist of aggregations of lymphoid tissue organized around small blood vessels (Fig. 15–6). They branch and anastomose freely with one another and, near

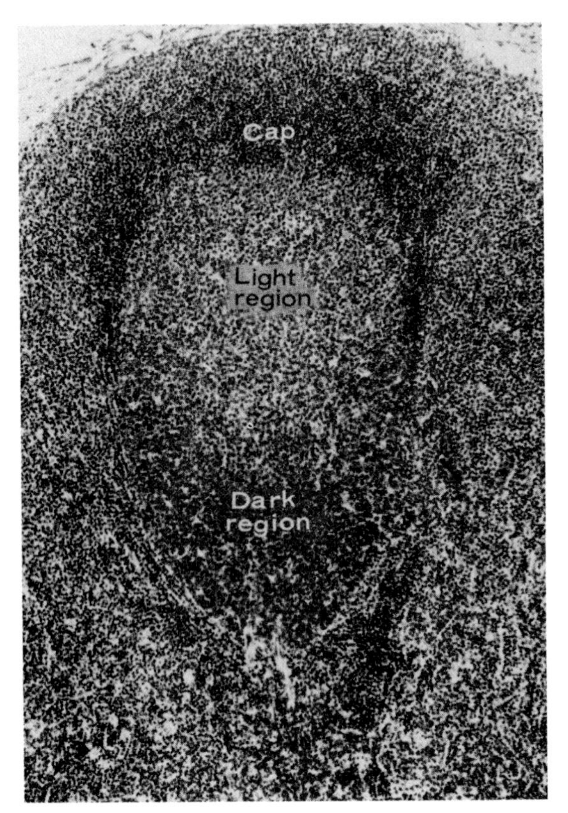

Figure 15–8. Histological section through the outer cortex of a mesenteric lymph node of the dog. Note the cap and the light and dark regions of the germinal center.

the hilus, they terminate or, more frequently, they form loops that establish continuity with other medullary cords converging upon the hilus. They are made up of small lymphocytes, plasma cells, and macrophages occupying the interstices of a rich network of reticular fibers and associated reticular cells. The parenchyma of the lymph node may normally contain small numbers of granulocytes and these may be greatly increased on stimulation or in pathological conditions.

BLOOD VESSELS AND NERVES

Nearly all of the blood vessels to the lymph node enter through the hilus, with only occasional small ones entering through the capsule elsewhere (Fig. 15–1). The larger arterial branches initially run within the trabeculae, but they soon enter the medullary cords and supply their capillary networks. Continuing along the medullary cords, the arteries reach the cortex where they supply capillary plexuses of the diffuse lymphoid tissue and those that surround the germinal centers. Special *postcapillary venules* with low cuboidal endothelium arise from these capillary plexuses and course radially through the deep cortex to enter the medullary cords. There they are continuous with small venules lined by normal squamous endothelial cells. These venules are tributaries of larger venous channels that accompany the major arterial trunks within the collagenous trabeculae of the medulla.

The postcapillary venules of the deep cortex (Fig. 15–9) are of special interest. Having taller endothelial cells and no muscular coat, their wall is traversed by great numbers of blood-borne small lymphocytes which migrate into the parenchyma by insinuating themselves between the endothelial cells. Because the emigration of lymphocytes from the blood into lymph nodes occurs at these *high-endothelial venules* and nowhere else, it was assumed that lymphocytes have receptors that recog-

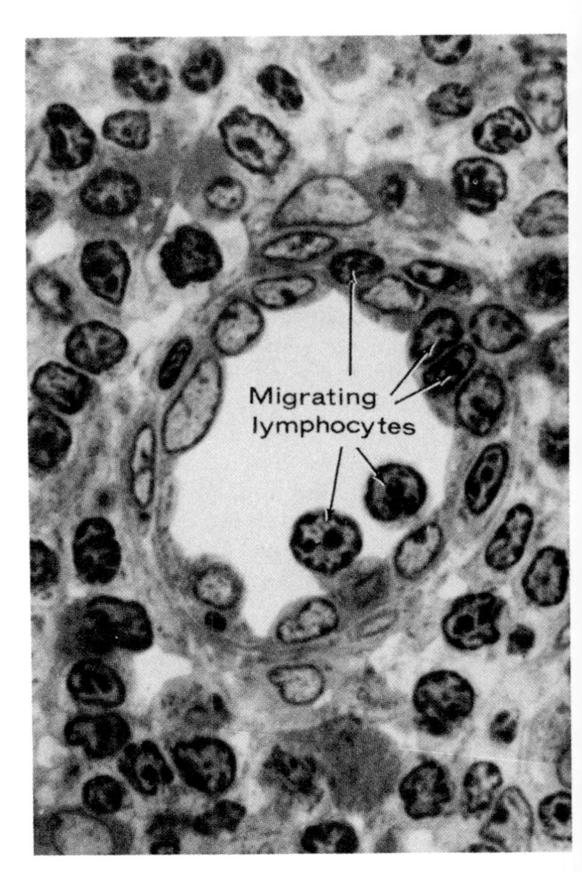

Figure 15–9. Cross section of a postcapillary venule in a popliteal lymph node of the dog. Note the thickness of the endothelium and the presence of lymphocytes migrating through it. (Courtesy of C. Compton.)

nize and bind to these endothelial cells. A glycoprotein has now been identified on the surface of virtually all lymphocytes that seems to be involved in recognition of high-endothelial cells. Similar postcapillary venules are found in the Peyer's patches of the gastrointestinal tract and in the tonsils and appendix.

Nerves enter the hilus of lymph nodes with the blood vessels forming perivascular plexuses. In the trabeculae and medullary cords, nerve fibers are observed that are independent of the vessels, but in the cortex all nerves are probably of the vasomotor type.

HISTOPHYSIOLOGY OF LYMPH NODES

Lymph nodes are highly effective filters interposed in series along the path of lymph drainage from nearly all regions of the body. One of their functions is to limit the dissemination of bacteria and malignant cells by their removal from the lymph before it reaches the blood via the thoracic duct. The delicate walls of lymphatic capillaries are easily penetrated by macromolecules, particulates, and microorganisms that have escaped destruction by macrophages and blood-borne granulocytes mobilized in the connective tissues. On reaching lymph nodes, they are filtered out and ingested by macrophages. The labyrinthine configuration and internal structure of the sinuses favor arrest of particles suspended in the lymph and facilitates their removal by macrophages in the wall of the sinuses and on the slender strands that traverse their lumen (Fig. 15–10).

The experiments involving perfusion of a lymph node with a known number of bacteria and collection of the perfusate from the efferent lymphatic, the filtration efficiency of a single node has been shown to be better than 95%. However, lymph nodes are a much less efficient barrier to lymph-borne cancer cells. These may accumulate in nodes and ultimately find their way into the efferent lymph to be carried to other sites in the body. Therefore, in surgical excision of a malignant tumor, an effort is made to prevent metastasis by removing the regional lymph nodes as well as the tumor. Viruses that are able to enter the lymphocytes of the lymph nodes are not destroyed and may actually be disseminated throughout the body by the recirculating population of lymphocytes.

In addition to their filtration and phagocytosis of invading microorganisms, lymph nodes have a very important role in the body's immunological defenses by virtue of the ability of their lymphocytes and plasma cells to generate specific antibodies. After injection of antigen into the footpad of an experimental animal, it can soon be detected around and within the lymphatic nodules in cortex of the popliteal lymph node. On interaction with antigen, lymphocytes are activated and undergo proliferation and differentiation. Large and medium-sized lymphocytes appear in the deep cortex. Plasma cells develop and antibody is synthesized and released into the efferent lymph together with lymphocytes that disseminate the humoral immune response to that antigen throughout the body. In a cellular immune response, such as that which may be initiated in the regional nodes by a skin graft, lymphocyte activation and differentiation lead to development and systemic dissemination of cytotoxic T-lymphocytes.

In unstimulated lymph nodes, the afferent lymph contains very few cells. Among these are lymphocytes, macrophages, and occasional granulocytes. The efferent lymph contains 20–75 times more cells than the afferent lymph and 98% of these are small lymphocytes. Only a very small fraction of the lymphocytes emerging in the efferent lymph arise from division of precursors in the lymph node. The vast majority (98%) are members of the recirculating pool that enter the node from the blood, through the cuboidal endothelium of the postcapillary venules in the deep cortex. As previously stated, blood-borne small lymphocytes selectively adhere to the endothelium of these vessels and migrate through the wall, whereas granulocytes and monocytes do not. Most of the recirculating cells are T-lymphocytes, and on entering the node, they localize in the deep cortex. Soon thereafter, they migrate into the sinus lymph and leave the organ through the efferent lymphatic vessels. The fate of the small component of the recirculating pool that consists of B-lymphocytes is less well understood. B-lymphocytes recirculate at a slower rate than T-cells. In small rodents, the transit time through the lymph node is 4–6 h for T-cells and somewhat longer for B-cells.

Lymph nodes are continuously seeded with new lymphocytes that have just emerged from the thymus. Neonatal thymectomy results in a deficit of small lymphocytes in the deep cortex of the lymph nodes, whereas the outer cortex and medullary cords are unaffected.

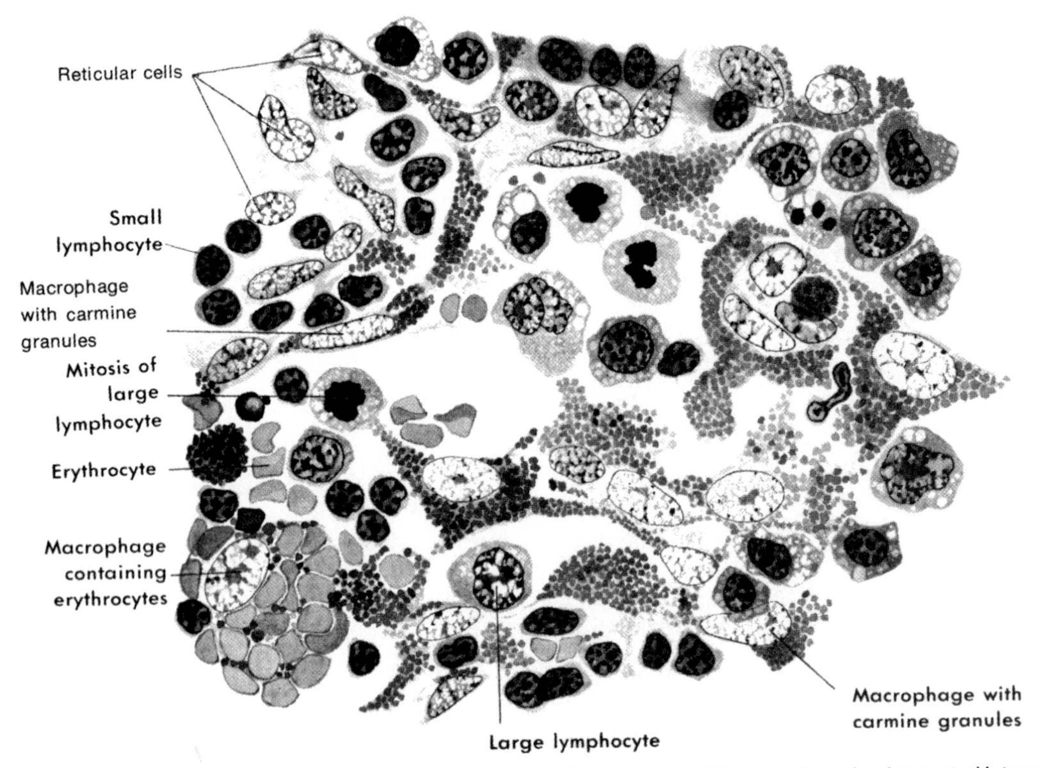

Figure 15–10. Drawing of a medullary sinus in a mesenteric lymph node of a rabbit that had received repeated intravenous injections of lithium carmine. Many macrophages in the sinus contain coarse granules of ingested lithium carmine. Small numbers of erythrocytes find their way into the sinuses. At the lower left is a macrophage filled with phagocytized erythrocytes. Sobotta, J. Atlas of Human Anatomy Vol. II. G.E. Stechert & Co., New York, 1936.

Moreover, experiments involving a careful infusion of radioactive label into the thymus verify that thymic lymphocytes specifically "home" into the deep cortex. Newly formed lymphocytes of bone marrow origin also appear to migrate continuously into unstimulated lymph nodes, but they do not seem to localize in specific regions of the organ but become distributed throughout the cortex and medulla. It is speculated that this direct inflow of lymphocytes from the thymus and bone marrow may endow the lymph node with a complement of newly formed, uncommitted elements, capable of reacting to antigens never previously experienced by the immune system.

Observations on the effects of thymectomy and the selective homing of both thymic and thoracic duct lymphocytes have given risen to the concept that the parenchyma of the lymph nodes consists of a thymus-dependent area, the deep cortex, and a marrow-dependent area which includes the medullary cords and the outer cortex with its germinal centers. This postulated compartmentation is understandable in view of the fact that the deep cortex is the major traffic area of the lymph node and the vast majority of the recirculating lymphocytes are T-lymphocytes. Less clear is the functional significance of the outer cortex and medullary cords that seem to be inhabited by a population of lymphocytes that are either sessile or only sluggishly motile, and whose function is still poorly defined.

The lymphocytopoietic activity of quiescent lymph nodes seems to be quite low, judging from the fact that 75% of the lymphocytes of the mesenteric lymph nodes of the rat are of the long-lived variety. The only sites of sustained lymphocyte proliferation in lymph nodes are the germinal centers, and the fate of the lymphocytes produced in these structures is still unclear. Of the remaining cell types of the resting node, the plasma cells of the medulla are sessile elements that either arise locally as a consequence of previous antigenic stimulation or differentiate from lymphocytes seeded throughout the body from a distant focus of immune activity. The macrophages of the lymph node parenchyma arise from blood-borne monocytes. Autoradiographic studies show that the turnover of reticular cells is extremely slow and not influenced by experimental procedures that deplete the lymphocyte population. Therefore, the earlier belief that they are precursors of lymphocytes, plasma cells, or macrophages has no experimental foundation and has been abandoned.

Until now, we have been describing the organization of the resting lymph nodes. Further insight into the histophysiology of these complex organs can be gained from studies of their response to antigen. During the first day after administration of an antigen that elicits antibody production, there is a transient increase in the number of granulocytes in the sinuses and the parenchyma. Large and medium-sized basophilic cells appear in the deep cortex, which is normally dominated by small lymphocytes. The antigen can be demonstrated in phagocytic vacuoles of the macrophages lining the sinusoids of the medulla and in intercellular clefts in the outer cortex. On days 2 and 3, granulocytes usually disappear and the large basophilic cells proliferate and greatly increase in number. The lymph node enlarges and the deep cortex seems to enlarge to extend throughout the organ. The preexisting germinal centers usually disappear and the medullary cords are greatly reduced in length or are no longer identifiable. With the electron microscope, the newly formed population of large basophilic cells appears to include lymphoblasts and transitional forms between large lymphocytes and plasma cells. The lymphoblasts have a pale nucleus with a prominent nucleolus and the cytoplasm contains a profusion of free polyribosomes. Cisternae of granular endoplasmic reticulum are very rarely found in these cells. Mitochondria are few but the Golgi complex is well developed. The transitional cells, on the other hand, display increasing amounts of granular endoplasmic reticulum, suggesting incipient differentiation into immature plasma cells. Both the lymphoblasts and the transitional cells can be shown to produce antibody.

In the days that follow, immature plasma cells with an eccentric nucleus, condensed chromatin, and large amounts of granular endoplasmic reticulum become more and more numerous. Antibody is actively synthesized at this stage and can be detected in both the efferent lymph and in the blood. Near the surface of the node, well-circumscribed nests of small and large lymphocytes appear. These probably represent early developmental stages of new germinal centers.

Toward the end of the first week after injection of antigen, the lymph node begins to revert to its normal architecture. Numerous newly formed germinal centers have appeared in the cortex, and medullary cords are again, prominent and contain abundant immature and mature plasma cells. During the second week, the number of plasma cells begins to decline and they become confined to the medullary cords. Antigen is still detectable in the node, localized both in residual bodies of the macrophages and in the intercellular clefts around the dendritic cells of the germinal centers.

Characteristic changes in the efferent lymph are associated with these events within the node. During the first 24 h following antigen administration, lymphocytes continue to enter the node from the blood, but the output of cells in the efferent lymph decreases. From 2 to 5 days after antigen injection, cells released by the node doubles because more lymphocytes are entering from the blood and are no longer retained in the node. However, lymphocytes that have been stimulated by antigen do not appear yet in the efferent lymph. After 5 days, cell output from the node declines, but the emerging population now contains a large proportion of activated lymphocytes. These are large lymphocytes having a euchromatic nucleus, prominent nucleolus, and abundant cytoplasm rich in polyribosomes. Although they are actively producing antibody, these cells have only a few cisternae of granular endoplasmic reticulum. They are motile and capable of incorporating DNA precursors into their chromatin. The remaining cells leaving the stimulated lymph node include antibody-producing small lymphocytes and immature plasma cells. The antibody-producing cells of the efferent lymph are thought to colonize successive lymph nodes along the chain. By entering the bloodstream via the thoracic duct, they may propagate the immune response throughout the body. If the efferent duct of a stimulated node is cannulated and its lymph drained off, antibody fails to appear in the blood and dissemination of the immune response is prevented. If the cells from a stimulated node are recovered from the efferent lymph, labeled radioactively in vitro, and reinfused into the afferent lymphatic of a quiescent node, they localize in the medullary cords, proliferate, and finally differentiate into plasma cells. Antibody-producing cells are present in the thoracic duct lymph. The fate of these cells has been studied after in vitro labeling and intravenous injection into a syngeneic animal. After being retained transiently in the lung and liver, they later localize in the spleen, lymph nodes, and the lymphoid structures in the lamina propria of the small intestine.

During a secondary humoral immune response, the lymph nodes undergo changes that resemble those observed following the first exposure to antigen, but they occur earlier and are much more pronounced.

When a lymph node is involved in a cellular immune response, it undergoes morphological changes that are not strikingly different from those typical of a humoral immune response. Examples of cell-mediated reactions are those that follow skin grafting or the delayed hypersensitivity induced by application to the skin of a chemical sensitizing agent. Grafting of skin from an individual of one strain to a member of another strain and, therefore, of different genetic composition (allograft) is followed by rejection of the graft. Rejection is mediated primarily by T-lymphocytes, but the exact mechanism is still not well understood. After applying such a graft, the lymph nodes draining the region become markedly enlarged and their deep cortex becomes very thick. Lymphoblasts that soon appear in this zone are actively dividing cells and their number increases rapidly, reaching a maximum toward the end of the first week. At the beginning of the second week, the number of lymphoblasts declines rapidly and a second phase of the response becomes apparent. Newly formed germinal centers appear in the outer cortex and immature and mature plasma cells become localized in the medullary cords. At this time, humoral antibody is detectable in the blood.

Shortly after the appearance of lymphoblasts in the inner cortex of the lymph nodes draining the region, lymphocytes and macrophages begin to infiltrate the skin graft. This response reaches its peak and the graft is rejected, at a time when the number of lymphoblasts in the inner cortex of the node has already begun to decline but before antibody is produced in significant amounts. The antibody response that accompanies the cellular immune reaction evidently contributes little to the rejection process. Antigens from the graft probably reach the nodes via the afferent lymph. Small lymphocytes in the inner cortex may react with the antigens and differentiate into proliferating lymphoblasts. These, in turn, give rise to lymphocytes of decreasing size, which emigrate from the regional lymph nodes and circulate in the blood to be disseminated throughout the immune system. Some of these lymphocytes are believed to invade the engrafted tissue and contribute to its destruction. The assumption that these are T-cells is supported by the observation that neonatal thymectomy prevents the appearance of lymphoblasts in the deep cortex of the regional lymph nodes in response to allogeneic transplantation, and prolongs the survival of the graft.

HEMAL NODES

In normal lymph nodes, a few erythrocytes are found. These have either entered in the afferent lymph or come from blood vessels in the node. Some of these pass with the lymph into the efferent lymphatics, but the great majority of them are phagocytized and destroyed by macrophages (Fig. 15–10). There are some nodes, however, called *hemal nodes* that have an exceptionally high content of erythrocytes. Such nodes are most numerous and have been most studied, in ruminants, especially in sheep. They probably do not occur in man. They vary from minute bodies that are scarcely noticable to nodes the size of a pea or slightly larger, and they are scattered along large blood vessels from the neck to the pelvis. They are also found near the kidneys and spleen.

Hemal nodes, in section, have a red color and a structure resembling that of lymph nodes, but the sinuses are filled with blood. They usually have no afferent or efferent lymph vessels. A single efferent lymphatic vessel has been reported in some hemal nodes of the rat. A sizable artery and vein enter and leave the hilus. Like lymph nodes, they have specialized postcapillary venules with high endothelium, and lymphocytes can be found migrating through their wall. In the pig, nodes have been described that have both lymphatics and blood vessels and the contents of both intermingle in the sinuses. These have been called *hemolymph nodes* and are considered, by some, to be intermediate between hemal nodes and lymph nodes. Other investigators regard hemal nodes as more closely associated with the vascular system than with the immune system and suggest that they may function as accessory spleens.

BIBLIOGRAPHY

Ada, G.L., G.J. Nossal, and J. Pye. 1964. Antigens in immunity. III. Distribution of iodinated antigens following injection into rats via the foot pad. Austr. J. Exp. Biol. Med. Sci. 42:295.

Anderson, A.O. and N.D. Anderson. 1976. Lymphocyte emigration from high endothelial venules in rat lymph nodes. Immunology 31:731.

Bailey, R.P. and L. Weiss. 1975. Light and electron microscopic studies of postcapillary venules in developing human fetal lymph nodes. Am. J. Anat. 143:43.

Brahim, F. and D.G. Osmond. 1973. The migration of lymphocytes from bone marrow to popliteal lymph nodes demonstrated by selective bone marrow labeling with H-thymidine in vivo. Anat. Rec. 175:737.

Cahill, R.N., H. Frost, and Z. Trinka. 1976. Effects of antigen on the migration of recirculating lymphocytes through single lymph nodes. J. Exp. Med. 143:870.

Claesson, M.H., O. Jorgensen, and C. Ropke. 1971. Light and electron microscopic studies of the paracortical postcapillary high-endothelial venules. Z. Zellforsch. 119:195.

Clark, S.J., Jr. 1962. The reticulum in lymph nodes of mice studied with the electron microscope. Am. J. Anat. 110:217.

Cohen, S., P. Vasalli, B. Benacerraf, and R.T. McCluskey. 1966. The distribution of antigenic and non-antigenic compounds within draining lymph nodes. Lab. Investig. 15:1143.

Downey, H. 1922. The structure and origin of the lymph sinuses of mammalian lymph nodes and their relations to endothelium and reticulum. Haematologica 3:431.

Drinker, C.K., M.E. Field, and H.K. Ward. 1934. The filtering capacity of lymph nodes. J. Exp. Med. 59:393.

Farr, A.G., Y. Cho, and P.P. DeBruyn. 1980. The structure of the sinus wall of the lymph node relative to its endocytic properties and transmural cell passage. Am. J. Anat. 157:265.

Ford, W.L. and J.L. Gowans. 1969. The traffic of lymphocytes. Semin. Hematol. 6:67.

Fossum, S. 1980. The architecture of rat lymph nodes. II. Lymph node compartments. Scand. J. Immunol. 12:411.

Fossum, S. 1980. The architecture of rat lymph nodes. IV. Distribution of ferritin and colloidal carbon in the draining lymph nodes after foot-pad injection. Scand. J. Immunol. 12:433.

Fujita, T., M. Miyoshi, and T. Murakami. 1972. Scanning electron microscope observations of the dog mesenteric lymph node. Z. Zellforsch. 133:147.

Gallatin, M., T.P. St. John, M. Siegelman, R. Reichert, E.C. Butcher, and I.L. Weissman. 1986. Lymphocyte homing receptors. Cell 44:673.

Gowans, J.L. and E.J. Knight. 1964. The route of recirculation of lymphocytes in the rat. Proc. Roy. Soc. London B 159:257.

Hall, J.B., B. Morris, G.D. Moreno, and M.C. Bessis. 1967. The ultrastructure and function of the cells of the lymph following antigenic stimulation. J. Exp. Med. 125:91.

Han, S.S. 1961. The ultrastructure of the mesenteric lymph node of the rat. Am. J. Anat. 109:183.

Harris, T.N., K. Hummeler, and S. Harris. 1966. Electron microscopic observations on antibody-producing lymph node cells. J. Cell. Med. 123:161.

Hay, J.B., M.J. Murphy, B. Morris, and M.C. Bessis. 1972. Quantitative studies on the proliferation and differentiation of antibody-forming cells in lymph. Am. J. Pathol. 66:1.

Leduc, E.H., A.H. Coons, and J.M. Connolly. 1955. Studies on antibody production. II. Primary and secondary responses in the popliteal lymph node of the rabbit. J. Exp. Med. 102:61.

Luc, S.C., C. Nopajaroonsri, and G.T. Simon. 1973. The architecture of the normal lymph node and hemolymph node. A scanning and transmission electron microscope study. Lab. Invest. 29:258.

Marchesi, V.T. and J.L. Gowans. 1964. The migration of lymphocytes through the endothelium of venules in lymph nodes: an electron microscope study. Proc. Roy. Soc. London B 159:283.

Millikin, P.D. 1966. Anatomy of germinal centers in human lymphoid tissue. Arch. Pathol. 82:499.

Moe, R.E. 1963. Fine structure of the reticulum and sinuses of lymph nodes. Am. J. Anat. 112:311.

Movat, H.Z. and N.V. Fernando. 1965. THe fine structure of lymphoid tissue during antibody formation. Exp. Mol. Pathol. 4:155.

Nieuwenhuis, P. and W.L. Ford. 1976. Comparative migration of T-and B-lymphocytes in the rat spleen and lymph nodes. Cell Immunol. 23:254.

Nopajaroonsri, C. and G.T. Simon. 1971. Phagocytosis of colloidal carbon in a lymph node. Am. J. Pathol. 65:25.

Nossal, G.J., A. Abbot, and J. Mitchell. 1968. Antigens in immunity. XIV. Electron microscopic radioautographic studies of antigen capture in the lymph node medulla. J. Exp. Med. 127:263.

Nossal, G.J., A. Abbot, J. Mitchell, and Z. Lummus. 1968. Antigens in immunity. XV. Ultrastructural features of antigen capture in primary and secondary lymphoid follicles. J. Exp. Med. 127:277.

Parrott, D.M., M.A. de Sousa, and J. East. 1966. Thymus-dependent areas in the lymphoid organs of neonatally thymectomized mice. J. Exp. Med. 123:191.

Sainte-Marie, G. and Y.M. Sin. 1968. Structures of the lymph node and their possible function during the immune response. Rev. Can. Biol. 27:191.

Sainte-Marie, G., F.S. Ping, and C. Bélisle. 1982. Overall architecture and pattern of lymph flow in the rat lymph node. Am. J. Anat. 164:275.

Schoefl, G.I. 1972. The migration of lymphocytes across the vascular endothelium. A reexamination. J. Exp. Med. 136:568.

Sorenson, G.D. 1960. An electron microscopic study of popliteal lymph nodes from rabbits. Am. J. Anat. 107:73.

Steinman, R.M. 1981. Dendritic cells. Transplantation 31:151.

Steinman, R.M. and M.C. Nussenzweig. 1980. Dendritic cells: features and functions. Immunol. Rev. 53:127.

Tew, J.G., G.J. Thorbecke, and R.M. Steinman. 1982. Dendritic cells in the immune response. Characteristics and recommended nomenclature. J. Reticuloendothelial Soc. 31:371.

16
SPLEEN

Elio Raviola

The spleen is an organ situated between the fundus of the stomach and the diaphragm, in the left upper quadrant of the abdominal cavity. It is elongated, has a somewhat irregular shape, and weighs about 150 g. It is invested by peritoneum and connected to the stomach, diaphragm, and left kidney by peritoneal folds called the gastrolineal, phrenicolienal, and lienorenal ligaments. The splenic blood vessels, lymphatics, and nerves are carried to it in the lienorenal ligament. The spleen serves as a complex filter interposed in the circulation to clear the blood of particulate matter and senescent blood cells. It is also concerned with immune defense against bloodborne antigens. In many animal species, but not in man, the spleen is also a hemopoietic organ involved in the formation of erythrocytes, granulocytes, and platelets. In some mammals, it acts as a reservoir of mature erythrocytes that can be added to the blood in response to unusual demands. The spleen possesses a peculiar type of blood vessels that allows the blood to come into contact with great numbers of macrophages. It also contains a large amount of lymphoid tissue that carries out its immunological functions.

HISTOLOGICAL ORGANIZATION

On the freshly sectioned surface of the spleen, elongated or rounded gray areas, 0.2–0.7 mm in diameter, are visible with the naked eye (Fig. 16–1). Together, these light areas constitute the *white pulp* of the spleen. They are scattered throughout a soft, dark-red mass, the *red pulp*. The lighter areas of white pulp, formerly called Malpighian bodies, consist of diffuse and nodular lymphoid tissue like that of the cortex of lymph nodes. The red pulp consists of irregularly shaped blood vessels of large caliber, the *venous sinuses,* together with cell-filled spaces between the sinuses which constitute the *splenic cords* (*cords of Billroth*). The color of the red pulp is due to the abundance of erythrocytes that fill the lumen of the venous sinuses and infiltrate the surrounding splenic cords.

The spleen has a collagenous *capsule* with inward extensions called *trabeculae* (Fig. 16–1). The capsule is continuous with a delicate reticular framework that occupies the interior of the organ and holds in its meshes the free cells of the splenic parenchyma. The capsule is thickened at the hilus of the organ, where it is attached to the folds of peritoneum (ligaments) through which the arteries and nerves enter, and the veins and lymphatic vessels leave the spleen.

The internal structure of the spleen and the relationships between the white pulp and the red pulp are based on the distribution of the blood vessels. The white pulp of the splenic parenchyma is organized around arteries, and the red pulp fills the interstices among the venous sinuses. The distribution and relative amount of red and white pulp differ significantly in different animal species and they change in the course of immune responses or disturbances of blood cell formation and destruction. Animal species with a large blood volume (ruminants, horse, carnivores) have scant white pulp and a robust framework of connective tissue and smooth muscle. Species with a relatively small blood volume (rabbit, laboratory rodents, man) have abundant white pulp, a less prominent connective tissue framework, and poorly developed smooth musculature.

WHITE PULP

The white pulp forms *periarterial lymphoid sheaths* (PALS) around the arteries where these leave the trabeculae to enter the parenchyma (Figs. 16–1 and 16–2). The periarterial

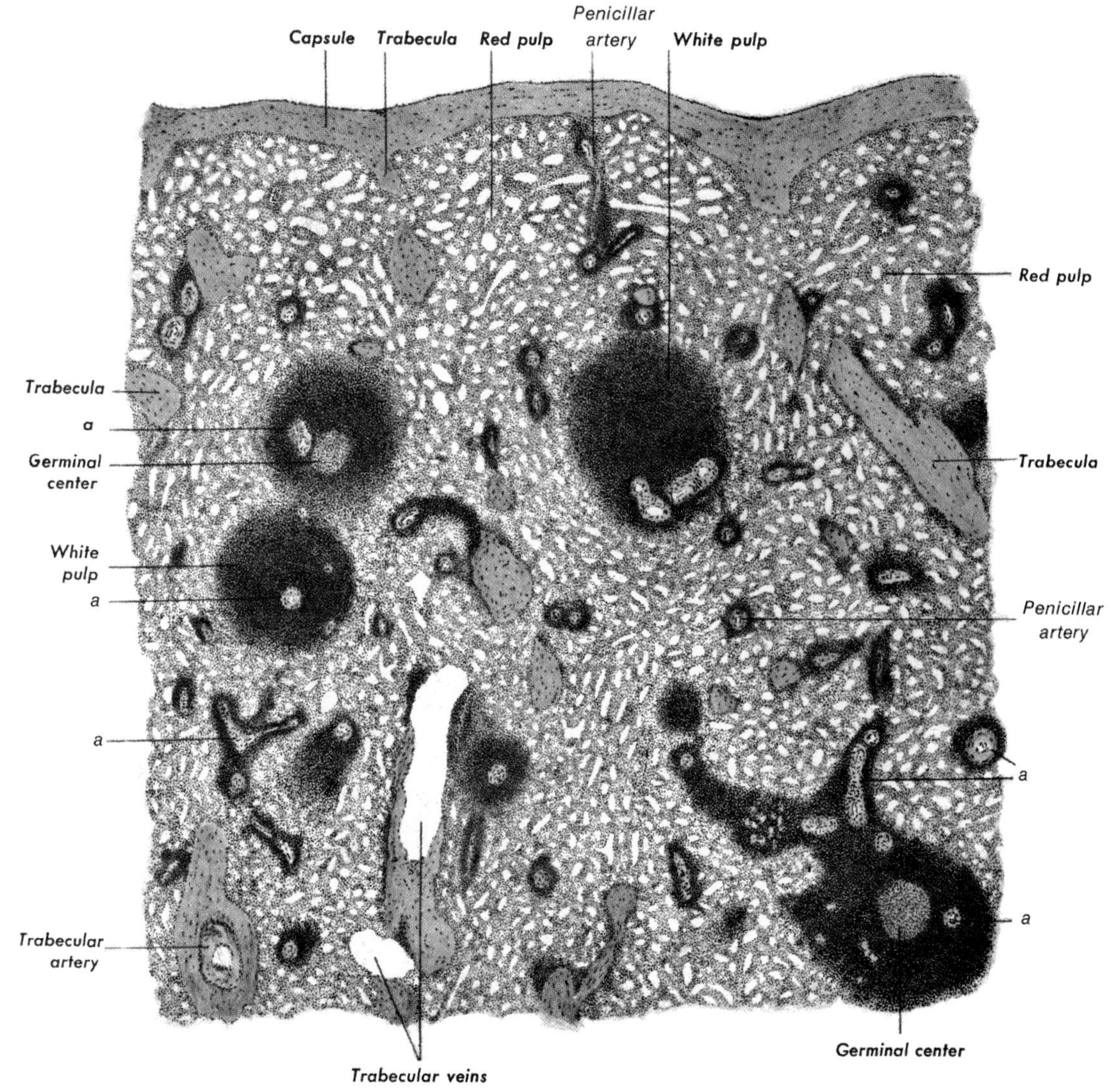

Figure 16–1. Drawing of a section of human spleen showing large dark areas representing the lymphoid tissue of the white pulp and lighter areas of red pulp.

lymphoid sheaths continue along the vessels nearly to the point where they break up into capillaries. In many places along their course, the sheaths contain germinal centers. Although both the sheaths and the germinal centers consist of lymphoid tissue they differ in their functional significance. The sheaths consist predominantly of T-lymphocytes of the recirculating pool, whereas the germinal centers are made up of B-lymphocytes. The germinal centers display the same architecture as those of the lymph nodes (see Chapter 13). They are eccentrically situated within the sheath and, when fully developed, their light region and cap of small lymphocytes are directed toward the red pulp. Their number varies in different animal species and tends to decrease progressively with age. The periarterial lymphoid sheaths, thus, have an organization similar to the cortex of the lymph nodes. They have a loose framework of reticular fibers with associated reticular cells. The meshes of this reticulum are occupied by small and medium-sized lymphocytes, sometimes associated with interdigitating cells. Plasma cells and macrophages are only occasionally found, but they increase in number toward the periphery of the sheath. In the course of immune responses to blood-borne antigens, great numbers of large lymphocytes, lymphoblasts, and immature plasma cells appear in the periarterial lymphoid sheaths and

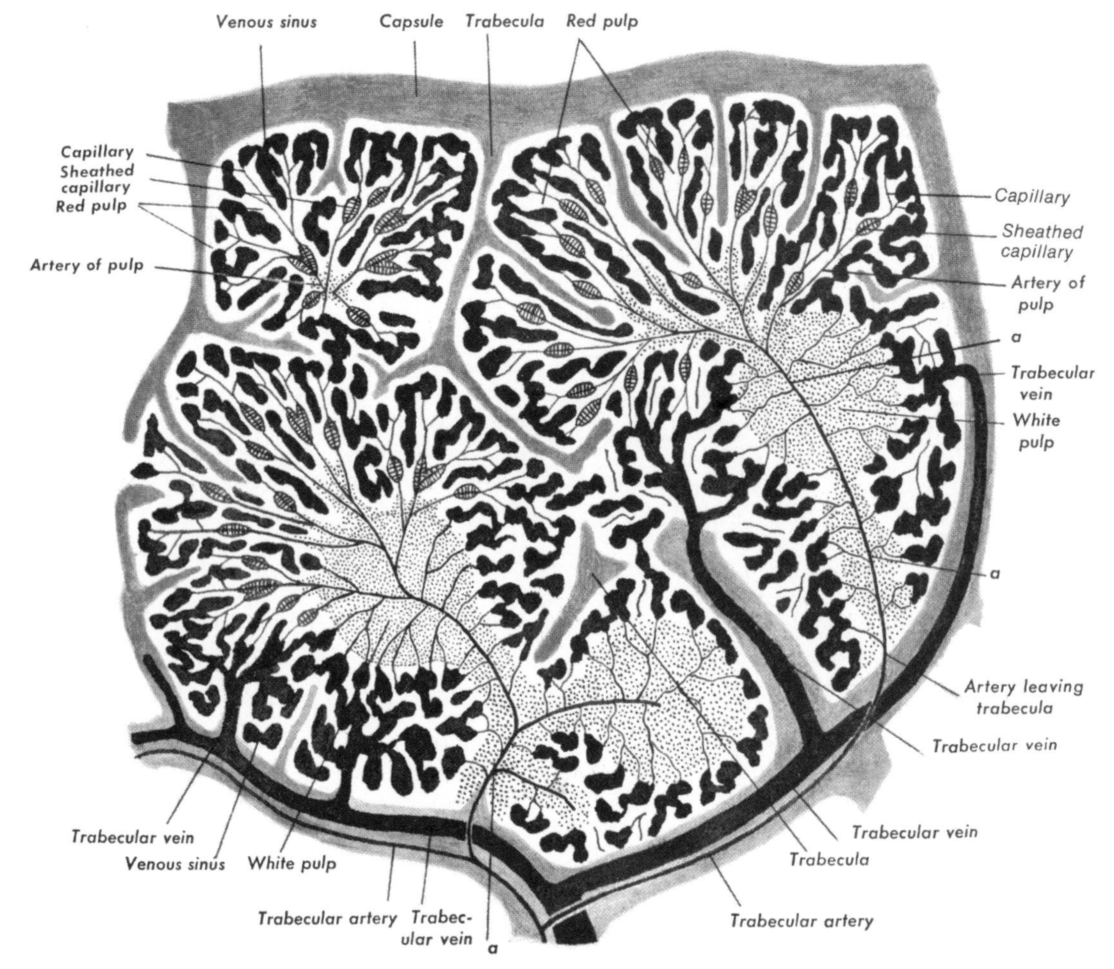

Figure 16–2. Diagram of the vascular tree of the spleen. The periarterial lymphoid sheaths of the white pulp are the stippled areas around the central arteries (a) leaving the trabeculae. A closed circulation is depicted here with the capillaries communicating with the sinuses, shown here as irregularly shaped black structures. Evidence now favors an open circulation with the capillaries opening into the interstitial spaces in the splenic cords of the red pulp.

soon become concentrated at their periphery. At the periphery of the sheath, the reticular fibers become arranged circumferentially and the flattened reticular cells associated with them form concentric layers that establish the boundary between the lymphoid tissue of the sheath and the surrounding red pulp.

Immediately peripheral to the periarterial lymphoid sheaths, there is an 80–100-μm transitional region between the white pulp and the red pulp, called the *marginal zone.* In this zone, the reticular fibers form a close network whose interstices are occupied by large numbers of small lymphocytes and plasma cells. The marginal zone receives the incoming arterial blood destined for the red pulp and is the site where blood-borne cells and particulate matter first contact the splenic parenchyma. It is here that the lymphocytes of the recirculating pool leave the blood in the venous sinuses to enter the periarterial lymphoid sheaths of the white pulp.

The artery in the axis of the periarterial sheath gives off radial branches along its course, and some of these extend beyond the boundary of the sheath to enter the marginal zone and red pulp. As the central artery diminishes in caliber toward its termination, the periarterial sheath also becomes thinner (Fig. 16–2) and loses the circumferential reticular fibers that mark its boundary. It ultimately comes to consist of a thin sleeve only a few lymphocytes in thickness. The resulting attenuated strands of white pulp, and equally thin surrounding marginal zone, then extend into the red pulp, forming so-called *bridging channels.*

RED PULP

The red pulp consists of an elaborate network of tortuous, branching, and anastomosing venous sinuses that drain into *pulp veins.* The interspaces between these sinuses are occupied by highly cellular *splenic* or *pulp cords* (Fig. 16–2). The sinuses will be discussed more fully later, with the blood vessels of the spleen. The splenic cords vary in thickness depending on the shape of the spaces between neighboring sinuses. They consist of a spongy mass of extravasated blood cells supported by a framework of reticular fibers. The reticular fibers merge with the coarser bundles of collagen fibers in the trabeculae and capsule of the spleen and with ribs of basal lamina material that support the endothelium of the venous sinusoids. The reticular fibers throughout the splenic cords are invested by stellate reticular cells. These cells are anchored to the walls of the sinuses by slender foot-like processes that are generally oriented perpendicular to the long axis of the sinuses. The meshes of the reticulum in the pulp cords are filled with great numbers of free cells, which include macrophages, a few plasma cells, and great numbers of erythrocytes and platelets (Figs. 16–3A and 16–4). With the light microscope, the macrophages are readily recognized as large rounded or irregularly shaped cells with a vesicular nucleus and abundant cytoplasm. They often contain engulfed erythrocytes, neutrophils, or platelets and they are loaded with masses of a yellowish-brown pigment that stains for iron with the Prussian blue reaction. This pigment represents the undigestible residues of phagocytized erythrocytes and other ingested material. Its iron, in the form of ferritin or hemosiderin, comes from the degradation of hemoglobin. In many mammalian species, and in the embryonic human spleen the red pulp contains groups of erythroblasts, myeloblasts, myelocytes, and megakaryocytes. In normal adult humans, these islands of hemopoietic tissue are lacking, but in certain infections, in some anemias, in leukemias, and in poisoning with blood-destroying agents, they may reappear—a condition described as *myeloid metaplasia.*

CAPSULE AND TRABECULAE

The spleen is covered on its external surface by a layer of mesothelium which is part of the general peritoneal lining of the abdominal cavity. The underlying capsule and the cylindrical or ribbon-like trabeculae that extend into the parenchyma consist of dense connective tissue, rich in elastic fibers. Its cellular elements are mainly fibroblasts. In man, rabbits, and laboratory rodents, there are few smooth muscle cells in the capsule and trabeculae, and any changes in volume of the spleen are attributable to variations in the flow of blood into the organ. In horses, ruminants, and carnivores, smooth muscle is abundant in the capsule and trabeculae, and rhythmic contraction of the spleen has been observed in these species, due apparently to contraction of the smooth muscle cells. Arteries, veins, and lymphatics are carried into the parenchyma in the trabeculae.

ARTERIES

Branches of the *splenic artery* enter the hilus of the spleen and decrease in diameter as they branch repeatedly within the connective tissue trabeculae (Fig. 16–2). They are muscular arteries with a rather loose adventitia. When they have been reduced by dichotomous branching to a diameter of about 0.2 mm, they leave the trabeculae. At this point, the adventitia is replaced by a relatively thick sheath of lymphoid tissue, and the vessel is then designated as the *central artery* of a periarterial lymphoid sheath. However, where lymphoid nodules and germinal centers occur in the sheath, the vessel may be displaced to one side, transiently losing its central position. The central artery is a small muscular artery with relatively tall endothelium and one or two layers of smooth muscle cells. Throughout its course, it gives off numerous lateral capillary branches that supply the lymphoid tissue of the sheath. The wall of these capillaries initially consists of a high endothelium, a basal lamina, and an investment of pericytes. Farther on, the endothelium becomes lower and the pericytes disappear. After coursing through the white pulp, these collateral capillaries pass into the surrounding marginal zone. Their mode of termination is uncertain.

As a central artery courses through the white pulp, its sheath of lymphoid tissue becomes progressively reduced in thickness. When the vessel reaches a diameter of 40–50 μm, it suddenly branches into several very slender vessels called *penicilli.* These radiate from their site of origin, still invested by one or two layers of lymphocytes that represent a

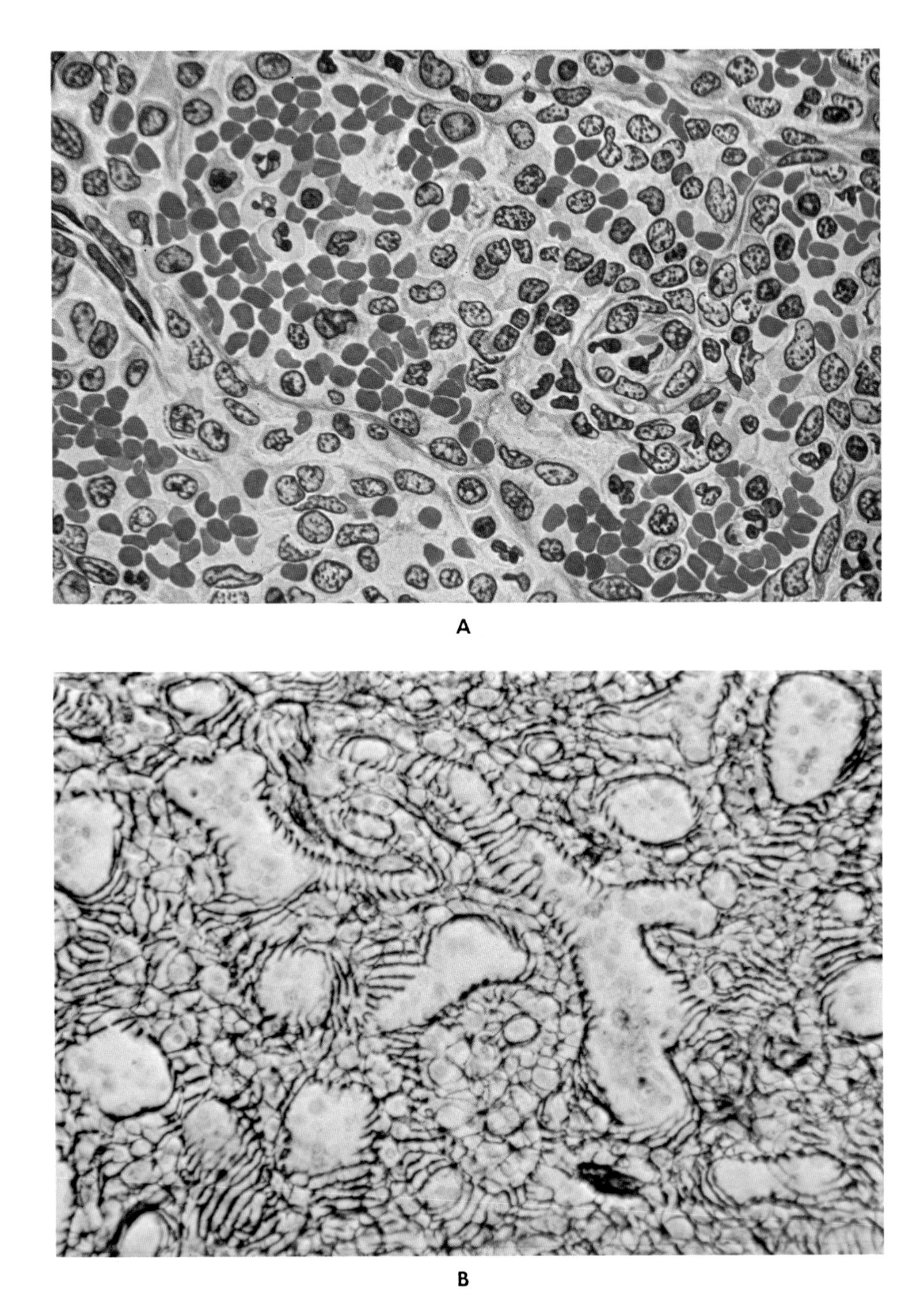

Figure 16–3. (A) A drawing of the red pulp of the human spleen. The splenic sinuses containing many erythrocytes are separated from each other by the cords of the red pulp. (B) Photomicrograph of a silver impregnation of the spleen, showing the reticular fibers and regularly spaced circumferential ribs around the endothelium of the sinuses (Preparation by K. Richardson.)

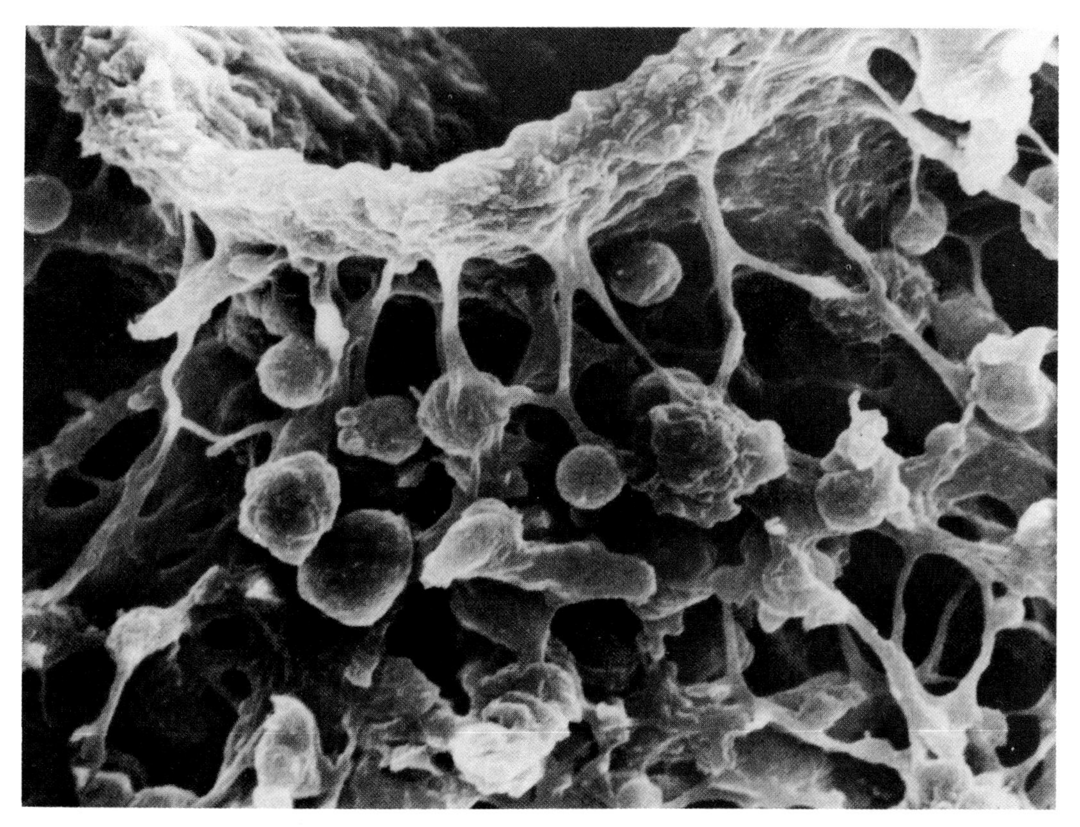

Figure 16–4. Scanning electron micrograph of a splenic cord adjacent to a pulp vein in the dog spleen. Prior perfusion of the spleen with physiological salt solution has removed most of the free cells, exposing the three-dimensional network formed by the reticular cells (From Miyoshi, M. and T. Fujita. 1971. Arch. Histol. Japan 33:225.)

greatly attenuated terminal extension of the periarterial lymphoid sheath of the central artery. The penicillar arteries are less than 1 mm in length and have a continuous basal lamina which is surrounded by a single layer of smooth muscle cells and a very thin adventitia. The branching of each penicillar artery gives rise to two or three *sheathed capillaries,* so called because they are surrounded by a local accumulation of reticular cells and macrophages, often referred to as the *Schweigger-Seidel sheath* or *ellipsoid* (Fig. 16–6). Usually only one or two of the branches of any given penicillar artery are sheathed. Other branches continue into the red pulp without sheaths. In the human, the sheath is quite thin, but in other species (pig, dog, cat), it is more prominent and ellipsoidal or cylindrical in shape. Sheathed capillaries are said to be lacking in the rabbit spleen.

In addition to very numerous macrophages, the sheaths may contain smaller numbers of granulocytes and erythrocytes. Many of the macrophages contain phagocytized erythrocytes and numerous residual bodies. As they move through the sheath and out into the red pulp, they are replaced by monocytes entering the sheath from the blood and differentiating there into macrophages. The sheaths actively remove particulates and senescent cells from the blood. After intravenous injection of particulate matter into an animal, it can be found in high concentration in macrophages in the ellipsoids of the spleen.

The atypical endothelium of the sheathed capillaries consists of fusiform cells oriented parallel to the long axis of the vessel and resting on a discontinuous basal lamina. At some sites, they are connected to adjacent cells at intercellular junctions, but over much of their length, they are separated by narrow intercellular clefts through which cells can pass from the blood into the sheath and on into the red pulp. The capillaries terminate beyond the sheathed region. Their exact mode of termination has long been a subject of controversy which will be discussed in a later section of this chapter.

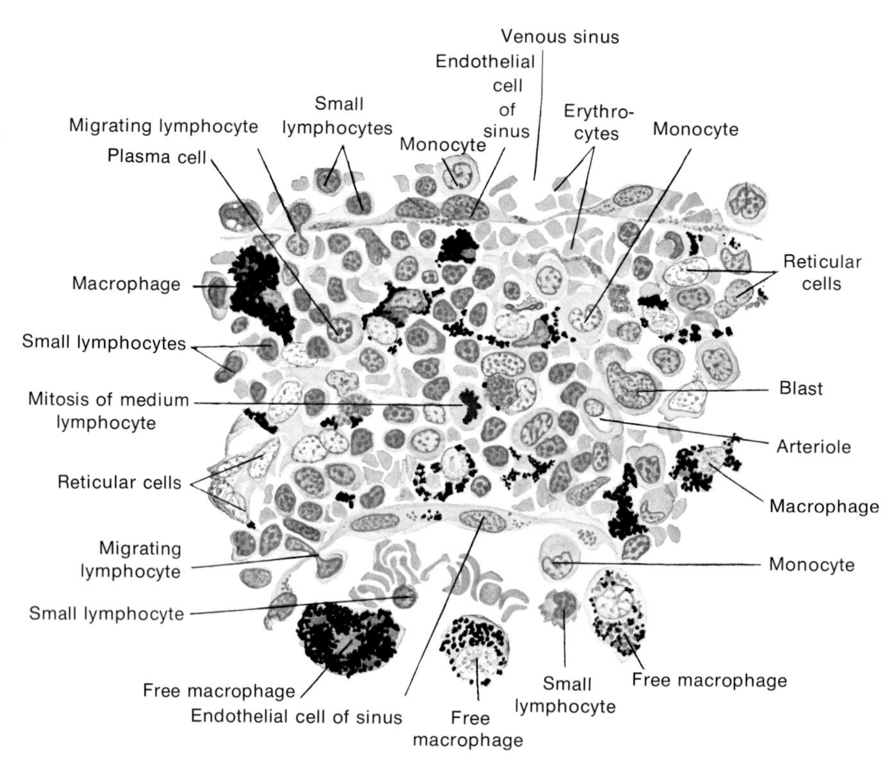

Figure 16–5. Drawing of a splenic cord between two venous sinuses, from the spleen of a rabbit injected with lithium carmine and India ink. Numerous macrophages containing phagocytosed carbon particles are seen among the reticular cells, lymphocytes, monocytes, and plasma cells. Many erythrocytes are also present.

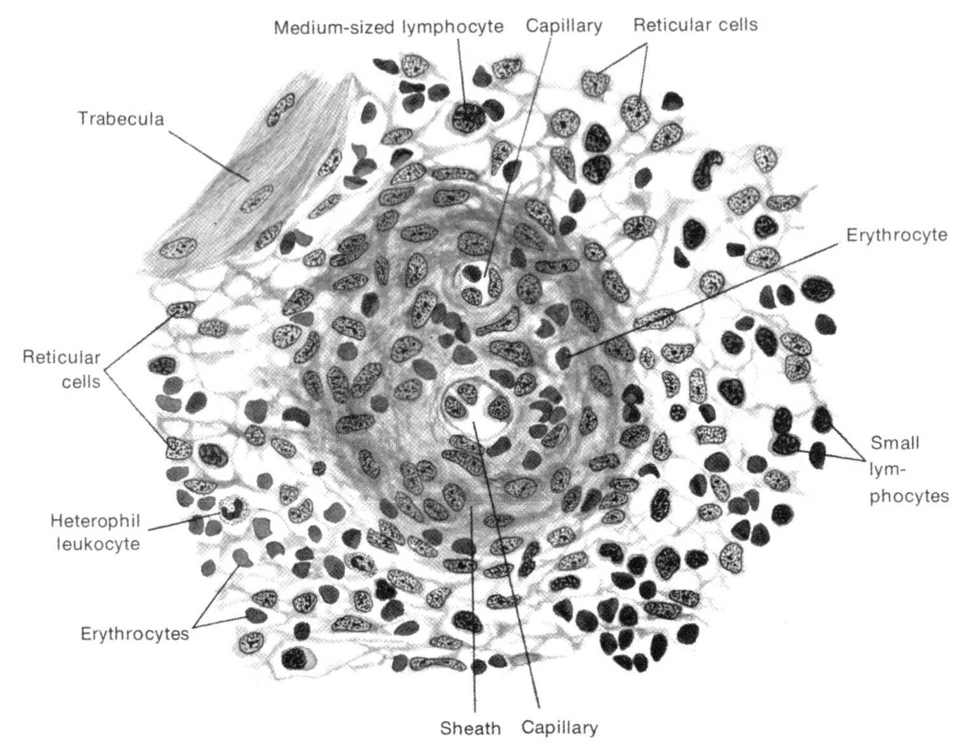

Figure 16–6. Drawing of a cross section through a Schweiger–Seidel sheath (ellipsoid) around two capillaries in the red pulp of the dog spleen. The surrounding network of reticular cells is also clearly depicted.

SPLENIC SINUSES AND VEINS

The red pulp of the spleen is permeated by an extensive system of thin-walled vessels called *sinuses* because they vary in shape and have a thin wall relative to the size of their lumen, which may be up to 40 μm in diameter (Fig. 16–8). The lumen varies in size depending on the volume of blood in the organ. Even when only moderately distended, the sinuses occupy more of the red pulp than the splenic cords between them. Unlike true veins, the walls of the sinuses lack a muscular coat and display a unique organization of the endothelial cells and the basal lamina. The endothelial cells are fusiform, up to 100 μm in length and are oriented parallel to the long axis of the sinus (Fig. 16–7). The central region containing the nucleus is relatively thick, but the cell tapers toward either end. After fixation for microscopic examination, the cells are usually in contact with one another laterally, but in the living organ, they are probably separated by narrow clefts. Occasionally junctional complexes can be found between the tapering ends of the cells. Micropinocytotic vesicles are abundant on the luminal and lateral surfaces of the endothelial cells. Intermediate filaments are found throughout the cell and thinner filaments are located in their basal cytoplasm. Except for their unusual shape, the paucity of lateral cell junctions, and the abundance of cytoplasmic filaments, the cells lining the sinuses resemble those of the endothelium of blood vessels elsewhere in the body. They have only a very limited capacity to take up particulate matter introduced into the bloodstream. Therefore, the traditional interpretation of the cells lining the sinuses as macrophages is no longer tenable.

A basal lamina is present but incomplete. It is reduced to slender bands that are deployed circumferentially around the endothelium like ribs or barrel hoops, but with anastomosing longitudinal or oblique strands connecting the successive hoops. Reticular cells are associated with the outer surface of these elements of the basal lamina. Their cell processes extend outward to join those of other reticular cells that form the cellular framework of the

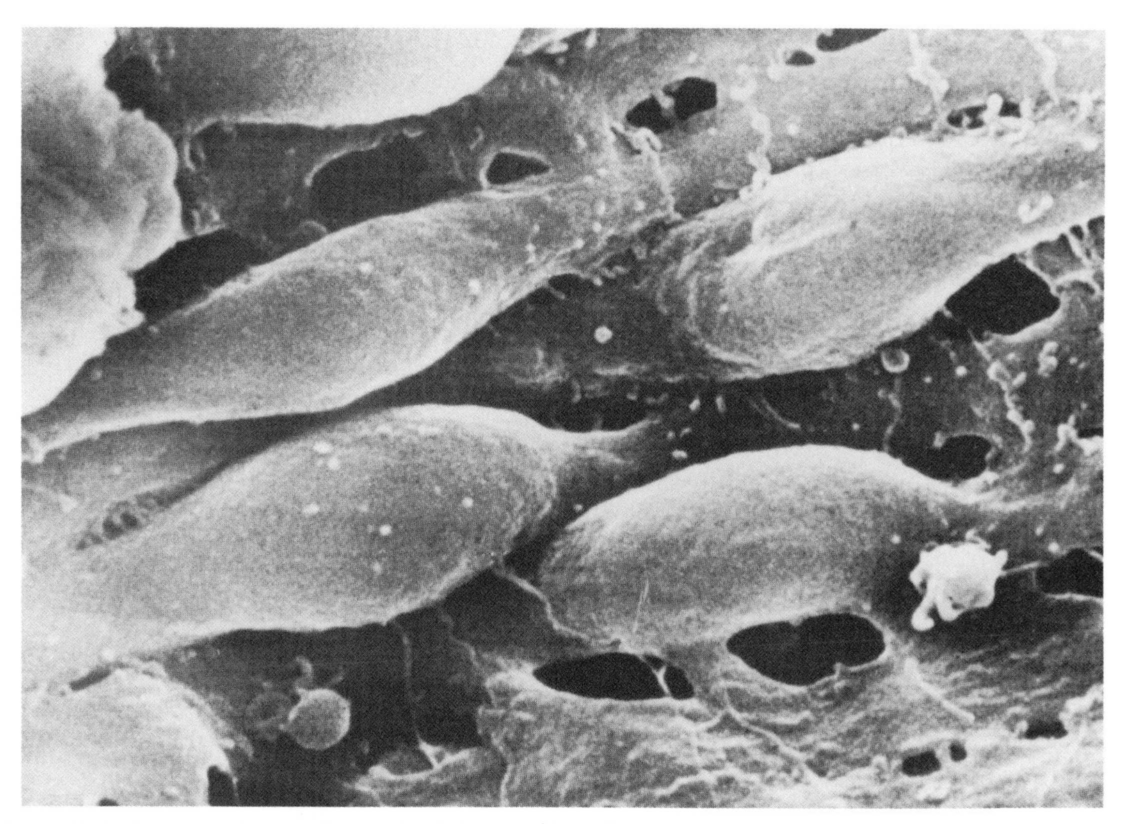

Figure 16–7. Scanning electron micrograph offering a surface view of the elongated endothelial cells of a sinus in the dog spleen. In air-drying of the specimen, the cells have separated slightly, exposing the fenestrations in the underlying basal lamina. (From Miyoshi, M., et al. 1970. Arch. Histol. Japan 32:289.)

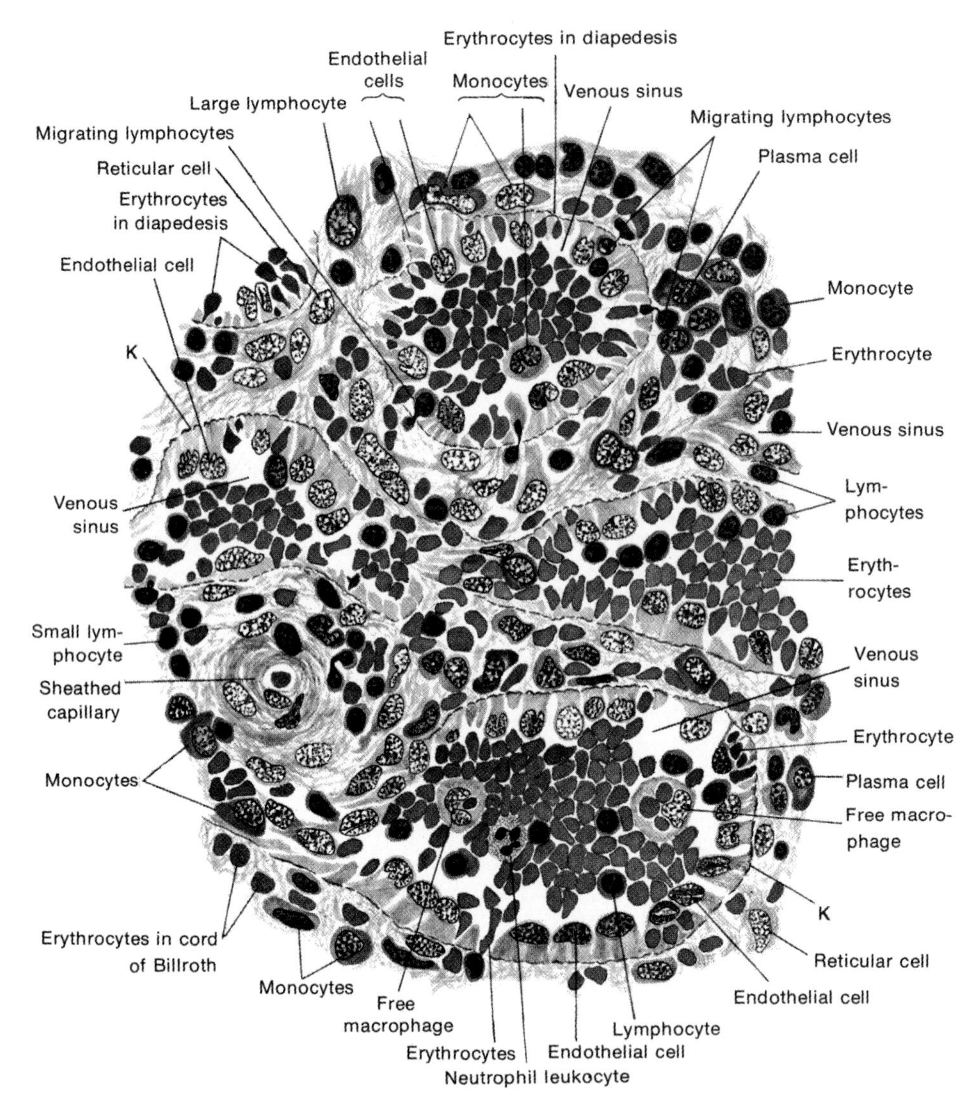

Figure 16–8. Drawing of four venous sinuses, a sheathed capillary, and surrounding red pulp of the human spleen. Note the tall profiles of the endothelial cells, in cross section, and their separation by narrow intercellular clefts. Many of the cell types of the red pulp are identified on the figure.

splenic cords. The unusual structure of the wall of the venous sinuses permits cellular elements of the blood to leave or reenter the circulation through the clefts between the endothelial cells.

The splenic sinuses conduct blood to *pulp veins* which have a conventional endothelium, a continuous basal lamina, and a thin layer of smooth muscle. They are supported externally by a few elastic fibers and a condensation of the reticulum of the red pulp. The pulp veins converge to form the veins of the trabeculae, and these, in turn, are drained by veins at the hilus of the spleen which are tributaries of the splenic vein.

SPLENIC CIRCULATION

In other organs of the body, blood flows from the arteries to the veins through a network of capillaries lined by a continuous endothelium. As indicated above, this does not appear to be the case in the spleen, but just how the blood gets from the penicillar arteries to the splenic sinuses has long been a subject of lively controversy that has generated three conflicting hypotheses.

(1) Proponents of the *open circulation hypothesis* contend that the capillaries arising from the penicillar arteries open at their ends into the interstitial spaces among the reticular cells

of the splenic cords and that blood slowly filters back into the circulatory system through the slit-like fenestrations in the walls of the splenic sinuses. (2) Proponents of the *closed circulation hypothesis* hold that capillaries do not terminate with open ends in the red pulp, but their lumen is continuous with that of the splenic sinuses. (3) Others offer the compromising interpretation that both types of circulation coexist, with some capillaries communicating directly with the sinuses and others opening into the spaces in the splenic cords.

The principal observations on which the conflicting interpretations are based are as follows:

1. There are always many erythrocytes scattered throughout the extracellular spaces of the splenic cords (Fig. 16–5). It is suggested, by proponents of an open circulation, that these erythrocytes have escaped from the blood through discontinuities in the vascular system between the penicillar arteries and the venous sinuses. Those who favor a closed circulation contend that the number of erythrocytes in the splenic cords is too low to be consistent with that interpretation. They insist that if the vessels were open, the red pulp would be completely filled with erythrocytes as it is in hemorrhages following trauma to the spleen. They also point out that over 95% of labeled erythrocytes entering the human spleen flow through it in 30 s and it is difficult to envision the red cells making their way through the spaces in the cords and the clefts between the endothelial cells of the sinuses this rapidly.

2. Proponents of the open circulation counter with experimental evidence that when dye solutions, carbon particles, or nucleated avian erythrocytes are injected at low pressure into the splenic artery, these foreign materials rapidly appear in the spaces of the splenic cords and, only somewhat later, do they appear in the sinuses (Fig. 16–5). Moreover, when these particulates are injected into the splenic vein in a retrograde direction, the splenic sinuses and the stroma of the cords are easily filled but not the arteries, and this is interpreted as evidence against continuity of the system. Those who favor a closed circulation discount this evidence arguing that injection of foreign matter is an artificial situation and that its retrograde injection might rupture the delicate walls of continuous vascular channels.

In histological sections of spleen, granulocytes, erythrocytes, and lymphocytes can be found passing through the wall of splenic sinuses. Proponents of an open circulation believe that these are cells returning to the bloodstream from the extravascular spaces of the splenic cords. Opponents of the open circulation insist that one cannot tell the direction of movement of cells in the sinus wall and argue that some cells may well migrate out into the cordal spaces from the arterial end of continuous capillaries and return to the circulation at the sinuses, possibly driven by a pressure gradient that may exist between these two segments of a closed circulation.

The complex organization and highly cellular nature of the splenic parenchyma made it impossible to resolve this controversy with the light microscope. However, with the electron microscope, branches of the penicillar arteries have been observed to open into the red pulp and no one has yet convincingly demonstrated direct endothelial continuity between the arterial and venous segments of the splenic circulation. There is increasing acceptance of an open circulation, with cells entering the extravascular spaces of the splenic cords from open ends of arterioles or capillaries and reentering the circulation through the slits between endothelial cells in the walls of the sinuses. It remains difficult to explain the rapid rate of circulation (30 s) through the organ. It has been speculated that the sheet-like processes of some reticular cells may be so arranged as to establish preferential pathways through the extravascular network, increasing efficiency of flow. There is evidence, however, that in some species, certain areas of the splenic cords have a slower transit time (8 min), and in those species that have areas of hemopoiesis in their red pulp, the transit time in those areas may be very slow, providing time for the cells to complete their differentiation before entering the circulation. It is clear that much remains to be learned about the circulation in the spleen.

LYMPHATIC VESSELS AND NERVES

Lymphatics are poorly developed in the human spleen and are found only in the capsule and the largest trabeculae, particularly those in the vicinity of the hilus. In some mammals, true lymphatics follow the arteries of the white pulp.

Networks of nerves that originate from the celiac plexus and consist almost entirely of unmyelinated fibers accompany the splenic artery and enter the hilus of the spleen. In the sheep and ox, these nerves form trunks of considerable size. The nerve bundles mainly follow the ramifications of the arteries and form networks that can be followed as far as the central arteries of the white pulp. The terminal branches usually end on the smooth muscle of the arteries and of the trabeculae. Many branches evidently penetrate into the red pulp, but their endings there are not definitely established.

HISTOPHYSIOLOGY

The spleen has a major blood-filtering function that depends on the large population of resident macrophages. On intravenous injection, macromolecular antigen or particulate matter first localize in the macrophages of the marginal zone and subsequently spread to those in the rest of the red pulp. Neither the endothelial cells of the sinuses nor the reticular cells of the splenic cords contribute significantly to clearing the blood of foreign matter. In such experiments, very little particulate matter enters the white matter, but if an animal possesses antibody from a previous exposure, injected antigen may be trapped for long periods of time in the germinal centers of the periarterial lymphoid sheaths. When the amount of lipid in the blood is increased, the macrophages of the spleen, as well as those of the rest of the body, have the capacity to remove it from the circulation. In this process, the macrophages enlarge and become filled with lipid drops, thus acquiring a foamy appearance in histological sections. This is observed in diabetic hyperlipemia in man and in experimentally induced hypercholesterolemia in rabbits.

The spleen also monitors the quality of the blood cells that pass through it. Aged, abnormal, or damaged blood cells and platelets are destroyed in the meshes of the cords of the red pulp. These cells are ingested by the macrophages, whereas the normal cells freely return to the intravascular compartment through the fenestrations of the basal lamina and the interendothelial clefts of the venous sinuses. The function of removing aged erythrocytes is evidently shared with the liver and bone marrow because splenectomy does not seem to affect the average lifespan of erythrocytes significantly. There is no doubt, however, that the spleen plays a major role in destroying pathological or defective cells of the blood. Splenectomy is followed by the appearance in the bloodstream of defective erythrocytes containing remanents of the nucleus or cytoplasmic organelles. Moreover, when experimentally damaged erythrocytes are perfused through the spleen, nearly all of them are retained within the organ. Granulocytes damaged by endotoxin have also been shown to be destroyed in the spleen. How the macrophages recognize old or abnormal cells is still unclear. It has been postulated that the immune system may react to age changes in the erythrocyte membrane and tag these cells with opsonizing antibody.

The walls of the sinusoids also constitute a barrier that tends to filter out abnormal cells. For erythrocytes to insinuate themselves through the interendothelial clefts they must be quite pliable. In certain anemias, the erythrocytes tend to be quite rigid. These have difficulty in reentering the circulation and tend to accumulate in the red pulp. Similarly, intraerythrocytic parasites, such as those of malaria, interfere with passage of the cells through the wall of the sinuses, and the spleen in such conditions may become greatly enlarged.

The spleen is involved in the recycling of iron in the body. The hemoglobin of erythrocytes ingested by macrophages is broken down to heme and globin. Iron is freed from heme and stored by the cell as ferritin or hemosiderin and made available as needed for synthesis of new hemoglobin by erythroblasts in the bone marrow. After release of iron from heme, the molecule is degraded by the macrophages to bilirubin, which is released into the blood where it binds to albumin and is carried to the liver. There it is conjugated with glucuronic acid and excreted in the bile.

In a number of mammalian species, in which the capsule and trabeculae are rich in smooth muscle, the spleen has an important storage function. Large numbers of erythrocytes can be retained in the red pulp and then given up to the circulation when a need arises. This function can be demonstrated by injection of drugs such as epinephrine, which induce contraction of the splenic smooth muscle. Although the storage capacity of the human spleen is limited to about 30 ml of erythrocytes, it is an important reservoir of platelets and is estimated to contain one-third of the body's supply. These are available for return to the circulation in emergencies.

During embryonic life, the spleen contains precursors of the blood cells, but in the adult human, hematopoiesis does not normally occur in this organ. However, in pathological conditions, especially in myeloid leukemia, the red pulp of the spleen undergoes *myeloid metaplasia,* after which large numbers of erythroblasts, myelocytes, and megakaryocytes appear, and the tissue comes to resemble the bone marrow. As previously mentioned, some erythroblasts and myelocytes may be found normally in the red pulp of other mammalian species. Megakaryocytes are consistently present in the spleen of rats and mice.

The spleen is of great importance in the immunological responses of the body to invasion of the circulation by bacteria and viruses. A large fraction of the splenic lymphocytes belong to the recirculating pool and they are specifically localized in the periarterial lymphoid sheaths. This has been verified by experiments involving drainage of thoracic duct lymph and reinjection of the lymphocytes after labeling them in vitro. Drainage of the thoracic duct initially affects the central portion of the periarterial lymphoid sheaths. Only after prolonged drainage do the peripheral regions of the white pulp become depleted of lymphocytes. This finding has been interpreted as evidence that the rapidly circulating T-lymphocytes localize close to the central artery, whereas the more sluggish B-cells assume a more peripheral position in the periarterial sheaths. After intravenous injection of labeled thoracic duct cells, which are predominantly T-lymphocytes, they first localize in the marginal zone of the red pulp, but a few hours later, they have migrated throughout the periarterial lymphoid sheaths. Labeled B-lymphocytes first appear in the marginal zone. After a few hours in the periphery of the sheaths, they finally migrate into the caps of the germinal centers. These findings are the basis of the current belief that the periarterial lymphoid sheaths consist of a central thymus-dependent region and a peripheral region occupied predominantly by B-lymphocytes. In neonatally thymectomize rodents, the periarterial lymphoid sheaths are very sparsely populated with lymphocytes, thus supporting the conclusion that the vast majority of their lymphocytes are T-cells.

On introduction into the bloodstream of an antigen that elicits a humoral immune response, morphological changes are first seen in the periarterial lymphoid sheaths. One day later, proliferating lymphoblasts appear, scattered through the sheaths. They increase in number in the next 2 days and become more concentrated at the periphery of the sheaths. Antibody first appears in the blood at this time. Lymphoblasts also occur around small arteries in the red pulp. These may have developed from lymphocytes in the terminal extensions of the periarterial sheaths that surround the penicillar arteries. On days 4 to 6, an increasing number of immature plasma cells appear at the periphery of the sheaths and along the penicillar arteries. Mature plasma cells are also found in limited numbers. At the end of the first week, lymphoblasts and immature plasma cells begin to decrease in the periarterial lymphoid sheaths, and mature plasma cells become more numerous at the boundary between the white and red pulp. They also occur in the cords of the red pulp and occasionally free in the lumen of sinuses. During the second week after introduction of the antigen, the structure of the spleen reverts to normal, except for the germinal centers, which continue to be prominent for about 1 month.

During a secondary immune response, the spleen undergoes changes similar to those following the first exposure to antigen, but they occur earlier and are much more dramatic. At the beginning of the response, the spleen is the most active antibody-secreting organ in the body, per unit weight, but it rapidly falls off in production as the response spreads throughout the peripheral lymphoid organs of the body.

BIBLIOGRAPHY

Barnhart, M.I. and J.M. Lusher. 1976. The human spleen as revealed by scanning electron microscopy. Am. J. Hematol. 1:243.

Blue, J. and L. Weiss. 1981. Periarterial macrophage sheaths (ellipsoid) in cat spleen—an electron microscope study. Am. J. Anat. 161:115.

Blue, J. and L. Weiss. 1981. Vascular pathways in nonsinusal red pulp—an electron microscope study of the cat spleen. Am. J. Anat. 161:135.

Blue, J. and L. Weiss. 1981. Species variation in the structure and function of the marginal zone—an electron microscope study of cat spleen. Am. J. Anat. 161:189.

Burke, J.S. and G.T. Simon. 1970. Electron microscopy of the spleen. I. Anatomy and microcirculation. Am. J. Pathol. 58:127.

Burke, J.S. and G.T. Simon. 1970. Electron microscopy of the spleen. II. Phagocytosis of colloidal carbon. Am. J. Pathol. 58:157.

Chen, L.T. and L. Weiss. 1972. Electron microscopy of the red pulp of the human spleen. Am. J. Anat. 134:425.

Chen, L.T. 1978. Microcirculation of the spleen: an open and closed circulation? Science 201:157.

Coons, A.H. 1959. Some reactions of lymphoid tissues to stimulation by antigen. Harvey Lecture Series 53:113.

Edwards, V.D. and G.T. Simon. 1970. Ultrastructural

aspects of red cell destruction in the normal rat spleen. J. Ultrastr. Res. 33:187.
Ernstrom, U. and G. Sandberg. 1968. Migration of splenic lymphocytes. Acta Pathol. Microbiol. Scand. 72:379.
Ford, W.L. and J.L. Gowans. 1969. The traffic of lymphocytes. Semin. Hematol. 6:67.
Fujita, T. 1974. A scanning electron microscope study of the human spleen. Arch. Histol. Japan 37:187.
Galindo, B. and T. Imaeda. 1962. Electron microscope study of the white pulp of the mouse spleen. Anat. Rec. 143:399.
Goldschneider, I. and D.D. McGregor. 1968. Migration of lymphocytes and thymocytes in the rat. I. The route of migration from blood to spleen and lymph nodes. J. Exp. Med. 127:155.
Irino, S., T. Murikami, and T. Fujita. 1977. Open circulation in the human spleen. Dissection scanning electron microscopy of conductive-stained tissue and observation of resin vascular casts. Arch. Histol. Japan 40:297.
Jacobsen, G. 1971. Morphological-histochemical comparison of dog and cat ellipsoid sheaths. Anat. Rec. 169:105.
Knisely, M.H. 1936. Spleen studies. I. Microscopic observations of the circulatory system of living unstimulated mammalian spleens. Anat. Rec. 65:23.
Langevoort, H.L. 1963. The histophysiology of the antibody response. I. Histogenesis of the plasma cell reaction in rabbit spleen. Lab. Investig. 12:106.
Lewis, O.J. 1957. The blood vessels of the adult mammalian spleen. J. Anat. 91:245.
MacKenzie, D.W. Jr., A.O. Whipple, and M.P. Wintersteiner. 1941. Studies on the microscopic anatomy and physiology of living transilluminated mammalian spleens. Am. J. Anat. 68:397.
Miyoshi, M. and T. Fujita. 1971. Stereo-fine structure of the splenic red pulp. A combined scanning and transmission electron microscope study on dog and rat spleen. Arch. Histol. Japan 33:225.
Nieuwenhuis, P. and W.L. Ford. 1976. Comparative migration of B-and T-lymphocytes in the rat spleen and lymph nodes. Cell Immunol. 23:254.
Pictet, R.L., L. Orci, W.G. Forssmann, and L. Girardier. 1969. An electron microscope study of perfusion-fixed spleen. I. The splenic circulation and the RES concept. Z. Zellforsch. 96:372.
Snook, T. 1950. A comparative study of the vascular arrangements in mammalian spleens. Am. J. Anat. 87:31.
Snook, T. 1950. A comprehensive study of the vascular arrangements in mammalian spleens. Am. J. Anat. 87:31.
Solnitzky, O. 1937. The Schweigger–Seidel sheath (ellipsoid) of the spleen. Anat. Rec. 69:55.
Weiss, L. 1962. The structure of the fine splenic arterial vessels in relation to hemoconcentration and red cell destruction. Am. J. Anat. 111:131.
Weiss, L. 1963. The structure of intermediate vascular pathways in the spleen of rabbits. Am. J. Anat. 113:51.
Weiss, L. 1974. A scanning electron microscopic study of the spleen. Blood 453:665.
Weiss, L. and M. Tavassoli. 1970. Anatomical hazards in the passage of erythrocytes through the spleen. Semin. Hematol. 7:372.
Wennberg, E. and L. Weiss. 1969. The structure of the spleen and hemolysis. Annu. Rev. Med. 20:29.

17 HYPOPHYSIS

In the evolution of multicellular organisms, it became necessary to develop mechanisms for coordinating the functions of various organs. Two mechanisms were evolved for achieving this integration—the *nervous system* and the *endocrine system.* The nervous system generates electrochemical signals that are transmitted over long-cell processes that synapse on the cells being regulated. The endocrine glands secrete chemical agents, called *hormones,* that are transported in the bloodstream to distant target cells that have specific surface receptors which bind the hormone and induce an intracellular response. The *hypophysis,* or *pituitary gland,* is an endocrine gland producing several hormones that have important functions in the regulation of metabolism, growth, and reproduction.

The hypophysis, located at the base of the brain, is about 1 cm in length, 1–1.5 cm in width, and 0.5 cm in depth (Fig. 17–1). The gland weighs approximately 0.5 g in men and slightly more in women. It has neural and vascular connections with the brain which give it a key role in the interplay of the nervous and endocrine systems. Two major subdivisions of the gland are the *neurohypophysis* (posterior lobe), which develops as a downgrowth from the diencephalon of the brain, and the *adenohypophysis,* which originates as a dorsal evagination from the roof of the embryonic pharynx. Three subdivisions of the adenohypophysis are distinguished: the *pars distalis* (anterior lobe), the *pars tuberalis* (also called the pars infundibularis), and the *pars intermedia* (Fig. 17–2). There are also three regions of the neurohypophysis: the *median eminence,* a funnel-shaped downward extension of the hypothalamus, the *infundibular stem,* which is continuous with the expanded *infundibular process* that forms the neural lobe of the hypophysis. A thin investment of glandular tissue that extends upward from the adenohypophysis to envelop the infundibular stem and median eminence is called the *pars tuberalis.* The infundibular stem and surrounding pars tuberalis together constitute the infundibular stalk (pituitary stalk).

In some species, the pars intermedia is a distinct layer, closely adherent to the infundibular process and separated from the pars distalis by a narrow cleft. In the human, the pars intermedia is rudimentary in the adult. Soon after its development in the embryo, its cells mingle with those of the pars distalis and it is no longer recognizable as a separate entity. The interlobar cleft in man is represented only by scattered colloid-filled vesicles along the boundary between the anterior and posterior lobes of the gland.

The hypophysis occupies a deep recess in the sphenoid bone, called the *sella turcia.* It is lined by the dura mater which forms a fibrous capsule around the intrasellar portion of the hypophysis and a layer over its upper surface, called the *diaphragma sellae.* This thin layer between the sella turcica and the cranial cavity is incomplete, having an opening 5 mm or more in diameter through which the *infundibular stalk* passes. Some of the pia arachnoid may also pass through this opening to occupy a narrow space between the diaphragma sellae and the gland. Elsewhere, the capsule of gland is separated from the periosteum of the sphenoid bone by a layer of looser connective tissue containing many small veins.

BLOOD VESSELS AND NERVES

Secretion by exocrine glands is dependent on stimulation by nerves. In contrast, the secretory activity of the adenohypophysis depends on activation of its cells by neurohumors, called *releasing factors,* produced by neurons in the median eminence and carried to the anterior lobe of the gland by a portal system of veins, called the *hypophyseoportal system.* The atypical vascular architecture of the gland is of cardinal importance to its function.

Two *inferior hypophyseal arteries,* branches of the internal carotid artery, arborize in the cap-

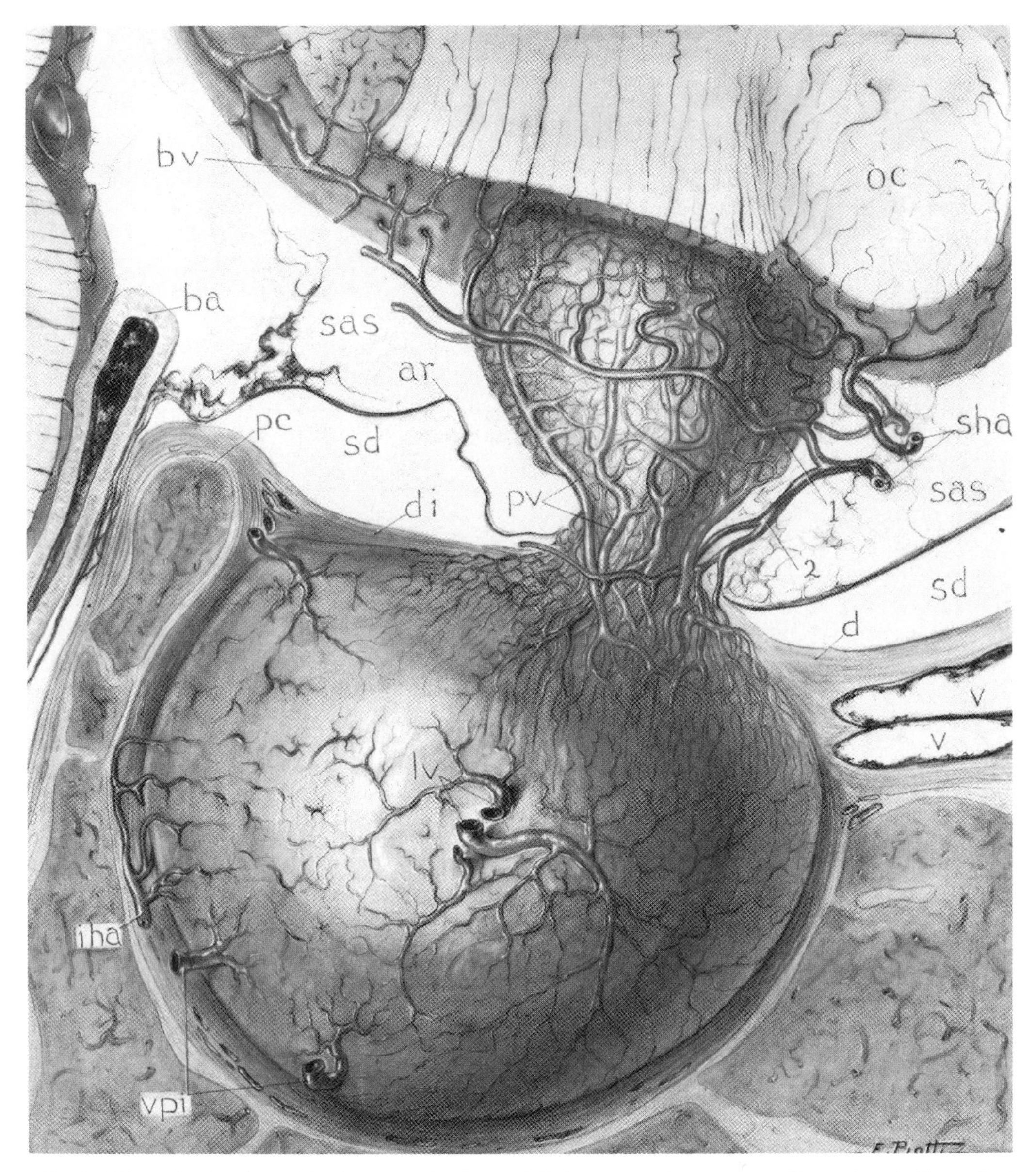

Figure 17–1. Schematic drawing of the hypophysis of an adult rhesus monkey showing its relation to the sella turcica of the sphenoid bone. Also depicted are the superior and inferior hypophyseal arteries (*sha* and *iha*) and the physiologically important portal venules (*pv*) coursing down the infundibular stalk. The superior hypophyseal artery usually sends an ascending branch (1) to the proximal part of the infundibular stalk and median eminence, and a descending branch (2) coursing downward. *ar,* arachnoid membrane; *ba,* basilar artery; *d,* dura; *di,* sellar diaphragm; *lv,* lateral hypophyseal veins; *oc,* optic chiasm; *pc,* posterior clinoid process; *sas,* subarachnoid space; *sd,* subdural space; *v,* dural vein; *vpi,* veins of the infundibular process. (After Wislocki, G.B. 1938. Proc. Assoc. Res. Nerv. Ment. Dis. 17:48.)

sule of the gland sending branches into the posterior lobe, and to a lesser extent into the anterior lobe. Several *superior hypophyseal arteries,* also arising from the internal carotid, anastomose freely around the median eminence. Capillaries arising from these vessels penetrate into the median eminence, forming the so called primary plexus (Fig. 17–1). These capillaries then return to the surface where they become confluent to form venules that course downward around the hypophyseal stalk to join an extensive network of thin-walled sinusoids within the adenohypophysis. The venules connecting the primary plexus in the median eminence with the secondary plexus of sinusoids in the anterior lobe constitute the *hypophyseoportal system* (Fig. 17–3). It supplies the major portion of the blood circulating in the anterior lobe and carries the releasing factors that stimulate its cells to secrete

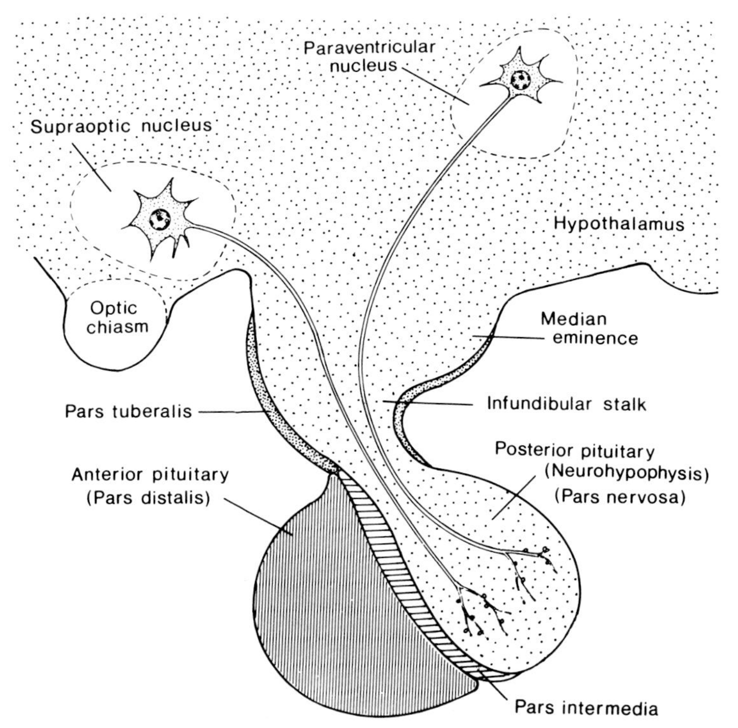

Figure 17–2. Diagram of a parasaggital section of the hypothalamus and pituitary presenting the relationships of their several components and their terminology. Two magnocellular neurones of the hypothalamo-hypophyseal tract are shown schematically.

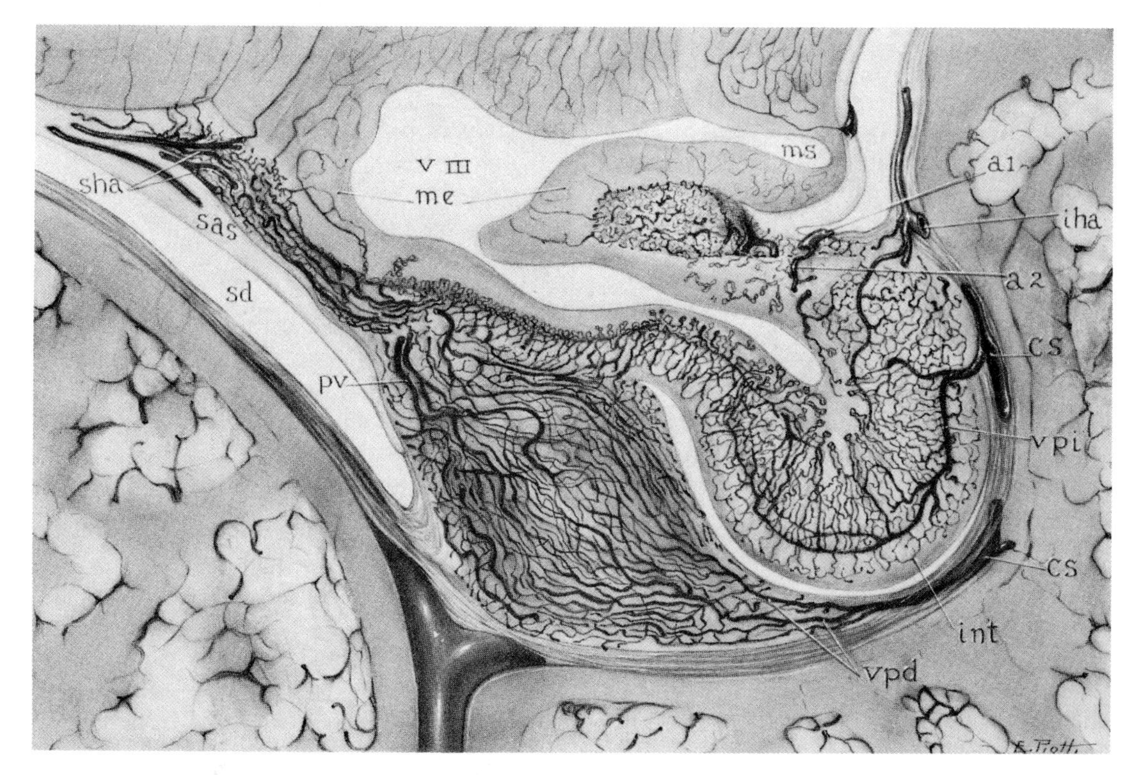

Figure 17–3. Drawing of a midsagittal section of a cat's hypophysis after injection of the blood vascular system with India ink. The main blood supply is via the superior hypophyseal artery (*sha*) and inferior hypophyseal arteries (*iha*). The venous drainage is via systemic veins from the pars distalis (*vpd*) and the pars nervosa (*vpi*). Portal veins arising in capillaries in the median eminence and pars tuberalis (*pv*) carry the neurohumoral releasing hormones from the median eminence of the hypothalamus (*me*) to the pars distalis. *sas,* subarachnoid space; *sd,* subdural space; *al* and *a2,* branches of the inferior hypophyseal artery; *cs,* capsular venous sinuses; *int,* pars intermedia. (From Wislocki, G.B. 1937. Anat. Rec. 69:361.)

their hormones. The venous drainage of the hypophysis is mainly via vessels that run in the vascular layer of the capsule toward the diaphragma sellae and then to the neighboring dural sinuses.

There are isolated reports in the literature of unmyelinated nerve axons being found in the perisinusoidal connective tissue and in the delicate septa between clusters of secretory cells. These are described as having varicosities containing small clear vesicles and somewhat larger dense-cored vesicles. It remains unclear as to whether these endings are functionally significant or represent an aberrant invasion of the pars distalis by nerves to the pars intermedia and pars tuberalis. There is, as yet, no supporting physiological evidence for neural control of secretion by the pars distalis of the hypophysis.

PARS DISTALIS

The pars distalis or anterior lobe is composed of irregular cords or clusters of glandular cells. The stroma of the gland is not abundant. Some connective tissue accompanying the superior hypophyseal artery and portal veins extends into the anterior lobe and the cords of parenchymal cells are surrounded by delicate reticular fibers. The thin-walled sinusoids throughout the lobe are also supported by reticular fibers. The endothelium lining the sinusoids is fenestrated and its pores no doubt facilitate the diffusion of blood-borne releasing factors into the gland and passage of the protein secretory products of its cells into the blood. The endothelium of the sinusoids was formerly considered to be phagocytic and was regarded as a component of the reticulo-endothelial system. This interpretation has now been abandoned because electron microscopic studies have shown that the uptake of particulate tracers is confined to extravascular macrophages.

The glandular cells have traditionally been classified as chromophilic or chromophobic on the basis of their avidity, or lack of affinity for the dyes commonly used is the routine staining of histological sections. The chromophilic cells were designated as *acidophils* or *basophils* according to their staining with acid or basic dyes (Fig. 17–4). Cells that showed little or no cytoplasmic staining were called *chromophobes*. The term basophilic, as applied to the cells of the pituitary, referred to the staining property of the secretory granules and is not to be confused with the basophilia attributable to cytoplasmic ribonucleoprotein in cells in general. This terminology served to distinguish two major classes of chromophilic cells, at a time when there were few dye combinations in general use for histological staining and the diversity of pituitary functions was not yet appreciated. The terminological problem was complicated by the fact that most of the staining procedures considered useful for the study of the adenohypophysis with the light microscope did not make use of an acid and a basic dye but involved mixtures of acid dyes. Staining with those methods does not depend on the binding of a dye by a tissue component of opposite charge and no conclusion could be drawn as to the chemical nature of the granules from their color in stained sections.

As more hypophyseal hormones were discovered, it became evident that there were probably more cell types than acidophils, basophils, and chromophobes, and this was confirmed when studies with the electron microscope revealed several cell types that were distinguishable on the basis of the size and shape of their secretory granules. It has since become possible to raise antibodies to each of the hormones and to conjugate the antibody with a fluorescent dye. When such a *labeled antibody* is applied to a histological section of the hypophysis, it binds to the secretory granules of the cell type that produces that hormone and causes those cells to fluoresce under the microscope when illuminated with ultraviolet light. Similarly, if an antibody conjugated to horseradish peroxidase is applied to an ultrathin section of the pituitary, the site of production of that hormone can be identified under the electron microscope by the localization of the reaction product of a histochemical method for peroxidase.

It is now common practice to refer to the cell types of the anterior pituitary, not by their staining properties but by terms that identify the target organ stimulated by the hormone produced. Thus, cells secreting *thyroid-stimulating hormone (TSH)* are called *thyrotrophs,* cells secreting *gonadotrophic hormone (GTH)* are called *gonadotrophs,* cells secreting *adrenocorticotrophic hormone* (ACTH) are called *corticotrophs,* and so on. Terms designating the hormone secreted may also be used by some authors, for example, *TSH cell, FSH/HS cell,* and *ACTH cell.*

The description of the ultrastructure of the various cell types that follows relies heavily on studies of the laboratory rat. Comparable

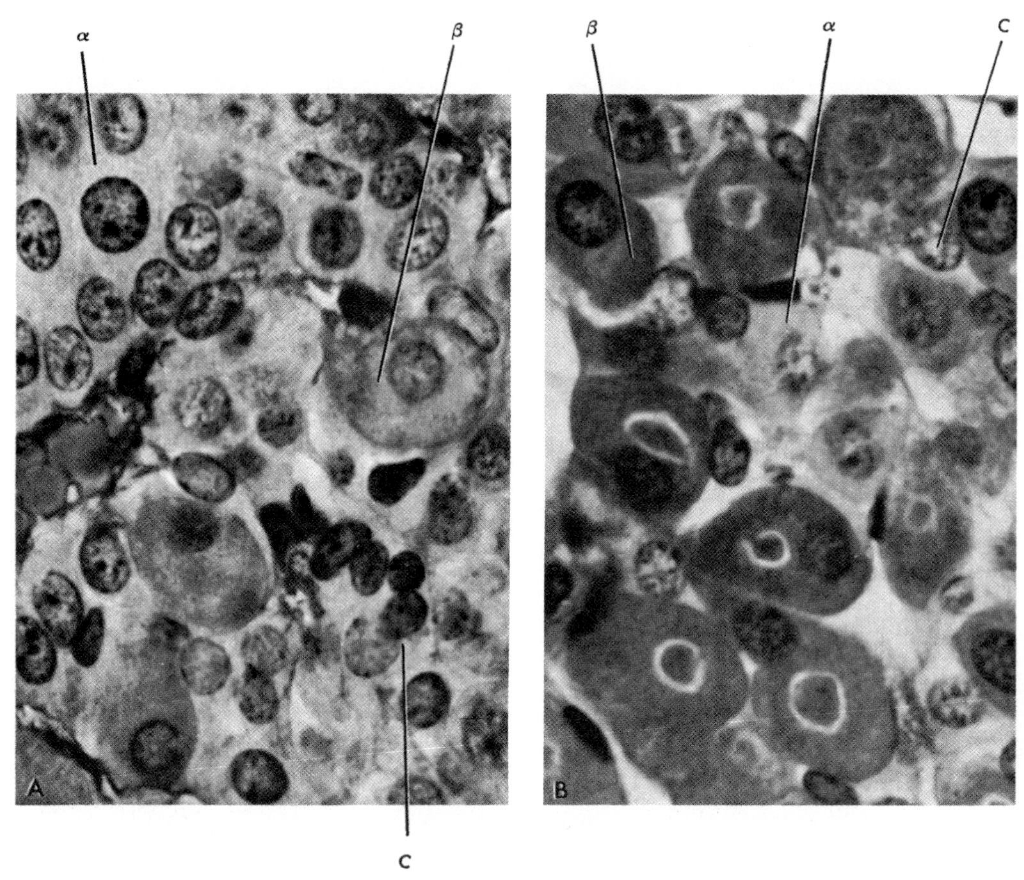

Figure 17–4. Photomicrographs of the anterior lobe of the rat hypophysis. Acidophils, basophils, and chromophobes are indicated. (A) Normal female rat; (B) castrated female rat of the same age. Castration has resulted in hypertrophy of the basophils and reduction in acidophhil and chromophobe cells. The clear circles are negative images of the greatly enlarged Golgi complexes of the hypertrophied basophil cells. (Courtesy of I. Gersh.)

studies of the human gland are not yet available. It can be assumed that the interspecific differences are relatively minor.

ACIDOPHILS

Acidophils are most numerous in the posterolateral portion of the anterior lobe. Their cytoplasm stains with eosin and other acid dyes and their granules are large enough to be resolved with the light microscope. They are relatively small rounded cells with a well-developed Golgi complex and small rod-shaped mitochondria. Two kinds of acidophils can be distinguished immunocytochemically and in electron micrographs.

Somatotrophs

Acidophils containing numerous, spherical granules 300–350 nm in diameter are now called *somatotrophs* or *STH cells*. The cisternae of their well-developed endoplasmic reticulum tend to be arranged parallel to the cell surface (Fig. 17–4 and 17–5). These cells are the most abundant cell type in the anterior lobe of the pituitary. Somatotrophs secrete *growth hormone* (*somatotrophin*), a protein with a molecular weight of about 22,000. They can be identified by immunocytochemical staining of their secretory granules with labeled antibody to somatotrophin. Their secretion is stimulated by *growth-hormone-releasing hormone* (GHRH) produced by neurones in the hypothalamus and carried to the anterior lobe of the pituitary via the hypophyseoportal system. Secretion is suppressed by another neurohumor, *somatostatin*.

Unlike other hormones of the anterior pituitary, somatotrophin does not have a specific target organ but has a generalized effect on cells throughout the body, increasing their uptake of amino acids and protein synthesis.

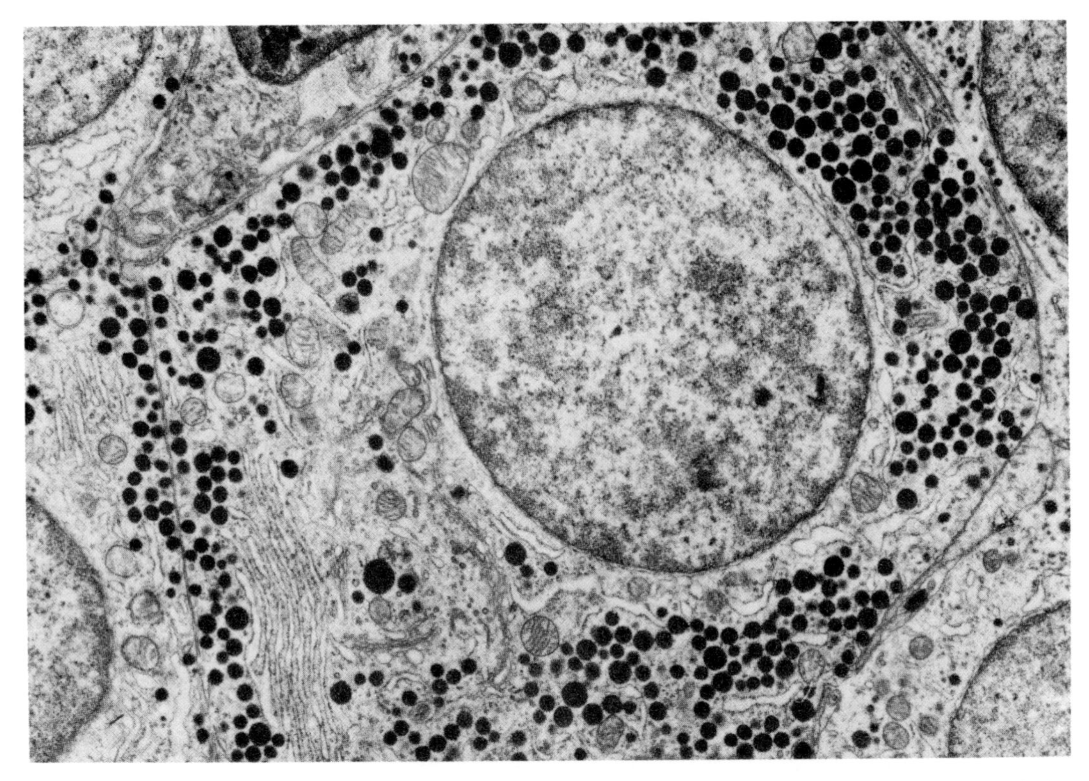

Figure 17–5. Electron micrograph of a typical somatotroph, showing parallel cisternae of endoplasmic reticulum, a juxtanuclear Golgi complex, and a great many secretory granules about 350 nm in diameter around the periphery of the cell. (Micrograph courtesy of M.G. Farquhar.)

Other metabolic effects include increased mobilization of fatty acids from adipose cells and a decreased rate of utilization of glucose. The most conspicuous effect of somatotrophin is on the rate of growth of young animals. This effect is mediated by smaller proteins, *somatomedins,* synthesized in the liver in response to growth hormone. The somatomedins, in turn, stimulate the proliferation of cartilage cells that is necessary for the growth in length of long bones. In children, a deficiency in secretion of growth hormones leads to *dwarfism* and an excess secretion by a rare tumor of the pituitary results in *gigantism.* Such a tumor in adult life results in *acromegaly,* characterized by a disproportionate thickening of the bones.

Mammotrophs

The second kind of acidophil, the *mammatroph* or *lactotroph,* tends to be distributed individually in the anterior lobe rather than in cords or clusters. They secrete the lactogenic hormone *prolactin,* a protein of 23,000 molecular weight that promotes mammary gland development during pregnancy and subsequent lactation. Mammotrophs are relatively small cells with an ovoid or polygonal shape. In males and cycling females, they usually have a few elongated cisternae of endoplasmic reticulum and a juxtanuclear Golgi complex of modest size, but during lactation these structures become much more highly developed, with numerous parallel cisternae of reticulum in the peripheral cytoplasm and a huge Golgi complex of a size approaching that of the nucleus. Mammotrophs are relatively easy to identify, owing to their distinctive large dense granules which range in size from 500 to 900 nm in diameter (Fig. 17–6). Small granules (100–150 nm), present within the inner cistern of the Golgi, bud off and subsequently aggregate and fuse to form the large granules.

During pregnancy, the anterior pituitary undergoes a twofold enlargement, due in large measure to hypertrophy and hyperplasia of the mammotrophs. The concentration of prolactin in the blood rises progressively from the fifth week of pregnancy to full term, when it reaches a level 10 times that of nonpregnant women. This elevated level of prolactin stimulates development of the mam-

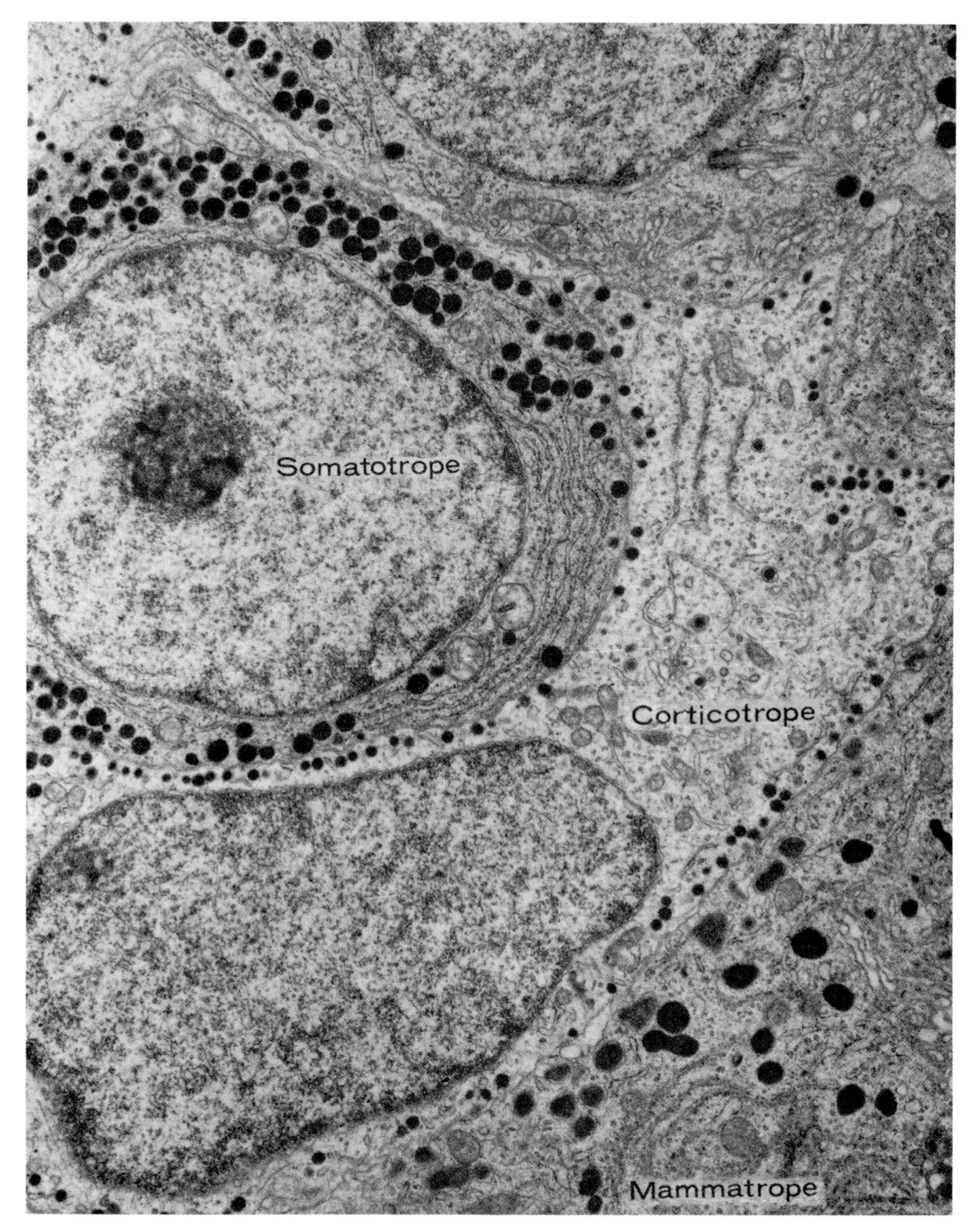

Figure 17–6. Electron micrograph of a rat mammotroph. Note the relatively large size and irregular shape of the secretory granules. Smaller granules in the Golgi complex, at the lower right, coalesce to form the large dense granules seen at the upper left. (Micrograph courtesy of M. Farquhar and T. Kanaseki.)

mary glands, but the lactogenic effect of the hormone is suppressed during pregnancy by high circulating levels of the ovarian hormones estrogen and progesterone. After birth of the baby, a precipitous fall in these steroid hormones allows the lactogenic effect of prolactin to be expressed in secretion of milk. Secretion of prolactin is stimulated by suckling. In experimental animals, increased numbers of mammotroph secretory granules can be found fusing with the cell membrane within minutes after initiation of suckling by the litter (Fig. 17–9). Nerve impulses generated in the nipples by suckling are transmitted to neurones in the hypothalamus that secrete the hormone oxytocin into the hypophyseoportal system. On reaching the anterior pituitary, this stimulates secretion of prolactin.

At the termination of lactation, the mammotrophs regress. Excess secretory granules fuse with lysosomes to form autophagic vacuoles within which they are degraded by hydrolytic enzymes. This mode of disposal of secretory products that are no longer needed is called *crinophagy* and is also observed in other glands. Excess organelles are also removed by autophagy and the mammotrophs revert to the relatively inactive state characteristic of the cycling female. It is considered likely that degeneration of whole cells is also involved. Mammotrophs account for about 50% of the total hypophyseal cell count in lactating rats and this percentage decreases to about 25% 7 days after removing the litter.

It was formerly believed that there was a different cell type for each hormone secreted by the pituitary. Although this is generally true, the gonadotrophs secrete two hormones (FSH and LH), and under certain circumstances, both growth hormone and prolactin can be found in the secretory granules of a cell type that has been designated the *somatomammotroph.* Moreover, it is now known that the corticotrophs synthesize a large prohormone of 38,000 molecular weight that undergoes posttranslational cleavage to yield three different hormones, namely, ACTH, β-endorphin, and β lipotropin. The latter two are of relatively minor physiological significance.

BASOPHILS

The basophils of the anterior pituitary are not easily identified in sections stained with hematoxylin and eosin, but they do stain well with the aniline blue of Mallory's trichrome stain. The secretions of two of the three types of basophils are glycoproteins and, therefore, those cells can be most easily distinguished from acidophils by their pink staining with the periodic-acid–Schiff reaction for carbohydrates.

Thyrotrophs

Thyrotrophs are commonly located in the anteromedial portion of the anterior lobe and make up about 15% of the cells of the adenohypophysis. They tend to be deeply situated in the cords of parenchymal cells and, therefore, are usually not in contact with the sinusoids. Basophils of this kind can be distinguished, at the light microscope level, by their staining with aldehyde thionin. In electron micrographs, the secretory granules are 140–160 nm in diameter, the smallest found in any cell type of the gland. They are usually located at the periphery of the cell. Thyrotrophs secrete *thyroid-stimulating hormone* (TSH), also called *thyrotrophin,* a glycoprotein of 28,000 molecular weight. It acts by binding to specific receptors on the cells of the thyroid follicles, stimulating their secretion of the thyroid hormones *thyroxine* and *triiodothyronine.* Activation of thyrotrophs depends on *thyrotrophin-releasing hormone,* a tripeptide generated in the hypothalamus and transported to the adenohypophysis via the hypophyseoportal system. Secretion of thyrotrophin is limited by a feedback mechanism wherein circulating thyroid hormones act back on the central nervous system to suppress generation of thyrotrophin-releasing hormone.

Corticotrophs

Corticotrophs are widely distributed in the anteromedial region of the pars distalis and a few may invade a short distance into the neural lobe. They are round or ovoid cells in man, but in rodents they may have a stellate form, with their processes extending between neighboring cells to end close to sinusoids. Their secretory granules are generally smaller than those of the somatotrophs and gonadotrophs (Fig. 17–7), but granule size varies from species to species and is not a reliable criterion for cell identification. More dependable is an immunocytochemical method, using labeled antibody against their secretory product. Corticotrophs secrete *adrenocorticotrophin* (ACTH), also called *corticotrophin,* a small peptide of molecular weight 4500, consisting of only 39 amino acids. Secretion is stimulated by *corticotrophin-releasing hormone* (CRH) produced in the hypothalamus. Adrenocorticotrophin, circulating in the blood, binds to receptors on the cells of the adrenal cortex and stimulates their secretion of the hormone *cortisol.*

Gonadotrophs

Gonadotrophs are rounded cells, usually situated close to sinusoids. In electron micrographs, they have a prominent Golgi complex and an endoplasmic reticulum of meandering

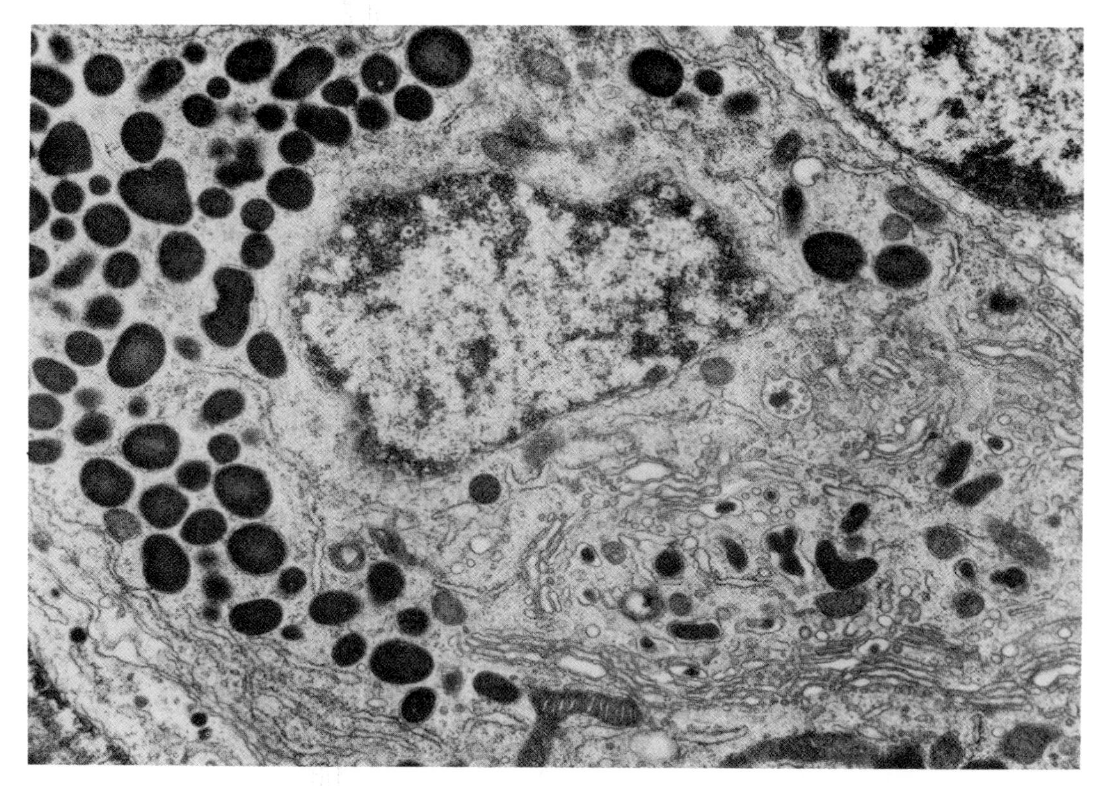

Figure 17–7. Electron micrograph of an area of the pars distalis of the rat hypophysis, illustrating the fine structure of a somatotroph, a corticotroph, and a portion of a mammotroph. Note the differing size of the secretory granules of the three cell types. (Micrograph from Nakayama, I., F.A. Nickerson, and F.R. Shelton. 1969. Lab. Investig. 21:169.)

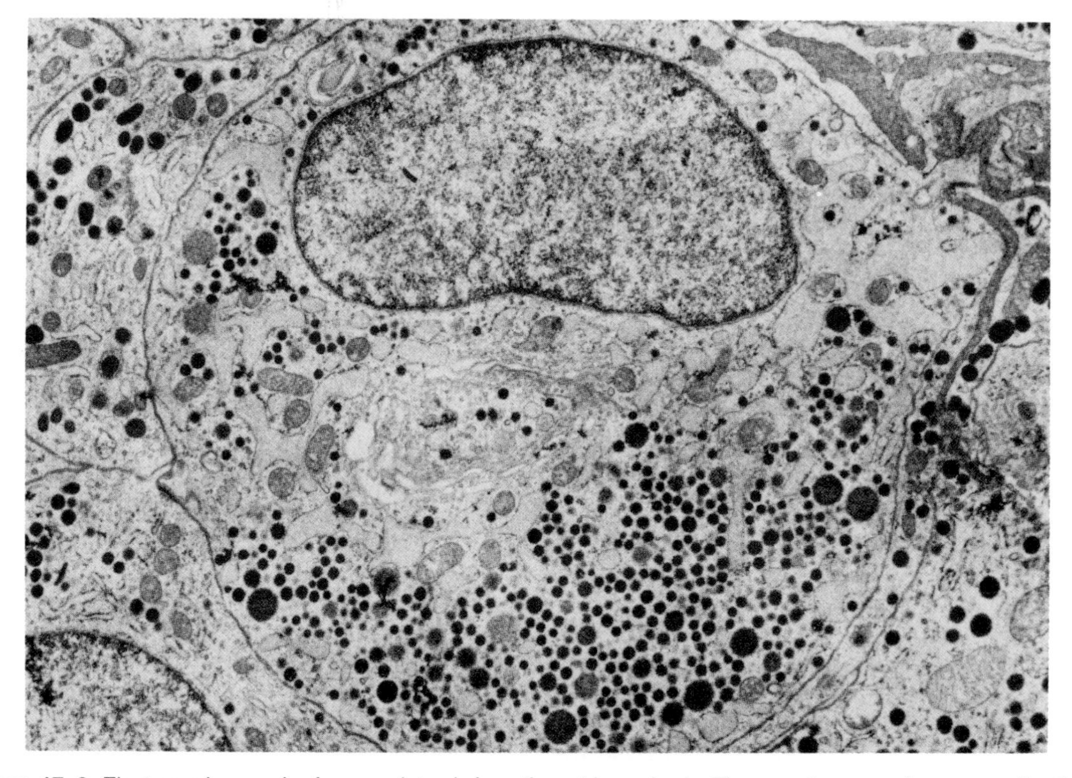

Figure 17–8. Electron micrograph of a gonadotroph from the rat hypophysis. The secretory granules are smaller than those of the somatotroph and mammotroph, but they exhibit considerable variation in size within the same cell. The endoplasmic reticulum is often distended with amorphous material of low density. (Micrograph courtesy of M. Farquhar.)

cisternae that are often distended with a homogeneous content of low electron density (Fig. 17–8). The secretory granules, within the same cell, vary in size over a wide range, from 200 to 400 nm in diameter. Gonadotrophs secrete *follicle-stimulating hormone* (FSH) and *luteinizing hormone* (LH), both are glycoproteins of about 30,000 molecular weight. Whether there are two kinds of gonadotrophs, one secreting FSH and the other LH, has been a subject of dispute. Some gonadotrophs stain immunocytochemically with anti-FSH antibody, others with anti-LH, and still others are reported to stain with both antibodies. It remains unsettled as to whether the two hormones are products of two subpopulations of gonadotrophs or are produced in different phases of the secretory cycle of a single cell type.

In the female, there is a cyclic increase and decrease in the secretion of FSH each month. The rising level stimulates the development of follicles in the ovary in preparation for ovulation. A midcycle surge in LH production triggers ovulation. After ovulation, it is necessary for development of the corpus luteum. In the pubescent male, FSH plays an important role in the initiation of spermatogenesis. Its role in the adult male is less clear, but it is known to act on the Sertoli cells of the testis to stimulate their production of androgen-binding protein. LH also stimulates steroid hormone production by the interstitial cells of the ovary and testis and, therefore, is sometimes called *interstitial cell-stimulating hormone* (ICSH).

CHROMOPHOBES

There are groups of small cells in the interior of the cords of the pars distalis that show little affinity for dyes in histological sections. They usually have less cytoplasm than the chromophilic cells but may occasionally reach the size of acidophils and basophils. These cells were called *chromophobes* by light microscopists and were estimated to make up 65% of the cells of the pars distalis. They were thought to be devoid of secretory granules and were considered to be reserve cells capable of differentiating into either acidophils or basophils. Studies of the pituitary with the electron microscope have now revealed that there are relatively few cells with no specific granules. The cells of the adenohypophysis are believed to have cyclic secretory activity, first accumulating and then releasing their product. It is likely that the cells, formerly identified as chromophobes, are actually partially degranulated acidophils or basophils. If chromophobes that are nonspecific stem cells do exist, they are much less numerous than they were formerly thought to be.

FOLLICULAR CELLS (STELLATE CELLS)

The principal nonsecretory cells of the pars distalis may adopt an epithelial pattern of association around the lumen of small cysts or follicles. In this form, the apices of the cells are joined laterally by juxtaluminal junctional complexes and they have microvilli and occasional cilia projecting into the lumen. Because of their tendency to form epitheloid aggregates around a small lumen, these cells have been called *follicular cells*. They may also take on a branching form with multiple processes extending between the chromophilic secretory cells to join other cells of the same type in a loose network throughout the anterior lobe. In this configuration, they were formerly termed *stellate cells*. To avoid the confusion of having separate descriptive terms for two forms of a single cell type, the term *folliculostellate cell* is now widely used. They contain the usual compliment of organelles, occasional lipid droplets, and a few beta granules of glycogen. Because they contain no secretory granules and bind little dye, they no doubt contributed to erroneously high estimates of the number of chromophobes in the anterior lobe.

The function of the folliculostellate cells is not known. They are thought to be able to undergo mitosis but there is no compelling evidence that they are stem cells capable of differentiating into acidophils and basophils. They contain a distinctive protein of unknown function designated S-100. The finding that their cytoskeletal filaments react with antibody to *gliofibrillar acid protein* has suggested the possibility that they may have a function comparable to that of the glial cells of the nervous system, providing a supportive framework and maintaining a favorable fluid and electrolyte environment for the secretory cells. It is interesting that the processes of the folliculostellate cells are connected by gap junctions that would provide a pathway for communication throughout the interstitial network.

PARS INTERMEDIA

In some mammals, the pars distalis is separated from the neurohypophysis by a cleft,

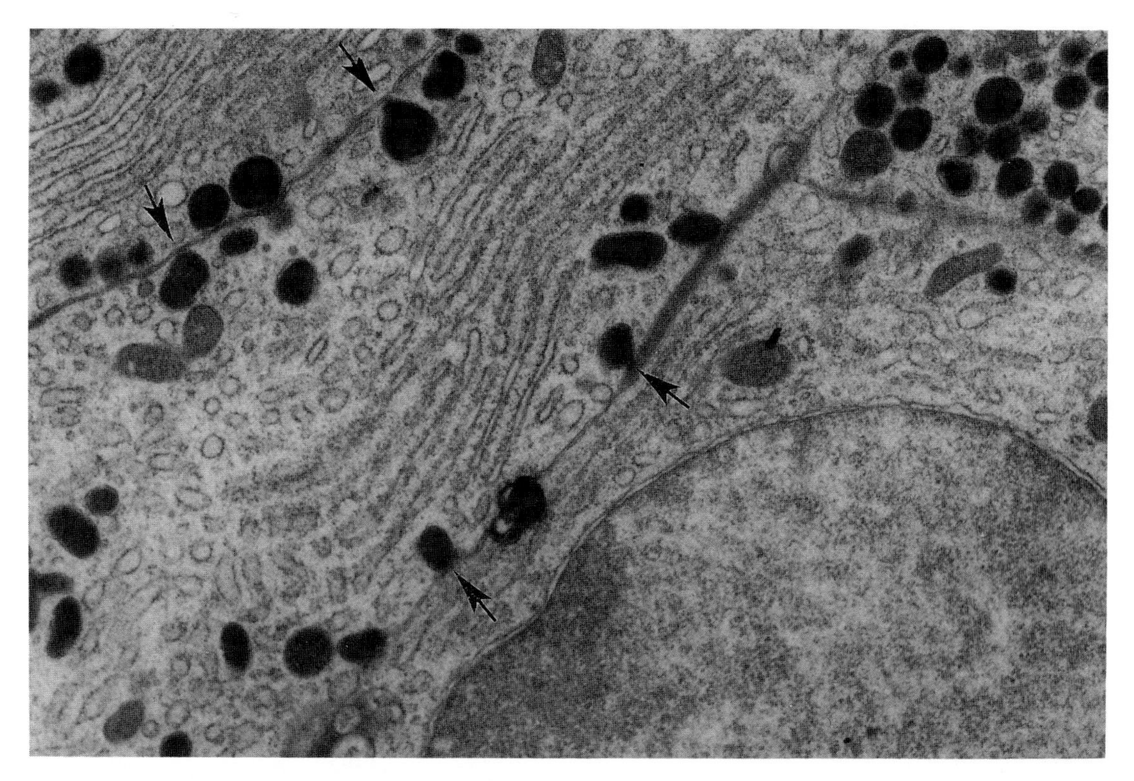

Figure 17–9. Electron micrograph of portions of three lactotrophs from the pituitary gland of a lactating rat. The cells are rich in rough endoplasmic reticulum. A number of secretory granules are in contact with the plasmalemma and some (at arrows) are in the process of exocytosis. (From Haggi, E., A. Torres, C. Maldonado, and A. Aoki. 1986. J. Endocrinol. 111:367.)

lined on the juxtaneural side by a stratified epithelium of basophilic cells that constitute the *pars intermedia.* There are considerable interspecific differences in the degree of development of this component of the hypophysis. In rodents, dogs, cats, and cattle, it is a conspicuous multilayered epithelium. In marsupials, it is reduced to a layer only one or two cells in thickness, and in cetacea, sirenia, and some birds it is absent. In the human fetus, there is a moderately thick pars intermedia making up as much as 3% of the adenohypophysis, but in the adult it is no longer identifiable as a distinct layer. The hypophyseal cleft usually becomes discontinuous in the postnatal period and is represented in the adult by a zone of cysts (Rathke's cysts). These are often lined by a ciliated epithelium and contain a pale-yellow viscous fluid. Concurrently with the disappearance of the cleft, the epithelium of the pars intermedia is dispersed into small cell groups and isolated individual cells. These may invade some distance into the neural tissue of the infundibular process where they are often overlooked in routine histological sections but can be detected by immunocytochemical methods. The description of these cells that follows is based on studies of the hypophysis of the laboratory rat, in which the pars intermedia is a distinct layer accounting for 19% of the volume of the gland.

The cells of the pars intermedia in this species are large polygonal epithelial cells, rich in mitochondria and possessing a well-developed endoplasmic reticulum and a conspicuous Golgi complex. Numerous secretory granules 200–250 nm in diameter are distributed throughout the cytoplasm. Some of these are electron-dense; others are pale, owing to extraction of some of their substance during specimen preparation. The cells secrete *melanocyte-stimulating hormone* (MSH). Like the corticotrophs of the anterior lobe, the cells of the pars intermedia synthesize a large glycosylated prohormone, *proopiomelanocortin* (POMC) which is cleaved to yield two forms of melanocyte stimulating hormone α-MSH, a molecule of 13 amino acids, and β-MSH, consisting of 22 amino acids. Both share amino-acid sequences with ACTH. It is now known that melanotrophs, corticotrophs, and certain neurones of the hypothalamus all synthesize the same prohormone but different modes of posttranslational processing of this molecule yield different ratios of the several possible cleavage products.

Melanocyte-stimulating hormone acts on the melanocytes in the skin of amphibians and reptiles, causing a dispersion of their melanin granules and a darkening of the skin. In mammals, this effect of the hormone is generally not detectable but it does induce synthesis of melanin in melanoma cells in tissue culture and administration of the hormone to humans over several days may result in slight darkening of the skin. The increased pigmentation observed in humans suffering from degeneration of the adrenal cortex (Addison's disease) is attributed to release of excess MSH and ACTH by the pituitary. The slight darkening of the skin sometimes observed during human pregnancy may also result from enhanced release of one or both of these hormones. There is suggestive evidence that melanocyte-stimulating hormone may have other metabolic and behavioral effects, but these are yet to be clearly defined.

PARS TUBERALIS

The *pars tuberalis* (pars infundibularis) forms a thin sleeve around the hypophyseal stalk. It is only 25–60 μm (Fig. 17–2) in thickness, with its thickest portion on its anterior aspect. It is frequently absent over some areas on the posterior surface of the stalk. The pars tuberalis is separated from the infundibular stalk by a thin layers of connective tissue that is continuous with the pia arachnoid and a similar layer covers the outer surface.

The pars tuberalis is the most highly vascularized subdivision of the hypophysis, containing the arterial supply to the anterior lobe and the venules of the hypothalamo-hypophyseal portal system. A distinctive morphological feature of the pars tuberalis is the longitudinal arrangement of its cords of epithelial cells, which occupy the interstices between those longitudinally oriented blood vessels. Its principal cells are 12–18 μm in size and are cuboidal or low columnar in form. In addition to short rod-like mitochondria, their cytoplasm contains small dense granules, numerous lipid droplets, and occasional colloid droplets. They are the only cells in the hypophyysis that contain significant amounts of glycogen. The cells may form follicle-like structures. Islands of squamous epithelial cells may also be found. Although some of the cells appear to contain secretory granules, no specific hormone has been identified and the function of the pars tuberalis remains unknown.

NEUROHYPOPHYSIS

The *pars nervosa* or neurohypophysis consists of the median eminence of the tuber cinereum, the infundibular stem, and the infundibular process (posterior lobe) (Fig. 17–2). The pars nervosa consists of glial elements and the axons and axon terminals of neurons whose cell bodies are located in the hypothalamus. Its organization cannot be adequately described without inclusion of the cell bodies that are located beyond its boundaries. The cell bodies are in the *supraoptic nucleus* located above and lateral to the optic chiasm, and in the *paraventricular nucleus* at a higher level in the lateral wall of the third ventricle. Unmyelinated axons of neurons in these nuclei form the *hypothalamohypophyseal tract* which de-

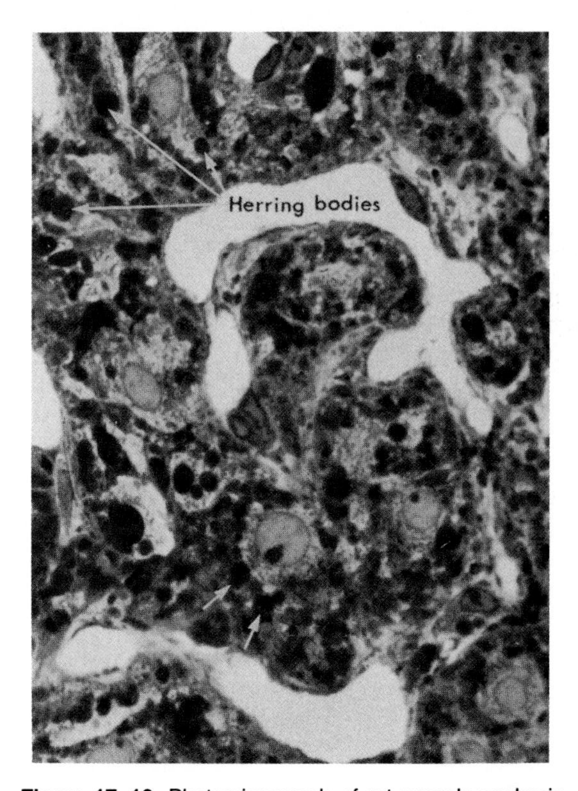

Figure 17–10. Photomicrograph of rat neurohypophysis fixed by perfusion. The large clear areas are capillaries. The dark rounded masses, at arrows, and elsewhere are what were traditionally called Herring bodies. In electron micrographs, these prove to be accumulations of neurosecretory material in dilations of hypothalamohypophyseal nerve axons. (Courtesy of P. Orkand and S. Palay.)

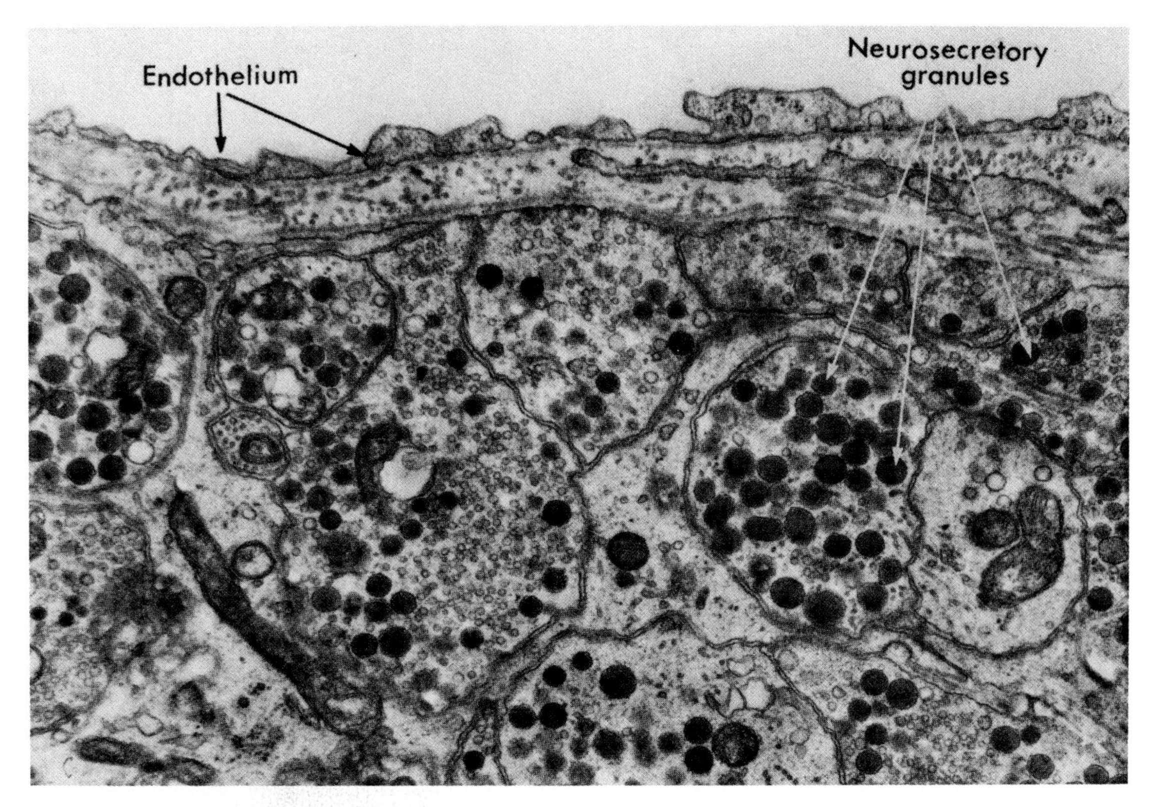

Figure 17–11. Electron micrograph of rat neurohypophysis showing many neurosecretory granules and small vesicles in the axoplasm of fibers of the hypothalamohypophyseal tract that are ending in close relation to a capillary. (Courtesy of P. Orkand and S. Palay.)

scends into, and makes up the bulk of, the substance of the neural lobe of the pituitary.

The hypothalamic neurons are large cells with an eccentric nucleus, abundant cytoplasm, and few processes. The endoplasmic reticulum occurs in arrays of parallel cisternae in the perikaryon and a prominent Golgi complex is the site of assembly of small (120–200 nm) neurosecretory granules. Neurotubules and neurofilaments converge to form an axial bundle that courses down the axon. The neurosecretory granules are continuously transported along these microtubules to the neural lobe of the hypophysis, at a rate of 4–8 mm per hour. Labeled hormone precursors injected intracisternally in experimental animals can be detected in the neural lobe in 1–2 h.

In histological sections of the posterior lobe stained with alum hematoxylin, aggregations of deeply stained material of varying size are found in dilations of the axons throughout the neural lobe. These were formerly called *Herring bodies* (Fig. 7–10). In electron micrographs, they are now found to be large aggregations of small neurosecretory granules (Fig. 17–11). The axons of the hypothalamohypophyseal tract are atypical in that they have numerous dilations along their length as well as at their terminations within the neurohypophysis (Fig. 17–12). It is estimated that each axon has about 450 of these expansions along its course containing, on average, over 2,000 neurosecretory granules. About 60% of the neurosecretory material resides in these axonal dilations and 40% in the axon endings that are associated with fenestrated capillaries throughout the neural lobe. The axon terminations are distinguishable from other axonal dilations by the presence of numerous small vesicles, in addition to the secretory granules. Although these are similar in appearance to the synaptic vesicles of cholinergic nerve endings, there is no evidence that they contain a neurotransmitter. Instead, they are interpreted as agents of retrieval of membrane added to the surface during exocytosis of the secretory granules.

The neural lobe also contains *pituicytes,* stellate cells with slender processes that are joined to the processes of neighboring cells of the

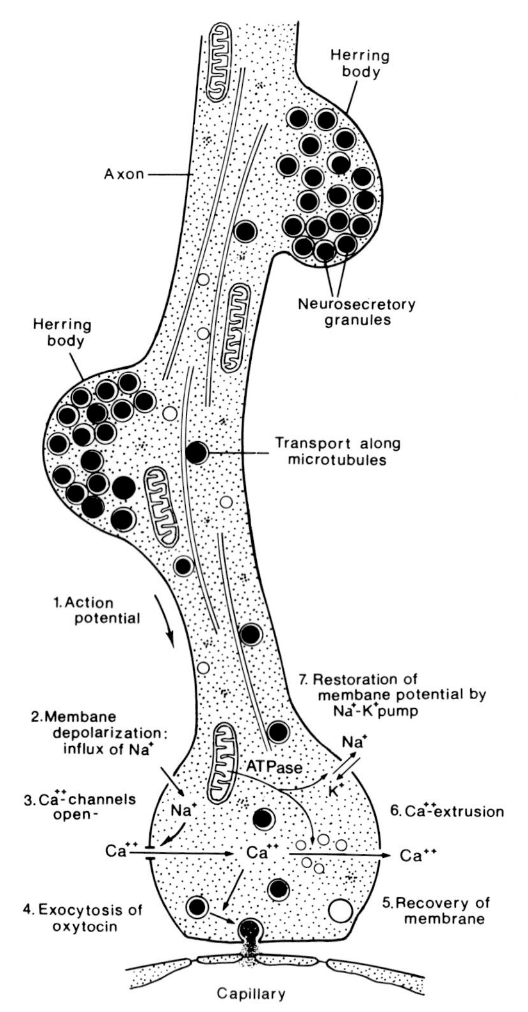

Figure 17–12. Schematic depiction of the terminal portion of an axon of the hypothalamohypophyseal tract in the neurohypophysis. The principal events in stimulus-secretion coupling are indicated. (Modified after Lincoln, D.W. 1984. *In* Hormonal Control of Reproduction. Cambridge, England, Cambridge University Press.)

same type to form a three-dimensional network among the axons of the hypothalamic neurosecretory cells. Their processes are connected by gap junctions which provide for their metabolic coupling. In the human, the pituicytes are highly variable in size and shape and commonly contain lipid droplets and deposits of lipochrome pigment. Their processes meander among groups of preterminal axons and often intimately ensheath the terminal dilations of the axons. The topographical relationship of pituicytes to the axons is, thus, similar to that of the neuroglial cells of the central nervous system. No physiological interaction between the pituicytes and the axons has yet been demonstrated. They seem to have no role in the secretory process but are believed to have a supportive and trophic function, possibly maintaining the ionic composition of the extracellular fluid compartment of the neural lobe.

The two hormones of the neural lobe are *oxytocin* (OT) and *arginine vasopressin* (AVP), also called *antidiuretic hormone* (ADH). They were formerly thought to be produced in separate hypothalamic nuclei—oxytocin in the paraventricular nucleus and vasopressin in the supraoptic nucleus. The two hormones are now known to be synthesized in different types of neurons, but these are present in both the supraoptic and paraventricular nucleus. The hormones are similar polypeptides, consisting of nine amino acids and differing from one another in only two amino acids. Each is synthesized as part of a large precursor molecule consisting of the hormone and a *neurophysin*, an associated protein of 10,000 molecular weight. The neurophysins associated with oxytocin and vasopressin are biochemically distinct. During axoplasmic flow in the hypothalamohypophyseal tracts, the prohormone is cleaved and, at the axon terminal, both the hormone and the neurophysin are released into the blood. The latter has no known physiological effect.

The principal target of oxytocin is the myometrium of the pregnant uterus. Its concentration in the blood increases during the late stages of labor and it is believed to have a significant role in parturition, stimulating contraction of the uterine smooth muscle. It is also responsible for milk ejection from the lactating mammary gland (Fig. 17–13). Stimulation of the nipple by the suckling infant sends afferent impulses to the brain that are relayed to the supraoptic and paraventricular nuclei, which respond by releasing oxytocin into the capillaries of the neurohypophysis. Blood-borne oxytocin then stimulates contraction of myoepithelial cells around the alveoli of the mammary gland, ejecting milk into the ducts. Flow of milk from the nipples begins about 1 min after the onset of suckling.

A major target of arginine vasopressin is the collecting ducts of the kidneys. The interstitium of the renal medulla is hypertonic to the glomerular filtrate in the lumen of the collecting ducts, creating an osmotic gradient that is necessary for conservation of water and concentration of the urine. Circulating vasopressin binds to specific receptors in the basolateral membranes of the cells lining the distal convoluted tubules and collecting ducts and stimulates cyclic AMP activity. This, in turn, activates a protein kinase that acts on a membrane protein to increase the permeability of the apical plasma membrane to water. This permits diffusion of water from the lumen of the tubules up the concentration gradient to the interstitium, thus decreasing the volume of urine and increasing its concentration (Fig. 17–14). This effect of AVP is the basis for its other name, antidiuretic hormone (ADP). In the absence of the hormone, the distal convoluted tubules and collecting ducts are relatively impermeable to water. Humans whose supraoptic and paraventricular nuclei have been invaded by a tumor are unable to secrete ADH and develop *diabetes insipidus* a condition characterized by constant thirst and drinking of large amounts of water (polydipsia) and by excessive urination (polyuria). Our understanding of the physiological basis of this disorder has been furthered by the availability of a convenient animal model, the Brattleboro rat.

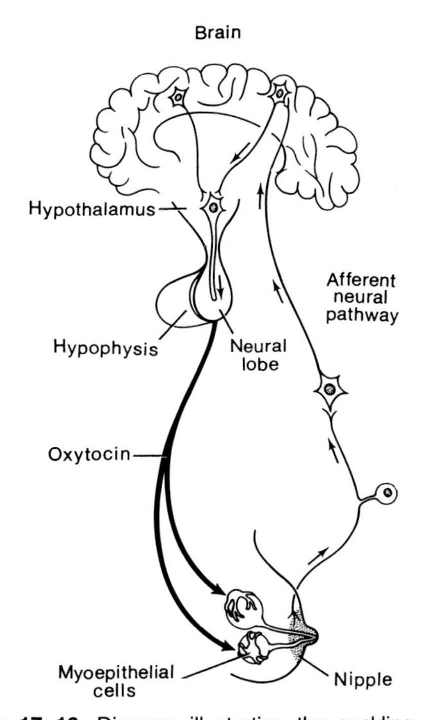

Figure 17–13. Diagram illustrating the suckling reflex. Stimulation of the nipples generates sensory impulses that pass to the brain via the dorsal root ganglia. In the brain, the impulses are relayed to the hypothalamus where they activate neurosecretory cells whose processes extend into the pars nervosa of the hypophysis. Activation of these cells results in the release of oxytocin which is carried in the blood to the mammary gland where it causes contraction of myoepithelial cells, resulting in outflow of milk from the glandular acini.

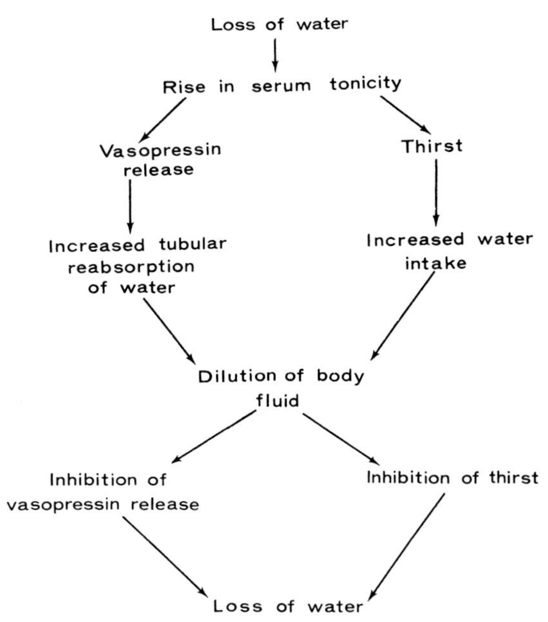

Figure 17–14. Diagram of the role of vasopressin (antidiuretic hormone) of the neurohypophysis in the regulation of body fluids. Interaction of the neurohypophysis, the thirst center of the hypothalamus, and the renal tubules ensures the maintenance of a constant osmolarity of the body fluids. (After Leaf, A. and C.H. Coggins. 19xx. *In* H.R. Williams, ed. Textbook of Endocrinology. Philadelphia, W.B. Saunders.)

This strain of rats inherits diabetes insipidus as a recessive trait. A single base-deletion in the vasopressin gene results in failure of their hypothalamic neurons to secrete the hormone. They excrete every day a volume of urine equivalent to 80% of their body weight and drink a corresponding amount of water. The posterior lobe of their pituitary is unusually large but contains little stainable neurosecretory material and no immunocytochemically detectable arginine vasopressin (Fig. 17–15).

Vasopressin is also involved in the control of blood pressure. Sudden decrease in blood volume is a potent stimulus for increased secretion of vasopressin. After severe hemorrhage, the hormone may be secreted at 50 times the normal rate. It acts on vascular smooth muscle, causing constriction of arterioles, thereby increasing peripheral resistance and raising the blood pressure. The action of the hormone on the kidneys to conserve water also plays a role in the long-term maintenance of blood volume.

HYPOPHYSEAL HORMONES IN OTHER ORGANS

It was long assumed that the hormones of the pituitary were produced exclusively by

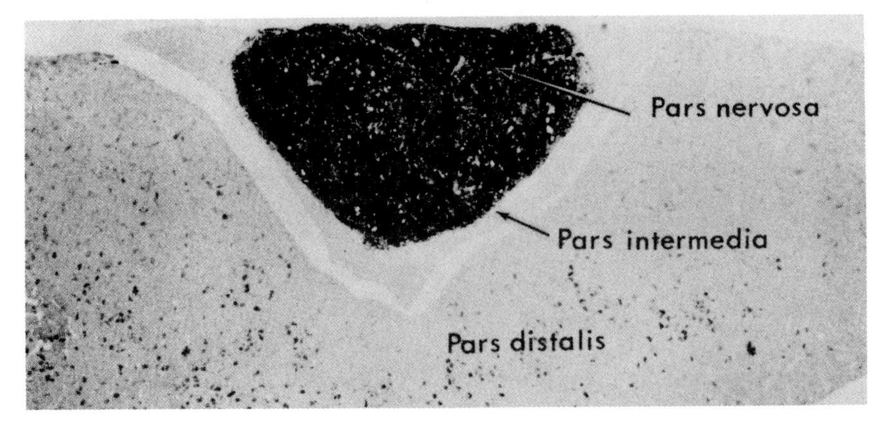

A

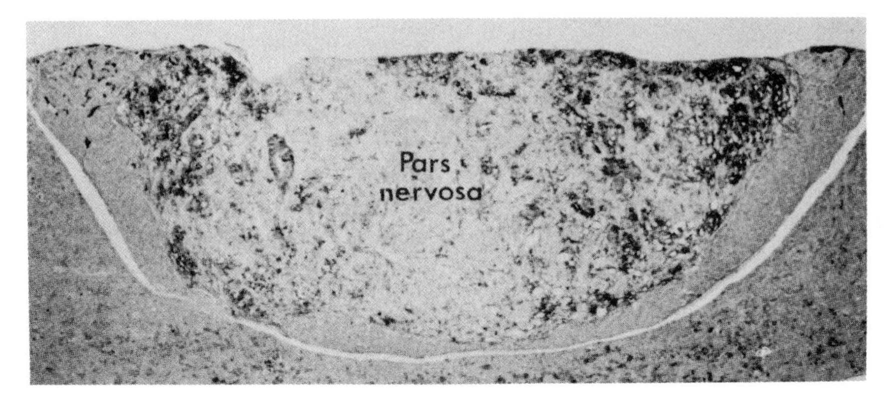

B

Figure 17–15. Photomicrographs of cross sections of the rat hypophysis stained with paraldehyde fuchsin. (A) Hypophysis of a normal rat showing abundant densely stained neurosecretory material in the neurohypophysis. (B) Hypophysis of a rat of the Brattleboro strain with congenital hypothalamic diabetes insipidus. The neurohypophysis is unusually large but contains very little neurosecretory material. (After Sokol, H.W. and H. Valtin. 1965. Endocrinology 77:692.)

specific cells in that gland. As radioimmunoassays for hormone detection and immunocytochemical methods for their localization have been developed, all of the hormones of the adenohypophysis except the gonadotrophins have been found in the central nervous system. These ectopic hormones were initially thought to be of pituitary origin, but evidence for their neural origin is accumulating. This interpretation is strongly supported by the finding that the concentration of ACTH, α-MSH, β-endorphin, and STH in certain areas of the brain remain unchanged or increase after hypophysectomy. There is now interest in the possible functions of these hormones within the nervous system. Some of these hormones have been reported to have effects on learning and behavior of experimental animals, and it is speculated that they may function as neurotransmitters or may modulate the effects of classical neurotransmitters on specific sets of target neurones.

Immunoreactivity for ACTH has been detected in certain cells of the gastrointestinal tract and in neoplasms of the lung derived from neuroepithelial bodies associated with the bronchial epithelium. β-endorphin, ACTH, α-MSH, vasopressin, and oxytocin have been found in the ovary. There is evidence that ovarian oxytocin is secreted into the general circulation but the others may exert paracrine effects within the ovary.

BIBLIOGRAPHY

PARS DISTALIS

Daughaday, W.H. 1983. The anterior pituitary. Nature (London) 301:568.

Duello, T.M. and N.S. Halmi. 1979. Ultrastructural immunocytochemical localization of growth hormone and prolactin in human pituitaries. J. Clin. Endocrinol. 49:189.

Farquhar, M.G. 1971. Processing of secretory products by cells of the anterior pituitary gland. Mem Soc. Endocrinol. 19:79.

Farquhar, M.G., E.H. Skutelsky, and C.R. Hopkins. 1975. Structure and function of anterior pituitary and dispersed pituitary cells in in vitro studies. *In* Anterior Pituitary. San Francisco, Academic Press.

Farquhar, M.G. 1977. Secretion and crinophagy in prolactin cells. *In* Comparative Endocrinology of Prolactin. H. Dellmann et al. eds. New York, Plenun Press.

Fumagalli, G. and A. Zanini. 1985. In cow pituitary, growth hormone and prolactin can be packed in separate granules of the same cell. J. Cell Biol. 100:2019.

Gershengorn, M.C. 1986. Mechanism of thyrotropin releasing hormone stimulation of pituitary hormone secretion. Annu. Rev. Physiol. 48:515.

Guillemin, R. 1975–1976. Control of adenohypophyseal functions by peptides of the central nervous system. Harvey Lecture Series 71. p. 24.

Guillemin, R. and R. Burgus. 1972. The hormones of the hypothalamus. Sci. Am. 227:24.

Haggi, E.S., A.I. Torres, C.A. Maldonado, and A. Aoki. 1986. Regression of redundant lactotrophs in rat pituitary gland after cessation of lactation. J. Endocrinol. 111:367.

Jones, T.H., B.L. Brown, and P.R. Dobson. 1990. Paracrine control of anterior pituitary hormone secretion. J. Endocrinol. 127:5.

Larsen, P.R. 1982. Thyroid-pituitary interaction. Feedback regulation of thyrotropin secretion by thyroid hormones. N. Engl. J. Med. 306:23.

Moriarty, G.C. 1973. Adenohypophysis: ultrastructural cytochemistry. A review. J. Histochem. Cytochem. 21:885.

Pelletier, G., F. Robert, and J. Hardy. 1978. Identification of human pituitary cell types by immunoelectron microscopy. J. Clin. Endocrin. Metab. 46:534.

Phifer, R.F., A.R. Midgley, and S.S. Spicer. 1973. Immunohistological and histological evidence that follicle stimulating and luteinizing hormones are present in the same cell types in the human pars distalis. J. Clin. Endocrin. Metab. 36:125.

Phifer, R.F. and S.S. Spicer. 1973. Immunohistochemical and histological demonstration of thyrotropic cells of the human adenohypophysis. J. Clin. Endocrin. Metab. 36:1210.

Rambourg, A., Y. Clermont, M. Chretien, and L. Oliver. 1992. Formation of secretory granules in the Golgi apparatus of prolactin cells in the rat pituitary: A stereoscopic study. Anat. Rec. 232:169.

Salpeter, M.M. and M.G. Farquhar. 1981. High resolution analysis of the secretory pathway in mammotrophs of the rat anterior pituitary. J. Cell Biol. 91:240.

Shiino, M., A. Arimura, A.V. Shalley, and E.G. Rennels. 1972. Ultrastructural observations of granule extrusion from rat anterior pituitary cells after injection of LH-releasing hormone. Z. Zellforsch. Mikrosk. Anat. 128:152.

Shiino, M., M.G. Williams, and E.R. Rennels. 1972. Ultrastructural observation of pituitary release of prolactin in the rat by suckling stimulus. Endocrinology 90:176.

Tixler-Vidal, A. and M.G. Farquhar. eds. 1975. The Anterior Pituitary. New York, Academic Press.

von Lauzewitsch, I., H. Dickman, L. Amezua, and C. Pardel. 1972. Cytological and ultrastructural characterization of the human pituitary. Acta Anat. 81:276.

PARS INTERMEDIA

Jackson, S., J. Hope, F. Estavarex, and P.J. Lowry. 1981. The nature and control of peptide release from the pars intermedia. *In* Peptides and the Pars Intermedia, Ciba Foundation Symposium 81. London, Pitman Medical.

Lerner, A.B. and J.S. McGuire. 1961. Effects of alpha- and beta-melanocyte stimulating hormones on skin color in man. Nature 189:176.

Lerner, A.B. and Y. Takahashi. 1956. Hormonal control of melanin pigmentation. Recent Progr. Horm. Res. 12:203.

Stoeckel, M.E., G. Schmitt, and A. Porte. 1981. Fine structure and cytochemistry of the mammalian pars intermedia. *In* Peptides of the Pars Intermedia, Ciba Foundation Symposium 81. London, Pitman Medical.

NEUROHYPOPHYSIS

Barer, R. and K. Lederis. 1966. Ultrastructure of the rabbit neurohypophysis with special reference to the release of hormones. Z. Zellforsch. 75:201.

Bargmann, W. 1966. Neurosecretion. Internat. Rev. Cytol. 18:183.

Bodian, D. 1963. Cytological aspects of neurosecretion in the opossum neurohypophysis. Bull. J. Hopkins Hosp. 113:57.

Bonner, T.I. and M.J. Brownstein. 1984. Vasopressin, tissue specific defects and the Brattleboro rat. Nature 310:17.

Brownstein, M., J.T. Russell, and H. Gainer. 1980. Synthesis, transport, and release of posterior pituitary hormones. Science 207:373.

Dierickx, K. and F. Vandesande. 1979. Immunocytochemical demonstration of separate vasopressin-neurophysis and oxytocin-neurophysin neurones in the human hypothalamus. Cell Tissue Res. 196:203.

Gainer, H., Y. Sarne, and M.J. Brownstein. 1977. Biosynthesis and axon transport of rat neurohypophyseal protein and peptides. J. Cell Biol. 73:366.

Guillemin, R. and R. Burgus. 1972. The hormones of the hypothalamus. Sci. Am. 227:24.

Sachs, H., P. Fawcett, and Y. Takabataka, and R. Portanova. 1969. Biosynthesis and release of vasopressin and neurophysin. Recent Progr. Horm. Res. 25:447.

Sokol, H.W. and H. Valtin. 1965. Morphology of the neurosecretory system in rats homozygous and heterozygous for hypothalamic diabetes insipidus (Brattleboro strain). Endocrinology 77:692.

BLOOD VESSELS

Bergland, R.M. and R.B. Page. 1979. Pituitary-brain vascular relations: a new paradigm. Science 204:18.

Farquhar, M.G. 1961. Fine structure and function in capillaries of the anterior pituitary gland. Angiology 12:270.

Green, J.D. and G.W. Harris. 1949. The neurovascular link between the neurohypophysis and the adenohypophysis. J. Endocrinol. 5:136.

Murakami, T., A. Kikuta, T. Taguchi, A. Ohtsuka, and O. Ohtani, 1987. Blood vascular architecture of the rat cerebral hypophysis and hypothalamus. A dissection/scanning electron microscopy of vascular casts. Arch. Histol. Japan 50:133.

18
THE THYROID GLAND

The hormones of the thyroid gland are essential for normal growth and development, and in the adult, its hormones, *thyroxin* and *triiodothyronine,* regulate the rate of metabolism in cells throughout the body. A third hormone, *calcitonin,* controls the concentration of calcium in the extracellular fluid and its deposition in bone. Thyroid function, in turn, is under control of the hypophyseal hormone, *thyroid-stimulating hormone* (TSH).

The gland is situated below the larynx in the anterior portion of the neck. It weighs 25–40 g and consists of two *lateral lobes* connected by a narrow *isthmus* that crosses the trachea just below the cricoid cartilage. About one-third of individuals also have a slender *pyramidal lobe* that extends upward from the isthmus near the left lobe. The gland is enclosed in a connective tissue capsule that is continuous with the cervical fascia. On its deep surface, this layer is connected to another layer of less dense connective tissue that is intimately adherent to the gland. This separation of the capsule into two layers creates a plane of cleavage between the two that facilitates surgical access to the gland when partial thyroidectomy is necessary.

HISTOLOGICAL ORGANIZATION

In most endocrine glands, limited amounts of hormone are stored in intracellular secretory granules. The thyroid is unique in having a histological organization that provides for extracellular storage of its product in the lumen of cyst-like *follicles.* In the human, the follicles are estimated to number (2–3) $\times 10^7$ and they contain several weeks supply of hormones. In section, they are nearly spherical and range from 0.2 to 0.9 mm in diameter. In other species, they are more uniform in size. The follicles are bounded by a simple cuboidal epithelium (Figs. 18–1 and 18–2). The cells are polarized toward the lumen, which is filled with a gelatinous or semifluid substance referred to as the *colloid.* Thyroxin and triiodothyronine are stored in the colloid as constituents of a large secretory glycoprotein called *thyroglobulin* (660,000 MW). Thyroglobulin must be hydrolyzed to release the thyroid hormones and this is achieved by its uptake from the lumen of the follicle by endocytosis and intracellular action of lysosomal proteases.

Each follicle is enveloped by a thin basal lamina, a delicate network of reticular fibers, and a plexus of capillaries (Fig. 18–3). In histological preparations, the follicles appear to be discrete structures, but when reconstructions are made from serial sections, the base of the epithelium of one follicle may, in some instances, be in direct contact with the epithelium of an adjacent follicle without an intervening basal lamina or layer of reticular fibers. However, continuity between the lumen of neighboring follicles has not been observed.

The epithelium of mammalian thyroid follicles contains two cell types: the *principal cells* that make up the greater part of the epithelium and the *parafollicular cells* that occur singly or in small groups between the bases of the principal cells. The epithelium is usually low cuboidal but varies somewhat in height from follicle to follicle and in different states of physiological activity. It may be predominantly squamous or cuboidal in relatively quiescent glands and columnar in hyperactive glands. However, an assessment of functional activity cannot be based on the height of the epithelium alone. The principal cells have a round or ovoid nucleus, poor in heterochromatin, and containing one or two nucleoli. The cytoplasm of the cells is basophilic, whereas the colloid stains with eosin and gives a strong periodic-acid–Schiff reaction for carbohydrates. The apical cytoplasm contains numerous small dense granules that give a positive reaction for acid hydrolases and are, therefore, identified as lysosomes rather than secretory granules. Vacuoles with a content that stains with aniline blue and with the PAS

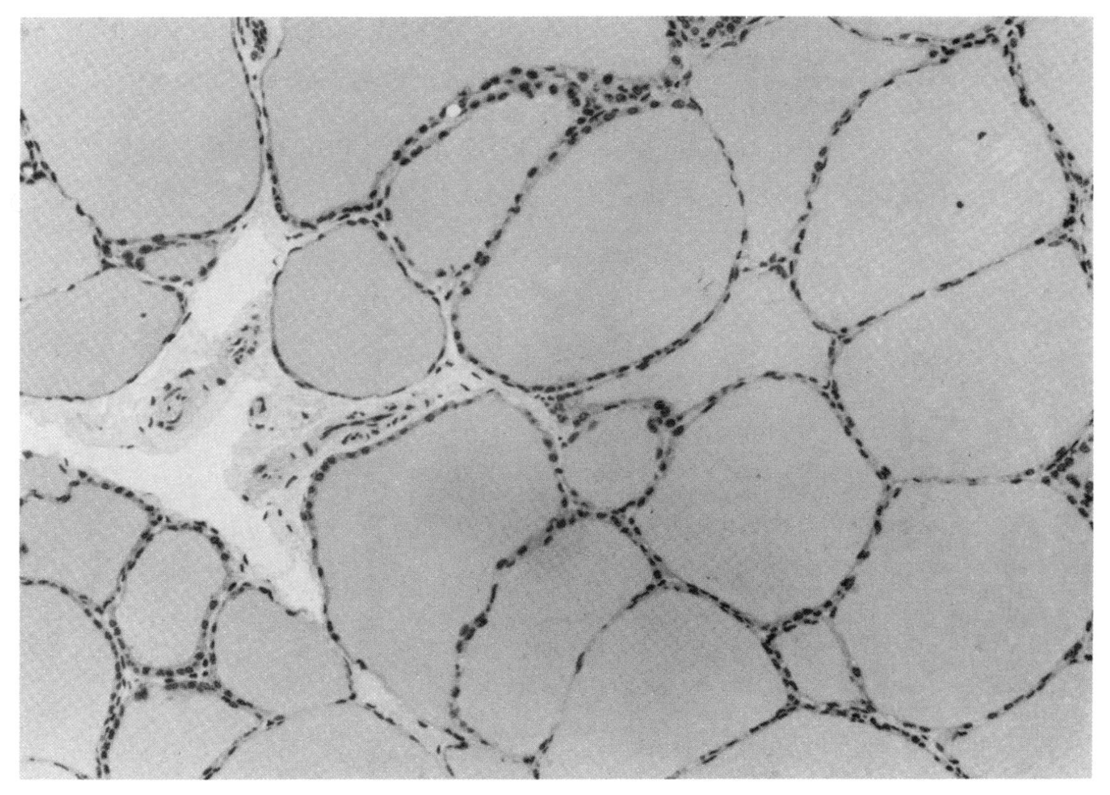

Figure 18–1. Photomicrograph of monkey thyroid showing the cuboidal epithelium of the follicles and their content of colloid.

reaction may be also be observed in the apical cytoplasm. These are interpreted as droplets of colloid that have been taken up by endocytosis in response to TSH stimulation.

In electron micrographs, the lumenal surface of the principal cells bears numerous short microvilli. The membrane at the base of the cell is smooth-contoured and rests on a thin basal lamina that is continuous around the entire follicle. The cells are in close apposition laterally and are joined by typical junctional complexes. The nucleus has no distinctive ultrastructural features. Granular endoplasmic reticulum is moderately well developed and its cisternae tend to be widely dilated by a content that is extracted in specimen preparation (Fig. 18–4). The juxtanuclear Golgi complex consists of stacks of flat, or slightly distended, cisternae and numerous associated small vesicles. Similar vesicles are found throughout the cytoplasm but are especially abundant near the apex of the cell. These are believed to be transporting thyroglobulin from the Golgi complex for exocytosis into the lumen of the follicle.

The large pale-staining parafollicular cells lie within the epithelium but do not reach its free surface, being separated from it by overarching portions of the neighboring principal cells. They occur singly or in small groups. Clusters of parafollicular cells have also been reported to occur in the interfollicular spaces, but it is now the consensus that this was a misinterpretation of tangential sections of follicles under the light microscope. In electron micrographs, all parafollicular cells appear to be within the epithelium.

Parafollicular cells are two to three times the size of the principal cells, but, in the human, they comprise only 0.1% of the epithelial mass of the gland. They tend to be more numerous in the central region of thyroid lobes. Their nucleus is round or ovoid and may be indented on one side. The cytoplasm is of low electron density and contains a moderate amount of endoplasmic reticulum, mainly tubular in form, but small stacks of cisternae may also be found. The secretory granules are not always retained by the common histological fixatives but are well preserved by the aldehyde fixatives employed for electron microscopy. They are small dense granules 0.1–

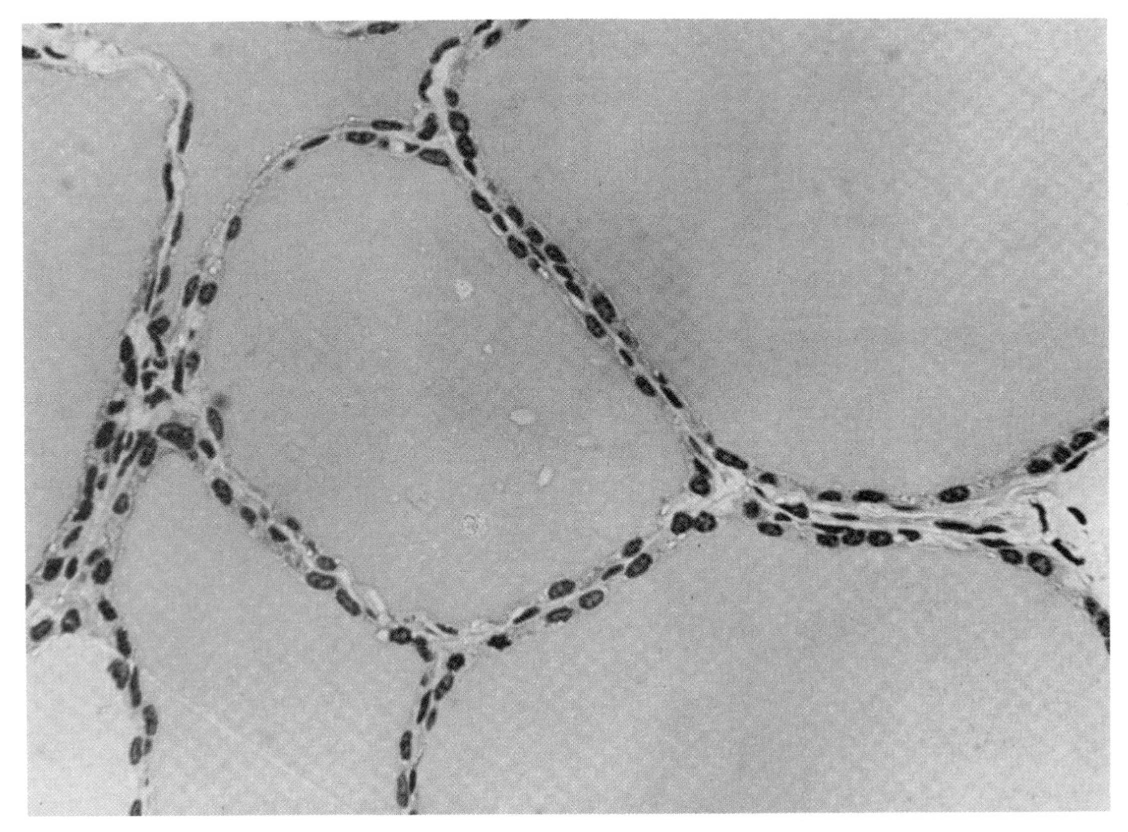

Figure 18–2. Photomicrograph of monkey thyroid gland, at higher magnification, to illustrate the character of the epithelium and the homogenous appearance of the colloid.

0.4 μm in diameter (Fig. 18–5), and they are usually congregated in the basal cytoplasm.

The secretory granules of parafollicular cells contain *calcitonin,* a peptide hormone of 32 amino acids that lowers the concentration of calcium in the blood by suppressing bone resorption. Experimentally induced hypercalcemia results in a marked degranulation of the parafollicular cells within 2 h. Calcitonin appears to be of less physiological significance in humans than in other mammalian species, because serum calcium is maintained within normal limits after total thyroidectomy. In fish, amphibians, reptiles, and birds, the calcitonin-secreting cells are not incorporated in the thyroid but form discrete epithelial cell masses called *ultimobranchial bodies,* located in the neck or mediastinum. Calcitonin extracted from the ultimobranchial bodies of salmon has a hypocalcemic effect 10 times as great as human calcitonin and has been used in treatment of Pagets disease and osteoporosis.

In a number of mammalian species, the parafollicular cells contain *serotonin* (5-hydroxytryptamine). In others, it is present in the fetal and postnatal periods but is not histochemically demonstrable in the adult. In all species, the cells take up exogenous amine precursors and deposit serotonin in the secretory granules, which contain a serotonin-binding protein. The physiological significance of serotonin in the parafollicular cells is unclear.

Immunocytochemical studies have established that the parafollicular cells of all species investigated contain *somatostatin,* a peptide of 14 amino acids that inhibits the secretion of growth hormone and thyroid-stimulating hormone by the pituitary, and secretion of insulin and glucagon by the pancreas. It is also present in cells of the hypothalamus and endocrine cells of the gastrointestinal tract. It is speculated that it may have a local effect in the thyroid and may be involved in regulation of secretion of calcitonin or thyroid hormone.

HISTOPHYSIOLOGY

The primary control of thyroid function is mediated by *thyroid-stimulating hormone* (TSH),

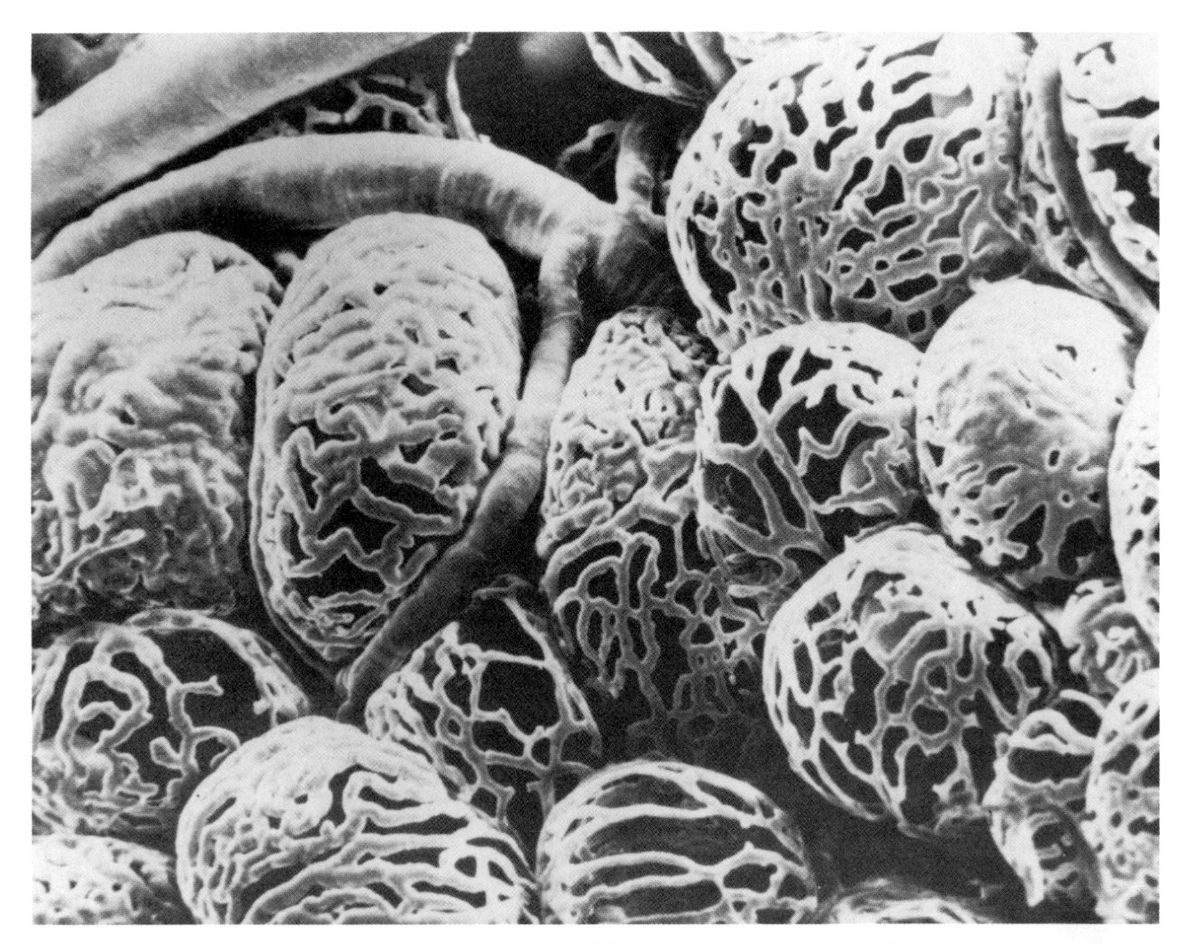

Figure 18–3. Scanning electron micrograph of a portion of the monkey thyroid in which the blood vessels have been injected with plastic and the tissue subsequently digested away. Each follicle is surrounded by a dense network of capillaries. (Micrograph from Fujita, H. and T. Murakami. 1974. Arch. Histol. Japan 36:181.

a glycoprotein secreted by the anterior pituitary in response to *thyrotropin-releasing hormone* (TRH). This tripeptide, secreted by cells in the hypothalamus, is carried in the hypothalamohypophyseal portal system to the anterior pituitary where it binds to specific receptors on the *thyrotroph* cells, stimulating their release of TSH. The ability of these cells to respond to TRH is under feedback control of thyroxin and triiodothyronine. An excess of circulating thyroid hormones diminishes the response of the thyrotrophs to TRH and a deficiency of these hormones increases their response. Thyroid-stimulating hormone binds to receptors on the basolateral domain of the follicular cell membrane and the cells rapidly respond with increased synthesis of cyclic AMP, accelerated iodine uptake and hormone synthesis.

Synthesis of thyroglobulin progresses along the same intracellular pathway described for other protein-secreting cells. Amino acids on ribosomes of the endoplasmic reticulum are assembled into polypeptides and then transported in vesicles to the Golgi complex. Thyroglobulin is a glycoprotein and the glycosyltransferases of the Golgi have an important role in synthesis and conjugation of its carbohydrate components. The product is not concentrated into secretory granules but is transported in small vesicles to the cell apex for discharge into the colloid by exostosis. Iodine is essential for thyroid hormone production and is utilized to iodinate tyrosines in the thyroglobulin molecule. The principal cells of the follicular epithelium have a remarkable capacity to take up iodide from the blood plasma and transport it to the lumen of the follicle, where thyroglobulin is iodinated by a membrane-bound enzyme, thyroid peroxidase (Fig. 18–6). Iodide is taken up at a higher rate than it is incorporated into thyroglobulin.

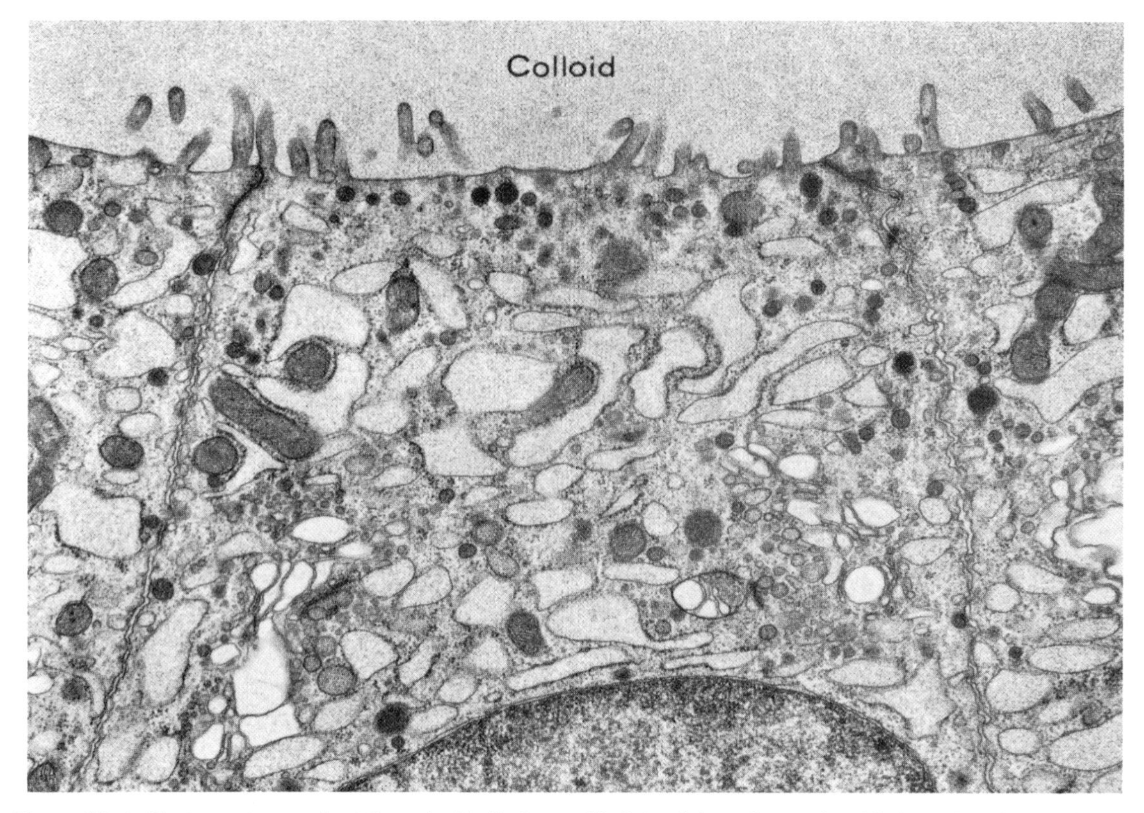

Figure 18–4. Electron micrograph of the apical half of an epithelial cell from the rat thyroid gland. The free surface of the cell bears numerous short microvilli that project into the colloid of the follicle. The endoplasmic reticulum is well developed and its cisternae are distended with an amorphous content of low density. The numerous small dense granules in the apical cytoplasm are lysosomes. (Micrograph courtesy of S. Wissig.)

After an injection of inorganic iodide, 40% of the circulating ion is concentrated within the thyroid within 10 min. When the dietary intake of iodine is deficient, as it may be in residents of certain geographical regions, little active thyroid hormone is produced but an excessive accumulation of colloid in the follicles results in enlargement of the gland, a condition called *colloid goiter*.

Because the thyroid gland stores its product extracellularly within the follicles, the mechanism for release of hormone into the blood is more complex than that of other endocrine glands. It begins by endocytosis of colloid at the cell apex. This normally takes place by micropinocytosis, but when the gland is strongly stimulated by administration of TSH, the cells exhibit macrocytosis, extending pseudopods into the lumen of the follicle to envelop droplets of colloid that are drawn into the cytoplasm in large vacuoles (Fig. 18–7). Hydrolysis of the thyroglobulin is necessary to liberate the hormones, and both the micropinocytic vesicles of the normal gland and the larger vacuoles of the overstimulated gland fuse with lysosomes and thyroxin and triiodothyronine are liberated by their acid hydrolases. Transfer of the hormones to the cell base cannot be observed in electron micrographs and the exact mechanism of their release into the interfollicular spaces is poorly understood.

As in other endocrine glands, the capillaries of the thyroid are fenestrated and offer little or no barrier to entry of the hormones. The blood vascular system, with its high rate of flow, is undoubtedly their principal avenue of egress, but their concentration in the lymph leaving the gland is as much as 100 times their concentration in the circulation. The lymphatics must, therefore, be considered a significant pathway for transport of the hormones to the blood vascular system. In the circulation, they are bound to a thyroid hormone-binding globulin and to albumin.

Thyroxin (tetraiodothyronine) is secreted at a rate nearly 10 times that of triiodothyronine, but the latter is 3 to 4 times as potent,

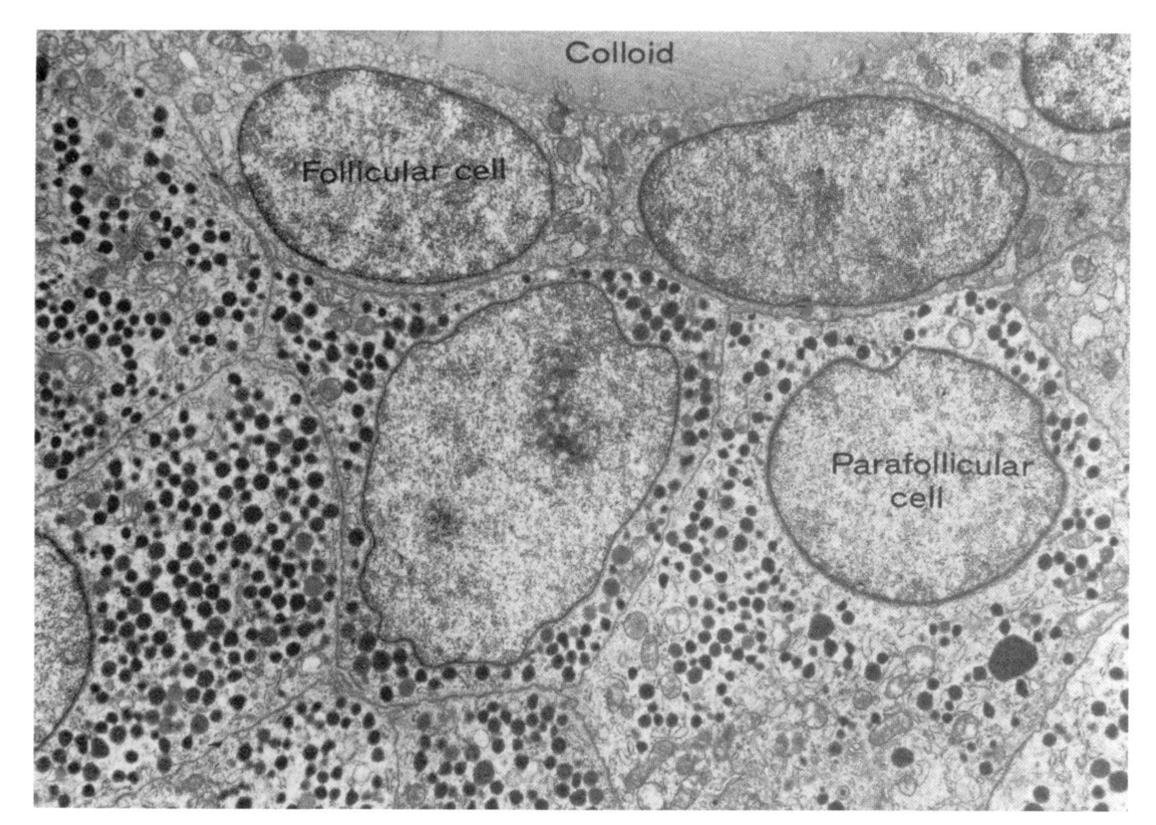

Figure 18–5. Electron micrograph of follicular cells (top) and parafollicular cells (bottom) from a normal cat thyroid. The parafollicular cells do not border on the lumen but are always separated from the colloid by follicular cells. When well fixed by glutaraldehyde, the parafollicular cells contain many dense secretory granules. (Micrograph courtesy of S. Wissig.)

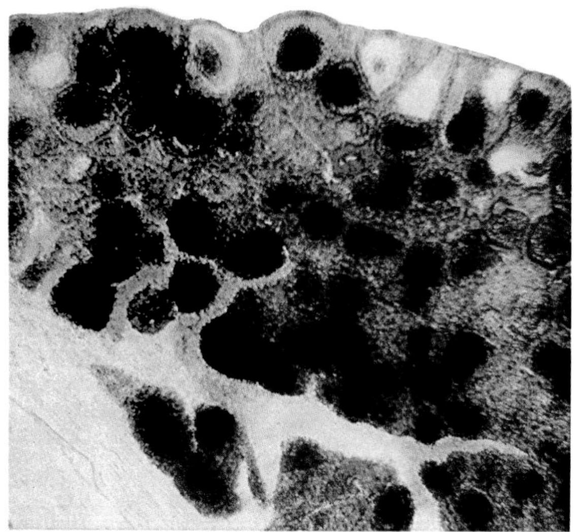

Figure 18–6. Low-power photomicrograph of thyroid gland of a rat previously injected with ^{131}I. The blackened areas represent sites of deposition of radioactive isotope in the colloid. There is great variation in the content of the isotope in the several follicles shown. (Courtesy of C. P. Leblond, D. Findlay, and S. Gross.)

and a large proportion of the circulating thyroxin is converted to triiodothyronine by monodeiodination in the liver, kidney, and other organs. The hormone exerts its effects by binding to nuclear receptors in the target organs and stimulating transcription of specific RNAs. The amount of Na^+,K^+-ATPase in the cells is significantly increased, and their protein synthesis and carbohydrate metabolism are enhanced.

Disturbances of thyroid function have striking effects on metabolism of the body as a whole. Deficiency of thyroid hormone, *hypothyroidism,* causes a fall in metabolic rate. When hypothyroidism begins in infancy and persists, it leads to *cretinism,* a condition characterized by stunting of growth and retarded mental development. Persistent hypothyroidism, in the adult, leads to *myxedema,* a disorder attended by a sallow, puffy appearance of the face, dry, sparse hair, lethargy, and slow cerebration. In both cretinism and myxedema, the basal metabolic rate can be raised and the symptoms relieved by administration of thyroid hormone.

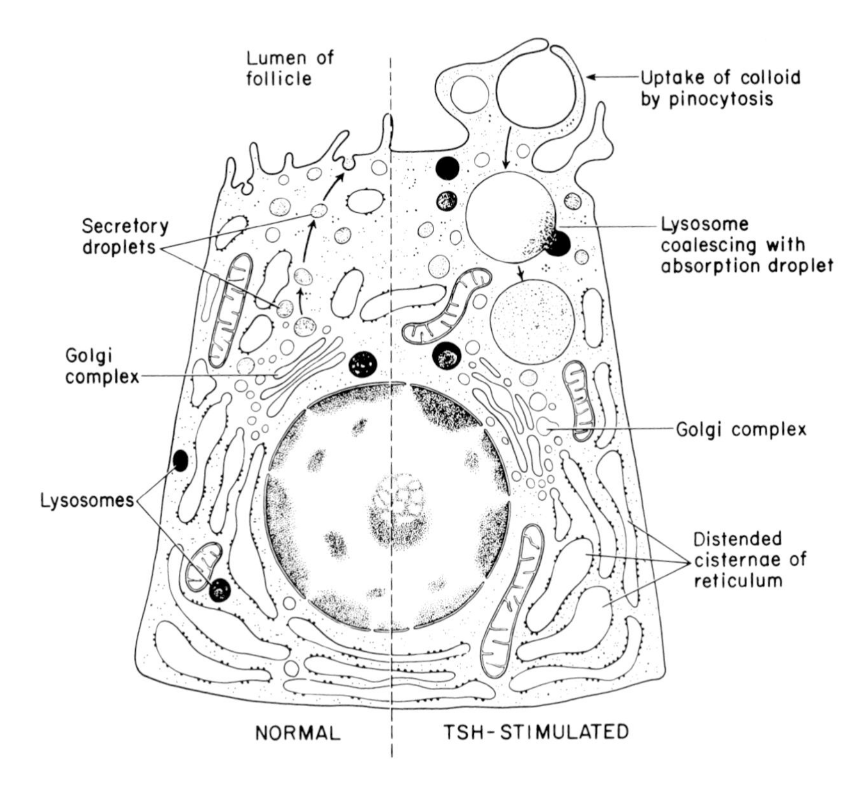

Figure 18–7. Left side: Diagram depicting the normal structure of a thyroid cell secreting thyroglobulin into the lumen of the follicle. **Right side:** The uptake of colloid by pinocytosis after heavy stimulation with thyroid-stimulating hormone, and the lysosomal degradation of thyroglobulin to release thyroxin and triiodothyronine. (From Fawcett, D. W., J. A. Long, and A. L. Jones. 1969. Recent Prog. Horm. Res. 25:315.)

Overproduction of thyroid hormones, *hyperthyroidism,* may result in elevation of the metabolic rate to dangerous levels. In its common form, *Grave's disease* (*exophthalmic goiter*), the principal cells of the thyroid follicles become very tall and papillary projections project into the lumen. Colloid is greatly diminished. Thyroid hormone may be secreted at 5 to 10 times the normal rate. The patient suffers weight loss, nervousness, fatigue, and rapid heart rate. The disease is caused by an immunoglobulin of the IgG class that interacts with the TSH receptors of the principal cells and results in prolonged stimulation of hormone production.

The secretion of calcitonin by the parafollicular cells of the thyroid is directly controlled by the level of calcium in the blood. The serum calcium level depends in large measure on the rate of demineralization of bone by the osteoclasts. Calcitonin is normally secreted at a low basal rate, but the parafollicular cells are markedly stimulated by any rise in serum calcium. Within a few minutes after augmented release of calcitonin, the osteoclasts in bone lose their ruffled borders and revert to a relatively inactive state. The resulting diminution in mineral resorption permits the serum calcium to fall to a normal level. There are also receptors for calcitonin in the kidney and their activation may increase the excretion of calcium in the urine.

BIBLIOGRAPHY

Austin, L. A. and H. Heath. 1981. Calcitonin: Physiology and pathophysiology. New Engl. J. Med. 304:269.

Bernd, P., M. D. Gershon, E. A. Nunez, and H. Tamir. 1981. Separation of dissociated thyroid follicular and parafollicular cells: Association of serotonin binding protein. J. Cell Biol. 88:499.

Bogdanove, E. M. 1962. Regulation of TSH secretion. Fed. Proc. 21:633.

Brazeau, P., W. Vale, R. Burgus, N. Long, M. Butcher, J. Rivier, and R. Guillemin. 1973. Hypothalamic polypeptide that inhibits secretion of pituitary growth hormone. Science 179:77.

Buffa, A., J. A. Chayvialle, P. Fontana, L. Uselini, C. Capella, and E. Solcia. 1979. Parafollicular cells of rabbit store both calcitonin and somatostatin and resemble gut D-cells ultrastructurally. Histochemistry 62:281.

Bussolati, G. and A. G. E. Pearse. 1967. Immunofluorescence localization of calcitonin in the C-cells of pig and dog thyroid. J. Endocrinol. 37:205.

Chambard, M., B. Verrier, J. Cambrion, and J. Mauchamp. 1983. Polarization of thyroid cells in culture: Evidence for basolateral localization of the iodide pump and the TSH receptor–adenyl cyclase complex. J. Cell Biol. 96:1172.

Daniel, P. M., L. G. Plaskett, and O. E. Pratt. 1967. The lymphatic and venous pathways for the outflow of thyroxine, iodoprotein and inorganic iodide from the thyroid gland. J. Physiol. (London) 188:25.

DeGroot, L. J. and H. Niepomniszeze. 1977. Biosynthesis of thyroid hormone: basic and clinical aspects. Metabolism 26:665.

DeGroot, L. J. 1965. Current views on formation of thyroid hormone. N. Engl. J. Med. 272:243.

Ekholm, R. and L. E. Ericson. 1968. Ultrastructure of the parafollicular cells of the rat. J. Ultrastr. Res. 23:378.

Ekholm, R. and U. Strandberg. 1967. Thyroglobulin biosynthesis in rat thyroid. J. Ultrastr. Res. 20:103.

Ekholm, R., G. Engstrom, L. E. Ericson, and A. Melander. 1975. Exocytosis of protein into thyroid follicle lumen: an early effect of TSH. Endocrinology 97:337.

Ericson, L. E. 1981. Exocytosis and endocytosis in the thyroid follicle cell. Mol. Cell. Endocrinol. 22:1.

Foster, G. V., A. Baghdiantz, M. A. Kumar, E. Slack, H. A. Soliman, and I. MacIntyre. 1964. Thyroid origin of calcitonin. Nature 202:1303.

Fujita, H. 1970. Outline of the fine structural aspects of synthesis and release of thyroid hormone. Gunma Symp. Endocrinol. 7:49.

Fujita, H. and T. Murakami. 1974. Scanning electron microscopy on the distribution of the minute blood vessels of the dog, cat, and Rhesus monkey thyroid. Arch. Histol. Japan 36:181.

Gershengorn, M. C. 1986. Mechanism of thyrotropin releasing hormone stimulation of pituitary hormone secretion. Annu. Rev. Physiol. 48:515.

Heimann, P. 1966. Ultrastructure of the human thyroid. A study of normal thyroid, untreated and treated toxic goiter. Acta Endocrinol. 53 (Suppl. 5):110.

Herzog, V. 1983. Transcytosis in thyroid follicle cells. J. Cell Biol. 97:601.

Hirsch, P. F. and P. L. Munson. 1968. Thyrocalcitonin. Physiol. Rev. 49:548.

Kameda, Y., H. Oyama, M. Endoh, and M. Horino. 1982. Somatostatin immunoreactive C-cells in thyroid glands of various mammalian species. Anat. Rec. 204:161.

Larsen, P.R. 1982. Thyroid-pituitary interaction. Feedback of thyrotropin secretion by thyroid hormones. N. Engl. J. Med. 306:23.

Nadler, N. J., B. A. Young, C. P. Leblond, and B. Mitmaker. 1964. Elaboration of thyroglobulin in the thyroid follicle. Endocrinology 74:333.

Nonidez, J. F. 1932. Further observations on the parafollicular cells of the mammalian thyroid. Anat. Rec. 53:339.

Nunez, E. A. and M. D. Gershon. 1978. Cytophysiology of thyroid parafollicular cells. Internat. Rev. Cytol. 52:1.

Nunez, E. A. and M. D. Gershon. 1983. Thyrotropin induced release of 5-hydroxytryptamine and accompanying ultrastructural changes in parafollicular cells. Endocrinology 113:309.

Seljelid, R. 1967. Exocytosis in thyroid follicular cells. II. A microinjection study of the origin of colloid droplets. J. Ultrastr. Res. 17:401.

Seljelid, R., A. Reith, and N. F. Nakken. 1970. Early phase of endocytosis in the rat thyroid follicle cell. Lab. Investg. 23:595.

Whur, P., A. Herscovics, and C. P. Leblond. 1969. Radioautographic visualization of the encorporation of galactose-^{3}H and mannose-^{3}H by rat thyroids in vitro in relation to the stages of thyroglobulin synthesis. J. Cell Biol. 43:289.

Wissig, S. L. 1960. The anatomy of secretion of the follicular cells of the thyroid gland. The fine structure of the gland in the normal rat. J. Biophys. Biochem. Cytol. 7:419.

Wissig, S. L. 1963. The anatomy of secretion in the follicular cells of the thyroid gland. II. The effect of acute thyrotropic hormone stimulation on the secretory apparatus. J. Cell Biol. 16:93.

19

PARATHYROID GLANDS

The *parathyroid glands* are endocrine glands producing *parathyroid hormone* (PTH) which acts on the kidneys, intestine, and bones to maintain the necessary concentration of calcium in the extracellular fluid of the body. Calcium is a very important element in mammalian physiology. It is required for muscular contraction, glandular secretion, blood coagulation, and activity of key enzymes involved in intermediary metabolism. Removal of the glands results in violent spasm of skeletal muscle (tetany) and ultimately to death.

The parathyroid glands are small ovoid bodies adhering to the posterior surface of the thyroid gland (Fig. 19–1). They are usually four in number, but accessory glands are not uncommon. They measure about 5 mm in length, 4 m in width, and 2 mm in thickness, and weigh 25–50 mg apiece. They are commonly associated with the middle third of the thyroid but may also be found on the lower third. In 5–10% of humans, one or more parathyroids may be found lower in the neck or in the mediastinum. The parathyroid glands and the thymus have a common origin from the third and fourth branchial pouches of the early embryo, and their occasional ectopic location appears to result from their failure to be arrested in the neck during their caudal migration with the anlage of the thymus during embryogenesis.

Each parathyroid gland is enclosed in a thin capsule from which trabeculae extend inward carrying the blood vessels nerves and lymphatics. The parenchyma of the gland consists of anastomosing cords and clusters of epithelial cells supported by a delicate framework of reticular fibers which also surrounds the rich network of capillaries (Fig. 19–2). The epithelial cells may rarely form isolated small follicles containing a colloidal material of unknown nature. The glands slowly increase in size from birth through adolescence, attaining their maximum weight at about 20 years of age. The connective tissue stroma of the adult gland contains variable numbers of adipose cells (Fig. 19–4). These increase in number, and in elderly individuals, may occupy 60% or more of the gland. Because the weight of glands remains relatively constant, there is evidently a decrease in the mass of the epithelial cells with advancing age. Two types of epithelial cells are found in the human parathyroid gland: *chief cells* and *oxyphil cells* (Fig. 19–3).

CHIEF CELL

In histological sections, the *chief cells* are 5–8 μm in diameter with a centrally placed nucleus and a pale, slightly eosinophilic cytoplasm. Coarse cytoplasmic granules of varying shape are of frequent occurrence and are interpreted as deposits of lipofuchsin pigment. Smaller granules that stain with iron hematoxylin and exhibit argyrophilia with the Bodian stain are evidently secretory granules. When stained with the periodic-acid–Schiff reaction, small aggregations of glycogen are scattered through the cytoplasm. Electron micrographs reveal a juxtanuclear Golgi complex, a moderate number of elongated mitochondria, and cisternal profiles of endoplasmic reticulum. The lipofuchsin pigment deposits consist of aggregations of pale spherical bodies of varying size in an electron-dense matrix. The secretory granules vary in shape and have a dense content. They appear to arise in the Golgi complex and accumulate near the cell surface. The chief cells are joined by occasional desmosomes. A single abortive cilium may be found projecting into the intercellular space. Some chief cells have a small Golgi complex, very few secretory granules, and areas of cytoplasm containing large accumulations of glycogen. Such cells may be quite numerous and are believed to be relatively inactive.

The first biologically active extracts of parathyroid glands were prepared some 75 years ago. Isolation and determination of the primary structure of the hormone were slow to follow because of the difficulty of obtaining

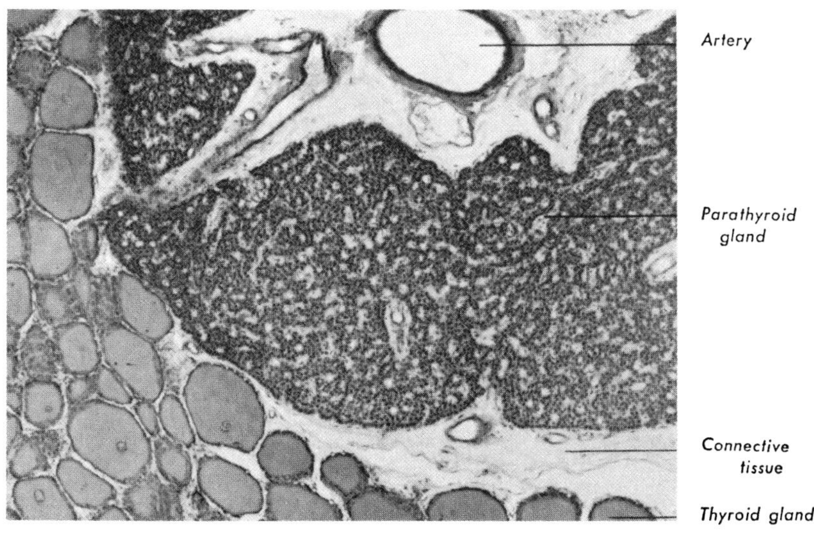

Figure 19–1. Low-power photomicrograph of a parathyroid gland and adjacent thyroid follicles of a rhesus monkey.

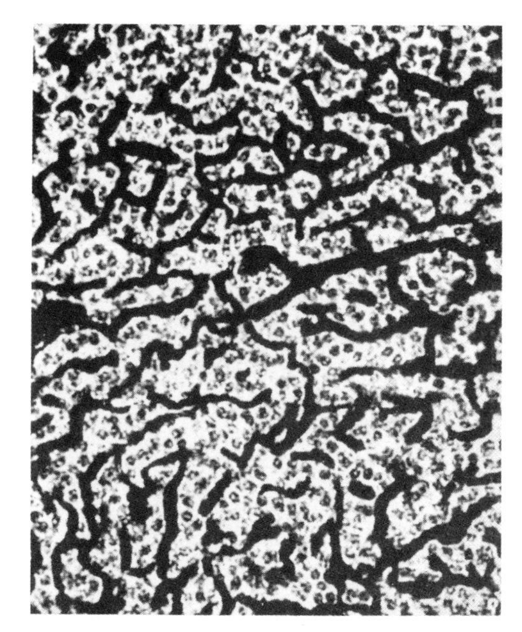

Figure 19–2. Low-power photomicrograph of a parathyroid gland of a monkey injected with India ink to reveal the rich network of capillaries and their intimate relation to the gland cells.

sufficient quantities of material for analysis. One or two milligrams of a precursor fraction were isolated and sequenced, in 1972, from several kilograms of bovine parathyroids. As in the genesis of other polypeptide hormones, a precursor of larger size was found to be synthesized and then shortened to the active hormone by enzymatic cleavage. Pulse-labeling experiments have since established the intracellular sites of the various steps in the process. A large precursor of 115 amino acids, *preproparathyroid hormone,* is synthesized on ribosomes associated with the endoplasmic reticulum. Within less than 1 min, 25 amino acids are cleaved off during translocation of the molecule into the lumen of the reticulum, forming *proparathyroid hormone,* consisting of 90 amino acids. On reaching the Golgi complex, some 15–20 min later, an additional 6 amino acids have been cleaved off, resulting in an 84 amino acid *parathyroid hormone,* with a molecular weight of 9500. This is packaged in the secretory granules that migrate to the cell surface for subsequent exocytosis.

OXYPHIL CELL

The *oxyphil cells,* 6–10 μm in diameter, are distinctly larger than the chief cells and stain more deeply with eosin. They are relative few in number and occur singly or in small groups. When stained with the aniline-acid fuchsin method, they are found to have many more mitochondria than the chief cells. This is borne out in electron micrographs which show a remarkable concentration of elongated mitochondria that have very numerous closely spaced cristae. The Golgi complex is small and the endoplasmic reticulum is sparse. Glycogen particles are found in the interstices between mitochondria but these do not form the conspicuous aggregates that are characteristic of the category of relatively inactive chief cells. The eosinophilic granulation of the oxyphil

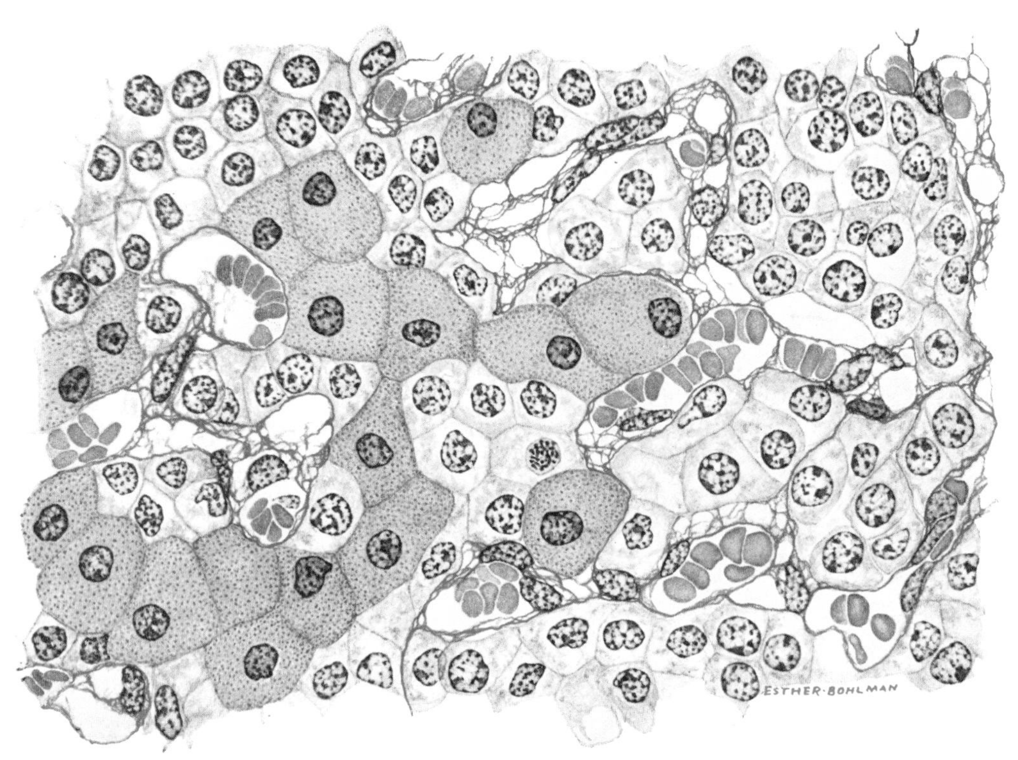

Figure 19–3. Drawing of a section of parathyroid gland showing the paler-staining vacuolated principal cells and the larger and more deeply staining oxyphil cells. The latter appear to contain many secretory granules, but in electron micrographs these prove to be unusually numerous mitochondria. Mallory azan stain.

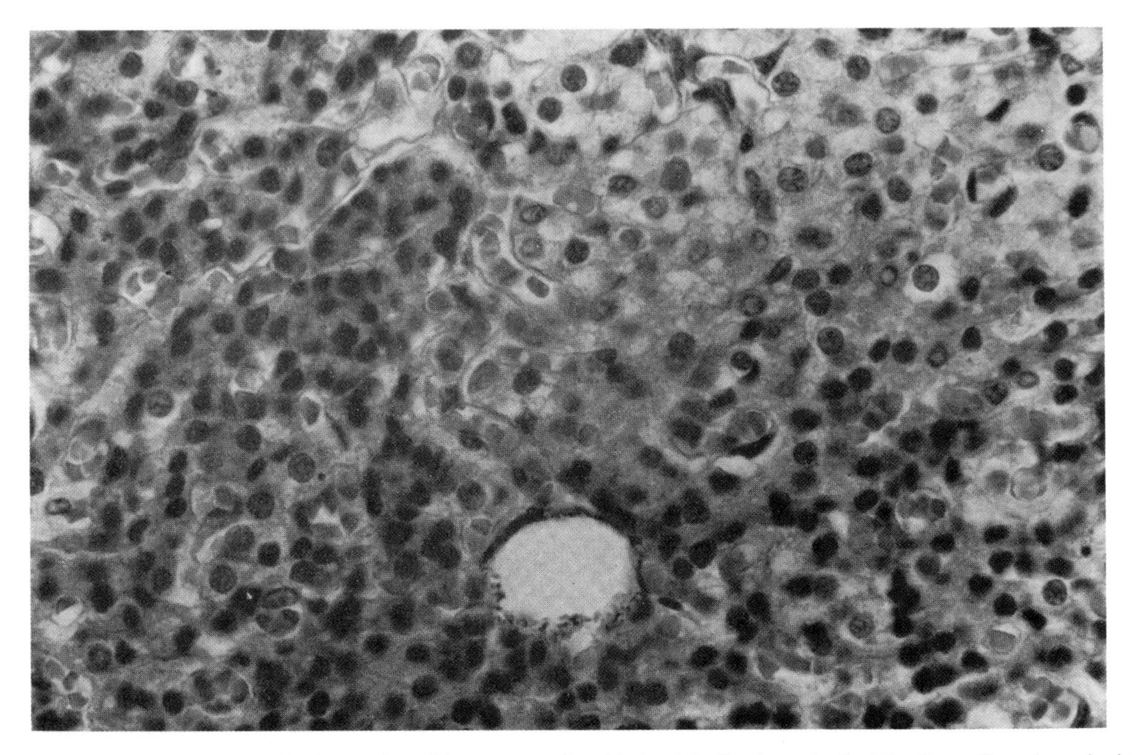

Figure 19–4. Photomicrograph of a section of human parathyroid gland. In the lower half of the figure there is a single adipose cell. In older individual adipose cells may be very abundant within the parathyroid gland. (Courtesy of S. I. Roth.)

cell cytoplasm described by light microscopists is now attributed to their abundant mitochondria.

A third cell type has been described, having cytological characteristics intermediate between those of the chief cell and of the oxyphil cell. This so-called *transitional cell* stains with acid dyes and has a nucleus that is somewhat smaller and more deeply staining than that of the other cell types. Because only one hormone is produced by the parathyroid glands, the three cell forms are widely believed to be different phases in the life cycle of a single cell type, with the chief cell being its physiologically active stage. This interpretation is supported by immunological studies localizing radioactive precursors of the hormone mainly over the secretory granules of the chief cells.

HISTOPHYSIOLOGY

The principal function of parathyroid hormone is to maintain the concentration of calcium ions in the body fluids within the narrow limits of 8.5–10.5 mg/100 ml. When calcium falls below this level, the parathyroids rapidly increase their secretion of parathyroid hormone to 5 to 10 times the basal rate. With prolonged hypocalcemia, the output of hormone may reach 50 times the basal rate. Parathyroid hormone acts on the osteocytes of bone, causing them to mobilize calcium ions from the bone mineral forming the walls of the lacunae that they occupy—a process called *osteocytic osteolysis*. This response is very rapid, resulting in a detectable rise in serum calcium within minutes. If hypocalcemia and increased PTH secretion persists, there is also a coalescence of precursor cells in bone to form additional osteoclasts which erode bone, liberating calcium. In contrast to osteocytic osteolysis, this process of *osteoclastic bone resorption* requires many hours to reach effective levels of calcium release.

In addition to its action on bone, parathyroid hormone acts on the distal convoluted tubules of the kidney to increase their resorption of calcium from the glomerular filtrate and its return to the blood. The hormone, thus, makes a very significant contribution to the maintenance of normal blood levels by reducing calcium loss in the urine.

Parathyroid hormone also influences the rate of uptake of calcium from the intestines. It does so by regulating the metabolism of vitamin D by the kidney. Pro-vitamin D (7-dehydrocholesterol), synthesized in the skin, is converted to vitamin D_3 (cholecalciferol). This is transported to the liver, where it undergoes initial hydroxylation to 25-$(OH)D_3$. This, in turn, is transported in the blood to the kidneys where it is further hydroxylated to form 1,25-$(OH)_2D_3$, the most potent vitamin D metabolite. The uptake from the diet of sufficient calcium to meet the body's needs is dependent on the action of 1,25-$(OH)_2D_3$ on the cells of the intestine. Parathyroid hormone is the principal regulator of the 1,25-$(OH)_2D_3$ production in the kidney.

Parathyroid hormone, thus, exerts its effects by acting directly on bone and kidney and indirectly on the intestine. The exact mechanisms by which the hormone exerts its effects on the cells of these target organs have yet to be worked out. However, there is increasing evidence that activation of adenyl cyclase and the resulting elevation of the intracellular concentration of cyclic AMP are involved. Within minutes after administration of the hormone to experimental animals, the concentration of cyclic AMP in their urine is elevated. And, on addition of the hormone to bone or kidney tissue in vitro, increased adenyl cyclase activity can be detected within 15 s.

The clinical condition called *primary hyperparathyroidism* often results from a benign tumor of one of the glands. Such patients secrete excessive amount of hormone and have high blood calcium, low blood phosphate, rarefaction of their bones, and a tendency to develop kidney stones and deposits of calcium in other soft tissues. Patients with *rickets* due to inadequate intestinal absorption of calcium may develop *secondary hyperparathyroidism* to compensate for the chronically low blood levels of calcium. Similarly, in severe kidney disease, there may be phosphate retention resulting in low blood calcium and consequent hypertrophy of the parathyroid glands.

BIBLIOGRAPHY

Abe, M. and L. M. Sherwood. 1972. Regulation of parathyroid secretion by adenyl cyclase. Biophys. Biochem. Res. Comm. 48:396.

Chang, H. Y. 1951. Grafts of parathyroid and other tissues to bone. Anat. Rec. 111:23.

Collip, J. B. 1925. The extraction of a parathyroid hormone which will prevent or control tetany and which regulates the level of blood calcium. J. Biol. Chem. 63:395.

Davis, R. and A. C. Enders. 1961. Light and electron microscope studies on the parathyroid glands. *In* R. O. Greep and R. V. Talmage, eds. The Parathyroids. Springfield, IL, Charles C Thomas.

Fetter, A. W. and C. C. Capen. 1970. The ultrastructure of the parathyroid gland of young pigs. Acta Anat. 75:359.

Grafflin, A. L. 1940. Cytological evidence of secretory activity in the mammalian parathyroid. Endocrinology 26:857.

Greep, R. O. and R. V. Talmage, eds. 1961. The Parathyroids. Springfield, IL, Charles C Thomas.

Habener, J. F. and J. T. Potts. 1978. Biosynthesis of parathyroid hormone. Parts I and II. New Engl. J. Med. 299:580, 635.

Habener, J. F., M. Amherdt, M. Ravazzolli, and L. Orci. 1979. Parathyroid hormone biosynthesis: Correlation of conversion of biosynthetic precursors with intracellular protein migration as determined by electron microscope autoradiography. J. Cell Biol. 80:715.

Munger, B. L. and S. I. Roth. 1963. The cytology of the normal parathyroid glands of man and Virginia deer: a light and electron microscopic study with morphologic evidence of secretory activity. J. Cell Biol. 16:379.

Potts, J. T., H. M. Kronenberg, J. F. Habener, and A. Rich. 1980. Biosynthesis of parathyroid hormone. Ann. N.Y. Acad. Sci. 343:38.

Roth, S. I. 1962. Pathology of the parathyroid glands in hyperparathyroidism with a discussion of recent advances in the anatomy and pathology of the parathyroid glands. Arch. Pathol. 73:492.

Trier, J. S. 1958. The fine structure of the parathyroid gland. J. Biophys. Biochem. Cytol. 4:13.

20
ADRENAL GLANDS

The *adrenal glands* are embedded in adipose tissue at the cranial pole of each kidney. They are relatively flat triangular organs, less than 1 cm in thickness, and ranging in width from 2 cm at the apex to 5 cm at their base. Their combined weight, in the adult, is from 15 to 20 g. On the cut surface of a transected adrenal, a thick yellow *cortex* is clearly distinguishable from a thin, gray *medulla* in its interior.

The cortex and medulla are both endocrine glands, but they differ in their embryological origin and in their functions. The cortex, which makes up 80–90% of the volume of the gland, is of mesodermal origin, whereas the medulla, constituting 10–20%, arises from ectoderm of the embryonic neural crest. In vertebrates other than mammals, the two components may intermingle to varying degrees, or they may be completely separated from one another, in which case the homologue of the cortex is called *interrenal tissue* and the homologues of the medulla are called *chromaffin bodies*.

The principal functions of the adrenal glands are to maintain the constancy of the internal environment of the organism and to make appropriate changes in its physiology in response to acute stress, injury, or prolonged deprivation of food and water. The cortex is controlled by the adrenocorticotrophic hormone (ACTH) of the anterior pituitary and secretes steroid hormones (*aldosterone, cortisol,* and *dehydroepiandrosterone*). These hormones have multiple regulatory effects on carbohydrate and protein metabolism and electrolyte balance. The medulla is controlled by preganglionic sympathetic nerves and secretes catecholamines (*norepinephrine* and *epinephrine*) which increase heart rate and blood pressure and mobilize glucose and fatty acids as energy sources in stressful emergency situations. The adrenal glands are indispensable. Their removal or destruction by disease is followed by death within a few days.

ADRENAL CORTEX

Three concentric zones are distinguishable in the adrenal cortex: a thin, outer *zona granulosa* immediately beneath the capsule; a broad, intermediate *zona fasciculata;* and an inner *zona reticularis,* adjacent to the medulla. In the human, these constitute, respectively, 15%, 78%, and 7% of the volume of the cortex. The transition from zone to zone is gradual in histological sections, but the boundaries become more apparent after injection of the blood vessels to reveal the distinctive vascular patterns of the three zones (see below).

ZONA GLOMERULOSA

In the zona glomerulosa, columnar epithelial cells form closely spaced arcades that bear a superficial resemblance to the acini of exocrine glands (Figs. 20–1 and 20–2). These are separated by thin connective tissue septa that extend inward from the capsule. The cells have heavily stained heterochromatic nuclei containing one or two prominent nucleoli. The acidophilic cytoplasm contains scattered clumps of basophilic material. The Golgi complex tends to be polarized toward the nearest blood vessel.

In electron micrographs, cells of the zona glomerulosa are joined by occasional desmosomes and a few small gap junctions. Where exposed to the intertitium, the cells bear a few short, irregularly oriented microvilli. The nuclei of the outer cells are often irregular in shape, whereas those deeper in the zone are spherical. There are a few parallel arrays of

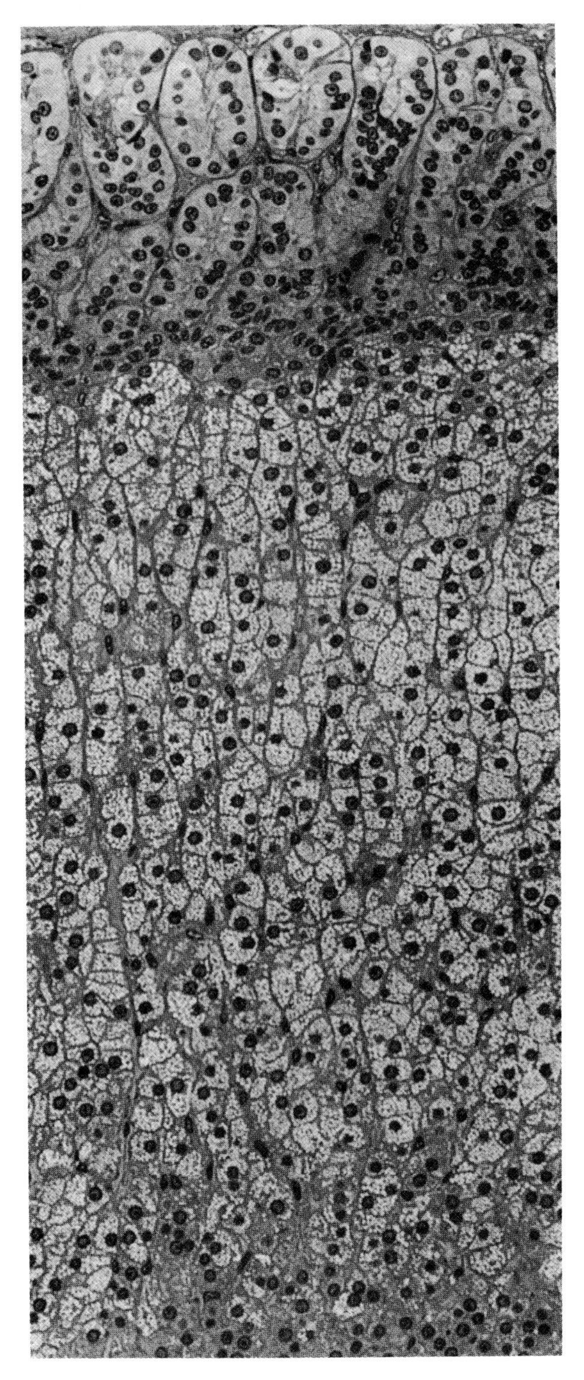

Figure 20–1. Photomicrograph of the full thickness of the adrenal cortex of a rhesus monkey, showing, from the top downward, the zona glomerulosa, zona fasciculata, and the zone reticularis.

rough endoplasmic reticulum and a relatively small Golgi complex. The mitochondria are elongated and contain sparse lamellar cristae. A network of smooth endoplasmic reticulum is found throughout the cytoplasm, but it is less extensive than in cells of the zona fasciculata. Lipid droplets are present but not numerous.

ZONA FASCICULATA

The zone fasciculata is made up of pale-staining polyhedral cells arranged in long columns that are oriented radially in relation to the medulla. The columns are one or two cells thick and separated from one another by capillaries of similar prevailing orientation. The faintly acidophilic cytoplasm of the cells has a highly vacuolated appearance owing to the extraction of abundant lipid droplets during specimen preparation (Fig. 20–3).

In electron micrographs, the cells are somewhat larger than those of the glomerulosa and have more numerous and larger gap junctions. The nucleus has a prominent nucleolus and a distinct fibrous lamina. The cytoplasm contains large numbers of lipid droplets of low electron density which are reported to occupy a large fraction of the cell volume in the human and rat adrenals. In the hamster and in bovids, lipid is less abundant. A distinctive feature of the cells of the zone fasciculata is a very extensive smooth endoplasmic reticulum which occupies 40–45% of the cell volume (Fig. 20–4). The rough endoplasmic reticulum is represented by occasional single or paired cisternal profiles. The juxtanuclear Golgi complex is unremarkable. Small dense bodies present in limited numbers in the cytoplasm are interpreted as lysosomes and microperoxisomes. Mitochondria occupy 25–30% of the cell volume and are shorter than those of the zona glomerulosa. Their internal structure is atypical and varies from species to species. In the human, the cristae are short tubules with vesicular dilatations along their length. In the hamster, the tubular cristae are of uniform diameter. In the rat, the mitochondria are spherical and cristae and replaced by large numbers of vesicles about 60 nm in diameter that are not attached to the inner membrane but are free in the mitochondrial matrix. The significance of these morphological differences in the ultrastructure of the mitochondria is obscure.

ZONA RETICULARIS

The parallel cell columns of the zona fasciculata give way to a three-dimensional net-

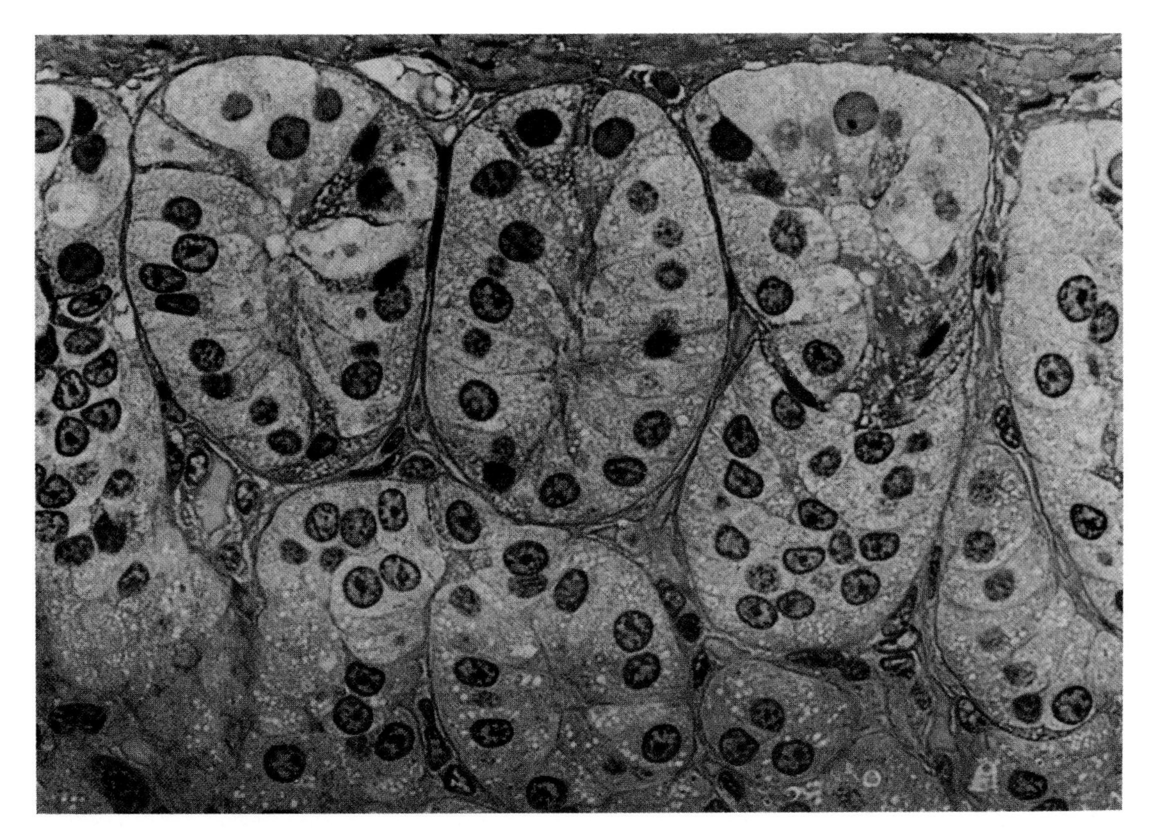

Figure 20–2. Photomicrograph of the zona glomerulosa, at higher magnification, showing the acinar or glomerular arrangement of the cells. Compared to the zona fasciculata, these cells have fewer cytoplasmic vacuoles resulting from extraction of lipid droplets during specimen preparation.

work of anastomosing cell cords, in the zone reticularis. The cells are somewhat smaller and stain more deeply because their cytoplasm contains fewer extracted lipid droplets. Intracellular accumulations of brown pigment are common.

In electron micrographs, the cells appear less active than those of the fasciculata. The endoplasmic reticulum is far less extensive, the Golgi complex is small, and lipid droplets are relatively few. Large aggregations of lipofucsin pigment are common (Figs. 20–5 and 20–6). Near the medulla, there are variable numbers of "dark cells" that have a more electron-dense cytoplasm and a shrunken hyperchromatic nucleus. The nuclear changes and the paucity of organelles and the accumulation of pigment in the cytoplasm suggest that cell degeneration is common in this zone.

The zonation of the adrenal cortex is reflected in production of different hormones in the three zones. Aldosterone is produced exclusively by the zona glomerulosa, cortisol is secreted mainly by the zona fasciculata, and the zona reticularis is believed to be the principal site of production of dehydroepiandrosterone. Surprisingly, when isolated from their natural location the cells of all three layers have similar products. This has led to the conclusion that the functional zonation is dependent on the arrangement of the cells in concentric zones. It is suggested that the steroids or metabolic by-products of their synthesis by the cells of the glomerulosa may inactivate certain enzymes in the fasciculata so that its cells cannot produce aldosterone. Similarly, steroids and peroxides of the fasciculata carried downstream in the blood may inhibit hydroxylases of the zona reticularis so that these cells are unable to secrete cortisol. Cortisol carried in the centripetal flow of blood from the cortex to the medulla may serve to maintain normal levels of secretion of catecholamines by the cells of the medulla.

ADRENAL MEDULLA

The boundary between the cortex and medulla in the human adrenal is usually irregu-

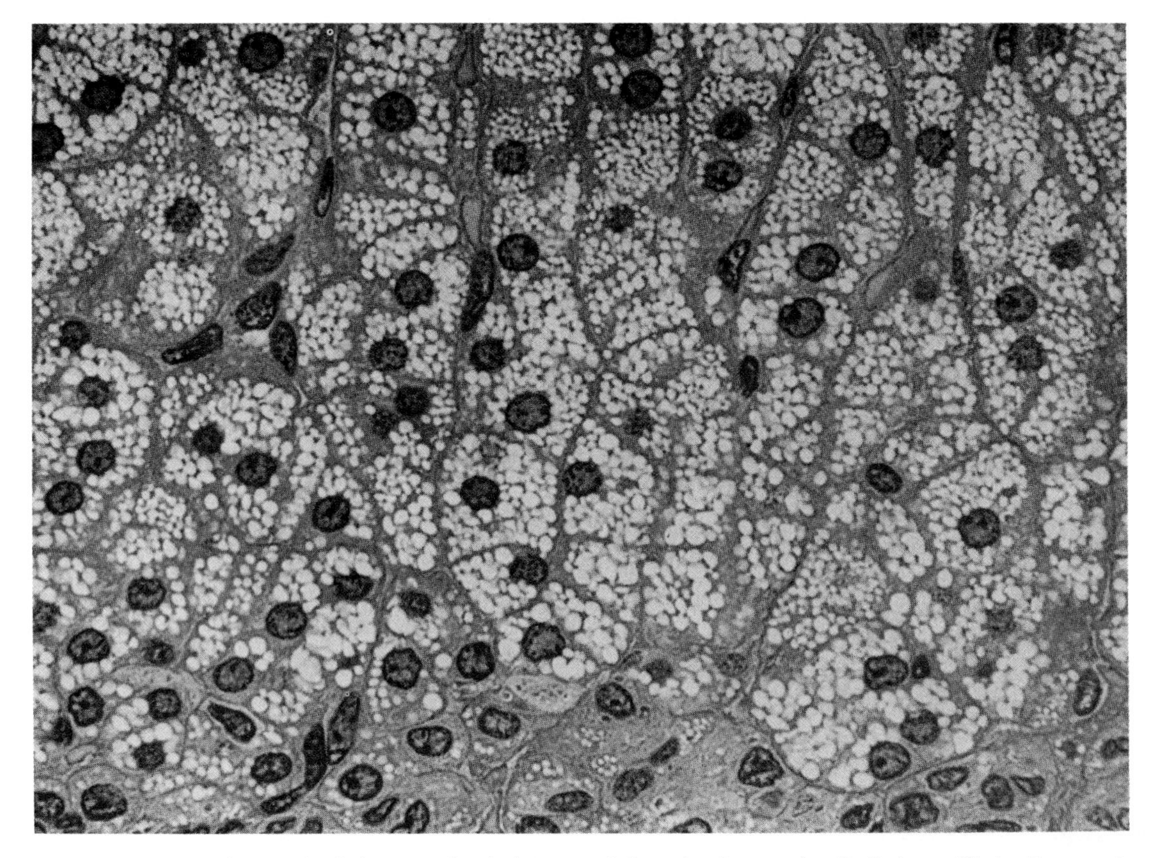

Figure 20–3. Photomicrograph of the zona fasciculata, consisting of columns of cells that are filled with vacuoles representing extracted lipid droplets.

lar, with some cords of the reticularis penetrating a short distance into the medulla. In other species, the boundary is more regular. The medulla is composed of large epithelioid cells arranged in rounded clusters or short cords that are in intimate relation to capillaries and venules (Fig. 20–7). In histological sections of tissue fixed in a solution containing potassium dichromate, the cells are crowded with small brown granules. These cells and isolated groups of similar cells in other organs that display this staining reaction are called *chromaffin cells*. The browning of the granules with chromium salts, the *chromaffin reaction*, results from oxidation and polymerization of catecholamines in the granules. Catecholamines are transmitters synthesized by cells of the sympathetic nervous system. The adrenal medulla can be thought of as a modified sympathetic ganglion made up of postganglionic cells that lack dendrites and axons. The catecholamines of the adrenal medulla are *norepinephrine* and *epinephrine*. They are secreted in response to stimulation by preganglionic fibers from the splanchnic nerves. Within the adrenal medulla, typical ganglion cells may also be found singly or in small groups among the chromaffin cells.

With histochemical staining reactions, two kinds of chromaffin cells can be distinguished. Those storing nonrepinephrine have a low affinity for the dye azocarmine, are autofluorescent, give argentaffin and potassium iodate reactions, and are negative for acid phosphatase. Those storing epinephrine have a strong affinity for azocarmine, are not fluorescent or reactive with silver or iodate, and exhibit a positive acid phosphatase reaction.

In electron micrographs, the most prominent feature of cells of the adrenal medulla is their content of very large numbers (up to 30,000) of small membrane-bounded dense granules (Fig. 20–8). The granules of cells that store norepinephrine have an electron-dense core that is often eccentric in its position within the limiting membrane. Cells that store epinephrine have granules with a more homogeneous content of lower density. The cytoplasm

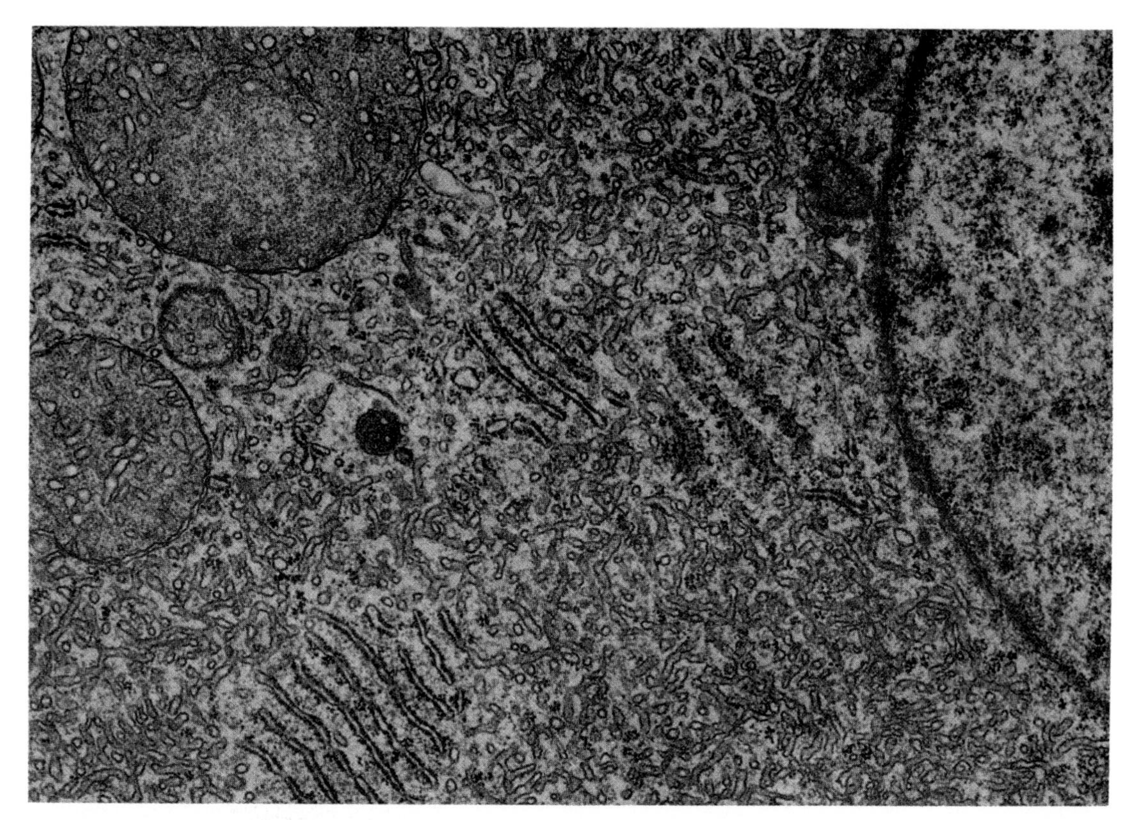

Figure 20–4. An electron micrograph of a portion of a cell of the human fetal adrenal cortex. Note the large spherical mitochondria with tubular cristae, the stacks of parallel cisternae of rough endoplasmic reticulum, and the abundant smooth endoplasmic reticulum. (Micrograph courtesy of A. L. Jones and S. McNutt.)

of both cell types contains short parallel arrays of rough endoplasmic reticulum and a moderate number of mitochondria with foliate cristae. Material interpreted as a precursor of the secretory granules is often present in the *trans*-cisternae of the juxtanuclear Golgi complex.

Norepinephrine or epinephrine account for as much as 20% of the volume of isolated medullary granules. The remainder is made up of a family of soluble proteins called chromagranins, together with ATP, and enkephalins. The catecholamines do not seem to be bound to a specific protein, as are hormones of other cells, and it is not entirely clear how substances of such low molecular weight are retained within the granules. It is the prevailing view that the catecholamines form high-molecular-weight aggregates with ATP and divalent cations within the granule. The uptake of catecholamines into the granules is attributed to an active transport mechanism dependent on magnesium-activated ATPase in their membrane. The depletion of catecholamines by the pharmacological agent *reserpine* may be the result of inhibition of an active transport mechanism required for retention of the hormones within the granules.

There was formerly some divergence of opinion as to how the catecholamines were released. Some investigators assumed that they were first released into the cytoplasm and then diffused through the membrane, whereas others believed that they were secreted by exocytosis of the granules. This has now been settled by morphological evidence for exocytosis of granules and by the finding that a perfusate of the stimulated adrenal contains not only catecholamines but also chromagranins and ATP in the same proportions as they are found in a lysate of isolated granules. It is now agreed that release of acetylcholine at the endings of preganglionic nerves depolarizes the membrane of the cells of the adrenal medulla, altering its permeability and permitting influx of calcium which triggers exocytosis.

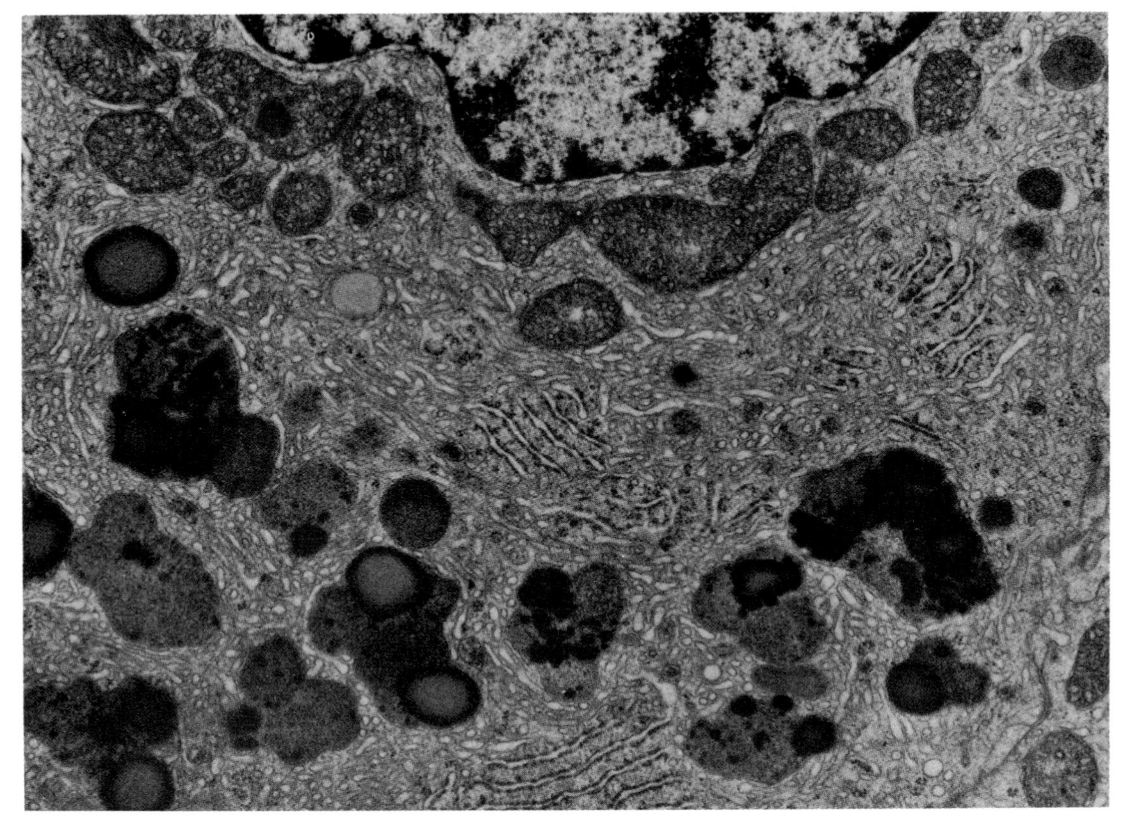

Figure 20–5. Electron micrograph of the juxtanuclear area of a cortical cell from the adrenal gland of an adult human. The smooth endoplasmic reticulum occupies the greater part of the cytoplasm. The mitochondria vary in their shape and usually have tubular cristae. Accumulations of dense masses of lipochrome pigment are common, especially in cells of the zona reticularis. (Micrograph courtesy of J. Long.)

BLOOD SUPPLY OF THE ADRENAL

The adrenal glands have a rate of blood flow per gram of tissue that is one of the highest in the body, and the unusual pattern of the blood vessels has important physiological correlates. Each gland receives its major blood supply from the inferior phrenic artery via *superior suprarenal arteries,* but *middle suprarenal arteries* from the aorta and *inferior suprarenal arteries* from the renal arteries are additional sources. These vessels ramify over the surface of the gland, giving rise to branches that pass through the capsule to form a dense *subcapsular plexus. Short cortical arteries* arising from this plexus give rise to a very extensive network of sinusoidal capillaries that occupy the interstices among clusters of parenchymal cells in the zona glomerulosa and among the cell columns of the zona fasciculata (Fig. 20–9). The endothelial cells lining these sinusoids are fenestrated, with pores ranging in size from 100 nm in the outer cortex to 250 nm, or more, in the inner fasciculata and reticularis. The sinusoids of the zona reticularis are confluent with a venous plexus from which small venules pass between the cords and clumps of medullary cells to veins in the center of the medulla. These, in turn, drain into the *suprarenal vein* which emerges from the hilus of the gland. From the right adrenal, this vessel joins the inferior vena cava, whereas on the left, the suprarenal vein drains into the left renal vein.

In addition to the short branches of the subcapsular arterial plexus that give rise to the cortical sinusoids, there are *long cortical arteries* that pass through the cortex unbranched and form networks of capillaries around the cells of the medulla. The medulla, thus, has a dual blood supply, receiving blood indirectly via the cortical sinusoids and di-

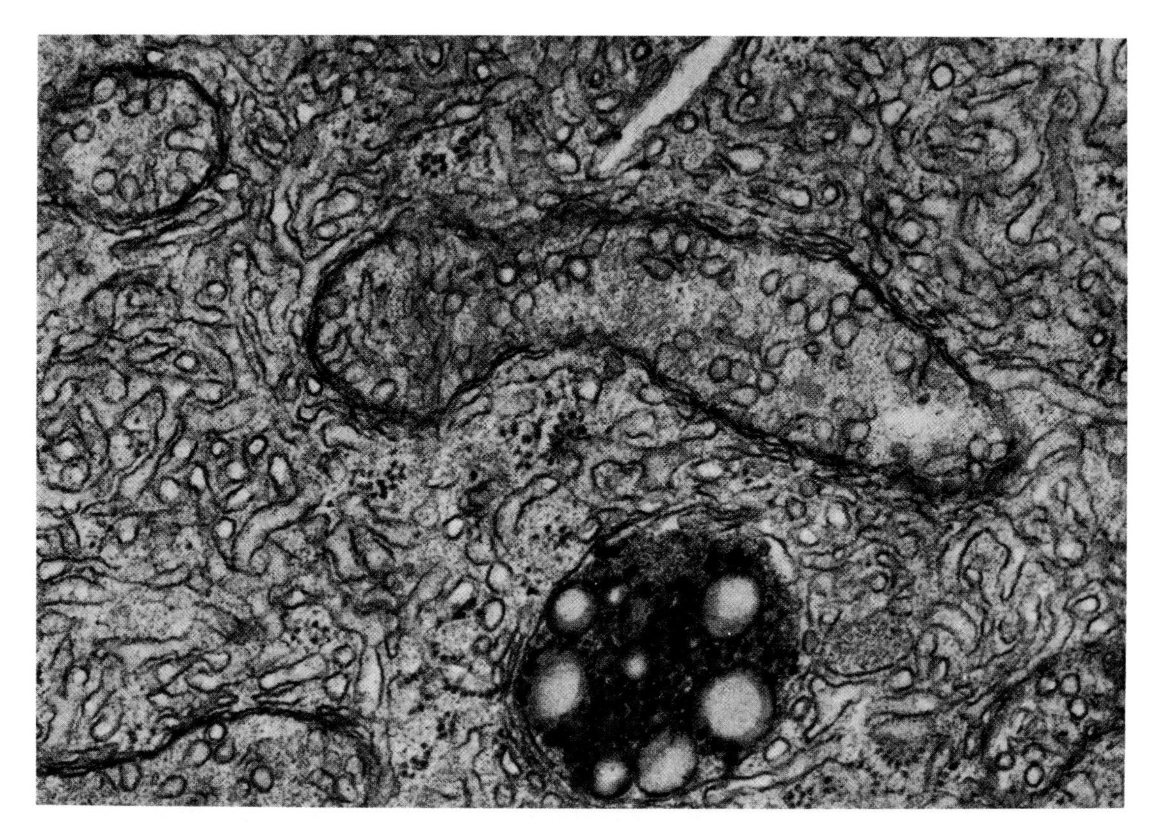

Figure 20–6. Electron micrograph of a small area of cytoplasm of an adrenal cortical cell from an adult. Note the tubular form of the abundant smooth endoplasmic reticulum and the unusual appearance of the mitochondrial cristae. (Micrograph courtesy of J. Long.)

rectly from the subcapsular plexus via the long cortical arteries.

In the older literature, there are a number of reports that the lining cells of the sinusoids take up colloidal vital dyes such as lithium carmine and trypan blue. On this basis, they were considered to belong to the reticuloendothelial system. More recent studies show that these dyes simply adhere to the surface of the endothelial cells or pass through the fenestrations and are taken up by macrophages lying between the endothelium and the parenchymal cells. Electron microscopic observations have failed to find any evidence of phagocytosis by cells of the sinusoidal endothelium.

HISTOPHYSIOLOGY OF THE ADRENAL CORTEX

Three classes of steroid hormones are produced by the adrenal cortex: *mineralocorticoids*, *glucocorticoids*, and *androgens*. Their biosynthetic pathways have been thoroughly studied. All are synthesized from cholesterol which is a major component of plasma low-density lipoprotein (LDL). LDL is taken up from the blood by receptor-mediated endocytosis, and cholesterol esters are stored in lipid droplets in the cytoplasm of the cortical cells. On stimulation of the cells, free cholesterol is released as a substrate for steroid synthesis. The majority of the enzymes involved are located in the extensive smooth endoplasmic reticulum of these cells, but those required for certain hydroxylation and oxidation steps reside in the inner mitochondrial membrane. Therefore, intermediate products must be transferred to-and-fro between the mitochondria and the reticulum several times before synthesis of the final product is completed. The mechanisms involved in these translocations are still not completely understood.

The principal mineralocorticoid is *aldosterone*, secreted by the zona glomerulosa. Its major function is to control body fluid volume by increasing the reabsorption of sodium by the kidneys. It is effective in very low concentration and its daily production is only 0.05–

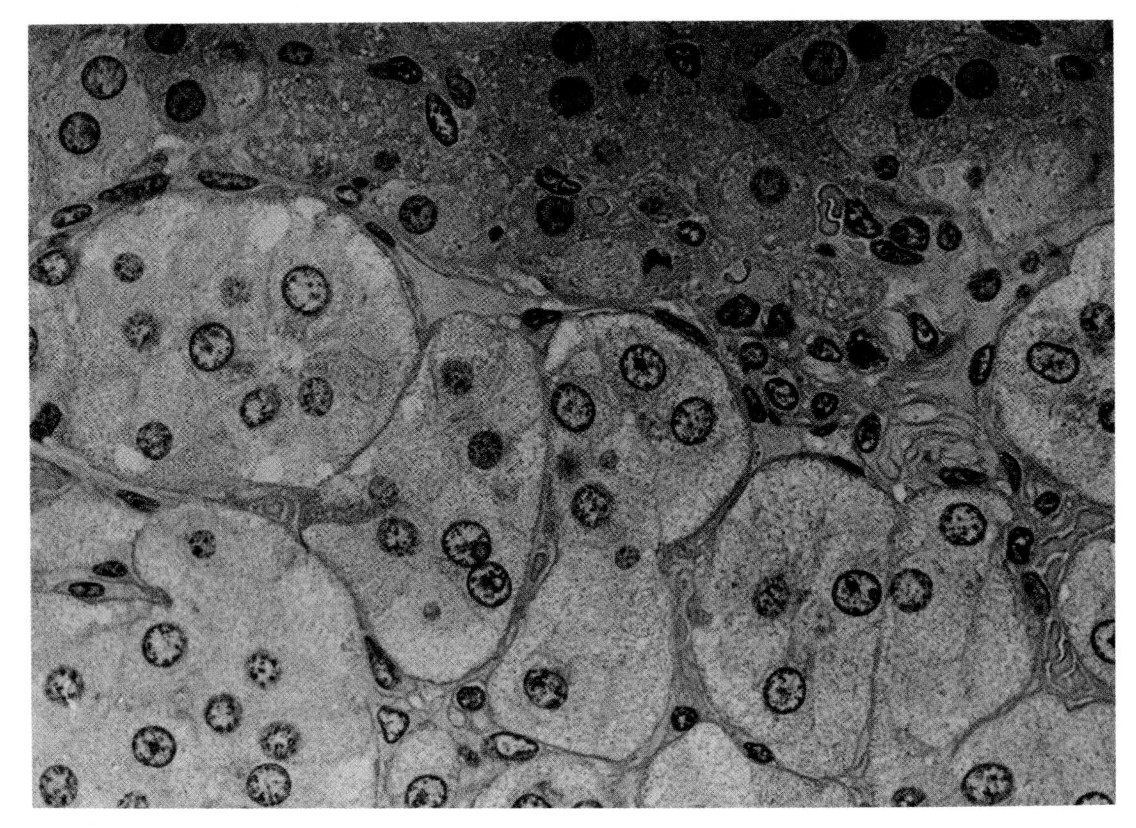

Figure 20–7. Photomicrograph of the junctional region between the zona reticularis (top) and the clusters of large pale cells of the adrenal medulla (bottom). With the light microscope, catecholamine granules are usually not visible, unless a special staining method has been used.

0.2 mg. The hormone is not stored but is produced as needed. The primary stimulus for its secretion is *angiotensin-II,* generated by the proteolytic enzyme *renin* secreted by the kidney in response to a fall in sodium or a rise in potassium concentration in the blood. Aldosterone acts on the distal tubules of the kidney, increasing their excretion of potassium and their resorption of sodium. Water is taken up with the sodium, restoring blood volume and normal electrolyte concentration in the extracellular fluid. Secretion of aldosterone is also influenced by adrenocorticotrophic hormone of the pituitary and by atrial natiuretic hormone of the heart but to a lesser extent than by the renin–angiotensin mechanism.

The principal glucocorticoid secreted by the zona fasciculata of the human adrenal is *cortisol,* produced in amounts of 20–30 mg daily. In rodents and some other species, *corticosterone* serves the same purpose and it is produced in very small amounts by the human adrenal. The activity of the cells of the zone fasciculata is controlled by adrenocorticotrophic hormone (ACTH) secreted by the pituitary. Binding of this trophic hormone to surface receptors activates release of cholesterol into the cytoplasm and initiation of steroid biosynthesis. Plasma levels of cortisol increase two- to fivefold within 30 min. Long-term administration of ACTH results in hypertrophy of cells of the zona fasciculata, with significant increase in their mitochondria and endoplasmic reticulum that may lead to a 10- to 20-fold increase in their secretion of cortisol.

Cortisol affects the metabolism of carbohydrate, protein, and fat. It decreases protein synthesis, thereby increasing the circulating level of amino acids. It enhances gluconeogenesis by acting on the liver to activate enzymes involved in the conversion of amino acids into glucose. It also mobilizes fatty acids and glycerol from adipose tissue, making more glycerol available for gluconeogenesis. In addition to these metabolic effects, cortisol has anti-inflammatory effects that make it useful to the clinician. It stabilizes lysosomal membranes reducing release of damaging proteolytic en-

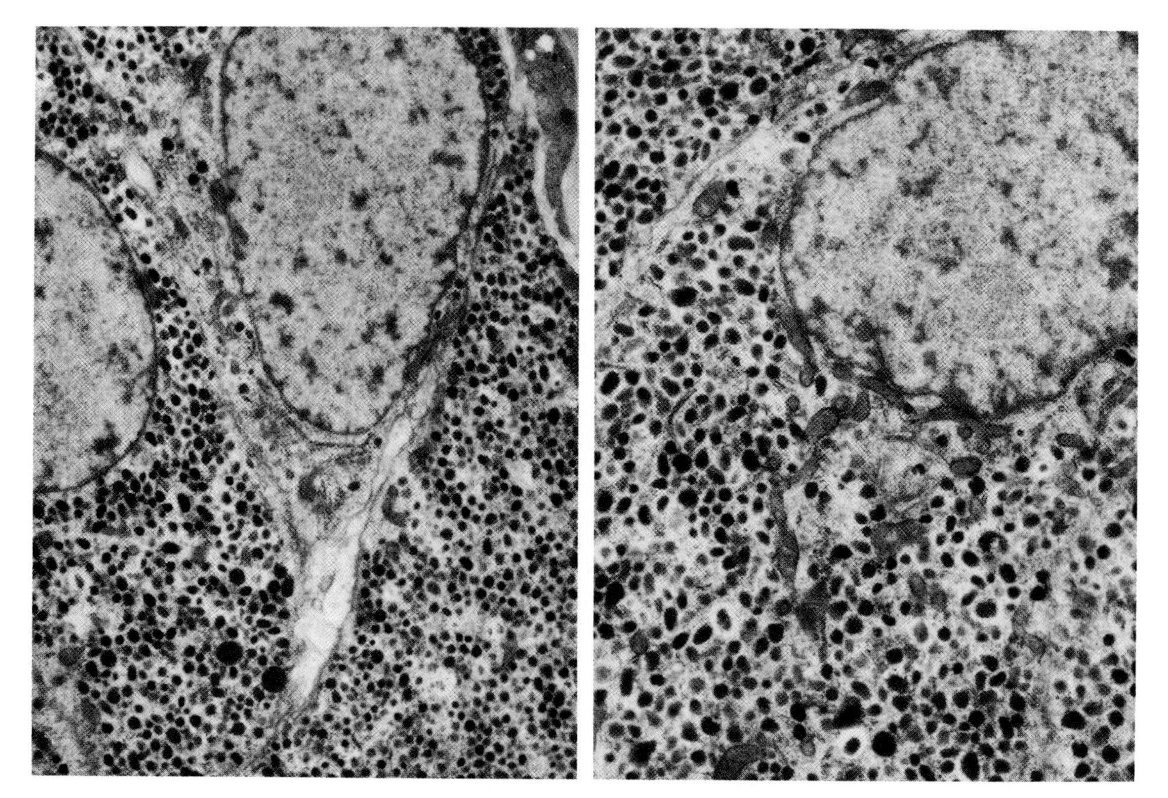

Figure 20–8. Low-power electron micrographs of cells from the adrenal medulla of the cat showing the abundant dense granules that are the sites of storage of catecholamines. (Micrographs courtesy of R. Yates.)

zymes at sites of inflammation. It decreases the permeability of capillaries, thereby reducing swelling. It is also beneficial to the surgeon because, when given in large doses, it causes atrophy of lymphoid tissue throughout the body, resulting in suppression of the immune response and decreasing the likelihood of rejection of transplanted tissues and organs.

The androgens secreted by the inner zone of the adrenal cortex are *dehydroepiandrosterone* (DHA) and its sulfate. These are produced in relatively small quantity and are of little physiological significance in normal humans. However, in rare individuals with *congenital adrenal hyperplasia,* an enzyme, 21-hydroxylase, is deficient and intermediates in cortisol synthesis are converted, instead, to androgens that result in virilization in girls and precocious development of the genitalia in boys.

The mechanism of release of steroids remains a subject of disagreement. In the absence of clear morphological evidence of exocytosis, a majority of investigators favor simple diffusion of steroids through the cytoplasm and across the cell membrane. The surface of unstimulated cells is relatively smooth, but on stimulation, large numbers of short filopodia appear. It is thought that the resulting increase in the area of membrane exposed to the interstitial fluid may facilitate release of steroids by diffusion. Other investigators believe that steroid release requires binding to a carrier molecule. Evidence has accumulated suggesting that small dense bodies that have previously been interpreted as lysosomes may instead be secretory granules. In support of this interpretation is the observation that these granules accumulate in the cytoplasm of ACTH-stimulated cells that have been exposed to vinblastin, a drug that blocks the microtubule-mediated transport commonly associated with secretion by exocytosis. There is also a 10-fold increase in the intracellular concentration of steroid in vinblastin-treated cells, further suggesting that exocytosis may be the mechanism of steroid release.

The clinical syndrome of *hyperadrenocorticism* (Cushing's disease) is associated with small tumors of pituitary basophils that produce excessive amounts of ACTH. The condition is characterized by obesity, largely confined to the face, neck, and trunk; hirsutism; impo-

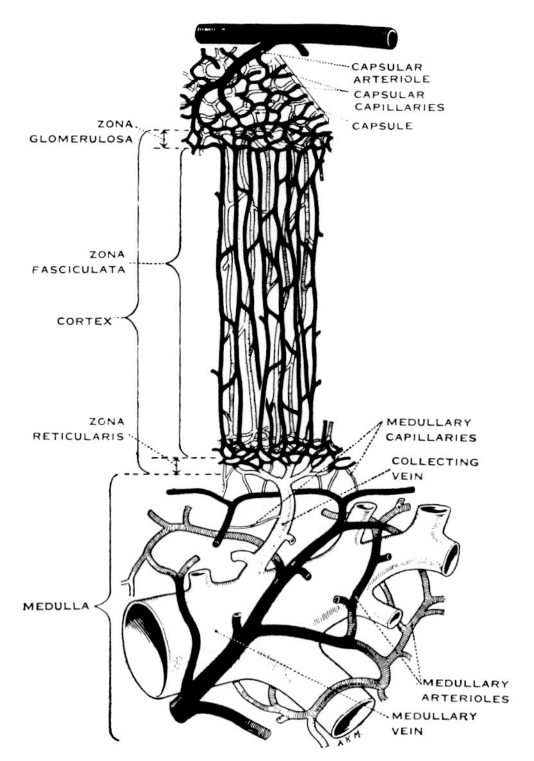

Figure 20–9. Schematic drawing of the blood supply of the adrenal showing how blood from the subcapsular plexus traverses the cortex and continues into the capillaries and venules of the medulla. (From Hamilton, W. J. ed. 1957. Textbook of Human Anatomy. London, St. Martin's Press.

tence in the male, and amenorrhea in the female; and peculiar striae in the skin of the abdominal wall similar to those seen late in pregnancy. The signs and symptoms of this disorder are due mainly to hypertrophy of the adrenal cortex, resulting in excess circulating cortisol.

Hypoadrenocorticism (Addison's disease) is usually due to destruction of the adrenal cortex by tuberculosis or some other infectious process. It is characterized by general weakness, weight loss, low blood pressure, and increased pigmentation of the skin. It culminates in death if not treated by hormone replacement.

HISTOPHYSIOLOGY OF THE ADRENAL MEDULLA

The cells of the adrenal medulla are modified postganglionic sympathetic neurons and their secretory activity is under nervous control. Centers in the posterior hypothalamus relay impulses to the adrenal medulla via the splanchnic nerves. On stimulation of these nerves, *norepinephrine* and *epinephrine* are detectable in increased amounts in the adrenal veins. Their secretion is prevented by section of the splanchnic nerves. Normally, about 25% of the secretion is norepinephrine and 75% is epinephrine. There is reason to believe that cells secreting norepinephrine and those secreting epinephrine are separately innervated and that they secrete their respective hormones independently. Emotional stimuli are especially effective in inducing release of norepinephrine, whereas other stimuli, such as pain or hypoglycemia, promote the release of epinephrone. In acute fear or stress, release of epinephrine prepares the body for combat or flight from the scene. Under such circumstances, plasma epinephrine may rapidly reach levels up to 300 times the normal concentration. Circulating epinephrine influences several target organs. Acting on the brain, it increases alertness. Acting on the vascular system, it increases heart rate and cardiac output; reaching the liver, it stimulates release of glucose to serve as an energy source for anticipated muscular exertion. Animals that have had their adrenals removed can survive, but they are unable to respond adequately to emergencies.

Although the two adrenal catecholamines are very closely related chemically, there are great qualitative and quantitative differences in their physiological effects. By increasing heart rate and cardiac output, epinephrine may augment the blood flow through some organs by as much as 100% and it is effective in very low concentrations. The denervated heart is accelerated by as little as 1 part epinephrine in 1.4 billion parts of perfusion medium. It may also increase metabolic rate by as much as 100%. On the other hand, norepinephrine has relatively little effect on metabolism, heart rate, or cardiac output but causes a marked elevation in blood pressure as a consequence of vasoconstriction of the peripheral blood vessels.

Production of norepinephrine is not confined to the adrenal medulla. It is also formed in the brain and peripheral nervous system, where it functions as a neurotransmitter, acting locally and being taken up, or destroyed enzymatically, before it can reach an effective concentration in the circulation. Norepinephrine released by the adrenal, on the other hand, does reach effective levels in the blood and, therefore, functions as a hormone acting on distant target organs. Unlike other long-acting neurosecretions, such as oxytocin and vasopressin, it is short acting, undergoing enzymatic degradation in the liver soon after its release.

Most of the constituents of the secretory granules of the medulla, including the chromogranins, proenkephalins, and the enzymes of their limiting membrane are synthesized in the rough endoplasmic reticulum. The granules are formed in the Golgi complex and subsequently become sites of synthesis and storage of catecholamines. Tyrosine is converted by tyrosine hydroxylase, in the cytosol, into dihydroxyphenylalanine (DOPA). This then enters the granules by a complex transport process during which norepinephrine is formed from DOPA by dopamine-B-hydroxylase, a major protein of the granule membrane. Synthesis of epinephrine requires transport of norepinephrine out of the granule for methylation by a cytosolic enzyme, phenyl-ethanolamine-*N*-methyl transferase (PNMT), followed by its return to the granule for storage. On sympathetic nerve stimulation, secretion involves release of Ca^{++} from the calcium-binding protein, calmodulin; movement of the granules to the surface; and fusion of their membranes with the plasmalemma. The membrane added to the surface in the process is recycled by endocytosis in clathrin-coated vesicles.

As stated in a foregoing section on blood vessels of the adrenal, the medulla is downstream from the cortex in the flow of blood through the gland. The synthesis of the key enzyme PNMT in the cells of the medulla is dependent on their being exposed to glucocorticoids carried in the blood reaching them from the cortex. Consequently, in hypophysectomized animals, which secrete very little glucocorticoid, the amount of epinephrine in the adrenal medulla is greatly reduced.

Of clinical interest are certain rare adrenal medullary tumors that release excessive amounts of catecholamines, resulting in attacks of "paraxysmal hypertension," characterized by sweating, hyperglycemia, and very high blood pressure, often terminating in death. Such attacks are ameliorated or abolished by intravenous injection of compounds blocking the action of epinephrine.

CELL RENEWAL AND REGENERATION IN THE ADRENAL CORTEX

Early studies on the mode of growth and renewal of the adrenal cortex led to differing interpretations. Some believed that the cells of all three zones arose by division of subcapsular cells in the zona glomerulosa which then migrated slowly through the zona fasciculata, ultimately degenerating in the zona reticularis. The dark-staining cells in this zone were interpreted as cells undergoing degeneration. The cells were believed to go through one cycle of secretion during their migration.

The concept of continual renewal of the cortex by a population of proliferating cells in the zona glomerulosa was not born out in later work, employing improved methods for studying cell dynamics. After administration of colchicine to arrest cell division at metaphase, mitotic figures were not confined to the glomerulosa but were found throughout the cortex, with the greatest number in the wide zona fasciculata. Moreover, study of autoradiographs at successive intervals after labeling of dividing cells with tritiated thymidine gave no clear indication of extensive cell migration. The bulk of the evidence now favors the view that, once formed, the cells of the three zones do not move appreciably and that they are replaced by local mitotic activity.

The adrenal cortex in laboratory animals has considerable capacity for regeneration. If the gland is incised and all of the tissue in its interior removed, leaving behind only the capsule and a few adherent cells of the zona glomerulosa, an entire cortex with normal structural and functional zonation will ultimately be regenerated. The medulla is not restored. Studies of the steroids elaborated during regeneration show that an adequate level of mineralocorticoid secretion is established early, with secretion of glucocorticoids following 2 to 3 weeks later. Thus, it is evident that cells functionally equivalent to those of the zona fasciculata and reticularis can differentiate from cells of the zona glomerulosa. However, in the untraumatized adult gland, cells of all three zones are apparently renewed by local mitotic activity. Hypertrophy of the cortical cells can be induced by ACTH, and their mitotic index is increased by growth hormone. Vasopressin and angiotensin-II have a mitogenic effect on cells of the zona glomerulosa.

THE PARAGANGLIA

The term *paraganglia* is used to describe small clusters of epithelioid cells that give a chromaffin reaction. They are found rather widely scattered in the retroperitoneal tissue.

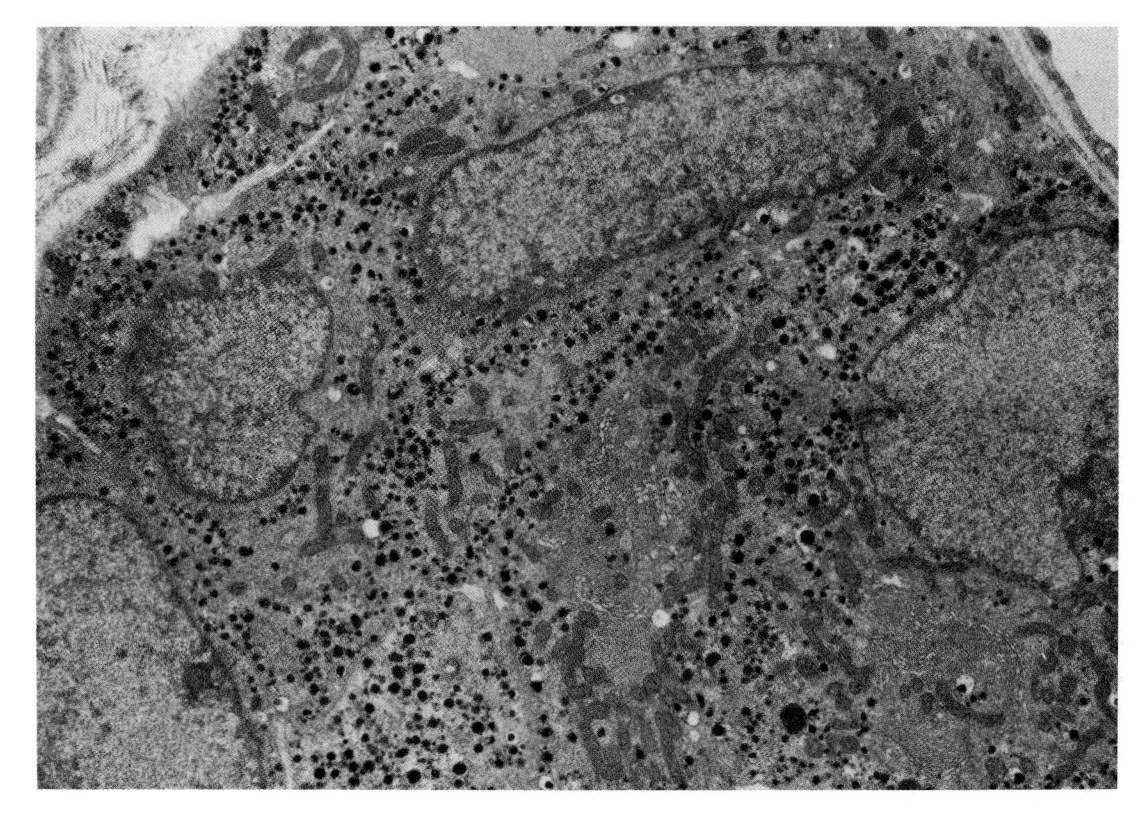

Figure 20–10. Electron micrograph of cells in a paraganglion from a rabbit showing chief cells containing numerous catecholamine granules resembling those of the adrenal medulla. (Micrograph courtesy of R. Yates.)

Some are associated with sympathetic ganglia, others with branches of the parasympathetic nerves. The cells of the paraganglia and those of the adrenal medulla are morphologically similar and of similar embryological origin. Together they make up the *chromaffin system.* In ordinary histological preparations, the cells of paraganglia appear pale or clear, but they can be stained with the chromaffin reaction.

These groups of cells found in ganglia or along nerves of the sympathetic nervous system have now been studied by electron microscopy and by histochemical procedures for identification of catecholamines. They are surrounded by a rather thick investment of connective tissue that extends inward between clumps of cells. Two types of parenchymal cells are distinguishable, *chief cells* and *supporting cells.* The chief cells are irregular in shape and have a single nucleus and a prominent Golgi complex. The endoplasmic reticulum is sparse, but occasional parallel associations of cisternae are observed. Glycogen particles, in small numbers, are scattered throughout the cytoplasm. In addition, there are numerous membrane-bounded electron-opaque granules, 50–200 nm in diameter, that closely resemble those of the adrenal medulla (Fig. 20–10). Histochemical staining methods indicate that these granules contain catecholamines, principally, if not exclusively, norepinephrine. The supporting cells partially or completely surround each of the chief cells. Their nucleus is elongated in section and often deeply infolded. The cytoplasm is devoid of secretory granules and is otherwise unremarkable.

The paraganglia are richly vascularized by capillaries lined with very attenuated endothelial cells, occasionally exhibiting fenestrated regions. The chief cells are usually separated from the blood by a barrier consisting of a thin supporting cell, two basal laminae, and the endothelium, but there are areas in which the supporting cell is absent and the chief cells are more intimately related to the capillary wall. The vascular relationships are of some significance because it is not yet clear whether the cells of the paraganglia have an endocrine function, releasing catacholamine into the blood, or whether the chief cells are essentially interneurons synapsing on sympathetic neurons and exerting an inhibitory effect on transmission in sympathetic ganglia.

The parasympathetic paraganglia often give a rather weak chromaffin reaction and they were formerly classified by light microscopists as "achromaffin paraganglia" to distinguish them from those associated with the sympathetic ganglia. This distinction between chromaffin and achromaffin paraganglia receives no support from electron microscopic studies and should probably be abandoned. The chief cells of vagal paraganglia contain 50–200-nm electron-opaque granules that tend to be at the cell periphery or in its processes. The supporting cells are somewhat less numerous than they are in sympathetic paraganglia, and chief cells may adjoin one another and be connected by desmosomes. The nerve terminals apposed to the surface of the chief cells contain numerous clear synaptic vesicles.

BIBLIOGRAPHY

ADRENAL CORTEX

Black, V. H., E. Robbins, E. McNamara, and T. Huima. 1979. A correlated thin section and freeze-fracture analysis of guinea pig adrenocortical cells. Am. J. Anat. 156:453.

Brown, M. S., P. T. Kovanen, and J. L. Goldstein. 1979. Receptor-mediated uptake of lipoprotein-cholesterol and its utilization for steroid synthesis in the adrenal cortex. Recent Progr. Horm. Res. 35:215.

Carey, R. M. and S. Sen. 1986. Recent progress in the control of aldosterone secretion. Recent Progr. Horm. Res. 42:251.

Fraser, R., J. J. Brown, A. F. Lever, P. A. Mason, and J. I. Robertson. 1979. Control of aldosterone secretion. Clin. Sci. 56:389.

Gill, G. N. 1976. ACTH regulation of the adrenal cortex. Pharmacol. Therap. (B) 2:313.

Griffiths, K. and E. H. D. Cameron. 1970. Steroid biosynthetic pathways in the human adrenal. Adv. Steroid Biochem. Pharm. 2:223.

Gwynne, J. T. and A. F. Strauss III. 1982. The role of lipoproteins in steroidogenesis and cholesterol metabolism in steroidogenic glands. Endocrine Rev. 3:299.

Hall, P. F. 1984: Cellular organization for steroidogenesis. Internat. Rev. Cytol. 86:53.

Long, J. A. and A. L. Jones. 1967. Observations on the adrenal cortex of man. Lab. Investig. 17:355.

Long, J. A. and A. L. Jones. 1970. Alterations in the fine structure of the opossum adrenal cortex following sodium deprivation. Anat. Rec. 166:1.

Neville, A. M. and M. J. O'Hara. 1982. The Human Adrenal Cortex. Berlin, Springer-Verlag.

Nussdorfer, G. G., G. Mazzochi, and V. Meneghelli. 1978. Cytophysiology of the adrenal zona fasciculata. Internat. Rev. Cytol. 55:291.

Pohorecky, L. A. and R. J. Wurtman. 1971. Adrenocortical control of epinephrine synthesis. Pharmacol. Rev. 27:1.

ADRENAL MEDULLA

Benedeczky, I. and A. D. Smith. 1972. Ultrastructural studies on the adrenal medulla of the hamster. Origin and fate of secretory granules. Zeitschr. Zellforsch. 124:367.

Bennett, H. S. 1941. Cytological manifestations of secretion in the adrenal medulla of the cat. Am. J. Anat. 66:333.

Burgoyne, R. D. 1984. Mechanisms of secretion from adrenal chromaffin cells. Biochim. Biophys. Acta 779:201.

Carmichael, S. 1983. The Adrenal Medulla, Vol. 3. Westmount, Quebec, Eden Press.

Coupland, R. E. 1965. Electron microscopic observations on the structure of the rate adrenal medulla. I. Ultrastructure and organization of chromaffin cells in the normal adrenal medulla. J. Anat. 99:231.

Trifaro, J. M., M. F. Bader, and J. P. Doucet. 1985. Chromaffin cell cytoskeleton. Its possible role in secretion. Can. J. Biochem. Cell Biol. 63:661.

Ungar, A. and J. H. Phillips. 1984. Regulation of the adrenal medulla. Physiol. Rev. 63:787.

Winkler, H., D. K. Apps, and R. Fischer-Colbrie. 1986. The molecular function of adrenal chromaffin granules: established facts and unsolved topics. Neuroscience 18:261.

Yates, R. D. 1964. A light and electron microscopic study correlating the chromaffin reaction and granule ultrastructure in the adrenal medulla of the Syrian hamster. Anat. Rec. 149:237.

PARAGANGLIA AND PARA-AORTIC BODIES

Bruden, T. 1865. Catecholamines in the pre-aortic paraganglia of fetal rabbits. Acta Physiol. Scand. 64:287.

Chen, I. and R. D. Yates. 1970. Ultrastructural studies of vagal paraganglia in Syrian hamsters. Zeitschr. Zellforsch. 108:309.

Coupland, R. E. and B. S. Weakley. 1970. Electron microscopic observations on the adrenal medulla and extraadrenal chromaffin tissue in the postnatal rabbit. J. Anat. 106:213.

Mascorro, J. A. and R. D. Yates. 1970. Microscopic observations on abdominal sympathetic paraganglia. Tex. Rep. Biol. Med. 28:59.

21 PINEAL GLAND

The *pineal gland* (*epiphysis cerebri*) is a small organ in the midline of the brain, projecting from the roof of the diencephalon. A shallow recess of the third ventricle extends into its short stalk (Fig. 21–1). In the human, the gland is a conical, grey body measuring 5 to 8 mm in length and 3 to 5 mm in its greatest width. The pineal was formerly considered to be a vestigial organ with little or no function, but it is now known to be an active endocrine gland. Its activity is influenced by the daily cycle of light and dark and it is an important link between the environment and the physiology of the organism. Responding to annual changes in day-length, it influences gonadal activity in seasonally breeding species and has a less apparent but nonetheless significant effect on the reproductive system in other species that breed throughout the year.

HISTOLOGICAL ORGANIZATION

The gland is invested by the *pia mater*, the delicate inner layer of connective tissue that covers the brain. In the human pineal, thin septa extend inward from this layer to surround cords or lobules of the parenchyma. Compartmentation by connective tissue septa is not a prominent feature in the gland of other species, but in some, cortical and medullary zones are distinguishable.

The parenchyma consists of pale-staining epithelioid cells, called *pinealocytes*. Their nucleus is spherical or indented on one side and they have a slightly basophilic cytoplasm that may contain a few lipid droplets (Fig. 21–4). Cell shape is difficult to discern in routine histological preparations, but with silver-impregnation methods, the cells can be shown to have one or more long processes that terminate in bulbous expansions (Fig. 21–2). Some of these end within the cords of parenchymal cells, but the majority appear to terminate on or near capillaries.

In electron micrographs, the irregularly shaped nuclei have a prominent nucleolus and small, peripheral clumps of heterochromatin. The cytoplasm contains both rough and smooth endoplasmic reticulum and a small Golgi complex (Fig. 21–5). Mitochondria are numerous and variable in form. Annulate lamellae are not uncommon. The cell processes contain microtubules and, at their ends, there are accumulations of small vesicles, some of which have electron-dense cores. In addition to the common organelles, pinealocytes contain *synaptic ribbons,* consisting of a dense rod or lamella perpendicular to the cell surface and surrounded by small vesicles. Similar structures are found at synapses in sensory cells of the retina and inner ear. In those cells, synaptic ribbons occur singly as components of the presynaptic complex and presumably play some role in directing the associated vesicles to sites of neurotransmitter release at the cell surface. In pinealocytes, there are multiple synaptic ribbons. They may be found anywhere in the peripheral cytoplasm of the cell body and do not appear to have a synaptic relationship to nerves, glial cells, or other *pinealocytes.* It has been reported that there is a two- to threefold increase in their number, in the dark phase of the diurnal cycle, and an increase in the length of their central dense rod. They are occasionally observed in aggregations of up to 20, referred to as synaptic-ribbon fields. The function of these structures remains a mystery.

The principal hormone of the pineal gland is the indolamine *melatonin,* but several biologically active peptides have also been identified and some of these may influence reproduction. The biosynthesis of melatonin has been studied, but the intracellular localization of the various enzymatic steps in the process remains unclear. Melatonin is not stored in the gland in secretory granules but is released as it is synthesized.

Cells of a second type, called *interstitial cells,* are found among the pinealocytes and in greater number in the stalk of the gland. They

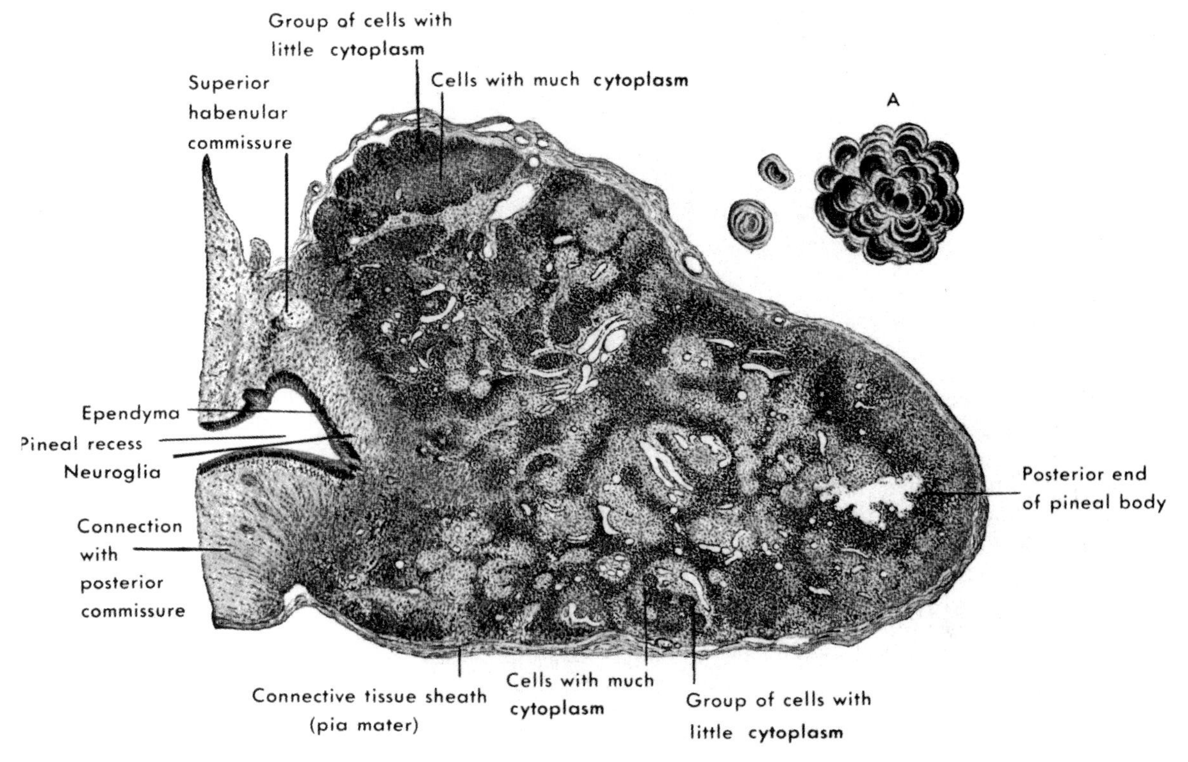

Figure 21–1. Median section through the pineal body of a newborn child. (A) Corpoa arenacea from the pineal body of a 69-year-old man. (After J. Schaffer Lehrbuch der Histologie und Histogenese. Engelmann, Leipzig, 1922.)

are considered to be comparable to the neuroglial cells of the brain. Their nuclei are elongated and stain more deeply than those of the pinealocytes. The endoplasmic reticulum is well represented in the cytoplasm and small deposits of glycogen are not uncommon. They resemble the astrocytes of the brain in having long-cell processes and an abundance of intermediate filaments throughout the cytoplasm.

The pineal gland of humans, and a few other species, contains peculiar extracellular concretions called *corpora arenacea* or "brain sand" (Fig. 21–3). These bodies consist of calcium phosphates and carbonates in an organic matrix deposited in concentric layers. Their mode of formation and their significance are poorly understood. They are not regarded as pathological for they appear in early childhood and increase in size and number with advancing age. Whatever the mechanism of their formation may be, it seems clear that their number is somehow linked to the metabolic activity of the gland, because when its secretory activity is increased by exposing animals to a short photoperiod, more concretions are formed and conversely, when pineal activity is reduced, fewer are formed. They may simply be accumulated by-products of secretory activity having no functional significance of their own. Calcified corpora arenacea are visible in X-rays or CAT scans of the head in 80% of individuals of 30 years of age. They are useful to the radiologist in the localization of tumors, or other expanding lesions of the brain, that may displace the pineal from its normal midline position.

PINEAL DEVELOPMENT

The pineal first appears at about 36 days of gestation as a prominent thickening of the ependyma in the posterior portion of the diencephalon. Cells migrate into this ependymal thickening to form a mantle layer within which the cells assume a follicular arrangement that is gradually transformed into the cell cords seen in the adult gland. By the sixth month, interstitial cells and pinealocytes have differentiated. The gland slowly increases in size until it reaches adult dimensions at about the age of 7. There is little subsequent change in the gland save for some increase in the prominence of the connective tissue septa.

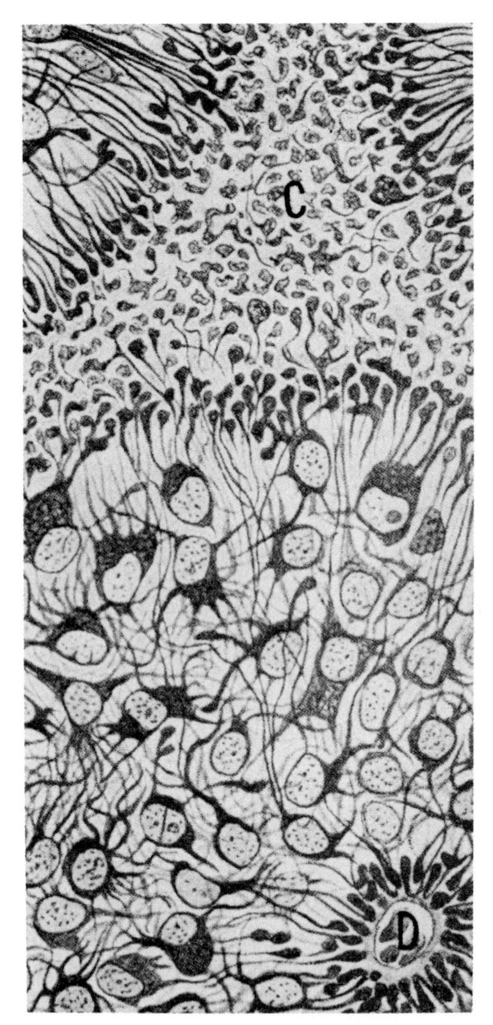

Figure 21–2. Drawing of a silver-impregnated section of the pineal of a young boy showing interlobular tissue (C) and blood vessel (D), with bulbous processes of pinealocytes ending in the adventitia. (After del Rio-Hortega, P. Arch. de Neurobiol. 3:359, 1922.)

INNERVATION OF THE GLAND

The innervation of the pineal gland is unusual in that there appears to be no afferent or efferent nervous connections with other parts of the brain. Its innervation is exclusively via sympathetic fibers that originate in the superior cervical ganglia and enter the skull with the major blood vessels supplying the brain. As the nerves enter the gland, their myelin sheaths terminate and the bare axons course among the parenchymal cells. In electron micrographs, aggregations of small vesicles in some of the axons are interpreted as sites of synaptic interaction with the pinealocytes. Release of norepinephrine at these sites controls the rate of melatonin synthesis.

PINEAL OF LOWER VERTEBRATES

In contrast to the compact organization of the gland in mammals, the pineal in lower vertebrates is a saccular organ. In most fish and amphibians the *pineal organ* or *intracranial epiphysis* is a single sac. In the more primitive fish, tailless amphibians, and lizards, there is a second component, the *parapineal organ* or *parietal organ* which arises as an anterior evagination of the intracranial epiphysis, or as a separate outgrowth of the roof of the diencephalon anterior to the main epiphyseal sac. In frogs, the distal end of the parapineal component lies just beneath the epidermis on the dorsum of the head, where it can be detected with the naked eye. It is joined to the intracranial epiphysis by a long stalk. Numerous nerves and nerve endings are found in the pineal organs of lower vertebrates, but as yet there is no evidence that they are of sympathetic origin.

Examination of the pineal organs of lower vertebrates with the electron microscope reveals the presence of photoreceptor cells that resemble those of the mammalian retina in having a lamellar portion of the apex and a receptor synapse at the base. The most elaborate pineal is found in the primitive lizard, Sphenodon. It contains a simple retina, consisting of photoreceptor cells backed by supporting cells that contain pigment, and its parietal component includes a lens-like structure. It, thus, constitutes a vestigial *parietal eye*. Experimental evidence of light perception by this organ in Sphenodon is still lacking but the large size of the pineal foramen in fossil reptiles strongly suggests that their parietal eye was functional.

The pinealocytes of mammals are believed to have evolved from the photoreceptor cells in the pineal organ of primitive vertebrates. It is speculated that in the course of their evolution from light-sensitive elements to endocrine cells, the region of the cell specialized for photoreception was lost, together with the sensory nerves connecting it to other regions of the brain. The synaptic ribbons of mammalian pinealocytes may be vestiges of the special synapses that are characteristic of photoreceptors. Whether they have acquired an alternate function related to secretion is not known.

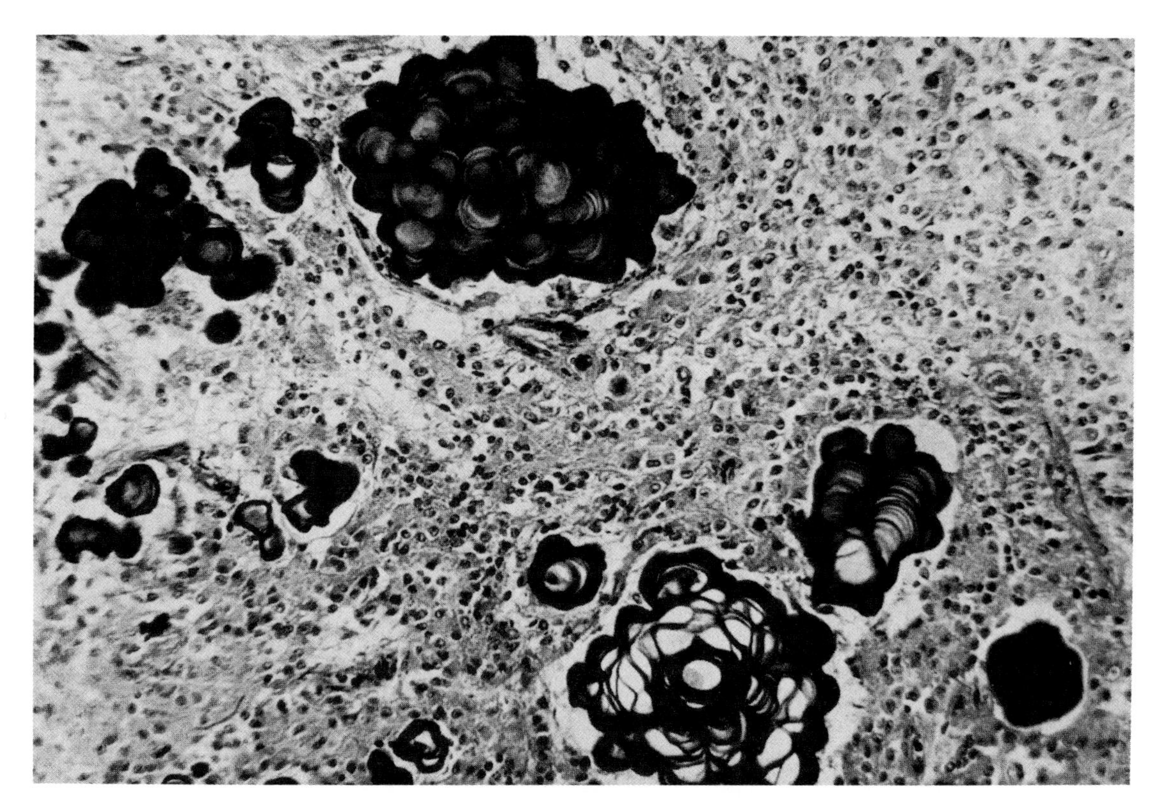

Figure 21–3. Photomicrograph of human pineal showing a number of corpora arenacea.

HISTOPHYSIOLOGY OF THE PINEAL

Long considered to be a vestigial organ of little functional significance, the mammalian pineal has now been firmly established as gland modulating gonadal function. A unique feature of this endocrine gland is that its biosynthetic activity exhibits a diurnal rhythmicity that is related to the periods of light and darkness. The concentration of its hormone in the blood increases in the dark phase of the cycle. Unlike endocrine glands that are controlled by blood-borne hormones from other endocrine glands, the pineal depends on its innervation and is, therefore, a neuroendocrine transducer converting nervous input into variations in hormone output. Synthetic activity is inhibited by light and favored by darkness. Information as to day or night, received by the eyes, is transmitted over retinohypothalamic nerve tracts to suprachiasmatic nuclei in the hypothalamus. From there, it is relayed over long cerebrospinal tracts to the intermediolateral column of the spinal cord in the upper thoracic region. Preganglionic sympathetic axons leave the cord and ascend in the sympathetic trunk to the superior cervical ganglia. Ascending postganglionic sympathetic fibers enter the skull and terminate in the pineal gland (Fig. 21–6). Release of norepinephrine at their endings among the parenchymal cells controls the rate of hormone synthesis.

Melatonin is an indolamine synthesized from the amino acid tryptophan, which is taken up from the blood and converted to 5-hydroxytryptophan and then to serotonin. Serotonin is converted, by the enzyme *N*-acetyltransferase (NAT), to *N*-acetyl serotonin and this, in turn, is transformed to melatonin by the enzyme hydroxyindole-*O*-methyl transferase (HIOMT). The hormone is released without prior storage.

The pineal is involved in reproduction to varying degrees in different species. Many species that inhabit temperate or arctic zones are seasonal breeders because it is important that the young be born in the spring to ensure the availability of food and tolerable ambient temperatures. In the winter, the gonads of these species regress and only regain reproductive competence with the approach of spring. The critical environmental factor reg-

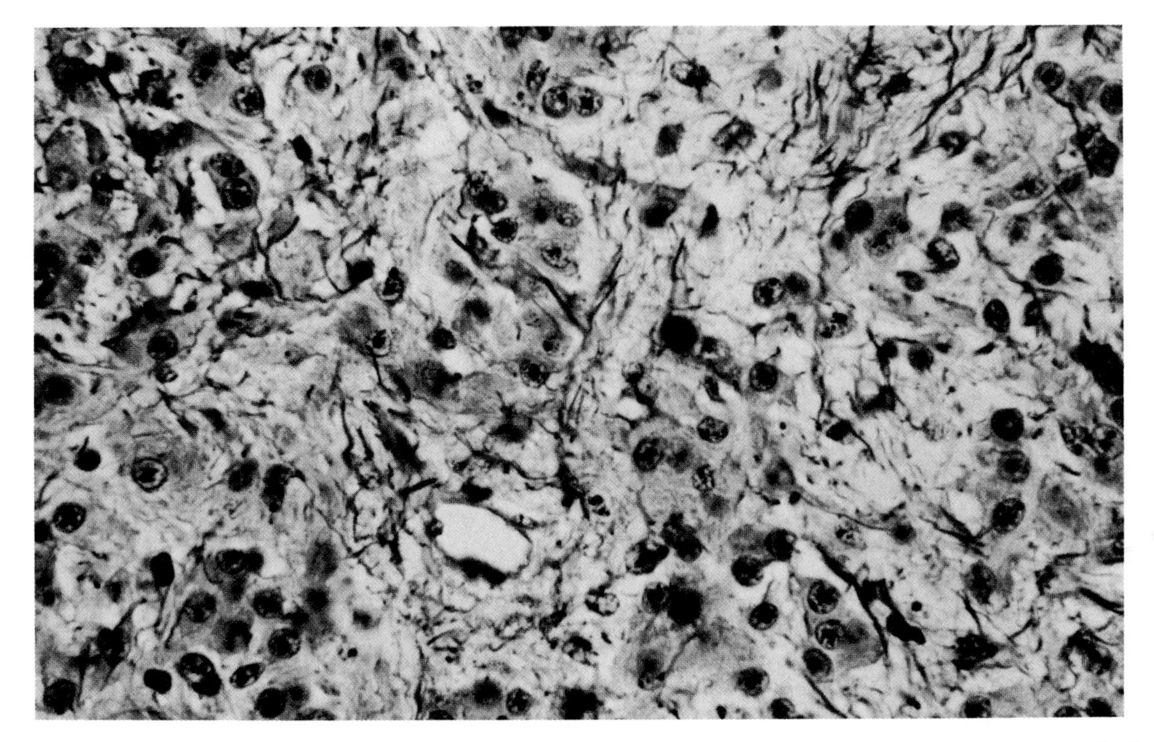

Figure 21–4. Photomicrograph of the bovine pineal gland. The pinealocytes have large nuclei with prominent nucleoli. The outlines of the stellate interstitial cells are not easily distinguished. Many densely stained cell processes are visible in this preparation but it is not possible to determine which belong to pinealocytes and which to interstitial cells. (Courtesy of E. Anderson.)

ulating this seasonal pattern of reproduction is day-length. The pineal mediates the response of the reproductive system to changing day length (Fig. 21–7).

The reproductive system of the laboratory rat responds little, and inconsistently, to experimental manipulation of pineal physiology. This may be a consequence of it having been inbred for many generations under unnatural conditions that may have led to the loss of mechanisms essential for the survival of a species in the wild. The heavy reliance of the scientific community on the laboratory rat contributed to slow progress in defining the role of the pineal in reproduction. The Syrian hamster, a species introduced into the laboratory more recently than the rat, has been especially useful in studies relating photoperiod to pineal function. Exposure of hamsters to a short photoperiod, for a few weeks, enhances melatonin secretion by the pineal and results in testicular atrophy. Under lighting conditions simulating long summer days, the combined testis weight is about 3000 mg. Simulation of long winter nights induces their atrophy to about 300 mg. Either pinealectomy or superior cervical ganglionectomy prevents the gonadal atrophy induced by short photoperiod. All of the effects of naturally occurring changes in photoperiod can be reproduced in the laboratory by administration of melatonin in appropriate dosage and at the right time. In seasonal breeders, the pineal continues to secrete at elevated levels throughout the winter, but the reproductive system seems to become refractory to its inhibitory effect and gonadal recrudescence begins as spring approaches. It is not yet known whether the pineal induces reproductive incompetence by acting on the hypothalamus or directly on the gonads.

Sunlight or artificial light of appropriate brightness and wavelength suppresses pineal melatonin production in all species studied, but the degree of pineal participation in reproductive activity of nonseasonally breeding species, including man, is unclear. The gland is active in young animals and children and it is postulated that a decline in its production of melatonin permits development of the gonads and onset of puberty. This is supported by animal experiments in which young rats subjected to pinealectomy or superior cervical galglionectomy were found to have acceler-

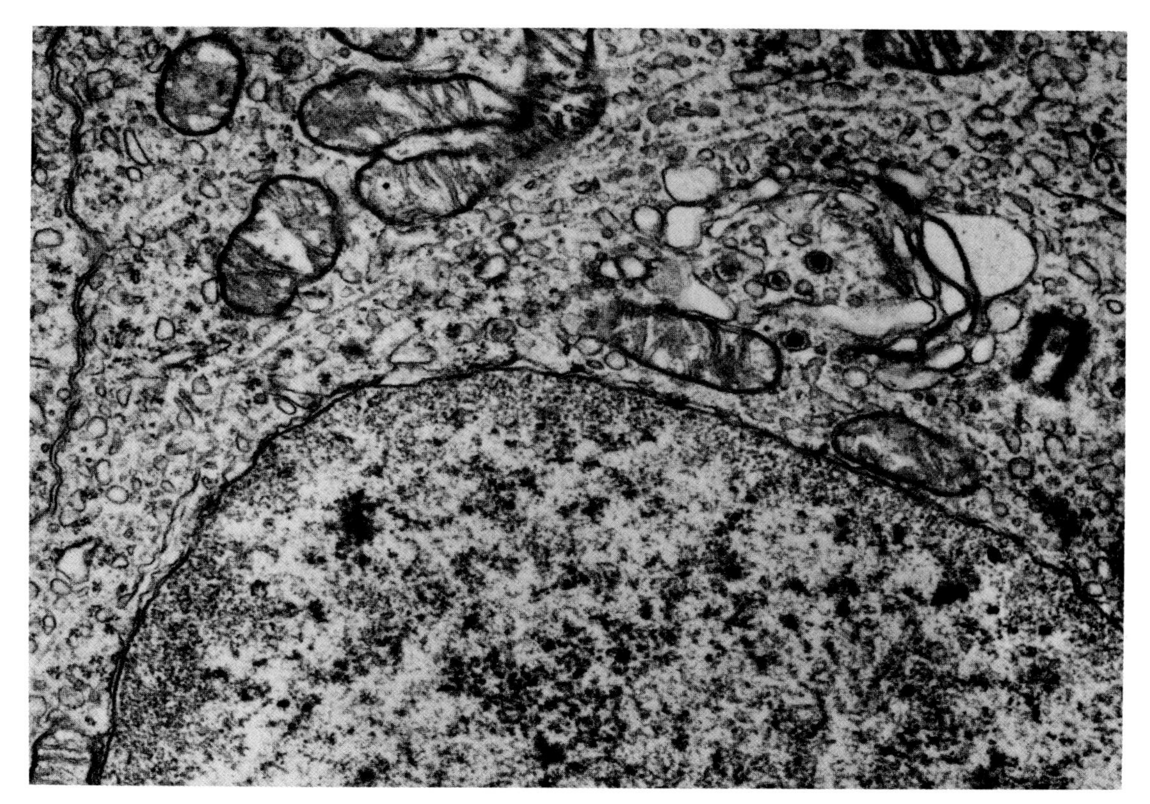

Figure 21–5. Electron micrograph of the juxtanuclear region of a pinealocyte, including a small Golgi complex and a centriole. Some of the vesicles associated with the Golgi have dense cores. A few microtubules are evident in the cytoplasm. (Courtesy of E. Anderson.)

ated growth of the gonads. Conversely, sustained administration of melatonin to young rats delayed puberty. Blood levels of melatonin in young boys are found to be high and to decline early in puberty. Further indirect support for the hypothesis has come from the observation that children with brain tumors that damage or destroy the pineal have precocious development of the reproductive organs, whereas tumors of the pineal itself may delay puberty if they secrete greater than normal amounts of melatonin.

An increasing volume of research is now centered on isolation and characterization of the peptides produced by the pineal. These include *arginine vasotocin, pineal antigonadotrophin,* and a *gonadotrophin-releasing factor* distinct from the gonadotrophin-releasing hormone (GnRH) of the hypothalamus. Of these, arginine vasotocin has been most thoroughly studied and is more effective than melatonin in suppressing gonadotrophic hormones. The site and mechanism of action of melatonin remain controversial and some investigators believe that the peptides are the principal pineal hormones influencing reproduction. It is suggested that the small dense-cored vesicles in the perivascular processes of the pinealocytes contain peptides conjugated to carrier proteins called *neuroepiphysins* to distinguish them from *neurophysins* associated with the hormones of the neural lobe of the pituitary. On exocytosis, the peptides are believed to dissociate from the neuroepiphysins and diffuse into the capillaries or the cerebrospinal fluid.

The amphibians have put the responsiveness of the pineal to light to a very different use, namely, to produce changes in skin color that have survival value for their larvae. This was the first pineal function to be established by laboratory studies. Seventy years ago it was found that feeding of desiccated bovine pineal to anuran tadpoles resulted in rapid lightening of their skin color due to aggregation of melanosomes in their melanophores. Forty years later, efforts to extract the active substance from the pineal were undertaken in the hope that it might be useful in the treatment of pigmentary disorders in humans. The

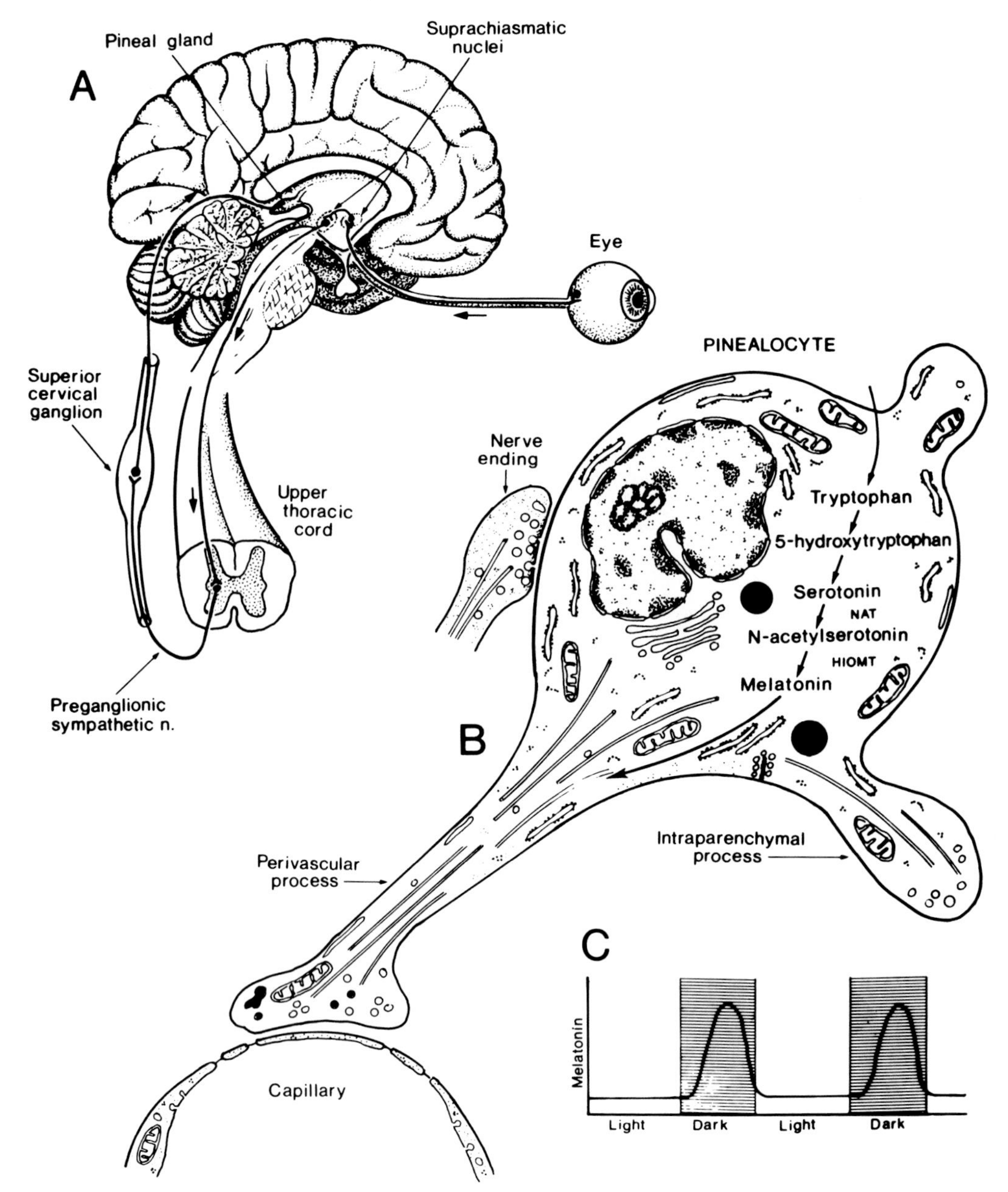

Figure 21–6. (A) Path of information transfer from eyes to pineal: via retinohypothalamic tracts to suprachiasmatic nuclei; relayed to intermediolateral column of spinal cord; then via preganglionic sympathetic fibers to superior cervical ganglion; and then via postganglionic sympathetic fibers to the pineal. (B) On sympathetic stimulation of the pinealocytes, tryptophan is taken up from the blood and converted to melatonin, which is transported to the ends of perivascular processes for release into the blood. (C) Graph of the light–dark cycle of melatonin concentration in the blood. (After R. J. Reiter, Groot's Endocrinology, Vol. I pp. 240–253, W. B. Saunders, Philadelphia, 1989.)

first purified extract, prepared from over 200,000 bovine pineals, was found to produce blanching of the skin of larval amphibia in a concentration as low as a trillionth of a gram per milliliter of water. It was concluded that a hormone of the pineal mediates the skin-lightening response of larval amphibia in a dark environment. Although the extract proved to have no pigmentary effect in mammals, these studies soon led to the identification of melatonin as an indole derivative and set in motion the pursuit of its function in mammals.

From the time of its discovery in the seventeenth century, when René Descartes assigned it the function of "seat of the rational soul,"

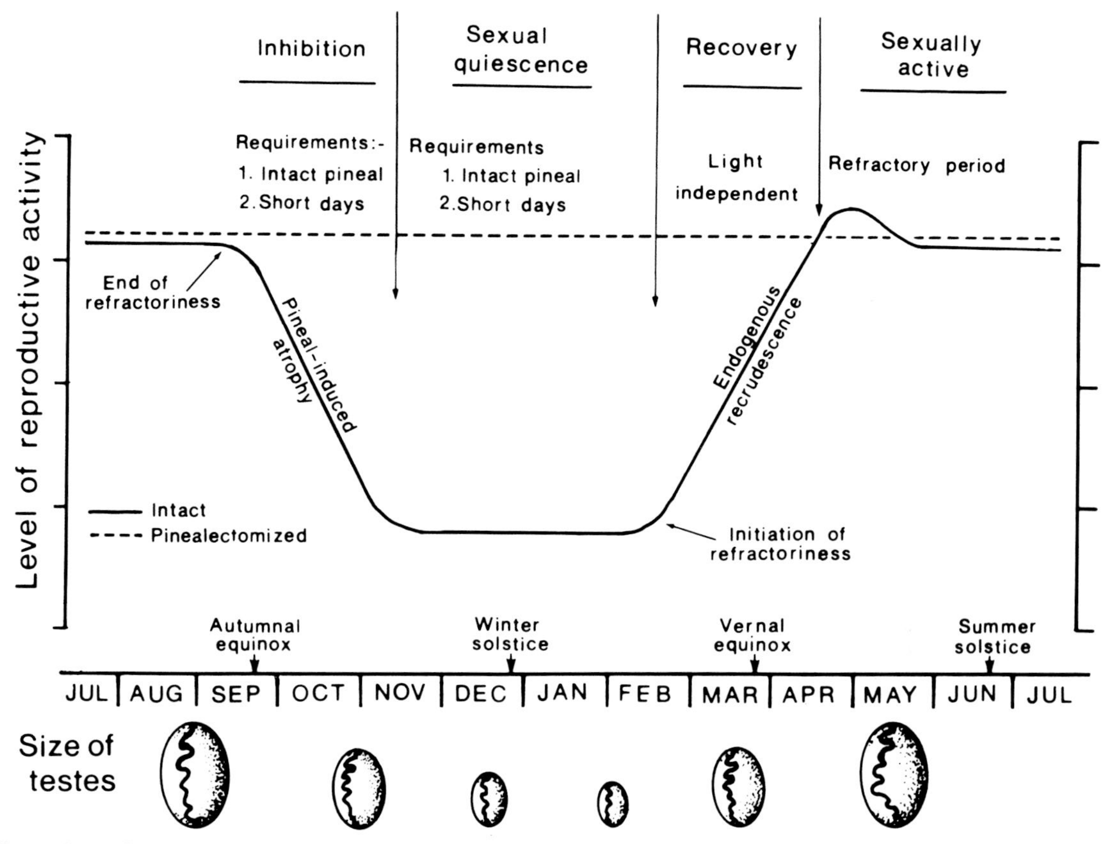

Figure 21–7. Schematic depiction of the relationships between the pineal gland and the annual reproductive cycle of a seasonal-breeding species. (From Reiter, R.J. 1980. Endocrinol. Rev. 1:109.)

the pineal has invited unrestrained speculation. This continues. There has been recent clinical interest in the possible involvement of the pineal in seasonal mood disorders and even in jet lag. Seasonal affective disorder (SAD) is a condition characterized by periods of depression, usually occurring in the winter months when the photoperiod is short and nocturnal peaks of melatonin secretion lengthened. The symptoms are claimed to be ameliorated by extending the photoperiod with exposure to artificial light and to be aggravated by administration of melatonin. It is also speculated that symptoms of jet lag, experienced by some individuals after long flights, may be due, in part, to a readjustment of the plasma melatonin rhythm to altered light–dark cycle, but the evidence is far from convincing. However, one cannot exclude the possibility that this interesting gland, linking the environment to mammalian physiology, may have functions in man that do not lend themselves to validation in laboratory animals.

BIBLIOGRAPHY

Arstila, A. U. 1967. Electron microscopic studies on the structure and histochemistry of the pineal gland of the rat. Neuroendocrinology (Suppl.) 2:1.

Bagnara, J. T. and M. E. Hadley. 1970. Endocrinology of the amphibian pineal. Am. Zoologist 10:201.

Benson, B. 1977. Current status of pineal peptides. Neuroendocrinology 24:241.

Kelly, D. E. 1962. Pineal organs: photoreception, secretion and development. Sci. Am. 50:597.

Kitay, J. L. and M. D. Altschule. 1954. The Pineal Gland; A Review of the Physiological Literature. Cambridge, MA, Harvard University Press.

Kumado, K. and W. Mori. 1977. A morphological study of the circadian cycle of the pineal gland of the rat. Cell Tissue Res. 182:565.

Lincoln, G. A. 1984. The pineal gland. *In* C. R. Austin and R. V. Short, eds. Hormonal Control of Reproduction. Cambridge, England, Cambridge University Press.

Lukaszyk, A. and R. J. Reiter. 1975. Histophysiological evidence for secretion of polypeptides by the pineal gland. Am. J. Anat. 143:451.

Matsushima, S., Y. Morisawa, I. Aida, and K. Abe. 1983. Circadian variations in pinealocytes of the Chinese hamster, *Cricetus griseus*. Cell Tissue Res. 228:231.

Reiter, R. J. 1973. Comparative physiology: pineal gland. Annu. Rev. Physiol. 35:305.

Reiter, R. J. 1973. Pineal control of seasonal reproductive rhythm in male golden hamsters exposed to natural daylight and temperature. Endocrinology 92:423.

Reiter, R. J. 1980. The pineal and its hormones in the control of reproduction in mammals. Endocrin. Rev. 1:109.

Reiter, R. J. 1988. Neuroendocrinology of melatonin. *In* A. Miles, D. R. S. Philbrick, and C. Thompson, eds. Melatonin: Clinical Perspectives. Oxford, Oxford University Press.

Reiter, R. J. 1989. The pineal gland. *In* L. J. DeGroot, ed. DeGroot's Endocrinology, Vol. I, 2nd ed. Philadelphia, W. B. Saunders Co.

Roth, W. D., R. J. Wurtman,, and M. D. Altschule. 1962. Morphological changes in the pineal parenchymal cells of rats exposed to continuous light or darkness. Endocrinology 77:888.

Soriano, F. M., H. A. Wether, and L. Volbrath. 1984. Correlation of the number of pineal "synaptic" ribbons and spherule with the level of serum melatonin over a 24 hour period in male rabbits. Cell Tissue Res. 236:555.

Theron, J. J., R. Biagio, and A. C. Meyer. 1981. Circadian changes in microtubules, synaptic ribbons, and synaptic ribbon fields in the pinealocytes of the baboon, *Papio ursinus*. Cell Tissue Res. 217:405.

Wartenberg, H. 1968. The mammalian pineal organ: electron microscopic studies on the fine structure of pinealocytes, glial cells, and on the perivascular component. Z. Zellforsch. 86:74.

Wurtman, R. J., J. Axelrod, and J. E. Fischer. 1964. Melatonin synthesis in the pineal gland: Effect of light mediated by the sympathetic nervous system. Science 143:1328.

22 SKIN

The skin covering the body is one of its largest organs, accounting for some 16% of the body weight. It has several important functions: It presents a barrier protecting the organism against injury and dessication; its tactile sense organs receive stimuli from the environment; and it plays an important role in thermoregulation and water balance.

The skin consists of two principal layers, the surface epithelium called the *epidermis* and a subjacent connective tissue layer, the *dermis* or *corium* (Figs. 22–1, 22–2). Beneath the dermis is a layer of loose connective tissue, the *hypodermis,* which, in some regions consists largely of adipose tissue. The hypodermis, in turn, is loosely attached to underlying deep fascia or to periosteum of bone. At the lips, nose, eyelids, vulva, and prepuce, the skin is continuous, at *mucocutaneous junctions,* with the mucous membranes lining those structures.

The specific functions of the skin depend mainly on the properties of the epidermis. This epithelium forms an uninterrupted investment over the entire surface of the body and is locally specialized for the production of the skin appendages, *hair* and *nails.* It also gives rise to two kinds of glands, one producing the watery secretion, *sweat,* and the other, an oily secretion, *sebum.*

Although the basic features of the structure of the skin are the same throughout, there are striking differences in its texture, fine structure, and function related to gender and to body region. For example, several local differences are apparent in the face alone. At the eyebrows, the skin is relatively thick and forms coarse hairs, whereas on the eyelids it is thin with very fine hairs. On the cheeks and forehead, it is soft with fine hairs and an oily texture, whereas over the chin and jowls of the male it lacks oil and forms the coarse hairs of the beard. On the lips, it is very thin and devoid of hair.

When magnified, the free surface of the skin is not smooth but is marked by shallow grooves that create varying patterns from region to region. These grooves and flexure lines are deeper on thick, hairless regions such as the knees, elbows, palms, and soles. The most familiar of these features are the alternating ridges and grooves on the finger pads that constitute the dermatoglyphs. There, the ridges form a distinctive pattern of arches, loops, or whorls that are responsible for the individuality of the fingerprints. A similar degree of individual variability holds for the skin in other areas where the pattern is less conspicuous.

The interface between the epidermis and the dermis is also highly irregular. An intricate pattern of ridges and grooves on the under side of the epidermis fits into a conforming pattern of grooves and ridges on the underlying dermis (Fig. 22–1). The projections of the dermis are called *dermal papillae* and the downgrowths of the epidermis have traditionally been called *interpapillary pegs.* Although the three-dimensional images afforded by the scanning microscope show that *peg* does not accurately describe their form, the term persists.

EPIDERMIS

Over much of the body surface, the epidermis varies in thickness from 0.07 to 0.12 mm, but it may reach a thickness of 0.8 mm on the palms and 1.4 mm on the soles of the feet. At these sites, it is already appreciably thicker in the fetus, but the continuous pressure and friction on these surfaces in postnatal life result in additional thickening. The histological organization of the skin is best studied in these regions where the epidermis attains its greatest thickness.

EPIDERMIS OF PALMS AND SOLES

The epidermis is a stratified squamous epithelium made up of multiple layers of cells

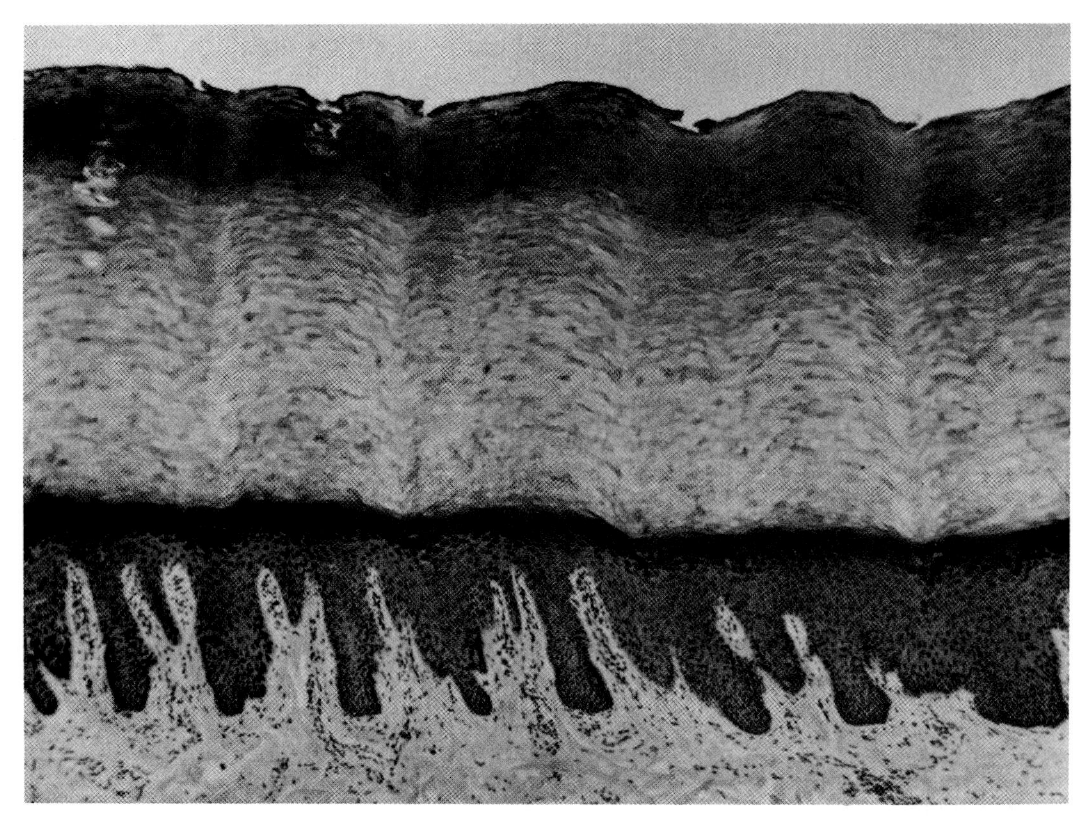

Figure 22–1. Photomicrograph of skin of the human finger tip, an example of thick skin, having a very thick stratum corneum.

called *keratinocytes.* These are continually renewed by mitosis of the cells in the basal layer. As new cells are formed, they are slowly displaced toward the surface of the epithelium by the proliferation of cells in the basal layer. In their transit, they differentiate, enlarging and accumulating increasing amounts of *keratin filaments* in their cytoplasm. As they approach the surface, they die and their flake-like lifeless cell bodies are continually shed. Their transit time from the base of the epithelium to the surface is 20 to 30 days. The structural modifications that they undergo during their passage are collectively described as the *cytomorphosis* of the epidermal cells. Their changing appearance at different levels in the epithelium makes it possible to distinguish four zones in histological sections perpendicular to the skin surface. These are the *stratum basale,* the *stratum spinosum* (stratum Malpighii), the *stratum granulosum,* and the *stratum corneum* (Figs. 22–2 and 22–2).

The *stratum basale* consists of a single layer of cells supported by a typical basal lamina and resting on the underlying dermis (Fig. 22–3). Its cells are cuboidal or low columnar. Their nucleus is large, relative to the size of the cell, and the cytoplasm is basophilic. In electron micrographs, there is a small Golgi complex, a few mitochondria and profiles of endoplasmic reticulum in a cytoplasmic matrix rich in ribosomes. Ten-nanometer intermediate filaments occur singly and in conspicuous bundles that often end in desmosomes on the lateral surfaces of the cell or in hemidesmosomes spaced at regular intervals along the membrane adjacent to the basal lamina. Mitotic figures are common in this layer, formerly called the *stratum germinativum,* because proliferation of its cells is responsible for the continual renewal of the epithelium. As the cells generated here move up into the overlying stratum spinosum, they assume a flattened polyhedral form with their long axis parallel to the surface of the epithelium and their nucleus somewhat elongated in the same direction.

The cells of the *stratum spinosum* (stratum Mapighii) have the same complement of organelles but are less intensely basophilic than

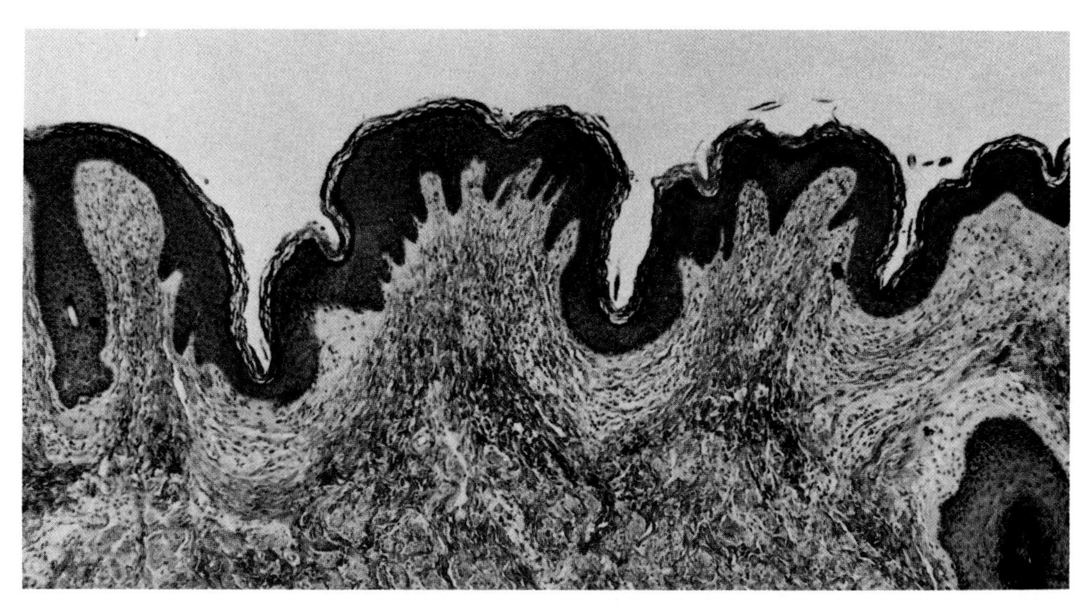

Figure 22–2. Photomicrograph of skin of the abdomen. Compare the thickness of the stratum corneum with that of the thick skin in Fig. 22–1.

those of the stratum basale. A prominent feature of these cells is the presence of numerous bundles of cytokeratin intermediate filaments that radiate from the perinuclear region, to end in the dense plague of numerous desmosomes along the highly interdigitated cell boundaries (Figs. 22–4 and 22–5). Also present in the cytoplasm are secretory granules, 0.1–0.4 μm in diameter, called *membrane-coating granules* or *lamellar granules*. These have a limiting membrane and a distinctive internal structure consisting of closely packed parallel lamellae. At high magnification, the alternating electron-dense and electron-lucent thin bands within these granules resemble those of myelin and other multilayered membrane systems. Pairs of dense bands are seen to be continuous with one another at their ends. This has led to the interpretation that these stacks are made up of discoid flattened vesicles with their outer surfaces tightly apposed.

The *stratum granulosum* consists of three to five layers of cells that are somewhat more flattened than those of the stratum spinosum. Their principal distinguishing feature is the presence of bodies of large size and very irregular shape that stain intensely with basic dyes (Fig. 22–6). Unlike secretory granules, these so-called *keratohyalin granules* do not have a limiting membrane. Bundles of the abundant keratin filaments in the cytoplasm may be incorporated in their periphery or may pass through them. Their exact chemical nature remains unclear, but they are believed to be precursors of an interfibrillar matrix that is distributed throughout the cytoplasm of fully keratinized cells in the overlying stratum corneum. The lamellar granules that first appeared in the stratum spinosum are present in greater number in the cells of the stratum granulosum, where they collect near the cell membrane. They may occupy as much as 15% of the cytoplasmic volume. They undergo exocytosis and their content coalesces to form a continuous multilayered coating of the cell membranes. Correlated with the release of these granules, there is an increase in the size of the extracellular spaces from less than 1% to 5–30% of the tissue volume, and this space is occupied by the lipid-rich secretory product of the cells, which is regarded as a kind of waterproof sealant that is a major component of the epidermal permeability barrier.

The *stratum lucidum* is a layer of thin, lightly staining, refractile cells located between the stratum granulosum and the stratum corneum in thick skin of the palms and soles (Fig. 22–3). This layer is usually not identifiable in the thinner skin of other regions. It consists of four to six rows of very flat cells. Nuclei begin to degenerate in the outer row of the stratum granulosum and are rarely seen in the cells of the stratum lucidum. In electron micrographs, the keratin filaments in the cytoplasm are closely aggregated and more consistent in their orientation parallel to the skin

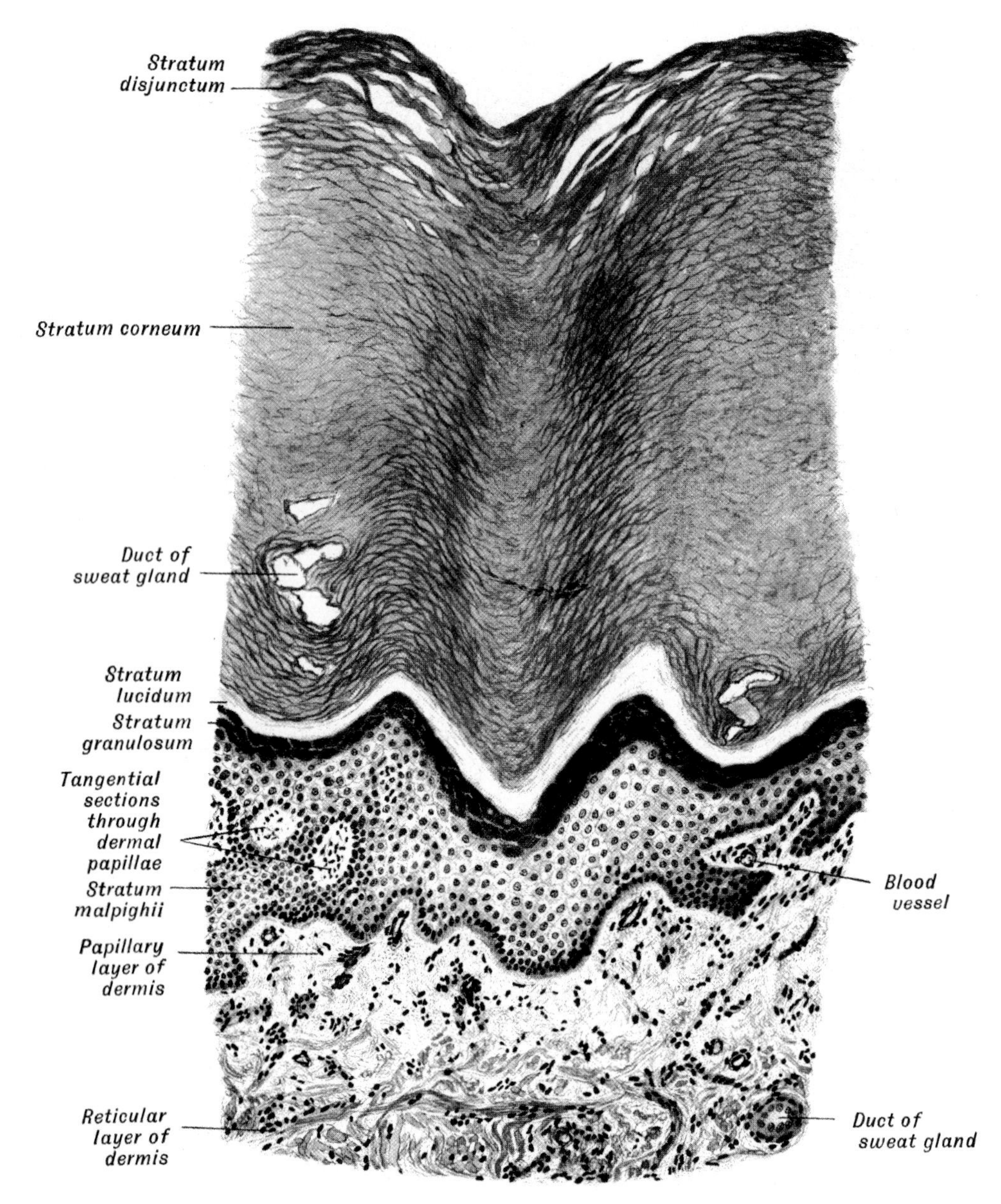

Figure 22–3. Drawing of a vertical section of skin from the sole of the human foot.

surface. The cell membrane appears thickened by deposition of dense material on its inner surface.

The *stratum corneum* consists of many layers of very flat, heavily keratinized cells containing no nucleus or cytoplasmic organelles (Figs. 22–1 and 22–3). The plasmalemma appears thickened and the entire cell is filled with keratin filaments embedded in an amorphous matrix. The cells of the lower layers of the stratum corneum are still closely adherent, but the desmosomes have been greatly modified (Figs. 22–7 and 22–8). In the outer layers, the fully keratinized, lifeless cells loosen and ultimately desquamate. This portion of the stratum corneum is sometimes referred to as the *stratum disjunctum,* but the cells are identical to those deeper in the stratum and its designation as a separate layer serves no useful purpose. As keratinocytes ascend through the several strata of the epidermis, they enlarge and become flattened to such an extent that a cell in the stratum corneum covers an area equivalent to that occupied by 15 or more of the cuboidal cells of the stratum basale.

The epidermis has a well-developed basal

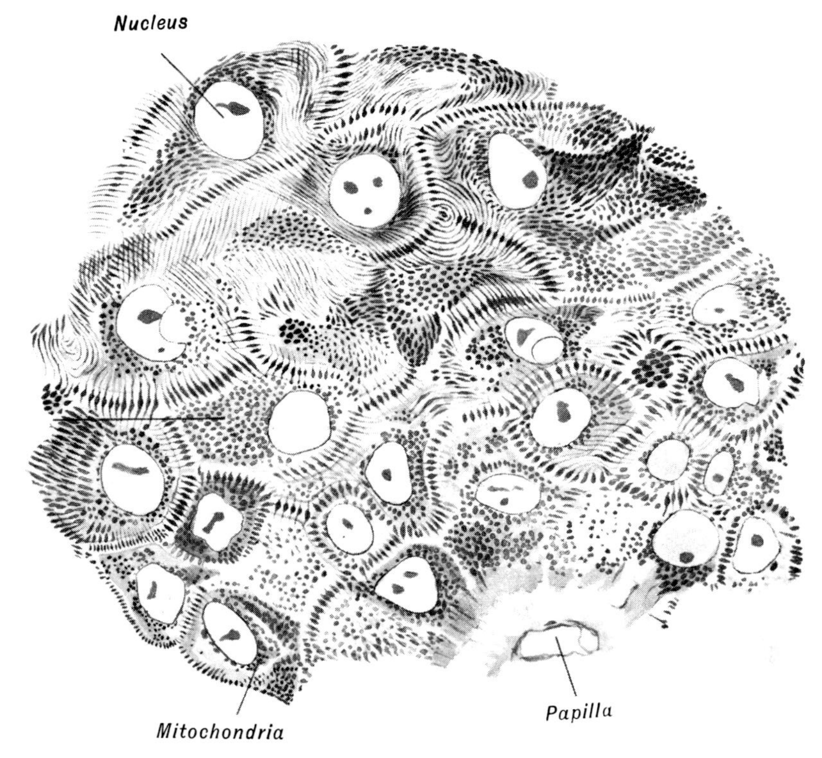

Figure 22–4. Drawing of an oblique section passing through the stratum spinosum of the epidermis showing bundles of filaments in neighboring cells converging on numerous closely spaced desmosomes at the cell boundaries. Before the advent of electron microscopy, these structures were interpreted as "intercellular bridges."

lamina. Recent studies of its mode of attachment to the underlying dermis have clarified the structural basis for the binding of all epithelia to their substrate. The basal lamina (formerly called the basement membrane) consists of a *lamina densa* parallel to the membrane of the basal cells of the epithelium and separated from it by a thin *lamina lucida,* which is traversed by exceedingly thin filaments crossing from the cell membrane to the lamina densa. The lamina densa is a fine meshwork of type-IV collagen, also containing heparan sulfate and glycoprotein. Slender *anchoring fibrils* extend from the lamina downward, arching around collagen bundles in the dermis and terminating in *anchoring plaques,* which are small bodies having the same density and substructure as the lamina densa. Other anchoring fibrils connect neighboring anchoring plaques (see Fig. 2–16). The loose network of anchoring fibrils around collagen bundles if believed to bind the epithelium firmly to the dermis. At high magnification, the anchoring fibrils have the beaded, or cross-striated, appearance characteristic of type-VII collagen, a rare member of the family of collagens that has not been found, to date, elsewhere.

The strength of attachment of the epidermis to the dermis is no doubt enhanced by the increase in total area of the interface, resulting from the deep interdigitation of the corrugated under surface of the epidermis with complimentary ridges and furrows on the upper surface of the dermis.

The epidermis is a remarkable epithelium, synthesizing a great variety of structural components that contribute to the protective function of the skin, and it may be useful here, to review some of its biosynthetic activities. Only the basal cells are capable of undergoing mitosis. Some of the daughter cells of their divisions leave the basal cell layer and begin an upward journey that will ultimately take them to the surface of the epithelium. In leaving the basal lamina, these cells become committed to a process of terminal differentiation that will lead to their transformation into flat, anucleate, lifeless, flakes (*squames*) that are sloughed from the skin surface.

The most abundant structural protein synthesized by the *keratinocytes,* during their differentiation, is *keratin* which forms increasing numbers of 10-nm cytoskeletal filaments in their cytoplasm. Biochemists have identified

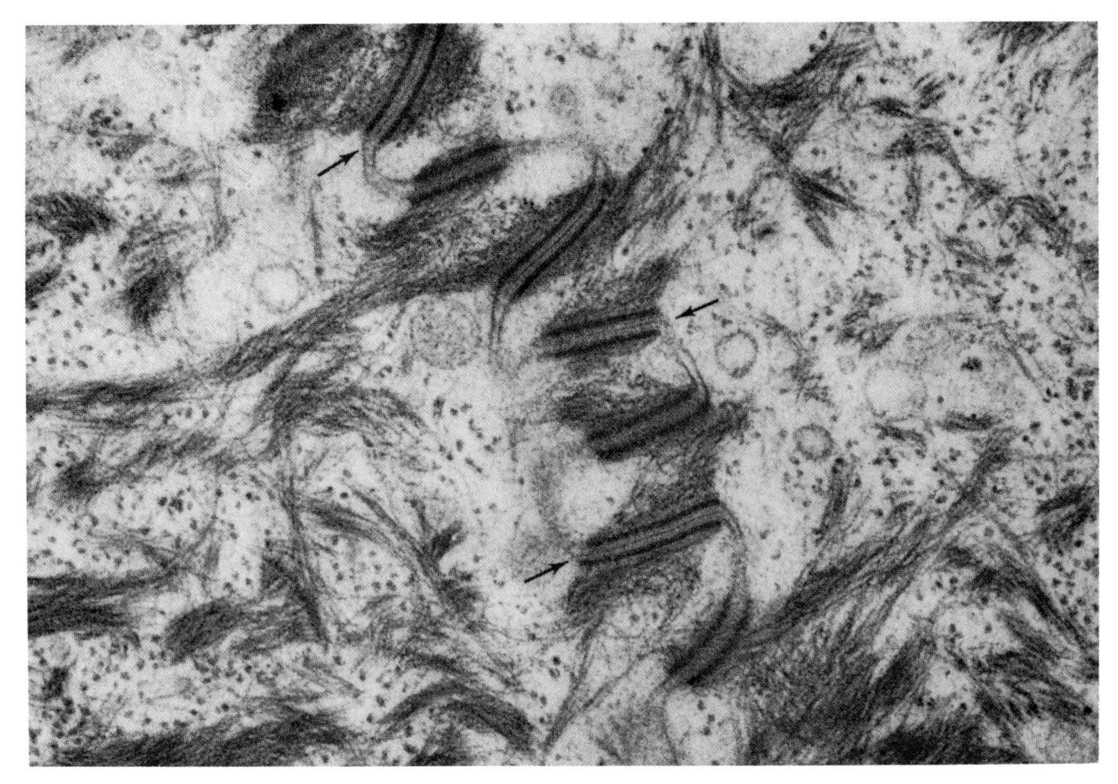

Figure 22–5. Electron micrograph of portions of two adjoining cells of the stratum spinosum. The junctional surface of the two cells runs diagonally across the field. Dense bundles of filaments in the cytoplasm terminate in the dense plaques of desmosomes on numerous short interdigitating processes. (Micrograph courtesy of G. Odland.)

more than a dozen molecular species of keratin in the tissues of the body and these are designated by the letter K and a number. At least four kinds occur in the keratinocytes of the skin. The cytoskeleton of the basal cells consists of a loose network of keratins K5 (58 kD) and K14 (50 kD). On reaching the metabolically active stratum spinosum, the cells synthesize two new keratins, K1 (67 kD) and K10 (56 kD), and these form coarser bundles of filaments than those in the stratum basal. The cells in this zone also produce *involucrin* and other "envelope proteins" that are deposited on the inner aspect of the plasmalemma. They also begin to form the *membrane-coating granules* that will later release complex lipid and lipoproteins into the intercellular spaces, where they will constitute a major component of the permeability barrier of the epidermis.

As the cells move on into the stratum granulare, they cease to produce keratins and envelop proteins and instead synthesize *filaggrin,* a basic protein that is believed to be involved in the assembly of keratin filaments into still coarser bundles. Also produced here is *loricin,* an additional component of the cell envelope with a function yet to be determined. During their sojourn in this zone, the cells become permeable to calcium ions that activate an enzyme which cross-links the various envelope proteins to form a very tough layer beneath the plasmalemma. Shortly thereafter, lysosomes release, into the cytoplasm, lytic enzymes that terminate all metabolic activity. The cells moving up into the stratum corneum are, thus, reduced to tough, inert shells packed with coarse bundles of keratin filaments. Between them, the intercellular spaces are filled with secreted lipid-rich compounds that render the epithelium relatively impermeable.

Studies of epidermal cells in tissue culture have revealed that their growth and differentiation are influenced by several cytokines. Among these are *epidermal growth factor* (EGF) and *interleukin-1 alpha* (Il-1α), which seem to be stimulatory, whereas *transforming growth factor* (TGF) suppresses keratinocyte proliferation and differentiation. Because epidermal cells can synthesize TGF, they may autoregulate their own growth to some extent. Their ability to both produce, and respond to,

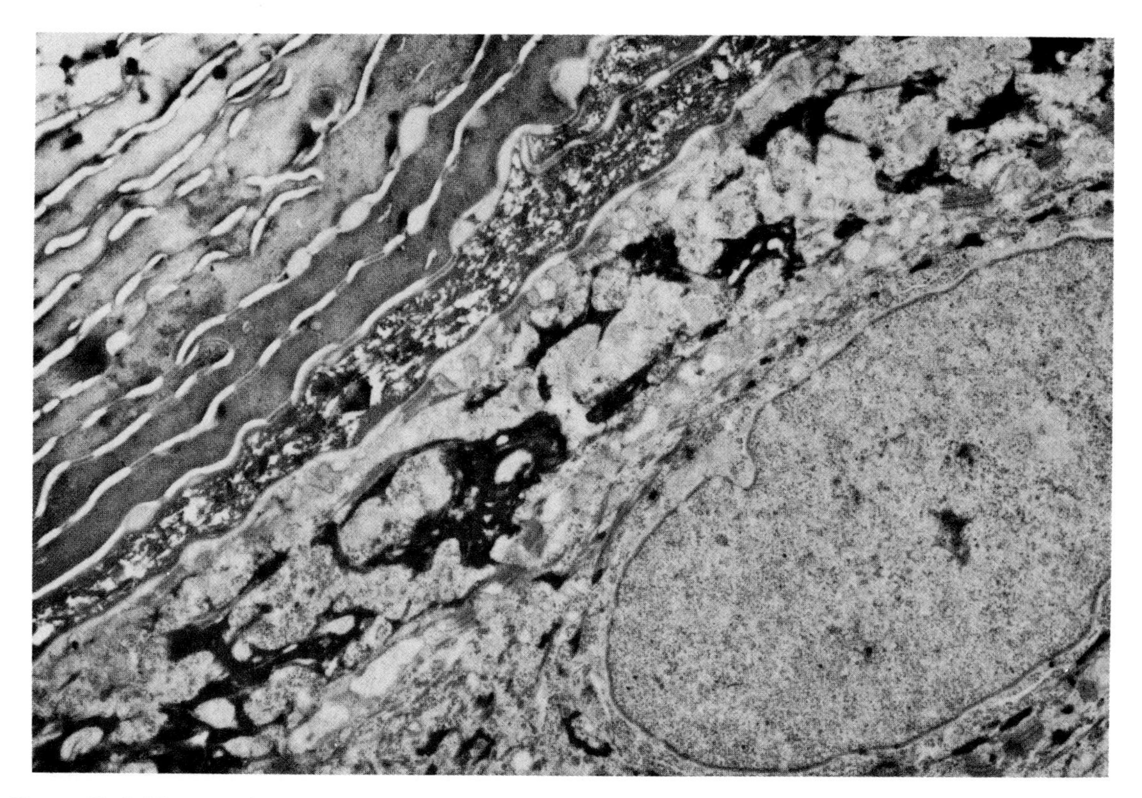

Figure 22–6. Electron micrograph at the junction of the stratum granulosum (lower right) and stratum corneum (upper left). Note the euchromatic nucleus and large irregularly shaped, dense keratohyalin granules in the cell of the stratum granulosum that occupies most of the field. (Courtesy of G. Odland.)

growth regulators may be significant in wound healing and in the genesis of skin cancers.

EPIDERMIS IN GENERAL

The epidermis over the rest of the body is similar to that of the palms and soles in its organization but has a much thinner stratum corneum. A thin stratum spinosum is always present and a stratum granulosum is usually identifiable but is only two or three cells thick. A distinct stratum lucidum is seldom found. The concavities on the underside of the epidermis, that are occupied by dermal papillae, are invariably shallower than those in the epidermis of the palms and soles. However, the contour of the dermoepidermal junction differs greatly from region to region. This becomes very apparent if the epidermis is dissociated from the dermis of skin from different regions, and its under surface is then examined at low magnification. The number, depth, and pattern of the concavities show striking regional variations.

LANGERHANS CELLS

Although keratinocytes are the dominant cell type, isolated dendritic cells can be found throughout the epidermis. These were first described in 1868 by Langerhans and have since been called *Langerhans cells.* They are usually located in the upper layers of the stratum spinosum. In routine hematoxylin and eosin preparations, they have a dark-staining nucleus and a pale, clear cytoplasm. Langerhans cells can be selectively stained with gold chloride, which blackens them and reveals more clearly their stellate or dendritic form (Fig. 22–9). Slender cell processes radiating from the cell body extend into the spaces between the surrounding keratinocytes. Other methods are available for their demonstration. They take up methylene blue and other supravital dyes. They also have an affinity for catecholamines and for 1,3,4-dihydroxyphenylalanine (L-DOPA) which are rendered fluorescent on subsequent exposure to formaldehyde vapor.

Langerhans cells are most numerous in the

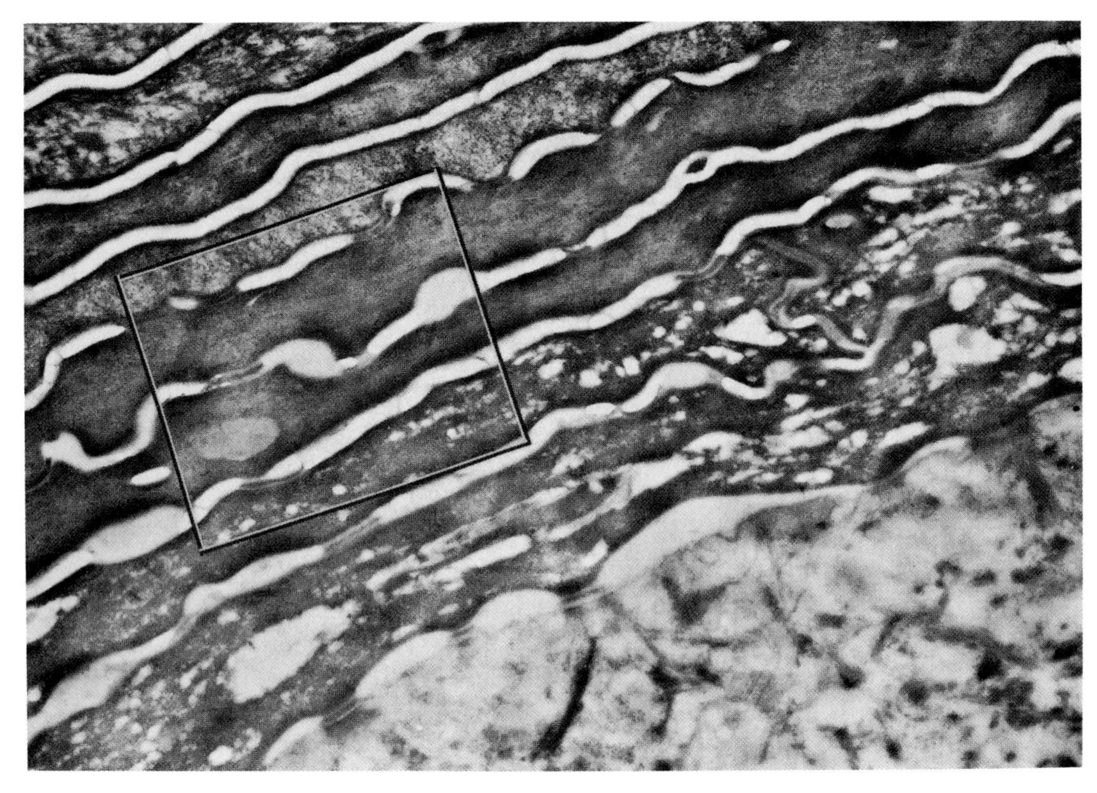

Figure 22–7. Electron micrograph of several layers of flattened cells of the stratum corneum, immediately above a cell of the stratum granulosum (lower right). No nuclei or organelles are seen in the cytoplasm of the heavily keratinized cells which remain attached at residues of desmosomes. The area in the box is seen at higher magnification in Fig. 22–8. (Courtesy of G. Odland.)

epidermis, but they are occasionally found in the dermis. They occur in other stratified squamous epithelia, including those of the oral cavity, esophagus, and vagina. Cells of similar form and staining properties are reported in the thymus, lymph nodes, and spleen. In the human epidermis, they make up from 3 to 8% of the cell population. Their number varies from region to region, but they may reach numbers as high as 800 per square millimeter of epidermis.

In electron micrographs, the nucleus of the Langerhans cell is highly irregular in outline. The cytoplasm is of low density and contains relatively few mitochondria and little endoplasmic reticulum (Fig 22–10). There are multivesicular bodies, lysosomes, and numerous small vesicles in the cytoplasm. They can be distinguished from the keratinocytes by their nuclear shape, the absence of desmosomes on their surface and the absence of conspicuous bundles of intermediate filaments in their cytoplasm. Their most reliable identifying feature is the presence of unique membrane-limited granules, called *Birbeck granules* or *vermiform granules*. These are discoid in their three-dimensional form but appear rod-like in section and are 15–50 nm in length and about 4 nm in thickness, with a central linear density from which faint striations radiate to the limiting membrane (Fig. 22–11). The profiles of Birbeck granules occasionally have an expanded end, giving them a racquet-like appearance. No enzymatic activity has been detected in these granules and their function remains unclear.

The function of the Langerhans cells was long a mystery, but it is now known that they participate in the body's immune responses. They possess surface receptors and immunological markers similar to those of macrophages. They bind the Fc fragment of IgG, and IgA and the C3 component of the complement. Like T-lymphocytes, they carry the T-4 antigen on their surface. At sites of allergic contact dermatitis, lymphocytes are observed to gather around Langerhans cells. It is believed that these cells take up foreign antigen and present it, on their surface, to T-lymphocytes in a form to which they can respond.

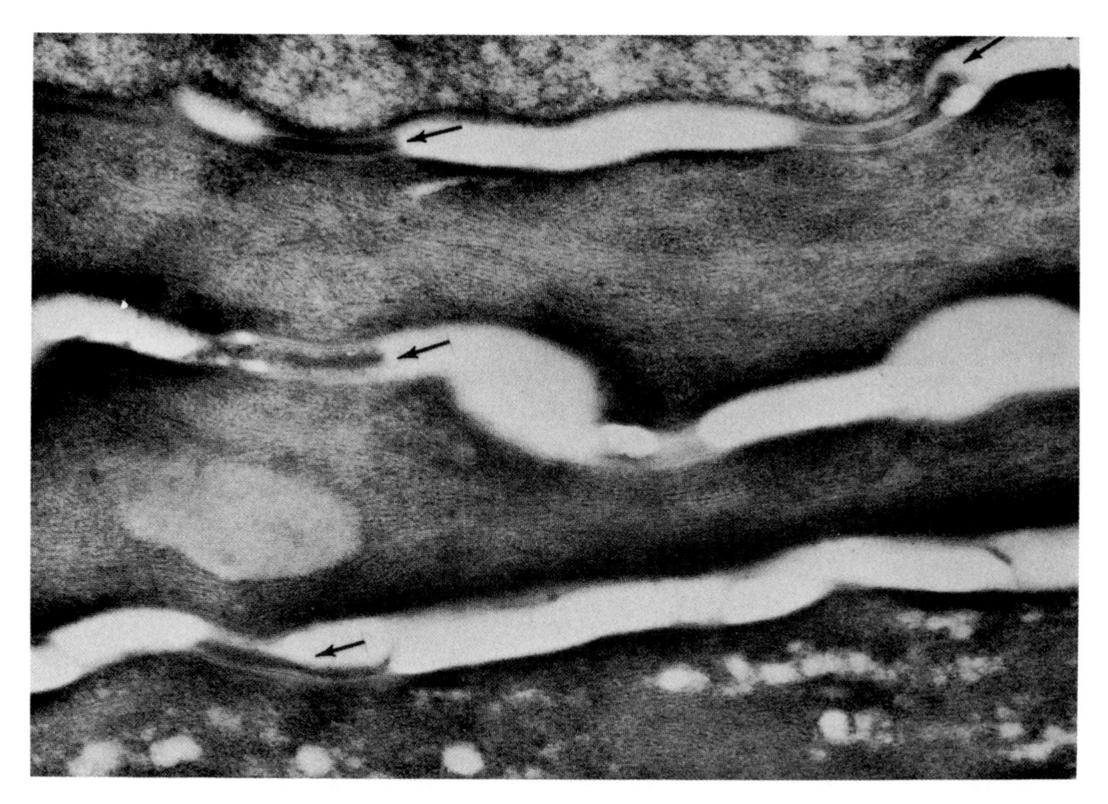

Figure 22–8. Micrograph of portions of four cells of the stratum corneum of human epidermis. The cytoplasm is filled with keratin filaments embedded in a dense matrix. The modified desmosomes (at arrows) have an unusually thick, dense, intermediate layer. The clear spaces between the cells are, in part, artifacts of specimen preparation. (Micrograph courtesy of G. Odland.)

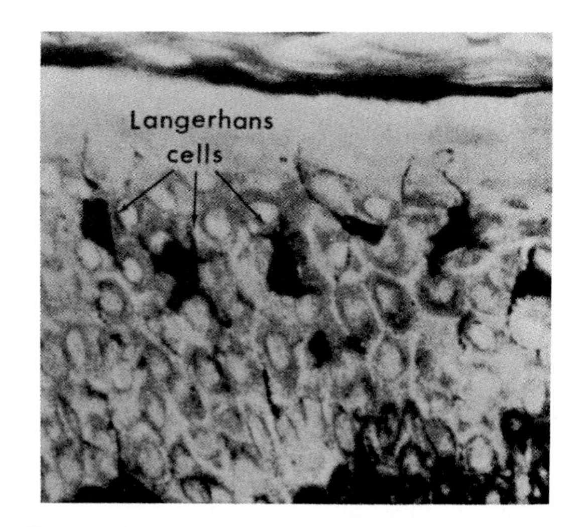

Figure 22–9. Photomicrograph of human epidermis stained with a gold chloride technique showing gold-impregnated Langerhans cells in the upper stratum spinosum. Their dendritic form is not apparent in routine histological sections of skin. (From Breathnach, A. S. 1965. Internat. Rev. Cytol. 18:1.)

Thus, the Langerhans cells are important agents in contact allergic responses and other cell-mediated immune reactions of the skin. Their role in the immune system, in general, will be discussed below.

Langerhans cells were formerly thought to be of neural crest origin, but unequivocal evidence has recently established that they come from a pool of precursors in the bone marrow. Those in the skin are continually replaced by blood-borne precursors that migrate into the epidermis and there differentiate into mature Langerhans cells. They have been shown to incorporate thymidine in vitro and are, therefore, capable of mitosis, but cell division probably makes only a very small contribution to maintenance of their numbers in the normal epidermis.

MERKEL CELLS

Small numbers of *Merkel cells* are found in the basal layers of the epidermis over the entire body, but they are more abundant in areas

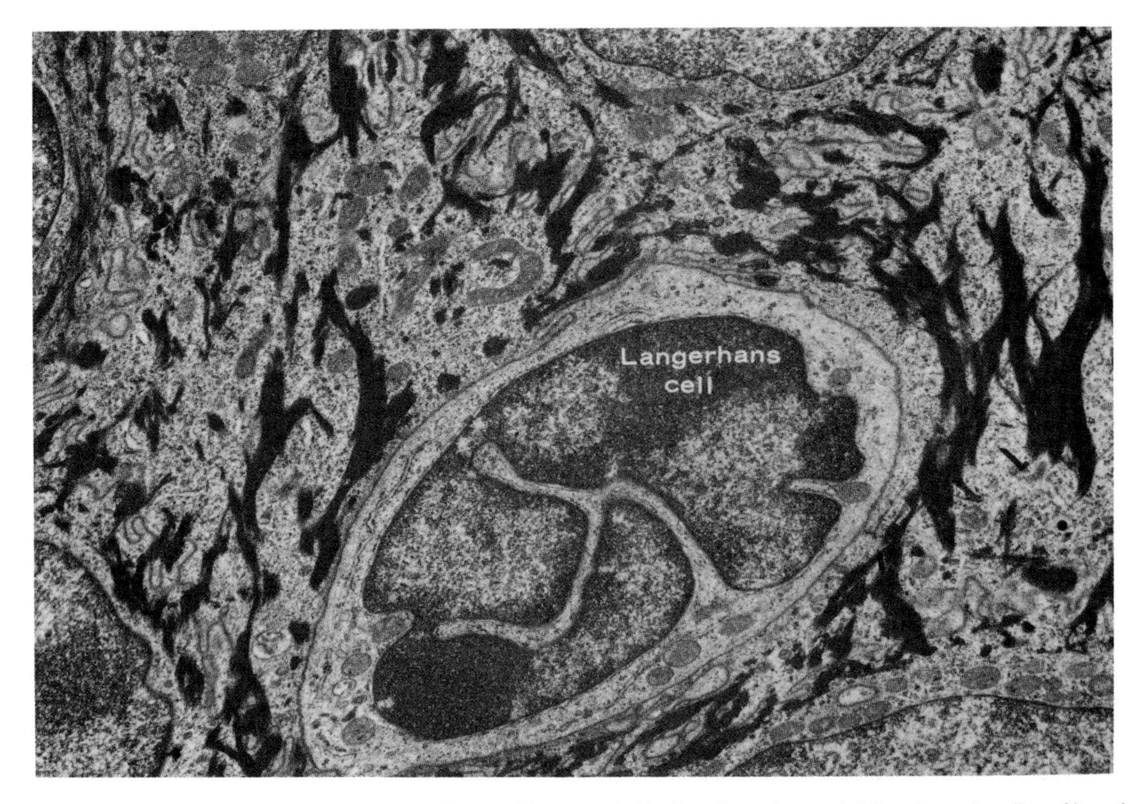

Figure 22–10. Electron micrograph of a Langerhans cell surrounded by keratinocytes containing dense bundles of keratin filaments. The polymorphous appearance of the nucleus is typical of these cells. None of the cell processes of this cell are included in this plane of section. (Courtesy of G. Szabo.)

such as the fingertips which have a special role in sensory perception. The basal lamina of the epidermis is traversed by the naked terminals of myelinated afferent nerves and these end in close apposition to these cells forming *Merkel cell-neurite complexes* that may have a mechanoreceptor function. For the most part, Merkel cells occur singly, but they may be clustered in certain specialized areas of the skin. Their long axis is usually parallel to the basal lamina and they often extend processes between the neighboring keratinocytes. In their ultrastructure, they bear a superficial resemblance to keratinocytes, to which they may be attached by desmosomes. Their nucleus is deeply invaginated and may contain a strange inclusion consisting of a bundle of short parallel filaments (Fig. 22–12). The cytoplasm is of low electron density and contains loose bundles of cytoskeletal filaments in the perinuclear region and at the cell periphery. These filaments contain cytokeratins K8, K18, and K19, which differ from those of the surrounding keratinocytes.

A distinctive ultrastructural feature of the Merkel cell is the presence of many dense-cored granules, 80–130 nm in diameter, located in the perinuclear cytoplasm and in the dendrite-like cell processes (Fig. 22–13). These closely resemble the granules seen in neuroendocrine cells elsewhere in the body, but efforts to detect catecholamines in them have been unsuccessful. Antisera against several neuropeptides have also yielded negative results. Detection of vasoactive intestinal peptide and metencephalin has been reported, but, to date, the chemical nature of the dense-cored granules remains uncertain, and the postulated mechanoreceptor function of the Merkel cell-neurite complex has yet to be firmly established. It is possible that they have a role in paracrine regulation of neighboring epidermal components, comparable to that of the neuroendocrine cells of the gastrointestinal and bronchopulmonary epithelia.

Merkel cells are also found in amphibian, reptilian, and avian skin. There are diverging views as to their origin with some investigators considering them derivatives of the neural crest, and others believing that they differenti-

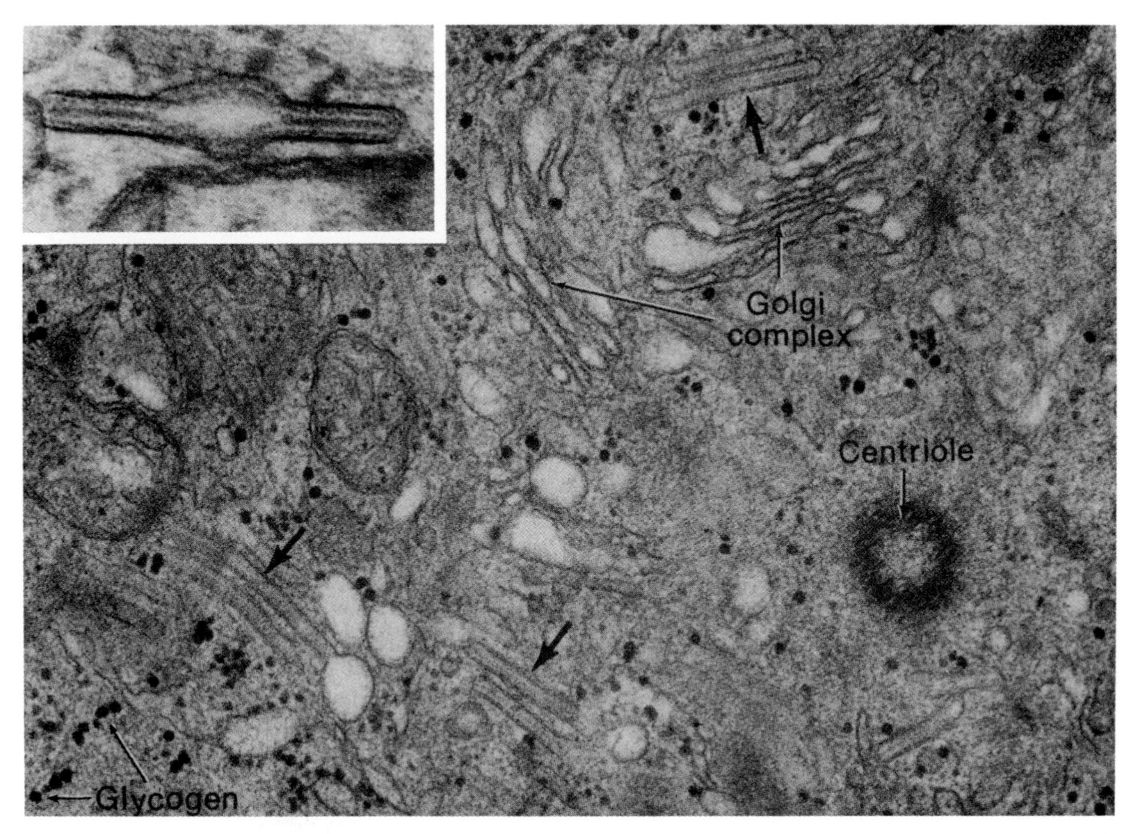

Figure 22–11. Micrograph of a small area of cytoplasm of a Langerhans cell including a centriole, small dense particles of glycogen, and several of the peculiar specific granules of this cell type (at arrows). One of these is shown at higher magnification in the inset. (Micrograph courtesy of G. Szabo.)

ate in the epidermis from cells of the stratum germinativum. They reappear rapidly following removal of segments of skin, and their regeneration does not seem to depend on migration of precursors from the dermis or on the presence of sensory nerves. Merkel cells are also found in the oral mucosa.

MELANOCYTES

The color of skin depends, in varying degrees, on three components. The tissue has an inherent yellowish color attributable in part to its content of *carotene*. The presence of oxygenated *hemoglobin* in the capillary bed of the dermis imparts a reddish tint, and shades of brown to black are due to varying amounts of the pigment *melanin*. Of these three colored substances, only melanin is produced in the skin. It is the product of *melanocytes*, specialized cells that are situated in the basal layer of the epidermis or in the underlying dermis and extend numerous branching cell processes between the surrounding keratinocytes (Fig. 22–14, 22–15). Melanin occurs in granules called *melanosomes* in the cytoplasm of melanocytes and in the cytoplasm of keratinocytes (Fig. 22–16). Melanin is formed only by the epidermal melanocytes because these cells alone possess the enzyme tyrosinase which is essential for synthesis of the pigment. However, fully formed melanosomes are transferred from the melanocyte dendrites to the keratinocytes in an unusual activity sometimes referred to as *cytocrine secretion*. Details of the process are incomplete, but vesicles containing multiple melanosomes are apparently pinched off from the tips of the melanocyte processes and incorporated in the cytoplasm of the keratinocytes. Each melanocyte has a number of associated epidermal cells to which it supplies melanin. A melanocyte and its satellite epidermal cells collectively constitute an *epidermal melanin unit*. Owing to their continuing transfer of pigment, the melanocytes may actually contain less melanin than the neighboring keratinocytes. Their cell shape is diffi-

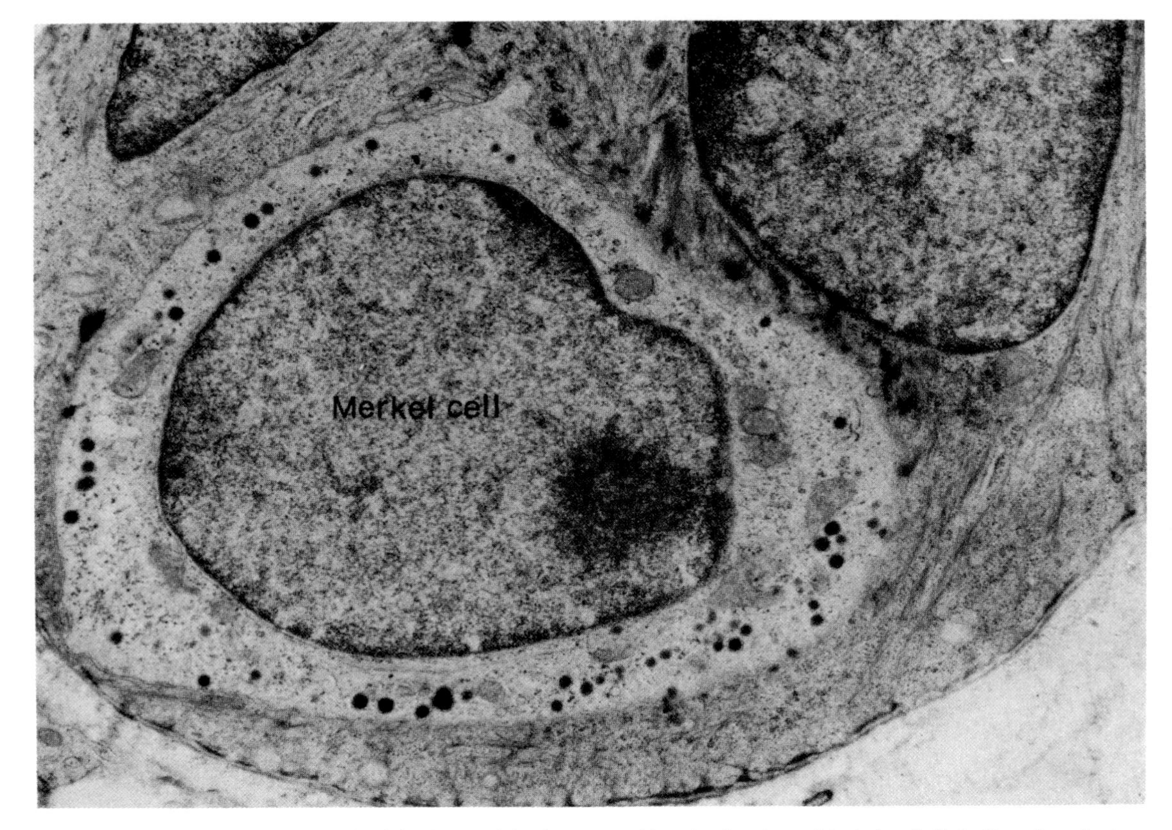

Figure 22–12. Electron micrograph of the base of the human epidermis showing a Merkel cell. Note its pale cytoplasm and characteristic dense secretory granules. (Courtesy of G. Szabo.)

cult to discern in sections stained with hematoxylin and eosin and they are best studied in whole mounts of epidermis separated from the underlying dermis and treated with 1,3,4-dihydroxyphenylalanine (DOPA). In such preparations, the melanocytes are blackened and their highly branched dendritic processes are then quite apparent (Fig. 22–14).

Not all areas of the body have an equal number of melanocytes. their ratio to basal epidermal cells ranges from 1:4 to 1:10. There may be as few as 1000/mm^2 on the arms and thighs and as many as 4000/m^2 on the face and neck. It is interesting that the number of melanocytes is approximately the same in all races. The racial differences in color are not attributable to differing numbers of melanocytes but to differences in the amount of melanin that these cells produce and transfer. In Caucasians, the melanosomes are largely confined to cells of the stratum germinativum, whereas in Negroids the melanosomes are larger, more numerous, and are found throughout the epidermis.

MUCOCUTANEOUS JUNCTIONS

Mucocutaneous junctions are the transitions from the skin to the mucous membrane lining the orifices of the body, namely, the mouth and the anus. They have a stratified squamous epithelium, but, in a number of respects, they more closely resemble the mucosa than the skin. They have a very thin stratum corneum but they contain no hairs, sebaceous glands, or sweat glands. Their surface is moistened by the products of mucous glands situated deeper in the orifices. Because the cornified layer at a mucocutaneous junction is very thin, the color of the blood in the underlying capillary bed shows through and gives this region a red tint, as seen in the lips.

THE DERMIS

Beneath the epidermis is the *dermis* or *corium,* a tough leathery layer of connective tis-

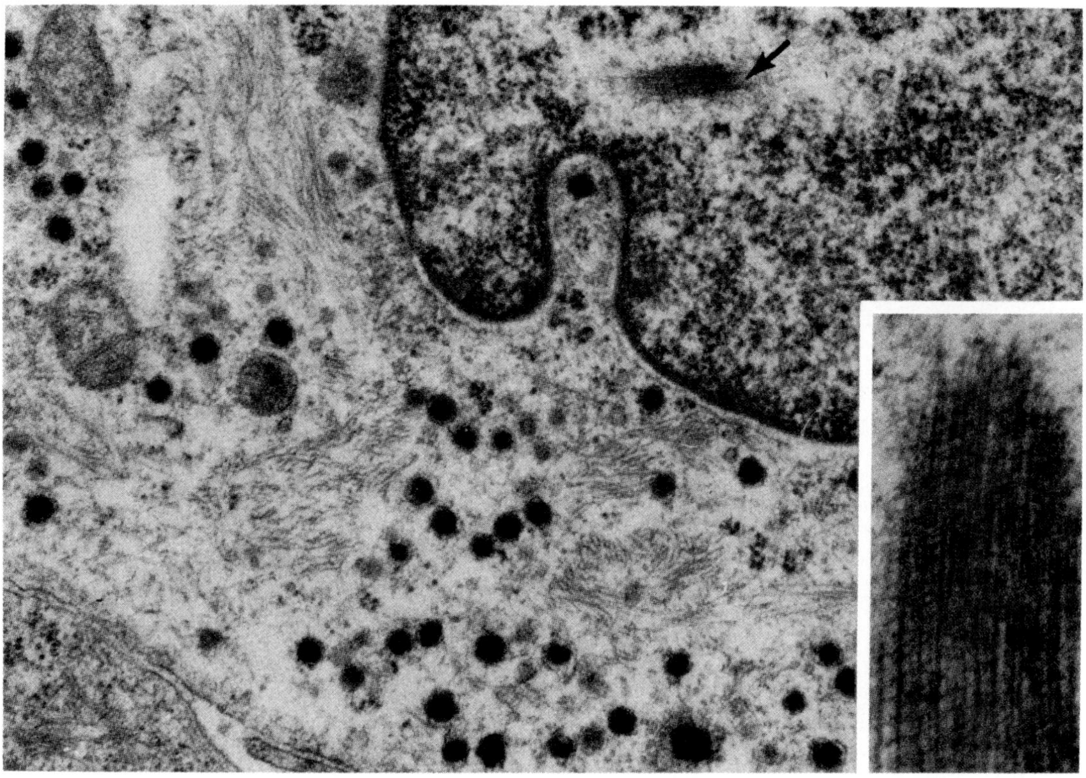

Figure 22–13. Micrograph of a portion of a Merkel cell from human gingival epithelium. The cytoplasm contains numerous dense granules and intermediate filaments. The nucleoplasm may contain an unusual inclusion (at arrow). As shown in the inset, these consist of a paracrystalline aggregation of slender filamentous subunits. (Micrograph courtesy of R. Winkelmann.)

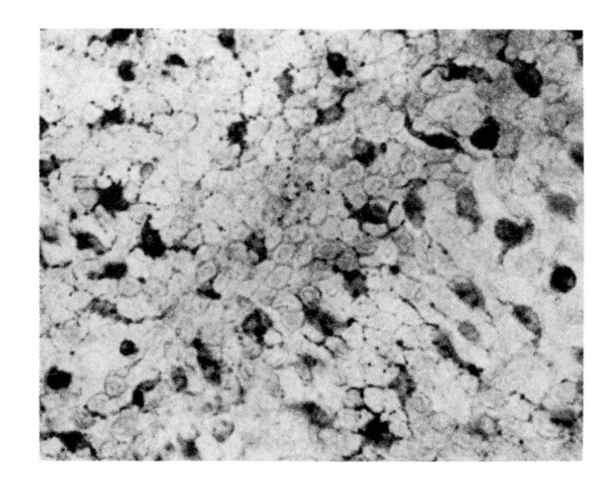

Figure 22–14. Photomicrograph of a sheet of intact epidermis from the thigh, spread upon a slide and viewed from the under side. The separated epidermis was incubated in 1,3,4-dihydroxyphenyl-alanine (DOPA), which selectively stains the melanocytes. Note their branching processes. (Courtesy of G. Szabo.)

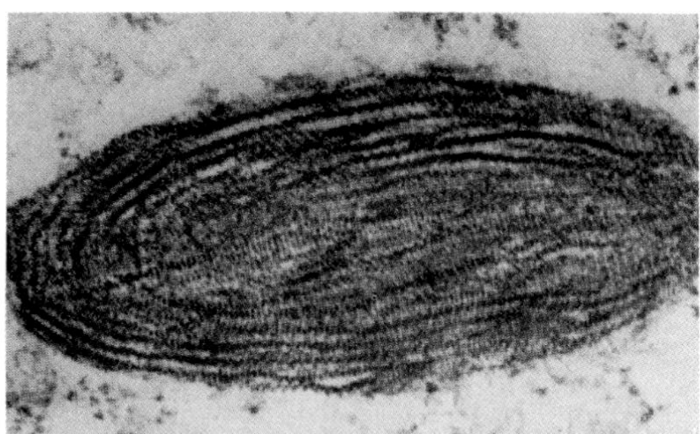

Figure 22–15. Electron micrograph of a developing human melanosome showing the periodicity in its internal framework. When the granule is fully developed, these structural components are obscured by the accumulated melanin. (Micrograph courtesy of A. Breathnach.)

sue that makes up the greater part of the thickness of the skin. Its depth cannot be measured with precision because it passes over into the subcutaneous tissue without a sharp boundary. The dermis ranges from 0.6 mm, in the thin skin of the eyelids and prepuce, to 3 mm or more on the palms and soles, but its average thickness is about 2 mm. It is thinner on the

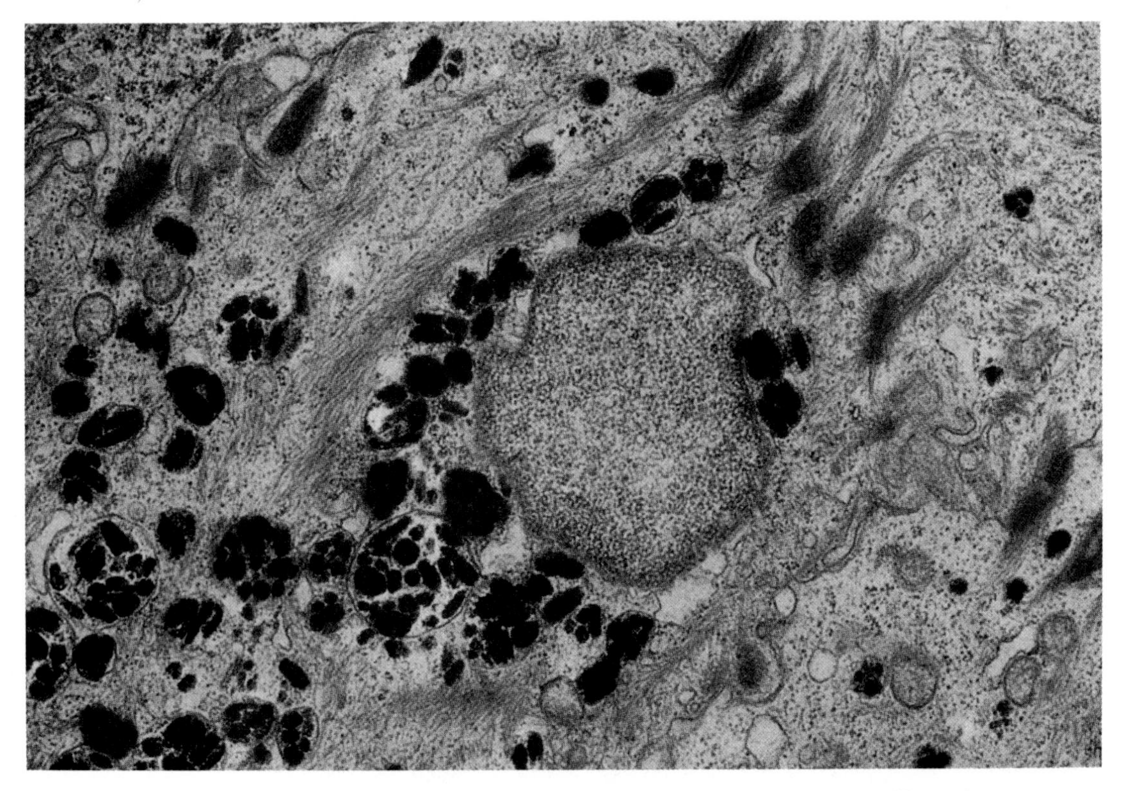

Figure 22–16. Electron micrograph of a keratinocyte from the stratum spinosum of human skin. The melanosomes occur individually in the cytoplasm of melanocytes, but after transfer to keratinocytes they occur in clusters of varying size enclosed in a membrane. (Courtesy of G. Szabo.)

ventral surface of the body and extremities than it is on the dorsum, and it is generally thinner in women than in men.

The interface of the dermis with the epidermis is quite irregular in contour and varies greatly in its pattern from region to region. The ridges forming the dermatoglyphic pattern on the surface of skin of the palm and sole are reflected in corresponding *primary ridges* on the upper surface of the dermis. These ridges are separated from one another by deep grooves into which processes of the epidermis project. Rows of conical *dermal papillae,* 0.1–0.2 mm in height, project upward from these ridges into conforming concavities on the underside of the epidermis. They number approximately 80 per square millimeter.

The complex topography of the dermo-epidermal junction cannot be fully appreciated from the study of histological sections. However, the epidermis can be separated from the dermis by incubating a sample of skin for 2 h in balanced salt solution containing the calcium-chelating agent EDTA. Lifting off the epidermis then exposes the surface of the dermis for scanning electron microscopy which provides three-dimensional images. In such preparations, the surface of the dermis is characterized by parallel dermal ridges separated by deep *primary grooves.* A slight thickening of the epidermis occupies a shallow *secondary groove* or sulcus along the midline of each primary ridge, flanked by two so-called *secondary ridges.* A row of dermal papillae runs along each secondary dermal ridge. Thus, each primary ridge bears two parallel rows of papillae separated by a shallow groove (Fig. 22–17). The papillae occur in groups of three or four sharing a common base (Fig. 22–18). In the intact skin, the primary groove is occupied by a long, ridge-like, downward projection of the epidermis that was inappropriately called an *interpapillary peg* before its three-dimensional form was revealed by scanning microscopy. Regularly spaced circular dark areas in the floor of the primary grooves represent the openings of channels that were occupied by the ducts of sweat glands which were pulled out of the dermis in removal of the epidermis (Fig. 22–19). In thin skin, lacking a dermato-

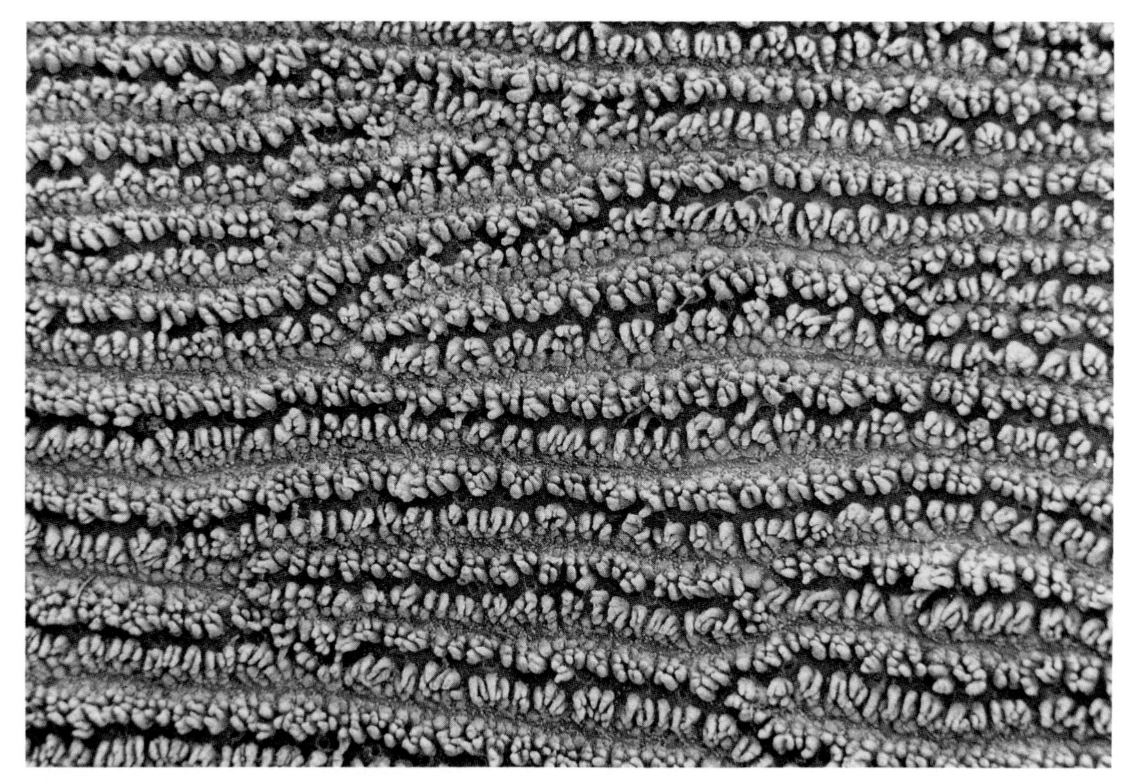

Figure 22–17. Low-power scanning micrograph human plantar dermis, after removal of the epidermis. The dark grooves are between primary ridges of the dermis. There is also a paler shallow groove on the crest of the ridges, between rows of dermal papillae. (Micrograph courtesy of MacCallum, D. K. 1985. Anat. Rec. 211:142.)

glyphic pattern, the configuration of the dermo-epidermal junction is much simpler than that just described. The dermal papillae are shorter, broader, and less numerous than those of the palms and they are not arranged in precise rows corresponding to ridges on the skin surface.

Two layers are identified in the dermis. A superficial *papillary layer* consists of fibroblasts and other connective tissue cell types widely dispersed among randomly interwoven bundles of thin collagen fibers, mainly type-III collagen. This layer also contains a loose network of elastic fibers and many capillaries. The deeper *reticular layer* is made up of closely packed coarse bundles of thicker fibers, predominately type-I collagen. Most of these bundles of collagen fibers are oriented more-or-less parallel to the skin surface, but some may run obliquely or nearly perpendicular to the majority. Intermingling with the collagen bundles is a network of elastic fibers which are especially abundant around the sebaceous and sweat glands that extend downward from the epidermis into the dermis. The interstices between the fibrous components are occupied by proteoglycans of which dermatan sulfate is a major component. The cells types of the dermis are those commonly found in connective tissues: fibroblasts, macrophages, lymphocytes, and mast cells. Occasional small clusters of adipose cells may be found in the deeper portion of the reticular layer. The dermis has a rich vascular bed from which networks of capillaries extend into the dermal papillae, permitting nutrients to diffuse into the avascular epidermis (Fig. 22–30).

In the skin of the penis, scrotum, and the areola around the nipples, the deeper portion of the reticular layer contains a loose plexus of smooth muscle cells. Skin in these areas is often somewhat wrinkled, owing to contraction of this smooth muscle. Other cells form the slender *arrector pili muscles* that insert into the body of the hair follicles (Figs. 22–20, 22–21). Their contraction is responsible for the erection of the hairs in a cold environment, which results in the so-called "goose-flesh" in the human. In animals, erection of hairs is also commonly associated with fear and anger. Cross-striated muscle fibers terminating in the dermis of the face, scalp, and the base of the

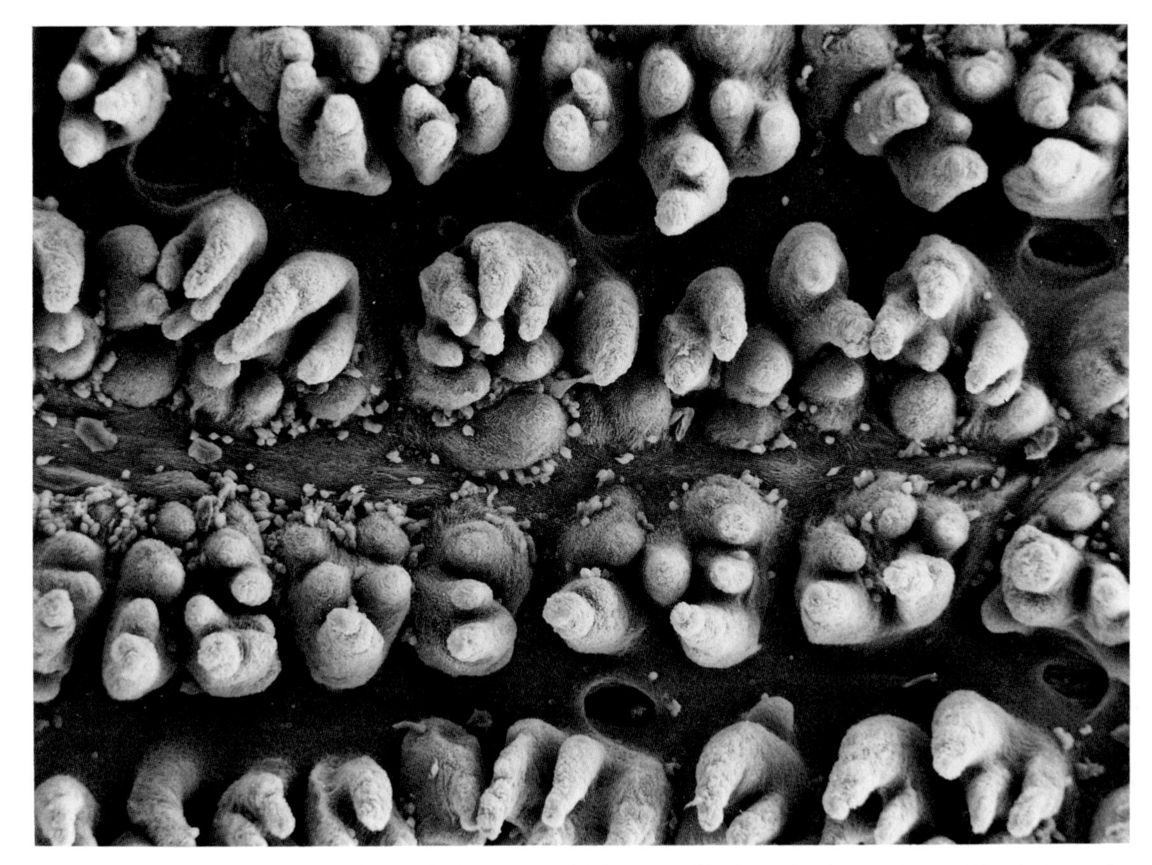

Figure 22–18. Scanning electron micrograph of 22–17, at higher magnification, showing a primary ridge between two primary grooves, viewed from above. Two rows of dermal papillae are shown on either side of a secondary groove on the crest of the ridge. The papillae are arranged in clusters sharing a common base. (Micrograph courtesy of MacCallum, D. F. 1985. Anat. Rec. 211:142.

ears constitute the *muscles of facial expression* which are involved in smiling, frowning, and voluntary movements of the ears and scalp. These muscles, in man, are vestiges of a more extensive subcutaneous layer of skeletal muscle, the *panniculus carnosus,* which is present in many animal species, permitting voluntary movements of large areas of skin when attempting to dislodge insects or to shake dry when emerging from the water.

A subcutaneous layer deep to the reticularis of the dermis is called the *hypodermis.* It is a looser connective tissue in which thin collagen fiber bundles are oriented mainly parallel to the skin surface, but a few are continuous with those of the dermis. In some regions, such as the back of the hands, this layer permits movement of the skin over the underlying structures. In other regions, the fibers crossing into the dermis are more numerous and the skin is relatively immobile. Adipose cells accumulate in far greater number in the hypodermis than in the dermis. Their abundance depends on the sex of the individual and the state of nutrition. Subcutaneous fat tends to occur preferentially in certain regions. Little or no fat is found in the subcutaneous tissue of the eyelids or penis, but on the abdomen, thighs, and buttocks, it may reach a thickness of 3 cm or more. Where it occurs, this layer of fat is referred to as the *panniculus adiposus.*

APPENDAGES OF THE SKIN

HAIRS

Hairs develop from cells lining deep invaginations of the epidermis called *hair follicles* (Fig. 22–20 and 22–25). Hairs vary in length and diameter in different regions of the body. Although humans appear to be largely hairless, the number of their hairs does not differ appreciably from the number on other primates, but over much of the body surface, they are very small and colorless and tend to

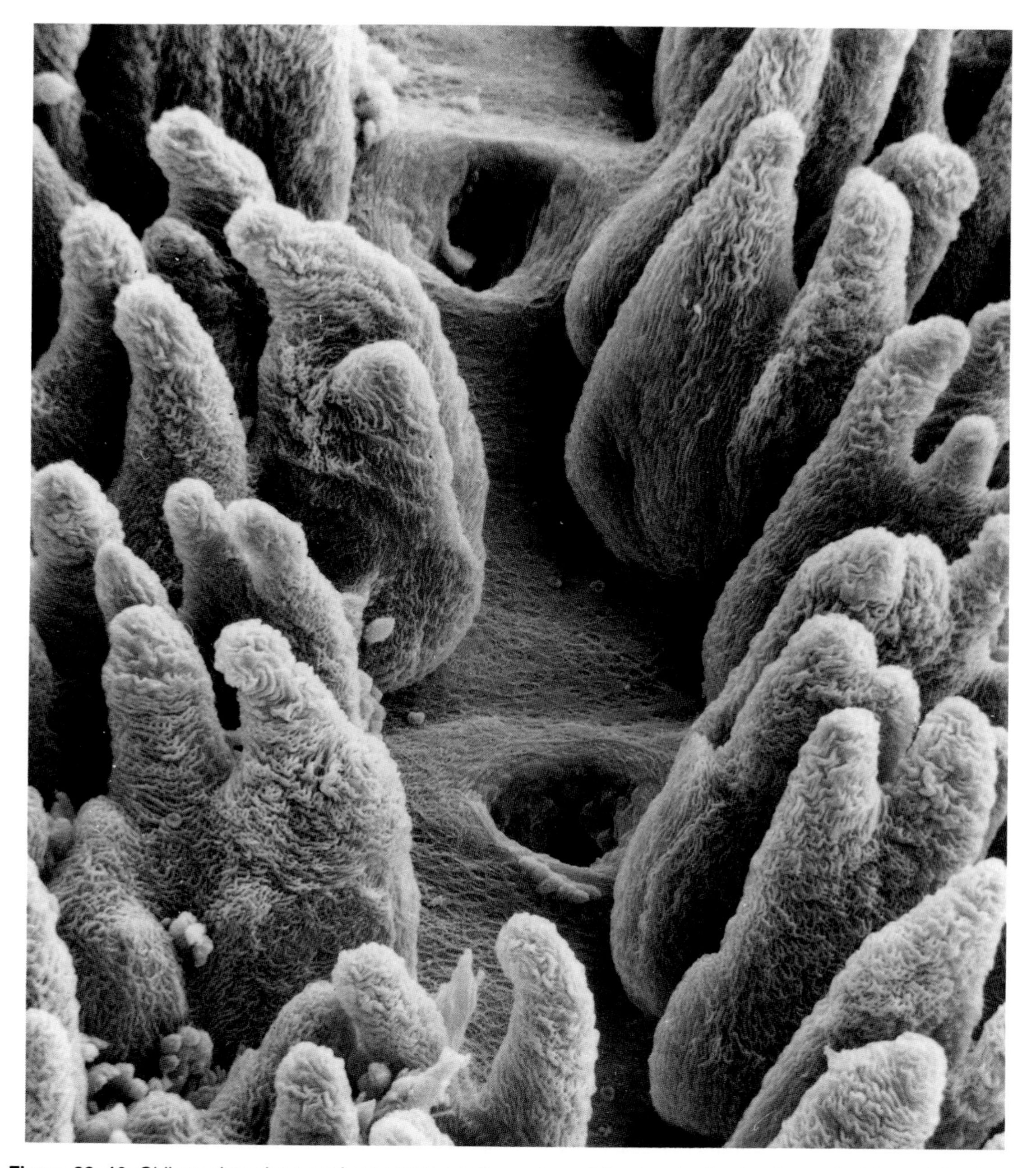

Figure 22–19. Oblique view along a primary groove in the surface of the dermis showing the conical form of the dermal papillae. The craters in the groove are openings of tubular channels formerly occupied by ducts of sweat glands. (Micrograph courtesy of MacCallum, D. K. 1985. Anat. Rec. 211:142.)

go unnoticed. Compared to the furry coat of animals, the vestigial hairs of humans provide little or no thermal insulation, but they are important in tactile sensation. They act as minute levers and when deformed they exert pressure that is detected by sensory nerves around the hair follicles. Hairs are absent only on the palms, soles, lateral surfaces of the feet, glans penis, clitoris, and the inner surface of the prepuce and labia minora and majora. On the eyelid, the hairs do not project beyond their follicles, whereas on the scalp, they may grow to well over 1 m in length.

An arrector pili muscle, originating in the papillary layer of the dermis, inserts into the connective tissue sheath of the hair follicle slightly above its midpoint. A hair and its follicle are always inclined at an angle to the sur-

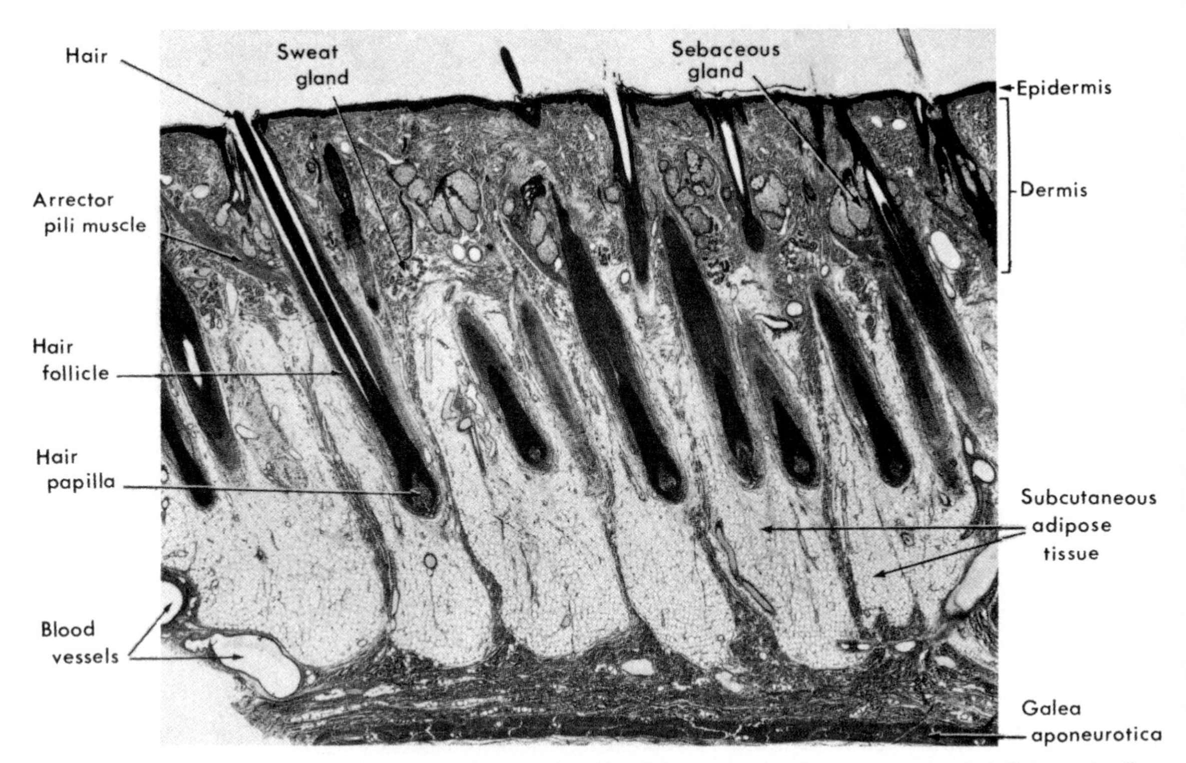

Figure 22–20. Photomicrograph of a section through the skin of the scalp showing numerous hair follicles extending downward into the subcutaneous adipose tissue. An arrector pili muscle is visible at the upper left. (Courtesy of H. Mizoguchi.)

face of the epidermis and contraction of the arrector pili muscle moves it into a more vertical position, resulting in depression of the skin over the muscle and elevation of the skin immediately around the hair, forming a "goose-pimple." One or more *sebaceous glands* are found immediately above the insertion of the arrector pili muscle. These discharge their secretion into the follicular canal (see below).

An active hair follicle has a terminal expansion called the *hair bulb* which has a deep recess in its under side occupied by a *papilla* of dermal connective tissue. The cells of the papilla have inductive properties influencing the activity of the follicle, and nutrients from its capillaries are essential for normal function. The epithelial cells covering the papilla are comparable to those of the stratum basale elsewhere in the epidermis. Together they form the *hair matrix,* and their proliferation is responsible for the growth of the hair at its base.

The hair follicle is surrounded by a condensation of the fibrous components of the dermis. Interposed between this and the follicular epithelium is a noncellular *vitreous layer* (glassy layer) which seems to be an exceptionally thick basal lamina of the outer layer of follicular epithelium, which is called the *external root sheath.* In the bulbous portion of the hair follicle, the external root sheath is only a single row of cells corresponding to the stratum basale of the epidermis. Nearer the surface of the skin, it becomes several layers thick and exhibits the strata typical of the epidermis of thin skin. The next of the concentric layers of the follicle is the *internal root sheath* which has three components: (1) *Henle's layer,* a single row of low elongated cells in close contact with the innermost cells of the external root sheath; (2) *Huxley's layer,* made up of two or three rows of less flattened cells; (3) the *cuticle of the inner root sheath* composed of flat, scale-like cells imbricated with their free edges directed downward (Figs. 22–22 and 22–23).

A mass of cells in the interior of the bulb, around the papilla, constitute the *cell matrix.* The proliferation, differentiation, and upward movement of these cells give rise to the hair. In some types of hair, those situated above the apex of the papilla produce large vacuolated cells that form the *medulla* of the hair, which contains relatively little keratin. More peripheral matrix cells give rise to the *cortex* of the hair. As these cells are displaced

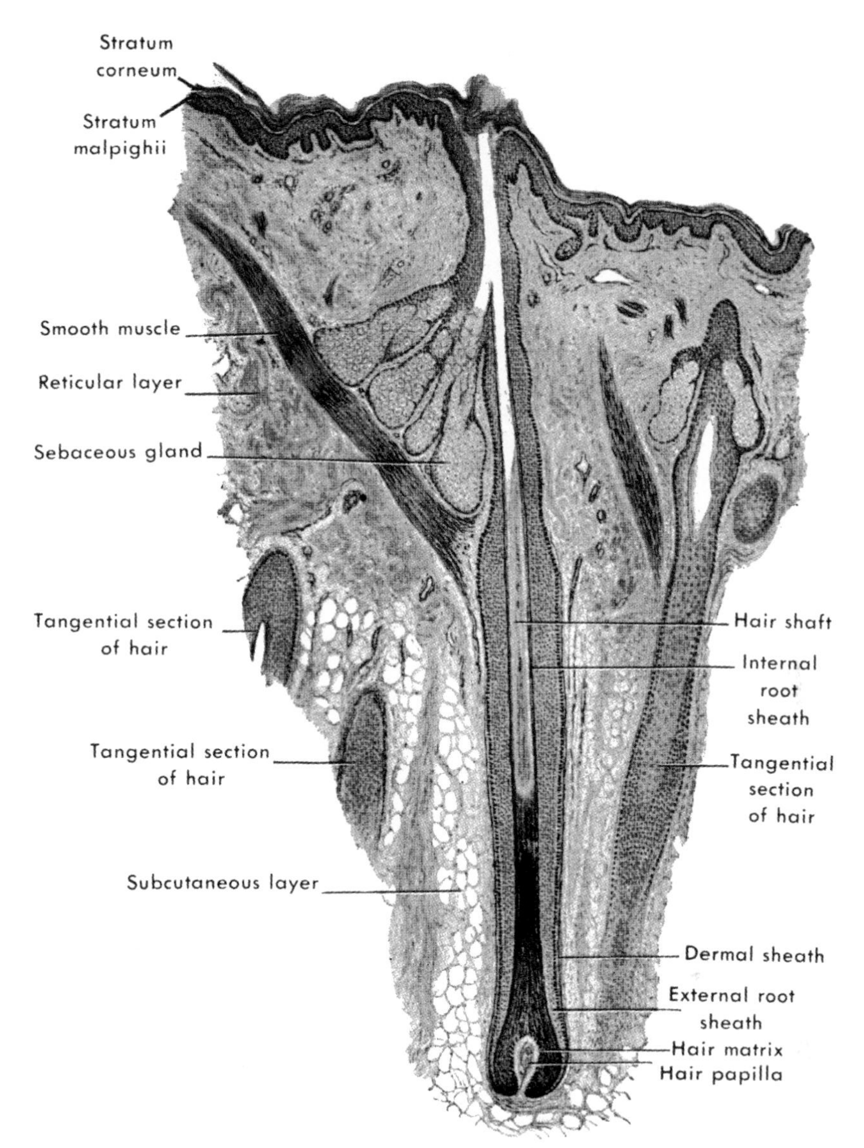

Figure 22–21. A drawing from a section of the human scalp showing the root of the hair and its follicle, the arrector pili muscle, and a sebaceous gland. (After Schaffer, J. Lehrbuch der Histologie und Histogenese. Wilhelm Engelmann Press, Leipzig, 1922.)

upward, they synthesize a great quantity of keratin filaments and many *trichohyaline granules.* The latter resemble the keratohyaline granules of the epidermis but differ in their staining properties and chemical constituents. Later in development, these granules coalesce into a hard, amorphous substance that obscures the keratin filaments. The insoluble proteins of this material have a high content of glutamic acid, glutamate, and citrulline. Matrix cells still farther toward the periphery of the bulb become very heavily keratinized and form the *hair cuticle.* Proliferation and differentiation of the most peripheral cells of the hair matrix give rise to the inner root sheath.

Among the cells of the matrix are a few large melanocytes whose long dendrites contribute melanosomes to the cells that will form the cortex of the hair. The graying of the hair in old age is attributed to a gradual loss in the capacity of these cells to produce tyrosine.

Certain differences between the life cycle of cells in the epidermis and those of the hair follicles deserves emphasis. Proliferation of cells, in the stratum basale, is continuous throughout the epidermis. As they move upward, the cells produce *soft keratin* consisting

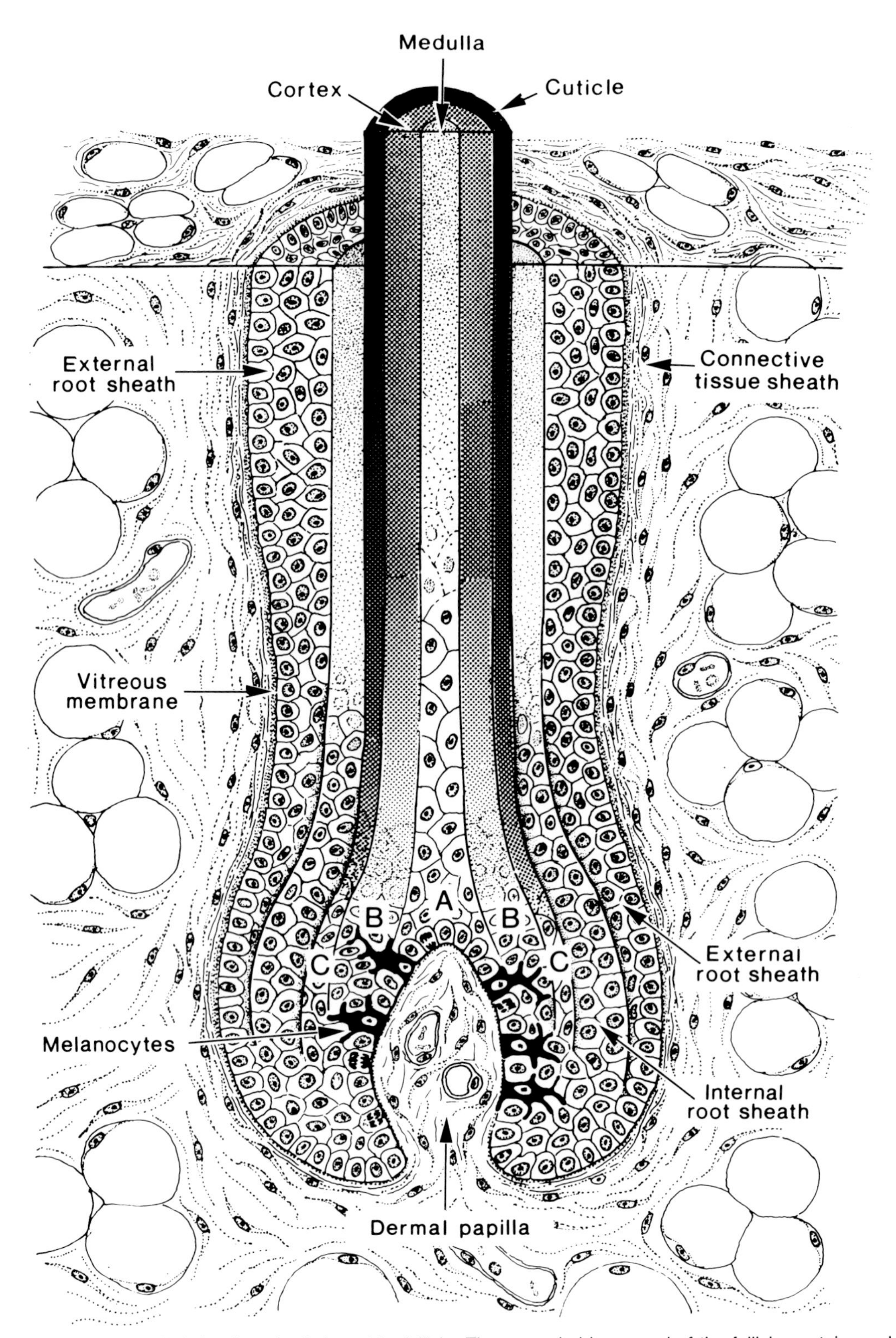

Figure 22–22. A simplified drawing of a hair and its follicle. The expanded lower end of the follicle contains a dermal papilla. Formation and growth of the hair depend on continuous proliferation and differentiation of cells around the tip of the dermal papilla that constitute the hair matrix. Cells over the tip of the papilla (A) give rise to the medulla of the hair. Those on the sides (B) give rise to its cortex, and cells situated lateral to these (C) form the cuticle. The peripheral cells of the hair bulb form the internal and external root sheaths. The color of the hair depends on the activity of melanocytes in the hair matrix. (After Junquiera, L. C. et al. 1971. Basic Histology. New York, Lange Medical Publications.)

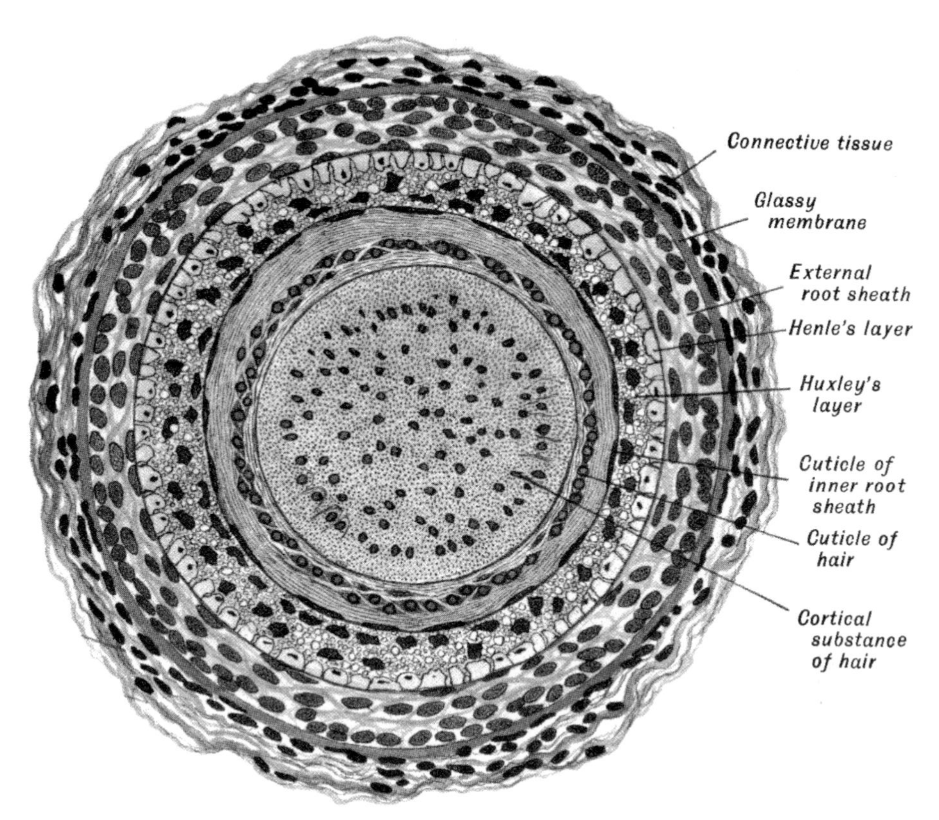

Figure 22–23. Drawing of a cross section of a hair follicle in pig skin at a level at which Henle's layer is completely cornified.

of filaments embedded in the basic protein, filaggrin, and they are continuously shed at the skin surface. In the hair follicle, proliferation is local and the cells have intermittent periods of mitotic activity and periods of rest. They produce a *hard keratin* with filaments embedded in the protein trichohyalin, and they are not shed but accumulate in concentric layers forming the hair shaft. Cell proliferation is induced by the underlying papilla, and if this is destroyed, a hair is not formed.

The alternating active and quiescent phases in the cycle are reflected in the histological appearance of the follicles (Fig. 22–24). In the resting phase, the follicle is shorter and its epithelium more closely resembles that of the epidermis. The melanocytes contain no melanin and are not identifiable. Below the shrunken bulb, there is a small cluster of cells that are remnants of the papilla. At the onset of the next period of activity, renewal of growth is heralded by resumption of melanin production, and the follicle soon takes on its fully differentiated form.

In young rodents, and probably in other species, waves of synchronous hair growth sweep over the body at regular intervals. In adults, this wave pattern is replaced by a mosaic pattern of hair growth, with activity confined to isolated islands of varying size scattered over the body. The mosaic pattern prevails in humans of all ages, and the duration of the resting and growing phases varies greatly from region to region. In the scalp, the growth phase is exceptionally long, being measured in years, whereas the resting phase is about 3 months in duration.

In the human, there are regional differences in the competence of the hair follicles to respond to male sex hormones. At the onset of male puberty, the area of the moustache and beard begins to produce thicker and more heavily pigmented hair. Although the comparable areas, in the female, contain the same number of hair follicles, they continue to produce fine hairs after puberty. In other areas, such as the axillae and pubis, coarse hairs appear in both sexes at puberty. In many men, there is a characteristic regression of scalp hair that varies in pattern and time of onset de-

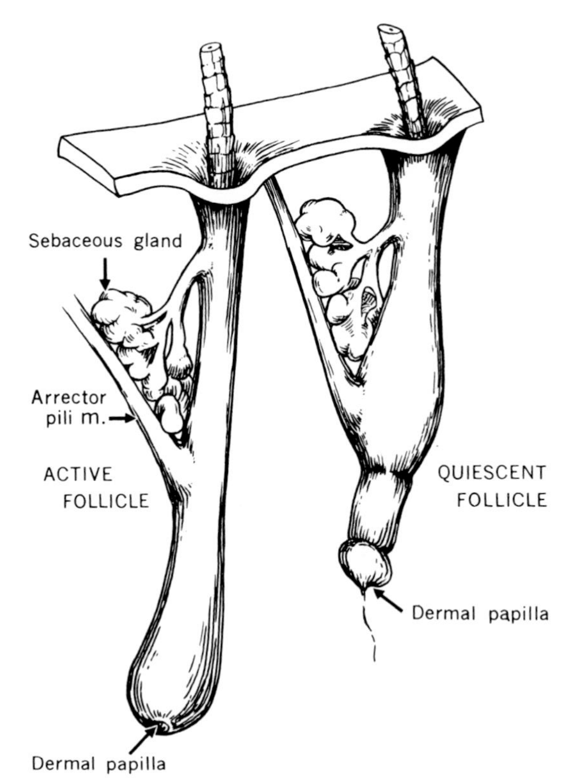

Figure 22–24. Diagram of an active hair follicle and a quiescent follicle. The hair bulb undergoes considerable regression during quiescence. Also shown is the position of the sebaceous glands, relative to the arrector pili muscle. (Redrawn after Montagna, W. 1956. *In* Structure and Function of Skin. New York, Academic Press.)

pending on the individual's genome. This may lead to baldness with loss of all hair follicles in the areas affected.

NAILS

The *nails* are plates of closely compacted hard keratin. They are formed by proliferation and keratinization of epithelial cells in a *nail matrix* that is comparable to the hair matrix but simpler in its organization (Fig. 22–26). The *nail root* and its matrix are located under a fold of skin called the *proximal nail fold.* The stratum corneum of the epidermis on this fold may extend for a short distance onto the upper surface of the nail, forming a thin covering of its proximal, 0.5–1 mm, that is called the *eponychium.* Where the *lateral nail folds* turn inward into the *lateral nail grooves,* their epidermis loses its stratum corneum and continues beneath the body of the nail plate as the *nail bed.* There the epidermis consists of a stratum basale and stratum spinosum, with the nail replacing the stratum corneum. Growth of the nail from the nail matrix at its proximal end slides the nail over the thin epidermis of the nail bed which makes no contribution to its formation. The anterior extent of the nail bed may be seen through the semitransparent nail as an opaque white crescent called the *lunula.* Quite often, however, the lunula is obscured by the proximal nail fold and eponychium.

Like those of the hair matrix, the cells of the nail matrix synthesize large amounts of keratin and many keratohyalin granules. As they are incorporated into the nail root, they are transformed into extremely flat anuclear elements consisting of keratin in a hard interfibrillar material. The dermis of the nail bed is highly vascular and this is reflected in the pale pink color transmitted through the translucent nail. This color is clinically useful as a very rough indication of the degree of oxygenation of the blood.

Nails grow continuously, at a rate of about 0.5 mm per week. Fingernails grow about four times as fast as toenails, and those on the middle fingers grow somewhat faster than the others. Bacteria entering via the lateral nail groove may cause *paronychia,* a painful inflammation and swelling of the lateral fold. Trauma to the nail bed often results in a subungual hematoma that may lead to loss of the nail. If the nail matrix has not been severely damaged, a new nail will usually be formed.

SEBACEOUS GLANDS

Sebaceous glands are found in the dermis of the entire integument except for the palms, soles, and sides of the feet, where hairs are lacking. They are appendages of the hair follicle, 0.2–2 mm in diameter, located above the insertion of the arrector pili muscle. Their ducts open into the upper third of the follicular canal. Where two or more are associated with the same follicle, they are at the same level. Sebaceous glands, independent of hairs, also occur on the lips, areola of the nipples, labia minora, and on the inner aspect of the prepuce. In these sites, they are located more superficially than those associated with hairs and their ducts open directly onto the skin surface. The secretion of the sebaceous glands, called *sebum,* is a mixture of lipids including triglycerides, cholesterol, and wax-like substances. It is believed to contribute to

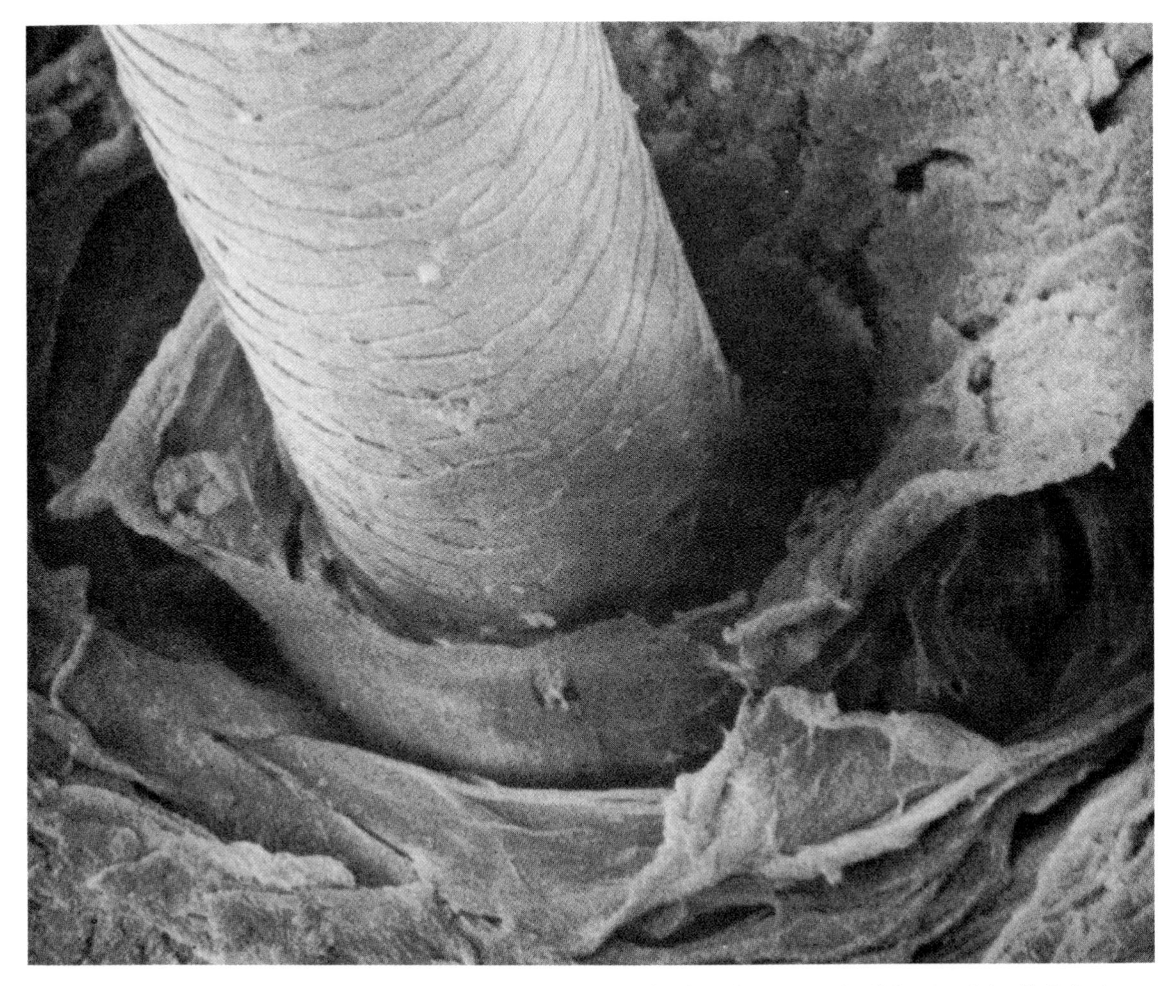

Figure 22–25. Scanning electron micrograph of a hair emerging from human scalp. (Micrograph by T. Fujita.)

the maintenance of the soft texture of thin skin and the flexibility of the hairs. In birds, the *uropygial gland* (preen gland) is a specialized sebaceous gland. Its oil secretion is spread over the surface of the feathers to make them more impervious to water.

Sebaceous glands have a lobular structure consisting of elongated acini that open into a short duct. The acini have a peripheral row of small basal cells having a spherical nucleus, the usual cytoplasmic organelles, and a few vacuoles. The acini have no lumen but are filled with large pale-staining cells with pycnotic nuclei (Fig. 22–27). In electron micrographs, the basal cells contain both rough and smooth endoplasmic reticulum, abundant glycogen, and a few small lipid droplets. The cells immediately above this layer are considerably larger and their cytoplasm is rich in smooth endoplasmic reticulum and crowded with lipid droplets. In the center of the acinus and in the portion nearest to the duct, the cells are in various stages of degeneration. Early in this process, they have dark-staining, pycnotic nuclei, disrupted membranes, and coalescing drops of lipid. Their cytoplasm is ultimately reduced to electron-dense strands among confluent masses of lipid. Thus, the production of sebum is an example of *holocrine secretion,* defined as the release of whole cells or the products of their degeneration. Continual proliferation of basal cells gives rise to larger cells in the center of the acinus. After a brief period of intense lipid synthesis, these cells become necrotic, releasing lipid and cell debris into a duct at the neck of the acinus. The ducts are lined by stratified squamous epithelium continuous with that of the external root sheath at their opening into the follicular canal.

Sebaceous glands are relatively inactive until puberty when they are stimulated by the

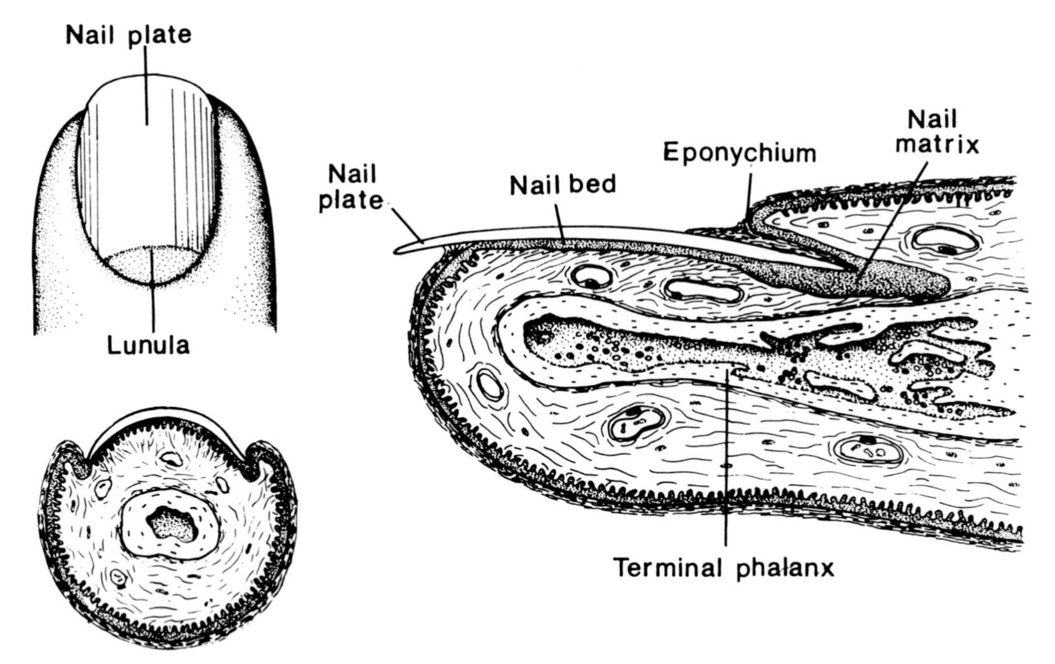

Figure 22–26. Drawing of fingernail, nail bed, nail matrix, and associated structures.

rising levels of sex hormones. Thereafter, they secrete continuously at a slightly greater rate. During puberty, boys and, to a lesser degree, girls suffer from *acne,* an inflammation of isolated sebaceous glands, usually on the face, chest, and upper back.

ECCRINE SWEAT GLANDS

Eccrine sweat glands are widely distributed throughout the integument. They are coiled tubular glands with their secretory portions usually located deep in the dermis, or more commonly in the hypodermis (Fig. 22–28). The slender duct ascends through the dermis and epidermis to open at a *sweat pore* on the surface of the skin. Owing to their diffuse distribution, we tend to underestimate their total mass and their physiological importance. They number from 3 to 4 million and, although each weighs only 30–40 μm, their aggregate weight is roughly equivalent to that of a kidney. Individuals engaged in vigorous exercise, in a warm environment, may perspire as much as 10 liters a day which is a volume of secretion exceeding that of some of the largest exocrine glands.

The secretory portion of the gland is lined by a cuboidal or low columnar epithelium containing two secretory cell types designated *dark cells* and *light cells.* Between these and the basal lamina are *myoepithelial cells* (Fig. 22–29). The clear cells have a broad apical region and a narrow basal region that extends down to the basal lamina. The dark cells have the form of an inverted pyramid with a broad adlumenal end and a narrower ablumenal portion occupying a conforming space between adjacent clear cells. They usually do not reach the basal lamina. The gland is enveloped by a thin connective tissue sheath containing the endings of cholinergic sympathetic nerves that control its secretory activity.

The dark cells owe their name to their appearance with traditional histological staining methods. In electron micrographs, they have a prominent Golgi complex, long mitochondria, a few cisternae of rough endoplasmic reticulum, and abundant free ribosomes. Their apical cytoplasm contains moderately dense secretory granules. Their chemical nature has yet to be defined, but histochemical staining reactions suggest a glycoprotein content.

The clear cells are devoid of secretory granules and, in electron micrographs, have little endoplasmic reticulum but usually contain conspicuous accumulations of glycogen. The only egress from the clear cells is via intercellular canaliculi between them and neighboring cells. The canaliculi are lined with microvilli and their commissures are closed by tight junctions. The narrow base of the clear cells is often elaborately infolded—a feature characteristic of cells involved in transepithelial fluid and electrolyte transport. The electrolyte composition of the primary secretion is the same as that of blood plasma, but most of the sodium, potassium, and chloride is reabsorbed as the secretion passes through the duct.

At the transition from the coiled secretory portion of the gland to the long duct, the tube narrows and its lumen takes on a star-shaped outline. Secretory and myoepithelial cells are replaced by a double layer of small cuboidal cells. The outer row of cells have a comparatively large dark-staining heterochromatic nucleus and abundant mitochondria (Fig. 22–29). The cells bordering on the lumen have an irregularly shaped nucleus and relatively little cytoplasm which contains few organelles. There is a conspicuous terminal web immediately beneath their apical plasma membrane.

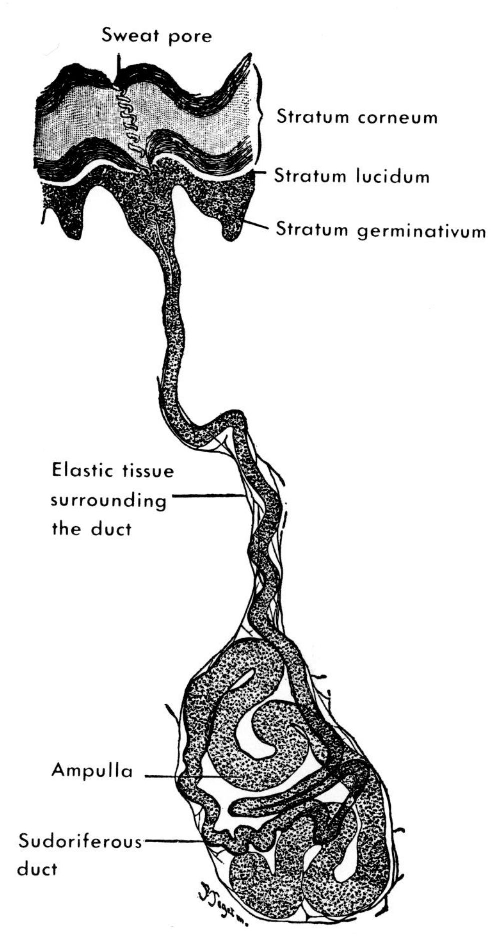

Figure 22–28. Drawing of a sweat gland from the palmar surface of an index finger showing the coiled secretory portion and the long relatively narrow duct. (Slightly modified from von Brunn.)

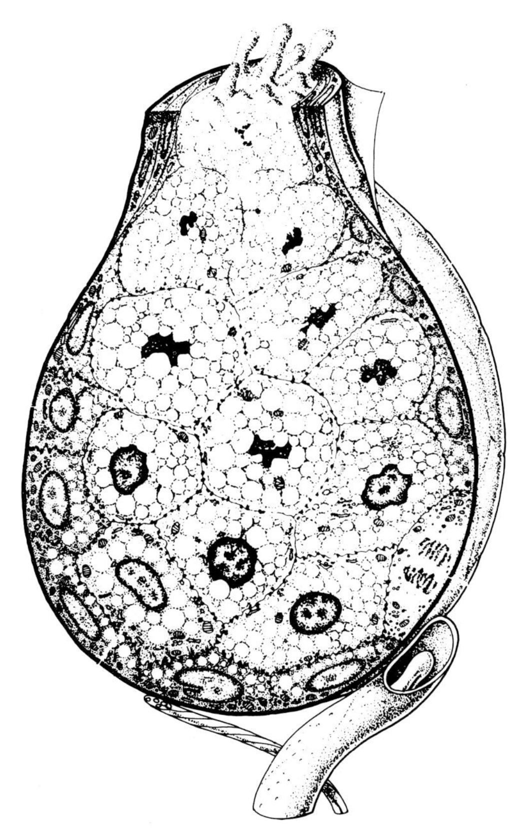

Figure 22–27. Drawing of a lobule of a human sebaceous gland showing actively synthesizing cells at the periphery and the highly vacuolated degenerating cells in the interior. (From Krstic, R. V. 1978. *In* Die Gewebe des Menschen und der Saugetiere. Berlin, Springer-Verlag.)

The ducts have a helical course through the dermis. In the epidermis, the duct is enveloped by concentrically arranged keratinocytes. On the volar surface of the fingers, their funnel-shaped openings on the epidermal ridges can easily be seen with a magnifying glass.

APOCRINE SWEAT GLANDS

A second kind of sweat gland is found in the axilla, on the mons pubis, and in the circumanal region. These *apocrine sweat glands* are larger than the eccrine glands. Their coiled secretory portion may be 3 mm in diameter, compared to 0.4 mm for eccrine sweat glands. They are located in the dermis and the duct of each opens into the canal of a hair follicle. The secretory cells are cuboidal or

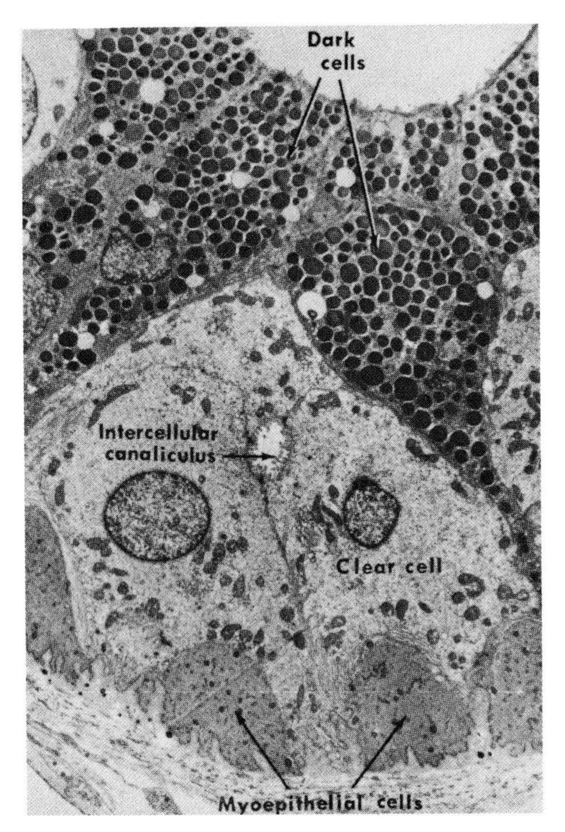

Figure 22–29. Low-power electron micrograph of a sector of the secretory coil of an eccrine sweat gland. Mucigenous "dark cells" border the lumen, whereas "clear" serous cells are more deeply situated and surround intercellular canaliculi. Myoepithelial cells form a discontinuous layer at the periphery of the tubular gland. (Courtesy of R. E. Ellis.)

low columnar but may be squamous when the gland is distended with secretory product. At their base, the secretory cells are associated with myoepithelial cells, as in the eccrine glands.

Eccrine sweat glands develop in fetal life from cords of cells that grow downward from the epithelium of the dermal ridges. Apocrine sweat glands arise as an epithelial bud growing from the side of a hair follicle. Eccrine sweat glands become functional soon after birth, whereas secretory activity of apocrine sweat glands does not begin until puberty.

Their designation as "apocrine" implies that a portion of the apical cytoplasm is shed in the secretory process and this was formerly believed to be true. However, the appearance of protruding blebs of apical cytoplasm that gave rise to this interpretation is now considered to be an artifact of specimen preparation. Their secretion is believed to be merocrine, but the traditional name apocrine sweat glands persists. In electron micrographs, the cells contain granules, usually separated from the apical membrane by a conspicuous terminal web. The composition of their product has been little studied. It is a slightly viscous fluid that is odorless when secreted, but when modified by the resident bacteria of the skin, it acquires an odor that has come to be considered socially offensive. The histology of the glands and their occurrence in sites where sex attractants are produced in lower animals has suggested that these glands evolved for a similar function in man, but the evidence supporting this interpretation is scant. In women, the apocrine sweat glands in the axilla show periodic cytological changes in the menstrual cycle. There is an enlargement of the cells and of the lumen, in the premenstrual period, followed by regression during menses.

The differences between the two kinds of sweat gland can be summarized as follows. The eccrine glands have no connection with hair follicles. They function throughout life producing a watery secretion, and they are innervated by cholinergic nerves. The apocrine sweat glands are appendages of hair follicles. They begin to function at puberty, producing a slightly viscous secretion, and they are innervated by adrenergic nerves. The mode of secretion of both glands is merocrine.

The *glands of Moll,* associated with the eyelids, are believed to be modified apocrine sweat glands, as are the *cerumenous glands* of the auditory canal that produce ear wax.

BLOOD AND LYMPH VESSELS

The arteries that supply the skin are branches of larger vessels in the subcutaneous tissue. These branches course upward and ramify to form the *rete cutaneum,* a plexus, parallel to the skin surface at the boundary between the dermis and the hypodermis. Descending branches from the rete cutaneum supply the subcutaneous tissue, and ascending branches traverse the reticular layer of the dermis. At the boundary between the reticular and papillary layers of the dermis, these small ascending arteries ramify to form a second plexus, the *rete subpapillare.* Branches from this network form capillary tufts in each dermal papilla to nourish the thick avascular epidermis (Fig. 22–30). Each hair follicle receives blood from two sources. A branch of one of the small ascending arteries forms a capillary

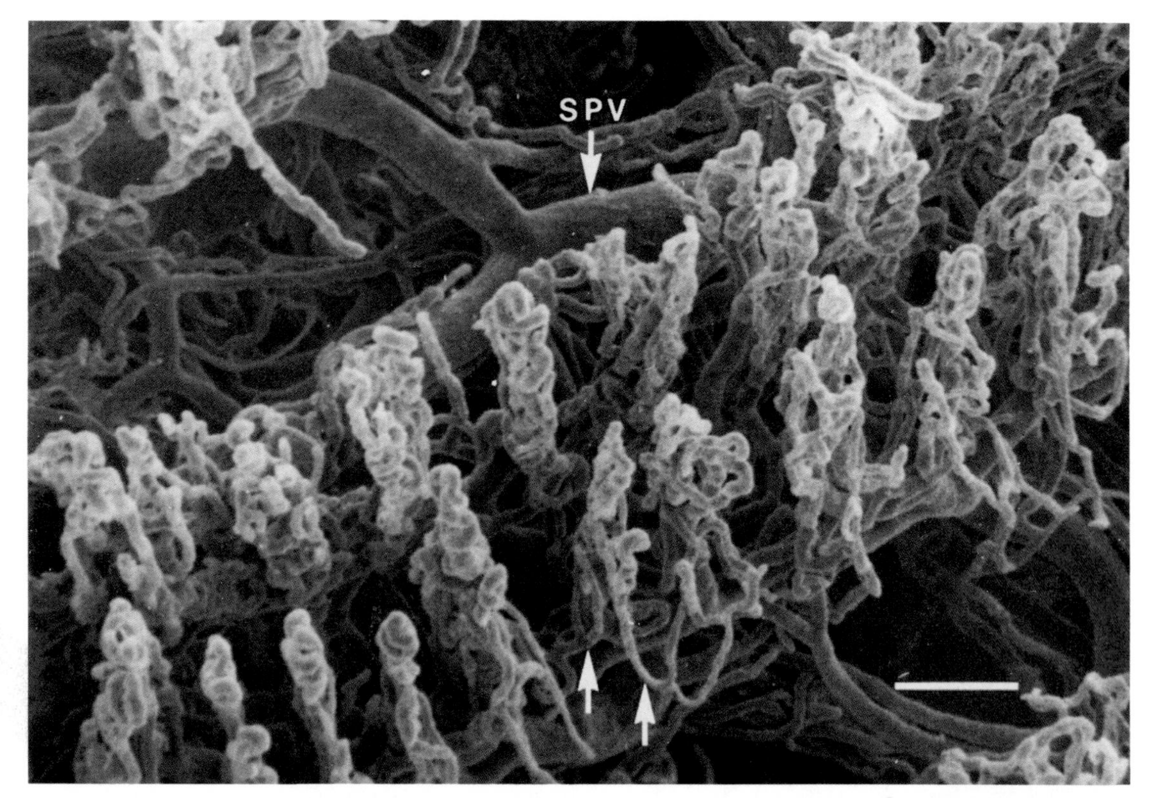

Figure 22–30. Scanning electron micrograph of the capillary network of digital dermal papillae of Macaca fusca, viewed at an angle of 45°. The vessels were injected with plastic and the tissue subsequently digested away. Afferent and efferent vessels (arrows below). Subpapillary venule SPV (top). (Micrograph courtesy of Umeda, N. and Ikeda, A. 1988. Acta Anat. 112:270.)

network in its papilla; other branches of the small artery, and branches from the rete subpapillare, contribute to a capillary network around the sebaceous gland and sheath of the follicle. A similar capillary network surrounds each sweat gland.

The venous limbs of the capillaries in the dermal papillae drain into a venous plexus beneath the rete subpapillare and veins from this drain into a venous plexus associated with the rete cutaneum. From this deeper plexus, veins descend to large veins in the subcutaneous tissue. Of more physiological interest are numerous *arteriovenous anastomoses* in the system. Under certain circumstances, these open, shunting blood directly from arteries to veins without an intervening capillary bed. They, thus, play an important role in thermoregulation by controlling blood flow to the superficial layers of the skin, where heat may be lost to a cold environment.

The skin has a rich lymphatic drainage, beginning in blind-ending lymphatic capillaries in the dermal papillae that join an extensive network underlying the dermo-epidermal junction. From there, branches descend through the reticular layer of the dermis to its boundary with the hypodermis, where they join a deeper network of larger lymphatics associated with the rete cutaneum. Larger lymph vessels, possessing valves, arise from this plexus and follow the course of the veins through the subcutaneous tissue.

NERVES

The skin is provided with abundant efferent nerves that activate its glands and control blood flow by changing the caliber of its vessels. It also has a variety of afferent sensory nerves that transmit tactile sensations. The endings of the sensory nerves fall into two broad categories: *free endings* and *encapsulated nerve endings* (Fig. 22–31). The term free ending does not necessarily imply that they are naked axons but simply that they lack morphologically recognizable receptor specializations at their ends. The commonest of these are in the epidermis. Myelinated nerves ap-

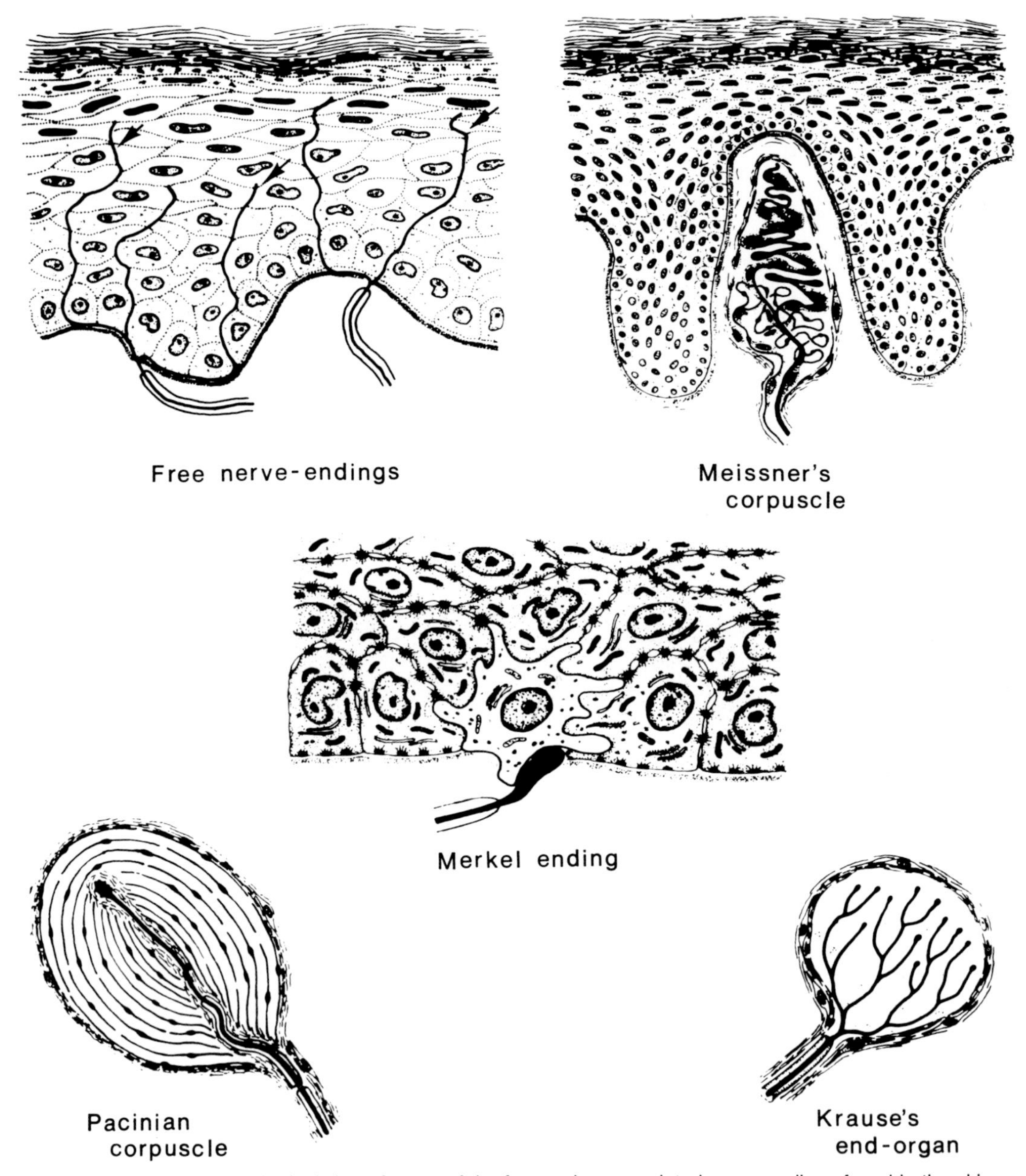

Figure 22–31. Schematic depiction of some of the free and encapsulated nerve endings found in the skin.

proaching the epidermis from below lose their myelin sheath and continue on a vertical course through interstices among the keratinocytes to terminate in blind endings in the stratum granulosum. At least some of these axons are ensheathed by processes of Schwann cells over part of their intraepidermal course. These free endings may be pain receptors or thermoreceptors. Other myelinated afferent nerves have disc-like expansions called *Merkel endings,* in contact with the plasmalemma of Merkel cells near the base of the epidermis. The function of these Merkel cell–neurite complexes is unknown.

The more complex encapsulated nerve endings have cellular and extracellular components that are organized so as to convey a mechanical stimulus to an axon in their interior. They are of several kinds: *Pacinian corpuscles, Meissner's corpuscles, Kraus's end bulbs,* and *Ruffini corpuscles.* Pacinian corpuscles are conspicuous ovoid structures up to a millime-

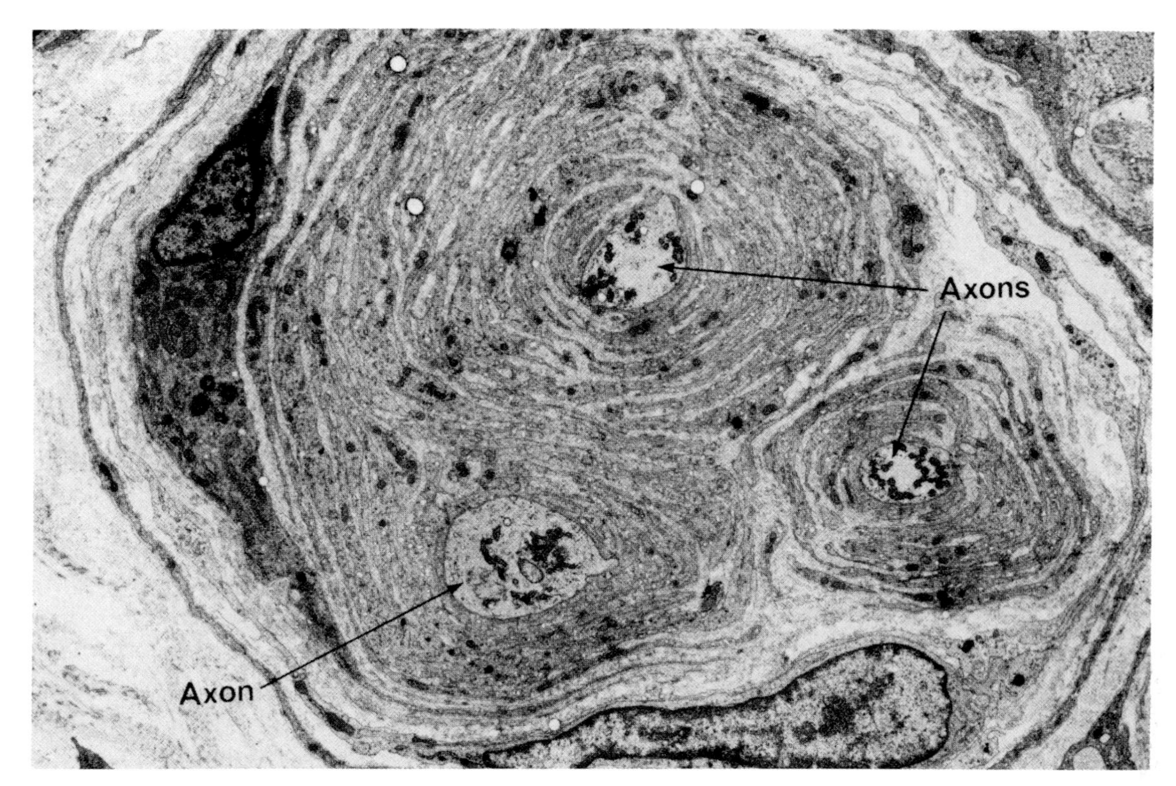

Figure 22–32. Electron micrograph of a cluster of three small encapsulated nerve endings with multiple layers of very thin cells surrounding an axon in the core of the corpuscle. (Micrograph courtesy of E. Weihe.)

ter in length. They are found in the dermis and hypodermis of the skin, in the periosteum of bone, and in the connective tissue stroma of some organs. A myelinated nerve enters one pole, loses its sheath, and its axon continues in the core of the corpuscle ending in several clavate processes. The axon and its processes are surrounded by 20 to 60 concentric lamellae consisting of very thin flat cells separated by narrow spaces filled with gel-like material of low viscosity (Fig. 22–32). this organization gives the corpuscle a cross-sectional appearance like that of an onion. The nerve and its surrounding lamellae are enclosed in a thin connective tissue capsule.

Meissner's corpuscles are pear-shaped structures, about 150 μm in length, found in a few of the dermal papillae of the glabrous skin of palms, soles, nipples, lips, and external genitalia (Fig. 22–33). The axon of a myelinated nerve, reaching the lower pole of the corpuscle, pursues a spiral or zigzag course in its interior, among flattened cells that are probably modified Schwann cells (Fig. 22–34). These are oriented transversely, resulting in a ladder-like cross-striation in routine hematoxylin and eosin preparations. The corpuscle

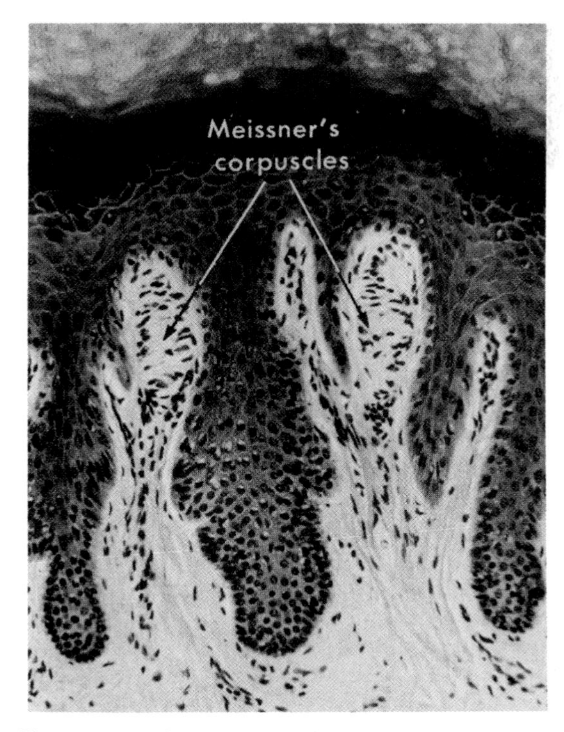

Figure 22–33. Photomicrograph of palmar digital epidermis showing Meissner's corpuscles in two neighboring dermal papillae.

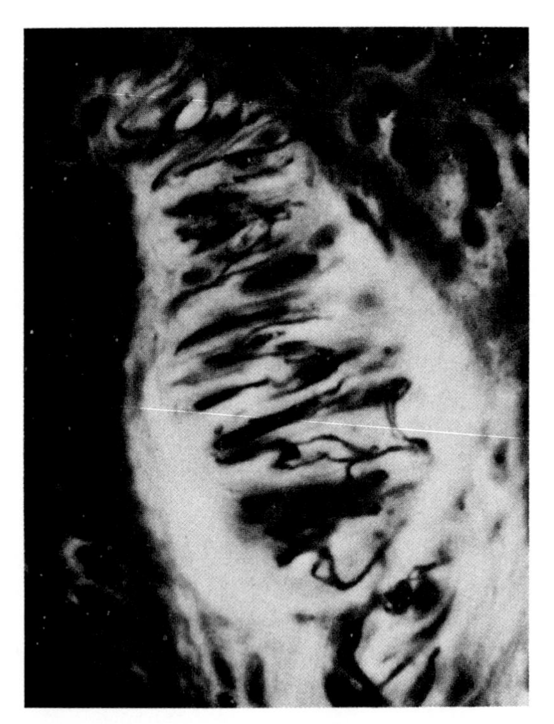

Figure 22–34. Meissner's corpuscle in which the nerve has been blackened with a silver stain. (Courtesy of N. Cauna.)

has a moderately thick capsule. Occurring in regions of considerable tactile sensitivity, Meissner's corpuscles are probably mechanoreceptors responding to slight deformation of the skin.

Kraus's end bulbs are small, more-or-less spherical bodies found in the papillary layer of the dermis, in the conjunctiva, the stratified squamous epithelia of the mouth, the tongue, and the external genitalia. the axon of a myelinated nerve enters the corpuscle and branches repeatedly in its interior. These corpuscles bear some resemblance to Pacinian corpuscles but are much smaller and the many orders of branching of the axon are its most distinctive feature.

Ruffini's corpuscles are small fusiform structures about 1 mm long and 0.2–0.5 mm wide with a relatively thin capsule. They are found deep in the dermis or hypodermis and are especially abundant beneath the skin on the plantar surface of the feet. They are usually oriented parallel to the surface of the skin and are unusual, in that bundles of collagen fibers run through the core of the corpuscle. Many terminal branches of the axon of a myelinated afferent nerve penetrate among the parallel fibers of the axial collagen bundles. Because the collagen in the corpuscle continues through it and intermingles with collagen bundles in the surrounding connective tissue, it is speculated that tension on the collagen bundles probably stimulates the nerve endings between them. The Ruffini corpuscles are, therefore, thought to be mechanoreceptors responding to tensional forces.

HISTOPHYSIOLOGY OF THE SKIN

PROTECTIVE FUNCTION

The human integument does not have the feathers, scales, or spines that have an obvious protective function in some lower animals, but the heavy keratinization of the cells and presence of lipid-rich extracellular material in the stratum corneum clearly provide some degree of protection against mechanical damage, fluid loss, and entry of noxious substances from the environment. Keratin filaments are components of the cytoskeleton of many epithelial cell types, but nowhere are they as abundant as in the epidermis, and the diversity of keratins in the skin suggests that they evolved to meet a specific need. Two keratins, K8 and K18, are commonly found in simple epithelia. In the epidermis, keratin synthesis is far more complex, yielding three type-I acidic keratins (K10, K11, K14) and three type-II basic keratins (K1, K2, K5). Moreover, different sets of keratins are synthesized at successive stages in the cytomorphosis of the epidermal cells. Cells near the base of the epithelium contain relatively small keratins (46–58 kD), whereas those in upper layers have these and larger keratins (63–67 kD). There appears to be a program of changing expression of keratin genes as the cells move from the stratum basale to the stratum corneum. There is also a specific high-molecular-weight keratin that is abundant in the palms and soles but only sparsely represented in the epidermis of other regions that are less subject to pressure and attrition. Thus, the amount and chemical nature of the keratins synthesized appear to depend on local needs. The keratin filaments and their filaggrin matrix are largely responsible for the skin's resistance to mechanical injury.

The skin has an important role in the photobiogenesis of vitamin D. When skin is exposed to sunlight, ultraviolet irradiation enters the epidermis and transforms 7-dehydrocholesterol to vitamin D. However, an excess of ultraviolet radiation can be very damaging and an important aspect of the skin's protective function is its ability to increase production of melanin on prolonged exposure to sunlight and, thus, minimize the potentially harmful effects of sunlight.

PERMEABILITY BARRIER

Maintenance of the normal internal environment of the body depends on the relative impermeability of the epidermis. Without this layer, there would very soon be an evaporative water loss equal to the total blood volume. Although the cells of the stratum corneum contribute to the barrier, it is now known that the complex intercellular lipids play a major role. The lipid bilayers liberated from the discoid granules released in the transition from the stratum granulosum to the stratum corneum coalesce to form continuous intercellular lamellae in which the dense and lucent layers, observed in the granules, are preserved. When carried up into the stratum corneum with the cells, these lipid lamellae constitute an essential component of the permeability barrier. They have an unusual composition, consisting of the sphingolipid, ceramine (40%), cholesterol (25%), and free fatty acids (25%), and this mixture is more resistant to bacterial attack and oxidation from exposure to the atmosphere than are other lipid bilayers in the body that are composed mainly of phospholipids.

In addition to protecting against loss of water and electrolytes, the barrier also prevents entry of water-soluble toxins from the environment. It does, however, permit entry of lipid-soluble substances. The rate of penetration of a substance depends on its oil/water partition coefficient; compounds that are equally soluble in oil and water penetrate best. Anything that can cross the epidermal barrier can enter the blood in the rete subpapillare. Advantage is now taken of this for percutaneous administration of some drugs. Enzymes of the epidermis are capable of transforming certain compounds from an inactive to an active form. For example, the anti-inflammatory drug, cortisone, applied to the skin would be ineffective were it not converted in the epidermis to hydrocortisone. Conversely, epidermal enzymes may break down certain potentially carcinogenic compounds to harmless products.

THERMOREGULATION

Heat produced continuously as a by-product of metabolism is lost by radiation and evaporation from the skin surface. When the ambient temperature is higher than body temperature, evaporation is the only mechanism of heat dissipation subject to physiological control, and it depends on the secretory activity of some 3 million sweat glands in the skin. During heavy exertion in a warm environment, these may produce 6 liters or more of sweat per day. Sweating usually begins on the forehead and spreads to the face and then over the rest of the body. The palms and soles are last to show an increase in sweating under these conditions. However, when sweating is induced by fear or other emotional stress, the palms start sweating first.

Sweating is controlled by centers in the preoptic area of the hypothalamus that function like a thermostat. Elevated body temperature may increase the rate of discharge of heat-sensitive neurons in these centers as much as 10-fold, resulting in profuse sweating. Impulses are conducted over autonomic pathways to postganglionic sympathetic fibers that terminate around sweat glands. These are cholinergic, for the most part, but sweat glands in the palms, soles, forehead, and axillae are thought to have an additional adrenergic innervation that would account for their selective activation in response to emotional stress.

Efficient temperature control also requires regulation of cutaneous blood flow because it is the blood that conducts deep body heat to the surface where it can be dissipated. The rate of blood flow is regulated, in part, by the same hypothalamic centers that control sweating. In addition to more general vasomotor effects, these centers control the degree of patency of numerous arteriovenous anastomoses that can shunt a large volume of blood into the capacious subcutaneous venous plexuses. Elevated temperature results in vasodilatation and opening of the arteriovenous anastomoses. Cooling results in vasoconstriction and return of the anastomoses to their normal state of contraction. In an extremely cold environment, blood flow through the skin may be as low as 50 ml/m^2/min, and in a hot environment, flow may increase to 2–3 liters/min.

SENSORY PERCEPTION

The rich sensory innervation of the skin transmits to the central nervous system information that triggers thermoregulatory mechanisms and pain that elicits avoidance of further injury. Firmly entrenched in the literature of physiology is the belief that the skin possesses four distinct types of sensory nerve endings, each responding to a specific kind of stimulus: *touch, heat, cold,* or *pain.* They are thought to occur in sensory spots having a punctate distribution, with each having specific *free nerve endings* for one of these four sensory modalities. Further complexity has been added by distinctions recently made between mechanosensitive, thermosensitive, and chemosensitive pain receptors and there is some evidence suggesting that there are endings that transmit only *itch* sensation. However, no ultrastructural differences have been described among free endings that can be related to the specific modalities of sensation defined by the physiologists. It is evident that our knowledge of the structural basis of sensation is far from complete.

There is agreement on the function of only one or two of the several kinds of encapsulated nerve endings. Tactile sensation is attributed to Meissner's corpuscles, but these are numerous only on the palms and soles, whereas the sense of touch is widely distributed over the whole body. It is interesting that in the gorilla which walks quadrapedally using the knuckles of the fore-limbs as weight-bearing surfaces, Meissner's corpuscles are also found on the dorsal aspect of the fingers, and in other primates that have a prehensile tail, they are found on its glabrous ventral surface. Touch sensation on the hair portions of the skin probably resides in networks of nerves around the hair follicles that are stimulated when anything comes in contact with the hair. It is likely that nerve networks at various levels in the skin may have free endings that function independently of organized sense organs recognizable with the microscope. The epithelium of the cornea, which is continuous with that of the skin, is exquisitely sensitive but contains only free nerve endings.

The distribution of Paccinian corpuscles deep in the dermis and in the subcutaneous tissue has suggested that they may sense pressure. It is true that a force applied to one side of the corpuscle elicits a receptor potential in its nerve, but the viscous interlamellar fluid redistributes the force within milliseconds so that it is the same on all sides of the core and the nerve ceases to be stimulated. Because of this rapid adaptation, the Pacinian corpuscle is poorly suited for detection of sustained pressure. However, experiments show that their rapid response to minute deformations enables them to detect vibrations of from 60 to 500 cycles per second. How this property would be advantageous in the normal activities of an animal is not apparent.

IMMUNOLOGICAL FUNCTION

The skin presents to the environment a large surface area continually exposed to irritants, toxins, viruses, and bacteria. In addition to its mechanically protective function, it has been shown, in recent years, to be an integral part of the body's immune system. The finding of cells in the epidermis that are located there to cope with antigenic substances in the environment should be no more surprising than the concentration of such cells in the lamina propria of the intestinal tract to defend against enteric antigens. For decades, the presence of small numbers of lymphocytes in the epidermis has been reported, but no special significance was attributed to this finding. The function of the keratinocytes was believed to be limited to synthesis of keratin and the extracellular components of the permeability barrier, and the significance of the Langerhans cells was unknown. All three of these cell types are now known to participate in the immune defenses of the body.

Although the number of lymphocytes observed in histological sections of skin is not impressive, their total number in this large organ may be as great as their number in the blood. For the most part, they are a population of immature T-lymphocytes that preferentially "home" to the skin and migrate into its epidermis. The early stages in their maturation took place in the thymus, but the kertinocytes of the epidermis evidently create a micrenvironment favorable for completion of the process. When sections of skin are exposed to fluorescein-labeled antibody to *thymopoietin,* a hormone that influences T-cell maturation in the thymus, the antibody binds to the cytoplasm of keratinocytes in the basal layers of the epidermis. The same cells also have three distinctive surface markers that are found in the plasmalemma of epithelial cells of the thymus. It is now believed that these keratinocytes produce thymopoietin, or a very similar molecule, that promotes the postthymic maturation of the resident T-lymphocytes. When reacting to an immunological challenge, they are also capable of producing *interleukin-1*, a cytokine that binds to T-lymphocytes and induces their release of *interleukin-2* which induces proliferation of T-lymphocytes. Such lymphocytes may enter the lymphatics and become distributed throughout the body. Thus, the keratinocytes are important participants in the immune defenses of the skin and of the body as a whole.

The Langerhans cells of the epidermis originate in the bone marrow and are carried in the blood to the skin, where they insinuate themselves among the keratinocytes and taken on a dendritic form. Like macrophages and reticular cells of the lymphoid tissue, Langerhans cells process antigen and present it to helper T-lymphocytes in a form capable of inducing an immune response. Interest in these cells has been heightened by the finding that the virus of AIDS binds to an antigen on the surface of T-cells and Langerhans cells. Although T-lymphocytes are destroyed, the Langerhans cells appear to be more resistant and are suspected of being a persistent reservoir of virus in patients suffering from this disease.

BIBLIOGRAPHY

GENERAL

Montagna, W. W. and P. F. Parakkal. 1974. The Structure and Function of the Skin, 3rd ed. New York, Academic Press.

Rothman, S. 1954. Physiology and Biochemistry of the Skin. Chicago, University of Chicago Press.

EPIDERMIS

Allen, T. D. and C. S. Pottan. 1975. Desmosomal form, fate, and function in mammalian epidermis. J. Ultratr. Res. 51:94.

Choi, Y. and E. Fuchs. 1990. TGF-B and retinoic acid regulators of growth and modifiers of differentiation in human epidermal cells. Cell Reg. 1:791.

Eichner, R., T-T. Sun, and U. Aebi. 1986. The role of keratin sub-families and keratin pairs in the formation of human epidermal intermediate filaments. J. Cell Biol. 102:1767.

Elias, P. J., J. Goerke, and D. S. Friend. 1977. Permeability barrier lipids: composition and influence on epidermal structure. J. Investig. Dermatol. 69:535.

Elias, P. J. 1983. Epidermal lipids, barrier function and desquamation. J. Investig. Dermatol. 80(Suppl.):44s.

Fuchs, E. and H. Green. 1980. Changes in keratin gene expression during terminal differentiation of the keratinocyte. Cell 19:1033.

Fuchs, E. 1990. Epidermal differentiation: The bare essentials. J. Cell Biol. 111:2807.

Kawabe, T. T., D. K. MacCollum and J. L. Lillie. 1985. Variations in basement membrane topography in human thick skin. Anat. Rec. 211:142.

Keene, D. R., L. Y. Sakai, G. P. Lunstrum, N. P. Morris, and R. E. Burgeson. 1987. Type VII collagen forms an extended network of anchoring fibrils. J. Cell Biol. 104:611.

Martinez, I. R. and A. Peters. Membrane-coating granules and membrane modifications in keratinizing epithelia. Am. J. Anat. 130:93.

Matoltsy, A. G. 1975. Desmosomes, filaments and keratohyalin granules: their role in stabilization and keratinization of the epidermis. J. Investig. Dermatol. 65:127.

Matoltsy, A. G. and P. E. Parakkal. 1965. Membrane coating granules of keratinizing epithelia. J. Cell Biol. 24:297.

Mehrel, T., D. Hohl, J. A. Rothnagel et al. 1990. Identification of a major keratinocyte cell envelope protein, loricin. Cell 61:1103.

Nelson, W. and T-T. Sun. 1983. The 50- and 58-kD keratin classes as molecular markers for stratified squamous epithelium. J. Cell Biol. 97:244.

Rice, R. H. and H. Green. 1979. Presence in human epidermal cells of a soluble protein precursor of the cross-linked envelope: activation of cross-linking by calcium ions. Cell 18:681.

MERKEL CELL

Fortman, G. J. and R. K. Winkelman. 1973. A Merkel cell nuclear inclusion. J. Investig. Dermatol. 61:334.

Gottschaldt, K. M. and C. Vahle-Hinz. 1981. Merkel cell receptors: structure and transducer function. Science 214:183.

Gould, V. E., T. Moll, I. Lee, and W. W. Franke. 1985. Neuro-endocrine (Merkel) cells of the skin: Hyperplasia, dysplasia, and neoplasms. Lab. Investig. 52:334.

Hartschuh, W., E. Weihe, N. Yanaihara, and M. Reinecke. 1983. Immunohistochemical localization of vasoactive intestinal peptide in Merkel cells of various mammals: Evidence for a neuromodulator function of the Merkel cell. J. Investig. Dermatol. 81:361.

Kurosumi, K., V. Kurosumi, and K. Inoue. 1979. Morphological and morphometric studies on the Merkel cells and associated nerve terminals of normal and denervated skin. Arch. Histol. Japan 42:243.

Mihara, M., K. Hashimoto, K. Ueda, and M. Kumakiri. 1979. The specialized junctions between Merkel cell and neurite: an electron microscopic study. J. Investig. Dermatol. 73:325.

Winkelmann, R. K. 1977. The Merkel cell system and a comparison between it and the neurosecretory of APUD cell system. J. Investig. Dermatol. 69:41.

LANGERHANS CELLS

Braathen, L. R., S. Bjercke, and E. Thorsby. 1984. The antigen presenting function of human Langerhans cells. Immunobiology 168:301.

Breathnach, A. S. 1965. The cell of Langerhans. Internat. Rev. Cytol. 18:1.

Edelson, R. I. and J. M. Fink. 1985. The immunologic function of the skin. Sci. Am. 252(6):46.

Friedmann, P. S. 1981. The immunology of Langerhans cells. Immunol. Today July:124.

Katz, S., K. Tamaki, and D. H. Sacks. 1979. Epidermal Langerhans cells are derived from cells originating in the bone marrow. Nature (London)282:324.

Rowden, G. 1977. Immunoelectron microscopic studies of surface receptors and antigens of human Langerhans cells. Br. J. Dermatol. 97:593.

MELANOCYTES

Billingham, R. E. and W. K. Silvers. 1960. The melanocytes of mammals. Quart. Rev. Biol. 35:1.

Drochmans, P. 1963. On melanin granules. Internat. Rev. Exp. Pathol. 2:357.

Snell, R. S. 1972. An electron microscopic study of melanin in the hair and hair follicles. J. Investig. Dermatol. 58:218.

Seiji, M., K. Shimao, M. S. C. Birbeck, and T. B. Fitzpatrick. 1963. Subcellular localization of melanin biosynthesis. Ann. N.Y. Acad. Sci. 100:497.

Szabo, G., A. B. Gerald, M. A. Pathak, and T. B. Fitzpatrick. 1969. Racial differences in the fate of melanosomes in human epidermis. Nature 222:1081.

SWEAT GLANDS

Cage, G. W. and R. L. Dobson. 1965. Sodium secretion and reabsorption by the human eccrine sweat glands. J. Clin. Investig. 44:1270.

Dole, V. P. and J. H. Thaysen. 1953. Variations in the functional power of human sweat glands. J. Exp. Med. 98:129.

Munger, B. L. 1961. The ultrastructure and histophysiology of human eccrine sweat glands. J. Biophys. Biochem. Cytol. 11:385.

Schaumberg-Lever, G. and W. F. Lever. 1975. Secretion from human apocrine glands: an electron microscopic study. J. Investig. Dermatol. 64:38.

Terzakis, J. A. 1964. The ultrastructure of monkey eccrine sweat glands. Z. Zellforsch. 64:493.

SEBACEOUS GLANDS

Bell, M. 1974. A comparative study of the ultrastructure of the sebaceous glands of man and other primates. J. Investig. Dermatol. 62:132.

Downing, D. T. and J. S. Strauss. 1982. On the mechanism of sebaceous secretion. Arch. Dermatol. Res. 272:343.

Hibbs, R. G. 1962. Electron microscopy of human axillary sebaceous glands. J. Investig. Dermatol. 38:329.

Jenkinson, D., H. Y. Elder, I. Montgomery, and V. A. Moss. 1985. Comparative studies of sebaceous gland ultra structure. Tissue Cell 17:683.

HAIR AND NAILS

Chase, H. B. 1954. Growth of the hair. Physiol. Rev. 34:113.

Ebling, F. J. 1976. Hair. J. Investig. Dermatol. 67:98.

Wyatt, E. H. and M. Riggott. 1977. Scanning electron microscopy of hair. Observations on surface morphology with respect to site, sex, and age in man. Br. J. Dermatol. 96:627.

Zaias, N. J. and J. Alvarez. 1968. The formation of the primate nail plate. J. Investig. Dermatol. 51:120.

INNERVATION

Breathnach, A. S. 1977. Electron microscopy of cutaneous nerves and receptors. J. Investig. Dermatol. 69:8.

Catton, W. T. 1970. Mechanoreceptor function. Physiol. Rev. 50:297.

Cauna, N. 1980. Fine morphological characteristics and microtopography of the free nerve endings of the human digital skin. Anat. Rec. 198:643.

Montagna, W. W. and J. M. Brookhart. 1977. Cutaneous innervation and the modalities of cutaneous sensibility. J. Investig. Dermatol. 60:3.

Munger, B., Y. Yoshida, S. Hayashi, T. Osawa, and C. Ide. 1988. A re-evaluation of the cytology of the cat Pacinian corpuscles. I. The inner core and clefts. Cell Tissue Res. 253:83.

Novotny, G. E. and E. G. Gommort-Novotny. 1988. Intraepidermal nerves in human digital skin. Cell Tissue Res. 254:111.

Wedell, G., W. Pallie, and E. Palmer. 1955. Nerve endings in mammalian skin. Biol. Rev. 30:159.

BLOOD VESSELS

Braverman, I. M. and A. Yen. 1977. Ultrastructure of the human dermal microcirculation. II. The capillary loops of the dermal papillae. J. Investig. Dermatol. 69:44.

Inoue, H. 1978. Three dimensional observations of microvasculature of human finger skin. Hand 10:144.

Umeda, N. and A. Ikeda. 1988. Scanning electron microscopic study of the capillary loops in the dermal papillae. Acta Anat. 132:270.

23

ORAL CAVITY AND ASSOCIATED GLANDS

The oral cavity is the entrance to the digestive tract, and a chamber in which food is mechanically fragmented by the teeth and chemically modified and lubricated by saliva before being transported via the pharynx and esophagus to the stomach for further processing. A narrow space between the inner surface of the lips and cheeks and the outer aspect of the gums and teeth is the *vestibule*. The *oral cavity proper* is bounded above by the hard and soft palate, anteriorly by the inner aspect of the gums and teeth and posteriorly by two *palatoglossal folds* of the mucous membrane on either side of the communication between the mouth and the pharynx. Much of the mouth is occupied by the *tongue*, a highly mobile muscular structure involved in mastication and swallowing. In man, it also has a role in speech.

The lips are made up of the orbicularis oris skeletal muscle and dense connective tissue, covered on their outer surface by skin with hair follicles and sebaceous and sweat glands (Fig. 23–1). At the free edge of the lips, this gives way to a hairless very thin skin, with an epidermis that is sufficiently transparent to permit the blood in the capillaries of the dermis to impart to it a red color. On the inner aspect of the lips, there is a gradual transition from skin to the mucous membrane lining the vestibule and the mouth proper.

MUCOUS MEMBRANE

The mucous membrane of the oral cavity differs from region to region in the character of its epithelium and the underlying lamina propria. The epithelium is stratified squamous throughout, but it does not keratinize completely as in skin. In the vestibule, on the floor of the mouth, and under side of the tongue, the epithelium is relatively thin and does not undergo keratinization. Its lamina propria is loose, permitting considerable mobility over the underlying structures. On the cheeks, it is somewhat thicker. These nonkeratinizing epithelia do not exhibit the zonation found in the epidermis. As cells move upward from the basal layer, they increase greatly in size and come to contain abundant tonofilaments, but they do not become greatly flattened as they approach the surface. Desmosomes are less numerous and smaller than in the epidermis. Where the red, freely mobile mucosa of the floor of the mouth is reflected onto the alveolar processes, there is an abrupt transition to a pink layer firmly fixed to the underlying bone by rather dense connective tissue. This is the *gingiva*. It covers the gums and extends between the teeth. In the roof of the mouth, it continues from the alveolar process, over the entire hard palate. It has a thick stratified squamous epithelium with numerous papillae penetrating deep into its lower surface. A stratum basale, stratum spinosum, stratum granulosum, and stratum corneum are distinguishable, as in the skin. The cells of the stratum corneum are keratinized, but they retain condensed nuclei and appear to be viable. They are continually exfoliated into the saliva. The cells of the stratum spinosum contain bundles of tonofilaments that terminate in conspicuous desmosomes that firmly attach neighboring cells. There are also hemidesmosomes at the base of the epithelium from which anchoring fibers loop around bundles of collagen fibers in the underlying lamina propria. The greater thickness, firmer attachment, and greater degree of keratinization of the epithelium on the gums and hard palate make these regions more resistant to attrition during chewing. The epithelium in different regions of the oral cavity differs not only in the degree of its keratinization but also in its permeability. The thin, nonkeratinized epithelium on the

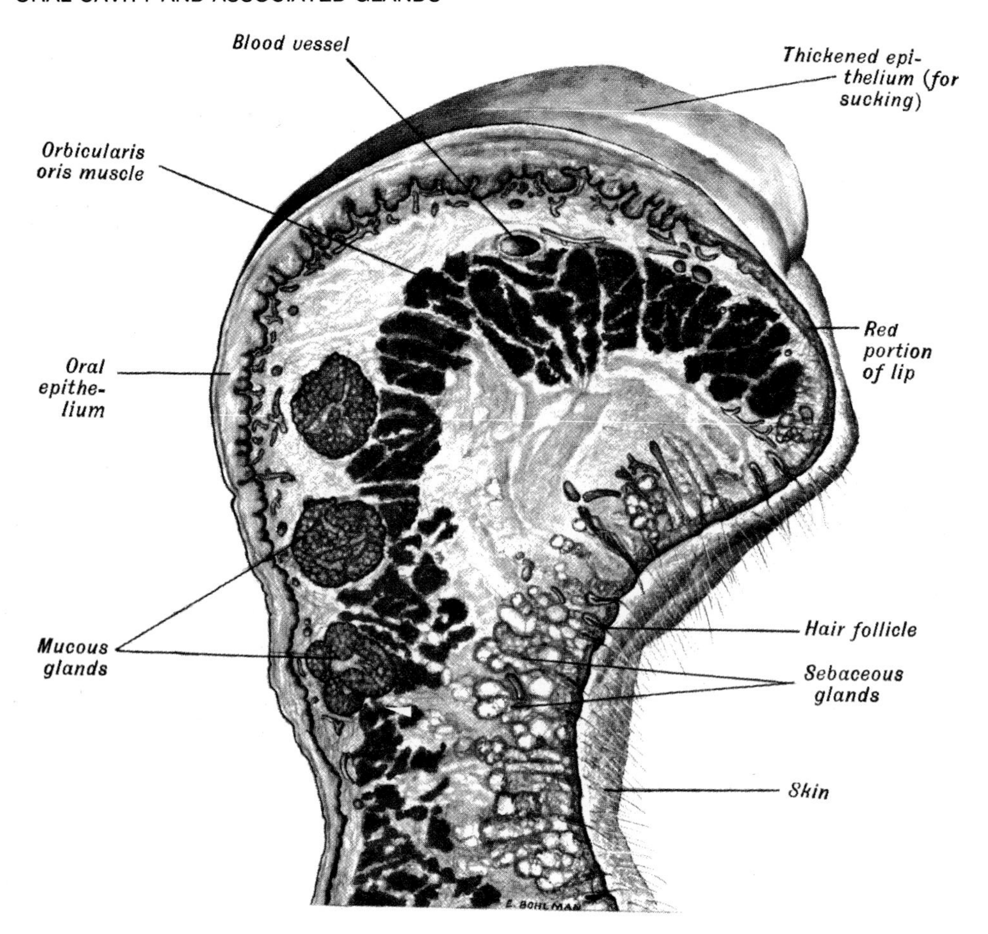

Figure 23–1. Camera lucida drawing of a saggital section through the lip of a newborn infant showing the transition from the thin pink epithelium to an epithelium thickened in preparation for suckling in the postnatal period. Also shown are some mucus-secreting labial glands.

floor of the mouth and under side of the tongue is more permeable. Advantage is taken of this clinically, in that certain medications, such as nitroglycerin for anginal heart attacks, can be placed in a tablet under the tongue, where it diffuses through the epithelium and into the circulation. In many animal species, especially ruminants that eat coarse grasses, the oral epithelium is much more heavily keratinized than in man.

The lamina propria of the epithelium extends into deep recesses in the under surface of the epithelium as connective tissue papillae like those found under the epidermis of the skin, but they are more delicate, with thinner collagen and elastic fibers. Large numbers of lymphocytes are found in the lamina propria of the mucosa in the posterior portion of the oral cavity and many of these migrate into the epithelium. In the floor of the mouth and on the cheeks, where the lamina propria is underlain by a loose submucosa, the mucosa can be moved or elevated into folds. But on the gums and hard palate, the mucosa is firmly bound to the periosteum of the underlying bone by dense connective tissue. The mucosa on the soft palate continues around its posterior margin for some distance onto its nasal surface, and there the stratified squamous epithelium gives way to pseudostratified, ciliated, columnar epithelium characteristic of the nasal and respiratory passages.

The blood supply to the oral mucosa is similar to that of the skin. A plexus of larger vessels in the submucosa contributes branches to a plexus of smaller vessels in the lamina propria, from which branches form capillary networks in the connective tissue papillae beneath the epithelium. The oral mucosa is richly innervated by sensory branches from the trigeminal nerve (V), and on that portion covering the tongue, by special sensory branches from the facial nerve (VII) to the specific organs of the sense of taste.

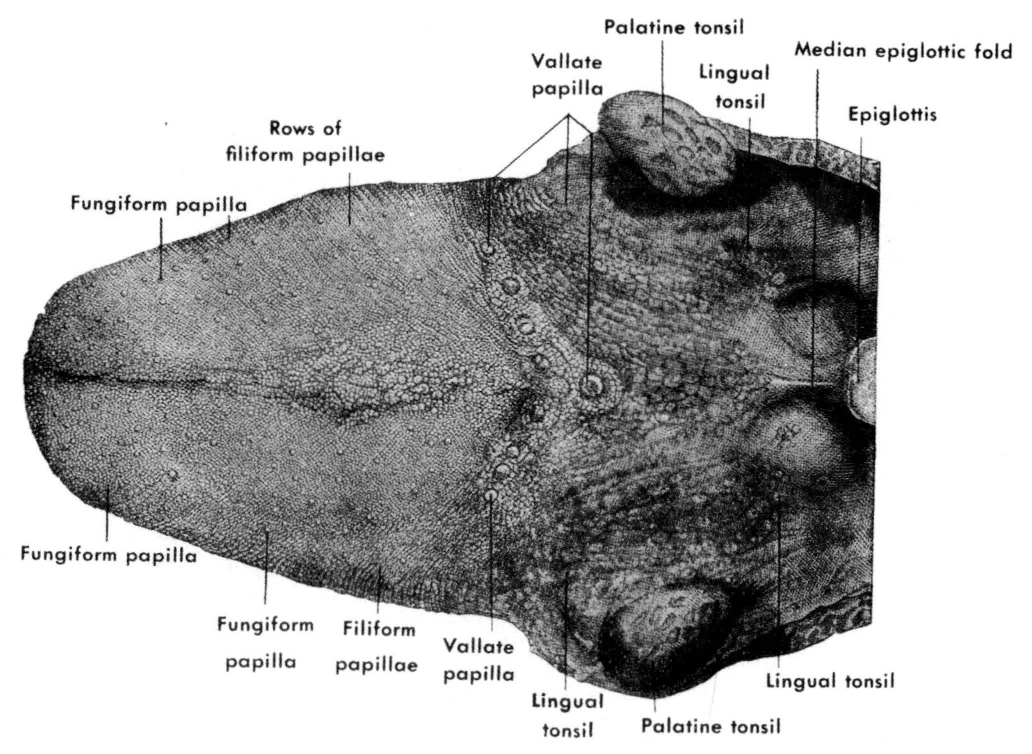

Figure 23–2. Surface view of the dorsum and root of the tongue. Note the circumvallate papillae along the sulcus terminalis separating the anterior and posterior portions of the tongue. (After Sappey.)

THE TONGUE

The bulk of the tongue consists of interlacing bundles of striated muscle oriented vertically, horizontally, and longitudinally and intersecting at right angles. This arrangement ensures a higher degree of mobility of the anterior portion of the tongue that is essential for mastication, phonation, and swallowing. The posterior portion of the tongue is less mobile owing to its continuity with the floor of the mouth and its attachment to the hyoid bone. The dorsal surface of the tongue is covered by a relatively thick epithelium, firmly bound to an underlying layer of dense connective tissue, from which septa extend downward between the underlying bundles of muscle fibers. The anterior two-thirds, and posterior one-third, of the tongue are of different embryological origin and the boundary between the two is marked by a shallow V-shaped groove, the *sulcus terminalis* (Fig. 23–2). The open part of the V is directed forward and at the apex of the V there is slight depression that is a vestige of the thyroglossal duct, an evagination of the floor of the mouth that gave rise to the thyroid gland early in embryonic life.

LINGUAL PAPILLAE

Anterior to the sulcus terminalis, the dorsum of the tongue is rough, being covered by a multitude of small excrescences called *lingual papillae*. These are of four types: *filiform papillae, fungiform papillae, foliate papillae,* and *circumvallate papillae*. The most abundant of these are the filiform papillae which are slender, conical in form, and slightly curved with their tip pointing toward the back of the tongue (Figs. 23–3 and 23–4). They are 2–3 mm in length and are arranged in more-or-less distinct rows coursing parallel to the diverging arms of the V-shaped sulcus terminalis. The heavily keratinized cells at the tips of the papillae are continuously exfoliated. In disturbances of gastrointestinal function, their normal shedding is delayed and they accumulate in a layer, mixed with bacteria, and form a gray film over the surface of the tongue. This is the "coated tongue" looked for by old physicians as a sign of illness. In animals, the filiform papillae are large and stiff resulting in the sandpaper texture of a cat's tongue.

The *fungiform papillae* have a narrow base and a slightly flattened hemispherical upper

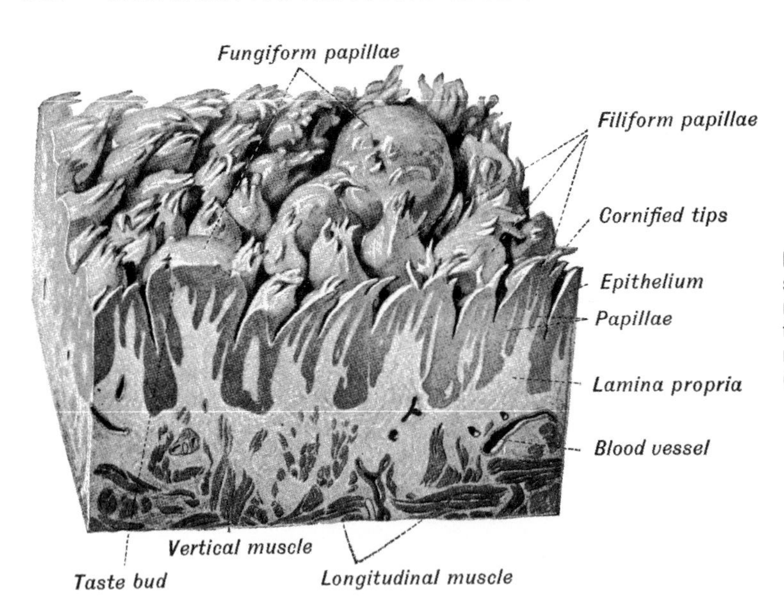

Figure 23–3. Oblique view of the dorsum of the tongue. The cut surface corresponds with the long axis, with the tip of the tongue to the left. Note the recurving tips of the filiform papillae. (After Braus.)

portion. They are 0.5–1.0 mm in diameter and stand slightly higher than the filiform papillae. Primary and secondary connective tissue papillae in their core project into conforming recesses in the under side of their epithelium which is essentially unkeratinized and has a smooth free surface (Figs. 23–3 and 23–5). Because their core is highly vascular and the overlying epithelium relatively thin, the fungiform papillae have a pink color.

Circumvallate papillae number only 6 to 14 and are confined to the posterior part of the tongue, where they are aligned just in front of the sulcus terminalis. They are considerably larger than the fungiform papillae (1–2 mm) and each occupies a recess in the mucosa so that it is surrounded by a circular furrow or sulcus (Figs. 23–6 and 23–7). The connective tissue core forms multiple secondary papillae. The epithelium on the free surface is smooth and that on the sides of the papilla contains numerous *taste buds*. Ten to twelve can often be found in a vertical section of a circumvallate papilla. A few may also be found on the lateral wall of the sulcus. The total number of taste buds in a single papilla is estimated to average 250. Deep in the connective tissue of the underlying muscle are the serous *glands of von Ebner* (Fig. 23–6). Their ducts open into the sulcus around the circumvallate papillae. This secretion is thought to function in rinsing out the furrow around the papilla.

The *foliate papillae* are rudimentary in the human but are well developed in rabbits, monkeys, and many other animals. In these species, a group of parallel ridges, separated by deep clefts, is found in a slightly elevated region on the sides of the tongue at the junction between its anterior and posterior portions. The epithelium on the sides of these ridges contains many taste buds (Fig. 23–8). Serous glands in the lamina propria discharge their secretion via ducts opening into the depths of the clefts. These topographic features are virtually absent in man, but a few taste buds are present in this region. Taste buds are also found in limited numbers on the glossopalatine arch, on the soft palate, on the posterior surface of the epiglottis, and on the posterior wall of the pharynx.

TASTE BUDS

There are about 3,000 taste buds on the human tongue. Taste buds appear, in histological sections, as pale ovoid bodies in the darker staining lingual epithelium (Fig. 23–9). Their vertical dimension is 50–80 μm and width 30–50 μm. They consist of 50–90 fusiform cells slightly wider at the base than at the apex. Their narrow apices converge on a small opening in the superficial layers of the epithelium called the *taste pore* (Fig. 23–10 and 23–11).

With the light microscope, two types of cells were distinguished in the taste buds. For lack of more precise identifying features, these were designated *light cells* and *dark cells*, based on the depth of their staining in histological sections. Small cells at the base of the taste

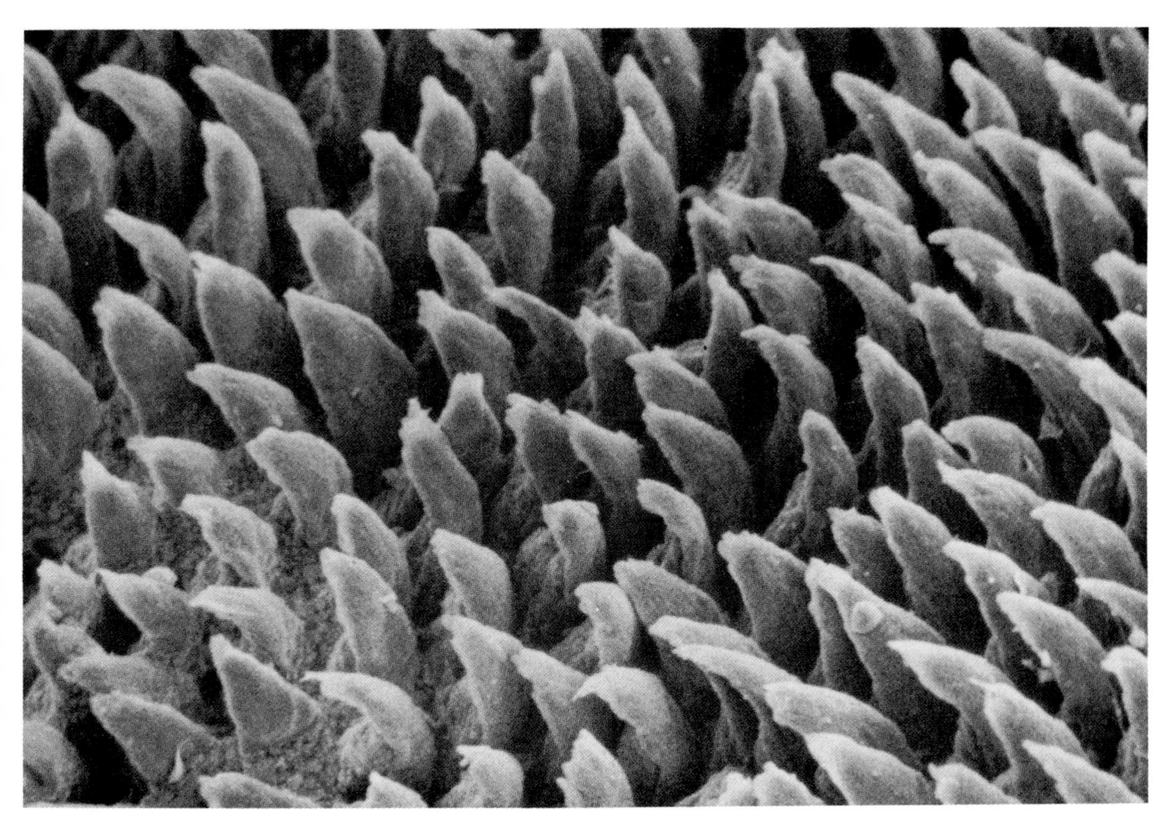

Figure 23–4. Scanning electron micrograph of the filiform papillae on the tongue of a rabbit. (Micrograph courtesy of F. Fujita.)

bud were later recognized and assumed to be stem-cell precursors of the gustatory cells.

The nomenclature of the cells types became somewhat more complicated with the advent of the electron microscope. Slender dark cells situated both at the periphery of the taste bud and in its interior were observed to have long microvilli projecting into the taste pore and to have small, dense secretory granules in their apical cytoplasm. These were designated *type-I cells* and were interpreted as supporting cells (Fig. 23–10). They appeared to largely sur-

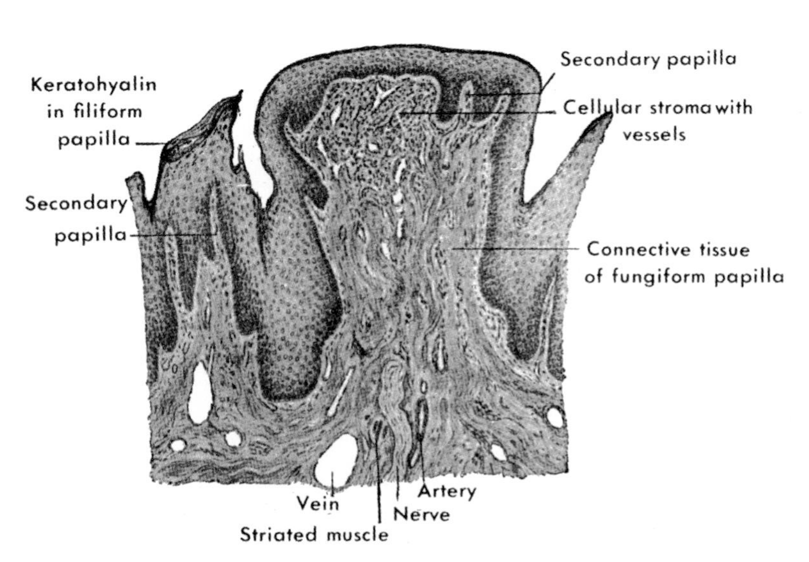

Figure 23–5. Drawing of a vertical section through a fungiform papilla. (After Schaffer, J., Lehrbuch der Histologie und Histogenese. Verlag. W. Engelmann, Leipzig, 1922.)

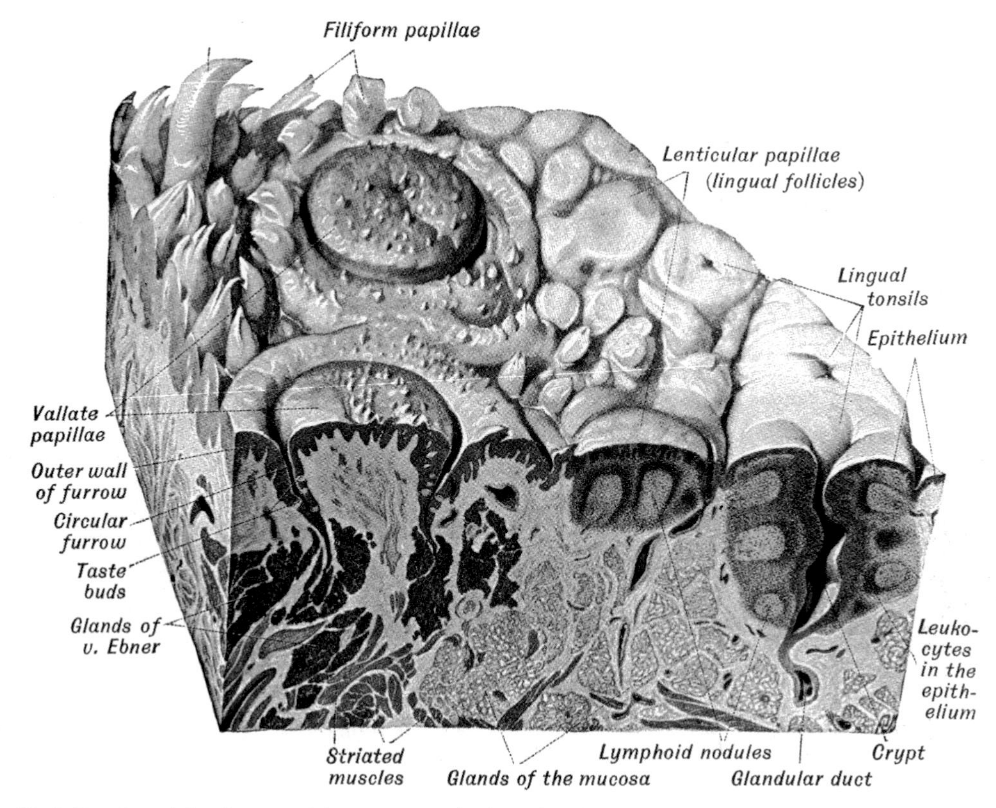

Figure 23–6. Drawing of the dorsum of the tongue at the boundary between the anterior portion of the so-called root of the tongue. (After Braus.)

round and isolate the other two cell types from each other and to secrete a dense amorphous material that surrounds the microvilli in the taste pore (Fig. 23–11). The more centrally situated *type-II cells* also have long microvilli but seem to lack secretory granules in their apical cytoplasm. They have abundant smooth endoplasmic reticulum but little rough endoplasmic reticulum. A *type-III cell*, which falls into the broad category of light cells, has also been identified. It has a long apical process, several times the diameter of a microvillus. This extends through the dense material in the pore to the free surface. The processes

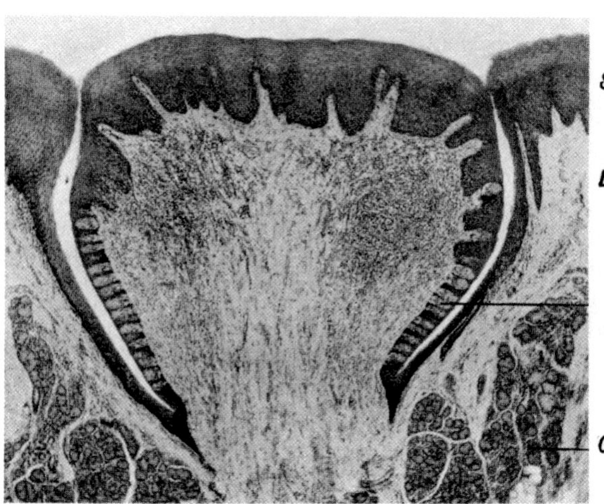

Figure 23–7. Histological section through a circumvallate papilla of *Macacus rhesis* showing taste buds and the neighboring glands of von Ebner.

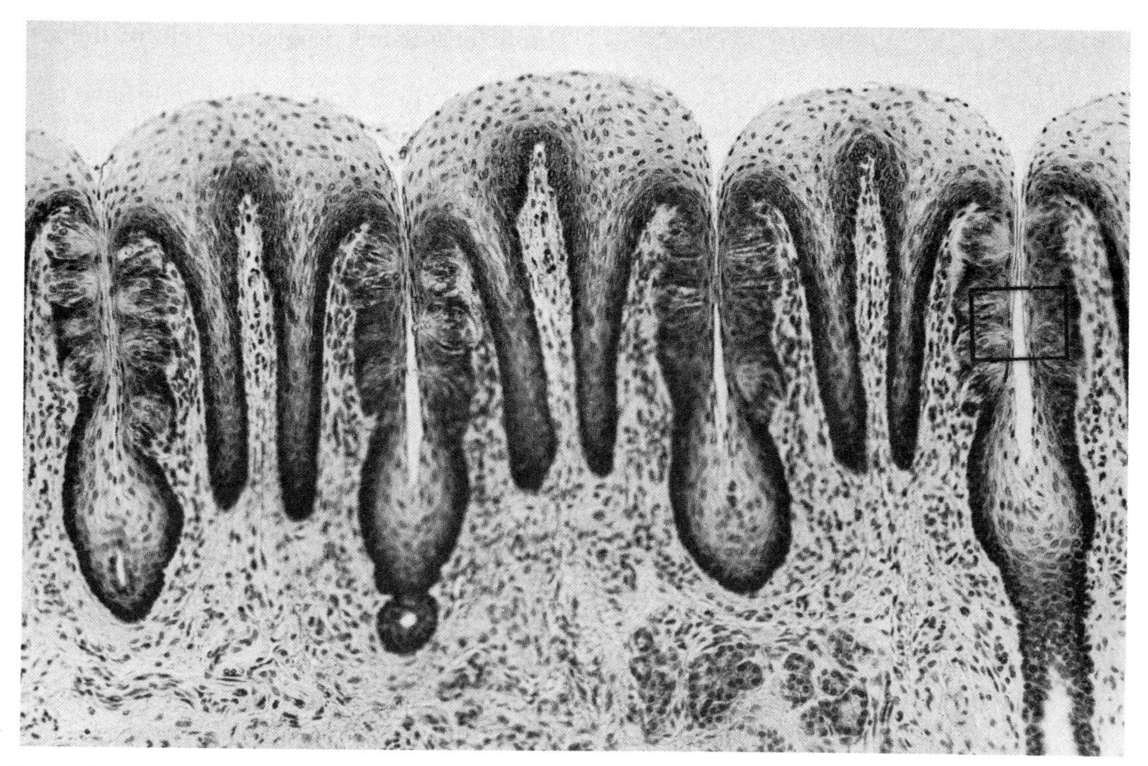

Figure 23–8. Photomicrograph of papillae of rabbit tongue showing the alternating ridges and deep clefts, with taste buds on either side of the clefts. The area in the box is shown at higher magnification in Fig. 23–9.

of this, and possibly those of other cell types projecting into the pore, are the receptor surface for the sense of taste. When exposed to a substance to which they can respond, the gustatory cells are depolarized and secrete a neurotransmitter that stimulates the endings of afferent nerves. The cytoplasm of the type-III cell contains small dense-cored vesicles that are most abundant near the cell base. Although nerves entering the taste bud are in contact with all three cell types, it is not clear which of these contacts are synaptic. Some investigators consider the type-III cell to be the primary gustatory receptor and suggest that the dense-cored vesicles in its basal cytoplasm contain a neurotransmitter.

Regrettably, no consensus has been reached as to how many taste cell types exist, or which cell types are gustatory and which are supportive. Four or more types have been described: dark (type I), light (type II), gustatory (type III), and basal (type IV). Some consider type III to be the only gustatory cell type, others believe both light and dark cells are sensory, based on the observation that both appear to synapse with intragemmal nerve fibers. The earlier belief that the cell types come from different cell lines has now been abandoned as a result of radioactive tracer studies. One day after injection of tritiated thymidine, label is found only over the nuclei of basal cells and type-I cells, but after four days, labelled light cells also appeared. These findings support the hypothesis that undifferentialed basal cells develop into dark cells and that these mature into light, Type II and Type III cells. The average life span of a cell in the mammalian taste bud is ten to twelve days.

There are four basic taste sensations: sweet, bitter, sour, and salty. Some studies suggest that taste buds for sweet and salty sensations are more abundant near the tip of the tongue, and those for sourness and bitterness are on the back of the tongue. However, no significant morphological differences have been detected in the taste buds in these locations and little is known about selectivity in taste cells. The evidence currently available indicates that there are different transduction mechanisms for each of the primary taste sensations. Sour taste appears to depend on the blocking of K^+ channels in the apical plasma membrane by acid (H^+ ions). Salty taste depends on apical Na^+ channels that can be blocked by amilor-

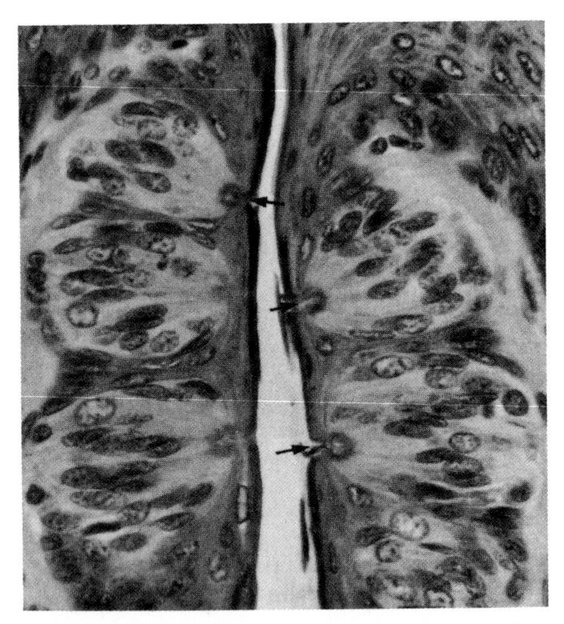

Figure 23–9. Photomicrograph of taste buds on foliate papillae of the rabbit. The arrows indicate the taste pores.

ide. Transduction of sweet taste appears to involve a subset of taste cells that have specific membrane receptors that bind sugars, resulting in a change in membrane conductance, depolarizing the cell and causing transmitter release. Similarly, bitter taste seems to involve bitter-specific receptors. It is the current view that the different primary tastes are localized in separate receptor cells, but there are indications that some cells may respond to more than one taste. Because the cells of the taste buds are joined by tight junctions near the taste pore, the receptors and the ion channels for K^+ and H^+ ions that are involved must be located in the apical membrane, which makes up only 1–2% of the total membrane area of the cell.

NERVES

Depending on their location on the tongue, taste buds may be innervated by sensory axons from the facial (VII), glossopharyngeal (IX), or vagal (X) cranial nerves. The general sensory innervation of the tongue, anterior to the sulcus terminalis, is via the lingual branch of the mandibular nerve (V), whereas gustatory sensation of this region, except for the circumvallate papillae, is via the chorda tympani branch of the facial nerve (VII), which accompanies the lingual nerve. Taste buds in the circumvallate papillae and the pharyngeal portion of the tongue are innervated by the lingual branch of the glossopharyngeal nerve (IX). Taste buds on the epiglottis and extreme posterior portion of the tongue are innervated by the superior laryngeal branch of the vagus nerve (X).

Nerves to the taste buds lose their myelin sheath and branch profusely to form a subepithelial plexus from which branches enter the epithelium. Some arborize between the taste buds as *intergemmal fibers*; others, called *perigemmal fibers*, closely surround the taste buds; still others enter them and have terminal dilatations in intimate contact with the cells of the taste bud. The viability of the cells is dependent on their innervation. Sectioning of the nerve results in their disappearance. The cells of a taste bud are continuously turning over, and it is likely that nerves associated with degenerating cells retract and reestablish synapses with newly formed sensory cells. It was formerly thought that some of the cells of the taste buds were sensory and others supportive. This has now been challenged by the observation that all of the cells, both "light" and "dark," synapse with intragemmal nerve fibers. However, any given nerve fiber appears to receive its sensory input from cells of the same type. This is consistent with the hypothesis that there is some degree of specificity in the response of the cell types to different kinds of gustatory stimuli, but this has yet to be conclusively demonstrated.

SALIVARY GLANDS

A number of different kinds of salivary gland secrete into the oral cavity. For convenience, these are considered in two categories: the *minor salivary glands* and the *major salivary glands*. The minor glands are located in the mucosa and open directly, or via short ducts, onto the surface of the oral epithelium. They seem to secrete continuously, contributing to the *saliva* that moistens and lubricates the oral cavity. The major salivary glands include the *parotid, submandibular*, and *sublingual glands*. These are situated at some distance from the oral epithelium and are connected to it by a branching system of ducts that have clusters of glandular acini at their ends. These glands produce a large volume of secretion on mechanical or chemical stimulation of nerve endings in the oral mucosa. Some may also secrete in response to certain olfactory stimuli.

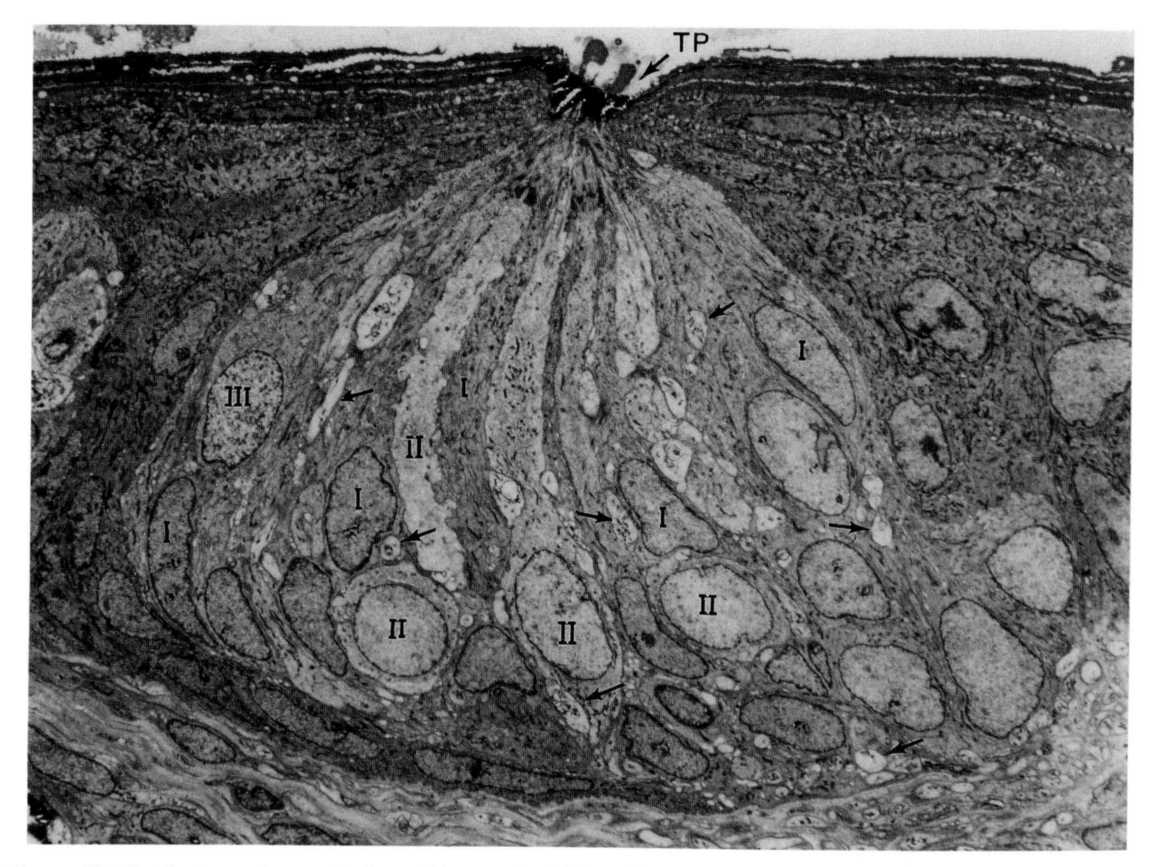

Figure 23–10. Electron micrograph of a rabbit taste bud. The cell types are indicated by Roman numerals and nerve axons by arrows. (Micrograph courtesy of S.M. Royer.)

Saliva is a mixture of the products of these several kinds of glands. It is a viscous, colorless, opalescent fluid containing water, mucoproteins, immunoglobulins, and inorganic ions, including calcium, potassium, sodium, chloride, and traces of iron. Among its protein constituents are enzymes such as amylase (ptyalin) which splits starch into smaller water-soluble carbohydrates. Also found in saliva are the so-called *salivary corpuscles* which are degenerating granulocytes and lymphocytes originating in the tonsils and lymph nodules on the back of the tongue.

The minor salivary glands are usually relatively short branching tubules lined with *mucous* cells. The major salivary glands are mixed glands in which the secretory portions are ovoid or elongated acini at the ends of a duct system with several orders of branching. Some acini are made up exclusively of *serous* cells; others entirely of mucous cells; and still others are *seromucous acini* in which the proximal pole consists of mucous cells and these are capped by a crescentic layer of serous cells, called a *serous demilune* (Fig. 23–12).

Many of the acini are continuous with the ends of secondary or tertiary branches of *intercalated ducts*, which are slender tubes lined by low cuboidal epithelial cells. Some acini on the sides of these ducts open into the lumen without an intervening short tertiary branch of the duct. The first order of intercalated ducts are continuous with *striated ducts* of larger diameter, lined by low columnar cells. These, in turn, converge on *excretory ducts* in each lobule that join the main duct opening into the oral cavity.

The secretions of the several salivary glands differ slightly. Saliva collected from the oral cavity may differ in its composition depending on the degree of participation of the several contributing glands, and the secretion from the same mixed gland may change somewhat with ingestion of different kinds of food.

MUCOUS ACINI

In mucous acini, a single layer of plump, pyramidal cells rest on a smooth basal lamina.

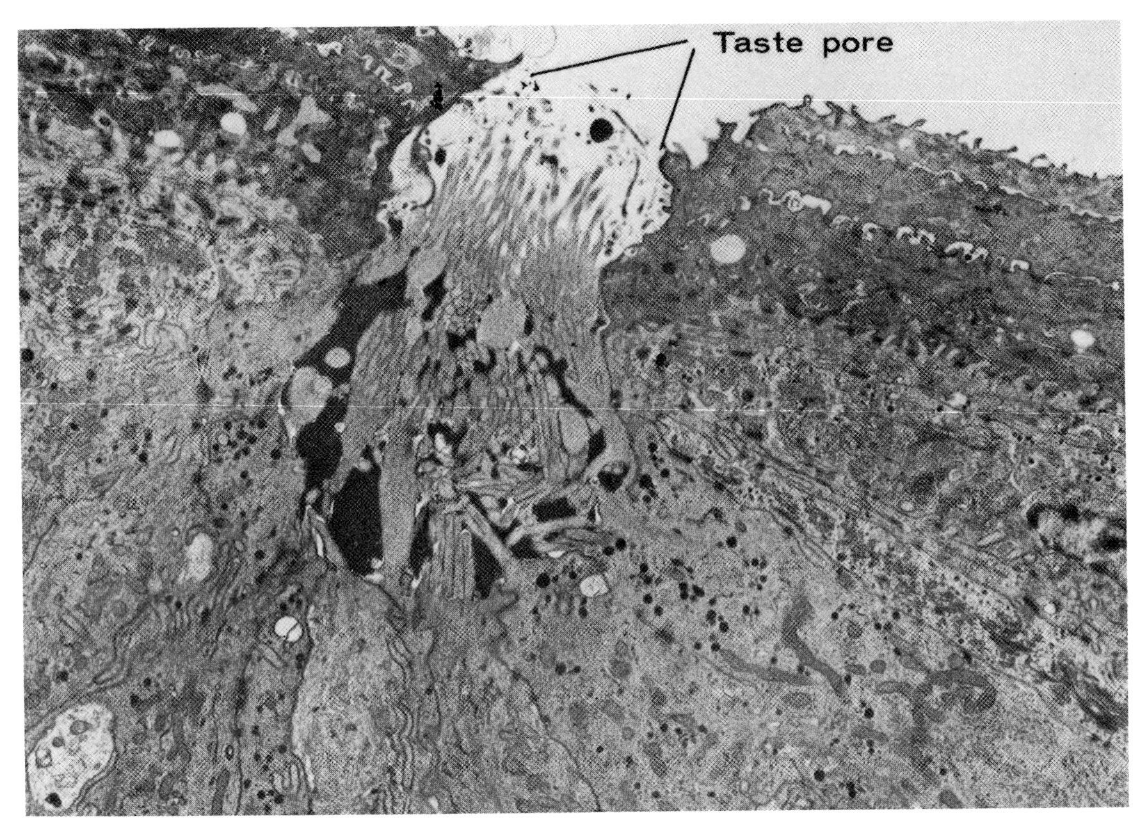

Figure 23–11. Electron micrograph of the pore region of a rabbit taste bud. Note the long microvilli on the sensory cells, surrounded by a dense amorphous secretory product. (Micrograph courtesy of M. Coppe.)

Their cytoplasm, in the fresh state, is filled with pale droplets of *mucigen*, the antecedent of mucus. In histological sections, the droplets of mucigen have usually been partially extracted during specimen preparation and appear as round clear areas outlined by a thin network of cytoplasm. Traces of mucigen that are preserved stain red with mucicarmine, or metachromatically with thionine. The nucleus is displaced far to the base of the cell and is often deformed by the accumulated secretory product that occupies the greater part of the cell volume. In preparation for electron microscopy, the mucigen is better preserved and appears as a pale gray content in membrane-limited droplets throughout the cytoplasm. The Golgi complex, a few mitochondria, and cisternae of rough endoplasmic reticulum are located in the basal cytoplasm with the compressed nucleus. The mucous cells are joined by juxtalumenal tight junctions and release their secretion from the apical cytoplasm into the slender lumen of the acinus. The lumen is often filled with precipitated mucin. The cells do not discharge all of their mucin under normal physiological conditions, but when strongly stimulated, only a few mucigen droplets may remain in the apical cytoplasm. They soon recover from this depleted state.

SEROUS ACINI

In serous acini, the cells have a columnar, or truncated pyramidal, form and surround a smaller lumen than that of mucous acini. Their apical cytoplasm is crowded with secretory granules. In some species, these have a homogeneous content of moderate electron density. In others, centrally or eccentrically placed dense areas are surrounded by material of lower density (Figs. 23–13 and 23–14). The disposition of the organelles is that typical of protein-secreting cells. A heterochromatic nucleus in the lower half of the cell is usually not deformed by accumulated secretory granules. The Golgi complex is in a supranuclear or paranuclear position and the surrounding basal cytoplasm contains mitochondria and numerous parallel cisternae of rough endo-

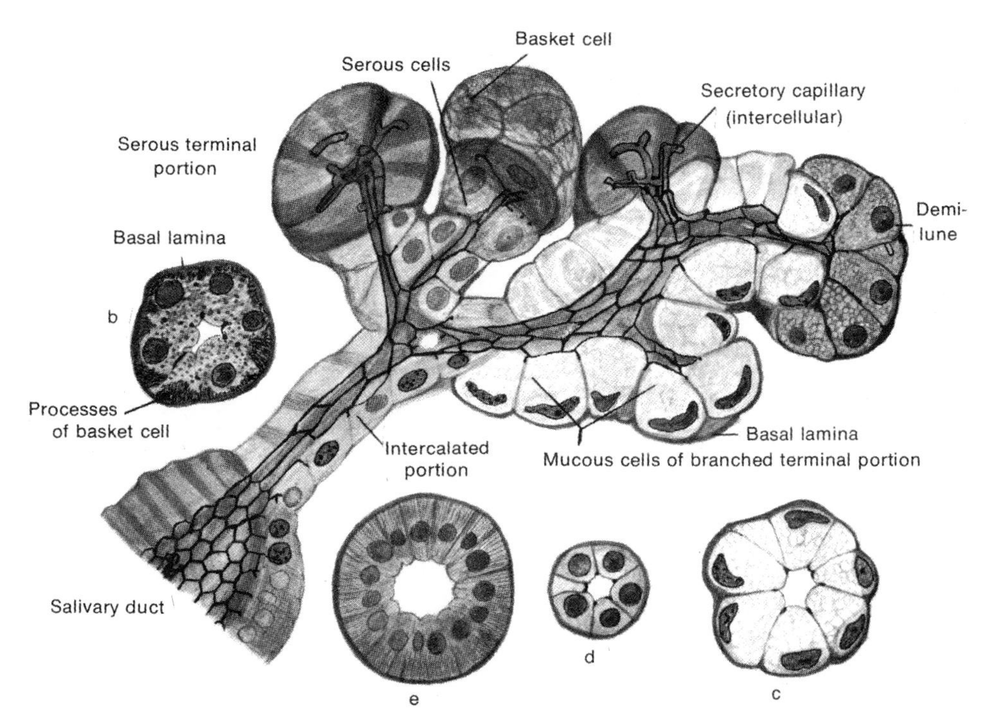

Figure 23–12. (A) Reconstruction of the terminal secretory portion of a major salivary gland and its ducts. (B) Cross section of a serous acinus; (C) cross section of a mucous acinus; (D) cross section of an intercalated duct; (E) cross section of a striated duct. (Redrawn and modified after a reconstruction by Vierling, from Braus, H. 1924. Lehrbuch der Anatomie, Vol 2, Berlin.)

plasmic reticulum. The serous cells of the human submandibular gland have slender radiating foot-processes that extend laterally and interdigitate with those of neighboring cells. This specialization greatly increases the surface area of the membrane nearest the blood supply and may increase the efficiency of their water and electrolyte transport. Another distinctive feature of the serous acini is the presence of *intercellular secretory canaliculi* that penetrate one-third to one-half the distance from the lumen to the basal lamina. The lumenal surface of the serous cells bears many short microvilli and these extend into the secretory canaliculi.

Although the organization of major salivary glands and the appearance of their cells in electron micrographs are much the same in different species, histochemical studies reveal differences that are correlated with interspecific variations in the composition of the saliva. The principal protein products of acinar cells are the enzymes amylase, lysozyme, peroxidase, desoxyribonuclease, and ribonuclease, but in some species, the secretory granules stain with the periodic-acid–Schiff reaction for carbohydrates and also contain sialomucin and sulfomucin in addition to enzymes. Such cells are termed *seromucous cells*. By this definition, the acini of the human parotid, usually identified as serous, are more correctly described as seromucous. Those of the submandibular gland are also seromucous, with some admixture of pure mucous acini. In the sublingual gland, the secretory end-pieces contain mainly mucous cells, but some seromucous cells are also present.

MIXED ACINI

Acini containing both serous and mucous cells were traditionally called *seromucous acini*, before the term seromucous came into use to describe a cell secreting both carbohydrates and protein. To avoid confusion, the term *mixed acini* may now be more appropriate. In such acini, the two types of cell are segregated, with the mucous cells occupying the proximal end and displacing the serous cells to the distal end, where they appear, in sections, as a crescentic cap of dark-staining cells called a *serous demilune* (demilune of Giannuzzi) (Figs. 23–15 and 23–16). The cells of this cap appear to be separated from the lumen of the acinus by the underlying mucous cells, but their se-

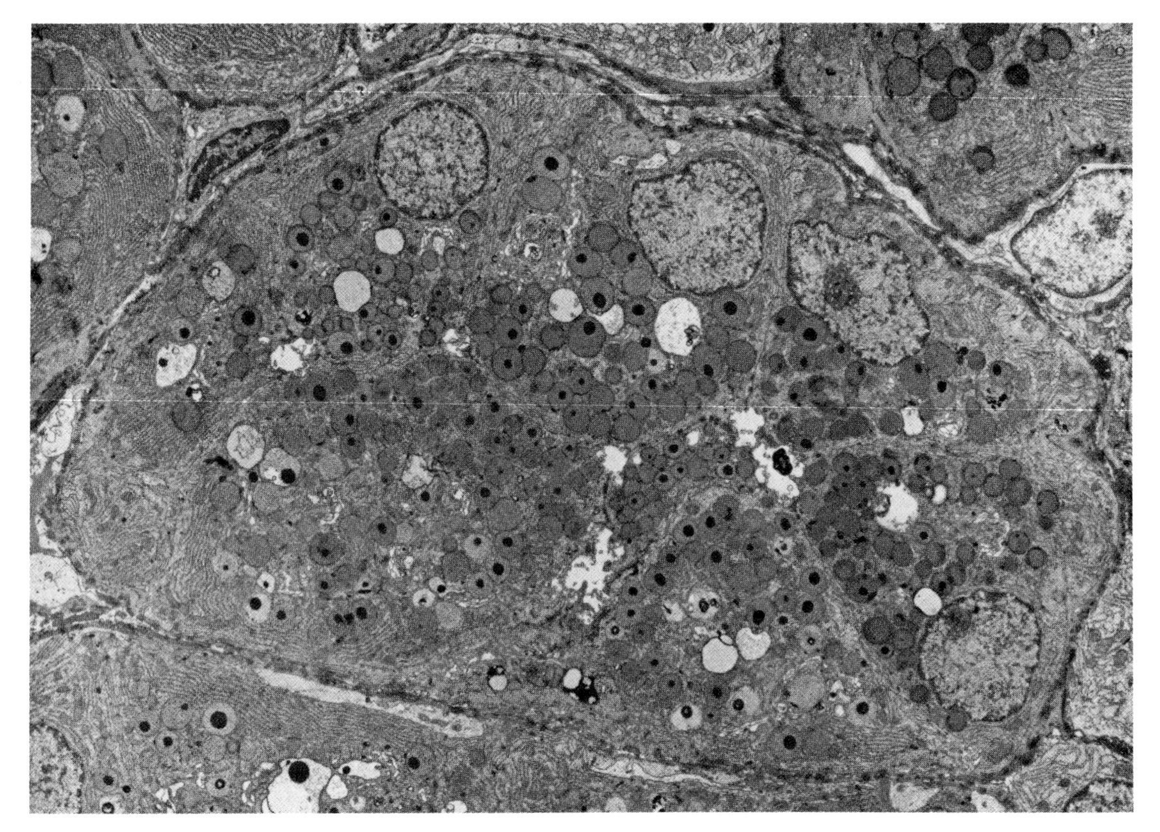

Figure 23–13. Electron micrograph of a serous acinus from human submandibular gland. The lumen of the acinus is not included in the section. (From Tandler, B. and R.A. Erlandson. 1972. Am. J. Anat. 135:419.)

cretion is conducted to the lumen of the acinus through narrow channels that can be found between the mucous cells.

Between the secretory cells and the basal lamina of all of the salivary acini, there are highly branched *myoepithelial cells*, formerly called basket cells. In sections, their radiating processes appear as rounded or fusiform anucleate profiles underlying the acinar cells. Their elaborate stellate form is appreciated only in whole mounts or scanning micrographs. In transmission electron micrographs, their cytoplasm resembles that of smooth muscle cells, containing many bundles of fine filaments oriented longitudinally in their processes. Their contraction is presumed to speed up the flow of saliva by constricting the lumen of the acini. They are also found around the intercalated ducts. Comparable cells are associated with the sweat glands in the skin and with the secretory portions of the mammary gland.

SALIVARY DUCTS

The intercalated ducts are lined by cuboidal epithelial cells devoid of significant ultrastructural specialization. Their complement of organelles is unremarkable and the plasma membrane shows only minimal surface amplification. In addition to serving as conduits for the fluid secretion, they may have a stem cell function. Cells at the junction of an intercalated duct with an acinus often contain a few secretory granules. These cells have been interpreted, by some investigators, as intermediates in the transformation of duct cells into acinar cells.

The much larger striated ducts, lined with a columnar epithelium, exhibit cytological specializations often associated with active electrolyte transport. The striation of the basal cytoplasm, noted with the light microscope, is found in electron micrographs to be due to the vertical alignment of numerous long mitochondria in narrow compartments formed, in part, by deep invaginations of the plasma membrane at the cell base. However, some of the compartments are not open at their top and these are evidently tall interdigitating processes of neighboring cells (Figs. 23–17 and 23–18). This elaborate basal specialization is like that seen in the epithelium lining certain segments of the nephron. By enor-

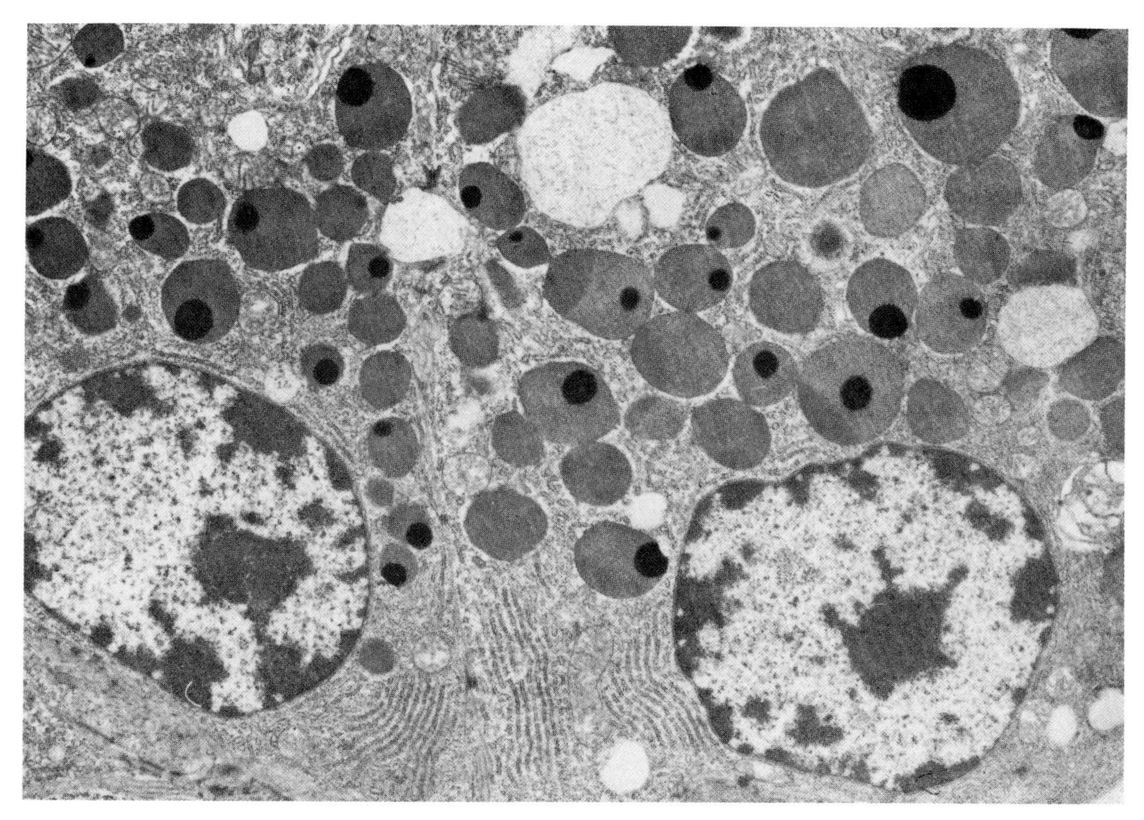

Figure 23–14. Electron micrograph of two serous cells from the submandibular gland of a rhesus monkey. Note the abundance of rough endoplasmic reticulum and the inhomogeneity of the secretory granules that have very dense and less dense regions. (Micrograph courtesy of A. Ichikawa.)

mously increasing the area of membrane associated with an energy source in the mitochondria, conditions are created for efficient active transport of water and ions to modify the primary secretion of the acini during its passage through the duct. In addition to altering the electrolyte composition of the saliva, the striated ducts are said to secrete lysozyme and kallikrein and to transport, into the saliva, immunoglobulin-A secreted by plasma cells.

The interlobular ducts course through the connective tissue stroma, becoming progressively larger and ultimately converge on the main duct that opens into the oral cavity. As the main duct approaches its opening onto the oral mucosa, its lining epithelium becomes stratified columnar for a short distance and then stratified squamous where it is continuous with the lining of the oral cavity.

DISTRIBUTION OF SALIVARY GLANDS

Having described the structural subunits and cytology of salivary glands, in general, we proceed now to additional remarks on specific glands in relation to the location of their openings into the oral cavity.

GLANDS OPENING INTO THE VESTIBULE

The narrow space between the gums and teeth, on the inside, and the cheeks and lips, on the outside, is commonly called the *vestibule* of the oral cavity. Several salivary glands open into this space. The largest of the major salivary glands are the *parotid glands* located subcutaneously on either side of the face below and anterior to the ears. They extend from the zygomatic arch above to below the angle of the jaw. Their long duct (Stenson's duct) passes through the facial muscles to open on a small papilla on the inside of the cheek, opposite the second upper molar. In the human, the cells of its acini are predominantly seromucous with mucous acini being relatively uncommon.

Among the minor salivary glands opening into the vestibule are *labial glands* between the

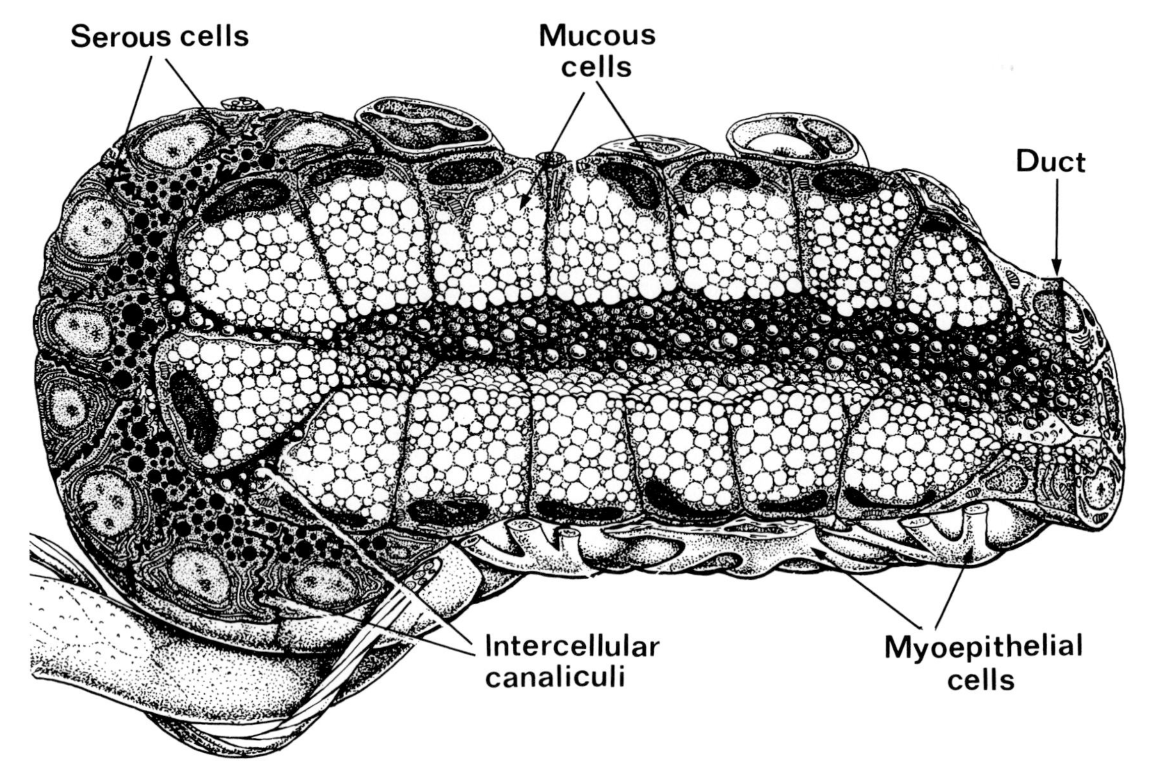

Figure 23–15. Drawing of a tubuloacinar end-piece in the human submandibular gland. Note the pale mucous cells capped by a serous demilune. (From Krstic, R.V. 1978. Die Gewebe des Menschen und Saugetiere. Berlin, Springer-Verlag.)

mucosa and the orbicularis oris muscle in the upper and lower lips and *buccal glands* distributed beneath the mucosa on the inner aspect of the cheek. Mucous cells predominate in both, but seromucous cells occur in demilunes at the ends of some acini. Intercalated ducts are very short or absent with mucus-secreting segments often passing directly into striated ducts.

GLANDS OPENING ON THE FLOOR OF THE MOUTH

The *submandibular glands* are situated, on either side, between the mandible and the muscles that form the floor of the mouth. Their duct (Wharton's duct) runs forward to open on the sublingual papilla at the side of the frenulum of the tongue. Like the parotid, this is a mixed gland with serous (seromucous) acini more numerous than mucous acini. Mixed acini with typical serous demilunes are less common in the human than in the submandibular gland of other species. The intercalated ducts are relatively short, whereas the striated ducts are longer than those of the parotid.

The *sublingual glands* are 3–4 cm long and located deep in the mucous membrane of the floor of the mouth on either side of the frenulum, and near the symphysis of the mandible. The duct often joins that of the submandibular gland but may open separately on the sublingual papilla. Like the other major glands, it is a mixed gland. About 60% of its acini are mucous and 30% serous. The striated ducts are poorly developed and may be represented only by small groups of basally striated cells in the epithelium of the interlobular ducts.

GLANDS OF THE TONGUE

The *anterior lingual glands* are located in the under side of the tip of the tongue, on either side of the frenulum. Their three or four ducts open on the under side of the tip of the tongue. The anterior portion of the gland is made up of tubules lined with serous cells (Fig. 23–19 B). In its posterior portion, branching tubules are lined with mucous cells but these

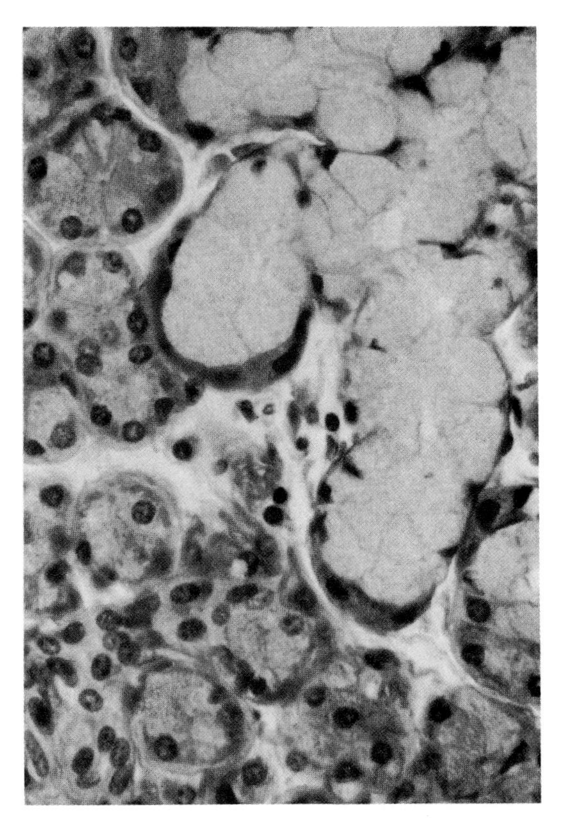

Figure 23–16. Photomicrograph of human submandibular gland showing serous acini at the lower left, and mixed acini of mucous cells and serous demilunes at the upper right.

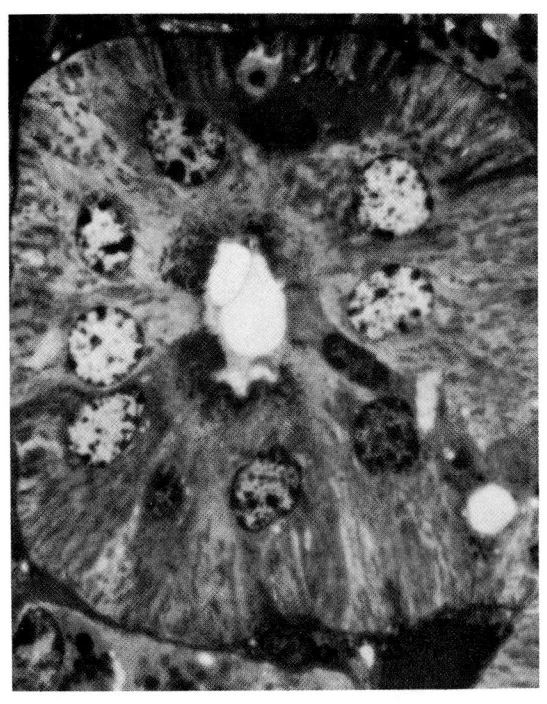

Figure 23–17. Photomicrograph of a striated duct from the parotid gland of a marmoset. Note the orientation of long mitochondria parallel to the cell axis, giving the basal cytoplasm a vertically striated appearance. (Micrograph courtesy of B. Tandler.)

may have thin demilunes of serous cells at their blind ends. The *glands of von Ebner* are serous glands associated with the circumvallate papillae (Figs. 23–6 and 23–7). Their watery secretion is released into the sulcus around the papilla where it may promote uniform diffusion of substances to the taste buds and may serve to wash out the sulcus. Other very small mucous and mixed glands are found in the back of the tongue.

HISTOPHYSIOLOGY OF THE SALIVARY GLANDS

The human salivary glands secrete continuously at a basal rate of about 0.5–1.0 ml/min, but the flow is increased many fold in response to the presence of food in the mouth. The total daily flow is estimated to be 1 liter or more. In addition to its function of moistening and lubricating ingested food, its enzyme α-amylase initiates the digestive process by hydrolyzing starch to soluble sugars.

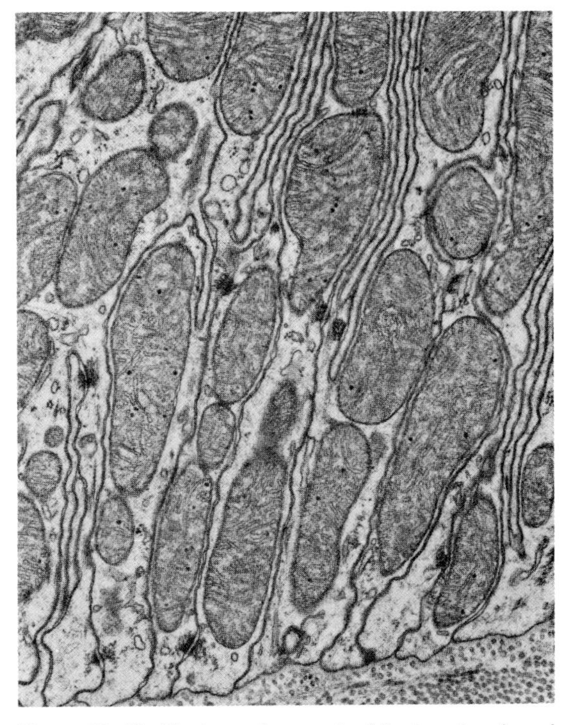

Figure 23–18. Electron micrograph of the basal region of a striated duct from cat submandibular gland. Note the desmosomes joining the interdigitating basal processes of neighboring cells. (Micrograph courtesy of B. Tandler.)

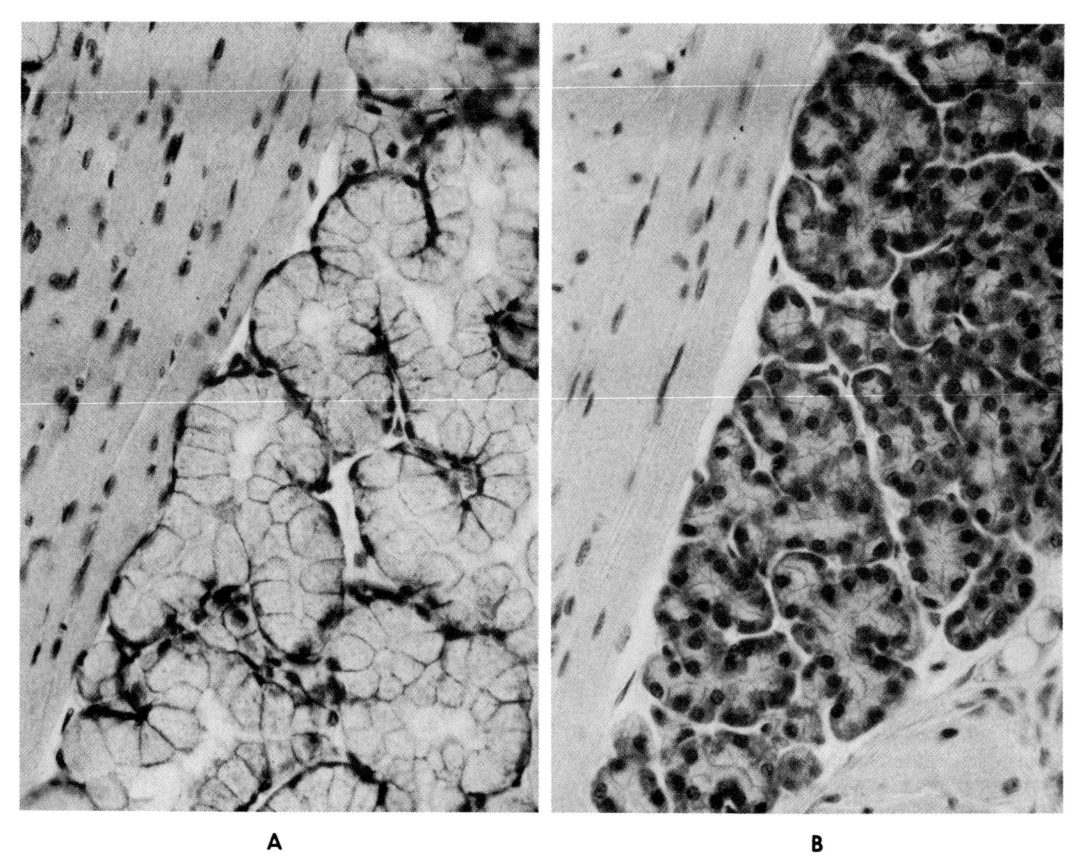

Figure 23–19. Lingual glands situated among bundles of striated muscle in rabbit tongue. (A) Mucous glands; (B) serous glands.

Saliva also has an important role in controlling the bacterial flora of the oral cavity. This cavity is normally inhabited by a very large number and variety of potentially pathogenic bacteria which contribute to dental caries and can initiate serious periodontal disease. Their numbers are held in check by the continual secretion and swallowing of saliva. In addition, saliva has bacteriostatic properties. The enzyme lysozyme, secreted by the serous cells of the salivary acini, has as its principal function the hydrolysis of bacterial cell walls. Deprived of their walls, bacteria are easily penetrated and destroyed by thiocyanate ions that are also present in saliva. Another bacteriostatic mechanism depends on the lymphocytes and plasma cells in the connective tissue stroma of the salivary glands. These produce immunoglobulin-A which forms a complex with a so-called secretory-piece that is synthesized by serous cells of the salivary acini. This complex, secreted in the saliva, is believed to participate in immunological defense against oral bacteria.

The primary secretion formed by the salivary acini has an ionic composition not significantly different from that of blood plasma or extracellular fluid. As it flows through the duct system, it is greatly modified by active transport of some ions and passive reabsorption of others. Sodium ions are actively reabsorbed and potassium ions are actively transported into the lumen. Bicarbonate ions are actively secreted and chloride ions are passively reabsorbed. As a result of these active transport processes and ion exchanges, the sodium and chloride concentration of the saliva is about one-eighth that of blood plasma, whereas bicarbonate is three times, and potassium is seven times, greater than that of plasma. The adrenal hormone, aldosterone, that controls absorption of sodium and excretion of potassium in the kidney also influences the electrolyte composition of the saliva. Act-

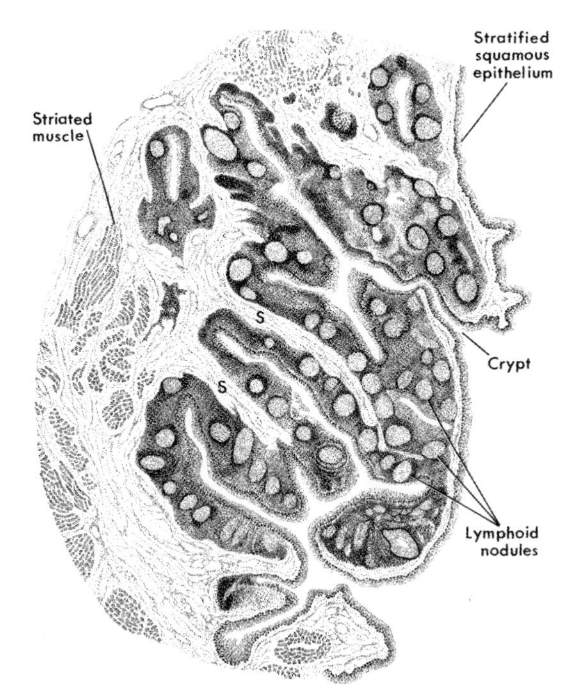

Figure 23–20. Drawing of a section through the human palatine tonsil showing crypts penetrating the tonsil from its free surface and connective tissue septa (S) penetrating the lymphoid tissue from beneath. (Redrawn and modified from J. Sobotta, Atlas of Human Anatomy, Vol. II. G.E. Stechert & Co, New York, 1936.)

ing on cells of the duct epithelium, it greatly increased reabsorption of sodium and excretion of potassium.

TONSILS

Between the glossopalatine and pharyngopalatine arches at the boundary between the mouth and the oropharynx are the *palatine tonsils,* two large ovoid accumulations of lymphoid tissue beneath the mucous membrane. The overlying stratified squamous epithelium is invaginated into the lymphoid tissue to form 15 or more *tonsillar crypts.* The crypts may be simple or branched and they extend nearly to a condensation of connective tissue that forms a capsule around the tonsil (Fig. 23–20). The lymphoid tissue consists of lymphatic nodules immediately beneath the epithelium along the sides of the crypts and these may have prominent germinal centers. Thin partitions of connective tissue may extend inward from the capsule, separating the masses of lymphoid tissue associated with the crypts. Mast cells and plasma cells abound in this connective tissue and there are varying numbers of polymorphonuclear leukocytes (Fig. 23–21). These may be very numerous when the tonsils are the site of serious inflammation. In the deeper portions of the crypts, the boundary between the epithelium and the lymphoid tissue is obscured by infiltration of the epithelium by very numerous lymphocytes which displace and distort the epithelial cells to such an extent that only a few epithelial cells at the surface are recognizable.

The lymphocytes and neutrophils that migrate through the epithelium are found in the saliva as *salivary corpuscles.* In the fresh state, these degenerating cells appear as vesicular structures containing a pycnotic nucleus and granules that show brownian movement. Those originating from polymorphonuclear leukocytes are distinguishable by their polymorphous nucleus and remanents of their specific granules.

Numerous small glands associated with the mucosa of the tonsil are outside of its capsule and their ducts open onto the surface. Few or none open into the crypts, where their secretion could wash detritus out of their lumen. The lumen of the crypts may, therefore, contain large accumulations of living and degenerating lymphocytes, exfoliated epithelial cells, and bacteria. These masses may increase in size to form cheesy plugs. As a rule, these are ultimately extruded, but if retained for a long time, they may become calcified.

In the midline of the roof and posterior wall of the nasopharynx is the unpaired *pharyngeal tonsil.* The epithelium covering this accumulation of lymphoid tissue is pseudostratified ciliated columnar epithelium like that in the rest of the nasopharynx. However, small patches of stratified squamous epithelium are not uncommon. Here, the epithelium is not invaginated to form crypts like those of the palatine tonsil but is plicated to form multiple surface folds. It is abundantly infiltrated with lymphocytes, especially on the crests of the folds. A 2-mm-thick layer of diffuse and nodular lymphoid tissue underlies the epithelium and participates in creation of the folds. The lymphoid tissue is surrounded by a thin connective tissue capsule which sends thin partitions into the core of each fold. Outside of this capsule are small mixed glands with ducts that are often markedly dilated. These traverse the lymphoid tissue and open onto the

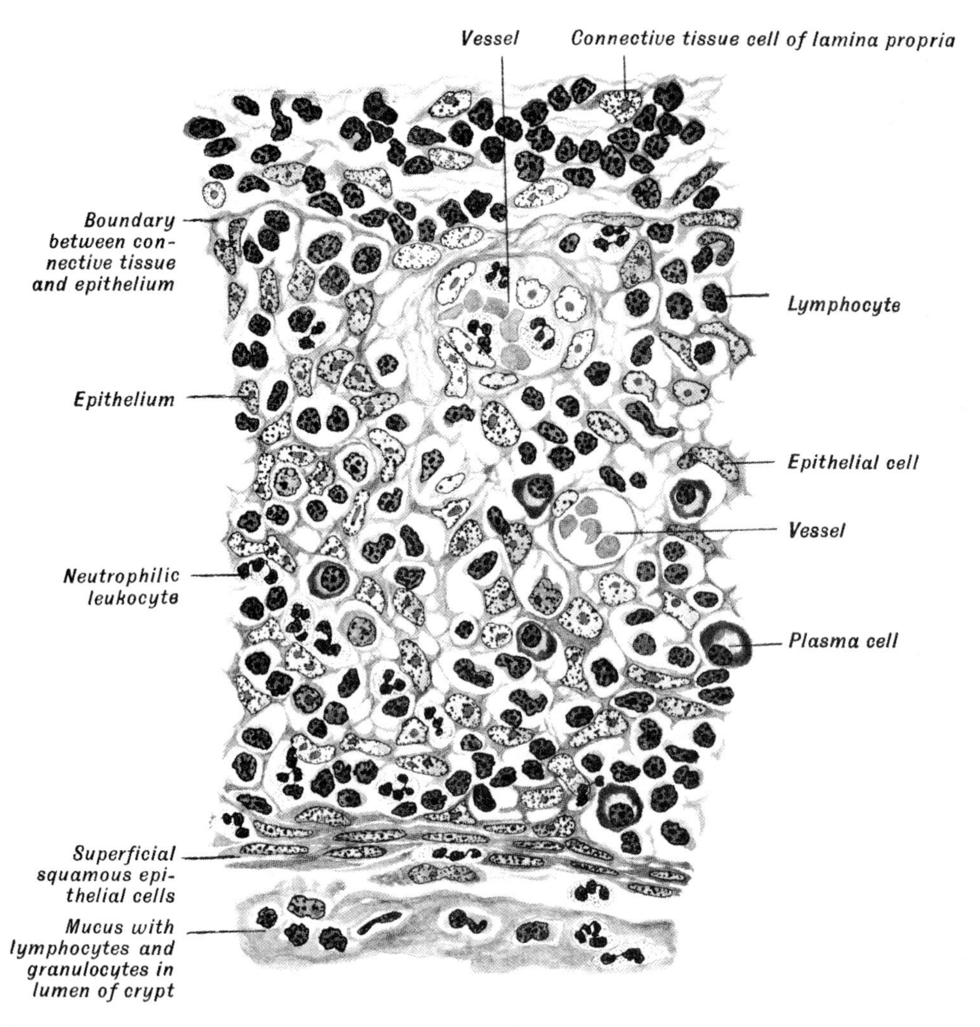

Figure 23–21. Drawing from a section of human palatine tonsil showing extensive infiltration of the epithelium of a crypt with lymphocytes, granulocytes, and plasma cells.

surface of the folds or into the furrows between them. Unlike lymph nodes, tonsils do not have lymphatic sinuses and lymph is not filtered through them. However, their outer surface is surrounded by blind-ending lymphatic capillaries.

Other small accumulations of lymphoid tissue occur in the mucous membrane of the pharynx, especially around the orifices of the eustachian tubes, on the pharyngeopalatine arches and in the posterior wall.

Tonsils generally reach their maximal development in childhood. Their involution begins around the age of 15 or earlier. In the adult, the pharyngeal tonsil is usually found in an atrophic condition with its ciliated epithelium largely replaced by stratified squamous epithelium.

THE PHARYNX

In the posterior continuation of the oral cavity, called the *pharynx*, the respiratory tract and the pathway for food merge and cross, so that, in breathing, air is conducted across this chamber to the larynx and, in eating, food passes through it to the esophagus. Three regions of this cavity are distinguished: the *nasopharynx*, the *oropharynx*, and the *laryngeal pharynx*. The mucosa in the nasopharynx is similar to that of the respiratory tract, whereas in the oropharynx and laryngeal pharynx, it corresponds to that of the digestive tract.

The pharyngeal mucosa lacks a muscularis mucosae and deep in the lamina propria there is a thick, dense fibrous layer rich in elastic fibers that rests on the underlying pharyngeal muscle which consists of inner longitudinal and outer oblique or longitudinal striated fibers. The fibroelastic layer is continuous with the interstitial connective tissue of the muscle, sending strands between the bundles of muscle fibers.

The oropharynx and laryngeal pharynx are lined by stratified squamous epithelium, and, in these regions, glands of a pure mucous type are found. They are always located beneath the elastic layer, and sometimes penetrate some distance into the muscle. Glands of mixed type, similar to those of the dorsal surface of the soft palate, are confined to the upper regions of the pharynx, covered by ciliated epithelium.

BIBLIOGRAPHY

GENERAL

Chen, S.Y. and C.A. Squier. 1984. *In* J. Meyer, C.A. Squier, and S.J. Gerson, eds. The Structure and Function of Oral Mucosa, pp. 7–30. Oxford, Pergamon Press.

TONGUE AND TASTE BUDS

Beidler, L.M. and R.L. Smallman. 1965. Renewal of cells within the taste buds. J. Cell Biol. 27:263.

Delay, R.J., J.C. Kinnamon, and S.D. Roper. 1986. Ultrastructure of mouse vallate taste buds: II. Cell types and cell lineage. J. Comp. Neurol. 270:1.

Farbman, A.I., G. Hellecant, and A. Nelson. 1985. Structure of the taste buds in foliate papillae of the Rhesus monkey. Am. J. Anat. 172:41.

Farbman, A.L. 1980. Renewal of taste bud cells in rat circumvallate papillae. Cell Tissue Kinetics 13:349.

Hodgson, E.S. 1961. Taste receptors. Sci. Am. 204:135.

Ide, C. and B. Munger. 1980. Cytological composition of laryngeal chemosensory corpuscles. Am. J. Anat. 158:193.

Kinnamon, J.C. 1987. Organization and innervation of taste buds. *In* T.E. Finger, ed. Neurobiology of Taste and Smell. New York, John Wiley and Sons.

Kinnamon, J.C. 1988. Taste transduction: A diversity of mechanisms. Trends Neurosci. 11:491.

Murray, R.G. 1986. The mammalian taste bud Type III cell: A critical analysis. J. Ultrastr. Res. 95:175.

Oakley, B. and R.P. Benjamin. 1966. Neural mechanisms of taste. Physiol. Rev. 46:173.

Zotterman, Y. 1963. Olfaction and Taste. New York, Macmillan Co.

SALIVARY GLANDS

Amsterdam, A., I. Ohad, and M. Schramm. 1969. Dynamic changes in the ultrastructure of the acinar cell of the rat parotid gland during the secretory cycle. J. Cell Biol. 41:753.

Castle, J.D., J.D. Jamieson, and G.E. Palade. 1972. Radioautographic analysis of the secretory process in the parotid acinar cell of the rabbit. J. Cell Biol. 53:290.

Leeson, C.R. 1967. Structure of the salivary glands. *In* Handbook of Physiology, Vol. 2, Sect. 6. Washington, DC American Physiological Society.

Munger, B.L. 1964. Histochemical studies on seromucous and mucus-secreting cells of human salivary glands. Am. J. Anat. 115:411.

Mason, D.K. and D.M. Chisholm, 1975. Salivary Glands in Health and Disease. London, W.B. Saunders Co.

Shackleford, J. and C.E. Klapper. 1962. Structure and carbohydrate histochemistry of mammalian salivary glands. Am. J. Anat. 111:25.

Tamarin, A. 1966. Myoepithelium of the rat submaxillary gland. J. Ultrastr. Res. 16:320.

Tandler, B. 1962. Ultrastructure of the human submaxillary gland. I. Architecture and histological relationships of the secretory cells. Am. J. Anat. 11:287.

Tandler, B. 1963. Ultrastructure of the human submaxillary gland. II. The base of the striated duct cells. J. Ultrastr. Res. 9:165.

Young, J.A. 1979. Salivary secretion of inorganic electrolytes. Internat. Rev. Physiol. 19:1.

Young, J.A. and E.W. VanLennep. 1977. Morphology and physiology of salivary myoepithelial cells. Internat. Rev. Physiol. 12:105.

24

THE TEETH

The adult human has 32 teeth of which 16 are in the alveolar process of the maxilla and 16 are in the mandible. These so-called permanent teeth are preceded by a set of 20 *deciduous teeth* that begin to emerge about 7 months after birth and reach their full complement at 6–8 years of age. These teeth are shed between the sixth and thirteenth year and are gradually replaced by the permanent, or *succedaneous teeth*. This process of tooth replacement extends over a period of about 12 years until full dentition is attained, usually by the eighteenth year, with the eruption of the third molars or wisdom teeth. Each of the several types of teeth has a distinctive shape adapted to its specific function. Thus, the chisel-like *incisors* are specialized for cutting or shearing; the pointed *canines* for puncturing and holding; and the *molars* for crushing and grinding.

All teeth consist of a *crown* projecting above the gums or gingiva and one or more tapering *roots* that occupy conforming sockets or *alveoli* in the bone of the maxilla or mandible. The junctional region between the crown and the root is called the *neck* or *cervix*. Incisors have a single root; lower molars have two; and upper molars have three. The tooth has a small central cavity or *pulp chamber* that corresponds roughly, in its shape, to the outer form of the tooth. This cavity continues downward into each root as a narrow *root canal* that communicates with the *periodontal membrane* through an *apical foramen* at the tip of the root. The blood vessels, nerves, and lymphatics enter and leave the tooth through the apical foramen.

The hard portions of a tooth consist of three different tissues: *dentin, enamel,* and *cementum* (Fig. 24–1). The bulk of the tooth is made up of dentin, which surrounds the pulp chamber. This layer is thickest in the crown and tapers to a thinner layer toward the apex of the root. In the crown, this is covered by a layer of *enamel* which is thinnest in the cervical region. On the root, the enamel is covered by a thin layer of *cementum* which extends from the neck to the apical foramen.

The soft parts associated with the tooth are the *pulp* which occupies the pulp chamber, the *periodontal membrane* which binds the cementum-covered surface of the root to the alveolar bone, and the *gingiva*, that portion of the oral mucous membrane surrounding the teeth and overlying the alveolar process. In young persons, the gingiva is attached to the enamel, but with increasing age it recedes from the enamel, and in old persons it is attached to the cementum.

For descriptive purposes, terms have been adopted for the various surfaces of teeth. The inner surface that faces the tongue is the *lingual surface*. The surface toward the cheek is the *buccal* surface, and for teeth in the anterior portion of the dental arch, it is the *labial* surface. On the sides of the arch, the anterior surface, that facing toward the midline of the arch, is its *mesial* surface, whereas the opposite side is its *distal* surface. At the front of the arch, the mesial surface is that facing toward

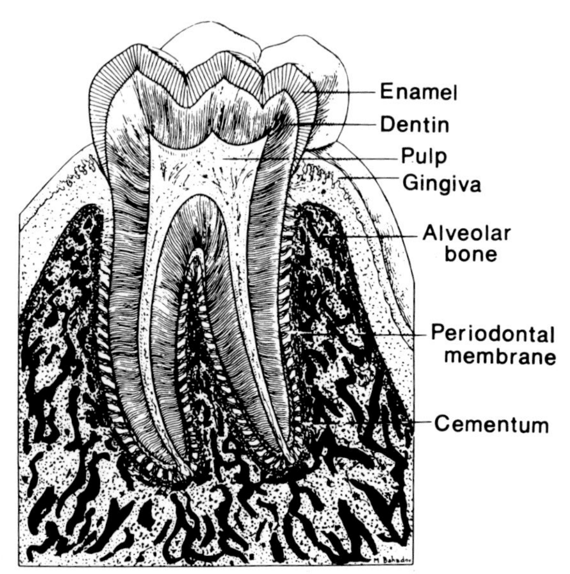

Figure 24–1. Diagram of a saggital section of a human lower first molar tooth. (Courtesy of I. Schour.)

the midline and the opposite side is its distal surface.

DENTIN

Dentin is semitranslucent, in the fresh condition, and slightly yellow in color. It is similar to bone in chemical composition but is considerably harder. It is 20% organic and 80% inorganic matter. The organic portion is 92% collagen and its inorganic portion consists mainly of crystals of hydroxyapatite. Teeth are studied in histological sections after removal of the hard inorganic constituents with acid, or in thin ground sections without decalcification.

In a ground section through the axis of a tooth, the dentin has a radially striated appearance due to the presence of innumerable minute parallel *dentinal tubules* that radiate from the pulp cavity toward the dentinoenamel junction. Each tubule contains the long apical process of an *odontoblast*. The dentin-producing odontoblasts are columnar cells that form an epithelial layer around the periphery of the pulp cavity immediately beneath the inner surface of the dentin. These cells are less closely adherent on their lateral surfaces than the cells of most epithelia, and capillaries can occasionally be found between them. The elongated nuclei are in the basal cytoplasm, but at different levels, resulting in a less uniform alignment than in most epithelia. The basal cytoplasm is basophilic in histological sections and, in electron micrographs, it contains many cisternae of rough endoplasmic reticulum. There is a large supranuclear Golgi complex. Dilated portions of its trans-cisterna, and vesicles associated with it, have a filamentous content believed to be *procollagen*. As these secretory vesicles, or granules, mature, their content becomes organized into parallel beaded strands. The apical portion of the cell tapers down to a slender *odontoblast process* that extends into a dentinal tubule (Fig. 24–2). The process may contain a few mitochondria, microtubules, thin filaments, and secretory granules. The latter can be found fusing with the plasma membrane to discharge their content. On discharge, the procollagen is cleaved to tropocollagen macromolecules and these polymerize to form the collagen fibers in the *predentin*, an unmineralized zone around the proximal portions of the odontoblast processes. At the base of the tapering apical portion of the cell, it is traversed by a terminal web and joined to neighboring cells by typical junctional complexes. Just above this region, the process may have short lateral branches. It is usually not possible to determine how far the odontoblast processes extend into the dentinal tubules. In de-

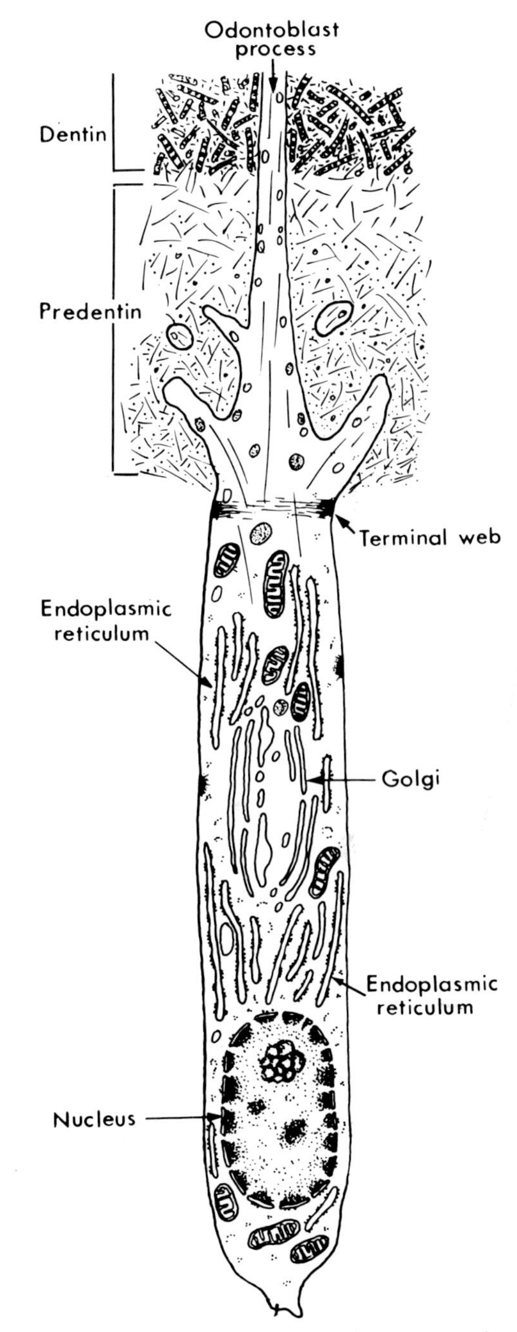

Figure 24–2. Drawing depicting the ultrastructure of a typical odontoblast from a developing rat incisor. (Redrawn after Weinstock, M. and C.P. Leblond. 1974. J. Cell Biol. 60:92.)

veloping teeth, and those of young individuals, they probably extend to their ends, but in older persons, the distal portion regresses and the lumen of the tubule beyond is filled with fluid.

There is an abrupt transition from the predentin to dentin that is called the *mineralization front*. Beyond this line, the collagen fibers are thicker and their cross-striation is masked by crystallites of hydroxyapatite. The fibers are randomly oriented except near the odontoblast process where they tend to run parallel to its surface and are the major component of the wall of the dentinal tubule. This area immediately surrounding the odontoblast process stains more intensely and is highly birefringent in polarized light owing to the close packing and parallel orientation of the collagen fibers. It is also stained with the periodic-acid–Schiff reaction indicating the presence of glycosaminoglycans. It also stains more intensely.

The dentinal tubules are not straight throughout their length, but have a slight S-shaped *primary curvature* and a helical *secondary curvature* with an amplitude of a few microns. Near their ends, they may branch and a few

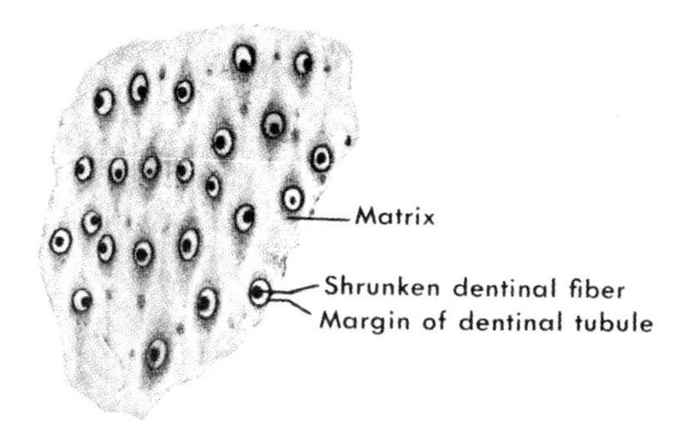

Figure 24–4. Tangential section through the dentin of a molar tooth showing cross sections of dentinal tubules. They are outlined by a denser zone and have a dot in the center which is the shrunken odontoblast process (Tome's fiber). (After Schaffer, J., Lehrbuch der Histologie und Histogenese. W. Engelmann Press, Leipzig, 1922.)

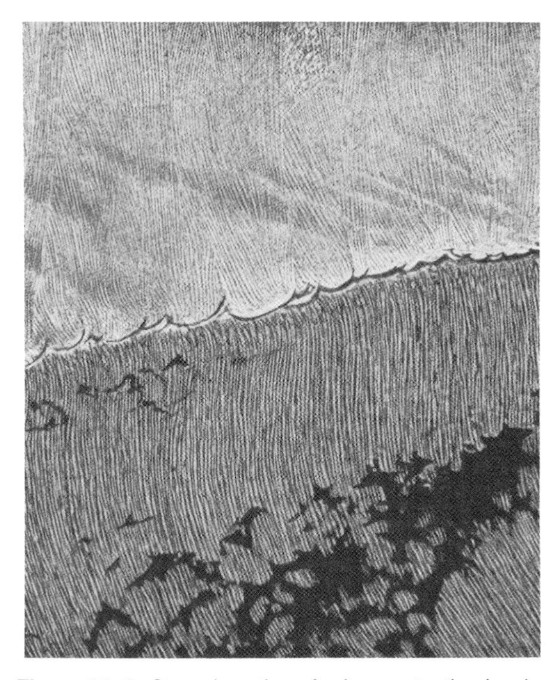

Figure 24–3. Ground section of a human tooth, showing enamel (top) and dentin (bottom). The enamel prisms appear as fine wavy striations. Tubules of the dentin appear darker. Note, in the dentin, the irregular, air-filled interglobular spaces which appear black. (After Braus, H. Lehrbuch der Anatomie. Vol 2. Berlin, 1924.)

branches may penetrate a short distance into the enamel as *enamel spindles*.

Calcification of developing dentin is not uniform. Mineral deposits initially appear as globular aggregations of apatite crystals that occur along, or within, collagen fibers. These nuclei of mineralization gradually enlarge and fuse, but occasional angular spaces containing only the organic matrix of dentin persist between them (Fig. 24–3). The dentinal tubules continue uninterrupted through the calcified globules and *interglobular spaces*. In the crown of adult human teeth, layers of sizable interglobular spaces persist in the deeper part of the dentin. In the root of the tooth, there is always a layer of small interglobular spaces, the *granular layer of Tomes*, immediate beneath the junction of the cementum with the dentin.

In sections of decalcified teeth, examined with the light microscope, cross sections of dentinal tubules appear as oval profiles each containing a central dot, surrounded by a clear area (Fig. 24–4). Before they were identified as the processes of odontoblasts, the dots were called *dentinal fibers* or *Tome's fibers*. The surrounding space, seen in histological sections, is now regarded as a fixation artifact. In the living tooth, the odontoblast process probably completely fills the lumen of the tubule.

Dentin continues to be formed slowly throughout life and the pulp cavity is progressively narrowed with advancing age. In old age, excessive calcification may completely obliterate the lumen of the dentinal tubules. The dentin then becomes more translucent. If dentin is exposed, by excessive abrasion of the overlying enamel, irregular masses of *secondary dentin* may be deposited on the wall of

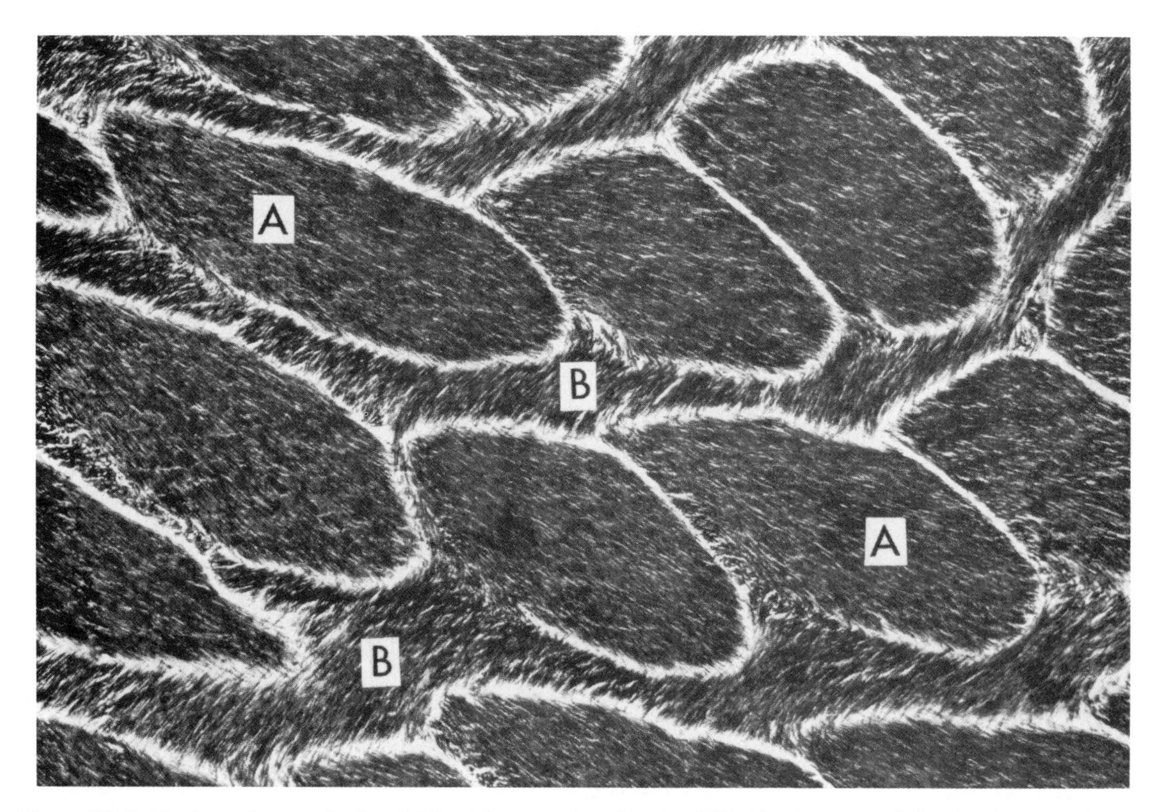

Figure 24–5. Electron micrograph of a slightly oblique section of undecalcified bovine enamel showing the enamel rods, or prisms (A) and the interprismatic enamel (B). Note the very regular orientation of the hydroxyapatite crystals within the rods and the differing orientation of the crystals in the interprismatic enamel. (Courtesy of E.J. Daniel and M.J. Glimcher.)

the pulp chamber. In rare instances, this may be so extensive as to completely replace the pulp.

The dentin is sensitive to touch, to cold, and to acid-containing foods. The pulp is richly innervated, but only a few nerves penetrate a very short distance into the dentin, and it has been suggested that the odontoblast processes may transmit sensory stimuli from the dentin to the pulp, but this remains to be demonstrated.

ENAMEL

Dental enamel is the hardest substance found in the body. It is bluish white and nearly transparent. Ninety-nine percent of its weight is mineral in the form of large hydroxyapatite crystals. The organic matrix makes up no more than 1% of its mass. Viewed with the light microscope, the enamel consists of thin *enamel rods* or *prisms* that stand upright on the dentin with a pronounced inclination toward the incisal or occlusal surface. Between groups of parallel enamel rods are angular spaces (interprismatic regions) occupied by interrod enamel that has a substructure very much like that of the rods, but its crystals of mineral are oriented in a different direction. Around each rod is a thin clear layer of organic matrix called the *enamel sheath* or *prismatic rod sheath*. Although the rods run through the entire thickness of the enamel layer, this is not obvious in ground sections because they have a sinuous course and soon leave the plane of the section.

Studies with the electron microscope show that the enamel rods and interrod regions are both made up of hydroxyapatite crystals in an organic matrix. The relation of the crystals in the rods to the interrod enamel is clearly shown in Figs. 24–5 and 24–6. In the human tooth, the rods in cross section are variously described as fluted semicircles, or keyhole-shaped prisms with their convex surfaces all facing in the same direction, resulting in an appearance reminiscent of the pattern of scales on reptilian skin (Fig. 24–7). The rod consists of groups of very long, thin, ribbon-

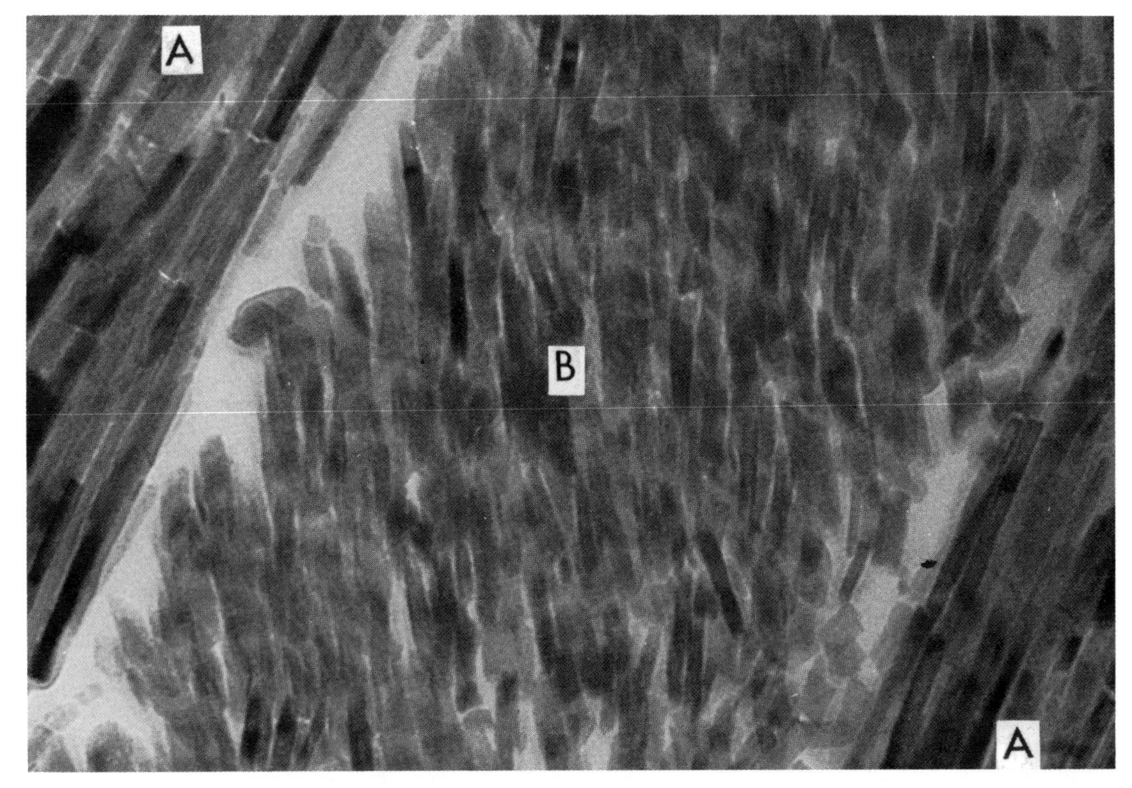

Figure 24–6. Electron micrograph, at higher magnification than that of Fig. 24–5, showing the longitudinal orientation of the prismatic crystals (A) and the interprismatic crystals which are oriented at approximately 30° to those of the enamel prisms. 100,000×. (Courtesy of E.J. Daniel and M.J. Glimcher.)

like crystallites of hydroxyapatite that run parallel to one another for its entire length. The relation of the organic matrix to the crystallites is not clear. After decalcification, a thin layer of stainable material outlines the spaces formerly occupied by hydroxyapatite. This material is presumed to be organic matrix, but whether it is on the surface of crystallites or within their periphery is unsettled.

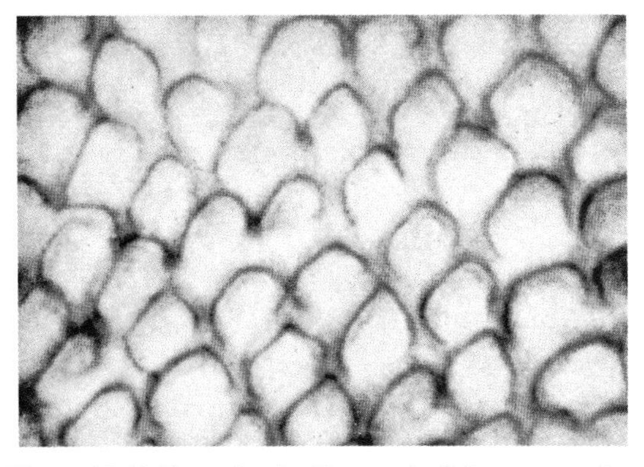

Figure 24–7. Enamel rods of human tooth in cross section. The dark lines are the interprismatic substance between the pale rods. Photomicrograph at high magnification. (Courtesy of B. Orban.)

The exact course of the enamel rods in human teeth is complex and still subject to differing interpretations. Each prism appears to undulate in the transverse plane of the tooth, but its undulations are slightly out-of-phase with those of the rod above and below it. Thus, there is also an undulation of columns of prisms in the vertical plane in addition to that in the transverse plane. As a consequence of this arrangement, the direction of curves in the rods at one level crosses that of rods at a deeper level. When a longitudinal section of a tooth is viewed by reflected light, there is an alternation of light bands with darker bands where directions of curvature cross. These bands traverse the enamel obliquely and are called the *lines of Schreger* (Fig. 24–8). In a cross section of the crown of a tooth, there are also concentric lines in the enamel that appear brown in transmitted light and colorless or bluish in reflected light. In undecalcified longitudinal sections, these are seen to run obliquely inward from the surface toward the pulp. These are called *lines of Retzius*, or

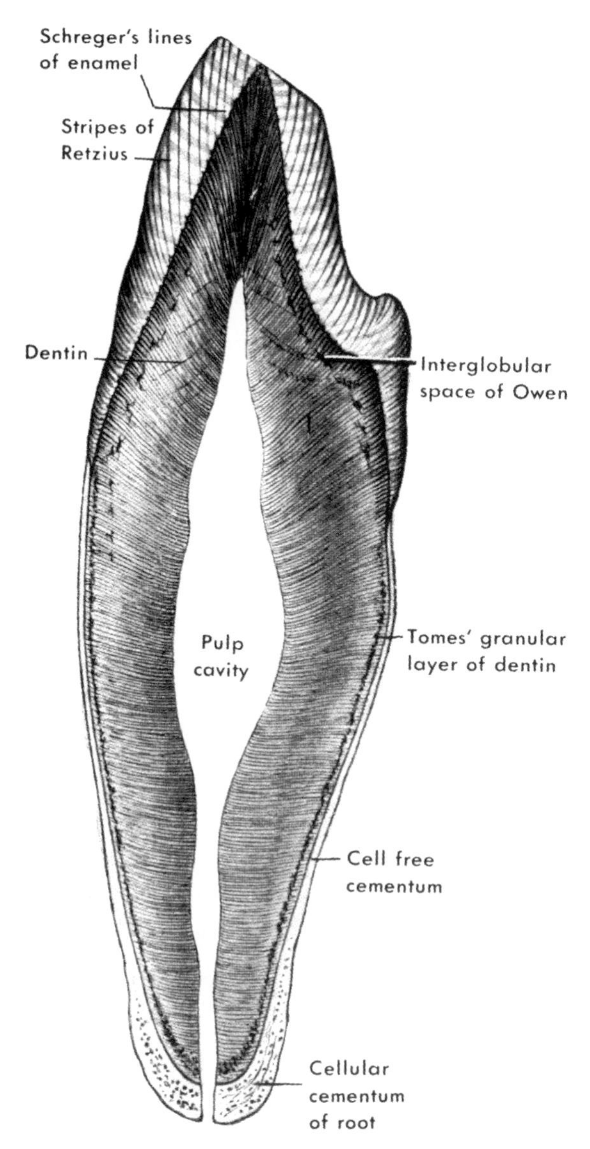

Figure 24–8. Longitudinal ground section of a human cuspid. The top of the crown has been abraded. The enamel shows Schreger's lines and Retzius bands. Interglobular spaces of Owen are seen in the dentin. (After von Ebner, from Schaffer, J., Lehrbuch der Histologie und Histogenese. W. Engelmann Press, Leipzig. 1922.)

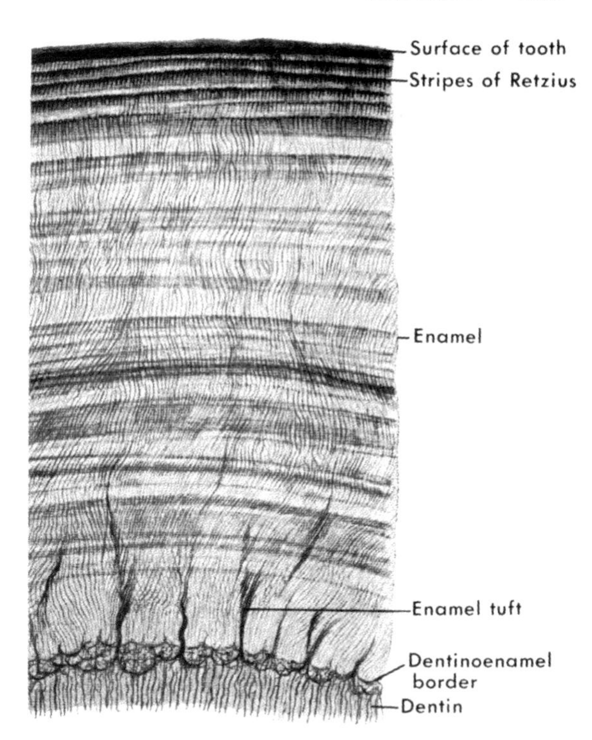

Figure 24–9. A portion of a ground cross section of the crown of a human cuspid showing the stripes, or bands, of Retzius in the enamel and enamel tufts extending into the enamel from the dentin. (After Schaffer, J., Lehrbuch der Histologie und Histogenese. W. Engelmann Press, Leipzig, 1922.)

striae of Retzius (Fig. 24–8). They are believed to result from rhythmic deposition and mineralization of enamel during development of the tooth. Where they reach the surface, they are just detectable as uniformly spaced, shallow, circumferential grooves that are soon obliterated by wear.

There are two thin superficial layers at the free surface of the enamel of recently erupted teeth. The inner, called the *enamel cuticle*, is about 1-μm thick and appears to be the final

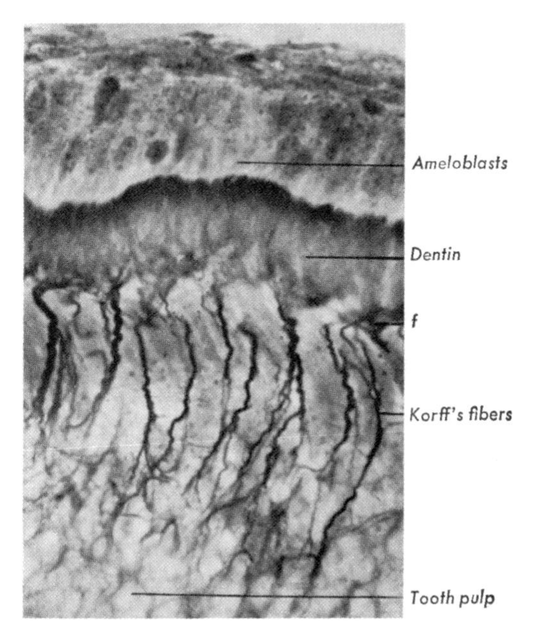

Figure 24–10. Photomicrograph of a silver-stained preparation showing Korff's fibers extending from the pulp into the matrix of the dentin. (Courtesy of B. Orban.)

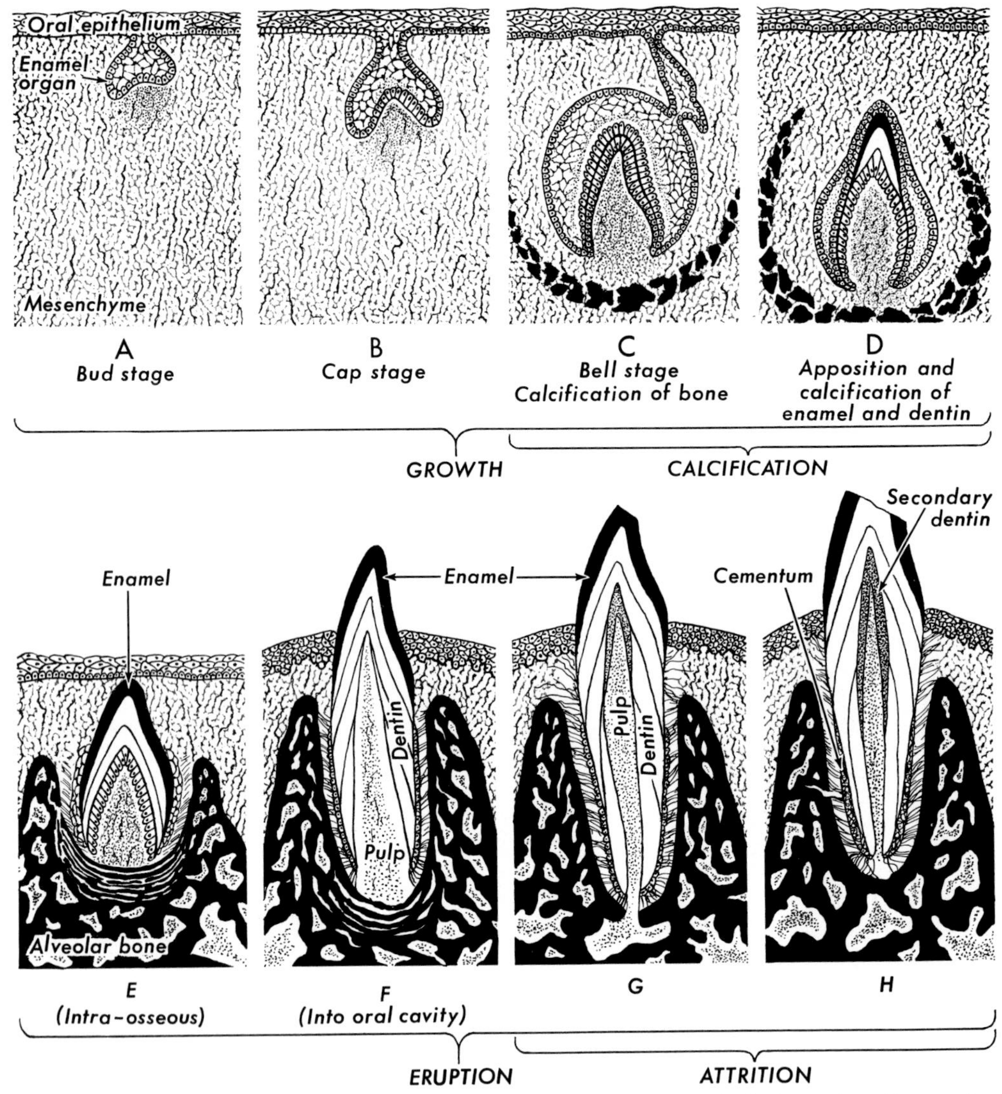

Figure 24–11. Diagram of the early development of a human deciduous incisor tooth, the formation of its root, its eruption, and beginning attrition. Enamel and bone are drawn in black. (Courtesy of I. Schour and S. Massler.)

product of the enamel-forming ameloblasts before they disappear. The outer layer is probably keratinized remanents of the dental sac of the developing tooth (see below). It is continuous below, with the cementum covering the root, and is similar to it in appearance and composition. This layer is tenaciously adherent to the tooth and is not part of the connective tissue of the gingiva. It may persist for some time after eruption of the tooth but is not present in older individuals.

The organic matrix that makes up a very small fraction of the enamel has been difficult to isolate and analyze and its composition and relation to the apatite crystals are still not well understood. However, it is clear that its protein component is not keratin or collagen because one-fourth of its amino acids are proline and it contains a relatively high concentration of bound phosphorus. The initial products of the ameloblasts that form the enamel are probably large protein or glycoprotein molecules that are broken down extracellularly to smaller molecules, collectively called *amelogenins*. The proteins extracted from mature enamel have a different amino-acid composition and are called *enamelins*. They are apparently bound to the crystallites of the enamel prisms.

In an axial section of a tooth, the *dentino-enamel junction* has a scalloped contour. Along this uneven junction, there are groups of dentinal tubules that extend for a short distance into the enamel. These are called *enamel spindles*. Local disturbances in enamel formation during tooth development may also result in so-called *enamel tufts* (Fig. 24–9). These extend from the dentino-enamel junction into the enamel for about one-third of its thickness and consist of groups of poorly calcified, twisted enamel rods with a greater than normal amount of matrix between them. Their tuft-like form is an optical illusion due to projection, into one plane, of distorted rods and fibers lying in slightly different planes. In longitudinal sections, linear markings may occasionally be seen extending inward from the surface of the enamel, nearly to the dentin. These are called *enamel lamellae* and are believed to be thin sheets of uncalcified matrix material. The three kinds of markings defined above are included in any thorough description of tooth structure, but they have little functional significance and are not important to students.

CEMENTUM

The root of the tooth is covered by a thin layer of *cementum*, a mineralized tissue closely resembling bone. The enamel meets this layer in an abrupt transition, the *cemento-enamel junction*, at the lower margin of the crown. The layer becomes somewhat thicker from there to the tip of the roots. In its physical and chemical properties, the cementum is more like bone than any of the other hard tissues of the tooth. It consists of a calcified matrix of collagen fibers, glycoprotein, and mucopolysaccharides. The cervical portion and a thin layer adjacent to the dentin are *acellular cementum*. The remainder is *cellular cementum*, within which osteocyte-like cells, *cementocytes*, are enclosed in lacunae in the matrix. A discontinuous layer of *cementoblasts* may be found on a thin layer of unmineralized matrix at the surface of the root. Haversian systems and blood vessels are usually lacking in the cementum, but as its thickness increases with age, blood vessels and haversian systems may appear. Cementum normally grows very slowly, but it may undergo hyperplasia in response to chronic irritation.

PERIODONTAL LIGAMENT

The roots of the tooth are each enveloped by a dense layer of collagen, forming the *periodontal membrane* or *periodontal ligament* between the cementum and the surrounding alveolar bone. The fibers run obliquely upward from the cementum to the bone so that pressure on the tooth applies tension to the fibers inserting into bone. Coarse bundles of collagen fibers penetrate the cementum just as Sharpey's fibers extend from the periosteum into bones. The orientation of the fibers of the periodontal ligament varies at different levels along the root. When the tooth is not in use, the fibers are slightly wavy but straighten when pressure is applied to the crown. Thus, the periodontal ligament firmly anchors the tooth to its socket while providing a limited degree of mobility. There are numerous fibroblasts between the bundles of collagen fibers and this tissue is more vascular and more metabolically active than other ligaments and tendons. There is radioautographic evidence for active synthesis of collagen by the fibroblasts, suggesting that there is a fairly rapid turnover of its fibrous and amorphous components.

PULP

The *pulp*, occupying the central cavity of the tooth, is derived from the tissue that formed the dental papilla during embryonic development. It retains some of the characteristics of mesenchyme, consisting of stellate cells in contact via their slender processes to form a three-dimensional cellular reticulum. The cells are in communication via gap junctions on their processes and they also make contact with the layer of odontoblasts that lines the pulp cavity. Other cells present in the pulp, in limited numbers, include lymphocytes, macrophages, plasma cells, and eosinophils. The interstitium between the pulp cells consists of a gelatinous ground substance that stains metachromatically and gives a positive PAS reaction. Within it are large numbers of randomly oriented thin fibrils of collagen that are best seen in electron micrographs. Adjacent to the layer of odontoblasts that line the pulp cavity, there is a relatively cell-free area

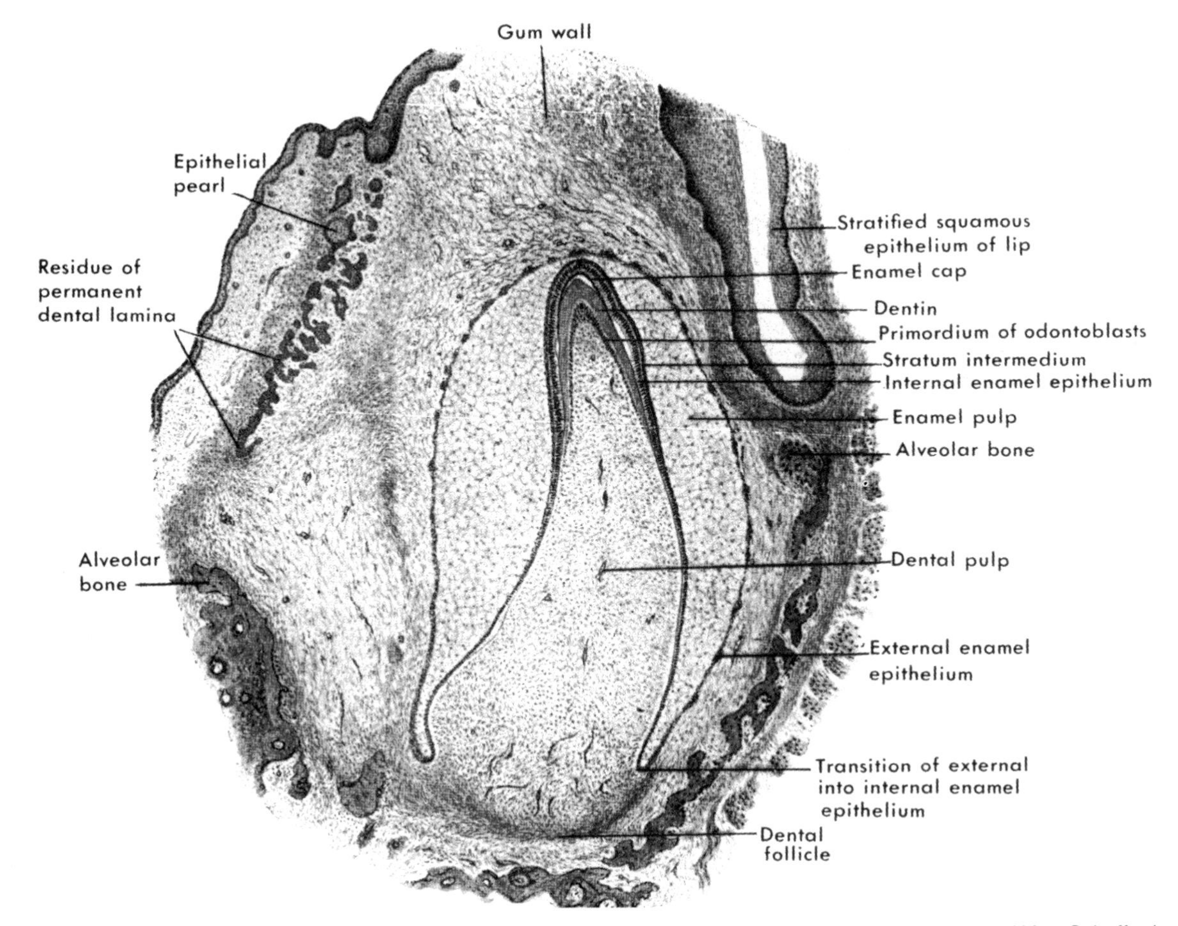

Figure 24–12. Primordium of a lower central incisor of a 5-month fetus and the surrounding structures. (After Schaffer.)

(*zone of Weil*). In preparations stained with silver-impregnation techniques, bundles of fibrils (Korff's fibers) are seen passing across this and between the odontoblasts. Their distal ends are incorporated in the dentinal matrix (Fig. 24–10).

Small arterioles enter the pulp through the apical foramen and their capillary branches ramify close to the bases of the odontoblasts and some may be found between them. These drain into small veins more centrally situated in the pulp. Arteriovenous anastomoses are common. Thin-walled veins leave the pulp cavity through the apical foramen. Owing to the unyielding wall of the pulp cavity, leakage of plasma and increased pressure associated with infection may compress the blood vessels resulting in necrosis of the pulp. There are also lymphatics in the pulp, but these are difficult to distinguish from the thin-walled veins.

Bundles of myelinated nerve fibers, originating from small cells in the gasserian ganglion, enter the pulp cavity through the apical foramen and form a plexus in the pulp. Branches from this form a plexus of finer unmyelinated fibers at the periphery of the pulp cavity. Nerve endings have been observed between the odontoblasts and some extend a short distance along the odontoblast cell processes, but there are believed to be no nerves deeper in the dentin. These nerves are sensory and are responsible for the pain experienced in toothache.

GINGIVA

The mucous membrane lining the vestibule of the oral cavity is reflected onto the outer surface of the alveolar bone. As it approaches the teeth, it is continuous with the lower margin of a firmer pink layer called the gum or *gingiva*, which is that part of the mucous membrane that is firmly bound to the periosteum of the crest of the alveolar bone. It is a stra-

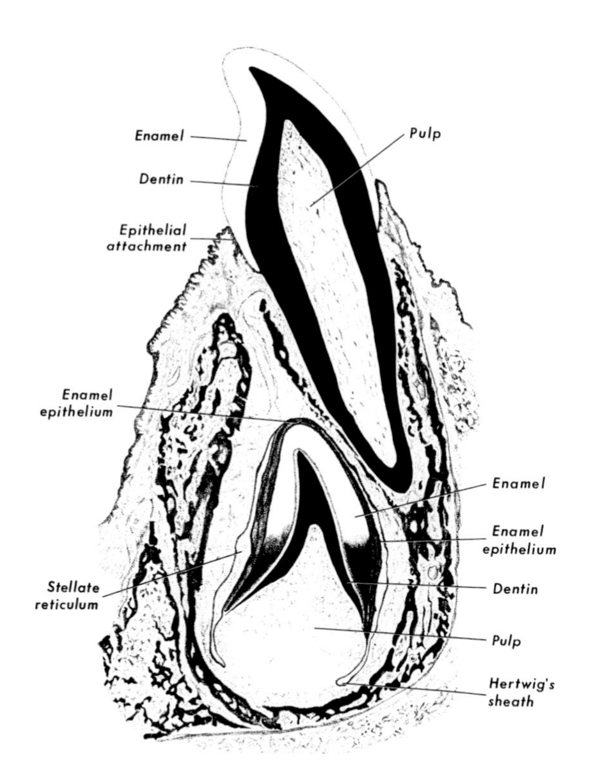

Figure 24–13. Diagram of the relationship between a deciduous tooth and the developing tooth germ of its corresponding permanent tooth in the alveolar bone below it. (Redrawn from a photograph by B. Orban.)

tified squamous epithelium with numerous connective tissue papillae projecting into its base. It is a keratinizing epithelium, but in this moist environment, it lacks a stratum granulosum and its superficial layer of flattened cells retain pycnotic nuclei. The term parakeratosis is sometimes used to distinguish the changes undergone by this epithelium from the more extreme changes observed in the epidermis (orthokeratosis). Over most of the gingiva, the lamina propria is firmly bound to the underlying periosteum and the mucosa is immobile. However, within 1 mm or so of a tooth, it is less firmly attached and is designated *free gingiva* or *marginal gingiva*. Around the crown of a tooth, the free gingiva is separated from the enamel by a shallow furrow called the *gingival crevice* or *gingival sulcus*. The epithelium lining this sulcus is relatively thin, it lacks connective tissue papillae at its base, and it is unkeratinized. The epithelium continues beyond the lower end of the gingival sulcus to attach to the cementum and periodontal ligament. This *junctional epithelium*, only a few cell layers in thickness, is attached at its surface to the enamel of the tooth. The superficial epithelial cells in this region appear to secrete, between the epithelium and the tooth, a layer of material having the same appearance in electron micrographs as a basal lamina. This layer is adherent to the tooth and the epithelium is bound to it by hemidesmosomes. This seal around the tooth normally prevents entry of bacteria into the peridontal tissues. The lamina propria, in this region, usually contains many lymphocytes and polymorphonuclear leukocytes. If the seal is seriously damaged, a persistent gingivitis may result.

ALVEOLAR BONE

The *alveolar bone* consists of cancellous bone between two layers of cortical bone. The outer

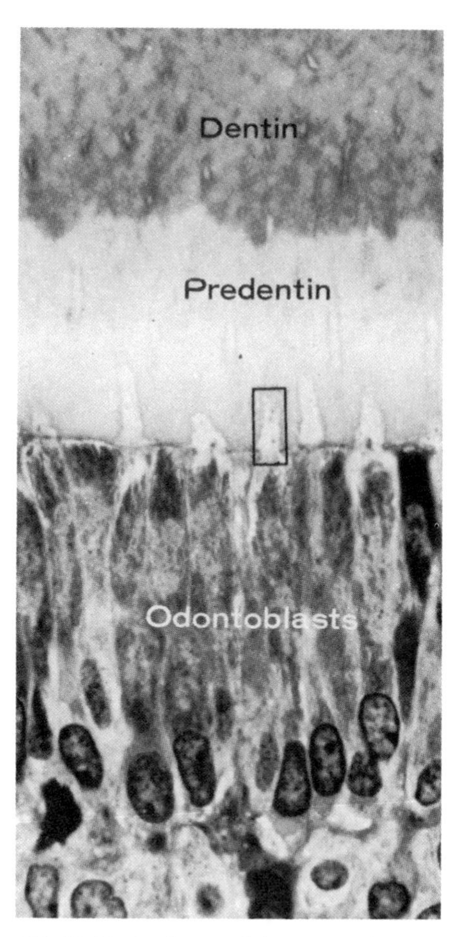

Figure 24–14. Photomicrograph from a growing rat incisor showing the relationships of the odontoblasts (bottom) to the predentin and dentin (top). An area such as that enclosed in the rectangle is shown at higher magnification in Fig. 24–15. (From Weinstock, M. and C.P. Leblond. 1974. J. Cell Biol. 60:92.)

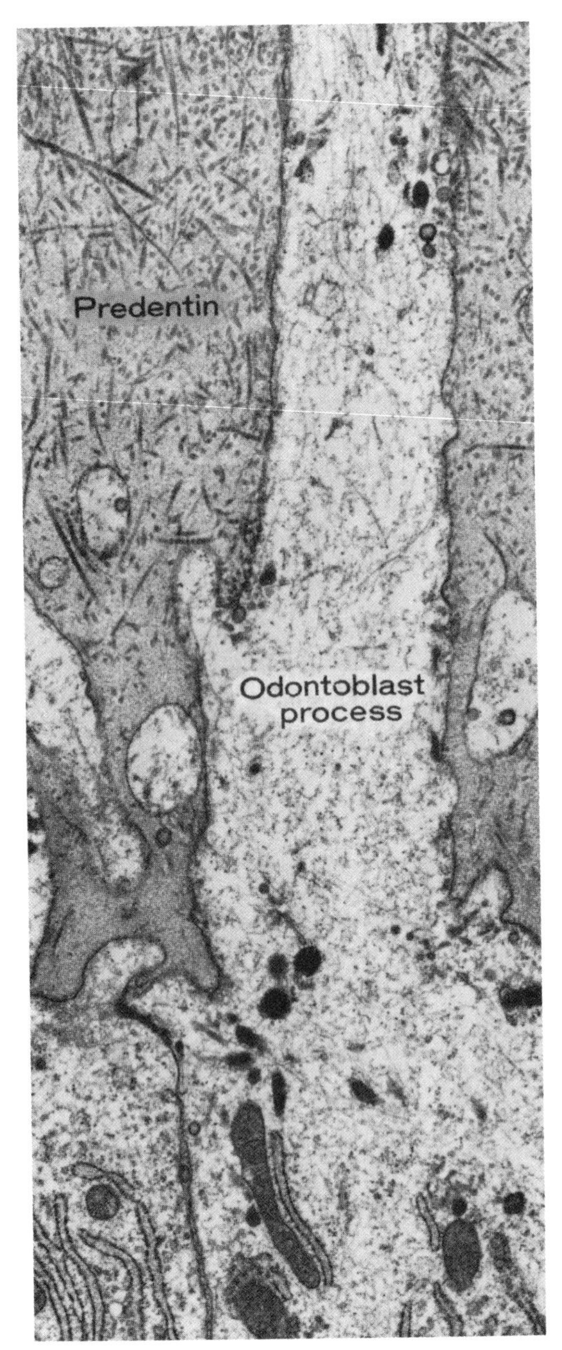

Figure 24–15. Electron micrograph of the apical region of an odontoblast showing the odontoblast process and the fibrous and amorphous components of the surrounding predentin. (From Weinstock, M. and C.P. Leblond. 1974. J. Cell Biol. 60:92.)

cortical plate is a continuation of the cortex of the mandible or maxilla. The inner cortical plate adjacent to the periodontal membrane of the teeth is called, by radiologists, the *lamina dura*. It surrounds the roots to form their sockets. The blood vessels and nerves to the teeth course through the alveolar bone to their apical foramina where they enter into the pulp cavity. The cancellous trabeculae, buttressed by the labial and lingual cortical plates, aid in resisting the pressure on the teeth during mastication. Alveolar bone is quite labile and serves as a readily available source of calcium to maintain blood levels of this ion. Considerable resorption of alveolar bone may occur after loss of the permanent teeth or after periodontitis.

HISTOGENESIS OF TEETH

In human embryos at the fifth week of gestation, the ectodermal epithelium lining the

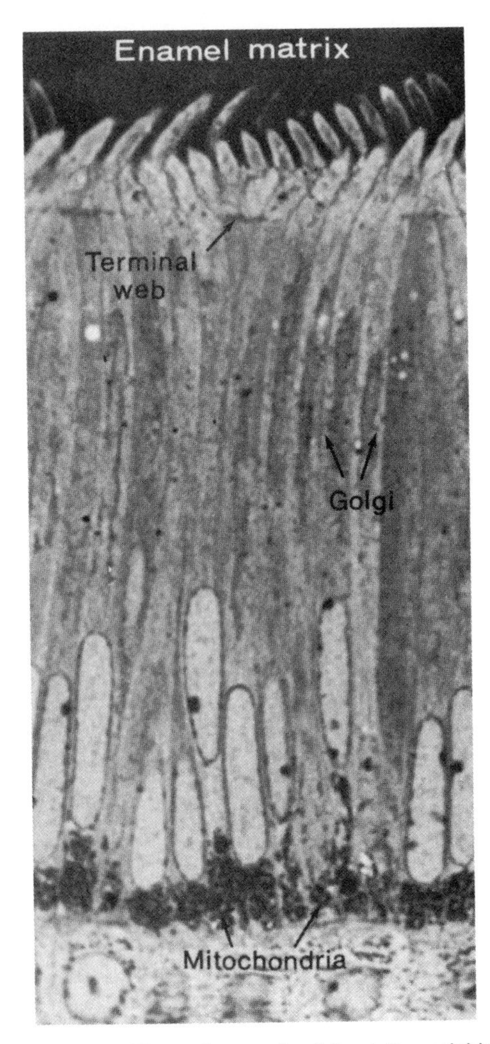

Figure 24–16. Photomicrograph of the tall ameloblasts and overlying enamel matrix of a rat maxillary incisor. Note the clustering of mitochondria at the base, the basal location of the ameloblast nuclei, the terminal web, and apical processes extending into the enamel. (From Weinstock, M. and C.P. Leblond. 1971. J. Cell Biol. 51:26.

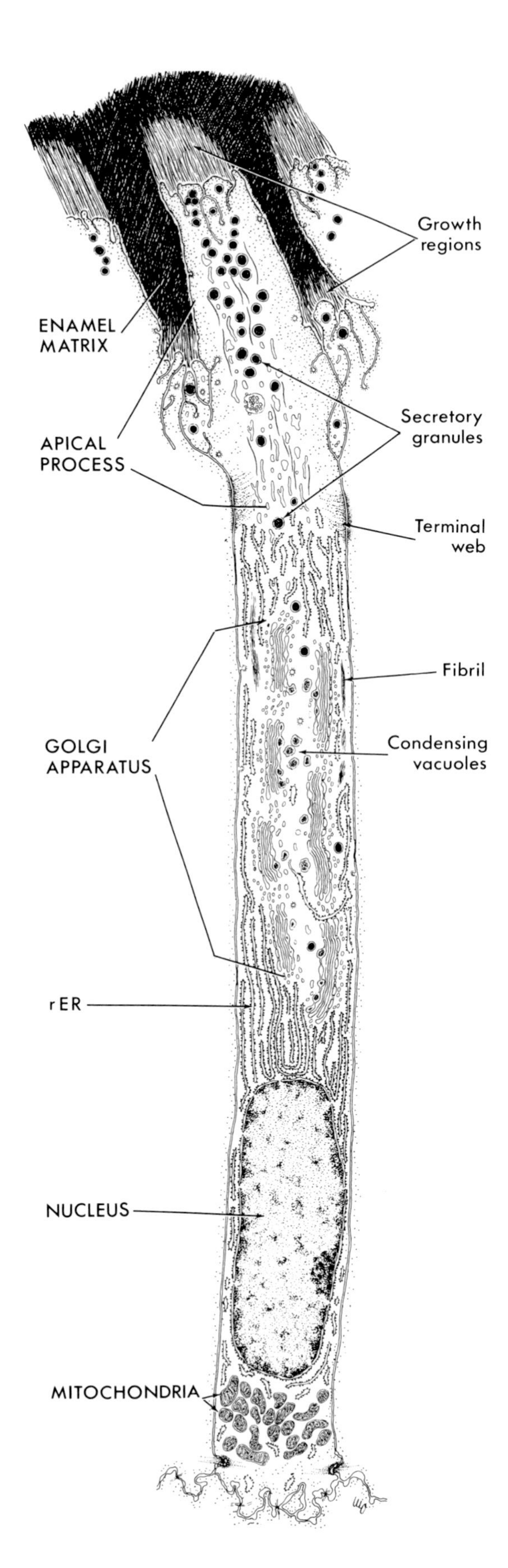

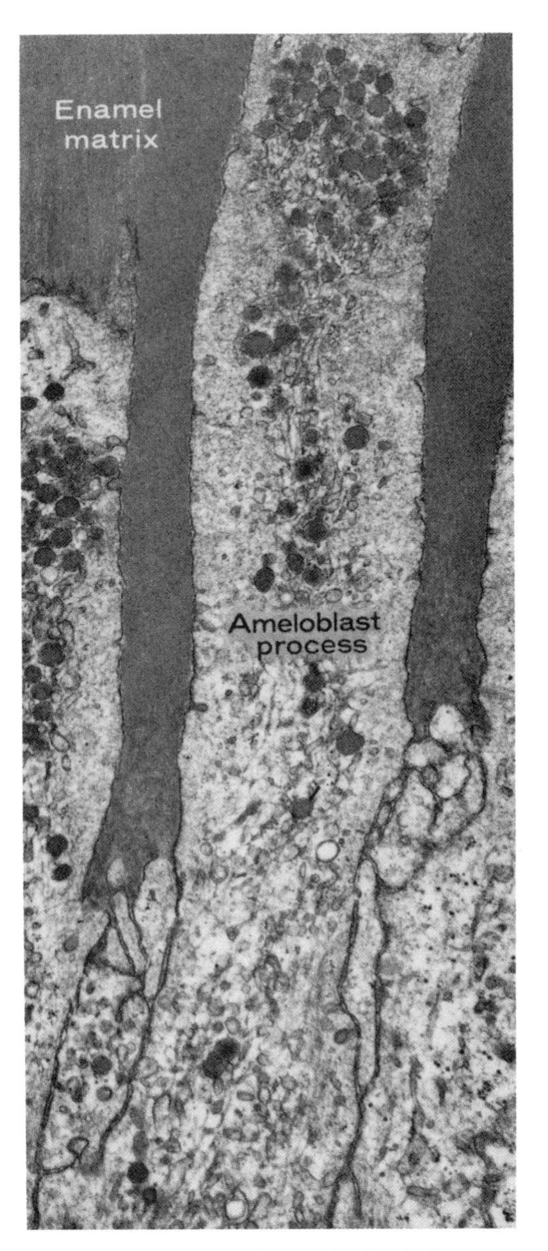

Figure 24–18. Electron micrograph of apical processes (Tome's processes) of ameloblasts from a developing rat incisor. (From Weinstock, M. and C.P. Leblond. 1971. J. Cell Biol. 51:26.)

Figure 24–17. Diagrammatic representation of the ultrastructure of a secretory ameloblast from a rat maxillary incisor. (From Weinstock, M. and C.P. Leblond. 1971. J. Cell Biol. 51:26.)

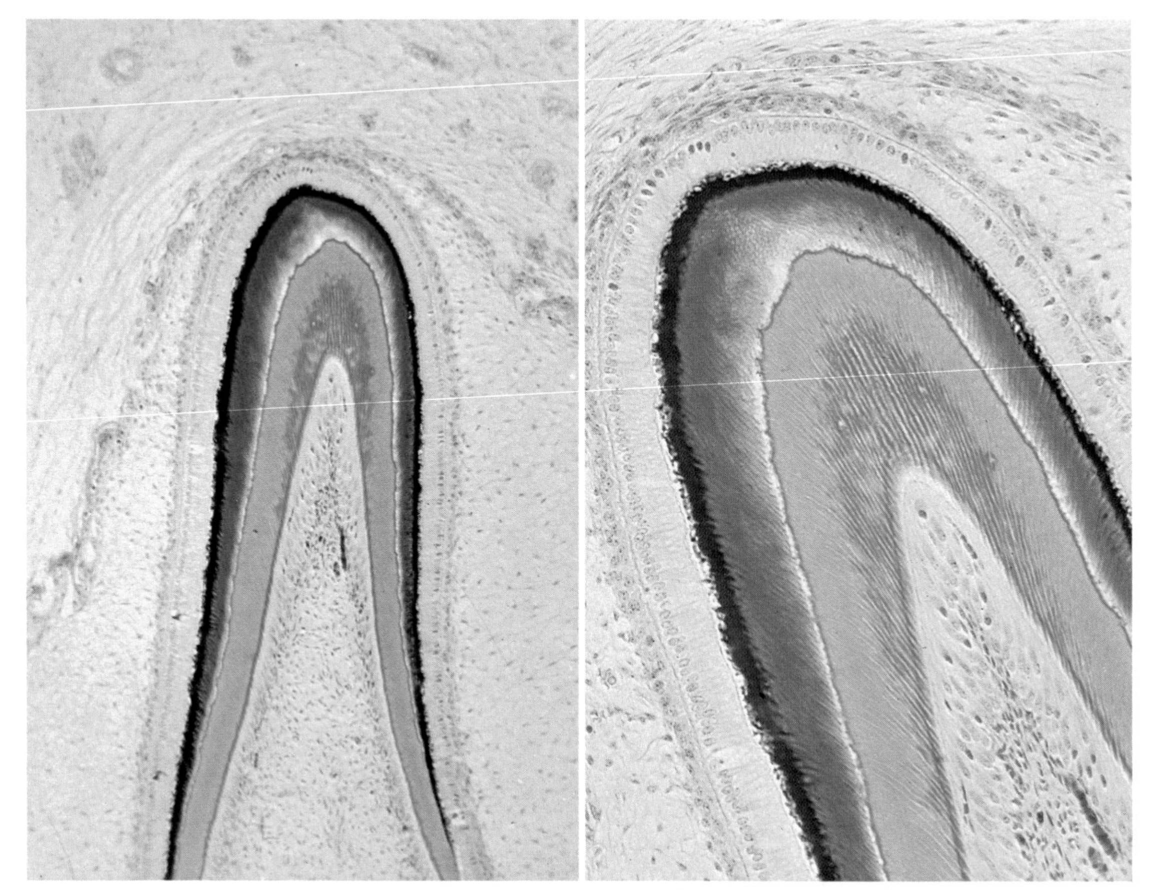

Figure 24–19. Photomicrographs ot a developing tooth in which the enamel is stained red and the dentin blue near the pulp and pink near the dentinoenamel junction. The faintly stained columnar epithelium of ameloblasts can be seen closely applied to the enamel. The dental pulp is lined by a faintly stained epithelium of odontoblasts.

oral cavity develops a thickening along the crest of the future alveolar arches of the upper and lower jaws. This layer of thickened epithelium overlies mesenchyme believed to have originated from the embryonic neural crest. The under surface of this thickened epithelium develops two parallel ridges that bulge into the mesenchyme. The outermost of these, called the labial ridge, subsequently splits to create the space between the lip and cheek on the outside and the alveolar arch on the inside. The lingual ridge, nearer the tongue, becomes the site of tooth formation.

At 10 sites beneath a thickening of the epithelium on the lingual ridge, called the *dental lamina*, mesenchymal cells aggregate and induce local proliferation of the overlying epithelium, resulting in the formation of 10 *tooth buds* that will give rise to the 10 deciduous teeth. Further proliferation of epithelial cells of each tooth bud forms a process that grows downward and becomes expanded and flattened at its deep end, forming the *enamel organ* (Fig. 24–11). The epithelial downgrowth later invaginates to accommodate the expanding population of underlying mesenchymal cells that will form the dental papilla. The cuboidal cells on the outer surface of the cap-shaped enamel organ constitute the *outer dental epithelium*, whereas those on its concave under surface are the *inner dental epithelium*. Between these layers, the epithelial cells are loosely packed, with long processes joined by desmosomes to form a stellate reticulum in the *enamel pulp* (Fig. 24–12). The outer dental epithelium is still connected to the oral epithelium by a slender stalk. The cells of the inner dental epithelium become columnar and later differentiate into *ameloblasts* that will produce the tooth enamel. The lower edge of the cap-like enamel organ, where the outer dental epithelium is continuous with the inner dental epithelium, will later mark the lower limit of the enamel at the neck of the tooth. As the enamel organ enlarges, it becomes bell-shaped and its under surface gradually takes on the contour of the crown of the tooth (Fig. 24–11).

Soon after formation of the enamel organ, local proliferation of cells in the stalk connecting it to the oral epithelium forms a small lateral bud on its lingual side that, years later, will be activated to initiate the formation of the permanent tooth to replace the deciduous tooth now forming during fetal life (Fig. 24–13). As development of the enamel organ and dental papilla progresses, the surrounding mesenchymal cells are compressed and form a layer of connective tissue termed the *tooth follicle (dental sac)* enveloping them. Concurrently with formation of the tooth follicle, the stalk connecting the enamel organ to the dental lamina of the oral epithelium is interrupted, but its lateral bud, destined to form the permanent tooth, remains associated with the epithelium of the dental lamina. Later, cells arising in the outer portion of the tooth follicle differentiate into osteoblasts that migrate some distance away from it and begin to lay down trabeculae of cancellous bone that will form the socket of the developing tooth.

In fetuses of about 20 weeks gestation, the dental pulp consists of mesenchymal cells in a loose meshwork of reticular fibers containing capillaries. Its peripheral mesenchymal cells, adjacent to the differentiating ameloblasts, then become transformed into tall, columnar odontoblasts, with their bases toward the interior of the pulp and their apical processes embedded in a layer of predentin. (Figs. 24–14 and 24–15). As indicated earlier in the chapter, these cells have an ultrastructure typical of cells actively synthesizing protein. However, they are unusual among collagen-secreting cells in that they are polarized. Procollagen is released only at the cell apex, in contrast to fibroblasts from which it is released over the entire cell surface.

Dentin first appears as a thin layer between the odontoblasts and the ameloblasts, sometimes called the *membrana perforata*. It gradually thickens as more dentin is continuously deposited on its inner surface. That first deposited is called the *mantle dentin* and this is followed by the *circumpulpar dentin*. Calcification follows soon after deposition of new dentin, but there is always a thin, uncalcified layer adjacent to the odontoblasts. As the odontoblasts recede, with the deposition of more dentin, their lengthening apical processes remain in the tubules within the dentin. The predentin around the apices of the odontoblasts is a soft fibrillar zone rich in collagen. It is traversed by fibers from deeper in the papilla, called *Korff's fibers* (Fig. 24–10). These spread out fan wise within the matrix of the dentin.

Soon after the first appearance of calcified dentin around the papilla, the ameloblasts begin to deposit layer after layer of enamel on its outer surface (Fig. 24–16, 24–20). On the sides of the developing tooth, the height of the layer of ameloblasts decreases toward the base of the enamel organ, and no enamel is deposited below this level. The columnar ameloblasts have an elongated nucleus in the basal cytoplasm and mitochondria are clustered in this region (Fig. 24–17). There is a long, more-or-less cylindrical Golgi complex in the supranuclear cytoplasm surrounded by numerous cisternae of rough endoplasmic reticulum. Distal to a conspicuous terminal web in the apical cytoplasm there is a broad apical process, *Tome's process*, which continues into the calcified enamel matrix (Fig. 24–18, 24–19). Numerous small membrane-bounded secretory granules containing glycoprotein precursors of the enamel matrix are found in the Golgi region and apical cytoplasm. These are transported into the apical process for release.

Development of the root of the tooth begins shortly before the eruption of the crown of the tooth. Continued downward growth of the inner and outer dentinal epithelium from the lower edge of the enamel organ gives rise to a bilayered fold, called the *sheath of Hertwig*, around a lengthening pulp cavity. The cells of this sheath induce neighboring pulp cells to differentiate into odontoblasts. These align themselves with the layer of differentiated odontoblasts in the cervical region of the tooth and begin to secrete a layer of predentin that is continuous with that already present in the crown. This is soon followed by the secretion of dentin by these odontoblasts, initiating the formation of the root of the tooth. Continuing downward growth of the sheath of Hertwig and its induction of more odontoblasts results in progressive elongation of the root until it reaches its definitive length. The sheath of Hertwig then disappears. After its disintegration, cells of the surrounding connective tissue sheath differentiate into *cementoblasts* and deposit an acellular layer of cement on the root. Further deposition of cement entraps bundles of collagen fibers that are incorporated, at their other end, in trabeculae of the alveolar bone. These fibers, and those that replace them in the continual turnover of the tissue, ultimately form the periodontal ligament that anchors the tooth to its bony socket.

In eruption of the tooth, the crown is moved through the overlying cellular remanents of the enamel organ which seem to disintegrate in its path. It then passes through the gingiva to emerge in the oral cavity. The source of the forces that elevate the tooth in this process is still not known.

BIBLIOGRAPHY

Miles, A.E.W. 1967. Structural and Chemical Organization of Teeth, Vols. I and II. New York, Academic Press.

Symonds, N.B., ed. 1967. Dentin and Pulp: Their Structure and Reactions. Edinburgh, Churchill Livingstone.

TenCate, A.R. 1985. Oral Histology: Development, Structure and Function, 2nd ed. St Louis, MO, C.V. Mosby.

DENTIN

Garant, P.R., G. Szabo, and J. Nalbandian. 1968. Fine structure of the mouse odontoblast. Arch. Oral Biol. 13:857.

Reith, E.J. 1968. Collagen formation in developing molar teeth of rats. J. Ultrastr. Res. 21:383.

Weinstock, A., M. Weinstock, and C.P. Leblond. 1972. Autoradiographic detection of H-fucose incorporation into glycoprotein by odontoblasts and its incorporation at the calcification front in dentin. Calcif. Tissue Res. 8:181.

Weinstock, A. and C.P. Leblond. 1974. Synthesis, migration, and release of precursor collagen by odontoblasts as visualized by radioautography after (^{3}H) proline administration. J. Cell Biol. 60:92.

Weinstock, M. 1981. Gap junctions in odontoblasts of rat incisor teeth. Anat. Rec. 199:270.

ENAMEL

Frank, R.M. 1979. Tooth enamel: current state of the art. J. Dent. Res. 58(B):684.

Glimcher, M.J., L.C. Bonar, and E.J. Daniel. 1961. The molecular structure of the protein matrix of bovine enamel. J. Mol. Biol. 5:541.

Glimcher, M.J., P.T. Levine, and L.C. Bonar. 1965. Morphological and biochemical considerations in structural studies of the organic matrix of enamel. J. Ultrastr. Res. 13:281.

Kallenbach, E. 1976. Fine structure of differentiating ameloblasts in the kitten. Am. J. Anat. 145:283.

Kallenbach, E. 1973. The fine structure of Tome's process of rat incisor ameloblasts and its relationship to the elaboration of enamel. Tissue Cell 5:501.

Leblond, C.P. and H. Warshawsky. 1979. Dynamics of enamel formation in the rat incisor tooth. J. Dent. Res. 58(B):844.

Matthiessen, M.E. and P. Romert. 1980. Ultrastructure of the human enamel organ. I. External enamel epithelium, stellate reticulum and stratum intermedium. Cell Tissue Res. 205:361.

Matthiessen, M.E. and P. Romert. 1980b. Ultrastructure of the human enamel organ. II. Internal enamel epithelium, preameloblasts and secretory ameloblasts. Cell Tissue Res. 205:371.

Smith, C.E. 1979. Ameloblasts: secretory and absorptive functions. J. Dent. Res. 58(B):695.

Warshawsky, H. 1968. The fine structure of secretory ameloblasts in rat incisors. Anat. Rec. 161:121.

Warshawsky, H. 1971. A light and electron microscopic study of the nearly mature enamel of rat incisors. Anat. Rec. 169:559.

Warshawsky, H., P. Bai, and A. Nanci. 1987. Analysis of crystallite shape in rat incisor enamel. Anat. Rec. 218:380.

Warshawsky, H., K. Josephsen, A. Thylstrup, and O. Fejerskov. 1981. The development of enamel structure in rat incisors as compared to the teeth of monkey and man. Anat. Rec. 200:371.

Weinstock, A. and C.P Leblond. 1971. Elaboration of the matrix glycoprotein of enamel by the secretory ameloblasts of the rat incisor as revealed by radioautography after galactose-^{3}H injection. J. Cell Biol. 51:26.

PERIODONTAL TISSUES

Beertsen, W., M. Brekelmans, and V. Everts. 1978. The site of collagen resorption in the periodontal ligament of the rodent molar. Anat. Rec. 192:305.

Listgarten, M.A. 1964. The ultrastructure of the human gingival epithelium. Am. J. Anat. 114:49.

Smuckler, H. and C.J. Dreyer. 1969. Principal fibers of the peridontium. J. Periodont. Res. 4:19.

Stern, L.B. 1964. An electron microscopic study of the cementum: Sharpey's fibers and periodontal ligament in the rat incisor. Am. J. Anat. 115:377.

Susi, F.R. 1969. Anchoring fibrils in the attachment of epithelium to connective tissue in oral mucous membrane. J. Dent. Res. 48:144.

25

THE ESOPHAGUS AND STOMACH

With this chapter we begin our description of the histology of the gastrointestinal tract, and it may be helpful, at the outset, to consider some general features of its organization and to define certain structural components that are found throughout its length. The wall of the alimentary tract is made up of four layers: the *mucosa*, the *submucosa*, the *tunica muscularis*, and the *serosa* (Fig. 25–1). The innermost of these, the mucosa, consists of a lining epithelium, its thin lamina propria, and a muscularis mucosae. The epithelium varies in type in different regions of the tract depending on whether the function of that segment is primarily conductive, secretory, or absorptive. Its lamina propria is a layer of highly vascular loose connective tissue interposed between it and the muscularis mucosae. In addition to fibroblasts, associated with a network of reticular and elastic fibers, it contains macrophages, local aggregations of lymphoid tissue, and wandering lymphocytes mobilized to protect the mucosa against invasion by microorganisms that are always present in great numbers in the lumen. The muscularis mucosae consists of two tenuous layers of smooth muscle, with the cells of the inner layer oriented circumferentially, and those of the outer layer having their long axis directed longitudinally. These layers permit independent movement of the mucosa to change its surface contour or to return it to the resting state after distension of the lumen.

The submucosa is a layer of moderately dense connective tissue containing many small blood vessels that supply the mucosa and a plexus of sympathetic nerves (*Meissner's plexus*) that control much of the intrinsic motility of the lining of the alimentary tract. In some segments of the tract, tubuloacinar glands extend from the mucosa into the submucosa.

The tunica muscularis is composed of two moderately thick layers of smooth muscle, with cells of the inner layer oriented circumferentially and those of the outer layer longitudinally. Between these layers is a second sympathetic nerve plexus (*Auerbach's plexus*), which coordinates the peristaltic contractions of the muscle that move the contents along the tract.

The outermost element of the wall, the serosa, consists of the *mesothelium*, a squamous epithelium that lines the abdominal cavity and covers the organs within it. The mesothelium is generally underlain by a very thin layer of loose connective tissue, but in some locations, adipose cells accumulate in this layer, making it much thicker. For most of its length, the gastrointestinal tract is suspended from the posterior wall of the abdomen by a *mesentery*, a very thin sheet of connective tissue covered on both sides by mesothelium that is continuous with that of the serosa covering the alimentary tract.

ESOPHAGUS

The esophagus is the tubular organ that conveys ingested food from the pharynx to the stomach (Fig. 25–2). The greater part of its length of 25 cm is within the thorax, but after passing through the diaphragm to join the stomach, its terminal is 2–4 cm in the abdominal cavity.

MUCOSA

The esophageal mucosa is 300–500 μm thick and has an epithelium that is a continuation of the stratified squamous epithelium lining the oropharynx (Fig. 25–3). Stratum germinativum, stratum spinosum, and stratum corneum are identifiable, but the thickness and degree of keratinization of the stratum

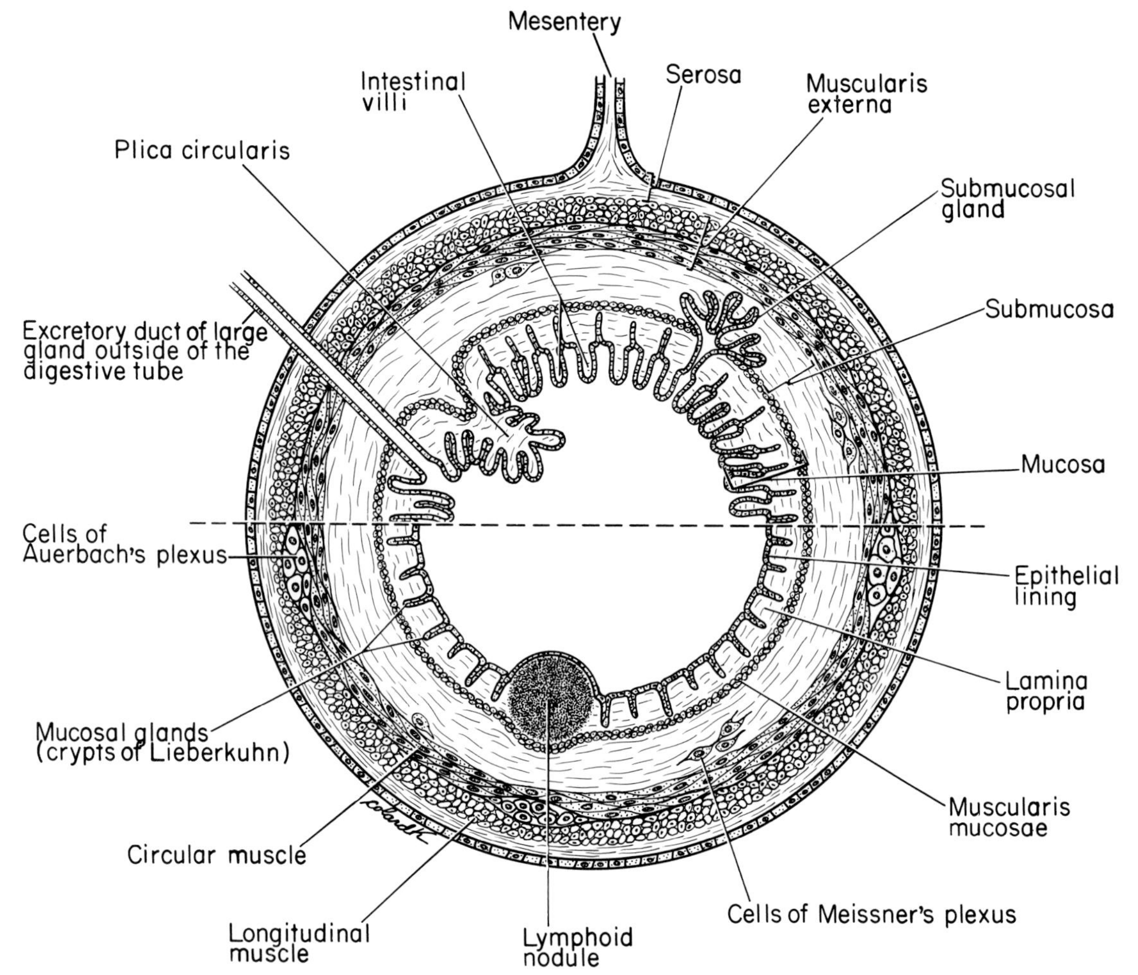

Figure 25–1. Schematic representation of the general organization of the gastrointestinal tract. The concentric layers, serosa, muscularis, and mucosa are common to all regions of the tract. In the upper half of the figure, the mucosa is depicted with glands and villi, as in the small intestine; in the lower half, it is shown with glands and no villi, as in the colon.

corneum vary greatly from species to species. In the human and other primates, this stratum is only two or three cells thick. The superficial cells retain their nucleus and have a few keratohyalin granules in their cytoplasm but show little evidence of heavy keratinization. Cells of the stratum spinosum have short microplicae that project into the intercellular spaces, and the processes of neighboring cells are attached by prominent desmosomes. In addition to their organelles, these cells contain bundles of intermediate filaments and 120–150-nm vesicles that contain eccentrically placed dense material. The base of the epithelium is quite irregular with closely spaced deep recesses in its under surface, occupied by papillae of the lamina propria. The cells of the stratum germinativum are cuboidal and have desmosomes on their interdigitating lateral surfaces and hemidemosomes at their base (Fig. 25–4).

In rodents and larger species that eat coarse grass and other abrasive fodder, the stratum corneum of the esophageal epithelium may consist of 7–12 layers of heavily keratinized cells. Degeneration of the nuclei is evident in the lower portion of this zone and none are present in the cells at the surface. The cell membrane appears unusually thick owing to the deposition of a layer of dense material on its surface. The intercellular spaces of the stratum corneum and outer portion of the stratum spinosum contain material that gives a strong staining reaction with Alcian blue at pH 2.5 and is deeply stained with the periodic-acid–Schiff reaction for glycoconjugates.

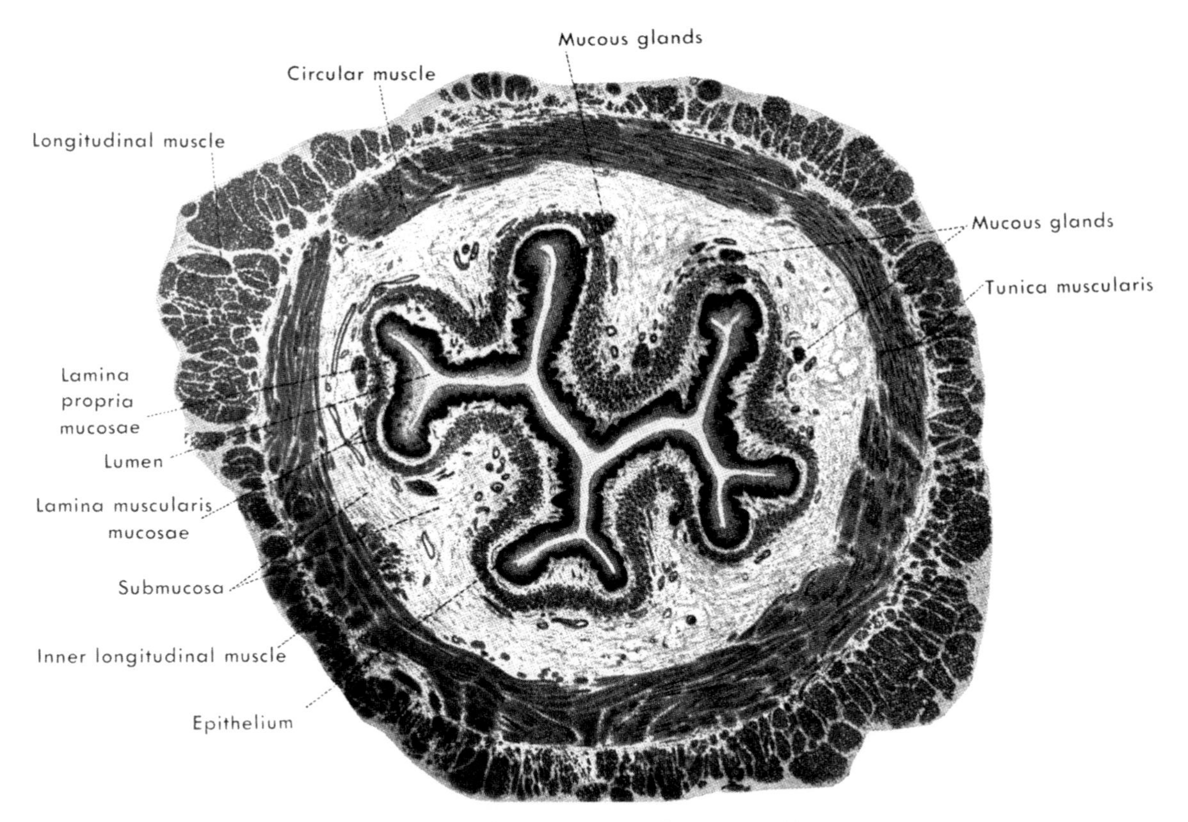

Figure 25–2. Cross section of the middle third of the esophagus of a 28-year-old-man showing the folds of the mucosa and the outer longitudinal and inner circular muscle. (After J. Sobotta, Atlas of Human Anatomie Vol. II. G.E. Stechert and Co., New York, 1936.)

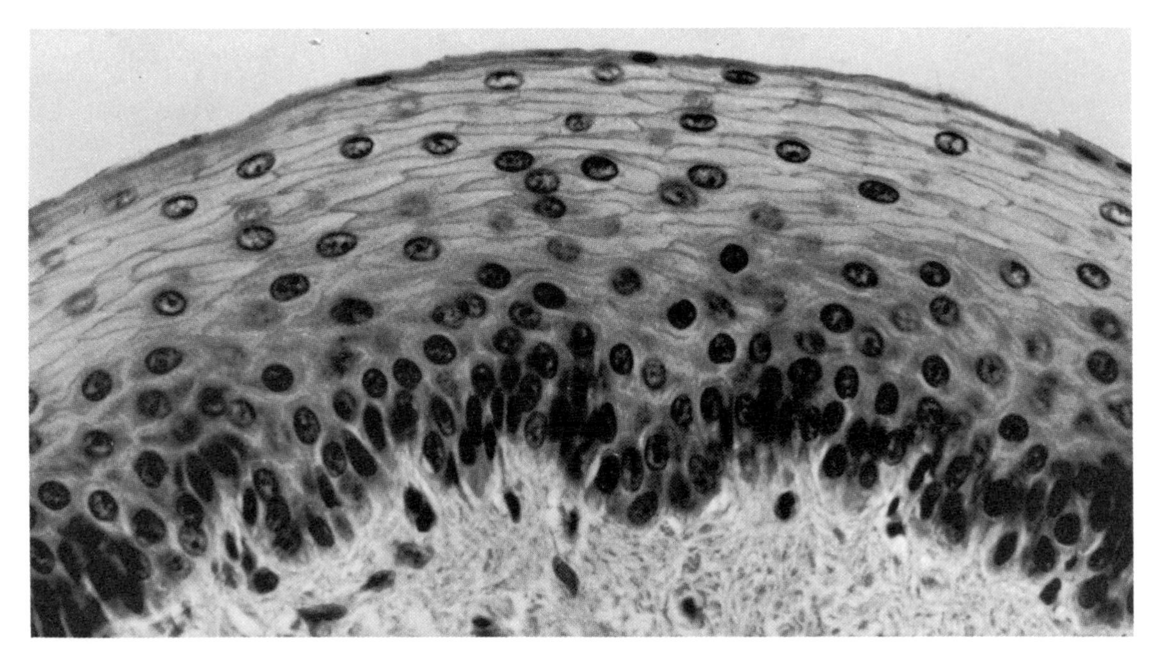

Figure 25–3. Epithelium of the esophagus of a monkey. It is a typical stratified squamous epithelium, without a conspicuous stratum corneum. The cells at the surface retain their nuclei.

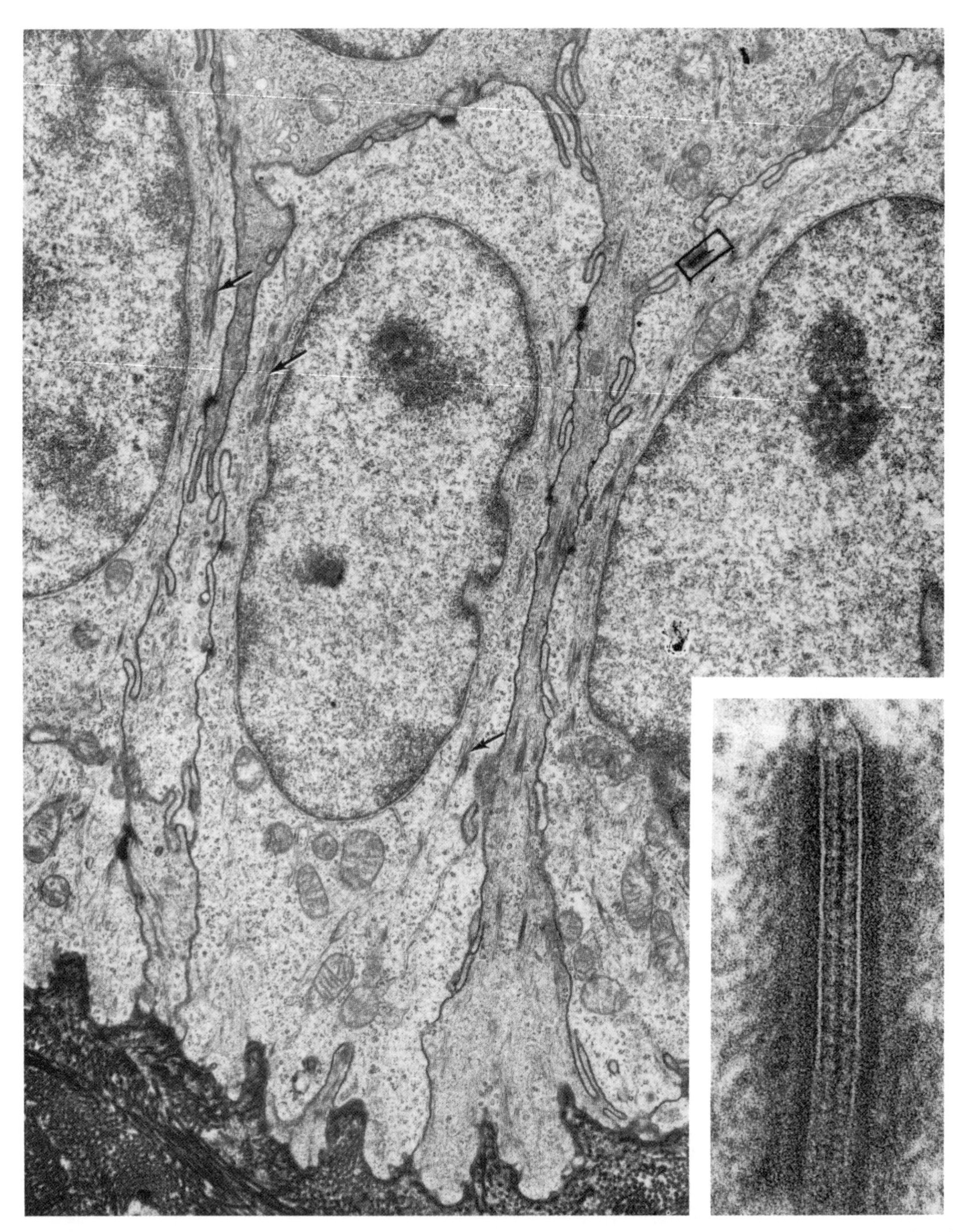

Figure 25–4. Electron micrograph of cells of the stratum germinativum of the rodent esophagus. The cells have abundant free ribosomes and occasional bundles of intermediate filaments (arrows). They are attached to neighboring cells by well-developed desmosomes. The desmosome in the inset is shown at higher magnification. Note the prominent intermediate dense line in the interspace between the two membranes. (Micrograph courtesy of Scott McNutt.)

Among the cells of the stratum germinativum in all species studied, there are occasional stellate cells that are not attached to neighboring cells by desmosomes. The cytoplasm contains fewer filaments than in the surrounding cells of the stratum germinativum and there are small numbers of distinctive rod-like granules with a laminar internal structure. The stellate shape of these cells and their possession of these characteristic granules serve to identify them as *Langerhans cells.* These antigen-presenting cells, in the esophagus, are no doubt involved in immunological responses to antigens in the lumen. At the lower end of the esophagus, there is an abrupt transition from stratified squamous epithelium to the simple columnar epithelium of the stomach.

In the upper portion of the esophagus, a muscularis mucosae is absent or is represented only by scattered slender fascicles of smooth muscle cells. Lower down in the esophagus, these come together to form a substantial continuous layer, attaining a thickness of 200–400 μm near the stomach. The muscle fibers are predominantly longitudinal in their orientation.

The submucosa is 400–600 μm in thickness and contains interlacing bundles of collagen fibers, abundant elastic fibers, and many small blood vessels. The mucosa and submucosa, in the undistended esophagus, form broad longitudinal folds that give the lumen a highly irregular outline (Fig. 25–2). As a bolus of food passes down the esophagus, these folds are transiently effaced, then promptly restored by the recoil of the elastic tissue of the submucosa.

The muscularis externa of the esophagus is 0.5–2.0 mm in thickness and consists of outer longitudinal and inner circumferential layers of muscle fibers. In the initial portion of the esophagus, both layers are striated muscle. In its middle third, smooth muscle fibers begin to appear deep to the striated muscle, and in the lower third, both layers of the muscularis consist entirely of smooth muscle. The orientation of the fibers of the muscularis is more variable in the esophagus than in the corresponding layers of the rest of the alimentary tract. Oblique fibers are common in both the inner and outer layers.

ESOPHAGEAL GLANDS

Esophageal glands are found in most mammals but are absent in rodents, equids, and cats. In the human, two kinds of esophageal glands are distinguished on the basis of their location. The superficial *mucosal glands* are limited to the lamina propria and are found in limited number in the upper esophagus and near its junction with the stomach. The *submucosal glands* are more widespread and extend into the submucosa (Fig. 25–5).

The submucosal glands are tubuloacinar glands arranged in small lobules that are drained by a single duct. The acini are made up of plump cells with their nucleus compressed to the base by droplets of mucus that occupy most of the cell volume. In electron micrographs, the limiting membrane of the mucus droplets appears fragmented or absent, possibly extracted during specimen preparation. A second cell type is cuboidal with a centrally placed nucleus, a basophilic cytoplasm, and somewhat smaller and denser secretory droplets or granules. These cells are considered by some to be an earlier stage in the secretory cycle of the mucous cell, but others regard them as a separated serous cell type. The histochemical demonstration of lysozyme and pepsinogen in their cytoplasm, and not in that of the mucous cells, favors their interpretation as a distinct cell type. The two cell types may occur together, but they tend to occur in different acini. Even more uncertain is the significance of occasional eosinophilic cells, called *oncocytes,* at the transition from acinus to duct. They have no obvious secretory granules. Their most notable feature is the presence of large numbers of closely packed mitochondria. The small ducts arising from the acini are lined by cuboidal epithelium. These converge on a straight main duct that traverses the muscularis mucosae and the epithelium to open into the lumen of the esophagus.

The more superficial *mucosal glands* are tortuous tubular glands lined with cuboidal or columnar epithelial cells that resemble those of the cardiac glands of the stomach. Owing to this resemblance, these glands are sometimes called *cardiac esophageal glands.* They are few in number and are interpreted by some as islands of ectopic gastric mucosa. Their small ducts join a larger duct that usually opens at the tip of a small papilla.

Like the minor glands of the oral cavity, the esophageal glands probably secrete, continuously maintaining a thin lubricating layer of mucus on the surface of the epithelium, but the rate of their secretion may be increased during the ingestion and swallowing of food.

HISTOPHYSIOLOGY OF THE ESOPHAGUS

Fluoroscopic observations on the junction of the pharynx with the esophagus have identified a region that appears to have higher muscular tone. Physiologists refer to this as

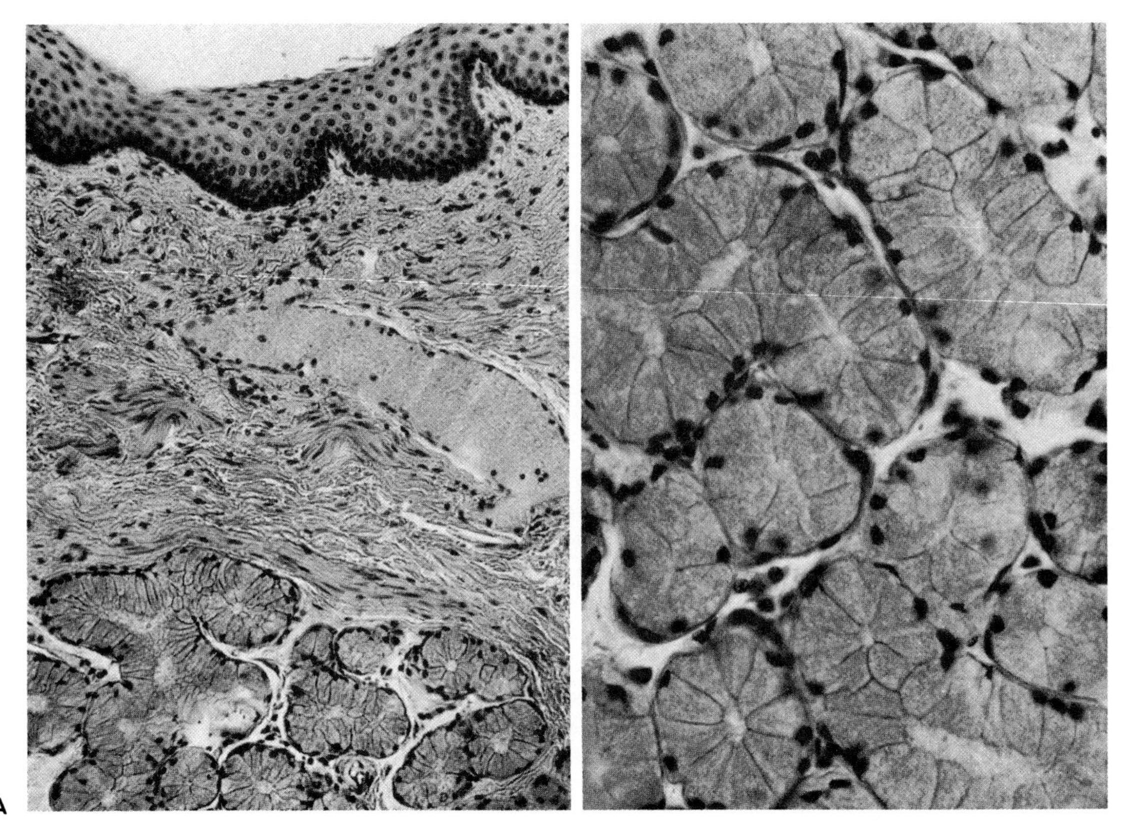

Figure 25–5. (A) Photomicrograph of the esophageal mucosa showing the epithelium at the top and glands in the submucosa. (B) Submucosal glands at higher magnification, illustrating that the dark-staining nuclei are displaced to the cell base by the accumulated mucigen in the apical region.

the *pharyngoesophageal sphincter*. Similarly, the terminal few centimeters of the esophagus serve as a *gastroesophageal sphincter*, normally maintaining an intraluminal pressure slightly higher than intragastric pressure. However, there is no thickening of the wall and no change in orientation of the muscle fibers in these segments. Thus, they are physiological rather than anatomical sphincters. The gastroesophageal sphincter is normally quite efficient in preventing reflux of gastric contents. However, in some individuals, the esophageal hiatus in the diaphragm fails to close completely around the esophagus during development, resulting in a *hiatus hernia* through which a portion of the stomach may protrude into the thoracic cavity. This often interferes with the normal sphincteric function of the terminal esophagus, permitting reflux of gastric contents. The esophageal epithelium is poorly equipped to resist the acidity of the gastric secretions, and the resulting inflammatory responses may cause difficulty in swallowing and may ultimately lead to fibrosis and stricture of the lower esophagus.

The innervation of the esophagus is via nerves from the cervical and thoracic sympathetic trunks that form plexuses in the submucosa and between the layers of the muscularis. These coordinate the movements involved in swallowing. Malfunctioning of this neuromuscular system is fairly common in older persons and may result in muscle spasm, severe substernal pain, and difficulty in swallowing.

In swallowing, the tongue propels food back into the pharynx. This sets in motion a train of voluntary and involuntary contractions of pharyngeal and esophageal muscle. These result in closure of the glottis, elevation of the larynx, constriction of the pharynx, and reflex relaxation of the pharyngeal sphincter. When the bolus of food enters the esophagus, the local stimulus of distension initiates a wave of peristalsis that is propagated toward the stomach at a rate of 4–6 cm/s. The gastroesophageal sphincter relaxes in anticipation of the arrival of the peristaltic wave, allowing the food to pass into the stomach.

The esophageal mucosa maintains a barrier to the passive diffusion of ions and toxic sub-

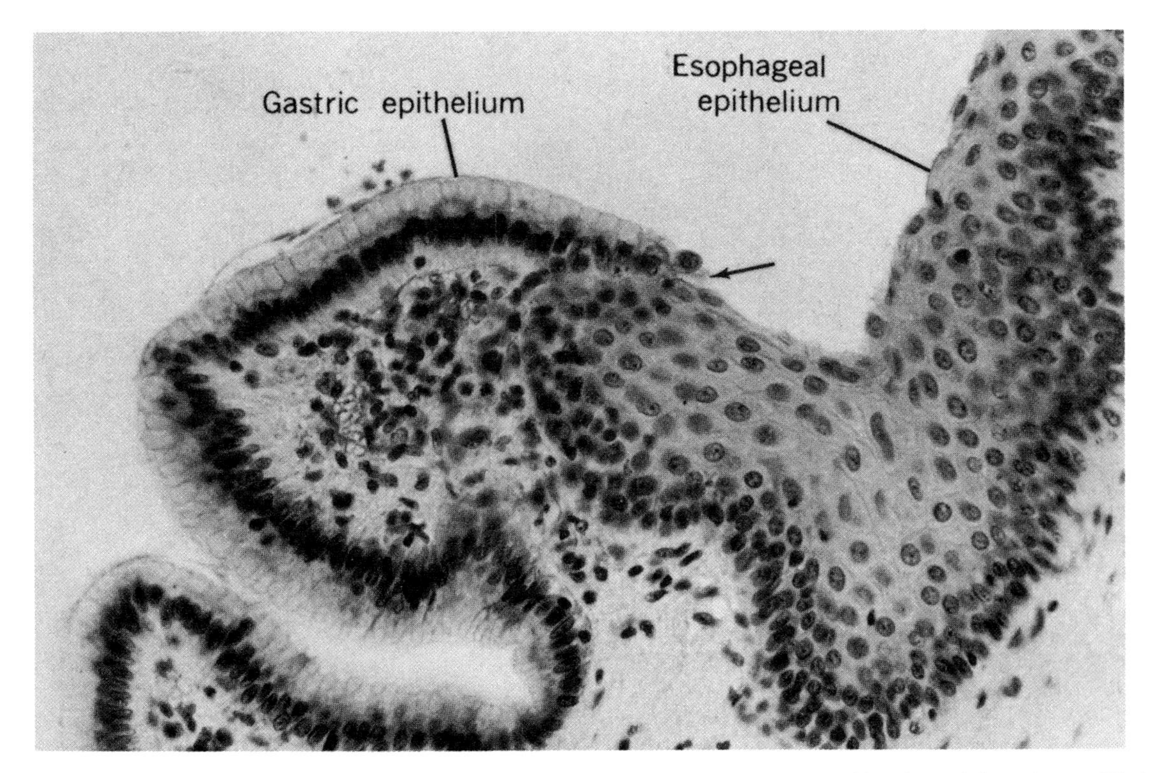

Figure 25–6. Photomicrograph of the gastoesophageal junction. Note the abrupt transition (arrow) from the stratified squamous epithelium of the esophagus to the simple columnar epithelium of the stomach.

stances from the lumen to the blood. This barrier function does not depend on tight junctions in the epithelium but appears to reside in the glycoconjugates that fill the intercellular spaces of the stratum corneum and the outer layers of the stratum spinosum. If the esophageal epithelium of a rabbit is exposed to tracers, such as horse radish peroxidase or lanthanum, from the luminal side, there is no penetration. On exposure from the basal side, where this intercellular material is lacking, the tracers penetrate about two-thirds of the way through the stratum spinosum and no further. In the thinner and less keratinized esophageal epithelium of humans, the barrier may be somewhat thinner than in rabbits, but there is, no doubt, enough of this intercellular material to provide an effective barrier.

STOMACH

The semisolid food swallowed is further homogenized by contractions of the muscular wall of the stomach and chemically processed

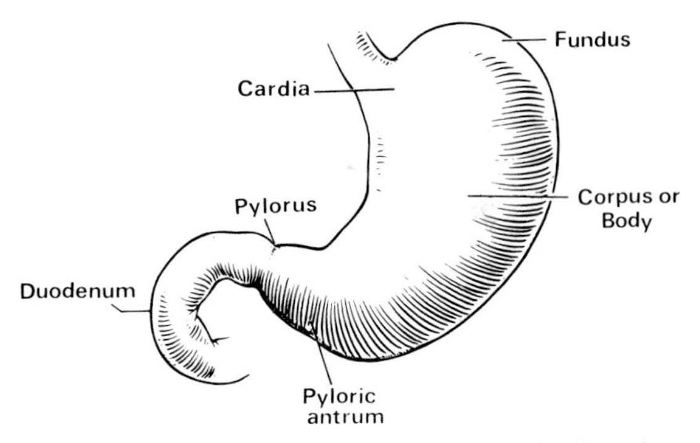

Figure 25–7. Sketch of the stomach labeled to introduce the terminology of its various regions.

by acid and enzymes secreted by the gastric mucosa. When reduced to a thick fluid, small quanta are expelled intermittently into the duodenum. In the *simple stomach* of man and many other mammalian species, the organ is capable of considerable expansion during a meal, without significant increase in internal pressure, but its storage function is quite limited. However, in ruminants, which have a *multichambered stomach*, food ingested during grazing, is stored for some time in the first

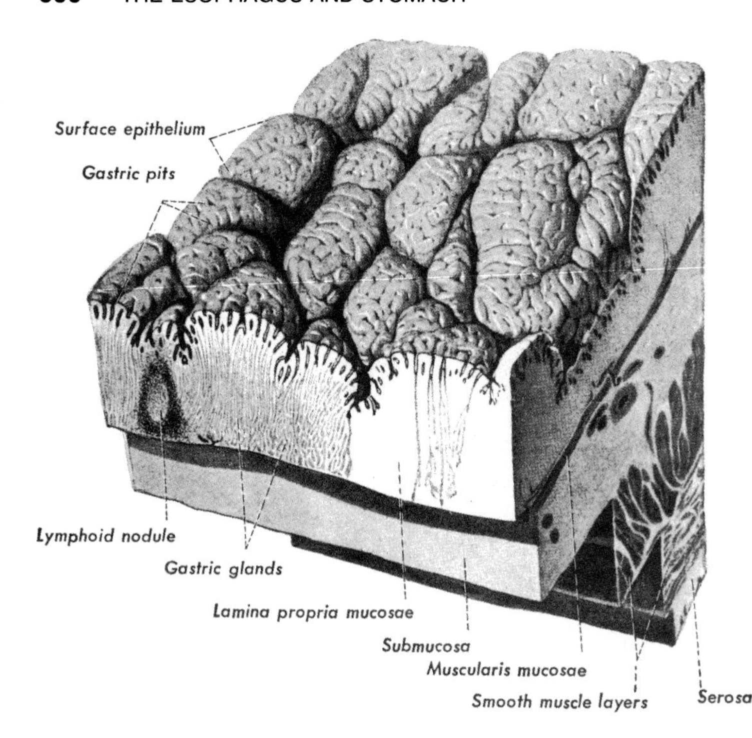

Figure 25–8. Surface topography of the human gastric mucosa as seen with the dissecting microscope.

chamber, the *rumen*. It is later returned to the oral cavity for further mastication, and when swallowed again, it proceeds through the *reticulum* and *omasum*, chambers lined with stratified squamous epithelium, to reach the final chamber, the *abomasum*, which is lined by a mucosa similar to that of simple stomachs.

In the human stomach, separate chambers do not exist, but four regions are distinguished. A narrow zone 2–3 cm wide around the esophageal orifice is called the *cardia*. A dome-shaped region bulging to the left above the level of the opening of the esophagus is the *fundus*. The capacious central region is the *corpus* and the tapering distal portion terminating at the gastroduodenal orifice is the *pyloris* (Fig. 25–7). There are significant differences in the mucosal glands of the cardia, corpus, and pyloris, whereas those of the fundus and corpus are very similar.

GASTRIC MUCOSA

There are conspicuous longitudinal folds, or *rugae*, of the mucosa in the empty stomach, but these flatten out in the full stomach where the surface appears relatively smooth. But, closer inspection reveals a pattern of narrow intercommunicating furrows that bound convex areas 2–4 mm in diameter. When these areas are examined at low magnification, each is found to be marked by numerous shallow *gastric pits* or *foveolae*. This topographical pattern of ridges, grooves, and pits is more clearly seen in scanning electron micrographs, which also resolve the rounded apices of the individual epithelial cells (Fig. 25–9).

In histological sections, the foveolae appear as funnel-shaped invaginations of the surface epithelium, and from the bottom of each, several slender, straight *gastric glands* continue downward to occupy the greater portion of the the depth of the mucosa (Fig. 25–10). The columnar epithelium covering the ridges and lining the foveolae consists of a single cell type over the entire mucosa, but the cell populations in the gastric glands of the cardia, corpus, and pyloris differ, and this is reflected in regional differences in chemical composition of the gastric secretions.

The gastric mucosa is normally covered by a lubricating layer of mucus that protects the epithelium from abrasion by ingested food. This blanket of mucus is the product of the mucus cells that make up the surface epithelium. The apical surface of these cells bears short microvilli decorated at their tips by delicate filaments of a sparse glycocalyx. The cells are attached by juxtaluminal tight junctions and have occasional gap junctions and desmosomes on their lateral surfaces. Although the

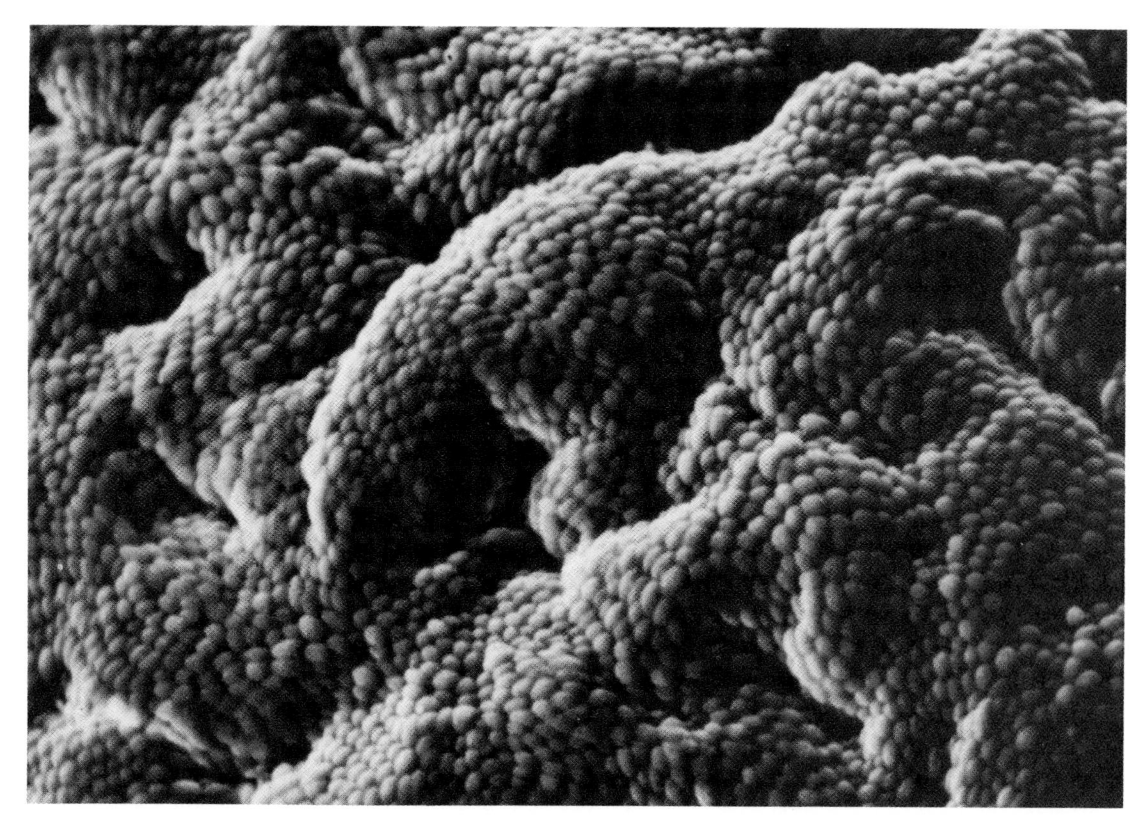

Figure 25–9. Scanning electron micrograph of the surface of the gastric mucosa. The convoluted pattern of ridges and pits is evident, as is the convex apical surface of each individual surface mucous cell. (Micrograph courtesy of J. Riddell.)

membranes of neighboring cells are closely apposed in the upper half of the epithelium, they diverge toward the base, bounding conspicuous intercellular spaces into which narrow lammellipodia extend from the side of the cells.

The apical cytoplasm of the surface mucous cells is filled with secretory granules that are only faintly stained in routine preparations but are intensely colored by the periodic-acid–Schiff reaction for carbohydrates. In electron micrographs, the secretory granules may appear homogeneous and electron-dense (Fig. 25–11), or pale with a uniformly stippled texture, depending on the method of specimen preparation. The cell nucleus is irregular in outline and displaced toward the cell base by the adluminal accumulation of secretory product. There is a prominent supranuclear Golgi complex in which the trans-cisternae and associated condensing vacuoles may contain material staining with the PAS reaction. The basal cytoplasm contains slender mitochondria and a moderate number of cisternae of rough endoplasmic reticulum.

If gastric mucosa is incubated in vitro with tritiated leucine and galactose, labeling of the Golgi complex of the surface mucous cells is observed in 40 min and maximal labeling of the secretory granules follows at 2 h. In vivo, exocytosis of secretory product normally goes on continuously at a slow rate, but under certain circumstances, massive expulsion of the stored mucus together with some of the apical cytoplasm may occur. The nature of the stimulus evoking this mode of secretion is not known.

In addition to its lubricating function, the thick blanket of mucus secreted by these cells constitutes a barrier that protects the mucosa from digestion by the acid and hydrolytic enzymes of the gastric juice. On reaching the end of their life span, the surface mucous cells are desquamated into the lumen. They are believed to be replaced by mitosis and differentiation of stem cells in the depths of the

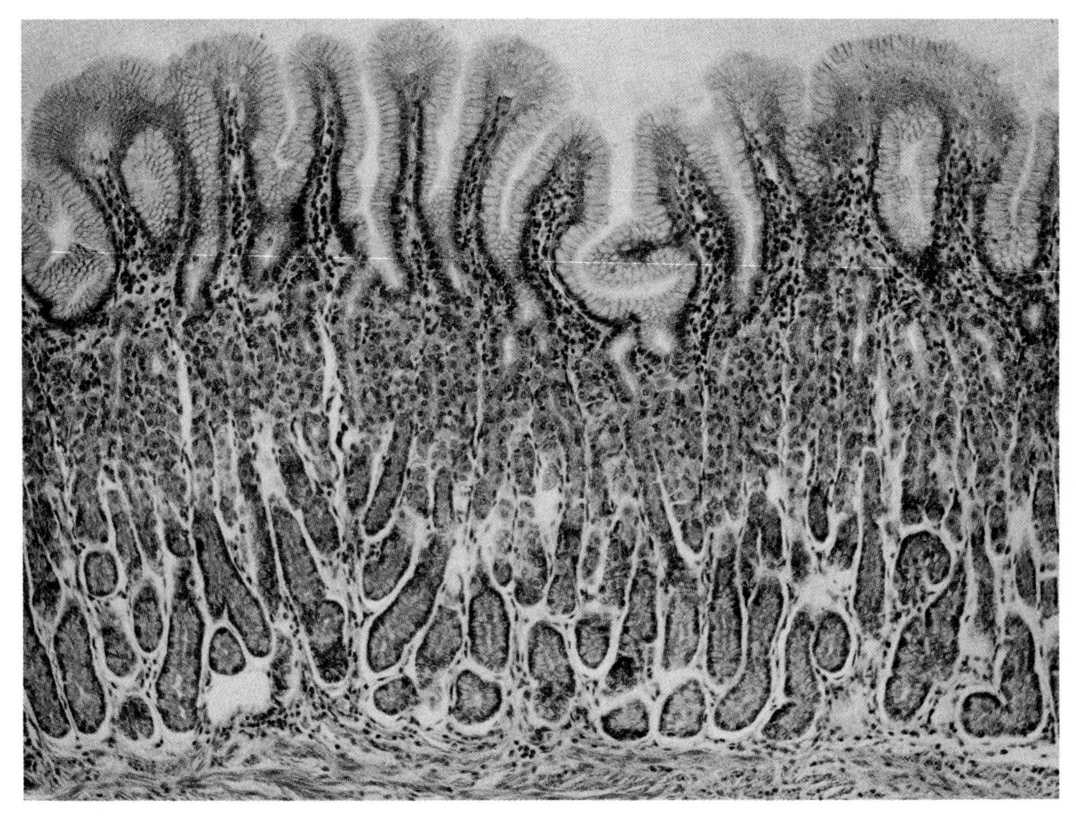

Figure 25–10. Photomicrograph of the gastric mucosa of a macaque showing the long, tubular gastric glands opening into the gastric pits or foveolae.

foveolae and necks of the gastric glands. The rate of cell renewal is evidently slow because mitosis of the undifferentiated precursors is seldom observed.

CARDIAC GLANDS

Slender tubular *cardiac glands* arise from shallow foveolae in a narrow zone (1–3 cm) around the gastroesophageal junction. These are tortuous at their lower end and some are branched. They are lined by mucus-secreting cells indistinguishable from those of the foveolae. A few relatively undifferentiated cells are found near the necks of the glands, and occasional endocrine cells occur among the mucous-secreting cells. The majority of these secrete *gastrin*, a polypeptide hormone that stimulates secretory activity of glands in the corpus and influences gastric motility. The area containing cardiac glands is very narrow in the human stomach, but it may occupy one-third of the stomach in swine.

OXYNTIC GLANDS

The glands of the fundus and corpus, called *oxyntic glands (gastric glands)*, make the greatest contribution to the gastric juice. In the human stomach, there is estimated to be 15 million of them associated with 3.5 million gastric foveolae. From one to seven arise from each foveola. They are 30–50 μm in diameter and extend downward for the greater part of the thickness of the mucosa (0.5–1.5 mm). Oxyntic glands contain five cell types: *mucous neck cells, stem cells, chief cells, (zymogenic cells), oxyntic cells (parietal cells)*, and *endocrine cells*. For descriptive purposes, three regions of the glands are defined (Fig. 25–12). Their confluence with the foveola, called the *isthmus*, consists mainly of surface mucous cells. A narrow segment be-

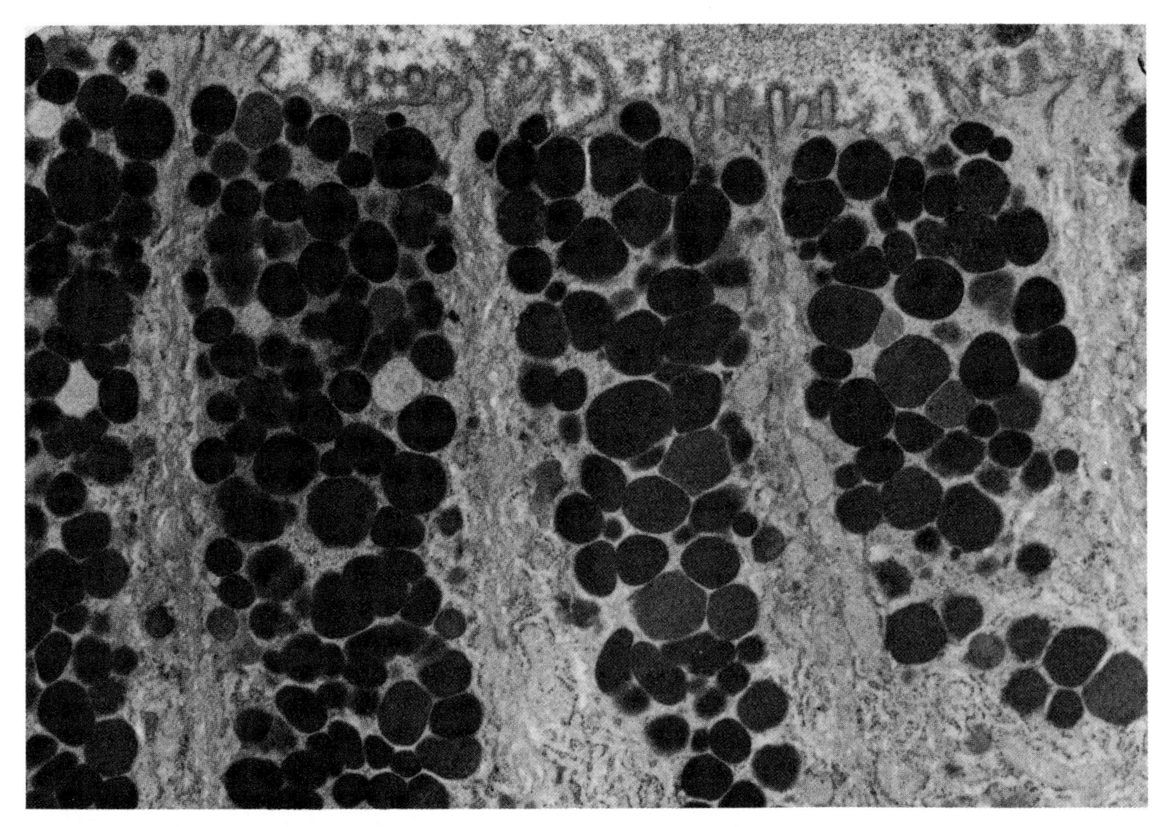

Figure 25–11. Electron micrograph of the apical portion of several surface mucous cells. The short microvilli have a conspicuous glycocalyx and the surface is covered by a layer of mucus. (Micrograph courtesy of S. Ito.)

low this is the *neck*, containing mucous neck cells, stem cells, and occasional oxyntic cells, followed by the *base* which makes up the greater part of the length of the gland and contains numerous chief cells, oxyntic cells, and occasional mucous neck cells. Isolated endocrine cells may be found in all segments of the glands. Mitotic activity is confined to a small number of stem cells in the neck of the glands.

At the necks of the glands, surface mucous cells give way to *mucous neck cells*. These are columnar cells, but being lodged between larger, rounded oxyntic cells, they are deformed to varying degrees. They may have a broad apex and a slender mid region, or a constricted apical region and a broader base. The nucleus is displaced to the cell base. The cytoplasmic organelles are not significantly different from those of the surface mucous cells, but polyribosomes are more abundant. These cells are not confined to the neck, as their name implies,. but are also scattered singly among the cells in deeper segments of the gland. There, they are less distorted by neighboring cells and may be difficult to distinguish from chief cells in routine histological sections, but after periodic-acid–Schiff staining, they stand out owing to the deep pink staining of their secretory granules. These are larger than those of the surface mucous cells and, in electron micrographs, they have a dense core and a lighter outer zone. However, their appearance varies considerably from species to species. The mucin in their apical cytoplasm has a stronger affinity for basic dyes at low pH than that of the surface cells. Uptake of radioactive sulfur by these cells suggests that they produce sulfated glycoproteins. The physiological significance of the production of two kinds of mucus by the gastric mucosa is not known.

Among the cells in the neck of the gastric glands are small numbers of stem cells, having a nucleus with a large nucleolus and a cytoplasm containing abundant polyribosomes. The continuous renewal of the gastric mucosa depends on their proliferation. As their daughter cells differentiate, they migrate either upward to replace surface mucous cells or downward in the gland to form new oxyntic

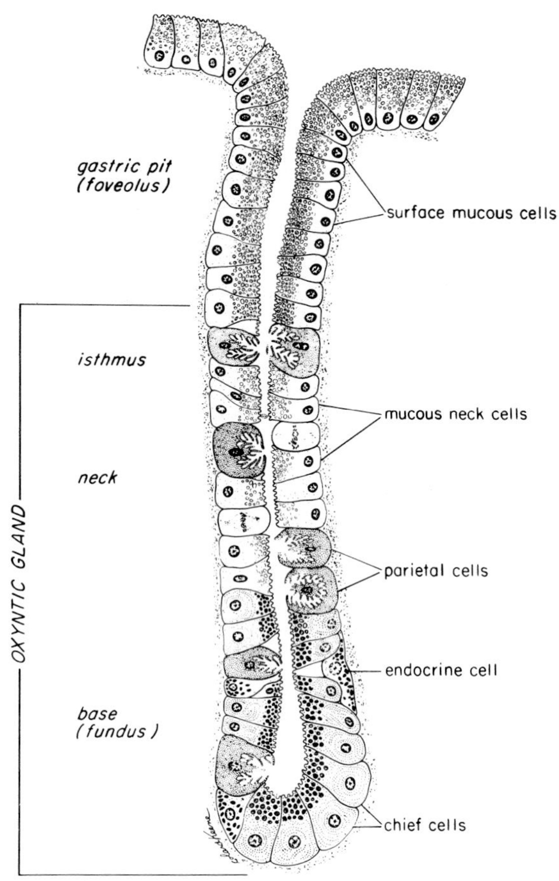

Figure 25–12. Diagram of an oxyntic gland from the corpus of a mammalian stomach showing the isthmus, base, and neck. (From Ito, S. *In* L.R. Johnson, ed. Physiology of the Gastrointestinal Tract. New York, Raven Press.

and chief cells. It is estimated that the surface mucous cells are replaced about every 4 days and the mucous neck cells about once a week. The turnover time of the oxyntic and chief cells is considerably longer.

The most conspicuous cells of the gastric mucosa are the *oxyntic* or *parietal cells* that produce the hydrochloric acid of the gastric juice. They are up to 25 μm in diameter and have broad, rounded bases that often bulge from the otherwise smooth outer surface of the gland. Their cytoplasm stains intensely with eosin or phloxine and their most distinctive feature is the presence of a meandering invagination of the apical surface called the *secretory canaliculus*. This may encircle the nucleus and extend nearly to the plasmalemma at the cell base (Figs. 25–13 and 25–14). The limiting membrane of the canaliculus is continuous with the apical plasmalemma around its opening into the lumen of the gland. Microvilli project into the lumen of the canaliculus and these vary in number in different phases of secretory activity. The cytoplasm of the oxyntic cell contains no secretory granules, and its paranuclear Golgi complex is smaller than that of other glandular cells. Large mitochondria occupy 40% of the cell volume. Their large number and elaborate internal structure reflect the high-energy requirement of acid secretion. Isolated oxyntic cells have been shown to have a rate of oxygen consumption five times that of the mucous cells.

A unique ultrastructural feature of the oxyntic cell is an abundance of membrane-bounded structures that do not appear to be elements of the endoplasmic reticulum. Their form was formerly a subject of dispute among electron microscopists, some describing them as vesicles and others insisting that they are tubules. The descriptive term *tubulovesicular system*, in current use, represents a compromise between these conflicting interpretations. Its appearance in electron micrographs is strongly influenced by the method of specimen preparation. Recent adoption of freezing in liquid helium followed by freeze-substitution has led to a consensus that the system is predominantly tubular in the living state (Fig. 25–15).

The internal organization of the oxyntic cells undergoes striking changes in different phases of their secretory activity. In the nonsecreting cell, the secretory canaliculus is relatively small and its microvilli are short and sparse, whereas the tubulovesicular system is very extensive. In the stimulated cell, there is a rapid elongation of the canaliculus and an increase in the number and length of its microvilli, resulting in a fivefold increase in surface area. Sixty to eighty percent of the protein in the membrane added is H^+,K^+-ATPase, a 95 kD proton pump involved in acid secretion. This amplification of surface area is accompanied by a dramatic reduction in the extent of the tubulovesicular system, and the most plausible explanation of this is that the membrane-bounded elements of the tubulovesicular system have fused with the membrane of the canaliculus, to greatly increase its area. A reorganization of the cytoskeleton is associated with these changes. The oxyntic cells contain more actin that other glandular cells, but in the resting cell, most of it is in the molecular form. However, on stimulation of acid secretion, it rapidly polymerizes to form actin filaments. Interaction of these filaments with myosin is believed to

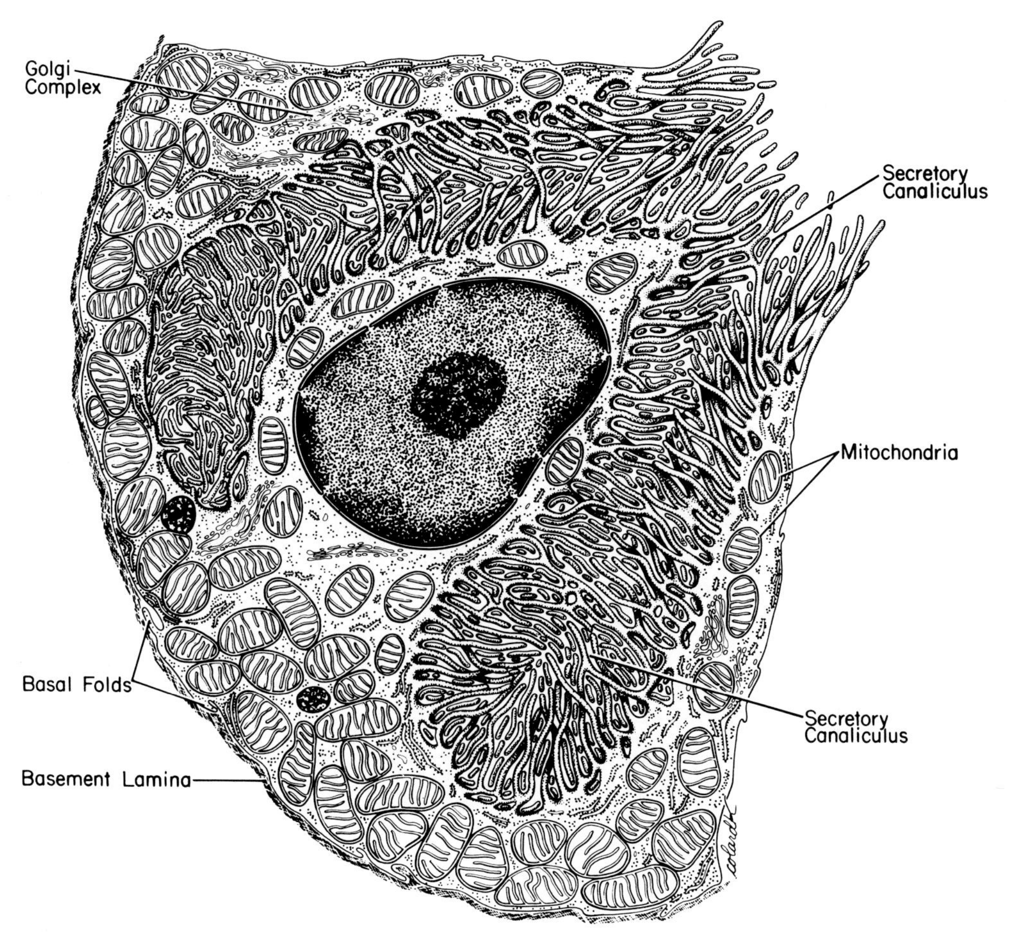

Figure 25–13. Drawing of the ultrastructure of an active parietal cell (oxyntic cell). It is a large cell with an exceptional number of mitochondria and a prominent intracellular canaliculus lined with microvilli. (Drawing courtesy of S. Ito.)

play a major role in movement of the tubules of the tubulovesicular system to the surface for fusion with the membrane of the canaliculus. In electron micrographs of the secreting oxyntic cell, actin filaments are abundant in the peripheral cytoplasm and they extend into the long microvilli stabilizing them and possibly contributing to their increase in length. After secretory activity has declined, the size of the canaliculus decreases as membrane is withdrawn from the surface in regeneration of a tubulovesicular system in the cytoplasm.

Although indirect evidence for recycling of membrane between the plasmalemma and the tubulovesicular system is persuasive, some slightly troubling inconsistencies remain. One is that certain enzymes demonstrable in the plasmalemma of the canaliculus, by histochemical methods, are not consistently demonstrable in the tubovesicular membranes. More puzzling is the fact that electron microscopic images of continuity between this system and the canaliculus, which one would expect to find in the stimulated cell, are rarely, if ever, observed. It is possible that the time course of such fusions is so brief that the probability of encountering one in a thin section, fusing is very small.

Organelles of the biosynthetic pathway for proteins are not prominent in oxyntic cells. The small Golgi complex and limited amount of rough endoplasmic reticulum are thought to be involved in synthesis of *gastric intrinsic factor*, a glycoprotein necessary for absorption of vitamin B-12. Extensive damage to these cells not only results in deficiency of hydrochloric acid in the gastric juice (*achlorhydria*) but also leads to anemia due to failure of erythrocyte production in a bone marrow deprived of vitamin B-12. Oxyntic cells differentiate from stem cells in the isthmus and slowly move downward as other cells are formed behind them. As they approach the base, the oxyntic cells degenerate and their residues are

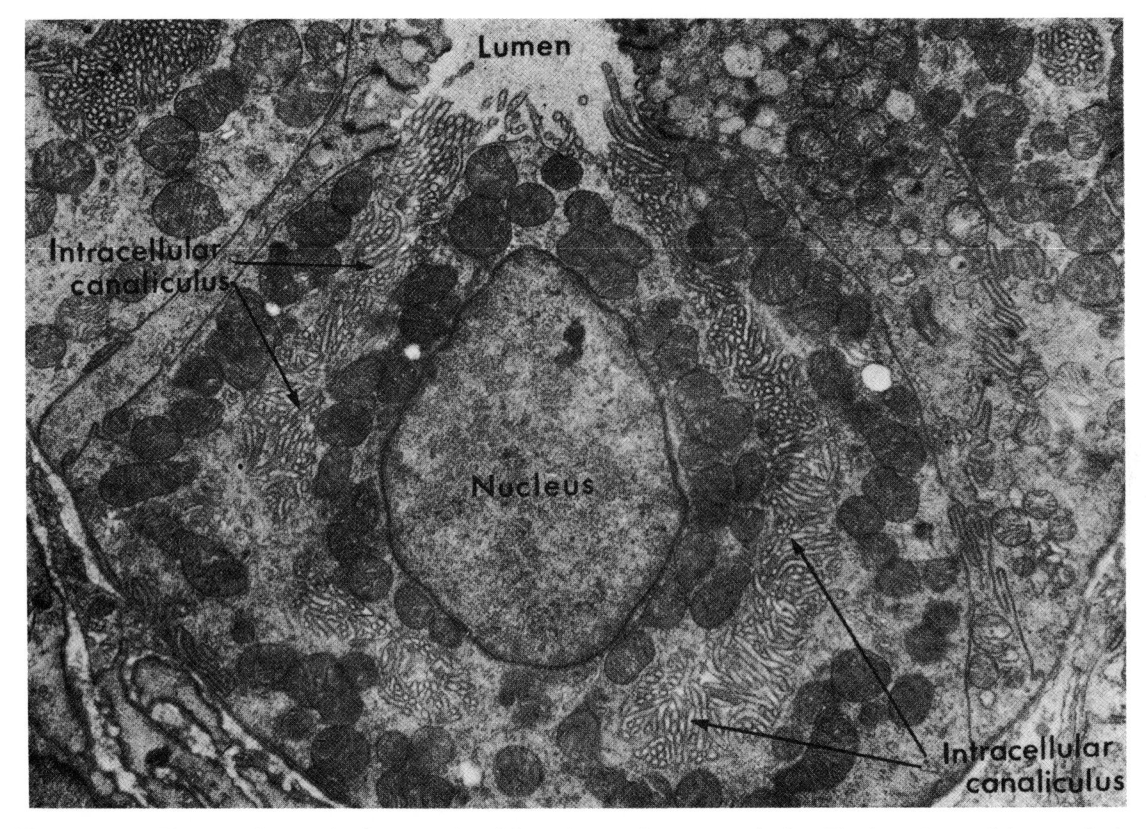

Figure 25–14. Electron micrograph of an oxyntic cell from the gastric mucosa of a bat. The large intracellular canaliculus is filled by its numerous microvilli. (Courtesy of S. Ito.)

eliminated by phagocytosis, or by extrusion into the gastric lumen.

The predominant cells in the lower third of oxyntic glands in the corpus of the stomach are the *chief cells*. They are absent from the cardiac glands, sparse in the glands of the fundus, and rare in those of the pyloris. They have strongly basophilic cytoplasm and numerous apical secretory granules that are hard to preserve and are often extracted during specimen preparation. In routine histological sections, the granules are usually pale and indistinct but they can be selectively stained with Bowie's Biebrich scarlet method. They are 1–3 μm in diameter and contain pepsinogen, the precursor of the proteolytic enzyme *pepsin*.

In electron micrographs, the chief cells have a structure similar to that of the zymogenic cells of the pancreas and other cells very active in protein synthesis (Fig. 25–16 and 25–17). The luminal surface of the cell bears short microvilli coated with a thin glycocalyx. There is a prominent supranuclear Golgi complex, and parallel cisternae of rough endoplasmic reticulum fill the basal cytoplasm. A few may extend into the apical cytoplasm. In the human, numerous lysosomes can be found among the secretory granules.

Exocytosis of the secretory product can be accelerated by feeding, after a period of fasting, or by administration of the gastrointestinal hormone *secretin*. Although the chief cells of the oxyntic glands are the principal source of pepsin, immunocytochemical studies suggest that small amounts may also be produced by mucous neck cells and, in some species, by the mucous cells of pyloric glands.

PYLORIC GLANDS

The pyloric glands occupy the distal 4 to 5 cm of the stomach, which represents about one-fifth of the surface area of the gastric mucosa. In this region, the gastric pits or foveolae are deeper than those of the body of the stomach, extending down through half the depth of the mucosa. The pyloric glands arising from them have a larger lumen and are more highly branched and tortuous than the oxyntic glands. For this reason, they are seldom seen in continuity in histological sections.

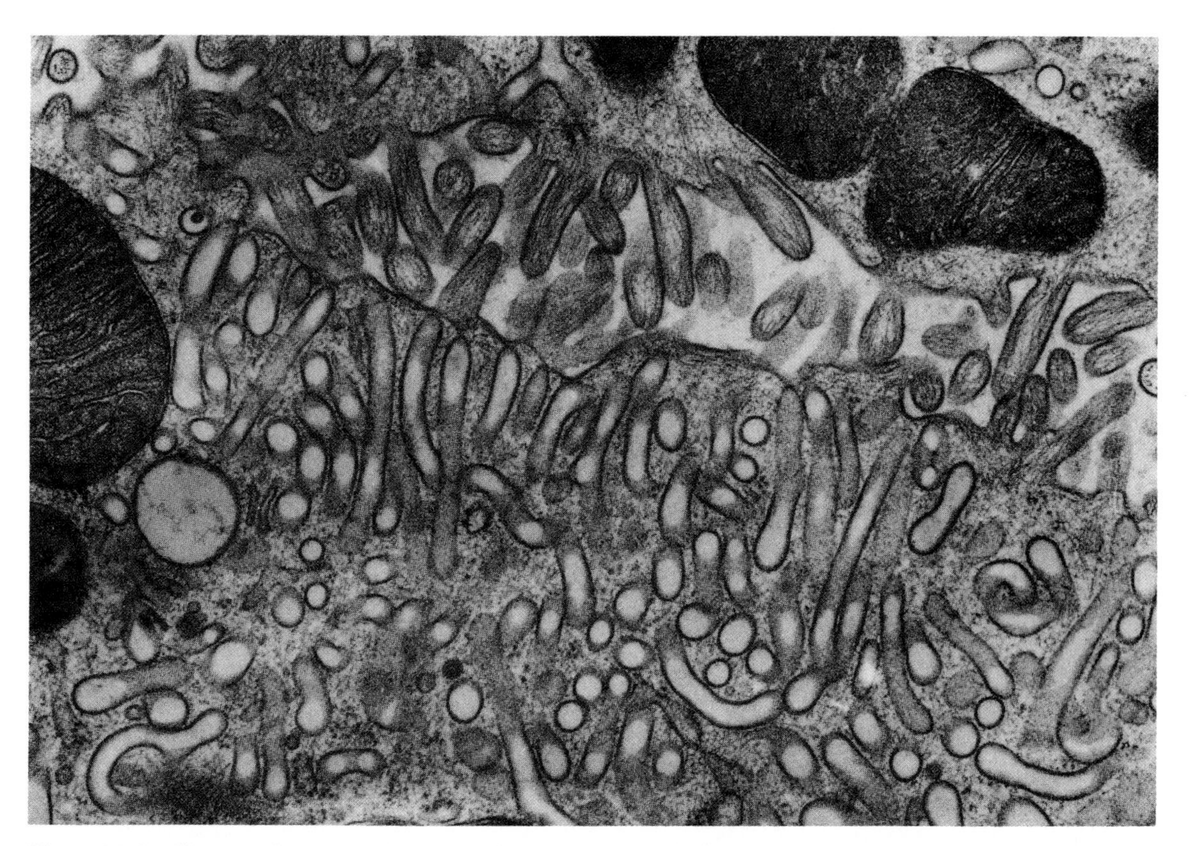

Figure 25–15. Electron micrograph of a portion of an oxyntic cell, including a segment of the secretory canaliculus (top). Numerous elements of the tubulovesicular system can be seen in the cytoplasm near the canaliculus. Specimen prepared by freezing in liquid helium followed by freeze substitution in osmium tetroxide and acetone. (Courtesy of N. Sugai and A. Ichikawa.)

The predominant cell type is a mucus-secreting cell that resembles the mucous neck cells of the oxyntic glands. The greater part of the cell is filled with large, pale, secretory droplets that flatten the nucleus and displace it to the base of the cell. There are mitochondria and cisternae of rough endoplasmic reticulum in this region. In addition to mucus, these cells secrete the enzyme lysozyme which is effective in lysing bacteria. In the dog, there is evidence for secretion of small amounts of pepsin. In the human stomach, occasional oxyntic (parietal) cells are also found in these glands, and enteroendocrine cells are abundant. Lymphoid cells containing coarse eosinophilic inclusions called Russell's bodies may be found between the epithelial cells of the glands. These occur in the normal mucosa but are more common in pathological conditions.

ENTEROENDOCRINE CELLS

Small granulated cells scattered individually among the cells of the glands have been recognized for more than a century. They could be stained selectively by silver or chromium salts and were, therefore, called *argentaffin* or *enterochromaffin cells.* These traditional staining methods permitted recognition of two or more categories of silver-reducing cells, but they shed no light on the chemical nature of their granules, or the physiological significance of their secretions.

In the past 20 years, advances in biochemical extraction techniques and radioimmunoassay procedures have led to the identification and purification of a large number of biogenic amines and peptide hormones. By using labeled antibodies to these substances, some of them have been localized to specific cell types widely distributed throughout the mucosa of the gastrointestinal tract. Immunocytochemical methods have now identified nine different endocrine or paracrine cell types in the tract, and the number continues to grow. All are small ovoid or pyramidal cells lodged between the bases of neighboring exocrine cells of the epithelium (Fig. 25–19, 25–20). Some have a narrow apex that extends to the lumen;

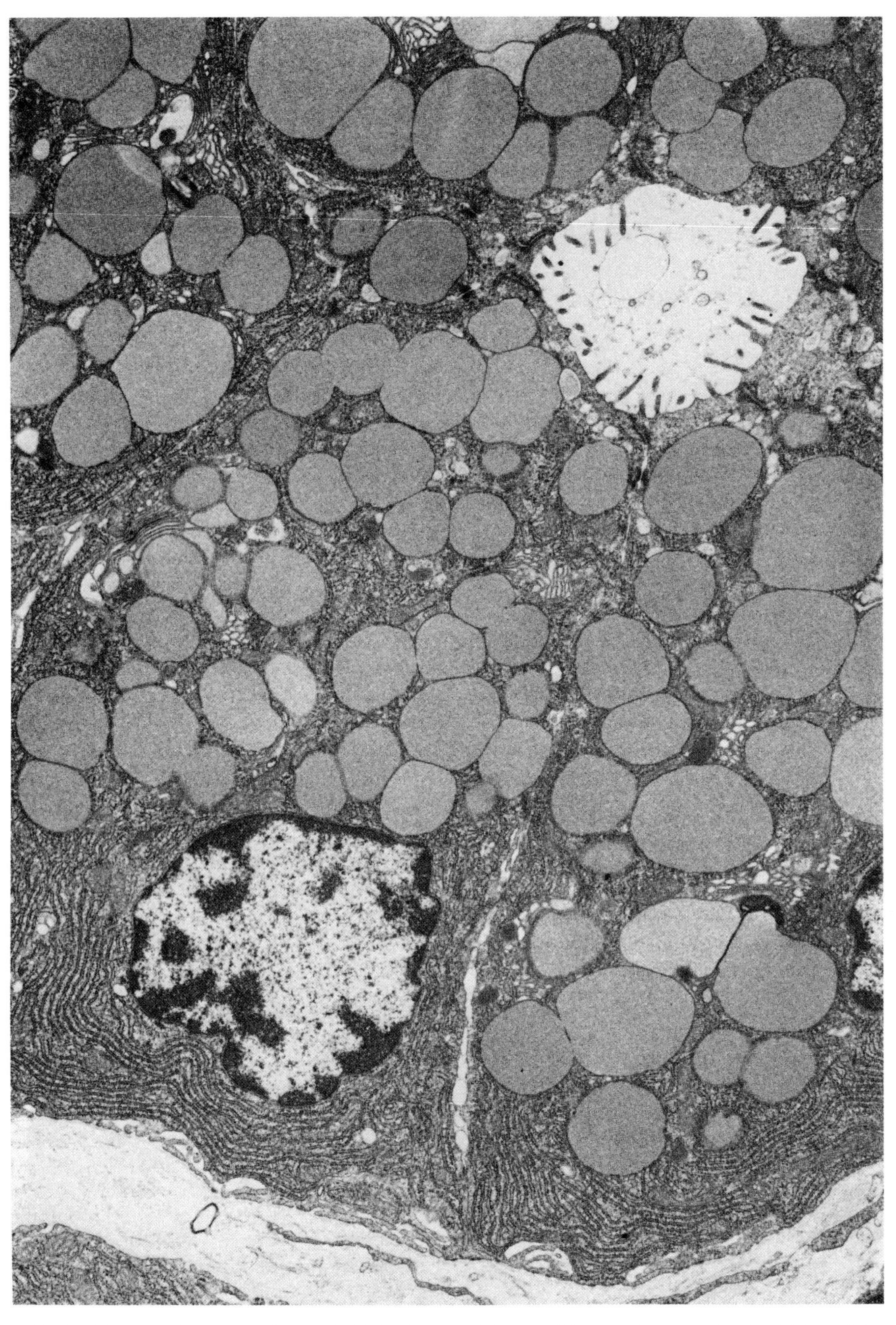

Figure 25–16. Electron micrograph of several chief cells around the small lumen of an oxyntic gland. The cell base is occupied by cisternae of rough endoplasmic reticulum and the apex is crowded with pale-staining secretory granules. (Courtesy of S. Ito.)

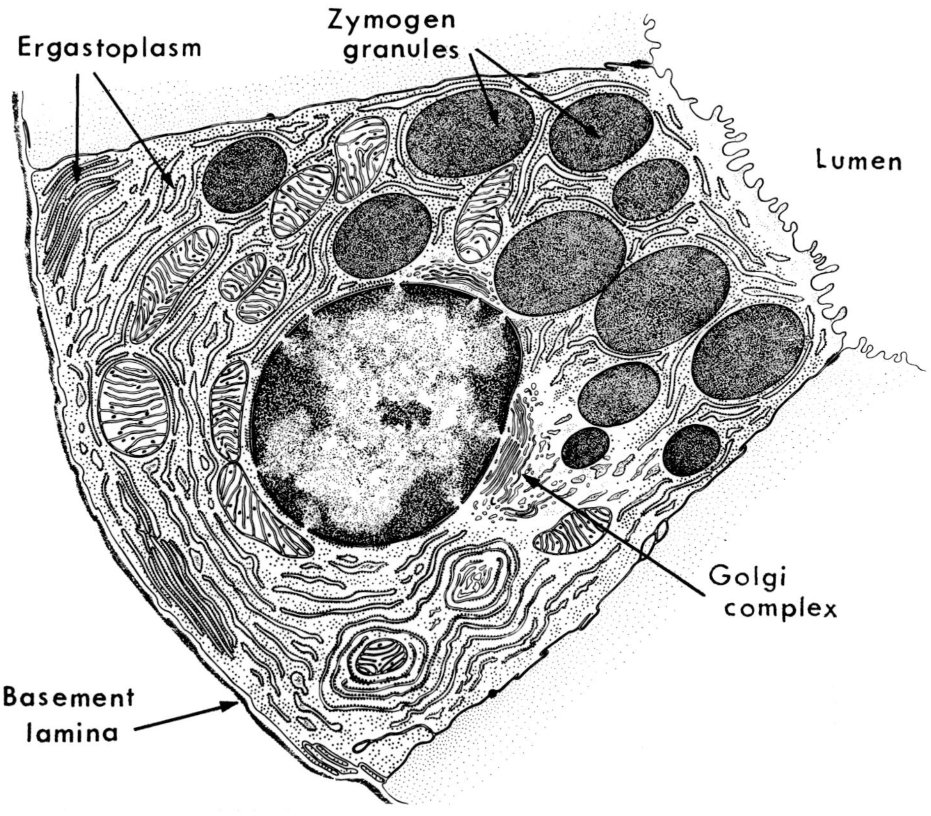

Figure 25–17. Drawing of a gastric chief cell (zymogenic cell), as seen with the electron microscope. (From Ito, S. and R.J. Winchester. 1963. J. Cell Biol. 16:541.)

others are confined to the base of the epithelium. All contain small secretory granules that are concentrated in the cytoplasm at the cell base. Some can be identified in electron micrographs on the basis of the size and substructure of the granules. Those containing monoamines exhibit a characteristic fluorescence, but the most reliable means of identification of the different cell types depends on the use of radiolabeled antibodies to their respective secretory products.

These cells are now referred to collectively as *enteroendocrine cells*. Several of them have cytochemical properties that are common to cells secreting peptide hormones and are grouped together, by some authors, under the term *APUD-cells*. This designation is based on their Amine Precursor Uptake and Decarboxylation. The APUD cells are not confined to the gastrointestinal tract but also occur in the respiratory tract and elsewhere in the body. Enteroendocrine cells will be considered again in the next chapter on the intestines; we are concerned here only with those in the stomach.

The enteroendocrine cells of the gastric mucosa include: *G-cells* secreting gastrin; *EC-cells* secreting serotonin; *D-cells* secreting somatostatin; and *A-cells* secreting enteroglucagon. Of these, the G-cells are of the greatest physiological importance. They are most abundant in the pyloric antrum where they may number $5 \times 10^5/cm^2$ of mucosa. They are pyramidal in form with a narrow apex bearing long microvilli. Secretory granules, 200–350 nm in diameter, are clustered at the cell base (Fig. 25–19). Some of these have dense cores, whereas others are vesicles largely devoid of contents. In response to vagal stimulation, or distension of the stomach, the G-cells secrete gastrin, a peptide hormone that stimulates gastric motility and is a potent stimulator of acid secretion by the oxyntic cells (parietal cells). It also acts on the stem cells in glands of the corpus, stimulating their proliferation and differentiation into oxyntic cells. Administration of gastrin to rats is reported to increase the number of these cells from 34 to 54 million. There is compelling indirect evidence that gastrin has a similar trophic ef-

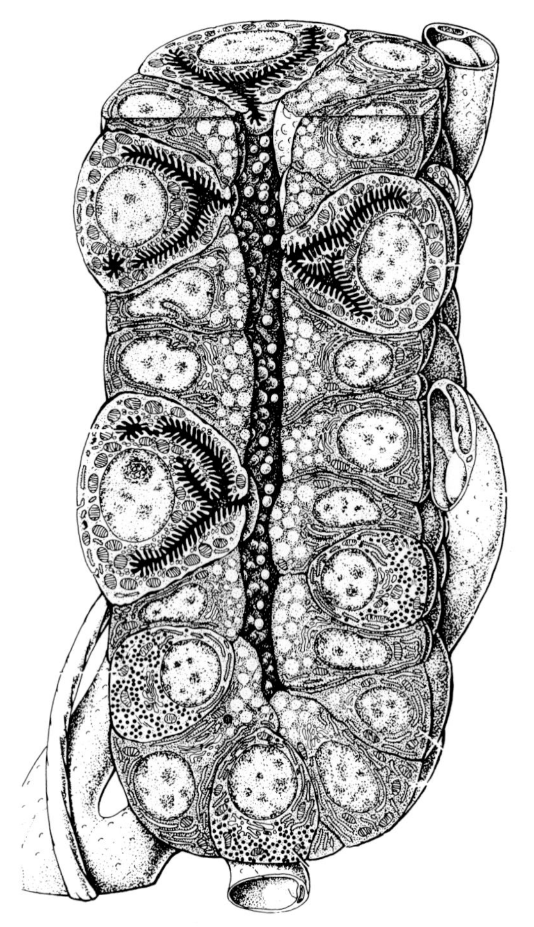

Figure 25–18. Drawing of the base of an oxyntic gland. Three cells with basally located small granules are enteroendocrine cells. (From Krstic, R.V. 1978. Die Gewebe des Menschen und Saugetiere. Berlin, Springer-Verlag.)

fect on the gastric mucosa in man. Resection of the antrum of the human stomach, which contains the majority of the G-cells, is followed by marked achlorhydria and hypoplasia of the mucosa. Overproduction of gastrin in patients with Zolliger–Ellison syndrome results in excessive acid secretion and mucosal hyperplasia. Thus, gastrin is probably a regulator of mucosal growth in all mammalian species.

The function of the other enteroendocrine cells of the stomach are less well understood but they seem to be less essential than the G-cells. Like the G-cells, the EC-cells are pyramidal with a narrow apex and have 300-nm secretory granules at their base. The granules have oval or elongated dense cores. Release of serotonin by these cells influences gastric motility. D-cells occur in glands near the pyloris but are more numerous in the duodenum. Their product, somatostatin, is believed to have an inhibitory effect on the other enteroendocrine cells. The ECL-cells have relatively large secretory granules (450 nm) containing one or more eccentrically placed dense cores. Histamine released by these cells stimulates gastric secretion and may mediate, or complement, the action of gastrin. A-cells have small granules (250 nm) with a clear halo around a dense core. They secrete enteroglucagon, a peptide hormone similar to the glucagon secreted by the α-cells of the pancreatic islets. It raises blood glucose levels by stimulating hepatic glycogenolysis.

LAMINA PROPRIA

The space around the glands and between their bases and the muscularis mucosae is occupied by the loose connective tissue comprising the lamina propria. It consists of a loose network of reticular and collagen fibers but very few elastic fibers. In addition to fibroblasts, the meshes of this fibrous network contains lymphocytes, eosinophils, mast cells, and a few plasma cells. A few slender strands of smooth muscle may be found running vertically in the lamina propria. Their contraction may compress the mucosa and facilitate discharge of secretions from the glands. Small accumulations of lymphoid tissue are normally present.

SUBMUCOSA

The submucosa is a moderately thick layer of denser connective tissue contain coarser bundles of collagen fibers and many elastic fibers. There are numerous wandering cells including lymphocytes, eosinophils, sessile mast cells, and plasma cells. A few adipose cells may occur in the submucosa. In this layer, there are also many arterioles, a venous plexus, and a network of lymphatics.

MUSCULARIS EXTERNA

The thick musculature of the stomach wall is usually said to consist of three layers of smooth muscle oriented longitudinally, circumferentially and obliquely, but these layers intermingle at the interfaces and are not clearly defined separate layers as they are in the muscularis of the intestine. Their relationships are not easily described. The longitudi-

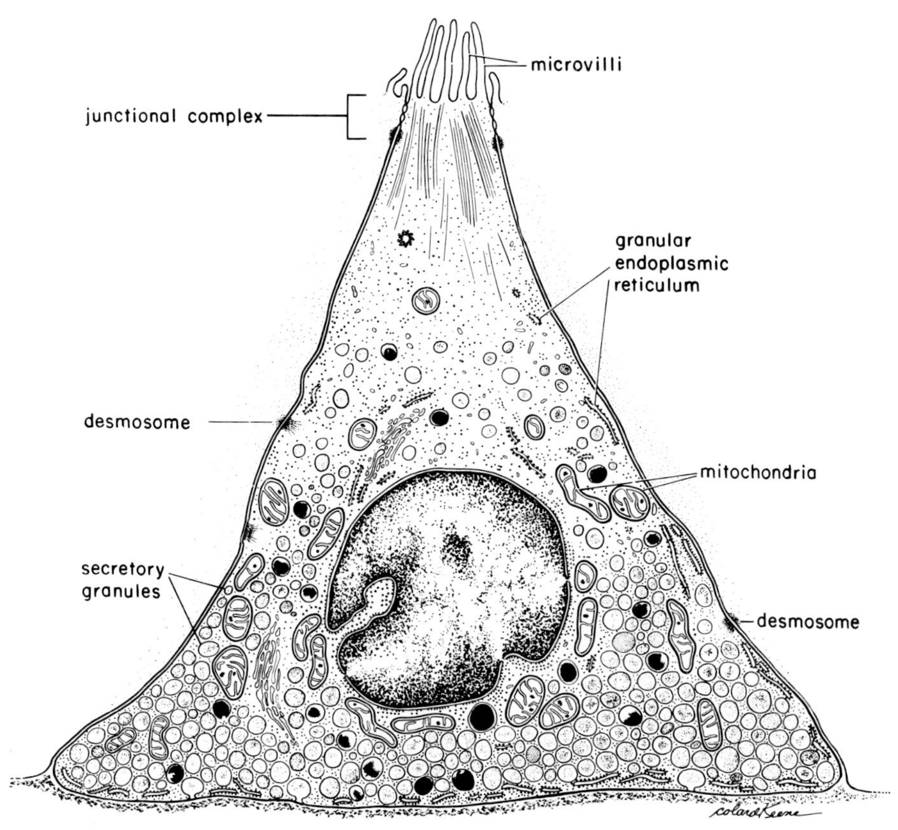

Figure 25–19. Drawing of a G-cell, an enteroendocrine cell type secreting gastrin. Note that secretory granules are concentrated at the vascular pole. The content of many of them has been extracted in specimen preparation. (From Ito, S. 1981. *In* L.R. Johnson ed. Physiology of the Gastrointestinal Tract. New York, Raven Press.

nal fibers immediately beneath the serosa are continuous above with the corresponding layer in the wall of the esophagus. They radiate from the cardia and are thickest along the greater and lesser curvatures of the stomach. They do not continue all the way to the pyloris. Thus, this layer is incomplete and cannot be found in some areas of the dorsal and ventral sides of the organ. The circular fibers, on the other hand, do form a complete layer over the whole stomach. It is continuous above with the circular smooth muscle of the lower esophagus and it is thickest in the pyloris, where it forms an annular *pyloric sphincter*.

The oblique smooth muscle fibers, lying deep to the circular layer, also do not form a complete layer. They are most concentrated at the cardia and sweep downward in broad thin bands running parallel to the lesser curvature, with some bands diverging toward the greater curvature and intermingling with fibers of the circular layer. Oblique fibers are generally lacking along the lesser curvature of the stomach.

Contraction of the muscularis is regulated with great precision by autonomic nerve plexuses between its layers. By varying the tonus of the smooth muscle in its wall, the stomach adapts to the volume of its contents with little or no change in the pressure in its lumen. Emptying of the stomach depends on intermittent peristaltic waves of contraction that sweep from the cardia to the pyloris and these are coordinated with relaxations of the pyloric sphincter.

BLOOD SUPPLY

The blood supply of the gastric mucosa comes from arterioles in the submucosa giving rise to capillaries that ascend in the lamina propria between the glands (Fig. 25–21). These fenestrated capillaries surround the

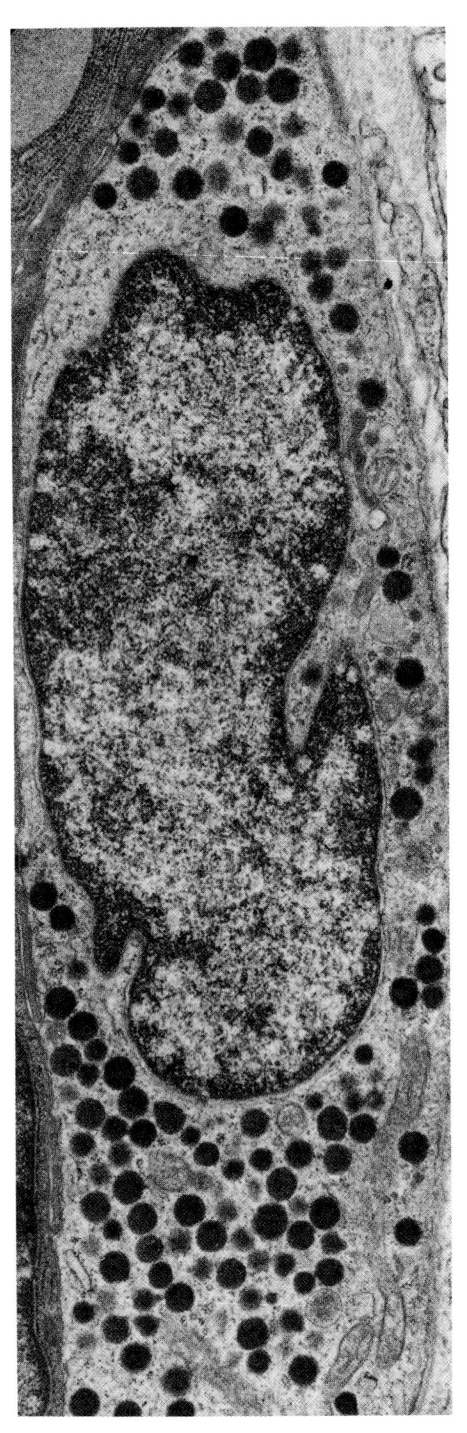

Figure 25–20. Electron micrograph of another kind of enteroendocrine cell. The exact cell type can only be determined by immunocytochemical methods.

glands and form a dense network beneath the surface epithelium. This capillary bed is drained by collecting venules that descend directly to the submucosal venous plexus. There appear to be no arteriovenous anastomoses in the gastric mucosa.

The upward flow of blood along the sides of the glands in intimate relation to the bases of the parietal cells encourages the speculation that bicarbonate produced as a by-product of acid secretion would diffuse into the blood and be transported to the capillaries beneath the surface epithelium (Fig. 25–22). There the bicarbonate would be favorably situated to neutralize any hydrogen ions diffusing into the mucosa from the lumen. One is tempted to believe that the microvascular architecture of the stomach, thus, provides the mucosa with maximal protection against potential damage from the hydrochloric acid content of the gastric lumen.

CELL RENEWAL AND REPAIR

As stated earlier in the chapter, the gastric mucosa has a rapid rate of cell turnover. Radiolabeling experiments on laboratory rodents have shown that the surface mucous cells are completely renewed in about 3 days. Although the rate is probably somewhat slower in the human stomach, it is still surprisingly rapid. Mitotic activity is largely confined to cells in isthmus and necks of the glands (Fig. 25–23). New cells migrating upward from this region replace superficial cells that are exfoliated into the lumen. Cells deeper in the glands are relatively long-lived and are renewed more slowly. Oxyntic cells probably arise by mitosis and further differentiation of stem cells but there is some reason to believe that chief cells are capable of division and their renewal may not depend on proliferation of undifferentiated cells in the neck of the glands.

The gastric mucosa also has a remarkable capacity to reestablish epithelial continuity after superficial injury. In humans, the stomach is frequently insulted by aspirin, strong alcoholic beverages, and other toxic substances that cause superficial erosion of the mucosa. Repair is due to migration of viable cells from the depths of the foveolae in a process now commonly called gastric *mucosal restitution*. In rodent gastric mucosa exposed to 20 mM aspirin or 40% ethanol (80 proof), the resulting injury to the surface epithelium is scarcely detectable after only 30 min. The time course of this repair is too short to have depended on cell proliferation. Instead, it is believed that undamaged epithelium in the lower third of the foveolae is stimulated to migrate over the vacated basal lamina of the surface epithelium. Within half an hour, the

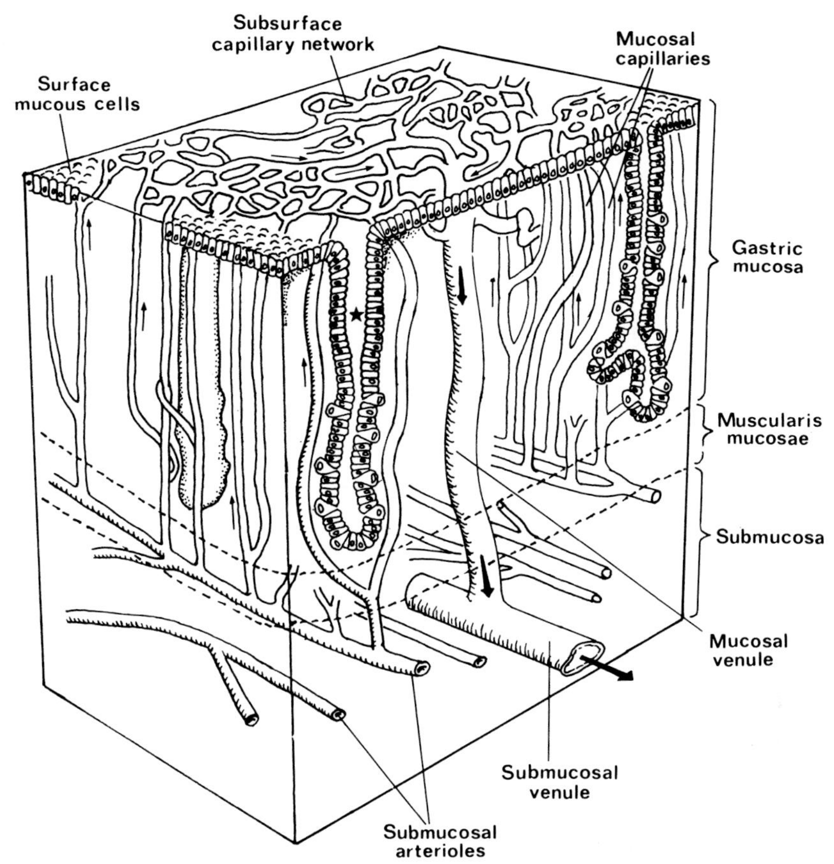

Figure 25–21. A diagramatic depiction of the blood vascular supply of the human gastric mucosa. Relationships of the gland marked with an asterisk are shown in greater detail in Fig. 25–22. (Redrawn after Gannon, B.J. J. Browning, and J.E. McGuigan. 1984. Gastroenterology. 86:866.)

basal lamina is covered by a thin continuous layer of squamous or cuboidal cells that later increase in height and resume secretory activity. It is concluded from these experiments that epithelial migration provides a rapid mechanism for coverage after chemical, thermal, or hyperosmolar injuries that do not extensively damage the basal lamina. Destruction of the basal lamina by very low pH in the gastric lumen greatly retards restoration of epithelial continuity. The capacity of the mucosa to withstand very low pH is quite remarkable. The high rate of blood flow to the mucosa and plasma leakage at a site of injury can maintain a pH of 6 to 7 even when acid of pH 1 is present in the lumen.

HISTOPHYSIOLOGY OF THE STOMACH

Having described the structural components of the stomach and some of their functional attributes, we proceed to a brief account of its physiology. The stomach is a distensible reservoir for accumulation of food and its processing by products of the glands in the mucosa. Its capacity is quite large. When empty, its luminal volume is only 50–75 ml, but 1.2 liters can be swallowed before intraluminal pressure begins to rise. The volume of secretions produced daily ranges from 500 to 1000 ml. Only a few milliliters are secreted per hour, between meals, but on ingestion of food, hundreds of milliliters are produced. The clear colorless *gastric juice* contains mucus, water, hydrochloric acid, and the enzyme pepsin. Secretion of acid maintains an optimal intraluminal environment for proteolysis by pepsin which is most active at pH 2.

One of the remarkable properties of the gastric mucosa is its ability to produce a secretion having a pH ranging from 2 to as low as 0.9. This corresponds to a concentration of hydrogen ions more than a million times that of blood. How this is accomplished was long

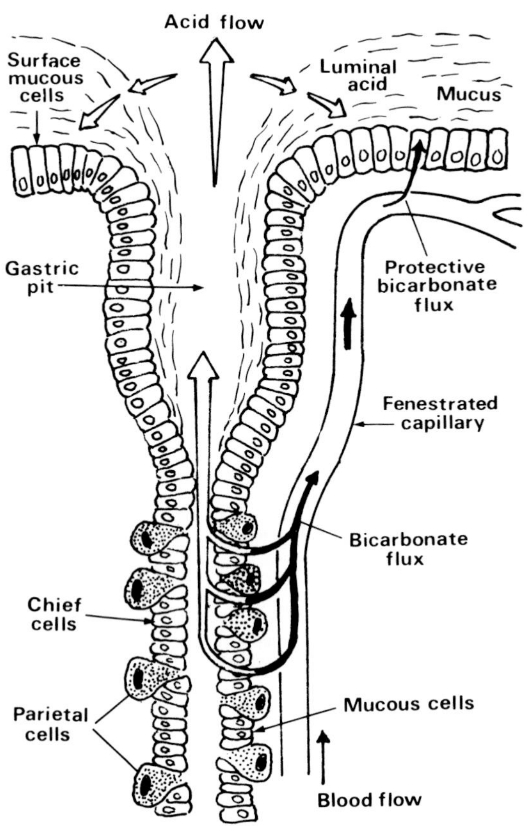

Figure 25–22. Diagram of the postulated diffusion of bicarbonate ions, generated by active parietal cells, to the subsurface capillary network, where they may protect the epithelium by neutralizing any back-diffusing hydrogen ions from the lumen. (Redrawn after Gannon, B.J. J. Browning, and J.E. McGuigan. 1984. Gastroenterology. 86:866.)

debated, but electron microscopic observations on the changes in ultrastructure of stimulated oxyntic cells and biochemical studies of cell fractions have led to a consensus on all by a few of the mechanisms involved. The membranes of the tubulovesicular system in the oxyntic cell cytoplasm contain a unique H^+,K^+-ATPase which is the proton pump that uses ATP to pump H^+ from the cell to the gland lumen, and K^+ from the lumen into the cell. In the unstimulated cell, the membrane of the tubulovesicular system is relatively impermeable to K^+ and Cl^- and there is little or no accumulation of H^+ in the vesicles. On stimulation of the oxyntic cells, polymerization of actin to form microfilaments and their interaction with myosin contribute to movement of the elements of the tubulovesicular system to the surface, where they fuse with the membrane of the canaliculus, resulting in a four- to fivefold increase in the cell surface area containing H^+,K^+-ATPase. By a mechanism that is still unclear, there is a concomitant opening of channels increasing the permeability of the membrane to ions. Flow of potassium chloride from the cell into the lumen provides K ions for which the H^+,K^+-ATPase pump exchanges H^+ and Cl^- ions, resulting in the secretion of hydrochloric acid. Water moves into the canaliculus along an osmotic gradient driven by the flux of ions (Fig. 25–24).

Gastric secretion is controlled by a complex interaction of neural and endocrine mechanisms that are still not well understood. The path of neural stimulation is via the vagus nerves to an intramural nerve plexus, from which, fibers ascend to the gastric glands and surface epithelium. Gastric secretory activity is greatly enhanced, early in a meal, when chemo- and mechanoreceptors in the oral cavity are stimulated by the chewing and tasting of food. Afferent impulses from these receptors travel to the brain and are relayed to efferent fibers in the vagus nerves which act directly on the oxyntic cells to increase their secretion of acid. Concurrently, neurones in

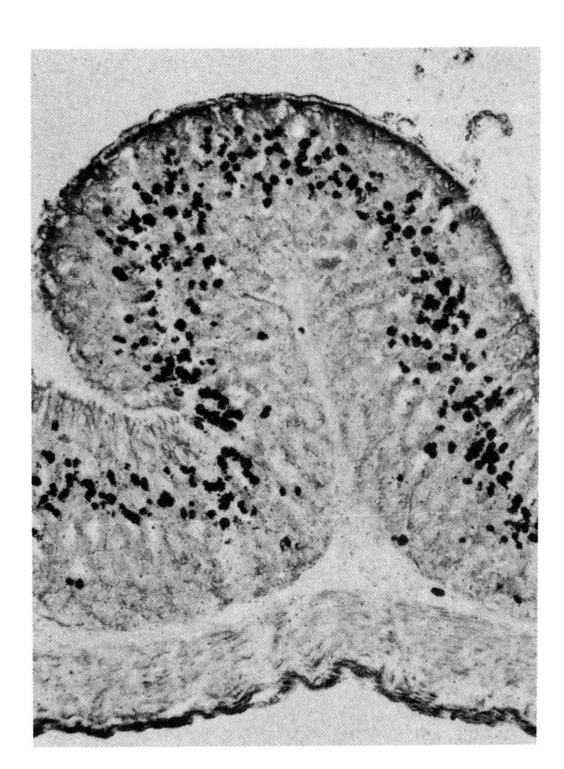

Figure 25–23. Autoradiograph of gastric mucosa of a mouse given three injections of tritiated thymidine over a 12-h period before fixation of the tissue. The distribution of the black deposits of silver demonstrates that the principal site of mitosis is in the necks of the glands. (Courtesy of A.J. Ladman.)

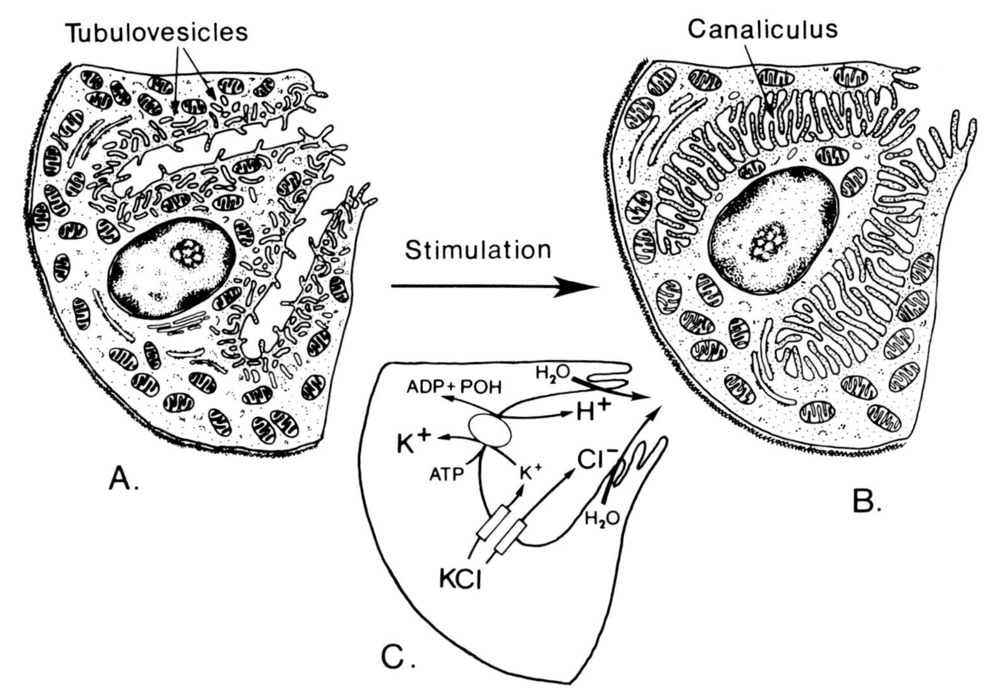

Figure 25–24. (A) Drawing of unstimulated oxyntic cell with extensive tubulovesicular system and small canaliculus. (B) Stimulated cell with long canaliculus, many microvilli, and a depleted tubulovesicular system. (C) Fusion of tubulovesicles transfers H^+,K^+-ATPase to surface and conductive channels for K^+ and Cl^-. This permits movement of K^+ and Cl^- into the canaliculus and the H^+/K^+ pump recycles K^+ back into the cytoplasm, with the net effect of HCl secretion and ATP turnover. Flux of water into the canaliculus is driven osmotically by net solute flux. [(C) redrawn from Forte, J.G. et al. 1989. *In* A. Garner and B.J. Whittle, eds. Advances in Drug Therapy for Gastrointestinal Ulceration. London, John Wiley and Sons Ltd.]

the intrinsic nerve plexus, stimulated by vagal efferents, generate impulses that induce the G-cells to release gastrin, which has a potent stimulatory effect on oxyntic cells. There is also evidence that release of gastrin may be stimulated by peptide and amino-acid products of digestion, by caffeine, and by low concentrations of alcohol ingested with the food. In the fasting stomach, the pH in the lumen is low and under these conditions the D-cells secrete somatostatin which exerts a paracrine inhibitory effect on release of gastrin by G-cells. In the full stomach, with a pH above 3, the D-cells are inactive. On emptying of the stomach after a meal and removal of the buffering effect of food, the pH of the stomach contents falls and inhibition of gastrin secretion, by D-cells, is resumed. The C-terminal tetrapeptide of gastrin, which is responsible for its activity, has been synthesized and is used clinically to promote acid secretion.

The secretion of pepsinogen by the chief cells is dependent on neural stimulation and is enhanced by the acid secreted following the ingestion of food. The low pH generated is also necessary for the conversion of pepsinogen to the active enzyme pepsin.

BIBLIOGRAPHY

ESOPHAGUS

Al Yassin, T.M. and P.G. Toner. 1976. Langerhans cells in the human esophagus. J. Anat. 122:435.

Edwards, D.A.W. 1971. The esophagus. Gut 12:984.

Geboes, K., C. DeWolf-Peeters, P. Rutgeerts, J. Janseen, J. VanTrappen and G. Desmet. 1983. Lymphocytes and Langerhans cells in human esophageal epithelium. Virchow's Arch. 401:45.

Hopwood, D., K.R. Logan, and I.A.D. Bouchier. 1978. The electron microscopy of normal human esophageal epithelium. Virchow's Arch. (Cell Pathol.) 26:345.

Hopwood, D., G. Coghill, and D.S.A. Sanders. 1986. Human esophageal submucosal glands. Their detection, mucin, enzyme, and secretory protein content. Histochemistry 86:107.

Orlando, R.C., E.R. Lacy, N.A. Tobey, and K. Cowart. 1992. Barriers to paracellular permeability in rabbit esophageal epithelium. Gastroenterology 102:910.

Parakkal, P. 1967. An electron microscopic study of the esophageal epithelium in the newborn and adult mouse. Am. J. Anat. 121:175.

STOMACH

Andrew, A. 1982. The APUD concept. Where has it led us? Br. Med. Bull. 38:221.

Baetens, D., C. Rufener, B.C. Srikant, R. Dobbs, R. Unger, and L. Orci. 1976. Identification of glucagon-producing cells (A cells) in dog gastric mucosa. J. Cell Biol. 69:455.

Berglindh, T., D.R. DiBona, S. Ito, and G. Sachs. 1980. Probes of parietal cell function. Am. J. Physiol. 238:G165.

Bertalanffy, F.D. 1962. Cell renewal in the gastrointestinal tract of man. Gastroenterology 43:472.

Black, J.A., T.M. Foote, and J.G. Forte. 1980. Structure of oxyntic cell membranes during conditions of rest and secretion of HCl as revealed by freeze-fracture. Anat. Rec. 196:163.

Forte, J.G. 1980. Mechanism of gastric H^+ and Cl^- transport. Annu. Rev. Physiol. 42:111.

Forte, J.G., J.A. Black, T.M. Forte, R. Machen, and J.M. Wolosin. 1981. Ultrastructural changes related to functional activity in gastric oxyntic cells. Am. J. Physiol. 241:G349.

Forssmann, W.G., L. Orci, R. Pictet, A.E. Renold, and C. Rouiller. 1969. The endocrine cells in the epithelium of the gastrointestinal mucosa of the rat. J. Cell Biol. 40:692.

Gannon, B.J., J. Browning, and P. O'Brien. 1982. The microvascular architecture of the glandular mucosa of rat stomach. J. Anat. 133:677.

Gannon, B.J., J. Browning, and P. O'Brien. 1984. Mucosal microvascular architecture of the fundus and body of the human stomach. Gastroenterology 86:866.

Goldstein, A.M.B., M.R. Brothers, and E.A. Davis. 1969. Architecture of the superficial layer of the gastric mucosa. J. Anat. 104:539.

Greider, M.H., V. Steinberg, and J.E. McGuigan. 1972. Electron microscopic identification of the gastrin cell of the human antral mucosa by means of immunocytochemistry. Gastroenterology 63:572.

Grossman, M.I. 1970. Gastrin and its activities. Nature 228:1147.

Hingson, D.J. and S. Ito. 1971. Effect of aspirin and related compounds on the fine structure of mouse gastric mucosa. Gastroenterology 61:156.

Ito, S. 1987. Functional gastric morphology. *In* L.R. Johnson, ed. Physiology of the Gastrointestinal Tract, 2nd ed. Chap. 26. New York, Raven Press.

Ito, S. and D. Lacy. 1985. Morphology of gastric mucosal damage, defenses, and restitution in the presence of luminal ethanol. Gastroenterology 88:250.

Ito, S. and R.J. Winchester. 1963. The fine structure of the gastric mucosa in the bat. J. Cell Biol. 16:541.

Leblond, C.P. and B.E. Walker. 1956. Renewal of cell populations. Physiol. Rev. 36:255.

Lee, E.P. and C.P. Leblond. 1985. Dynamic histology of the antral epithelium in the mouse stomach. IV. Ultrastructure and renewal of gland cells. Am. J. Anat. 172:241.

Lillibridge, C.B. 1964. The fine structure of normal human gastric mucosa. Gastroenterology 47:269.

Lipkin, M., P. Sherlock, and B. Bell. 1963. Cell proliferation kinetics in the gastrointestinal tract of man. II. Cell renewal in stomach, ileum, colon, and rectum. Gastroenterology 47:721.

Silen, W. and S. Ito. 1985. Mechanisms for rapid epithelialization of the gastric mucosal surface. Annu. Rev. Physiol. 47:271.

Sugai, N., S. Ito, A. Ichikawa, and M. Ichikawa. 1985. The fine structure of the tubulovesicular system in mouse gastric parietal cells processed by cryofixation. J. Electron Micras. 34:113.

Walsh, J.H. and M.I. Grossman. 1975. Gastrin. N. Engl. J. Med. 292:1324.

VanGolde, L.M.G., J.J. Batenburg, and B. Robertson. 1988. Regulation of gastrointestinal mucosa growth. Physiol. Rev. 68:456.

26
INTESTINES

THE SMALL INTESTINE

Digestion of food that is begun in the stomach is continued in the small intestine by enzymes produced in its mucosa and assisted by emulsifying agents and enzymes secreted into its lumen by the liver and pancreas. Little or no absorption of nutrients takes place in the stomach. This is the principal function of the small intestine, which is 4–7 m in length and arbitrarily divided into three successive segments: the *duodenum,* the *jejunum,* and the *ileum.*

The duodenum, about 25 cm in length, is firmly fixed to the dorsal wall of the abdomen and is largely retroperitoneal. It has a C-shaped course around the head of the pancreas and is continuous at its distal end with the jejunum, which is suspended from the dorsal wall of the cavity on a mesentery. The jejunum is freely moveable on its mesentery and occupies the proximal two-fifths of the length of the small intestine, whereas the ileum occupies about three-fifths. The convolutions of the jejunum occupy the central region of the abdomen, whereas the ileum is situated in the lower portion of the cavity. There are minor differences in the histology of the mucosa in the three segments of the small intestine, but there are no distinct boundaries between them. Throughout its length of 5–6 m, the wall of the intestine consists of four concentric layers: the mucosa, submucosa, muscularis, and serosa.

INTESTINAL MUCOSA

The efficiency of the absorptive function of the small intestine is augmented by a number of structural devices that increase the total area of the mucosa. The most obvious of these are the *plicae circulares* (valves of Kerkring) that are visible to the naked eye as crescentic folds that extend for one-half to two-thirds of the distance around the lumen (Fig. 26–1). These are permanent structures including both mucosa and submucosa. The larger plicae are 8–10 mm in height, 3–4 mm in thickness, and up to 5 cm in length. They are absent from the first portion of the duodenum but begin about 5 cm distal to the pyloris and reach their greatest abundance in the terminal portion of this segment and the first portion of the jejunum. From there onward, they gradually diminish in size and number and are seldom found beyond the middle of the ileum.

A second and more effective means of augmenting the surface area of the mucosa is the presence of enormous numbers of *intestinal villi* (Fig. 26–2 and 26–3). These finger-like projections of the mucosa have a length of 0.5 to 1.5 mm, depending on the degree of distension of the intestinal wall and the degree of contraction of smooth muscle fibers in their interior. Villi cover the entire inner surface of the intestine and give it a characteristic velvety appearance in the freshly opened organ. Their number varies from 10 to 40 per square millimeter. They are most numerous in the duodenum and proximal jejunum. A further amplification in surface area is achieved by invaginations of the mucosa between the bases of the villi, called the *crypts of Lieberkuhn* or *intestinal glands* (Fig. 26–4). These tubular glands, 320 to 450 μm in length, extend downward nearly to the muscularis mucosae. Between the intestinal glands is loose connective tissue forming the *lamina propria* of the intestinal mucosa.

Absorptive Cells

The surface of the mucosa is a simple columnar epithelium in which three cell types can be distinguished: *absorptive cells, goblet cells,* and *enteroendocrine cells* (Fig. 26–5). The absorptive cells (enterocytes) are columnar, and 20 to 26 μm in height with a centrally situated,

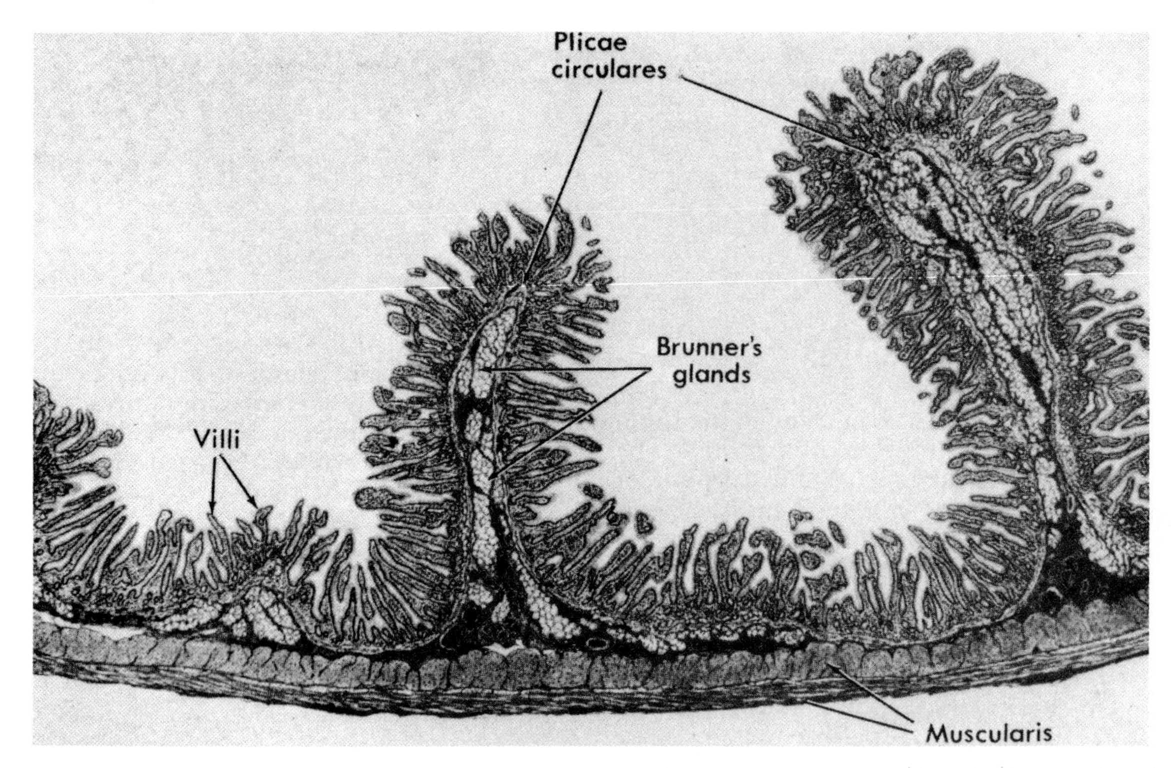

Figure 26–1. Longitudinal section through the wall of the human duodenum, showing the plicae circulares (valves of Kerkring), the villi, and the submucosal glands of Brunner. (From Bargmann, W. 1962. Histologie und Mikroskopische Anatomie des Menschen, 6th ed. Stuttgart, Georg Thieme Verlag.)

vertically elongated nucleus. The luminal surface has a prominent *brush border* (*striated border*), beneath which is a clear zone devoid of organelles but containing a distinct *terminal web*, a layer of transversely oriented fine filaments that exhibit birefringence under a polarizing microscope. It can be selectively stained by a method employing tannic acid, phosphomolybdic acid, and the dye amido black.

In electron micrographs, the striated border consists of closely packed microvilli, numbering up to 3000 per cell, and resulting in a 30-fold amplification of the surface area exposed to the lumen. Each is 1 to 1.4 μm in length and about 80 nm in diameter (Figs. 26–6 and 26–7). Exceedingly thin filaments radiating from the tips of the microvilli intermingle to form a continuous *surface coat* or *glycocalyx* that varies from 0.1 to 0.5 μm in thickness, depending on the species. The filaments comprising the surface coat are of molecular dimensions, each consisting of the core polypeptide and oligosaccharide side-chains of a glycoprotein that is an integral part of the plasmalemma. The layer they form is resistant to mucolytic and proteolytic agents and may, thus, protect the striated border. There is some evidence, however, that it may also form a substrate for the digestive process because it has been found that pancreatic amylase, and other intraluminal enzymes, are adsorbed to the large surface presented by its filaments. Thus, some of the lytic events that take place in the fluid in the gut lumen may actually be occurring very near the tips of the microvilli.

The ultrastructure of the intestinal brush border has been very thoroughly studied. In the core of each microvillus, there is a bundle of about 20 parallel actin filaments (Fig. 26–8). These are anchored in a cap-like subplasmalemmal density at the tip of the villus and they extend downward into the apical cytoplasm, where they intermingle with the transversely oriented cytoskeletal filaments of the terminal web. (Fig. 26–9). The actin filaments of the villus core are cross-linked by two proteins, *fimbrin* (68 kD) and *villin* (95 kD), and the bundle, as a whole, is attached to the membrane by a helical array of lateral arms or bridges that are visible, in electron micrographs, at 33-nm intervals along its length. These bridges consist of *brush-border myosin-I*,

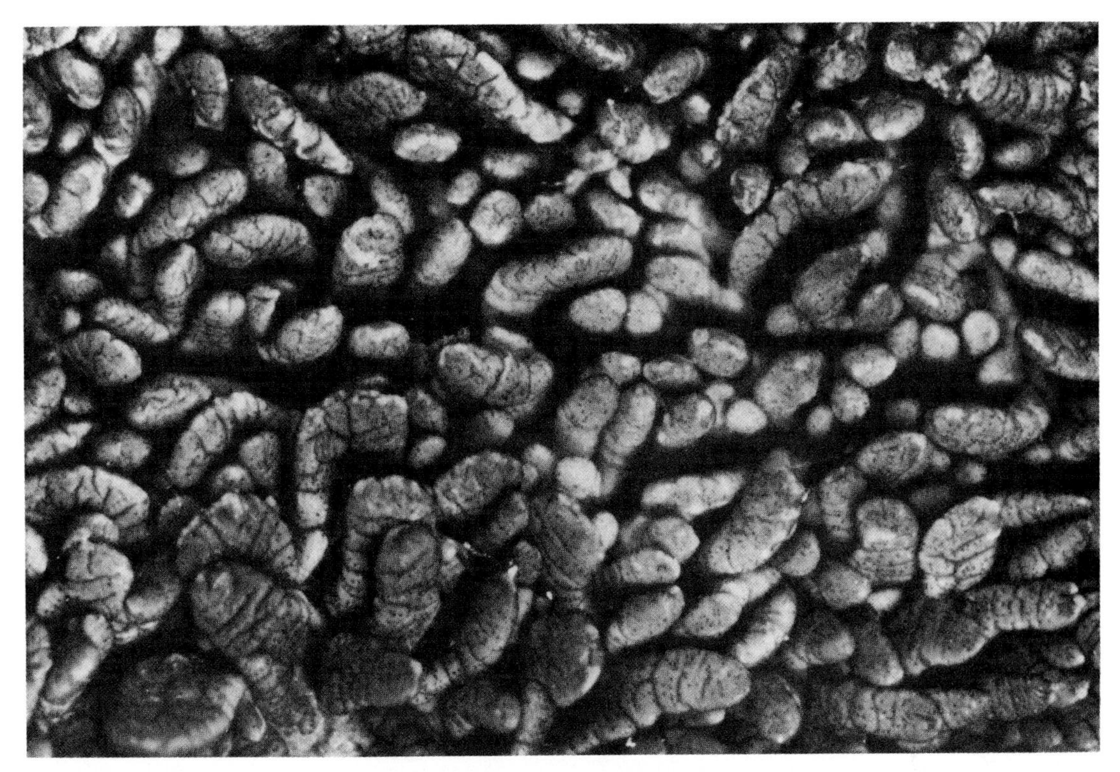

Figure 26–2. Photograph of the mucosal surface of a human jejunal biopsy showing intestinal villi of both finger-like and foliate form. (From Poulsen, S. 1977. Scand. J. Gastroenterol. 12:235.)

a complex of the Ca^+-binding protein *calmodulin* and a single-headed myosin molecule that is bound by its short tail to the membrane. Where the actin filaments of the cores splay out at their lower end, they are surrounded by actin filaments, tropomyosin and fodrin of the terminal web. Confidence in the above interpretation of the internal organization of the microvilli has been strengthened by the observation that, if highly purified actin, fimbrin, and villin are incubated together in vitro, typical cores are reconstituted, and on addition of the calmodulin–myosin-I complex, arms appear, spaced at appropriate intervals along the bundle of core filaments.

The intestinal brush border has been widely studied to gain insight into the relationship of the cytoskeleton to the plasmalemma of cells in general, but it is apparent that this is a special case of unusual complexity and its functional implications are still not entirely clear. It was originally thought that the actin filaments of the microvillus cores interacted with myosin in the terminal web, resulting in intermittent shortening that might favor movement of absorbed material into the cell body. Although isolated brush borders, which include the terminal web, do contract somewhat in the presence of Ca^+ ions and ATP, it is now believed that the microvilli do not shorten. The lateral contraction of the terminal web probably increases the convexity of the cell apex and spreads the tips of the microvilli apart. This would provide access to the membrane on the sides, as well as the tips, of the microvilli. Whether this is important for intestinal absorption is not known.

The cytoplasm below the terminal web contains a number of mitochondria, occasional lysosomes, and a few small lipid droplets. Highly branched profiles of smooth endoplasmic reticulum are also abundant in this region. This organelle plays an important role in absorption of fat because its membrane contains enzymes essential for synthesis of triglycerides from fatty acids and monoglycerides. Cisternae of rough endoplasmic reticulum may also be found in the supranuclear cytoplasm, but they are more plentiful near the cell base. The Golgi complex is moderately well developed but shows little morphological evidence of activity except during lipid absorption.

A juxtaluminal junctional complex bars access to the intercellular clefts from the lumen.

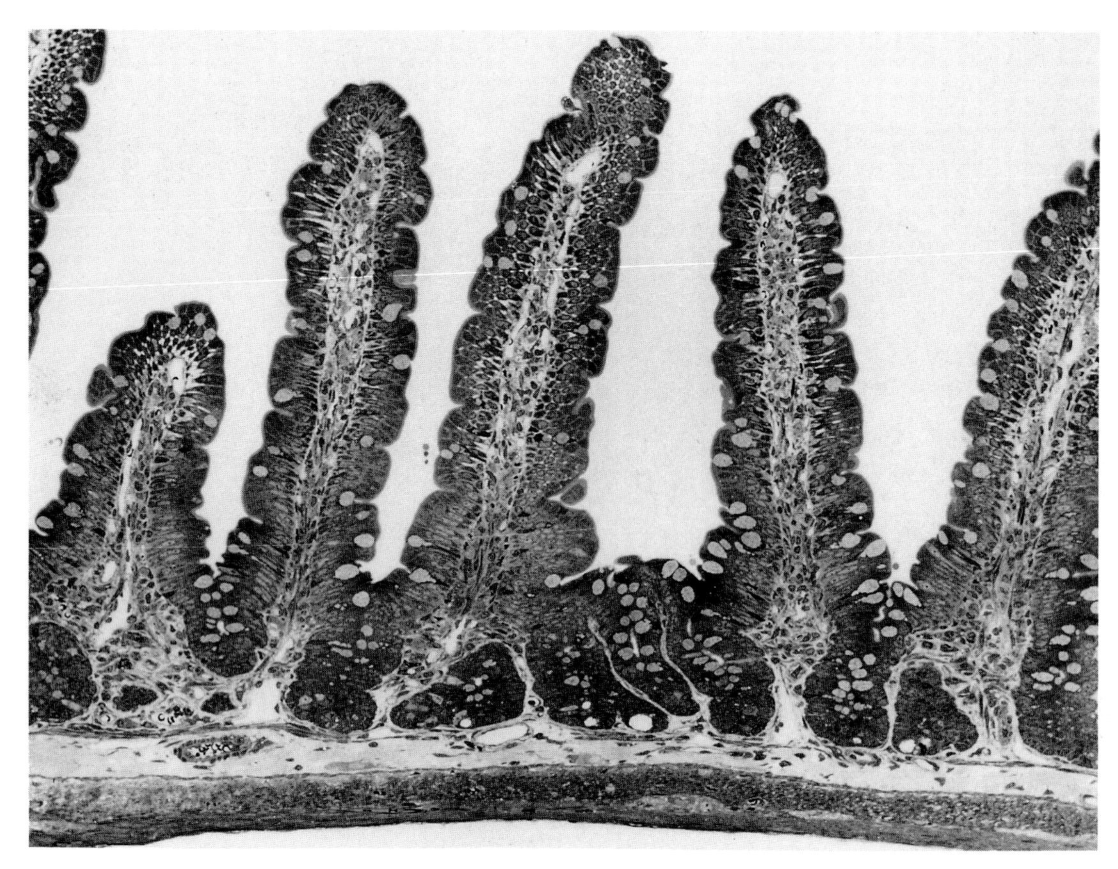

Figure 26–3. Photomicrograph of rat intestinal mucosa showing the prominent villi and short intestinal glands opening between the bases of the villi. (Courtesy of Komuro, T. 1990. Cell Tissue Res. 239:183.)

An occluding junction completely encircling each cell ensures that products of digestion must traverse the brush border, the apical cytoplasm, and the lateral cell membranes below the tight junction to gain access to the intercellular spaces and move on to capillaries of the lamina propria. As in many other transporting epithelia, the apical domain differs from the lateral domain of the plasmalemma in its biochemical composition. The adluminal membrane is rich in glycolipid and *peptide hydrolases* (aminopeptidase, *N*-dipeptidylpeptidase-IV, and *p*-aminobenzoic acid peptide hydrolase) and in *disaccharidases* (sucrase-isomaltase, lactase-phlorizin hydrolase, maltase-glucoamylase), as well as carrier proteins for amino acid and carbohydrate transport. These enzymes are absent from the basolateral membrane which contains Na^+, K^+-ATPase and receptors for various molecules taken up from the blood.

As in the stomach, the epithelium lining the intestinal tract is covered by a lubricating and protective layer of mucus. Nevertheless, the surface membrane of the cells is occasionally disrupted by abrasive contents of the lumen, and the cells need considerable potential for repair. Contrary to the traditional belief that breaking the membrane of a cell inevitable resulted in its death, the intestinal epithelial cells have a remarkable capacity to close tears in their membrane and survive.

Goblet Cells

The *goblet cells* are mucus-secreting unicellular glands scattered among the absorptive cells of the intestinal epithelium. Their name is descriptive of the shape of the cell in routine histological preparations. The apex has an expanded cup-shaped rim of cytoplasm, called the *theca,* filled with secretion, and a narrow base extending downward to the basal lamina (Fig. 26–5). The secretory material is in the form of large pale granules that may be more-or-less confluent. The shape that gives the cell its name is now known to be an artifact. The common fixatives alter the permeability of the

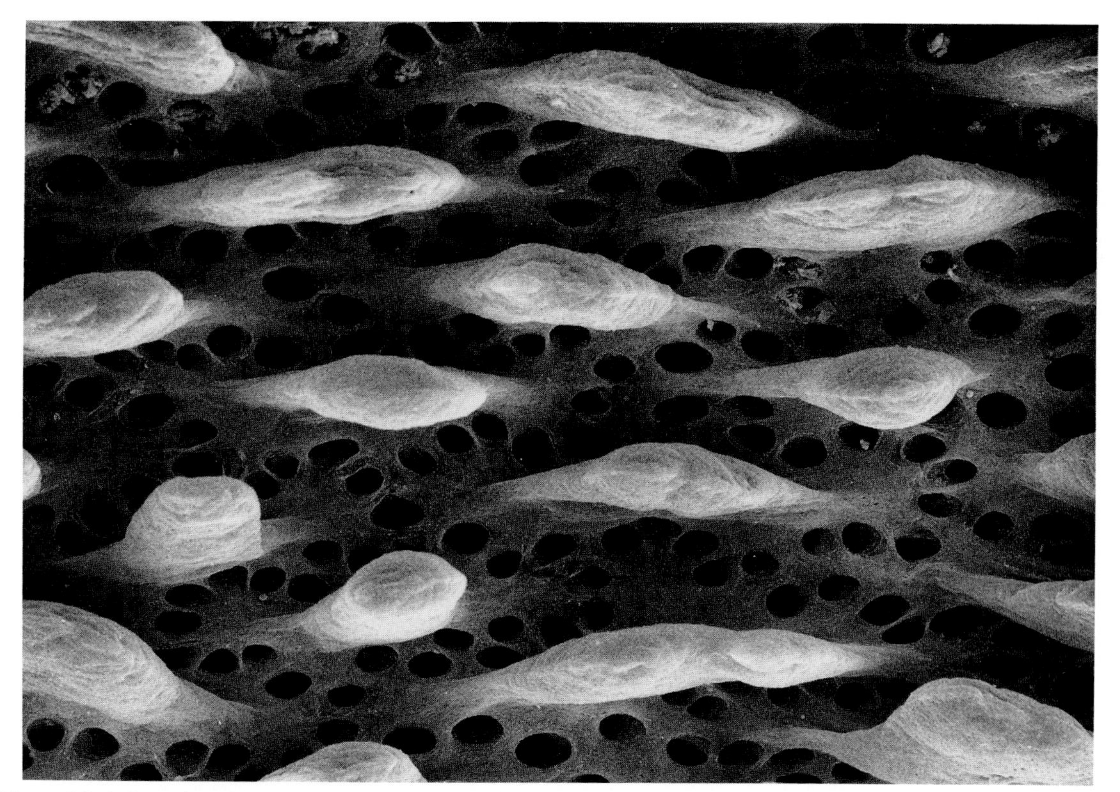

Figure 26–4. Scanning electron micrograph of rat intestinal mucosa, viewed from the lumen after removal of the epithelium. Between the foliate villi, one can see the openings of the recesses occupied by the glands. (Micrograph from Komuro, T. and Y. Hashimoto. 1990. Cell Tissue Res. 239:183).

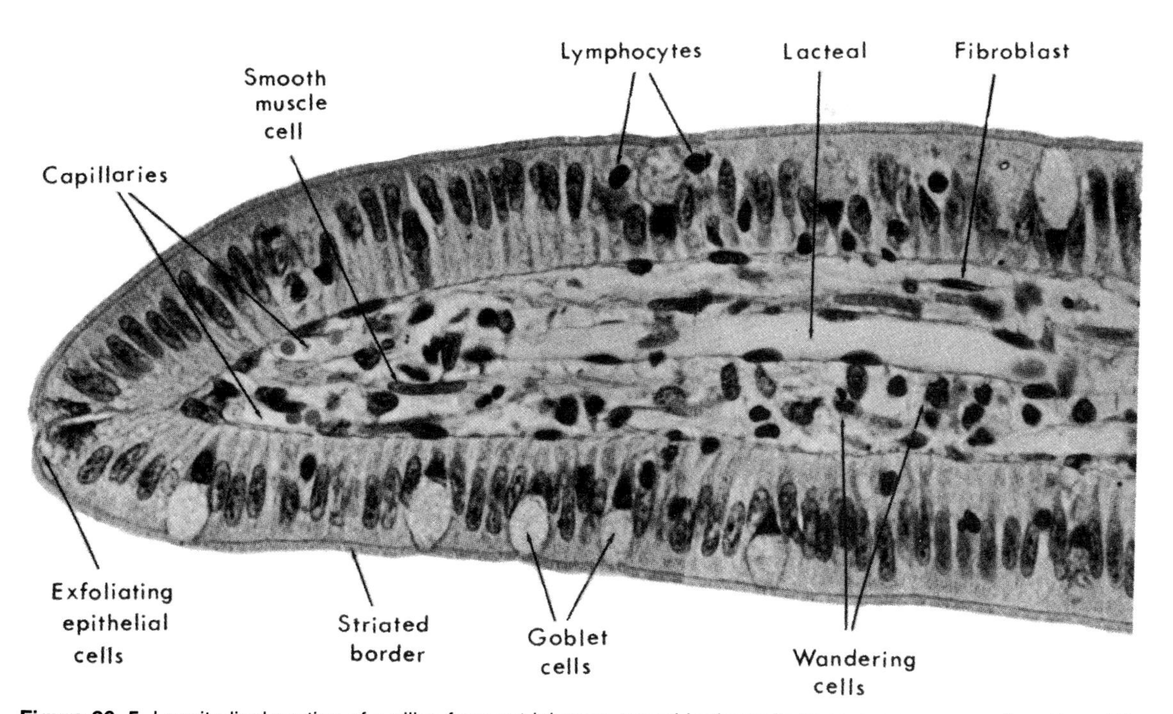

Figure 26–5. Longitudinal section of a villus from cat jejunum, turned horizontally to save page space. A portion of the central lacteal is included.

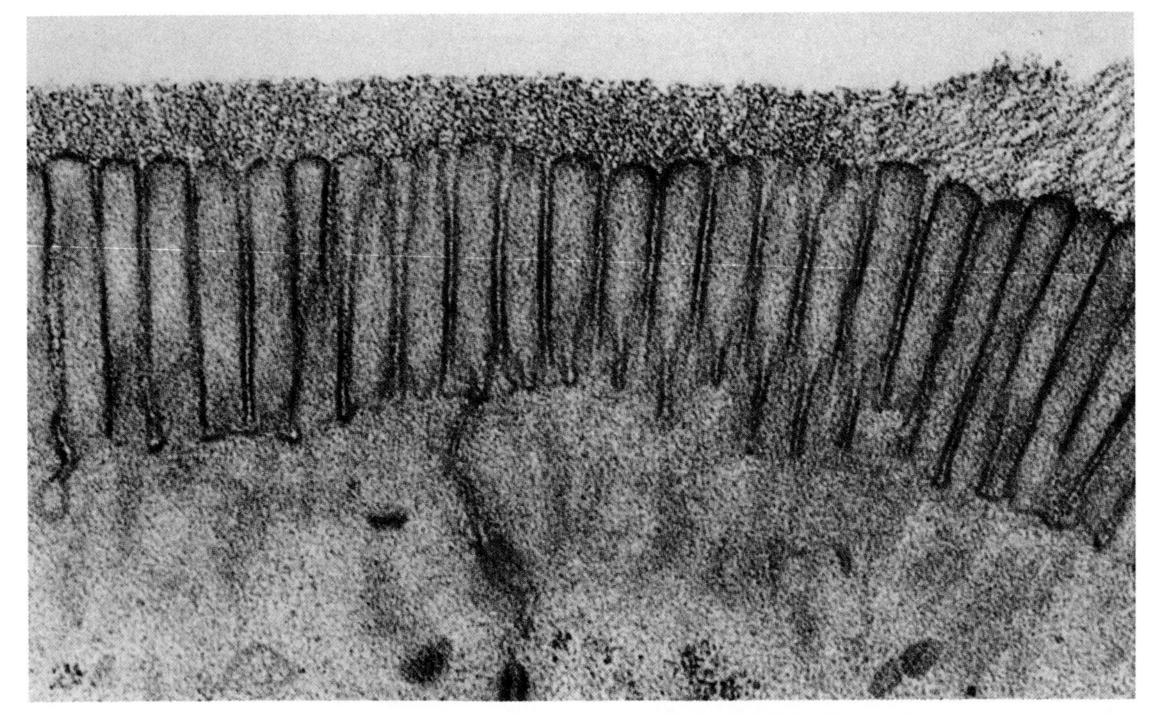

Figure 26–6. Electron micrograph of the striated border of an intestinal epithelial cell, showing the prominent surface coat (glycocalyx) consisting of oligosaccharide chains of integral glycoproteins of the plasma membrane. (Micrograph courtesy of S. Ito.)

cell membrane and the hydrophilic mucin takes up water, resulting in swelling of the apical portion of the cell. In specimens prepared by quick-freezing and cryosubstitution, the secretory granules are smaller and electron-dense and show little or no coalescence. With this method, which better preserves their normal form, the cells are not goblet-shaped but are columnar or ovoid. But the name goblet cell is so firmly fixed in the literature it will persist.

The luminal surface of the cell bears a few microvilli around the periphery, but it is usually smooth and convex over the secretory granules. Goblet cells are firmly attached to neighboring absorptive cells by junctional complexes and there may be a few shallow interdigitations on their otherwise smooth lateral surfaces. Cisternae of rough endoplasmic reticulum are abundant in the basal and lateral cytoplasm, and mitochondria are scattered throughout these regions. A large Golgi complex, situated between the nucleus and the secretory granules, consists of multiple stacks of cisternae and associated small vesicles.

The goblet cell has a well-developed cytoskeleton. Intermediate filaments are abundant in the theca. An inner basket-like layer is surrounded by circumferential bundles of filaments arranged like barrel hoops around the mass of secretory granules. Between the inner layer of filaments and the mucin granules, there are numerous vertically oriented microtubules. These may play a role in the upward movement of newly formed mucin granules from the Golgi complex to the cell apex. The basket-like framework of filaments in the theca contains little or no actin and there is no evidence that its contraction is involved in release of the cells secretory product.

Mucus is a viscid fluid, or thin gel, consisting of glycoprotein macromolecules ranging in size from 250,000 to 2×10^6 daltons. It is about 20% peptides and 80% carbohydrate. The peptide moiety is synthesized in the rough endoplasmic reticulum and transported to the Golgi complex, where a variety of oligosaccharides are added. Mucin is synthesized and secreted at a relatively constant basal rate throughout the limited life span of the goblet cells. It is normally released by exocytosis of one granule at a time, but in accelerated secretion there may be fusion of granule membranes resulting in chains of intercommunicating granules opening at the cell

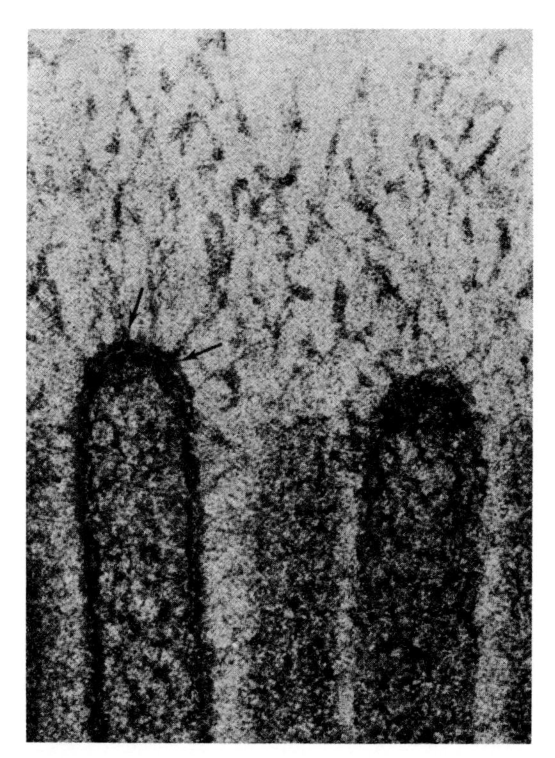

Figure 26–7. Electron micrograph of several microvilli from cat ileum showing the branching oligosaccharide chains emerging from the outer leaflet of the plasma membrane. (Courtesy of Ito, S., from Fawcett, D. 1965. J. Histochem. Cytochem. 13:75.)

surface, a process called *compound exocytosis*. Within a few seconds of release, the content of the granules undergoes a several-hundred-fold expansion in volume due to its rapid hydration. The resultant gel forms a layer over the surface that protects the epithelium from abrasion and prevents adherence and invasion by pathogenic bacteria.

Enteroendocrine Cells

In 1870, Heidenhain described small cells near the base of the intestinal epithelium that had staining reactions similar to those of the chromaffin cells of the adrenal medulla. These came to be called *enterochromaffin cells*. Their basal location in the epithelium and the presence of secretory granules concentrated at the cell base suggested that they were endocrine cells releasing their secretion into the lamina propria and not into the intestinal lumen.

In addition to their ability to bind alkaline bichromates (chromaffinity), some of these cells also precipitated silver salts in the absence of a reducing agent (argentafinity) and were called *argentaffin cells*. It was then found that if sections were treated with a reducing agent prior to their exposure to silver nitrate, a greater number of basal granular cells could be demonstrated. Cells stainable with this method were termed *argyrophilic cells*. The differences in number of argyrophilic and argentaffin cells and the fact that some of these granulated cells exhibited fluorescence in ultraviolet light while others did not led to the conclusion that not all enteroendocrine cells were the same. Indeed, it is now known that they are a highly heterogeneous cell population. In recent years, correlation of their ultrastructure with immunocytochemical staining has produced a surge of new information about their secretory products and probable functions. More than 15 different endocrine cell types have now been identified in the gastrointestinal tract.

They occur as rather widely scattered individual cells and, therefore, appear to be a minor component of the epithelium, but their

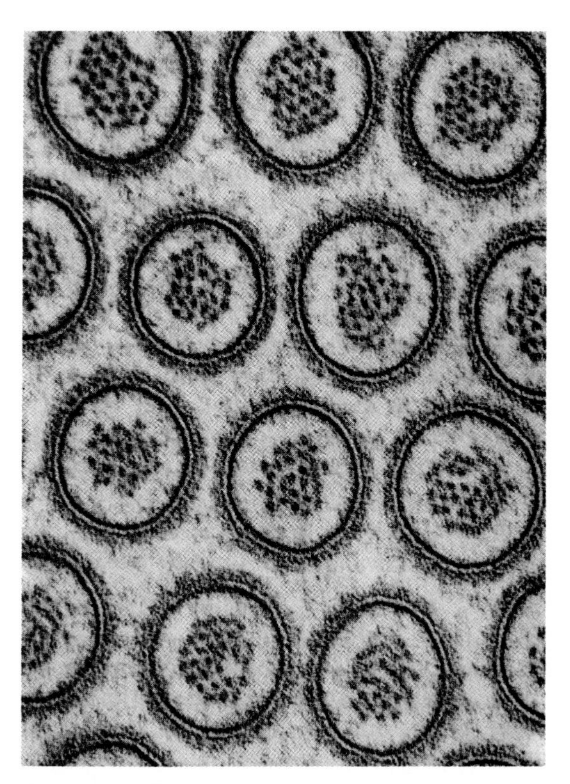

Figure 26–8. Electron micrograph of cross sections of microvilli from the brush border of an intestinal epithelial cell showing the bundle of actin filaments in the core of each microvillus. Specimen prepared by quick-freezing in liquid helium followed by freeze-substitution. (Micrograph courtesy of A. Ichikawa.)

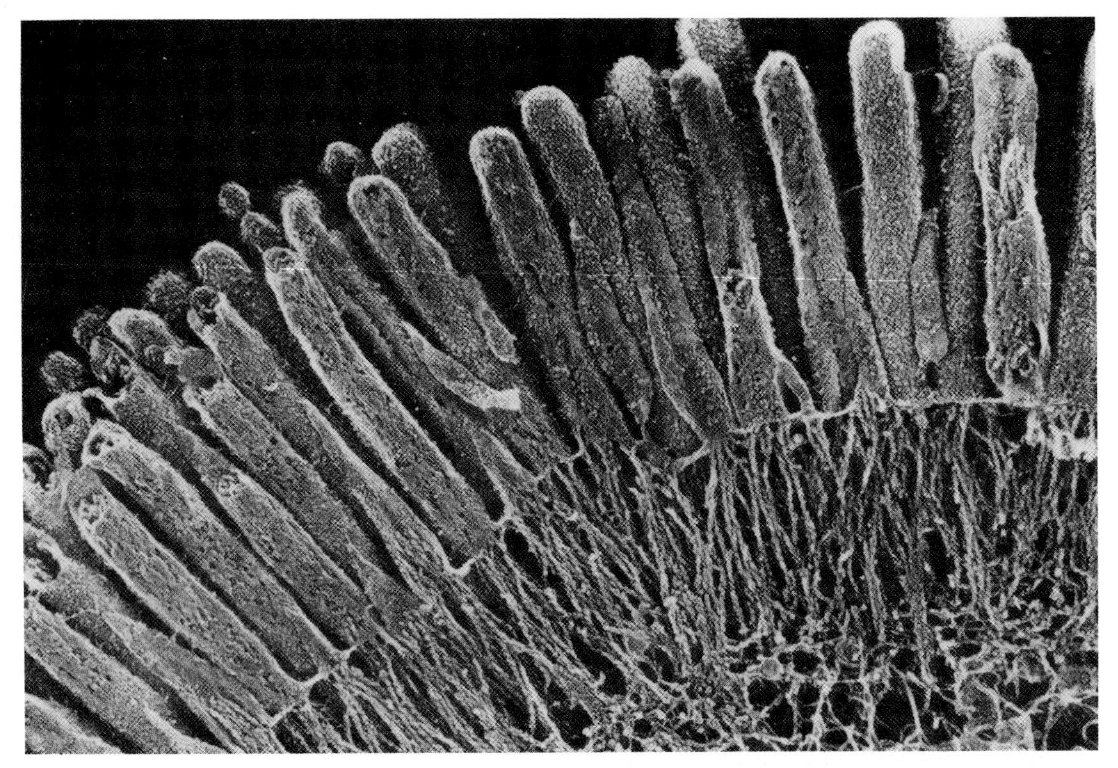

Figure 26–9. Brush border of an intestinal absorptive cell prepared by quick-freezing, deep-etching, and rotary-shadowing. Bundles of actin filaments can be seen extending from the cores of the microvilli downward into the meshwork of filaments that make up the terminal web. (Micrograph courtesy of N. Hirokawa and J. Heuser.)

number in the human intestine is estimated to be about 3×10^9. They share a number of morphological features. They are highly variable in form. Those in the crypts tend to be ovoid or pyramidal, whereas those on the villi may be more nearly columnar. The bulk of the cell body is always in the lower half of the epithelium, but a narrow apical region usually extends to the lumen and has a brush border. The nucleus is round and generally poor in heterochromatin. The cytoplasm is paler than that of the surrounding enterocytes. The secretory granules vary in size from cell to cell and are always in the basal cytoplasm.

In electron micrographs, the microvilli of the enteroendocrine cells may be longer and thicker than those of the adjacent absorptive cells—a finding that has suggested to some that they may have a chemoreceptor function. The cytoplasm is relatively electron-lucent and the organelles do not differ significantly from those of other epithelial cells. The rough endoplasmic reticulum varies in amount from one cell type to another, but in no case is it highly developed. Morphological identification of the several types of enteroendocrine cells depends mainly on differences in size, shape, electron density, and substructure of their secretory granules but can only be made with confidence by their immunocytochemical staining with fluorescein-labeled antibodies specific for their amine or peptide products.

The substances that have been identified in enteroendocrine cells include: *5-hydroxytryptamine* (serotonin), *somatostatin, glucagon/glicentin, cholecystokinin, gastrin, motilin, secretin, neurotensin, substance-P, gastric inhibitory polypeptide,* and *B-endorphin.* In general, one cell type contains one hormone but there are one or two exceptions in which the same cell may contain two different hormones.

The distribution of intestinal endocrine cells has been studied in the human. They are found in the greatest number and variety in the duodenum and jejunum. Serotonin containing cells (*EC-cells*) are found throughout the intestinal tract and constitute the largest single endocrine cell population. The second largest population is made up of cells containing glucagon/glicentin (*GLI-cells*), which are most numerous in the distal ileum, colon, and rectum. Cells containing somatostatin (*D-cells*) occur throughout the intestine. Gastrin-containing cells (*G-cells*) are few in number and confined to the proximal duodenum. Cells storing cholecystokinin (*I-cells*), motilin (*Mo-cells*), secretin (*S-cells*), neurotensin (*N-cells*), and gastric inhibitory peptide (*K-cells*) are most numerous in the proximal and midportion of the intestine and are only very rarely found in the colon and rectum (Fig. 26–10).

Much remains to be learned about the factors controlling release of these endocrine, or paracrine, secretions and about their role in intestinal physiology. It is known that the presence of food in the stomach results in release of gastrin from the G-cells in the antrum and first portion of the duodenum, and this stimulates the cells of the gastric glands to secrete hydrochloric acid and digestive enzymes. The acid chyme from the stomach discharged into the duodenum and jejunum stimulates release of secretin which is carried in the blood to the pancreas where it stimulates secretion of fluid with a high bicarbonate content that serves to neutralize the acid from the stomach. Similarly, the presence of fats and protein breakdown products in the upper intestine induces release of cholecystokinin, which stimulates secretion by the pancreas and promotes emptying of the gall bladder. Other hormones, gastric inhibitory peptide, vasoactive intestinal polypeptide, and somatostatin inhibit gastric secretion and motility. It is speculated that these effects may be advantageous in slowing the discharge of additional gastric content into an upper intestine that is already full.

A puzzling aspect of the enteroendocrine system is the fact that several of the peptide hormones found in the gut (gastrin, cholecystokinin, vasoactive intestinal peptide, and motilin) have also been localized in certain cells of the central nervous system. Conversely, some polypeptide hormones originally isolated from the central nervous system (somatostatin, neurotensin, substance-P) have also been found in intestinal or pancreatic endocrine cells. The physiological significance of such a diffuse distribution of isolated endocrine cells in organ systems of such disparate function awaits explanation.

CRYPTS OF LIEBERKUHN AND CELL TURNOVER

The epithelium covering the villi continues into the *intestinal glands* or *crypts of Lieberkuhn* (Figs. 26–3 and 26–4). Approximately the upper half of the wall of the crypts is lined with low columnar epithelium containing absorptive cells and goblet cells. In the lower half of the crypts, the cells are less differentiated except for groups of secretory cells called Paneth cells. Numerous cells in the crypts are found in mitosis. It is here that new cells are formed to replace those that are continually lost at the tips of the villi.

The epithelial lining of the intestinal tract is continuously being renewed by proliferation of cells in the crypts, their migration up onto the villi, and the exfoliation of effete or dying cells at the villus tips. This process of renewal is referred to as the *cell turnover* of the epithelium and its duration is the *cell turnover time*. The mucosa of the jejunum has the fastest rate of turnover of any tissue in the body. If tritiated thymidine is given to an animal, biopsies taken at later time intervals show that label incorporated into the nuclei of dividing cells in the crypts gradually moves upward onto the villi. About one day after administration of the thymidine, labeled cells are found on the sides of the villi, and by the fifth day, labeled cells are being exfoliated at the tips of the villi. The time course of these events in humans may differ slightly, but it is evident that billions of cells are being shed each day from our gastrointestinal tract and are being replaced by upward migration of cells from localized regions of cell proliferation in the crypts of Lieberkuhn. In the small intestine, this mitotic activity is confined to the crypts of Lieberkuhn.

The cells in the lower part of the crypts are rich in enzymes involved in nucleic acid synthesis and they have a shorter interphase than cells in more slowly proliferating tissues. Synthesis of DNA takes place in 6–11 h. The premitotic and postmitotic stages of the mitotic cycle are brief and the mitotic phase itself takes about 1 h. The complete cell cycle occupies 10–17 h in rodents and about 24 h in humans. The intestinal epithelium is completely replaced in 2 to 3 days in laboratory rodents and in 3 to 6 days in humans.

The discovery of this rapid turnover of cells in the lining of the intestine has altered our interpretation of the function of some of the cell types. For example, it was formerly thought that the goblet cells accumulated secretory product, discharged it, and then refilled, and that this cycle was repeated many times in the life of the cell. It is now realized that the lifespan of intestinal goblet cells is only four to six days—the time required for them to differentiate in the crypts, move up onto the villi, and be exfoliated at the villus tips. Thus, it is probable that goblet cells secrete continuously while passing through only one secretory cycle. This cycle has an initial phase in the crypt when the rate of synthesis of mucus exceeds the rate of discharge and mucin accumulates; there follows an intermediate phase when the cells are in the upper portion of the crypt and on the lower half of the villus, where synthesis and discharge are approximately in equilibrium and the cells appear engorged; and, then, a final phase when rate of discharge exceeds synthesis as the cells approach the tip of the villus appearing depleted. This normal course of events can be modified by irritants that cause accelerated expulsion of mucus. If mustard-seed oil is applied locally to the mucosa of an experimental animal, the goblet cells expel nearly all of their store of mucus. Under these abnormal conditions, they are found to initiate a new cycle of mucus accumulation.

In the colon, villi are lacking, but the pattern of cell renewal is much the same. The proliferative zone in the crypts is somewhat more extensive and the cells are extruded when they reach the mucosal surface between crypts. Cell division and migration are slightly slower, resulting in a turnover time of 4 to 8 days in humans.

The finding of a continual upward migration of epithelial cells poses a number of puzzling morphogenetic questions. Do the cells move with respect to a relatively stationary basal lamina, or does the epithelium, as a whole, move with respect to the underlying lamina propria? The answer to this question remains in doubt, but valuable new insight into the problem has been gained from autoradiographic studies on the crypts of the colon. These reveal that there is also a continuous renewal and upward migration of the pericryptal fibroblasts. This surprising finding probably also applies to the crypts of the small intestine.

The intestine has a remarkable capacity to adapt to changing conditions of alimentation. Starvation or protein deficiency results in atrophy of both muscular and mucosal components of the small intestine. The mitotic cycle in the crypts is prolonged and migration is slowed. These changes are reversed by refeeding. Food intake above normal levels results in hypertrophy of the intestinal villi and enhanced absorption of nutrients. The intestine also responds dramatically to surgical excision of large segments of bowel. After such an operation, there is a compensatory increase in the height of the villi and the depth of the crypts in the remaining intestine. This is accompanied by growth in the muscularis and an increase in length of the remaining small intestine. The hyperplastic response is proportional to the length of small intestine resected. Much less is known about the adaptive capacity of the large intestine.

Paneth Cells

Paneth cells do not participate in the upward migration of cells. Groups of them remain at the bottom of the crypts (Fig. 26–11). They are pyramidal in form with a round or ovoid nucleus near their base. The basal cytoplasm is basophilic and the numerous secretory granules, at the cell apex, stain with acid dyes such as eosin and orange-G. They are long-lived, are not observed in mitosis, and do not incorporate tritiated thymidine.

Paneth cells have an ultrastructure typical of cells active in protein synthesis. The supranuclear Golgi complex is large and the basal and paranuclear cytoplasm is rich in parallel arrays of cisternae of rough endoplasmic reticulum. In the rat, the cisternae may contain a thin layer of material having a regular 50 Å periodicity. This feature has not been observed to date in other species. Lysosomes and irregularly shaped granules of lipochrome pigment are usually abundant. In the human, the large secretory granules of Paneth cells are homogeneous and electron-dense, but in rodents, they have a pallid core and a dense outer zone (Fig. 26–12).

Paneth cells evidently secrete continuously, but the rate of secretion is enhanced by feeding. It can also be increased experimentally by administration of pilocarpine. Despite decades of study, the functional role of Paneth cells is still unknown. Research on the chemical nature of their secretory product has been hampered by the difficulty of obtaining their secretion free from contamination by products of other cell types in the crypts. Immunocytochemical studies have identified *lysozyme* in their prominent phagolysosomal system. Lysozyme is a highly charged cationic protein that is capable of digesting the wall of certain bacteria. Under some circumstances, Paneth cells have been observed to phagocytize and digest intestinal flagellates and certain spirilliform microorganisms commonly found in the

CELL TYPE	SECRETION GRANULES	LOCALIZATION Pancreas	Stomach	Intestines	PRODUCT
A	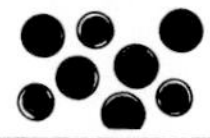 250 nm	Islets			Glucagon, Glicentin
B	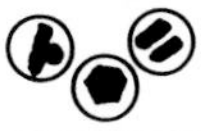 350	Islets			Insulin
D	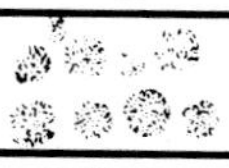 350	Islets	Fundic Pyloric	Jejunum Ileum Colon	Somatostatin
D1	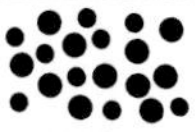 160	Islets	Fundic Pyloric	Jejunum Ileum Colon	Unknown
EC	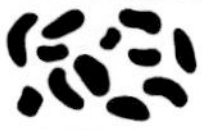 300	Islets	Fundic Pyloric	Jejunum Ileum Colon	Serotonin Various peptides
ECL	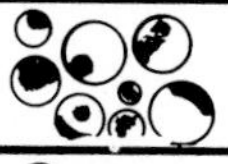 450		Fundic		Histamine
G	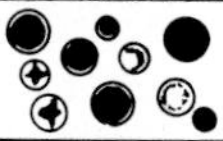 300		Pyloric	Duodenum	Gastrin
I	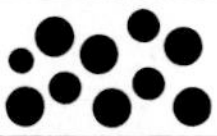 250			Jejunum Ileum	Cholecystokinin
K	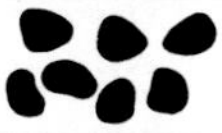 350			Jejunum Ileum	Gastric inhibitory peptide
L	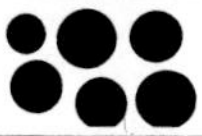 400			Jejunum Ileum Colon	Glucagon-like immunoreactivity
Mo				Jejunum Ileum	Motilin
N	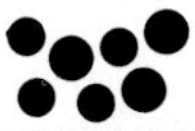 300			Ileum	Neurotensin
P	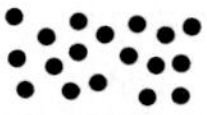 120		Fundic Pyloric	Jejunum	Unknown
PP	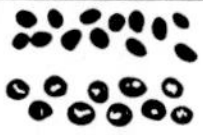 180	Islets	Fundic Pyloric	Colon	Pancreatic polypeptide
S	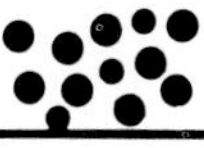 200			Jejunum Ileum	Secretin
TG				Jejunum	C-terminal gastrin immunoreactivity
X	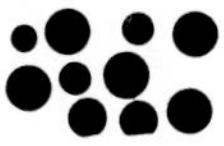 300		Fundic Pyloric		Unknown

Figure 26–10. Summary of the enteroendocrine cell types thus far described, including their nomenclature, distribution, ultrastructure of their granules, and their amine or peptide contents. (Modified after Grube, H. and G. Forssmann. 1979. Horm. Metab. Res. 11:603.)

crypts of Lieberkuhn of the rat intestine. This has led to the suggestion that they may play a role in controlling the microbial flora of the intestinal glands. However, this alleged phagocytic role is inconsistent with their obvious structural specialization as secretory cells. Equally puzzling is the observation that a subpopulation of Paneth cells contain IgA, suggesting a cooperation between them and antibody-producing cells in the lamina propria.

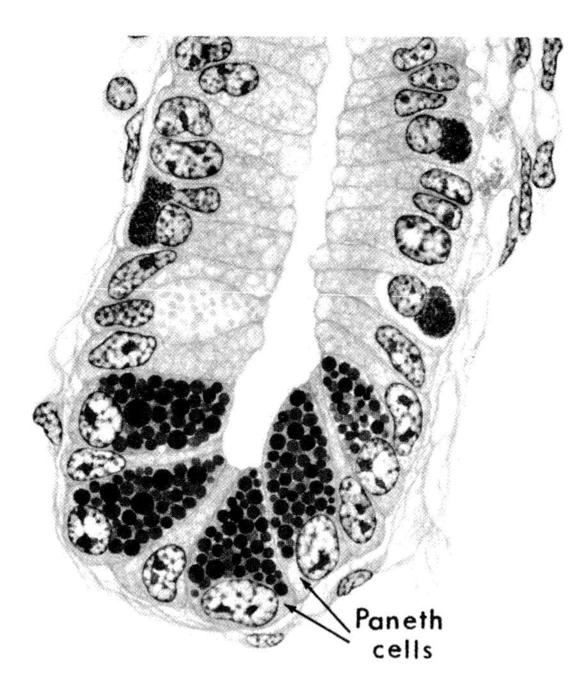

Figure 26–11. Drawing of a crypt of Lieberkuhn illustrating the Paneth cells at the base of the crypt. Higher in the crypt are four argentaffin (enteroendocrine) cells.

It is clear that the principal function of these cells is yet to be discovered. Paneth cells are abundant in the intestine of man, mice, rats, guinea pigs, and ruminants, but they are reported to be absent in dog, cat, pig, and raccoon.

Lamina Propria

The *lamina propria* is a loose connective tissue that occupies the interstices between the crypts of Lieberkuhn and the cores of the intestinal villi. It consists of fixed and wandering cells in a delicate network of reticular and elastic fibers and contains a rich network of capillaries subjacent to the epithelium. Fibroblast-like cells are found immediately beneath the epithelium. These appear fusiform in sections and are commonly referred to as subepithelial fibroblasts. But in preparations examined by scanning electron microscopy, after removal of the epithelium, these cells are found to be stellate in form (Fig. 26–13), and they are attached to one another via gap junctions on their multiple radiating processes. In addition to the usual organelles, the cytoplasm

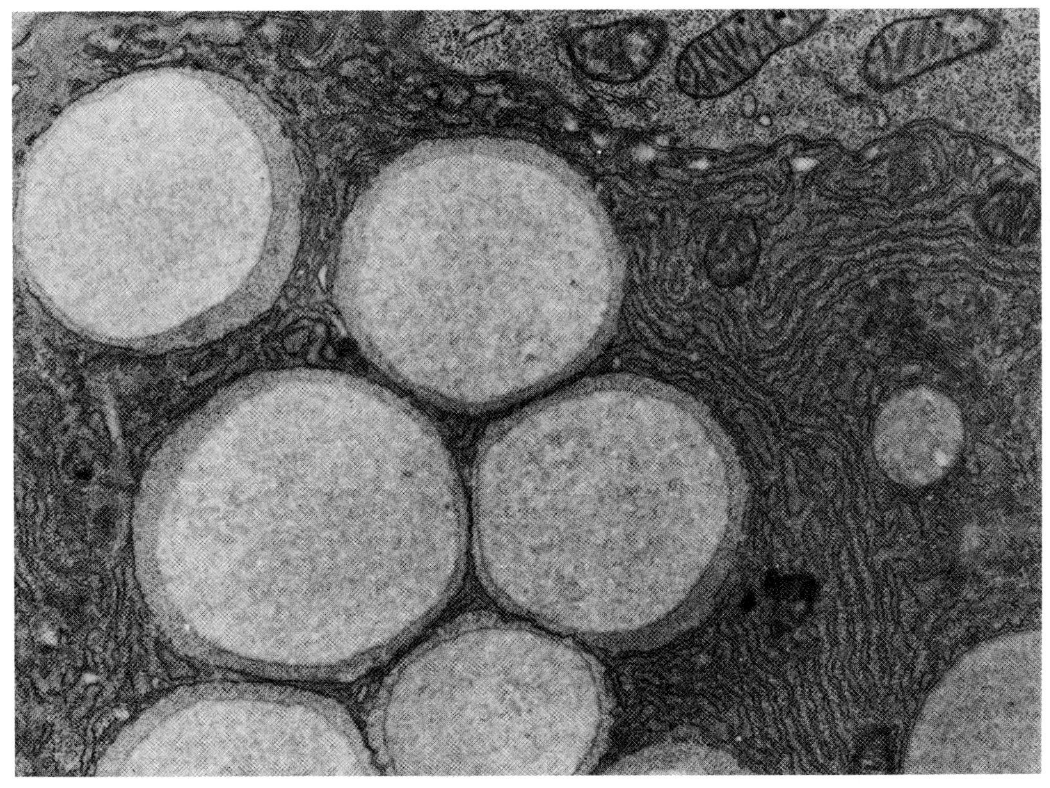

Figure 26–12. Electron micrograph of a portion of a Paneth cell showing the abundance of rough endoplasmic reticulum and the heterogeneity of the secretory granules. (Micrograph from Staley, M. and J. Trier. 1965. Am. J. Anat. 117:365.)

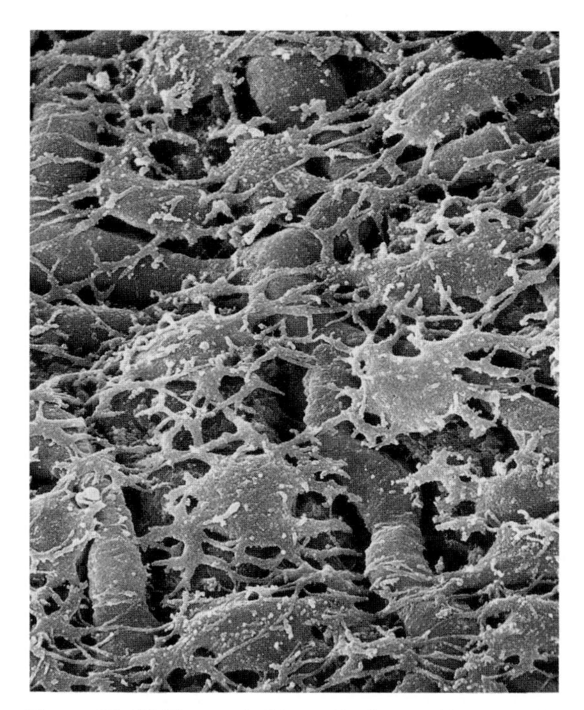

Figure 26–13. Removal of the epithelium and basal lamina from an intestinal villus reveals a fenestrated layer of highly branched fibroblast-like cells overlying the subepithelial capillaries. (Scanning micrograph from Komuro, T. and Y. Hashimoto. 1980. Cell Tissue Res. 239:183.)

of these cells contains bundles of filaments that are not commonly seen in typical fibroblasts. Actin and myosin have been demonstrated in them histochemically. It is speculated that this network of cells, interposed between the epithelium and the subepithelial capillaries, are contractile and may contribute to the intermittent shortening and lengthening of the villi observed in vivo. However, the principal agents of villus motility are very thin strands of smooth muscle that extend vertically from the muscularis mucosae into the core of the villus where they run parallel to the central *lacteal,* a slender lymphatic vessel that ends blindly near the tip of each villus. The lacteals are terminal branches of a *submucous lymphatic plexus.* They are important pathways for the transport of absorbed lipid and other nutrients. The periodic contractions of the smooth muscle in the lamina propria of the villi empty their lacteals and propel lymph toward the plexus, from where it flows onward to the mesenteric lymph nodes and ultimately to the thoracic duct.

The intestinal mucosa is exposed to a lumen containing potentially harmful ingested substances and an immense and varied bacterial flora. The constant threat of penetration of the epithelial barrier by toxins and pathogenic bacteria has been countered by the development of special immunological defenses, in which the major participants are the lymphocytes, plasma cells, macrophages, and mast cells that infiltrate the lamina propria.

Macrophages vary in number and location in the different segments of the intestine. In the small intestine, they are located mainly in the lamina propria of the upper half of the villi. In the colon, they are found in greatest number immediately beneath the surface epithelium. They contain levels of lysosomal hydrolases (nonspecific esterase, acid phosphatase, β-glucuronidase, and N-acetyl-β-D-glucosamidase) four to six times higher than in the monocytes from which they arise. They are avidly phagocytic and are the first line of defense against any microorganisms that may invade the mucosa from the lumen. In addition to ingesting and digesting bacteria, macrophages process antigens and incorporate them into their surface in a form that is highly effective in inducing an immune response by associated lymphocytes. Relatively weak antigens are hundreds of times more immunogenic after processing by macrophages. Lymphocytes take advantage of this by gathering around macrophages in lymphoid nodules and elsewhere in the lamina propria and synthesizing specific antibodies to the antigens they present. Many of the lymphocytes go on to differentiate into plasma cells that are even more productive in antibody synthesis.

Two kinds of mast cells are identifiable in the intestinal mucosa: *typical mast cells* that are found in connective tissues throughout the body and *atypical mast cells* (*mucosal mast cells*) of more restricted distribution. Typical mast cells predominate in the submucosa, whereas those in the lamina propria are the atypical mucosal mast cells. They differ in the ultrastructure of their granules and in certain histochemical reactions, but the functional significance of these differences is not yet known. The number of mast cells in the human duodenum is estimated at 20,000/mm^3. They have, on their surface, Fc receptors for the IgE class of immunoglobulins. Their exposure to specific antigen results in cross-linking of their IgE receptors and this activates the mast cell to secrete histamine. 5-hydroxytryptamine, and chemotactic agents for neutrophils and eosinophils. Intestinal mast cells are thought to be involved in local defenses against enteric parasites. Perhaps more important than any direct effect of their products on the parasites is their release of chemotactic factors that mobilize eosinophils and neutrophils that can attack the invading parasites or bacteria.

The most abundant of the free cells of the lamina propria are the lymphocytes, which constitute a ready reserve of immunocompetent cells. Some T-lymphocytes stimulate the immune response of B-lymphocytes and some of the B-lymphocytes differentiate into the antibody-producing plasma cells found in the lamina propria. Other T-lymphocytes invade the intercellular spaces in the epithelium. These are most numerous in the colon and they were formerly believed to migrate, in great numbers, through the epithelium to be lost in the discharge of the intestinal contents. Autoradiographic observations on lymphocytes labeled with tritiated thymidine provide no support for this interpretation. Over 95% of the lymphocytes are located in the basal third of the epithelium and the great majority of them are cytotoxic T-lymphocytes. Their function there is not clear.

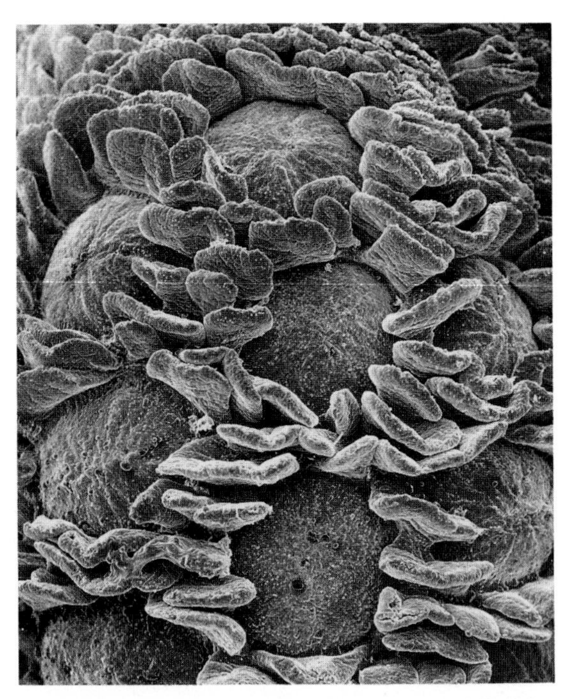

Figure 26–14. Surface view of a group of lymphoid follicles in the intestinal mucosa. Villi are lacking over the domes of the follicles. (Scanning micrograph from Komuro, T. and Y. Hashimota. 1990. Cell Tissue Res. 239:183.)

IMMUNOLOGICAL SURVEILLANCE OF LUMINAL ANTIGENS

The intestinal epithelium with its intercellular tight junctions normally provides an effective barrier to entry of bacteria deeper into the tissues, but in addition to this barrier function, certain cells take up samples of intraluminal foreign matter, including bacterial antigens, and pass these on to the mucosal immune system. This system consists of great numbers of individual lymphocytes found in the epithelium and its lamina propria and *solitary lymphoid nodules*, or *lymphoid follicles*, in the lamina propria. These dense aggregations of lymphocytes are scattered along the entire intestinal tract but are larger and more numerous in the ileum. The smaller lymphoid nodules are confined to the portion of the mucosa superficial to the muscularis mucosae, but the larger ones may occupy its entire thickness, extending down into the submucosa. Their presence can be detected with the naked eye, as round or oval bulges on the luminal surface (Fig. 26–14). In sections, the intestinal crypts are distorted by the underlying lymphoid aggregations or may be absent.

In some areas, groups of lymphoid nodules coalesce to form *aggregated lymphoid nodules*, also called *Peyer's patches* (Fig. 26–15). Although these may occur in the jejunum, some 30 to 40 are consistently found along the length of the ileum. They are usually located in the mucosa opposite the line of attachment of the mesentery. They are 12 to 20 mm in length and 8 to 12 mm across. In sections, they are seen to be made up of a number of lymphoid nodules, each having a large pale *germinal center* consisting of proliferating lymphoblasts that differentiate into IgA-producing B-lymphocytes. Also present are helper T-lymphocytes, antigen presenting macrophages, and dendritic cells. Cytotoxic T-lymphocytes are common in the surrounding mucosa. Solitary lymphoid nodules are also found, in smaller numbers, in the mucosa of the respiratory and urinary tracts. It is now believed that the total number of antibody-producing cells in the mucosal tissues of the body exceeds that in the spleen, lymph nodes, and bone marrow combined.

The intestinal epithelium covering the dome of the larger lymphoid nodules and Peyer's patches contains specialized *M-cells* that are not found elsewhere in the mucosa. They are relatively broad cells with a few short thick microvilli that are more widely separated than those forming the brush border of the other enterocytes (Figs. 26–16 and 26–17). Their basal surface is invaginated forming deep re-

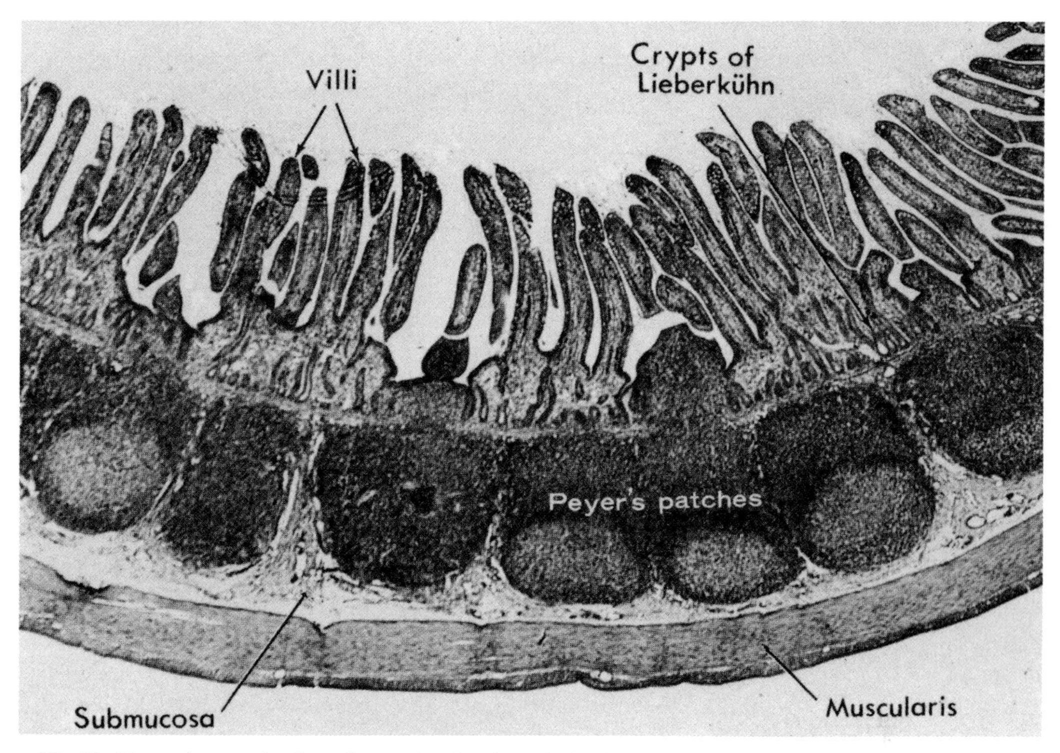

Figure 26–15. Photomicrograph of cat ileum showing intestinal villi, crypts of Lieberkuhn, and submucosal lymphoid nodules (Peyer's patches).

cesses or pockets between basal plasma membrane and the basal lamina. These invaginations are usually occupied by lymphocytes and pseudopodia of macrophages of the underlying lymphoid nodule (Fig. 26–18). It is believed that the M-cells are continuously sampling antigens in the intestinal lumen and transporting them to the cells of the mucosal immune system to induce an appropriate immune response. Long overlooked, the M-cells have now been thoroughly studied. If soluble proteins, lectins, or tracers such as cationized ferritin are infused into the intestinal lumen, they are rapidly taken up in clathrin-coated vesicles at the luminal surface of the M-cells and transported across its cytoplasm. All tracers taken up by endocytosis accumulate transiently in endosomes, but these appear to bypass the usual lysosomal pathway and go directly to the ablumenal surface to release their content into the interstices among the lymphocytes occupying the invagination of the cell base. No component of the glycoconjugates on the cell surface that is unique to the M-cells has yet been identified, but it is observed that certain gram-negative bacteria and viruses adhere selectively to these cells. Immediately below the epithelium, there are MHC–class-II positive dendritic cells and macrophages, as well as helper T-cells and these are believed to complete the processing and presentation of antigens to antibody producing B-lymphocytes.

Secretory Immune System of the Intestine

The general immunological defenses of the body depend on the IgG class of immunoglobulins present in the blood and tissue fluids. The very large mucosal surface of the gastrointestinal tract exposed to a lumen inhabited by a host of potentially invasive microorganisms require special protective mechanisms. A major component of these defenses is the *secretory immune system* which produces immunoglobulins of the IgA class. Antibodies of this class are present in the secretions of the salivary glands, the glands of the tracheobronchial mucosa, and those of the gastrointestinal tract. When the stroma of these glands and the lamina propria of the intestines are surveyed with fluorescein-labeled anti-sera against IgG and IgA, the great majority of plasma cells are found to be producing IgA. The mean population density of IgA reactive plasma

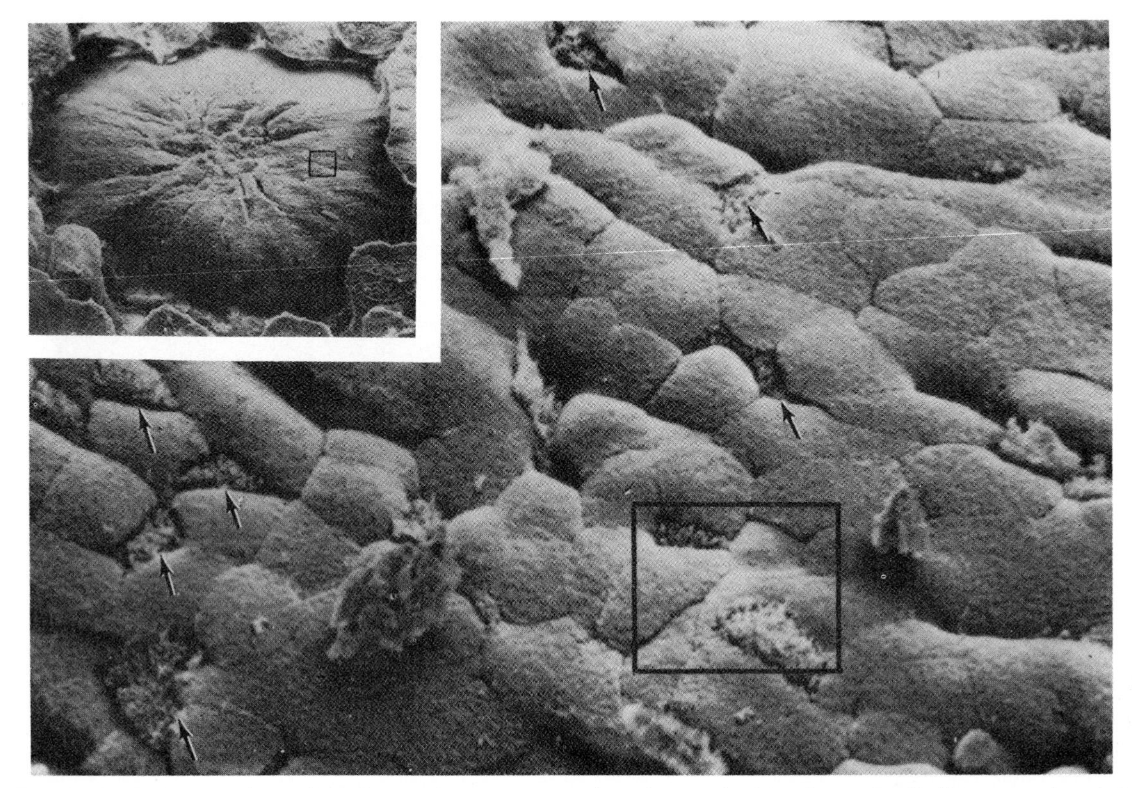

Figure 26–16. The inset (upper left) shows a low-power scanning micrograph of the dome of epithelium over a lymphoid follicle. The area in the superimposed small square is shown at higher magnification in the main micrograph. The polygonal outlines of the cells are evident. Certain cells (at arrows) differ from the majority in their surface texture. This is seen more clearly in Fig. 26–17 (a higher magnification of the area in the rectangle). (Micrograph from Owen, R. and A. Jones. 1974. Gastroenterology 66:189.)

cells in the intestine is reported to be 400,000/mm as compared to 18,000 for IgG.

Lymphocytes that have interacted with antigen in the lymphoid nodules do not immediately begin to produce antibody in the lamina propria. Instead, they migrate to the mesenteric lymph nodes and, after further maturation there, are carried in the lymph via the thoracic duct to the general circulation. In the circulation, they "home" back to the intestine and become widely distributed as free cells in the lamina propria (Fig. 26–19). There they differentiate into plasma cells that produce specific IgA antibodies to the antigen previously presented to them in the mucosal lymphoid tissue.

IgA produced by mucosal plasma cells binds to receptors on the base of the epithelial cells. It is taken up by endocytosis, transported across the cells in combination with a carrier protein called the *secretory component* (*secretory piece*) and discharged at the luminal surface. There, it is adsorbed onto the glycocalyx of the epithelium where it is strategically situated to inhibit bacteria adherence and to neutralize viruses and toxins—a process called *immune exclusion.*

Only a portion of the IgA destined for the intestinal lumen takes the direct pathway from the lamina propria across the epithelium. Much of the antibody produced by the plasma cells in the mucosa and the mesenteric lymph nodes is carried via the thoracic duct to the general circulation. Liver cells also produce secretory component and take up IgA from blood in the hepatic sinusoids and transport it to the bile canaliculi. The bile is subsequently discharged into the intestinal lumen. In biliary obstruction, the level of IgA in the blood rises and that in the small intestine falls to a fraction of its normal level. Thus, it is apparent that a significant percentage of the newly synthesized IgA antibodies reach the intestinal lumen via the hepatobiliary route.

The mystery that long enshrouded the function of the free cells and lymphoid aggregations in the lamina propria has now been solved by advances in immunology which have

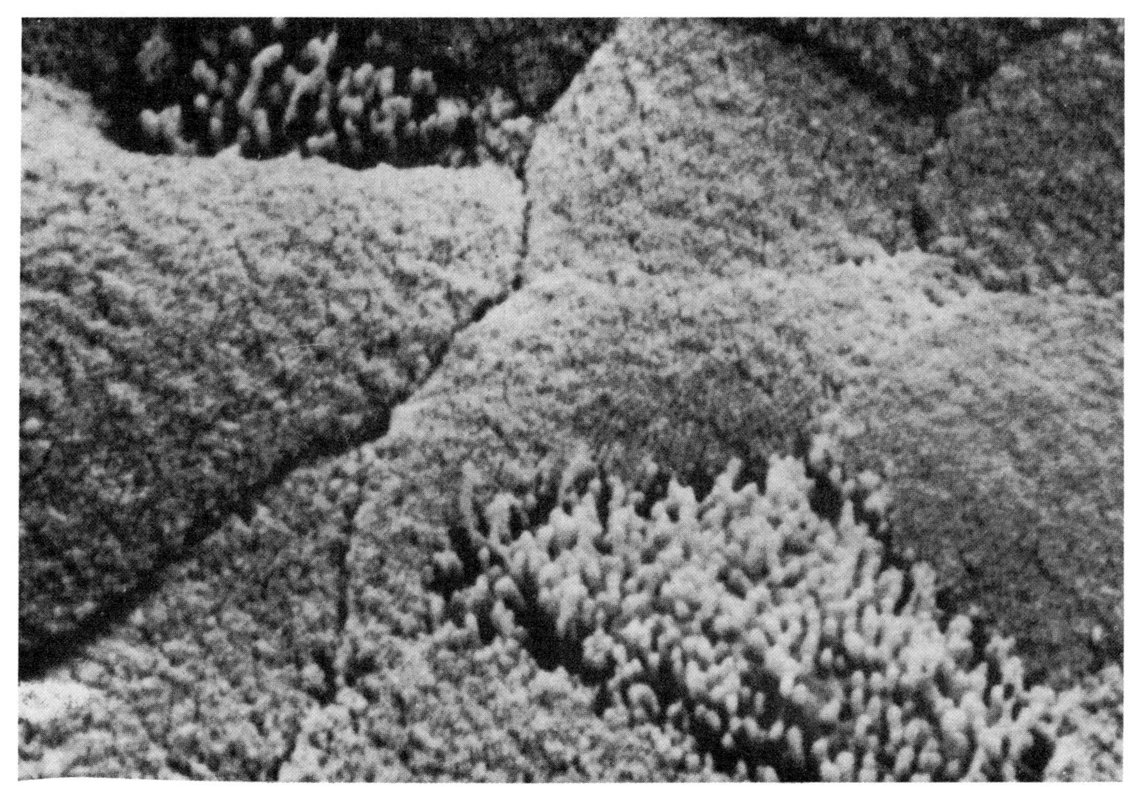

Figure 26–17. Scanning micrograph of the area boxed in Fig. 26–16. Two of the cells bear loosely packed microvilli that are longer and broader than those of the brush border of the surrounding cells. These are the so-called M-cells. (Micrograph from Owen, R. and A. Jones. 1974. Gastroenterology 66:189.)

shown that they constitute an efficient local immune system supporting the epithelium in its role as a barrier to penetration of toxins and pathogenic microorganisms from the external environment.

It is interesting to note that in the ongoing "arms race" between microbes and higher organisms, a few species of bacteria have evolved a counterweapon, *IgA proteases*—enzymes that cleave IgA immunoglobulins. No other substrate for their activity has yet been identified. These proteases may play a part in the pathogenesis of certain human diseases by interfering with the immunological defenses mediated by IgA.

MUSCULARIS MUCOSAE

The muscularis mucosae averages 38 μm in thickness and consists of thin inner and outer layers of smooth muscle together with networks of elastic fibers. Its contraction increases the height of folds of the mucosa. In fixed preparations, it is usually contracted, slightly exaggerating the irregularity of the outline of the lumen. It is conceivable that such changes in the surface topography of the mucosa may play a minor ancillary role in the mixing of the contents of the gut.

SUBMUCOSA

The submucosa consists of moderately dense connective tissue rich in elastic fibers. It may also contain small clusters of adipose cells. In the duodenum, it is largely occupied by the *glands of Brunner.*

Submucosal Glands (Brunner's Glands)

At the pyloris of the mammalian stomach, there is an abrupt transition from pyloric glands to *Brunner's glands,* which are an identifying histological feature of the initial portion of the duodenum. In the human, a few of these glands may also be found in the pyloric antrum. Pyloric glands are usually confined to the lamina propria, whereas Brunner's glands

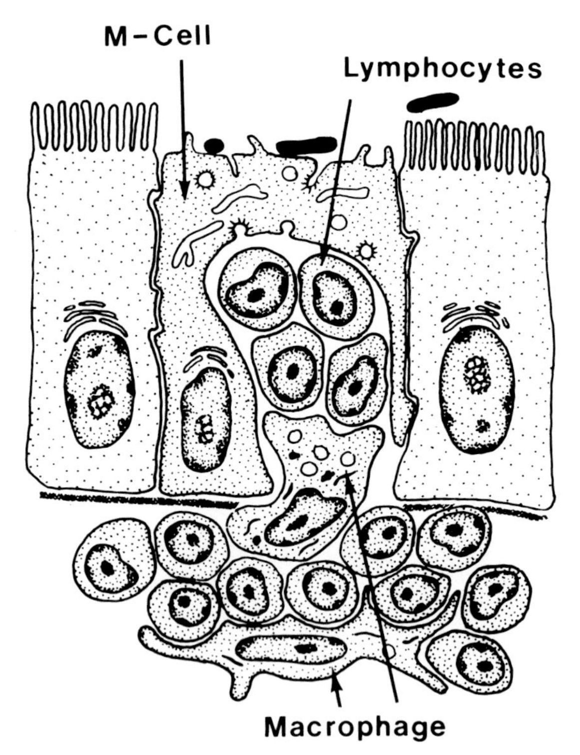

Figure 26–18. Diagram of an M-cell showing lymphocytes and macrophages occupying a deep recess in the base of the cell. Gram-negative bacteria adhere selectively to M-cells which transport antigen into the basal pocket. (Redrawn after Neutra, M.R. and J.P. Kraehenbuhl. 1992. Trends Cell Biol. 2:134.)

are found in the submucosa of the plicae circulares (Fig. 26–2). The secretory portions of the glands are coiled tubules forming small lobules 0.5–1.0 mm in diameter. The ducts ascend through the muscularis mucosae to open into crypts of Lieberkuhn, or occasionally onto the surface between villi (Fig. 26–20). Under the light microscope, the gland cells have the pale appearance of mucus cells, but in electron micrographs, they bear a superficial resemblance to pancreatic acinar cells in having dense secretory granules, a large Golgi complex, and abundant rough endoplasmic reticulum.

The secretion of the duodenal glands is a clear, viscous, and distinctly alkaline fluid (pH 8.2 to 9.3). Its principal function is to protect the duodenal mucosa against the potentially damaging effects of the strongly acidic gastric juice periodically discharged through the pyloric sphincter. The mucoid nature of the secretion, its alkaline pH, and the buffering capacity of its bicarbonate content make it well suited to this role.

Another function has emerged in recent years with the discovery that Brunner's glands synthesize and secrete a low-molecular-weight polypeptide that was originally called *urogastrone* when first detected in human urine and later found to stimulate cell division and to inhibit gastric acid secretion. It has since been found to be the human form of *epidermal growth factor* (EGF) which has been widely studied in animals. It is implicated in the regulation of a variety of physiological processes including growth, tissue repair, and regeneration. Although secreted by Brunner's glands, the submandibular salivary glands are an even richer source. It is secreted into the oral cavity in the saliva and into the intestinal lumen by the Brunner's glands. Receptors for urogastrone (EGF) are found on many cells types including those of the gastric glands, the liver, and the mucosa of the small intestine. The polypeptide is resistant to trypsin, chymotrypsin, and pepsin digestion. In the gastrointestinal tract, it is believed to modulate the secre-

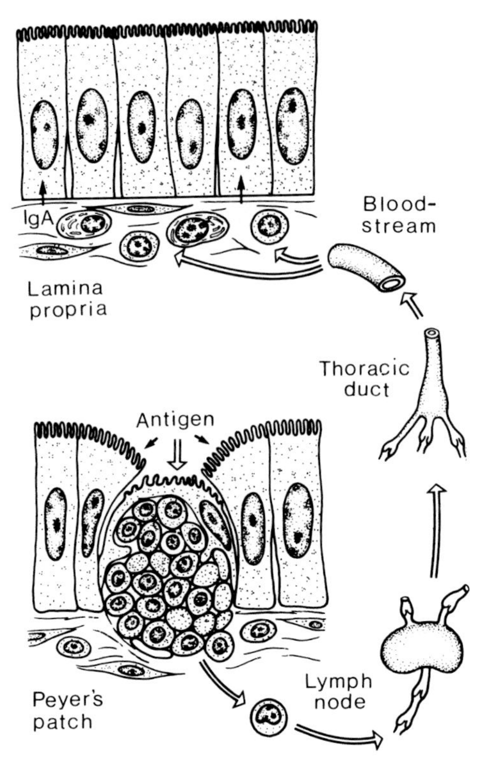

Figure 26–19. Schematic of the pathways involved in the secretory immune system. Lymphocytes in Peyer's patches, exposed to antigens from the lumen, migrate to regional lymph nodes, then to the thoracic duct and the bloodstream. Carried in the circulation, they home into the lamina propria of the gut and there develop into plasma cells secreting IgA, which acquires a secretory piece in the epithelium and is released into the gut lumen. (Redrawn from Walker, W.A., and K.J. Isselbacher. 1977. N. Engl. J. Med. 297:767.)

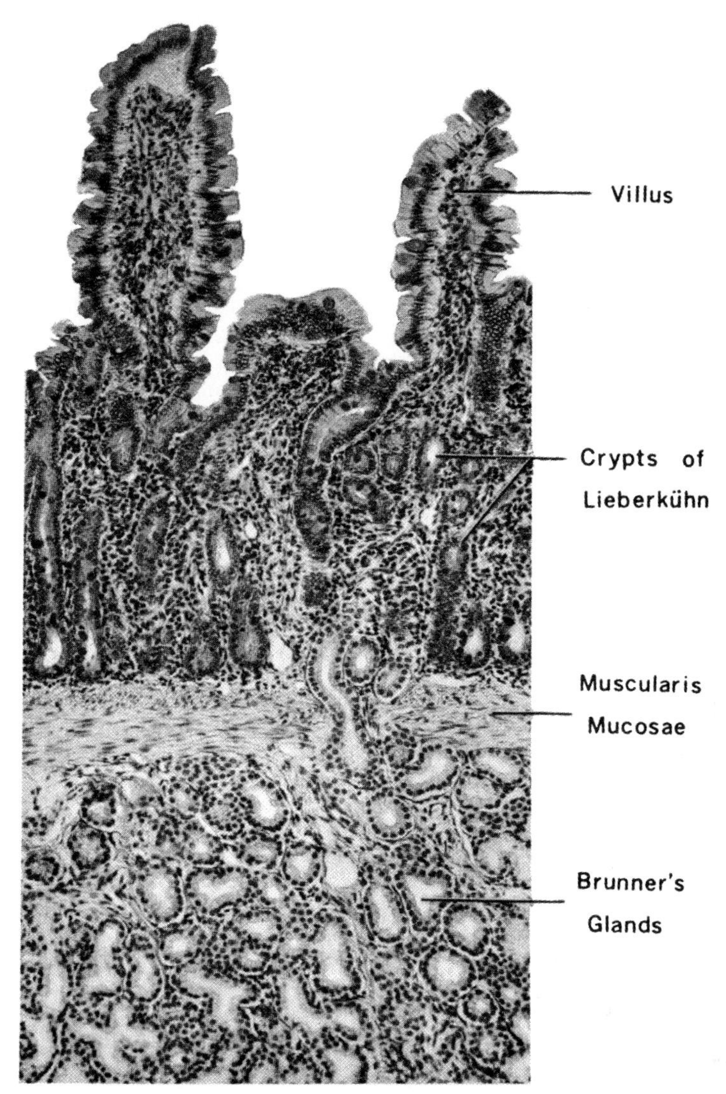

Figure 26–20. Photomicrograph the duodenal mucosa of the macaque. The villi, crypts of Lieberkuhn, and Brunner's glands are shown. A duct of the gland is seen traversing the muscularis mucosae to empty into one of the crypts.

tion of acid by the oxyntic cell of the stomach and to influence the rate of cell proliferation in the intestinal crypts, but its effects are much more widespread. It is found in significant concentrations in urine, gastric juice, saliva, bile, and milk. It is interesting that nearly all animals persistently lick any superficial wounds, and with EGF in the saliva, this may have a beneficial effect in accelerating healing. The mechanism by which EGF stimulates DNA synthesis and cell division is still unknown.

MUSCULARIS

The muscular coat of the small intestine consists of outer longitudinal and inner circular layers of smooth muscle, but some strands of smooth muscle fibers pass from one layer into the other. Between these layers is the sympathetic *myenteric nerve plexus*. The smooth muscle of the muscularis was formerly regarded as a static population, but autoradiographic studies have now shown that there is a slow rate of cell replication throughout the external layer and the rate differs in different portions of the alimentary tract.

The muscularis is responsible for *peristalis,* a wave-like contraction that travels along the intestine at a rate of a few centimeters per second and propels the luminal contents onward. The peristaltic waves are propagated for short distances along the intestine and then die out, to be followed a few minutes later by another wave. Several waves may be in progress at the same time in successive segments of the small bowel, but it is rare for a single wave to pass along its entire length. In addition to these traveling waves of contraction, there are *segmental movements,* consisting of alternative constriction and relaxation of short segments. These do not advance the content toward the large intestine but result in to-and-fro movements that serve to agitate and mix the material in the lumen.

In the terminal portion of the ileum, the muscularis is somewhat thickened, forming the *ileocecal sphincter.* This normally remains partially contracted, delaying emptying the contents of the small intestine into the cecum, the blind pouch at the beginning of the large intestine. Some time after a meal, there is a reflex activation of ileal peristalsis and a relaxation of the ileocecal sphincter, permitting the intestinal contents to advance into the large intestine. Folds of mucosa that project into the cecum at the ileocecal valve act as a bicuspid valve, closing when the cecum fills and preventing reflux into the ileum.

SEROSA

The outermost layer of the gut wall, the *serosa,* consists of a continuous sheet of squamous cells, the *mesothelium,* separated from the underlying muscularis by a very thin layer of loose connective tissue. For most of its length, the gastrointestinal tract is suspended from the dorsal wall of the abdomen by a *mesentery,* a thin bilaminar sheet of mesothelium through which the blood vessels reach the gut. Along the line of attachment of the mesentery, the serosa of the intestine is continuous with the two apposed leaves of the mesentery, and at the base of the mesentery these are, in turn, continuous with the serous lining of the abdominal cavity. Thus, the inner aspect of the abdominal wall and the surface of all of the organs suspended from it are covered by a continuous layer of mesothelium, usually referred to as the *peritoneum.* That portion lining the cavity is called the *parietal peritoneum* and that covering the organs is the *visceral peritoneum.* The transudation of fluid from the underlying capillaries moistens the smooth serous surfaces of organs and facilitates frictionless sliding of the loops of the intestine over one another during peristalsis. Bacterial contamination of the abdominal cavity due to perforating lesions of the gut wall results in *peritonitis,* a severe inflammatory process that is often fatal.

LARGE INTESTINE

The large intestine includes several successive segments: the *cecum,* the *ascending, transverse,* and *descending colon,* the *sigmoid colon,* the *rectum,* and the *anus.* The cecum is a blind-ending pouch at the proximal end of the ascending colon. At the junction of the cecum and the ascending colon, the ileum joins it on its medial side and the orifice between the two is closed by the *ileocecal valve.* Projecting from the cecum posteromedial to the ileocecal valve is the vermiform *appendix.*

THE APPENDIX

The appendix, arising from the blind end of the cecum, ranges in length from 2 to 8 cm. Its wall has all of the layers typical of the intestinal wall, but it is thickened by an extensive accumulation of lymphoid tissue which forms a nearly continuous layer of large and small lymphatic nodules (Fig. 26–21). The lymphatic tissue of the appendix, like that of the tonsils, often shows chronic inflammatory changes. The small lumen of the appendix has an angular outline in cross section and is often filled with dead cells and detritus. It is difficult to make a distinction between the normal structure of the appendix and common pathological conditions of this rudimentary organ. Villi are usually absent. The crypts of Lieberkuhn are irregular in shape and are largely embedded in the underlying lymphoid tissue. The glandular epithelium contains only a few goblet cells and consists mainly of columnar cells having a brush border. The zone of mitotically active cells in the crypts is shorter than in the small intestine. Enteroendocrine cells and Paneth cells are regularly found in the depths of the crypts. The later are more numerous than in the crypts of the small intestine and 5 to 10 may be found in a single gland.

The muscularis mucosae is poorly developed and the submucosa is a relatively thick layer containing blood vessels, nerves, and occasional lobules of adipose tissue. The muscularis externa is reduced in thickness, but its two layers are still identifiable. The serosa is the same as that covering the rest of the intestines.

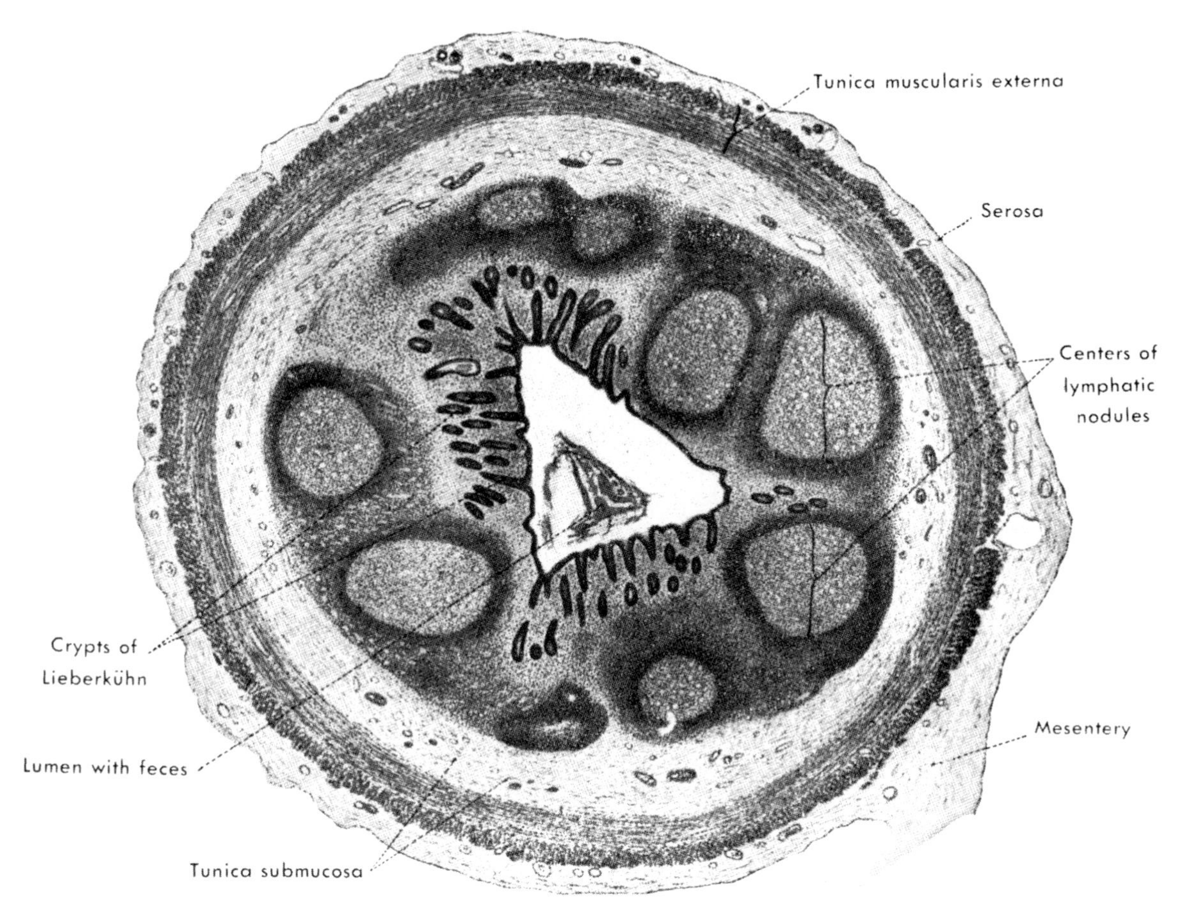

Figure 26–21. Cross section of the appendix of a 23-year-old man. (After J. Sobotta. Atlas of Human Anatomy. G.E. Steckert & Co. New York, 1936.)

CECUM AND COLON

The mucosa of the large intestine does not form folds comparable to the plicae circulares, and intestinal villi are not found beyond the ileocecal valve. The mucosa of the colon has a smooth surface when examined with the naked eye but may be somewhat irregular in outline in histological sections due to agonal contraction of the muscularis (Fig. 26–22). At low magnification, one can see the openings of innumerable crypts or glands of Lieberkuhn (Fig. 26–23). These are straight tubular glands about 0.5 mm in length and, thus, somewhat longer than their counterparts in the small intestine. In the rectum, they attain a length of 0.7 mm. They differ from crypts of the small intestine in the absence of Paneth cells and in the greater abundance of goblet cells (Fig. 26–24). Enteroendocrine cells are present in small numbers. Goblet cells are the most conspicuous cell type, but actually the majority of cells in the middle and upper portions of the crypts are columnar absorptive cells and these are also the principal cell type in the epithelium at the surface of the mucosa. As in the small intestine, the epithelium is constantly being renewed. Undifferentiated cells in the depths of the crypts divide and their progeny differentiate into columnar, goblet, and enteroendocrine cells which slowly move up the wall of the crypt and onto the surface. There they slough off into the lumen in *extrusion zones* situated about midway between the openings of neighboring crypts. The life span of most of the cells in the epithelium is about 6 days, but the endocrine cells appear to be an exception, having a life span measured in weeks rather than days. This implies that they must migrate independently and at a different rate from the surrounding cells. Little is known about the mechanism of cell migration in the walls of the crypts. The fibroblasts that ensheath the intestinal crypts also proliferate at the base and move upward with the epithelial cells.

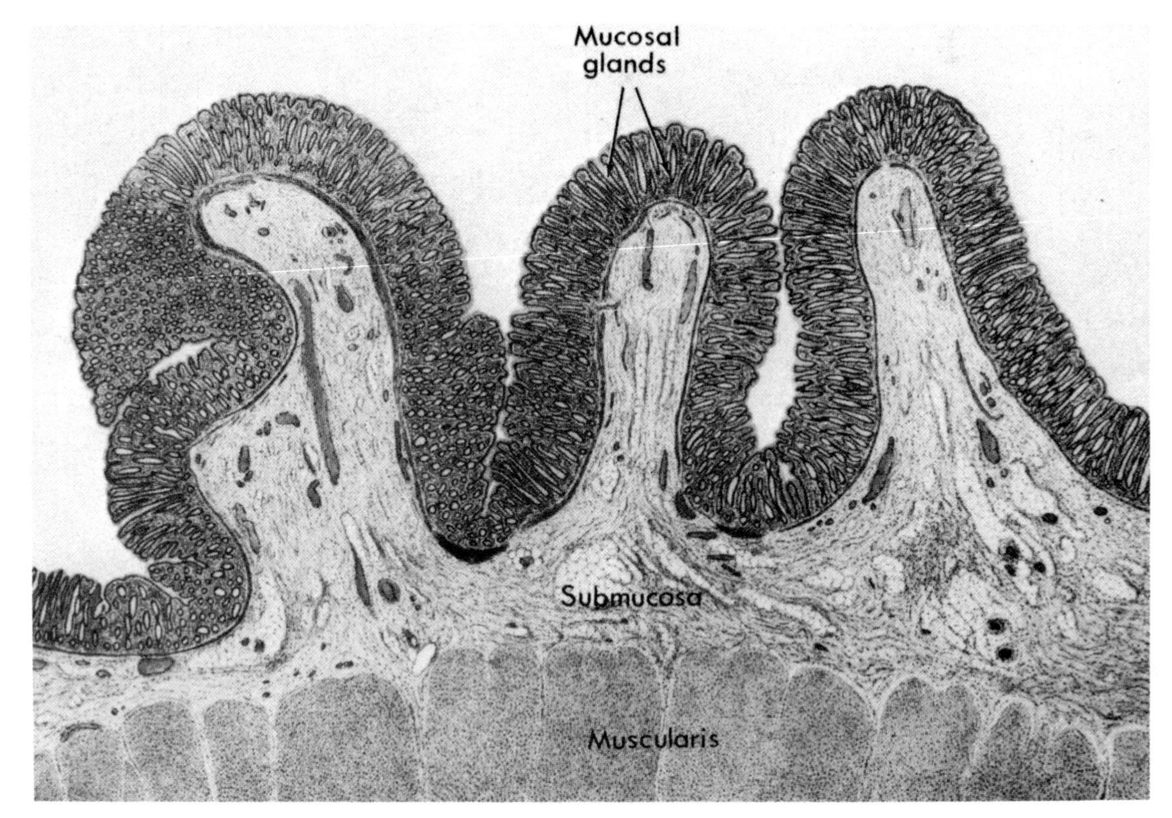

Figure 26–22. Longitudinal section of the wall of the human colon. (From Bargmann, W. 1962. Histologie und Mikroskopische Anatomie des Menschen, 6th ed. Stuttgart, Georg Theime Verlag.)

The lamina propria of the colon is similar to that of the small intestine. Scattered lymphoid nodules are always present and may extend deep into the submucosa. The muscularis mucosae is well developed, consisting of longitudinal and circular fibers, and it may send slender fascicles of fibers upward toward the surface. The submucosa presents no unusual features.

The muscularis of the colon differs in organization from that of the small intestine. Instead of forming a continuous layer of uniform thickness, the longitudinal fibers are aggregated into three evenly spaced longitudinal bands called the *taenia coli.* Between the taenia, longitudinal smooth muscle fibers form a very thin, and often discontinuous layer. The inner circular layer is similar to that of the small intestine. In the living, the taenia are in a state of partial contraction which causes the intervening portions of the wall to bulge outward, forming shallow sacculations called the *haustrae.* These are conspicuous in the ascending, transverse, and descending colon and in the sigmoid flexure. However, in the rectum, the muscularis externa again forms a continuous layer of uniform thickness, and haustrae are not present.

The serosa of the colon is unusual in having conspicuous accumulations of adipose cells beneath the mesotheium that form pendulous protuberances called *appendices epiploicae.*

THE RECTUM

The rectum is the terminal portion of the intestinal tract, about 12 cm in length and extending from the sigmoid colon to the pelvic diaphragm. It is slightly dilated in its lower portion to form the *rectal ampulla.* Two or three transversely oriented folds of mucosa are found above the rectal ampulla. The rectal mucosa is similar to that of the colon, but its crypts are somewhat longer (Fig. 26–25). The rectum narrows rather abruptly at the lower end of the ampulla and continues as the *anal canal,* about 4 cm in length. The mucosa here exhibits longitudinal folds, the *rectal columns of Morgagni.* The crypts of Lieberkuhn in this

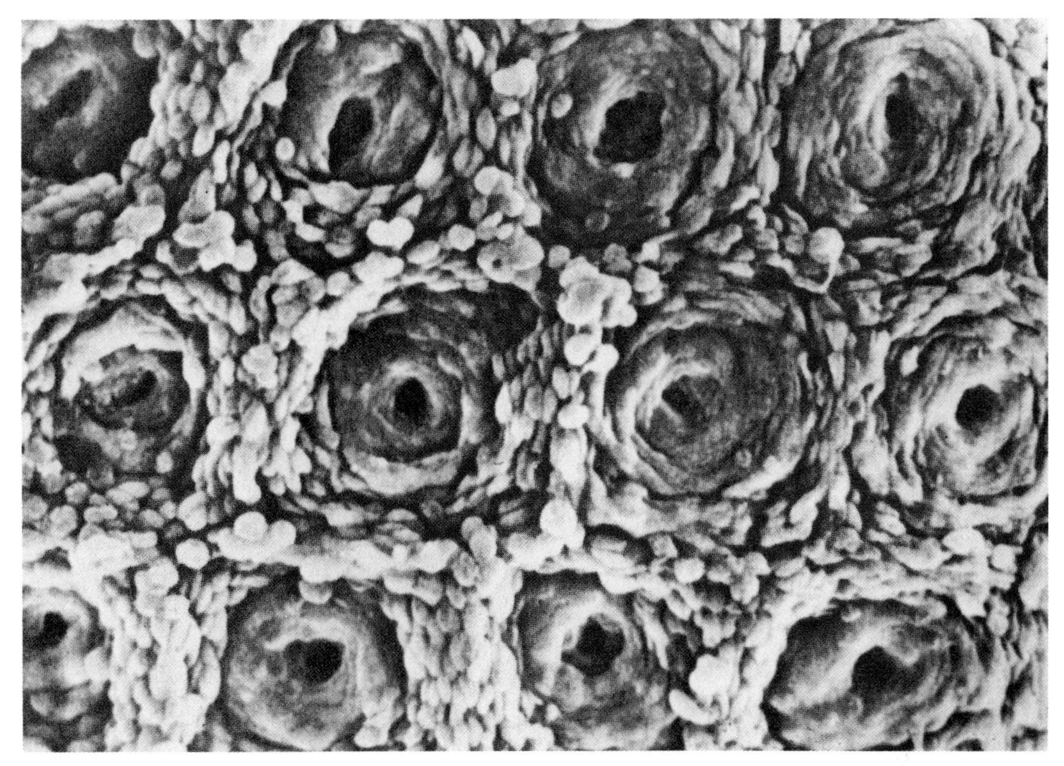

Figure 26–23. Scanning electron micrograph of the surface of the descending colon of a monkey (Macaca mulatta) showing the regular array of openings of the crypts. (From Specian, R. and M.R. Neutra. 1981. Am. J. Anat. 160:461.)

region suddenly become short and disappear all together along an irregular line about 2 cm above the anal opening. Here, there is an abrupt transition from simple columnar to stratified squamous epithelium. Thus, at the level of the external muscular sphincter of the anus, the lining of the canal has the appearance of skin with typical sebaceous glands and also large circumanal apocrine glands. The lamina propria here contains a plexus of large veins that often become distended and varicose and may protrude from the anus as hemorrhoids.

The circular layer of smooth muscle of the anal canal is considerably thickened, forming the *anal sphincter*. Distal to this, there is a circumferential annulus of striated muscle, the *external anal sphincter*.

HISTOPHYSIOLOGY OF THE INTESTINE

The function of the alimentary tract is to reduce ingested carbohydrates, fats, and proteins to molecules that can be absorbed by the cells of the mucosa. Each day some 8–9 liters of water, 100 g of fat, 50–100 g of amino acids, and several hundred grams of carbohydrate are absorbed from the small intestine.

Many of the physiologically important processes of living organisms take place at cell surfaces and at the interfaces between membrane-limited intracellular compartments. The rate of metabolic activity per unit area of surface probably cannot be increased above a certain limit. Therefore, at all levels of organization, there are architectural devices for increasing surface area, without increasing the overall size of the organism. This design principle is dramatically exemplified in the structure of the alimentary tract (Fig. 26–26). The absorptive surface is first increased by elongation and convolution of the tubular intestine. The mucosal surface is increased by plication to form the plicae circulares. At higher magnification, the surface is found to be amplified by some 40 intestinal villi per square millimeter. In electron micrographs, the surface of every absorptive cell in the epithelium covering the villi is found to be augmented another 30-fold by 2 to 3 thousand microvilli per cell. At the molecular level, the polysaccharide chains of the membrane

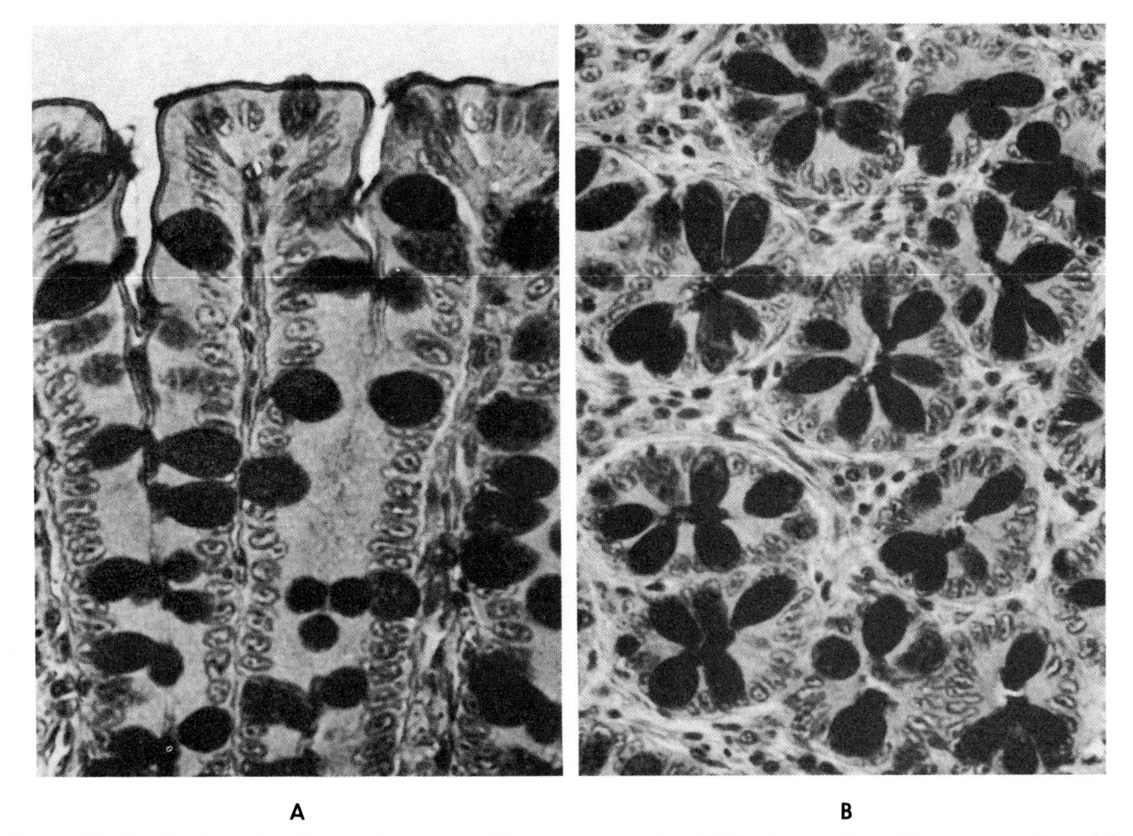

Figure 26–24. Histological sections of the crypts of the macaque colon. (A) Vertical section of the upper portion of the mucosa showing the columnar epithelial cells and goblet cells; (B) horizontal section through several crypts showing the radial distribution of goblet cells around the lumen and the highly cellular lamina propria between the crypts.

glycoproteins form a surface coat of highly branched polymers that add still further to the enormous area of surface exposed to the intestinal contents. Within the cell, convolution is again seen in the configuration of the tubular and cisternal endoplasmic reticulum, and plication to increase surface is seen in the cristae of the mitochondria. These are but a few of Nature's strategems for increasing the efficiency of the metabolic machinery, with minimal increase in body mass.

The secretions of the liver and pancreas delivered to the duodenum are essential for digestion in the small intestine. The bile from the liver and gall bladder, together with the mechanical mixing action of peristalsis, reduces ingested fat to a fine emulsion of triglycerides. The intestinal mucosa itself contributes intestinal juice called *succus entericus*.

Several digestive enzymes were formerly thought to be secreted by cells of the crypts of Lieberkuhn, but it has become clear from biochemical studies of isolated brush borders of these cells that some of the enzymes believed to be secreted into the lumen are actually incorporated into the membrane of the brush border of the absorptive cells. Among these are *leucine aminopeptidase, sucrase,* which cleaves sucrose to glucose and fructose, *lactase,* cleaving lactose to glucose and galactose, and *maltase,* which hydrolyzes maltose derived from starch to glucose. These enzymes residing in the membrane and surface coat of the microvilli reduce dietary carbohydrates in the gut lumen to hexoses that are actively transported into the absorptive cells by carrier proteins present in the brush border. Thus, the brush border is not only a device for increasing the surface area for absorption but is also the site of enzymes involved in the terminal steps in digestion of carbohydrates and proteins, and it possesses the carriers necessary for transport of glucose and amino acids into the cell. Infants suffering from a rare genetic defect are unable to tolerate milk, and feeding milk results in bloating and copious diarrhea. These symptoms have been traced to the absence of a single enzyme, lactase, from their

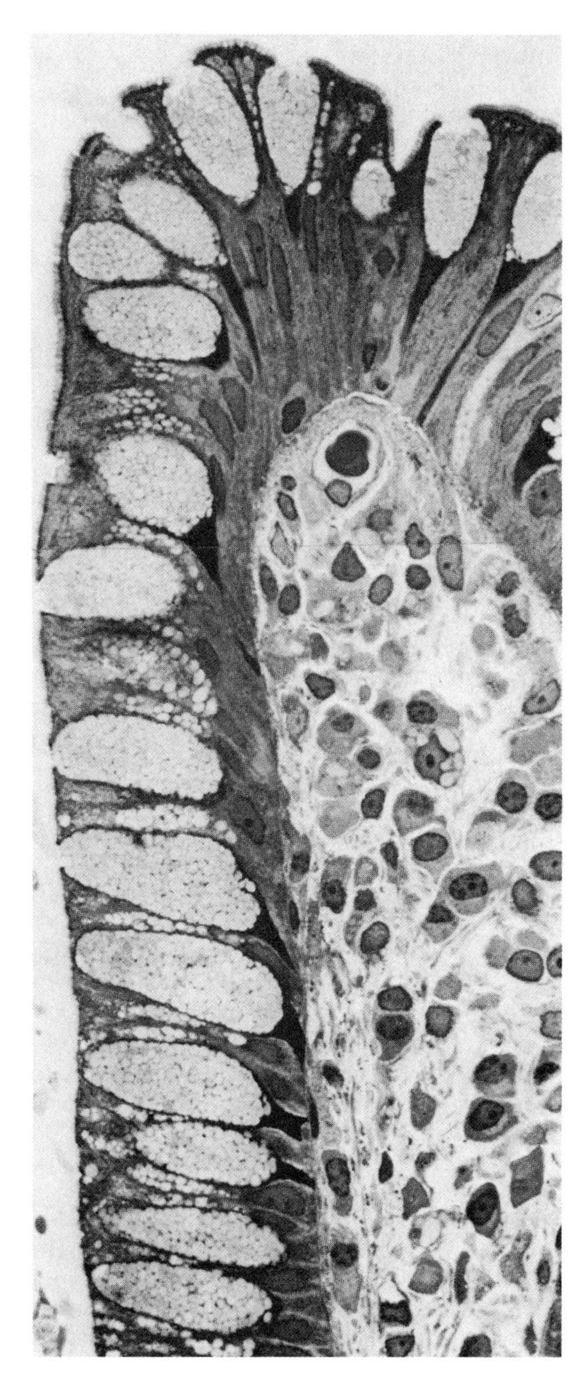

Figure 26–25. Photomicrograph of the epithelium on one side of a crypt in the human rectal mucosa joining the surface epithelium (top). (Photomicrograph from Neutra, M. 1977. Lab. Invest. 36:535.)

intestinal brush border. If lactase is eliminated from the diet, these infants do very well.

Intraluminal digestion of most food reduces it to units of molecular size, whose path of absorption cannot be followed by microscopy. Fat lends itself best to morphological study because lipid can be preserved in the tissue and intensely stained by fixatives containing osmium tetroxide (Figs. 26–27 and 26–28). Dietary fat in the intestinal lumen is hydrolyzed by pancreatic lipase to free fatty acids and monoglycerides. These products combine with bile salts to form minute micelles, about 2 nm in diameter (Fig. 26–29). When myriads of these come into contact with the microvilli of the absorptive cells, the fatty acids and monoglycerides diffuse across the plasma membrane and accumulate in the apical cytoplasm. Membranes of the smooth endoplasmic reticulum there contain the enzymes for resynthesis of triglycerides. The resynthesized triglycerides form numerous readily visible lipid droplets in the lumen of the reticulum in the apical cytoplasm. From there, the lipid appears to be transported to the Golgi complex for further processing that converts it into *chylomicra,* complex glycolipoprotein droplets that leave the cells and are transported via the intestinal lymphatics to the bloodstream. The precise role of the Golgi complex in the process has not been established, but it seems likely that the carbohydrate moiety of the chylomicra is added there to the triglyceride synthesized in the smooth endoplasmic reticulum. In their passage through the Golgi complex, the chylomicra also acquire a membranous investment that enables them to coalesce with the basolateral plasma membrane of the columnar absorptive cells during their discharge into the intercellular clefts and into the lymphatic capillaries in the lamina propria of the intestinal villi (Fig. 26–30).

The absorptive cells of the intestine are able to respond rapidly and to change their internal structure. In the fasting state, the apical cytoplasm contains some profiles of granular reticulum, a limited amount of smooth reticulum, and a relatively quiescent Golgi complex. Ingestion of lipid stimulates the formation of a more extensive smooth reticulum to provide for resynthesis of triglyceride and its transport to the Golgi. The rapid turnover of Golgi membranes during lipid absorption also requires accelerated synthesis of new membrane to replace that lost to the cell surface in discharge of chylomicra. If protein synthesis is blocked, by administration of puromysin, membrane replacement in smooth reticulum and Golgi complex is prevented, as is the synthesis of protein constituents of the chylomicra. Lipid absorption and transport is, therefore, inhibited, and large amounts of lipid

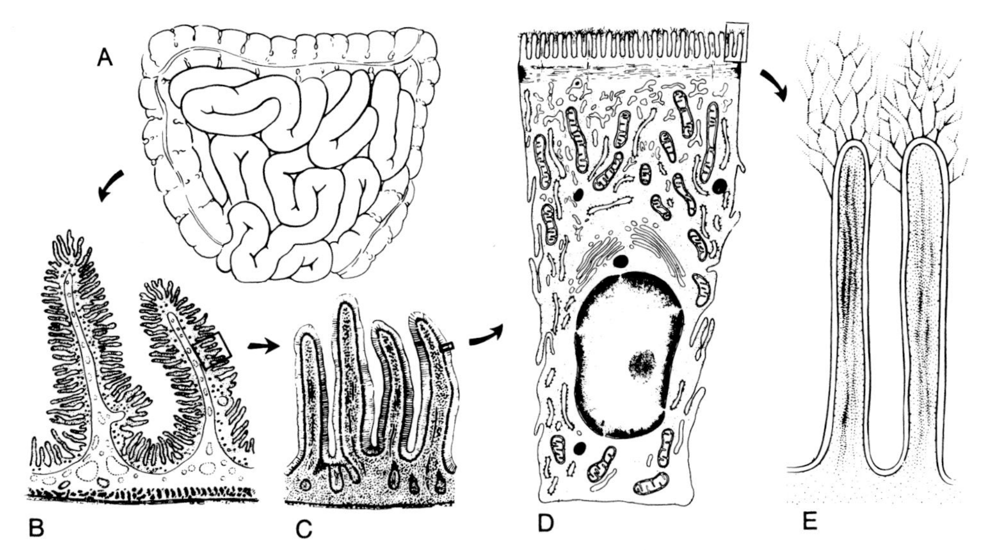

Figure 26–26. Drawing illustrating the several levels of amplification of the absorptive surface of the intestine. (A) Convolution of a long gut; (B) plicae circulares; (C) villi of the mucosa; (D) microvilli of the cells; (E) oligosaccharide chains of integral glycoproteins of the microvillar membrane. (From Fawcett, D. 1981. The Cell, 2nd ed. Philadelphia, W.B. Saunders Co.)

accumulates in the cytoplasm of the absorptive cells.

An important part of the mechanism of absorption in the intestine is the movement of the villi. This can be observed in a living animal if a loop of intestine is opened and studied under a dissecting microscope. A villus is seen to suddenly shorten to about half its length with an appreciable increase in its diameter, and it then slowly extends to its original length. Each villus contracts about six times a minute. During contraction, its volume is reduced and the contents of the central lacteal are forwarded to the submucous lymphatic plexus. Contraction results from shortening of the slender strand of smooth muscle in the core of the villus. Contraction of the villi is believed to be under control of Meissner's submucous nerve plexus. Direct mechanical stimulation of the base of a villus with a bristle also induces contraction, and the stimulus radiates from the affected villus to the surrounding villi.

In addition to the absorption of water and nutrients, the small intestine has an essential function in the absorption and conservation of ions. About 6 g of sodium is taken in daily in the diet and 20–30 g are secreted into the lumen in the succus entericus, but little or none is lost in the feces. Sodium is constantly reabsorbed in the intestine. It diffuses through the membrane of the absorptive cells and is actively transported through the lateral membranes, creating, in the intercellular clefts, a standing gradient that draws water through the epithelium and into the capillaries of the villi. Chloride ions diffuse along the electrochemical gradient with the sodium. The importance of this reabsorption of ions becomes evident in cholera and other forms of severe diarrhea, in which the sodium reserves of the body can be reduced to lethal levels in a few hours.

Absorption of water and electrolytes continues in the colon. About 1 liter of chyme passes through the ileocecal valve daily, but normally less than 100 ml is lost in the feces. The bulk of the feces consists of dead bacteria and the undigestible fibrous constituents of ingested vegetable matter. The bacterial flora of the intestine, in humans, digest only small amounts of cellulose, but in herbivorous mammals, cellulose is an important nutritional source, the digestion of which depends on the bacteria in their digestive tract. In humans, the major contribution of the intestinal flora is the production of vitamin B_{12}, needed for haemopoiesis, and vitamin K, which is essential for maintenance of the clotting mechanism of the blood.

BLOOD VESSELS OF THE INTESTINAL TRACT

The arrangement of the blood and lymph vessels in the wall of the stomach and intestine are basically similar. In the stomach, the arter-

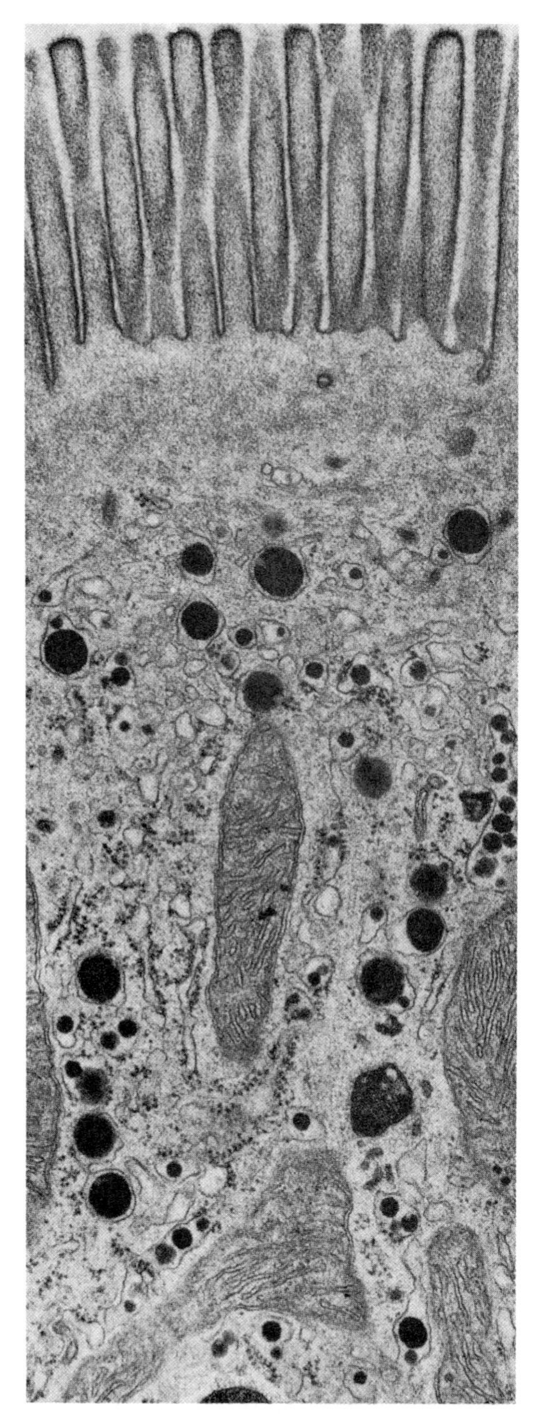

Figure 26–27. Electron micrograph of an intestinal epithelial cell of the rat. Lipid accumulates in sizable droplets in the smooth endoplasmic reticulum, but very little is seen in invaginations of the surface membrane or in vesicles traversing the terminal web. Pinocytosis is not the principal mechanism for lipid absorption. (Courtesy of S.L. Palay and J.P. Revel.)

ies arise from two arterial arches along the lesser and greater curvatures and are distributed to the ventral and dorsal surfaces. In the intestine, the vessels reach the organ from the mesentery and break up into large branches that penetrate the muscularis externa to enter the submucosa, where they form a large plexus. In the small intestine, the submucous arterial plexus gives off two kinds of branches. Some of these ramify on the inner surface of the muscularis mucosae and break up into capillary networks that surround the crypts of Lieberkuhn. Other branches are destined for the villi, each villus receiving one, and sometimes two or three, such small arteries. In the villi, they form a dense capillary network immediately beneath the epithelium (Fig. 26–31). Near the tip of the villus one or two small veins arise from the capillary network and run downward to anastomose with the venous plexus around the glands, and then pass on into the submucous venous plexus. These small veins of the intestine have no valves. However, their continuations that pass though the muscularis externa with the arteries are provided with valves.

LYMPH VESSELS OF THE INTESTINAL TRACT

In the stomach and colon, the lymphatics begin as an extensive system of large lymphatic capillaries in the superficial portion of the mucosa between the glands. They are always situated below the blood capillaries. They anastomose extensively around the glands and take a downward course to the inner surface of the mucosa where they form a plexus of lymphatics that are provided with valves. From the submucous plexus, larger lymphatics run through the muscularis externa. Here, they receive numerous lymphatics from the lymphatic plexus in the muscular coat and then follow the blood vessels into the retroperitoneal tissues.

Lymphatics are very important for the absorption of fat in the small intestine. During digestion, they become filled with milky white lymph, a fine emulsion of neutral fats. This white lymph draining from the intestine is called *chyle,* and the lymphatics that carry it away from the epithelium are called the *lacteals.* The most interesting of the lymphatics of the small intestine are the central lacteals in the core of the villi. Each conical villus has an

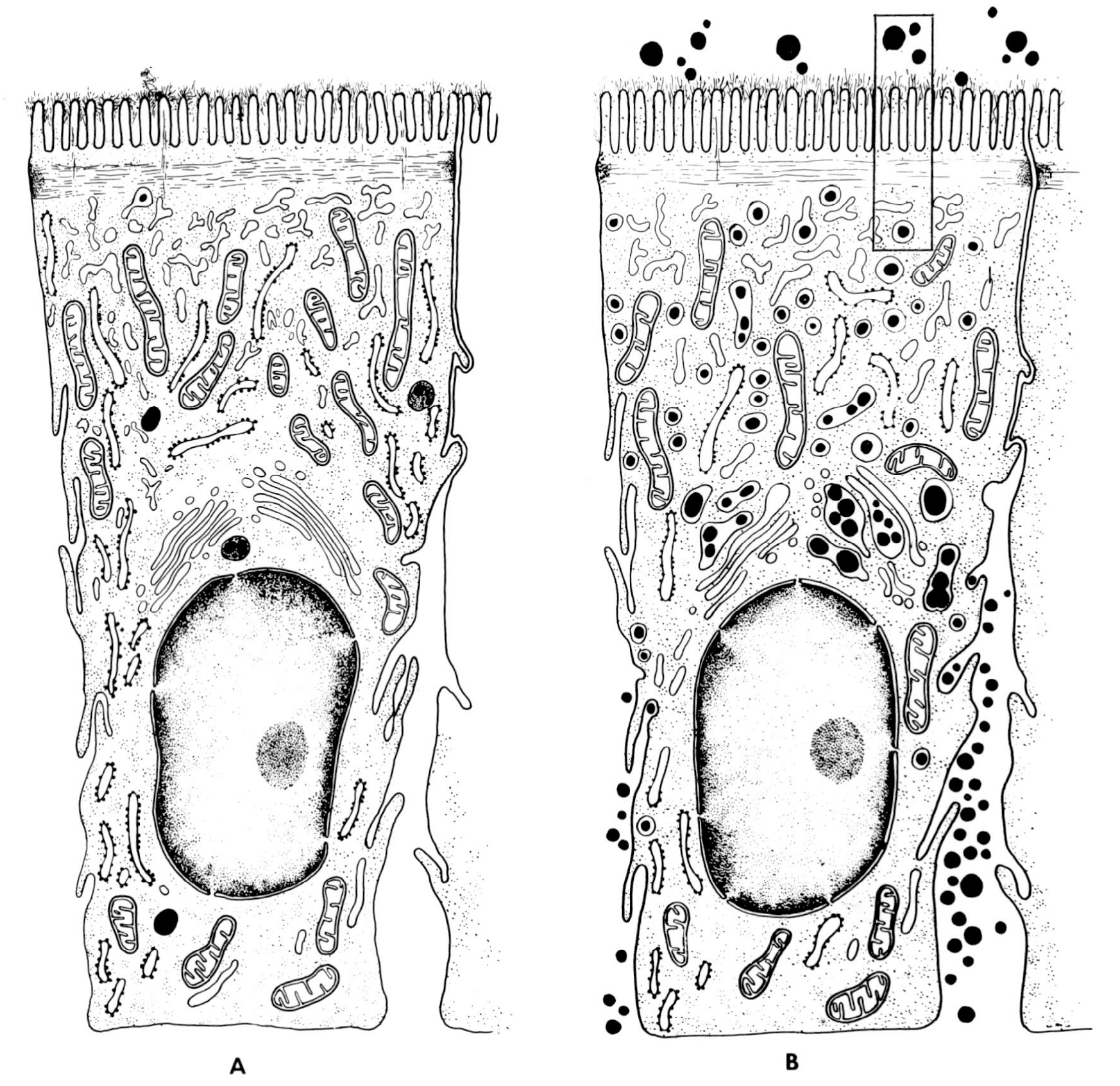

Figure 26–28. Schematic representation of the ultrastructure of an intestinal absorptive cell (A) in the fasting state and (B) after a lipid-rich meal. The area in the rectangle is shown at higher magnification in Fig. 26–29. (Redrawn after Cardell, R., S. Badenhausen, and K.R. Porter. 1967. J. Cell Biol. 34:123.)

axial lacteal that ends blindly near its tip. The broader villi of the duodenum may contain two or more lacteals that intercommunicate. When distended, their lumen is considerably larger than that of a blood capillary. The wall consists of very thin endothelial cells supported by an argyrophilic reticulum and surrounded by thin longitudinal strands of smooth muscle.

At the base of the villi, the central lacteals join the lymphatic capillaries around the glands and continue downward to form a plexus on the inner surface of the muscularis mucosae. From this plexus, branches provided with valves penetrate the muscularis mucosae and form a second loose plexus of larger lymphatics in the submucosa. These vessels receive tributaries from the dense networks of thin-walled lymphatics that surround the solitary and the aggregated lymphoid follicles.

NERVES OF THE INTESTINAL TRACT

The gastrointestinal tract is innervated by the autonomic nervous system, which consists

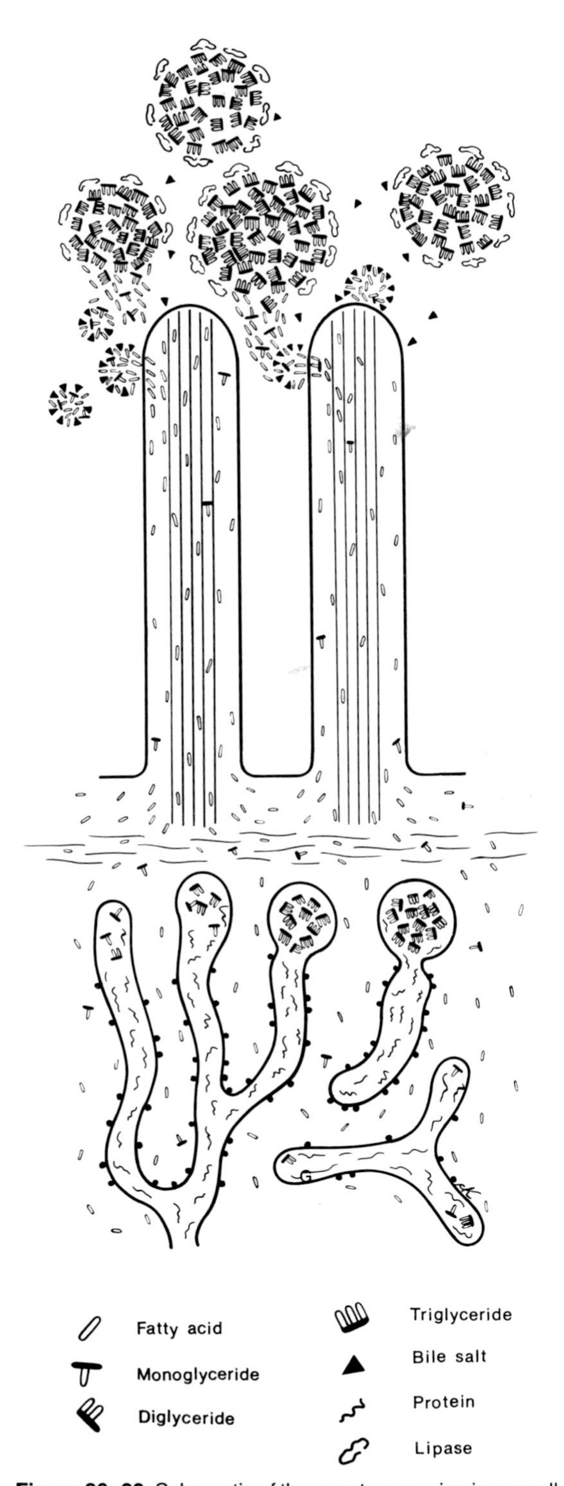

Figure 26–29. Schematic of the events occurring in a small area of the apex of an intestinal absorptive cell (see Fig. 26–28). An emulsion of fine droplets of lipid in the lumen is broken down by pancreatic lipase to fatty acids and monoglycerides. These diffuse into the microvilli and apical cytoplasm where they are esterified to form triglycerides in the smooth endoplasmic reticulum. (Redrawn after Cardell, R., S. Badenhausen, and K.R. Porter. 1967. J. Cell Biol. 34:123.)

of three subdivisions: sympathetic, parasympathetic, and enteric. All three play a role in regulating the activity of the intestines, but the enteric system is the most important. The sympathetic and parasympathetic nerves to the tract are its *extrinsic* nerve supply and exert their influence on digestive function through the *intrinsic* enteric nervous system, which consists of nerve cell bodies and their processes located within the wall of the tract. The extrinsic nerves are preganglionic fibers from the vagus nerve and postganglionic sympathetic fibers that arise mainly in the celiac ganglion. They are distributed to the intestine with the blood vessels via the mesentery. The enteric nervous system consists of ganglia and interconnecting bundles of nerve fibers that form extensive plexuses in various layers of the digestive tract. They extend throughout its length, from the lower esophagus to the internal anal sphincter. The enteric system is estimated to contain from 10^7 to 10^8 neurons, including sensory neurons, interneurons, and motor neurons which form reflex pathways that are intrinsic to the digestive tract. Unlike other subdivisions of the autonomic nervous system, the enteric system is largely autonomous and can carry out many of its functions without input from the central nervous system.

The sympathetic and parasympathetic nerves do have some effect on the digestive tract, but cutting the extrinsic nerves results in surprisingly little impairment of digestive function. If the intestine is detached from the mesentery and immersed in warm physiological salt solution, it will show normal peristaltic movements when the mucosa is stimulated by the introduction of material into the lumen. Thus, intestinal movements are determined by local neuromuscular mechanisms that are only modulated by input through the extrinsic nerves.

The most superficial neural elements in the gut wall form a *subserous plexus* which generally lacks ganglia and is made up of a loose network of fine nerve fibers that connect the extrinsic nerves with the more deeply situated intrinsic nerve plexuses. The majority of the nerves coursing from the mesentery to the deeper enteric plexuses traverse the longitudinal muscle layer near the attachment of the mesentery.

The most conspicuous enteric plexus is found between the longitudinal and circular layers of the muscularis. This *myenteric plexus* (Auerbach's plexus, plexus entericus externa)

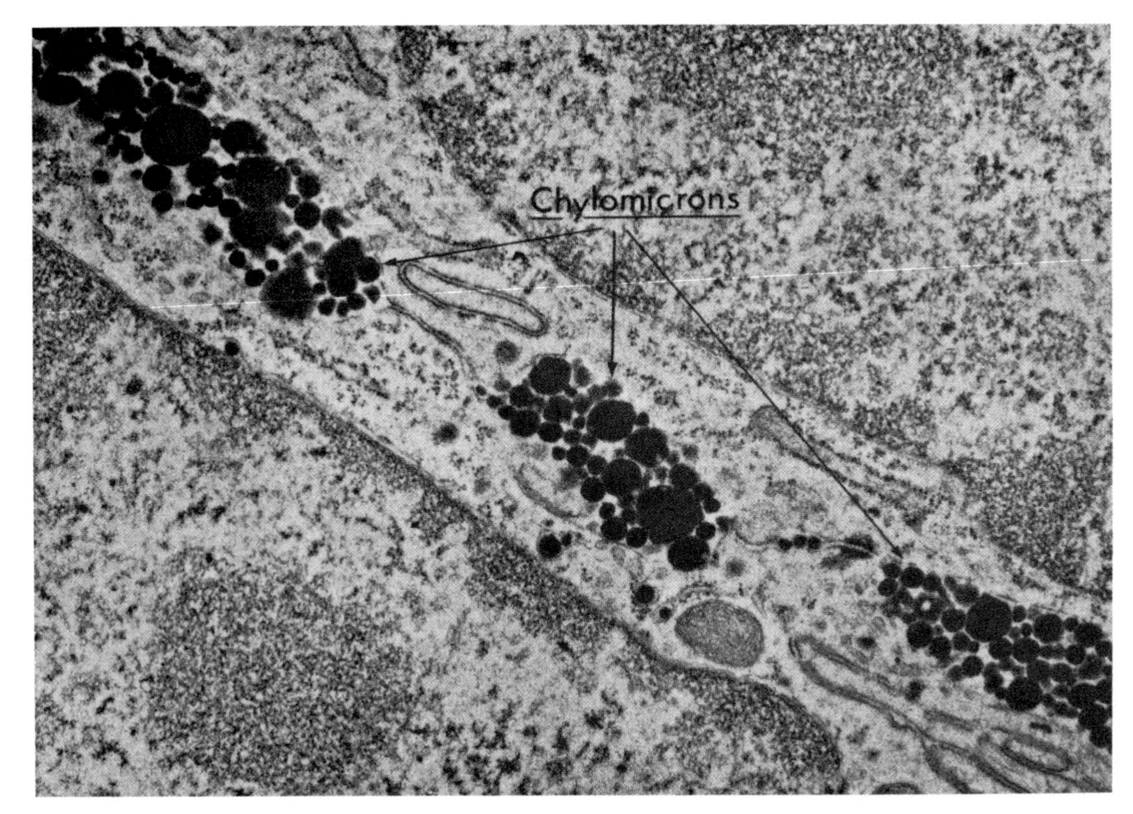

Figure 26–30. Micrograph of portions of two adjacent rat intestinal epithelial cells during lipid absorption. The absorbed lipid has been released at the lateral cell surfaces and is seen here to have accumulated in aggregations of chylomicrons in the intercellular space. (Micrograph courtesy of S.L. Palay and J.P. Revel.)

consists of ganglia containing from 3 to 50 or more nerve cell bodies and bundles of unmyelinated axons that connect the ganglia to form a continuous network (Fig. 26–32). The cells of the ganglia are of two morphological types. One is a multipolar cell with short dendrites in contact with the bodies of similar cells within the same ganglion, whereas the axon can be traced for a considerable distance to sites of synaptic contact with cells of the second type in neighboring ganglia (Fig. 26–33). Cells of the second type are far more numerous and more variable in form. The dendrites are diffuse receptor endings related to cells of the first type, or to the same type, in the same or in other ganglia. The axon enters one of the fiber bundles associated with the ganglion and its fibers terminate in the circular or longitudinal muscle layers. Thus, cells of the first type appear to be associative, whereas those of the second type are motor. A third cell type called the *interstitial cell* has short branching processes that intermingle with those of the other cell type. It does not contain demonstrable neurofibrils and may be a form of glial cell.

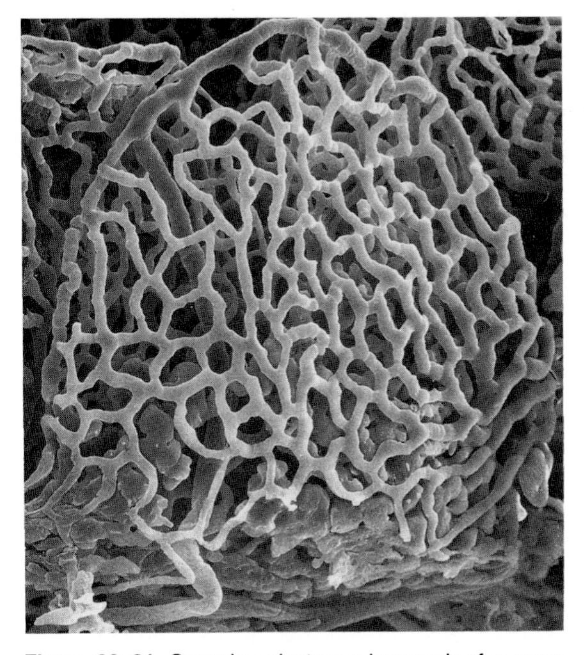

Figure 26–31. Scanning electron micrograph of a corrosion cast of the microcirculation of a rat intestinal villus showing a dense capillary network arising from an arteriole at the margin of the villus. (From Komuro, T. 1990. Cell Tissue Res. 239:183.)

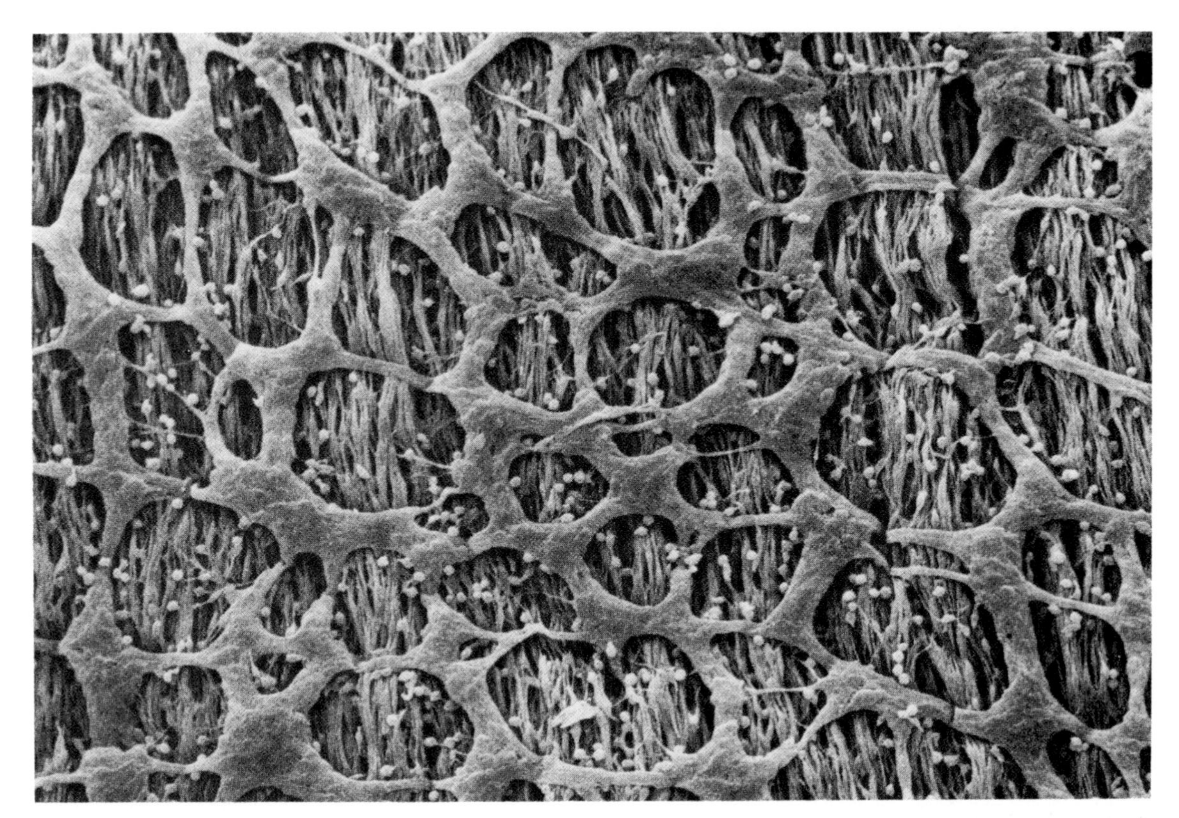

Figure 26–32. Scanning electron micrograph of the myenteric plexus of rat intestine. The overlying longitudinal muscle and connective tissue have been removed by dissection and enzymatic digestion. (Micrograph from Fujiwara, T. and Y. Uehara. 1980. J. Electron Microsc. 29:397.)

Most of the unmyelinated fibers in the ganglia and in the internodal strands of the plexus are processes of enteric neurons. The remainder are axons of extrinsic vagal or sympathetic origin. The vagal fibers terminate as perikaryal arborizations on ganglion cells of the second type. The sympathetic fibers do not seem to have synaptic relationships with the nerve cells of the ganglia but are thought to terminate in the muscularis and on blood vessels.

A *deep muscular plexus* (plexus muscularis profundus) is situated on the mucosal aspect of the circular muscle layer. It is devoid of ganglia and consists of thin anastomosing nerve bundles with their prevailing orientation parallel to the muscle fibers. Branches from this plexus penetrate into the muscle layer and some are connected with the myenteric plexus.

The *submucous plexus* (Meissner's plexus, plexus entericus interna) is a network of ganglia and interconnecting nerve bundles within the connective tissue of the submucosa (Fig. 26–34). Its fibers innervate the muscularis mucosae and smooth muscle fibers in the cores of the intestinal villi. Fibers from the submucous plexus also form a mucosal plexus situated in the lamina propria and sending components between the intestinal glands and into the villi.

Although these several plexuses are distinguished on the basis of their architecture and location in the intestinal wall, they do not function independently. Connections can be traced from the subserous to the myenteric plexus; from the myenteric plexus to the submucous plexus; and from the latter to the mucosal plexus and to paravascular nerves along the submucosal arteries.

Detailed investigation of the "wiring diagram" of the enteric nervous system, using the traditional neuroanatomical methods, is difficult, and our information is far from complete. Recent investigations have focused on histochemical and pharmacological definition

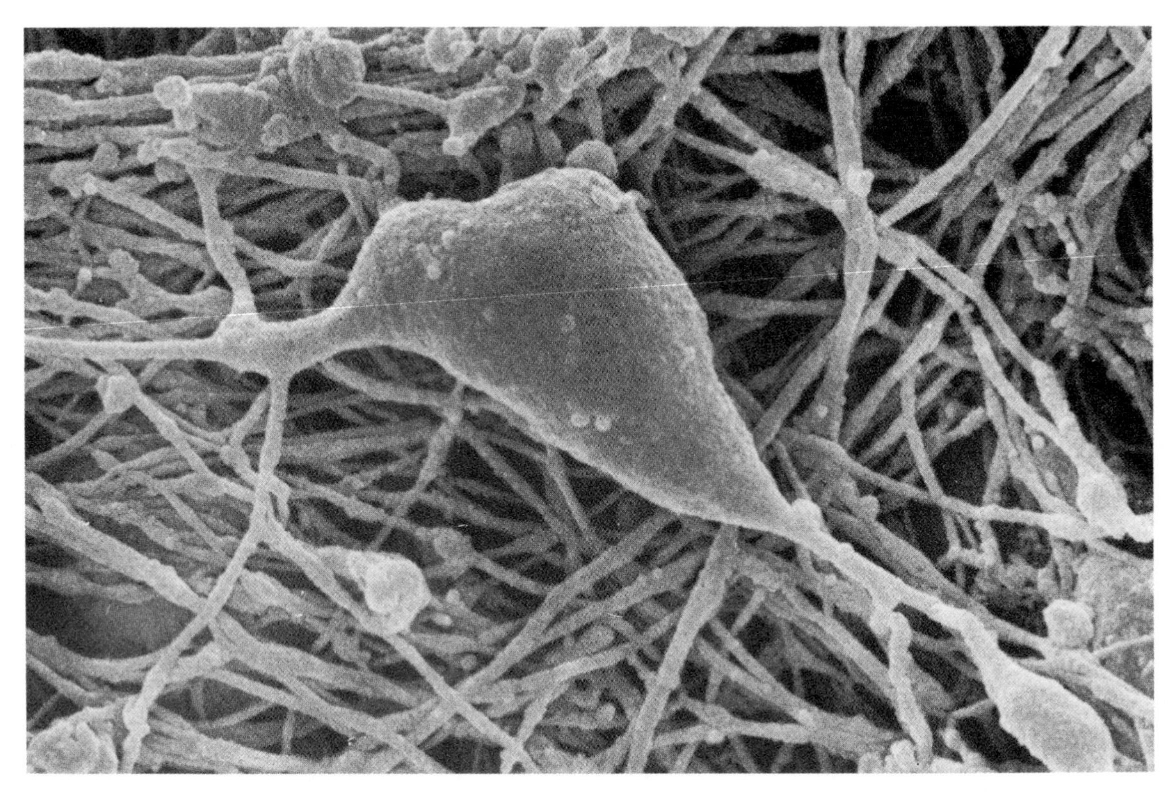

Figure 26–33. Scanning micrograph of a multipolar neurone in the myenteric plexus of a newborn rat. (Micrograph courtesy of T. Fujiwara and Y. Uehara.)

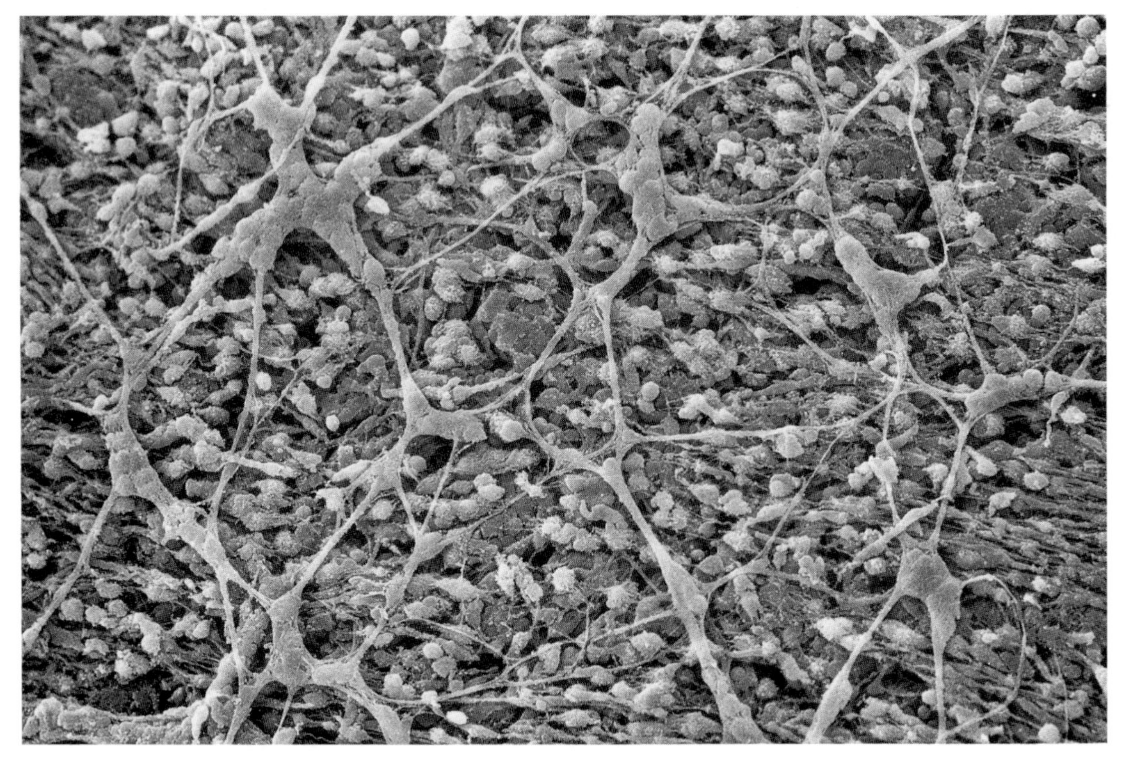

Figure 26–34. Scanning electron micrograph of the submucous nerve plexus of rat intestine showing small ganglia connected by slender strands of nerve fibers. (Micrograph from Komuro, T. and Y. Hashimoto. 1990. Cell Tissue Res. 239:183.)

of cell types on the basis of the neurotransmitters and neuromodulators that mediate their functions, and it is evident that there are many more functionally distinct cell types than have been identified to date on the basis of purely morphological criteria.

Cholinergic neurons in the intestine are the only intrinsic nerves for which both the transmitter and the functions are known. The cholinergic neurons of the enteric plexuses supply both longitudinal and circular muscle and are of prime importance in the peristaltic reflex. Another class of neurons is responsible for relaxation of intestinal smooth muscle. These are noncholinergic and nonadrenergic inhibitory neurons. The nature of their transmitter is a subject of debate. Some investigators insist that they release adenosine-5-triphosphate and refer to them as *purinergic neurons*. Others favor a *vasoactive intestinal polypeptide* as the more likely transmitter. These enteric nerves are believed to be responsible for inhibitory reflexes that relax smooth muscle in advance of a wave of peristaltic contraction, thus facilitating passage of the intestinal contents along the tract.

The presence of other excitatory and inhibitory nerves has been postulated on the basis of neurophysiological and pharmacological experiments, but their location in the enteric plexuses and the nature of their transmitters have yet to be established. Recent immunohistochemical studies have localized a variety of biologically active peptides in nerve cells of the enteric plexus. These include *substance-P, somatostatin, enkephalins, vasoactive intestinal polypeptide, bombesin,* and *neurotensin*. It is not known whether these serve as neurotransmitters or as neuromodulators.

BIBLIOGRAPHY

ABSORPTIVE CELLS

Bretscher, A. and K. Weber. 1978. Localization of actin and microfilament associated proteins in the microvilli and terminal web of the intestinal brush border by immunofluorescence microscopy. J. Cell Biol. 79:839.

Brunser, O. and J. Luft. 1970. Fine structure of the apex of absorptive cells from rat small intestine. J. Ultrastr. Res. 31:291.

Coluccio, L.M. and A. Bretscher. 1989. Reassociation of microvillar core proteins: Making a microvillar core in vitro. J. Cell Biol. 108:495.

Drenckhahn, D. and R. Dermietzel. 1988. Organization of the actin filament cytoskeleton in intestinal brush border: a quantitative and qualitative immunoelectron microscope study. J. Cell. Biol. 107:1037.

Ito, S. 1974. Form and function of the glycocalyx on free cell surfaces. Trans. R. Soc. London (Biol.) 268:55.

Komura, T. and Y. Hashimoto. 1990. Three dimensional structure of rat intestinal wall (mucosa and submucosa). Arch. Histol. Cytol. 53:1.

Madara, J.L., J.S. Trier, and M.R. Neutra. 1980. Structural changes in the plasma membrane accompanying differentiation of epithelial cells in human and monkey small intestine, Gastroenterology 78:963.

McNeil, P.L. and S. Ito. 1989. Gastrointestinal plasma membrane wounding and resealing in vivo. Gastroentrology 96:1238.

Mooseker, M.S. 1983. Actin binding proteins of the brush border. Cell 35:11.

Mooseker, M.S. 1985. Organization, chemistry, and assembly of the cytoskeletal apparatus of the intestinal brush border. Annu. Rev. Cell Biol. 1:209.

Trier, J.S. 1963. Studies on small intestine crypt epithelium. I. The fine structure of the crypt epithelium of the proximal small intestine of fasting humans. J. Cell Biol. 18:599.

GOBLET CELLS

Berlin, J.D. 1967. The localization of acid mucopolysaccharides in the Golgi complex of intestinal goblet cells. J. Cell Biol. 32:760.

Freeman, J.A. 1966. Goblet cell fine structure. Anat. Rec. 154:121.

Hollman, K. 1963. The fine structure of the goblet cells in the rat intestine. Ann. N.Y. Acad. Sci. 106:545.

Neutra, M.R. and J.F. Forstner. 1987. Gastrointestinal mucus: Synthesis, secretion, and function. *In* L.R. Johnson, ed. Physiology of the Gastrointestinal tract, 2nd ed., p. 875. New York, Raven Press.

Sandoz, D., G. Nicolas, and M.C. Lane. 1985. Two mucous cell types revisited after quick freezing and cryosubstitution. Biol. Cell 54:79.

PANETH CELLS

Benke, O. and H. Moe. 1964. An electron microscopic study of mature and differentiating Paneth cells in the rat. J. Cell Biol. 22:633.

Erlandsen, S.L., J.A. Parsons, and T.D. Taylor. 1974. Ultrastructural immunocytochemical localization of lysozme in the Paneth cells of man. J. Histchem. Cytochem. 22:401.

Erlandsen, S.L. and D.G. Chase. 1972. Paneth cell function: phagocytosis and intracellular digestion of microorganisms. J. Ultrastr. Res. 41:296.

Erlandsen, S.L., C.B. Rodning, C. Montero, J.A. Parsons, C.A. Lewis, and I.D. Wilson. 1976. Immunocytochemical identification and localization of immunoglobulin-A within Paneth cells of the rat small intestine. J. Histochem. Cytochem. 24:1085.

Rodning, C.B., S.L. Erlandsen, I.D. Wilson, and A.M. Carpenter. 1982. Light microscopic morphometric analysis of rat ileal, mucosa. II. Component quantitation of Paneth cells. Anat. Rec. 204:33.

ENTEROENDOCRINE CELLS

Fujita, T.S. and S. Kobayashi. 1977. The structure and function of gut endocrine cells. Internat. Rev. Cytol. (Suppl.) 6:187.

Grube, D. and W.G. Forssmann. 1979. Morphology and

function of the enteroendocrine cells. Horm. Metabol. Res. 11:603.

Helmstaedter, V., G.E. Feurle, and W.G. Forssmann. 1977. Ultrastructural identification of a new cell type—The N-cell as the source of neurotensin in the gut mucosa. Cell Tissue Res. 184:445.

Johnson, L.R. 1976. The trophic action of gastrointestinal hormones. Gastroenterology 70:278.

Pearce, A.G.E., J.M. Polak, and S.R. Bloom. 1977. The newer gut hormones. Cellular sources, physiology, pathology, and clinical aspects. Gastroenterology 72:746.

Sjolund, K., G. Sanden, R. Hakanson, and F. Sundler. 1983. Endocrine cells in the human intestine: An immunocytochemical study. Gastroenterology 85:1120.

INTESTINAL IMMUNE SYSTEM

Brandtzaeg, P., and K. Baklein. 1977. Intestinal secretion of Ig-A and Ig-G: a hypothetical model. *In* Immunology of the Gut, Ciba Foundation Symposium 46, p. 77. Amsterdam, Elsevier.

Bye, W.A., C.H. Allan, and J.S. Trier. 1984. Structure distribution and origin of M-cells in Peyer's patches of mouse. Gastroenterology 86:789.

Hashimoto, Y. and T. Komuro. 1988. Close relationship of cells of the immune system with the epithelial cells in rat small intestine. Cell Tissue Res. 254:41.

Neutra, M.R., T.R. Phillips, E.L. Mayer, and D. Fishkind. 1987. Transport of membrane bound macromolecules by M-cells in follicle associated epithelium of rabbit Peyer's patch. Cell Tissue Res. 247:537.

Owen, R.L. and A.L. Jones. 1974. Epithelial cell specialization with human Peyer's patches: an ultrastructural study of intestinal lymphoid follicles. Gastroenterology 66:189.

Walker, W.A. and K.J. Isselbacher. 1977. Intestinal antibodies. N. Eng. J. Med. 297:767.

SUBMUCOSAL GLANDS OF BRUNNER

Friend, D.S. 1965. The fine structure of Brunner's glands in the mouse. J. Cell Biol. 25:563.

Marti, U., J.J. Burwen, and A.L. Jones. 1989. Biological effects of epidermal growth factor, with emphasis on the gastrointestinal tract and liver. Hepatology 9:126.

Moe, H. 1960. The ultrastructure of Brunner's glands of the cat. J. Ultrastr. Res. 4:58.

Skov, Olsen, P., S.S. Poulsen et al. 1985. Exocrine secretion of epidermal growth factor from Brunner's glands. Stimulation by VIP and acetylcholine. Regul. Pept. 7:367.

INTESTINAL ABSORPTION

Cardel, R.R., S. Badenhausen, and K.R. Porter. 1967. Intestinal absorption in the rat. An electron microscopic study. J. Cell Biol. 34:23.

Crane, R.K. 1962. Hypothesis for mechanism of intestinal active transport of sugars. Fed. Proc. 21:891.

Hauri, H.P., E.E. Sterchi, D. Bienz, J.A. Fransen, and A. Marxer. 1985. Expression and intracellular transport of microvillus membrane hydrolases in the human intestinal epithelial cells. J. Cell Biol. 101:838.

Ockner, R.K. and K.J. Isselbacher. 1974. Recent concepts of intestinal fat absorption. Rev. Physiol. Biochem. Pharmacol. 71:107.

Palay, S.L. and L.J. Karlin. 1959. An electron microscopic study of the intestinal villus. I. The fasting animal. II. The pathway of fat absorption. J. Biophys. Biochem. Cytol. 5:363, 373.

Strauss, E.W. 1966. Electron microscopic study of intestinal fat absorption from mixed micelles containing linolenic acid, monoolein, and bile salt. J. Lipid Res. 7:307.

CELL TURNOVER AND RENEWAL

Chang, W.W. and C.P. Leblond. 1971. Renewal of the epithelium in the descending colon of the mouse. Parts I, II, and III. Am. J. Anat. 131:73, 101, 111.

Cheng, H. and C.P. Leblond. 1974. Origin, differentiation and renewal of the four main epithelial cell types in the mouse small intestine. Parts I to IV. Am. J. Anat. 141:461.

Eastwood, G.L. 1977. Gastrointestinal epithelial renewal. Gastroenterology 72:962.

Leblond, C.P. 1981. Life history of cells in renewing systems. Am. J. Anat. 160:113.

Leblond, C.P. and B. Messier. 1958. Renewal of chief cells and goblet cells in the small intestine as shown by radioautography after injection of thymidine-H^3 into mice. Anat. Rec. 132:247.

Lipkin, M. 1965. Cell replication in the gastrointestinal tract of man. Gastroenterology 48:616.

Parker, F.G., E.N. Barnes, and G.I. Kaye. 1974. The pericryptal fibroblast sheath. IV. Replication, migration, and differentiation of the subepithelial fibroblasts of the crypts and villus of the rabbit jejunum. Gastroenterology 67:607.

Tsubouchi, S. and C.P. Leblond. 1979. Migration and turnover of the enteroendocrine cells in the epithelium of the descending colon, as shown by radioautography after continuous infusion of ^{3}H-thymidine into mice. Am. J. Anat. 156:431.

LARGE INTESTINE

Essner, E., J. Schreiber, and R.A. Griewski. 1978. Localization of carbohydrate components in rat colon with fluoreceinated lectins. J. Histochem. Cytochem. 26:452.

Garry, R.C. 1934. The movements of the large intestine. Physiol. Rev. 14:103.

Kaye, G.I., N. Lane, and R.R. Pascal. 1968. Colonic pericryptal fibroblast sheath. Replication, migration, and differentiation, of a mesenchymal cell system in the adult. II. Fine structural aspects of normal rabbit and human colon. Gastroenterology 54:852.

Lineback, P.E. 1925. Studies on the musculature of the human colon, with special reference to the taeniea. Am. J. Anat. 36:357.

Loenzonn, V. and J.S. Trier. 1968. The fine structure of the human rectal mucosa. The epithelial lining at the base of the crypt. Gastroenterology 55:88.

Martin, B.F. 1961. The goblet cell pattern of the large intestine. Anat. Rec. 140:1.

Neutra, M.R., R.J. Grand, and J.S. Trier. 1977. Glycoprotein synthesis, transport, and secretion by epithelial cells of the human rectal mucosa: normal and cystic fibrosis. Lab. Investig. 36:535.

INNERVATION

Burnstock, G. 1972. Purinergic nerves. Pharmacol. Rev. 24:509.

Fujiwara, T. and Y. Uehara. 1980. Scanning electron microscopy of the myenteric plexus: a preliminary communication. J. Electron Microsc. 29:397.

Furbess, J.B. and M. Costa. 1980. Types of nerves in the enteric nervous system. Neuroiscience 5:1.

Richardson, K.C. 1958. Electron microscopic observations on Auerbach's plexus in the rabbit with special reference to the problem of smooth muscle innervation. Am. J. Anat. 103:99.

Richardson, K.C. 1958. Studies on the structure of the autonomic nerves in the small intestine correlating the silver impregnated image in light microscopy with the permanganate-fixed ultrastructure in electron microscopy. J. Anat. (London) 94:457.

27
THE LIVER AND GALLBLADDER

LIVER

The liver is an accessory gland of the gastrointestinal tract but it has a remarkable diversity of other functions unrelated to alimentation. It is the largest gland in the body, weighing about 1500 g in the adult. It is situated in the right upper quadrant of the abdominal cavity with its rounded upper surface conforming to the dome of the diaphragm. Its thin investment of connective tissue, *Glisson's capsule,* is covered over most of its surface by peritoneal mesothelium. On its under side, blood vessels enter, and the right and left *hepatic ducts* leave the organ at its *hilum,* also called the *porta hepatis.*

The liver has an indispensable role in the metabolism of absorbed nutrients that depends on its unique relationship to the two major subdivisions of the vascular system. It has a dual blood supply, receiving well-oxygenated blood from the general circulation via the *hepatic artery* (25%) and a larger volume of poorly oxygenated blood coming from the intestinal tract via the *portal vein* (75%). Blood from these two sources mingles in the hepatic sinusoids, where its solutes have direct access to the hepatic cells. The blood leaving the organ is carried via the hepatic veins to the inferior vena cava. Thus, interposed between the intestinal tract and the general circulation, the liver receives absorbed nutrients and stores or degrades them to smaller molecules that are released into the systemic circulation for distribution to the other tissues and organs of the body.

The liver continuously produces *bile,* a fluid that is ultimately secreted into the duodenum via the *common bile duct.* As much as 1 liter is produced daily, but the greater portion is diverted to the gall bladder where it is concentrated up to 10-fold and stored until released in response to the ingestion of food. Bile facilitates digestion by emulsifying dietary fats and reducing them to micelles that are more readily absorbed by the intestinal epithelium. In addition to its exocrine function, the liver synthesizes plasma proteins and delivers them directly into the blood. It also exercises considerable control over the general metabolism of the body through its ability to store carbohydrate in the form of glycogen and to release glucose as needed to maintain the normal concentration of this important energy source in the blood. The liver also takes up drugs and other potentially harmful substances absorbed by the intestines and degrades them by oxidation or forms harmless conjugates that are excreted back into the intestines in the bile.

ORGANIZATION OF THE LIVER

The majority of exocrine glands are partitioned by connective tissue into distinct lobes and smaller lobules, and their parenchyma is made up of groups of epithelial cells forming bulbous acini at the ends of a branching system of ducts. The liver is quite different, in that there is little connective tissue in its interior. Its epithelium presents a remarkably uniform appearance throughout the organ and structural subunits are not easily identifiable. It is possible, however, to detect a repeating pattern of roughly hexagonal areas, in which fenestrated plates of parenchymal cells are arranged radially around a central vein (Fig. 27–1). At three corners of these polygonal areas there is a small triangular area of connective tissue enclosing a small bile duct, a branch of the hepatic artery, and a branch of the portal vein. This complex is referred to as the *portal triad* or *portal area* (Figs. 27–2 and 27–3). Lateral branches of these vessels, occurring at short intervals along their length,

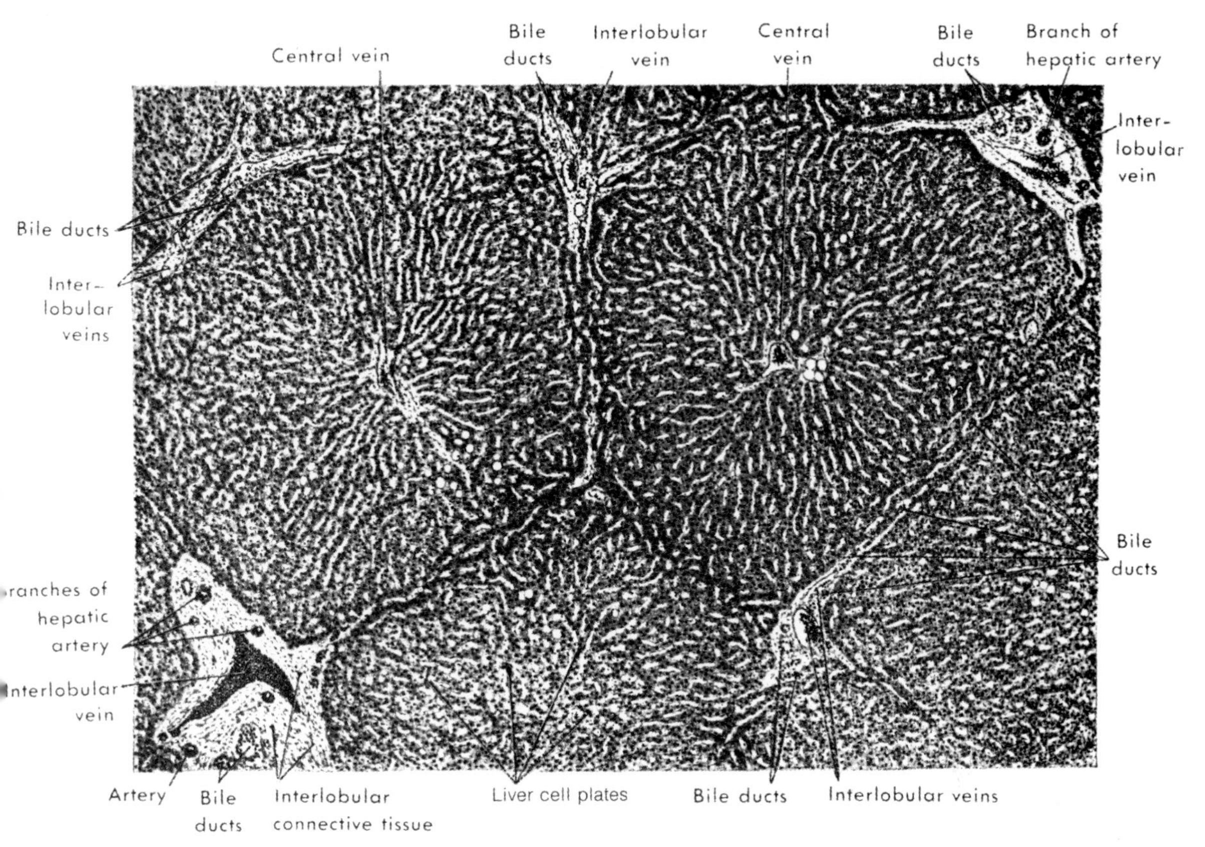

Figure 27–1. Portion of a histological section of the liver of a 22-year-old man showing the radiating pattern cell plates in two classical liver lobules and portions of other lobules. (After J. Sobotta. Atlas of Human Anatomy. Vol. II. G.E. Stechert & Co. New York, 1936.)

are confluent with thin-walled *hepatic sinusoids* that occupy the spaces between the radially arranged trabeculae and drain into the central vein. The fenestrated plates of hepatic cells are, thus, exposed to a large volume of blood flowing centripetally in the labyrinthine system of sinusoids. Bile is continuously secreted into a network of intercellular *bile canaliculi* within the cell plates and flows outward to bile ductules in the portal areas at the periphery. This polygonal unit, about 0.7 mm in diameter and 2 mm long, was called the hepatic lobule and for a century or more was considered to be the structural and functional unit of the liver. It is now commonly referred to as the *classical lobule* to distinguish it from other subunits described in more recent interpretations of liver architecture.

Around the turn of the century, an alternative interpretation of liver organization was proposed. In this, the liver lobule was considered to consist of the mass of parenchyma around each portal area, including all of those cells secreting into its bile ductule. This structural unit was called the *portal lobule.* In section, it is roughly triangular in shape and includes sectors of three neighboring classical lobules. Its proponents argued that it is more consistent with the organization of other glands, in having a blood supply radiating from axial vessels and its secretory product draining to a central duct, but it has not been widely accepted. Since the 1950s, the majority of investigators have preferred the *hepatic acinus* as the structural and functional unit of the liver. This is a roughly ovoid mass of parenchymal cells around each terminal arteriole, venule, and bile duct that branch laterally from the portal area. At either end of the acinus is a vessel that was called the central vein in the classical lobule but is now referred to as the *terminal hepatic venule* in reference to the acinus. The acinus is a smaller unit including a sector of two neighboring classical lobules (Fig. 27–4).

The classical lobule, portal lobule, and the acinus are not conflicting interpretations but alternative ways of visualizing its organization.

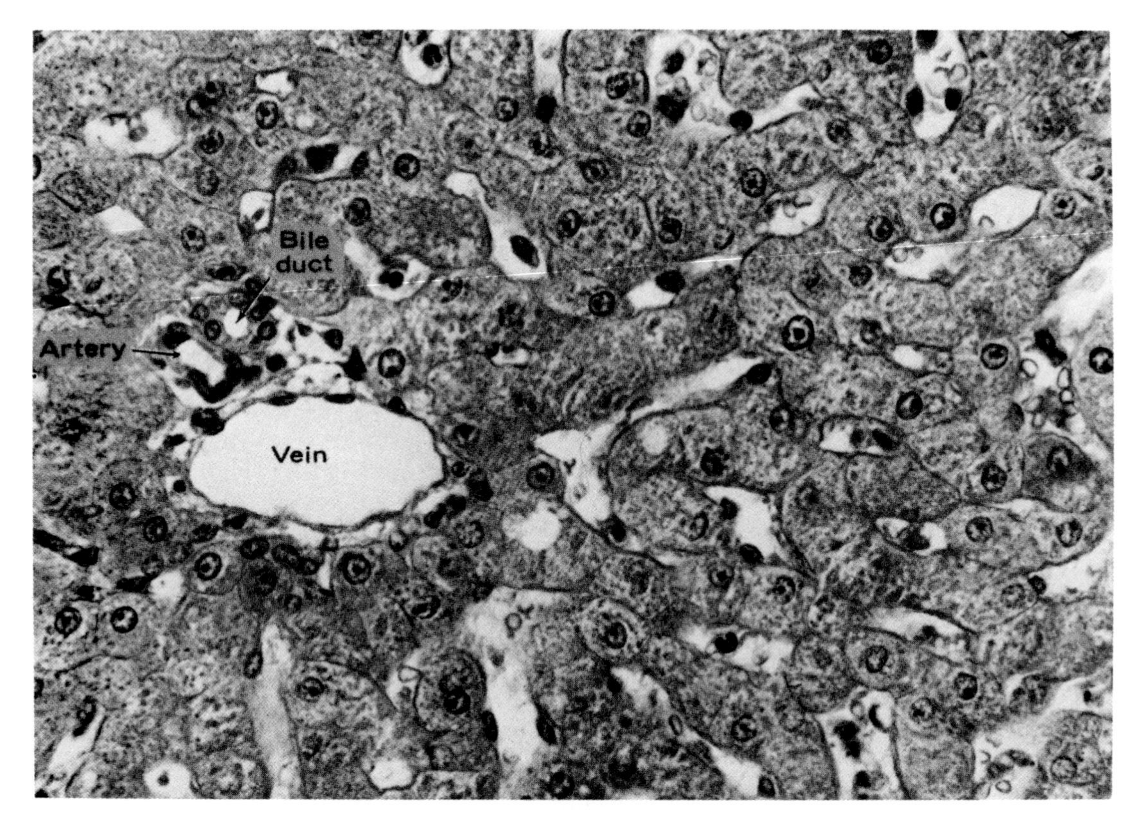

Figure 27–2. Photomicrograph of a peripheral portion of two traditional liver lobules showing a typical portal triad, consisting of branches of the hepatic artery, the portal vein and a small bile duct.

The acinus was adopted, in part, because it facilitated explanation of the pattern of cell degeneration seen in hypoxic and toxic damage to the liver, and it has become the basis for most contemporary considerations of liver function. However, the interpretation of the classical polygonal lobule as the true anatomical subunit derives support from the observation that this unit is clearly demarcated by connective tissue septa in the liver of pig, camel, bear, and raccoon. Although the basic architecture of the liver, in these species, conforms to the classical concept of polygonal lobules with a hexagonal cross section, pentagonal cross sections are common, and reconstruction from serial sections has shown that neighboring units are often continuous at their base to form compound lobules.

BLOOD SUPPLY

To understand the physiology of the liver, it is essential to understand some unusual features of its blood supply. As previously stated, the processing and metabolism of absorbed nutrients depends on the unique position of the liver between the portal vascular system and the general circulation. Its principal afferent blood supply is via the *portal vein* which carries poorly oxygenated blood that has already circulated through the intestine, the pancreas, and the spleen. Entering the porta hepatic, it divides into *interlobal veins* and these, in turn, divide into *conducting veins* that are about 400 μm in diameter and have thinner walls than vessels of comparable size elsewhere in the body. Their branching gives rise to *interlobular veins*. Smaller veins arising from these are 280 μm in diameter and very thin walled. These, accompanied by a branch of the hepatic artery and a bile ductule, are components of the portal triads or portal areas that course parallel to the *central vein* at the corners of the classical lobules. Small lateral branches of these, called *terminal portal venules* or *perilobular venules,* given off at short intervals along their length, course along the boundaries between classical lobules and give off short *inlet venules* that empty into the sinusoids.

On entering the porta hepatis, the *hepatic*

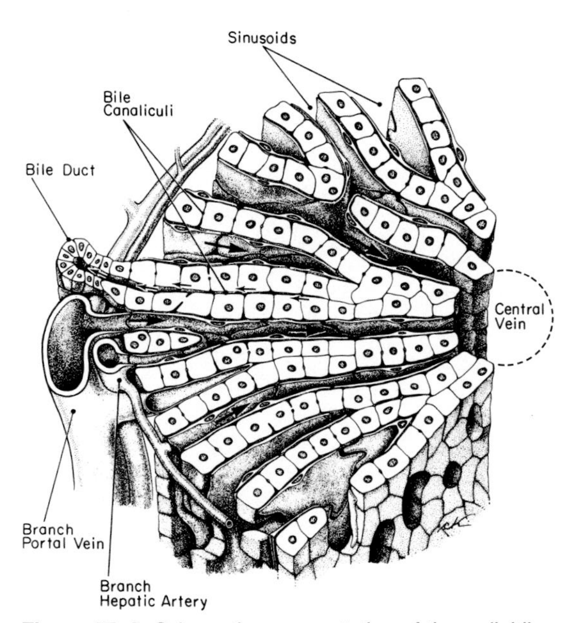

Figure 27–3. Schematic representation of the radial liver cell plates around the central vein (terminal hepatic venule), the centripetal flow of blood from branches of the hepatic artery and vein and the centrifugal flow of bile (small arrows). (Redrawn and modified from Ham, A.W. 1965. Textbook of Histology, 5th ed. Philadelphia, J.B. Lippincott Co.)

artery branches into *interlobar* and *interlobular arteries*. The bulk of the flow in these vessels is distributed to capillaries of the connective tissue stroma of the organ, but a smaller volume continues into the *hepatic arterioles* of the portal triads. These give off lateral branches emptying into the sinusoids and numerous small branches to a dense network of capillaries that surround the bile ductule (Fig. 27–5). This *peribiliary* or *periductal plexus* was formerly thought to drain into the portal venules, but scanning micrographs of vascular casts have now clearly shown that the efferent vessels of the plexus empty into the sinusoids (Fig. 27–6). Thus, much of the arterial blood reaches the sinusoids indirectly via the peribiliary plexus. This rich vascularity of the smallest bile ducts suggests the possibility that some constituents of the bile may be reabsorbed in their passage through the intrahepatic bile ducts.

The primary function of the hepatic circulation is carried out in the sinusoids that form an elaborate three-dimensional plexus within the lobules, presenting an enormous surface area for exchange of metabolites between the blood and the hepatic parenchyma. Every cell in the radially arranged cellular trabeculae is

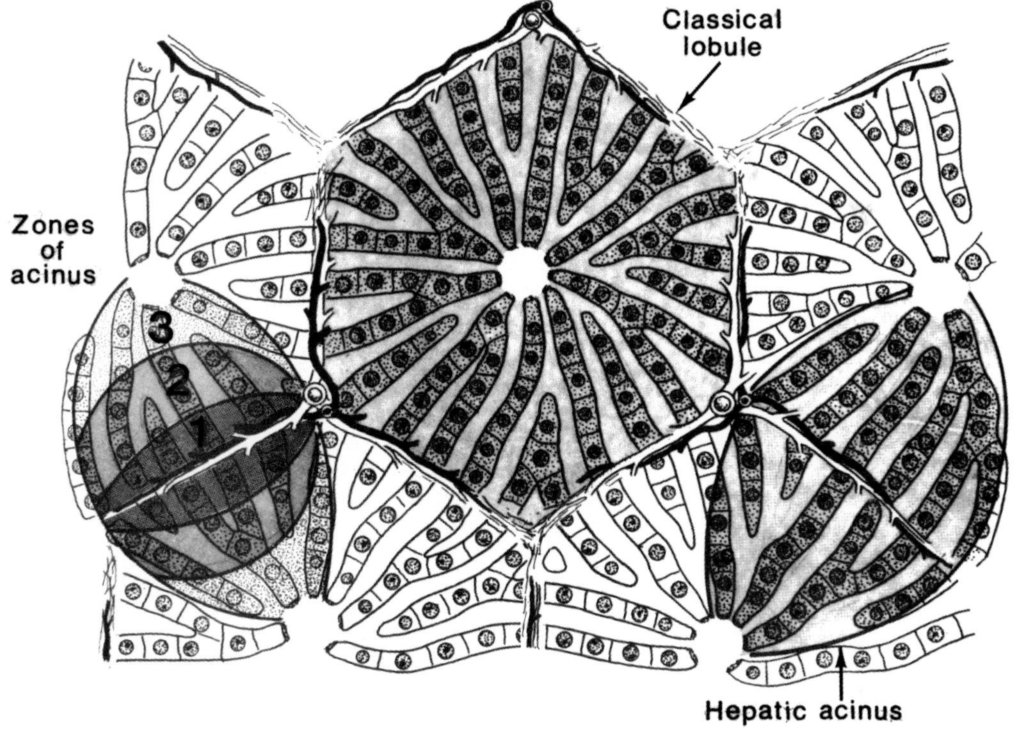

Figure 27–4. Schematic depiction of the classical polygonal lobule and the ellipsoidal hepatic acinus. At the left, three zones are designated, indicating the relative position of the cells in the acinus with respect to a gradient in oxygen concentration of blood flowing from branches of the hepatic artery and portal vein.

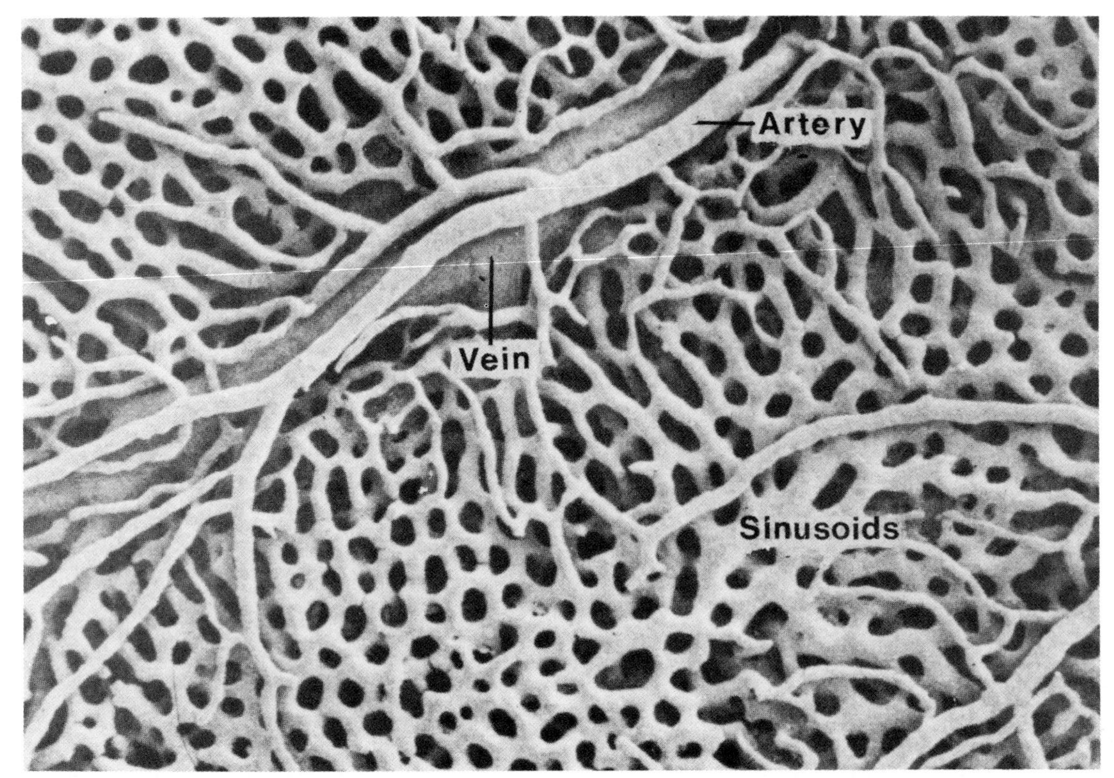

Figure 27–5. Scanning micrograph of a vascular cast of monkey liver from which the cells have been digested away. Crossing the figure diagonally are a terminal branch of the hepatic artery and portal venule supplying an extraordinarily rich network of hepatic sinusoids. (Micrograph by T. Murikami, from Johari, O. and I. Corvin, eds. Scanning Electron Microscopy 1978, Part II. Chicago, SEM Inc. AMF O'Hare, 1978.)

exposed on at least one, and usually on two, sides to blood flowing through the sinusoids. Vascular casts viewed with the scanning microscope reveal the richness of the vascularity of the hepatic parenchyma. Blood leaves the sinusoids through numerous openings in the thin wall of the central vein (terminal branch of the hepatic vein) (Fig. 27–7) and continues into *sublobular veins* and then to *collecting veins.* The numerous collecting veins converge to give rise to two or more large *hepatic veins* that emerge from the porta hepatic and join the inferior vena cava.

Hepatic Sinusoids

The hepatic sinusoids are wider than capillaries and their walls conform to the surface of the plates of hepatocytes on either side but are separated from them by a narrow space. The boundaries of the endothelial cells do not blacken with silver nitrate as those of capillaries do. This led investigators to suggest that the endothelium was a syncytium. However, later studies with the electron microscope established that the wall is made up of individual endothelial cells. Physiological studies on the rate of clearance of solutes from the blood during its passage through the liver and observations on the size of colloidal particles that pass through the wall of the sinusoids suggested that there were discontinuities in the wall that permitted direct access of blood plasma to the hepatic cells. This has been confirmed in electron micrographs which show that the endothelial cells have typical overlapping cell junctions in some areas, but in other areas, the thin margins of cells may be separated by 0.1–0.5 μm. In addition, the thin peripheral portions of the cells have fenestrations that are more variable in size and shape than the pores in the endothelium of fenestrated capillaries elsewhere in the body. These fenestrae often occur in groups that have been called "sieve-plates" (Fig. 27–8). Thus, the wall of the sinusoids have both discontinuities between cells and transcellular fenestrations.

There are significant interspecific differences in the sinusoidal endothelium. In sheep, goats, and calves, the sinusoidal endothelium

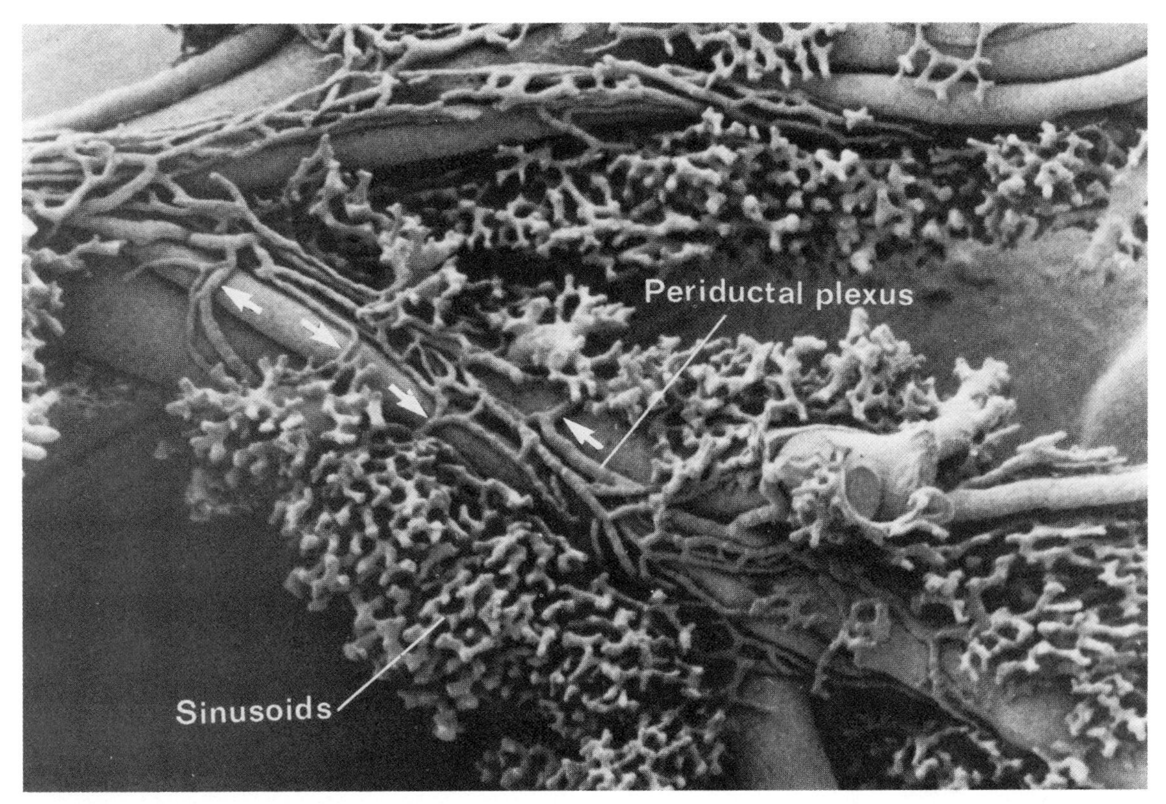

Figure 27–6. Scanning micrograph of a methacrylate cast of the blood vessels forming a plexus around the small bile ducts. Blood from the periductal plexus flows into the sinusoids (at arrows). The sinusoids are only partially filled with plastic in this specimen. (From Murikami, T. 1974. Arch. Histol. Japan 37:245.)

is reported to have a distinct basal lamina and relatively few fenestrations. In rats, a basal lamina is lacking and there is, therefore, no significant barrier to passage of particulate tracers through the openings in the wall of the sinusoids. In as short a time as 30 s after injection of colloidal thorium dioxide into the portal vein, the electron-dense particles can be found between the wall of the sinusoids and the surface of the hepatic cells.

Kupffer Cells

In 1898, von Kupffer observed stellate cells in the hepatic sinusoids that could be selectively stained with gold chloride. They were depicted with processes crossing the lumen and were thought to lie within the sinusoid but fixed to its endothelium. These Kupffer cells frequently contained engulfed erythrocytes and deposits of iron-containing pigment. They actively took up Trypan blue and other particulates injected into the bloodstream (Fig. 27–9). Some later investigators thought they could recognize intermediates between endothelial cells and Kupffer cells and there was disagreement as to whether endothelial cells and Kupffer cells were separate cell types or different functional states of a single cell type. We now know that they are distinct cell types, having different origins and functions.

Repeated injection of particulates into the blood leads to an increase in the number of these phagocytic cells. Their ability to undergo mitotic division is demonstrated by their uptake of tritiated thymidine, under these conditions. Their numbers are also increased by recruitment of precursors from the blood and their differentiation into Kupffer cells. If bone marrow cells bearing a chromosomal marker are injected into an animal that has been irradiated to prevent division of its own cells, Kupffer cells in the liver of the recipient can later be shown to have originated from the donor marrow cells. Like the sessile macrophages in other organs, Kupffer cells are derived from circulating monocytes and are members of the body's mononuclear phagocyte system.

Kupffer cells are situated on the surface of

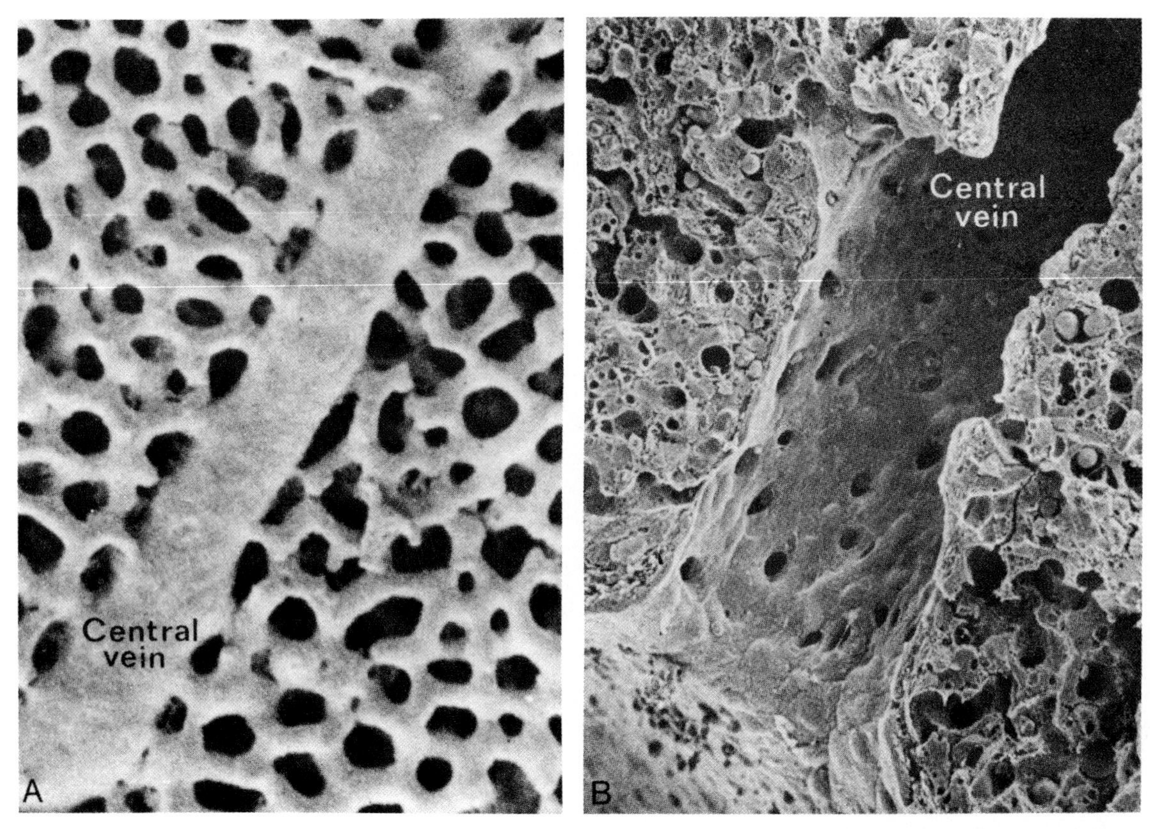

Figure 27–7. (A) Scanning micrograph of a plastic cast of the central portion of a classical lobule showing the confluence of the hepatic sinusoids with the central vein. (B) A comparable scanning micrograph of this region of a lobule cut longitudinally through the central vein showing numerous openings of the sinusoids into its lumen. (A) Courtesy of T. Murikami. (B) From Mota, P.M., M. Muto, and T. Fujita. 1978. The Liver. Tokyo, Igaku Schoin.)

the endothelial cells with processes extending into the lumen and between the underlying endothelial cells. They do not form desmosomes or other specializations for cell-to-cell attachment, and their variable form and relationship to the endothelium suggests that their location may continually change. Electron micrographs show that they have slender villi and undulant lamellipodia projecting from the surface exposed to the blood. Narrow invaginations of the plasmalemma extend into the cytoplasm. These form sinuous *vermiform bodies* consisting of two parallel membranes with a dense line between them and faint transverse striations. This structure is occasionally seen in macrophages in other organs. Its functional significance is unknown.

The Kupffer cell has a small juxtanuclear Golgi complex and numerous mitochondria. There are short profiles of endoplasmic reticulum that can be stained with the histochemical method for peroxidase. This reaction serves to distinguish Kupffer calls from endothelial cells which lack this enzyme. The cytoplasm is crowded with clear vacuoles, phagosomes, lysosomes, and lipochrome pigment deposits (Fig. 27–10). The Kupffer cells are able to recognize and phagocytize effete and damaged erythrocytes and they clear the blood of colon bacilli that manage to get into the portal blood during its circulation through the intestines.

Perisinusoidal Space

In early studies of the human postmortem liver, a narrow space was observed between the sinusoids and the parenchymal cells. This was called the *perisinusoidal space* (*space of Disse*). Such a space was not apparent in biopsies of human liver or in the liver of laboratory animals, and it was dismissed, by many, as a postmortem artifact. However, its reality has now been firmly established by electron microscopy. The endothelium rests lightly on the tips of numerous irregularly oriented hepatocyte microvilli that project into a narrow perisinusoidal space (Fig. 27–11). Slender

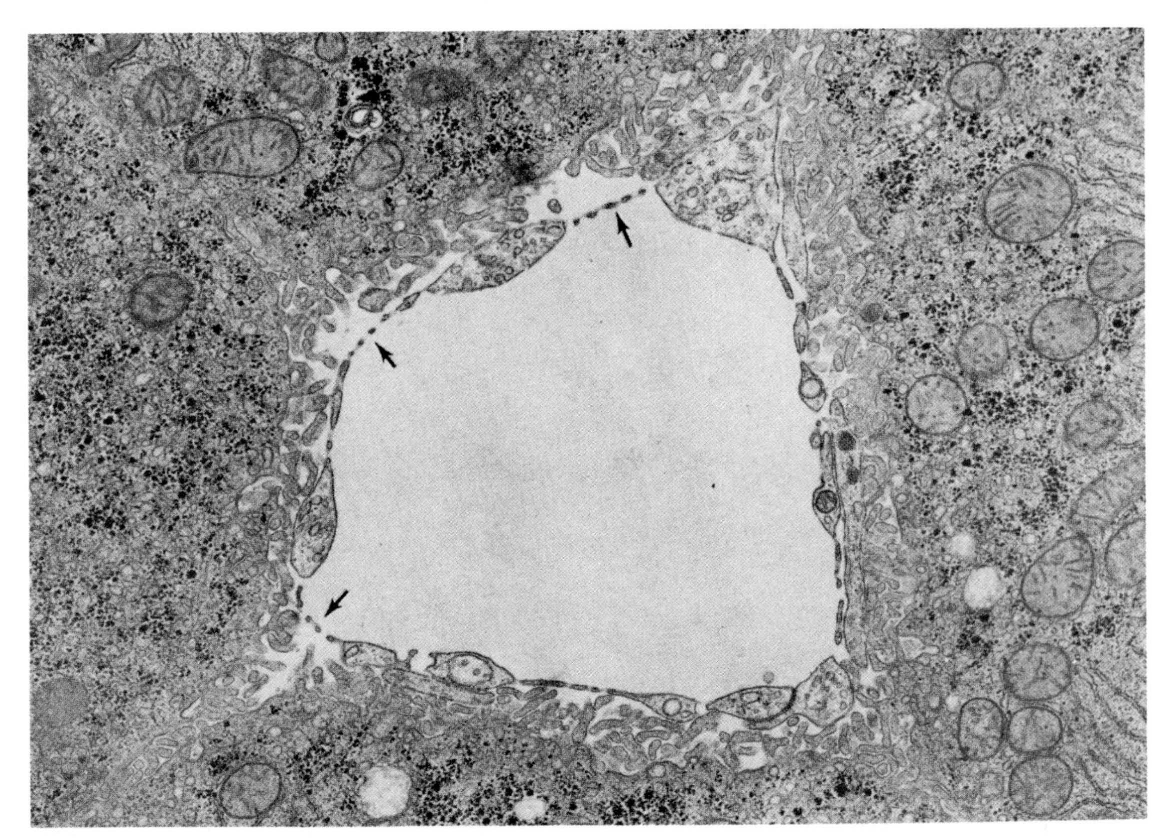

Figure 27–8. Electron micrograph of a sinusoid in rat liver fixed by vascular perfusion. The endothelium is extremely thin, and in some areas, there are groups of fenestrations, sometimes referred to as "sieve-plates" (at arrows). (Micrograph from Wisse, E. 1970. J. Ultrastr. Res. 31:125.)

bundles of collagen fibers in this space form a loose network that corresponds to the argyrophilic reticulum demonstrable around the sinusoids by silver-impregnation methods for light microscopy. The networks of reticular fibers around neighboring sinusoids are connected by coarser bundles of collagen that pass between the cells of the intervening liver cell plate. Occasional unmyelinated nerve axons are found in the perisinusoidal space.

The gel-like extracellular matrix commonly associated with connective tissue appears to be lacking in the perisinusoidal space, and plasma escaping through fenestrations in the endothelium of the sinusoids has direct access to the surface of the hepatocytes. This, no doubt, facilitates exchange of metabolites between the blood and the liver cells. The efficiency of this interchange is also enhanced by a sixfold amplification of surface area achieved by the microvilli on the liver cells.

Typical fibroblasts are rarely found in the perisinusoidal space, but there are sparse populations of two other cell types: *fat-storing cells* and *pit cells*. The fat-storing cells occupy shallow recesses between hepatic cells and usually have processes that contact the endothelial cells. They can be selectively stained with gold chloride (Fig. 27–12), but their distinguishing feature in routine histological preparations is the presence of multiple lipid droplets in their cytoplasm. Several other names have been given to these cells: *stellate cells, interstitial cells,* and *lipocytes*. They are more common near the center of the classical lobule than they are at its periphery. Their origin and functional significance remain obscure. When exogenous vitamin A is administered, it is stored in these cells owing to its lipid solubility. There is reason to believe that the "stellate cells" originally described by von Kupffer, after gold chloride staining, and believed to be intravascular, were actually fat-storing cells (Ito cells). The intravascular phagocytic cells that now bear his name do not stain selectively with gold.

The so-called pit cells are found in small numbers in the liver of rodents, but they have

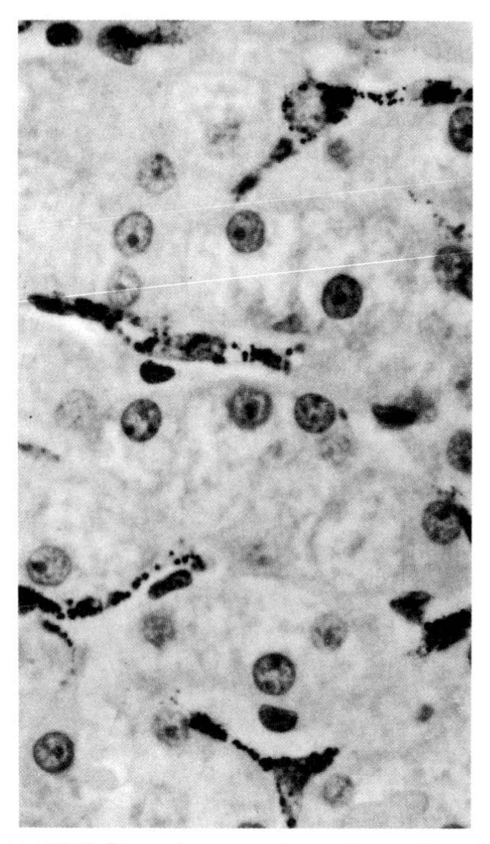

Figure 27–9. Photomicrograph of a small area of liver from a dog that had been injected with dilute India ink. The Kupffer cells are clearly distinguished by their content of carbon particles taken up by phagocytosis. (Courtesy of A.J. Ladman.)

not yet been reported in the human liver. They are small cells with short pseudopodia, but they are not phagocytic. Their cytoplasm contains small dense granules and vesicles containing a rod-like inclusion. These cells were formerly thought to be related to the enteroendocrine cells of the intestine, but more recent evidence suggests that they belong to the immune system and are large granule-containing lymphocytes of a kind that immunologists call natural killer cells. Similar cells are found in the lung, small intestine, epididymis, and mammary gland.

ZONATION WITHIN THE LIVER LOBULE

Some 70 years ago, histologists using the light microscope noted minor differences in the appearance of hepatic cells in three concentric zones within the classical lobule. These variations were believed to reflect differences in the degree of metabolic activity of the cells in these three zones. A region at the periphery of the lobules was, therefore, designated a "zone of permanent function"; an intermediate region, a "zone of variable function"; and the area around the central vein, a zone of "permanent repose." Knowing that the afferent blood enters the periphery of the classical lobule and exits via the central vein, it was reasoned that the activity of the hepatocytes depended on their location with respect to a gradient in concentration of oxygen along the length of the sinusoids. Cells at the periphery would be most favorably situated, those midway, less so, and those near the central vein would be exposed to blood largely depleted of oxygen and other metabolites. This interpretation derived support from the observation by pathologists that "centrilobular necrosis" occurs in disease states attended by hypoxemia.

The cytological heterogeneity of hepatocytes in different regions of the lobule is no longer believed to depend entirely on their position with respect to a gradient of available oxygen, but the concept of zonation within the microvascular unit is still a basic tenet of hepatology. The three concentric zones of the classical lobule have been replaced in our thinking by three comparable zones in the hepatic acinus: *zone-1*, an ellipsoidal area immediately surrounding the hepatic arteriole and terminal portal venule; *zone-2*, intermediate; and *zone-3*, cells near ends of the acinus. Blood flows sequentially through these zones and exits via the terminal branches of the hepatic vein at either end of the acinus (Fig. 27–4, 27–13).

Along the plates of parenchymal cells, differences in cell ultrastructure and in enzyme activity can be demonstrated from zone to zone. In zone-1, enzymes involved in oxidative metabolism and gluconeogenesis predominate, whereas in zone-3, the cells are especially rich in enzymes involved in glycolysis and lipid and drug metabolism. Cells of zone-2 have a mixed complement of enzymes. All hepatocytes probably have the same potentialities, but they express differences in ultrastructure and function depending on the blood oxygen and solute concentration prevailing in their zone of the acinus. Their ability to alter their structure and function in response to a change in their microenvironment indicates that the cells in the three zones are not intrinsically different. Brief administration of the drug phenobarbital induces an hypertrophy of the smooth endoplasmic reticulum that is initially

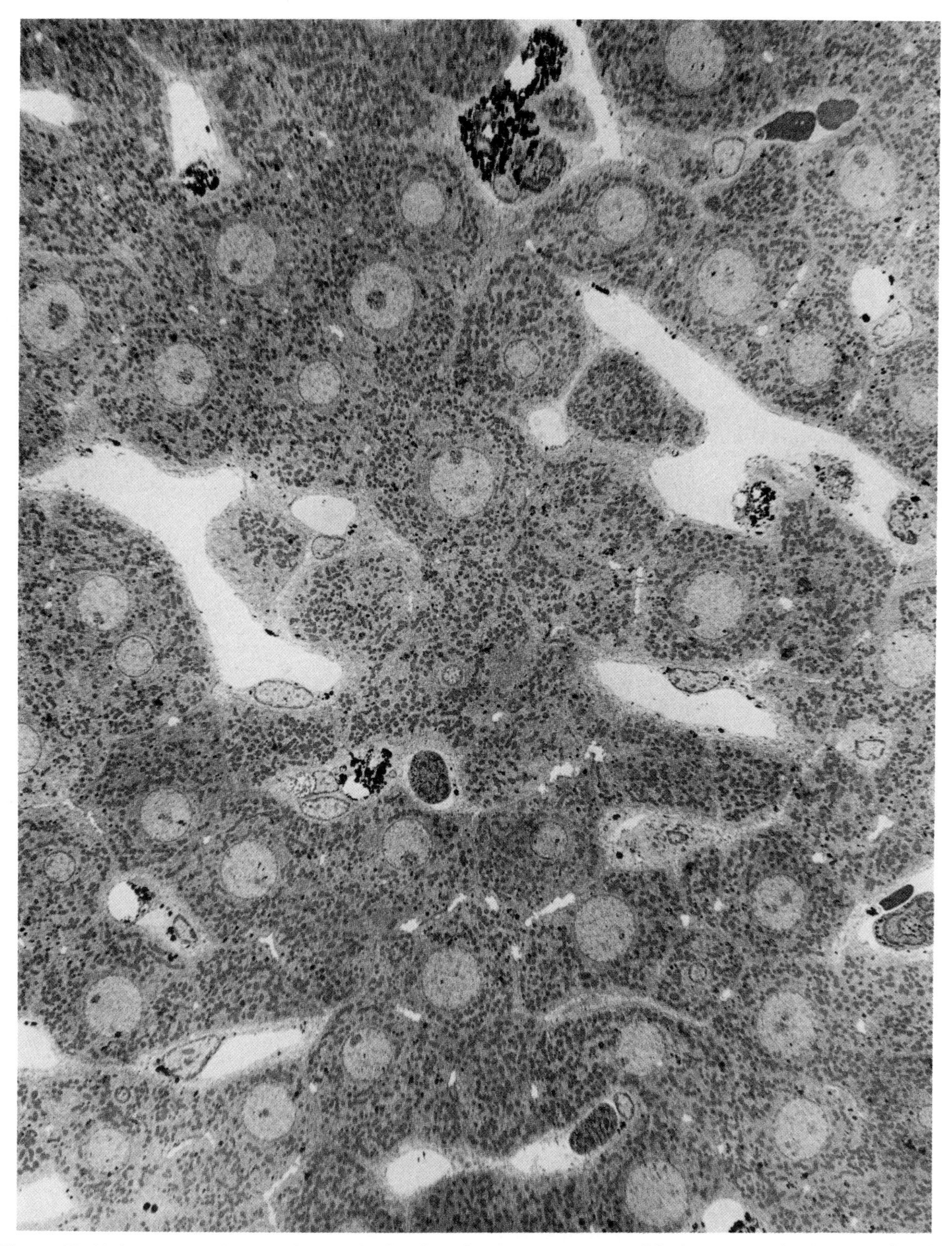

Figure 27–10. Low-power electron micrograph of rat liver showing arrangement of the hepatocytes in plates or trabeculae and their content of very numerous mitochondria. Several of the sinusoids contain Kupffer cells recognizable by their lipochrome pigment deposits and dense phagocytized material. (Micrograph courtesy of E. Wisse.)

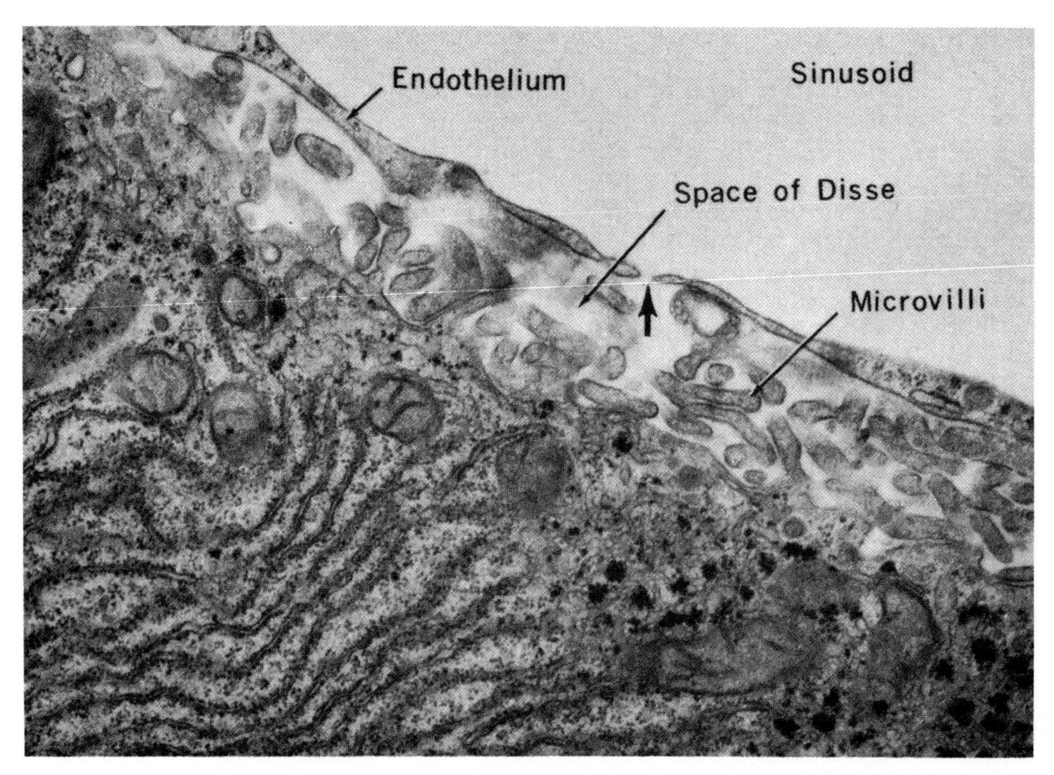

Figure 27–11. Electron micrograph of a portion of a liver cell bordering on a sinusoid. Numerous irregularly oriented microvilli project into the space between the hepatocyte and the endothelium of the sinusoid. This perivascular space is also called the space of Disse. Note the single fenestration in the endothelium at the arrow. (Micrograph courtesy of K.R. Porter and G. Millonig.)

confined to cells of zone-3, but if the drug is continued over a period of 10 days, hypertrophy of smooth reticulum and an attendant increase in drug metabolizing enzymes takes place in cells of zone-2 and finally in zone-3 as well.

CYTOLOGY OF THE HEPATOCYTES

Hepatocytes make up approximately 80% of the cell population of the liver. Because they are polygonal and arranged in plates or trabeculae between sinusoids, they do not have surfaces that can appropriately be described as apical and basal. For descriptive purposes, the sides of the cell exposed to the sinusoids are called the *sinusoidal domain* of the plasmalemma, and the sides in contact with neighboring hepatocytes are the *lateral domain.* A portion of the lateral membrane that forms the wall of the intercellular bile canaliculi is the *bile canalicular domain.* The sinusoidal and bile canalicular domains bear sparse microvilli. The other surfaces of the cell are planar.

The nucleus is round, with peripheral clumps of heterochromatin and one or two prominent nucleoli (Fig. 27–14). The nuclei vary somewhat in size, with 40–60% being polyploid. The majority of hepatocytes have a single nucleus, but as many as 25% are binucleate. The perinuclear cisterna has a thin, filamentous nuclear lamina on its inner surface. Examined with the light microscope, the cytoplasm contains conspicuous basophilic bodies that were traditionally referred to as the *ergastoplasm* (Figs. 27–15 and 27–16). In electron micrographs, these bodies are found to be aggregations of cisternae of the rough endoplasmic reticulum, and it is the ribosomes on its membranes that are responsible for its basophilia in histological sections. The cisternae are spaced further apart than in comparable arrays of reticulum in pancreatic acinar cells. There are also meandering tubular elements of the reticulum and free polyribosomes are abundant throughout the cytoplasm. The rough endoplasmic reticulum is the site of synthesis of protein constituents of the cytoplasm and the plasma proteins of the blood.

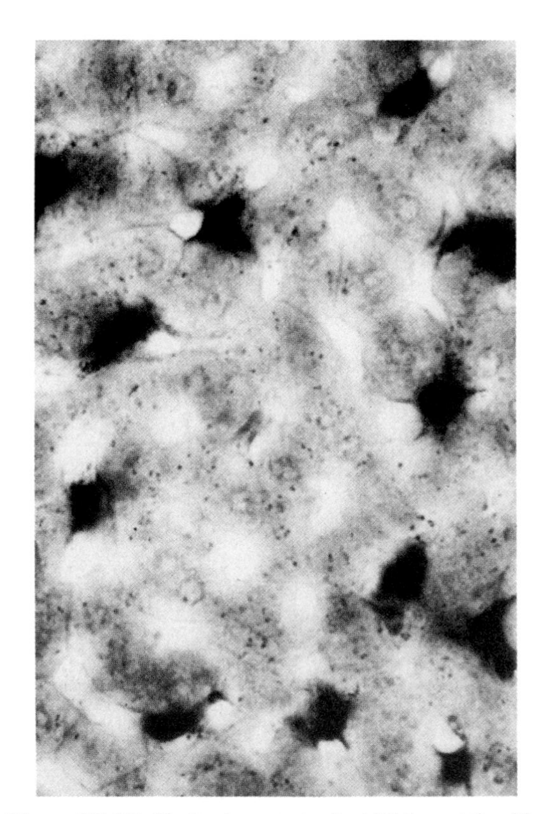

Figure 27–12. Photomicrograph of rabbit liver stained by gold chloride. The cells in the perivascular spaces that are selectively stained by this method are variously called stellate cells, fat-storing cells, lipocytes, or Ito cells. (Photograph from Wake, K. 1971. Am. J. Anat. 132:429.)

Smooth endoplasmic reticulum is present in varying abundance. It consists of a network of branching and anastomosing tubules, but the continuity of these elements is not always apparent in the thin sections required for electron microscopy (Fig. 27–17). Sites of continuity between the smooth and the rough endoplasmic reticulum are often observed (Fig. 27–18). Smooth reticulum is not well developed in cells of the periportal region (zone-1), but it is abundant in cells of zone-3 which are active in lipid metabolism. Small, dense globules, 30–40 μm in diameter, are often present in its lumen. These are very low-density serum lipoprotein (VLDL) that is synthesized in the liver and released into the blood as a carrier for cholesterol. The membranes of this organelle are rich in a family of enzymes called cytochromes-P450 that are involved in the synthesis of prostaglandins and other biologically active agents. They also have an important role in the catabolism of drugs and other potentially toxic exogenous compounds.

The mitochondria of hepatocytes are elongated, with lamellar or tubular cristae projecting into their interior, which is occupied by a matrix of relatively low density containing a few dense matrix granules. Thus, the ultrastructure of the mitochondria is not unusual, but there are striking regional differences in their size and number. In cells of the periportal region (zone-1), they are fewer in number, but nearly twice the size of those in the centrilobular region (zone-3 of the acinus).

The Golgi complex of the liver cell is not a single juxtanuclear organelle as in other glandular cells but consists of multiple stacks of five to nine cisternae slightly expanded at their ends. These are located along both sides of the cell near the bile canaliculi. Numerous small vesicles associated with the trans-Golgi cisterna, no doubt, transport constituents of the bile to the nearest bile canaliculus. There are usually several membrane bounded dense bodies, 0.2–0.5 μm in diameter, in the vicinity of the Golgi bodies. These give positive staining reactions for acid hydrolases and are, therefore, identified as lysosomes. Other membrane-limited spherical bodies, 0.2–0.8

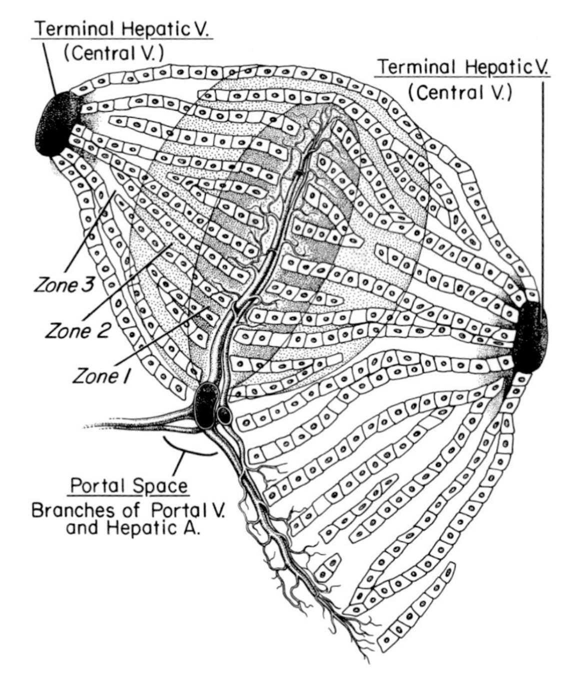

Figure 27–13. Diagram of the acinus, consisting of parenchyma centered around the terminal branches of the hepatic artery and portal vein. The cells in zone-1 have first call on the incoming oxygen and nutrients. The cells of zone-2 are less favored, and those of zone-3 are least favorably situated. (Redrawn after Rappaport, A.M. et al. 1954. Anat. Rec. 119:11.)

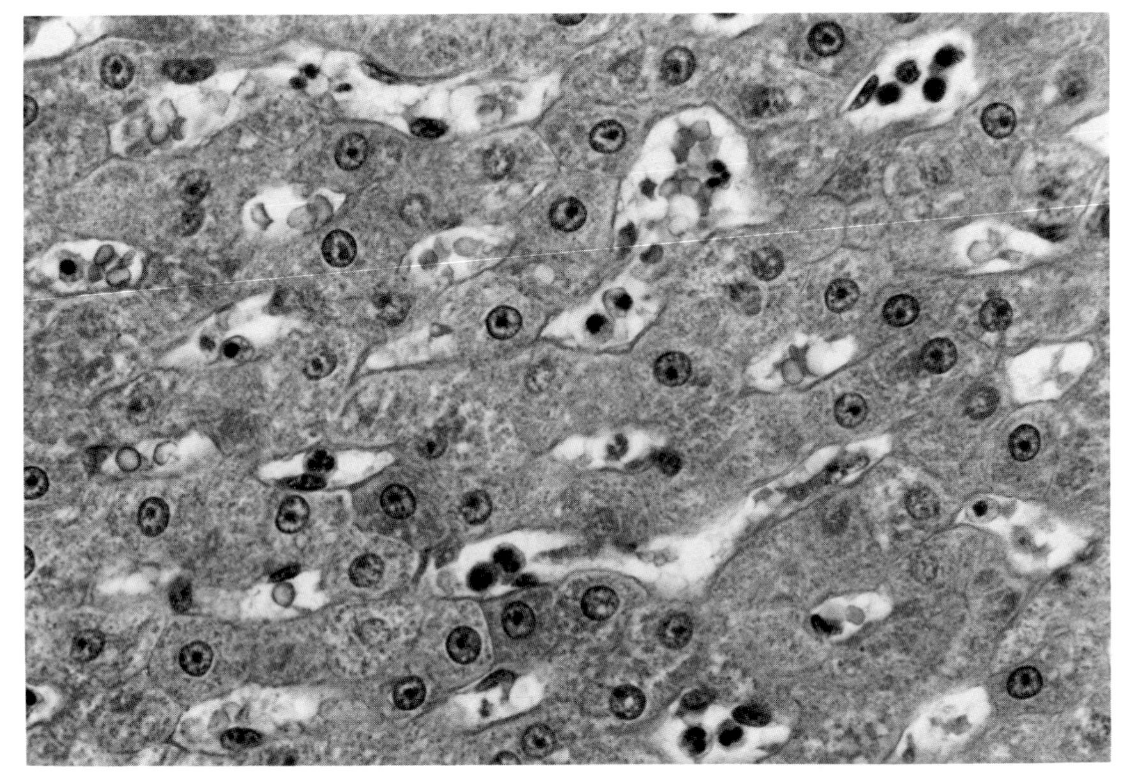

Figure 27–14. Electron micrograph of rat liver showing the round nuclei and prominent nucleoli.

μm in diameter, that are scattered through the cytoplasm are peroxisomes (Figs. 27–19 and 27–20). These contain catalase and other hydrogen peroxide generating oxidases. In laboratory rodents, a crystalline nucleoid is eccentrically placed in the finely granular matrix of the peroxisome. Nucleoids isolated from liver homogenates have been found to consist of the enzyme uricase. The nucleoid is lacking in the peroxisomes of human liver and the functional significance of liver peroxisomes is poorly understood.

In routine histological sections of liver, many of the cells have irregularly shaped unstained areas of cytoplasm free of organelles. In preparations stained with the periodic-acid–Schiff reaction for carbohydrates, these areas are found to contain deposits of glycogen (Fig. 27–21). In electron micrographs, the glycogen is in the form of electron-dense particles up to 0.1 μm in diameter called α-particles (Fig. 27–22). These are aggregates of smaller subunits, 20–30 nm in diameter, called β particles. Glycogen is a storage form of carbohydrate that can be drawn on to maintain the normal glucose concentration in the blood.

Hepatocytes contain varying amounts of lipid in electron-dense droplets that are not enclosed in a membrane. They are few in number in the normal liver but are dramatically increased after consumption of alcohol or other hepatotoxic substances. Accumulation of lipid usually begins in cells of zone-3 with multiple small droplets that later coalesce, and in severely toxic states the cells may become distended by a single very large lipid drop.

The cytoskeleton of the hepatic cell consists of a subplasmalemmal layer of cytokeratin and actin filaments. This layer is identifiable around the entire periphery of the cell, but it is thicker under the bile canalicular domain of the plasmalemma, where it helps to maintain the patency of the bile canaliculus. Bundles of intermediate filaments extend inward from the cortex, converging on the centrosome and the pore complexes of the nuclear envelope to form a resilient cytoskeletal framework within the cytoplasm.

The cell membrane has the same ultrastructural appearance over the entire surface, but functionally distinct domains are identifiable by cytochemical methods. With labeled anti-

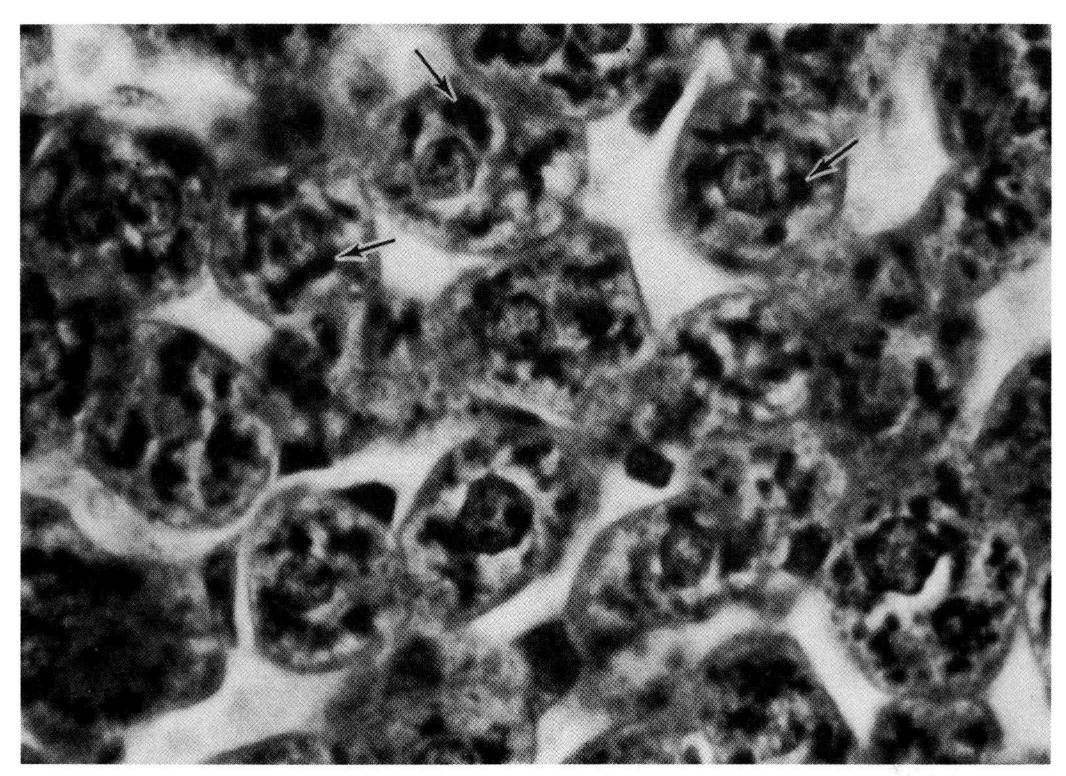

Figure 27–15. Photomicrograph of rat liver stained with eosin and methylene blue. The deeply stained basophilic bodies in the cytoplasm (at arrows) were traditionally called the ergastoplasm. They correspond to aggregations of rough endoplasmic reticulum in electron micrographs.

bodies, receptors for sialoglycoproteins, mannose-6-phosphate, and other substances taken up by receptor-mediated endocytosis can be localized in the sinusoidal domain. The bile canalicular domain contains aminopeptidase, phosphatases, and three glycoproteins that are not found elsewhere on the cell surface. Adenyl cyclase and Na^+,K^+-ATPase are found in both the sinusoidal domain and the lateral domains that interface with adjacent cells. The functional significance of some of these membrane proteins is yet to be elucidated.

HEPATIC DUCTS

A *bile canaliculus* is located midway along the interface between adjoining hepatic cells. These minute channels, 0.5–1.5 μm in diameter, form a network within the plates of hepatocytes, with a single cell in each of its polygonal meshes (Fig. 27–23). Owing to the branching and anastomosis of the cell plates, the network is continuous throughout the lobule and, in most species, into neighboring lobules.

In early descriptions of the histology of the liver, the bile canaliculi were assumed to be distinct entities, having a wall of their own, and it was thought that the network they formed contributed to the structural stability of the liver. This view was abandoned when the electron microscope revealed that the wall of the canaliculus is merely a specialization of the surfaces of adjoining cells, and its lumen is a local expansion of the intercellular cleft. Over most of their length, the apposed lateral membranes of contiguous cells are planar and separated by about 15 nm. Near the middle of this interface, the membranes diverge to bound a wider intercellular space that constitutes the lumen of a bile canaliculus (Fig. 27–24). Along either side of the lumen, the closely apposed membranes form a tight junction comparable to the zonulae occludentes of other epithelia. These junctions isolate the lumen of the canaliculus and prevent escape of bile. A few short microvilli project into its lumen and the membrane bounding the canaliculus is reinforced by a thickening of the underlying cortical layer of cytoskeletal filaments.

At the periphery of the classical hepatic lob-

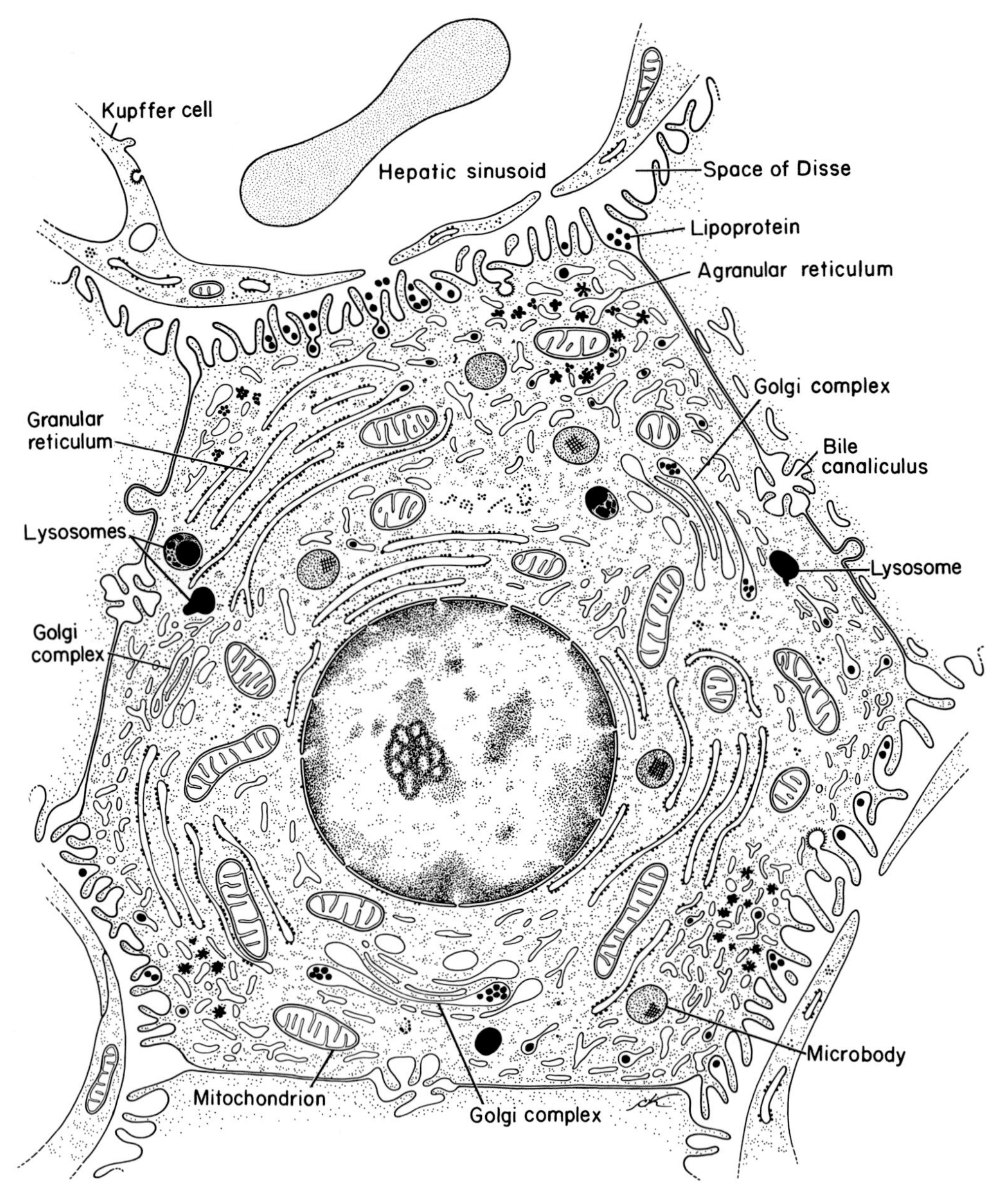

Figure 27–16. Drawing depicting the relationships of the hepatic cells to each other and to the sinusoids and showing the principal organelles and inclusions in the cytoplasm. (Drawing by Sylvia Colard Keene.)

ule (the axis of the acinus), the bile canaliculi are confluent with *terminal ductules* (*canals of Hering*) that drain into *interlobular bile ducts* associated with the branches of the hepatic artery and portal vein in the portal areas (Fig. 27–25). Their wall is initially made up of squamous cells, but these give way to low cuboidal cells as the ductules approach the interlobular ducts. This transitional region of the duct system is seen clearly with the light microscope only when the ductules are distended, as they are following occlusion of a bile duct. The interlobular ducts, 30–40 μm in diameter, continue into a system of progressively larger ducts that converge on the porta hepatis. They are lined by cuboidal to low columnar epithelium and, in the larger ducts, the epithelium contains occasional clusters of mucus-secreting cells. These ducts are enveloped by moderately dense connective tissue.

The extrahepatic portion of the duct system consists of *right* and *left hepatic ducts* emerging from corresponding lobes of the liver, and the *common bile duct* formed by their convergence.

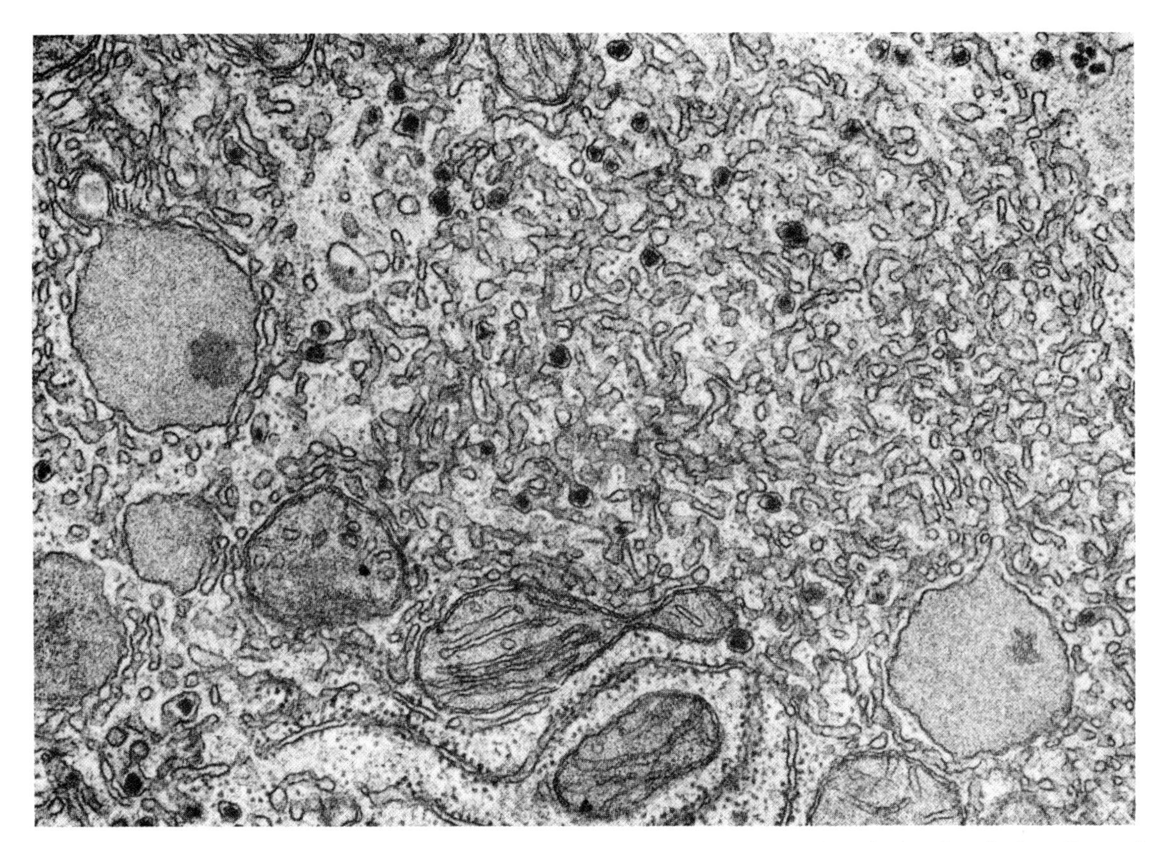

Figure 27–17. Electron micrograph of an area of hepatocyte cytoplasm rich in smooth endoplasmic reticulum. Some of the tubular elements of this organelle contain small, dense, spherical particles representing newly synthesized very low-density serum lipoprotein. Also present in this field are two peroxisomes with eccentrically placed nucleoids. (Micrograph by R. Bolender.)

The *cystic duct* from the gallbladder joins the common duct, which continues to the duodenum. These ducts are lined by columnar epithelium and have a moderately thick wall which includes a thin submucosa, muscularis, and adventitia. At intervals along their length, tubular glands extend down into the submucosa. Lymphocytes are common in the submucosa and may migrate through the epithelium into the lumen. Bundles of smooth muscle first appear in the wall of the common duct. They are oriented longitudinally and obliquely but do not form a complete layer. Smooth muscle becomes more prominent as the common duct approaches the duodenum and, in its intramural portion, it forms a sphincter that exercises control over the flow of bile into the duodenum.

CONNECTIVE TISSUE STROMA

The liver has remarkably little stroma for an organ of such large size. Beneath the peritoneal mesothelium that covers all but a small area of its diaphragmatic surface, there is a layer of dense connective tissue, 70–100 μm thick, called *Glisson's capsule*. This is thickest at the porta hepatis and from there connective tissue continues inward with the large vessels and ducts and ensheathes the intrahepatic branches of these structures in their arborization throughout the organ to the level of the interlobular portal tracts where it is continuous with the more delicate stroma of the classical hepatic lobules (Fig. 27–26).

With silver-staining methods for light microscopy, the intralobular stroma appeared as a network of reticular fibers between the sinusoids and the plates of parenchymal cells (Fig. 27–27). In the ultrathin sections required for electron microscopy, the stromal network is not apparent, but slender bundles of collagen can be seen in the perisinusoidal space (space of Disse). The three-dimensional organization of the intralobular stroma is more profitably studied in scanning electron micrographs of tissue, from which the cellular elements have been removed by maceration

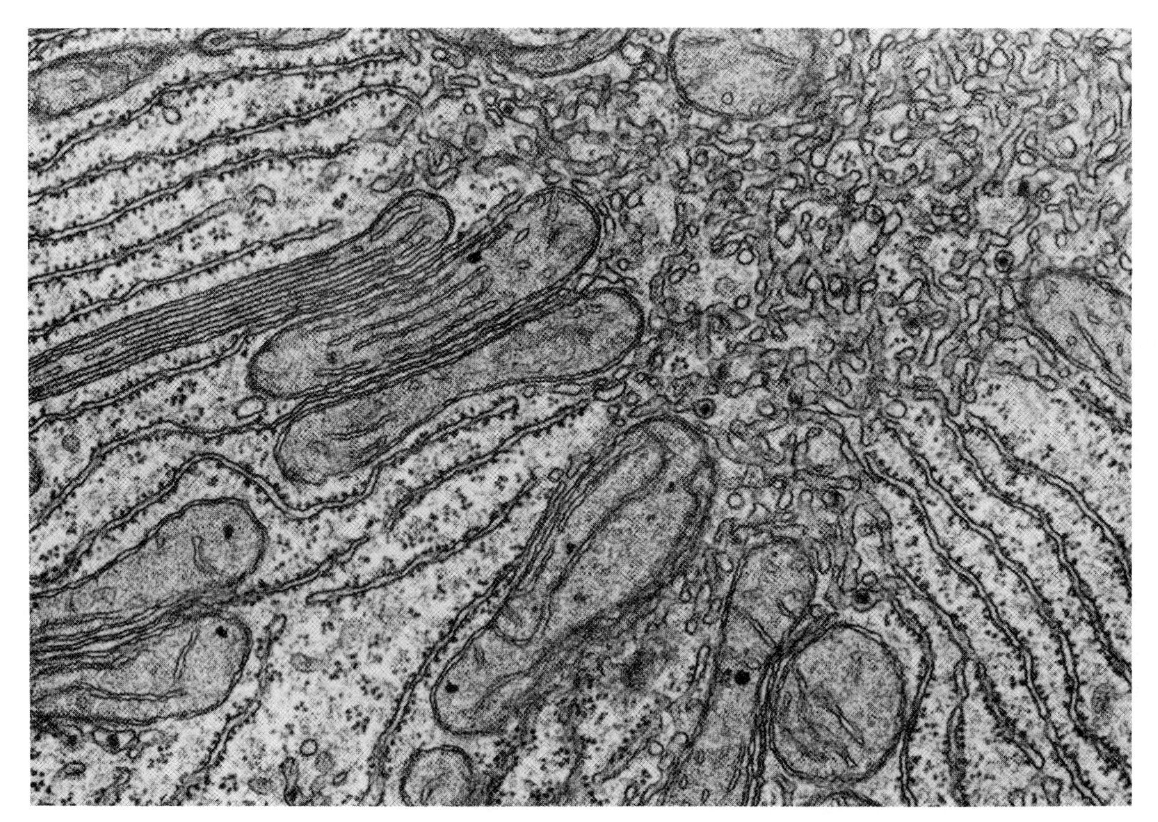

Figure 27–18. Electron micrograph of a small area of hepatocyte cytoplasm including several mitochondria, and profiles of rough endoplasmic reticulum in continuity with a close-meshed plexus of smooth endoplasmic reticulum (at upper right). (Micrograph courtesy of R. Bolender.)

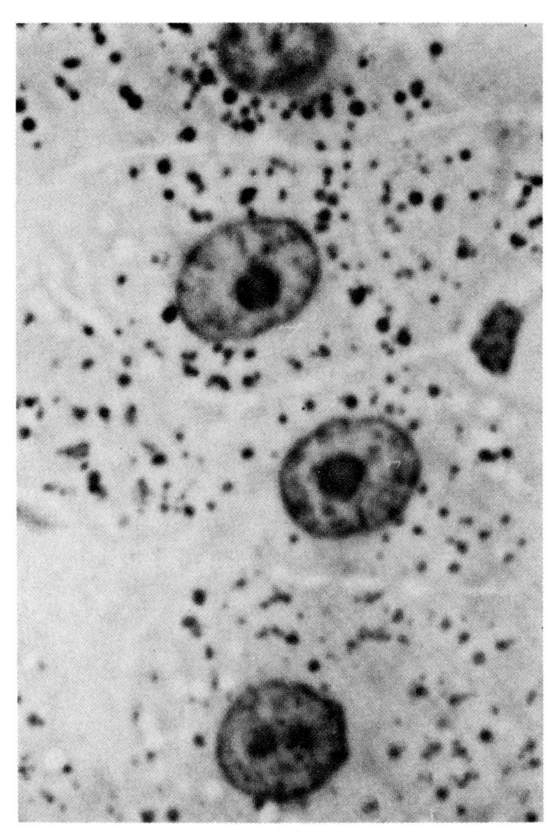

Figure 27–19. Photomicrograph of rat liver stained by a histochemical reaction for the enzyme peroxidase. The distribution of the reactive bodies corresponds to that of peroxisomes in electron micrographs. (Micrograph from Fahimi, D. 1969. J. Cell Biol. 43:275).

in strong alkali (Fig. 27–28). Coarse bundles of 60-nm collagen fibrils in the portal areas are continuous with a network of very thin bundles of fibrils surrounding the sinusoids. The delicate network of fibrils surrounding neighboring sinusoids are interconnected by larger bundles of collagen fibrils that cross the plates, passing between the parenchymal cells (Fig. 27–29). The bundles of collagen in the portal areas are larger than those forming the perisinusoidal networks, but the unit fibrils of both are of the same diameter. In view of this finding, there is no reason to perpetuate the traditional distinction between "reticular fibers" and collagen fibers that was based on nonspecific silver-staining methods for light microscopy.

In the absence of typical fibroblasts in the space of Disse, the origin of the collagenous framework of the liver lobules is a subject of debate. There is reason to believe that the fat-storing cells (Ito cells) may be involved. Endothelial cells have been implicated and liver cells in culture are reported to produce small amounts of collagen. Thus, more than one cell type in the liver is a candidate, but which one is principally involved in production of stroma is not known. The question is of some importance because of the prevalence of fibrosis in chronic liver disease. Excessive proliferation of connective tissue often impedes the flow of blood and bile and may interfere with the growth of nodules of regenerating liver cells.

LYMPHATICS

The liver produces a large volume of lymph. From one-quarter to one-half of the lymph of the thoracic duct comes from the liver. Hepatic lymph differs from that from other regions in containing a large amount of plasma protein. The ratio of albumen to globulin is somewhat higher than in the plasma.

The network of lymphatics parallels the branches of the portal vein from the interlobular portal areas to the porta hepatis. Lymphatics have not been demonstrated within the hepatic lobules. Plasma escaping through fenestrations in the sinusoidal epithelium is believed to move along the spaces of Disse in a direction counter to the flow of blood, seeping into the tissue spaces around the terminal twigs of the portal vein and hepatic artery at the periphery of the classical lobules (axis of the acini). There it enters lymphatic capillaries that accompany the blood vessels and ducts of the portal tracts.

NERVES

The liver is innervated mainly by efferent autonomic nerves. These are regularly found in the connective tissue around the portal triads and adrenergic endings can be found in the space of Disse in close apposition to hepatocytes (Fig. 27–30). In the rat and mouse, nerves appear to contact only cells in the periportal region of the classical lobule, but in other species, including the human, they are found throughout the lobule. It has been suggested that in those species in which nerves do not penetrate deeply into the lobules, there may be more extensive electrotonic coupling

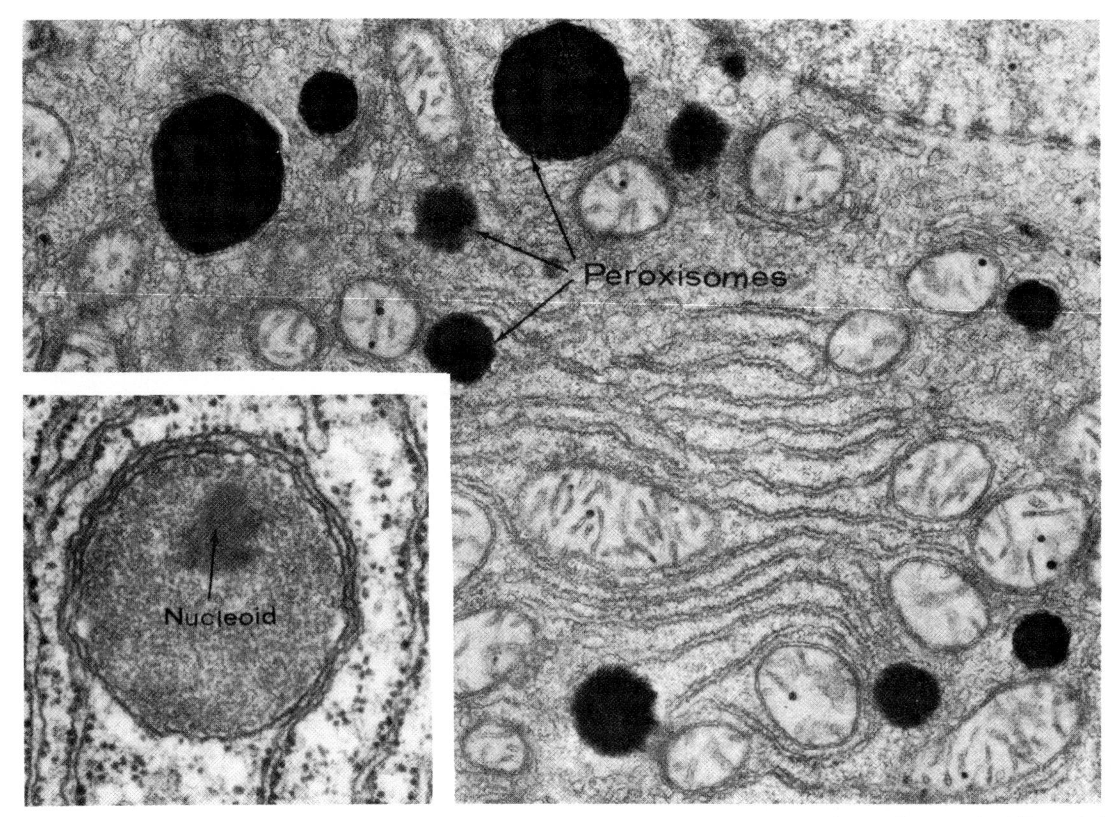

Figure 27–20. Peroxisomes, or microbodies, of rodent liver are limited by a membrane and contain a "nucleoid" consisting of a paracrystalline array of tubular subunits (inset). When stained for peroxidase activity, the matrix reacts intensely, but the nucleoid remains unstained. (From Fahimi, D. 1969. J. Cell Biol. 43:275. Inset: courtesy of R. Wood.)

of the hepatocytes by gap junctions (Fig. 27–31).

The automatic innervation of the liver plays an important role in the short-term regulation of cell metabolism, influencing glucose and lactate output. There is less convincing evidence that the nerves may be involved in the longer-term induction of enzymes.

LIVER REGENERATION

Compared to other organs that are constantly being renewed, the hepatic parenchyma is a rather stable cell population. The life span of hepatocytes is in excess of 150 days and cells in division are seldom seen in the normal liver. However, the organ has an exceptional capacity for regeneration. In laboratory rodents, two-thirds of the liver can be removed and, in a few days, most of it will have been replaced. Similar rapid regeneration occurs after destruction of a substantial part of each lobule following administration of chlorinated hydrocarbons. Most of the research on liver regeneration has been done on the rat and mouse in which the amount restored is usually as great as the volume removed. Regeneration in other species is roughly in inverse relation to the size of animal. Although the human liver has considerable regenerative capacity, it falls far short of that seen in laboratory animals.

Some of the pathological changes characteristic of chronic liver disease in humans can be reproduced in rats and mice. A toxic dose of carbon tetrachloride produces a central necrosis involving one-third to one-half of the each lobule. Only the parenchymal cells are killed, leaving the sinusoids intact so that circulation of blood through the lobule is maintained. The damaged central cells undergo autolysis and the remaining cells proliferate rapidly, completely restoring normal architecture of the lobule in 5 or 6 days. If the hepatotoxic agent is administered repeatedly while the regeneration is still in progress, resulting in new injury before the old has been repaired, there is extensive fibrosis comparable to that seen in *cirrhosis* of the liver in man.

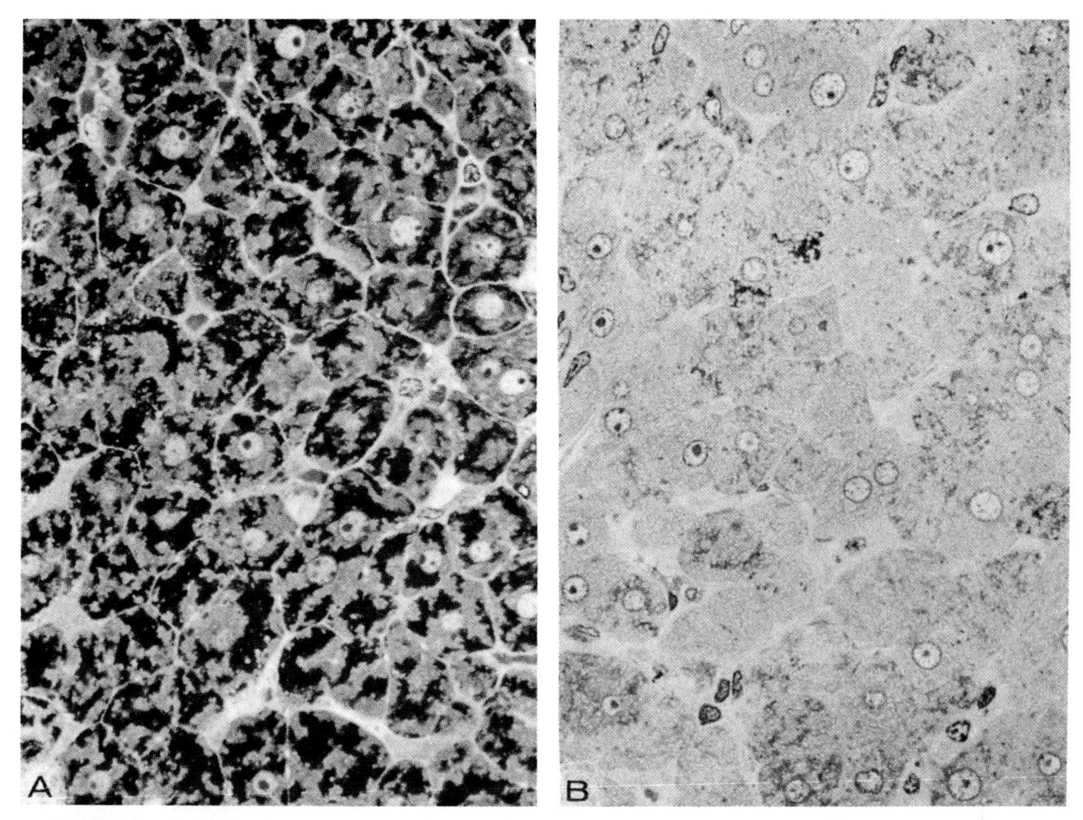

Figure 27–21. Dietary differences in the amount of glycogen in the hepatocytes are clearly demonstrated in these two photomicrographs (A) Liver of an animal fasted for 2 h and containing 8.2% glycogen. (B) Liver of an animal fasted 24 h and containing 0.9% glycogen. (From Cardell, R., J. Larner, and M.B. Babcock. 1973. Anat. Rec. 177:23.)

There has been much investigative interest in what factors initiate cell proliferation and terminate it when regeneration is complete, but answers have proven elusive.

HISTOPHYSIOLOGY OF THE LIVER

The principal contribution of the liver to the digestive process is its secretion of bile, a complex fluid consisting of cholesterol, lecithin, fatty acids, and bile salts. Of these, the most important are the bile salts. The latter are synthesized from cholesterol by conversion to cholic and chenocholic acids which then combine with glycine or taurine in salt linkage. About 0.5 g of these conjugated bile acids are secreted daily. They have an emulsifying action on ingested fat that promotes absorption of fatty acids and monoglycerides. In the absence of bile secretion, much of the dietary fat is not absorbed and passes out in unusually fatty feces.

An important excretory function of the liver, associated with the secretion of bile, is the elimination of *bilirubin* from the blood. This toxic, greenish pigment originates from the degradation of the hemoglobin of senescent erythrocytes that are removed from the circulation by Kupffer cells of the liver and by other phagocytes in the spleen. It is taken up by the liver cells and conjugated with glucuronide in the endoplasmic reticulum. The greater part of the conjugate, bilirubin glucuronide, is excreted into the bile, but some is released into the blood. An abnormal accumulation of bilirubin in the blood results in *jaundice*. This may occur when bilirubin production exceeds the capacity of the normal liver to excrete it or when either bilirubin uptake or conjugation is impaired by liver disease. Determination of the relative amounts of conjugated and unconjugated bilirubin in a sample of blood is commonly used as a measure of liver function and to determine the probable cause in a patient with jaundice.

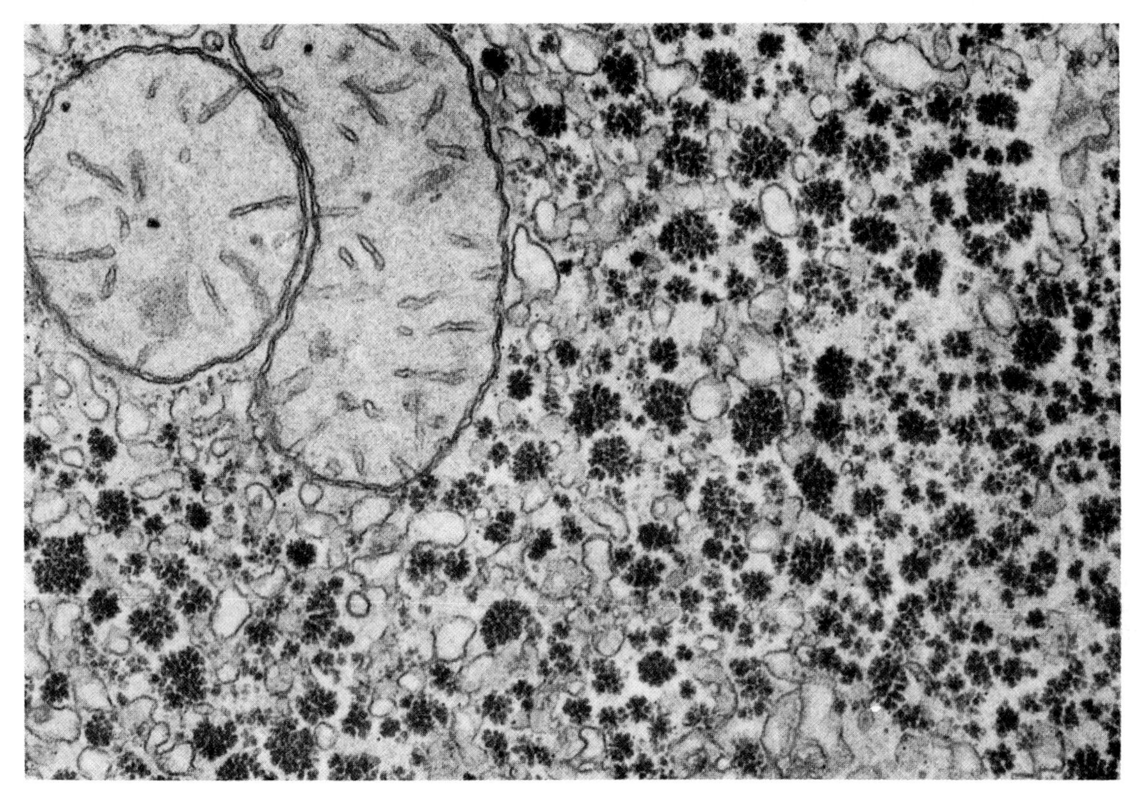

Figure 27–22. Electron micrograph of an area of hepatocyte cytoplasm containing a high concentration of α- granules of glycogen. On close inspection, the smaller β- particles can be seen within the α-particles.

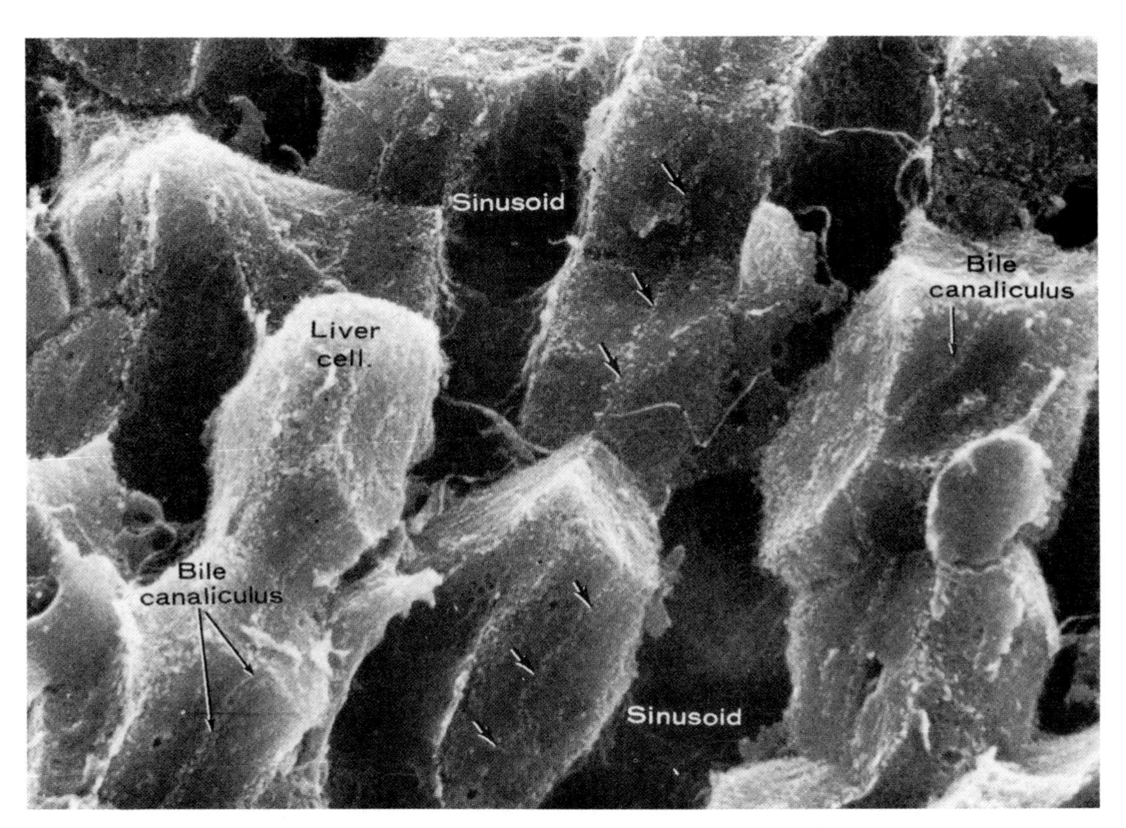

Figure 27–23. Scanning electron micrograph of rat liver fixed by perfusion and then broken open to provide a three-dimensional view of the polygonal hepatic cells alternating with sinusoids. Where adjoining cells have been separated, half of a bile canaliculus can be seen coursing along the middle of the exposed cell face (at arrows). (Micrograph courtesy of M. Karnovsky.)

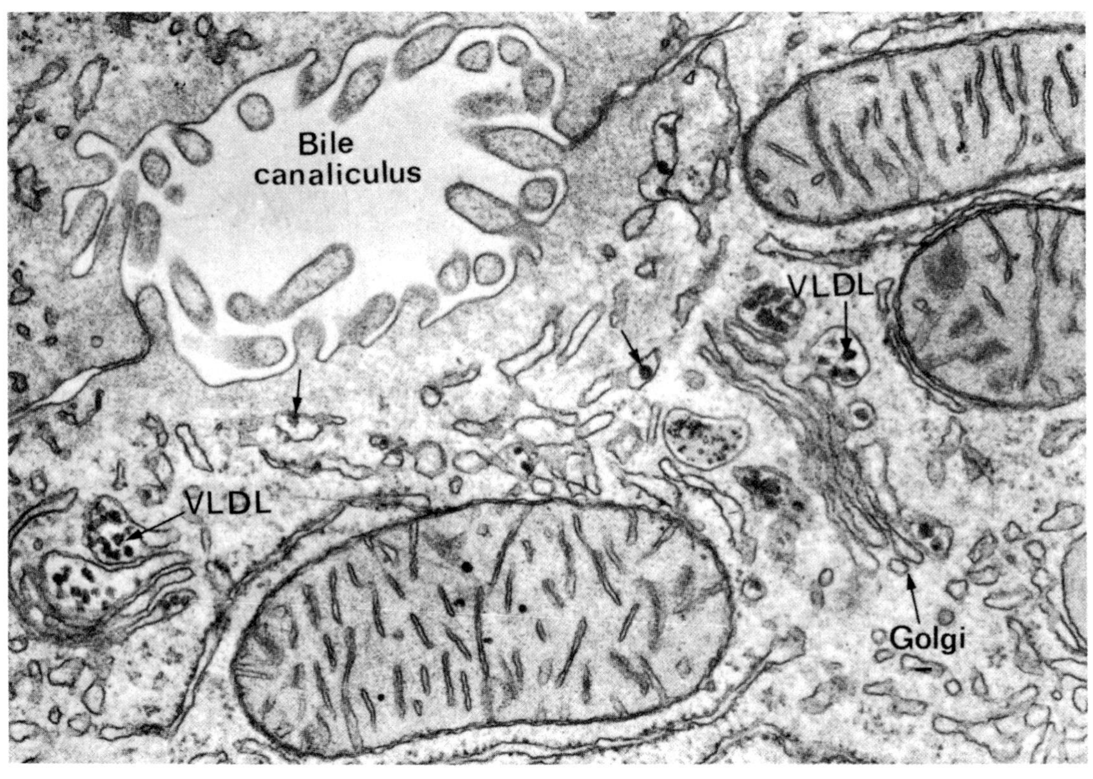

Figure 27–24. Electron micrograph of a bile canaliculus. Note the tight junctions between cells along either side of the lumen. Particles of very low-density lipoprotein can be seen in the lumen of the smooth endoplasmic reticulum and in vesicles associated with the juxtacanalicular Golgi complex. (Micrograph courtesy of R. Bolender.)

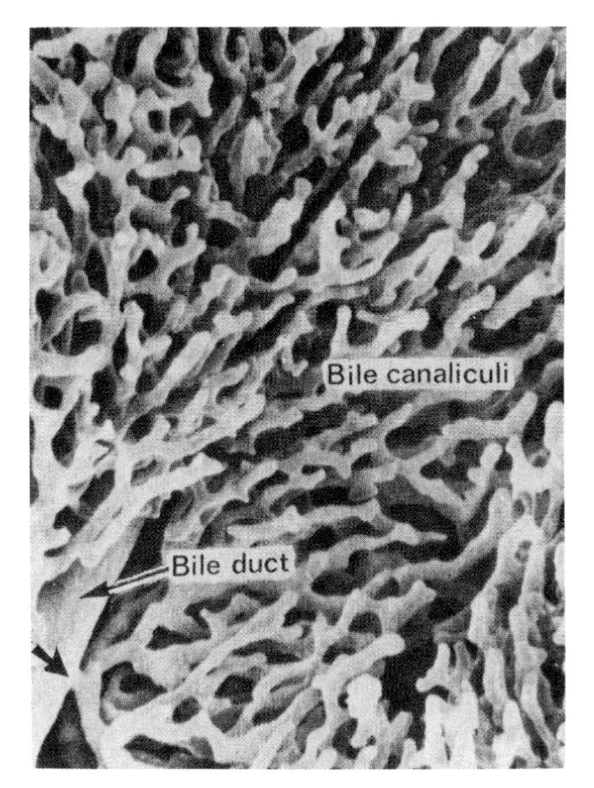

Figure 27–25. Scanning micrograph of a cast of branches of the biliary tree showing the arborizing pattern of bile canaliculi. At the arrow is a canal of Herring communicating with the duct of a portal triad. (Micrograph from Murikami, T. 1980. Digest. Dis. Soc. 25:609.)

Situated between the portal system and the general circulation, the liver is strategically located to process nutrients absorbed by the intestine. One of its most important functions is to maintain the normal concentration of glucose in the blood. Absorbed glucose is taken up from the portal blood and polymerized by a series of enzymatic reactions into glycogen, the storage form of carbohydrate. Other compounds such as lactic acid, glycerol, and pyruvic acid can be converted by the liver cells into glucose and then to glycogen. As needed, glycogen is broken down to glucose in a process catalyzed by the enzyme phosphorylase. This enzyme, normally present in an inactive form, is specifically activated by the hormones epinephrine and glucagon which induce release of glucose into the blood. These functions cannot be attributed to any particular organelle because the enzymes involved in gluconeogenesis and glycogenolysis are free in the cytoplasm. However, in electron micrographs, glycogen is usually located in areas of cytoplasm rich in smooth endoplasmic reticulum.

Superimposed on the enduring ultrastructural and functional differences in hepatocytes from zone to zone, there are, in rats and mice, transient changes that are related to food intake. After a large meal, glycogen is deposited first in the cells of zone-1 that are particularly rich in enzymes concerned with gluconeogenesis and glycogen synthesis. As assimilation progresses, glycogen deposition spreads through zone-2 and into zone-3 until all but the cells immediately adjacent to the central vein are heavily laden. Between meals, glucose is released into the blood beginning at zone-3 and progressing to zone-1. Thus, in rodents, which normally feed at night, there is a diurnal tide of glycogen within the lobules (Fig. 27–21). In other species, including man, these changes are less easily demonstrated.

The liver also plays a major role in the metabolism of lipids and in the maintenance of normal lipid levels in the circulating blood. The blood lipids are derived from ingested food, or from mobilization of fat reserves in the adipose tissue. Lipid is transported in the blood in the form of lipoprotein and it is in the liver that lipid is transformed into serum lipoprotein. In electron micrographs, small, dense particles, 30–100 nm in diameter, are seen in the terminal expansions of cisternae of rough endoplasmic reticulum, in the tubular elements of the smooth reticulum, in small transport vesicles, and in the space of Disse. These are *very low-density lipoprotein* (VLDL) formed in the liver and released by exocytosis into the space of Disse. Triglycerides are first generated from fatty acids in the smooth reticulum and combined there with protein synthesized in the rough reticulum to form these lipoprotein particles (Figs. 27–24 and 27–32). The smooth reticulum is evidently also the site of synthesis of cholesterol. When hypertrophy of this organelle is experimentally induced, the liver can be shown to have an enhanced capacity for synthesis of cholesterol from acetate.

The liver is the site of synthesis of *plasma proteins*. The organelle principally involved is the rough endoplasmic reticulum. In electron micrographs, a fine flocculent material can sometimes be observed in the lumen of its cisternae, and albumen has been detected in the microsome fraction of liver homogenates. Other proteins produced in the liver include *fibrinogen, thrombin,* and *Factor III,* substances essential for blood clotting. Impaired synthesis of these clotting factors in liver disease may result in a tendency to bleed excessively from

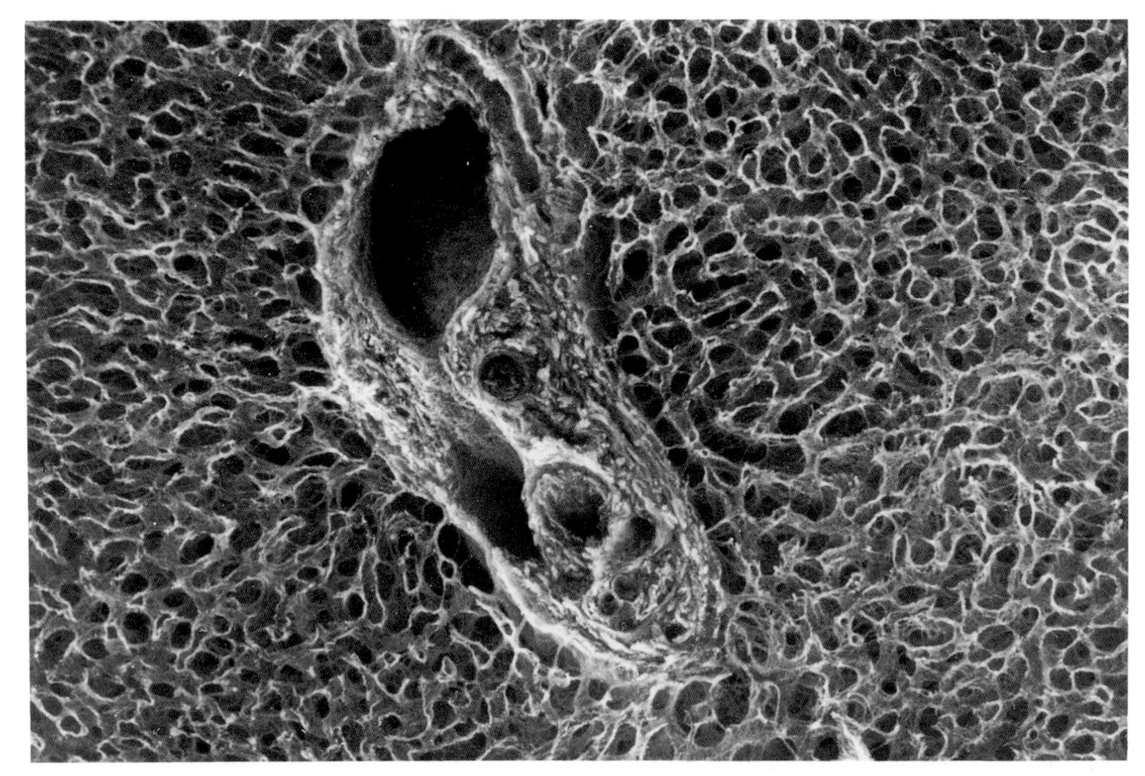

Figure 27–26. Low-power scanning micrograph of human liver from which the cells have been digested away. Collagen fibers associated with a portal area, in the center, are continuous with a network of fibers surrounding the sinusoids. (Micrograph from Ohtani, O. 1988. Arch. Histol. Cytol. 51:473.)

minor injuries. The concentration of these substances in the blood is used as a measure of liver cell function.

The hepatocytes have an important accessory function in the immune system of the intestine. As stated in an earlier chapter, immunoglobulin-A synthesized by plasma cells in the lamina propria of the gut is complexed with *secretory component* in cells of the intestinal epithelium and secreted into the lumen. However, only a fraction of the antibody produced in the lamina propria takes this direct route to the lumen. The remainder is carried in the lymph to the thoracic duct and then to the general circulation. Much of the IgA in the blood is destined to reach the lumen of the intestine via the hepatobiliary pathway described in a foregoing paragraph. The secretory component is continuously synthesized by the liver cells and inserted as a transmembrane receptor protein at the surface facing the space of Disse. IgA is taken up by receptor-mediated endocytosis and transported in vesicles to the bile canaliculi where the secretory component is cleaved releasing the antibody into the bile for transport to the intestinal lumen. IgA is present in bile at four times its concentration in the blood. If the bile duct is surgically occluded in experimental animals, the amount of IgA in the blood rises markedly, whereas the amount in the lumen of the gut falls to one-tenth its normal concentration. It is, therefore, evident that biliary IgA makes a major contribution to the level of antibody in the intestinal lumen.

The liver takes up, by receptor-mediated endocytosis, a number of the hormones produced by the endocrine glands and excretes them into the bile. Some of these proteins and steroids traverse the cell by a direct pathway in which they are released intact into the bile by fusion of their transport vesicles with the membrane of the bile canaliculus. Others follow an *indirect path* in which the vesicles fuse, en route, with small primary lysosomes that degrade the contents. The breakdown products are then released into the bile.

Metabolism of the barbiturates that are commonly used as sedatives and of many other lipid soluble drugs takes place in the liver. The enzymes that degrade these compounds are localized mainly in the smooth

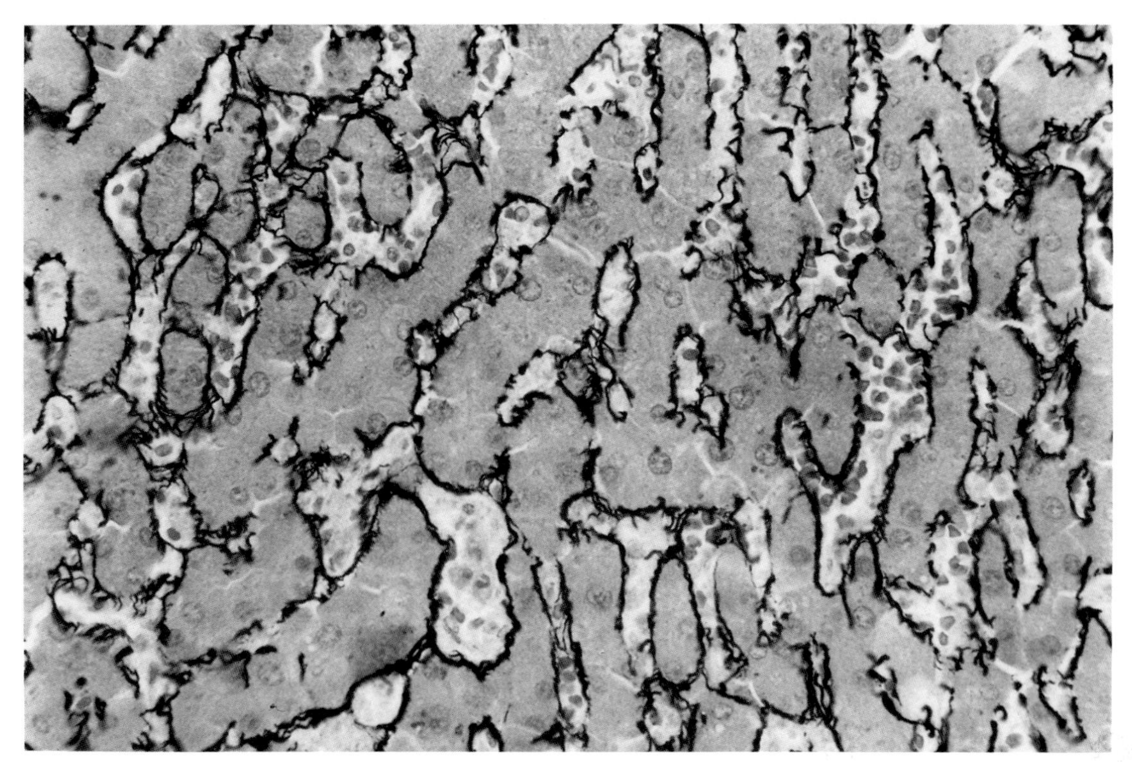

Figure 27–27. Photomicrograph of liver stained with a silver method for "reticular fibers." The fibers are in the perisinusoidal spaces of Disse.

endoplasmic reticulum. Administration of such drugs induces a marked hypertrophy of this organelle with a concomitant increase in the drug-metabolizing enzymes. This proliferation of smooth membranes is not a toxic effect of the drug but an adaptive response that enhances the ability of the liver cells to eliminate the inducing drug. These ultrastructural and biochemical changes are the basis of *drug tolerance*—the progressive loss in the effectiveness of a drug with continued use.

The liver has an important blood-filtering function. It is a highly vascular organ, receiving each minute about 1000 ml of blood from the portal vein and 350 ml from the hepatic artery. As it flows through the sinusoids, the blood is exposed to some 1.2×10^7 phagocytic Kupffer cells per gram of tissue, and these remove cellular debris and foreign particulate matter including microorganisms than may invade the blood from the intestinal lumen. The Kupffer cells have surface receptors for immunoglobulins and for complement, and they secrete the cytokines, interleukin-1, and the tumor necrosis factor. They are, therefore, active participants in the body's immunological defenses.

THE GALLBLADDER

The gallbladder is a pear-shaped hollow organ occupying a shallow fossa on the inferior surface of the liver. It consists of a fundus, a body, and a neck that continues into the cystic duct. Normally, it measures about 10 by 4 cm and has a capacity of 40–70 ml. It is subject to considerable variation in shape and is frequently the site of pathological processes that change its size and thickness of its wall. The functions of the gallbladder are to store, concentrate, and release into the duodenum the bile secreted by the liver.

All but the hepatic surface of the gallbladder is covered by a serosa continuous with that covering the liver. Its wall consists of a thin subserosal layer of connective tissue overlying a layer of smooth muscle. Deep to this is the mucosa, composed of the epithelium and its highly vascular lamina propria. The mucosa is plicated into convoluted folds of varying height that delimit narrow bays or clefts. The mucosal folds are tall and closely spaced in the contracted gallbladder but are short and more widely spaced when the organ is distended. These differences are most dramati-

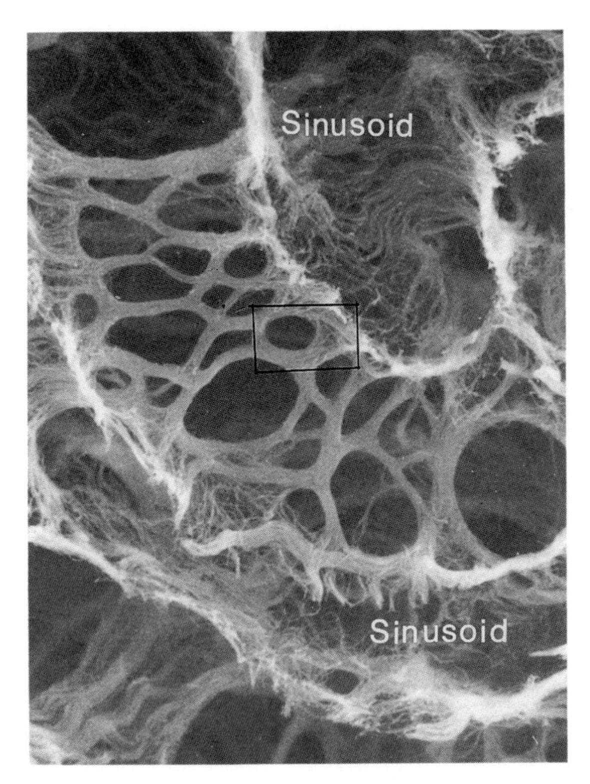

Figure 27–28. A scanning micrograph of the collagenous framework around a column of hepatocytes and the adjacent sinusoids. The cells have been digested away. Note that the delicate networks of fibrils around the sinusoids are connected by a network of coarser strands that pass between the liver cells. The area in the rectangle is shown at higher magnification in Fig. 27–29. (Micrograph courtesy of T. Ohtani.)

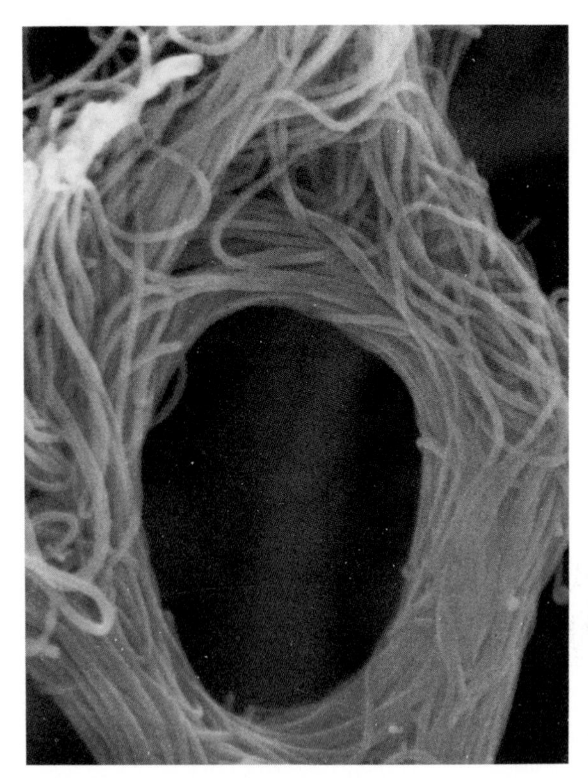

Figure 27–29. High-magnification micrograph of the area enclosed in a rectangle in Fig. 27–28. The fibrils making up the coarser interconnecting strands are of the same diameter as those of the finer networks around the sinusoids. Therefore, there is no intrinsic difference in those that stain with silver and those that do not. (Micrograph courtesy of T. Ohtani.)

cally revealed in surface views with the scanning electron microscope. In the contracted gallbladder, the folds follow a generally parallel course (Fig. 27–33). In the distended state, the folds are reduced to low ridges and it becomes apparent that they branch and anastomose to form a network outlining shallow polygonal recesses (Fig. 27–34). A loose organization of the collagenous and elastic fibers of the lamina propria provides the flexibility to accommodate these changes in surface topography.

The epithelium is a single layer of tall columnar cells, with oval nuclei and a faintly eosinophilic cytoplasm (Fig. 27–35). In histological sections, an inconspicuous striated border is detected, but in electron micrographs, the micovilli are shorter and less regular in their orientation than are those of the striated border of the intestine (Fig. 27–36). The tips of the microvilli bear minute filiform appendages similar to those comprising the glycocalyx on other absorbtive epithelia. The lateral cell boundaries are relatively straight in their apical portion but may be plicated and interdigitated from the level of the nucleus to the basal lamina. The intercellular cleft in the upper half of the epithelium is 15–20 nm wide and sealed, near the lumen, by a zonula occludens. The width of the intercellular cleft in the lower half of the epithelium depends on the functional state of the gallbladder. It is narrow in the inactive condition but distended when bile is being concentrated by transport of water across the epithelium.

Near the neck of the gallbladder, there are simple tubuloalveolar glands in the lamina propria and extending into the muscular layer. Their epithelium is cuboidal with an unstained apical region and nucleus that is compressed at the base by accumulated secretion, which is a form of mucus. Larger inpocketings of the mucosa in this region have sometimes been mistaken for glands. They extend through the lamina propria and muscular

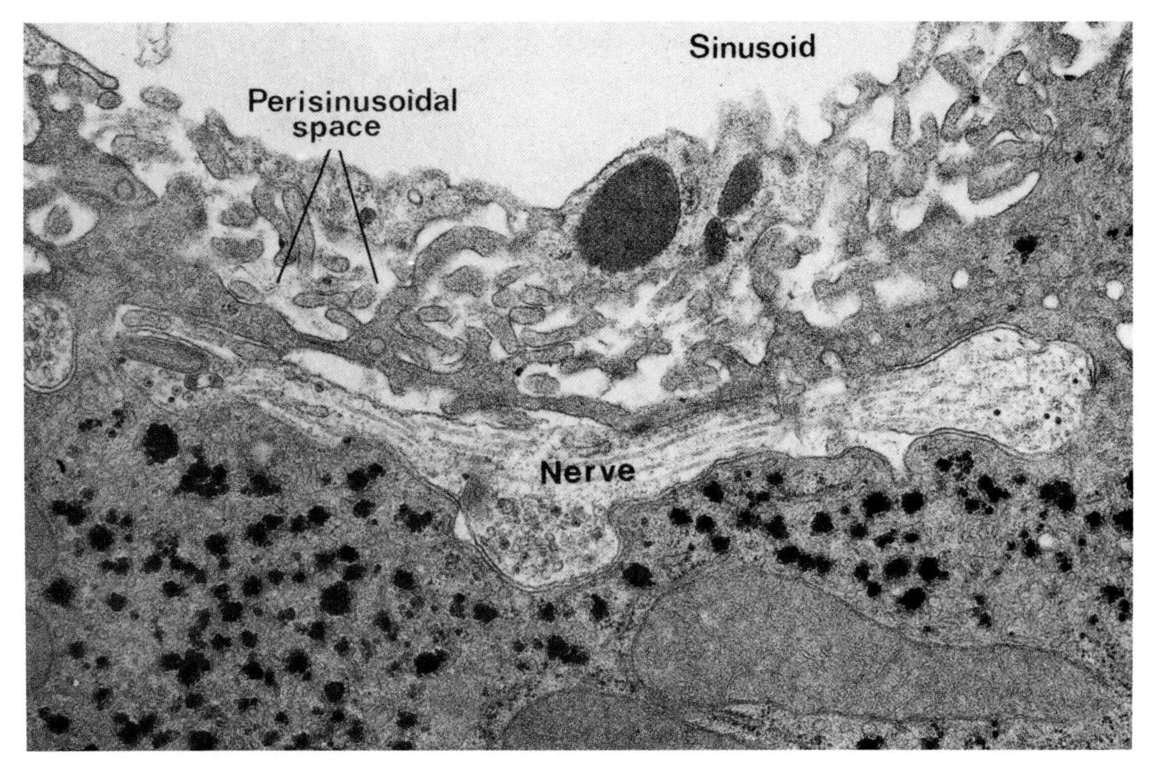

Figure 27–30. In some species, nerve axons terminating on hepatic cells can be found in the space of Disse. Note the synaptic vesicles in the nerve adjacent to the hepatocyte. (Micrograph courtesy of E. Weihe and G. Metz.)

layer, with a lining that is continuous with the surface epithelium. They are called *Rokitansky–Aschoff sinuses* and may represent a pathological change in the gallbladder wall that permits evagination of the mucosa though enlarged meshes of the submucosal smooth muscle.

The muscle layer of the gallbladder wall is an irregular loose network of longitudinal transverse, and oblique bundles of smooth muscle cells. Spaces between the bundles are occupied by collagenous and elastic fibers and occasional fibroblasts. External to the muscularis is a fairly dense connective tissue layer, rich in collagen and elastin and containing fibroblasts, macrophages, and occasional clusters of adipose cell. The blood vessels, nerves, and lymphatics of the organ run in this layer and send branches through the muscular layer to the mucosa.

Not infrequently, peculiar duct-like structures may be found on the hepatic surface of the gallbladder near its neck. They can be traced in the connective tissue for a considerable distance but none open into the lumen. Some appear to connect with the bile ducts. They are called *Luschka ducts* and may be aberrant bile ducts formed during embryonic life and persisting in the adult.

The *cystic duct* continues from the neck of the gallbladder for 3–4 cm and joins the *common hepatic duct* (common bile duct) which courses downward behind the head of the pancreas, approaching the pancreatic duct. The two pass together through the muscularis of the duodenum. In their oblique course through the submucosa, the two ducts unite to form the *ampulla of Vater* (*hepatopancreatic ampulla*) which opens into the lumen of the duodenum at the tip of a small papilla. In the wall of the duodenum, the bile and pancreatic ducts are encircled by a band of smooth muscle called the sphincter of Oddi. This muscle complex consists of four parts: (1) a strong circular band of smooth muscle, the *sphincter choledochus* around the terminal portion of the bile duct; (2) a corresponding *sphincter pancreaticus* around the pancreatic duct; (3) longitudinal bundles of smooth muscle, the fasciculus longitudinalis in the space between the ducts; and (4) a meshwork of muscle fibers around the ampulla, the *sphincter ampullae*. The de-

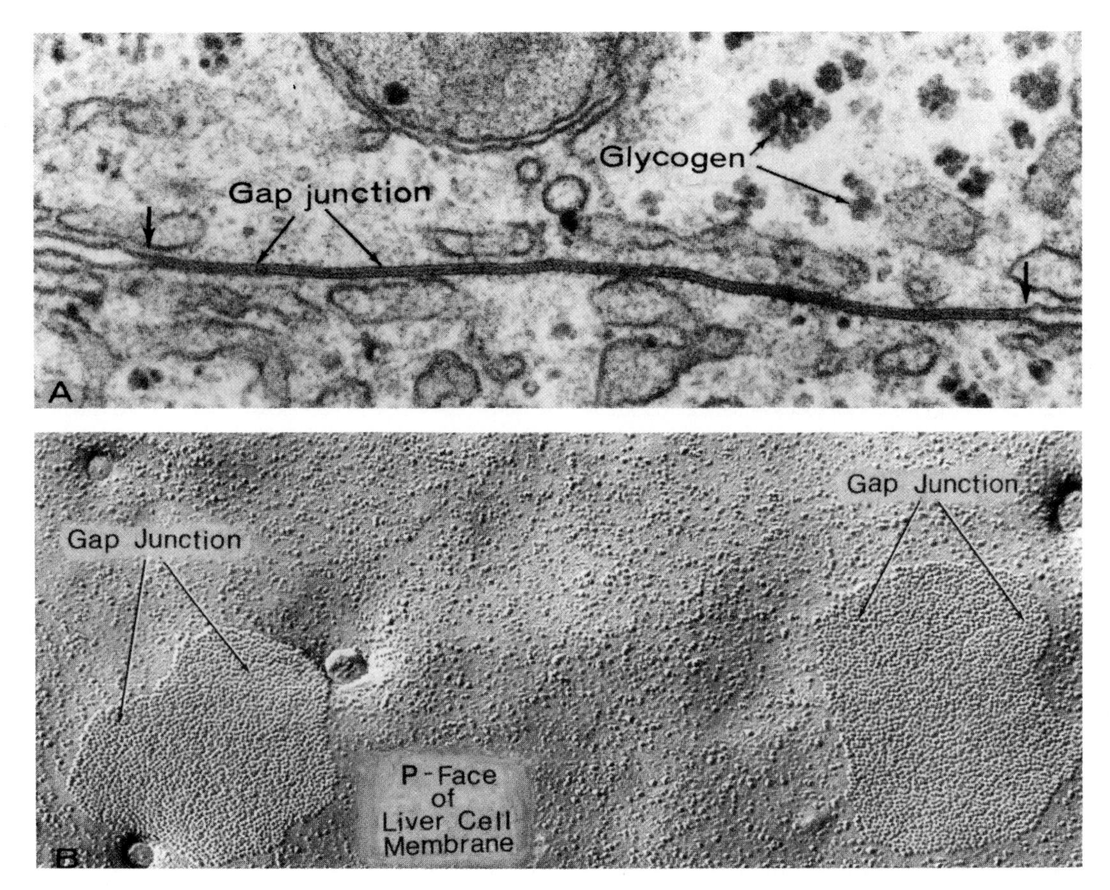

Figure 27–31. Hepatocytes are in communication via gap junctions. (A) Boundary between two hepatocytes showing the membranes converging (at arrows) and coming into close apposition at a nexus, or gap junction. (B) Replica of a liver cell membrane freeze-fractured to show its P-face. In addition to the randomly distributed intramembrane particles, there are two gap junctions exhibiting closely packed particles of uniform size. [(A) Micrograph by R. Wood; (B) micrograph by A. Yee.)]

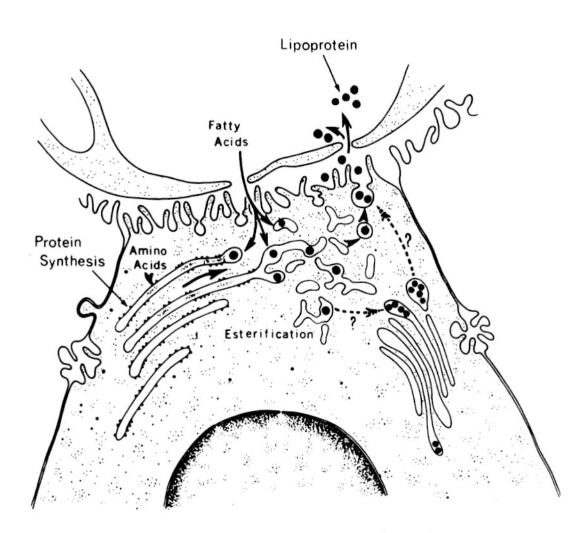

Figure 27–32. Diagram of the intracellular pathway of synthesis and release of very low-density serum lipoprotein. Fatty acids from the blood are esterified in the smooth endoplasmic reticulum to form triglycerides. These are combined, in the Golgi, with protein synthesized in the rough endoplasmic reticulum and the resulting particles are released into the blood via the space of Disse.

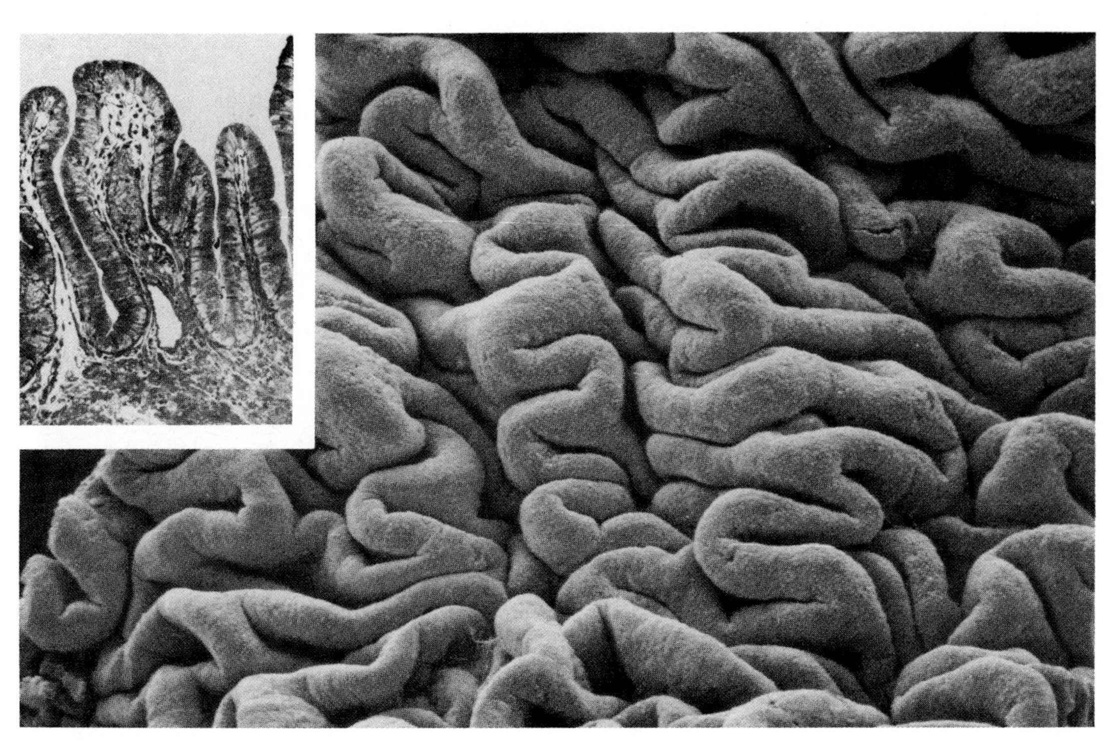

Figure 27–33. Scanning micrograph of the contracted gallbladder. The mucosa is in the form of highly convoluted folds. A histological section has the appearance shown in the inset. Compare with the distended gallbladder, Fig. 27–34. (Micrographs from Castellucci, M. 1980. J. Submicrosc. Cytol. 12:375.)

gree of development of these components of the sphincter of Oddi are subject to great individual variation. Normally, contraction of the sphincter choledochus stops the flow of bile. The longitudinal fasciculi shorten the intramural portion of the ducts and probably facilitate the flow of bile into the duodenum. When the sphincter ampullae is unusually well developed, its contraction may have the undesirable effect of causing reflux of bile into the pancreatic duct, resulting in pancreatitis.

BLOOD VESSELS, LYMPHATICS, AND NERVES

The gallbladder is supplied with blood by the cystic artery. The venous blood is collected

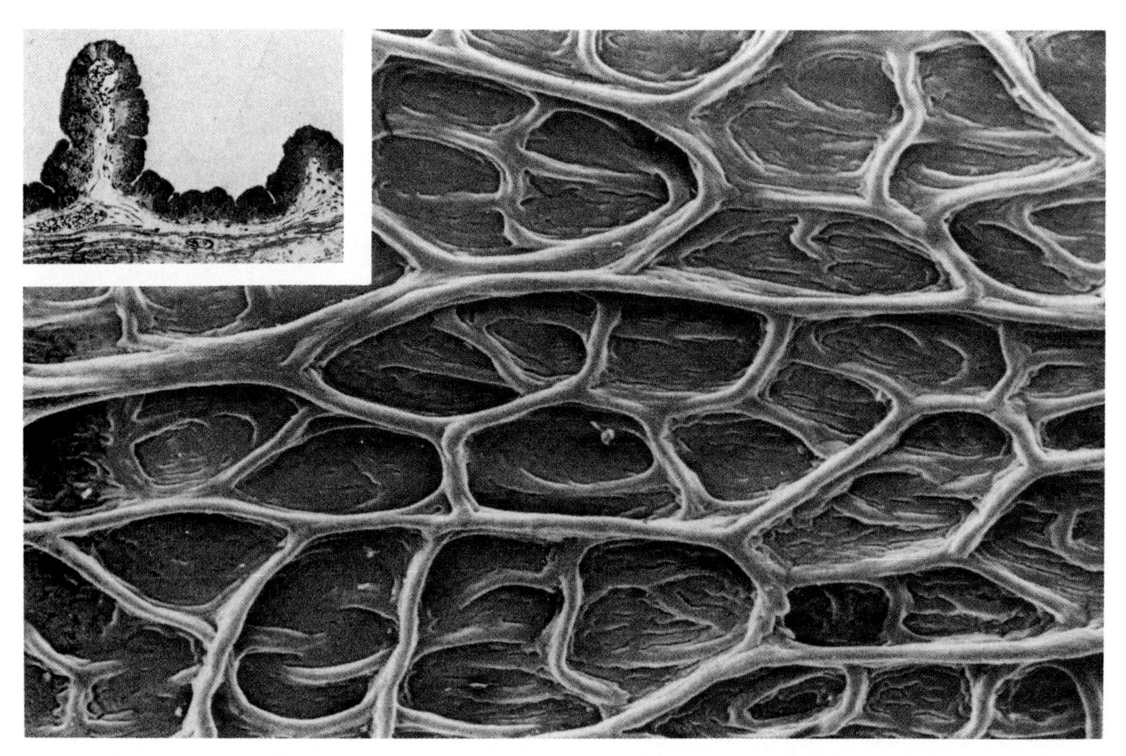

Figure 27–34. Scanning micrograph of the mucosa of a normally distended gallbladder. Relatively low folds form a network with polygonal meshes. A histological section has the appearance shown in the inset. Compare with Fig. 27–33. (Micrograph from Castellucci, M. 1980. J. Submicrosc. Cytol. 12:375.)

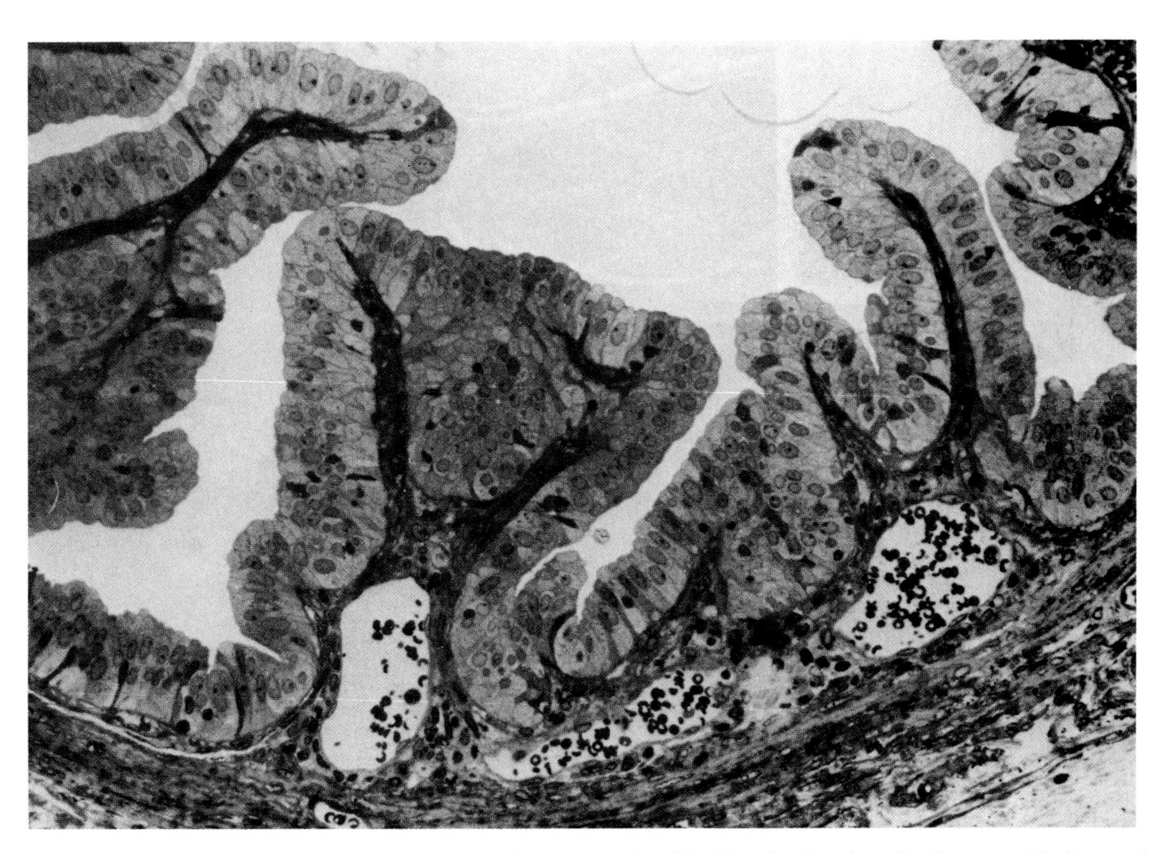

Figure 27–35. Photomicrograph of the mucosa of the contracted gallbladder showing the tall columnar epithelium and the thin-walled blood vessels in the lamina propria. (Photomicrograph from Castellucci, M. 1980. J. Submicrosc. Cytol. 12:375.)

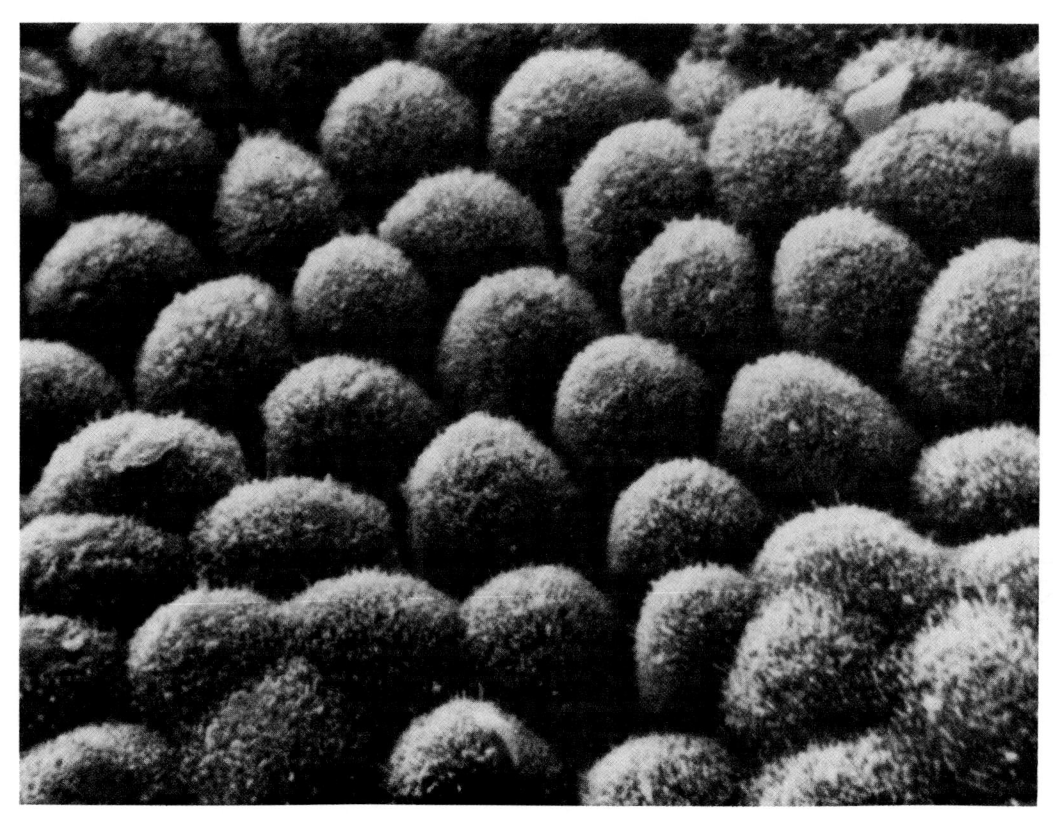

Figure 27–36. Scanning electron micrograph of the luminal surface of the gallbladder epithelium. The convex apical ends of the cells are covered with short microvilli. (Micrograph from Mueller, J.C., A.L. Jones, and J. Long. 1972. Gastroenterology 63:856. Copyright © The Williams and Wilkins Co., Baltimore, MD.)

by veins that empty, for the most part, into small veins of the liver with only a few joining the cystic branch of the portal vein. There is a rich supply of lymphatic vessels deployed in two plexuses, one in the lamina propria and the other in the outer connective tissue layer. The latter receives tributaries from the liver, thus affording a pathway that accounts for the cholecystitis often associated with hepatitis. These lymphatic plexuses drain into larger lymphatics that pass to the lymph node or nodes at the neck of the gallbladder. The efferent lymph from these flows in lymphatics that accompany the cystic and common ducts and, after traversing several nodes near the duodenum, empties into the cisterna chyli.

The nerves of the gallbladder are branches of the splanchnic sympathetic and vagus nerves. Reports of the effects of stimulating these nerves have been contradictory but it is probable that both contain excitatory and inhibitory fibers. Of greater clinical importance are the sensory nerve endings because overdistension of the gallbladder or spasm of the extrahepatic biliary tract may initiate reflex disturbances in the gut.

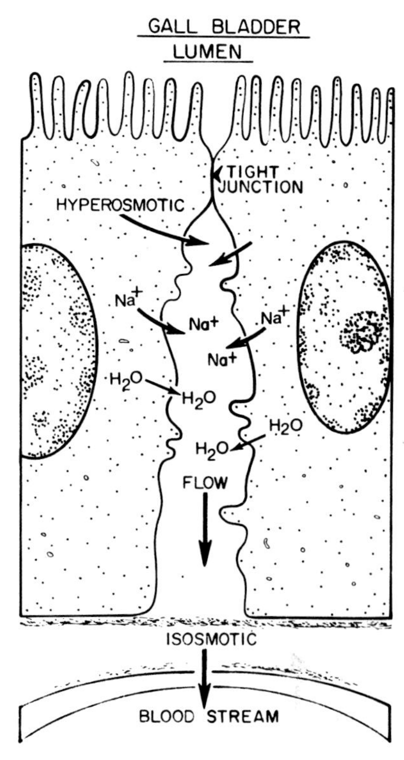

Figure 27–37. Diagram illustrating the mechanism of concentration of the bile. Sodium is actively pumped into the intercellular cleft below the occluding junction, creating a standing gradient that moves water from the lumen to blood vessels in the lamina propria.

HISTOPHYSIOLOGY OF THE GALLBLADDER

The function of the gallbladder is to store and concentrate the bile that is continually secreted by the liver and to release it in response to hormones signaling the presence of food in the duodenum. The entry of food causes certain enteroendocrine cells in the intestinal mucosa to release *cholecystokinin.* Carried in the blood to the gallbladder, this hormone induces rhythmic contractions of its wall. As waves of smooth muscle relaxation pass the ampulla of Vater in duodenal peristalsis, the sphincter of Oddi relaxes, permitting intermittent outflow of bile.

The mechanism by which the gallbladder concentrates bile has much in common with that in other epithelia that transport ions and water at high rates, namely, renal proximal tubule, small intestine, and choroid plexus. This function of the epithelium depends on differences in the biochemical properties of the apical and basolateral membranes of its cells. Ion channels present in the apical membrane permit free passage of Na^+ ions and the basolateral membranes contain Na^+K^+-pumps that actively transport Na^+ into the extracellular space (Figs. 27–37 and 27–38). The increased concentration of solute there creates a concentration gradient that moves water across the epithelium, thereby concentrating the bile in the lumen.

The functional capacity of the gallbladder is assessed clinically by observing its ability to concentrate halogen salts of phenophthalein that are radio-opaque. Failure to clearly visualize the gallbladder in X-rays, taken in the course of this test, indicates that the organ has lost its concentrating power.

BIBLIOGRAPHY

LIVER

Lobule and Its Zonation

Elias, H. 1949. A re-examination of the structure of the mammalian liver. I. Parenchymal architecture. II. The hepatic lobule and its relation to the vascular and biliary systems. Am. J. Anat. 84:311; 85:379.

Gumucio, J.J. and D.L. Miller. 1981. Functional implications of liver cell heterogeniety. Gastroenterology 80:393.

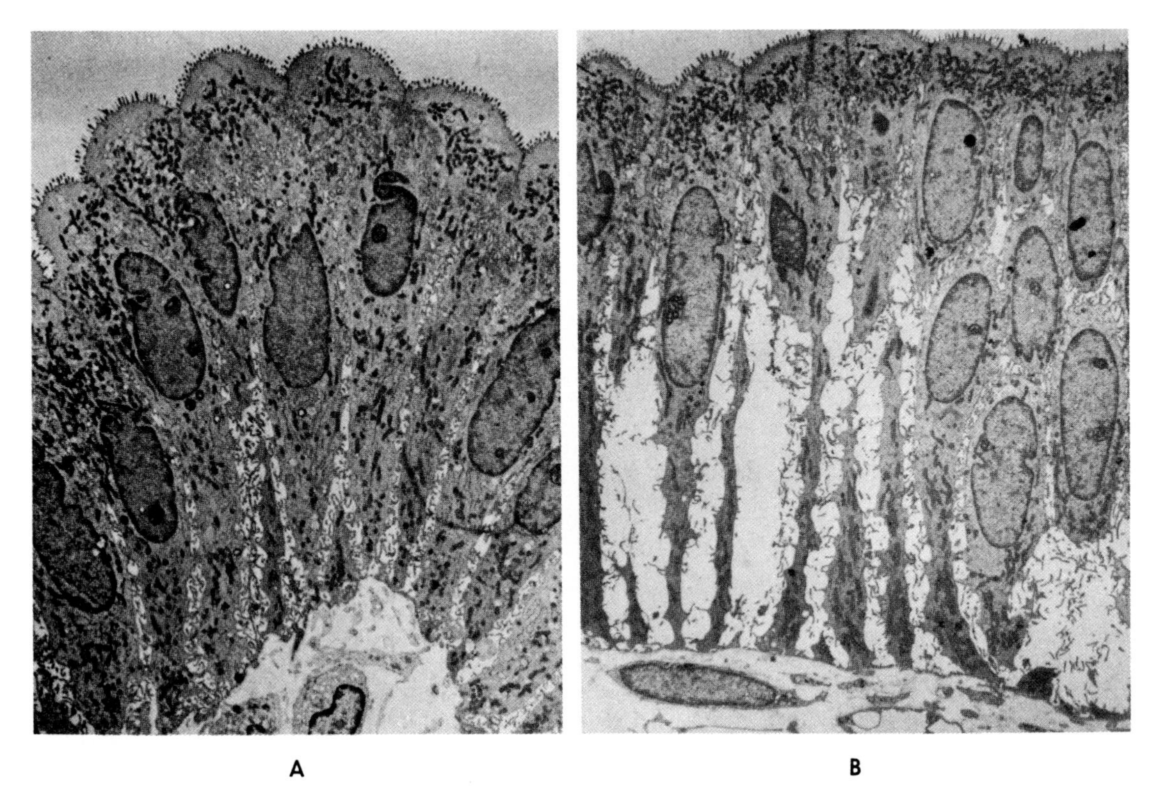

Figure 27–38. Photomicrograph of rabbit gallbladder epithelium. (A) With hyperosmotic solution in the lumen, the net water flux is very low and the intercellular clefts are relatively inconspicuous. (B) In a gallbladder actively moving water and concentrating the bile, the intercellular spaces are greatly distended. (From Kaye, G. 1966. J. Cell Biol. 30:237.)

Jungermann, K. and N. Katz. 1989. Functional specialization of different hepatocyte populations. Physiol. Rev. 49:708.

Lamers, W.H., A. Hilberts, E. Furt et al. 1989. Hepatic enzyme zonation: A reevaluation of the concept of the liver acinus. Hepatology 1:72.

Mall, F.P. 1906. A study of the structural unit of the liver. Am. J. Anat. 5:227.

Noel, R. 1923. Recherches histo-physiologique sur la cellule heparic des mammiferes. Arch. Anat. Micr. 19:1.

Rappaport, A.M., Z.J. Borowy, W.M. Lockheed, and W.N. Lotto. 1954. Subdivision of hexagonal liver lobules into a structural and functional unit: Role in hepatic physiology and pathology. Anat. Rec. 119:11.

Blood Supply

Brawer, R.W. 1963. Liver circulation and function. Physiol. Rev. 43:115.

Burkel, W.E. 1970. The fine structure of the terminal branches of the hepatic arterial system of the rat. Anat. Rec. 167:329.

Greenway, C.V. and R.D. Stark. 1971. Hepatic vascular bed. Physiol. Rev. 51:23.

Murikami, T., T. Itoschima, and Y. Schimada. 1974. Peribiliary portal system in the monkey liver as evidenced by the injection replica scanning method. Arch. Histol. Japan 37:245.

Parenchymal Cell

Bruni, C. and K.R. Porter. 1965. The fine structure of the parenchymal cell of the normal rat liver. I. General observations. Am. J. Pathol. 46:691.

Fahimi, H.D. 1969. Cytochemical localization of peroxidatic activity of catalase in rat hepatic microbodies (peroxisomes). J. Cell Biol. 43:275.

Fawcett, D.W. 1955. Observations on the cytology and electron microscopy of hepatic cells. J. Natl. Cancer Inst. 15 (Supp.):1475.

Katsuma, Y., N. Marceau, M. Ohta, and S.W. French. 1988. Cytokeratin intermediate filaments of rat hepatocytes: Different cytoskeletal domains and their three-dimensional structure. Hepatology 8:559.

Novikoff, P.M. and A. Yam. 1978. Sites of lipoprotein particles in normal rat hepatocytes. J. Cell Biol. 76:1.

Ohtani, O. 1988. Three-dimensional organization of the collagen fibrillar framework of human and rat livers. Arch. Histol. Cytol. 51:473.

Stow, J.L., L. Kjellen, E. Unger, M. Hook, and M. Farquhar. 1985. Heparan sulfate proteoglycans are concentrated on the sinusoidal plasmalemmal domain and intracellular organelles of hepatocytes. J. Cell Biol. 100:975.

Kupffer Cell

Crofton, R.W., M.M. Dieselhoff-den-Dulk, and R. van Furth. 1978. The origin, kinetics, and characteristics of Kupffer cells in the normal steady state. J. Exp. Med. 148:1.

Fahimi, H.D. 1970. The fine structural localization of endogenous and exogenous peroxidase activity in Kupffer cells of rat liver. J. Cell Biol. 47:247.

Howard, J.G. 1970. The origin and immunological significance of Kupffer cells. *In* R. van Furth, ed. Mono-

nuclear Phagocytes, p. 178. Oxford, Blackwell Scientific Publications.
von Kupffer, C. 1876. Uber Sternzellen der Leber. Arch. Mikr. Anat. 12:353.
von Kupffer, C. 1899. Uber die sogenannte Sternzellen der Saugethierleber. Arch. Mikr. Anat. 54:254.

Hepatic Sinusoids

Montesane, R. and P. Nicolescu. 1978. Fenestrations in the endothelium of the rat liver sinusoids revealed by freeze–fracture. Anat. Rec. 190:861.
Motta, P. and K.R. Porter. 1974. Structure of the rat liver sinusoids and associated tissue spaces as revealed by scanning electron microscopy. Cell Tissue 148:111.
Vidal-Vanaclocha, F. and E. Barabera-Guillem. 1985. Fenestration pattern in endothelial cells of rat liver sinusoids. J. Ultrastr. Res. 90:115.
Wisse, E. 1970. An electron microscope study of fenestrated endothelial lining of rat liver sinusoids. J. Ultrastr. Res.
Wisse, E. and D.I. Knook. 1982. Investigation of sinusoidal cells: a new approach to the study of liver function. Progr. Liver Res. 6:153.
Wright, P.F., K.F. Smith, W.A. Day, and R. Fraser. 1983. Hepatic sinusoidal endothelium in sheep: an ultrastructural reinvestigation. Anat. Rec. 207:385.

Perisinusoidal Space

Ito, T. 1951. Cytological studies on stellate sells of von Kupffer and fat-storing cells in the capillary wall of the human liver. Acta. Anat. Nippon 26:2.
Ito, T. and S. Shibasaki. 1968. Electron microscopic study of the hepatic sinusoidal wall and the fat-storing cells in the normal human liver. Arch. Histol. Japan 29:137.
Wake, K. 1971. "Sternzellen" in the liver: perisinusoidal cells with special reference to storage of vitamin A. Am. J. Anat. 132:429.
Wake, K. 1980. Perisinusoidal stellate cells (fat-storing cells, interstitial cells, lipocytes), their related structures in and around the liver sinusoids, and vitamin A storing cells in extrahepatic organs. Internat. Rev. Cytol. 66:303.

Lymphatics

Lee, F.C. 1923. On the lymph vessels of the liver. Carnegie Contrib. Embryol. 15:63.
Magari, S., K. Fujikawa, and A. Nishi. 1981. Form, distribution, fine structure, of hepatic lymphatics with special reference to blood vessels and bile ducts. Asian Med. J. 24:254.

Nerves

Forssmann, W.G. and S. Ito. 1977. Hepatic innervation in primates. J. Cell. Biol. 74:299.
Reilly, F.D., A.P. McClusky, and R.S. McClushy. 1978. Intrahepatic distribution of nerves in the rat. Anat. Rec. 191:55.

Liver Regeneration

Bucher, N.L.R. 1967. Experimental aspects of hepatic cell regeneration. N. Engl. J. Med. 277:686.
Harkness, R.D. 1957. Regeneration of liver. Br. Med. Bull. 13:87.

Histophysiology of the Liver

Babcock, M.B. and R.R. Cardell. 1974. Hepatic glycogen patterns in fasted and fed rats. Am. J. Anat. 140:229.
Brown, T.A., M.W. Russell, and J. Mestecky. 1984. Elimination of intestinally absorbed antigen into the bile by IgA. J. Immunol. 132:780.
Cardell, R.R., J. Larner, and M.B. Babcock. 1973. Correlation between structure and glycogen content of livers from rats on a controlled feeding schedule. Anat. Rec. 177:23.
Deane, H.W. 1944. A cytological study of the diurnal cycle of the liver of the mouse in relation to storage and secretion. Anat. Rec. 88:39.
Fischer, M.M., H. Bazin, B. Nagy, and B.J. Underdown. 1979. Biliary transport of IgA; role of secretory component. Proc. Nat. Acad. Sci. USA 76:2008.
Forker, E.L. 1977. Mechanisms of hepatic bile formation. Annu. Rev. Physiol. 39:323.
Hamashima. Y., J.G. Harter, and A.H. Coons. 1964. The localization of albumin and fibrinogen in human liver cells. J. Cell Biol. 20:271.
Jones, A.L. and D.W. Fawcett. 1966. Hypertrophy of the agranular reticulum in hamster liver induced by phenobarbital (with a review of the functions of this organelle in the liver). J. Histochem. Cytochem. 14:251.
Jones, A.L., N.B. Ruderman, and M.G. Herrera. 1967. Electron microscopic and biochemical study of lipoprotein synthesis in isolated perfused rat liver. J. Lipid Res. 8:429.
Jones, A.L. and D.L. Schmucker. 1977. Current concepts of liver structure as related to function. Gastroenterology 73:833.
Jones, A.L. and S.J. Burwen. 1985. Hepatic receptors and their ligands: Problems of intracellular sorting and vectorial movement. Semin. Liver Dis. 2:136.
Mostov, K.E., J.P. Kraehenbuhl, and G. Blobel. 1980. Receptor mediated transcellular transport of immunoglobulin: Synthesis of secretory component. Proc. Natl. Acad Sci. USA 77:7257.
Orrenius, S., J.L. Erickson, and L. Ernster. 1965. Phenobarbital induced synthesis of microsomal drug metabolizing enzyme system and its relationship to the proliferation of the endoplasmic reticulum. J. Cell Biol. 25:627.
Peters, T.B., B. Fleischer, and S. Fleischer. 1971. The biosynthesis of rat serum albumin. IV. Apparent passage through the Golgi apparatus during secretion. J. Biol Chem. 246:240.
Remmer, H. and H.J. Merker. 1965. Effect of drugs on the formation of smooth endoplasmic reticulum and drug metabolizing enzymes. Ann. N.Y. Acad. Sci. 123:79.
Sztyl, E.S., K.E. Howell, and G.E. Palade. 1983. Intracellular and transcellular transport of secretory component and albumin in rat hepatocytes. J. Cell Biol. 97:1583.

GALL BLADDER AND BILE DUCTS

Banfield, W.J. 1975. Physiology of the gall bladder. Gastroenterology 69:770.
Boyden, E.A. 1957. The anatomy of the choledochoduodenal junction in man. Surg. Gyn. Obs. 104:641.
Castellucci, M. and A. Caggiati. 1980. Surface aspects of rabbit gallbladder mucosa and their functional implications. J. Submicrosc. Cytol. 12:375.
Chapman, G.B., A.J. Chiardo, R.J. Coffey, and K. Weineke. 1966. The fine structure of the human gall bladder. Anat. Rec. 154:579.
Diamond, J.M. 1964. Transport of salt and water in rabbit and guinea pig gall bladder. J. Gen. Physiol. 48:1.
Evett, R.D., J.A. Higgins, and A.L. Brown, Jr. 1964. The fine structure of normal mucosa in the human gall bladder. Gastrenterology 47:49.

Hayward, A.F. 1968. The structure of the gall bladder epithelium. Internat. Rev. Gen. Exp. Zool. 3:205.

Kaye, G.I., H.O. Wheeler, R.T. Whitlock, and N. Lane. 1966. Fluid transport in rabbit gall bladder. A combined physiological and electron microscope study. J. Cell Biol. 30:237.

Mueller, J.C., A.L. Jones, and J.A. Long. 1972. Topographical and subcellular anatomy of the guinea-pig gall bladder. Gastroenterology 63:856.

Reves, L. 1989. Ion transport across gall bladder epithelium. Physiol. Rev. 69:503.

28 PANCREAS

The pancreas is a pinkish-white organ lying retroperitoneally on the posterior wall of the abdominal cavity, at the level of the second and third lumbar vertebrae (Fig. 28–1). It is commonly described as having a head, body, and tail. The head is lodged in the concavity of the C-shaped duodenum and its narrower body and tail extend traversely across the posterior wall of the abdomen to the hilus of the spleen. In the adult, it measures 20–25 cm in length and weighs from 100 to 150 g. It is covered by a thin layer of connective tissue which does not form an opaque capsule. The gland is lobulated and the outlines of the larger lobules can be seen with the naked eye.

The pancreas is the second largest gland associated with the alimentary tract. It consists of (1) an *exocrine* portion that secretes daily about 1200 ml of an enzyme-rich fluid required for the digestion of dietary fats, carbohydrates, and proteins and (2) an *endocrine* portion, secreting hormones essential for the control of carbohydrate metabolism.

THE EXOCRINE PANCREAS

ACINAR TISSUE

The pancreas is a compound acinous gland made up of many small lobules bound together by loose connective tissue, through which course the blood vessels, nerves, and interlobular ducts. The acini are round or slightly elongated and consist of 40 to 50 pyramidal epithelial cells around a narrow lumen. The size of the lumen varies with the physiological state of the gland, becoming somewhat wider during active secretion.

In histological sections, the cytoplasm near the base of the acinar cells is strongly basophilic owing to its high concentration of ribonucleoproteins (Fig. 28–2). The spherical nucleus has a prominent nucleolus and peripheral clumps of heterochromatin. There is a less deeply stained supranuclear Golgi region that varies in size in different phases of the secretory cycle. The apical cytoplasm is filled with large numbers of secretory granules containing the precursors of the pancreatic digestive enzymes (Fig. 28–3). These *zymogen granules* are most abundant in acinar tissue fixed during fasting and are noticeably reduced in number after the copious secretion induced by a meal. After depletion of the zymogen granules, the Golgi region enlarges while new secretory granules are being formed.

The intensely basophilic lower portion of the acinar cell is found, in electron micrographs, to be crowded with closely spaced parallel cisternae of granular endoplasmic reticulum (Fig. 28–4). In morphometric studies, this organelle has been shown to occupy about 20% of the cell volume and to present a surface area of some 800 μm^2. The surrounding cytoplasm is rich in free polyribosomes. Here and there, the cisternae diverge to accommodate long mitochondria that have numerous cristae and many matrix granules. The supranuclear Golgi consists of several short stacks of parallel cisternae that have numerous small vesicles associated with the convex cis-face. At the concave trans-face of the stacks, there are a few larger vesicles and condensing vacuoles with a homogeneous content of low density. These represent formative stages of new secretory granules. Occasional lipid droplets and lysosomes may also be found in this region.

Dense membrane-bounded zymogen granules completely fill the apical portion of the cell (Fig. 28–5). In actively secreting cells, these may be found in the process of discharging their content into the lumen of the acinus. Although the term zymogen "granule" implies a solid or semisolid consistency, it is evident in electron micrographs that their content is fluid at the time of release because it appears to flow through the opening formed

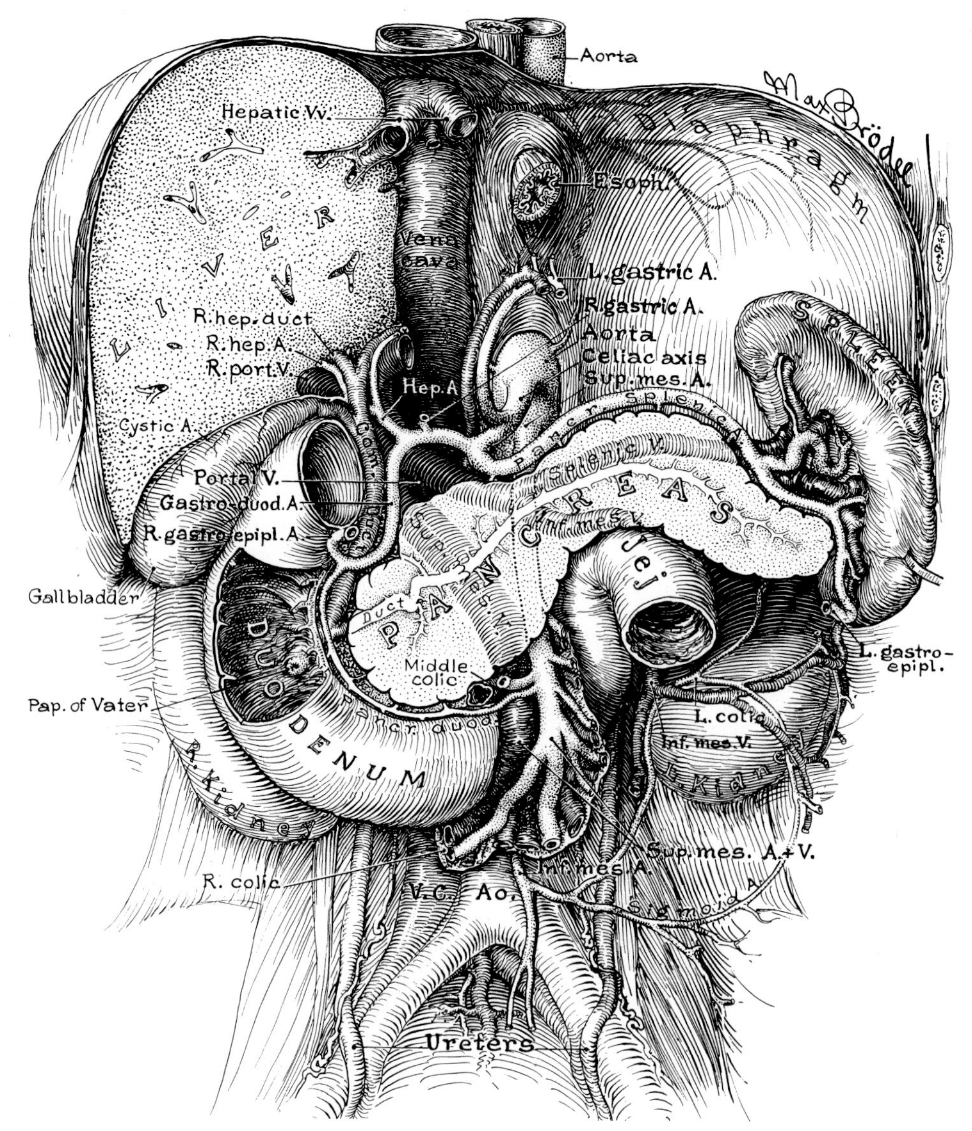

Figure 28–1. Drawing of the upper abdominal viscera, with most of the anterior portion of the liver cut away, to show the location and relationships of the pancreas. (Drawing by M. Brödel, from Trimble, I.R., J.W. Parsons, and C.P. Sherman. 1941. Surg. Gyn. Obstet. 73:711. By permission of Surgery, Gynecology and Obstetrics.)

by fusion of the limiting membrane with the plasmalemma. No granules are seen in the lumen, only a diffuse material of moderate density. Secretory vesicle might be a more appropriate descriptive term than secretory granule. However closely these are crowded together in the apical cytoplasm, they normally remain discrete, but during very active secretion, a second zymogen vesicle may fuse with one engaged in exocytosis, and a third may fuse with the second, so that a series of intercommunicating secretory vesicles is formed that extends some distance down into the apical cytoplasm (Fig. 28–6).

DUCT SYSTEM

The pancreas is unique among compound acinous glands in that low cuboidal or squamous cells lining the duct extend a short distance into the acinus. These so-called *centroacinar cells* are easily identified by their pale staining in histological sections and by their very low density and paucity of cytoplasmic organelles in electron micrographs (Figs. 28–3 and 28–7). The centroacinar cells are continuous with the lining epithelium of slender *intercalated ducts* that drain the acinus (Fig. 28–8). These slender tubes converge to form

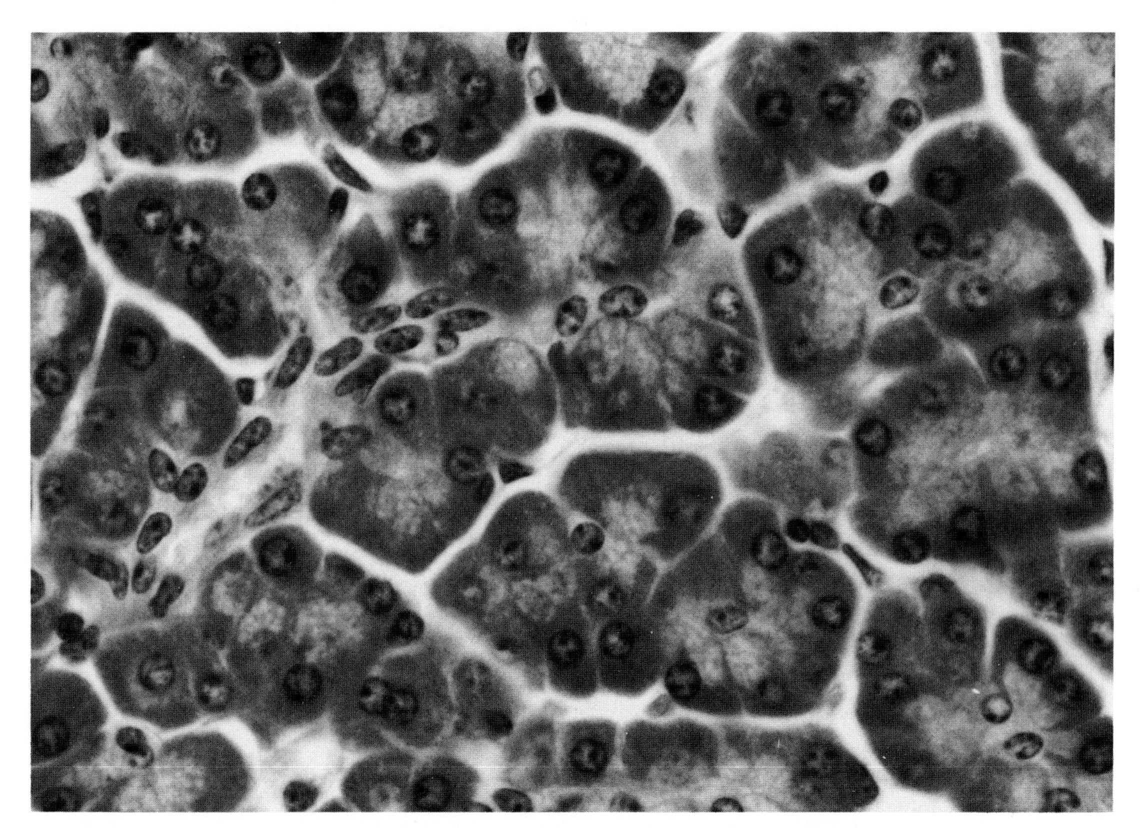

Figure 28–2. Photomicrograph of a section of exocrine pancreas showing the glandular acini and, at the left, a small duct draining three or four acini. Note the intense basophilia of the basal cytoplasm of the cells.

larger *intralobular ducts* that are, in turn, tributaries of *interlobular ducts* in the connective tissue septa between lobules. The latter are lined by a low columnar epithelium containing occasional goblet cells (Fig. 28–9). The smaller ducts of the gland are not simply conduits for the secretory products of the acini. Their lining epithelium is active in transporting water and bicarbonate ions into the lumen, and they make a major contribution to the total volume of pancreatic secretion.

The interlobular ducts join the main pancreatic ducts, of which there are two. The larger, the *duct of Wirsung,* begins in the tail and runs through the length of the gland, gradually increasing in diameter as it is joined by numerous interlobular ducts. In the head of the pancreas, it runs parallel to the common bile duct (ductus choledochus), with which it may have a common opening into the duodenum at the *ampulla of Vater.* The opening and closing of this common outlet is controlled by the *sphincter of Oddi* in its wall. An accessory *duct of Santorini* is nearly always present. It lies cranial to the duct of Wirsung and is about 6 cm in length. These larger pancreatic ducts are lined by a low columnar epithelium containing a moderate number of goblet cells and occasional argentaffin cells. They are enveloped in a substantial layer of connective tissue, containing some smooth muscle fibers and many mast cells.

BLOOD VESSELS, LYMPHATICS, AND NERVES

The pancreas receives its blood supply from numerous branches of the splenic artery and from pancreaticoduodenal branches of the hepatic and superior mesenteric arteries. The larger vessels course through the interlobular septa and give off branches that arborize into rich capillary networks surrounding the acini. The walls of the capillaries, in the exocrine pancreas, have a continuous endothelium, whereas the capillaries of the islets of the endocrine pancreas are fenestrated. The capillary bed of the gland is drained by veins that

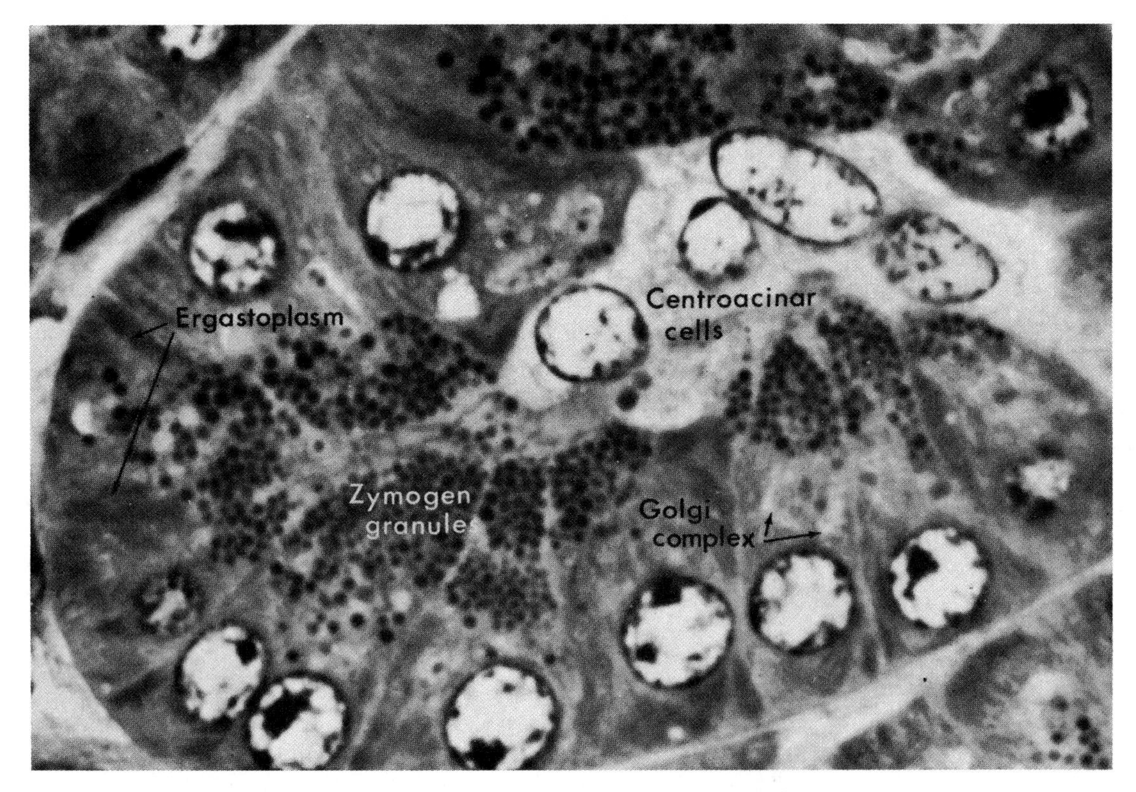

Figure 28–3. Photomicrograph of an acinus from human pancreas. The ergastroplasm, Golgi complex, and zymogen granules are clearly shown, and a few pale centroacinar cells are seen at the upper right. (Courtesy of S. Ito.)

join the portal, splenic, and superior mesenteric veins.

There are lymphatic capillaries that end blindly among the acini and drain via larger lymphatics that follow the course of the blood vessels to reach pancreaticosplenic lymph nodes distributed along the upper border of the gland.

The nerve supply is from the vagus and splanchnic nerves via the splenic nerve plexus. Small clusters of autonomic ganglion cells are sometimes encountered in histological sections of the acinar tissue. In electron micrographs, axons are occasionally observed penetrating the basal lamina and ending in intimate contact with the base of an acinar cell. These are probably terminations of branches of the vagus nerve because stimulation of the vagus results in exocytosis and accumulation of secretion in the lumen of the acini and in small ducts. However, there is little outflow of secretion from the gland under these circumstances because only very small amounts of water and electrolytes are added to the secretion. Nervous regulation of pancreatic secretion is thought to be of less importance than its hormonal regulation.

HISTOPHYSIOLOGY OF THE EXOCRINE PANCREAS

Few cells produce as great a quantity and variety of proteins as do those of the exocrine pancreas. For this reason, the acinar cells have been the subject of intensive ultrastructural and biochemical study to establish the respective roles of the cell organelles in the synthesis of protein. The findings of these investigations have been presented in some detail in Chapter 3 on glands and secretion and need only be briefly reviewed here.

The sites of synthesis are the *ribosomes* bound to the membrane of the endoplasmic reticulum. In polyribosomes, these units are joined together by their binding to a thin strand of *messenger RNA* that encodes the information necessary for the sequential assembly of amino acids into a specific protein. As the ribosomes move along the messenger RNA molecule, its base sequence is translated by *transfer RNA* into the amino-acid sequence of the protein. The nascent protein molecule is directed vectorially from the ribosome and, traversing the underlying membrane of the reticulum, it is ultimately set free in its lumen.

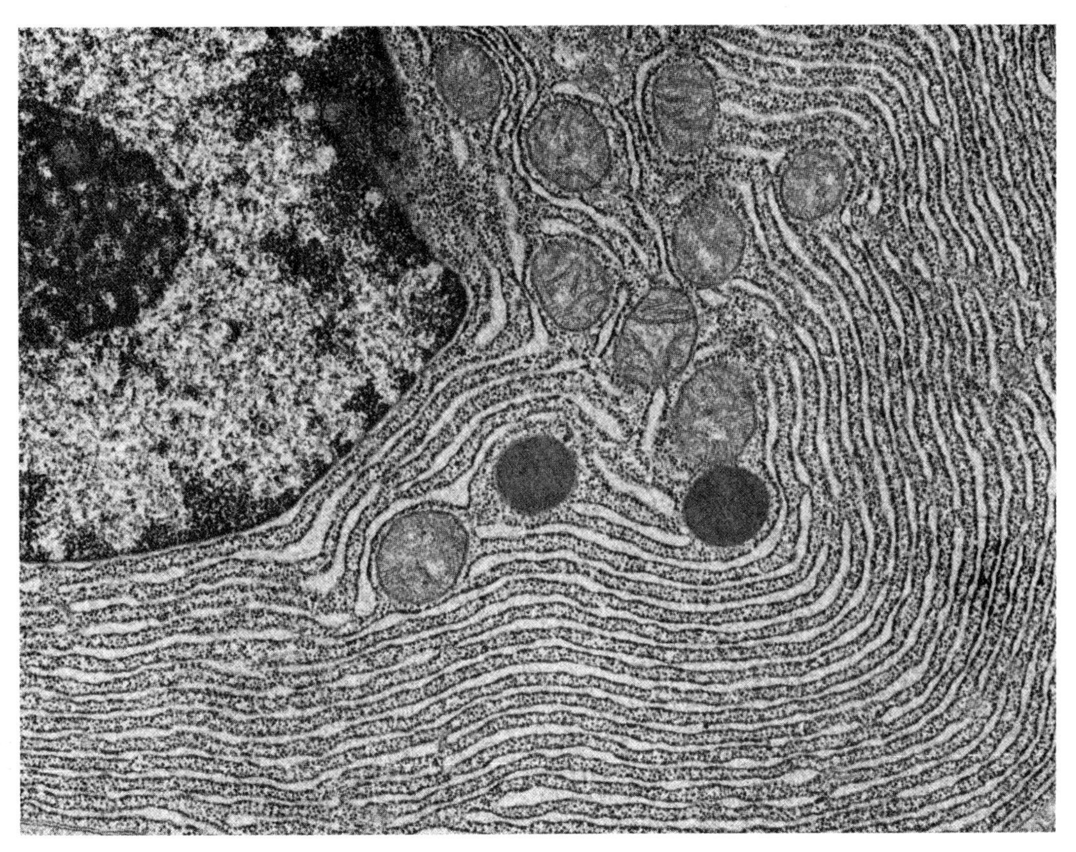

Figure 28–4. Electron micrograph of the basal region of a pancreatic acinar cell showing a portion of the nucleus and the closely packed cisternae of rough endoplasmic reticulum characteristic of these cells. (Micrograph courtesy of A. Like and S. Ito.)

In the pancreatic acinar cell, translation of a dozen or more different messenger RNAs yields a great variety of protein products, including the proenzymes and enzymes: *trypsinogen, chymotrypsinogen, procarboxypeptidase, ribonuclease, deoxyribonuclease, lipase, elastase, amylase, trypsin inhibitor,* for secretion. The completed protein molecules are packaged in small vesicles that bud from ribosome-free transitional domains of the endoplasmic reticulum. These vesicles fuse with a cistern on the cis-face of the Golgi stacks. In transit through this organelle, some proteins are converted into glycoproteins by glycosyl transferase; others are not significantly modified. Sorting of the products of protein synthesis takes place in the trans-Golgi network, where certain glycoproteins are segregated in vesicles targeted to the plasmalemma to contribute to its protein constituents. Other proteins, destined to be secreted, are enclosed in vesicles that coalesce to form condensing vacuoles. These gradually take on the appearance of mature zymogen granules and move into the apical cytoplasm for temporary storage.

The acinar cells secrete enzymes for digestion of protein, lipid, carbohydrate, and other constituents of the food ingested. To protect the integrity of the gland itself, it is essential that these be produced in an inactive form and be activated only after they are secreted into the lumen of the intestine. Thus, trypsin, which is the most abundant pancreatic enzyme, is synthesized as inactive trypsinogen, and so also for the other enzymes. As an additional safeguard, the cytoplasm of the acinar cells contains *trypsin inhibitor,* a protein produced concurrently with the digestive enzymes. However, in rare instances, these security measures may fail leading to *acute pancreatitis,* a condition in which proteolytic enzymes are activated and the pancreas is rapidly digested by its own enzymes, often with fatal outcome.

The secretory activity of the pancreas has a rhythmical cycle, with a low basal rate of

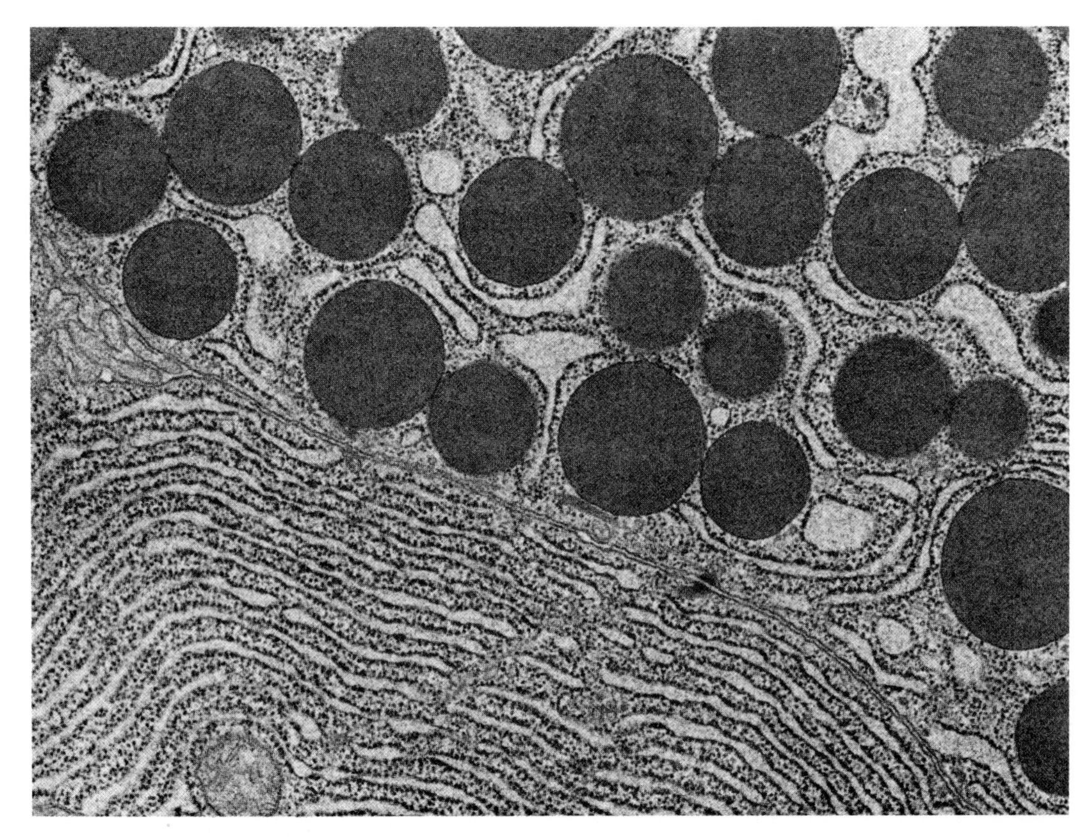

Figure 28–5. Micrograph of portions of two adjacent human pancreatic acinar cells. Below is the endoplasmic reticulum of the paranuclear region of one cell, and above is the apical region of the other cell, filled with zymogen granules and tubules of the reticulum. (Micrograph courtesy of A. Like and S. Ito.)

continuous secretion, which is greatly increased periodically by hormonal stimulation associated with the ingestion of food. The presence of food in the gastric antrum and the passage of acidic products of gastric digestion into the duodenum stimulate release of two intestinal hormones, *secretin* and *cholecystokinin*. Secretin is a small peptide of 27 amino acids. When carried in the bloodstream to the pancreas, it stimulates the secretion of a large volume of fluid, containing a high concentration of bicarbonate. It does not stimulate the acinar cells. Instead, this fluid is produced mainly by the epithelial lining of the smaller ducts and it has little or no enzymatic activity. The copious alkaline fluid produced serves to neutralize the acidic chyme entering the intestine from the stomach and creates the neutral or alkaline pH required for optimal activity of digestive enzymes secreted under the influence of cholecystokinin.

Cholecystokinin is a peptide hormone of 33 amino acids secreted by the mucosa of the duodenum and upper jejunum. Food entering these segments of the intestine stimulates its release. When transported, in the blood, to the pancreas it binds to specific receptors in the basolateral membranes of the acinar cells and induces their release of highly concentrated digestive enzymes. Acting alone, it does not significantly increase the outflow from the pancreatic ducts, but its coordinated action with secretin results in secretion of a large volume of enzyme-rich pancreatic juice.

THE ENDOCRINE PANCREAS

ISLETS OF LANGERHANS

The endocrine tissue of the pancreas is segregated in relatively small aggregations of cells forming the *islets of Langerhans* (Fig. 28–10). These are not distinguishable with the naked eye, but if the gland is perfused with a dilute solution of the dye neutral red, the islets are selectively stained and their number and distribution can be studied. They are scattered

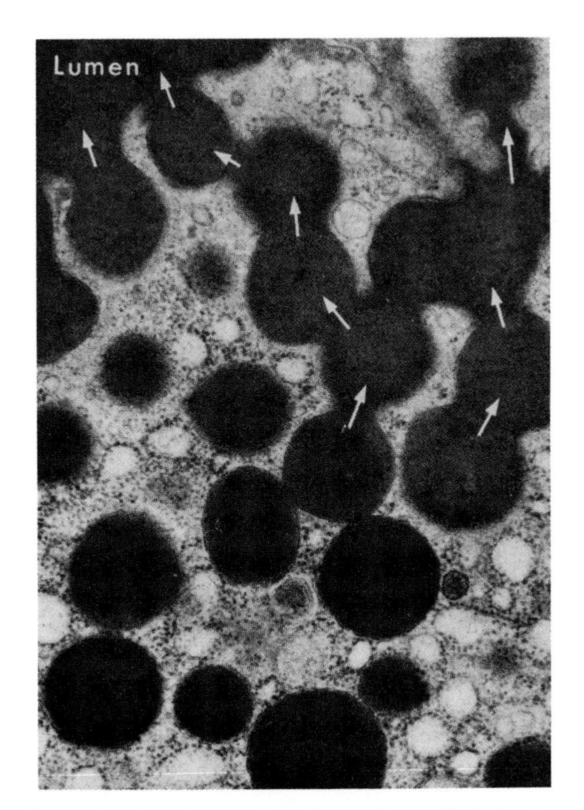

Figure 28–6. Apical portion of an acinar cell of the dog pancreas. In the strongly stimulated cell, a zymogen droplet opening into the lumen may be confluent with a second, and this with a third, so that their contents are discharged through several intercommunicating secretory vacuoles. Normally, the zymogen granules are probably discharged individually. (After Ichikawa, A.J. 1965. J. Cell Biol. 24:369.)

throughout the gland but are somewhat more numerous in the tail than in the body and head of the gland. There is estimated to be over a million islets in the human pancreas, but owing to their small size, they constitute only 1–2% of the volume of the gland. Each islet is composed of 2 to 3 thousand cells which have been described as being arranged in anastomosing cords or plates. However, three-dimensional reconstruction of islets from serial sections reveals no such architecture. They are simply a compact mass of epithelial cells pervaded by a labyrinthine network of capillaries. The cells are polarized toward the capillaries. The islets are demarcated from the surrounding acinar tissue by a thin layer of reticular fibers that extend inward to form a delicate investment around the capillaries.

The islets of Langerhans contain four principal types of cells, each secreting a different hormone: *α-cells* (A-cells) secreting *glucagon; β-cells* (B-cells) secreting *insulin*; *δ-cells* (D-cells) secreting *somatostatin;* and *F-cells* (PP-cells) secreting *pancreatic polypeptide.* These cannot be distinguished in routine hematoxylin and eosin preparations, but separate methods have been devised for selectively staining the α-, β-, and δ-cells. In islets stained by the aldehyde-fuchsin trichrome method, the beta cells are deeply colored (Fig. 28–11) With the Grimelius silver-impregnation technique, the α-cells are blackened (Fig. 28–12A), and with the Hellerstrom–Hellman silver method the δ-cells are selectively impregnated (Fig. 28–12B). These classical techniques are now seldom used. In their stead, it is common practice to use fluorescein-conjugated antibodies to the three hormones for definitive identification of their cells of origin.

The α-cells are located mainly at the periphery of the islet, but a few are scattered along the capillaries in its interior. The β-cells are the predominant cell type in the islet, occupying its center and making up 70% of its mass. The F-cells are widely scattered, very few in number, and may occur among the acini as well as in the islets.

The ultrastructure of the major cell types of the islets has been studied in some detail. They all have the complement of organelles we have come to expect of protein-secreting epithelial cells, but the granular endoplasmic reticulum is far less extensive than that of the acinar cells. The mitochondria vary somewhat in length but have the usual internal structure. Small vesicles and nascent secretory granules are associated with a juxtanuclear Golgi complex. The only distinctive features that permit identification of the cell types in electron micrographs are differences in size, density, and internal structure of the secretory granules.

After aldehyde fixation, the numerous granules of the α-cells have homogeneous cores of high electron density surrounded by a narrow outer zone of lower density. After primary osmium tetroxide fixation, the material of the outer zone is extracted leaving a clear space between the dense core of the granule and its limiting membrane (Fig. 28–13). The β-cell granules in the human, cat, and dog are quite distinctive, containing one or more dense crystals in a matrix of low density. The crystals are rectangular or polygonal in section and, at very high magnification, have a very regular periodic substructure. The amorphous matrix in which they are embedded is often extracted in specimen preparations, in which case the crystals stand out

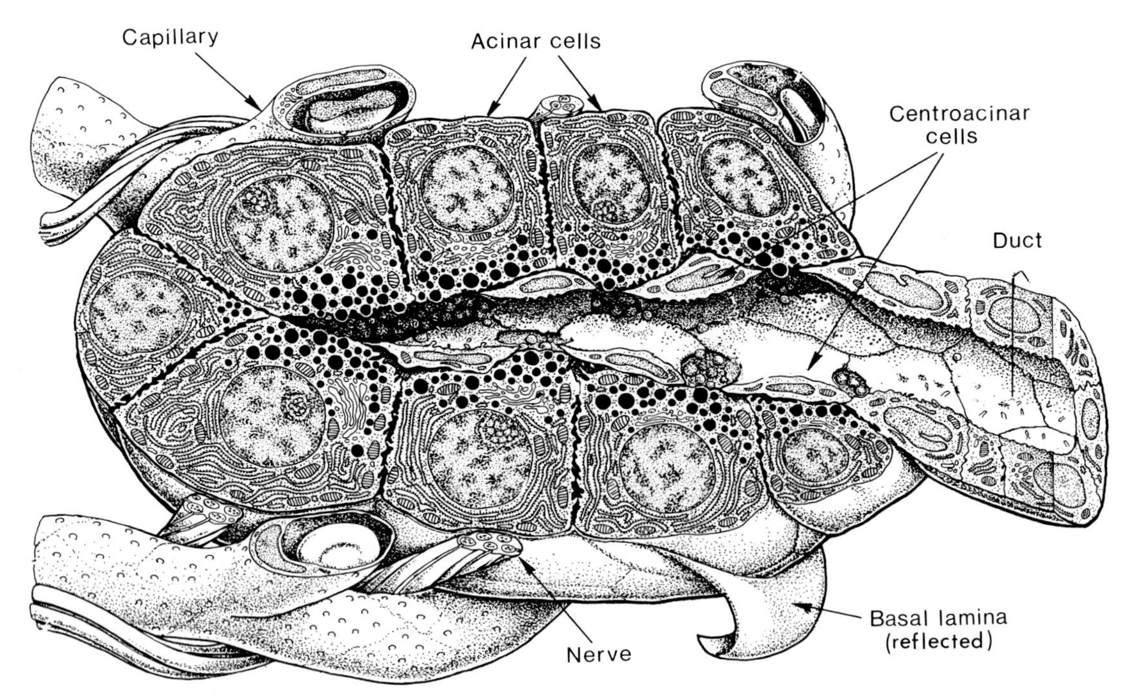

Figure 28–7. Drawing of a pancreatic acinus and its associated capillaries and nerve. Note an incomplete layer of centroacinar cells lining the distal portion of the lumen. (Reproduced from Krstić, R.V. 1978. Die Gewebe des Menschen und Saugetiere. Berlin, Springer-Verlag.)

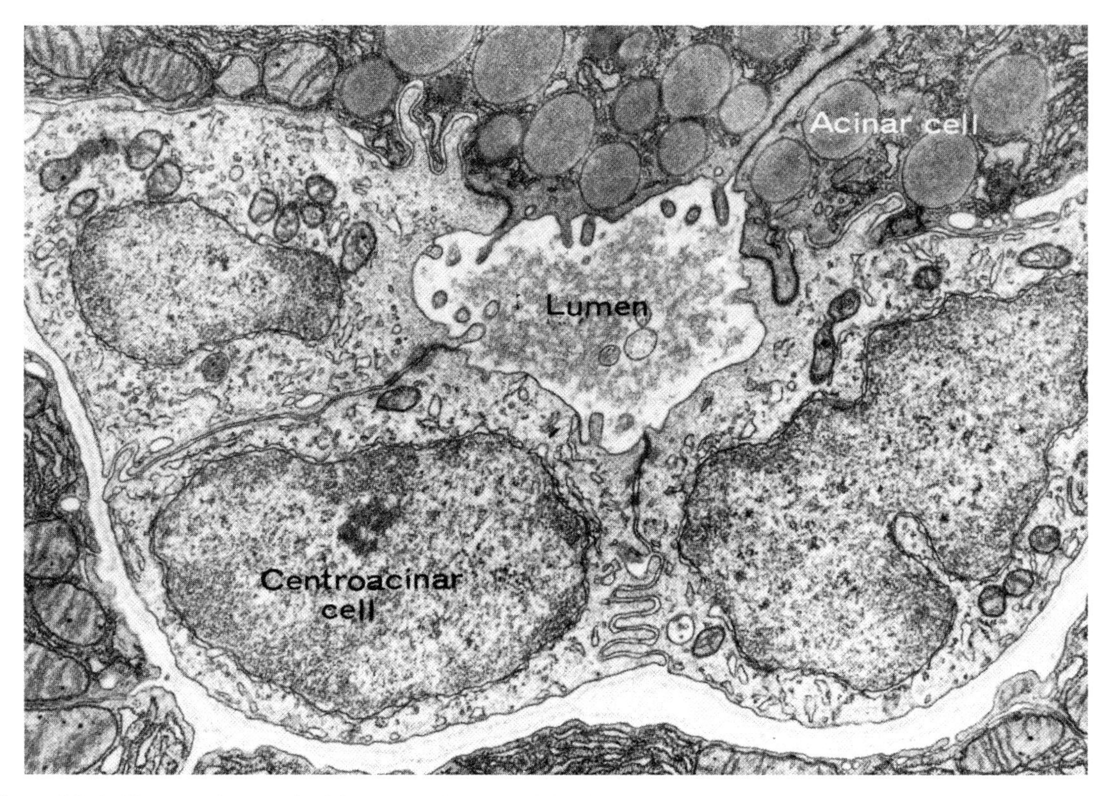

Figure 28–8. Electron micrograph of the terminal portion of the duct system of the guinea pig pancreas showing a lumen bounded, on one side, by acinar cells and, on the other side, by centroacinar cells. (From Bolender, R.P. 1974. J. Cell Biol. 61:269.)

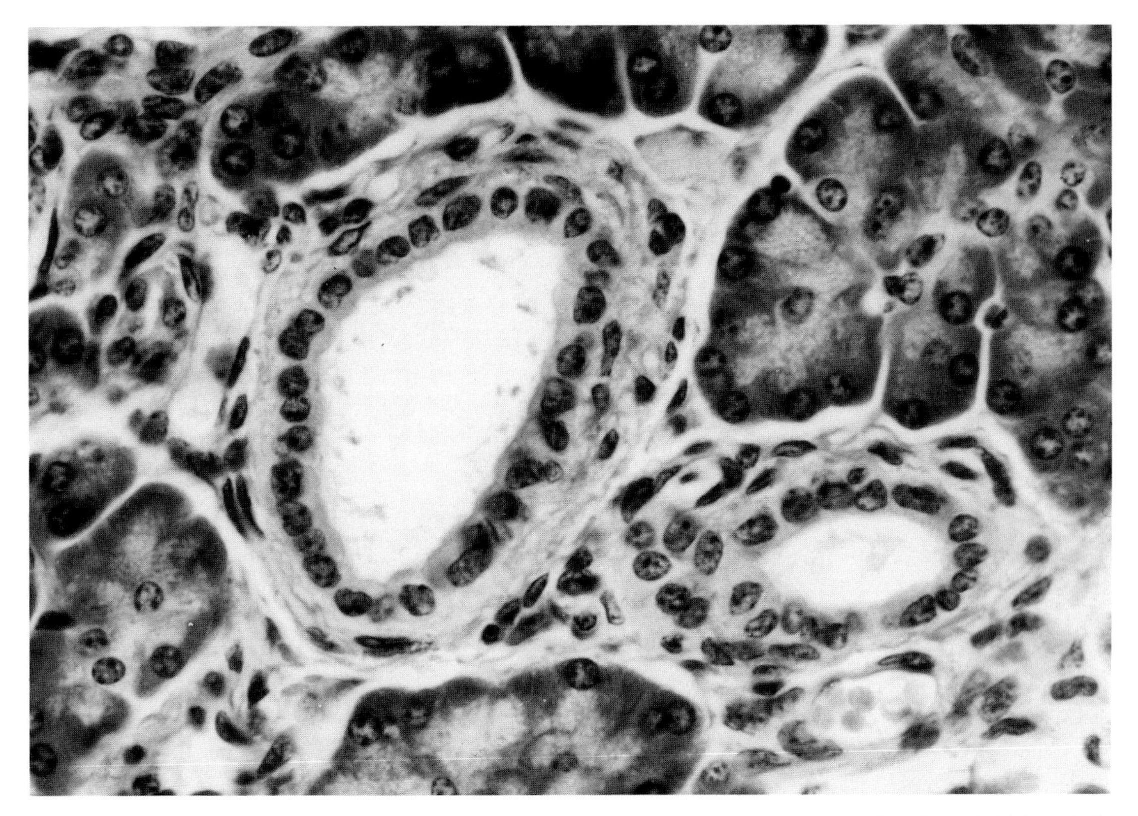

Figure 28–9. Photomicrograph of a section of pancreas including two small interlobular ducts lined by cuboidal epithelium.

in sharp contrast against a clear background within their loose-fitting limiting membrane (Fig. 28–14). There is considerable interspecific variation in the appearance of the β-cell granules. In a number of animal species, no crystals are discernible and the granules are difficult to distinguish from those of the β-cells which exhibit more variation in size and in the electron density of their homogeneous content than those of the α-cells (Fig. 28–15). In all islet cell types, the content of the secretory granules is released by exocytosis into the extracellular space where it disperses to act on neighboring islet cells or to enter the blood through the pores in the adjacent capillaries.

Axons of sympathetic and parasympathetic nerves can be found terminating among the cells of the islets of Langerhans. In animal experiments, sympathetic stimulation is reported to diminish secretion of insulin and parasympathetic stimulation to promote secretion. However, it is questionable whether the autonomic nervous system plays an important role in islet cell function under physiological conditions.

HISTOPHYSIOLOGY OF THE ENDOCRINE PANCREAS

The major product of carbohydrate digestion in the alimentary tract is *glucose,* which is utilized as an energy source in cell metabolism throughout the body. The hormones secreted by the principal cell types in the islets of Langerhans are all involved in the control of the level of glucose in the blood.

Insulin is a polypeptide consisting of a chain of 21 amino acids (α-chain) and a chain of 30 amino acids (β chain) linked together by two disulfide bridges. It is an essential hormone directly or indirectly affecting cell function in nearly every organ. Research in recent years on the β-cells of the islets has provided a rather clear picture of the intracellular pathway of insulin production. A much larger precursor, *pre-proinsulin,* is assembled on the ribosomes of the endoplasmic reticulum. A short amino-acid sequence on this polypeptide participates in its translocation across the membrane of the reticulum. In the lumen, this sequence is removed by *cleaving enzymes* to

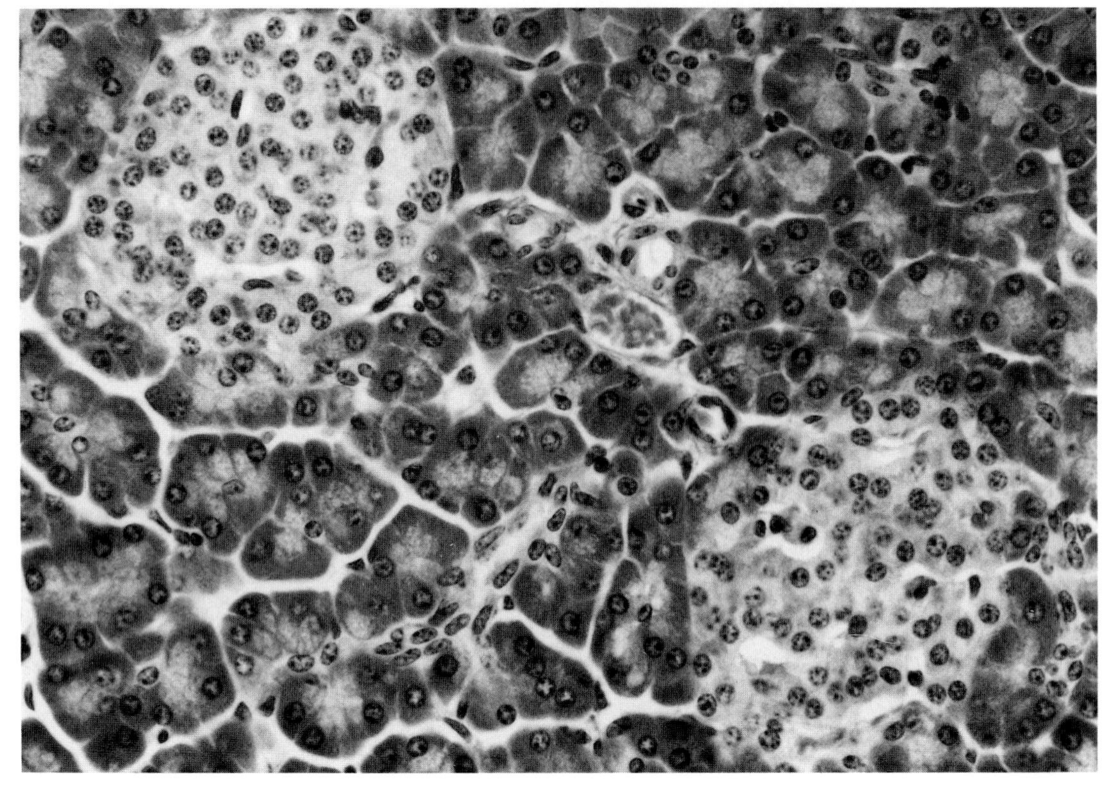

Figure 28–10. Photomicrograph of a section of pancreas including two islets of Langerhans.

yield *proinsulin,* a single polypeptide chain of 73 amino acids made up of the α-and β-chains of insulin and an intervening *connecting peptide* (C-peptide). Proinsulin, together with its cleaving enzymes, is transported to the Golgi apparatus in small vesicles that bud off the cisternae of the endoplasmic reticulum and fuse with a cistern on the cis-face of the Golgi. During transport through this organelle, there appears to be little processing of the proinsulin molecule because immunocytochemical studies comparing the localization of precursor and product indicate that little or no insulin is present in the Golgi complex. The conversion of proinsulin to insulin takes place in small clathrin-coated vesicles budded off from the trans-Golgi cisternae. These vesicles containing insulin, C-peptide, and cleaving enzymes then lose their clathrin coat, concentrate their contents, and give rise to secretory granules that are ultimately discharged by exocytosis. For reasons that are still poorly understood, not all of the insulin produced is destined to be secreted. Some of the secretory granules fuse with primary lysosomes and are degraded by lysosomal enzymes. This process called *granulolysis* or *crinophagy* has also been described in α-cells of the pancreatic islets and in the mammotrophs of the anterior pituitary.

Secretion of insulin is stimulated by the elevation of blood glucose that follows a meal rich in carbohydrates. It is also promoted by certain gastrointestinal hormones released during digestion. The circulating insulin diffusing to cells throughout the body binds to receptors in their membrane that facilitate entry of glucose into their crytoplasm. The tissues most affected are liver, muscle, and fat. In the liver, glucose is encorporated in glycogen from which it is later released to maintain the blood glucose level between meals. In active muscle, it is used as an energy source, and in resting muscle, it is transiently stored as glycogen for subsequent use. In adipose cells, it is used in the synthesis of fatty acids and glycerol.

The *insulin receptor* has been purified, sequenced, and shown to be present in the membrane of most cells. The immediate effects of insulin binding to its receptor have been elucidated. The entry of glucose into cells is dependent on the presence in their membrane of a specific transport protein called

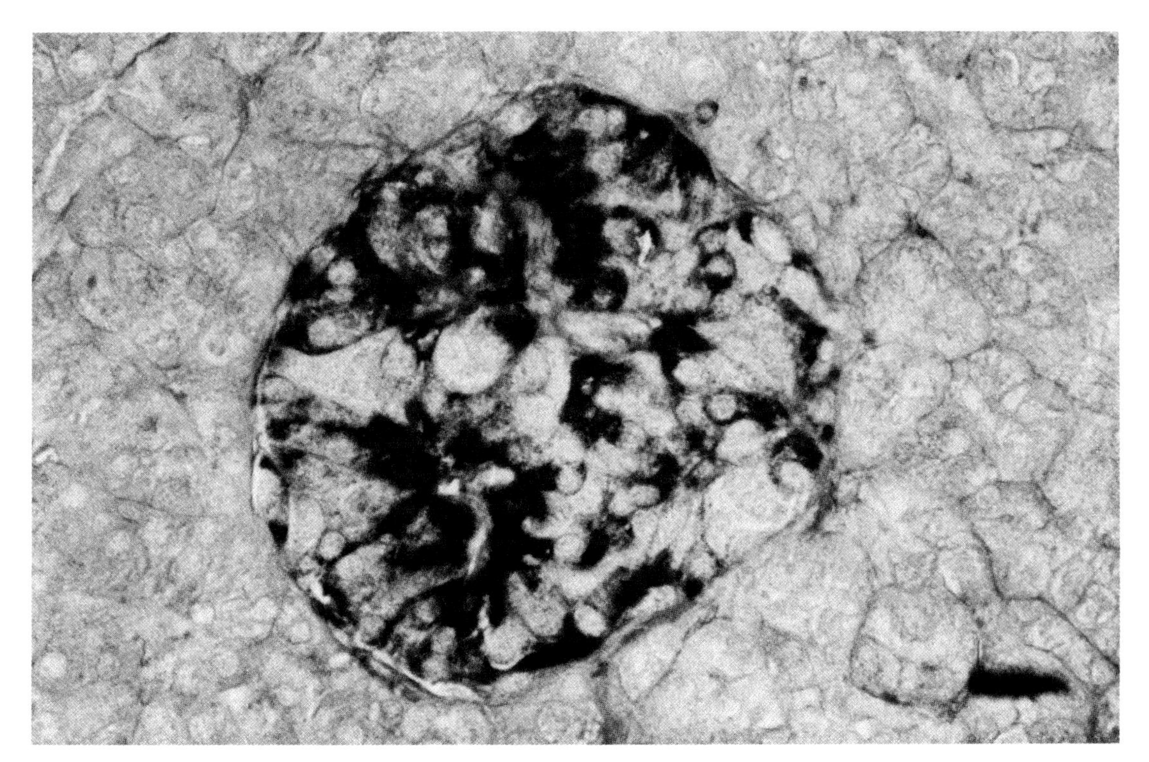

Figure 28–11. An islet of Langerhans from the human pancreas stained with aldehyde-fuchsin, which selectively stains secretory granules in the insulin-secreting B-cells. The cells are polarized, with the secretory material in the portion of the cell nearest a capillary. (Micrograph from Hellerström, C. 1977. Acta Paediatr. Scand. Suppl. 270:7.)

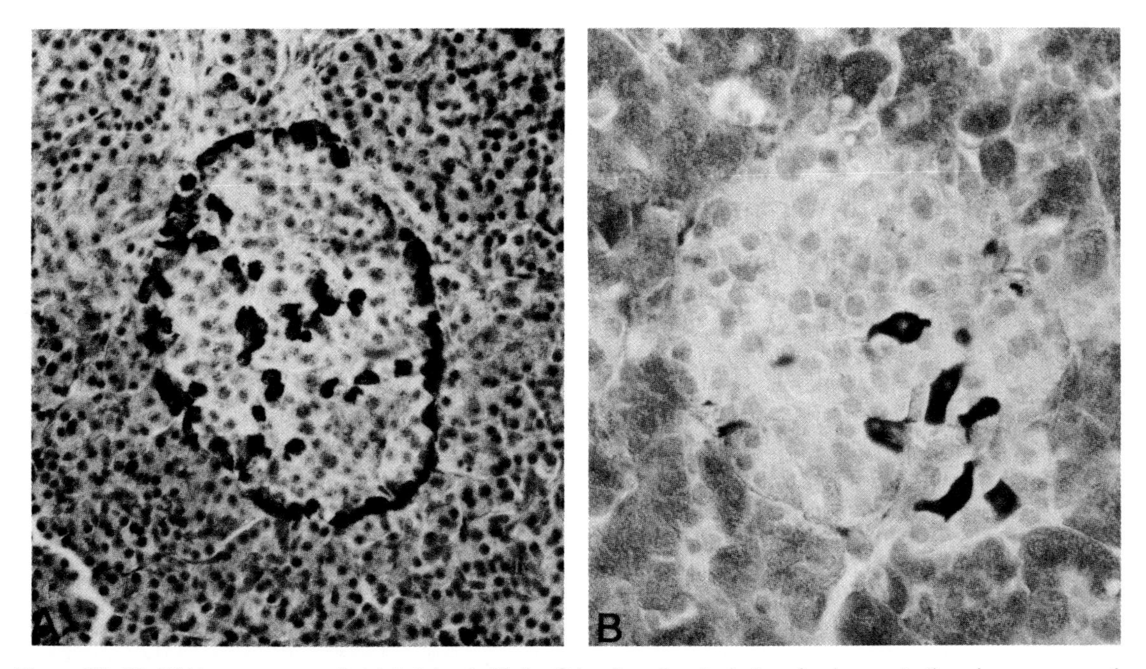

Figure 28–12. (A) Human pancreatic islet stained with the Grimelius silver technique for demonstrating glucagon-secreting A-cells (A_2-cells). These cells are preferentially located near capillaries around the periphery of the islet. (B) Human pancreatic islet stained with the Hellerstrom–Hellman silver technique for demonstrating somatostatin-producing D-cells. These cells are few in number and irregular in shape. (Photomicrographs from Hellerström, C. 1977. Acta Paediatr. Scand. (Suppl) 270:7.)

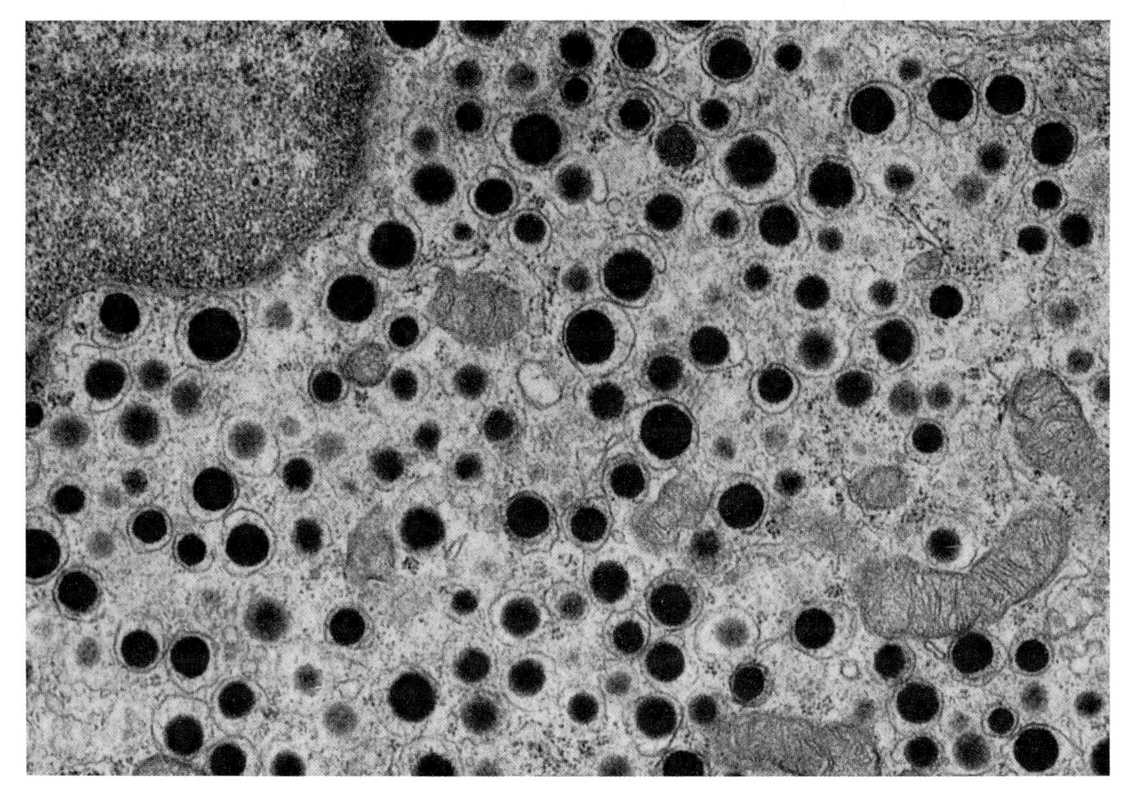

Figure 28–13. Electron micrograph of the juxtanuclear area of an α-cell in a human islet of Langerhans. The α-cell granules have a very dense core surrounded by a less dense region beneath the limiting membrane. (Micrograph courtesy of A. Like.)

glucose permease. Binding of glucose to the permease induces a change in its conformation that permits passage of the glucose into the cytoplasm. The number of permease molecules in the cell membrane is normally rather limited, but there are vesicles in the subjacent cytoplasm bounded by membrane rich in permease. The binding of insulin to its receptors is believed to induce rapid fusion of these vesicles with the plasma membrane greatly increasing its permease content. Insulin stimulation of adipose cells has been shown to result in a 10-fold increase in the glucose permease in the membranes within a few minutes. Reduction in the concentration of insulin is presumably followed by aggregation of permease molecules and their interiorization in the membrane of pinocytosis vesicles.

The disease *diabetes* is a consequence of a chronic deficiency in insulin production. In the absence of insulin, glucose cannot enter cells outside of the nervous system. The resulting excess of glucose in the blood (hyperglycemia) leads to excretion of an abnormal volume of urine (polyuria), which, in turn, causes dehydration with excessive thirst and intake of water (polydipsia). Cells of the hypothalamus that normally control appetite are activated, leading to eating in excess (polyphagia). Unable to use glucose as an energy source, fat and muscle protein are metabolized with rapid weight loss, despite increased food intake. Increased metabolism of fat generates excess plasma ketones and their excretion in the urine (ketonuria). The loss of sodium involved in excretion of ketone salts lowers the buffering capacity of the blood, which becomes excessively acid (acidosis). If not treated by administration of exogenous insulin, the diabetic patient is at risk of becoming comatose and dying from metabolic acidosis and dehydration.

Histologic examination of the pancreas of diabetic humans reveals hyalinization or fibrosis of the islets of Langerhans with destruction of a large portion of the β-cells. Less common than diabetes is the occurrence of tumors of islet cells resulting in *hyperinsulinism.* Such patients are at risk of insulin shock. Massive release of insulin in such episodes results in

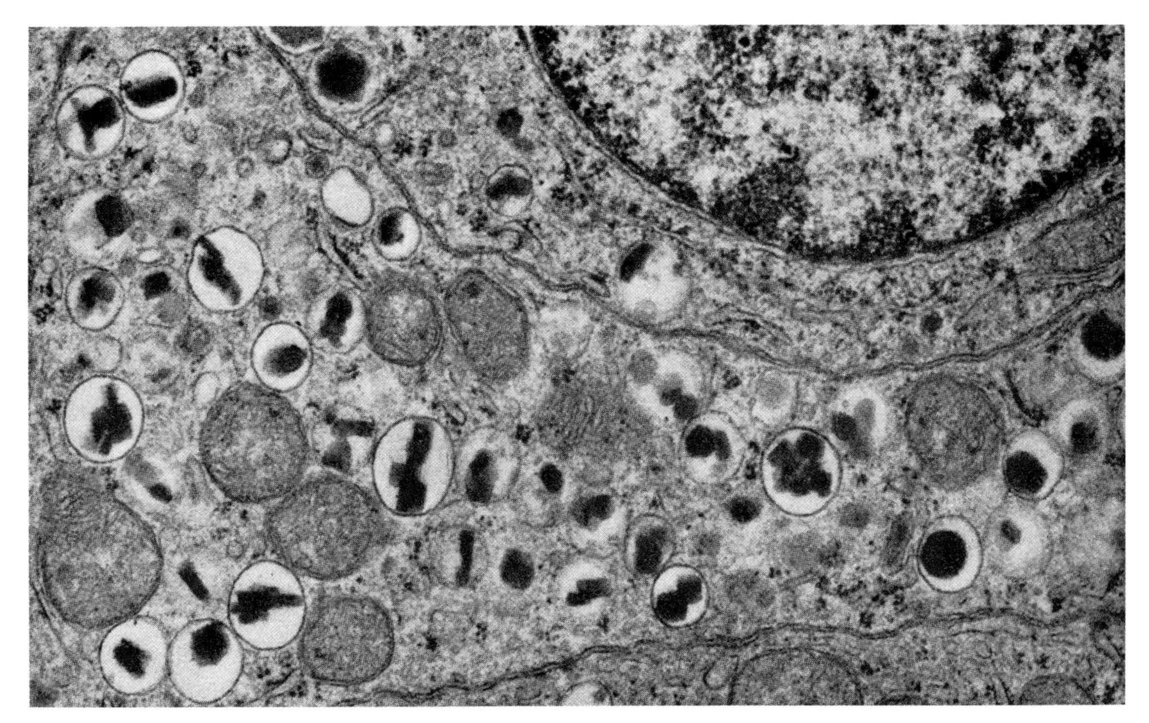

Figure 28–14. Electron micrograph of portions of two adjoining β-cells. The β-cell granules, in man and certain other species, are membrane-bounded vesicles containing dense crystals of varying size and shape. (Micrograph courtesy of A. Like.)

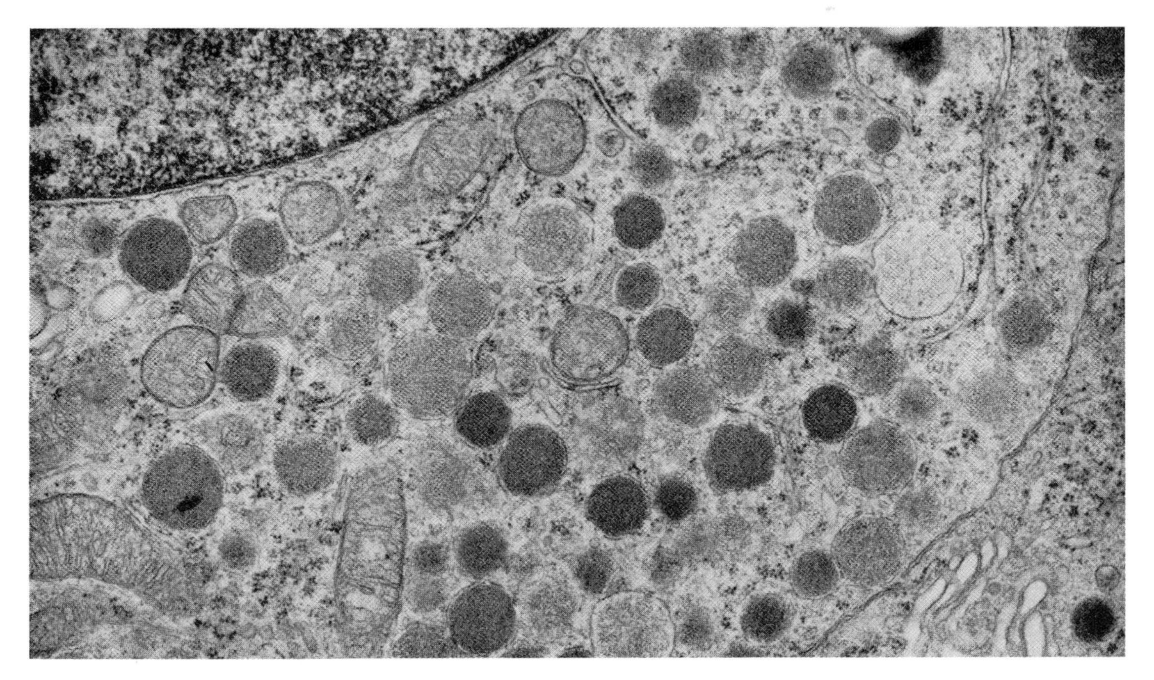

Figure 28–15. Electron micrograph of a portion of a δ-cell of an islet of Langerhans. The content of the granules varies considerably in its density. (Courtesy of A. Like.)

precipitous fall in blood glucose. The central nervous system becomes hyperactive with extreme agitation, tremor, sweating, and convulsions, culminating in coma. Timely administration of intravenous glucose will arrest insulin shock and even restore comatose patients to consciousness.

The other two major peptide hormones of the islets are also involved in control of blood glucose. *Glucagon,* the hormone produced by the α-cells, is secreted in response to a fall in blood glucose concentration. It acts mainly upon the hepatic cells, increasing the degradation of glycogen to release glucose into the blood. When the glycogen is depleted, glucagon is also capable of increasing gluconeogenesis by the hepatic cells.

Somatostatin, the hormone secreted by the δ-cells, is a small polypeptide of only 14 amino acids. Its secretion is stimulated by the postprandial increase in blood glucose, amino acids, or fatty acids. Its local effects within the islets are inhibitory, decreasing the rate of secretion of both insulin and glucagon. Its distant effect is to diminish the motility of the stomach, small intestine, and gallbladder. The overall effect of its secretion seems to be to slow the uptake of nutrients from ingested food and make the products of assimilation available over a longer period of time. Production of somatostatin is not limited to the δ-cells of the pancreatic islets. It is also produced by cells in the hypothalamus, where it serves to reduce the secretion of growth hormone by the somatotrophs of the anterior pituitary.

The F-cells (PP-cells) that are present in very small numbers in the islets secrete *pancreatic polypeptide.* To date, little is known about its function or the control of its release.

BIBLIOGRAPHY

EXOCRINE PANCREAS

Caro, L.G. and G.E. Palade. 1964. Protein synthesis, storage and discharge in the pancreatic exocrine cell, an autoradiographic study. J. Cell Biol. 20:4.

Herzog, V. and M. Farquhar. 1977. Luminal membrane retrieved after exocytosis reached most Golgi cisternae. Proc. Natl. Acad. Sci. USA 74:5073.

Herzog, V. and H. Reggio. 1980. Pathways of endocytosis from luminal plasma membrane in rat exocrine pancreas. Eur. J. Cell Biol. 21:141.

Ichikawa, A. 1965. Fine structural changes in response to hormonal stimulation in the perfused canine pancreas. J. Cell Biol. 24:239.

Jamieson, J.D. and G.E. Palade. 1971. Condensing vacuole conversion and zymogen granule discharge in pancreatic exocrine cells: metabolic studies. J. Cell Biol. 48:503.

Janawitz, H.D. 1966–67. Pancreatic secretion of fluid and electrolytes. *In* C.F. Code and M.I. Grossman, eds. Handbook of Physiology, Sect. 6. Washington, DC, American Physiological Society.

Palade, G.E., P. Siekevitz, and L. Caro. 1962. Structure, chemistry, and function of the pancreatic exocrine cell. *In* A.V. de Reuch and M.P. Cameron, eds. The Exocrine Pancreas, Ciba Foundation Symposium. Boston, Little Brown & Co.

Rothman, S.G. 1977. The digestive enzymes of the pancreas: a mixture of inconstant proportions. Annu. Rev. Physiol. 39:373.

Sarles, H. 1977. The exocrine pancreas. Internat. Rev. Physiol. 12:173.

Stroud, R.M., A.A. Kossiakoff, and J.L. Chambers. 1977. Mechanism of zymogen activation. Annu. Rev. Biophys. Bioeng. 6:177.

ENDOCRINE PANCREAS

Baetens, D., J. De Mey, and W. Gepts. 1977. Immunohistochemical and ultrastructural identification of the pancreatic polypeptide producing (PP-cell) in the human pancreas. Cell Tissue Res. 185:239.

Baetens, D., F. Maisse-Lagae, A. Perrelet, and L. Orci. 1979. Endocrine pancreas: three dimensional reconstruction shows two types of islets of Langerhans. Science 206:1323.

Banting, F.G., J.B. Best, W.R. Campbell, and A.A. Fletcher. 1922. Pancreatic extracts in the treatment of diabetes. Can. Med. Assoc. J. 12:141.

Baum, J.G., R.H. Simmons, R.H. Unger, and L.L. Madison. 1962. Localization of glucagon in the alpha cells of the pancreatic islet by immunofluorescent techniques. Diabetes 11:371.

Björkman, N., C. Hellerstrom, B. Hellman, and B. Petersson. 1966. The cell types in the endocrine pancreas of the human fetus. Zeitschr. Zellforsch. 74:425.

Bloom, W. 1931. A new type of granular cell in the islets of Langerhans of man. Anat. Rec. 49:363.

Cooperstein, G.J. and D.T. Watkins, ed. 1981. The Islets of Langerhans. New York, Academic Press.

Czech, M.P. 1980. Insulin action and the regulation of hexose transport. Diabetes 29:399.

Dubois, M.P. 1975. Immunoreactive somatostatin is present in discrete cells of endocrine pancreas. Proc. Natl. Acad. Sci. USA 72:1340.

Erlandsen, G.L. 1980. Types of pancreatic islet cells and their identification. Internatl. Acad. Pathol. 21:140.

Goldstein, M.B. and E.A. Davis. 1968. Three dimensional architecture of the islets of Langerhans. Acta Anat. 71:161.

Gomez-Acebo, J., R. Parrilla, and J.L. Candella. 1968. The fine structure, of the A and D cells of rabbit endocrine pancreas in vivo and incubated in vitro. I. Mechanism of secretion of A cells. J. Cell Biol. 36:33.

Lacy, P.E. 1975. Endocrine secretory mechanisms. J. Pathol. 79:170.

Larson, L.I., F. Sundler, and R. Hakansson, 1976: Pancreatic polypeptide. A postulated new hormone: Identification of its storage site by light and electron immunocytochemistry. Diabetologia 12:211.

Like, A.A. 1967. Ultrastructure of the secretory cells of the islets of Langerhans in man. Lab. Investig. 16:937.

Orci, L., M. Ravazolla, M. Amherdt, O. Madsen, L.D. Vassali, and A. Perrelet. 1985. Direct identification of prohormone conversion site in insulin secreting cells. Cell 42:671.

Orci, L., J.D. Vassali, and A. Perrelet. 1988. The insulin factory. Sci. Am. 85:259.

Reichlin, S. 1983: Somatostatin, N. Eng. J. Med. 309:1495. 309:1556.

Unger, R.H., R.E. Dobbs, and L. Orci. 1978. Insulin, glucagon, and somatostatin secretion in the regulation of metabolism. Annu. Rev. Physiol. 40:307.

29

RESPIRATORY SYSTEM

All higher animals require oxygen to maintain their metabolism. The respiratory system provides for the intake of oxygen in the inspired air and for the elimination of carbon dioxide produced by metabolism of cells throughout the body. Carbon dioxide is carried to the lungs, and oxygen is carried from them to the tissues by the circulatory system. The respiratory tract is thought of as having a *conducting* portion, proximally, which connects the exterior with a *respiratory* portion, distally, where the exchange of gases between the blood and the inspired air takes place. The conducting portion includes the cavity of the *nose,* the *pharynx,* the *larynx,* the *trachea,* and a branching system of *bronchi* of progressively diminishing caliber. Their smallest branches, the *bronchioles,* are continuous with the respiratory portion of the lungs. This consists of the *respiratory bronchioles, alveolar ducts,* and *alveoli,* which together make up the greater part of the volume of the lungs.

THE NOSE

The nose consists of a framework of bone and cartilage covered by connective tissue and skin. It is divided into right and left *nasal cavities* by a median *nasal septum.* The nasal cavities open anteriorly at the *nares* and posteriorly into the *pharynx.* Their surface area is increased by three thin scroll-like projections from the lateral walls, called the *superior, middle,* and *inferior conchae.* The skin covering the nose bears very fine hairs and is provided with unusually large sebaceous glands. The interior of the nose is lined by four types of epithelium. The stratified squamous epithelium of the skin continues through the nares into the *vestibule,* where a few large stiff hairs project into the airway. These are believed to help exclude large dust particles in the inspired air. A few millimeters into the vestibule, stratified squamous epithelium gives way to a narrow transitional band of nonciliated cuboidal or columnar epithelium. This is continuous with ciliated pseudostratified columnar epithelium that lines the remainder of the nasal cavity, save for a small area in the dorsal wall, where it is replaced by the sensory *olfactory epithelium.*

The nasal epithelium consists of ciliated columnar cells, goblet cells, and small basophilic cells at the base of the epithelium that are regarded as stem cells for the replacement of the more differentiated cell types. In the human, the number of goblet cells gradually increases from anterior to posterior. In addition to mucus, the epithelium secretes a thin fluid that forms a layer between the blanket of mucus and the surface of the epithelium. The cilia beat within this layer of fluid, continuously moving the overlying layer of mucus toward the pharynx. Beneath the epithelium, there is a thick lamina propria containing *submucosa glands* made up of both mucous and serous cells. Also present in the lamina propria are plasma cells, mast cells, and aggregations of lymphoid tissue. Beneath the epithelium over the lower conchae are extensive venous plexuses that are a common site of nosebleed.

THE OLFACTORY EPITHELIUM

The receptors for the sense of smell are located in the *olfactory epithelium,* a specialized region of the nasal mucosa that occupies the roof of the nasal cavity and extends downward to 8–10 μm on either side of the septum, and a short distance onto the upper nasal conchae. This specialized area of epithelium is irregular in outline and has a total area of about 500 mm^2.

The olfactory epithelium is a tall pseudostratified epithelium about 60 μm thick (Fig. 29–1). It consists of three kinds of cells: *sustentacular cells, basal cells,* and *olfactory cells.* The olfactory cells are bipolar neurons, evenly distributed among the sustentacular cells. Their round nuclei occupy a zone below those of

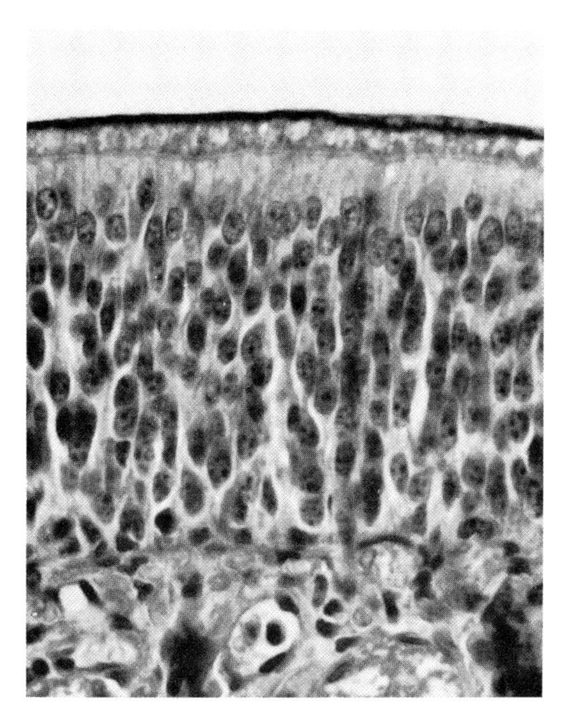

Figure 29–1. Photomicrograph of mammalian olfactory epithelium.

the supporting cells (Fig. 29–2). There is a small supranuclear Golgi complex and some tubulovesicular elements of the smooth endoplasmic reticulum. The apical portion of the cell is narrowed to a thin cylindrical process that extends upward to the surface of the epithelium, where it ends in a terminal expansion, called the *olfactory bulb* or *knob* (Fig. 29–2B). This projects somewhat above the surface of the surrounding supporting cells and contains the basal bodies of six to eight *olfactory cilia* that radiate from it parallel to the surface of the epithelium. The cilia are nonmotile and atypical in their internal structure. They are very long, attaining a length of 70 μm in the cat and 150 μm in the frog. The basal portion of the ciliary shaft is of normal diameter (250 nm) and contains the usual 9 plus 2 arrangement of longitudinal microtubules. A few micrometers from the base, there is an abrupt narrowing of the shaft to about 150 nm and this slender portion continues to the tip, occupying about 80% of the length of the cilium. The axoneme in this narrow portion of the shaft consists of 11 single microtubules instead of the usual doublets. This is subject to interspecific variation and, in some species, the narrow portion of the cilia may contain only one or two microtubules. The basal portion of the olfactory cell tapers down to a smooth process about 0.5 μm in diameter which is the axon of the nerve cell. This passes through the basal lamina into the underlying connective tissue where it joins others to form fascicles of unmyelinated axons surrounded by Schwann cells. Passing through the cribriform plate of the ethmoid bone, these assemble into about 20 macroscopically visible *fila olfactoria* that enter and synapse in the *olfactory bulb* of the brain.

The tall columnar sustentacular cells bear many closely packed micovilli that project into the overlying blanket of mucus. Beneath them is a conspicuous terminal web traversing the cell between junctional complexes that attach it to adjoining olfactory or supporting cells. These cells have a pale-staining nucleus, a prominent Golgi complex, and their apical cytoplasm is rich in smooth endoplasmic reticulum and contains a few pigment granules that are responsible for the yellowish-brown color of the olfactory epithelium.

The basal cells are small deeply basophilic cells between the bases of the olfactory sensory and supporting cells. The olfactory epithelium can regenerate following its partial destruction. By labeling with tritiated thymidine, basal cells have been shown to divide and differentiate into either sustentacular cells or olfactory cells. This is the only known example of nerve cells being replaced from stem cells in adult animals. On the basis of experiments in rodents, it is widely believed that the olfactory epithelium is constantly renewed by division and differentiation of basal cells. It has been reported that the sensory cells may survive for only 2 to 3 weeks in mice. However, this surprisingly rapid rate of turnover may have been due, in part, to an ongoing regeneration following destruction of receptor cells by rhinitis. In other experiments on mice protected against infection, the number of labeled cells remained relatively constant over 12 months, suggesting that fully differentiated receptor cells may be quite long-lived in the absence of disease-related destruction. No data are available on the rate of renewal in the human olfactory epithelium.

The lamina propria of the olfactory mucosa overlies the dense connective tissue forming the periosteum of the cribriform plate. It includes some pigment cells, lymphoid cells, and a rich plexus of blood capillaries. In its deeper portion, there is a plexus of large veins and numerous lymphatics which drain toward lymph nodes on either side of the head. If dye is injected into the subarachnoid space of

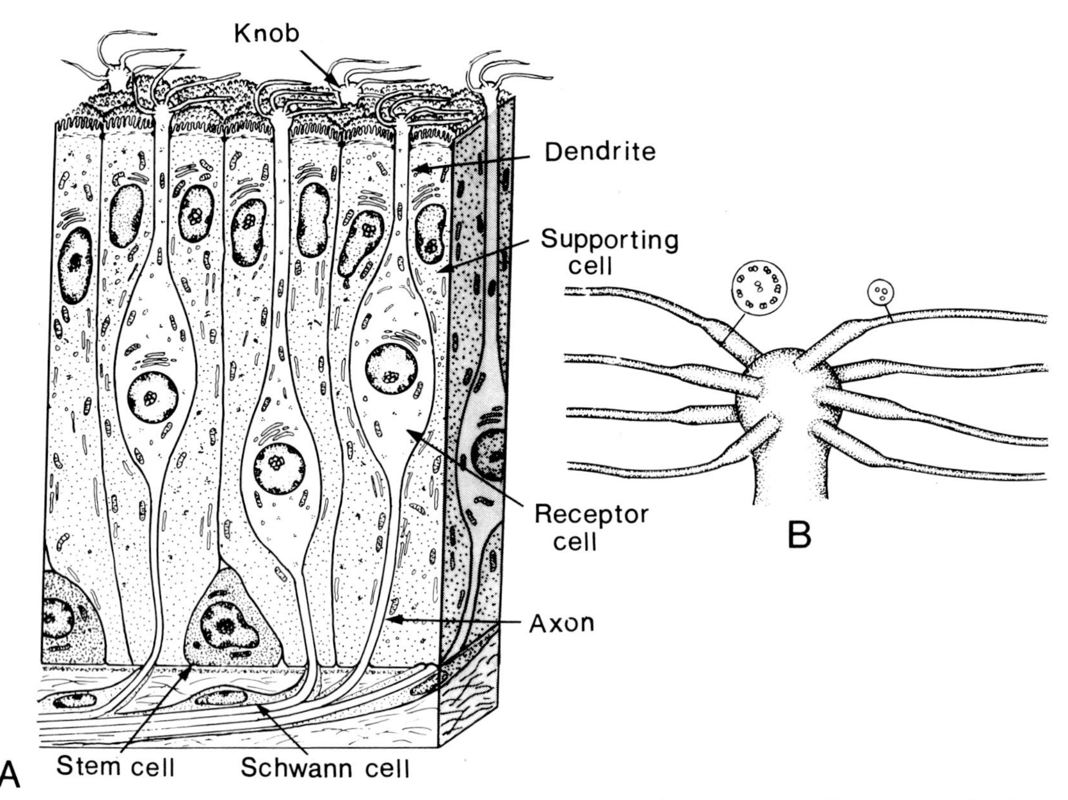

Figure 29–2. (A) Drawing of olfactory epithelium showing the receptor cells, basal stem cells, and sustentacular cells. (B) Drawing of the knob at the exposed end of the dendrite of the neuron, more highly magnified to illustrate the modified cilia that bear the receptors for various odorants.

the brain, it can be found in lymph capillaries of the olfactory region and in the sheaths of the fila olfactoria. This demonstrates a possible pathway for infections to spread, in the opposite direction, from the nasal cavity to the meninges, resulting in meningitis.

The lamina propria also contains the *olfactory glands of Bowman,* branched tubuloalveolar glands made up of pyramidal serous cells containing pale secretory granules. They continuously secrete a watery fluid that is probably essential for the solubilization of air-borne odorants.

HISTOPHYSIOLOGY OF THE NOSE

While acting as a pathway for the inspired air, the nose provides other services that tend to protect the delicate acini of the lung. The vascularity of the nasal mucosa, and particularly the venous plexus in the inferior concha, warms the air. The moving blanket of mucus entraps dust particles and carries them to the pharynx where they are swallowed instead of being inhaled.

The function of the mucosa is not limited to the secretion and transport of mucus. Plasma cells in the lamina propria produce IgA that binds to secretory component on the basal surface of cells of the submucous glands and is transported together with their secretory product to the surface of the nasal mucosa. Serum albumin, IgA, IgE, and IgG that diffuse from fenestrated capillaries around the submucous glands also reach the surface of the epithelium where they provide local protection against bacterial infection. In individuals suffering from the common cold or allergic rhinitis (hay fever), IgE binds to mast cells causing their release of histamine and other mediators that result in increased nasal secretion and edema of the submucosa that are responsible for the partial obstruction of the nasal passages that is a distressing symptom of these disorders.

Just how odors are distinguished by the olfactory epithelium has long puzzled physiologists, but there has been some recent progress toward understanding the mechanism of olfactory perception. The existence of specific receptors for a wide range of odor molecules was first suggested by the occurrence of individuals with an inherited inability to detect a particular odor. Because several dozen different specific anosmias have been reported in humans, it was reasonable to believe that there were at least that many different receptors, and it seemed likely that the number might be in the thousands. Now, a large family of odor receptors has recently been cloned. They are encoded by at least 100 genes, and possibly more, making this one of the largest, and most diverse, gene families discovered to date. The genes are expressed only in the olfactory epithelium and the receptors are located in the membrane of the specialized olfactory cilia. Like a number of other receptors that have been extensively studied, these receptors have seven transmembrane domains and the ligand probably binds deep within the area bounded by the transmembrane domains of the receptor.

Olfactory perception, thus, appears to employ an extremely large number of receptors, each capable of recognizing a very small number of odorous ligands. It is not yet known whether a single neuron expresses a number of different receptors or whether a single neuron expresses a single type of receptor. The thin layer of mucus moistening the olfactory cilia is probably essential for uptake of airborne odorants and a tissue-specific 2 kD *olfactory binding protein* has been identified in the mucus that may present hydrophobic odorants to the receptors on the cilia. The continuous secretion and transport of mucus over the epithelium may serve to remove residues of odorants to which the epithelium was previously exposed, and thus keep receptors available to new chemical stimuli.

It is reported that the specific activity of several enzymes that are capable of metabolizing foreign molecules is often higher in the cells of the nasal epithelium than in the liver. This has led to the speculation that certain inhaled xenobiotics may be detoxified by the nasal mucosa. This possibility takes on added interest in this period of increasing concern over the pollution of the atmosphere with smoke and industrial toxins.

PARANASAL SINUSES

Connected with the nasal cavity and forming cavities in the respective bones are the *accessory nasal sinuses:* the frontal, ethmoidal, sphenoidal, and maxillary sinuses. These are lined with a ciliated epithelium similar to that of the nose. The cilia beat in a direction that moves a blanket of mucus toward the nasal cavity. The mucosa of the sinuses is relatively thin and contains fewer and smaller mucous glands than that of the nose. The lamina propria cannot be differentiated as a layer separate from the periosteum of the bones to which it is tightly adherent. The paranasal sinuses are often a site of painful inflammation, *sinusitis,* and they occasionally require surgical drainage.

THE LARYNX

The larynx is a hollow organ, about 42 mm in length and 40 mm in diameter, interposed between the pharynx and the trachea. It is designed to produce sound and to close the trachea during swallowing to prevent food and saliva from passing down the airway to the lungs. Its wall is made up of the *thyroid* and *cricoid* hyaline cartilages and a thin leaf of fibroelastic cartilage, the *epiglottis,* that projects obliquely, upward and backward, over the lumen. During swallowing, the epiglottis is pressed forward by the base of the tongue, closing the larynx and presenting a smooth surface over which the bolus of food slides into the esophagus. *Extrinsic muscles,* attaching the larynx to the hyoid bone, raise it during deglutition, and *intrinsic muscles* join the thyroid and cricoid cartilages and their contraction changes the tension on the vocal cords and, thus, influences phonation.

Projecting inward from the wall of the larynx, on either side, are two folds of the mucosa. The upper pair are called the *vestibular folds* (*false vocal cords*) and the lower pair are the *vocal folds* or *vocal cords.* Between them is a narrow recess, called the *sinus of the larynx.* The space between the vocal cords is called the *rima glottis.* The vestibular fold is merely a plication of the mucosa and underlying lamina propria, but the vocal fold contains, in its margin, a dense band of elastic tissue, the *vocal ligament,* and lateral to this is a bundle of striated muscle, sometimes referred to as the *vocalis muscle* (Fig. 29–3). The space between the vocal folds varies in different phases of respiration and in phonation. In forced inspiration, the folds are abducted, widening the interspace for the passage of air to the lungs. In phonation, they are strongly adducted, reducing the interspace to a linear slit. Production of sound is due to vibration of the free

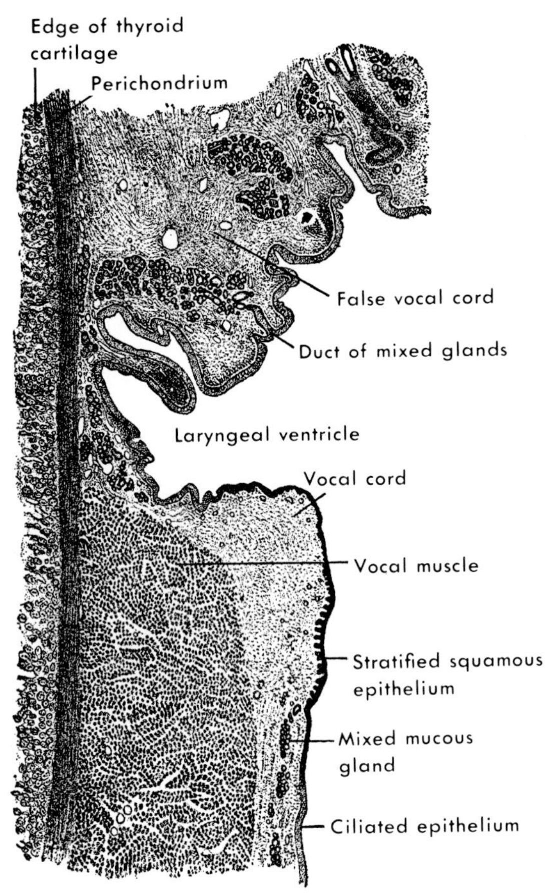

Figure 29–3. Frontal section through the middle of the glottis of a boy showing the vocal cord, false vocal cord, and, between them, the sinus of the larynx, also called the laryngeal ventricle. (After V. von Ebner in A. Kolliker's Handbuch der Gewebelehre, Vol. III. Leipzig 1899–1902).

edges of the cords resulting from passage of air between them. Contraction of intrinsic muscles of the larynx increases tension on the cords, changing the pitch of the sound produced.

The anterior surface of the epiglottis and the vocal folds are covered by stratified squamous epithelium. All the rest of the lining of the larynx is ciliated pseudostratified epithelium, and the direction of ciliary beat is toward the pharynx moving foreign particles, bacteria, and mucus toward the exterior. Tubuloacinar mucus-secreting glands with serous crescents are present in the lamina propria, in limited numbers. Glands are absent on the vocal folds.

The blood supply of the larynx is from the middle and lower laryngeal arteries which arise from the superior and inferior thyroid arteries. The veins drain into the thyroid veins. Rich plexuses of lymphatics drain to the upper cervical lymph nodes and to nodes along the trachea. Sensory innervation of the larynx is via the superior laryngeal nerve and motor innervation of its intrinsic muscles from the inferior laryngeal nerve.

CONDUCTING PORTION OF THE RESPIRATORY TRACT

Beyond the larynx, the respiratory tract continues as the *trachea,* a flexible tube about 11 cm long and 2 cm in diameter, which then divides into two *primary bronchi.* Continuing dichotomy through 16 generations of branching forms an arborescent system of tubules that constitute the *conducting portion* of the respiratory tract. This pattern of branching results in a progressive decrease in the diameter of the individual tubules and an increase in the total cross-sectional area of the portion of the airway conducting the inspired air to and from the respiratory portion of the system. The branches immediately distal to the trachea are *bronchi* and those more distal are *bronchioles,* but it should be noted that there are several generations of branching within these categories so that, at the level of the *terminal bronchioles,* which are bout 0.2 mm in diameter, their number has reached about 65,000. Beyond the terminal bronchioles, the thin-walled *respiratory bronchioles, alveolar ducts,* and *alveoli* constitute the respiratory portion of the tract, where the exchange of oxygen and carbon dioxide with the blood takes place.

TRACHEA

The wall of the trachea is reinforced by a series of 16 to 20 C-shaped hyaline cartilages that encircle it on its ventral and lateral sides (Fig. 29–4). These incomplete cartilaginous rings are separated by interspaces that are bridged by fibroelastic connective tissue. This arrangement gives the trachea great pliability, whereas its cartilaginous rings enable it to resist external forces that might otherwise constrict the airway. External to the cartilages, there is a layer of dense connective tissue rich in elastic fibers. The posterior wall of the trachea is devoid of cartilages. In their place is a thick band of transversely oriented smooth muscle that intermingles at its ends with the dense connective tissue layer outside of the cartilages.

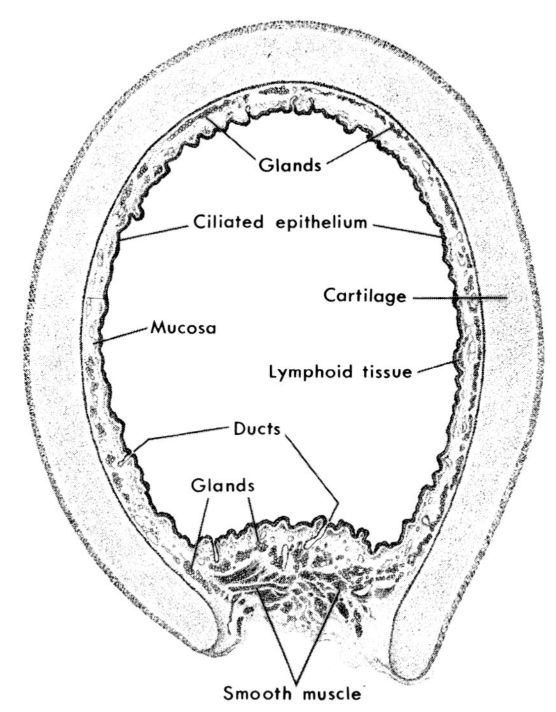

Figure 29–4. Drawing of a cross section through the trachea. (Modified after V. von Ebner in A. Kolliker's Handbuch der Gewebelehre, Vol. III. Leipzig 1899–1902.)

The trachea is lined by a ciliated, pseudostratified columnar epithelium that has an unusually thick basal lamina. Numerous goblet cells are scattered throughout the epithelium. In electron micrographs, the ciliated cells have a microvillous border through which the cilia project into the lumen (Fig. 29–5). The apical cytoplasm contains a number of mitochondria and a small Golgi complex. The endoplasmic reticulum is not extensive and there are relatively few free ribosomes. The *goblet cells* are similar in appearance to those in the nasal and gastrointestinal epithelium. Their expanded apical region is occupied by closely packed mucigen granules of low electron density and these tend to compress the underlying Golgi complex. The narrower basal region of the cell contains numerous cisternae of rough endoplasmic reticulum.

Less abundant than the ciliated and goblet cells is the *brush cell,* a slender columnar cell with a luminal border of microvilli 2 μm in length. The actin filaments in the core of the microvilli extend downward some distance into the apical cytoplasm. There are no secretory granules but small aggregations of glycogen may be scattered through the cytoplasm. The function of the brush cells and their relation to the other cell types of the epithelium remain unknown. They have been variously interpreted as depleted goblet cells or intermediate stages in the differentiation of basal cells to replace ciliated cells. The occasional observation of intraepithelial nerve endings associated with them has led to the speculation that they may function as sensory receptors, but physiological validation of this suggestion is lacking.

Another nonciliated cell type that has been described in the epithelium is the *serous cell.* It appears to be identical to serus cells found in the acini of the bronchial submucosal glands. It has electron-dense apical granules and is believed to produce a secretion of lower viscosity than that of the mucous cells.

Small, pyramidal *basal cells* are intercalated between the bases of the columnar cells. The alignment of their nuclei below those of the columnar cells gives the epithelium its characteristic pseudostratified appearance. The basal cells have few organelles and are interpreted as a reserve of stem cells capable of differentiating to replace damaged or exfoliated ciliated and goblet cells.

A second type of basally situated cell is sparsely distributed in the tracheobronchial epithelium. It has an electron-lucent cytoplasm and contains numerous dense-cored vesicles with a clear halo between the core and the limiting membrane. The vesicles are often concentrated near the basal lamina. These cells, called *bronchial Kulchitsky cells,* resemble the argentaffin cells found between cells lining the crypts of the intestinal mucosa and are presumed to have a neuroendocrine function. There may be more than one category of these cells. Some have the staining properties and fluorescence characteristic of cells containing catecholamines. Others resemble the peptide hormone-secreting cells of the enteroendocrine system. To date the small, granule-containing cells of the respiratory tract have attracted less investigative interest than those of the intestinal epithelium.

In the epithelium of the upper trachea, ciliated cells comprise about 30% of the total cell population, goblet cells 28%, and basal cells 29%. From the upper to the lower trachea, there is an increase in the percentage of ciliated cells and a decrease in the number of goblet and basal cells.

Small numbers of migratory cells are found in the tracheal and bronchial epithelium. These include *lymphocytes* and *globule leukocytes.* The latter bear some resemblance to the mast

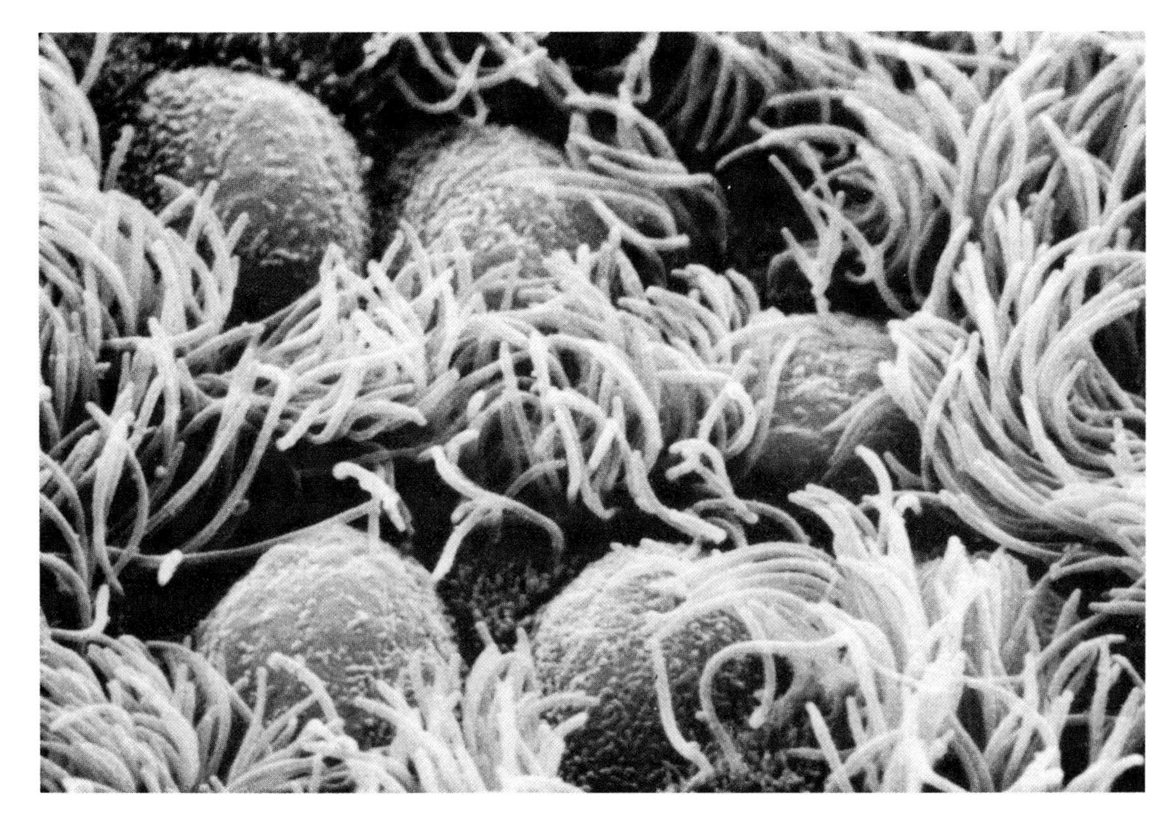

Figure 29–5. Scanning electron micrograph of a small area of the surface of the tracheal epithelium of a horse. The dome-shaped apices of goblet cells, with very short microvilli, can be seen among the tufts of cilia on the ciliated epithelial cells. (Micrograph courtesy of P. Gehr.)

cells that are present in the lamina propria. They contain a variable number of metachromatic granules that range in size from 0.1 to 0.3 μm in diameter and may be round or somewhat irregular in outline. Their content is finely granular and may show local variations in density, but they do not contain the lamellar or scroll-like formations characteristic of the granules of human connective tissue mast cells. The origin and function of globule leukocytes are not known.

The lamina propria, between the epithelium and the cartilages in the wall of the trachea and bronchi, is a loose connective tissue unusually rich in elastic fibers. It contains numerous *bronchial submucosal glands* whose ducts open onto the surface of the epithelium. The first part of the duct is lined by epithelium identical to that lining the bronchial tree. This short *ciliated duct* about 350 μm in length is continuous with a *collecting duct* about 800 μm long, from which the secretory tubules of the gland arise. This segment of the duct is lined by columnar cells that interdigitate along their lateral borders. There are a few dense apical granules and a well-developed Golgi complex. Their most striking feature is a cytoplasm packed with large mitochondria having numerous cristae. This exceptional concentration of mitochondria has led to the suggestion that these cells have high metabolic activity and probably regulate the water and electrolyte composition of the glycoprotein secretory product of the gland. A dozen or more secretory tubules arise from the collecting duct. These usually branch and terminate in a cluster of short tubules or acini. The secretory tubules are lined by columnar mucous cells, and the acini, by serous cells. The serous cells are pyramidal in form with a nucleus situated near the cell base and secretory granules occupying the apex. The granules of the serous cells are discrete and electron-dense, whereas those of the mucous cells are electron-lucent and tend to be confluent. Myoepithelial cells are found between the bases of the secretory cells in both the mucous and serous regions of the gland.

Secretion of a blanket of mucus onto the surface of the epithelium has an important role in entrapping inhaled dust and other particulate matter, and it also protects the conducting portion of the lungs from potentially damaging toxic fumes. The beating of the cilia continuously moves the layer of mucus toward the pharynx, where it is swallowed with the saliva. When the airway is chronically exposed to tobacco smoke or other irritants, the goblet cells increase in number and the submucous glands are enlarged. The composition of the secretory products also undergoes some modification. These changes are usually reversed within a few months after removal of the irritant.

Beneath the tracheal epithelium, there is a delicate network of lymphatics that communicate with a much coarser plexus of lymphatics in the submucosa. This drains into lymph nodes scattered along the entire length of the trachea. The blood supply comes mainly from the inferior thyroid artery. Innervation is from the recurrent branch of the vagus nerve and from the sympathetic chain. Small ganglia are found along the trachea, from which nerve fibers distribute to the smooth muscle in its posterior wall. Sensory nerves terminating in the mucosa are the afferent pathways for the cough reflex.

THE BRONCHI

The two main branches of the trachea are called *primary bronchi* or *main stem bronchi.* These enter the hilus of the lungs and, coursing downward and outward, they divide into *lobar bronchi.* The left lung has upper and lower lobes, whereas the right has upper, middle, and lower lobes. Thus, there are two lobar bronchi on the left and three on the right. These, in turn, divide into *segmental bronchi* to the several bronchopulmonary segments in each lung. There are three such segments in the right upper lobe, two in the middle lobe, and five in the lower lobe. In the left lung, there are five in the upper and five in the lower lobe. The segmental bronchi divide into *subsegmental bronchi.* The blood supply to the lungs follows the same pattern of branching. The parallel course of the bronchi and the blood vessels is of great importance to the surgeon because it makes lobectomy or segmental resection technically feasible.

The structure of the primary bronchi is very similar to that of the trachea up to point where they enter the lungs. There the rings of cartilage in their wall are replaced by cartilage plates of irregular outline distributed around the circumference of the tube (Fig. 29–6). The intrapulmonary bronchi are, therefore, cylindrical and not flattened posteriorly as are the trachea and extrapulmonary bronchi. Farther distally along the airway, the intramural cartilaginous plates become reduced in size and number and disappear altogether in subsegmental bronchi about 1 mm in diameter.

As cartilage in the wall of the bronchial tree diminishes, smooth muscle becomes more prominent. It is organized in interlacing bundles, some of which have a prevailing circular or spiral course. In the larger intrapulmonary bronchi, the bundles of smooth muscle are packed closely enough to form a continuous layer. In the distal portions of the bronchial tree, smooth muscle is less abundant and more loosely organized. In histological sections, the bronchial mucosa exhibits longitudinal folds, presumable due to agonal contraction of the smooth muscle layer during fixation (Fig. 29–6).

The bronchial epithelium is not significantly different from that of the trachea, consisting of ciliate columnar epithelium with many goblet cells and submucosal glands. The glands diminish in number and end at the level of the bronchioles. The height of the epithelium gradually decreases along the tract, becoming sparsely ciliate cuboidal epithelium in the bronchioles and low cuboidal in the terminal bronchioles. The lamina propria, which is separated from the epithelium by a thick basal lamina, is a loose connective tissue rich in reticular and elastic fibers. It normally contains lymphocytes, mast cells, and occasional eosinophils.

BRONCHIOLES

The bronchioles, about 0.3–0.5 mm in diameter, are the twelfth to fifteenth generations of branching of the bronchial tree. There are no cartilaginous plates in their wall, and no glands in the lamina propria. Smooth muscle does not form a continuous circumferential layer but is represented by discrete bundles of varying orientation that form a loose network with connective tissue occupying the spaces between bundles. The muscle is innervated by parasympathetic nerve fibers. Although smooth muscle is not a conspicuous component of the wall, its contraction does constrict the lumen of the bronchioles. It is said to relax during inspiration and to contract

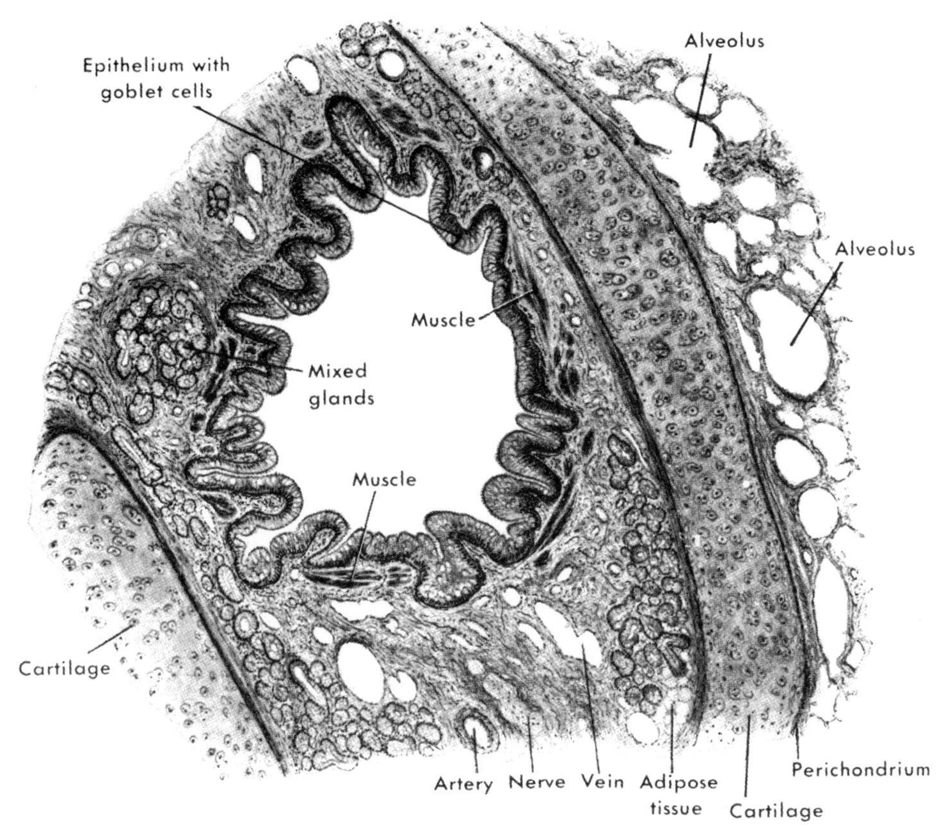

Figure 29–6. Cross section through a small bronchus of the human lung. Note the plates of cartilage and the folds of the mucosa that are probably due to agonal contraction during fixation. (After J. Schaffer, Lehrbuch der Histologie und Histogenese, W. Englemann Press, Leipzig 1922.)

at the end of expiration. When contraction is abnormally persistent, as it is in individuals suffering an asthma attack, constrictio ı of the bronchioles makes it difficult to er ıpty the lungs during exhalation.

Goblet cells are no longer prese ıt at the level of the bronchioles and the ep ithelium consists of ciliated cells and nonciliat d bronchiolar cells, called *Clara cells.* These are columnar with a rounded apex that may project above the other cells of the epitheli m. Its surface is covered with microvilli, and the apical cytoplasm contains a small number of dense secretory granules with a mean diameter of 0.3 μm. Near the free surface, the Clara cell is joined to neighboring cells by zonulae occludentes, but below this, the membranes diverge and short processes project into the intercellular space. The centrally located nucleus is ovoid or slightly indented and a Golgi complex is located above it or at one side. In the Clara cells of the human and other primates, there are long slender mitochondria and strands of rough reticulum distributed throughout the cell, but no smooth reticulum. This is surprising because in several rodent species, smooth endoplasmic reticulum is abundant. This suggests that there may be species differences in the composition of the secretory product. Efforts to establish the chemical nature of the product have been contradictory. ^{3}H-leucine is incorporated into the secretory granules, suggesting that they contain protein, and this is supported by the observation that the granules are digested by pretreatment of histological sections with the proteolytic enzyme pepsin. They do not incorporate galactose or glucosamine and, therefore, are probably not glycoprotein. Clara cells are distributed from major bronchi to the distal bronchioles. In some species, they make up more than 50% of the cells of the terminal bronchioles. Their function remains obscure.

Fixation of lung by perfusion preserves a lining layer in the bronchioles that is continuous with the layer of surfactant lining the alveoli. The hypophase of this fluid layer is electron-dense and it is thought that it may consist, in part, of a basic protein secreted by the Clara cells. A viscous mucus in the bronchioles might result in their closure due to adherence of opposing walls late in expiration. The absence of goblet cells, and the abundance of Clara cells, in the bronchioles may reflect a need for a nonsticky proteinaceous lining layer to ensure the patency of these minute tubes that are less than 0.4 mm in diameter.

RESPIRATORY PORTION OF THE LUNGS

RESPIRATORY BRONCHIOLES

The bifurcation of the terminal bronchioles gives rise to *respiratory bronchioles,* short tubes 0.5–0.2 mm in diameter. In the human, there are three successive generations of respiratory bronchioles that constitute the transition from the conducting to the respiratory portion of the lung. Their lining is initially cuboidal becoming low cuboidal and nonciliated in subsequent branches. Unlike more proximal bronchioles, their walls are interrupted at intervals by very thin saccular out-pocketings, called *alveoli.* Gas exchange can take place in these thin-walled appendages, hence the name respiratory bronchioles. With each branching, the number of these alveoli increases, until much of the bronchiolar wall is replaced by their openings.

ALVEOLAR DUCTS

The respiratory bronchioles continue into the *alveolar ducts.* Here the alveoli are so numerous and so closely spaced that the limits of the ducts are discernible in sections only by the alignment of thickenings of the free edges of the septa between adjacent alveoli (Fig. 29–7). The thickened adluminal edges of these interalveolar septa are covered by a few bronchiolar epithelial cells overlying delicate strands of smooth muscle within the septal connective tissue. After two or three branchings, each alveolar duct ends in a small space. This is sometimes called the *atrium,* but it is debatable whether it deserves a separate designation (Figs. 29–8). It is simply a common lumen or vestibule at the end of the alveolar duct into which clusters of four or more alveoli open.

ALVEOLI

The most physiologically important components of the lung are the *pulmonary alveoli,* the very thin-walled saccular compartments at the termination of the arborescent branching of the bronchioles and respiratory bronchioles (Figs. 29–9; 29–10 and 29–16). It is here that the exchange of oxygen and carbon dioxide takes place between the blood and the inspired air. Estimates of the number of alveoli in the two human lungs range from 200 to 500 million. The figure most widely accepted is 300 million, presenting a total area of about 140 m^2 for gas exchange. In histological sections, the alveoli are rounded or polygonal and about 200 μm in diameter, but their size and shape vary greatly depending on the degree of postmortem collapse of the lungs and the amount of distortion of their thin walls during specimen preparation.

The septa between adjacent alveoli contain a dense network of capillaries supported by delicate collagenous and elastic fibers. This layer of vessels and connective tissue is covered on either side by an exceedingly thin pulmonary epithelium. The epithelium is made up of two cell types the *squamous alveolar cells* (*type-I alveolar cell*) (Fig. 29–11) and the *great alveolar cells* (*type-II alveolar cells*) (Figs. 29–12 and 29–13). Except for a slightly thickened area accommodating the nucleus, the squamous alveolar cells are less than 0.2 μm in thickness. The perinuclear cytoplasm contains a small Golgi complex, a few mitochondria, and occasional profiles of rough endoplasmic reticulum, but the cytoplasm in the broad thin portion of these cells is largely devoid of organelles. Although they make up only 10% of the cell population of the lung, these cells occupy 95% of the total alveolar surface. They are attached, by occluding junctions, to each other and to the great alveolar cells which make up 12% of the cell population but occupy only about 5% of the alveolar surface. Over the capillaries, connective tissue is lacking and the epithelium is separated from the vessel wall only by the apposed basal laminae. These thin areas are especially favorable for gas exchange.

The great alveolar cells (type-II alveolar cells) are commonly located near the angles between neighboring alveolar septa. They are somewhat thicker than the squamous alveolar cells and have a rounded apical surface that projects above the level of the surrounding epithelium. The free surface of the great alve-

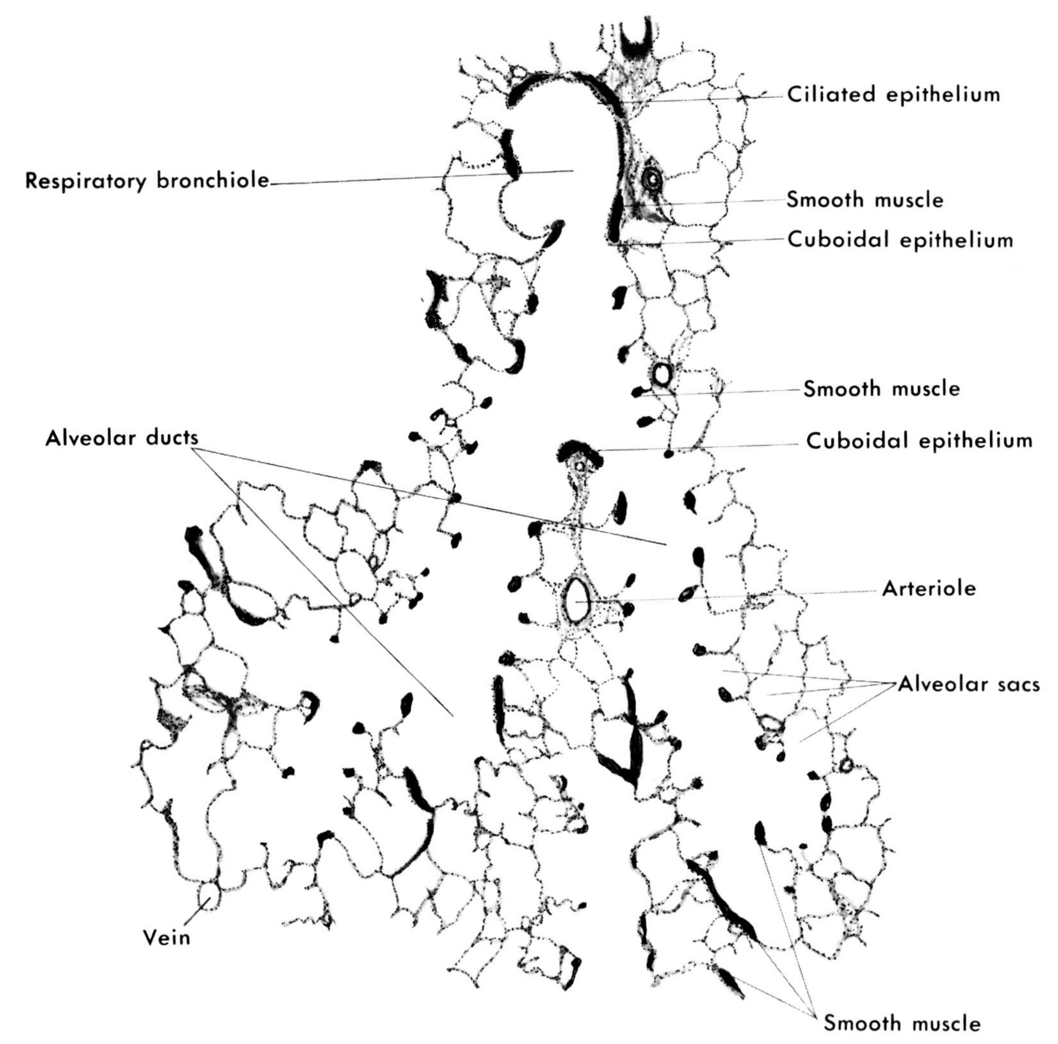

Figure 29–7. Drawing of a section through a respiratory bronchiole and two alveolar ducts of human lung. The wall of the alveolar duct is interrupted by the mouths of multiple alveoli. Between these, the wall contains some smooth muscle.

olar cell is covered by short microvilli, whereas the surface of the squamous epithelial cells is smooth. The nucleus is slightly irregular in outline with small clumps of heterochromatin on the inner side of the nuclear envelope. The cell organelles include a small Golgi complex and a few plump mitochondria. Dense, ovoid, membrane-bounded granules are the most conspicuous feature of the cytoplasm (Fig. 29–13). These are called *lamellar bodies,* a term descriptive of their distinctive internal structure, which consists of closely spaced, thin lamellae that have a thickness comparable to that of a lipid bilayer. However, in freeze–fracture preparations, these do not contain the protein particles seen in fractured membranes. With cytochemical staining methods, lamellar bodies have some of the same enzymatic activities as lysosomes, but these are associated with the limiting membrane and not with their contents.

The great alveolar cells synthesize and secrete *pulmonary surfactant* and the lamellar bodies are their secretory granules. The surfactant is released by exocytosis (Fig. 29–14) and spreads, as a monolayer, over a thin film of fluid that normally coats the wall of the alveoli. In doing so, it lowers the surface tension at the air/liquid interface and thereby reduces the tendency of the alveoli to collapse at the end of expiration. The thin film of surfactant that normally lines the alveoli cannot be seen in electron micrographs because no fixative has yet been found that adequately preserves it. However, excess surfactant is often observed at a level deep to the surface film

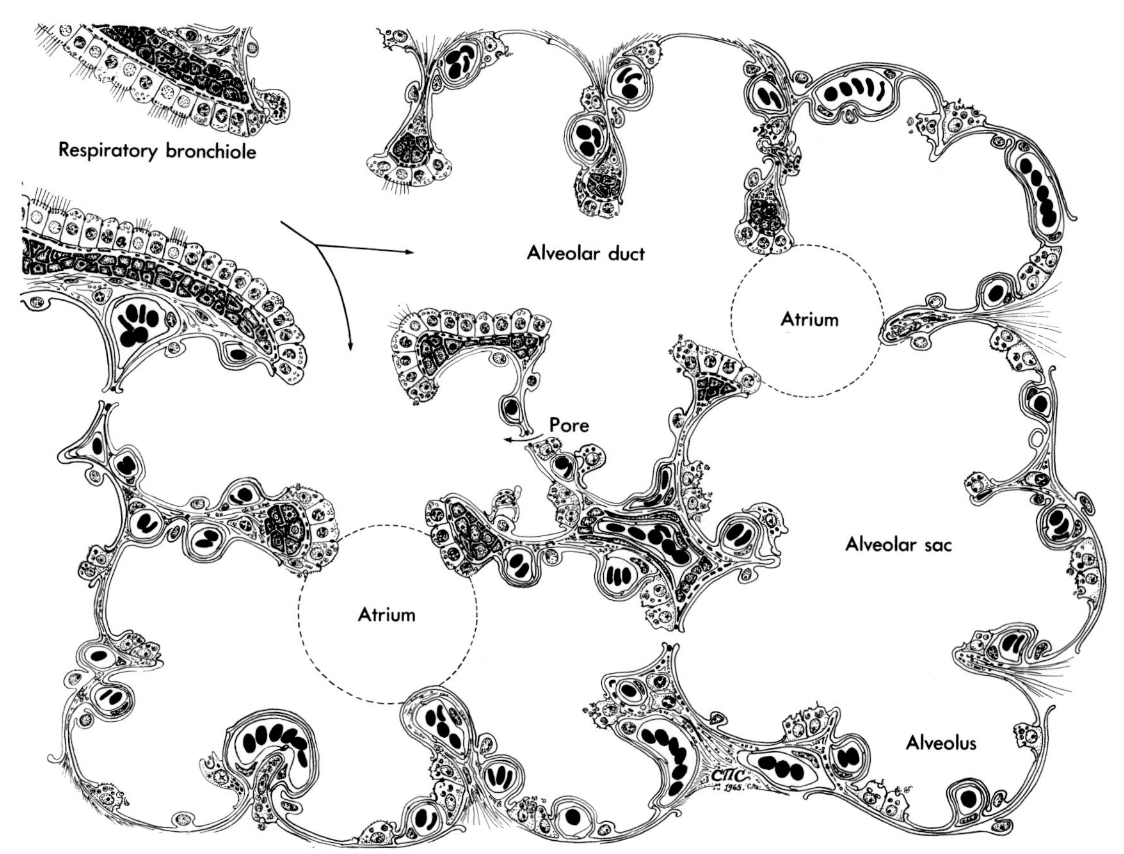

Figure 29–8. A somewhat more idealized schematic representation of a respiratory unit of the lung. The epithelium and smooth muscle of the wall of the alveolar ducts can be seen here more clearly than in the section depicted in Fig. 29–7. The atria, indicated here by dotted circles, are spaces bounded on one side by the termination of the alveolar duct and, on the other, by the openings of the alveolar sacs. (Slightly modified after Sorokin, S. 1966. *In* R.O. Greep, ed. *Histology,* 2nd ed. New York, McGraw-Hill Book Co.

where it forms patterns typical of hydrated phospholipids (Fig. 29–15).

Surfactant purified from bronchoalveolar lavage is 80–90% phospholipid, mainly phosphatidylcholine, but it also contains a small amount of surfactant-specific protein (10%). Its biosynthetic pathway has been traced with radioactively labeled choline. In such experiments, the label is first localized over the endoplasmic reticulum, then over the Golgi complex, and finally over the lamellar bodies. Continuous secretion of surfactant creates a pressure gradient in the surface film that favors flow of the film from the alveoli into the bronchioles and upward to the mucociliary escalator that carries mucus up to the pharynx where it is swallowed. Some surfactant may also be degraded by alveolar macrophages, but there is evidence suggesting that a major portion of it may be cleared by uptake of phospholipid by the great alveolar cells and its reutilization in surfactant synthesis.

The tissue between the two layers of epithelium on the *alveolar septa* is called the *interstitium* of the lung (Fig. 29–17). In addition to the capillaries and fibrous components, it contains *septal cells* (*interstitial fibroblasts*), mast cells, and a few lymphocytes. In some species, there may be occasional smooth muscle cells but they are rarely found in the human lung. The septal cells are the most abundant cell type of the interstitium. They resemble ordinary fibroblasts but have some distinguishing features. They have long branching processes, and gap junctions have been reported between processes of neighboring septal cells. They contain from one to several lipid droplets, and bundles of actin filaments are more prominent, in their cytoplasm, than in that of fibroblasts elsewhere in the body. Excised strips of lung tissue contract slightly, in vitro, in response to hypoxia, and it has been speculated that contraction of septal cells may decrease alveolar size under similar conditions

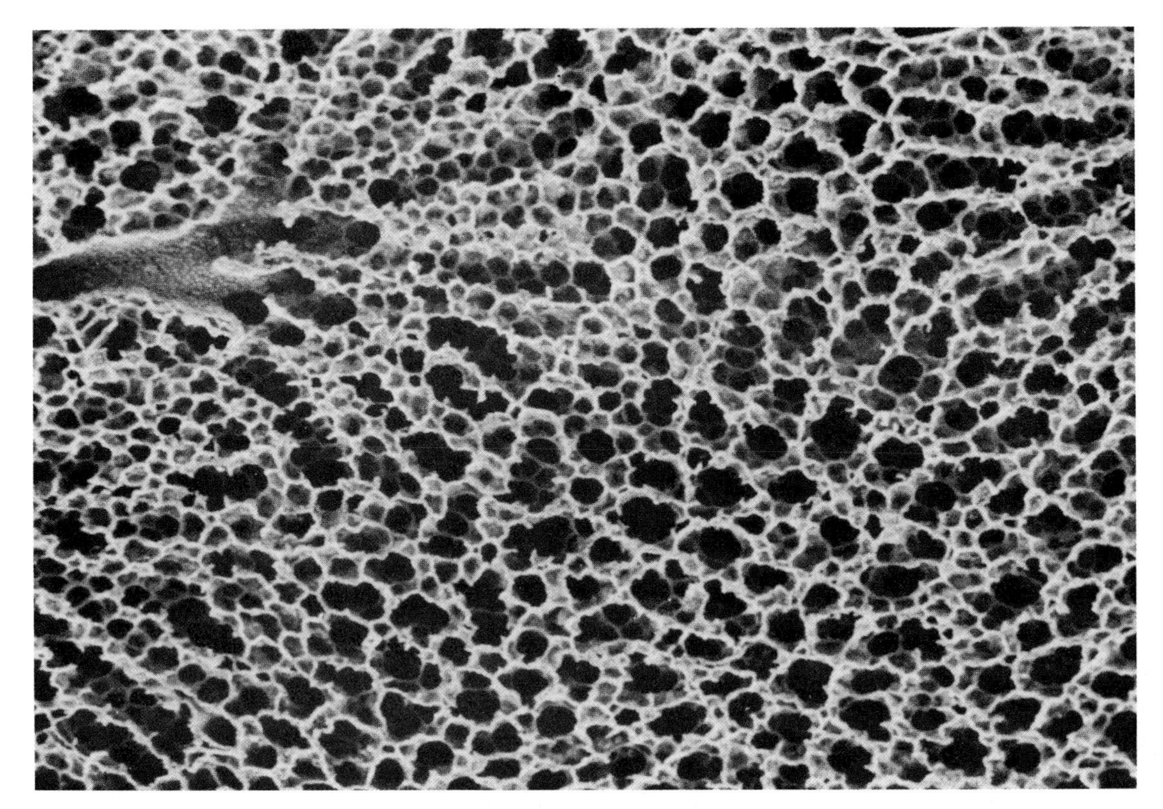

Figure 29–9. Scanning micrograph of the lung of a gazelle, prepared by instillation of the fixative into the bronchi to prevent the collapse of the alveolar ducts and acini that commonly occurs with simple immersion fixation. A terminal bronchiole can be identified at the upper left. (Micrograph courtesy of P. Gehr.)

in vivo. Some investigators have called them *myofibroblasts,* but the evidence for their contractility is not sufficiently compelling to justify this descriptive term. Like fibroblasts, their principal function is production of type-III collagen, elastin, and proteoglycans of the extracellular matrix of the alveolar septa. In the early phases of pulmonary pathology, there is leakage of fluid from the capillaries resulting in interstial edema and accumulation of fluid in the alveoli.

The thin septa between adjacent alveoli are traversed by small openings, the *alveolar pores* (*pores of Kohn*) (Fig. 29–18). There are from one to six of these but larger numbers have been reported. Their origin is unclear. From our knowledge of the development of the lungs as progressively branching tubular outgrowths from the embryonic foregut, no communication would be expected between the terminal branches of one bronchus and those of neighboring bronchi. One must conclude that the alveolar pores arise by a late formation of openings in the interalveolar septa both within the branches of the same bronchiole and also within septa formed by fusion of alveoli associated with adjoining bronchioles. The alveolar pores observed in histological sections are 8–10 μm in diameter, but studies of human lung that involved infusion of a suspension of polystyrene beads of graded size into one alveolus and their recovery in the outflow from a neighboring bronchus suggest that openings up to 60 μm in diameter also occur. These communications are physiologically significant. Owing to their presence, blockage of a small bronchus does not result in collapse of its associated alveoli because these can continue to be ventilated from adjacent unobstructed respiratory units. This is called *collateral respiration* by analogy with collateral circulation in the vascular system.

Around the mouths of the alveoli, the interstitium contains a wreath of collagen fiber bundles. Each of these contains fibers that are continuous with those encircling the mouths of neighboring alveoli, and they, therefore, tend to give some stiffness and support to the wall of the alveolar duct. During inspiration, the wavy collagen fibers no doubt straighten

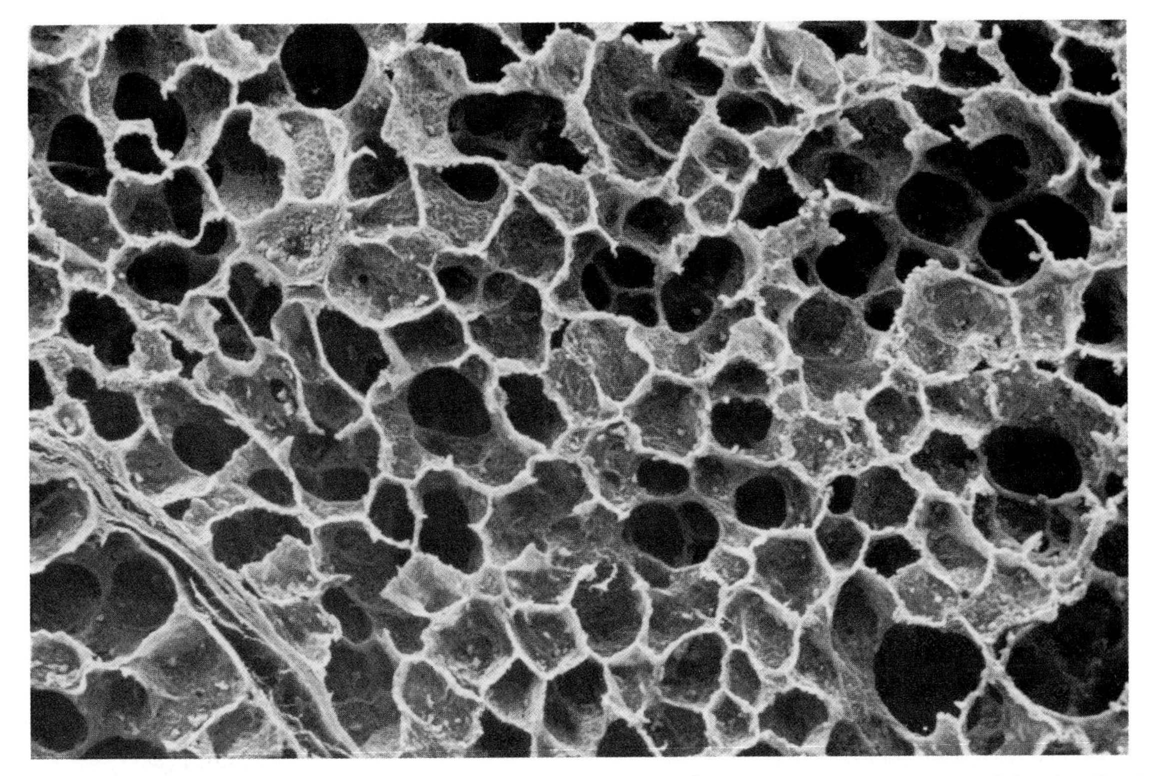

Figure 29–10. Scanning micrograph of the cut surface of the human lung illustrating the saccular form of the alveoli and the very thin alveolar septa. (Micrograph courtesy of P. Gehr.)

out as the alveoli expand. The collagen bundles that encircle the mouths of the alveoli also mingle with collagen fibers in the walls of the bronchioles and in the adventitia of small arteries and venules that accompany them.

Alveolar Macrophages

The principal mononuclear phagocytes of the lungs are the *pulmonary alveolar macrophages.* These are not part of the alveolar wall but are free cells migrating over its luminal surface. In this location, they are directly exposed to any inhaled dust or bacteria that may have escaped entrapment by the mucus blanket in the proximal portions of the airway.

Alveolar macrophages vary in size from 15 to 40 μm in diameter and have an irregularly shaped nucleus and prominent nucleolus. The cytoplasm is highly vacuolated and contains a small Golgi complex, a number of mitochondria and occasional profiles of endoplasmic reticulum. Free ribosomes and glycogen particles are present in moderate numbers. The most striking ultrastructural features of the cell are the prominent filopodia and lamellipodia on it surface and the large number of membrane-bounded inclusions in its cytoplasm (Fig. 29–19). Many of the latter are primary lysosomes, 0.5 μm or less in diameter and round or ovoid in form. These are rich in hydrolytic enzymes. The specific activities of acid phosphatase, glucuronidase, and lysozyme are reported to be substantially higher in alveolar macrophages than in macrophages from the peritoneal cavity.

In cigarette smokers, the cytoplasm of these cells is crowded with large irregularly shaped, membrane-limited bodies, that represent undigestible residues of phagocytosed material (Fig. 29–20). These heterogeneous inclusions have electron-dense and electron-lucent areas and contain lipid, myelin figures, and occasionally, crystals of unknown provenance. In persons with heart disease, attended by pulmonary congestion, the alveolar macrophages contain many vacuoles filled with *hemosiderin* resulting from phagocytosis of extravasated erythrocytes and degradation of their hemoglobin.

The origin of alveolar macrophages was formerly a subject of controversy, with some workers insisting that they arose by transfor-

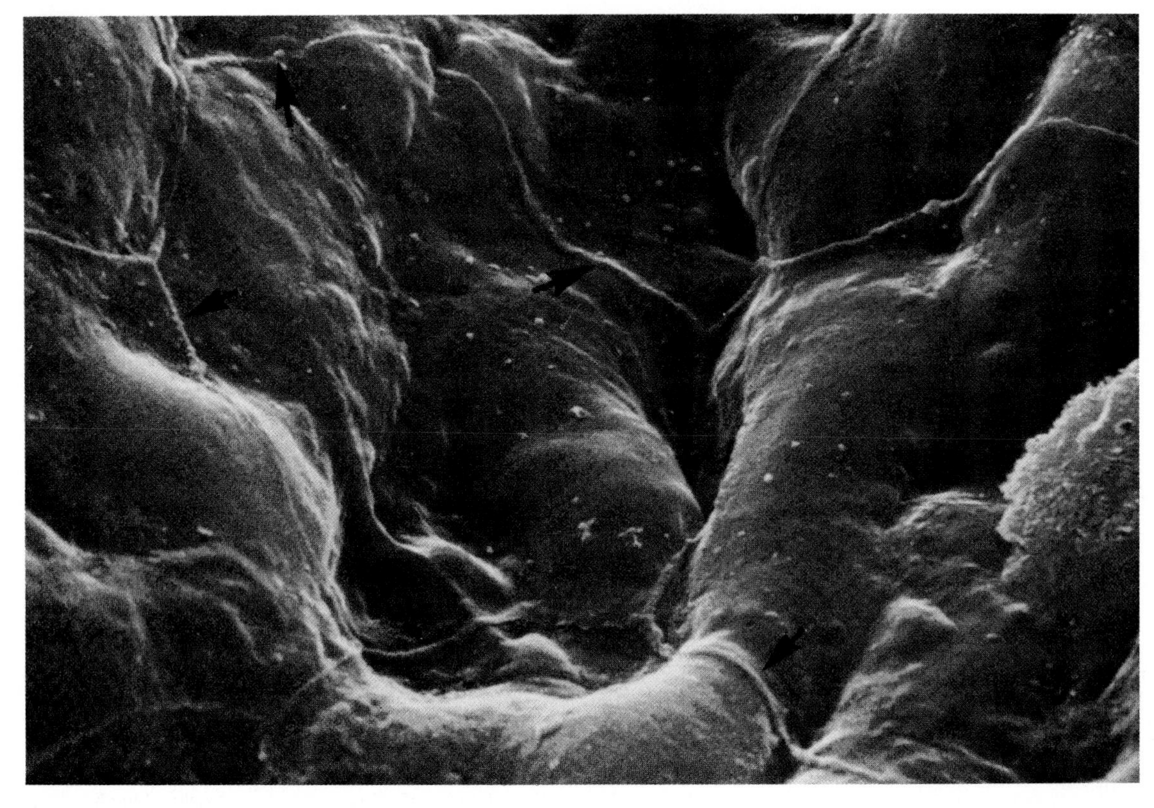

Figure 29–11. A high magnification of the interior of an alveolus from bovine lung. The very thin type-I alveolar cells conform to the contours of the underlying capillaries. The polygonal boundaries of adjacent squamous cells appear as linear ridges (at arrows). (Micrograph courtesy of P. Gehr.)

mation of exfoliated epithelial cells and not from the general mononuclear phagocyte system. This dispute has now been resolved with DNA-labeling techniques and chromosome markers for identifying cells and tracing their origins. It is now generally accepted that the pulmonary macrophages originate from stem cells in the bone marrow and are transported in the blood as monocytes. These enter the interstitium of the lung and are there transformed into macrophages that migrate into the lumen of the alveoli. Although most of the proliferative activity giving rise to macrophages takes place in the marrow, monocytes in the interstitium of the lung also have a limited capacity for division.

Alveolar macrophages form the first line of defense against infection of the lung and they are remarkably efficient. They have surface receptors for IgG and the C3b component of complement. Their ability to ingest bacteria is enhanced in the presence of specific antibody. Intracellular destruction of bacteria is carried out by their phagolysosomal system and by the generation of superoxide ions. Although large numbers of bacteria are continually carried into the lungs in the inspired air, the alveolar surface usually remains sterile. Macrophages incessantly cleanse the extracellular lining layer of the alveoli by removing inhaled particulate matter. In addition to their phagocytic activity, they secrete lysosomal hydrolases, prostaglandins, and components of complement. When stimulated by metabolic products of bacteria, they release chemotactic factors that induce transendothelial migration of polymorphonuclear leukocytes to join them in combating the invading microorganisms.

Alveolar macrophages greatly outnumber all other cell types in the lung and are constantly being eliminated and replaced. Many of them migrate from the alveoli to the surface of the bronchi and are carried by ciliary action through the upper airway to the pharynx where they are swallowed with the saliva. The mechanism of their movement to the bronchioles is not entirely clear, but the continuous production of surfactant and the transudation of fluid from the capillaries probably form a moving surface film that contributes to their

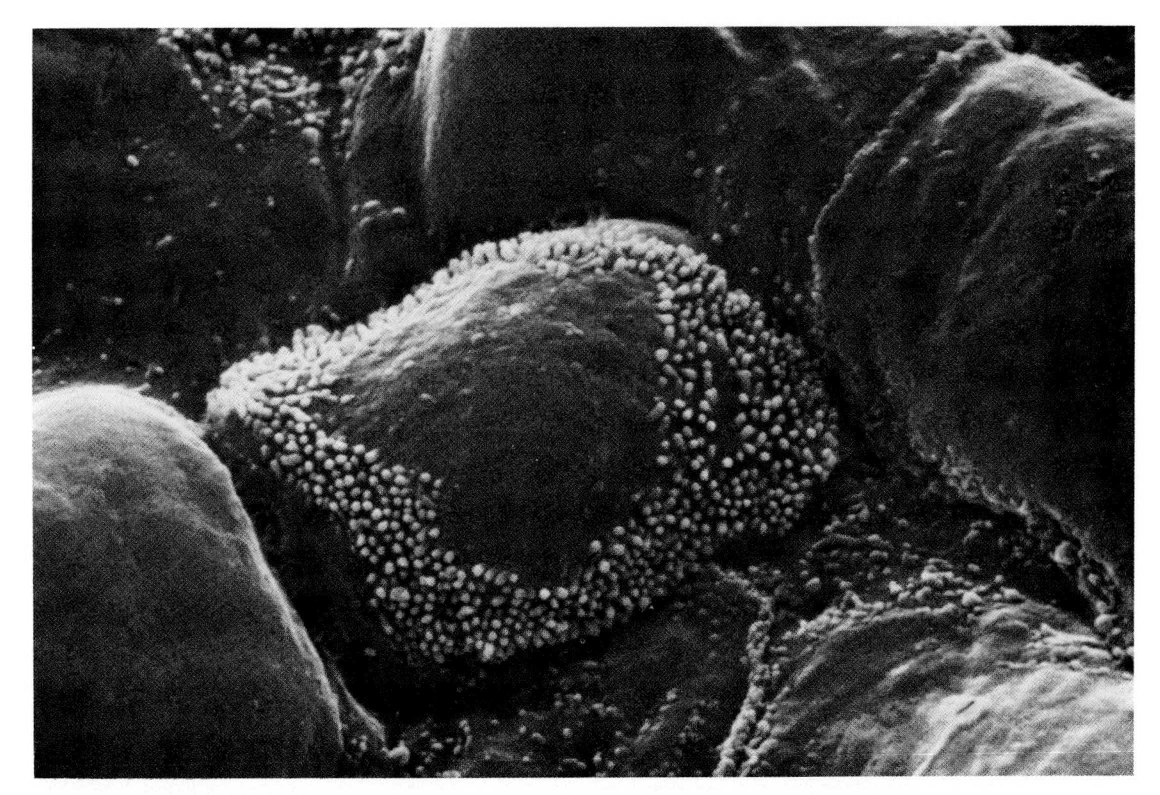

Figure 29–12. Scanning electron micrograph of a small area of the interior of a human pulmonary alveolus showing a great alveolar cell (type-II alveolar cell) with very short microvilli at the periphery of its bulging free surface. (Micrograph courtesy of P. Gehr.)

directed movement. The number cleared from the lungs each day is astronomical. On the basis of counts of mononuclear cells in the fluid from a cannula introduced into the trachea of a cat, it is estimated that the rate of clearance is about 2×10^6 alveolar macrophages per hour. Comparable measurements for humans would no doubt give much higher numbers.

THE PLEURA

The thoracic cavities containing the lungs are lined by a serous membrane, the *pleura,* which consists of a thin layer of connective tissue containing some fibroblasts as well as collagen fibers and several layers of elastic fibers. On its inner surface, it is covered by a layer of mesothelial cells like those lining the peritoneal cavity. The layer of this tissue that is applied to the wall of the cavity is called the *parietal pleura,* whereas that reflected over the surface of the lungs is the *visceral pleura.* A noteworthy feature of the pleura is the great number of capillaries and lymphatics it contains. The few nerves found in the parietal pleura are branches of the phrenic and intercostal nerves. The nerves to the visceral pleura are believed to be branches of the vagus and of the sympathetic nerves that supply the bronchi.

INNERVATION OF THE LUNGS

The lung is innervated by parasympathetic nerves via the vagus and by sympathetic nerves arising from the second to fourth thoracic sympathetic ganglia. Nerves from these sources form a plexus around the hilus of the lungs and give rise to intrapulmonary nerves that accompany the ramifications of the bronchial tree and its associated blood vessels. Parasympathetic and sympathetic nerves to the lung contain both afferent and efferent fibers. The bronchoconstrictor fibers are from the vagus and the bronchodilator fibers are sympathetic.

Sensory and motor nerves have been identi-

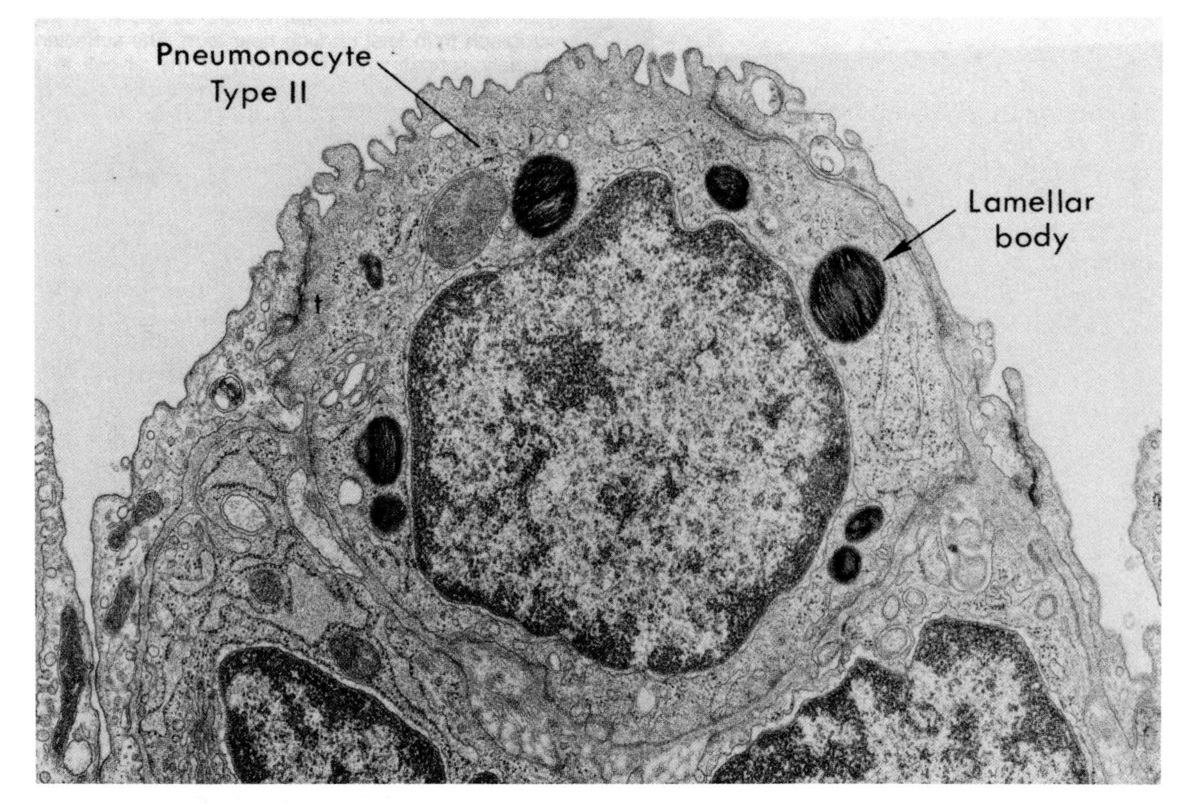

Figure 29–13. Electron micrograph of a type-II alveolar cell (type-II pneumonocyte) illustrating the characteristic lamellar bodies in the cytoplasm. (Micrograph courtesy of M.C. Williams.)

fied extending as far peripherally as the terminal bronchioles. Electron microscopic studies have revealed nerve endings in the alveolar ducts and alveolar walls of laboratory rodents and they probably also occur in these sites in the human. These endings are of two types. One, located in the interstitium and containing many small mitochondria but no synaptic vesicles, is considered to be sensory. It may correspond to the juxtacapillary receptor postulated by physiologists and believed to be stimulated by an increase in pulmonary capillary pressure. The second type of ending is of less common occurrence and contains many dense-cored vesicles. It is closely associated with the type-II alveolar cells. It is speculated that it may be the morphological basis for the reported effect of the nervous system on the secretion of pulmonary surfactant.

SMALL GRANULE CELLS AND NEUROEPITHELIAL BODIES

The epithelium lining the conducting airways contains solitary *small granule cells* and clusters of similar cells with associated nerves constituting *neuroepithelial bodies.* The small granule cells are argyrophilic and some of them emit a fluorescence at a wavelength characteristic of serotonin, whereas others do not. Thus, they appear to be a heterogeneous population comparable to the cells of the diffuse endocrine system previously described in the gastrointestinal epithelium. They occur at all levels in the conducting airways and are tall cells with a broad base and a narrow apex bearing short microvilli exposed to the lumen. Their nucleus and cytoplasmic organelles are in no way unusual. Their centrioles and Golgi complex are in a supranuclear position, but they contain numerous 100–300-μm dense-cored granules that are concentrated near the cell base. There is little firm evidence bearing on the function of the small granule cells, but their fine structure and location suggest that they are adapted to receive stimuli from the lumen and to respond by release of one or more regulatory amines and peptides.

The neuroepithelial bodies occur in the epithelium of the airway as far distally as the terminal bronchioles. They seem to be prefer-

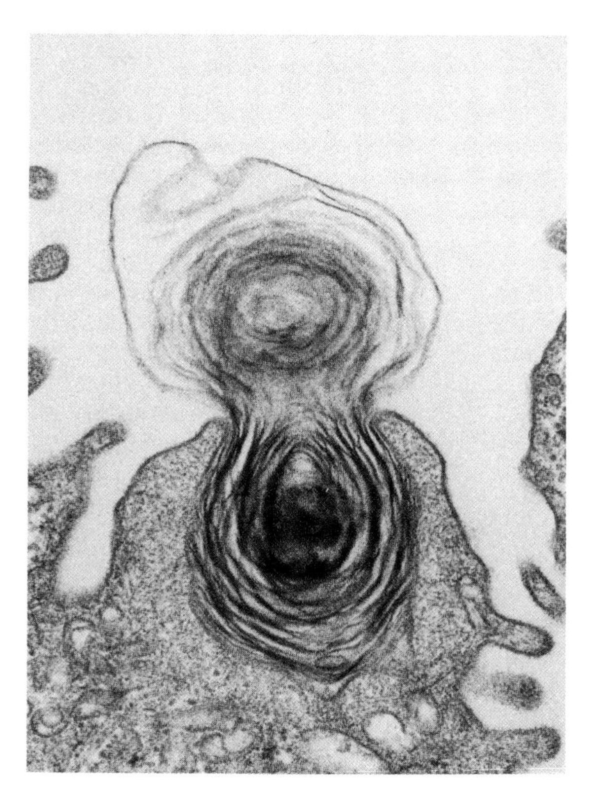

Figure 29–14. Micrograph of a lamellar body being released by exocytosis from a type-II alveolar cell in a 21-day fetal rat lung. (Micrograph by M.C. Williams.)

entially located at or near sites of bifurcation of the tract. They consist of from 3 to over 50 cells about 15 μm in height that resemble the small granule cells in their nuclear and cytoplasmic characteristics. In the hamster, there are about 10 such bodies per millimeter of axial airway length and they may be as numerous in the human airway, but no comparable quantitative studies have been done. All cells contact the lumen, but the basal surface is at least five times greater in area than that exposed to the lumen. Dense-cored vesicles or granules may be found throughout, but they are most numerous in the basal cytoplasm. In the rabbit and rat, nerve axons penetrate the basal lamina and ramify among the cells of the neuroepithelial body. Bulbous dilatations along their length contain synaptic vesicles. Cell processes may also extend from the cell base through the basal lamina to contact nerves in the lamina propria. Which nerves are afferent and which are efferent is not certain.

Physiologists have long postulated the existence of chemoreceptors in the airway that are sensitive to variations in the concentration of oxygen in the inspired air. It is now speculated that the neuroepithelial bodies may fulfill this role. Some support for this interpretation comes from the finding that, in acute hypoxia, there is a significant reduction in the number of dense-core vesicles in the cells of the neuroepithelial bodies and a concomitant decrease in their serotonin fluorescence. The paracrine release of their secretory products is assumed to activate the associated nerves, with an effect that is generally assumed to be regulatory. But much remains to be learned about how they affect respiratory functions.

BLOOD SUPPLY

The lung receives deoxygenated blood from the right side of the heart via the pulmonary trunk which branches into right and left *pulmonary arteries.* These, in turn, branch into arteries of progressively diminishing caliber

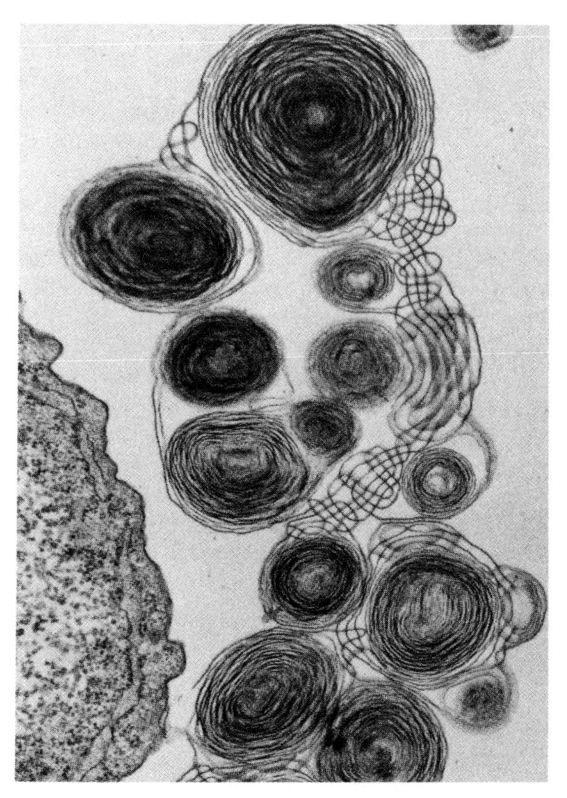

Figure 29–15. After release from the type-II alveolar cells, the phospholipid of the lamellar bodies forms complex myelin figures in the alveolar lumen. Some of the surfactant ultimately forms a monomolecular film over the surface of the alveolus. (Micrograph from M.C. Williams. Reproduced from J. Cell Biol. 72:260, 1977, by copyright permission of the Rockefeller Institute Press.)

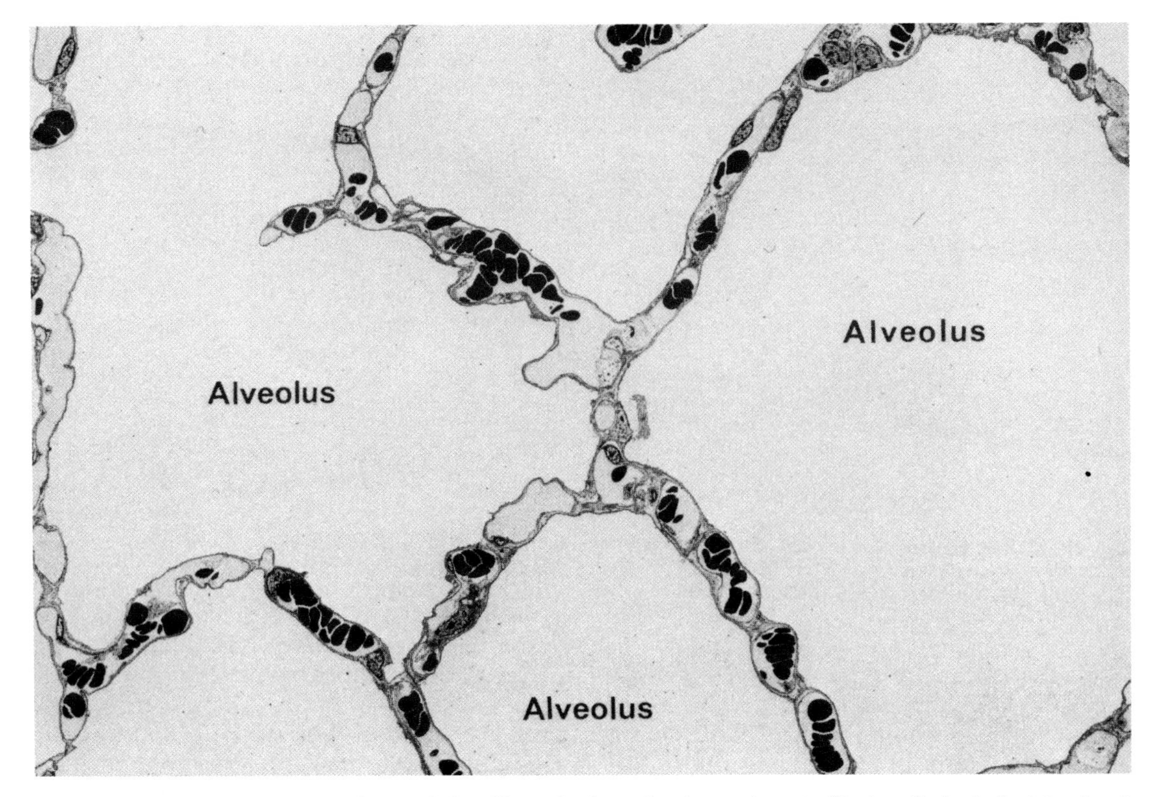

Figure 29–16. Electron micrograph of several alveoli in equine lung showing erythrocyte-filled capillaries in the interalveolar septa. (Micrograph courtesy of P. Gehr.)

that accompany the branches of the intrasegmental bronchi as far as the respiratory bronchioles. Branches to each alveolar duct then give rise to capillary networks in the septa between the alveoli. Oxygenated blood from the alveolar capillaries is carried by venules that converge to form veins of increasing size that run in the pleura and intersegmental connective tissue independently of arteries. As they approach the hilus, they course along branches of the bronchi and join to form a single large vein draining each lobe in the lung. Two veins from each lung ultimately open into the left atrium of the heart.

The lung also receives oxygenated blood and nutrients from *bronchial arteries* that arise from the descending aorta and upper intercostal arteries. These supply the wall of the bronchial tree as far distally as the respiratory bronchioles as well as the pleura and interlobular connective tissue. The bronchial veins returning blood from these latter structures and the hilar lymph nodes join the azygos and superior intercostal veins. However, there are numerous capillary anastomoses between the terminal branches of the pulmonary and bronchial arteries and between small bronchial and pulmonary veins. Most of the blood carried by the bronchial arteries is returned by the pulmonary veins.

The respiratory function of the lungs depends on the exchange of oxygen and carbon dioxide between the blood and the alveolar air. It is the unusually dense capillary network in the walls of the alveoli that makes this possible by making available a total endothelial surface of 126 m^2 for gas exchange. The lumen of the capillaries is only about 8 μm in diameter, making it necessary for erythrocytes to flow in single file, thus reducing the diffusion distance. The ultrastructure of the pulmonary capillaries is not significantly different from that of capillaries elsewhere in the body, but the endothelium has metabolic properties that enable it to carry out certain important nonrespiratory functions. These will be discussed below.

LYMPHATICS

The lymphatics of the lung fall into two main divisions, one in the pleura and the other

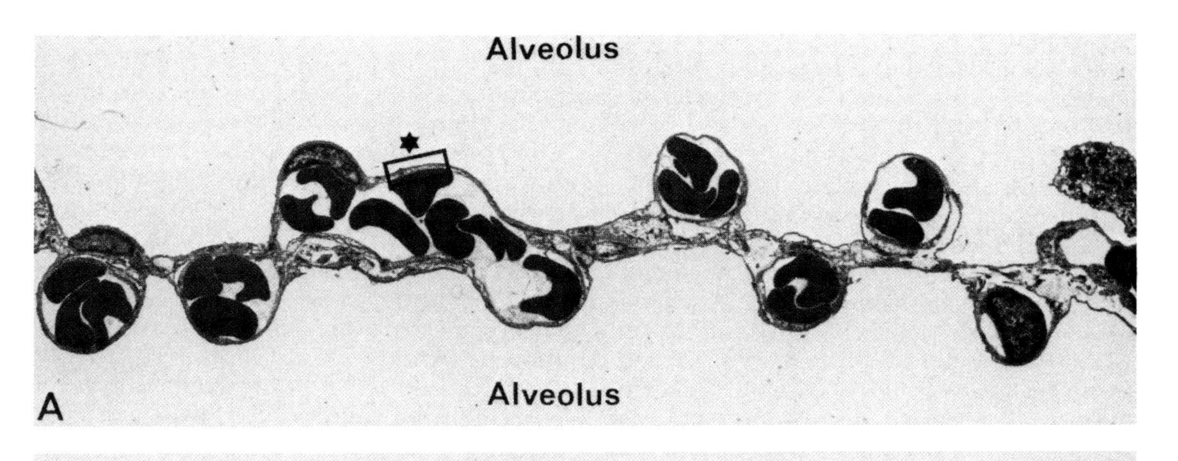

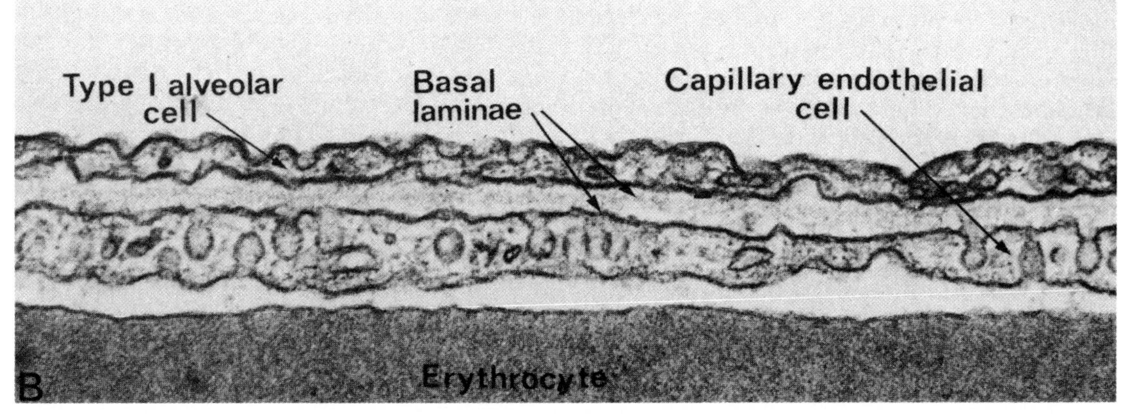

Figure 29–17. (A) Micrograph of the septum between two alveoli of rabbit lung. Capillaries covered by type-I alveolar cells bulge into the lumen, exposing a large surface to the inspired air. (B) A higher magnification of an area such as that enclosed in the rectangle in (A), showing the layers making up the diffusion barrier to gas exchange. (Micrographs courtesy of P. Gehr.)

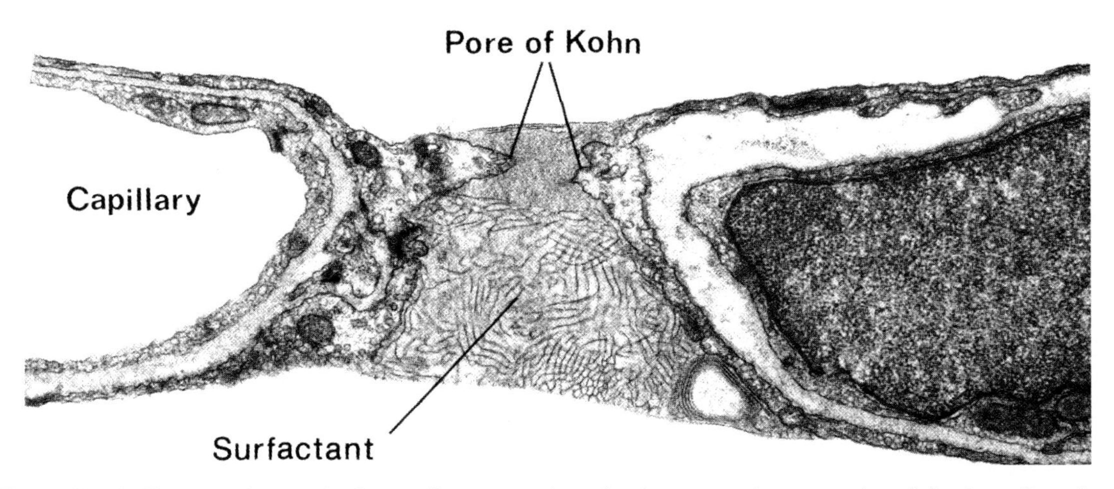

Figure 29–18. Electron micrograph of a small segment of an alveolar septum from a section of dog lung. Occasional small openings, called the pores of Kohn, traverse the thin wall between adjacent alveoli. The pore shown here is partially obstructed by an accumulation of surfactant. (Micrograph courtesy of P. Gehr.)

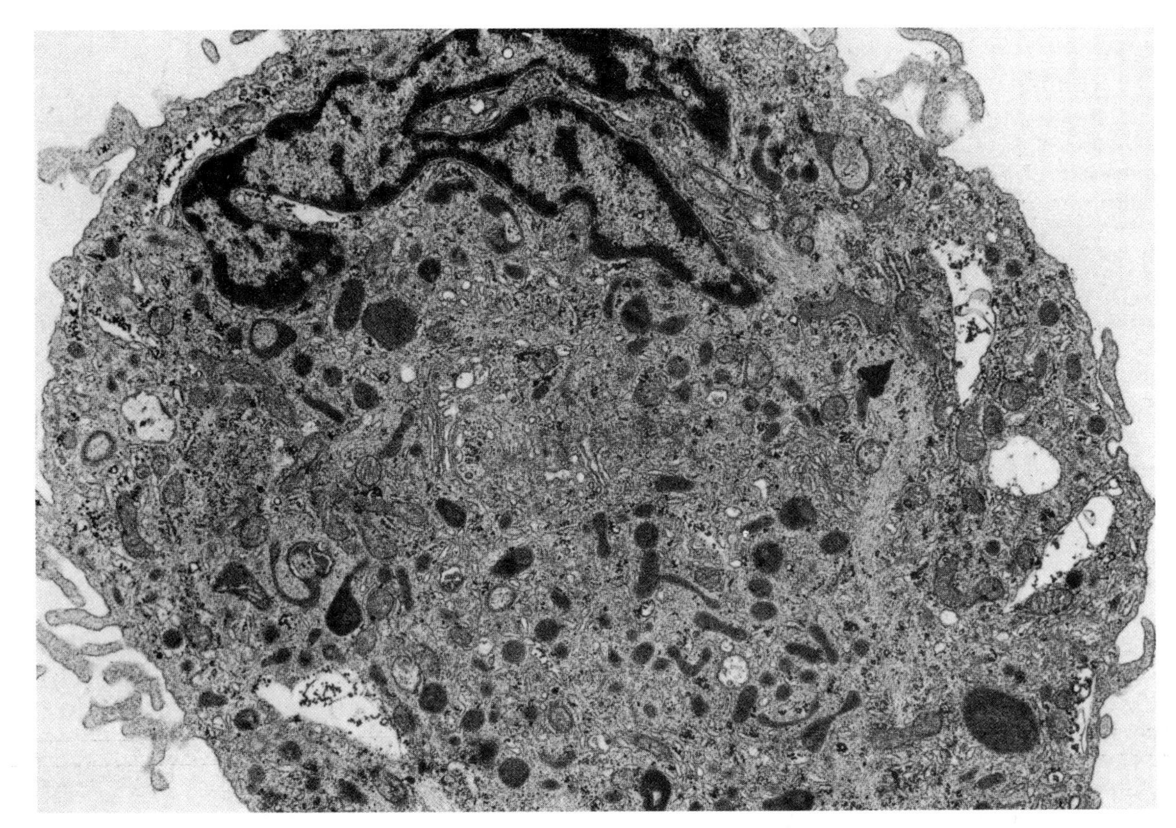

Figure 29–19. Electron micrograph of a human alveolar macrophage from a nonsmoker. The cell contains numerous small lysosomes but relatively few heterophagic vacuoles. (Compare with Fig. 29–20.) (Micrograph courtesy of S. Pratt and S.J. Ladman.)

in the pulmonary parenchyma. There are many communications between them. Both drain into lymph nodes in the hilus of the lungs. The lymphatics of the pleura form a dense network with larger and smaller polygonal meshes. The larger meshes demarcate the lobules and the smaller network tend to outline the smaller anatomical units. The pleural lymphatics join to form several main trunks that drain into the hilar lymph nodes.

Three main groups of pulmonary lymphatics are distinguishable namely, those associated with the bronchi, the pulmonary artery, and the pulmonary vein. Two or three main lymphatic trunks accompany the pulmonary artery. The lymphatics associated with the bronchi extend peripherally as far as the alveolar ducts. Their terminal branches join small branches of the lymphatics around the pulmonary artery and vein. There are no lymphatics beyond the alveolar ducts. Lymphatics accompanying the pulmonary vein begin in small branches in the alveolar ducts and pleural. The efferent trunks from the hilar nodes join to form the right lymphatic duct which is the principal channel of lymph drainage from both the right and left lungs. The intrapulmonary lymphatics lack valves, except in a few vessels in the interlobular connective tissue near the pleura. These lymphatics connect the pulmonary and the pleural lymphatic plexuses, and because their valves point toward the pleura, they provide a pathway through which lymph can flow from the lung parenchyma to the pleural lymphatics if the normal flow toward the hilus is interrupted.

HISTOPHYSIOLOGY OF THE RESPIRATORY TRACT

The function of the nasal passages in warming and humidification of the inspired air has already been pointed out. The importance of partial saturation of the air with water vapor is especially apparent in patients with a tracheostomy, who are obliged to take air directly into the trachea. Under these conditions, ex-

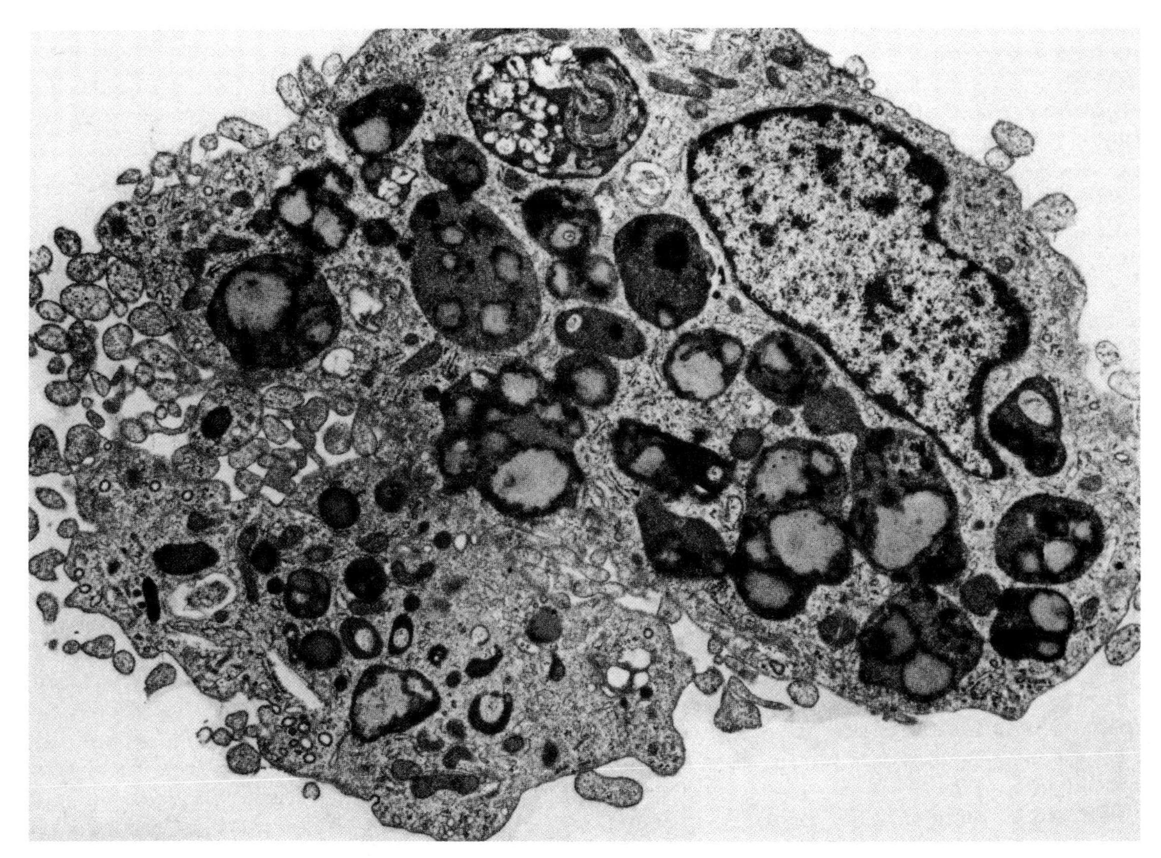

Figure 29–20. Electron micrograph of an alveolar macrophage from an 18-year-old smoker. The cytoplasm is crowded with masses of lipochrome pigment, representing undigestible residues of material phagocytized from the lumen of the alveoli. (Micrograph courtesy of S. Pratt and A.J. Ladman.)

cessive drying of the mucosa may lead to encrustation, interference with clearance of mucus from the upper airway and ultimately to severe infection. Similarly, if one nostril of a dog is surgically closed, the increased ventilation of the other nasal cavity exceeds its humidifying capacity and the drying of the mucosa may result in transformation of the ciliated columnar epithelium into stratified squamous epithelium, a change called *squamous metaplasia*.

Equally important is the clearing of the respiratory passages by the secretion of mucus and the coordinated beating of the epithelial cilia. Constant beating of the cilia at about 14 cycles per second moves the blanket of mucus at a speed of as much as 2 cm per minute, carrying dust, cellular debris, bacteria, and chemical pollutants toward the pharynx to be disposed of by swallowing. The physiological significance of this process is dramatically revealed in patients with the rare inherited condition known as *Karagener's syndrome* or *immobile cilia syndrome*. These individuals lack the dynein arms on the microtubules of the ciliary axonemes that are essential for motility. In the absence of motile cilia to clear their respiratory tract, these individuals suffer from chronic sinusitis, bronchitis, and bronchiectasis.

Another important device for removal of particulate matter and chemical irritants is the *cough reflex*, which depends on the presence of sensory nerve endings in the mucosa of the upper airway. Afferent impulses pass from these nerve endings to the central nervous system, triggering an involuntary sequence of events that involves deep inspiration, closure of the glottis, and forceful contraction of the abdominal and intercostal muscles that raises the pressure on the air impounded in the lungs. The epiglottis and larynx are then suddenly opened and the air, under pressure, bursts out, attaining velocities as high as 100 mph. The rush of air carries with it the irritant matter, removing it from the trachea and bronchi. The *sneeze reflex* involves a similar train of events that clears the nasal passages.

The primary life-sustaining function of the

lungs is to provide for uptake of oxygen from the inspired air and removal of carbon dioxide from the body. In inspiration, contraction of the diaphragm lowers intra-alveolar pressure, drawing air into the lungs. The rich network of capillaries in the walls of the alveoli are separated from the air by a very thin moist sheet of pulmonary epithelium that permits rapid diffusion of oxygen into, and carbon dioxide out of, the blood. The exchange of gases takes place by passive diffusion, but the liberation of carbon dioxide from carbonic acid is accelerated about 5000-fold by the enzyme *carbonic anhydrase* in the erythrocytes of the blood. Alcohol, ether, and other volatile substances are also eliminated via the lungs. In addition to the gas exchange there is a loss of about 800 ml of water a day in the expired air.

Expiration results mainly from a relaxation and elevation of the diaphragm that diminishes the volume of the thorax. But, a significant component of expiration is attributable to the inherent elastic properties of the lungs. As emphasized earlier in the chapter, the parenchyma of the lungs contains delicate networks of elastic fibers that are stretched during inspiration and recoil during expiration. In addition, the intermolecular forces within the thin film of fluid coating the walls of the alveoli maintain a surface tension that tends to reduce the surface area of the alveoli. This surface tension is thought to be responsible for about two-thirds of the recoil of the lungs during expiration and the elastic fibers account for the rest. The resistance to alveolar expansion during inspiration would be much greater were it not for the surfactant secreted by the type-II alveolar cells (type-II pneumonocytes) which lowers surface tension and thereby facilitates expansion. Pulmonary surfactant is especially important during the late fetal and early postnatal period. As the end of gestation approaches, the production and secretion of surfactant increases in preparation for air-breathing after birth. Premature infants in which this process is incomplete, often succumb to *respiratory distress syndrome* (hyaline membrane disease) caused by a deficiency in surfactant production. Administration of exogenous surfactant to infants with this disease results in dramatic improvement in oxygenation of their blood. Measurement of the amount of surfactant in the amniotic fluid late in pregnancy can be used to assess the degree of maturity of the lungs in the fetus.

Destruction of elastic fibers and diminished elastic recoil of the lungs are prominent features of the pathophysiology of *pulmonary emphysema*, a disease characterized by destructive changes in the alveolar walls, resulting in great enlargement of the air spaces distal to the terminal bronchioles, and attendant inefficiency of gaseous exchange. A number of environmental factors, including excessive cigarette smoking and air pollution, contribute to the development of the disease. However, it may occur in certain susceptible individuals in the absence of these factors. Susceptible individuals lack normal blood levels of α-antitrypsin, a versatile inhibitor of various proteases, including elastase. Such patients may be unable to control the effects of hydrolytic enzymes released from the lysosomes of pulmonary macrophages and polymorphonuclear leukocytes that accumulate in chronic pulmonary infections, and enzymatic destruction of the connective tissue framework of the alveolar walls results.

BIBLIOGRAPHY

GENERAL

Bettalanffy, F.D. 1964. Respiratory tissue: Structure, histophysiology, and cytodynamics. Internat. Rev. Cytol. 16:233.

Bryant, C. 1979. The Biology of Respiration. Baltimore, MD, University Park Press.

Buck, L. and R.A. Azel. 1991. A novel multigene family may encode receptors for odor recognition. Cell 65:175.

Comroe, J.H. 1974. Physiology of Respiration. Chicago, IL, Yearbook Medical Publishers.

Lancet, D. 1986. Vertebrate olfactory reception. Annu. Rev. Neurosci. 9:329.

Morrison, E.E. and R.M. Costanza. 1990. Morphology of the human olfactory epithelium. J. Comp. Neurol. 297:1.

Murray, J.F. 1976. The Normal Lung. Philadelphia, W.B. Saunders Co.

Thurlbeck, W.M. 1977. Structure of the lungs. Internat. Rev. Physiol. 14:1.

NOSE, PHARYNX, LARYNX

Allison, A.C. 1953. The morphology of the olfactory system of vertebrates. Biol. Rev. 28:195.

Cauna, N. 1982. Blood and nerve supply of the nasal lining. *In* B.F. Procter and I. Anderson, eds. The Nose: Upper Airway Physiology and the Atmospheric Environment, p. 45. New York, Elsevier Biomedical Press.

Cauna, N. and K.H. Hinderer. 1969. Fine structure of the blood vessels of the human nasal respiratory mucosa. Ann. Ontol. 78:865.

Fink, B.R. 1975. The Human Larynx. A Functional Study. New York, Raven Press.

Polyzonis, B.M., P.M. Kafandaris, P.I. Gigis, and T. Demi-

triou. 1979. An electron microscopic study of human olfactory mucosa. J. Anat. 128:77.
Reese, T.G. 1965. Olfactory cilia of the frog. J. Cell Biol. 25:209.

TRACHEA, BRONCHI, BRONCHIOLES

Baert, J. and M. Frederix. 1985. Globule leukocytes in the respiratory epithelium of the human upper airways. Anat. Rec. 212:143.
Boyd, M.R. 1977. Evidence for the Clara cell as a site of P450-dependent mixed function oxidase activity of the lung. Nature 269:713.
Breeze, R.G. and E.G. Wheeldon. 1977. The cells of the pulmonary airways. Am. J. Resp. Dis. 116:705.
Hoyt, R.F., S.P. Sorokin, and H. Feldman. 1983. Number, subtypes, and distributions of small granule neuroendocrine cells in the hamster lung. Exp. Lung Res. 3:273.
Lauweryns, J.M. and M. Cokelaere. 1973. Hypoxia-sensitive neuroepithelial bodies. Intrapulmonary secretory neuro-receptors modulated by the CNS. Z. Zellforsch. 145:521.
Lauweryns, J.M., M. Cokelaere, P. Theunyck, and M. Delearsnyder. 1974. Neuroepithelial bodies in mammalian respiratory mucosa: light optical, histochemical, and ultrastructural studies. Chest 65 (Suppl.):228.
Nadel, J. 1981. Regulation of fluid and mucous secretions in airways. J. Allergy Clin. Immunol. 67:417.
Plopper, C.G., L.H. Hill, and A.T. Mariassy. 1980. Ultrastructure of the non-ciliated bronchiolar epithelial (Clara) cell of mammalian lung III. A study of man with a comparison of 15 mammalian species. Exp. Lung Res. 1:171.
Sleigh, M.A. 1981. Ciliary function in mucus transport. Chest 80 (Suppl.):791.
Sleigh, M.A., J.R. Blake, and N. Liron. 1988. The propulsion of mucus by cilia. Annu. Rev. Resp. Dis. 137:726.

RESPIRATORY PORTION OF THE LUNG

Boyden, E.A. 1971. The structure of a pulmonary acinus in a child of 6 years. Anat. Rec. 169:282.
Chevalier, G. and A.J. Collet. 1972. In vivo incorporation of choline-^{3}H and galactose-^{3}H Into alveolar type-II pneumonocytes in relation to surfactant synthesis. A quantitative radioautographic study in mouse by electron microscopy. Anat. Rec. 174:289.
Clements, J.A. 1977. Function of the alveolar lining. Am. Rev. Resp. Dis. 115:67.
Gehr, P., M. Bachofen, and E.R. Weibel. 1978. The normal human lung: ultrastructure and morphometric estimation of diffusion capacity. Respir. Physiol. 32:121.
Gil, J. 1980. Organization of the microcirculation of the lung. Annu. Rev. Physiol. 42:177.
Post, M. and L.M. VanGolde. 1988. Metabolic and developmental aspects of pulmonary surfactant system. Biochim. Biophys. Acta 947:249.
Ryan, U.S., J.W. Ryan, and D.S. Smith. 1975. Alveolar type II cells: Studies on the mode of release of lamellar bodies. Tissue Cell 7:587.
Sorokin, S.P. 1967. A morphological and cytochemical study of the great alveolar cell. J. Histochem. Cytochem. 14:884.
Stratton, J.C. 1978. The ultrastructure of the multilamellar bodies and surfactant in human lung. Cell Tissue Res. 193:219.
Strum, J.M. and A.F. Junod. 1972. Radioautographic demonstration of 5-hydroxytryptamine-^{3}H uptake by pulmonary endothelial cells. J. Cell Biol. 54:456.
Weibel, E.R. 1973. Morphological basis of alveolar-capillary gas exchange. Physiol. Rev. 53:419.
Weibel, E.R., P. Gehr, D. Haies, and J. Gil. 1976. The cell population of the normal lung. *In* A. Bouhuys, ed. Lung Cells in Disease. Amsterdam, Elsevier/North Holland Biomedical Press.

PULMONARY MACROPHAGES AND MAST CELLS

Hocking, W.G. and D.W. Golde. 1979. The pulmonary alveolar macrophage. N. Engl. J. Med. 301:580.
Sorokin, S.G. 1977. Phagocytes in the lungs: incidence, general behavior, and phylogeny. *In* J.D. Brain, D.F. Proctor, and L. Reid, eds. Respiratory Disease Mechanisms, p. 711. New York, Marcel Dekker.
Wasserman, G.I. 1980. The Lung mast cell: its physiology and potential relevance to defense of the lung. Environ. Health Perspect. 35:153.

30

THE URINARY SYSTEM

The urinary system consists of the *kidneys, ureters,* the *urinary bladder,* and the *urethra.* In producing urine, the kidneys excrete excess water and the waste products of metabolism. This fluid is transported in the ureters, to the bladder for temporary storage, and is later voided via the urethra. In the female, the urethra is solely a urinary duct, but in the male, it also serves as the pathway for ejaculation of the semen. In addition to their excretion of the waste products of metabolism, the kidneys play an important role in maintenance of the body's normal extracellular fluid volume, and in the control of acid–base balance. They also have an endocrine function, releasing into the blood two hormones, *erythropoietin,* which acts on the bone marrow to stimulate production of erythrocytes, and *renin,* which is important in the regulation of blood pressure. They are also involved in the metabolism of vitamin D to yield a compound that controls the level of calcium in the body fluids.

KIDNEYS

The human kidneys are situated retroperitoneally on the posterior wall of the abdomen on either side of the vertebral column. They are bean-shaped organs 10–12 cm in length, 5–6 cm in width, and 3–4 cm in thickness. On the medial border of each kidney, there is a fissure, called the *hilus,* which leads inward to the *renal sinus,* a deep recess in the organ that contains the renal artery and vein, some adipose tissue, and a funnel-shaped expansion of the upper end of the ureter called the *renal pelvis.* The renal pelvis divides into two long branches, the *major calyces,* and these, in turn, have short branches called the *minor calyces* (Fig. 30–1).

When the cut surface of the hemisected kidney is viewed with the naked eye, a dark reddish-brown *cortex* is readily distinguishable from a lighter colored *medulla.* The latter is made up of 6 to 10 conical sectors, called the *renal pyramids,* each having its broad base toward the cortex and its apex, called a *renal papilla,* projecting into the lumen of a minor calyx. The lateral boundaries of each pyramid are defined by darker inward extensions from the cortex, the *renal columns.* One renal pyramid and its bounding renal columns constitute a *renal lobule.* Each lobule develops, in the embryo, in association with a separate minor calyx, and the lobules are clearly outlined by grooves on the surface of the fetal kidney, but they fuse completely as development progresses and they are no longer recognizable on the postnatal kidney which has a smooth surface. In the *multilobular* human kidney, each lobule corresponds to an entire *unilobular* kidney of laboratory rodents.

The parenchyma of the kidney is made up of myriad, minute *uriniferous tubules* that are its functional units. Along the length of these tubules, successive segments are specialized for different roles in the formation of the urine. Corresponding segments of the many parallel tubules are in register at the same level of the renal medulla, resulting in transverse bands or zones which differ slightly in color or texture. Thus, the *outer medulla* can be distinguished from the *inner medulla,* and the outer medulla is further divisible into a thin light-colored *outer stripe* and a slightly thicker and darker *inner stripe.* A fine radial striation, detectable in each pyramid, is attributable to the convergence of the straight portions of the uriniferous tubules, on the papilla. On the so-called *area cribrosa* at the end of the papilla, one can see about 25 pores, which are the openings of the terminal segments of the uriniferous tubules into the minor calyx. From the base of the medullary pyramids, bundles of straight segments of the tubules extend for some distance upward into the cortex, forming pale vertical striations described as the *medullary rays* (Fig. 30–1).

The structural basis for the pattern seen on the cut surface of the normal kidney will be better understood after the description of the

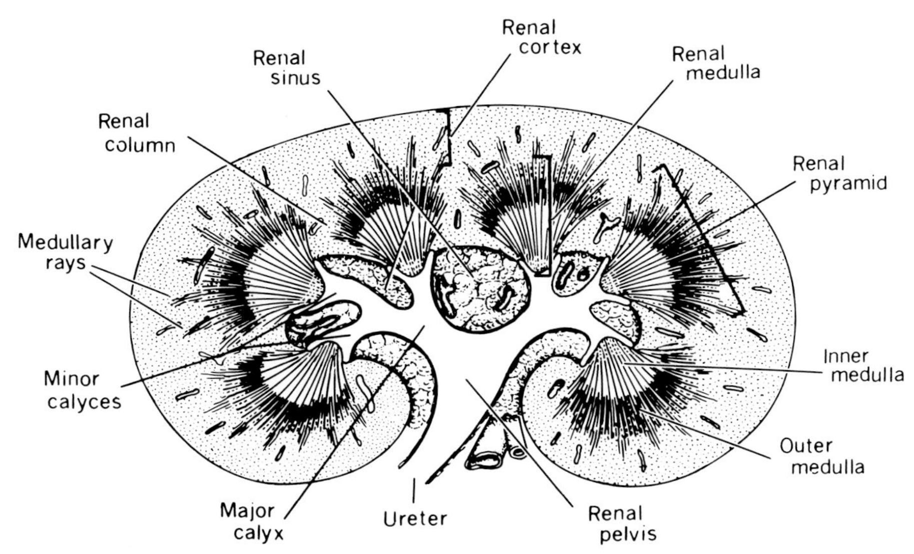

Figure 30–1. Schematic delineation of the structural components identifiable with the naked eye on the cut surface of a hemisected kidney.

microscopic organization of the uriniferous tubules. Conversely, description of their form and location will be facilitated by reference to the visible landmarks on the hemisectioned kidney, presented in the foregoing paragraph. Familiarity with these markings is also useful to the pathologist because their pattern is often distorted, in characteristic ways, in different disease states.

URINIFEROUS TUBULES

The uriniferous tubule consists of two functionally distinct portions. The first, called the *nephron,* collects a filtrate of the blood created in a spherical mass of tortuous capillaries, at its proximal end (Fig. 30–5), and modifies the composition of this fluid by adding nitrogenous wastes to it and by reabsorbing from it certain components that need to be conserved. The second portion, the *collecting tubule,* absorbs water from the filtrate to concentrate its solutes, resulting in a hypertonic urine which is conveyed to the renal pelvis. These two portions arise in the embryo from separate primordia that become connected later in development. This contrasts with the development of glands, where the ducts and the secretory portions arise from a single primordium that branches repeatedly and later becomes secretory in the distal portions of its arborescence.

The Nephron

There are approximately 1.5 million uriniferous tubules in a human kidney. Along the length of the nephron in each of these, there are six morphologically distinguishable segments, each occurring at a particular level in the cortex or medulla. The epithelium lining of each segment has a characteristic microscopic structure related to its specialization for a specific function in the formation of urine.

Traditionally, only four segments of the renal tubule were recognized, namely, the *proximal convolution,* the *loop of Henle,* the *distal convolution,* and the *collecting duct.* With the rapid increase in knowledge that followed the introduction of the electron microscope, and the development of sophisticated physiological methods for assessing the function of short segments of the renal tubule, the traditional description of the nephron no longer sufficed and a proliferation of new terms led to inconsistencies in usage. In an effort to resolve the resulting confusion, a standard nomenclature for the components of the kidney was developed by the Renal Commission of the International Union of Physiological Sciences. In what follows, we adopt this terminology but enclose in parentheses older terms or abbreviations that are still in general use.

Four major subdivisions of the uriniferous tubule are now recognized: the *proximal tubule, intermediate tubule, distal tubule,* and the *collecting system.* Each of these is further subdivided into two or more segments. At the proximal end of each nephron, there is a closed, thin-walled expansion of the tubule that is deeply invaginated to form a cup-shaped hollow structure called *Bowman's capsule.* The concavity of this blind end of the nephron is occupied by a globular tuft of highly convoluted capillaries, the *glomerulus.* This mass of capillaries and its surrounding chalice-shaped epithelial capsule, together, constitute the *renal corpuscle.* It has a vascular pole where the afferent and efferent vessels enter and leave the glomerulus, and a urinary pole where the slit-like cavity between the layers of the invaginated Bowman's capsule (*urinary space* or *Bowman's space*) is continuous with the lumen of the proximal tubule. Two segments of the proximal tubule are distinguished: the *proximal convoluted tubule* (PCT, *pars convoluta*), situated in the cortex, and the *proximal straight tubule* (PST, *pars recta*), extending from the cortex into the outer stripe of the medulla. This is followed by the *intermediate tubule* which forms a long loop which is subdivided into the *descending thin limb* (DTL, *pars descendens*), traversing the inner stripe of the outer medulla and extending deep into the inner medulla, and a recurrent portion, the *ascending thin limb* (ATL, *pars ascendens*). At the junction of the inner and outer medulla, the ascending thin limb is continuous with the *distal straight tubule* (DST, *thick ascending limb*) which traverses the outer medulla and continues into the cortex, where it becomes the *distal convoluted tubule* (DCT). In the cortex, the distal convoluted tubule is joined by a *connecting tubule* (CT), to a *collecting duct* (CD), which passes downward through the cortex and medulla to the area cribrosa of the renal papilla, where it opens into a minor calyx (Fig. 30–2).

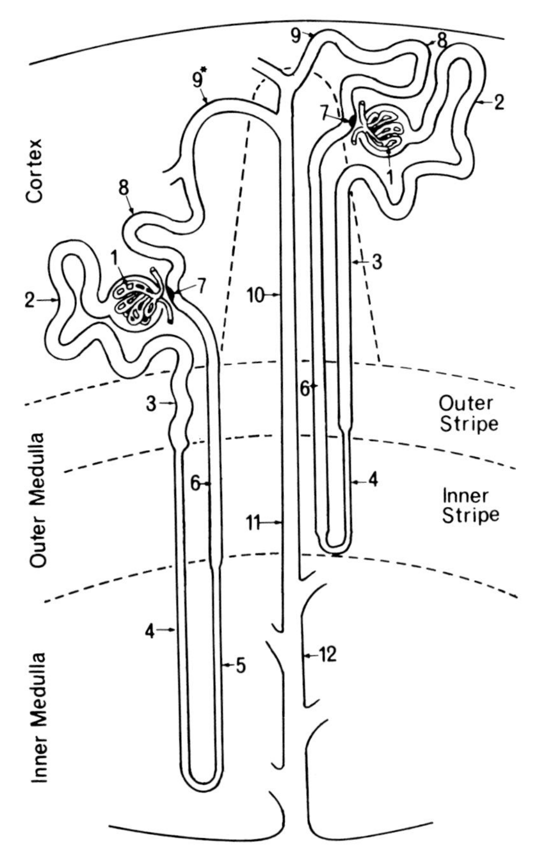

Figure 30–2. Drawing depicting the principal segments of a uriniferous tubule and their approximate location in the cortex, outer medulla, or inner medulla. A long-looped nephron is depicted on the left and a short-looped nephron on the right.

The portion of the nephron, traditionally called the *loop of Henle,* includes the segments now called the thick descending limb of the proximal tubule, the thin descending and ascending limbs of the intermediate tubule, and the thick ascending limb of the distal tubule. These several segments are represented in the same sequence in all nephrons, but the length of the loop of Henle varies. In addition to *long-looped nephrons* described above, there are *short-looped nephrons,* in which the loop turns back in the outer medulla (Fig. 30–2), and *cortical nephrons,* which have a very short loop that does not extend into the medulla but turns back in the inner cortex. The renal corpuscles also vary in their location. Some may be near the renal capsule, others midcortical, and still others are juxtamedullary (Fig. 30–2). Surprisingly, the length of the loop of Henle of a nephron is not closely correlated with the position of its glomerules in the cortex.

The intermingling of the serpentine convoluted tubules within the cortex makes it impossible, in histological sections, to relate their cross sections to a particular renal corpuscle. What is known of the three-dimensional configuration of the nephron has been gained by their reconstruction from serial sections, or by maceration of the tissue followed by teasing out intact individual nephrons with a micromanipulator. It has also been possible, by micropuncture, to impale individual glomerular capsules and to observe directly the progress of injected contrast medium through the lumen of an entire uriniferous tubule.

Renal Corpuscle

Bowman's capsule around a glomerulus is a double-walled cup composed of squamous epithelial cells. Although it is not strictly true, it is conceptually useful to envision that in development of the renal corpuscle, the glo-

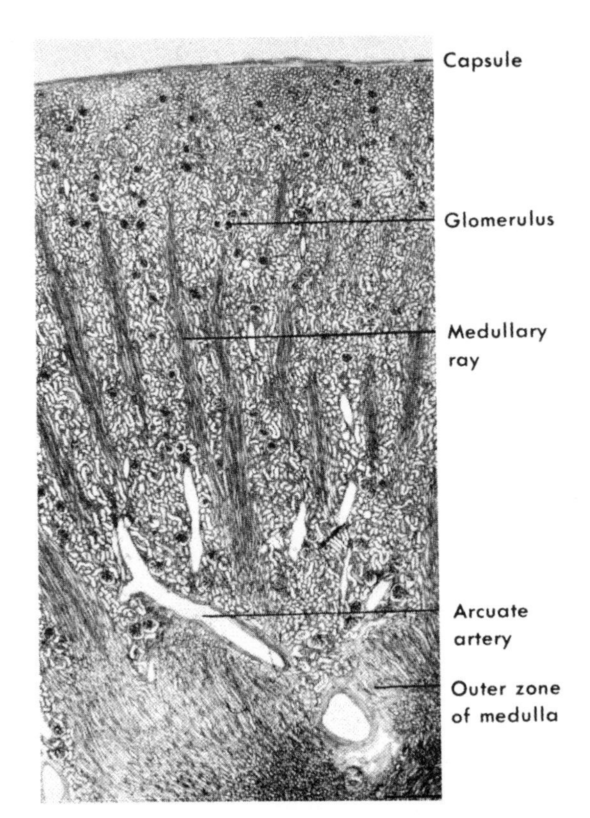

Figure 30–3. A low-power photomicrograph of monkey kidney showing the glomeruli distributed through the cortex and the medullary rays extending upward from the medulla.

merulus is pushed into and deeply indents a blind terminal expansion of the uriniferous tubule. There is, therefore, a *visceral layer* of epithelium (the *glomerular epithelium*) closely applied to the capillaries and a *parietal layer* (the *capsular epithelium*), with the two separated by a narrow cavity, the *capsular space* (*Bowman's space*). At the vascular pole of the renal corpuscle, the visceral layer is reflected off of the afferent and efferent vessels and is continuous with the parietal layer of epithelium. At the urinary pole, the squamous epithelium of the parietal layer is continuous with the cuboidal epithelium lining the neck of the proximal convoluted tubule (Fig. 30–4).

In the development of the renal corpuscle, the cells of the visceral layer become so extensively modified that they bear little resemblance to those of any other epithelium in the body. The individual cells, called *podocytes,* are basically stellate in form with several radiating primary processes that embrace the underlying capillaries and give rise to very numerous secondary branches called *foot-processes* or *pedicels.* These interdigitate with corresponding processes of neighboring podocytes but are not closely adherent to them. An extraordinarily elaborate system of intercellular clefts is thus formed through which a filtrate of the blood plasma can enter the capsular space. These relationships go undetected with the light microscope but are clearly seen in scanning electron micrographs (Figs. 30–6, 30–7 and 30–8). The secondary processes of the podocytes are closely applied to the basal lamina of the underlying capillary but the cell body is usually separated from it by 1–3 μm. The cell body and primary processes of one podocyte may arch over processes of neighboring podocytes. As a result of this intermingling and crossing of primary processes, their terminal branches appear always to interdigitate with those of another cell rather than with foot-processes arising from another primary process of the same cell. The separation of the cell bodies from the underlying capillaries permits the greater part of the capillary surface to be carpeted by small interdigitating foot-processes, an arrangement maximizing the total area of intercellular clefts available for filtration (Fig. 30–9).

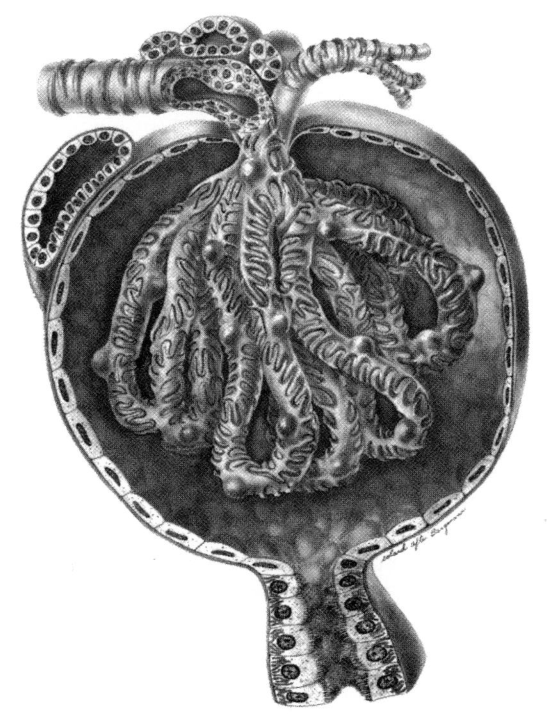

Figure 30–4. A highly schematic drawing of a renal corpuscle. The parietal layer of Bowman's capsule is not as thick as depicted here. Although the glomerulus was formerly described as a cluster of capillary loops as shown here, the capillaries are now known to branch and anastromose forming a complex network. (Redrawn and modified after Bargmann, Zeitschrift Zellforschung 8:765, 1929.)

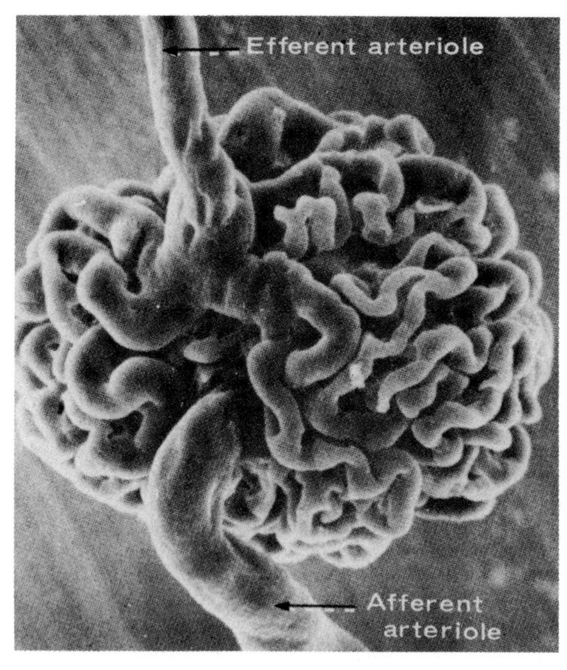

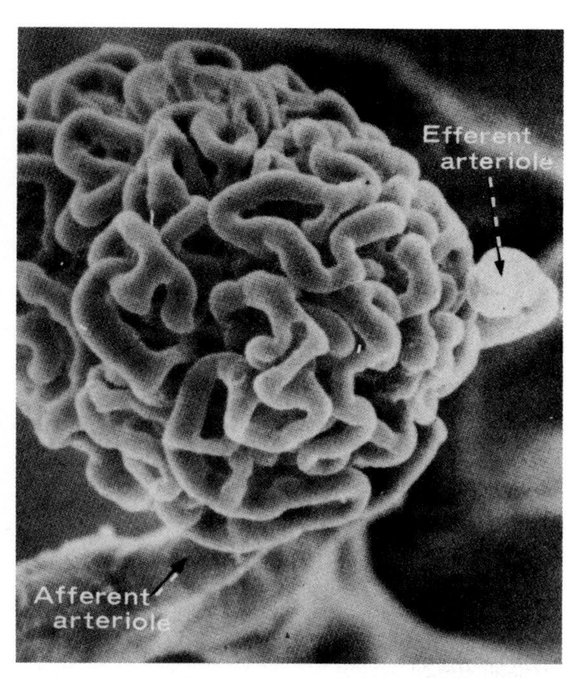

Figure 30–5. Scanning micrographs of plastic casts of two glomeruli, one viewed from the vascular pole (left) and the other from the capsular side (right). Observe that the capillaries branch and anastomose. Note also that the caliber of the afferent arteriole is smaller than that of the efferent arteriole, which no doubt ensures an adequate filtration pressure in the capillaries. (Micrographs from Takizawa, J. et al. 1979. Lab. Investig. 40:519.)

In electron micrographs of thin sections, the nucleus of the podocytes is often infolded and irregular in outline. The cytoplasm contains a small Golgi complex, a moderate number of cisternal profiles of rough endoplasmic reticulum, and abundant free polyribosomes. Intermediate filaments and microtubules are plentiful, both in the cell body and in its primary processes. Actin filaments and heavy meromyosin have been localized cytochemically in the bases of the foot-processes. In sections that pass longitudinally through a glomerular capillary, cross sections of foot-processes of rather uniform size are aligned on the unusually thick basal lamina of the endothelium (Fig. 30–10). The bases of the foot-processes are somewhat expanded, giving them a characteristic bell-shaped profile. Adjacent foot-processes are separated by *filtration slits* 25–35 nm wide. At the level of the basal lamina, the slits are spanned by a 4–6 nm *slit-diaphragm.* In surface view, the diaphragm has a porous substructure with a central linear density connected to the membrane of adjacent foot-processes by cross-bridges spaced about 4 nm apart. The resulting pores between them are believed to be small enough to prevent passage of albumin and larger molecules from the blood into the glomerular filtrate. The plasma membrane of the foot-processes has a prominent glycocalyx that is negatively charged and stains intensely with ruthenium red (Fig. 30–11). This coat has now been isolated and identified as a 140 kD sialoglycoprotein that is called *podocalyxin.* In the living state, the filamentous molecules forming the glycocalyx on adjacent foot-processes, probably largely fill the filtration slits. Because both molecular size and charge play a role in determining what substances can enter the filtrate, the high negative charge of the surface coat could be a significant component of the filtration barrier.

The basal lamina between the glomerular epithelium and the endothelium of the capillaries is 0.1–0.15 μm in thickness and has the same three layers seen in other basal laminae, namely, a *lamina rara externa* adjacent to the foot-processes, a darker central zone, the *lamina densa,* and a *lamina rara interna* adjacent to the endothelium. These show little resolvable substructure, in routine electron micrographs, but when stained with ruthenium red or cationized ferritin, the density of the lamina densa is enhanced, and regularly spaced densities are revealed in the laminae rarae. These coincide with the immunocytochemical localization of fibronectin, which may serve to an-

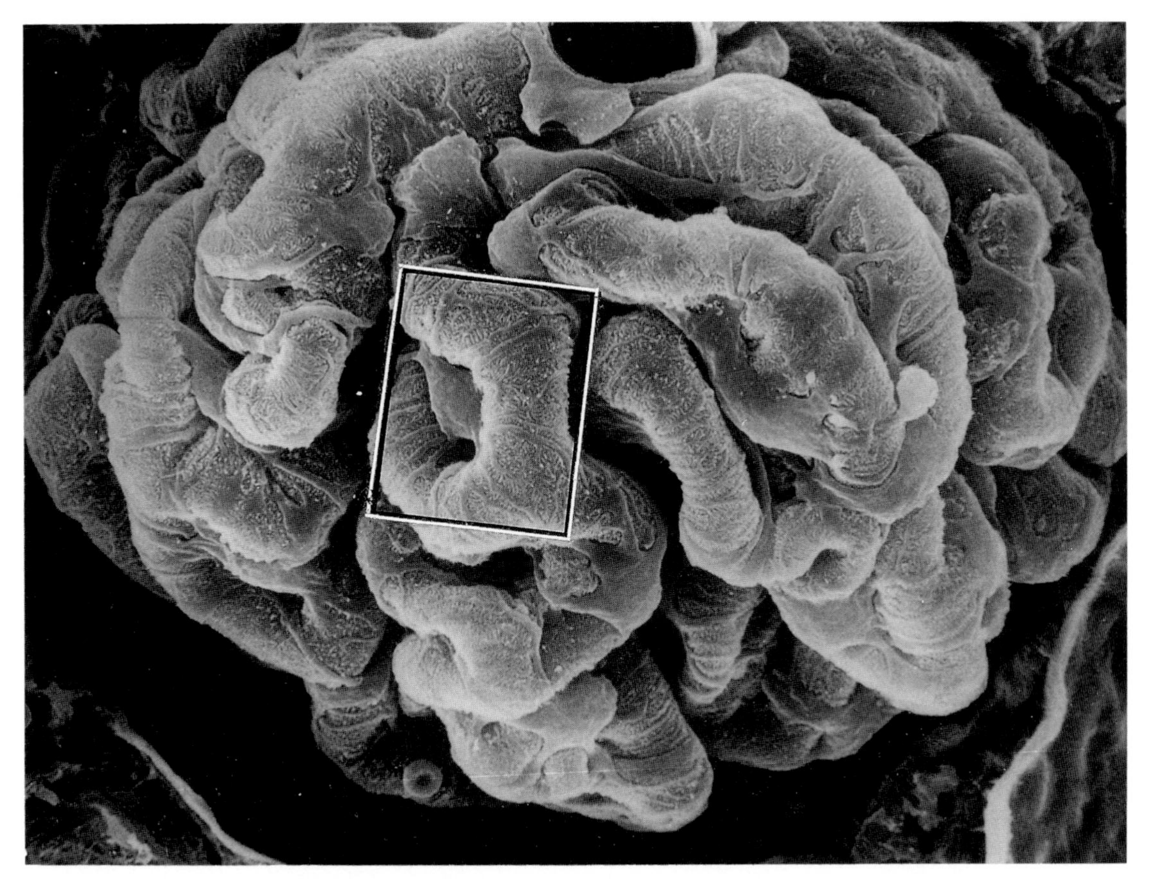

Figure 30–6. Scanning micrograph of a renal glomerulus. The area enclosed in the rectangle is shown at higher magnification in Fig. 30–7. (Micrograph courtesy of Andrews, P. 1988. J. Electr. Microsc. Tech. 9:115.)

chor the epithelial and endothelial cells to the lamina densa, which consists of a meshwork of type-IV collagen and laminin in a matrix rich in heparan sulfate proteoglycan. The negatively charged proteoglycan is believed to contribute to the electrostatic barrier of the glomerular filter (Fig. 30–11).

The endothelium of the glomerular capillaries is thin and perforated by pores 70–90 nm in diameter. The freeze–fracture method of specimen preparation often provides extensive *en face* views of the pores (Fig. 30–12). Their abundance and uniform distribution are also clearly seen in scanning electron micrographs of glomeruli dissociated by enzymatic digestion, which removes the basal lamina (Fig. 30–13). Unlike those of other fenestrated capillaries, the pores of the glomerular capillaries do not have a pore diaphragm. The thicker portion of the endothelial cell bodies, containing the nucleus, is usually located on the side of the capillary away from the capsular space.

The spaces between the glomerular capillaries is occupied by *mesangium,* a connective tissue consisting of *mesangial cells* in an extracellular matrix that is relatively free of fibrous elements other than fibronectin. The mesangial cells are considered to be a specialized type of pericyte providing structural support for the capillary loops. Unlike other pericytes, they are phagocytic and it is speculated that they may participate in the continuous turnover of the basal lamina by removing its outer portion containing residues of filtration, while the lamina is renewed on its inner surface by the endothelial cells. Studies of mesangial cells in culture have directed attention to other properties that may be of physiological significance. They have been shown to be contractile and to respond to angiotensin-II and other vasoconstrictors that are known to reduce the area of the intraglomerular filtration barrier by reducing the blood flow through some of the capillary loops. The mesangial cells that are most favorably situated to regulate the number of open loops are those near the vascular pole of the glomerulus. Vasodila-

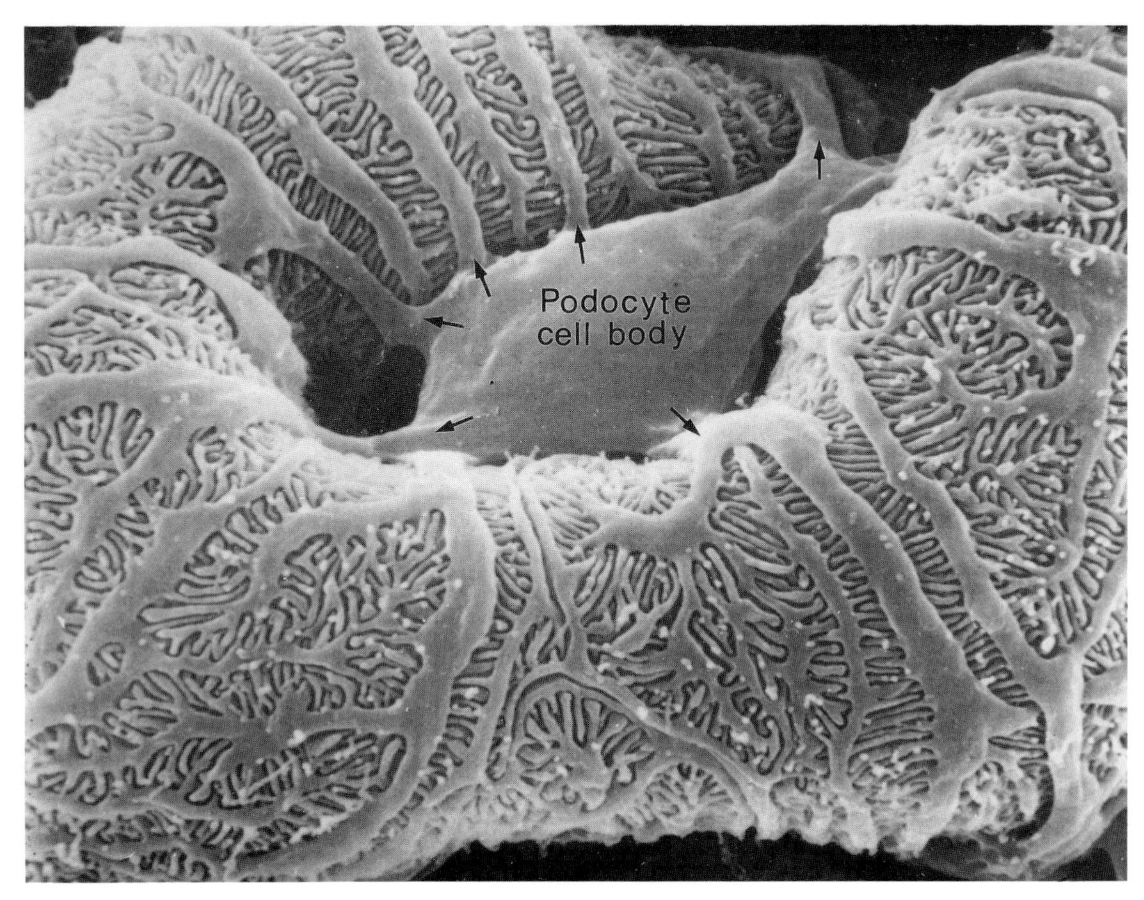

Figure 30–7. Higher magnification of the area in the rectangle on Fig. 30–6, which includes a glomerular capillary loop and a podocyte cell body, its primary processes (at arrows), and the labyrinthine system of interdigitating secondary processes (pedicels) that bound the filtration slits. (Micrograph courtesy of Andrews, P. J. Electr. Microsc. Tech. 9:115, 1988.)

tation increasing the filtration rate is one of the principal effects of hormones, called atriopeptides, that are secreted by certain cells of the myocardium. The mesangial cells have been found to have specific receptors for these hormones, suggesting that it is these cells that mediate their effects on flow through the glomeruli.

The continuous filtration of the blood plasma in the renal glomeruli is a process that is essential for the elimination of nitrogenous wastes and control of the extracellular fluid composition and of blood volume. The structural components of the filter are (1) the fenestrated endothelium, (2) the basal lamina, and (3) the filtration slits between the foot-processes of the podocytes. Which of these components is the primary filter serving to retain plasma proteins in the circulation is still debated, but it is the prevailing view that the endothelial pores are only a coarse sieve holding back the formed elements of the blood and that the basal lamina is the main filter. The mesangial cells may serve to unclog and recondition the filter by disposing of filtration residues that may accumulate within it.

The Proximal Tubule

At the urinary pole of the renal corpuscle, the squamous parietal epithelium of Bowman's capsule is continuous with the cuboidal epithelium of the proximal tubule of the nephron (Fig. 30–4). After a few short convolutions near the glomerulus, this tubule forms a longer loop directed toward the surface of the kidney. The recurrent limb of this loop returns to the vicinity of the renal corpuscle and enters the nearest medullary ray, where it straightens out to become the *pars recta* of the proximal tubule, coursing inward toward the medulla. The proximal tubules are the longest segment of the nephron and together

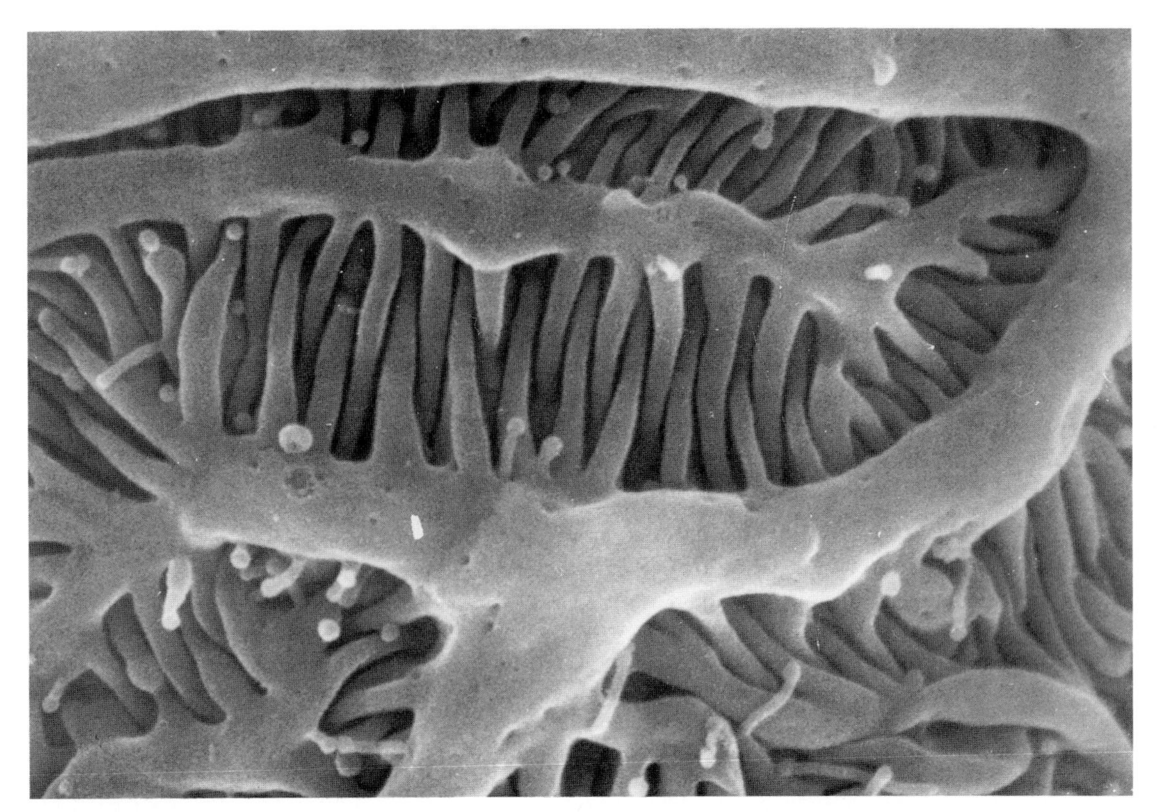

Figure 30–8. High-magnification scanning micrograph of primary processes and foot processes (pedicels) of a podocyte. Note the narrow filtration slits between the foot processes. (Micrograph courtesy of Andrews, P. 1988. J. Electr. Microsc. Tech. 9:115.)

they make up the greatest part of the renal cortex.

The epithelium of the proximal tubule has a prominent bush border. In histological sections, the lumen of this segment often appears occluded by approximation of the brush borders of the cells around it. It was formerly thought that this was the normal condition and that the glomerular filtrate percolated through the interstices between the microvilli of the brush border. This apparent obliteration of the lumen is now known to be a fixation artifact. If the kidney is fixed by perfusion and an agonal fall of intravascular pressure is prevented, all proximal tubules will have an open lumen (Figs. 30–14 and 30–15). The cells have a single spherical nucleus in an eosinophilic cytoplasm. The Golgi complex forms a crown around the upper pole of the nucleus, and numerous long mitochondria, in the basal half of the cells, tend to be oriented parallel to the cell axis. This orientation of the mitochondria results in a faint vertical striation of the basal cytoplasm in histological sections.

The tips of the thousands of closely spaced microvilli forming the brush border are limited by a membrane with a prominent glycocalyx. Opening into the clefts between the microvilli are tubular invaginations of the plasma membrane called *apical canaliculi* (Fig. 30–16). On the cytoplasmic surface of their limiting membrane, there are short spiny projections resembling those seen on the clathrin-coated vesicles of other cell types engaged in receptor-mediated endocytosis. In the cytoplasm around the ends of the canaliculi, there are numerous small vesicles and larger vacuoles. Some of the latter are no doubt early endosomes resulting from receptor-mediated endocytosis.

The lateral boundaries of the cells usually are not resolved with the light microscope, due, in part, to their extensive interdigitation. The very complex shape of the proximal tubule cells can only be fully appreciated in the three-dimensional reconstructions from electron micrographs (Fig. 30–17). A number of alternating ridges and grooves extend the full length of the cell, as on the fluted columns of classical architecture. The ridges become increasingly prominent from apex to base,

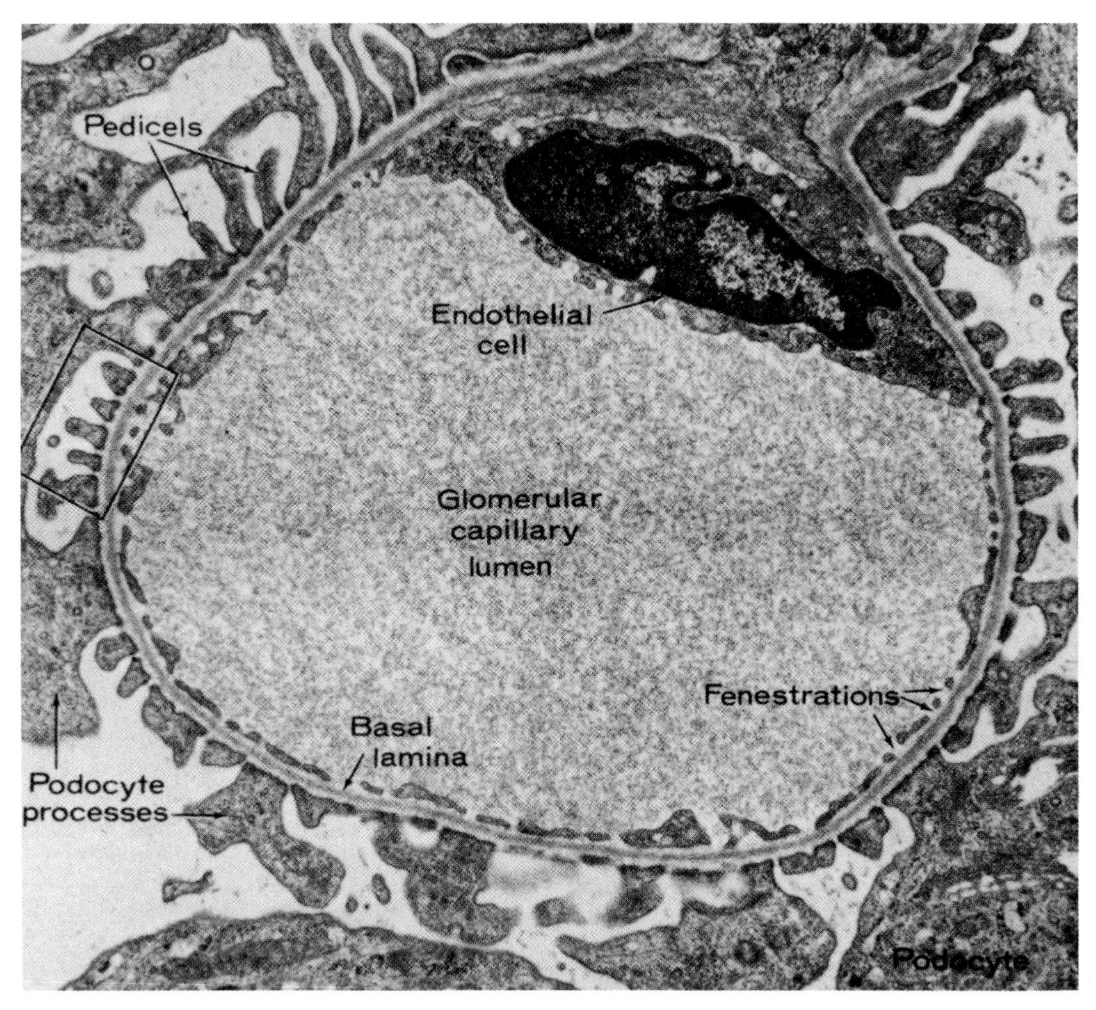

Figure 30–9. Electron micrograph of a transverse section through a glomerular capillary showing the basal lamina interposed between the fenestrated endothelium and the slit pores between pedicels of the visceral epithelium of Bowman's capsule. An area comparable to that in the rectangle is shown at higher magnification in Fig. 30–10. (Micrograph from Tyson, G., and R. Bulger. 1972. Anat. Rec. 172:669.)

and near the basal lamina they become elongated into branching processes that extend beneath the bodies of neighboring cells (Figs. 30–18 and 30–19). In thin sections, paired membranes run from the basal lamina up into the cell, compartmentalizing the basal cytoplasm. The membranes were initially interpreted as simple infoldings of the plasmalemma, but it was noted that some of the basal compartments are not open to the cytoplasm at any point. It is now clear that these compartments are not part of the overlying cell but are cross sections of undermining processes of neighboring cells. This elaborate interdigitation of the basal portions of the cells greatly amplifies the area of the cell surface exposed to the fluid in a labyrinthine system of intercellular clefts.

The proximal tubule reabsorbs nearly all of the glucose and amino acids in the glomerular filtrate, while allowing other substances of no nutritional value to be excreted in the urine. As in other transporting epithelia, the apical and basolateral domains of the plasma membrane differ in the nature of their integral proteins. The membrane of the brush border contains the transport systems for glucose and amino acids. Peptidases, also present in this membrane, are also believed to be involved in the regulation of circulating levels of small peptide hormones. The efficiency of the mechanisms residing in the apical membrane is greatly enhanced by the brush border's 20-fold amplification of the area of membrane exposed to the glomerular filtrate. Similarly, the efficiency of transport mechanisms in the

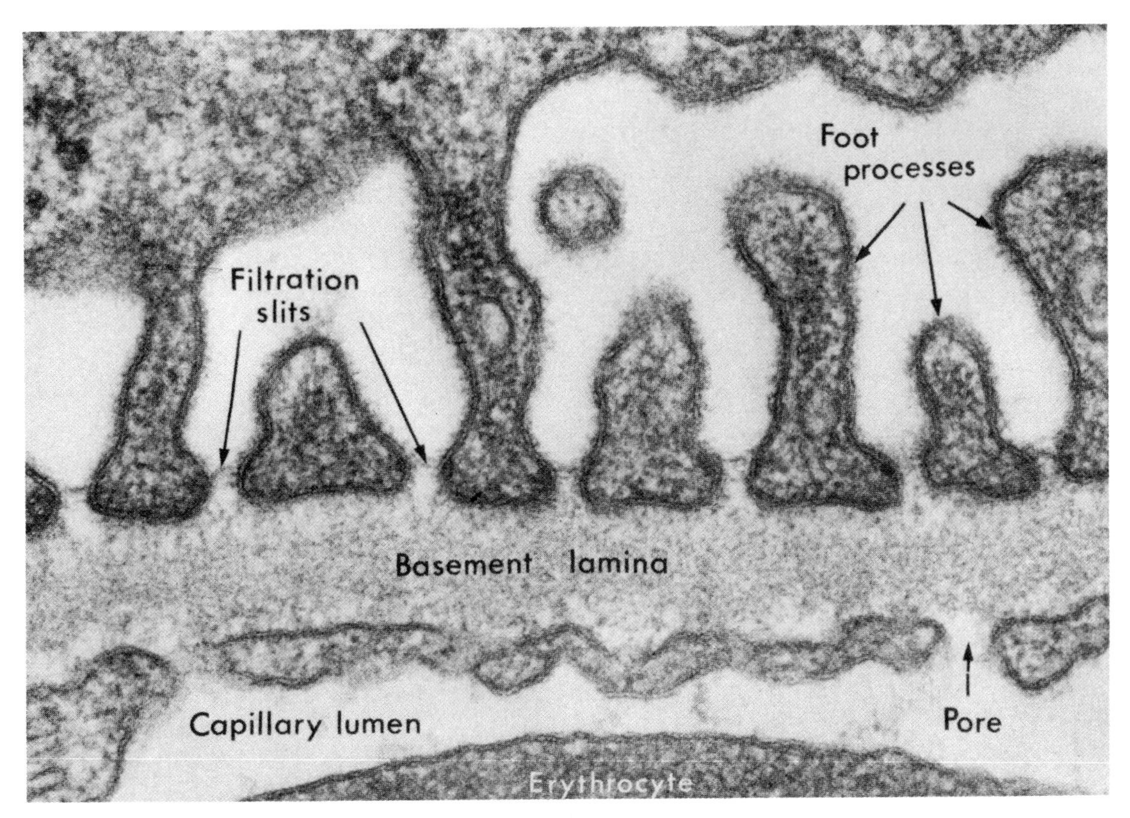

Figure 30–10. Electron micrograph of a portion of the wall of a glomerular capillary showing the foot processes of a podocyte on the outer surface of the basal lamina and the fenestrated endothelium on its inner aspect. (Micrograph courtesy of D. Friend.)

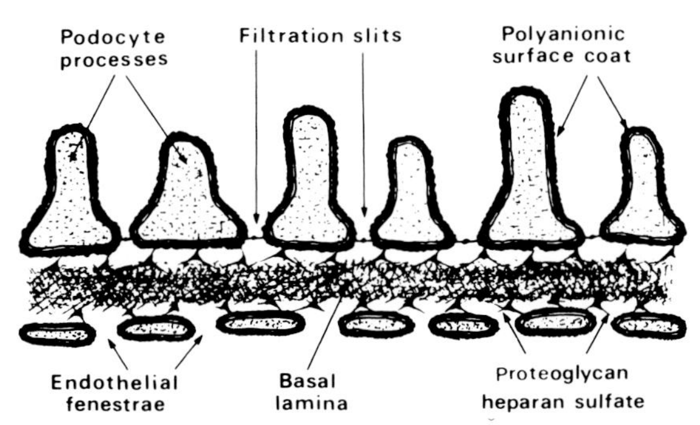

Figure 30–11. Diagram of the glomerular filtration barrier. Anionic sites reside in the surface coat of the endothelium and of the podocyte processes and in proteoglycan macromolecules, rich in heparan sulfate, that form a network of angular particles in the laminae rara interna and externa of the basal lamina. (From Farquhar, M. 1979. J. Cell Biol. 81:137. By permission of Rockefeller Institute Press.)

basolateral domain of the plasmalemma is enhanced by the lateral cell processes that amplify the area exposed to the interstitial fluid. Nearly 70% of the water and sodium ions in the glomerular filtrate is reabsorbed in the proximal tubule. The principal pump involved in Na^+,K^+-ATPase in the basolateral membrane. Pumping of sodium, accompanied by chloride, into the interstitial fluid creates an electrochemical gradient that moves water from the tubule lumen to the peritubular capillaries.

The traditional subdivision of the proximal tubule into a pars convoluta, located in the cortical labyrinth, and a pars recta, in the medullary rays and outer stripe of the medulla, was based on their location and macroscopic form in teased preparations. With the light microscope, the epithelium lining the tubule appeared the same throughout. However, with the electron microscope, three ultrastructurally distinct segments are identifiable in the proximal tubule of all mammalian species studied to date. These are designated S1, S2, and S3. In S1, which includes the initial and midportion of the pars convoluta, the cells are taller than those of more distal segments, their basolateral interdigitation with neighboring cells is very extensive, and their mitochondria are large and numerous. There is also clear evidence that these cells are active in endocy-

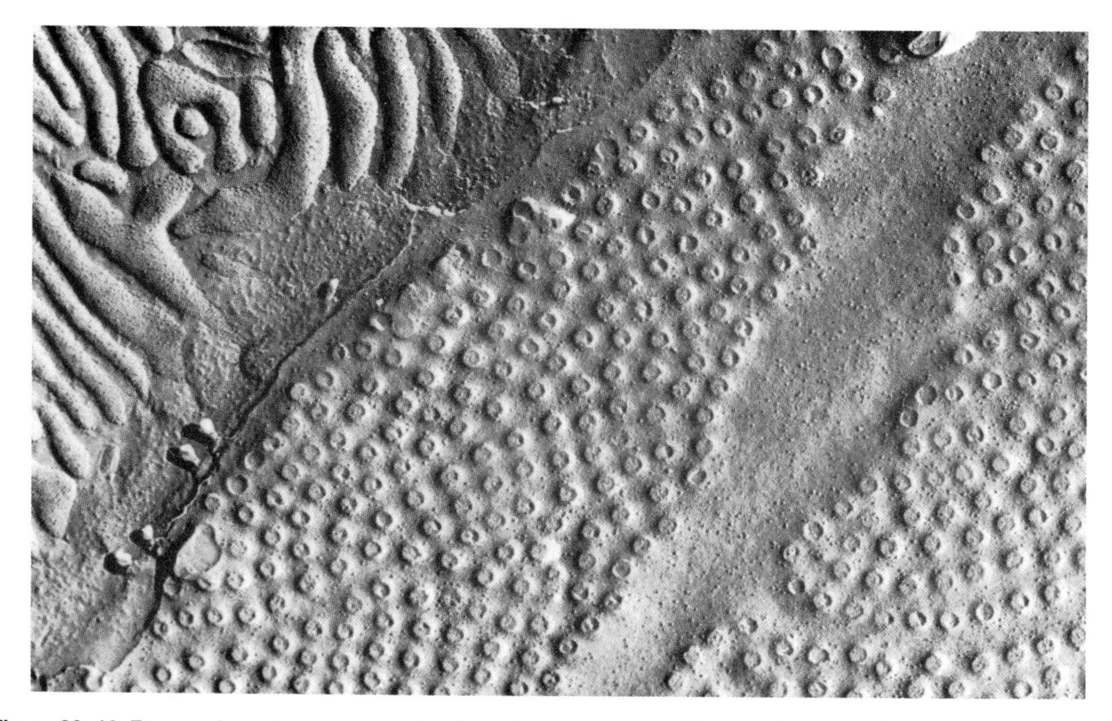

Figure 30–12. Freeze–cleave preparation of rat kidney glomerulus. At the right, the membrane of the capillary endothelium has been cleaved, showing the uniform size and distribution of the endothelial pores. At the upper left, the membranes of a number of podocyte foot processes have been cleaved. (Micrograph courtesy of D. Goodenough.)

tosis. There is a gradual transition to S2, which includes the distal portion of the pars convoluta and the beginning of the pars recta. In this region, cell height is lower, there is less basolateral interdigitation of cells, and their mitochondria are shorter. The transition to S3, which makes up the remainder of the pars recta, is rather abrupt. The cells here are cuboidal and have only a few interdigitating lateral processes. Their mitochondria are relatively small and randomly oriented. Although the cells of all three segments have a brush border, the microvilli in S3 are noticeably longer. Physiological studies on isolated proximal tubules yield results consistent with the observed structural differences along their length. The rate of sodium transport is highest in S1 and decreases progressively in S2 and S3.

Intermediate Tubule (Thin Segment)

The descending straight portion of the proximal tubule, 60 μm in diameter, abruptly narrows in the outer medulla and continues as the *descending thin limb* (DTL) of the loop of Henle, with a diameter of 15 μm (Fig. 30–20). At this transition, the prominent brush border ends and the cuboidal epithelium gives way to a squamous epithelium bearing a few short microvilli. This epithelium is only 0.5–2.0 μm thick, with the central portion of the cells containing the nucleus bulges slightly into the lumen. In short-looped nephrons, the cells (type-I cells) are polygonal in outline and do not have interdigitating lateral processes. The shape of the cells and the small caliber of the tubules result in a cross-sectional appearance resembling that of a capillary or venule. In short-looped nephrons, the lining epithelium of the thin limb has the same appearance throughout its length. In such nephrons, there is no ascending thin limb. The descending thin limb is continuous at the bend of the loop, with the straight ascending limb of the distal tubule (Fig. 30–22).

In long-looped nephrons, on the other hand, three cytologically distinct segments are identifiable in electron micrographs of the thin limb of the loop of Henle. In its initial descending portion, the squamous lining cells (type-II cells) have long radiating processes that interdigitate with similar processes of neighboring cells, and there are shallow infoldings of the basal plasma membrane. The highly irregular outlines of these cells are best seen in scanning electron micrographs of isolated tubules from which the basal lamina has

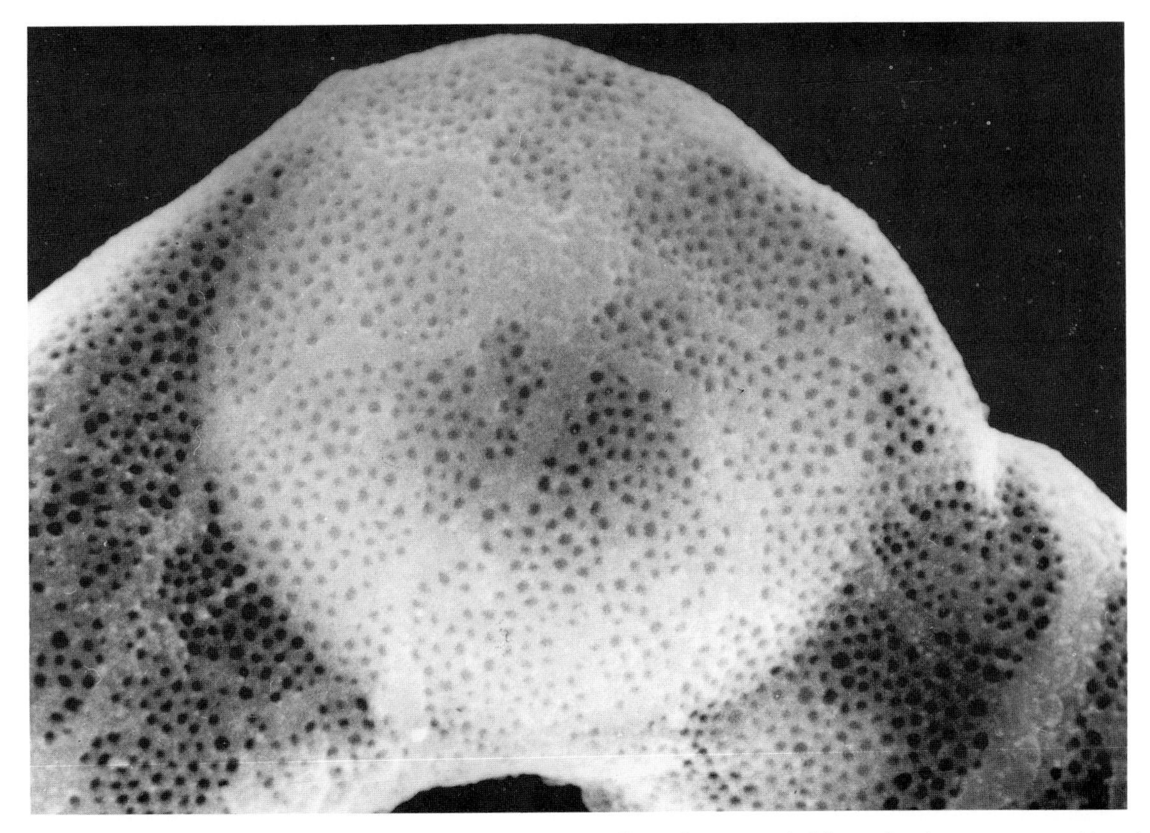

Figure 30–13. Scanning electron micrograph of a glomerular capillary after removal of the podocyte processes and basal lamina by enzymatic digestion. The round pale region beneath the fenestrated endothelium is an erythrocyte in the lumen. (Courtesy of Jones, D.B. 1985. Lab. Investig. 52:453.)

been extracted with sodium hydroxide. In thin sections of this segment, cell profiles containing a nucleus make up only a fraction of the epithelium. The rest is made up of 1–3-μm anucleate profiles which are cross sections of the numerous interdigitating cell processes. Between their lateral membranes are narrow intercellular clefts closed at their adluminal end by shallow occluding junctions.

As the thin limb of a long-loop descends to the inner medulla, there is a progressive decrease in the number and length of the lateral processes of the cells (type-III cells). These ultimately become irregularly polygonal. In the ascending thin limb, the cells (type-IV cells) again have interdigitating processes like those of the initial portion of the descending limb, but basal infoldings of the plasmalemma are lacking (Fig. 30–21). The physiological significance of these differences in cell form along the thin limb of long loops of Henle is less clear than in the proximal tubule. There is no active transport of sodium in the thin limb, but there is some passive sodium efflux that contributes to concentration of the urine. The descending thin limb has a high permeability to water, possibly related to the amplification of the intercellular pathway that results from the extensive interdigitation of the cells. The ascending thin limb of long-looped nephrons has a somewhat lower water permeability.

The foregoing description of cell form and relationships along the length of the thin segment is based on studies of the kidney of laboratory rodents. The intermediate tubule of the human kidney has been less thoroughly studied, but there appear to be comparable differences in the pattern of interdigitation of cells in the descending and ascending thin limbs of long-looped nephrons.

In the human kidney, zonation of the medulla is less obvious than in species having a unipyramidal kidney. The boundary between the outer and inner zones is the site of the transition of the thin limb to the ascending thick limb of the long-looped nephrons. The boundary between the outer and inner stripes

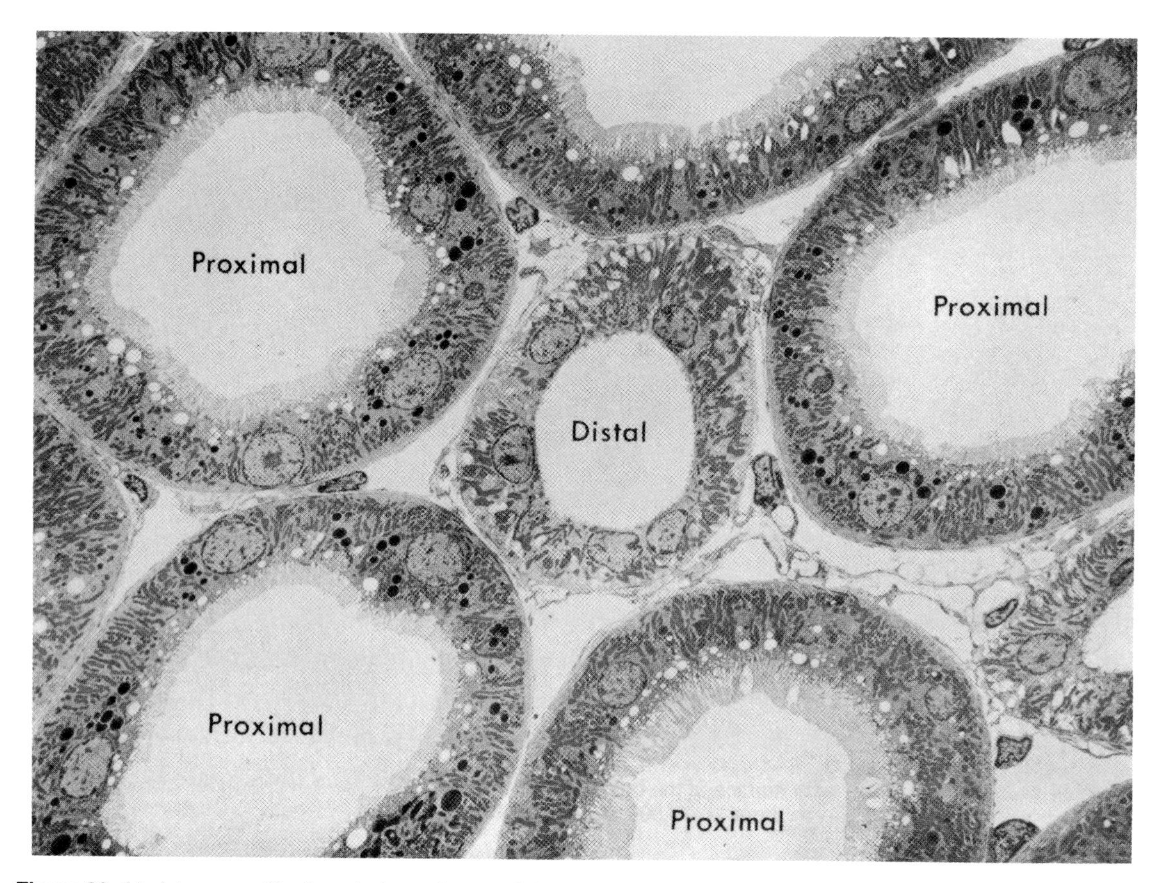

Figure 30–14. A low-magnification electron micrograph from the cortex of the rat kidney. The field includes cross sections of five proximal convoluted tubules and one distal tubule. Two distinct segments of the proximal convolution can be recognized. The first portion (lower right) has a thicker brush border. The second segment has a thinner brush border and prominent dense bodies in the cytoplasm (three other labeled sections). (From Maunsbach, A. 1966. J. Ultrastr. Res. 15:252.)

in the outer medulla is somewhat obscured by variations in the level at which this transition occurs in short-looped nephrons. The length of the short thin segment of such nephrons varies, and, in rare instances, a thin segment is entirely lacking and the descending straight portion of the proximal tubule continues directly into the ascending thick limb of the distal tubule. In long-looped nephrons, the thin segment may be 10 mm or more in length, extending nearly to the apex of the papilla. Short-looped nephrons are seven times as numerous as long-looped nephrons.

Distal Tubule

The distal tubule begins in the inner stripe of the outer medulla at an abrupt transition from the thin limb of the loop of Henle to its *thick ascending limb* (TAL, pars recta) (Fig. 30–22). Its initial portion is designated the *medullary thick ascending limb* (MTAL) and its continuation becomes the *cortical thick ascending limb* (CTAL). Where the latter contacts the vascular pole of the renal corpuscle of the same nephron, its epithelium contains a plaque of specialized cells called the *macula densa*. Distal to this point, the tubule pursues a tortuous course and is called the *distal convoluted tubule* (DCT, pars convoluta).

The epithelium of the distal tubule is cuboidal and 7–8 μm in height in its medullary thick ascending limb, gradually diminishing in height to about 5 μm in the cortical thick ascending limb. The lumen is generally wider than that of the proximal tubule. A brush border is lacking but short microvilli are found on some cells, whereas others have a smooth surface. Cells with a smooth surface predominate in the medullary portion of the thick ascending limb. A pair of centrioles is located beneath the apical plasma membrane with one

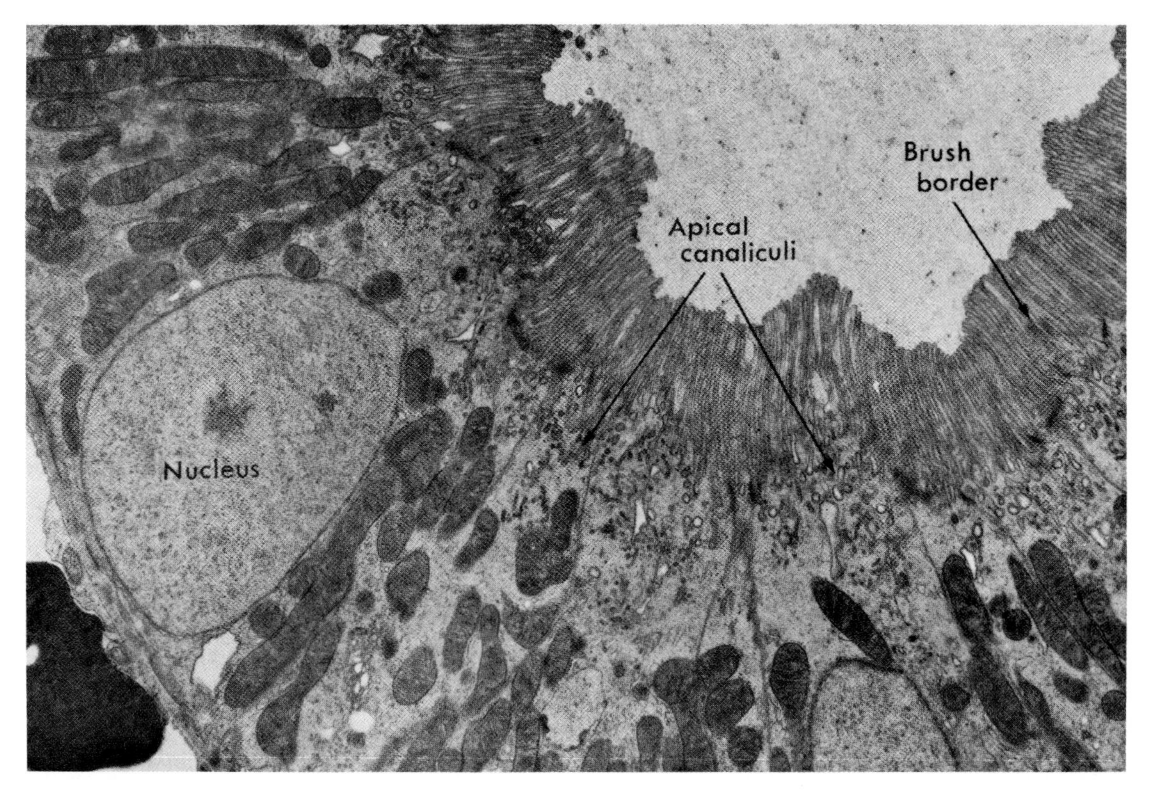

Figure 30–15. Electron micrograph of a portion of the wall of a proximal tubule of rat kidney showing the thick brush border, the abundance of canaliculi and vesicles in the apical cytoplasm, and the numerous large mitochondria. (Micrograph courtesy of R. Bulger.)

serving as the basal body of a single short flagellum that projects into the lumen. Vesicles are present in moderate numbers in the apical cytoplasm, but the clathrin-coated vesicles and canaliculi that are a prominent feature of cells of the proximal tubule are not found in the distal tubule. There are a few cisternae of rough endoplasmic reticulum and a small Golgi complex. The nucleus is round or ovoid and tends to be displaced toward the lumen by deep infoldings of the basal plasmalemma that bound narrow compartments, occupied by long mitochondria (Fig. 30–23). While some compartments are formed by invagination of the basal plasma membrane and are open to the cytoplasm above, others are closed above and are cross sections of undermining processes of neighboring cells. These are somewhat less numerous than in the proximal convoluted tubule.

The thick ascending limb is nearly impenetrable to water. Its principal function is resorption of sodium and chloride from the glomerular filtrate. Its Na^+-K^+-ATPase activity and its resorptive capacity are greatest in the inner stripe of the outer medulla. This correlates well with morphometric data, indicating that the surface area of the basolateral membrane and the volume of the mitochondria are greatest in the inner stripe and diminish toward the cortex.

The epithelium of the distal convoluted tubule closely resembles that of the thick ascending limb. The cells are slightly taller. The membrane invaginations and interdigitation of the lateral cell processes near the cell base are somewhat more extensive, resulting in a greater total area of basolateral membrane.

About 85% of the sodium in the glomerular filtrate has already been reabsorbed before it reaches the distal convoluted tubule, but this segment is capable of reabsorbing nearly all of the remaining sodium if this is necessary to maintain the normal electrolyte composition of the body fluids. The distal convoluted tubule has a higher Na^+-K^+-ATPase activity than any other segment of the nephron. Delivery of an excess of sodium and chloride to this segment induces an increase in its basolateral membrane area and in its Na^+-K^+-ATPase activity.

A unique protein, *Tamm–Horsfall protein,* is

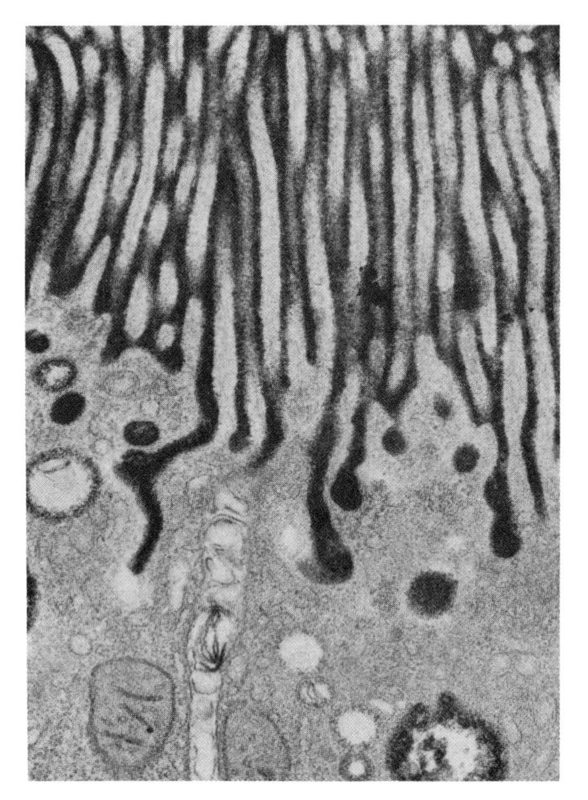

Figure 30–16. Electron micrograph of a portion of the brush border of two adjacent cells of a proximal convoluted tubule a few seconds after intravenous injection of myoglobin. The electron-dense myoglobin has already passed through the glomerular filtration barrier and can be seen between the microvilli and in the apical canaliculi. (Micrograph courtesy of W. Anderson.)

associated with the ascending thick limb of the loop of Henle and it is also detectable in the urine. Its functional significance is unknown. It contributes to the formation of intratubular casts that occlude the tubules in some diseases of the kidney and is, therefore, of interest to pathologists.

Collecting Tubules

A short transitional segment called the *connecting tubule* joins the distal convoluted tubule to the *collecting duct*. Three successive segments of the collecting ducts are distinguished on the basis of their location in the zonation of the renal pyramids (Figs. 30–24 and 30–25). These are the *cortical collecting duct* (CCD), the *outer medullary collecting duct* (OMCD), and the *inner medullary collecting duct* (IMCD). The ducts course inward in the medullary rays and when they reach the inner medulla, pairs of them approach at an acute angle and become confluent. About seven such convergences, in the inner medulla, result in the formation of larger straight ducts 100–200 μm in diameter, called the *papillary ducts* (*ducts of Bellini*). It is these that open into a minor calyx of the renal pelvis on the area cribrosa of each renal papilla.

Connecting tubules are lined by an epithelium that exhibits considerable interspecific variation in the number of cell types. In most species, four types are distinguishable with the electron microscope: *distal convoluted tubule cells* (DCT cells), *connecting tubule cells* (CTC cells), *principal cells* (P-cells), and *intercalated cells* (I-cells). Distal convoluted tubule cells have already been described.

The *connecting tubule cell* has a round or ovoid nucleus in an electron-lucent cytoplasm, a small paranuclear Golgi complex, and numerous small mitochondria. Other organelles are poorly represented. The luminal surface of the cell is relatively smooth and there are few vesicles in the apical cytoplasm. There is less lateral interdigitation of cells than in the distal convoluted tubule.

The *intercalated cells* are recognizable by distinctive microplicae on their free surface (Fig. 30–26) and by the presence of an extraordinary abundance of vesicles in the apical cytoplasm. The majority of the vesicles are 50 nm in diameter, but there may be a few larger ones up to 200 nm in diameter. Short, plump mitochondria are distributed throughout the cytoplasm. There is no basal compartmentation of the cell, but many slender villi or folds of the plasmalemma may be interposed between the cell body and the basal lamina in varying orientation.

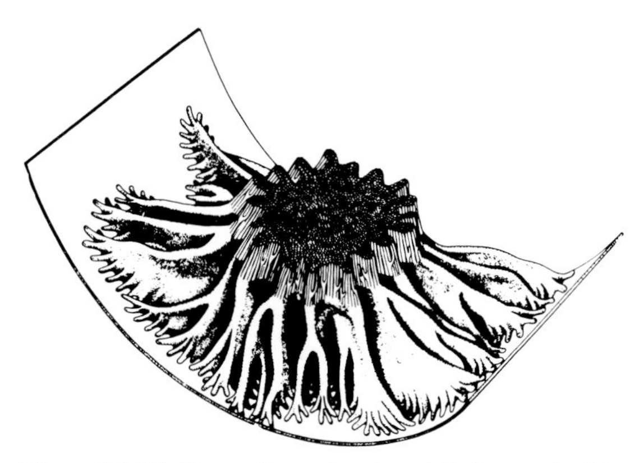

Figure 30–17. Three-dimensional model of a proximal tubule cell showing the long lateral ridge-like processes and their smaller branches at the cell base. (From Evans, A.P., et al. 1976. Anat. Rec. 191:397. After Welling, L.W., and D.J. Welling. 1976. Kidney Internat. 9:385.)

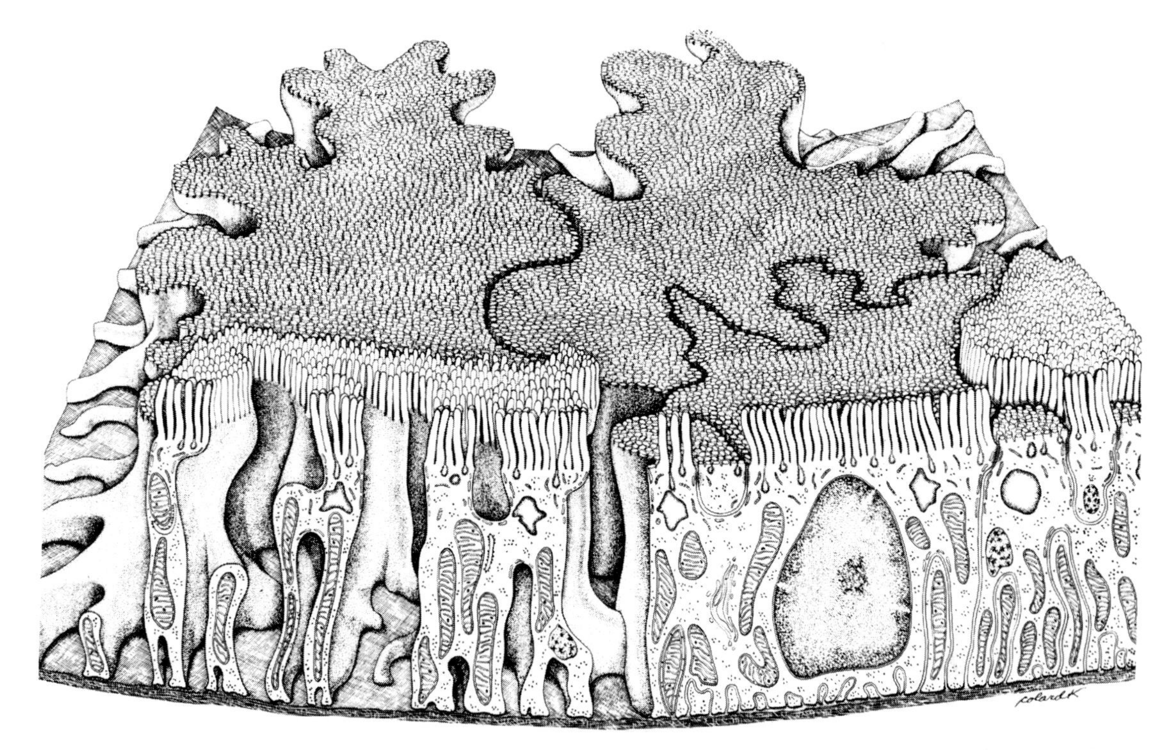

Figure 30–18. Drawing of the shapes and interrelationships of cells of the proximal convoluted tubule. Some of the interdigitating lateral ridges extend the full height of the cell, whereas branches of these are confined to the base and extend beneath adjacent cells. (From Bulger, R. 1965. Am. J. Anat. 116:237.)

Principal cells have a simpler ultrastructure than the other cell types. There are short, stubby microvilli and a centrally located single flagellum (Fig. 30–26). The ovoid nucleus is centrally located and the mitochondria are quite small and randomly oriented. At the cell base, there are many folds of the basal membrane that are closely compacted in varying orientation. There is less space between these peculiar basal folds than there is between those of the intercalated cells. The function of these cells is not known.

The cellular heterogeneity that is characteristic of the epithelium of the connecting tubule diminishes in the cortical and outer medullary collecting ducts, where only principal cells and intercalated cells are found. In rat kidney, intercalated cells gradually decrease from about 35% of the cell population in the ducts of the outer medulla to 10% in the inner medulla. No intercalated cells have been reported in the inner medulla of the human kidney. Intercalated cells are believed to be involved in the control of acid–base balance by resorption of bicarbonate. They have a high carbonic anhydrase activity and their basolateral membranes contain the anion-channel protein, *band-3,* linked to the membrane skeletal proteins *ankyrin* and *spectrin.* In animals subjected to chronic bicarbonate loading, the number of intercalated cells in the collecting ducts increases dramatically.

Collecting ducts were formerly thought to be relatively inert conduits conveying urine from the distal tubules to the renal pelvis. But since the development of isolated-perfused-tubule techniques for studying the various segments of the uriniferous tubules, the collecting ducts have been found to participate in secretion of potassium and in acidification of the urine.

RENAL INTERSTITIUM

The contents of the spaces external to the basal laminae of the tubules constitute the *renal interstitium.* Its volume, in the cortex, is relatively small, but it increases in the medulla. It includes fibroblast-like cells, mononuclear cells, and small bundles of collagen fibers in a highly hydrated proteoglycan matrix. In the cortex, the fibroblasts have long tapering processes that are in contact with processes of like cells. Their elongate nucleus is often indented and small clumps of chromatin are evenly

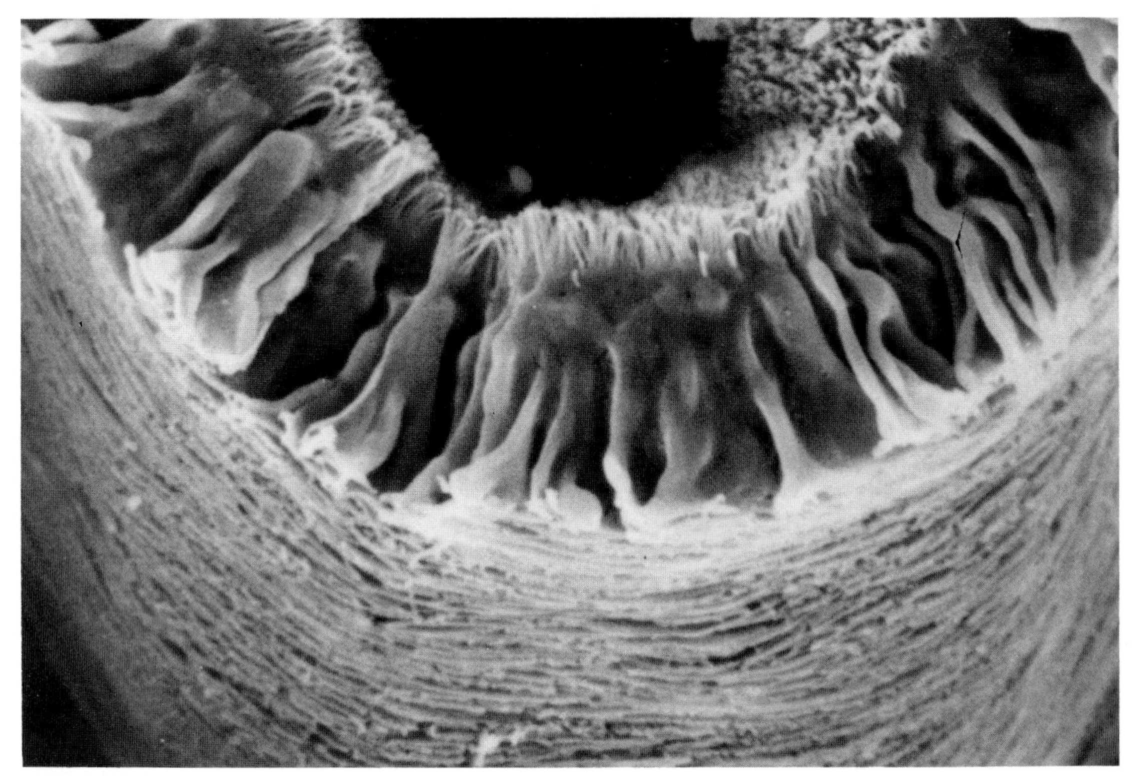

Figure 30–19. Scanning micrograph of a slightly oblique view of a proximal convoluted tubule of a rat nephron illustrating the long ridges on the sides of the epithelial cells. Note also that the small secondary processes at the cell base are oriented perpendicular to the axis of the tubule. (Micrograph courtesy of Takahashi-Iwanaga, H. 1989. Cells and Tissues: A Three-Dimensional Approach. New York, Alan R. Liss, Inc.)

spaced along the nuclear envelope. Actin filaments are abundant in the peripheral cytoplasm and subplasmalemmal densities, resembling those of smooth muscle, are not uncommon. The cytoplasm contains occasional small lipid droplets and dilated cisternae of rough endoplasmic reticulum that may contain flocculent material of low electron density. Like the fibroblasts of other organs, these interstitial cells are believed to produce the fibrous and amorphous components of the extracellular matrix.

The so-called *mononuclear cells* are more-or-less spherical and have a large heterochromatic nucleus surrounded by a relatively thin rim of cytoplasm that contains a few mitochondria and abundant free ribosomes but little or no endoplasmic reticulum. They are often located in close proximity to the fibroblasts. There has been some reluctance about identifying these cells, but it is likely that they are early stages of the monocyte-macrophage lineage.

The *medullary interstitial cells* are fibroblast-like cells that differ from those of the cortex in their orientation and in their ultrastructure. They are highly pleomorphic cells, generally oriented perpendicular to the axis of the tubules and, thus, presenting an appearance reminiscent of the rungs of a ladder. Their long processes are more slender than those of the fibroblasts in the renal cortex and their tips are closely apposed to the tubules and to the walls of blood vessels. A conspicuous feature of these cells is the presence of multiple lipid droplets (Fig. 30–27). These may be surrounded by smooth endoplasmic reticulum. A few expanded cisternae of rough endoplasmic reticulum may also be found. A few mononuclear cells are present in the outer zone of the medulla, but they are rare or absent in the inner zone and papilla.

The observation that the size and number of lipid droplets in the medullary interstitial cells vary in different states of salt and water balance, prompted much speculation as to the function of these cells. In water-loaded animals, the volume density of lipid droplets is more than twice that seen in dehydrated animals. The finding that prostaglandins can be

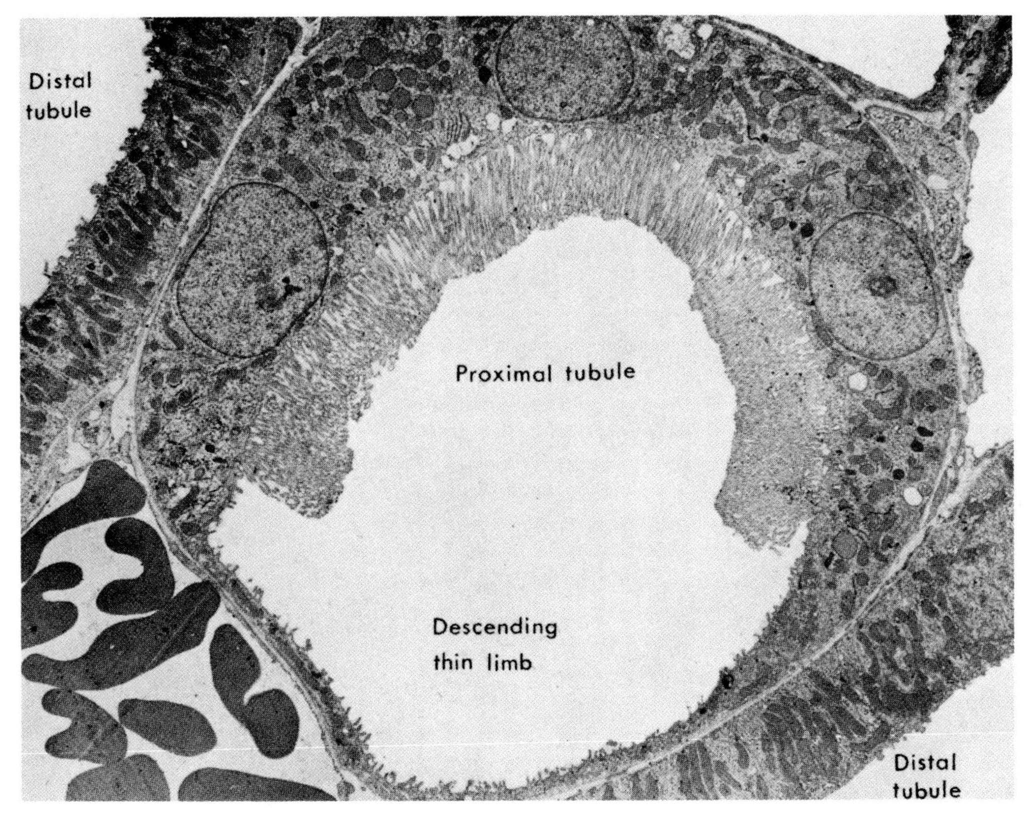

Figure 30–20. Electron micrograph of a slightly oblique section of the abrupt junction of a proximal convoluted tubule with the thin limb of the loop of Henle. The brush border stops suddenly and the epithelium becomes very thin. (From Osvaldo, J. and H. Latta. 1966. J. Ultrastr. Res. 15:144.)

extracted in considerable amount from the renal medulla but not from the cortex led to the suggestion that the interstitial cells might synthesize prostaglandin and store it in their lipid droplets. However, on analysis, the lipid droplet fraction consisted of triglycerides, rich in arachidonic acid and polyunsaturated fatty acids, but contained no significant amount of prostaglandin or prostaglandin synthetase. Thus, there is no evidence to support the speculation that the medullary interstitial cells are specialized for secretion of prostaglandins.

More plausible is the suggestion that these cells have an endocrine function in the regulation of systemic blood pressure. This interpretation had its origin in the observation that the lipid droplets in interstitial cells are significantly reduced in number in animals with experimentally induced hypertension. Moreover, when normal medullary tissue is transplanted subcutaneously in such animals, it forms nodules that are interpreted as proliferating interstitial cells, and the blood pressure of the hypertensive host is significantly lowered. On removal of the nodules, the blood pressure rises again to hypertensive levels. It is speculated that the lipid droplets of the medullary interstitial cells contain the substrate for synthesis of a hormone, *medullipin-I*. This substance has been extracted from the renal papilla and purified chromatographically. When injected intravenously, it causes vasodilatation of major vascular beds and lowering of blood pressure of hypertensive animals. This action of the extract is prevented if the liver is excluded from the circulation. It is, therefore, concluded that the hormone must traverse the liver to be converted to an active vasodilator, *medullipin-II*. The secretion of medullipin-I by the interstitial cells is believed to be influenced by renal artery perfusion pressure. How an increase in pressure stimulates secretion remains unclear. There is growing support for the concept of a dual control of blood pressure in which secretion of medullipin in the medulla is antihypertensive and the secretion of *renin* by the juxtaglomerular cells in the cortex is prohypertensive.

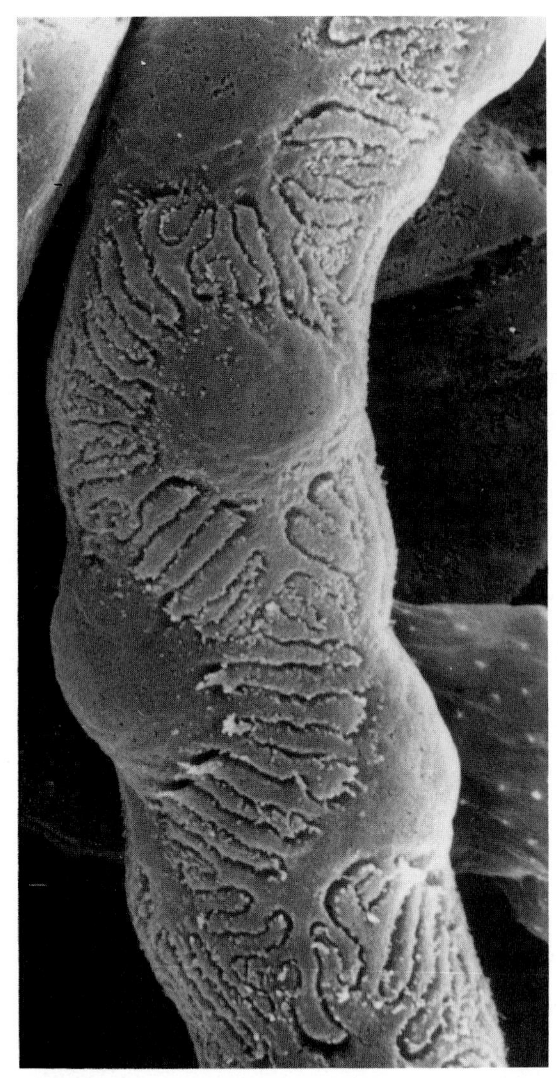

Figure 30–21. Scanning micrograph of an isolated thin limb of a long-looped nephron from rat kidney showing the interdigitation of radiating cell processes of the squamous epithelial cells. (Courtesy of Takahashi-Iwanaga, H. 1987. Cells and Tissues. A Three-Dimensional Approach. New York, Alan R. Liss, Inc.)

JUXTAGLOMERULAR COMPLEX

The juxtaglomerular complex is made up of tubular and vascular elements of the nephron that have interactive functions influencing systemic blood pressure and the rate of glomerular filtration. In histological sections, the distal convoluted tubule of the nephron is located at the vascular pole of the glomerules, between the afferent and efferent arterioles (Fig. 30–28, 30–29). On the side of the tubule nearest to the afferent arteriole, the epithelial cells are slender and more crowded than elsewhere. This sector of the wall of the tubule is conspicuous owing to the close packing and intense staining of its nuclei and is, therefore, called the *macula densa.* The media of the afferent arteriole adjacent to the macula densa contains the *juxtaglomerular cells,* modified smooth muscle cells that have round nuclei and a cytoplasm containing secretory granules. The angular interspace between the glomerulus and the diverging afferent and efferent arterioles is occupied by irregularly shaped cells with pale-staining nuclei, called *extraglomerular mesangial cells* (*lacis cells* or *Goormaghtigh cells*). The macula densa, juxtaglomerular cells, and extraglomerular mesangial cells constitute the *juxtaglomerular complex* (Fig. 30–29).

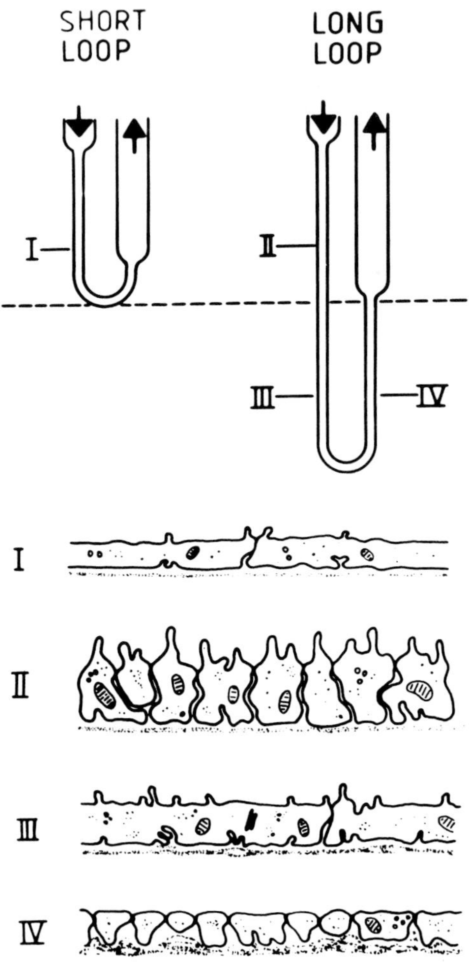

Figure 30–22. Schematic drawing of the typical profiles of cell processes as seen in longitudinal sections of the epithelium in four segments of the loop of Henle. The nuclear region of the cells is not included. (Modified after Kriz, W., et al. 1980. eds. Functional Ultrastructure of the Kidney. London, Academic Press.)

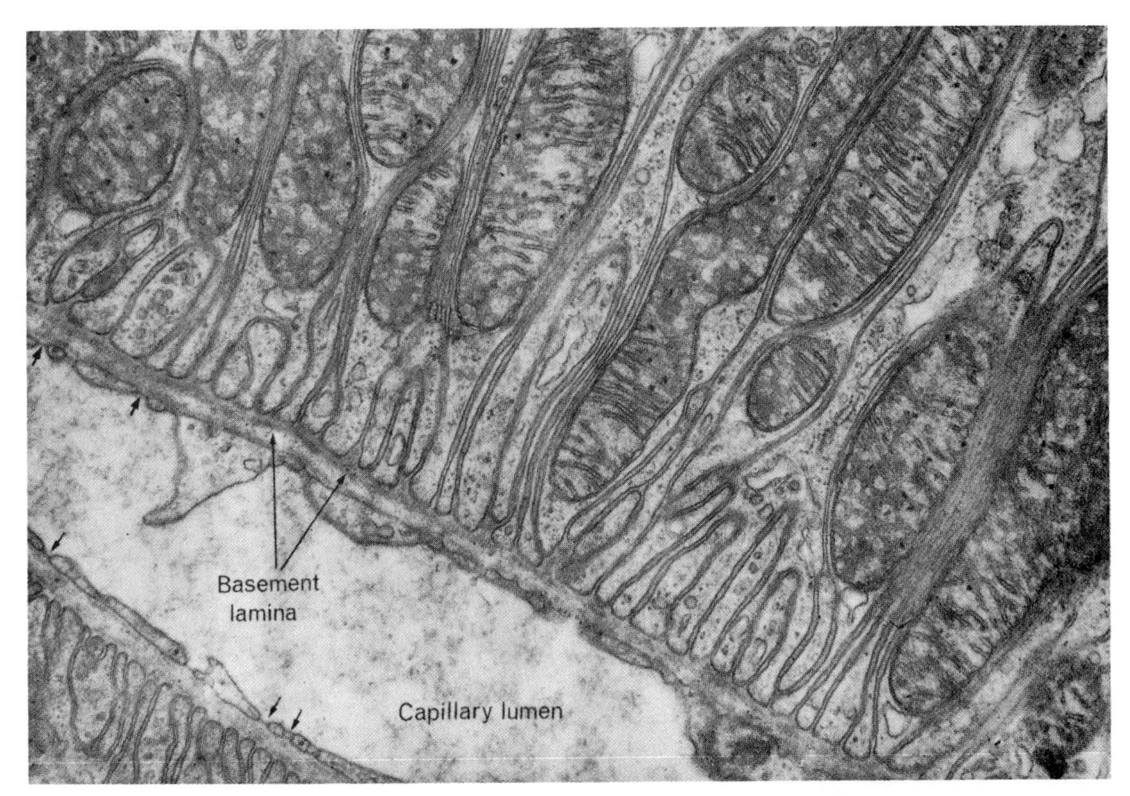

Figure 30–23. Electron micrograph of the base of the epithelium in a distal convoluted tubule of guinea pig kidney illustrating the small and large compartments. The large compartments contain long mitochondria oriented perpendicular to the basal lamina. The peritubular capillary at the lower left is fenestrated (at arrows). (Micrograph courtesy of A. Ichikawa.)

The cells of the macula densa have numerous microvilli on their lumenal surface and a single centrally located cilium. The mitochondria are short and randomly oriented because the compartmentation of the cell base by incursions of the basal membrane that is characteristic of the distal tubule is lacking in cells of the lamina densa. The Golgi complex is usually located between the nucleus and the cell base. Thus, the polarity of these cells is opposite that of cells elsewhere in the tubule. The basal lamina is thin and discontinuous, and blunt cell processes are reported to extend through it toward the juxtaglomerular cells in the afferent arteriole. These relationships strongly suggest that the macula densa has a sensory function that influences the activity of the juxtaglomerular cells.

Juxtaglomerular cells vary in abundance from nephron to nephron and may be absent from some. They are located in the terminal segment of the afferent arteriole near the glomerulus and may extend for 10–40 μm, but single cells or small groups of cells may be found up to 100 μm upstream. They are rarely found in the efferent arteriole. In electron micrographs, juxtaglomerular cells vary in their fine structure. Some have few secretory granules and retain features typical of smooth muscle, including bundles of myofilaments and dense bodies at their sites of attachment to the plasma membrane (Fig. 30–30). Others have more numerous granules, a well-developed endoplasmic reticulum, prominent Golgi complex, and few or no myofilaments. These variations appear to be different stages in the transformation of contractile smooth muscle to secretory juxtaglomerular cells.

When first formed, the secretory granules are small and fusiform or rhomboid in shape and have a paracrystalline interior with a periodicity of 5–10 nm. These later coalesce into irregularly shaped conglomerates that are gradually transformed into spheroidal mature granules having a homogeneous content devoid of crystalline order. The granules contain the hormone *renin,* an acid protease that catalyzes the cleavage of plasma *angiotensinogen* to *angiotensin-I.* During subsequent pas-

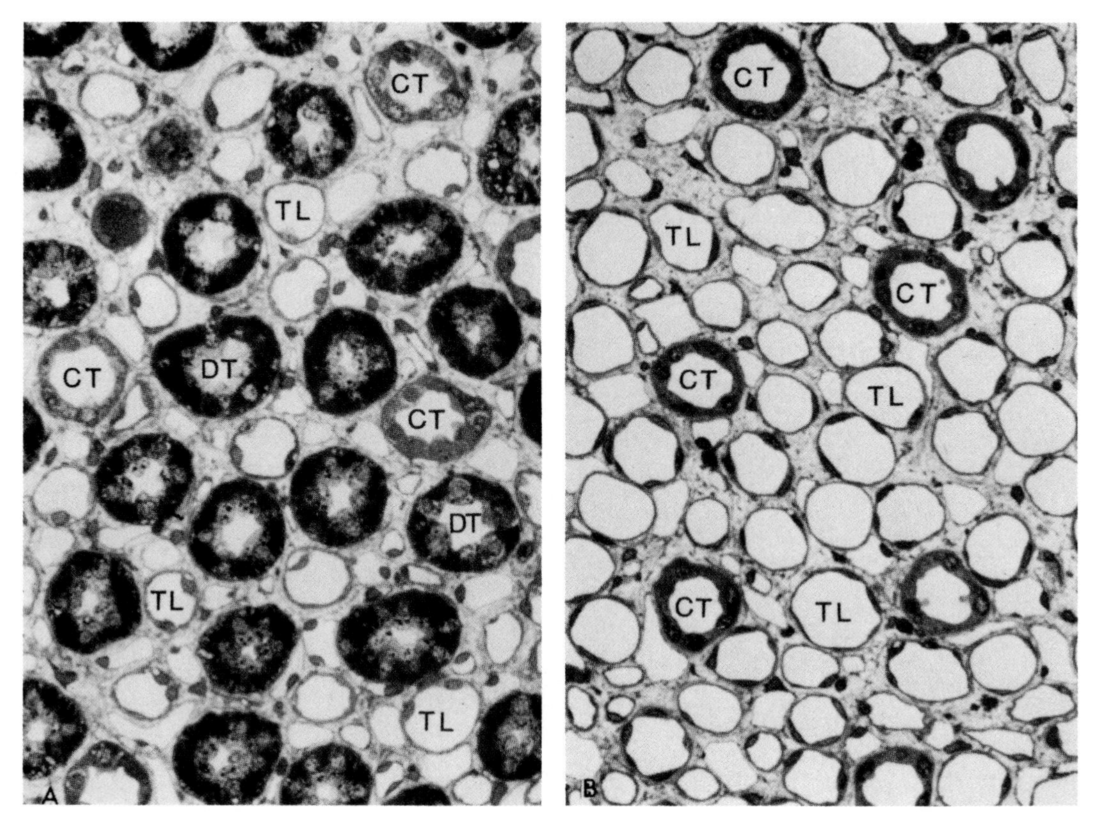

Figure 30–24. (A) A photomicrograph of a transverse section through the outer medulla, which is made up of thin segments of the loop (TL), ascending straight portions of the distal tubule (DT), and collecting tubules (CT). (B) A comparable section through the inner medulla made up of thin limbs of the loop of Henle (TL) and collecting ducts (CT).

sage through the lung, a *converting enzyme* on the surface of the endothelium rapidly cleaves *angiotensin-I* to yield *angiotensin-II,* a potent vasoconstrictor that raises blood pressure and indirectly influences renal blood flow.

Synthesis in the reticulum, concentration in the Golgi, and progranule formation in a trans-Golgi cistern are widely accepted, but two puzzling observations have prompted alternative interpretations of later events in granulopoiesis. Exogenous tracers such as horseradish peroxidase and ferritin are taken up and incorporated in the secretory granules, and histochemical studies have revealed that they contain the enzymes acid phosphatase, cathepsin-B and -D, and α-glucosidase. The secretory granules of these cells, therefore, share some of the properties of secondary lysosomes. The significance of these findings for interpretation of the events in granule maturation remain unclear. However, it is speculated that cathepsin-B may be involved in activation of renin in the course of granulopoiesis prior to its release by exocytosis.

In addition to its systemic effect, renin is believed to have an important local action in the kidney, regulating the rate of glomerular filtration. There is now immunocytochemical and other evidence for the presence of angiotensin-I, converting enzyme, and angiotensin-II, as well as renin, in the juxtaglomerular cells. This raises the possibility that local release of angiotensin-II may influence filtration rate by causing constriction of glomerular vessels. In the tubuloglomerular feedback mechanism postulated, the macula densa is envisioned as a sensor detecting changes in salt concentration or flow rate through the renal tubule and transmitting signals to other elements of the juxtaglomerular complex that alter glomerular filtration rate. It is known that mesangial cells are contractile and have receptors for angiotensin-II and other vasoconstrictors and for atriopeptide vasodilators. The contraction or relaxation of the glomerular mesangial cells induced by these vasoactive agents may modulate flow through the glomerular capillaries. Extraglomerular mesangial cells in the angle between the afferent and efferent arterioles are in communication

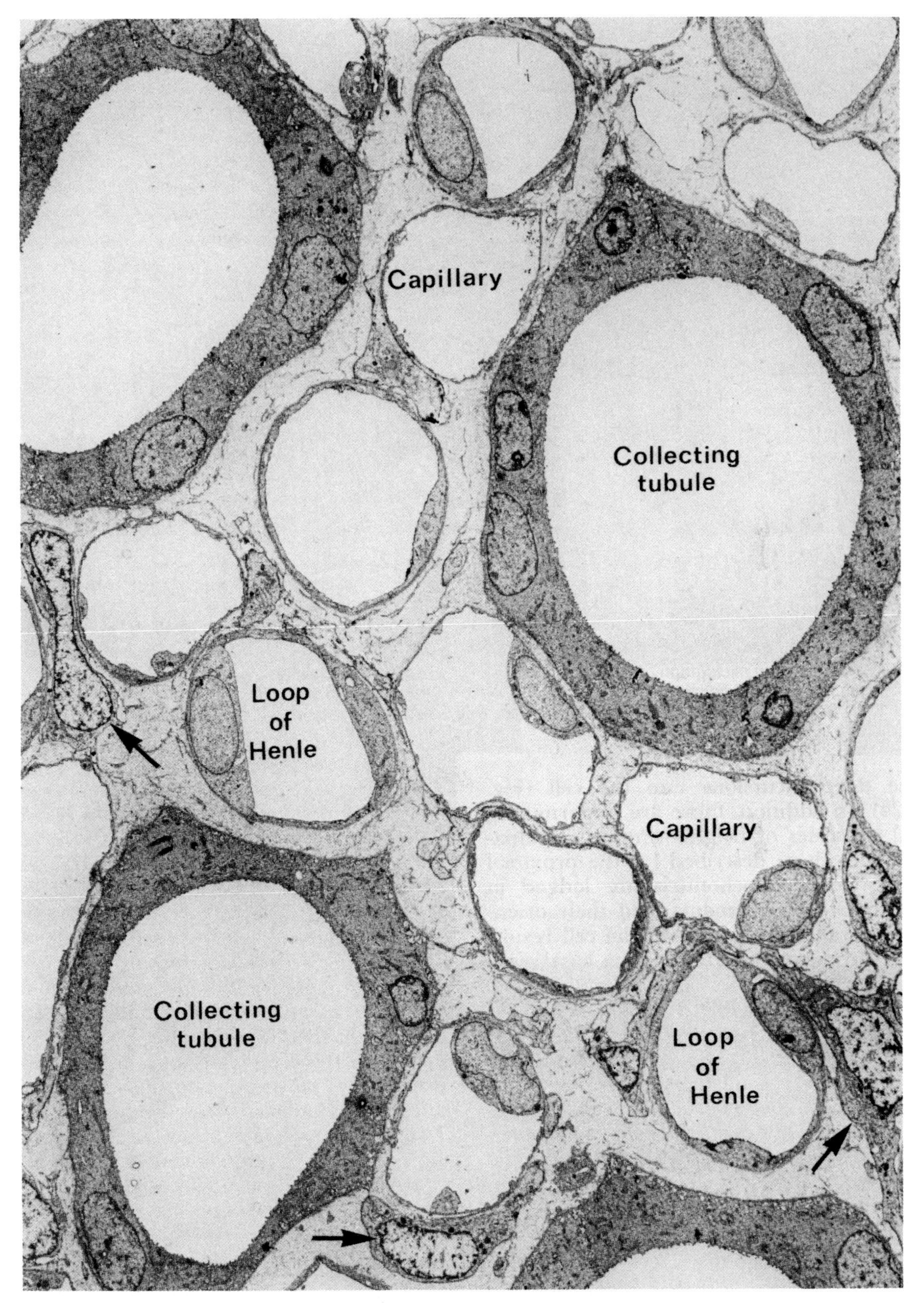

Figure 30–25. Low-power electron micrograph of a transverse section through the inner zone of the medulla of rat kidney showing the simple cuboidal epithelium of the collecting ducts. Between them are thin limbs of the loop of Henle and capillaries. These are surrounded by an extracellular matrix of low electron density. (Micrograph from Bohman, S. 1974. J. Ultrastr. Res. 47:329.)

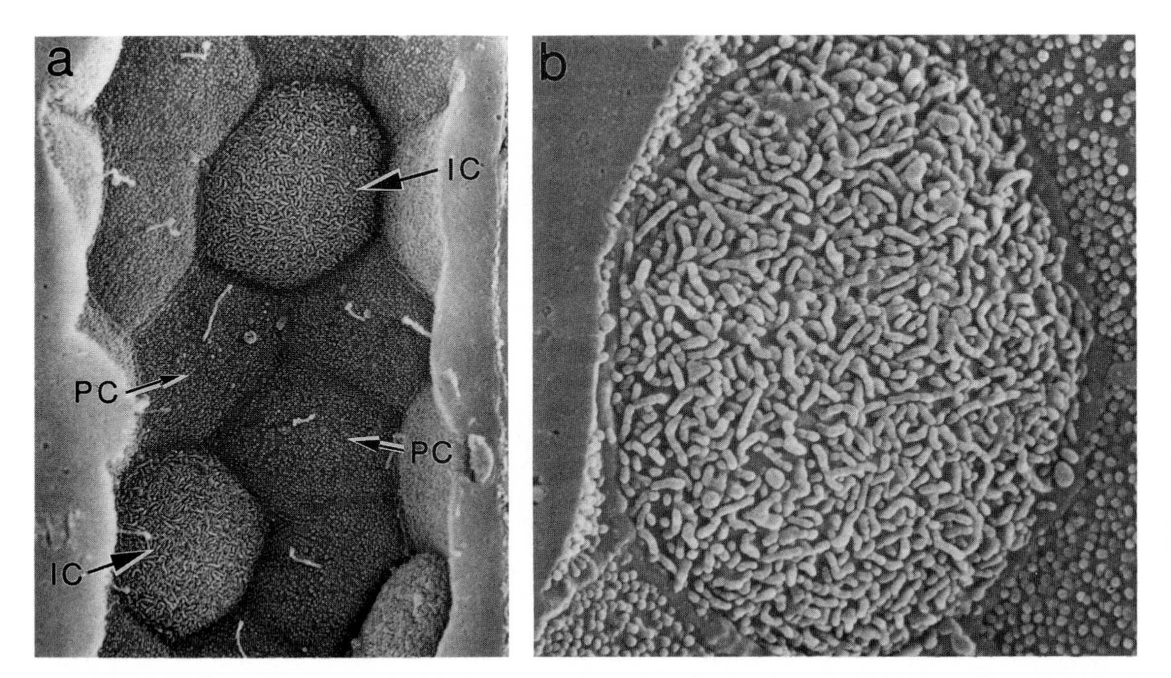

Figure 30–26. (A) Scanning micrograph of the lumenal surface of a collecting duct of rabbit kidney. The principal cells (PC) bear a single short flagellum; the interstitial cells (IC) have closely packed microplicae. (B) High magnification of the apical surface of an interstitial cell. Its closely spaced microplicae can be compared to the short microvilli on the principal cells at the right of the figure. (Courtesy of Evans, A.P. 1989. Cells and Tissues: A Three-Dimensional Approach. New York, Alan R. Liss, Inc.)

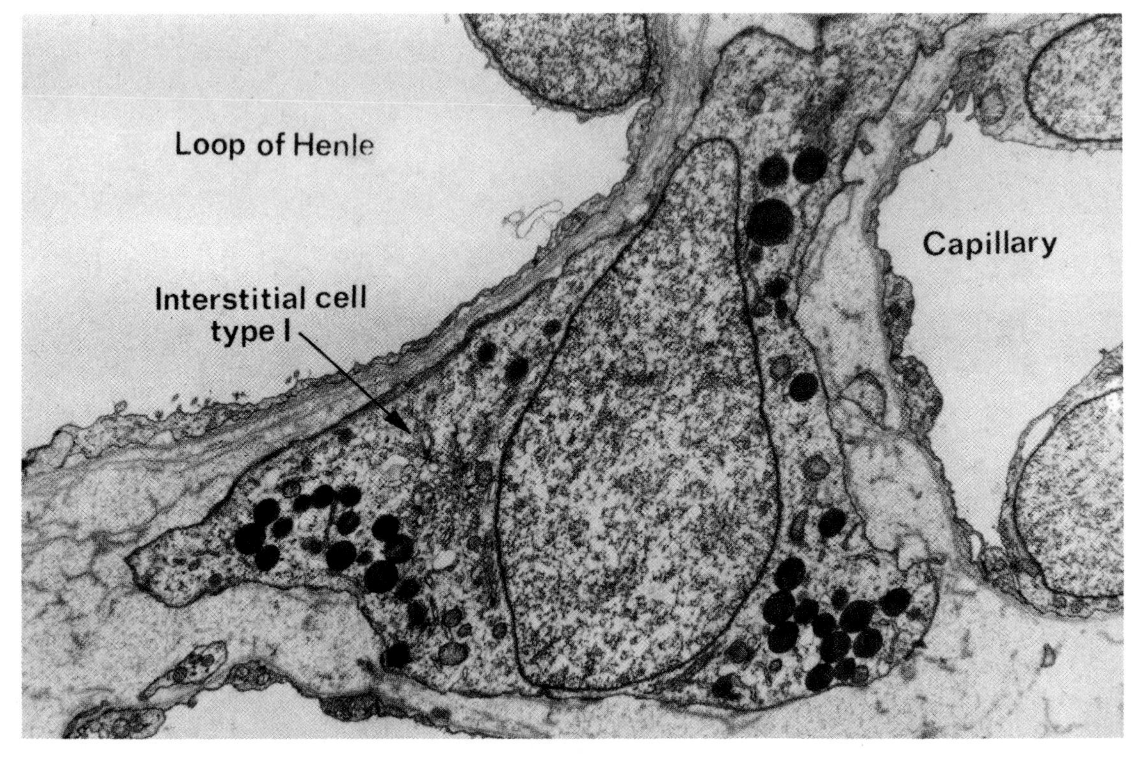

Figure 30–27. Micrograph of a medullary interstitial cell between a capillary and a thin limb of the loop of Henle. The cytoplasm contains multiple small lipid droplets. (Micrograph from Bohman, S-O. 1972. J. Ultrastr. Res. 38:225.)

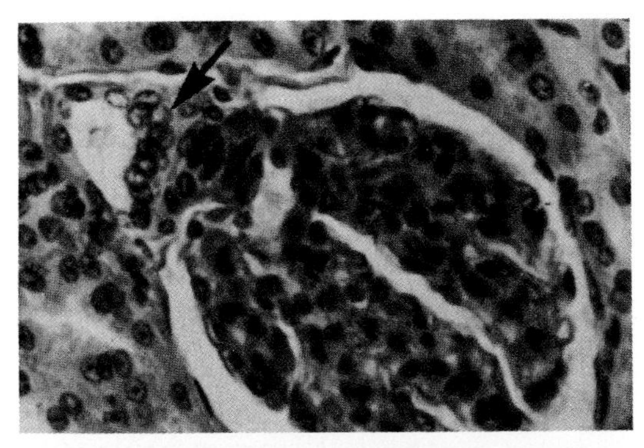

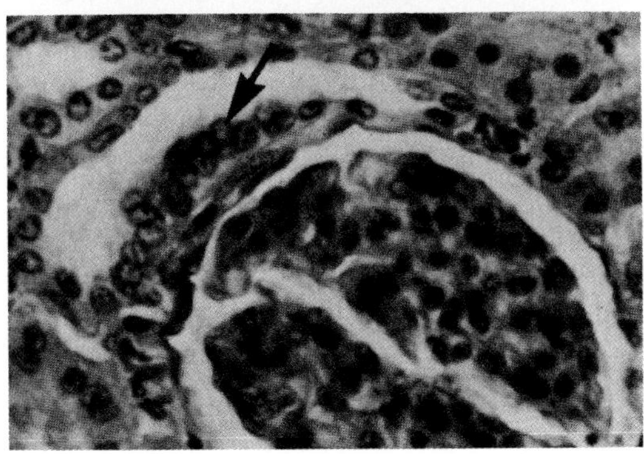

Figure 30–28. Photomicrograph of two renal corpuscles from monkey kidney showing (at arrows) two typical examples of the macula densa of the juxtaglomerular complex. Note the close crowding of nuclei of the distal convoluted tubule adjacent to the vascular pole of the renal corpuscle.

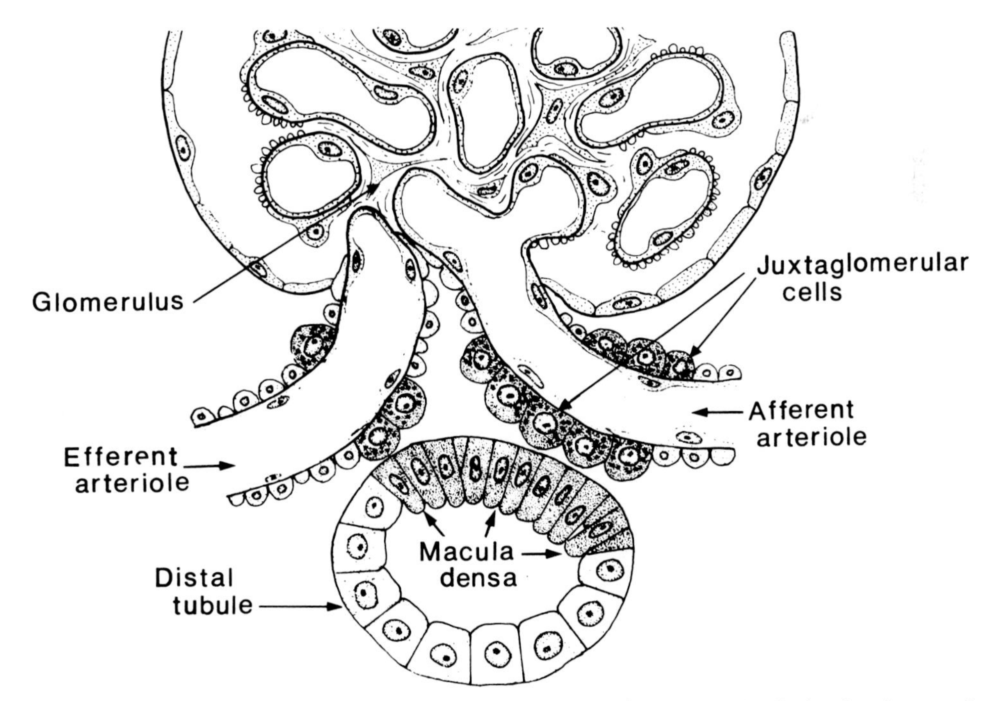

Figure 30–29. Diagram of the juxtaglomerular complex, which consists of specialized cells forming the macula densa in the wall of the distal convoluted tubule and modified smooth muscle cells in the wall of the afferent and efferent arterioles of the renal corpuscle.

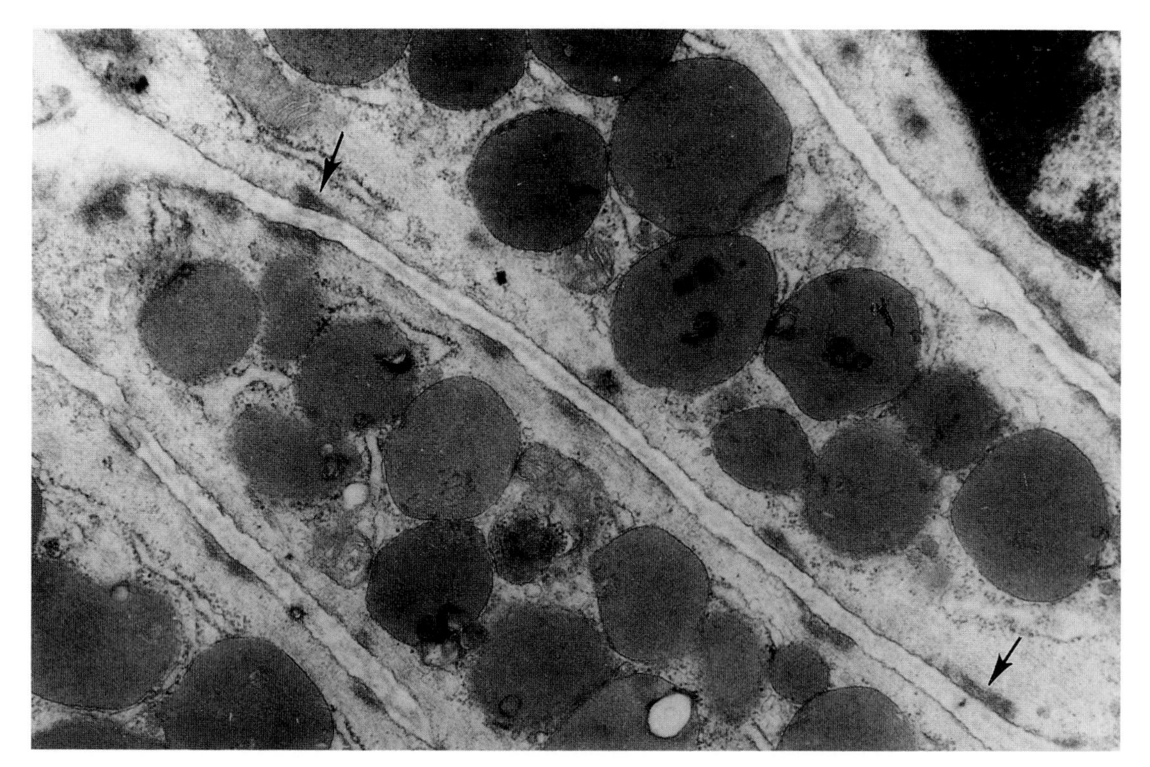

Figure 30–30. Electron micrograph of modified smooth muscle cells of a renal vessel containing large renin-containing secretory granules that resemble lipid droplets. Note that the cells retain characteristics of smooth muscle in their peripheral myofilaments and subplasmalemmal dense bodies (at arrows). (From Hackenthal, E., M. Paul, D. Ganten, and E. Taugner. 1990. Physiol. Rev. 70:1067. Micrograph courtesy of R. Nobiling.)

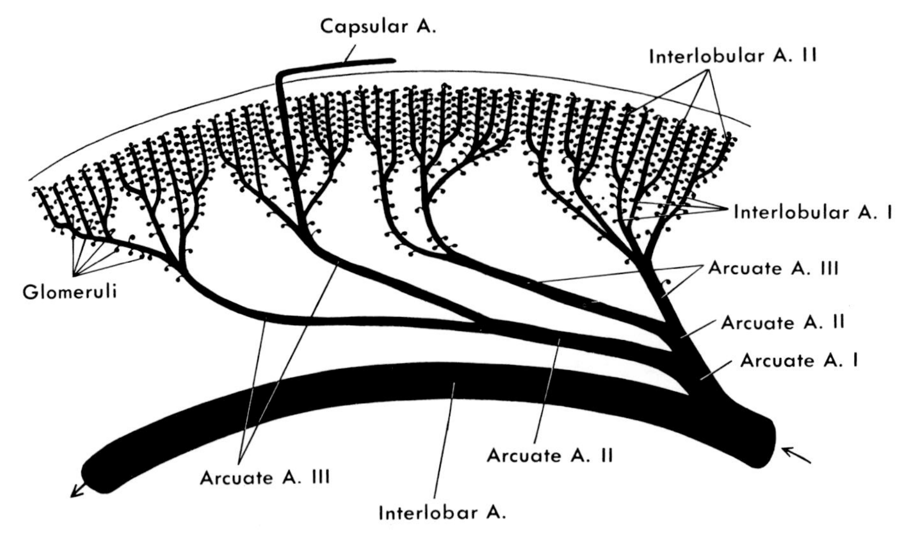

Figure 30–31. Schematic representation of the finer branches of the arterial blood supply of the kidney. (After Kugelgen, A. and K.J. Otto. 1959. *In* Zwanglos Abhandlungen aus dem Gebiet der normalen und pathologischen Anatomie, Vol. 5. Stuttgart, Georg Thieme.)

with each other and with glomerular mesangial cells via gap junctions. Similar junctions have been reported among these cells, juxtaglomerular cells, and smooth muscle cells of the afferent arteriole. Thus, pathways would seem to exist for integration of vasomotor activities of the afferent arteriole and the glomerular capillaries. The nature of the signals from the macula densa to the juxtaglomerular cells has yet to be discovered.

BLOOD SUPPLY

The kidneys have a very large blood flow, averaging about 1200 ml/min. Some familiarity with their complex vascular architecture is essential to an understanding of renal function.

The *renal artery* enters the hilus and divides in the adipose tissue of the renal sinus into anterior and posterior divisions which give rise to *segmental arteries*. These, in turn, provide *lobar arteries* to each renal pyramid. Just before entering the substance of the kidney, these divide into two *interlobular arteries* that course toward the cortex in the renal columns on either side of a pyramid. These divide dichotomously at the level of the corticomedullary boundary, forming *arcuate arteries* running parallel to the surface of the kidney (Fig. 30–31). Small *cortical radial arteries,* arising at regular intervals from the arcuate arteries, course radially in the cortex. These provide the *afferent arterioles* to juxtamedullary, midcortical, and superficial glomeruli (Fig. 30–31). Blood leaves the glomeruli via *efferent arterioles*. Efferent arterioles of superficial glomeruli are of small caliber and ramify to form the cortical *intertubular capillary network*. In the renal cortex, the endothelium of the peritubular capillaries is fenestrated and rapid-freeze, deep-etched preparations reveal that the pore diaphragms have a complex hub-and-spoke pattern with the openings between the radial spokes (Fig. 30–34). The larger efferent arterioles of juxtamedullary glomeruli course into the medulla, branching into many vessels somewhat larger than capillaries, called the *vasa recta* (Fig. 30–32). The efferent vessels of juxtamedullary glomeruli and the vasa recta both contribute to the intertubular capillary network of the medulla.

Continuing deeper into the medulla, the vasa recta form hairpin loops at various levels in the medulla, turning back and coursing parallel and close to the descending limb of

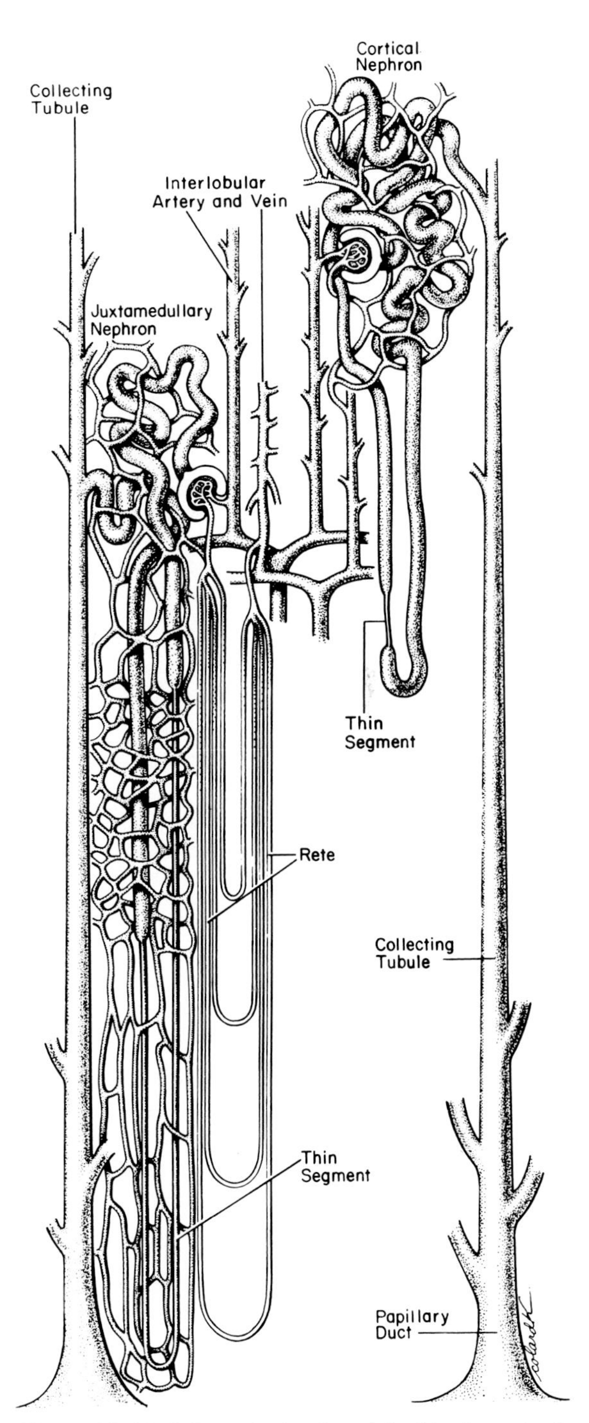

Figure 30–32. Schematic drawing of the blood supply of cortical and juxtamedullary nephrons. In the latter, the efferent arteriole courses downward into the medulla, where it gives rise to a bundle of vasa recta. These, together with their recurrent venules, form long bundles of parallel vessels called retia mirabilia. In this drawing, the arterial and venous elements of the rete have been separated to show their continuity in long loops. In life, the arterial and venous limbs of the loops intermingle as shown in Fig. 30–33.

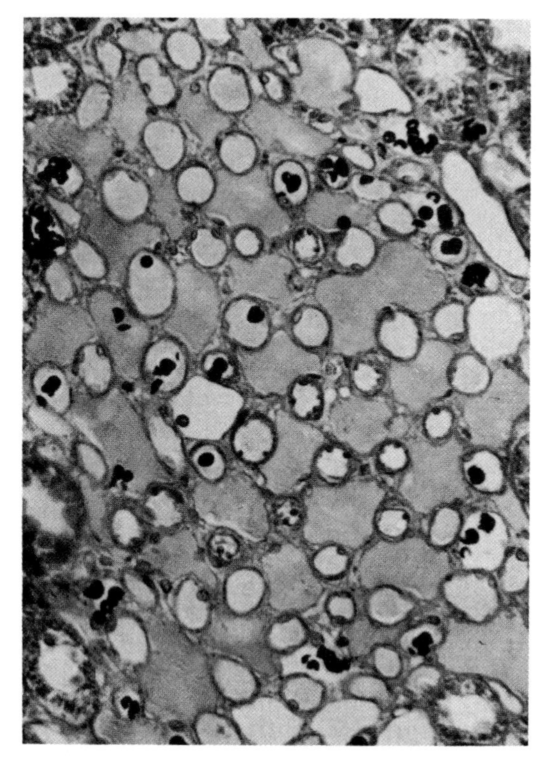

Figure 30–33. Photomicrograph of a rete mirabile from dog kidney. The descending arterial limbs of the loops are capillaries with a round cross section and walls of appreciable thickness. The ascending venous limbs are larger, more irregular in outline, and have exceedingly thin walls. In this micrograph, they are filled with a gray precipitate of plasma, whereas the descending capillaries appear empty or contain a few erythrocytes.

the loop of Henle. The descending and ascending limbs of these numerous loops form a countercurrent system of vessels referred to as a *vascular bundle* or *rete* (Fig. 30–32). The descending arterial limbs and the ascending venous limbs differ in diameter and in the character of their wall (Fig. 30–33). The descending limbs are smaller and have a continuous endothelium, whereas the larger ascending limbs of the loops have thin walls and a fenestrated endothelium. The proximity of the vessels in the vascular bundles and the large surface area they present to one another facilitate diffusion of ions and small molecules between blood in the ascending and descending limbs. The vascular bundles, thus, serve as efficient countercurrent exchangers for diffusable substances.

The capillaries of the outermost zones of the cortex are drained toward the surface by radially arranged branches, the *superficial cortical veins,* which join vessels on the surface of the kidney, *stellate veins,* that have a characteristic radial pattern. This outer mantle of venous channels is drained by a relatively small number of *interlobular veins* that are confluent at their inner end with *arcuate veins* that accompany arteries of the same name. Capillaries in the deeper portion of the cortex empty into radially oriented *deep cortical veins,* of which there are 400 per square centimeter, running parallel to a corresponding number of interlobular arteries. The blood in these veins flows inward to the arcuate veins and then into *interlobal veins* that join to form the *renal vein.*

LYMPHATICS

The distribution of lymphatics in the kidney has been controversial. Some have contended that intrarenal lymphatics are found only in association with the larger blood vessels and that they extend peripherally only as far as the interlobular vasculature. Others report that there are lymphatic capillaries among the tubular elements making up the parenchyma of the renal lobules and that these are tributaries of larger interlobar lymphatics. This latter interpretation has been strongly supported by light and electron microscopic studies employing improved methods for their identification. It is now accepted that there are lymphatics in the renal cortex in addition to those accompanying the larger arterial vessels. These drain mainly into interlobular lymphatics and then to lymphatic plexuses in the hilus of the kidney. Some in the outer cortex drain to a plexus in the renal capsule. The volume of lymph in the cortex is estimated to be only about 1% of volume of the blood in peritubular capillaries.

NERVES

The sympathetic celiac plexus sends many nerves into the kidney, but their distribution within the organ has not been worked out in detail. Myelinated and unmyelinated fibers can be traced along the course of the larger blood vessels. These provide sensory endings to the adventitia of the vessels and motor endings in their muscular coat. Nerve fibers can be traced to the afferent arterioles of the renal corpuscles and some seem to terminate there. Some investigators have reported a plexus of fine fibers surrounding, and seeming to penetrate, the basal lamina of the uriniferous tu-

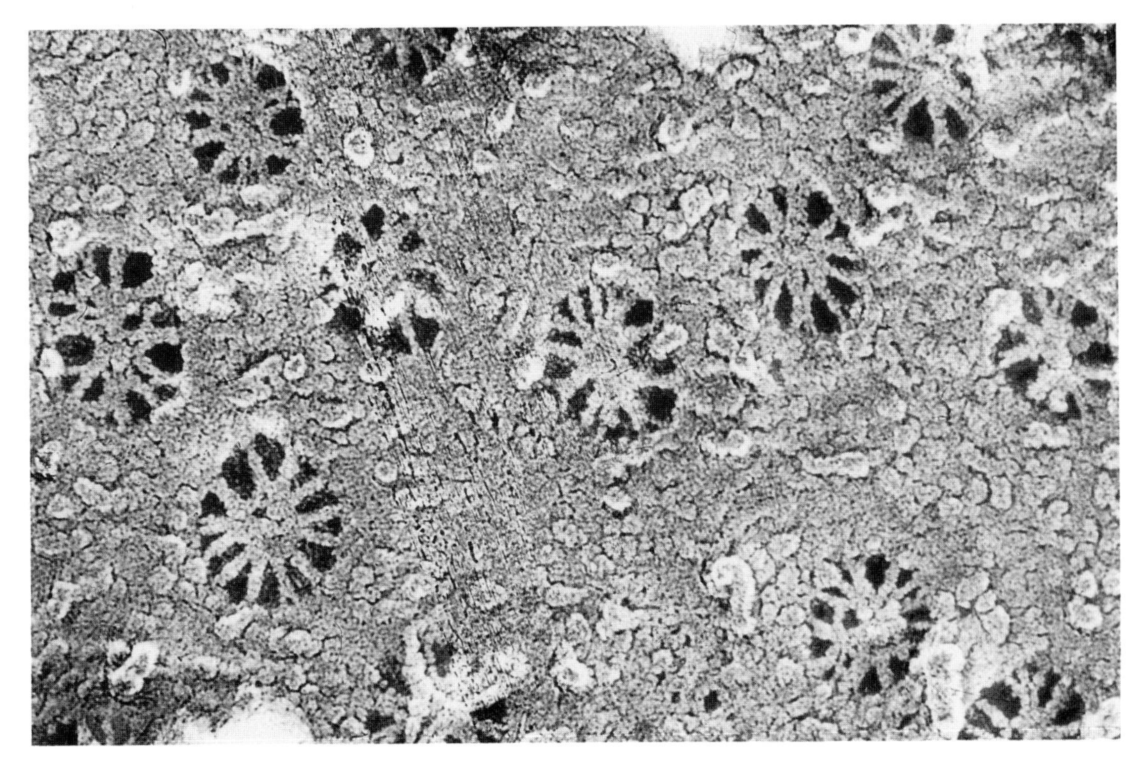

Figure 30–34. A high-magnification micrograph of a rapid-freeze, deep-etched preparation of a peritubular capillary of the renal cortex showing the hub-and-spokes pattern of radial strands forming the diaphragms of the endothelial pores. (Micrograph courtesy of Orci, L. 1985. J. Cell Biol. 100:418.)

bules to end among the epithelial cells. However, it is possible that the silver-impregnation methods used were impregnating reticular fibers rather than nerves. To date, there has not been a convincing demonstration of a nerve supply to the renal tubules. A systematic investigation of the finer innervation of the kidney with the electron microscope might settle this matter.

HISTOPHYSIOLOGY OF THE KIDNEYS

In addition to their *excretory* function, the kidneys have important *conservative* functions by which they retain water, electrolytes, and nutrients in the amounts needed by the body. The kidneys carry out these functions by a combination of filtration, passive diffusion, active secretion, and selective reabsorption. Many of the unusual features of the cells, described in the foregoing pages, are structural specializations that increase the efficiency of these processes.

Blood circulates through the glomerular capillaries with a hydrostatic pressure (~70 mm Hg) that forces fluid constituents of the plasma through the fenestrated endothelium, basal lamina, and filtration slits between podocyte processes and into Bowman's capsule. The hydrostatic pressure in the capillaries is opposed by the colloid osmotic pressure of the plasma (~32 mm Hg) and the intracapsular pressure (~20 mm Hg), resulting in a net filtration pressure of ~18 mm Hg. With blood flowing through the glomeruli of both kidneys at a rate of ~1300 ml/min, glomerular filtrate is produced at a rate of ~125 ml/min. From this volume of filtrate, urine is produced at a rate of only ~1 ml/min. The rest of the water is reabsorbed during passage through the renal tubules, and the composition of the filtrate is further modified by addition of some substances through active secretion, and removal of others by active transport and osmotic forces.

Fluid aspirated from Bowman's capsule by micropuncture is an ultrafiltrate of blood plasma that contains only small molecules such as uric acid, urea, creatine, and small amounts of albumen. Substances of molecular weight over 70,000 are excluded. The filtration barrier is not only size selective but also has selectivity based on charge, with anionic molecules being more limited in their passage than neutral molecules of the same size. The principal negatively charged components responsible for charge selectivity are heparan sulfate proteoglycan and type-IV collagen in the basal lamina and the sialoglycoprotein, podocalyxin, in the surface coat of the podocyte processes (Fig. 30–11). Electrostatic repulsion prevents other negatively charged protein molecules from passing through the barrier.

In the proximal tubule, 70% of the sodium and water of the glomerular filtrate is reabsorbed, together with chloride, calcium, phosphate, glucose, and amino acids. Although some water and solutes may pass from the lumen to the interstitial spaces via a paracellular route through the juxtaluminal cell junctions, most of the traffic takes a transcellular route. Sodium enters the cells from the lumen by facilitated diffusion through the apical plasma membrane and is actively pumped out of the cells through their basolateral membranes into the interstitial fluid. In the electrochemical gradient so created, water and chloride follow to maintain osmotic equilibrium. Glucose and amino acids are conserved by being carried through the lumenal membrane in cotransport with the sodium and then diffusing through the basolateral membrane and into the peritubular capillaries. The efficiency of the proximal tubule in conserving these useful constituents of the filtrate is attributable to the remarkable structural devices for maximizing the area of the physiologically significant domains of the cell surface. The waste products of metabolism, urea, uric acid, and creatine that are not needed are allowed to remain in the tubule fluid and are voided in the urine.

The ability of the human kidneys to excrete a hypertonic urine depends on the loop of

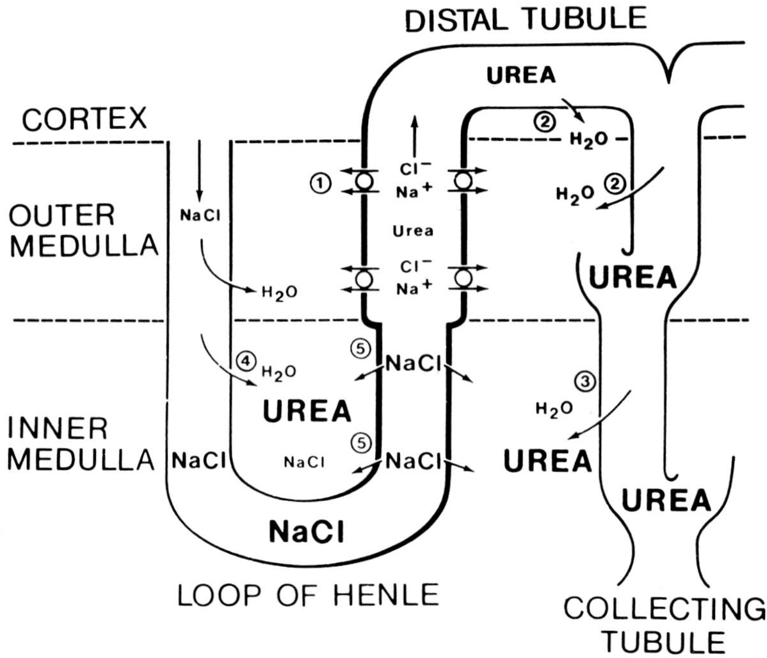

Figure 30–35. Countercurrent multiplier mechanism. The thin ascending limb in the inner medulla and the thick ascending limb in the outer medulla, as well as the first part of the distal tubule, are all impermeable to water, as indicated here by their thickened wall. In the thick ascending limb, active chloride resorption, accompanied by passive sodium movement (1), renders the tubule fluid dilute and the outer medullary interstitium hyperosmotic. In the last part of the distal tubule and in the collecting tubule in the cortex and outer medulla, water is reabsorbed down its osmotic gradient (2), increasing the concentration of urea that remains behind. In the inner medulla, both water and urea are reabsorbed from the collecting duct (3). Some urea reenters the loop of Henle (not shown). This medullary recycling of urea and the trapping of urea by countercurrent exchange in the vasa recta (not shown) causes urea to accumulate in large quantities in the medullary interstitium (indicated by large type), where it osmotically extracts water from the descending limb of the loop (4) and thereby concentrates sodium chloride in fluid in the descending limb. When fluid, rich in sodium chloride, enters the sodium-chloride-permeable (but water-impermeable) thin ascending limb, sodium chloride moves passively down its concentration gradient (5) rendering the tubule fluid relatively hypo-osmotic to the surrounding interstitium. (From Jamieson, R.L. and R.H. Maffly. 1976. N. Engl. J. Med. 295:1059.)

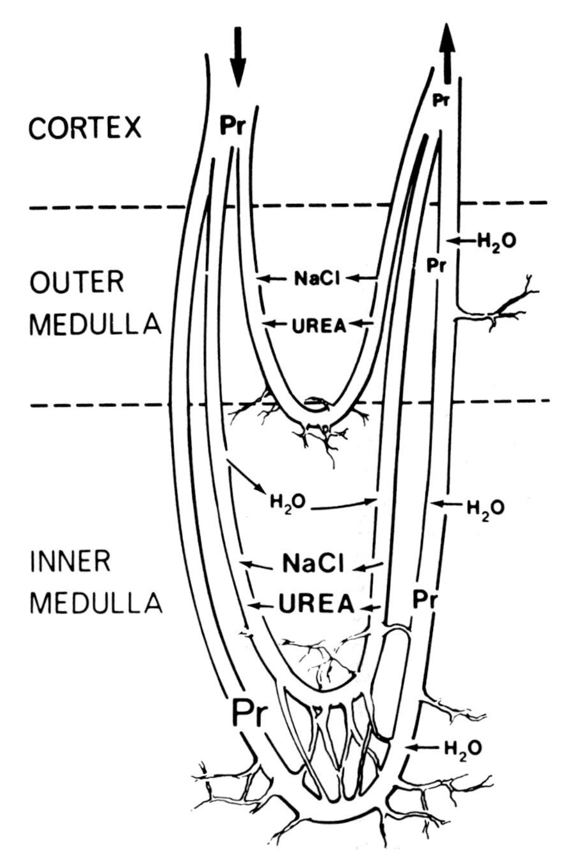

Figure 30–36. Diagram of countercurrent exchange in the rete mirabile. The blood supply of the medulla comes from the vasa recta and their branches. In this diagram, Pr stands for plasma protein. The size of type indicates relative concentration of each solute in relation to its location in the medulla, but not necessarily with respect to other solutes. The progressive rise in the concentration of sodium chloride and urea in the medullary interstitium, toward the pelvis, is due to the loop of Henle and the collecting tubules. Because the vessels are permeable to sodium chloride and urea, these solutes enter descending vasa recta and leave ascending vasa recta. This exchange helps to "trap" the solutes in the medulla. Conversely, water leaves the descending vasa recta, causing the plasma protein concentration in their lumen to increase. In the ascending vasa recta, the sum of the osmotic pressure due to plasma protein and other nonprotein solutes results in uptake of water into the intravascular fluid. Thus, water reabsorbed from the collecting tubule and Henle's descending limb is removed from the medullary interstitium and returned to the general circulation. Vasa recta of the rete, thus, function in a dual capacity, "trapping" solute and removing water to preserve the hyperosmolarity of the renal medulla. (From Jamieson, R.L. and R.H. Maffly. 1976. N. Engl. J. Med. 295:1059.)

Henle. Only those species that have a thin segment in the loop, excrete urine that is hypertonic to blood plasma. The degree to which the glomerular filtrate is concentrated is correlated with the extent of the thin segment and with the length of the renal papilla in which it is located. Mammals living in an aqueous environment have little need to conserve water and have short loops and papillae. They excrete a relatively dilute urine. Desert-dwelling species, on the other hand, have a well-developed thin segment in long loops of Henle and have long renal papillae. They are able to concentrate their urine up to 20 times the osmolarity of plasma. The maximum concentration achieved by the human kidney is about fivefold.

The interstitial fluid in the outer renal cortex is approximately isomotic with plasma, but there is a continuous increase in its osmolarity from the corticomedullary junction to the tip of the papilla. The maintenance of this gradient is essential for excretion of concentrated urine. It depends, in large measure, on distinctive permeability properties of the successive segments of the loop of Henle. The vasa recta of the medullary vasculature also contribute to maintenance of the gradient by serving as a countercurrent exchanger that minimizes washout of solutes from the interstitial fluid (Fig. 30–35).

The thin descending limb of the loop is highly permeable to water but not to salt. The thin ascending limb is impermeable to water but permeable to salt. Water diffusing from the descending limb creates an increased intratubular concentration of solute, mainly salt. After the fluid rounds the bend of the loop, the permeability of the ascending limb permits salt to diffuse into the interstitium contributing *passively* to the high osmolarity of the inner medulla.

The thick ascending limb of the loop of Henle is relatively impermeable to diffusion but it *actively* transports chloride out of the tubule accompanied by passive movement of sodium, thus rendering the tubule fluid dilute and the interstitium hyperosmotic. In the water-permeable portion of the distal tubule in the cortex and in the collecting duct, the osmotic gradient draws water from the tubule increasing the intratubular concentration of urea (Fig. 30–35).

On a diet of average protein content, the body produces about 25 g of urea per day as a waste product. Its concentration in the tubule fluid is increased nearly 100-fold during passage through the renal tubules. In the lower part of the collecting ducts, a considerable amount of urea is reabsorbed into the medullary interstitium. Much of this reenters the thin limb of the loop of Henle and recirculates repeatedly through the distal nephron before being excreted in the urine. This recirculation of urea makes a significant contribution to the hyperosmolarity of the interstitium and helps conserve water.

If blood circulated through the medulla in large volume, solutes in the interstitial fluid would be washed out and the high osmolarity of the medulla would not be maintained. Actually, the flow to the medulla is less than 2% of the total renal blood flow. Moreover, the unusual configuration of its vascular supply creates a countercurrent exchange system that further reduces solute extraction. The hairpin loops formed by the vasa recta permit free exchange of water and solutes between the highly permeable descending and ascending segments of the loops. As blood flows down the descending limb, salt and urea diffuse into the blood, increasing their concentration toward the bend. As blood flows back toward the cortex in the ascending limb, water moves into the blood, and salt and urea diffuse back out into the interstitium. Thus, very little solute is lost due to blood flow through the medulla, and high interstitial osmolarity is maintained (Fig. 30–36).

The conservation of water and electrolytes by the kidney is strongly influenced by hormones. Sodium reabsorption in the distal tubule and collecting duct is controlled by *aldosterone,* a hormone secreted by the adrenal cortex. The hormone binds to specific receptors on the cells and, by a mechanism still poorly understood, affects sodium transport across the basolateral membranes of the cells. Because movement of sodium across cells is accompanied by movement of potassium in the opposite direction, aldosterone controls potassium secretion at the same time that it controls sodium reabsorption. When the hormone is present in excess, almost no sodium is found in the urine.

The permeability of the connecting tubules and collecting ducts to water is regulated by *antidiuretic hormone* (*vasopressin*) secreted by the pars nervosa of the pituitary. When present in the blood in greater than normal amounts, the permeability of the collecting ducts is increased, permitting reabsorption of large amounts of water and excretion of a highly concentrated urine. The permeability of the ducts to urea is unaffected by the hormone.

An increase of blood or extracellular fluid volume results in release of *atrial natiuretic peptide* from secretory cardiac myocytes in the atrium of the heart. The peptide directly increases the excretion of sodium and water by an increase in glomerular filtration rate and by inhibition of salt resorption in the medullary collecting ducts. It may also affect salt and water excretion indirectly by inhibiting the release of aldosterone and vasopressin. The peptide has been localized immunocytochemically in the intercalated cells of the collecting ducts, but it is not known whether it is produced by these cells or whether it is taken up by receptor-mediated endocytosis. The role of these cells, if any, in salt and water excretion is not known.

In addition to their function in regulation of blood pressure and electrolyte balance, the kidneys play an important role in the control of the oxygen-carrying capacity of the blood through their secretion of *erythropoietin.* Because the kidneys receive a large portion of the cardiac output of blood (20–25%), they are favorably situated to monitor the oxygen saturation of the blood. Hemorrhage, high altitude, impaired pulmonary function, or any other condition causing a low partial pressure of oxygen in the blood results in increased synthesis and release of erythropoietin by the kidneys. Erythropoietin acts on the bone marrow, increasing the rate of division of erythroid progenitors and accelerating the release of new erythrocytes, thereby enhancing the oxygen-carrying capacity of the blood. Patients with severe renal disease requiring dialysis are invariably anemic. Such patients now benefit from advances in molecular biology that have made it possible to produce erythropoietin by recombinant DNA technology.

The location of the oxygen-sensor in the renal cortex and the identity of the cells producing erythropoietin have long evaded detection. The erythropoietin gene has now been isolated and in situ hybridization of erythropoietin mRNA suggests that the endothelial cells of the peritubular capillaries around the straight and convoluted tubules are the site of its synthesis. Whether they respond directly to changes in oxygen concentration or are activated by products of other cells having a sensory function is not clear.

RENAL PELVIS AND URETER

The excretory passages of the urinary tract are lined by transitional epithelium throughout, but there are regional differences in its thickness. In the calyces, it is only two to three

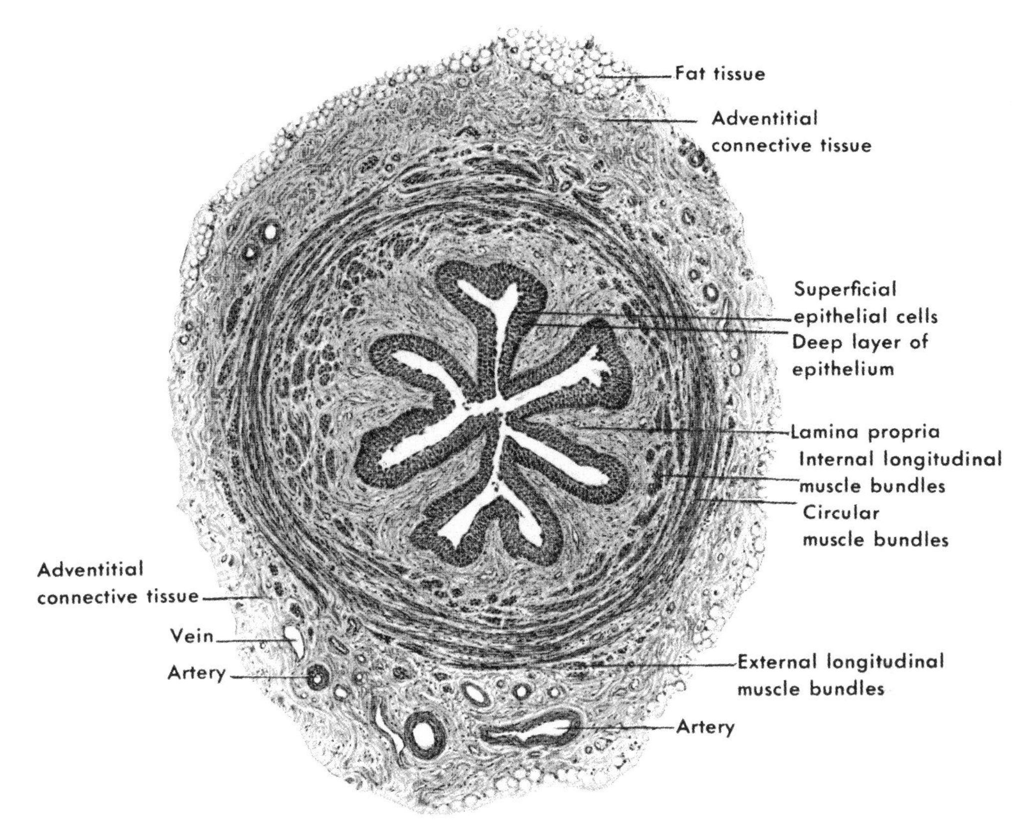

Figure 30–37. Cross section of a greatly contracted human ureter, with the mucosa thrown up into several longitudinal folds that nearly obliterate the lumen. (After J. Schaffer Lehrbruch der Histologie und Histogenese, Verlag von W. Engelmann, 1922.)

cells thick; in the ureters, four to five. The connective tissue of the lamina propria is abundant and rich in networks of elastic fibers. It may contain small lymphoid nodules. Its deeper portion has a loose arrangement, permitting the mucosa of the empty ureter to be thrown up into several longitudinal folds that give the lumen a highly irregular outline (Fig. 30–37). There is no distinct submucosa, the lamina propria blending with the connective tissue of the surrounding muscular layer.

The walls of the renal calyes, pelvis, and ureter are all provided with a well-developed layer of smooth muscle. In contrast to the muscularis of the intestinal tract, the muscular coat of the urinary tract is not arranged in clearly defined longitudinal and circular layers. Instead, it is made up of anastomosing bundles of muscle fibers of varying orientation. Although the inner bundles are predominantly longitudinal and the outer mainly circumferential, they grade into one another with no clearly defined boundary. The thickness of the wall gradually increases along the tract and, beginning in the lower third of the ureter, an additional layer of predominantly longitudinal fibers is added.

In the small calyces capping the papillae of the renal pyramids, the bundles of inner longitudinal smooth muscle terminate at the attachment of the calyx to the papilla. The outer bundles, predominantly circumferential in orientation, extend farther up and form a muscular ring around the papilla. In the living, this region of the calyces exhibits periodic contractions. This muscular activity may assist in expelling urine from the papillary ducts into the calyces. In the pelvis and ureter, the muscular coat creates a slow peristalsis with waves of contraction proceeding from the renal pelvis toward the bladder.

URINARY BLADDER

The transitional epithelium of the contracted urinary bladder is six to eight cells thick and those at the lumenal surface are rounded or club-shaped (Fig. 30–38). In the distended bladder, the epithelium is much

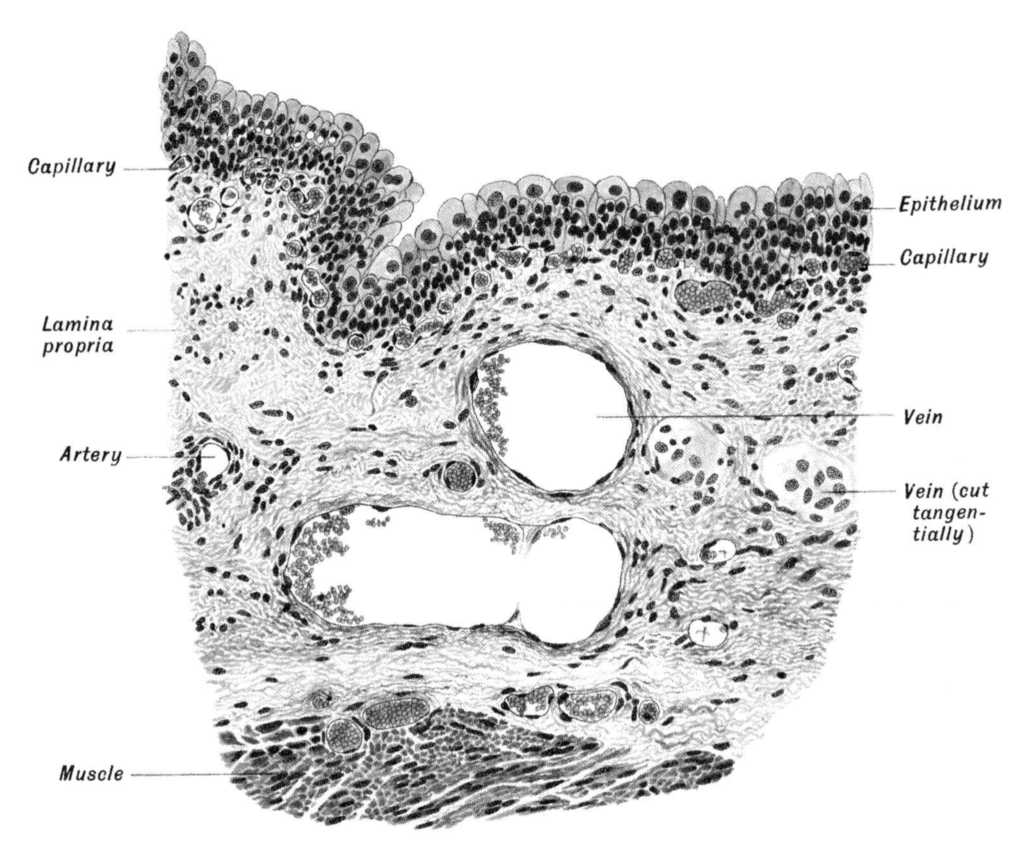

Figure 30–38. Section of the wall of the human urinary bladder in the contracted state. The large superficial cells of the transitional epithelium bulge into the lumen. Capillaries are abundant in the lamina propria immediately beneath the epithelium.

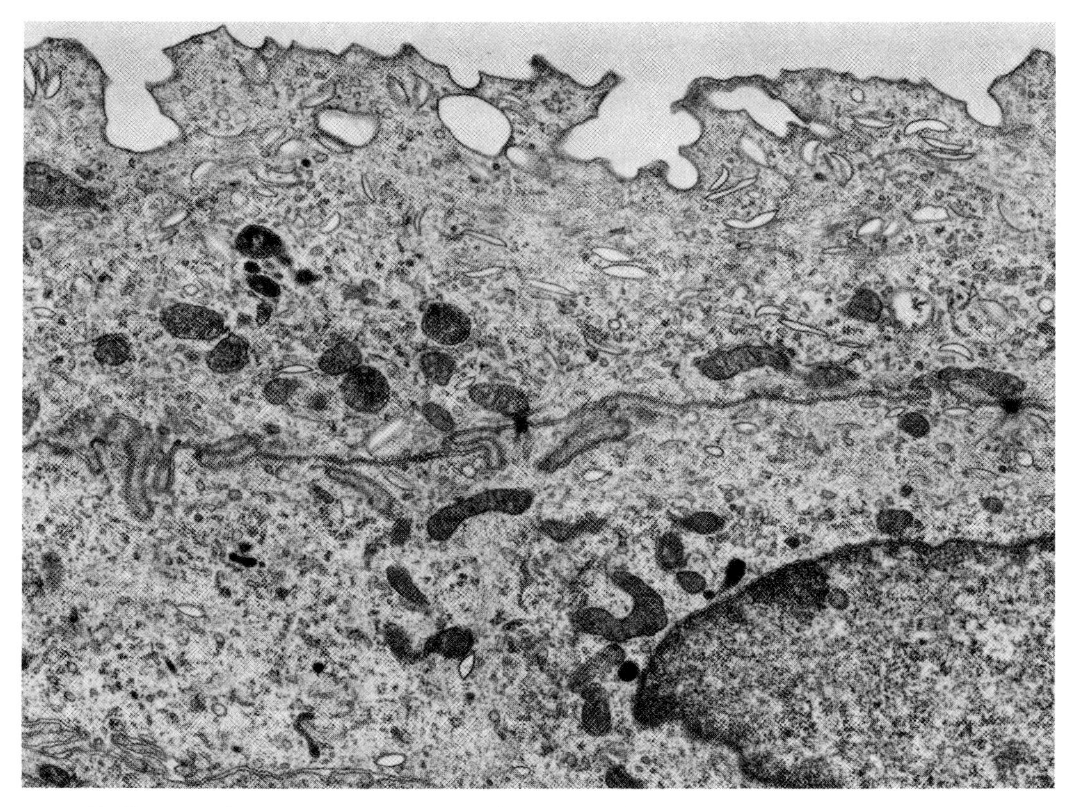

Figure 30–39. Electron micrograph of transitional epithelial cells of the bladder. The lumenal surface has a peculiar angular contour which is apparently due to insertion of relatively stiff plaques of membrane into it when lenticular vesicles in the apical cytoplasm fuse with the plasma membrane. (Micrograph from Hicks, M. and B. Ketterer. 1970. J. Cell Biol. 45:452.)

thinner and the cells are flattened. In electron micrographs, their lumenal surface has a characteristic scalloped appearance. The cell membrane is thicker than that of other cells (12 nm) and asymmetrical, with the outer dense line of the unit membrane noticeably thicker than the inner dense line. The membrane is made up of plaques of thick membrane connected by thinner interplaque regions. In section, the plaques appear as segments of fairly uniform length that are straight or slightly concave and seemingly stiff (Fig. 30–39). Neighboring plaques are so oriented that they produce angular surface contours seen in no other epithelium. Beneath the membrane, there is a conspicuous ectoplasmic layer of microfilaments with some filament bundles extending deeper into the cell. In the apical cytoplasm, there are numerous discoidal vesicles that are lenticular or elliptical in section. These are bounded by thick membrane identical to that at the lumenal surface of the cell. Vesicles of this unusual shape are unique to the transitional epithelium of the bladder. They appear to be formed by interiorization of adjoining plaques of the surface membrane and they are subsequently reinserted into the membrane to provide for rapid expansion of its surface area during bladder distension. Morphometric studies indicate that a large percentage of the membrane surface area is translocated in and out of the cells during the expansion–contraction cycles of the bladder. When the surface membrane is isolated and examined by negative staining and optical diffraction, the plaques are found to have a highly ordered substructure consisting of hexagonally arranged particulate subunits. Each subunit seems to be a hexamer of smaller subunits arranged in a stellate configuration (Fig. 30–40). The functional significance of this lattice structure is by no means clear. Membranes of the superficial cells, other than the lumenal membrane, do not appear to differ from those of other cells. There are juxtalumenal tight junctions between adjoining cells and numerous desmosomes elsewhere on the lateral surfaces.

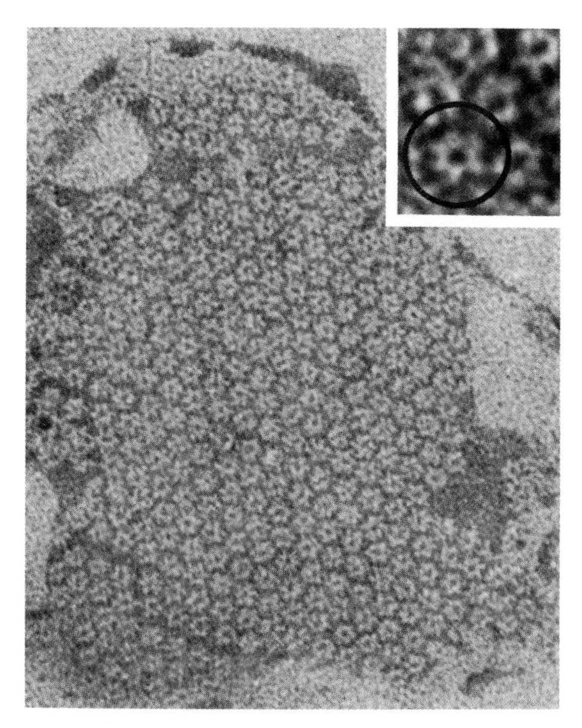

Figure 30–40. Electron micrograph of a negatively stained plaque within the cell membrane at the free surface of the transitional epithelium of the bladder. These regions of the membrane have a unique structure consisting of hexagonally arranged subunits (see inset). It is not clear how these are related to the unusual permeability characteristics of this epithelium. (Micrograph from Hicks, M. and B. Ketterer. 1970. J. Cell Biol. 45:542.)

The dense network of filaments in the apical cytoplasm is reported to be attached to the plaques in the lumenal membrane and to the discoid vesicles in the cytoplasm. The cross-linking of adjacent plaques by filaments may lead to an orderly infolding of membrane and pinching off of discoid vesicles during bladder contraction. It is further speculated that, during stretching produced by bladder distension, the discoid vesicles are drawn to the surface by the stretched filament network and there fuse with the cell membrane expanding its surface area.

The specializations of the bladder epithelium have significance beyond adaptation to changes in bladder volume. It is known that in man the tonicity of bladder urine is two to four times higher than that of plasma in the capillaries of the lamina propria. If the epithelium were permeable to water, the content of the bladder would be diluted by movement of water from the blood to the urine. Because this does not occur, it is evident that the epithelium is an effective permeability barrier against water loss. This function is diminished or lost after chemical or mechanical damage to the surface of the epithelium. The barrier is, thus, believed to reside in the occluding junctions between the superficial cells and in special properties of the thick lumenal membrane.

The thick muscular coat of the bladder is composed of sizable strands of smooth muscle

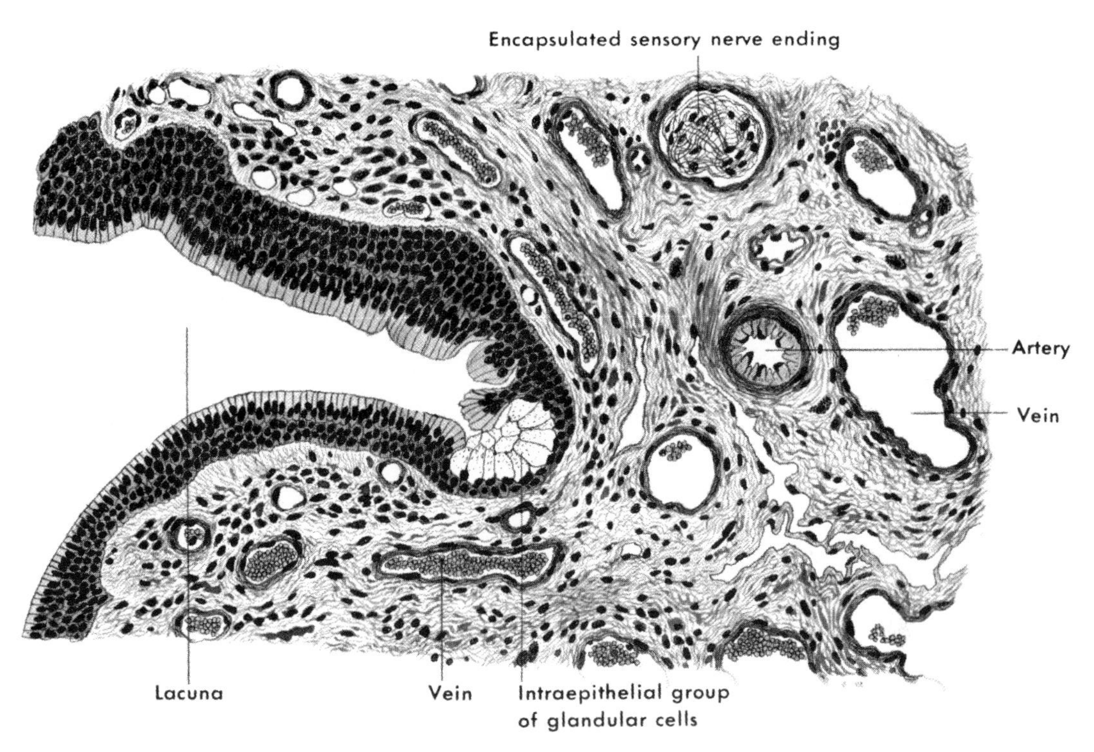

Figure 30–41. Section of the pars spongiosa of the human male urethra. Stratified columnar epithelium lines a small diverticulum called a lacuna (at left). At the right are several vessels of the highly vascular submucous layer which become engorged during erection.

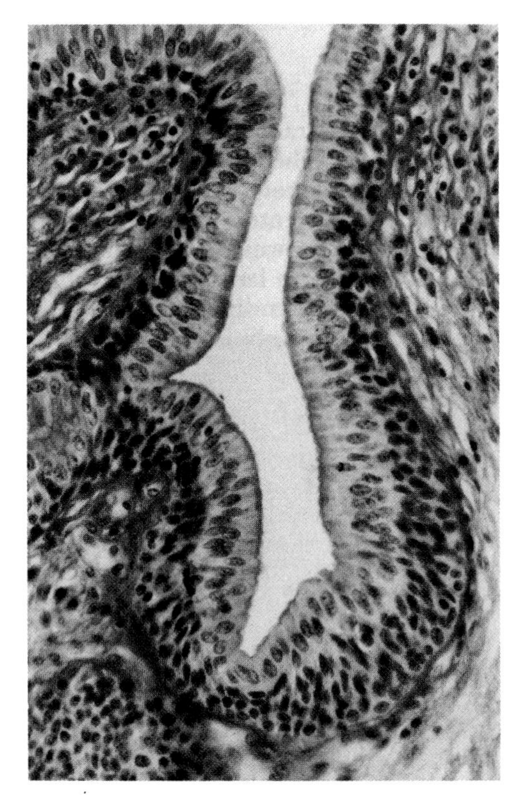

Figure 30–42. Photomicrograph of the stratified columnar epithelium that lines the pars spongiosa of the male urethra.

cells that form three layers. These intermingle at their interface so that the layers cannot be clearly separated from one another. The outer longitudinal layer is most prominent and compact on the dorsal and ventral surfaces of the bladder, whereas, elsewhere, longitudinal fiber bundles are more widely separated. Of the three layers, the middle circular or spiral layer is the thickest. In the body of the bladder, the inner layer consists of relative sparse longitudinal and oblique muscle strands. In the region of the trigone, at the base of the bladder, dense bundles of smooth muscle encircle the transmural portion of the urethra, forming the *internal sphincter* of the bladder.

BLOOD VESSELS, LYMPHATICS, AND NERVES

The blood vessels of the excretory passages provide capillaries to the muscle coat as they pass through it and then form a plexus in the outer portion of the lamina propria. From there, small arteries pass inward to form a richer plexus immediately beneath the epithelium.

A well-developed network of lymphatic capillaries is found in the lamina propria and muscularis of the renal pelvis and ureters. In the bladder, lymphatics have been reported only in the muscularis.

Nerve plexuses and small ganglia are present in the adventitial and muscular layers of the ureter. Most of the fibers supply the muscle, but some, thought to be sensory, have been traced through the lamina propria to the epithelium. A sympathetic nerve plexus in the adventitial coat of the bladder, the *plexus vesicalis,* arises from the hypogastric plexus. The efferent parasympathetic fibers arise from sacral segments of the spinal cord and synapse with nerve cells in the wall of the bladder. These neurones send motor fibers to the muscle and inhibitory fibers to the internal sphincter. The sympathetic efferent fibers of the plexus arise from lower thoracic and upper lumbar segments of the cord and synapse on cells in the hypogastric plexuses and in the wall of the bladder. These neurones send inhibitory fibers to the muscle coats and motor fibers to the sphincter.

MALE URETHRA

The urethra in the male is about 18 cm in length and serves as the terminal portion of both the urinary tract and the reproductive tract. Three successive segments are distinguished: the *prostatic urethra* (pars prostatica), the *membranous urethra* (pars membranacea), and the *spongiose* or *penile urethra* (pars spongiosa).

The prostatic urethra is about 3 cm long and runs through the prostate from its base to its apex. On its posterior wall, there is a medial longitudinal ridge, the *urethral crest,* and, in it a slight elevation, called the *colliculus seminalis* (verumontanum). In the midline of the colliculus is the opening of the *prostatic utricle* (utriculus prostaticus), a blind pouch extending upward and backward into the substance of the prostate. This is the rudimentary homologue of the uterus in the male. On either side of its orifice are the slit-like openings of the two *ejaculatory ducts* (ductus ejaculatorius). In grooves on the posterior wall of the prostatic urethra on either side of the colliculus seminalis are numerous minute openings of the ducts of the prostate gland.

The lining of the urethra, proximal to the

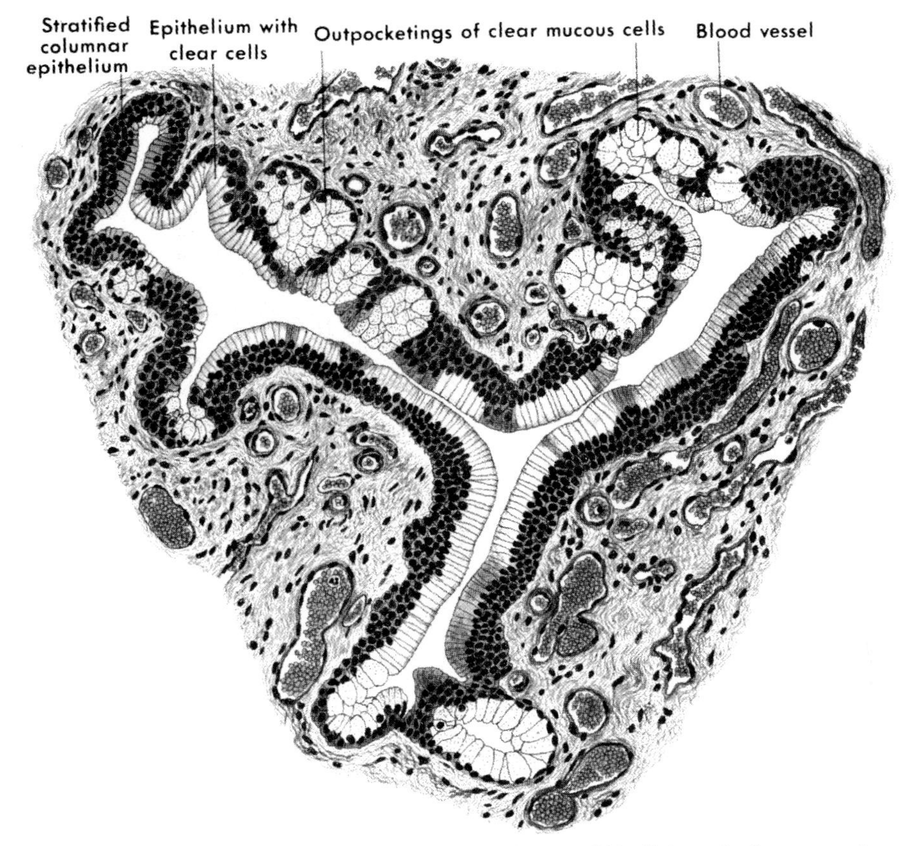

Figure 30–43. Section of a mucus-secreting urethral gland (gland of Littré) from the human penile urethra.)

ejaculatory ducts, is a typical transitional epithelium, but distal to this, it becomes pseudostratified or stratified columnar epithelium and contains occasional mucus-secreting goblet cells (Figs. 30–41 and 30–42). When viewed in scanning electron micrographs, the lumenal surface shows considerable variation in cell size and membrane specialization. Most of the cells are polygonal in outline and have abundant short microvilli. Others have a convex apex bulging into the lumen. Microvilli are few and largely confined to the periphery, leaving the central area smooth. Still other cells are nearly twice as large and have a surface exhibiting a labyrinthine pattern of microplicae. Rare cells bear numerous cilia.

There is no significant change in the character of the epithelium in the membranous urethra, which is 1–2 cm in length and passes through the urogenital diaphragm (perineal membrane) postero-inferior to the pubic symphysis. Striated muscle surrounding the urethra in the urogenital diaphragm constitutes the *external sphincter urethrae*. It is supplied by the peroneal branch of the pudendal nerve and is under voluntary control.

The penile urethra, 12–14 cm in length, courses through the corpus spongiosum from the urogenital diaphragm to the external opening of the urethra on the glans penis. It is lined by stratified columnar epithelium up to the *fossa navicularis,* the slightly expanded terminal 6–7 mm of the urethra which is lined by stratified squamous epithelium like that covering the glans penis.

Two glands, the *bulbourethral glands,* about 1 cm in diameter, lie on the urogenital diaphragm on either side of the membranous urethra. Their long ducts penetrate the diaphragm and, about 2.5 cm below it, open into the floor of the penile urethra. Along the entire length of the urethra, there are many shallow recesses in the mucous membrane, the *lacunae of Morgani.* Opening into these out-pocketings are the *glands of Littré* (Fig. 30–43). These run obliquely in the lamina propria, with their blind ends directed toward the base of the penis. The largest of them are on the dorsal aspect of the pars spongiosa and a few may penetrate into the corpus spongiosum. Their lining epithelium is similar to that on the surface of the mucous membrane but contains nests of pale

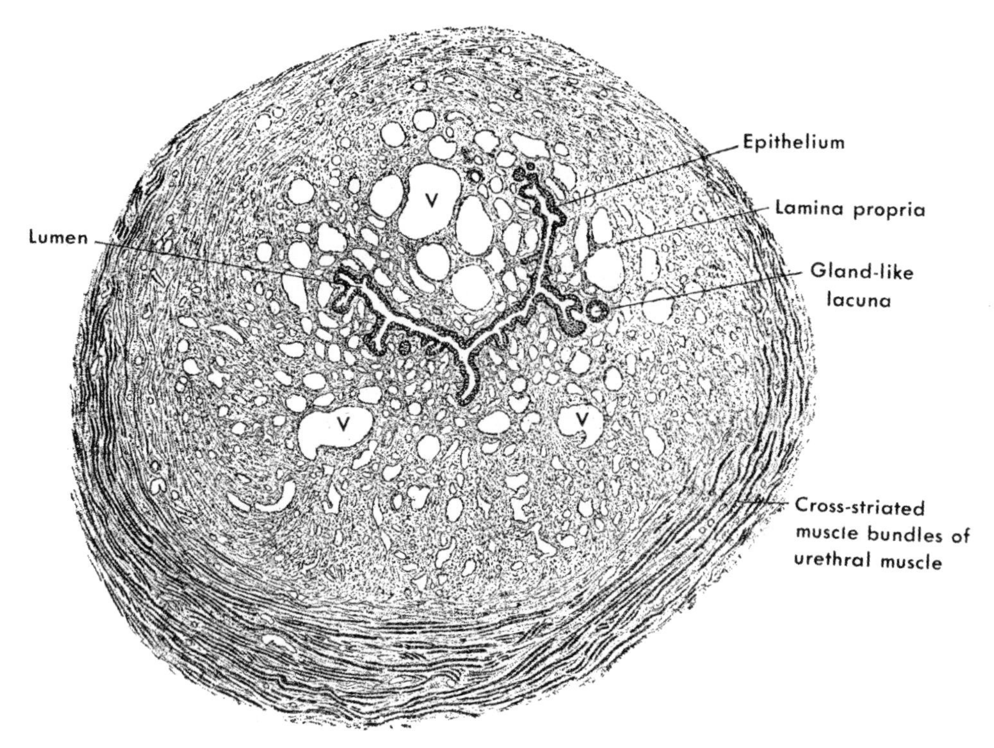

Figure 30–44. Cross section through the human female urethra, which corresponds to the proximal portion of the prostatic urethra of the male.

cells that have staining reactions for mucus. In old age, some of these recesses in the urethral mucosa may contain concretions similar to those found in the prostate.

FEMALE URETHRA

The female urethra is 25–30 mm long. Its mucosa is covered with stratified squamous epithelium and it is plicated to form longitudinal folds. There are numerous shallow invaginations of the epithelium, having walls lined, in many places, with mucous cells like those of the glands of Littré in the male urethra (Fig. 30–44). These invaginations may accumulate colloidal material in their lumen, and may even contain more solid concretions. The lamina propria is a loose connective tissue containing abundant elastic fibers. It includes a complex system of venous plexuses that give it an architecture resembling that of the corpus cavernosum of the male. The mucous membrane and its venous plexuses are surrounded by a thick mass of smooth muscle, within which inner longitudinal and outer circumferential fibers can be distinguished. Distal to the smooth muscle, there is a sphincter of striated muscle.

BIBLIOGRAPHY

GENERAL

Rouiller, C. 1969. General anatomy and physiology of the kidney. *In* C. Rouiller and A.F. Miller, eds. The Kidney, Vol. 1. New York, Academic Press.

Smith, H.W. 1969. The Kidney. New York, Oxford University Press.

RENAL CORPUSCLE

Caulfield, J.P. and M.G. Farquhar. 1974. The permeability of glomerular capillaries to graded dextrans. J. Cell. Biol. 63:883.

Courtoy, P.J., Y.S. Kanwar, R.O. Hines, and M.G. Farquhar. 1980. Fibronectin localization in the rat glomerulus. J. Cell Biol. 87:691.

Farquhar, M.G. 1975. The primary glomerular filtration barrier–basement membrane or filtration slits? Kidney Internat. 8:197.

Farquhar, M.G. 1983. The glomerular basement membrane. A selective macromolecular filter. *In* E.B. Hay, ed. Cell Biology of the Extracellular Matrix, p. 335. New York, Plenum Publishing Co.

Farquhar, M.G. and G.E. Palade. 1962. Functional evidence for the existence of a third cell type in the renal glomerulus. Phagocytosis of filtration residues by a distinctive "third" cell. J. Cell. Biol. 13:55.

Jones, D.B. 1985. Enzymatic dissection of the glomerulus. Lab. Investig. 52:453.

Latta, H.W., W.H. Johnston, and T.M. Stanley. 1975. Sialoglycoproteins and filtration barriers in the glomerular capillary wall. J. Ultrastr. Res. 51:354.

Michael, A.F., W.F. Keane, L. Rau et al. 1980. The glomerular mesangium. Kidney Internat. 17:141.

Mene, P., M.S. Simonson, and M.J. Dunn. 1989. Physiology of the mesangial cell. Physiol. Rev. 69:1347.

RENAL TUBULES

Andrews, P.M. and K.R. Porter. 1974. A scanning electron microscopic study of the nephron. Am. J. Anat. 140:81.
Bulger, R.E. 1965. The shape of rat kidney tubule cells. Am. J. Anat. 116:237.
Bulger, R.E. and B.F. Trump. 1966. The fine structure of the rat renal papillae. Am. J. Anat. 118:685.
Jones, D.B. 1985. Scanning electron microscopy of basolateral surfaces of rat renal tubules isolated by sequential digestion. Anat. Rec. 213:121.
Kriz, W. and H. Koepsell. 1974. Structural organization of the mouse kidney. Z. Anat. Entwichlungs. 144:137.
Madsen, K.R., J.W. Verlander, and C.C. Tisher. 1988. Relationship between structure and function in distal tubule and collecting duct. J. Electron. Microsc. Tech. 9:187.
Maunsbach, A.B. 1966. Observations on the segmentation of the proximal tubule of the rat kidney. J. Ultrastr. Res. 16:239.
Meyers, C.E., R.E. Bulger, C.C. Tischler, and B.F. Trump. 1966. Human renal ultrastructure IV. Collecting duct of healthy individuals. Lab. Investig. 15:1921.
Oswaldo, L. and H. Latta. 1966. The thin limb of the loop of Henle. J. Ultrastr. Res. 15:144.
Pricam, C., F. Humbert, A. Perrelet, and L. Orci. 1974. A freeze etch study of the tight junctions of the rat kidney tubules. Lab. Investig. 30:286.
Rhodin, J. 1958. Anatomy of the kidney tubules. Internat. Rev. Cytol. 7:485.
Tisher, C.C. 1976. Morphology of the ascending thick limb of Henle. Kidney Internat. 9:8.
Tisher, C.C., R.E. Bulger, and B.F. Trump. 1966. Human renal ultrastructure I. Proximal tubule of healthy individuals. Lab. Investig. 15:1357.
Tisher, C.C., R.E. Bulger, and B.F. Trump. 1968. Human renal ultrastructure III. The distal tubule in healthy individuals. Lab. Investig. 18:655.
Welling, L.W. and D.J. Welling. 1975. Surface areas of brush border and lateral cell walls in rabbit proximal nephron. Kidney Internat. 8:343.
Welling, L.W. and D.J. Welling. 1976. Shape of epithelial cells and intercellular channels in the rabbit proximal nephron. Kidney Internat. 9:385.
Welling, L.W. and D.J. Welling. 1988. Relationship between structure and function in renal proximal tubule. J. Electron Micros. Tech. 9:171.

RENAL INTERSTITIUM

Bulger, R.E. and R.B. Nagle. 1973. The ultrastructure of the interstitium of the rabbit kidney. Am. J. Anat. 136:183.
Schifferli, J., A. Grandcamp, and F. Chatelanat. 1975. Ultrastructure of the interstitial cells of the rat renal papilla. Kidney Internat. 7:336.

JUXTAGLOMERULAR APPARATUS

Barajas, L. 1970. The ultrastructure of the juxtaglomerular apparatus as disclosed by three-dimensional reconstructions from serial sections. J. Ultrastr. Res. 33:116.
Barajas, L. and E. Salido. 1986. Juxtaglomerular apparatus and the renin-angiotensin system. Lab. Investig. 54:361.
Edelman, R. and P.M. Hartroft. 1961. Localization of renin in the juxtaglomerular cells of the rabbit and dog by the fluorescent antibody technique. Circ. Res. 9:1069.
Hackenthal, E., M. Paul, D. Ganten, and R. Taugner. 1990. Morphology, physiology and molecular biology of renin secretion. Physiol. Rev. 70:1067.
Hartroft, P.M. 1963. Juxtaglomerular cells. Circ. Res. 12:525.

BLOOD VESSELS

Beeuwkes, R. 1980. The vascular organization of the kidney. Annu. Rev. Physiol. 42:531.
Bialstock, D. 1957. The extraglomerular arterial circulation of the renal tubules. Anat. Rec. 129:53.
Brenner, B.M. and R. Beeuwkes, 1978. The renal circulation. Hosp. Pract. 13(7):35.

LYMPHATICS

Albertine, K.H., and C.G. O'Morchoe. 1979. Distribution and density of canine renal cortical lymphatic system. Kidney Internat. 16:470.

HISTOPHYSIOLOGY

Brenner, B.M., J.L. Troy, and T.M. Daugharty. 1971. The dynamics of glomerular ultrafiltration in the rat. J. Clin. Investig. 29:336.
Gottschalk, C.W. 1961. Micropuncture studies of tubular function in the mammalian kidney. Physiologist 4:35.
Jamieson, R.L. and R.L. Maffly. 1976. Urine concentrating mechanism. N. Engl. J. Med. 295:1059.
Leninsky, N.G. and R.W. Berliner. 1959. The role of urea in the urine concentrating mechanism. J. Clin. Investig. 38:741.
Stephensen, J.L. 1978. Countercurrent transport in the kidney. Annu. Rev. Biophys. Bioeng. 7:315.

URINARY BLADDER

Hicks, R.M. 1965. The fine structure of the transitional epithelium of the rat ureter. J. Cell Biol. 26:25.
Hicks, R.M. 1966. The permeability of rat transitional epithelium, keratinization, and the permeability to water. J. Cell Biol. 28:21.
Hicks, R.M. and B. Ketterer. 1970. Isolation of the plasma membrane of the lumenal surface of rat bladder epithelium, and the occurrence of a hexagonal lattice of subunits both in negatively stained whole mounts and in sectional membranes. J. Cell Biol. 45:542.
Staehelin, A., F.J. Chlapowski, and M.A. Bonneville. 1972. Luminal plasma membrane of the urinary bladder. I. Three-dimensional reconstruction from freeze-etch images. J. Cell Biol. 53:73.

31

MALE REPRODUCTIVE SYSTEM

The external genitalia of the male consist of the *penis*, a copulatory organ, and two *testes* suspended in a cutaneous and fibroelastic sac, the *scrotum* (Fig. 31–1). The excurrent ducts of the testes, the *ductuli efferentes*, join the *ductus epididymidis*, a long convoluted duct coiled to form the *epididymis*, an organ on the posterior surface of the testis. From the epididymis, a long straight *ductus deferens* ascends from the scrotum and passes through the inguinal canal into the pelvis, where it is continuous with the *ejaculatory duct*, a terminal segment of the duct system that opens into the prostatic urethra. Associated with the duct system are three accessory glands, the *seminal vesicles*, the *prostate*, and the *bulbourethral glands*. Spermatozoa from the epididymis, together with the secretory products of these glands, constitute the *semen* that is discharged via the penile urethra.

The human testes are ovoid in form, 4–5 cm in length, 2.5 cm in width, and 3 cm in anteroposterior diameter. They have an average weight of 14 g. There is little correlation between body weight and testicular size in primates. The chimpanzee, which is one-quarter the weight of a gorilla, has a testis four times heavier. There are significant differences among the human races. The average weight of the testis in Scandinavian caucasians (21 g) is more than twice the weight of the testis in Chinese (8.8 g). Daily production of spermatozoa, in humans, is relatively inefficient, being about 4.2×10^6, compared to some non-human species which range 12×10^9 to 25×10^9.

The testes develop early in embryonic life beneath the peritoneum on the dorsal wall of the abdominal cavity. They later descend into the scrotum, each carrying with it an out-pocketing of the peritoneum, the *tunica vaginalis propria testis*. This becomes detached from the peritoneal cavity in the descent of the testes and forms an independent serous cavity enveloping the anterior and lateral surfaces of the testis. Its visceral layer is closely adherent to the capsule of the testis and separated by a narrow cleft from its outer or parietal layer. Where the vessels and nerves enter the testis, on its posterior surface, the visceral layer of the tunica vaginalis is continuous with its parietal layer. The closed cavity so formed is an isolated vestige of the embryonic coelom and is lined by mesothelium like that lining the peritoneal cavity. There is a thin film of fluid within this cavity. The limited amount of movement of the pressure-sensitive testis that is permitted within this cavity and within the elastic scrotum helps to prevent damage to the organ. Although descent into the scrotum places the gonads at risk of injury, this provides an environment a few degrees lower in temperature than the abdominal cavity, and this lower temperature is a necessary condition for spermatogenesis.

The testis is enclosed in a thick fibrous capsule, the *tunica albuginea*. On its posterior surface, dense connective tissue extends a short distance inward from the tunica albuginea, forming the *mediastinum testis* through which the blood vessels enter and its ductuli efferentes leave the organ. Thin fibrous partitions, called the *septula testis*, radiate from the mediastinum to the tunica albuginea, dividing the interior of the testis into about 250 pyramidal compartments, the *lobuli testis* (Fig. 31–2). Near the periphery of the testis, the lobules may intercommunicate through fenestrations in the septula, but where these converge on the mediastinum the lobules are completely separated.

Each lobule contains from one to four *seminiferous tubules*. These are 150–250 μm in diameter, 30–70 cm long, and extremely tortuous. The majority of these form highly convoluted loops, but some may branch and a few may end blindly. At the narrow apex

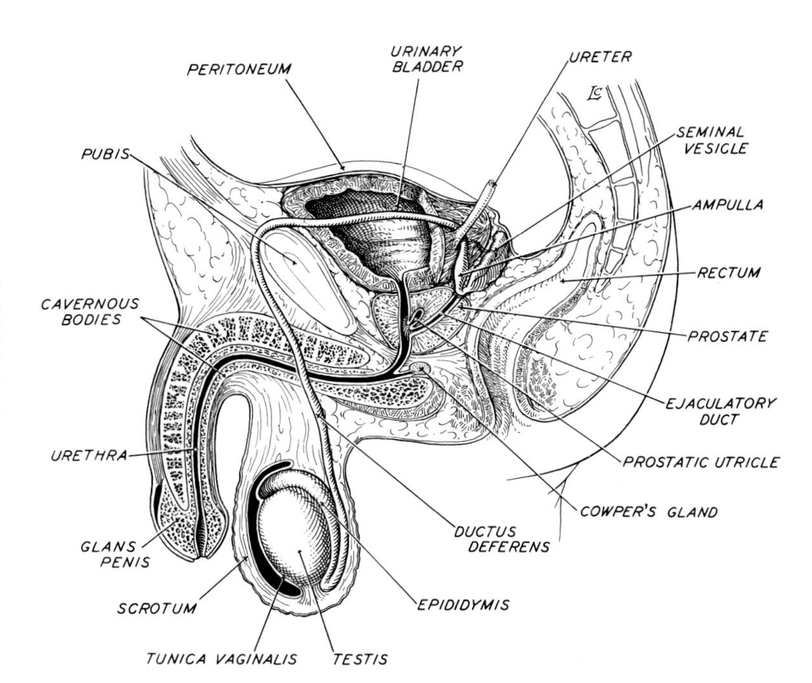

Figure 31–1. Diagram of the male reproductive system. Midline structures are shown in sagittal section; bilateral structures such as the testis, epididymis, vas deferens, and seminal vesicles are depicted intact. (After C.D. Turner.)

of each pyramidal lobule, there is an abrupt transition of its seminiferous tubules to short straight *tubuli recti* that converge on the *rete testis*, a plexus of epithelium-lined spaces in the connective tissue of the mediastinum testis. From there, a number of *ductuli efferentes* emerge from the testis conducting the spermatozoa to the *ductus epididymidis* (Fig. 31–2).

The interstices among the seminiferous tubules are occupied by a highly vascular loose connective tissue. Each seminiferous tubule is enclosed in a rich capillary network (Fig. 31–3), and the surrounding connective tissue contains perivascular mesenchymal cells, fibroblasts, and a few macrophages in a meshwork of fine reticular fibers. Within this loose stroma, there are clusters of *Leydig cells (interstitial cells)* occupying the angular interstices between the seminiferous tubules. These cells are the endocrine component of the testis, secreting the male sex hormone *testosterone*.

SEMINIFEROUS TUBULES OF THE TESTIS

BOUNDARY TISSUE

The seminiferous tubules are ensheathed in a layer of adventitial cells derived from mesenchymal cells of the interstitium. The organization of this boundary layer varies from species to species. In the laboratory rodents, it is a single layer of flat polygonal cells joined edge-to-edge to form a continuous sheet around each tubule. These cells have some of the ultrastructural features of smooth muscle cells and are contractile, but because of their atypical shape and epithelioid organization, they are called *myoid cells*. They are responsible for the rhythmic shallow contractions observed in the seminiferous tubules of these species. Bundles of actin filaments in their cytoplasm are oriented at right angles to one another, suggesting that contraction of the myoid cells results in reduction of their area and a consequent slight constriction of the tubule. No nerve endings have been found in or near this layer and their contraction is apparently generated intrinsically. The myoid cells have surface receptors for testosterone and there is recent evidence that they produce a protein that influences the synthetic activities of supporting cells within the epithelium of the seminiferous tubules. The myoid cell layer is also a significant component of the blood-testis permeability barrier which will be discussed later in the chapter.

In larger species, such as ram, boar, and bull, the seminiferous tubules are ensheathed in multiple layers of adventitial cells. The innermost cells resemble myoid cells but do not form a continuous epithelioid layer, and the outer cells appear to be fibroblasts. In monkey and man, none of the adventitial cells resemble smooth muscle and no contractility of the

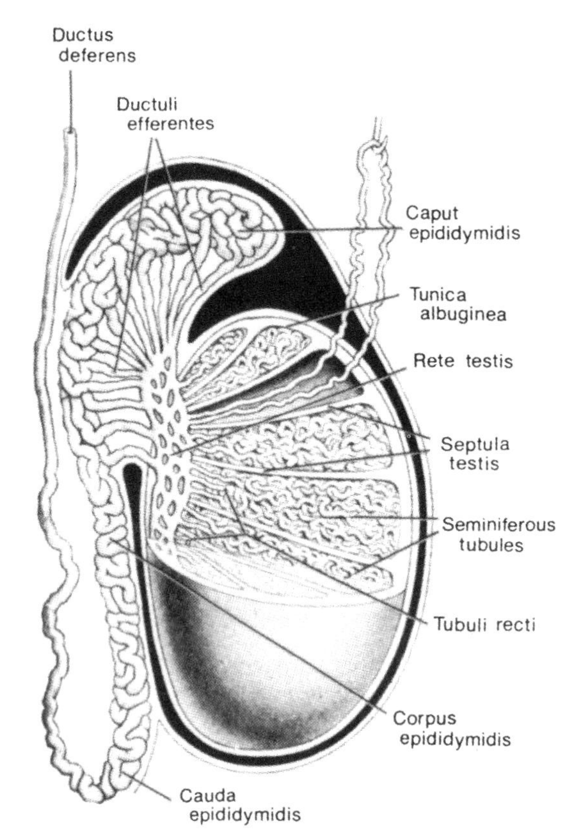

Figure 31–2. Cut-away diagram of the testis and its excurrent ducts. Septula divide the organ into a number of compartments occupied by highly convoluted seminiferous tubules. One of these has been drawn out to show that it is a long loop with both ends terminating in the rete testis. (Modified from Hamilton, W.J. 1957. Textbook of Human Anatomy. London, Macmillan & Co.)

seminiferous tubules has been observed. In human cases of infertility the boundary tissue of the seminiferous tubules is often greatly thickened.

SEMINIFEROUS EPITHELIUM

The seminiferous tubules are lined by a very complex stratified epithelium containing spermatogenic cells and supporting cells (Fig. 31–3). Supporting cells are of a single type, the *Sertoli cells*. The spermatogenic cells include several morphologically distinguishable types: *spermatogonia, primary spermatocytes, secondary spermatocytes, spermatids,* and *spermatozoa*. These are not ontogenetically distinct cell types but represent successive stages in a continuous process of germ cell differentiation (Fig. 31–4).

Sertoli Cells

The lateral boundaries of the Sertoli cells are not resolved by the light microscope and this led some early histologists to believe that they formed a syncytium. This erroneous interpretation was abandoned when the electron microscope revealed pairs of apposed membranes at the interface between adjacent Sertoli cells, as well as between them and the germ cells. They are now known to be separate cells that extend from the basal lamina to the free surface of the epithelium. They are basically columnar, but the germ cells between them occupy deep recesses of varying shape in their lateral surfaces (Fig. 31–5). Slender lateral processes of the Sertoli cells fill all of the interstices between the germ cells. The seminiferous epithelium, thus, consists of population of nonproliferating Sertoli cells and a population of germ cells that proliferate near the base and slowly move upward toward the free surface as they differentiate into spermatozoa. This dynamic relationship between the two cell populations is a unique feature of the seminiferous epithelium.

The Sertoli cells provide nutritional and mechanical support and, by their shape changes, they actively participate in the upward movement of the differentiating germ cells and in the release of spermatozoa at the free surface of the epithelium. Their nucleus is usually ellipsoidal in outline but may have one or two deep invaginations of its surface. The nucleoplasm is relatively homogeneous save for a large centrally located nucleolus flanked by two rounded masses of centromeric heterochromatin. This tripartite nucleolar apparatus is characteristic of this cell type in most mammalian species. The cytoplasm contains numerous mitochondria that have the usual internal structure and are remarkable only for their length and their tendency to be oriented parallel to the vertical axis of the cell. The Golgi complex is large but has no associated secretory vesicles or granules. Granular endoplasmic reticulum is sparse, but smooth endoplasmic reticulum is abundant, especially near the cell base. It is usually in the form of a network of tubules but may occasionally form concentric arrays of cisternae around lipid droplets. At certain stages of the spermatogenic cycle, dense aggregations of smooth endoplasmic reticulum may be found in the Sertoli cell cytoplasm adjacent to the developing acrosome of an associated spermatid. The significance of this striking

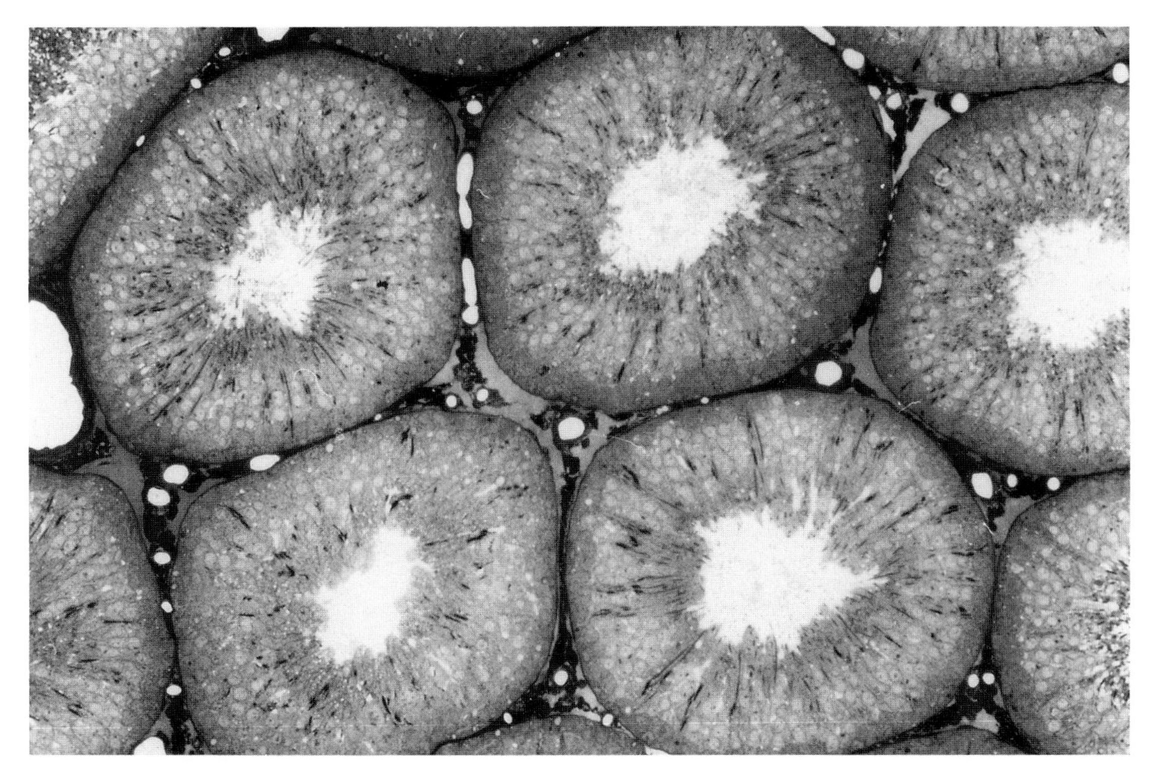

Figure 31–3. Photomicrograph of cross sections of several seminiferous tubules in a rodent testis. Between the tubules are clusters of interstitial cells of Leydig and blood vessels that have been cleared of their contents by perfusion of the fixative and, therefore, appear as round white spots.

localization is unexplained, but it suggests that the Sertoli cell contributes, in some way, to the development of this organelle of the spermatozoan.

Sertoli cells have a well-developed cytoskeleton. A meshwork of actin filaments forms a thin ectoplasmic layer immediately beneath the plasmalemma, and a similar layer of filaments also ensheaths the nucleus, excluding organelles from this region. Occasional fascicles of 10-nm intermediate filaments are oriented more-or-less parallel to the cell axis. Microtubules in similar orientation are abundant in the paranuclear and supranuclear cytoplasm at certain stages of the spermatogenic cycle. These cytoskeletal elements no doubt participate in the changes in cell shape that are involved in the movement of the germ cells toward the lumen of the tubule.

The digestive system of the cell is represented by numerous primary lysosomes, dense pleomorphic secondary lysosomes, and irregularly shaped conglomerates of lipochrome pigment. Although these organelles are conspicuous in the basal cytoplasm, the amount of accumulated lipochrome pigment is not large when one considers that these cells ingest and degrade a large volume of residual cytoplasm discarded by generation after generation of late spermatids.

An inclusion peculiar to the human Sertoli cells is the *crystalloid of Charchot-Bottcher*. These slender fusiform structures are 10–25 μm long and consist of a bundle of filaments about 15 nm in diameter that are generally parallel but converge toward the ends. Although originally described as crystals by light microscopists, their subunits appear rather poorly ordered in electron micrographs and there may be discontinuities in the subunits in their interior. Their chemical nature and significance are unknown.

Little is known about the contribution of the Sertoli cells to the nutrition and differentiation of the germ cells, but analysis of supernates of Sertoli cell enriched cultures has detected 10 or more proteins, many of which are increased by hormonal stimulation. The function of only a few of these has been identified. Some seem to be transport proteins essential for maintenance of spermatogenesis. The most thoroughly studied, to date, is *androgen-binding pro-*

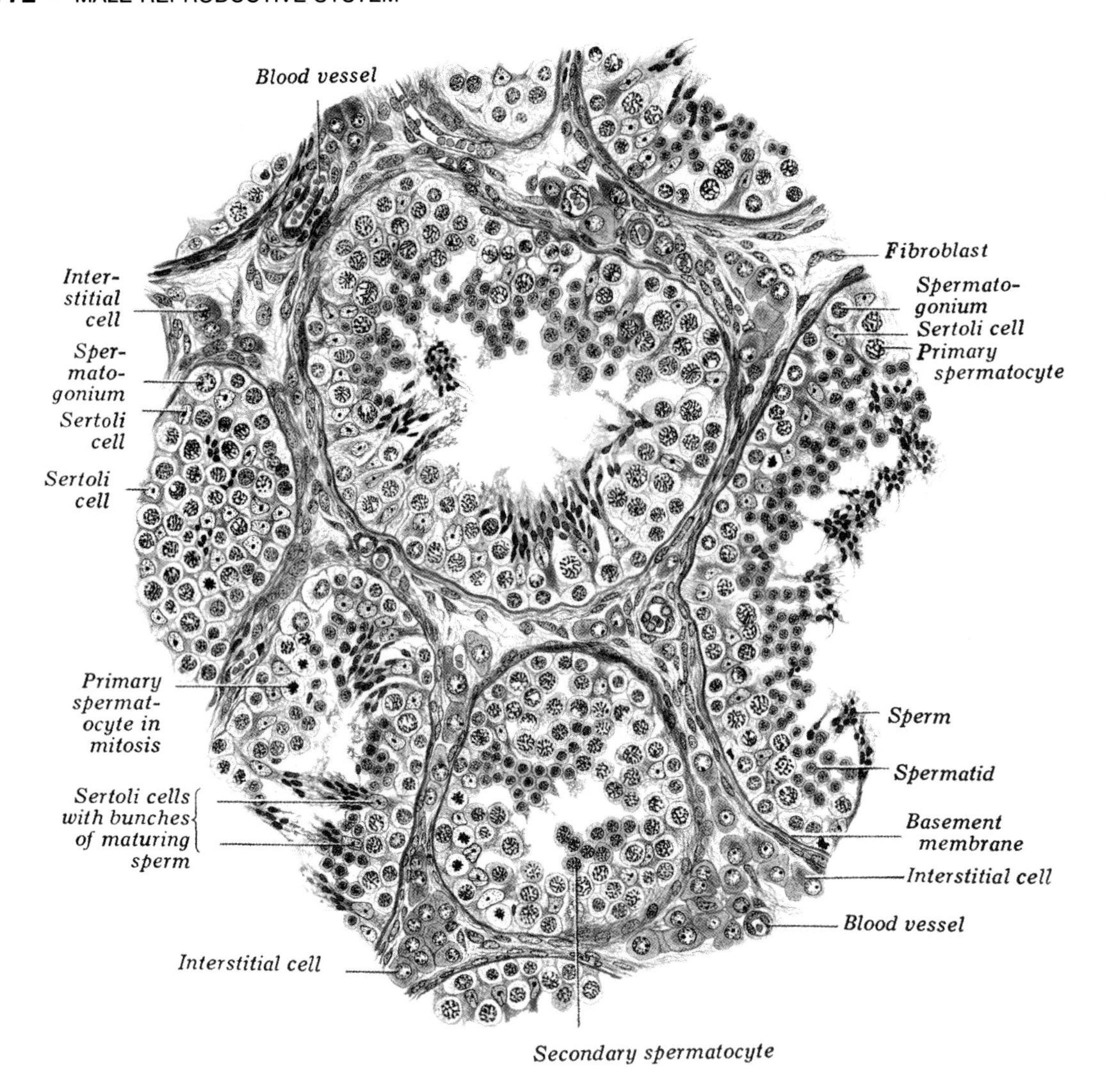

Figure 31–4. Drawing of a small area from a section of human testis showing the interstitium and various stages of spermatogenesis in the seminiferous tubules.

tein (ABP) which binds the testosterone secreted by the interstitial cells of Leydig and transports it to the lumen of the tubules and onward to the epididymis. Another is *testicular transferrin*, a protein believed to transport iron to the germ cells. A related iron-transporting protein in the blood, serum transferrin, binds to specific receptors at the base of the Sertoli cells and is taken into the cytoplasm. There, iron is transferred from serum transferrin to testicular transferrin which delivers it to the developing germ cells in the adluminal compartment of the seminiferous epithelium.

Spermatogenesis

The term *spermatogenesis* encompasses the entire sequence of proliferative events and cytological changes from the early male germ cells, *spermatogonia*, to mature *spermatozoa*. For descriptive purposes, it is customary to consider the process in three phases. In the first of these, *spermatocytogenesis, type A spermatogonia* undergo a series of divisions that expand their numbers and give rise to *type-B spermatogonia*. Division of this last generation of spermatogonia produces *primary spermatocytes*. In the second phase of spermatogenesis, *meiosis*, the spermatocytes undergo two maturation divisions that reduce the chromosome number by half and produce a cluster of *spermatids*. In the third phase, called *spermiogenesis*, the spermatids go through a remarkable sequence of cytological transformations culminating in the release of *spermatozoa* into the lumen of the seminiferous tubule.

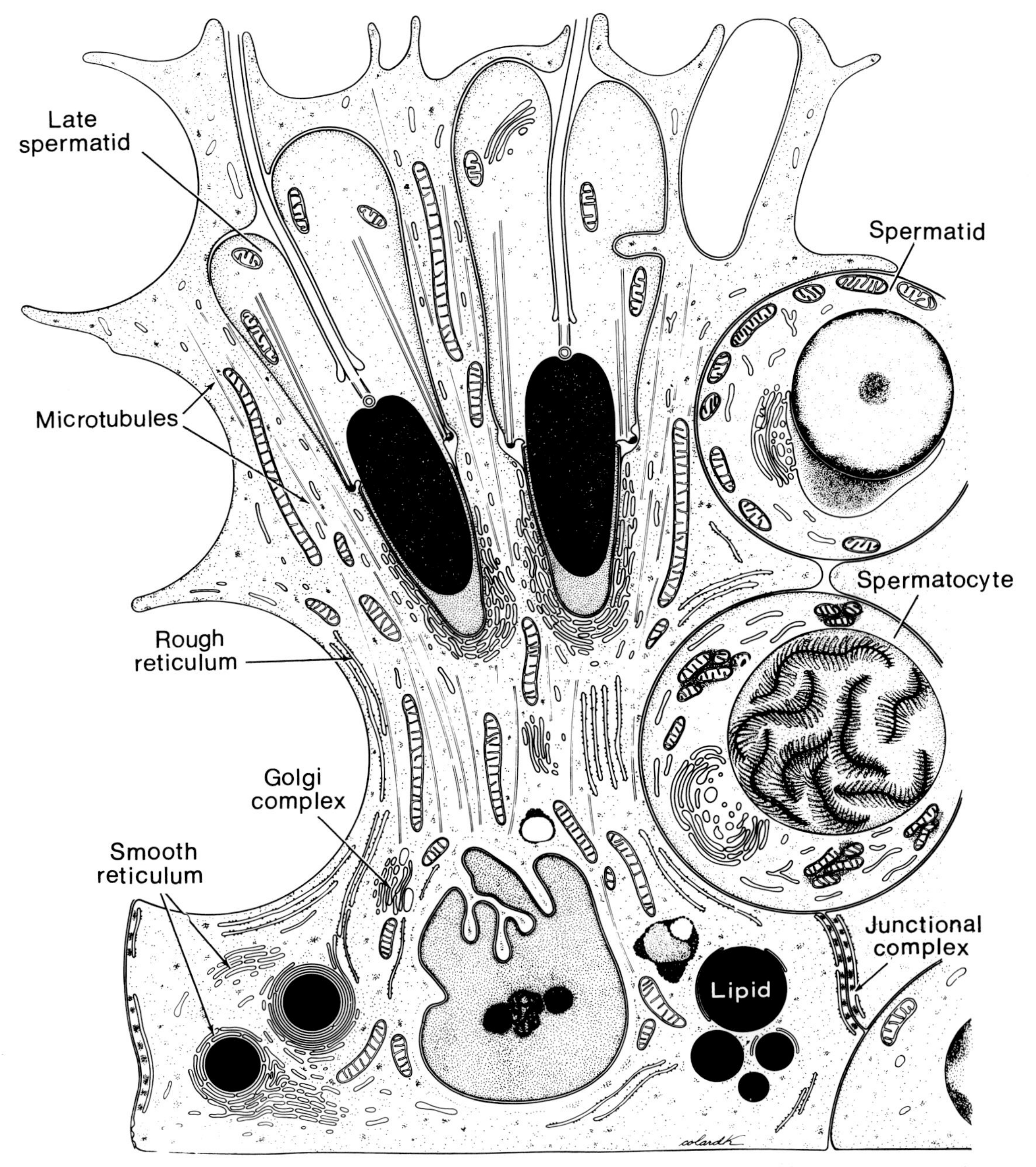

Figure 31–5. Drawing depicting the elaborate shape and ultrastructure of the Sertoli cell and its relationship to the germ cells. Spermatocytes and early spermatids occupy niches in its lateral surfaces, and late spermatids reside in deep invaginations in its apical surface. (From Fawcett, D.W. 1974. *In* Male Fertility and Sterility, R.E. Mancini, ed. Academic Press, New York.)

The type-A spermatogonia are dome-shaped cells resting on the basal lamina of the seminiferous epithelium (Fig. 31–6). They have an ovoid nucleus containing scant heterochromatin and two nucleoli that are usually located adjacent to the nuclear membrane. Type-B spermatogonia can be distinguished by their more rounded nucleus with coarser clumps of marginated heterochromatin and a single centrally placed nucleolus. The primary spermatocytes are larger round cells above the spermatogonia. Soon after they arise by division of type-B spermatogonia, they enter prophase of the first meiotic division. Several stages of meiosis are distinguishable on the basis of differences in the

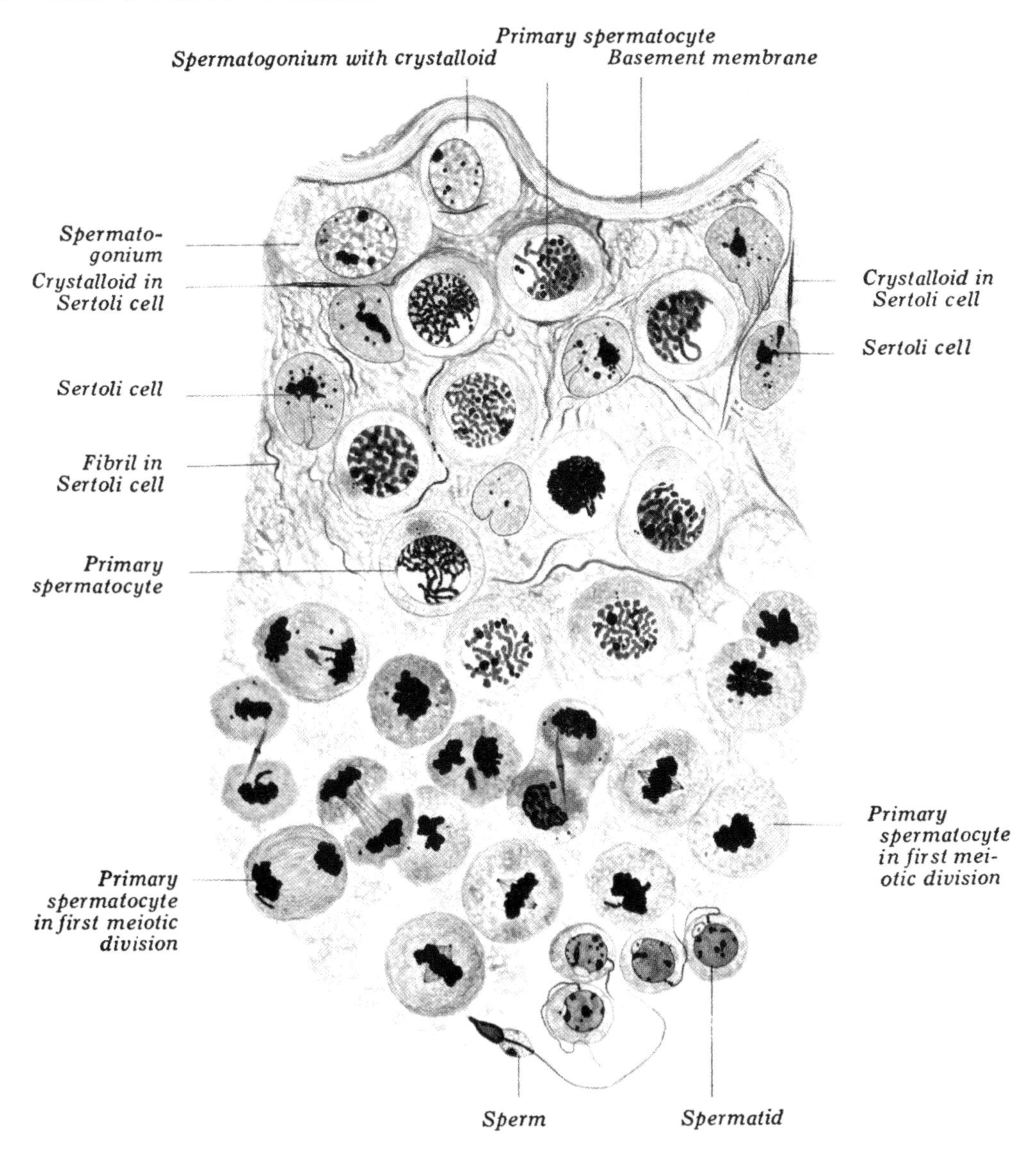

Figure 31–6. Drawing of the seminiferous epithelium of the human testis showing spermatogonia at the base of the epithelium (top) and some primary spermatocytes in an early stage of meiosis and others, near the lumen, in the metaphase and anaphase of the first meiotic division.

form and relationships of the pairs of homologous chromosomes and their degree of condensation. In the *leptotene* stage, they are long slender threads that pursue a meandering course throughout the spermatocyte nucleus and are difficult to identify in histological preparations. During the succeeding *zygotene* stage, the homologous chromosomes come together, forming the haploid number of synaptic pairs and these are easier to identify in routine preparations. In the *pachytene* stage, the pairs of chromosomes contract longitudinally, becoming thicker and more conspicuous. The two members of each synaptic pair also split longitudinally, forming tetrads consisting of four parallel chromatids. In the following *diplotene* stage of prophase, corresponding segments of the paired chromosomes are exchanged in a process unique to meiosis, called crossing-over. The parental genes are, thus, mixed and rearranged in new combinations.

Prophase of the first meiotic division is very prolonged, extending over about 22 days. Therefore, more than one generation of spermatocytes, in different stages of prophase, are seen in sections of the epithelium. At the end of prophase, the nuclear membrane disappears and the tetrads assemble on a metaphase equatorial plate. At anaphase, the members of each homologous pair of chromosomes separate and move to opposite ends of the spindle. Thus, at telophase, the number of chromosomes in each daughter cell is reduced to the haploid number 23 and they differ from both the maternal and paternal chromosomes because of the exchanges that took place in crossing-over.

The secondary spermatocytes resulting from the first meiotic division remain in interphase only very briefly and are, therefore, encountered infrequently in sections of seminiferous tubules. Prophase of the second meiotic division is brief. At metaphase, the centromeres of the chromosomes divide as in mitosis, permitting the chromatids to migrate to opposite poles at anaphase. Telophase results in two spermatids with the haploid number of chromosomes.

Meiosis also involves a mechanism that ensures about equal numbers of male and female offspring. Of the 23 pairs of chromosomes in human primary spermatocytes, 22 are *autosomes* and one pair consists of *sex chromosomes* that differ from one another in size and genetic complement. One is the female-determining X-chromosome, and the other is the male-determining Y-chromosome. Separation of the paired chromosomes at anaphase of the first meiotic division ensures that the spermatids, and the spermatozoa that develop from them, will be of two kinds, one bearing an X-chromosome and the other a Y-chromosome. Thus, in the human, male is the *heterogametic sex,* whereas the female which produces only X-bearing ova is the *homogametic sex.* Fertilization of an ovum by an X-bearing spermatozoan results in a female child (XX), whereas fertilization by a Y-bearing spermatozoan results in a male child (XY).

Research on the early phases of spermatogenesis was long focused on the events in nuclear division (*karyokinesis*) and it was assumed that cytoplasmic division (*cytokinesis*) in germ cells did not differ from that observed in somatic cells. Studies with the electron microscope have now shown that this assumption was incorrect. In all divisions of the male germ cells subsequent to the self-renewing divisions of the type-A spermatogonia, the daughter-cells remain connected by an *intercellular bridge*, where the constricting cleavage furrow encounters the bundle of spindle microtubules that extend from pole to pole at anaphase. Such bridges occur as transient structures in telophases of somatic cell mitosis. However, in the divisions of the male germ cells, communication between the daughter cells persists after disassembly of the microtubules of the spindle. Intercellular bridges are found between pairs of spermatogonia, in chains of primary and secondary spermatocytes, and connecting large groups of spermatids (Fig. 31–7, 31–8). The progeny of a conjoined pair of spermatogonia, thus, form a large group of germ cells that remain in cytoplasmic continuity throughout their differentiation. This no doubt accounts for the synchrony of development observed in the cells of any one area of the seminiferous epithelium. Individual spermatozoa are separated from the syncytium at the time of their release into the lumen of the tubule.

SPERMIOGENESIS

The term *spermiogenesis* refers to the sequence of postmeiotic changes by which spermatids are transformed into spermatozoa. The major events in this process can be followed with the light microscope, but many of the finer details that will be described below can only be seen with the electron microscope.

Spermatids are smaller than spermatocytes and are located higher in the epithelium. They are round cells, often mutually deformed to polygons by their close packing. The nuclei are devoid of coarse clumps of heterochromatin and their cytoplasm contains short mitochondria, vesicular and tubular profiles of endoplasmic reticulum, and a prominent Golgi complex. The first sign of their differentiation into spermatozoa is the appearance of small membrane-bounded *proacrosomal granules* at the trans-face of the juxtanuclear Golgi complex (Fig. 31–9A). As development progresses, these coalesce into a single large granule within a larger *acrosomal vesicle.* The limiting membrane of this vesicle becomes adherent to the nuclear envelope. The point of its initial adherence marks the future apex of the condensed sperm nucleus (Fig. 31–9B). The Golgi complex remains closely associated with the surface of the acrosomal vesicle and continues to form condensing vacuoles that fuse with it, adding to its contents. As the volume of the acrosomal vesicle increases, the area of its membrane adhering to the nuclear envelope spreads laterally from the point of initial contact and it becomes hemispherical in shape. This marks the end of the so-called *Golgi phase* of spermiogenesis.

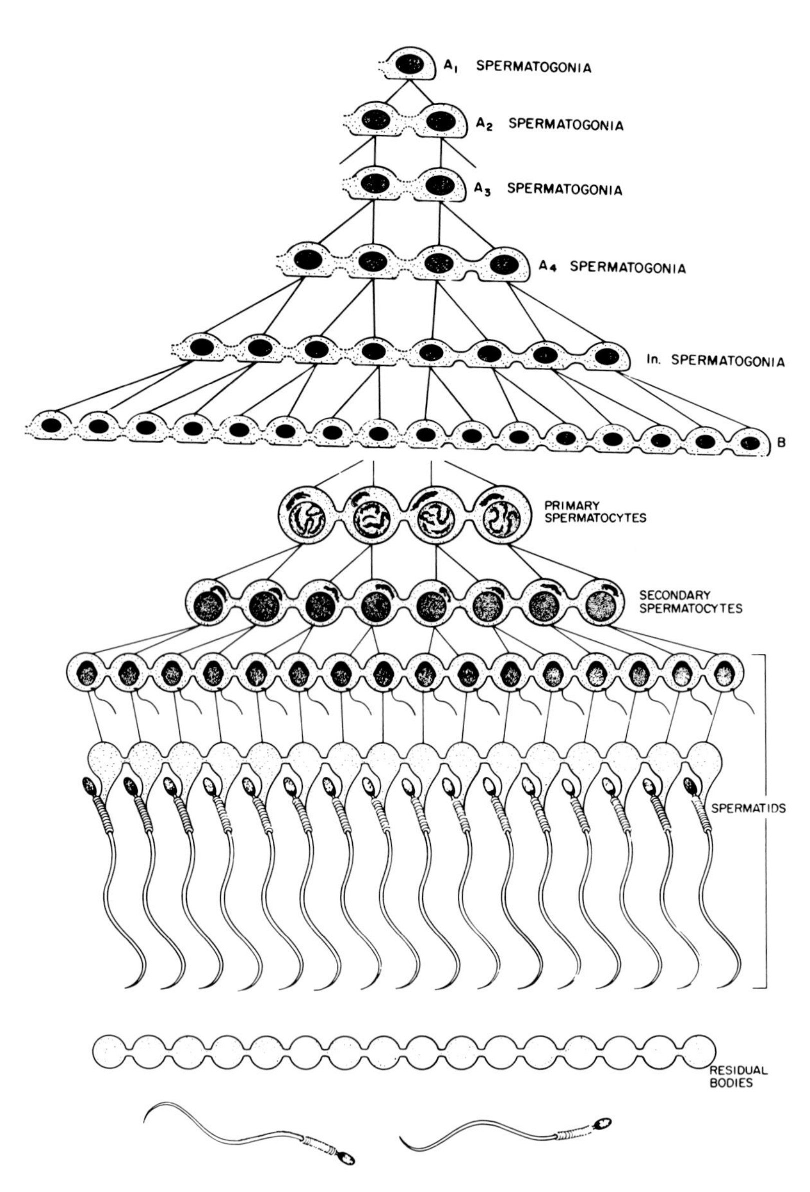

Figure 31–7. Diagram of the syncytial nature of the clones of developing male germ cells. Only the type-A spermatogonia, dividing to replace the stem cell population, complete cytoplasmic division and give rise to separate daughter cells. The daughter cells of all subsequent spermatogonial and spermatocyte divisions remain connected by intercellular bridges. Individual spermatozoa are ultimately separated from syncytial chains of residual bodies that remain connected by bridges. The number of interconnected cells in the clones is much larger than shown here.

In the ensuing *cap phase*, the dense acrosomal granule remains at the pole of the nucleus while the surrounding vesicle further expands its area of attachment to the nuclear envelope by forming a thin fold that extends laterally and posteriorly until it covers the whole anterior hemisphere of the nucleus (Fig. 31–9C).

In the *acrosome phase* that follows, the greater part of the substance of the acrosomal granule becomes redistributed throughout the interior of the cap formed by the acrosomal vesicle. With these changes, the formation of the *acrosome* or *acrosomal cap* is completed. In the human, the acrosomal cap is only slightly thicker at its pole than elsewhere, but in the guinea pig and several rodents that form an unusually large acrosomal granule, the acrosome extends 3 μm or more beyond the pole of the nucleus. Late in development, it takes on a shape typical of that species.

Concurrent with the later stages of acrosome formation, there is a condensation of the nucleoplasm beginning with the appearance of thin filaments that then shorten and thicken to form coarse granules of chromatin. These increase in size and ultimately coalesce, transforming the chromatin to a dense homogeneous state devoid of resolvable substructure (Fig. 31–10). The considerable decrease in volume of the nucleus, due to condensation of the chromatin, is accompanied by a change in its shape to a form characteristic of the

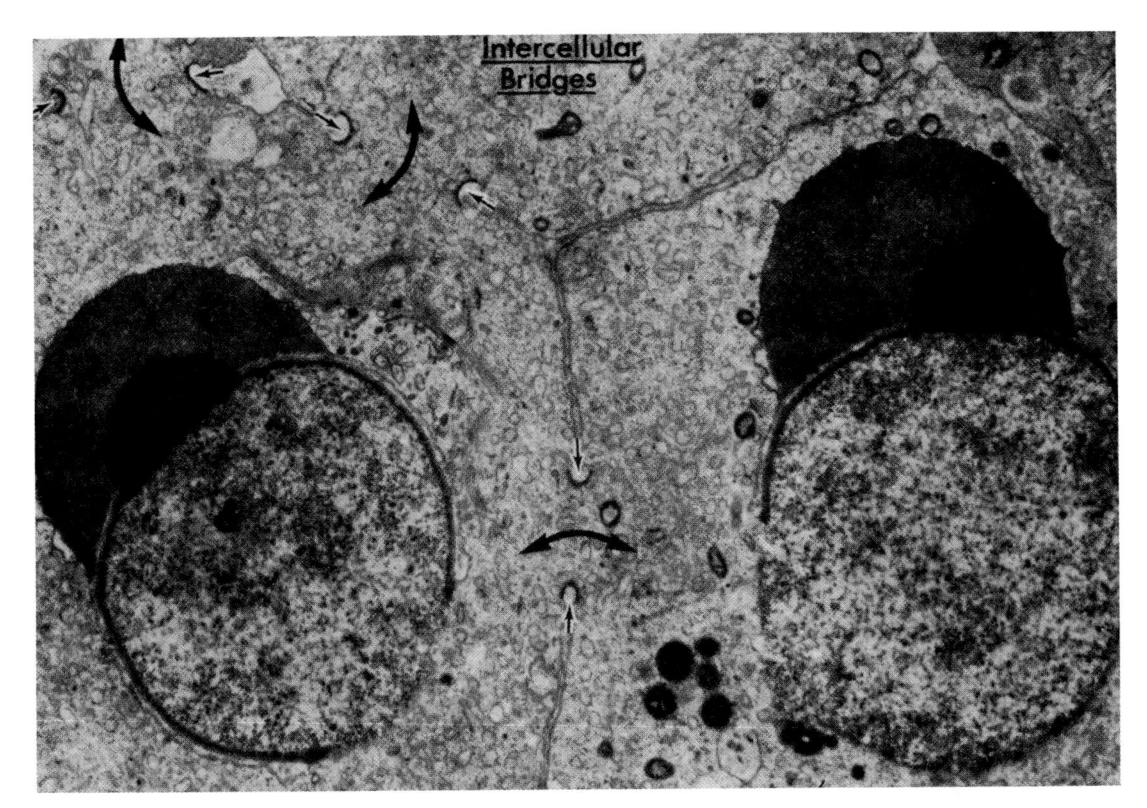

Figure 31–8. Electron micrograph of two guinea pig spermatids showing the intercellular bridges by which they are connected to one another and to neighboring spermatids of the same clone. The large arrows passing through the bridges indicate the sites of cytoplasmic continuity between cells. Small arrows point to a local thickening of the cell membrane encircling the bridges.

species. In the guinea pig, it becomes discoid; in the rat, scimitar-shaped; and in the human, pyriform.

While the acrosome is forming at the anterior pole of the nucleus, the centrioles move to the cell surface at the posterior pole of the spermatid. There, one of the centrioles becomes oriented perpendicular to the cell membrane and the triplet microtubules in its wall serve as templates for assembly of doublet microtubules, initiating the formation of the *axoneme* of the sperm flagellum (Fig. 31–11). The lengthening flagellum grows out into the space between the spermatid and its supporting Sertoli cell. At about the time that nuclear condensation begins, the pair of centrioles moves inward to the posterior pole of the nucleus. In doing so, the initial portion of the flagellum and its enveloping membrane are drawn into a deep tubular recess in the cell surface (Fig. 31–12, 3–13).

In the spermatid cytoplasm, microtubules increase in number and become associated in a roughly cylindrical array forming the *manchette*, which extends caudally from a circumferential specialization of the nuclear envelope at the posterior margin of the acrosomal cap (Fig. 31–13B, C). With the formation of the manchette, there is a marked elongation of the spermatid, with the bulk of the cytoplasm moving behind the posterior pole of the nucleus where it surrounds the proximal portion of the flagellum. As a consequence of this shift, the membrane at the anterior end of the cell becomes closely applied to the outer membrane of the acrosome with no intervening cytoplasm (Fig. 31–13 C, D).

Until this stage of spermatid differentiation, the tail of the future spermatozoon is represented only by the axoneme enclosed in a flagellar membrane. Where the flagellar membrane is continuous with the membrane of the cell body, dense material adhering to its cytoplasmic face condenses to form a ring that is the precursor of the *annulus* that will later be situated at the junction of the midpiece and principal piece of the sperm tail. The annulus and its adherent membrane then move caudad along the axoneme obliterating the tubular invagination of the cell surface

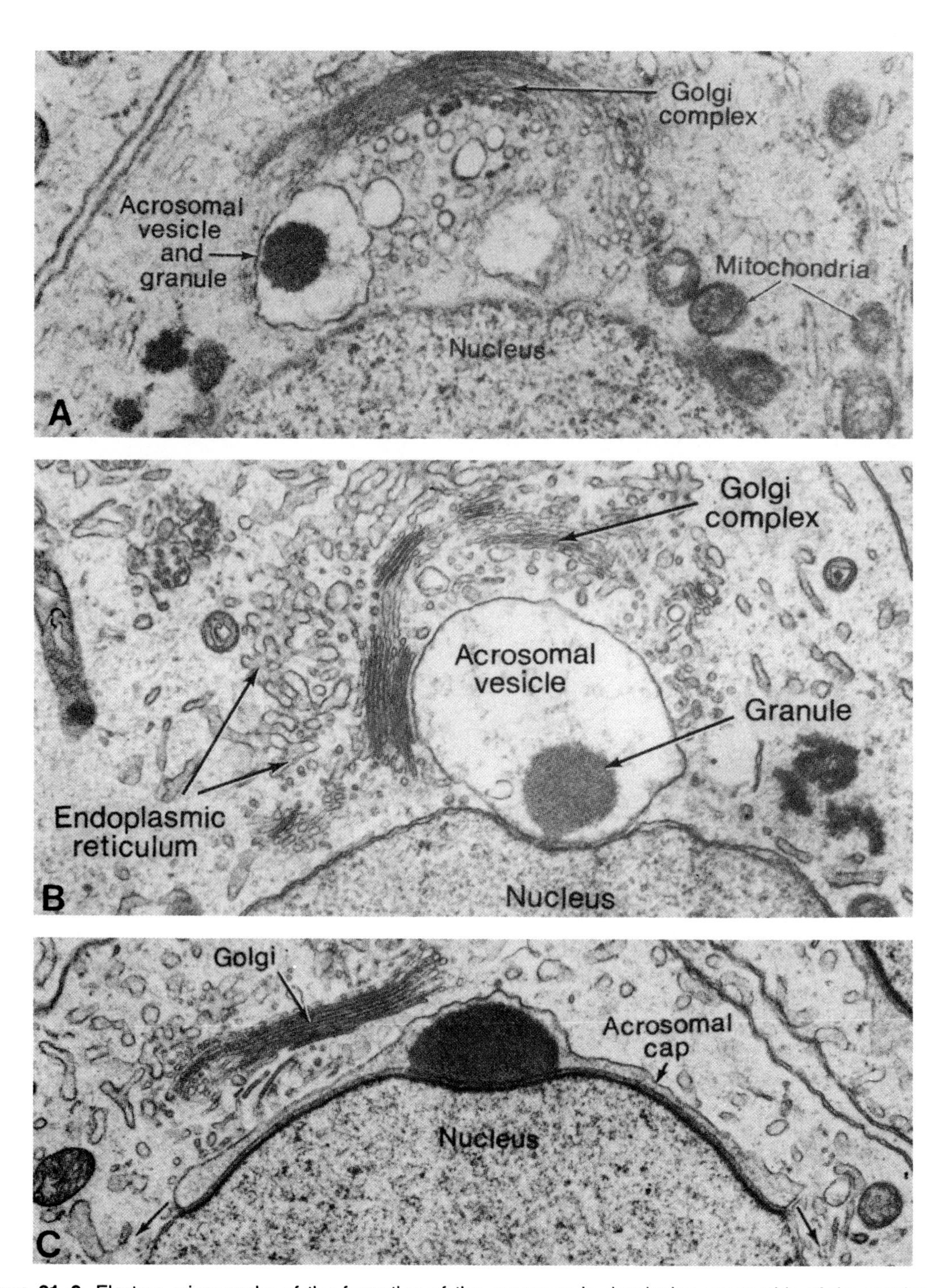

Figure 31–9. Electron micrographs of the formation of the acrosome in developing spermatids of the monkey. (A) Appearance of a proacrosomal granule in an acrosomal vesicle associated with the Golgi complex. (B) Enlargement of the acrosomal vesicle and its adherence to the pole of the nucleus. (C) Spreading of the acrosomal vesicle over the anterior hemisphere of the nucleus to form an acrosomal cap. The substance of the granule subsequently spreads laterally to occupy the entire interior of the acrosomal cap. (Micrographs courtesy of M. Dym.)

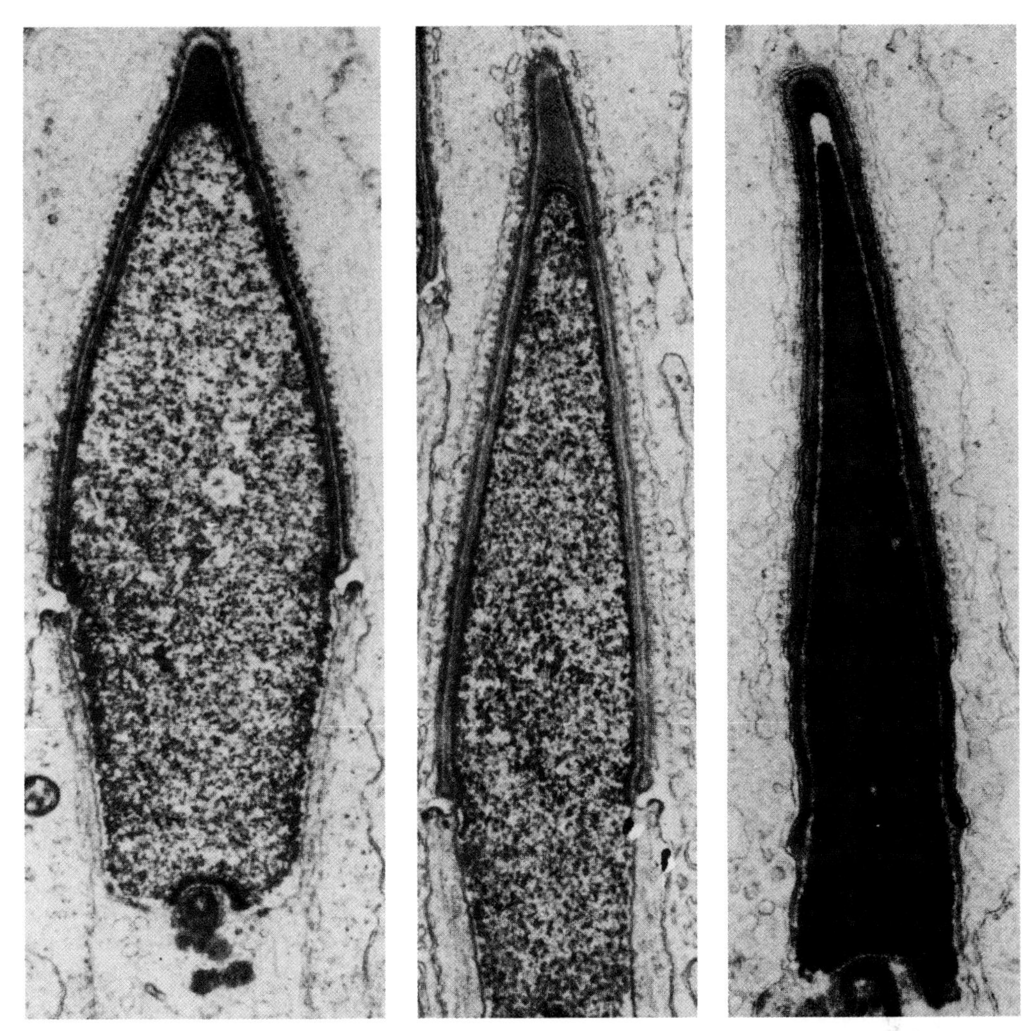

Figure 31–10. Micrographs showing the completed acrosome, the successive stages in condensation of the chromatin, and the accompanying change in shape of the nucleus to that of the mature spermatozoon. (Micrographs courtesy of M. Dym.)

and exposing the first few microns of the axoneme to the cytoplasm. Concurrently, the microtubules of the manchette disperse and mitochondria gather around the initial segment of the axoneme, where they become arranged end-to-end in a tight helix, forming the *mitochondrial sheath* of the sperm middle-piece.

While these events are in progress, nine longitudinal *dense fibers* form immediately outside of the nine doublets of the axoneme. These are continuous at their proximal end with nine cross-striated columns of the *connecting piece* that surrounds the centrioles and attaches to the rim of a shallow depression in the posterior surface of the condensed nucleus. The outer dense fibers course parallel to the doublets of the axoneme from the connecting piece to the caudal end of the principal piece of the future spermatozoon. After formation of the dense fibers, a succession of circumferentially oriented *ribs* form around that portion that is distal to the annulus. At their ends, these semicircular ribs are joined to two longitudinal dense columns that run along the dorsal and ventral aspects of the tail. Together, the ribs and the longitudinal columns make up the *fibrous sheath* of the principal piece of the sperm tail.

SPERMIATION

Spermiation is the term referring to the release of the spermatozoa from the seminifer-

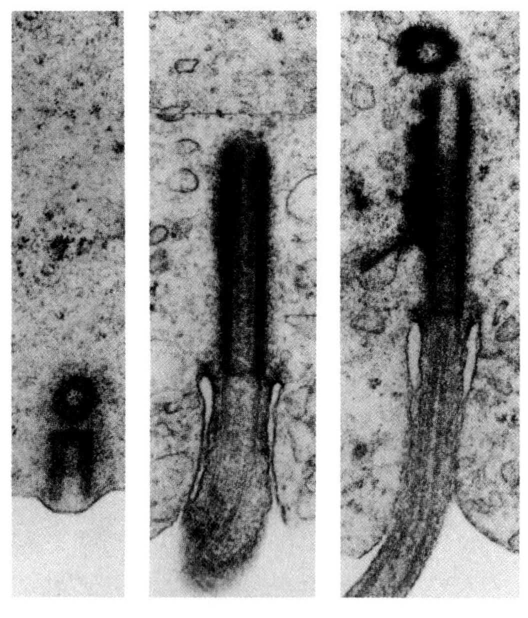

Figure 31–11. Early events in the formation of the flagellum. Polymerization of microtubule protein on the template provided by the distal centriole results in formation of a flagellum with the typical 9+2 axoneme. The axoneme elongates by accretion of molecules to the tips of its microtubules.

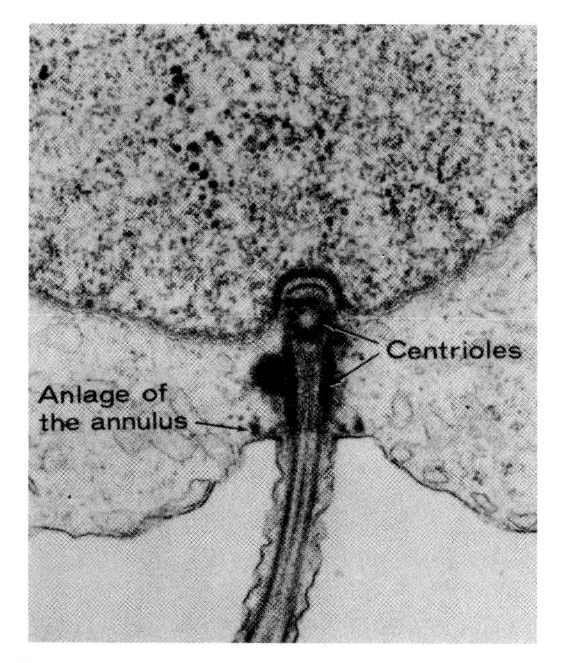

Figure 31–12. The centrioles and base of the flagellum move deeper into the cytoplasm, and the proximal centriole occupies a shallow groove, the implantation fossa, in the posterior pole of the spermatid nucleus. The anlage of the future annulus then appears as a ring-like density adjacent to the membrane at its site of reflection onto the flagellum.

ous epithelium. As the spermatids differentiate, they are slowly moved toward the surface of the epithelium by the proliferation of succeeding generations of germ cells behind them. In their final stages of development, their tails project into the lumen. The acrosome-capped nucleus and a retort-shaped appendage of excess cytoplasm occupy conforming recesses in the apical surface of Sertoli cells (Fig. 31–14). During release of a spermatozoon, the head appears to be actively extruded by the Sertoli cell, and the flask-shaped appendage of excess cytoplasm is pinched off, freeing the spermatozoon and leaving behind an anucleate mass of spermatid cytoplasm, called a *residual body* that is still enveloped by the Sertoli cell. The residual bodies contain lipid droplets and leftover organelles not used in the formation of the spermatozoon. Because the cell bodies in each group of spermatids were connected by intercellular bridges, so too are the residual bodies. However, soon after spermiation, the bridges are severed and the individual residual bodies are phagocytosed by the Sertoli cells and digested by their lysosomal hydrolases.

SPERMATOZOON

Head

The mature spermatozoon has a *head* consisting of the condensed nucleus, that contains all the genetic traits that a father can transmit to his offspring, and a *tail* that provides the motility necessary to transport the sperm to the site of fertilization and to assure that it is appropriately oriented to penetrate the coatings of the ovum (Figs. 31–15, 31–16). The size and shape of the sperm head vary greatly in different mammalian species. In the human it is ovoid in frontal view, and pyriform when seen from the side, being thicker near the base and tapering toward the tip. It is 4–5 μm in length and 2.5–3.5 μm in width. The nucleus forms the greater part of the head. It is covered on its anterior two-thirds by the *acrosome*—a membrane-limited cap-like organelle containing enzymes that digest a path through the zona pellucida of the ovum during sperm penetration. Enzymes that have been identified in the acrosome include hyaluronidase, neuraminidase, aryl sulfatase, and a protease called *acrosin* that is closely related to trypsin.

The acrosome is interposed between the plasma membrane and the condensed nu-

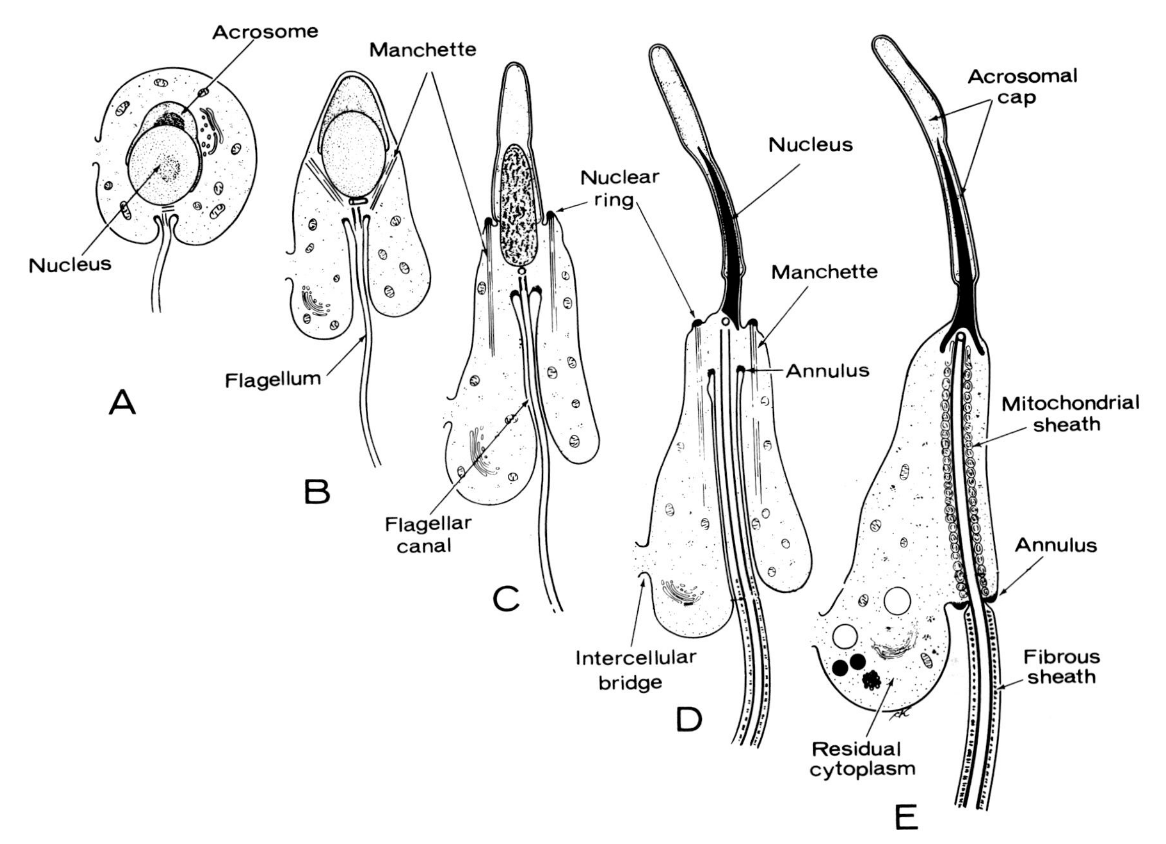

Figure 31–13. Diagram of successive stages in guinea pig spermatid differentiation. The principal morpohogenetic events include nuclear condensation; appearance of the manchette; elongation of the cell; appearance of the fibrous sheath; caudal migration of the annulus; and formation of the mitochondrial sheath. (From Fawcett, D.W., W.A. Anderson, and D.M. Phillips. 1971. Develop. Biol. 26:220.)

cleus, with its inner membrane adherent to the nuclear envelope. In the human spermatozoon, the acrosome does not extend much beyond the leading edge of the nucleus, but in some other mammals, an *apical segment* of the acrosome projects for some distance beyond the nucleus (Figs. 31–17 and 31–18). The portion of the acrosome covering the tapering anterior portion of the condensed nucleus is called its *principal segment*. Behind this is an *equatorial segment* where the thickness of the cap abruptly diminishes and its content appears slightly more condensed. Proximity to an ovum induces an *acrosome reaction* during which the outer acrosomal membrane fuses at multiple sites with the overlying plasma membrane, creating openings through which the enzyme-rich contents of the acrosome escape. This is a process comparable to exocytosis of the secretory product of a glandular cell. Release of these enzymes enables the spermatozoon to penetrate the zona pellucida of the ovum. The equatorial segment of the acrosome remains intact and its function in fertilization is unclear.

The sperm nucleus, in most species, is of the same electron density throughout. The human spermatozoon is atypical in that the degree of chromatin condensation is variable. The nucleus of some sperm is uniformly dense, whereas in others, the chromatin appears as a conglomerate of coarse granular subunits, and, not uncommonly, there are one or two irregularly shaped clear areas of varying size. Although these spaces are not membrane-bounded, they have traditionally been called *nuclear vacuoles*. They are rarely found in species other than man and are apparently randomly occurring defects in the process of chromatin condensation during spermatogenesis. There is no evidence that they impair fertilizing capacity. Despite the absence of resolvable order in the fine structure of the nucleus, there are indications that the chromosomes retain their identity and have a consistent arrangement within the condensed

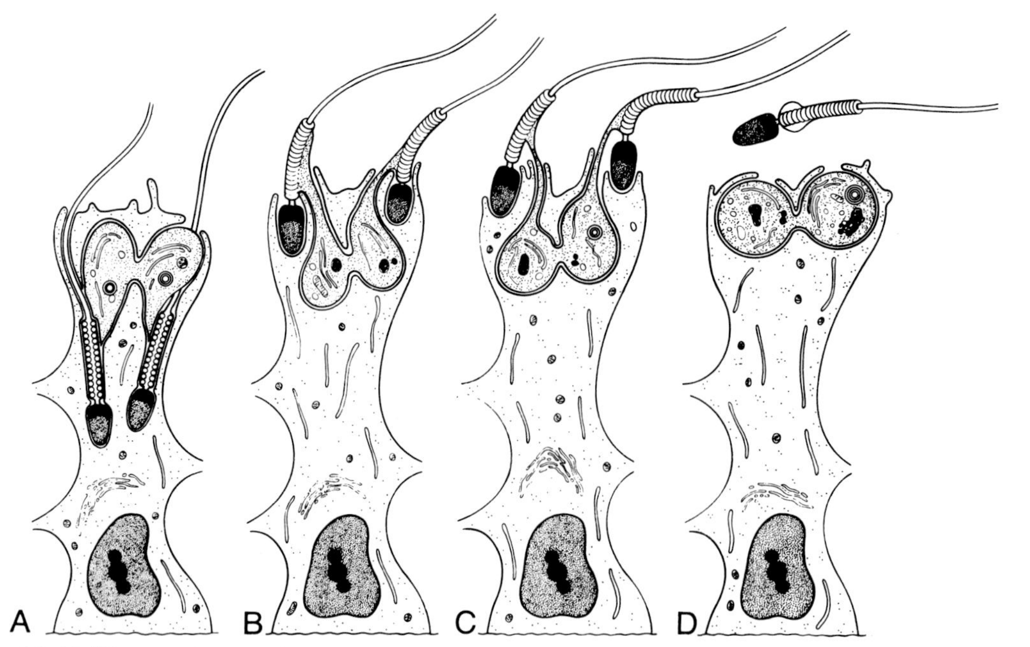

Figure 31–14. Diagram of successive stages in release of spermatozoa from the epithelium. Axial components of the sperm are gradually extruded by the Sertoli cell while the syncytial chain of spermatid cell bodies is retained in the epithelium. The attenuated stalk connecting the sperm to the residual cytoplasm finally gives way, freeing the spermatozoon. (From Fawcett, D.W. 1973. *In* S.J. Segal et al. eds. The Regulation of Mammalian Reproduction. Springfield, IL, Charles C Thomas.)

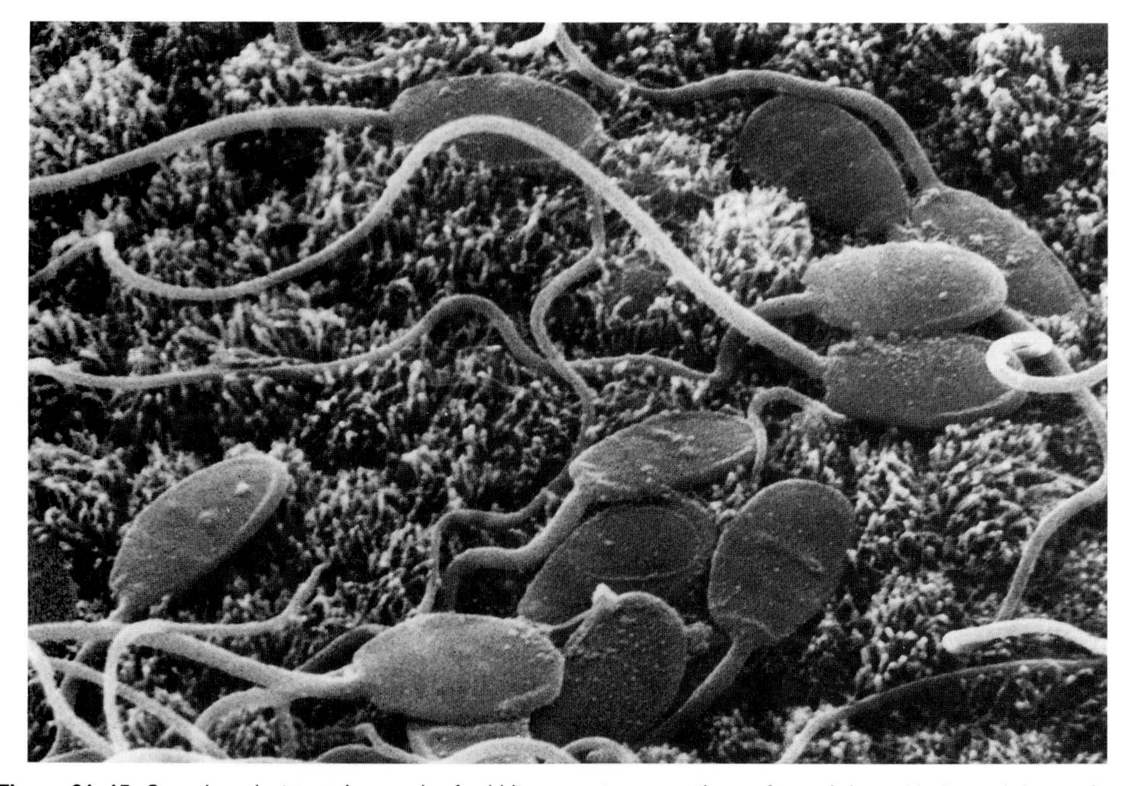

Figure 31–15. Scanning electron micrograph of rabbit spermatozoa on the surface of the epithelium of the vagina. (Micrograph courtesy of D. Phillips.)

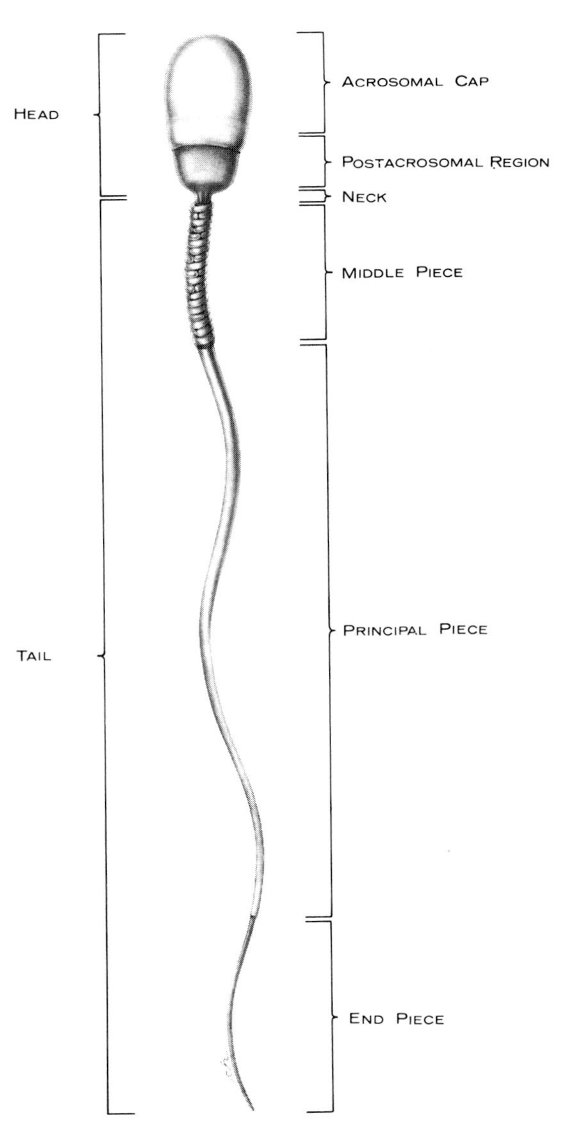

Figure 31–16. Drawing of a mammalian sperm, defining the terms used in describing its various regions.

nucleus. The human Y-chromosome can be stained selectively with quinacrine mustards. When this method is applied to intact human spermatozoa, a fluorescent yellow spot is located in approximately the same position in all of the male determining spermatozoa.

Posterior to the acrosome, a thin dense layer with a distinctive fine structure is interposed between the plasma membrane and the nucleus. This is called the *postacrosomal dense lamina* (Fig. 31–19). Although its chemical nature is not known, it may have functional significance because it is in this region that the sperm head first fuses with the oolemma during fertilization. At the posterior margin of this layer, the nucleus is encircled by the *posterior ring*, a circumferential line of fusion of the plasmalemma with the underlying nuclear envelope. Behind this ring, the cell membrane and nuclear envelope are no longer adherent to the condensed chromatin and they may form a fold or small scroll of membrane extending back into the neck region of the spermatozoon. Pores are absent from that portion of the nuclear envelope that is adherent to the condensed chromatin, but they are abundant in this fold or scroll of redundant nuclear envelope caudal to the posterior ring.

Connecting Piece

Four regions of the sperm tail are recognizable by the nature of the structures that ensheath their axoneme. From its base to its tip, these are the *connecting piece, middle-piece, principal piece*, and *end-piece*. The connecting piece consists of a basal plate, or capitulum, that

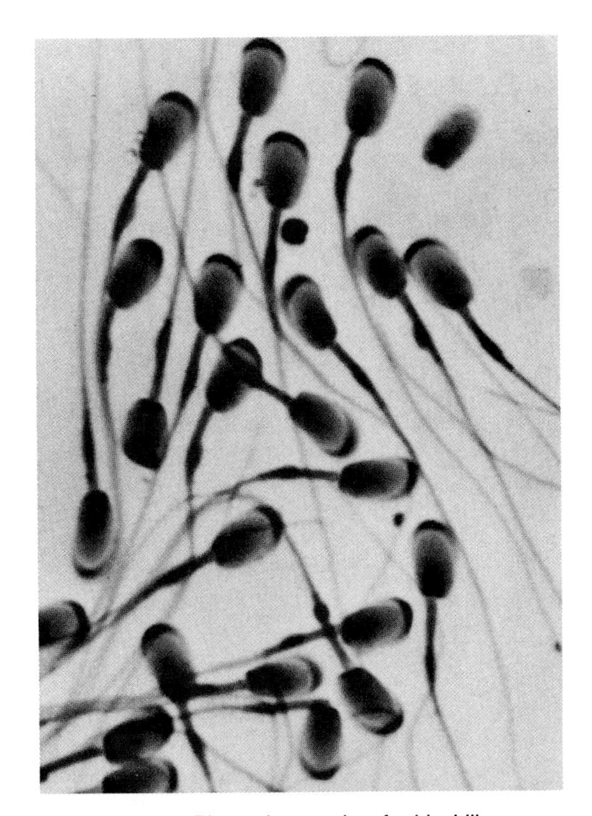

Figure 31–17. Photomicrograph of chinchilla sperm, stained by the Feulgen reaction and counterstained with Light Green. The crescentic apical segment of the acrosome can be seen at the leading edge of the sperm head.

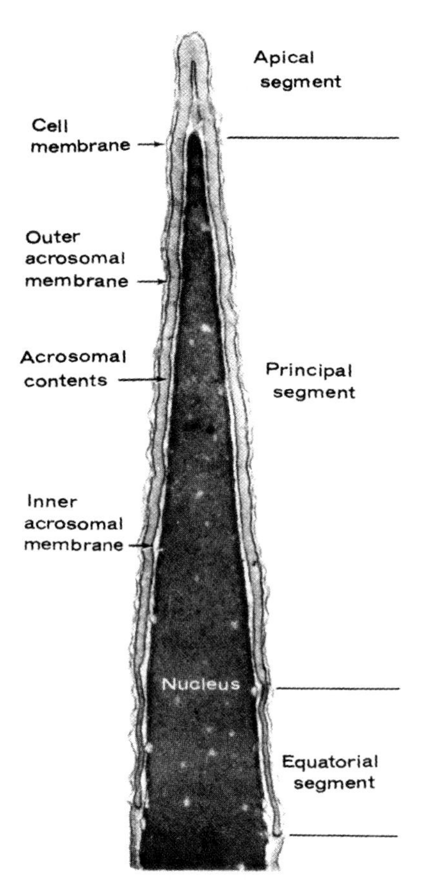

Figure 31–18. Electron micrograph of a monkey sperm head, illustrating the relationship of the acrosomal cap to the condensed nucleus, and its apical, principal, and equatorial segments.

conforms to the implantation fossa in the posterior surface of the nucleus, and nine columns that extend caudad from it for a distance of 1–5 μm (Fig. 31–20B). The columns of the connecting piece are cross-banded and are continuous at their caudal end with the nine outer dense fibers that run parallel to the nine doublets of the axoneme for the greater part of the length of the tail. A transversely oriented *proximal centriole* is found within the connecting piece just distal to the basal plate and often partially embedded within it. A *distal centriole,* oriented in the axis of the flagellum, is usually absent in the mature spermatozoon, but remanents of it may be found adhering to the inner surface of one or two of the columns. A small bulbous mass of residual cytoplasm, called the *cytoplasmic droplet,* is commonly found at the neck of the human spermatozoon, but in other mammalian species, this is either absent or is located farther caudad.

Middle-Piece

The middle piece of the spermatozoon is the segment of the tail surrounded by circumferentially oriented mitochondria (Fig. 31–19). Its organization is similar in all mammalian species, but the length of the mitochondrial helix ranges from about 15 gyres, in man, to over 200 in some rodents. In the human, the midpiece is 5–7 μm in length and 1–1.5 μm in diameter. Immediately caudal to the last gyre of the mitochondrial sheath is the *annulus,* a thick ring of dense material to which the flagellar membrane is firmly attached (Fig. 31–21). The adherence of the membrane to the annulus is assumed to prevent caudal displacement of the mitochondria during tail movements.

Running through the core of the middle-piece is the *axoneme,* consisting of two central microtubules surrounded by nine doublet microtubules, in the same arrangement previously described for cilia (Chapter 2). The axoneme runs through the entire length of the sperm tail from the connecting piece to its tip. In the midpiece, nine *outer dense fibers* are evenly spaced around the axoneme in register with its nine doublets. In cross section, the dense fibers are narrower near the corresponding doublet and thicker toward their outer surface, so that in cross sections they resemble the petals radiating from the carpel of a flower (Fig. 31–22). The thickness of the dense fibers is greatest in the middle-piece and gradually diminishes along their length to their termination at the caudal end of the principal piece. The mitochondrial sheath of the middle-piece provides the energy for motility of the axoneme. The dense fibers are believed to be merely resilient supporting elements. Two of these fibers terminate at the annulus, but the others continue into the principal piece.

Principal Piece

The principal piece is about 45 μm in length and 0.5 μm in diameter, gradually tapering toward the end-piece. In this segment, the axoneme and outer fibers are enclosed in the *fibrous sheath* made up of dorsal and ventral longitudinal columns connected by numerous regularly spaced ribs. In cross section, the tapering inner edges of the dorsal and ventral columns project into the spaces occupied by dense fibers 3 and 8 in the midpiece, and they attach to doublets 3 and 8 of the axoneme.

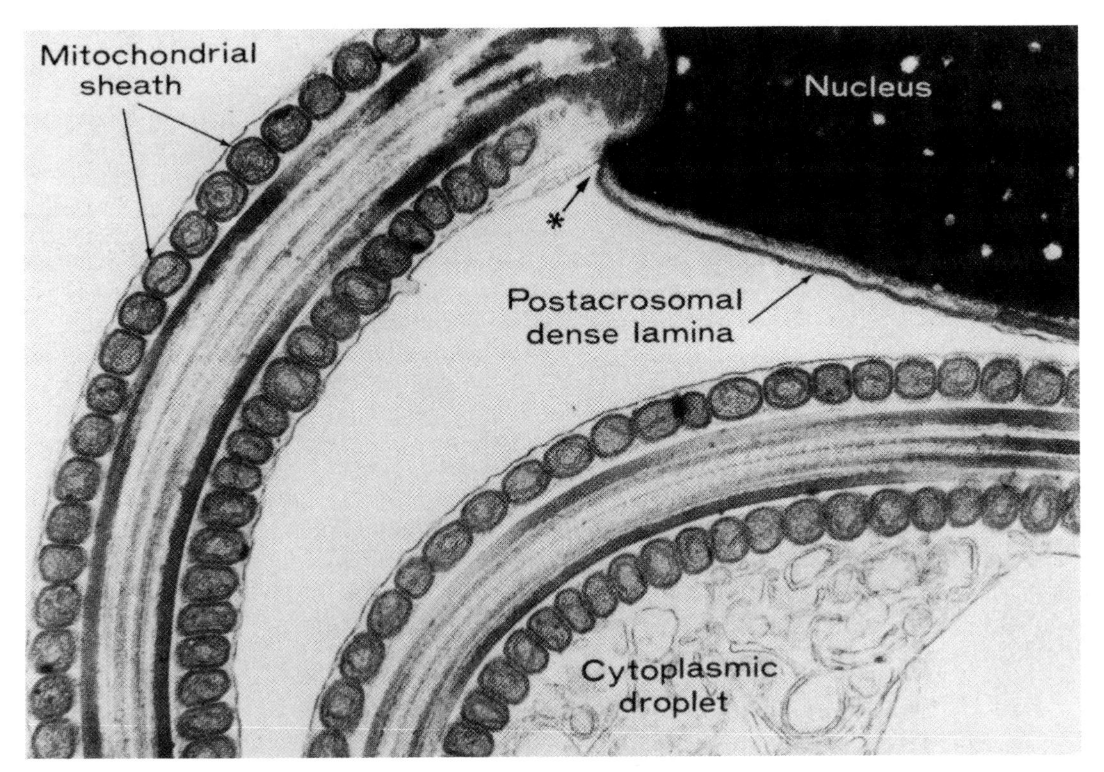

Figure 31–19. Electron micrograph of portions of two rodent spermatozoa. A dense layer beneath the plasma membrane is visible behind the acrosome of the upper spermatozoon. This is called the *postacrosomal dense lamina*. It may be important for fertilization because it is this region of the sperm head that first fuses with the egg membrane. The asterisk points to the *posterior ring*, a circumferential line of fusion of the plasmalemma with the outer and inner membranes of the nuclear envelope. (Micrograph by D. Phillips, from Fawcett, D.W. 1970. Biol. Reprod. 2 (Suppl. 2):90.)

Thus, a plane through the dorsal and ventral columns of the fibrous sheath would pass through the central pair of microtubules and divide the flagellum asymmetrically into a minor compartment, containing three outer dense fibers (numbers 2, 1 and 9) and a major compartment containing four outer dense fibers (numbers 4, 5, 6, and 7) (Fig. 31–23). This asymmetry in the distribution of the axonemal doublets and outer fibers is reflected in the bending movements of the proximal part of the tail, in which the "power stroke" is toward the side having the larger number of doublets and dense fibers. The exact mechanism of tail movements has yet to be worked out in detail, but it is thought that the axoneme generates propagated waves of bending by a sliding mechanism depending on the dynein arms that project from the subunit-A of each doublet microtubule toward subunit-B of the next doublet. (See Cilia, Chapter 2.)

End-Piece

The distal end of the principal piece is marked by the abrupt termination of the fibrous sheath. The portion of the tail beyond this point is the *end-piece*. It is from 5 to 7 μm long and consists of the axoneme covered only by the flagellar membrane (Fig. 31–22 G, H). It, therefore, resembles a cilium. There is some interspecific variation in the way the axoneme ends. In some species, the doublet microtubules terminate at different levels in the tapering tip of the flagellum, but in primates, the 9 doublets dissociate into 18 single microtubules in addition to the central pair. Thus, cross sections of the terminal ½ μm of the tail may contain sections of 20 microtubules.

THE CYCLE OF THE SEMINIFEROUS EPITHELIUM

Spermatogenesis has been most thoroughly studied in the common laboratory rodents, where it displays a degree of order that facilitates analysis of the process. The several stages of germ cell development are found at different levels in the germinal epithelium. The stem cells and early stages of their differentia-

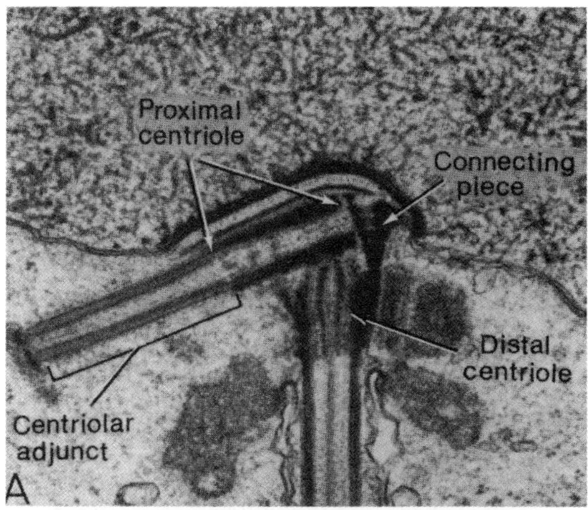

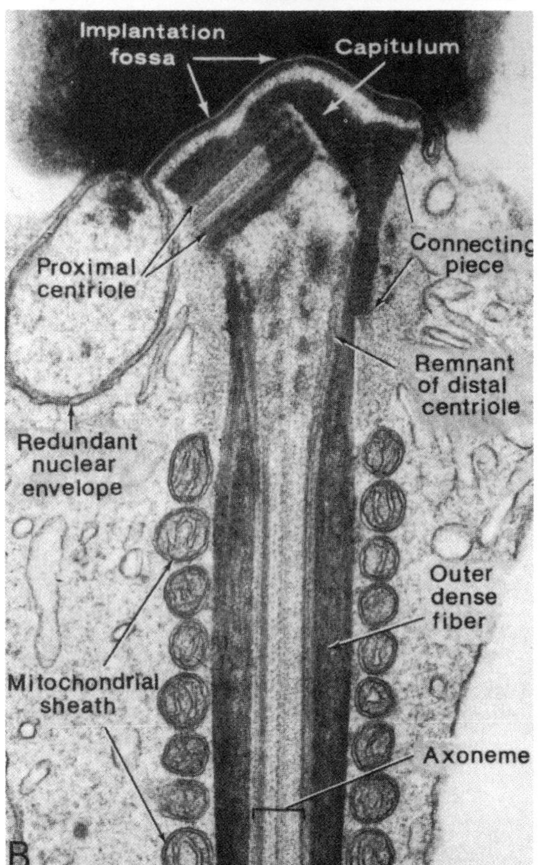

Figure 31–20. (A) Micrograph of the neck region of a late spermatid showing an extension of the proximal centriole, called the centriolar adjunct. This is a transient structure not found in the mature sperm. Also visible is the beginning formation of the striated columns of the connecting piece. (B) A mature spermatozoon showing the fully formed capitulum and striated fibers of the connecting piece continuous with the outer dense fibers. Note the absence of the centriolar adjunct and distal centriole.

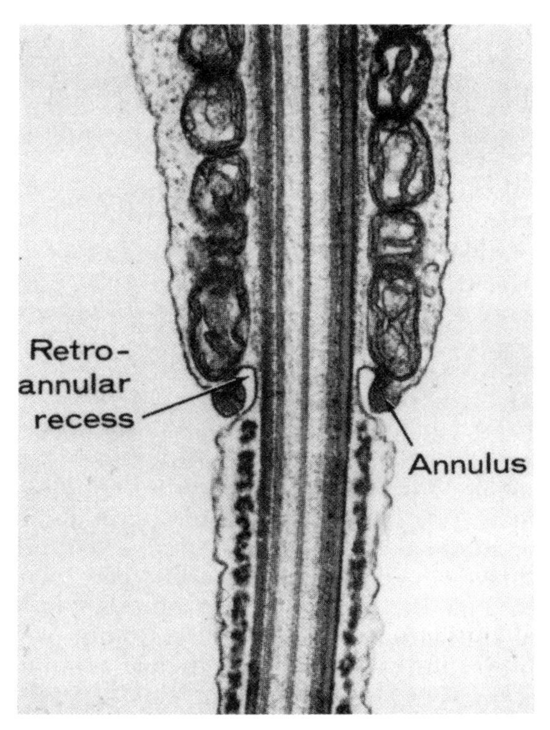

Figure 31–21. Electron micrograph of the junction of the midpiece and principal piece of a rodent spermatozoon. At this site, the plasma membrane is bound to a dense ring, called the annulus. In some species, the plasma membrane turns inward behind the annulus to form a deep groove, called the retroannular recess. In other species, the membrane is relatively smooth in this region.

tion are found near the base, and the more differentiated cells are found at higher levels (Fig. 31–4 and 31–25). The development of two or three successive generations of germ cells goes on concurrently. The cells of different generations are not randomly distributed within the epithelium but occur in a number of well-defined and easily recognizable associations. The number of distinguishable associations varies with the species. In the guinea pig, 12 distinct associations or *stages of spermatogenesis* are identified. These are illustrated in the 12 vertical columns of Fig. 31–25 and are designated by the Roman numerals at the bottom of each column. In any histological section of the guinea pig testis, the cross sections of neighboring tubules will differ in their appearance because of they contain different associations of cells (compare Figs. 31–26 and 31–27). If enough tubules are examined, all 12 cell associations, or stages of spermatogenesis, corresponding to the vertical columns in Fig. 31–25, can be found. In studying this figure, it should be realized that, in the course of its development into spermatozoa, a spermatogonium passes through all of the stages

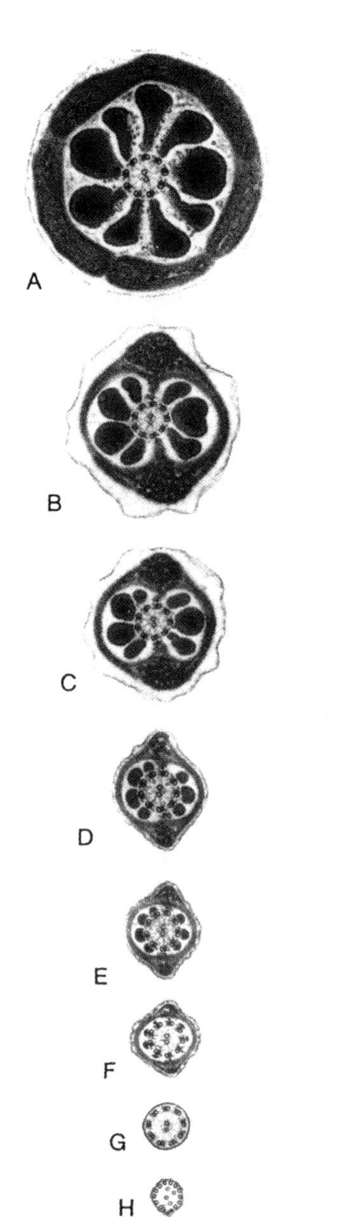

Figure 31–22. Cross sections at successive intervals along the length of the Chinese hamster sperm tail illustrating the reduction in diameter of the outer dense fibers and the tapering of the tail as a whole. (A) Section at the level of the midpiece: (B)–(F) Sections of the principal piece; and (G) and (H) Sections in the end-piece. (Micrographs by D. Phillips.)

encountered in reading from left to right along the horizontal rows from the bottom to the top row of the figure.

Spermatids at different phases of differentiation are always associated with specific phases of development of spermatocytes and spermatogonia, as illustrated in the figure. At any point along the length of a seminiferous tubule, the cell types change with the passage of time, ultimately passing through all 12 stages and then repeating the same sequence. The *cycle of the seminiferous epithelium* is defined as the series of changes occurring in a given area of the epithelium, between two successive appearances of the same cell association. The duration of the cycle has not been determined for the guinea pig, but it is about 12 days in the rat, and a spermatogonium takes about 4 cycles, or 48 days, to complete its differentiation and be released as a spermatozoon.

The various cell associations also occur in orderly sequence along the length of the seminiferous tubule. Thus, instead of considering the changes at a given point in the tubule, one can think of the sequence of cell associations found along the length of the same tubule. From this perspective, the *wave of the seminiferous epithelium* is the distance between two identical associations. Stated differently, the sequence of associations along a wave is similar to the sequence of developmental events taking place in any given area during the cycle of the seminiferous epithelium. In the rat, there are said to be about 12 waves along the length of each tubule.

In contrast to this precise order in the germinal elements of the rodent testis, the appearance of the seminiferous epithelium in sections of human testis, at first, suggests a haphazard arrangement of the developmental stages of the germ cells. Owing to this apparent disorder, it was formerly believed that there was no synchronicity of germ cell development in man and that no "cycle of the seminiferous epithelium" was identifiable. This has now been found to be erroneous. Six well-defined stages can be recognized, but instead of each occupying the entire cross section of the tubule, as in rodents, the recognizable cell associations occupy smaller, wedge-shaped areas of the cross section (Fig. 31–28). The human germinal epithelium is a mosaic of such areas representing six different cell associations, and three or more stages of the cycle can be seen in a single cross section of a seminiferous tubule. The situation is further complicated by the fact that there may be some intermingling of cells at the borders of these areas, resulting in apparently atypical associations. The six typical associations are depicted in Fig. 31–29.

The duration of the cycle of the human seminiferous epithelium has been determined by autoradiographic analyses of testicular biopsies from volunteers. Within 1 h of local injection of tritiated thymidine, the label was found in the nuclei of preleptotene spermatocytes of Stage III, but not in pachytene sperm-

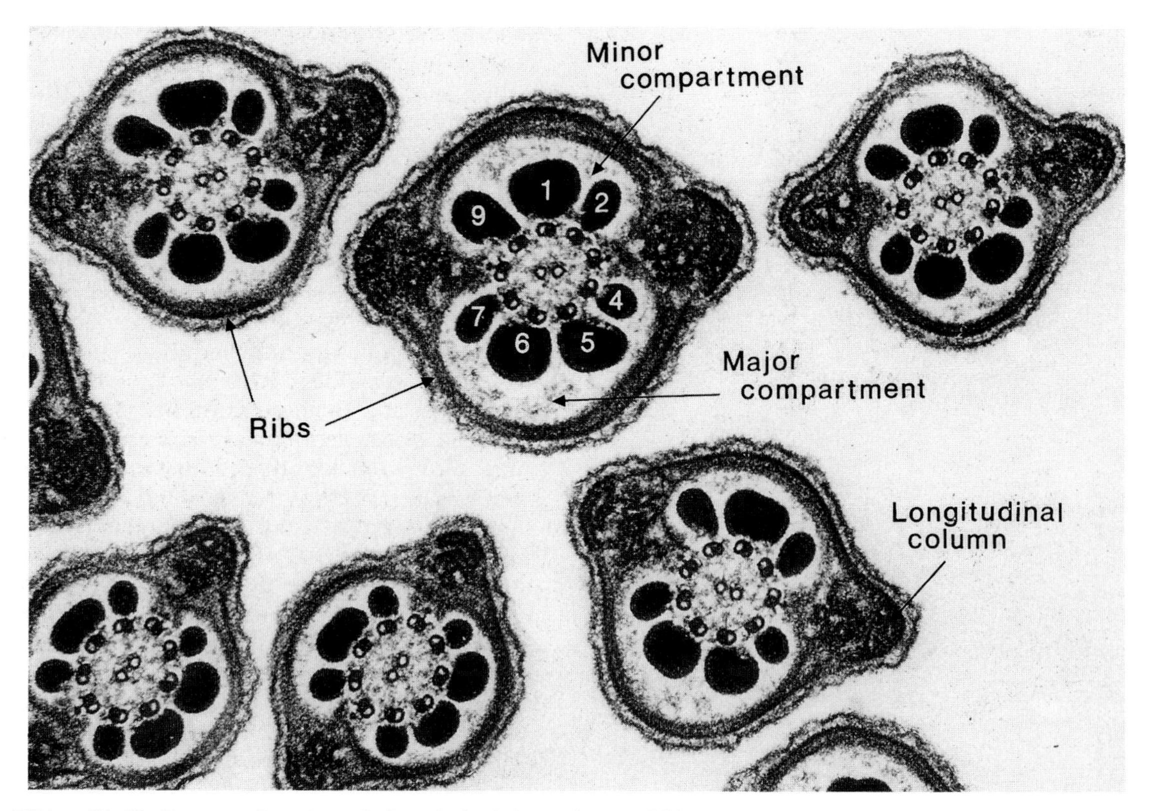

Figure 31–23. Cross sections through the principal piece of several Chinese hamster spermatozoa. Outer dense fibers 3 and 8 have terminated and their place has been taken by inward extentions of the dorsal and ventral longitudinal columns of the fibrous sheath. The cross sections are asymmetrical with a major compartment, containing four outer fibers, and a minor compartment containing 3. (Micrograph by D. Phillips.)

atocytes of that stage or in any other cells more advanced in their development. With passage of time, these labeled cells would be expected to pass through leptotene, zygotene, and early pachytene stages of meiotic prophase and reappear at the end of the cycle in a Stage III cell association as midpachytene spermatocytes. Serial biopsies revealed that these midpachytene spermatocytes of Stage III first showed label 16 days after the initial injection of thymidine. It was, thus, established that the duration of one cycle is 16 days. As expected, labeled spermatids in Stage III were found at 32 days (two cycles). Assuming one cycle for the cells to develop from spermatogonia to preleptotene spermatocytes and one to advance from spermatids to spermatozoa, the total duration of spermatogenesis in man is estimated to be four cycles or 64 days.

Atrophy and Regeneration

In seasonally breeding mammals, spermatogenesis begins at puberty but is discontinued and resumed periodically throughout the life of the animal. At each resumption, it continues only during a period of rut, after which most of the spermatogenic cells are eliminated by maturation depletion or by degeneration. The seminiferous tubules come to contain only Sertoli cells and limited numbers of spermatogonia. In this state, they resemble the seminiferous tubules of the prepubertal testis. At the beginning of the next period of sexual activity, spermatogonia multiply and rapidly regenerate the full complement of spermatogenic cells. Such seasonal changes in the testes are even more prominent in the lower vertebrates.

In man and other mammals that are not seasonal breeders, spermatogenesis is continuous. However, scattered degenerating cells are found in the normal seminiferous epithelium and may occur in segments in which active spermatogenesis is in progress. In the human, abnormal cells are also common. Giant forms of spermatogonia and spermatocytes occur and large multinucleate spermatids are infrequently observed. These abnormalities

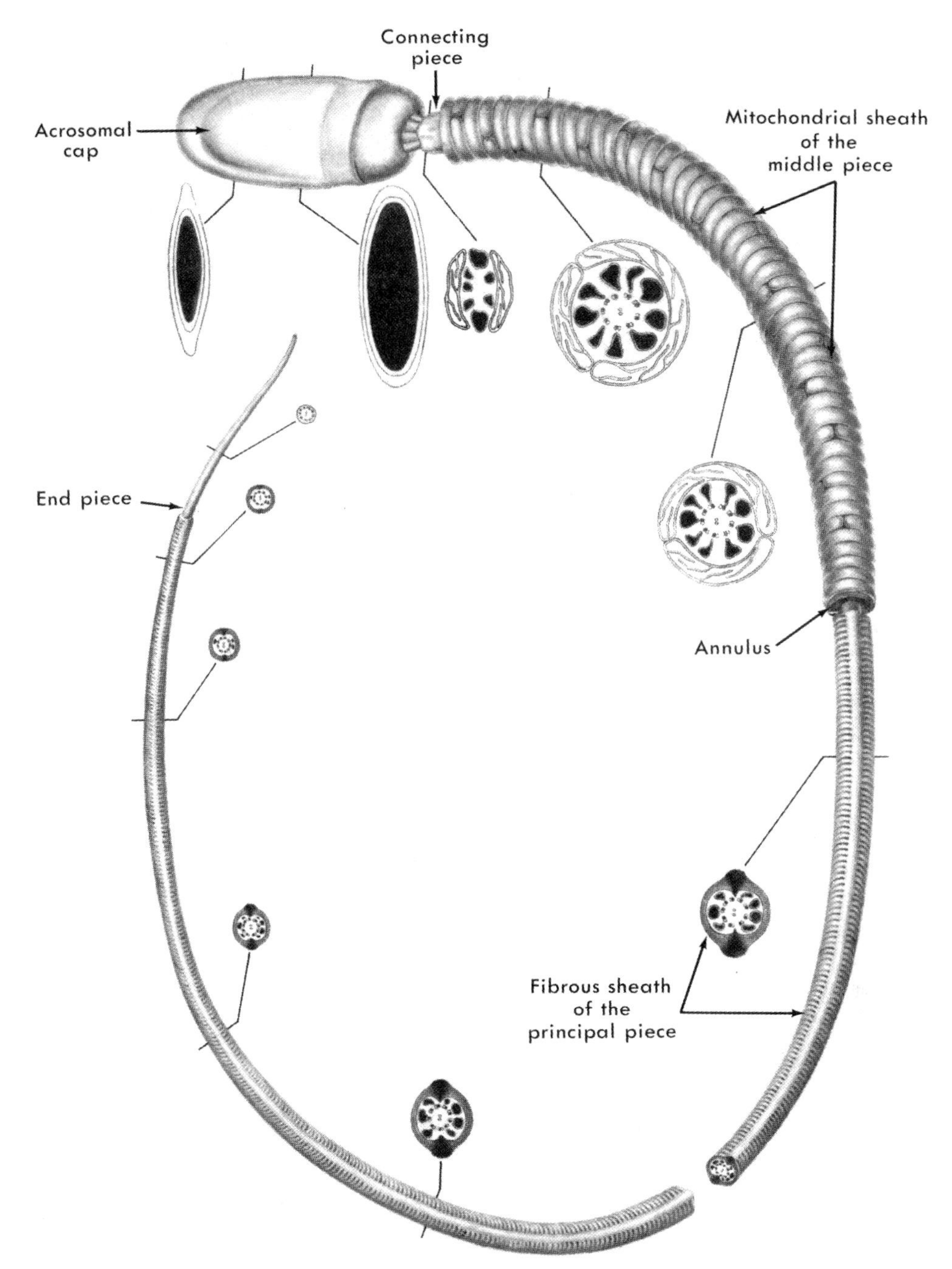

Figure 31–24. Drawing summarizing the ultrastructure of the mammalian spermatozoon. The plasma membrane has been omitted.

are related to the peculiar mode of cytokinesis of the germ cells, which normally leaves the daughter cells connected by a slender intercellular bridge. A subsequent enlargement of the bridges between two or more cells may lead to their coalescence to form multinucleate spermatocytes or spermatids. Spermatids with two nuclei may continue to differentiate, leading to the formation of spermatozoa with two tails or with one tail and two heads. These abnormal sperm are carried, with the normal sperm, into the epididymis, where some degenerate but others persist and can be found in the ejaculate. Such abnormalities are of widespread occurrence but are more common in the human than in other species.

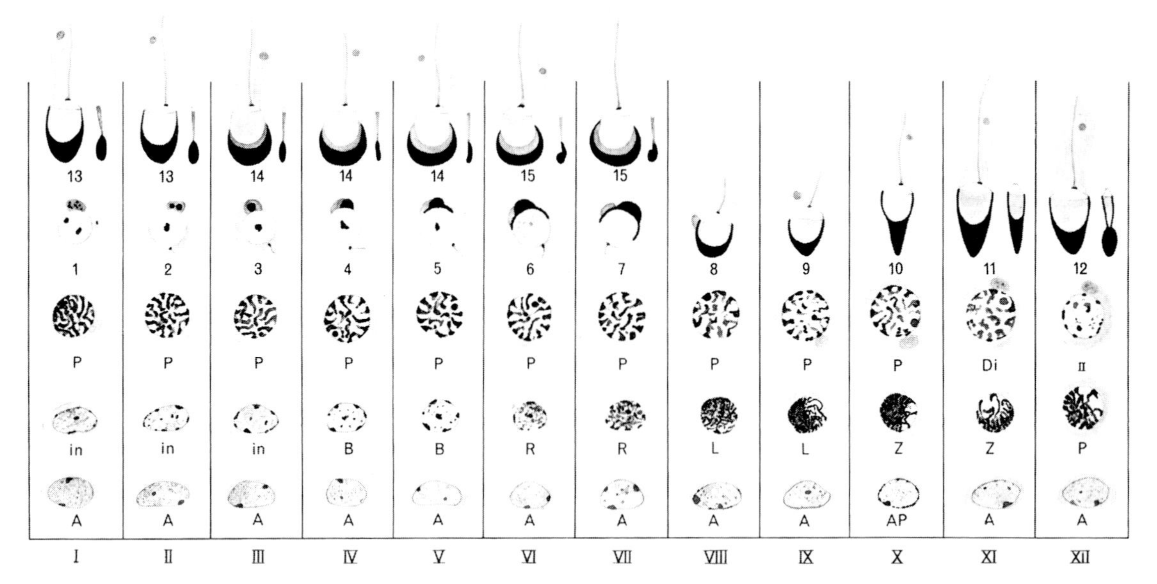

Figure 31–25. The vertical columns of this diagram illustrate all 12 cell associations, or stages, found in sections of guinea pig seminiferous tubules. They have been assembled in the correct sequence, so that reading from lower left to right, and from the bottom row through each of the four upper rows, one progresses through all of the events of germ cell differentiation from spermatogonium to the release of mature spermatozoa. The time from the appearance of any one of these associations, at a given point along the tubule, to the reappearance of same cell association is defined as one cycle of the seminiferous epithelium. (From Clermont, Y. 1960. Fertil. Steril. 6:563.)

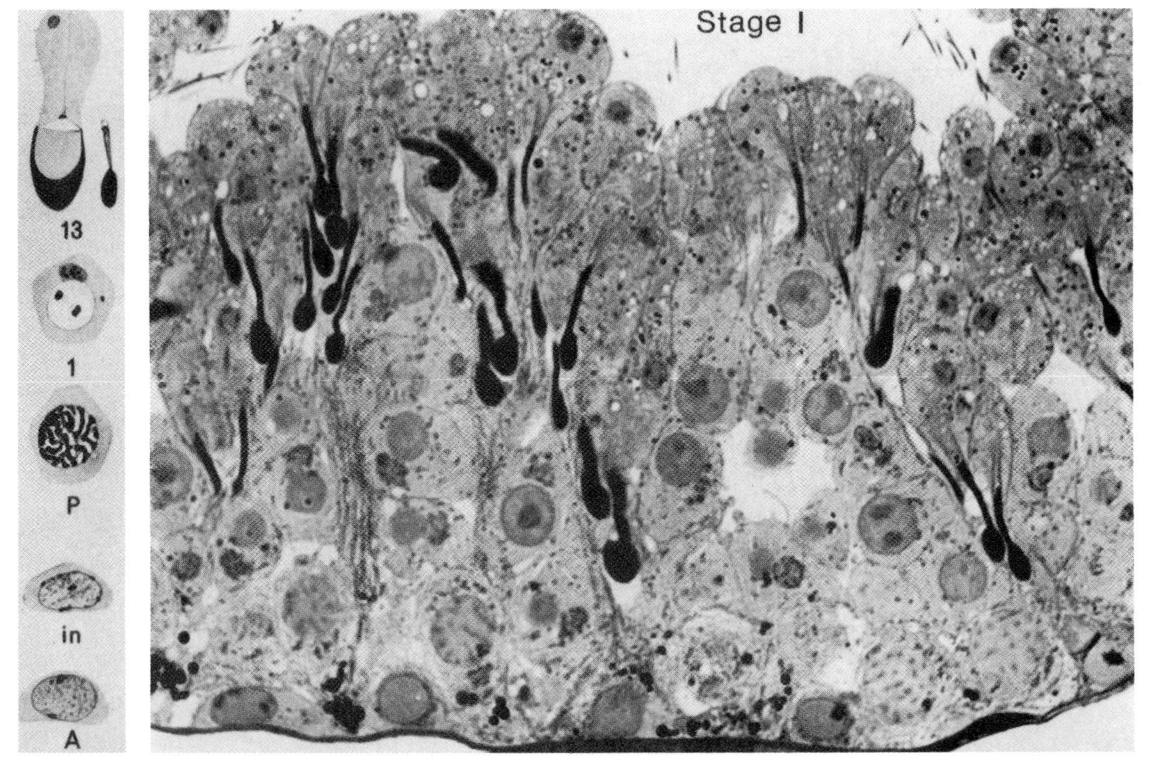

Figure 31–26. Photomicrograph of Stage I of guinea pig spermatogenesis, which includes type-A spermatogonia (A); intermediate spermatogonia (in); pachytene spermatocytes (P); spermatids at the beginning of acrosome formation (1); and a more advanced generation of elongated spermatids with flattened condensed nuclei (13). (Inset: Clermont, Y. 1960. Fertil. Steril. 6:563.)

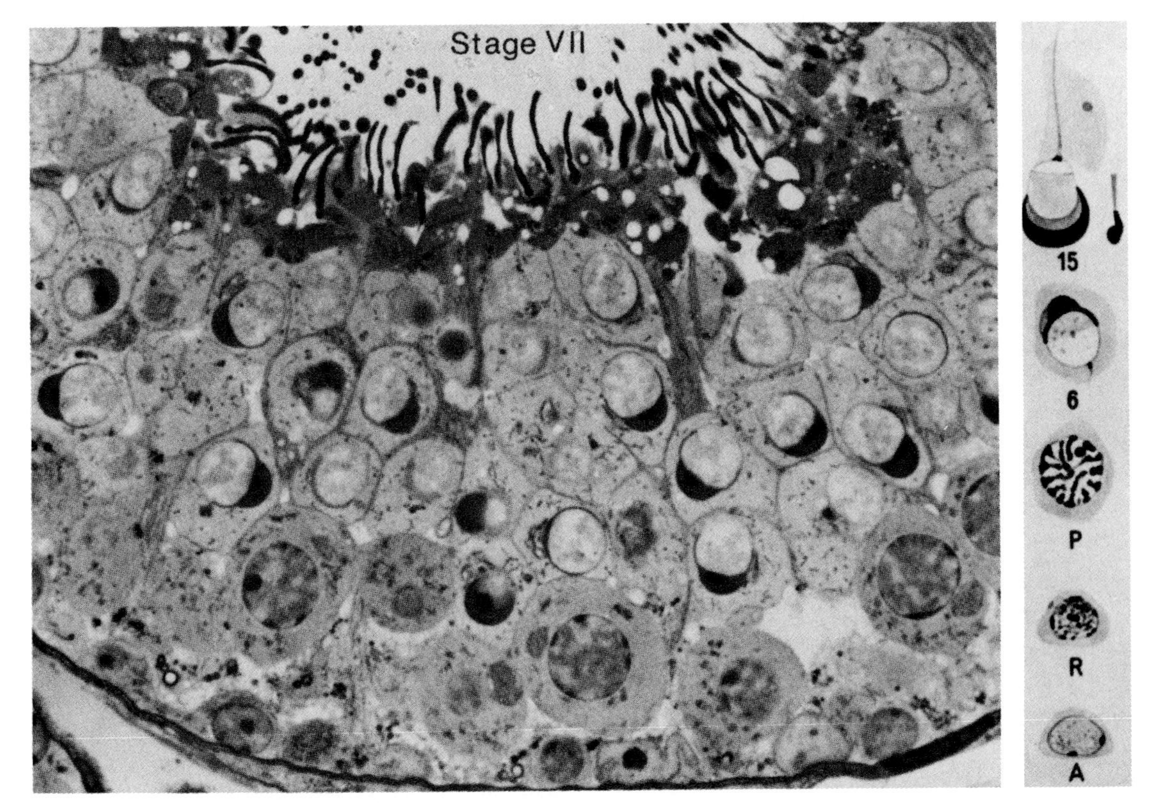

Figure 31–27. Photomicrograph of Stage VII of guinea pig spermatogenesis, characterized by the presence of spermatogonia (A), large pachytene spermatocytes (P); spermatids in the cap phase of acrosome formation (6); nearly mature spermatids projecting into the lumen (15); and dense residual bodies forming a layer adjacent to the lumen (Inset: Clermont, Y. 1960. Fertil. Steril. 6:563.)

The seminiferous epithelium is sensitive to a variety of toxic agents, including alcohol, infectious diseases, and dietary deficiencies. Degenerating cells become more common, and formation of multinucleate giant cells by coalescence of spermatids is a prominent feature of these toxic effects. Exposure of the testis to more then minimal doses of X-rays causes extensive cell degeneration and may result in sterility. The germ cells are also sensitive to elevated temperatures. Even the normal internal temperature of the body is incompatible with normal spermatogenesis. Therefore, in the majority of mammals, the testes are lodged in a scrotum which has a temperature a few degrees below that of the rest of the body. Testes that fail to descend into the scrotum during development and remain in the abdomen never produce mature spermatozoa. The seminiferous tubules are atrophic and contain only Sertoli cells and rare spermatogonia. Failure of descent of the testes is called *cryptorchidism*.

In all conditions, the Sertoli cells are more resistant than the spermatogenic cells. Of the latter, a few spermatogonia usually remain. Therefore, when the noxious agent is removed or the vitamin E or A deficiency is corrected, a more-or-less complete regeneration of the seminiferous epithelium can be expected. In mammals with a short life span, spermatogenesis continues undiminished until death. In man, although some spermatogenesis continues into senility, the seminiferous tubules do undergo a gradual involution with advancing age. Scattered atrophic tubules may be found in the testis of men over 45, and in very old men, all of the tubules may be largely depleted of spermatogenic cells.

INTERSTITIAL TISSUE

In the angular interstices between the seminiferous tubules are the *Leydig cells*, which constitute the principal endocrine component of the testis. The organization of the interstitium

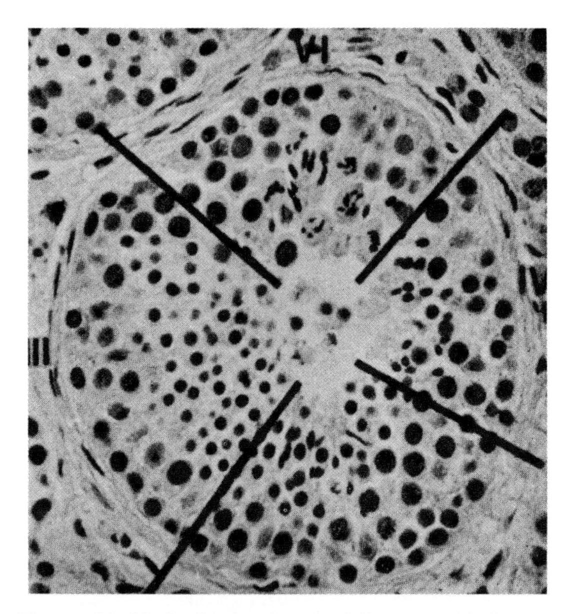

Figure 31–28. In the human seminiferous epithelium, a single stage of the cycle does not extend around the entire circumference of the tubule, as in rodents. In this photomicrograph, for example, four different associations of cells are found in the same cross section. (From Clermont, Y. 1963. Am. J. Anat. 112:50.)

varies considerably from species to species. In the human, it is a very loose connective tissue containing small clusters of Leydig cells, occasional fibroblasts, macrophages, and mast cells (Fig. 31–30). In addition, there are relatively undifferentiated cells of mesenchymal origin that are capable of developing into additional Leydig cells in response to stimulation by gonadotropic hormones. In other species, such as the pig, horse, and opossum, the Leydig cells are very abundant, occupying nearly all of the extravascular space of the interstitium (Fig. 31–31).

In the human, the Leydig cells are in clusters of varying size usually closely associated with blood vessels. Where closely packed, they are irregularly polyhedral and 14–20 μm across, but at the periphery of the clusters, where they occur individually, they may be spindle-shaped. Binucleate cells are common. Adjacent to the nucleus is a well-developed Golgi complex which responds to gonadotropic stimulation by enlargement. There are no secretory granules in the Leydig cells. They evidently secrete constitutively, without accumulation and storage of their product in the cytoplasm. Mitochondria are abundant and variable in size and shape. Their cristae tend to be tubular instead of lamellar in form, but this is not true of all species. The acidophilic cytoplasm may contain a number of clear vacuoles where lipid droplets have been extracted. In common with other steroid-secreting endocrine glands, the most striking ultrastructural feature of the testicular interstitial cell is its extensive smooth endoplasmic reticulum (Fig. 31–32). Cisternal profiles of rough endoplasmic reticulum may also be present in limited numbers. The membranes of the smooth reticulum contain the enzymes necessary for several steps in the biosynthesis of androgenic steroids. Peroxisomes and lysosomes are also present in the cytoplasm, and golden brown deposits of lipochrome pigment are present in the Leydig cells in men of all ages, but they become increasingly prominent with advancing age (Fig. 31–33).

A feature peculiar to the human Leydig cell is the presence, in the cytoplasm, of conspicuous crystals, 3 μm or more in thickness and up to 20 μm in length, called the *crystals of Reinke*. These are highly variable in size and shape and may be either rounded or pointed at the ends (Fig. 31–33). They have little affinity for the common histological strains and appear nearly colorless in routine preparations. However, they can be stained with azocarmine. They are isotropic in polarized light and have solubility properties of protein. In electron micrographs, they present a highly ordered crystalline lattice that differs somewhat in appearance depending on the plane of section. Such crystals occur in the testes of most men, from puberty to senility, but their abundance is highly variable. They are found in no other mammalian species and their significance is unknown.

Leydig cells first appear in the testis in the eighth month of gestation and increase in number for a few weeks; then, for reasons that are poorly understood, they decline until few remain at birth. They slowly increase in number in childhood and adolescence, and early in adult life they show abundant evidence of being active in synthesis of androgenic steroid hormones. With advancing age, they slowly decline in number. A 60-year-old man usually has fewer than half as many Leydig cells as the average 20-year-old. Surprisingly, in the 30 years, while a man is slowly losing half of the cells he had at the end of puberty, there is not a proportional decrease in the level of circulating testosterone. In men between 50 and 90, there is no linear relationship between the number of Leydig cells and the daily sperm production.

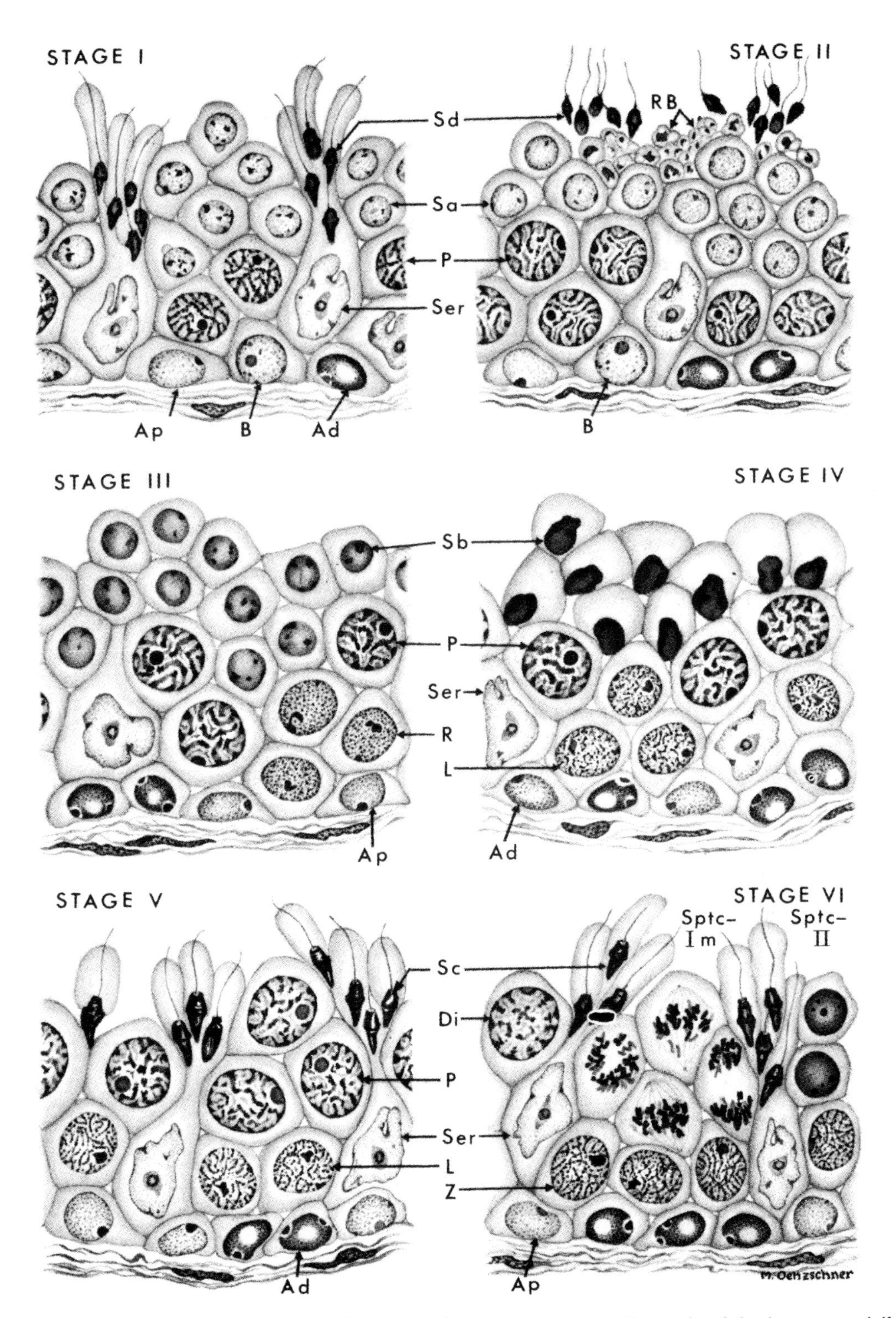

Figure 31–29. Drawing of the six recognizable stages of spermatogenesis in the cycle of the human seminiferous epithelium. Sertoli cell (Ser); dark and pale type-A spermatogonia (Ad and Ap); type-B spermatogonia (B); resting primary spermatocyte (R); leptotene spermatocyte (L); zygotene spermatocyte (Z); pachytene spermatocyte (P); diplotene spermatocyte (Di); primary spermatocyte in division (Sptc-Im); primary spermatocyte in interphase (Sptc-II); spermatids in various stages of differentiation (Sa, Sb, Sc, and Sd); residual bodies of Regaud (RB). (From Clermont, Y. 1963. Am. J. Anat. 112:35.)

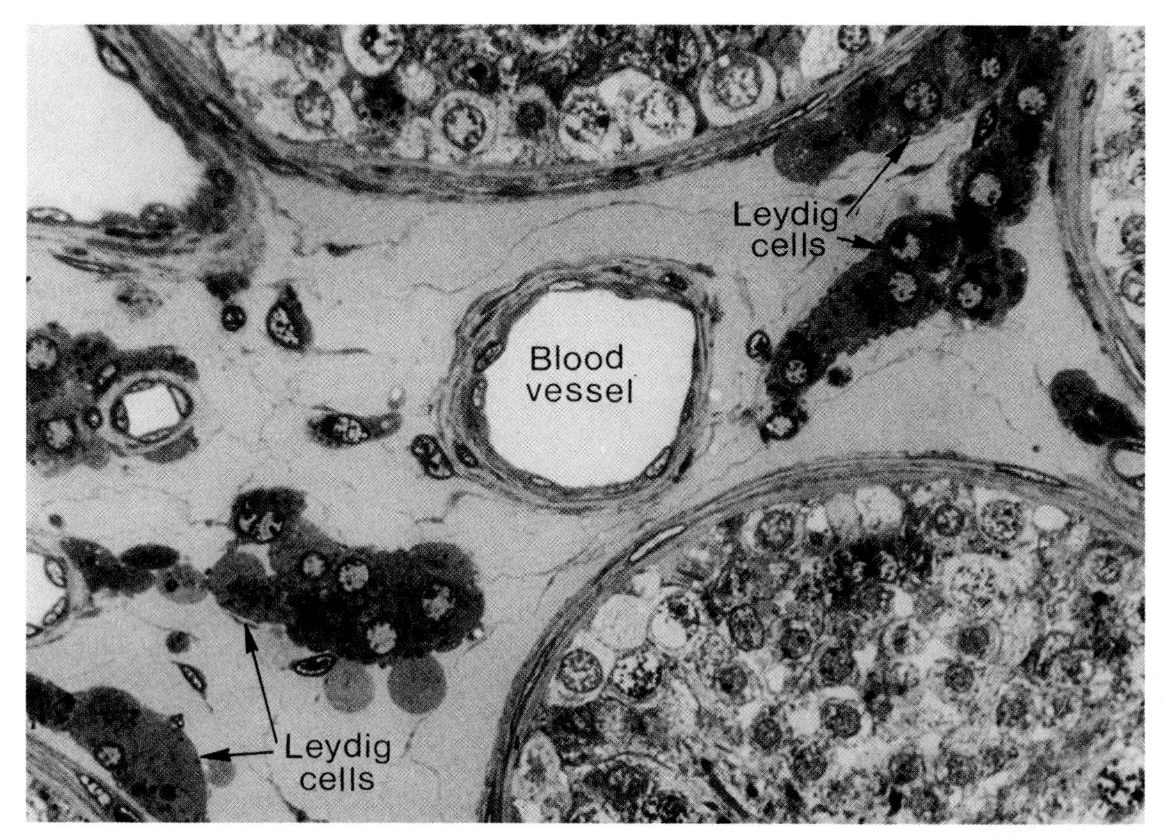

Figure 31–30. Low-power micrograph an interstitial space of the human testis, showing several groups of Leydig cells. Most of the extravascular space of the interstitium in this species is occupied by a protein-rich fluid, which appears a uniform gray in this figure. There is relatively little collagen in the interstitium of the human testis. (Micrograph courtesy of W. Neaves.)

BLOOD VESSELS AND LYMPHATICS

The blood supply to the testis is from a branch of the aorta, the *internal spermatic* or *testicular artery*. It divides before reaching the testis, giving rise to several branches that penetrate the capsule of the organ and form *centripetal branches* that course toward the rete testis. Major branches of these vessels run in the opposite direction from the parent vessel as *centrifugal arterioles*, located in the columns of interstitial tissue between seminiferous tubules. *Intertubular capillaries* derived from these form networks in the interstitium. The capillaries in neighboring interstitial columns are connected by ladder-like, circumferentially oriented *peritubular capillaries* (Fig. 31–34).

Postcapillary venules join to form collecting venules. Their confluence forms veins that course toward the tunica albuginea (*centrifugal veins*) or toward the rete testis (*centripetal veins*). The former drain into the veins of the tunica albuginea, whereas the latter, running in the septula testis, converge on a venous plexus associated with the rete testis. On reaching the surface, these veins join those of the tunica in forming the *pampiniform plexus* of veins surrounding the ductus deferens in the spermatic cord. The right pampiniform plexus drains directly into the inferior vena cava via the *internal spermatic vein*. The corresponding vein on the left joins the left renal vein. This junction evidently results in some resistance to flow because the left pampiniform plexus is often more distended than the right, and the left testis is situated lower in the scrotum than the right. The vessels of the left pampiniform plexus are often quite tortuous and varicose, a condition described as *varicocele*.

In many animal species, and possibly in man, the arrangement of blood vessels in the spermatic cord, with the internal spermatic artery surrounded by the pampiniform plexus, constitutes a countercurrent heat-exchange system that allows the arterial blood to lose heat to the cooler venous blood in the pampiniform plexus. This precooling of the

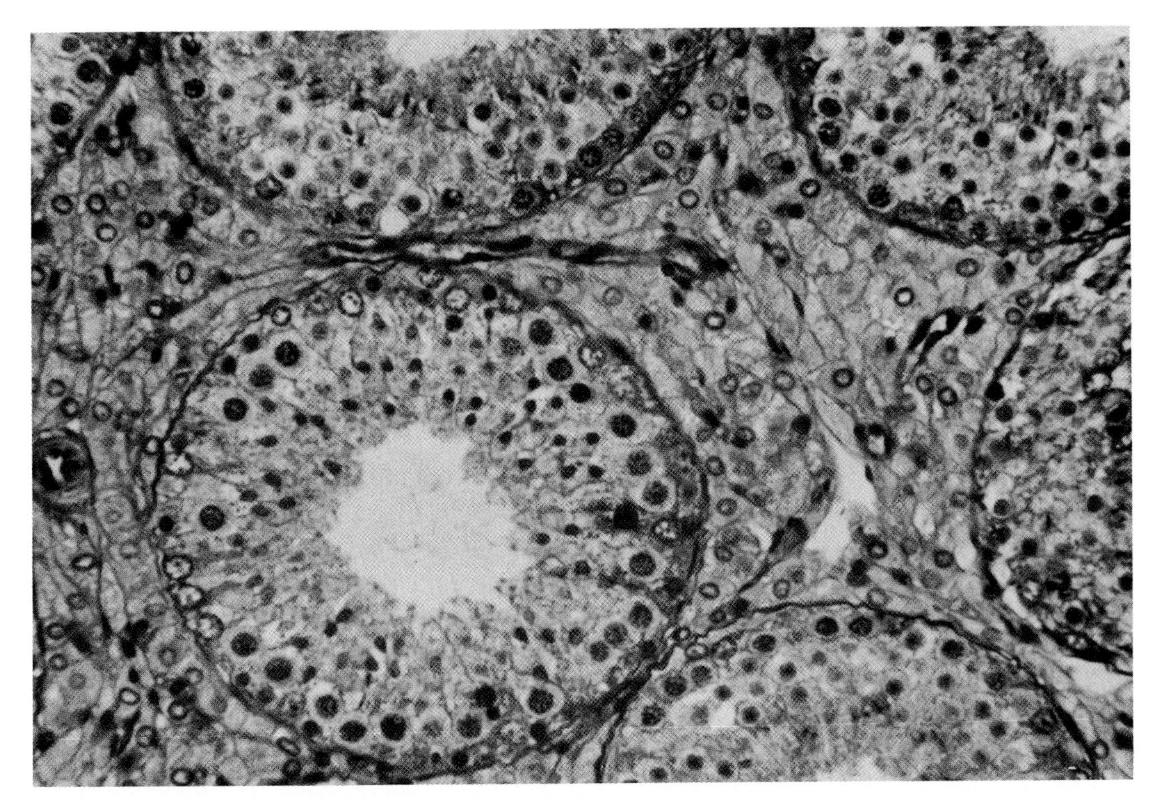

Figure 31–31. Photomicrograph of opposum testis for comparison with Fig. 31–30. In contrast to the human testis, the interstitial spaces here are almost completely filled by Leydig cells. The significance of the striking species differences in volume of testicular endocrine tissue is poorly understood.

arterial blood helps to maintain the temperature of the testis a few degrees below deep body temperature. This lower temperature is essential for continued spermatogenesis.

The intertubular areas of the testis also contain thin-walled lymphatic vessels that drain into larger lymphatics in the septula testis and tunica albuginea and then upward in lymph vessels of the spermatic cord to para-aortic lymph nodes and nodes associated with the renal blood vessels. The lymphatics show considerable variation in pattern from species to species. In the laboratory rodents, they form very extensive peritubular sinusoids. In these species, the clusters of Leydig cells are centrally located in the intertubular spaces and closely associated with the walls of the blood vessels. They are surrounded by the sinusoidal lymphatics. The steroid-secreting cells are, thus, interposed between the blood vessels, on the inside, and the lymphatics around their outside, and they presumably release their hormones into both. In larger species such as the ram, bull, and man, the lymphatics are not sinusoidal, but form thin-walled vessels, more-or-less centrally located in the intertubular spaces. The Leydig cells are not intimately related to either the blood or lymphatic vessels, but evidently release their hormone into the abundant extracellular fluid of the interstitium, from which it diffuses to the tubules to exert its local effect on spermatogenesis, and into the blood and lymphatic vessels for its effects on distant target organs.

HISTOPHYSIOLOGY OF THE TESTIS

ENDOCRINE FUNCTION

The endocrine function of the testis resides in the interstitial cells of Leydig. These synthesize and release the male sex hormone *testosterone*, which is required in high local concentrations to sustain spermatogenesis in the seminiferous tubules. In addition to its local action, testosterone circulating in the blood is essential for maintenance of the function of the accessory glands of male reproduction—the seminal vesicles, prostate, and bul-

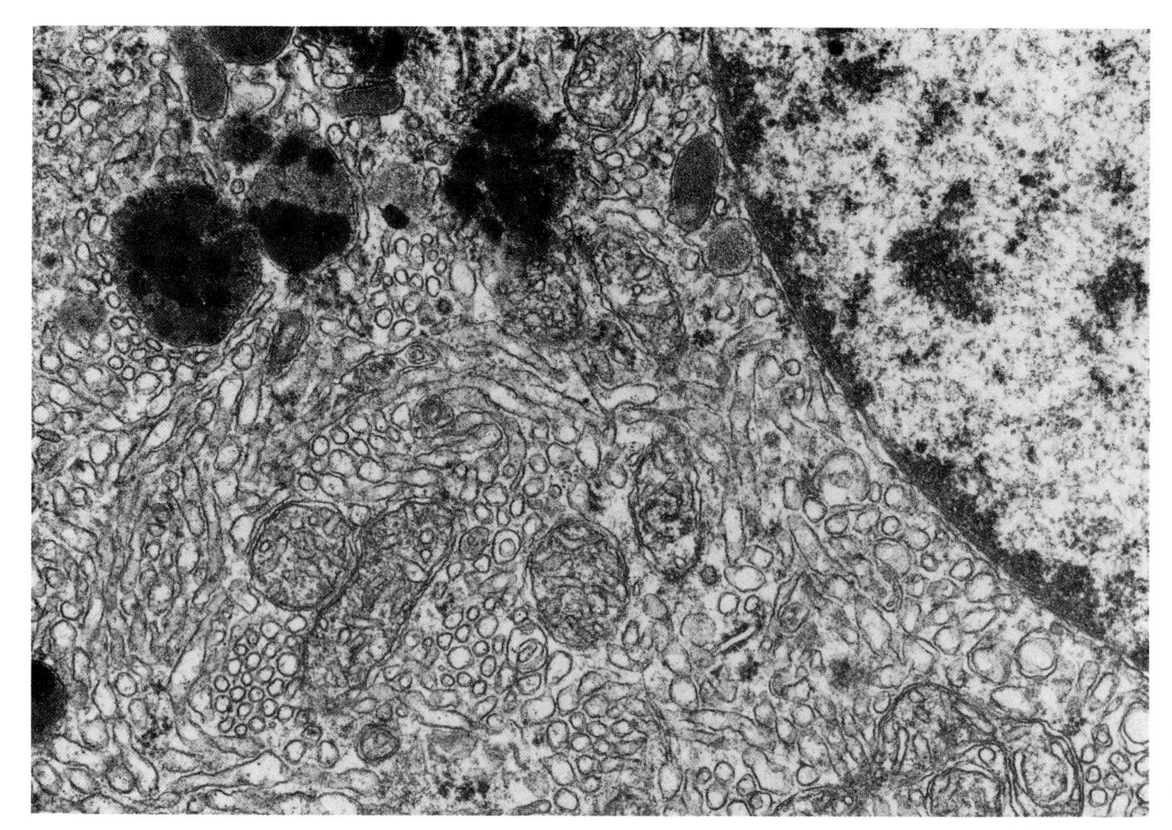

Figure 31–32. Electron micrograph of a juxtanuclear region of cytoplasm in a human Leydig cell. As in most other steroid secreting cells, its most striking ultrastructural feature is an abundance of smooth endoplasmic reticulum. The dense bodies at the top of the figure are deposits of lipofuchsin pigment that accumulates with advancing age. (Micrograph courtesy of W. Neaves.)

bourethral glands. It is also responsible for maintenance of the male secondary sex characteristics—male pattern of pubic hair, growth of beard, low-pitched voice, and muscular body build.

Production of testosterone by the Leydig cells depends primarily on *luteinizing hormone* (LH) secreted by the anterior pituitary. This hormone binds to specific receptors on the plasma membrane of the Leydig cells. This leads to cyclic AMP formation and activation of protein kinases. Cholesterol esterase liberates free cholesterol from cholesterol esters in cytoplasmic lipid droplets of the Leydig cells. Mitochondrial enzymes cleave off the side-chain of cholesterol to form pregnenolone and enzymes of the smooth endoplasmic reticulum, then carry out several biosynthetic steps in the transformation of pregnenolone to testosterone.

Although Leydig cells make up only a small percentage of the total volume of the testis, their steroidogenic potential is impressive. In the rat, where they constitute only 1% of the testis volume, there is an estimated 22 million Leydig cells per gram of testis. Their mitochondria number about 600 per cell and the smooth reticulum, which contains the steroidogenic enzymes, has a surface area estimated at 10,500 μm^3. It is calculated from this morphometric data that an average Leydig cell can produce about 10,000 molecules of testosterone per second. The hormone is not stored in secretory granules as in many other secretory cells but is produced and released as needed. Comparable stereological analysis of the human testis has not been carried out, but it is estimated that Leydig cells occupy less than 3% of the total volume of the organ.

The hypophyseal control of Leydig cell function has proven to be more complex than it was formerly thought to be. Release of LH from pituitary gonadotropes is now known to be a discontinuous process, occurring mainly at night, in pulses at intervals of about 90 min. Moreover, hormones other than LH have been found to influence testosterone production. Prolactin binds to surface receptors on

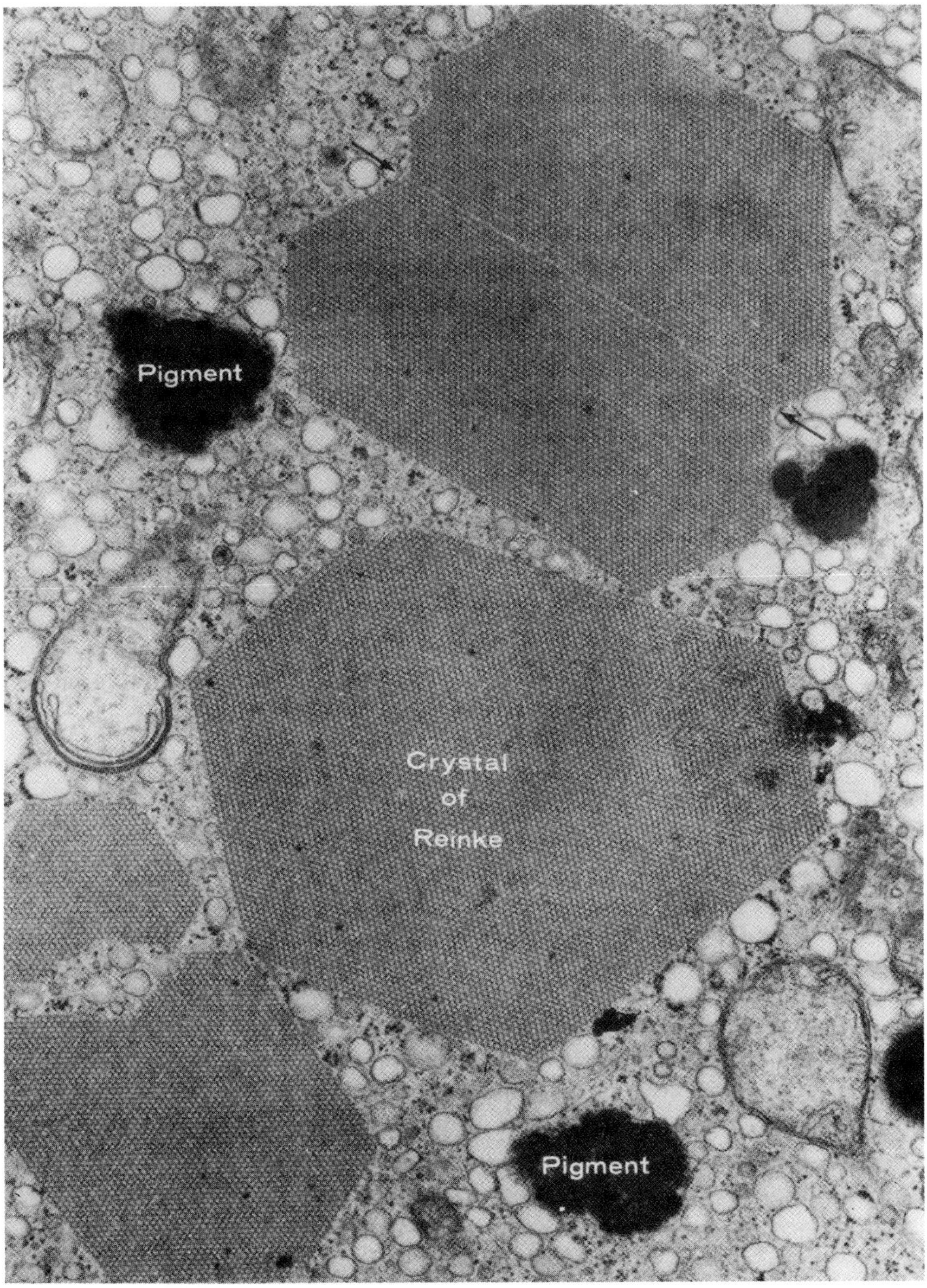

Figure 31–33. Electron micrograph of Leydig cell cytoplasm from human testis showing lipochrome pigment deposits and several crystals of Reinke, which are peculiar to human Leydig cells. (Micrograph from Nagano, T., and I. Ohtsuki. 1971. J. Cell Biol. 51:148.)

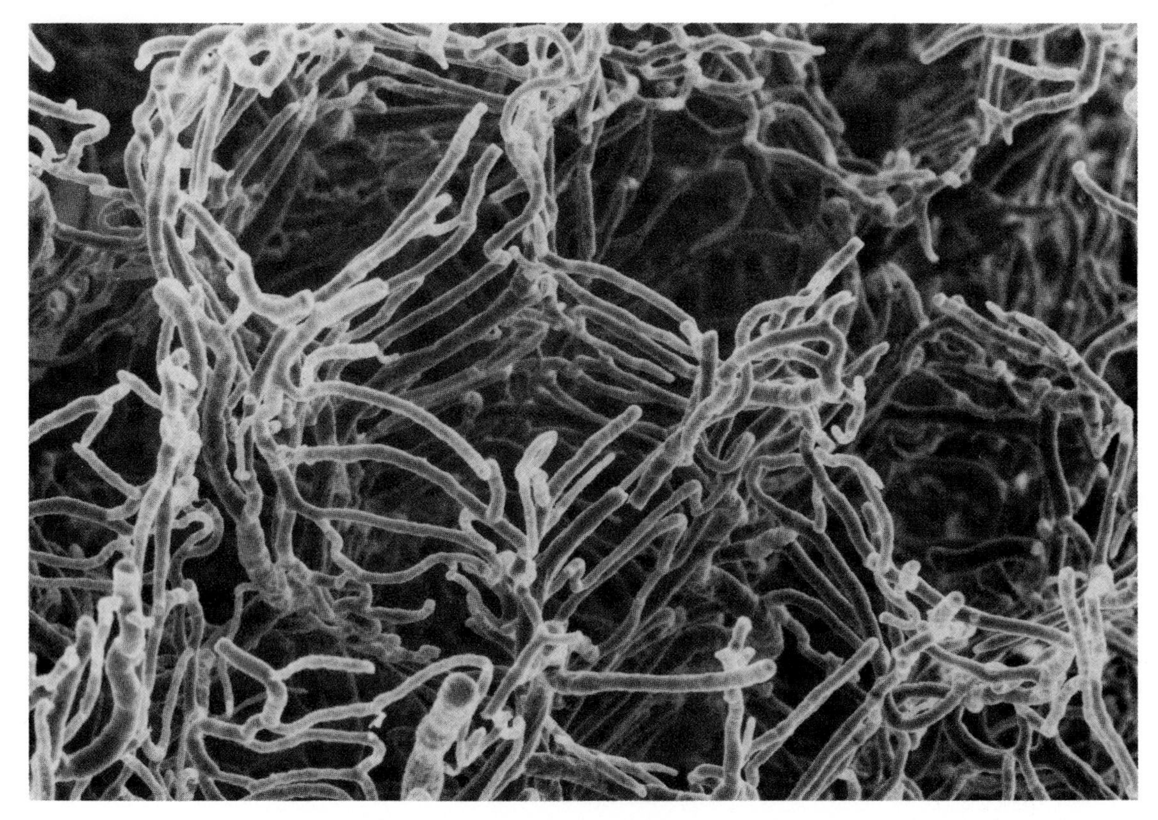

Figure 31–34. Scanning micrograph of a plastic cast of the microvasculature surrounding several seminiferous tubules that have been removed from the preparation by enzymatic digestion. Vessels coursing parallel to the tubules are interconnected by closely-spaced peritubular capillaries to form a circumferential ladder-like pattern. (Micrograph from Susuki, F. 1982. Am. J. Anat. 163:309.)

the Leydig cells, affecting the number of LH receptors and impairing the capacity of the cells to store cholesterol esters as precursors of testosterone. *LH-releasing hormone* (LHRH) not only affects pituitary gonadotropes but is now reported to act directly on Leydig cells affecting their LH binding and their steroidogenic responsiveness.

There is increasing evidence that the seminiferous tubules also exert a local regulatory effect on the ultrastructure and function of the Leydig cells. A peptide, thought to be produced by the Sertoli cells, is inhibitory to Leydig cells. Local damage to seminiferous tubules appears to diminish this inhibition and induces hypertrophy of the neighboring Leydig cells.

EXOCRINE FUNCTION

Spermatozoa can be thought of as a holocrine secretory product of the seminiferous epithelium. The numbers of sperm produced are astronomical. Improved methods for estimating daily sperm production, in the human, yield a mean value of 94.6×10^6 per testis, or 5.6×10^6 per gram of testicular tissue. Although this seems a very large number, it is low compared to other species. Daily sperm production per gram of testis in the rat is at least 20×10^6; in the rabbit, 25×10^6; and in the boar, 23×10^6. Taking into account the weight of the testis in the boar, the daily production of the two testes would be 16.2×10^9 spermatozoa.

The production of such large numbers of spermatozoa is less surprising if one considers the enormous surface area of the seminiferous epithelium. In the human, the two testes contain 800–1200 seminiferous tubules, each 30–70 cm long. In the aggregate, these add up to one-third of a mile of continuously proliferating seminiferous epithelium. The normal ejaculate is 2–5 ml in volume and contains 40–100 million sperm per milliliter. Men with counts below 20 million per milliliter are usually infertile. The reserves of mature sperm available for ejaculation, in man, are small relative to those of other animals. Reserves in the ram are equivalent to about 95 ejaculates, in rabbits about 30, and in man no more than 2.

Spermatogenesis depends on *testosterone* produced by the Leydig cells in response to stimulation by *luteinizing hormone* (LH) released from the pituitary gland. The other gonadotropic hormone, *follicle stimulating hormone* (FSH), binds specifically to Sertoli cells of the seminiferous tubules. It is suggested that FSH is necessary for the initiation of spermatogenesis, but whether it is required for its maintenance is unclear. It is known to increase Sertoli cell synthesis of certain proteins that transport substances to the germ cells and into the fluid in the lumen of the seminiferous tubules. One of these is *androgen-binding protein* (ABP) which is secreted at the apical and lateral surfaces of the Sertoli cells and binds testosterone. Another is an iron-binding protein, *transferrin*. In addition to contributing to germ cell development, these proteins, released into the lumen, are carried downstream in the excurrent ducts of the testis and are believed to contribute to the maintenance of normal epididymal function.

The release of LH by the cells of the pituitary is regulated by negative feedback. Increased levels of testosterone synthesis by the Leydig cells, suppresses release of LH and conversely, low levels of circulating testosterone result in increased release of LH. A similar feedback regulation of FSH release by the pituitary involves a hormone *inhibin*, produced by the Sertoli cells in the male and by the granulosa cells of the ovarian follicle in the female. Inhibin is a glycoprotein consisting of a heterodimer of two subunits, inhibin-α and inhibin-β. It is believed to be of greater physiological importance in the female than in the male.

Given a normal complement of germ cells in the seminiferous epithelium, inhibin is believed to be continuously released and to act on the hypophysis to suppress FSH production. Depletion of the germ cells results in an increase in circulating FSH. The secretory functions of the seminiferous epithelium thus include synthesis and release of androgen-binding protein, an RHLH-like peptide, transferrin, and inhibin. It also produces a considerable volume of fluid that serves as a vehicle for transport of the spermatozoa to the rete testis and epididymis. This fluid is rich in glutamate, inositol, and potassium ions, constituents that are probably important for the maintenance of spermatozoa in their transit through the excurrent ducts.

The peritubular myoid cells, in some species, are observed to generate shallow rhythmic contractions that may contribute to sperm transport. It now appears that their function goes beyond this mechanical function. They have been shown to have androgen receptors and may mediate androgen effects on the Sertoli cells. A protein produced by the myoid cells has been shown to stimulate synthesis of transferrin and androgen-binding protein by Sertoli cells in vitro.

BLOOD-TESTIS PERMEABILITY BARRIER

It has long been known that vital dyes and other substances introduced into the blood stream readily leave the vessels and enter the extracellular spaces of most tissues and organs except the brain. This vital organ is protected by a *blood-brain barrier* that resides in the tight endothelial junctions of the brain capillaries. More recently, a *blood-testis barrier* has been described. The barrier in this case is not in the walls of the blood vessels of the interstitial tissue, which are actually unusually permeable. Instead, the exclusion of vital dyes and other large molecules from the seminiferous tubules is due to the presence of special junctional complexes between adjacent Sertoli cells near the base of the seminiferous epithelium. These consist of many parallel lines of fusion of the apposed cell membranes, which effectively prevent entry of these substances into the system of intercellular clefts higher in the epithelium. These occluding junctions are situated at the interface between overarching Sertoli call processes, just above the spermatogonia (Fig. 31–35). Thus, they divide the epithelium into a *basal compartment* containing spermatogonia and an *adluminal compartment*, containing the more advanced stages of germ cell differentiation. Substances in the extracellular spaces of the interstitium have relatively unimpeded access to the basal compartment but are barred from deeper penetration into the epithelium by the Sertoli cell junctional specializations. At the appropriate stage of the spermatogenic cycle, newly formed spermatocytes must move from the basal compartment into the adluminal compartment. This is accomplished without disruption of the permeability barrier. Undermining processes are ex-

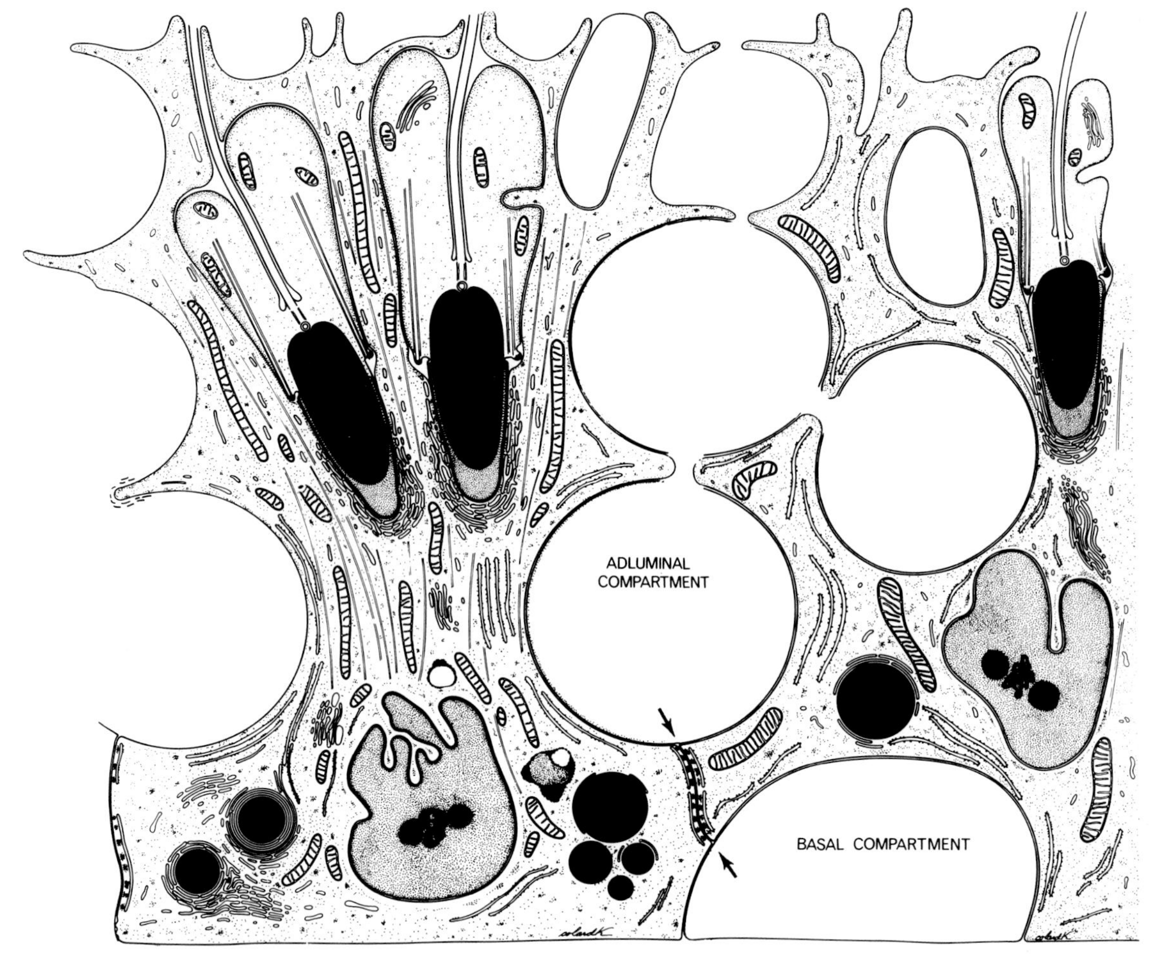

Figure 31–35. Drawing illustrating how occluding junctions between overarching processes of the Sertoli cells (at arrows) divide the epithelium into basal and adluminal compartments. Substances diffusing from the interstitium have direct access to the spermatogonia in the basal compartment but are excluded from the adluminal compartment by the junctional complexes. These constitute the main structural basis of the blood-testis permeability barrier. (From Fawcett, D.W. 1975. *In* Handbook of Physiology, Vol. 3. Baltimore, MD, Williams and Wilkins Co.)

tended from the Sertoli cells to join between the spermatocytes and form new occluding junctions. The preexisting Sertoli junctions above the spermatocytes then dissociate, permitting upward movement of this cohort of conjoined germ cells.

The full significance of these unusual cell relationships is still being studied, but it is clear that the existence of a barrier near the base of the epithelium enables the Sertoli cells to maintain, in the adluminal compartment, a unique microenvironment especially favorable for germ cell differentiation. Because the postmeiotic germ cells are genetically different from the parent cells, it is conceivable that the blood-testis barrier may serve to prevent foreign protein from these cells from reaching the blood and inducing formation of antibodies which might result in autoimmune infertility.

EXCRETORY DUCTS OF THE TESTIS

THE TUBULI RECTI AND RETE TESTIS

The several seminiferous tubules in each lobule of the testis converge toward a plexus of epithelium-lined channels in its mediastinum that form the *rete testis* (Fig. 31–2). As the seminiferous tubules approach the rete, the germ cells disappear and their epithelium then consists only of Sertoli cells. There is an abrupt narrowing beyond which each tubule is joined to the rete testis by a short, straight *tubulus rectus*. The tubuli recti and rete testis are lined by a simple cuboidal epithelium that does not appear to be secretory. Its free surface bears numerous microvilli and a majority of the cells have a single flagellum that projects into the lumen. The flagella are presumed to be motile but it is not obvious what function they could serve other than to produce some degree of agitation of the fluid contents of the lumen.

In the guinea pig, the cells of the tubuli recti and rete testis store a remarkable amount of glycogen which displaces the nucleus toward the lumen and all other organelles to the periphery. Glycogen accumulation to the same degree has not been reported in other mammalian species.

DUCTULI EFFERENTES

Twelve or more *ductuli efferentes* arise from the rete testis and traverse the tunica albuginea to emerge on the posterosuperior surface of the testis. These segregate and become very highly convoluted, forming a number of *lobuli epididymidis* corresponding to the number of ductuli. These extend from the testis to the head of the epididymis, a distance of about 10 mm. There, the ductuli become confluent with the *ductus epididymidis*.

The ductuli efferentes are lined by an epithelium that has a distinctive scalloped outline in sections because it consists of groups of columnar ciliated cells alternating with groups of short nonciliated cells. The cytoplasm of the nonciliated cells contains granules that were formerly interpreted as secretory material. These have now been identified as lysosomes. Conspicuous invaginations of the surface of these cells are taken to be evidence of endocytosis. This is reaffirmed in experiments demonstrating their uptake of vital dyes. The tall ciliated cells are broader at the apex than at their base and their cilia beat toward the epididymis, moving the luminal fluid and spermatozoa in that direction.

DUCTUS EPIDIDYMIDIS

The highly convoluted ductus epididymidis constitutes the *epididymis*, an organ about 7.5 cm long running along the posterior surface of the testis from its upper to its lower pole. The dimensions of the epididymis do not adequately reflect the very large surface area of its epithelium to which the spermatozoa are exposed. If the ductus epididymidis were to be freed from surrounding connective tissue and straightened out, it would be over 6 m in length.

The epididymis is considered to have three regions: the *caput* (head) at the upper pole of the testis, the *corpus* (body), and the *cauda* (tail) at its lower pole (Fig. 31–2). At the distal end of the cauda, the duct straightens and turns upward as the *ductus deferens*, which ascends in the spermatic cord to the ejaculatory duct in the pelvic cavity.

The epididymis is the site of accumulation, maturation, and storage of spermatozoa. When the spermatozoa leave the testis, they are physiologically immature, but during the 3–5 days that they are in transit through the caput and corpus of the epididymis, they acquire motility and the capacity to feritilize ova. The epithelium lining this organ is believed to contribute to their maturation.

The ductus epididymidis is lined by a pseudostratified columnar epithelium in which two types of cells, *principal cells* and *basal cells*, are easily distinguishable (Fig. 31–36). The principal cells are very tall in the caput, but they gradually decrease in height along the duct, becoming low columnar in the corpus and cuboidal in the cauda. The principal cells each have on their free surface a tuft of very long microvilli. Although these are as long as cilia, they are nonmotile and are commonly called *stereocilia* (Fig. 31–37). Like microvilli, they have in their interior an axial bundle of actin filaments that extends downward into a terminal web in the apical cytoplasm. The cell surface between stereocilia is quite irregular in contour with numerous invaginations, suggesting that these cells take up fluid from the lumen by pinocytosis. This is further indicated by the presence of numerous coated vesicles and larger multivesicular bodies in the apical cytoplasm. If an electron opaque particulate tracer is injected into the rete testis, it is taken into vacuoles and multivesicular bodies of the principal cells of the epididymal epithelium. It is now known that over 90% of the volume of fluid leaving the testis is absorbed in the ductuli efferentes and ductus epididymis.

The nuclei of the principal cells are somewhat irregular in outline and are situated in the lower third of the cell. The relatively small amount of heterochromatin occurs in small clumps adjacent to the nuclear envelope. The cytoplasm contains lysosomes that may be quite numerous and large in some species. These are visible with the light microscope and formerly were erroneously interpreted as secretory granules. These cells do, however,

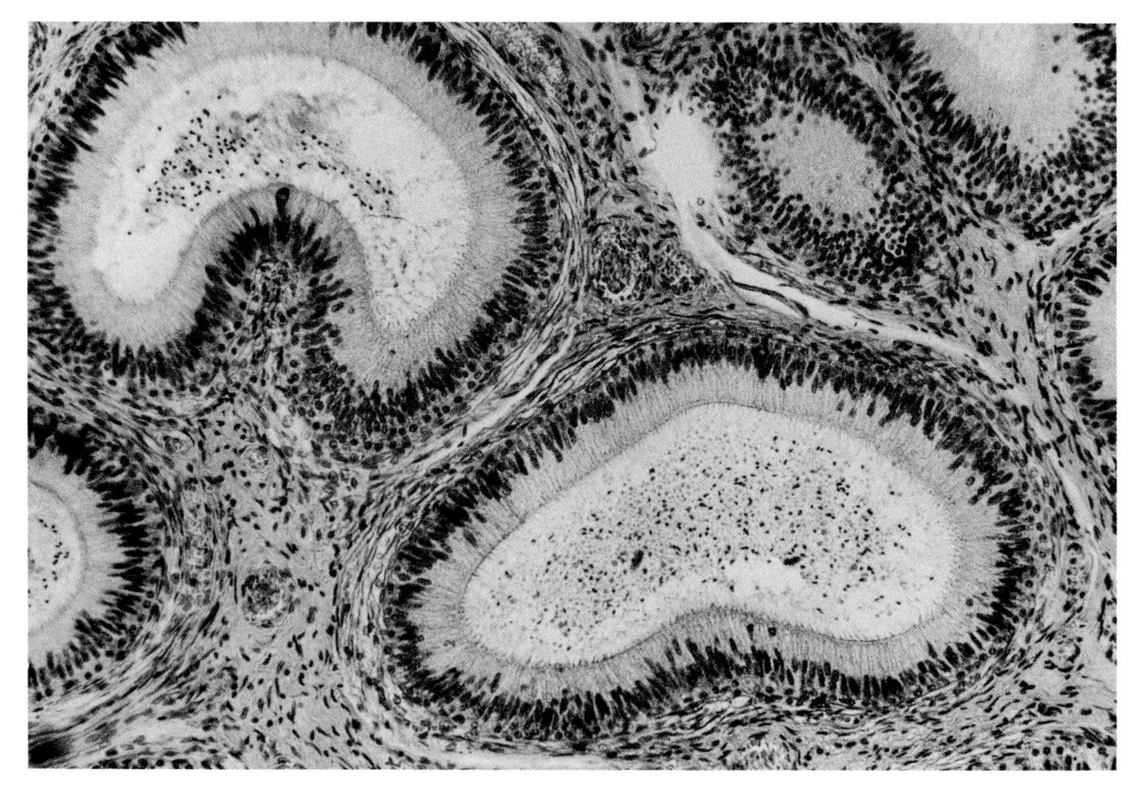

Figure 31–36. Histological section of the ductus epididymidis from an adult man. Many spermatozoa are visible in the lumen.

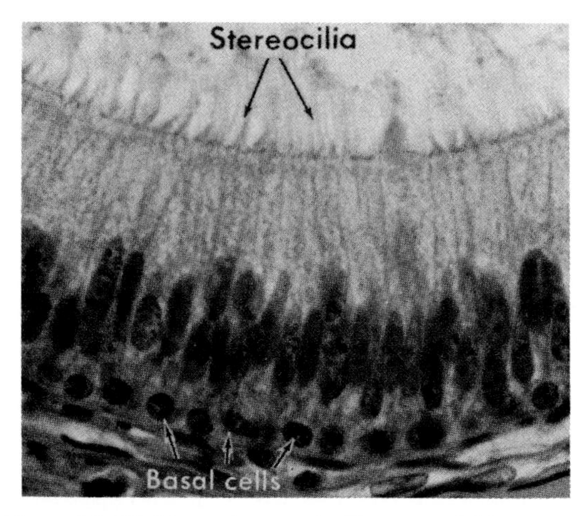

Figure 31–37. Photomicrograph of human epididymal epithelium showing the characteristic row of basal cells and the long tufts of stereocilia projecting into the lumen.

have some of the ultrastructural characteristics of secretory cells. Cisternae of rough endoplasmic reticulum are abundant in the basal cytoplasm and profiles of smooth or sparsely granulated reticulum are found in the apical cytoplasm. Some of these appear distended with a homogeneous content of low electron density. The supranuclear Golgi complex is one of the largest found anywhere in the body, but surprisingly it shows little ultrastructural evidence of being involved in segregation and packaging of a secretory product. However, it has been clearly established that these cells incorporate labeled amino acids and carbohydrate into a glycoprotein secretory product that is released into the lumen. It has also been shown that glycoproteins are adsorbed onto, and possibly incorporated into, the membrane of spermatozoa during their passage through the ductus epididymidis. It is now widely accepted that secretions of the principal cells are necessary for sperm maturation.

The second cell type of the epididymal epithelium is the *basal cell*. These are small rounded or pyramidal cells lodged between the bases of the columnar cells (Fig. 31–37). Their cytoplasm has little affinity for stains and is of low density in electron micrographs. The nucleus contains coarser clumps of marginated chromatin than does that of the principal cells. The cytoplasmic organelles are few.

Their surface may interdigitate extensively with the bases of neighboring principal cells. In their location, the basal cells resemble the stem cells of renewing epithelia, but there is no evidence that they have such a role here. Their function remains obscure.

Scattered among the principal cells are columnar cells of a different appearance that have been called *clear cells* because of their pale staining. They have few of the long stereocilia that are characteristic of the principal cells. The apical cytoplasm is crowded with small endocytic vesicles, and the basal cytoplasm contains numerous small lipid droplets. These aberrant columnar cells were formerly interpreted as principal cells in an inactive phase. Recent studies showing that they have greater endocytotic activity, a different glycoprotein content, and distinctive intramembrane particles in freeze–fracture preparations have suggested that they may be a distinct cell type. Their physiological significance is unknown.

External to the epithelium of the excurrent ducts there is a layer of contractile cells. From the ductuli efferentes to the ductus deferens, there is a gradual increase in the thickness of this coat and a change in ultrastructure of its cells. In the caput epididymidis, they are very slender and loosely organized in circumferential bundles. Myofilaments are inconspicuous in these slender cells. (Fig. 31–38A). In the corpus, sparse bundles of longitudinally and obliquely oriented cells form an incomplete outer layer. These cells are larger and they have the structure typical of smooth muscle fibers elsewhere in the body. Their numbers increase in the transition from the corpus to the cauda epididymidis where they form a more distinct and continuous second layer (Fig. 31–38B). In the distal portion of the cauda, an additional layer is added to form the three-layered muscle coat characteristic of the ductus deferens. The proximal segments of the duct system are very sparsely innervated, whereas the smooth muscle layers of the cauda and ductus deferens have a profuse adrenergic innervation.

Regional differences in motility of the duct system are correlated with these differences in cytology and organization of the musculature. In the caput and upper corpus where slender fibers with few myofilaments predominate, the ductus epididymidis exhibits rhythmic, perstaltic contractions that slowly move the spermatozoa along the tract. These contractions are largely independent of nervous stimulation because they continue when the duct is excised and maintained in vitro. Such spontaneous contractions are much reduced in the cauda, which is the principal site of sperm storage. The larger smooth muscle cells that predominate in this region evidently require adrenergic sympathetic nervous stimulation. The sympathetic nerve network increases in density in the cauda and reaches its maximum in the intrapelvic portion of the ductus deferens which undergoes powerful contractions that expel spermatozoa during the ejaculatory reflex.

DUCTUS DEFERENS

The *ductus deferens* (vas deferens), the spermatic artery, nerves, and pampiniform plexus of veins constitute the *spermatid cord.* The spermatic cord is surrounded by the *cremaster muscle* which consists of slender fascicles of striated muscle fibers that arise from the inguinal ligament and internal oblique muscle of the abdominal wall and form long loops that are incorporated in the connective tissue of the sac-like cremaster fascia in which the testes are suspended. Reflex contraction of the cremaster muscle in response to cold or fear raises the testes and is believed to have a protective and thermoregulatory function.

In the transition from the ductus epididymidis to the ductus deferens, the lumen widens and the wall thickens. The epithelium and its lamina propria form longitudinal folds that give the lumen a highly irregular outline in cross section (Fig. 31–40 and 31–41). The height of the pseudostratified columnar epithelium is lower and there is an extensive network of elastic fibers in underlying loose connective tissues. The muscular coat is 1 mm thick and consists of inner and outer layers of longitudinal smooth muscle and an intermediate circular layer. The muscle is enveloped in an adventitial layer of connective tissue. The thick-walled ductus deferens is palpable through the thin skin of the scrotum and is easily accessible for vasectomy in individuals desiring sterilization.

After crossing the ureter in the pelvic cavity, the ductus expands into a fusiform *ampulla.* In histological sections, numerous branching and intersecting folds of its mucosa give it a spurious appearance of compartmentation. Tortuous out-pocketings that arise between the folds extend some distance into the surrounding muscle and are lined by a low columnar epithelium of pale-staining secretory cells.

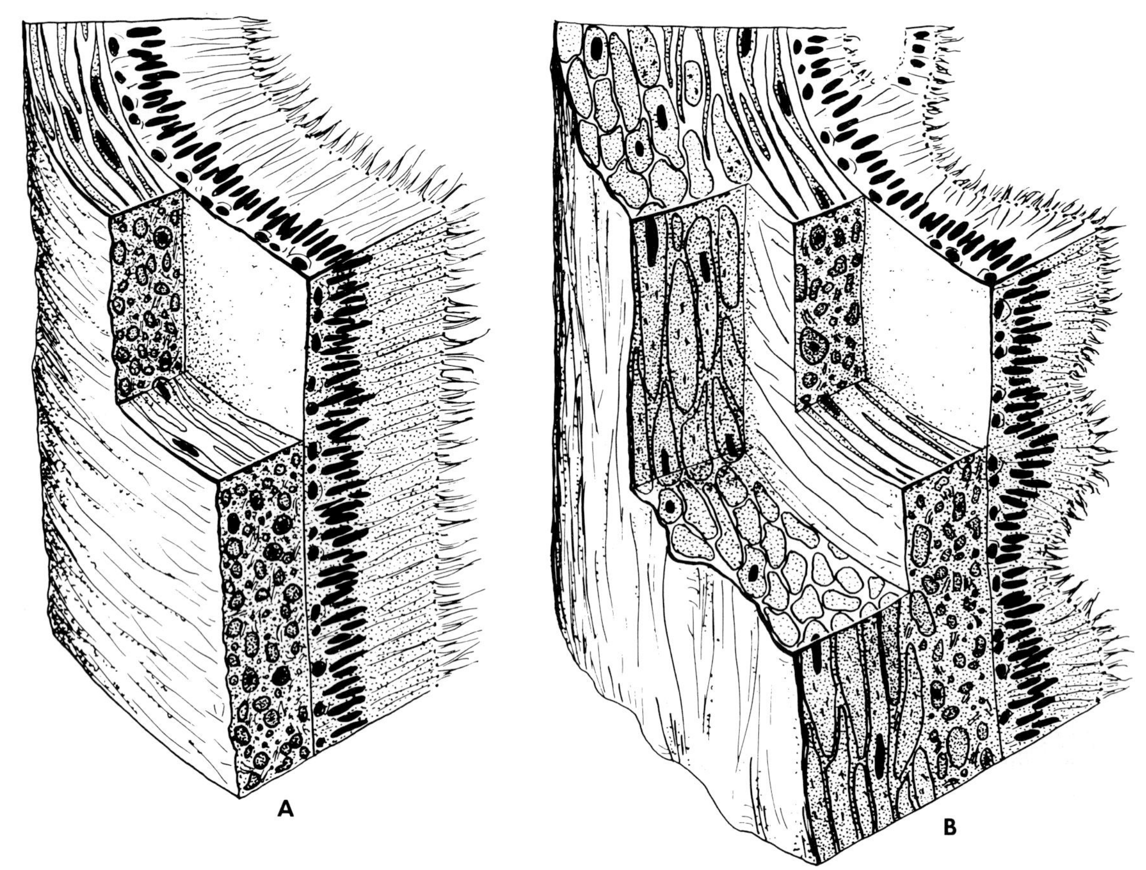

Figure 31–38. (A) Drawing showing the circumferentially oriented thin contractile cells underlying the epithelium of the initial portion of the ductus epididymidis. (B) Corresponding illustration of the transitional zone between the corpus and the cauda of the epididymis. Slender contractile cells are still found immediately subjacent to the epithelium, but peripheral to these, there are several rows of more typical, large smooth muscle cells. (From Baumgartner, H., A. Holstein, and E. Rosengren. 1971. Zellforsch. 120:37.)

EJACULATORY DUCTS

Lateral to the ampulla of each ductus deferens is a *seminal vesicle* and each ampulla is joined at its distal end by the duct of the corresponding seminal vesicle to form a short, straight *ejaculatory duct.* The ejaculatory ducts penetrate the prostate gland and open through a narrow slit onto a thickening of the posterior wall of the prostatic urethra called the *colliculus seminalis (verumontanum).* Between the openings of the ejaculatory ducts there is a blind invagination of the surface of the colliculus, the *utriculus masculinus*, which is the homologue of the uterus in the female.

The mucosa of the ejaculatory ducts forms folds projecting into the lumen and there are a number of small out-pocketings on the dorsomedial wall that resemble the seminal vesicles. The ducts are lined by a simple columnar epithelium, but near their termination, this becomes stratified taking on the characteristics of the transitional epithelium that lines the bladder and urethra.

ACCESSORY GLANDS OF THE MALE REPRODUCTIVE TRACT

SEMINAL VESICLES

The seminal vesicles are a pair of diverging saccular structures about 5 cm in length situated behind the neck of the bladder and between the ampullae of the ductus deferens, above, and the prostate gland, below. Their lower ends taper to a narrow straight duct that opens into the ampullae of the ductus deferens where these continue as the ejaculatory ducts. The wall of the vesicles is composed of a connective tissue capsule with an

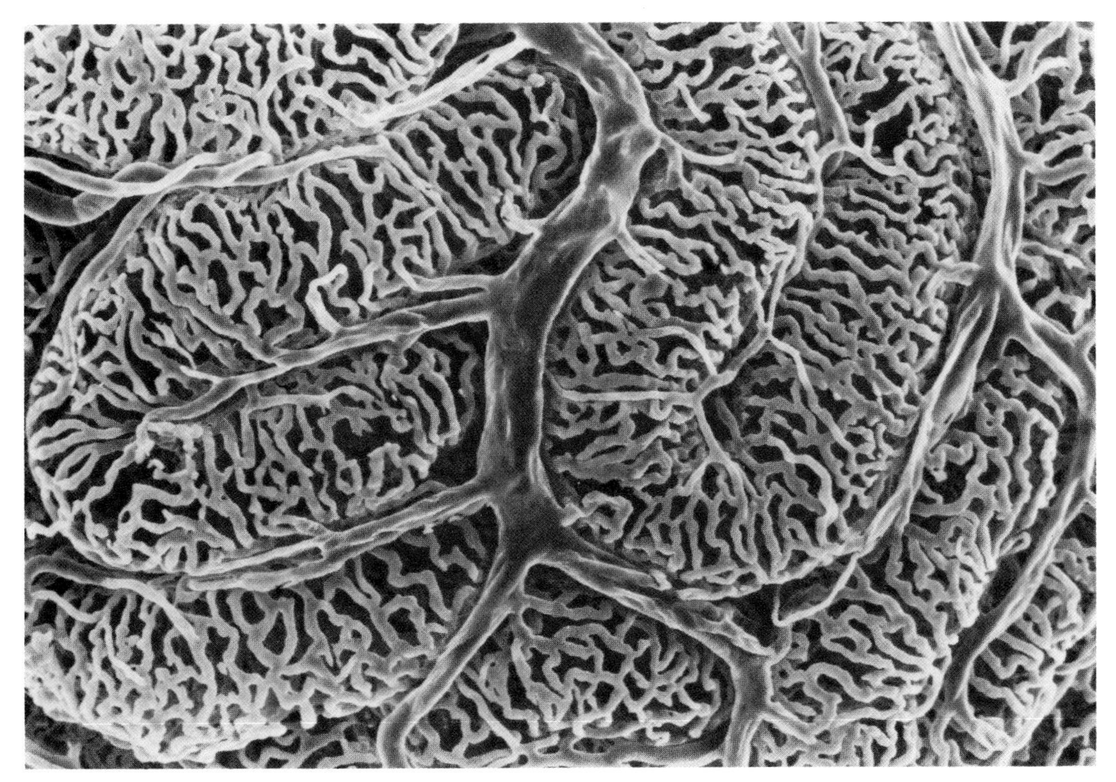

Figure 31–39. Scanning micrograph of a resinous cast of the vascular supply of the initial segment of the mouse epididymis. (Micrograph from Suzuki, F. 1982. Am. J. Anat. 163:309.

underlying layer of smooth muscle that is thinner than that of the ductus deferens. A plexus of sympathetic nerve fibers and small ganglia can be found in the vesicle wall.

Seminal vesicle structure can best be described as a coiled or convoluted tube with numerous diverticula along its length that result in a lumen of labyrinthine complexity. In sections, the mucosa forms thin folds from which secondary and tertiary folds project into the lumen, bounding narrow recesses that may give a spurious appearance of being cross sections of epithelium-lined tubules (Fig. 31–42). However, all of these recesses open into a wider central portion of the lumen. The pseudostratified epithelium consists of low columnar or cuboidal cells with smaller numbers of rounded cells between their bases. The surface of the epithelium bears sparse microvilli, and some of the cells have a single flagellum projecting into the lumen from a pair of centrioles in their apical cytoplasm. The cells contain numerous slender mitochondria, a well-developed granular endoplasmic reticulum, and abundant secretory granules. Small lipid droplets and aggregations of lipochrome pigment are commonly found in the basal cytoplasm. The pigment first appears at puberty, and in older adults may be sufficiently abundant to give the interior of the vesicles a brownish color in the fresh state.

As their name implies, the seminal vesicles were long thought to be reservoirs for the storage of semen. This is now known to be incorrect. Although their secretion accounts for the greater part of the volume of the ejaculate, spermatozoa are not normally found in their lumen. There are considerable species differences in the consistency of their secretion, but it is usually described as a clear, viscous, or gelatinous fluid.

PROSTATE GLAND

The prostate is the largest of the accessory glands of the male reproductive tract. Its secretion together with that of the seminal vesicles contributes to the volume of the ejaculate. The gland is about the size of a horse chestnut and surrounds the urethra at its origin from the urinary bladder. Dense connective tissue forms a thin capsule around the gland and extends into it as its stroma. Both capsule and

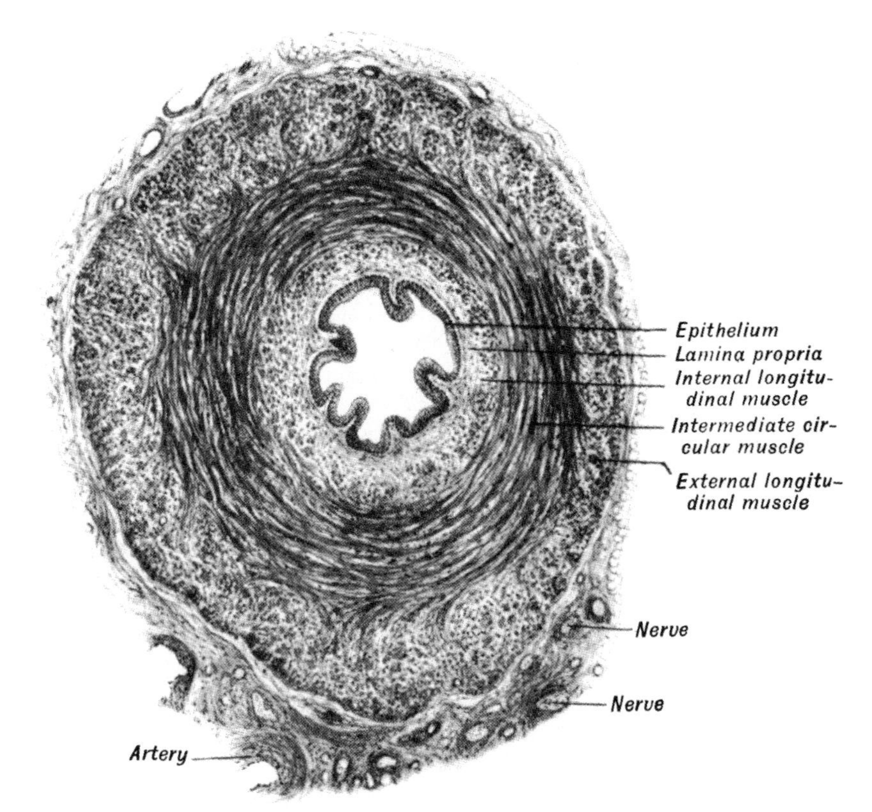

Figure 31–40. Cross section of the human ductus deferens (After J. Schaffer. Lehrbuch der Histologie und Histogenese, Verlag von W. Engelmann, 1922.)

the stroma contain smooth muscle as well as fibroblasts and collagen. Septa of this fibromuscular stroma radiate from the colliculus seminalis toward the capsule partioning the parenchyma into more-or-less distinct lobes.

Compound tubuloacinar glands, differing in length and degree of branching, are arranged in three concentric zones. Thirty to forty short glands immediately around the urethra discharge their secretion through separate openings on either side of the colliculus seminalis. These are called the *mucosal glands*. Peripheral to these is a zone of longer, branching *submucosal glands* that share a smaller number of ducts. Outside of these are the *main glands* that make up the greater part of the prostate (Fig. 31–43). For reasons that are not known, the mucosal and submucosal glands undergo hyperplasia in older men, producing adenomatous nodules that narrow the urethra—a condition called *nodular prostatic hyperplasia*. This disease has its onset at about 45 years of age and by the age of 80, 80% of men have varying degrees of obstruction of the bladder neck and urinary retention.

The tubuloacinar units of the gland are quite variable in form, being narrow in some places, wider in others, and sometimes having cystic dilatations. Branching folds or papillae of the mucosa project into the lumen (Fig. 31–44A). The epithelium is usually simple or pseudostratified columnar but may be reduced to low cuboidal or even squamous in dilated or cystic regions. The cells contain abundant rough endoplasmic reticulum, a conspicuous Golgi complex, and numerous secretory granules. The secretion of the prostate contains acid phosphatase, amylase, and fibrinolysin.

Ovoid or spherical bodies called *corpora amylacea* or *prostatic concretions* are often found in the lumen of the glands (Fig. 31–44B). These are glycoprotein in composition but may become a site of calcium deposition. They are more common in the prostate of older men. Their significance is not known.

BULBOURETHRAL GLANDS

The paired bulbourethral glands (Cowper's glands), partially embedded in the muscle of

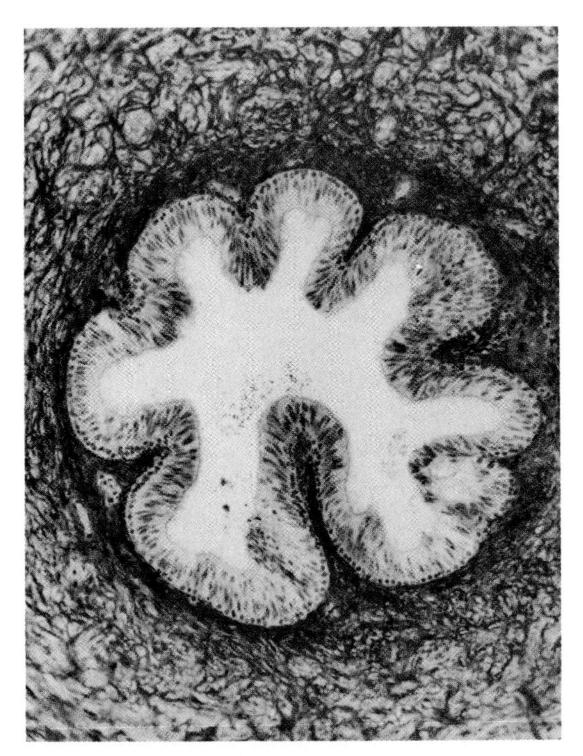

Figure 31–41. Histological section of the human ductus deferens showing its irregular lumen, pseudostratified epithelium, lamina propria, and surrounding bundles of smooth muscle. (Micrograph courtesy of A. Hoffer.)

the urogenital diaphragm, are compound tubuloalveolar glands less than 1 cm in diameter (Fig. 31–45). Each opens by a single duct into the floor of the proximal portion of the cavernous urethra. Their secretion is emitted at the onset of ejaculation and makes a small contribution to the initial fraction of the semen.

The glands consist of branched and contorted tubules whose blind ends are often dilated to form alveoli. The tubules comprising the small lobules of the gland converge on wider channels called ampullae. The duct arises from confluence of the ampullae of the several lobules. Prominent connective tissue partitions between the lobules contain collagenous and elastic fibers and both striated and smooth muscle fibers. Some of the latter extend into the lobules.

The glandular epithelium is quite variable in appearance. In the alveoli, the cells are cuboidal, whereas in the tubules, they are pyramidal or low columnar. Their nuclei are irregular in outline and displaced toward the base by the large number of secretory droplets in the apical cytoplasm. There is a prominent Golgi complex, a moderate number of short profiles of endoplasmic reticulum, and a few lipid droplets near the nucleus. The abundant secretory droplets have the staining properties of an acidic mucin. In electron micrographs, they are electron-lucent but may include an eccentrically placed spherical area of greater density. Closely associated with the secretory droplets near the nucleus are a few membrane-bounded spindle-shaped inclusions that have a content of parallel fine fibrils. Coalescence of these fibrillar bodies with the secretory droplets has been reported and it is suggested that their content is secreted with the mucus. Similar filamentous inclusions have been described in the mucous cells of human Bartholin glands, urethral glands, and in the salivary glands. Their nature and exact relationship to mucus secretion remain unknown. Nerve endings containing both clear and dense-cored vesicles occupy recesses in the base of the secretory cells of the gland.

The small ducts and ampullae are lined by cuboidal or columnar epithelial cells. Their lumenal surface is irregular and bears short microvilli. The basolateral surfaces are corrugated and interdigitate with similar irregularities on adjacent cells. Patches of mucous cells in the epithelium are not uncommon. In addition, there are a few cells that contain in their apical cytoplasm limited numbers of electron-dense secretory granules resembling those of serous cells. Such cells have also been described in the ducts of von Ebner's glands and in Bartholin's glands in the female. The chemical nature of their product is unknown. The larger excretory ducts of the bulbourethral gland are lined by pseudostratified epithelium resembling that of the urethra but, here too, patches of mucous cells may be found.

The secretion of the bulbourethral glands in the human is a clear, mucus-like, viscous fluid that, on contact, can be drawn out into a long thin thread. It is thought to have a lubricant function. Unlike true mucus, it does not form a precipitate with acetic acid. In the boar, the secretion is extremely viscous and rubbery and is believed to play an important role in the gelation of the seminal plasma that takes place soon after ejaculation in this species.

HISTOPHYSIOLOGY OF DUCTS AND ACCESSORY GLANDS

On leaving the testis, the spermatozoa are nonmotile and incapable of fertilization. As

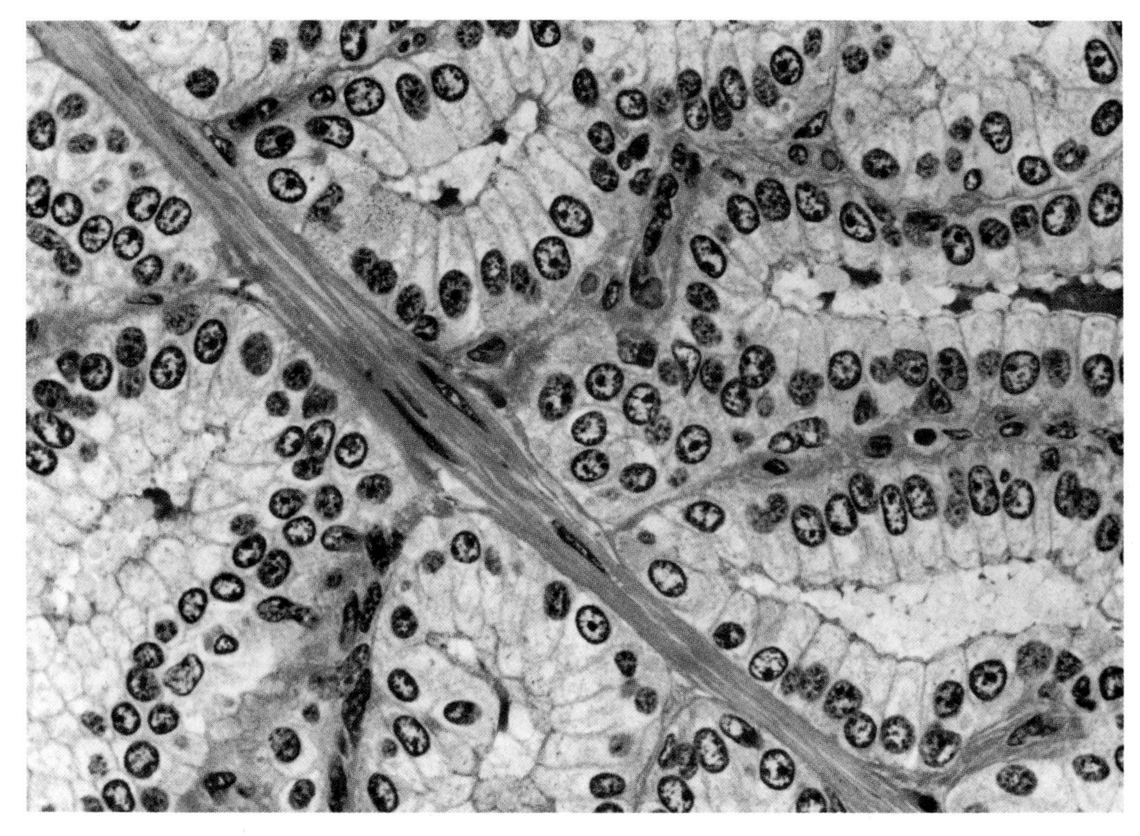

Figure 31–42. Photomicrograph of a section of monkey seminal vesicle.

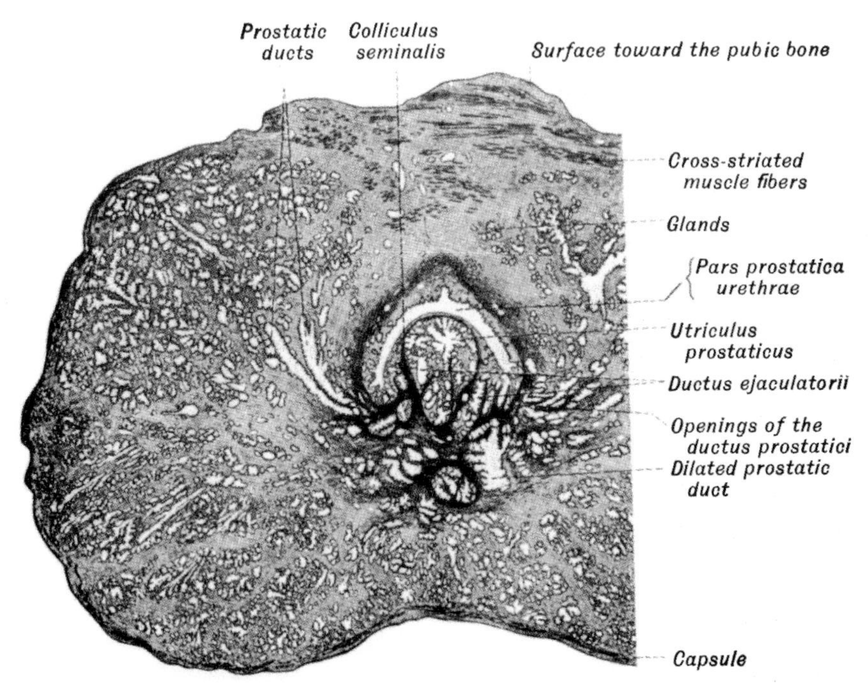

Figure 31–43. A cross section through the human prostate showing its relation to the urethra and the openings of the ejaculatory ducts on the utriculus prostaticus. (After H. Braus Lehrbuch der Anatomie. Vol II. Berlin, 1924)

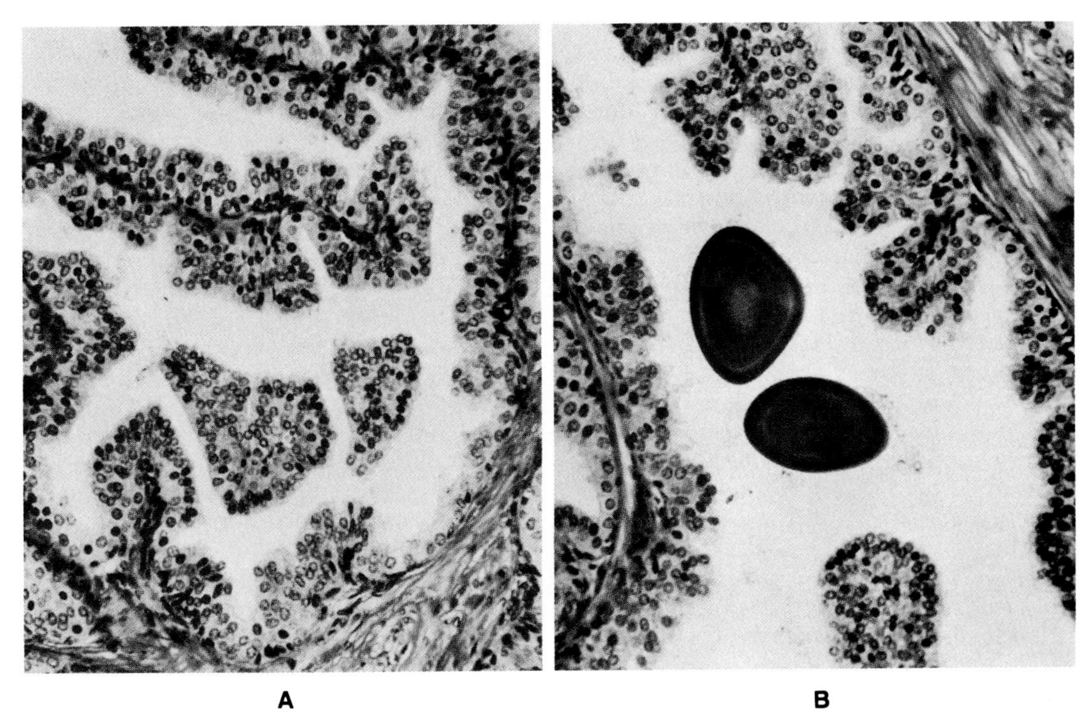

Figure 31–44. Photomicrograph of human prostate. (A) Branching folds of mucosa projecting into the lumen of the tubuloacinar units. (B) Two corpora amylacea in the lumen.

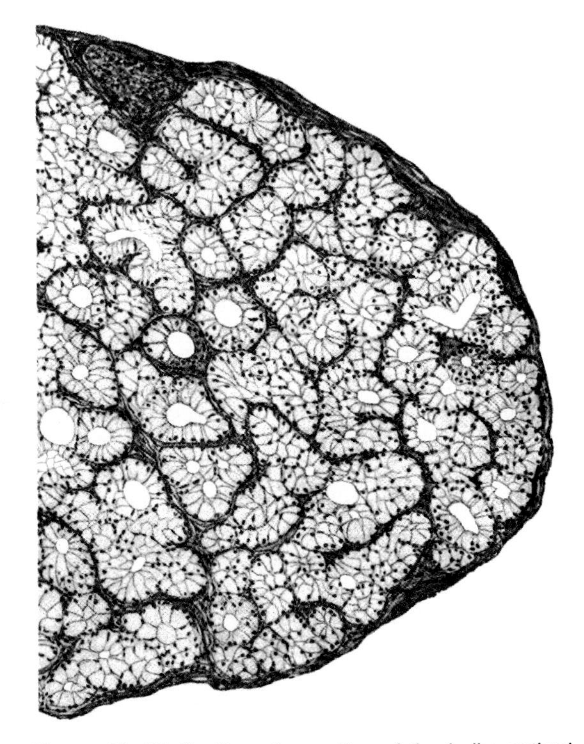

Figure 31–45. Section of a portion of the bulbourethral gland of a 23-year-old man. (Slightly modified after H. Stieve in W. von Möllendorff, Handbuch der Mikroskopischen Anatomie des Menschen, Vol. VII. Verlag von J. Springer. Berlin, 1930.)

they pass through the epididymis, they undergo biochemical and minor morphological modifications and gradually acquire fertilizing capacity. These changes appear to depend on the specific environment maintained in the lumen of the ductus epididymidis by the secretory activity of its epithelium. The functions of the epididymis are controlled by testosterone secreted by the Leydig cells of the testis and carried downstream in the duct system, bound to androgen-binding protein secreted by the Sertoli cells. Few of the secretory products of the epididymal epithelium have been identified and how these influence sperm maturation is largely unknown. Spermatozoa are moved along the tract by continued production of testicular fluid, the beating of the cilia in the ductuli efferentes, and the shallow peristaltic contractions of the ductus epididymidis. The duct is more quiescent in the cauda of the epididymis where the sperm are stored. The thick muscular wall of the ductus deferens is of primary importance in expulsion of the spermatozoa during emission.

The urethral glands of Littré and the bulbourethral glands produce a small volume of slippery secretion that is believed to have a lubricating function. These glands are the first to be activated during sexual arousal, their secretion appearing as clear droplets at the urethral meatus of the erect penis. The secretions of the other accessory glands are believed to be discharged in a definite sequence during emission. The fibromuscular capsule and stroma of the prostrate contract expelling its secretion into the urethra. Prostatic fluid has a stimulating effect on the progressive motility of the spermatozoa which are discharged concurrently from the ductus deferens. Finally, the viscous secretion of the seminal vesicles is added and makes a major contribution to the volume of the ejaculate. It is rich in fructose which is the principal carbohydrate of the semen and serves as an energy source for sperm motility. It also contains a small amount of a yellowish flavin pigment that gives the semen a strong fluorescence in ultraviolet light—a property useful in medicolegal detection of semen stains. Evidence for sequential release of the products of the accessory glands comes from analysis of split ejaculates in humans and is strongly supported by studies on rodents in which the abundant secretion of the seminal vesicles is coagulated by an enzyme in the prostatic fluid, forming a solid plug in the vagina that occludes its lumen and prevents the escape of the foregoing fluid components of the semen.

Thus, the semen is a mixture of the suspension of spermatozoa ejected from the ampulla of the ductus deferens and the secretions of the bulbourethral glands, prostate, and seminal vesicles. In addition to spermatozoa, it contains occasional epithelial cells exfoliated from the lining of the tract, minute droplets of cytoplasm of degenerating cells, lipid droplets, and small corpora amylacea from the prostate. The average volume of the human ejaculate is about 3 ml. The spermatozoa, numbering from 200 to 300 million, account for less than 10% of its volume.

FERTILIZATION

The *maturation* of spermatozoa during their transit through the epididymis and the *activation* of their motility by secretions of the accessory glands have already been mentioned. After ejaculation, their motility becomes more vigorous and their capacity for fertilization is enhanced during their transit through the uterus and oviducts to the ovum. These changes occurring in the female reproductive tract are called *capacitation.*

At the site of fertilization, the spermatozoa become associated with the thick extracellular coating of the ovum called the *zone pellucida.* Egg-binding protein constituents of the plasma membrane covering the sperm head then become bound to sperm receptors on the zona pellucida. These receptors are species-specific and, thus, prevent interspecific fertilization. The zone pellucida is composed of three glycoproteins that have been designated ZP1, ZP2, and ZP3. These are assembled into 7-nm filaments composed of ZP2 and ZP3 cross-linked by molecules of ZP1 to form a porous coat around the ovum 10–14 μm thick. The sperm receptors are oligosaccharide side chains on ZP3. Binding of a spermatozoon to these receptors induces it to undergo the *acrosome reaction.* The plasma membrane covering the anterior portion of the sperm head fuses at many sites with the underlying outer acrosomal membrane, creating openings through which the enzyme-rich content of the acrosome flows out and digests a passageway through the zona. When the vigorously motile spermatozoon has made its way through this opening and into the perivitelline space, the intact plasma membrane behind the acrosome fuses with the egg membrane, permitting the sperm to sink into the ooplasm to complete fertilization. This event triggers the *cortical reaction* in which the limiting membrane of thousands of cortical granules in the peripheral cytoplasm of the ovum fuse with the egg membrane, releasing their enzymes into the perivitelline space. These enzymes are believed to alter the structure of ZP3 in such a way as to destroy its sperm-receptor activity and prevent binding and entry of other spermatozoa.

THE PENIS

The penis is formed of three cylindrical bodies made up of cavernous erectile tissue, namely the two *corpora cavernosa* and the unpaired *corpus spongiosum (corpus cavernosum urethrae)* (Fig. 31–46). The corpora cavernosa, arising from the ascending rami of the pubis, converge at the pubic angle and adhere side to side. From there they run together to their conical distal ends, forming the dorsal two-thirds of the shaft of the penis. On the upper surface of the penis, there is a shallow groove occupied by the dorsal artery and vein. Between the lower surfaces of the corpora cavernosa there is a deeper groove occupied by the corpus cavernosum urethrae. The *penile urethra* runs longitudinally through the corpus

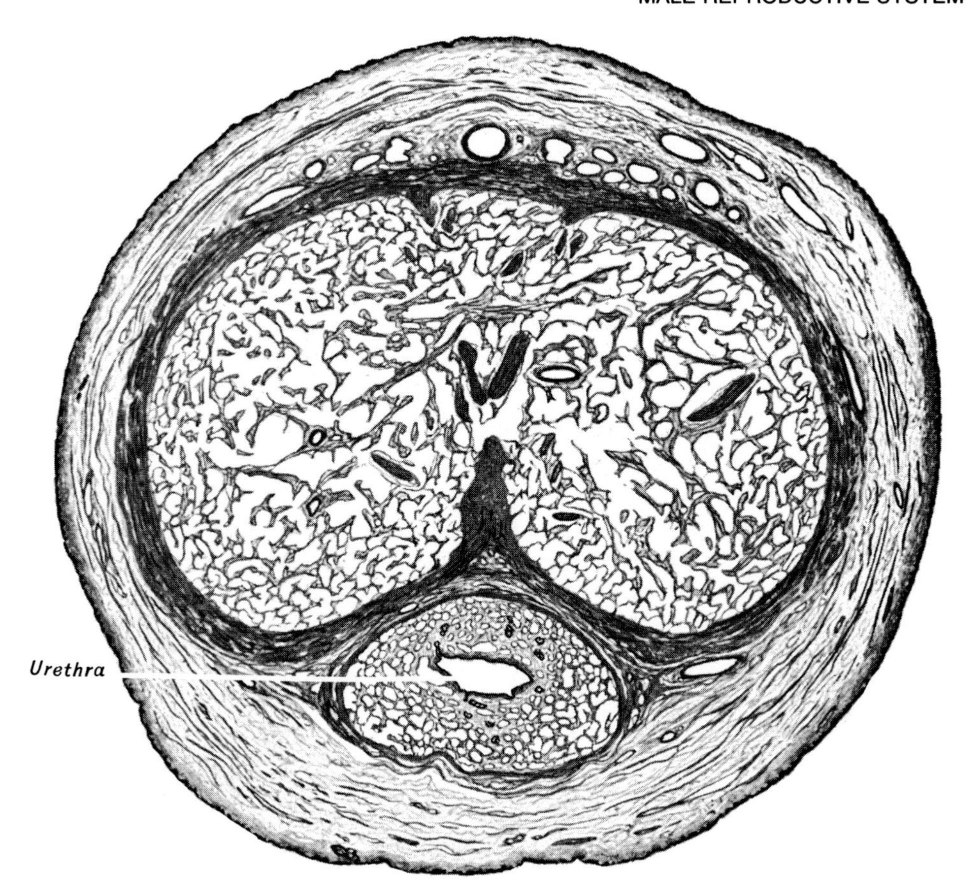

Figure 31–46. Cross section of the penis of a 21-year-old man. The medial septum between the corpora cavernosa penis is incomplete in this figure because the section is from the distal part of the organ. (Slightly modified from H. Stieve in W. von Möllendorff, Handbuch der Mikroskopischen Anatomie des Menschen, Vol. VII. Verlag von J. Springer. Berlin, 1930.)

cavernosum urethrae, which ends in an acorn-shaped expansion, the *glans penis*. On the posterior aspect of the glans penis, there are two concavities that cap the conical ends of the two corpora cavernosa penis.

The erectile tissue of the corpora cavernosa is a sponge-like system of irregularly shaped vascular spaces fed by afferent arteries and drained by efferent veins. In the flaccid penis, these cavernous spaces contain very little blood and appear as irregular narrow clefts. During erection, they expand as they become engorged with blood under pressure. The increased inflow of blood and relative restriction of outflow results in enlargement and rigidity of the erect penis. The three cavernous bodies making up the shaft of the penis are surrounded by a thick, fibrous capsule, the *tunica albuginea*. In the flaccid penis, the tunica is about 2 mm in thickness, but in erection, it is reduced to about 0.5 mm. Its bundles of collagen fibers are arranged mainly longitudinally in its outer layer and circularly in its inner portion. In the flaccid state, the collagen fiber bundles have a wavy course, but they straighten out during erection to accommodate the considerable increase in volume of the corpora cavernosa. Elastic fibers are relatively sparse. The few elastic fibers in the tunica may play a role in the recoil of the collagen bundles to their wavy course.

The tunica albuginea also forms a fibrous partition between the two corpora cavernosa. In the distal half of the shaft, this septum is fenestrated so that the cavernous spaces of the two corpora communicate. Dense fibrous trabeculae extend inward from the tunica albuginea, branching and rejoining to form an elaborate framework around the vascular spaces of the corpora cavernosa. This meshwork is continuous with a dense connective tissue sheath that surrounds the deep artery which is centrally located in each corpus. Thin bundles of smooth muscle fibers run longitudinally in the sheath of the central artery and in the trabecular meshwork throughout the corpus and insert on the inner aspect of the tunica albuginea. The abundance of smooth muscle in the organ has not been fully appreciated, but recent studies indicate that it is the predominant constituent of the parenchyma of the corpora cavernosa.

The central artery of the corpora gives off helicine arteries that course through the trabeculae, terminating in end arteries that open into the cavernous spaces. These spaces are largest in the central portion of the corpora and gradually diminish in size toward the cavernous venules on the inner aspect of the tunica albuginea. These veins are continuous with larger veins that penetrate the tunica to join circumflex veins that are tributaries of the deep dorsal vein of the penis.

The tunica albuginea of the corpus cavernosum urethrae is much thinner than that of the corpora cavernosa penis and it contains circularly arranged smooth muscle cells in its inner layer. It also contains elaborate networks of elastic fibers. The vascular spaces, unlike those of the corpora cavernosa, are of the same size throughout. The trabeculae between them contain abundant elastic fibers, but smooth muscle fibers are relative few. The cavernous spaces communicate with a venous plexus beneath the urethral mucosa.

The glans penis consists of dense connective tissue containing a plexus of large anastomosing veins with both circular and longitudinal smooth muscle in their walls. The longitudinal strands of smooth muscle often bulge into the lumen.

The skin covering the penis is thin and provided with an abundant subcutaneous layer containing some smooth muscle. It is devoid of adipose tissue. The skin is devoid of hair and has only a very limited number of sweat glands. The glans is covered by a fold of skin called the *prepuce*. The dermis of the skin of the glans penis is fused with the deeper dense connective tissue of the glans. In this region, there are peculiar sebaceous glands, *glands of Tyson*, which are not associated with hairs. They show great variations in number and distribution.

MECHANISM OF ERECTION

Erection of the penis is controlled by complex neural pathways activated by both psychic and tactile stimuli. Reflex erection results from afferent sensory input carried via the pudendal nerve to the spinal cord, where vasomotor impulses are generated in parasympathetic fibers of the nervi erigentes. These produce vasodilatation of the arteries of the penis, filling the cavernous spaces in the corpora cavernosa and thereby causing erection. In addition to this simple reflex arc, there is a thoracolumbar pathway that can be activated by psychic stimuli including memory and imagination as well as visual input to the cerebral cortex. Higher neural centers appear to control vasodilator fibers originating in thoracic sympathetic ganglia. These can cause erection independently of tactile reflex stimulation. An adrenergic nerve supply to the corpora from sacrococcygeal sympathetic ganglia is believed to be involved in the vasoconstriction that results in detumescence.

The hemodynamics of erection continues to be a subject of debate. There is general agreement that erection involves rapid filling of the corpora following vasodilatation of the deep arteries and their helicine branches, accompanied by relaxation of the intrinsic smooth muscle of the parenchyma. A majority of investigators believe that this is sufficient to explain erection and experiment evidence, obtained mainly in dogs, seems to support this view. Others believe that there must also be constriction of venous outflow. Noninvasive measurements of intracavernosal pressure, in man, during erection indicate that it is several times higher than sytolic blood pressure. It is argued that because the helicine arteries open mainly into the larger axial cavernous spaces, the expansion of these may compress the smaller peripheral spaces and the thin-walled veins underlying the relatively unyielding tunica adventitia. The outflow of blood would, thus, be throttled down as blood accumulates in the corpora under increasing pressure. Contraction of the intrinsic smooth muscle is also thought to contribute to the high intracavernous pressure and rigidity of the erect penis. In further support of the concept of restriction of outflow is the observation that the walls of the circumflex veins are unusually muscular. Moreover, these vessels consistently exhibit specializations of their intima called *polsters* (Fig. 31–47). These are local accumulations of fibroblasts and smooth muscle cells that form longitudinal ridges that can be followed through hundreds of serial sections. These are believed to have a role in constricting the lumen and retarding venous outflow during erection.

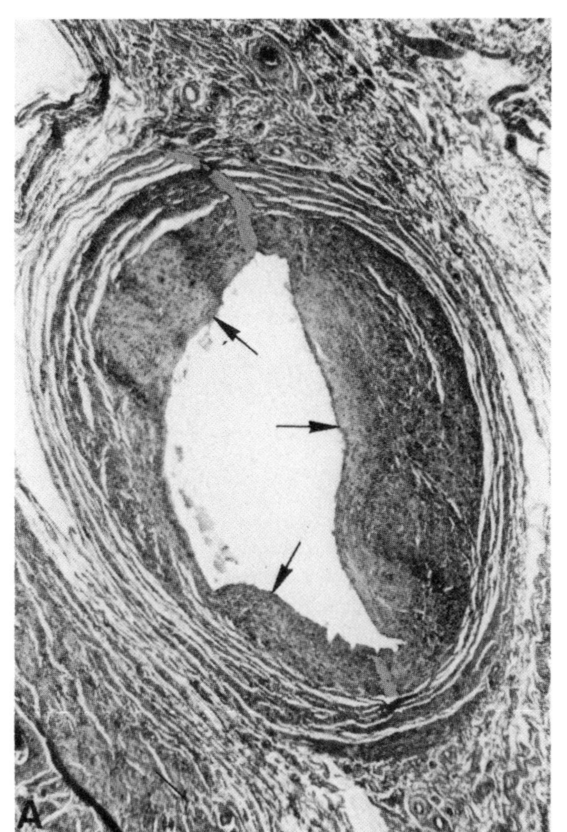

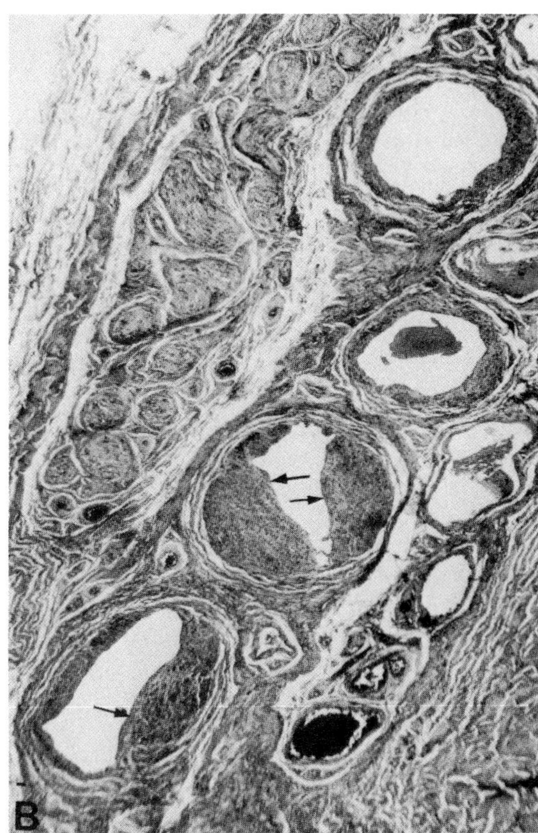

Figure 31–47. Photomicrographs of cross-sectioned specialized veins of the penis that some believe to be involved in the hemodynamics of erection. (A) Section through a circumflex vein at the proximal end of the corpora cavernosa of a 68-year-old man, showing (at arrows) thick muscular polsters. (B) Sections of circumflex veins near the distal end of the corpora cavernosa. The polsters are indicated by arrows. (Photomicrographs from Goldstein, A.M.B., et al. 1982. Urology 20:259.)

NERVES OF THE PENIS

The nerves of the penis come from the sacral plexus via the pudendal nerve and from the pelvic sympathetic system. Branches of the pudendal nerve supply the bulbocavernosus muscle and other striated muscles associated with the penis and also provides sensory nerve endings in the skin and the urethral mucosa. Free nerve endings can be demonstrated in the epithelium of the glans, the prepuce, and the urethra. There are also free nerve endings in the subepithelial connective tissue of the skin. In addition, there are numerous encapsulated nerve endings of various kinds. *Corpuscles of Meissner* are found in the papillae of the skin of the prepuce and glans; *genital corpuscles* are located in the deeper layers of the stratum papillare of the dermis of the glans and in the mucosa of the urethra; and *corpuscles of Vater Pacini* occur along the dorsal vein, in the deeper connective tissue of the glans, and under the tunica albuginea of the corpora cavernosa. The sympathetic nerve plexuses are connected to smooth muscle of the blood vessels and form extensive unmyelinated nerve networks among the smooth muscle bundles of the trabeculae in the corpora cavernosa.

BIBLIOGRAPHY

Bardin, C.W. and R.J. Scherins, eds. 1982. Cell biology of the testis. Ann. N.Y. Acad. Sci. 383:1 New York. Academy of Science, New York

DeKretser, D.M. and J.F. Kerr. 1988. The cytology of the testis. *In* E. Knobil et al., eds. Physiology of Reproduction p. 121 New York, Raven Press.

Hamilton, D.W. and F. Naftolin. 1982. Basic Reproductive Medicine, Vol. 2. Reproductive Function in Men. Cambridge, MA, MIT Press.

SPERMATOZOA

Bedford, J.M. 1970. Sperm capacitation and fertilization in mammals. Biol. Reprod. (Suppl.) 2:128.

Bishop, D. 1962. Sperm motility. Physiol. Rev. 42:1.
Bleil, D. and S.S. Howards. 1980. Mammalian sperm–egg interaction: Identification of a glycoprotein in mouse egg zona pellucida possessing receptor activity for sperm. Cell 20:873.
Fawcett, D.W. 1970. A comparative view of sperm ultra structure. Biol. Reprod. (Suppl 2) 2:90.
Fawcett, D.W. 1975. The mammalian spermatozoon. Develop. Biol. 44:394.
Florman, H.M. 1985. O-Linked oligosaccharides of mouse egg ZP-3 account for its sperm receptor activity. Cell 41:313.
Friend, D.S. and D.W. Fawcett. 1974. Membrane differentiations in freeze-fractured mammalian sperm. J. Cell Biol. 63:466.
Friend, D.S., L. Orci, A. Perrelet, and Y. Yanagimachi. 1977. Membrane particle changes attending the acrosome reaction in guinea pig spermatozoa. J. Cell Biol. 74:561.
Parrish, R.F. and K.L. Polakoski. 1979. Mammalian sperm pro-acrosin-acrosin system. Internat. J. Biochem. 10:391.
Soupart, P. and L.L. Morgenstern. 1973. Human sperm capacitation and in vitro fertilization. Fertil. Steril. 24:462.
Wasserman, F.M. 1987. Early events in mammalian fertilization. Annu. Rev. Cell Biol. 3:109.
Wasserman, F.M. 1987. The biology and chemistry of fertilization. Science 235:553.
Zamboni, L., R. Zemjanis, and M. Stefanini. 1971. The fine structure of monkey and human spermatozoa. Anat. Rec. 169:129.
Zamboni, L. 1992. Sperm structure and its relevance to infertility: an electron microscope study. Arch. Pathol. Lab. Med. 116:325.

SEMINIFEROUS EPITHELIUM

Clermont, Y. 1963. The cycle of the seminiferous epithelium in man. Am. J. Anat. 112:135.
Clermont, Y. 1966. Renewal of spermatogonia in man. Am. J. Anat. 118:509.
Clermont, Y. 1972. Kinetics of spermatogenesis in mammals. Seminiferous epithelium cycle and spermatogonial renewal. Physiol. Rev. 52:198.
DeKretser, D.M., J.B. Kerr, and C.A. Paulsen. 1975. Peritubular tissue in the normal and pathological human testis. Biol. Reprod. 12:317.
Dym, M. 1973. The fine structure of the monkey Sertoli cell and its role in maintaining the blood-testis barrier. Anat. Rec. 175:639.
Dym, M. and D.W. Fawcett. 1970. The blood-testis barrier in the rat and the physiological compartmentation of the seminiferous epithelium. Biol. Reprod. 3:309.
Dym, M. and D.W. Fawcett. 1971. Further observations on the numbers of spermatogonia, spermatocytes, and spermatids connected by intercellular bridges in the mammalian testis. Biol. Reprod. 4:195.
Fawcett, D.W. 1975. The ultrastructure and functions of the Sertoli cell. *In* D.W. Hamilton and R.O. Greep, eds. Handbook of Physiology: Endocrinology, Vol. 5, Sect. 7, Male Reproductive System. Washington, DC, American Physiological Society.
Fawcett, D.W. and D.M. Phillips. 1969. Observations on the release of spermatozoa and on changes in the head during passage through the epididymis. J. Reprod. Fertil. (Suppl.) 6:405.
Flickinger, C.J. and D.W. Fawcett. 1970. The junctional specializations of Sertoli cells in the seminiferous epithelium. Anat. Rec. 158:207.
Gilula, N.B., D.W. Fawcett, and A. Aoki. 1976. The Sertoli cell occluding junctions and gap junctions in mature and developing mammalian testis. Devel. Biol. 50:142.
Setchell, B.P. 1980. The functional significance of the blood-testis barrier. J. Androl. 1:3.
Tindall, D.J. et al. 1985. Structure and biochemistry of the Sertoli cell. Internat. Rev. Cytol. 94:127.
Ying, S.Y. 1988. Inhibins, activins, and follistatins gonadal proteins modulating the secretion of follicle stimulating hormone. Endocrine Rev. 9:267.

INTERSTITIAL TISSUE

Christensen, A.K. 1975. Leydig cells. *In* Hamilton, D.W. and R.O. Greep, eds. Handbook of Physiology: Endocrinology, Vol. 5, Sect. 7, Male Reproductive System. Washington, DC, American Physiological Society.
Christensen, A.K. 1965. The fine structure of the testicular interstitial cells of the guinea pig. J. Cell Biol. 26:911.
Fawcett, D.W., W.B. Neaves, and N.M. Flores. 1973. Comparative observations on the intertubular lymphatics and the organization of interstitial tissue of the mammalian testis. Biol. Reprod. 9:500.
Kaler, L.W., and W.B. Neaves. 1978. Attrition of the human Leydig cell population with advancing age. Anat. Rec. 192:513.
Mori, H. and A.K. Christensen. 1980. Morphometric analysis of Leydig cells in the normal testis. J. Cell Biol. 84:340.

BLOOD VESSELS AND LYMPHATICS

Fawcett, D.W., P. Heidger, and L.V. Leak. 1969. Lymph vascular system of the interstitial tissues of the testis as revealed by electron microscopy. J. Reprod. Fertil. 19:109.
Kormano, M. and H. Suoranta. 1971. Microvascular organization of the adult human testis. Anat. Rec. 170:31.
Suzuki, F. and T. Nagano. 1986. Microvasculature of the human testis and excurrent duct system. Cell Tissue Res. 243:79.

EXCRETORY DUCTS OF THE TESTIS

Dym, M. 1976. The mammalian rete testis—a morphological examination. Anat. Rec. 186:493.
Flickinger, C.J. 1983. Synthesis and secretion of glycoprotein by the epididymal epithelium. J. Androl. 4:157.
Flickinger, C.J., S.S. Howard, and H.F. English. 1978. Ultrastructural differences in efferent ducts and several regions of the epididymis of the hamster. Am. J. Anat. 152:557.
Hoffer, A., D.W. Hamilton, and D.W. Fawcett. 1973. Ultrastructure of the principal cells and intraepithelial leukocytes in the initial segment of the rat epididymis. Anat. Rec. 175:169.
Jones, R.D., D.W. Hamilton, and D.W. Fawcett. 1979. Morphology of the rete testis, ductuli efferentes, and ductus epididymidis of the rabbit. Am. J. Anat. 156:373.
Nagano, T. and F. Suzuki. 1983. Cell junctions in the seminiferous tubule and the excurrent ducts of the testis. Internat. Rev. Cytol. 81:163.
Nicander, L. 1958. Studies on the regional histology and cytochemistry of the ductus epididymis in stallions, rams, and bulls. Acta. Morphol. Neerl. Scand. i:337.
Olsen, G.E. and B.J. Danzo. 1981. Surface changes in

rat spermatozoa during epididymal maturation. Biol. Reprod. 24:431.

Orgebin-Crist, M.C. and S. Fournier-Delpech. 1982. Sperm-egg interaction. Evidence for maturational changes during epididymal transit. J. Androl. 3:429.

Sun, E.L. and C.J. Flickinger. 1980. Morphological characteristics of cells with apical nuclei in the initial segment of the rat epididymis. Anat. Rec. 196:285.

ACCESSORY GLANDS OF MALE REPRODUCTION

Brandes, D., D. Kirchheim, and W.W. Scott. 1964. Ultrastructure of the human prostate:normal and neoplastic. Lab. Investig. 13:1541.

Harbitz, T.B. and O.A. Haugen. 1972. Histology of the prostate in elderly men. Acta Pathol. Microbiol. Scand. (Sect. A) 80:756.

Hellgren, L., E. Mylius, and J. Vincent. 1982. The ultrastructure of the human bulbourethral gland. J. Submicros. Cytol. 14:683.

McNeal, J.E. 1973. The prostate and prostatic urethra—a morphological synthesis. J. Urol. 197:1008.

Riva, A., P. Sirigu, F. Testa-Riva, and E. Usai. 1981. Fine structure and histochemistry of the epithelial cells of human bulbourethral glands. Acta Anat. 11:125.

Riva, A., E. Usai, M. Cossu, R. Scarpa, and F. Testa-Riva. 1988. The human bulbourethral glands. A transmission electron microscopy and scanning electron microscopy study. Andrology 9:133.

PENIS

Goldstein, A.M., J.P. Meehan, R. Zachary, P.A. Buckley, and F.A. Rogers. 1982. New observations on the microarchitecture of the corpora cavernosa in man and their possible relationship to the mechanism of erection. Urology 21:259.

McConnell, J., C.S. Benson, and W.A. Schmidt. 1982. The vasculature of the human penis: a reexamination of the morphological basis for the polster theory of erection. Anat. Rec. 203:475.

Meehan, J.P. and A.M.B. Goldstein. 1983. High pressure within the corpus cavernosum in man during erection. Its probable mechanism. Urology 21:385.

Schirai, M. and N. Ishii, 1981. Hemodynamics of erection in man. Arch. Androl. 6:27.

Weiss, H. 1972. The physiology of human penile erection Ann. Int. Med. 76:793.

32

FEMALE REPRODUCTIVE SYSTEM

The female reproductive system includes both external and internal genitalia. The internal organs are the *ovaries, uterus,* and the *vagina*. The external genitalia are the *clitoris*, the *labia majora*, and *labia minora* (Fig. 32–1). The development of these is not complete until gonadotrophic hormones of the pituitary gland initiate *puberty*. Somatic changes associated with puberty include an acceleration of skeletal growth and increased muscle mass, an increase in adipose tissue over the hips and buttocks, development of the breasts (*thelarche*), growth of axillary and pubic hair (*pubarche*), and growth and differentiation of the ovaries and uterus that culminate in the first menstrual flow (*menarche*), at about age 13. Thereafter, throughout the woman's reproductive life, the ovaries and uterus undergo repeated 28-day cycles of hormonally controlled histological change. At about 50 years of age, the menstrual cycles gradually become irregular and finally cease (*menopause*).

OVARY

The human ovary is a slightly flattened amygdaloid organ measuring 3 cm in length, 1.5 cm in width, and 1 cm in thickness. It is suspended from the broad ligament of the uterus in a fold of peritoneum called the *meso-*

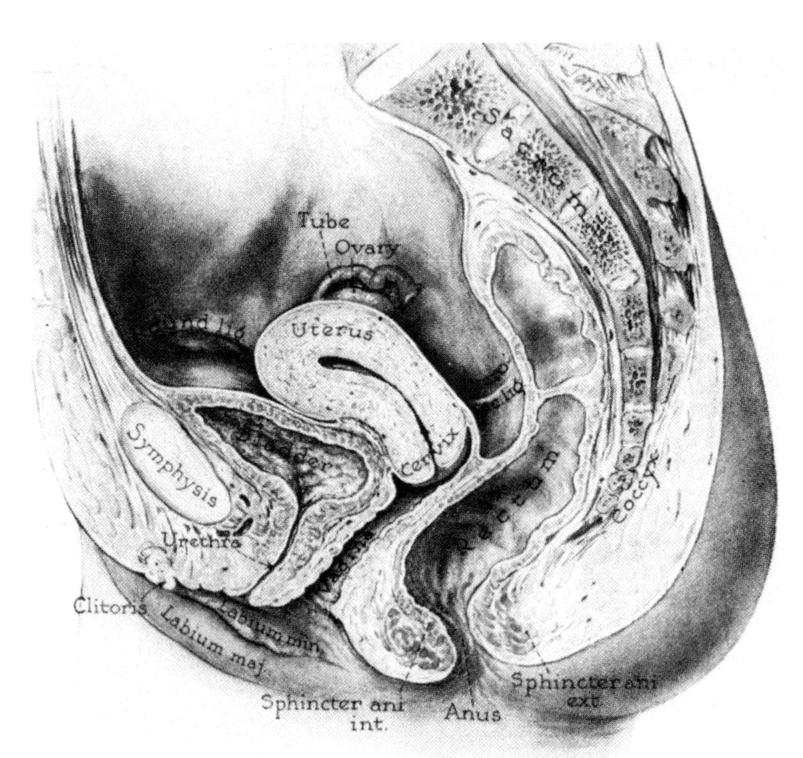

Figure 32–1. Drawing of a saggital section of the female pelvis showing the reproductive organs and their relationship to the bladder, urethra, and rectum. (From Anson, B.J. 1963. Atlas of Human Anatomy, 2nd ed. Philadelphia, W.B. Saunders Co.)

varium, through which the blood vessels pass to enter the ovary at its *hilum*. The organ is covered by a low cuboidal epithelium originally called the *germinal epithelium* in the mistaken belief that the oocytes originated from it. Although it is now known that the primordial germ cells have an extragonadal origin, the term persists. Beneath the germinal epithelium there is a pale-staining avascular layer of connective tissue, the *tunica albuginea*, which consists of collagen fibers that are oriented mainly parallel to the surface of the organ. An outer zone of the ovary, the *cortex*, is highly cellular and composed of fibroblast-like cells in a meshwork of thin collagen fibers. A smaller inner zone of the ovary, the *medulla*, is paler staining and consists of a looser connective tissue containing more elastic fibers, occasional smooth muscle cells, and numerous tortuous arteries and veins from which small branches radiate to the cortex (Fig. 32–2). The cortex and medulla grade into one another without a clearly defined line of demarcation.

In the cortex, there are large numbers of *follicles* exhibiting a wide range of sizes. The vast majority are *primordial follicles* consisting of a large spherical oocyte enveloped by a single layer of squamous or low cuboidal cells (Fig. 32–3). At birth, these are the only kind of follicles present. In the months and years that follow, a few of these at a time undergo further development to form *primary follicles*, in which the oocyte is somewhat larger and is surrounded by two or more layers of follicular cells (Fig. 32–4). After puberty, a number of these primary follicles enter a phase of rapid growth, in each menstrual cycle. The oocyte enlarges further and the cells around it, now called *granulosa cells*, proliferate, rapidly increasing the diameter of the follicle. The oocyte is displaced to one side by the development of an eccentrically placed fluid-filled cavity in the mass of granulosa cells, called the *antrum*. At this stage of development, the follicles are called *secondary follicles* or *antral follicles*. One of this cohort of growing follicles becomes dominant, continuing its development, attaining a diameter of up to 20 mm, and bulging from the surface of the ovary. At *ovulation* in midcycle, its thin wall ruptures and an ovum is released. The other large antral follicles undergo a natural process of degeneration called *follicular atresia*.

The factors that determine which primary follicles will enter a growth phase and which of the 5 to 10 resulting antral follicles will become dominant and go on to ovulation are not known. The ovaries of a young woman are estimated to contain 400,000 primordial and primary follicles. During her reproductive life, fewer than 500 of these will complete their maturation and release an ovum. All the others will undergo atresia at one stage or another of their development. As a result of this continual follicular degeneration, the number in the ovaries progressively declines until few remain at menopause.

PRIMORDIAL FOLLICLE

In the fetal ovary, the oogonia proliferate and advance to prophase of the first meiotic division where they are arrested in the dictyate stage. In the primordial follicles of the postnatal ovary, the oocyte is a large spherical cell, up to 25 μm in diameter, enveloped by several squamous follicular cells (Fig. 32–3). Its pale, eccentrically placed nucleus contains a conspicuous nucleolus, and in well-preserved specimens, the meiotic chromosomes can sometimes be resolved in the nucleoplasm. There is a dense aggregation of mitochondria near the nucleus. In electron micrographs, a small juxtanuclear Golgi apparatus consists of short parallel cisternae with numerous associated small vesicles. The endoplasmic reticulum is represented by widely dispersed vesicular or tubular profiles bearing relatively few ribosomes. One or two annulate lamellae are not uncommon and a few multivesicular bodies may be found in the peripheral cytoplasm.

PRIMARY FOLLICLE

The transition from a quiescent primordial follicle to a primary follicle involves changes in the oocyte, the follicular cells, and the adjacent stromal cells. The oocyte grows larger and the follicular cells lose their squamous epithelial configuration, first becoming cuboidal, then proliferating to form two or three layers of irregularly shaped granulosa cells (Fig. 32–4). The follicle is surrounded by an unusually thick basal lamina called the *membrana limitans externa*. As these changes in the follicle progress, the surrounding stromal cells become more closely packed around it and form a layer with ill-defined outer limits, called the *theca folliculi*.

As the oocyte increases in size, there are noticeable changes in its organelles. The single Golgi complex gives rise to multiple com-

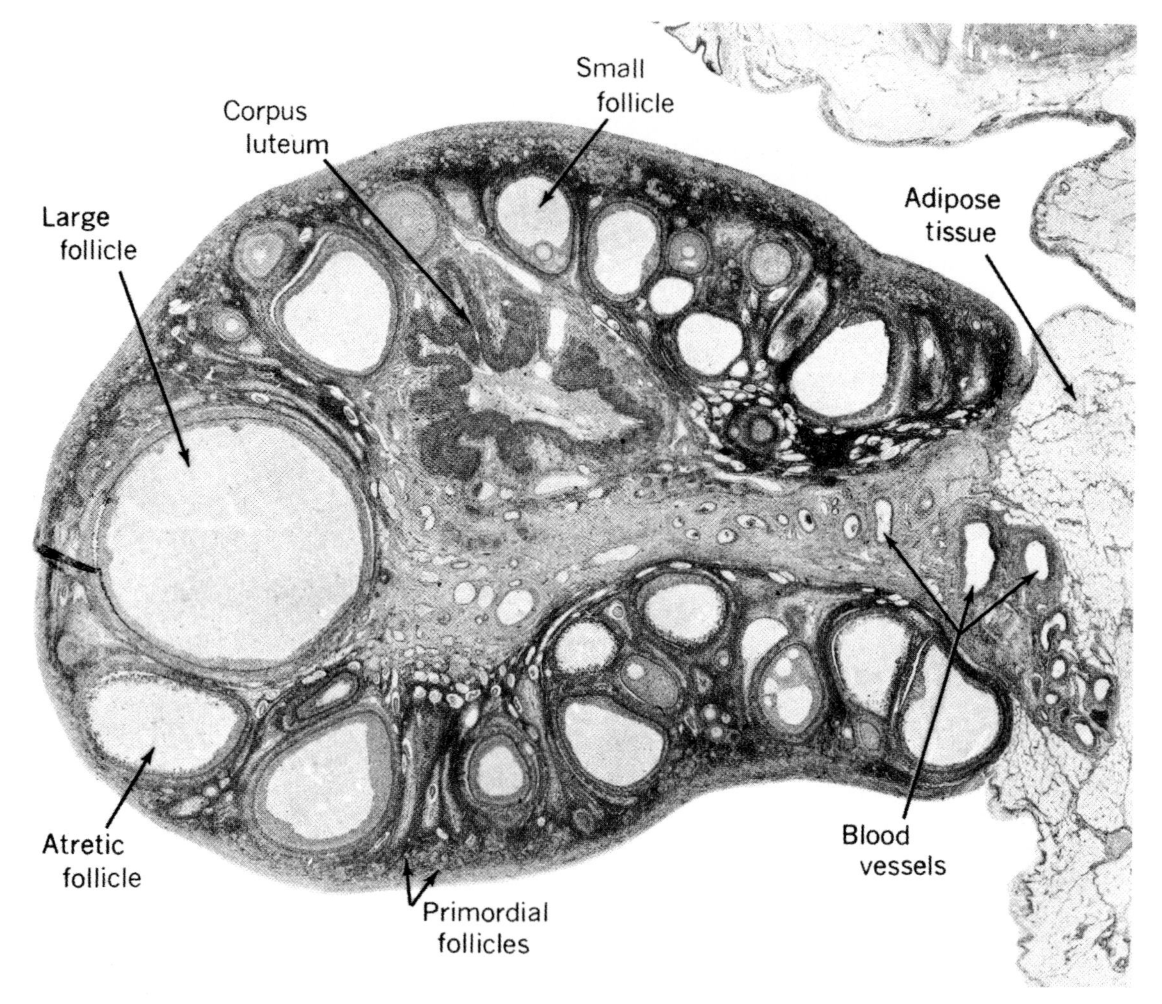

Figure 32–2. Photomicrograph of a longitudinal section of a macaque ovary showing the fibrous medulla and a cortex containing numerous follicles and a single corpus luteum. (Courtesy of H. Mizoguchi.)

plexes widely dispersed in the ooplasm. The endoplasmic reticulum becomes more extensive and is enriched in ribosomes. Free ribosomes also become more abundant. Mitochondria proliferate and disperse throughout the cytoplasm. The oocyte and the surrounding granulosa cells become separated by a narrow space into which microvilli, and larger processes, project from both cell types (Fig. 32–5). An amorphous material, secreted into this space, gradually condenses to form the *zona pellucida*, a highly refractile layer of glycoprotein that stains intensely with the periodic-acid–Schiff reaction for carbohydrates (Figs. 32–6 and 32–7). Throughout subsequent follicular development, the oocyte and the granulosa cells are believed to remain in communication via gap junctions on the processes that tranverse the zona pellucida. This highly refractile layer of glycoproteins was formerly thought to be secreted by the granulosa cells. Recent studies with labeled antibody to zone pellucida antigens reveal that these proteins first appear in the peripheral cytoplasm of the oocyte at an early stage of follicular development. Later in development, specific zona pellucida, antigens appear transiently in the innermost row of follicular cells. It is now believed that it is the oocyte that secretes the precursors of the zona pellucida. The possibility that the follicular cells may make a minor contribution to its formation cannot be excluded.

ANTRAL FOLLICLE

When primary follicles begin their growth, early in a menstrual cycle, the granulosa cells

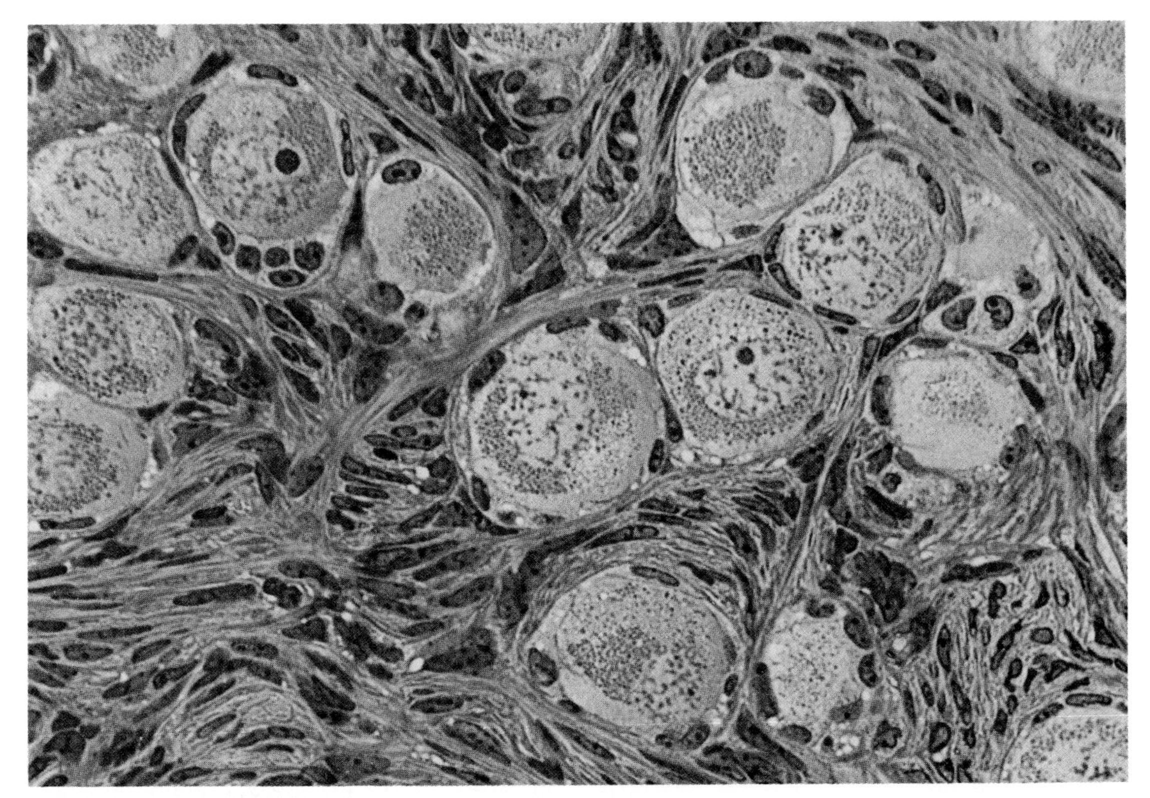

Figure 32–3. Photomicrograph of a number of primordial follicles in the cortex of a monkey ovary. The oocytes are surrounded by a single layer of squamous follicular cells. Chromosomes, in the dictyate stage of meiosis, are visible in the oocyte nuclei.

proliferate rapidly and when the follicles are about 200 μm in diameter with 6–10 rows around the oocyte, a clear fluid begins to accumulate in intercellular spaces of varying size and shape among the granulosa cells. This fluid, called the *liquor folliculi*, is mainly a transudate of blood plasma, but it is rich in hyaluronate and contains growth factors, steroids, and gonadotrophic hormones at several times their concentration in the blood. As it increases in amount, the spaces it occupies become confluent, forming a single crescentic *antral cavity* (Figs. 32–9 and 32–10). After its appearance, the follicle is called a secondary follicle or antral follicle.

Although the multilayered portion of a follicle is often described as a stratified epithelium, the cells are more loosely organized than in typical epithelia, and as fluid accumulates in the intercellular spaces, the granulosa cells take on a variety of angular or stellate shapes while maintaining contact via short processes. In growing follicles, a few small accumulations of densely staining material may be found among the granulosa cells. These are called *Call-Exner bodies* (Fig. 32–7, 32–8). Their chemical nature and significance are not known. The oocyte of the antral follicle is located in the *cumulus oophorus*, a local thickening of the mass of granulosa cells that projects into the antrum. Immediately surrounding the zona pellucida there is a layer of closely adherent cuboidal granulosa cells, called the *corona radiata* (Fig. 32–11). Slender processes of these cells traverse the zona pellucida and contact the oocyte.

The granulosa cells have deeply staining nuclei rich in heterochromatin. The cytoplasm contains a small Golgi complex, occasional meandering cisternae of granular endoplasmic reticulum, and a few mitochondria. Free ribosomes are abundant and some cells contain a few droplets of lipid. Their ultrastructural appearance is not that of a cell making protein for export nor do they have characteristics of cells secreting large amounts of steroids.

At the antral stage of follicular growth, the theca folliculi becomes more conspicuous and consists of a dense network of perifollicular

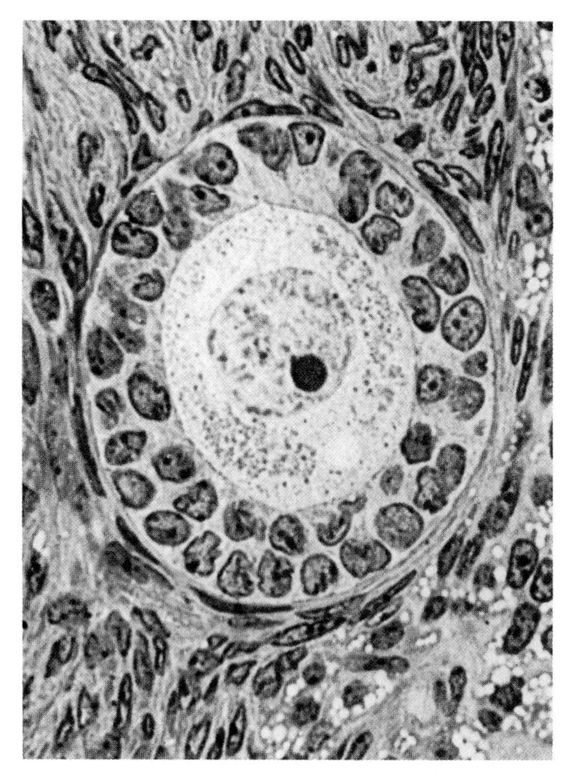

Figure 32–4. Photomicrograph of a bilaminar primary follicle from monkey ovary. Note the large size of the oocyte and the numerous mitochondria in its cytoplasm. A few fusiform cells around the periphery of the follicle represent an early stage in the development of the theca interna.

capillaries and plump fusiform stromal cells. A wedge-shaped thickening of the theca interna, called the *theca cone*, extends from the follicle toward the surface of the ovary. As development progresses, two layers become recognizable in the theca, namely, the *theca interna*, a highly vascular layer of capillaries and epithelioid cells that later acquire features typical of steroid-secreting cells and the *theca externa* which consists predominantly of fusiform stromal cells and connective tissue. The boundaries between the theca interna and externa, and between the latter and the surrounding ovarian stroma are indistinct. The thick granulosa cell layer of the follicle remains avascular throughout follicular development and is nourished by diffusion from the capillaries of the theca interna.

MATURE FOLLICLE (GRAAFIAN FOLLICLE)

In the second half of the follicular phase of the cycle, the majority of the cohort of follicles that have developed to the antral stage begin to undergo atresia, but the dominant follicle goes on. There is no further enlargement of its oocyte, which has already reach a diameter of 100 μm, but the follicle as a whole continues to grow over the next 2 weeks with its granulosa cells increasing in number from 0.5×10^6 to 50×10^6. Thus, a follicle that was only 2 mm in diameter on day 1 of the cycle comes to measure 15–20 mm in diameter at the time of ovulation on day 14.

The oocyte that began meiotic division in the embryo and arrested in prophase resumes division shortly before ovulation. This long interruption in meiosis, lasting from 12 to 40 years, is one of the most remarkable phenomena in reproductive biology and is one of the least understood. Agonists to switch the primordial germ cells from mitosis to meiosis and inhibitors to account for the arrest in prophase have been postulated, but experimental evidence for such factors is scant.

Several hours before ovulation, the oocyte nucleus moves to a position immediately beneath the oolemma. The later stages of prophase are completed and the chromosomes assemble on the metaphase plate of a spindle oriented tangential to the oolemma (Fig. 32–12). The spindle then rotates 90° and a small rounded mass of ooplasm around the pole of the spindle projects above the surface of the oocyte as division begins. A unique feature of meiosis in the female is that the daughter cells are of unequal size, one being the huge *secondary oocyte* and the other a tiny spherical cell with little cytoplasm, called the *first polar body*, which remains within the zona pellucida in contact with the oocyte. The secondary oocyte then proceeds quickly to metaphase of the second meiotic division, where it is again arrested (Fig. 32–13). This division is not completed, with formation of a *second polar body*, until after ovulation and fertilization.

The mature follicle is a large translucent vesicle that occupies the full thickness of the cortex and bulges 1 cm or more above the surface of the ovary. Its wall appears tense, as though the fluid within it were under pressure, but this impression is not borne out by direct measurements. Thus, the thinning of its wall in preparation for ovulation is not due to pressure but to rearrangements of its cells during the terminal phase of its growth. Accompanying these changes, there is a coalescence of fluid-filled intercellular spaces among the cells at the base of the cumulus oophorus. This results in detachment of the

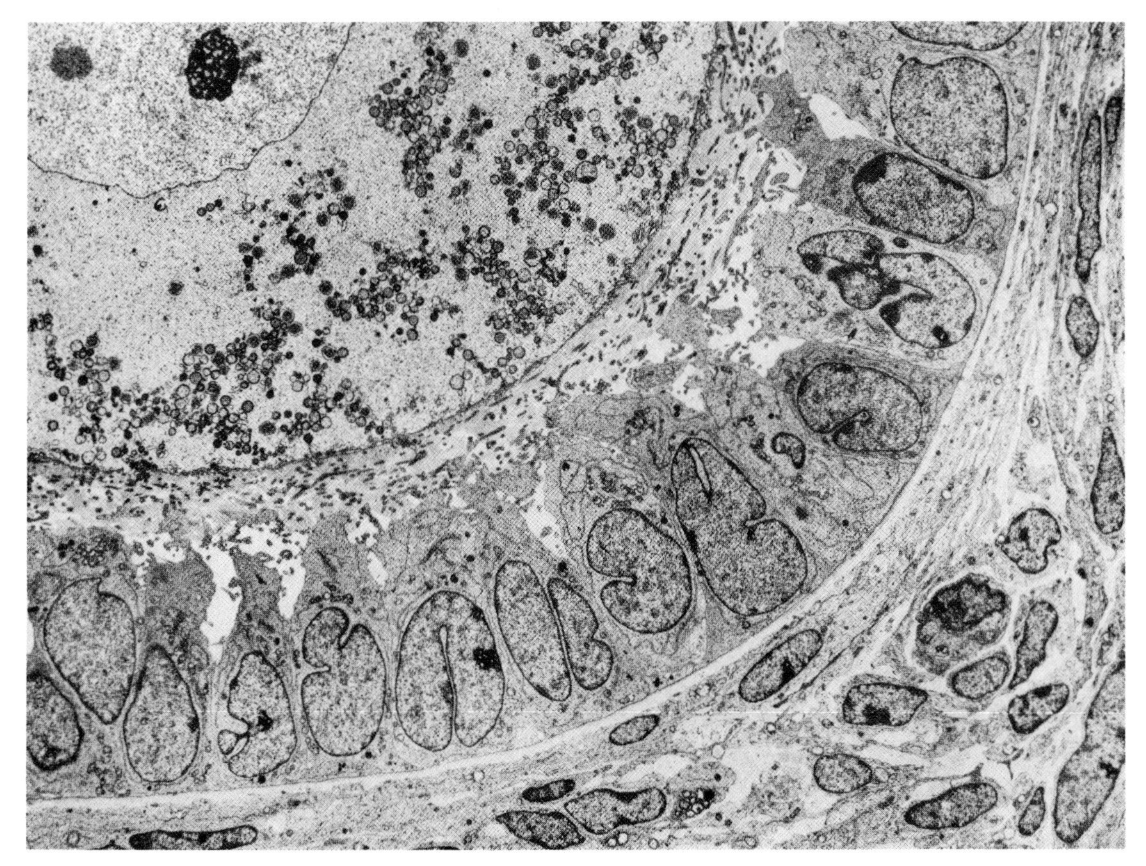

Figure 32–5. Electron micrograph of a quadrant of a primary follicle. Numerous mitochondria are evident in the oocyte. A space has appeared between it and the follicular cells, in which amorphous material is accumulating to form the zona pellucida. (Micrograph courtesy of P. Motta.)

oocyte, its corona radiata, and a few adherent granulosa cells, which then float free in the liquor folliculi.

OVULATION

Ovulation has been directly observed in living anaesthetized animals and in the human. The first indication of impending ovulation is the appearance of a pale oval area on the bulging outer pole of the follicle. The change in color and translucency of this area, called the *stigma* or *macula pellucida*, is due to local cessation of blood flow in the capillaries of the theca interna. Discontinuities in the germinal epithelium and the connective tissue of the tunica albuginea soon appear, and the thin stigma bulges outward, forming a clear vesicle. Within a minute or two after its formation, the vesicle ruptures and the ovum and its adherent cumulus cells pass through the opening, followed by a small gush of follicular fluid (Fig. 32–14). Usually only one ovum is released in each cycle, but occasionally two follicles, and very rarely three, may complete their maturation and ovulate, resulting in twins or triplets. Anovulatory cycles, in which no ovum is released, are not uncommon.

The thinning of the tissue at the stigma, from 80 μm to 20 μm or less, involves both cellular translocation and dissociation and fragmentation of collagen fibrils in the theca and tunica albuginea. A preovulatory increase in *collagenase* can be detected in follicles and this appears to be necessary for ovulation. Other enzymes may be involved. Like the blood plasma, the follicular fluid contains *plasminogen*, the inactive form of an enzyme, *plasmin*. In response to a preovulatory increase in LH, the granulosa cells produce increasing amounts of *plasminogen activator*, which converts the inactive proenzyme to plasmin which is capable of degrading the basal lamina around the follicle and of converting procolla-

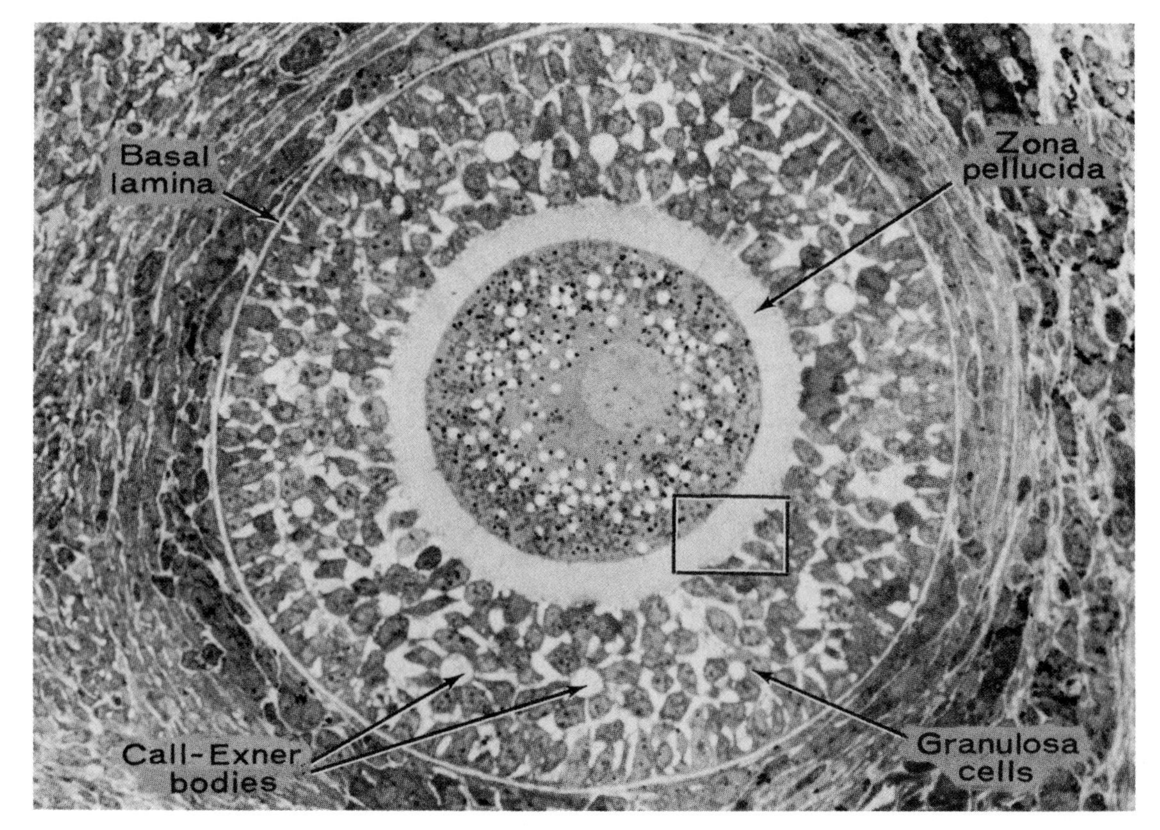

Figure 32–6. Photomicrograph of a follicle with a stratified follicular epithelium, a prominent basal lamina, and a thick zona pellucida. The spherical unstained areas among the follicular cells are Call–Exner bodies. The development of the theca interna is now more advanced. (Photomicrograph courtesy of E. Anderson.)

genase to the active enzyme. Together these mechanisms facilitate escape of the ovum.

FERTILIZATION

Hormonal activation of the *oviduct* (Fallopian tube) has prepared it for reception of the ovum, and while ovulation is in progress, the turgid fronds, or *fimbriae*, around its *ostium* become closely applied to the ovary. Their active movements sweeping over its surface and the currents created in the overlying film of fluid by the beating of cilia in their epithelium draw the ovum into the ostium of the oviduct.

Human ova are not available in the numbers necessary for biochemical studies of fertilization. Our understanding of its molecular events has been gained mainly from studies on the sperm and ova of laboratory rodents, but the mechanisms involved are, no doubt, much the same in all mammals. A successful outcome of the encounter of the ovum with spermatozoa in the oviduct depends on the presence of a specific protein in the membrane covering the sperm head that is recognized by receptors on the zona around the ovum. The granulosa cells adhering to the recently ovulated ovum are quickly dispersed, leaving it surrounded only by the zona pellucida. This layer, about 12 μm thick, is composed of three glycoproteins that have been designated *ZP1* (200,000 MW), *ZP2* (120,000 MW), and *ZP3* (83,000 MW). In the developing follicle, these proteins are secreted, presumably by the oocyte, and molecules of ZP2 and ZP3 copolymerize to form microfilaments that are cross-linked by molecules of ZP1 to form a firm meshwork that makes up the zona pellucida. Certain of the oligosaccharides of ZP3 constitute the *sperm receptors* that bind to the specific membrane protein on the sperm head (Fig. 32–15). This binding event triggers the *acrosome reaction* in the spermatozoon.

The acrosome reaction involves fusion of the acrosomal membrane with the overlying plasmalemma at multiple sites, creating open-

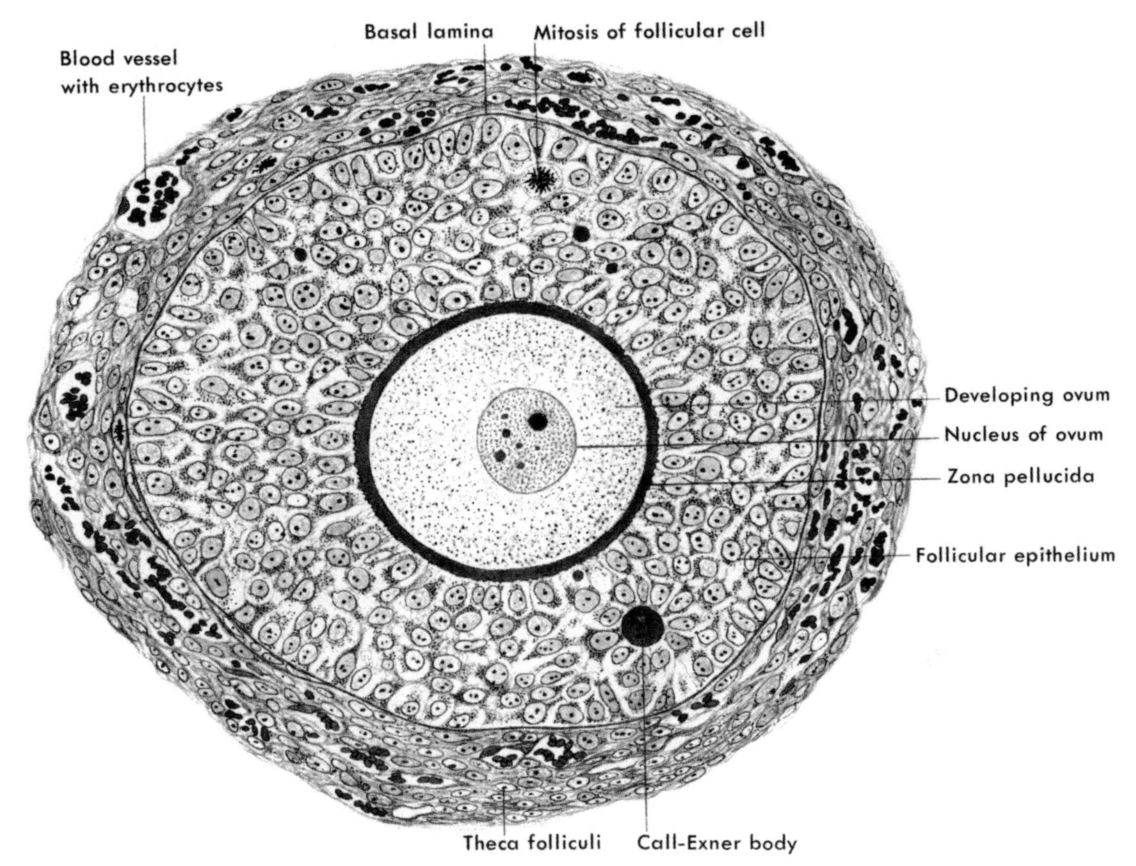

Figure 32–7. Drawing of a large primary follicle in the human ovary with its various components labeled. There is a heavily stained Call–Exner body at the lower right.

ings through which the contents of the acrosome are released. The acrosomal enzymes digest the zona pellucida beneath the sperm head forming a channel through which the vigorously motile spermatozoon enters the *perivitelline space* between the zona and the oolemma. The membrane on the postacrosomal region of the sperm head then fuses with the oolemma and the sperm head penetrates into the ooplasm, where its chromatin begins to decondense. Fusion of the membranes triggers the *cortical reaction* of the ovum in which several thousand *cortical granules* in its peripheral cytoplasm undergo exocytosis, releasing their content into the perivitelline space (Fig. 32–16). The enzymes of the cortical granules, acting on the glycoproteins of the zona pellucida, destroy its sperm-receptor properties, thus preventing the binding and entry of other spermatozoa. Thus, the zona pellucida is responsible (1) for sperm-binding, (2) for initiating the acrosome reaction, and (3) after its modification by the cortical reaction, for the block to polyspermy.

Entry of the spermatozoon triggers completion of the second meiotic division of the ovum with production of a second small polar body. This is followed by fusion of the nucleus of the ovum with the decondensed sperm nucleus, restoring the diploid chromosome number in the resulting zygote. How long the ovum remains fertilizable after ovulation is not known, but it is probably less than 24 h. If not fertilized, it gradually fragments and its residues are phagocytized.

ENDOCRINE CONTROL OF OVARIAN FUNCTION

Ovarian function is dependent on the gonadotrophic hormones of the anterior pituitary: *follicle-stimulating hormone* (FSH) and *luteinizing hormone* (LH). Secretion of these hormones is, in turn, controlled by the *gonadotrophin-releasing hormone* (GnRH) produced by hypothalamic neurones. The ovary itself has important endocrine functions, in that the

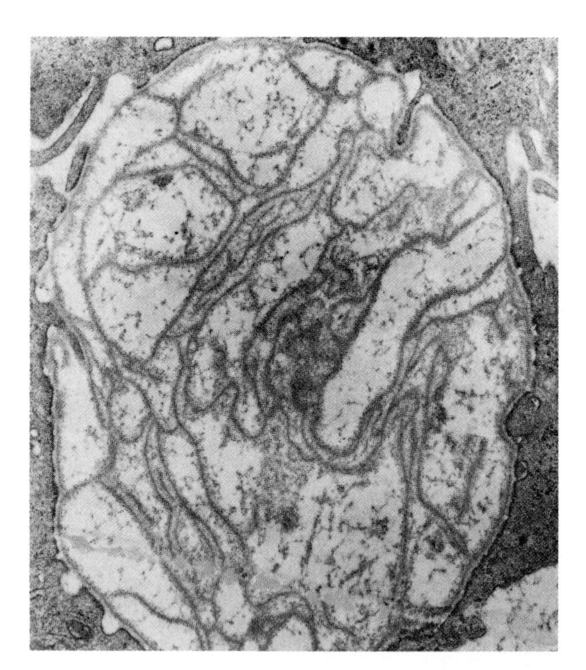

Figure 32–8. Electron micrograph of a Call–Exner body. It appears to consist of a cavity lined by a distinct basal lamina and with a filagree of excess basal lamina in its interior. There is also a sparse flocculent precipitate of proteinaceous material of unknown origin. (Courtesy of E. Anderson.)

granulosa cells and thecal cells secrete steroid hormones that act back on the hypothalamo-hypophyseal system to modulate the release of gonadotrophic hormones.

The formation of primary follicles, in the first half of the cycle, is independent of gonadotrophic hormones, but their further development to antral follicles and beyond requires FSH. At the onset of the follicular phase of the cycle, an elevation of circulating FSH stimulates growth of a cohort of primary follicles. The receptors for FSH are exclusively in the granulosa cells. Under its influence, these cells proliferate, increase the number of their FSH receptors, and activate an enzyme, *aromatase*, that is essential for their production of the steroid hormone *estradiol*. Receptors for LH are located predominantly on the cells of the theca interna, which are stimulated to differentiate and to secrete the hormone *testosterone*. This steroid diffuses through the basal lamina of the follicle and into its expanding granulosa layer where it is taken up by the granulosa cells and converted by their aromatase to *estradiol*. The increasing intrafollicular concentration of estradiol is a further stimulus to granulosa cell proliferation. Estradiol diffuses into the capillaries of the theca interna and its concen-

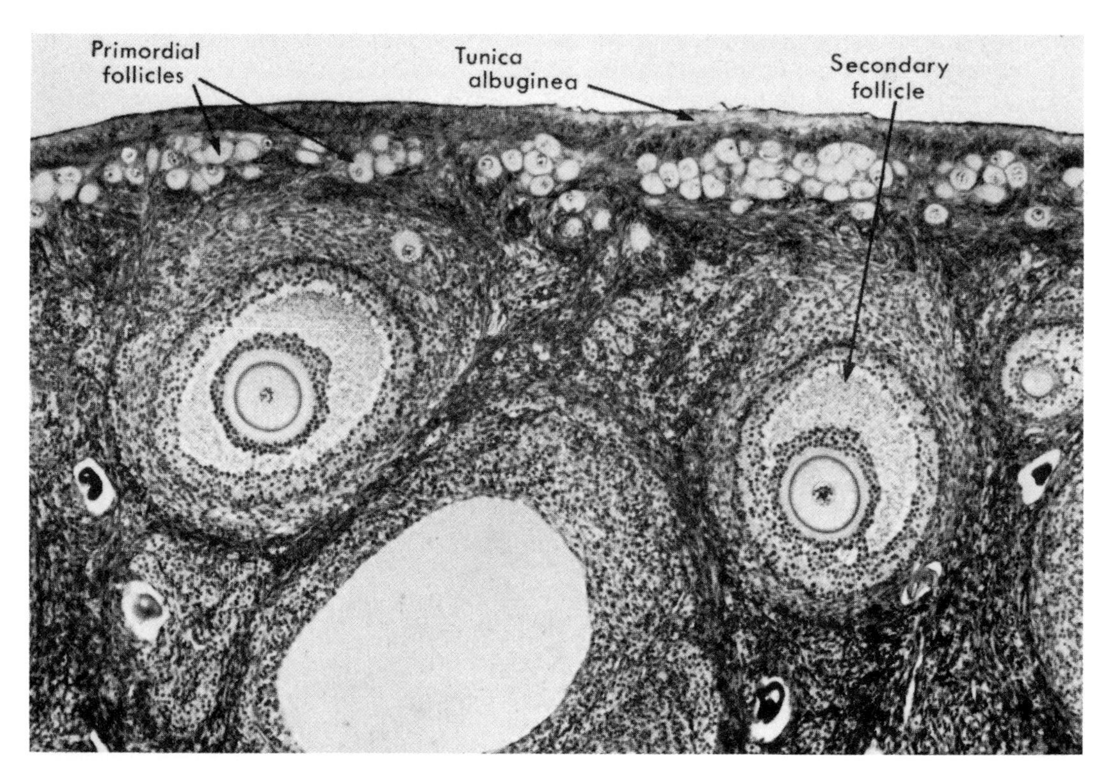

Figure 32–9. Low-power photomicrograph of the cortex of a cat ovary showing a layer of primordial follicles beneath the tunica albuginea and two secondary follicles with a fluid-filled antrum.

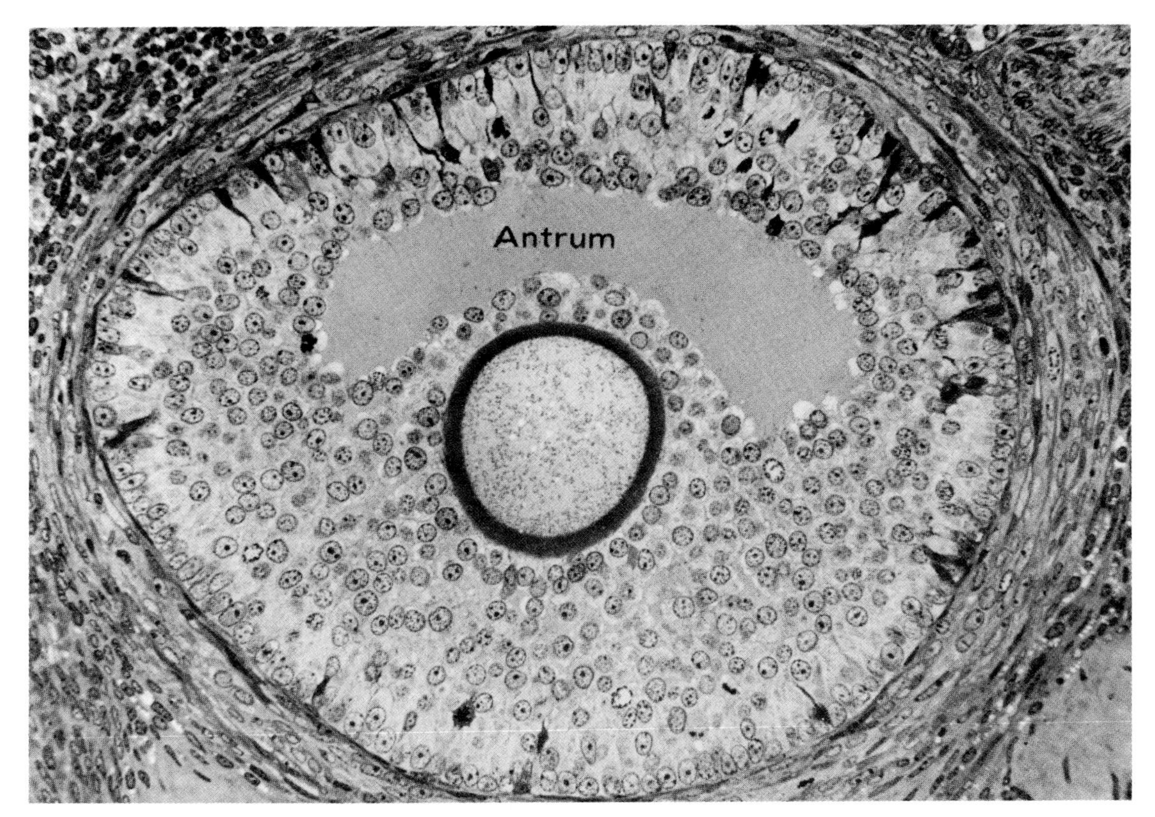

Figure 32–10. Photomicrograph of a secondary follicle from monkey ovary with a small antrum and cumulus oophorus. Note that the theca folliculi is now quite thick.

tration in the general circulation rises. Late in the follicular phase of the cycle, estradiol in the plasma reaches a level that has a positive feedback on the pituitary, increasing its sensitivity to GnRH and resulting in a midcycle surge of LH release that induces ovulation 16–20 h after the LH peak.

In the preovulatory period, the granulosa cells have acquired LH receptors and, responding to this hormone after ovulation, they decrease their production of estradiol and their principal product becomes *progesterone*, the steroid hormone that is responsible for preparing the endometrium of the uterus for reception of the fertilized ovum. The loss of the ovum from the follicle, at ovulation, and the elevated level of LH initiate the transformation of its granulosa cells into lutein cells of the *corpus luteum*.

In addition to steroid hormones, the ovary secretes proteins and polypeptides with functions that are less well known but nonetheless significant. A protein called *follicular regulatory protein* is credited with establishing the dominance of one follicle in the cohort recruited at the beginning of the cycle and retarding the growth of the others. It is believed to be secreted by the dominant follicle and to suppress the response of the others to gonadotrophic stimulation. It can be detected in the venous blood from the ovary containing the dominant follicle but not in blood from the other ovary. A small polypeptide called *relaxin* is secreted in small amounts by the ovulating follicle and in larger amount by the corpus luteum of pregnancy. It promotes relaxation of the uterus during gestation and induces relaxation of the pelvic ligaments, and softening of the cervix of the uterus in preparation for parturition. Another hormone, *inhibin*, secreted by the ovary appears to have an ancillary inhibitory effect, similar to that of estradiol, on the secretion of FSH and LH.

CORPUS LUTEUM

After ovulation and discharge of the liquor folliculi, the wall of the follicle collapses and becomes deeply infolded (Fig. 32–17). The basal lamina that formerly separated the granulosa from the theca interna breaks down

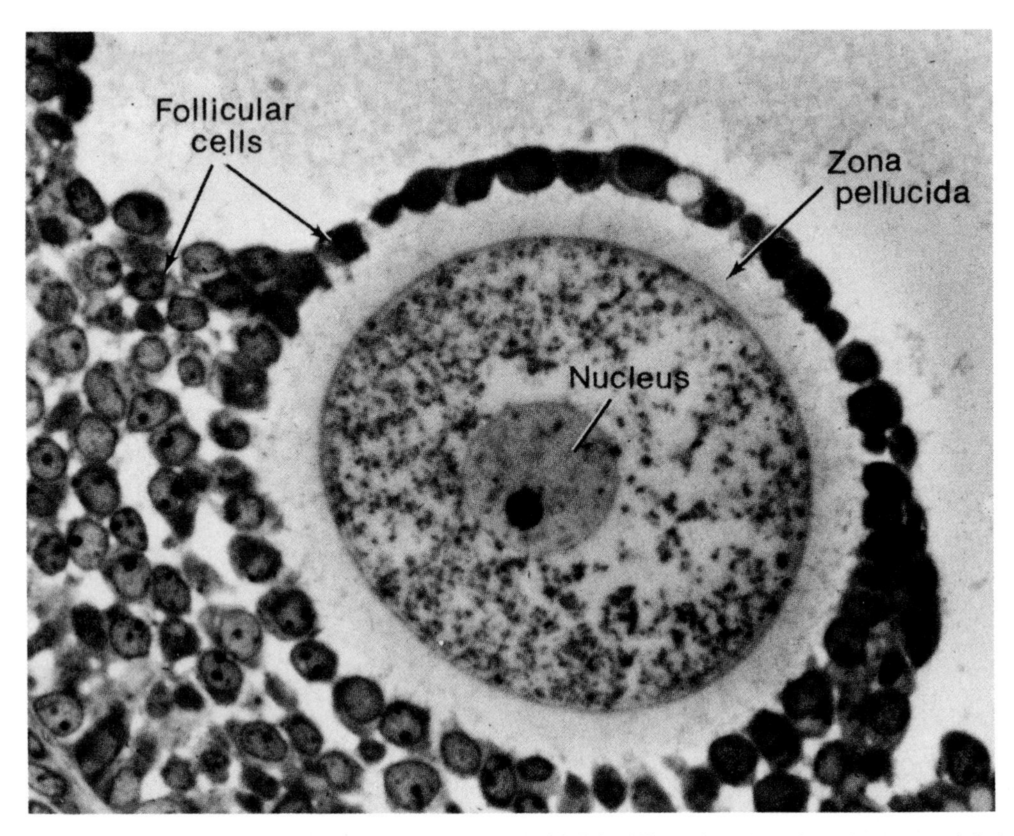

Figure 32–11. Photomicrograph of a human oocyte in an antral follicle. Where it projects into the antrum, it is invested by a single layer of granulosa cells, whose processes are anchored within the zona pellucida. Note the very great number of mitochondria in the oocyte. (Photomicrograph courtesy of L. Zamboni.)

and there may be some extravasation of blood from the capillaries of the theca, resulting in the formation of a central clot. The cells of the granulosa layer and those of the theca interna then undergo stiking cytological changes. They hypertrophy, accumulate lipid droplets, and become plump, pale-staining *lutein cells*. After completion of this postovulatory transformation, the former follicle is called a *corpus luteum*. While the cells of the collapsed follicular wall are becoming lutein cells, capillaries of the theca interna sprout and new vessels, accompanied by fibroblasts, rapidly invade the previously avascular granulosa layer. A delicate reticulum is deposited around the lutein cells and the blood clot in the central cavity is gradually converted to a fibrous core in the interior of the corpus luteum.

In the development of the human corpus luteum, two kinds of lutein cells are distinguishable. Those in its interior, developing from the granulosa cells and making up the bulk of the lutein tissue, are called *granulosa lutein cells*, whereas smaller, more deeply staining cells at the periphery are called *theca lutein cells*, in the belief that they originate from the cells of the theca interna (Fig. 32–18 and 32–19). These two morphologically and ontogenetically distinct cell types differ in their response to LH and in the steroids that they secrete. Theca lutein cells are not found in all mammalian species. The principal secretory product of the corpus luteum is *progesterone*, but in man and other primates, estradiol and other steroids are also secreted.

In histological sections, the cells of the corpus luteum occur in clusters separated by a minimal amount of connective tissue stroma. The cells may be ovoid but are more often polygonal due to mutual deformation. The granulosa lutein cells are 30 μm in diameter in the corpus luteum of a cycle in which the ovum was not fertilized, and up to 50 μm in diameter in a corpus luteum of pregnancy. The smaller theca lutein cells are only 15–20 μm in diameter.

In electron micrographs, granulosa lutein cells have numerous long microvilli projecting into the intercellular clefts and occasionally into deep invaginations of the cell surface.

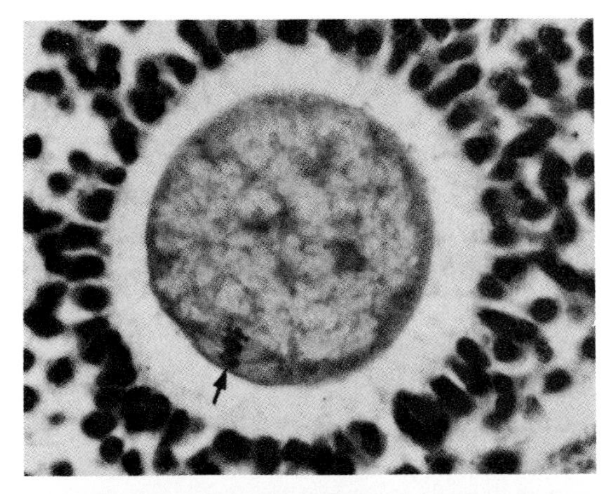

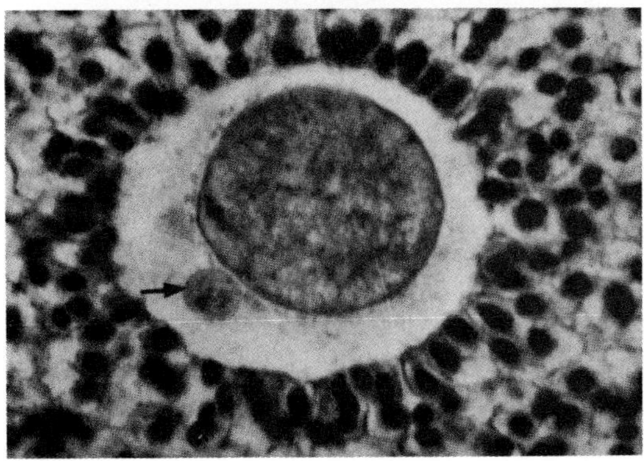

Figure 32–12. Photomicrographs of two stages in the maturation of the rat ovary. (A) Ovum shortly before ovulation, showing diploid chromosomes on the metaphase plate of the first polar spindle; (B) ovulated ovum recovered from the ampulla of the oviduct before sperm penetration. The first polar body lies in the perivitelline space (arrow) and the second maturation spindle can be seen above it. (Photomicrographs courtesy of R.J. Blandau.)

The nuclei have a prominent nucleolus but relatively little heterochromatin. Mitochondria are abundant and pleomorphic. Rod-shaped forms predominate, but in corpora lutea of pregnancy, large spherical mitochondria are not uncommon. The cristae mitochondriales are mainly tubular and the matrix often contains irregularly shaped granules considerably larger than the matrix granules of other cell types. A striking feature of the lutein cells is the abundance of their smooth endoplasmic reticulum which is in the form of close-meshed networks of anastomosing tubules (Fig. 32–20). Rough endoplasmic reticulum is represented by scattered cisternae occurring singly or in small parallel arrays. There are multiple small Golgi complexes distributed in different regions of the cytoplasm. Numerous lipid droplets occur singly or in clusters and tend to be associated with concentrations of smooth endoplasmic reticulum. Irregularly shaped dense granules, interpreted as lysosomes, are present in moderate numbers and increase during involution of the corpus luteum. Other small dense granules, in lutein cells of the corpus luteum of pregnancy, are believed to be sites of storage of the peptide hormone *relaxin*. These are not found in the theca lutein cells.

The theca lutein cells share most of the ultrastructural features of the granulosa lutein cells, but they lack the long microvilli and their nuclei have a bolder pattern of heterochromatin. The mitochondria are more consistent in size and internal structure. The large spherical mitochondria with pleomorphic matrix granules seen in the granulosa lutein cells are not found in these cells. The Golgi complexes are fewer and somewhat larger. Smooth endoplasmic reticulum occupies most of the cytoplasm (Fig. 32–21). The ultrastructural differences in the two types of lutein cells are related to differences in their function, with the granulosa lutein cells primarily producing progesterone and the theca lutein cells secreting estradiol and estrone in addition to progesterone. In the human, the amount of estradiol secreted by the corpus luteum is nearly as great as that of the preovulatory follicle.

If the ovulated ovum is not fertilized, the corpus luteum begins to regress after 9 or 10 days. The lutein cells undergo autolysis and the region is invaded by macrophages that phagocytize the cellular debris. A pale-staining hyaline scar, called a *corpus albicans*, is left at the site, and this may persist in the ovary for many months. If the ovum is fertilized and successfully implants in the uterine endometrium, the cells of the rapidly developing placenta begin to secrete *chorionic gonadotrophins* in time to replace the declining levels of LH from the pituitary. The corpus luteum, therefore, survives and continues to enlarge. The corpus luteum is the predominant source of the steroids needed to sustain the pregnancy for about 2 months. Thereafter, the placenta becomes the major source of the steroids required.

FOLLICULAR ATRESIA

About 98% of the oocytes originally present in the ovary are destined to degenerate. Their depletion begins in intrauterine life, increases from birth to puberty, and continues on a smaller scale throughout reproductive life.

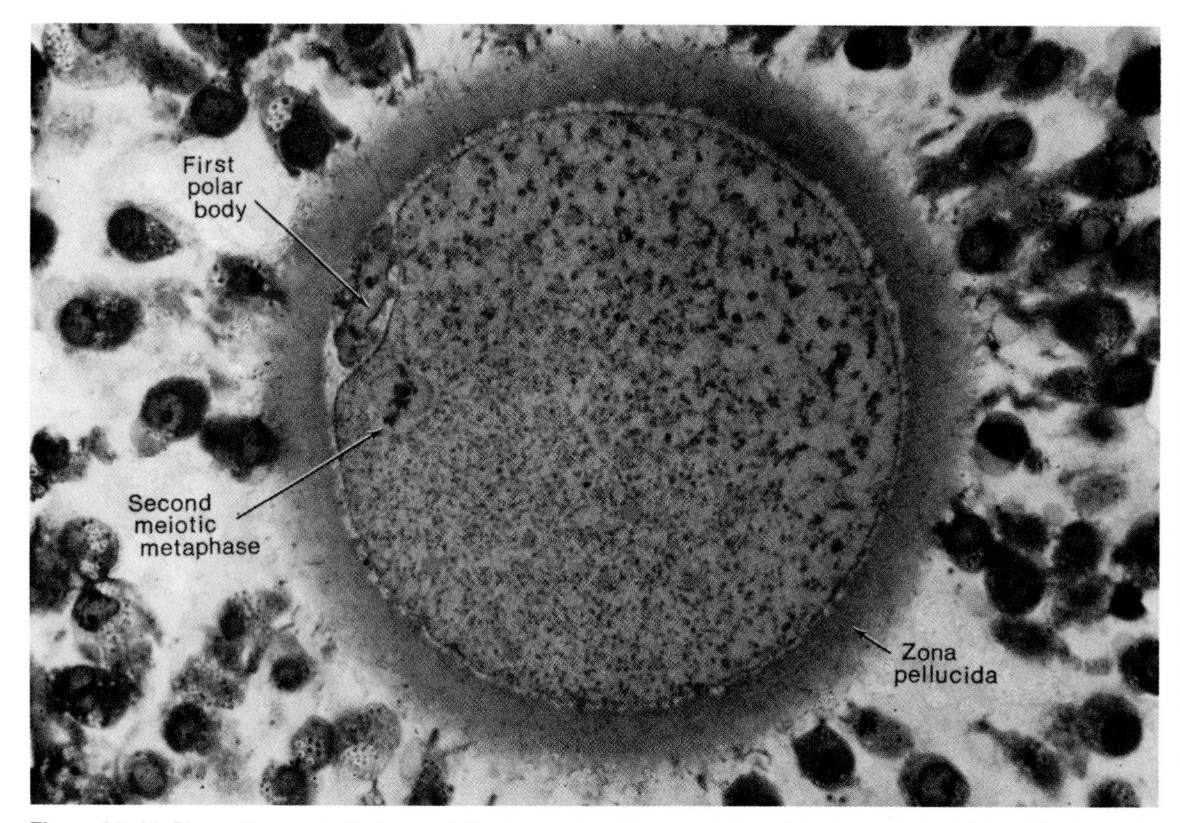

Figure 32–13. Photomicrograph of a human follicular oocyte at the completion of the first meiotic division. The first polar body has been extruded and the chromosomes and spindle of the second meiotic metaphase are visible. (Photomicrograph courtesy of L. Zamboni.)

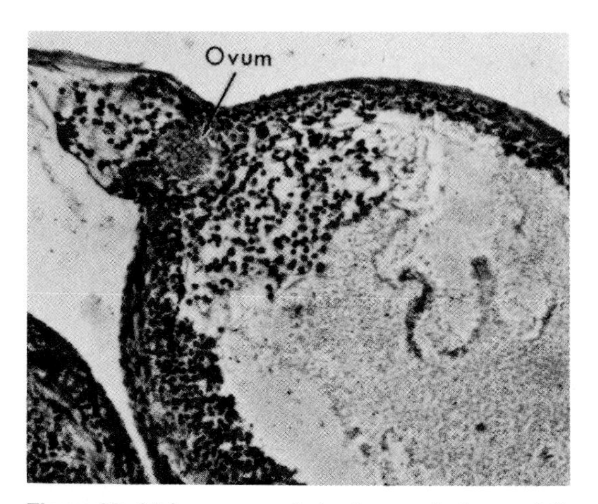

Figure 32–14. Low-power photomicrograph of an ovulating follicle from rat ovary. The ovum and associated cumulus oophorus can be seen in passage through the ruptured stigma. (Courtesy of R.J. Blandau.)

Every normal ovary, therefore, contains degenerating follicles. Atresia may begin at any stage of their development. In the elimination of primary follicles, the oocyte degenerates, followed by breakdown of the granulosa cells. The resulting small cavity in the ovarian stroma is rapidly closed without leaving a trace. The sequence of events is much the same in degeneration of more advanced follicles.

In the atresia of large follicles in the cycle of the adult human ovary, the process appears to begin in the wall of the follicle with secondary effects on the oocyte. One of the earliest changes is the invasion of the granulosa layer by capillaries and accompanying connective tissue. This is followed by a loosening and shedding of the granulosa cells into the cavity of the follicle. Cells of the theca interna hypertrophy and the basal lamina thickens to form a conspicuous "glassy membrane" that is characteristic of atretic follicles. The oocyte degenerates soon thereafter. As the dissolution of the exfoliated granulosa cells progresses, the follicle collapses, its wall becomes undulant, and its cavity is invaded by fibroblasts. The empty and collapsed zona pellucida may persist for some time within the invading connective tissue. Hypertrophied thecal cells become arranged in radial columns separated by strands of connective tissue. They accumulate lipid droplets and come to resemble theca lu-

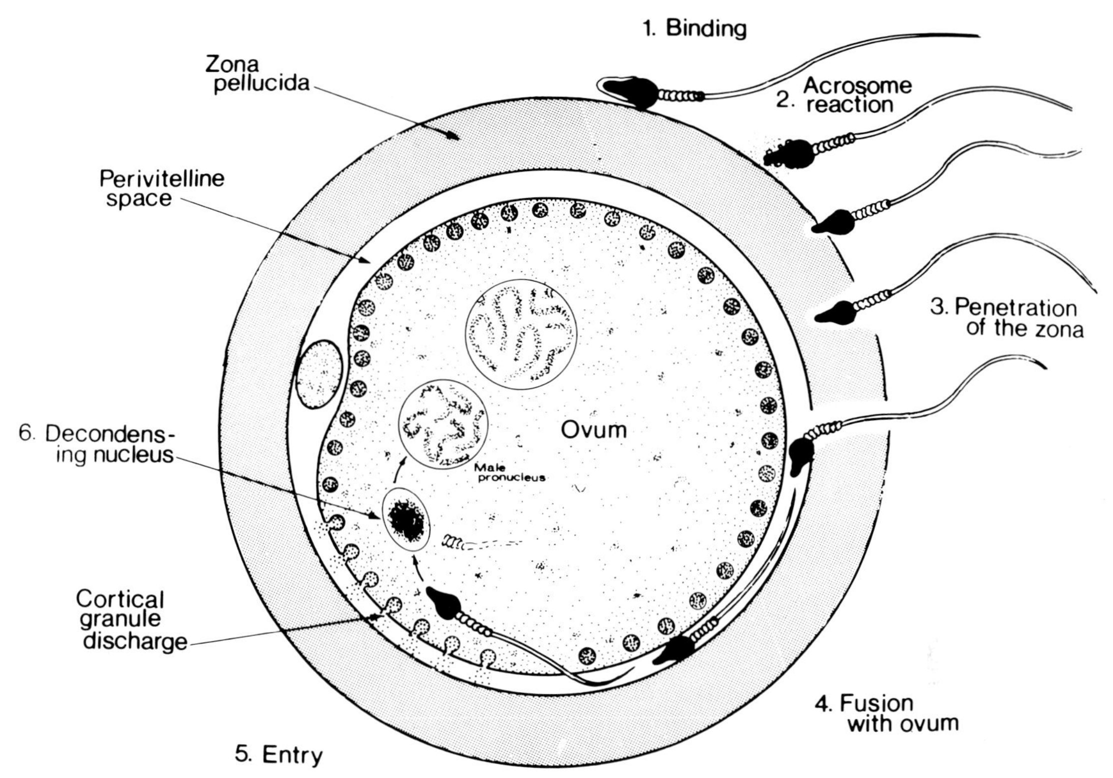

Figure 32–15. Diagram of the various steps leading to fertilization of the ovum. (1) Sperm head binds to zona. (2) Acrosome reaction of sperm is induced in sperm head. (3) Zona is penetrated. (4) In perivitelline space, sperm head binds to oolemma and fuses with it. (5) Sperm sinks into the ooplasm (6) Sperm nucleus decondenses in preparation for conjugation with oocyte nucleus.

tein cells. These degenerating follicles bear some resemblance to regressing corpora lutea but can be distinguished by their so-called glassy membrane and by the presence of a collapsed zona pellucida. The glassy membrane is finally broken down and the surrounding columns of hypertrophied theca cells are broken up into cell groups of varying size scattered throughout the ovarian stroma. The residues of the follicle are reduced to a small fibrous scar.

The activation and development of several primary follicles each month when only one goes on to ovulate would seem to be wasteful and unproductive, but it is speculated that they make a significant contribution to the level of circulating estrogens up until the time they begin to degenerate.

INTERSTITIAL TISSUE

The spindle-shaped cells of the ovarian stroma have potentialities different from those of fibroblasts as evidenced by their differentiation into the hormone-secreting cells of the theca interna. They are supported by a meshwork of fine collagen fibers but no elastic fibers. The stroma of the ovarian medulla, on the other hand, consists of fibroblasts in collagen-rich loose connective tissue containing many elastic fibers.

In many mammalian species, the ovarian stroma also contains clusters and cords of epithelioid *interstitial cells* which are reported to secrete estrogens. Because of their epithelioid appearance and presumed secretory activity, these cells are referred to, collectively, as the *interstitial gland,* even though they are widely dispersed in the stroma. The gland is very extensive in species that have large litters. As new cells are added to it from the theca of regressing follicles, it gradually becomes a more-or-less continuous mass of closely packed cells resembling lutein cells. In older rodents, the follicles are surrounded by masses of these cells. In the human ovary, the interstitial gland is much less extensive. Clusters of interstitial cells are common in the first few years of life but they involute with the onset of menstrual cycles. In the adult, they are found only in small numbers widely scattered in the ovarian stroma.

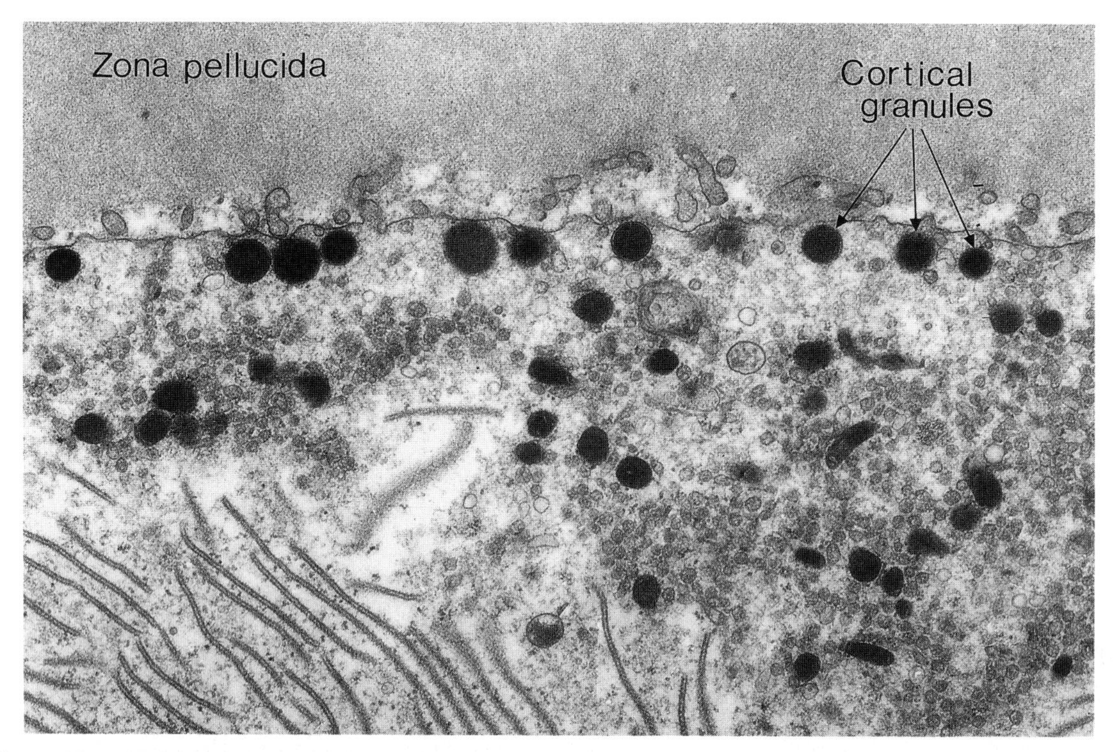

Figure 32–16. Electron micrograph of the peripheral cytoplasm of an ovulated, but unfertilized, hamster ovum showing the cortical granules that undergo exocytosis after fusion of the sperm and egg membranes. Their content modifies the zona in such a way as to prevent binding of another spermatozoon. (Micrograph courtesy of Oura, C. and K. Toshimori. 1990. Internat. Rev. Cytol. 122:105.)

Another kind of large epithelioid cell, the *hilus cell*, is found in small groups in the hilus of the ovary and in the mesovarium. These cells bear a striking resemblance to the Leydig cells of the testis. They contain multiple droplets of lipid, rich in cholesterol esters, and numerous irregular granules of lipofuchsin pigment. Some may even have crystals in their cytoplasm that appear identical to the crystals of Reinke found in Leydig cells. Other features of their ultrastructure are consistent with secretion of steroids. The suggestion that they may secrete androgens is supported by the clinical observation that women with hilus cell hypertrophy, or tumors of these cells, often exhibit varying degrees of masculinization.

VESTIGIAL ORGANS ASSOCIATED WITH THE OVARY

Several parallel or diverging tubules can be found in the mesovarium, running from the hilus of the ovary toward the oviduct and fusing with a longitudinal tubule that courses parallel to the oviduct. These tubules end blindly and are lined by cuboidal epithelium which is sometimes ciliated. They are enveloped by a condensed connective tissue layer containing occasional smooth muscle fibers. The upper end of the longitudinal tubule may end in a cyst-like expansion, the *hydatid of Morgagni*, whereas its other end extends some distance toward the uterus as the so-called *duct of Gartner*. Taken together, the transverse tubules and the longitudinal duct of Gartner comprise the *epoophoron*. In the broad ligament, between the epoophoron and the uterus, there is another group of vestigial epithelium-lined tubules, the *paroophoron*. The epoophoron is a rudiment of the embryonic mesonephros and is the homologue of the ductuli efferentes and epididymis in the male. The paroophoron is a remanent of the caudal portion of the mesonephros and corresponds to the vestigial paradidymis of the male.

VESSELS AND NERVES

The principal arterial blood supply of the ovary comes from the *ovarian arteries*, which arise bilaterally from the aorta below the level of the renal vessels and reach the ovary

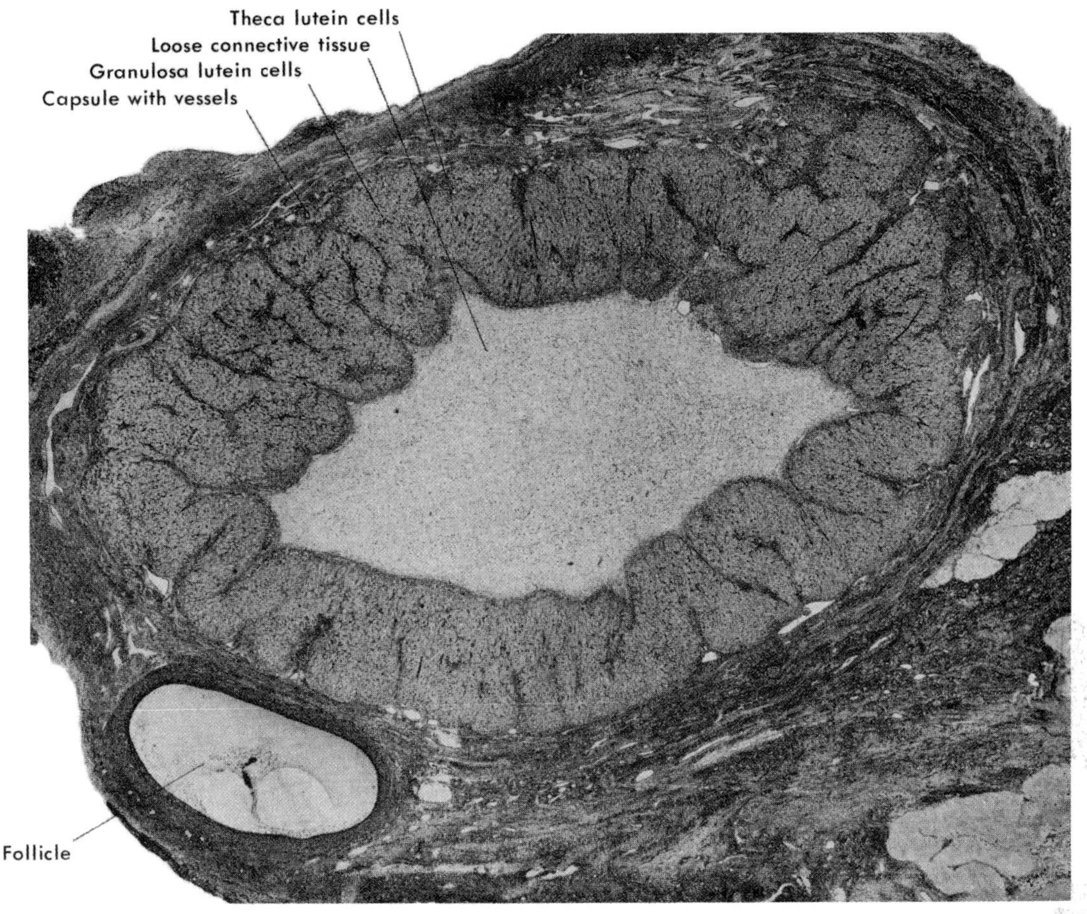

Figure 32–17. Photomicrograph of a corpus luteum in the human ovary showing the folding of the thick layer of granulosa lutein cells and invasion of some of the folds by theca lutein cells.

through the infundibulopelvic ligament. Along the mesovarial border of the ovary, each ovarian artery anastomoses with the *uterine artery*, which courses upward along that side of the uterus. Relatively large branches enter the hilus of the ovary from the region of anastomosis of the uterine and ovarian arteries, and branch repeatedly as they course through the medulla. Because of their tortuosity, these are called the *arteriae helicinae* (helicine arteries). They contribute to formation of a plexus in the medulla from which smaller radial branches pass between the large follicles to enter the cortex, where they break up into loose networks of capillaries. Tortuous veins accompany the larger arteries and form a plexus in the hilus.

The nerves of the ovary are from the ovarian plexus, which accompanies the ovarian artery. The plexus is formed by branches of the renal and aortic plexuses which are derived from the coeliac plexus, the largest of the three large autonomic nerve plexuses. Branches of the ovarian plexus enter the ovary with the blood vessels and they are mainly vasomotor in their function. Nerve fibers penetrate the cortex and can be found around the follicles and under the germinal epithelium. It is doubtful that they penetrate into the follicles. Sensory fibers ending in Pacinian corpuscles have been described in the ovarian stoma.

THE OVIDUCT OR FALLOPIAN TUBE

The *oviduct* or *Fallopian tube* is the portion of the female reproductive tract that receives the ovum released from the ovary, provides the appropriate environment for its fertilization, and transports it to the uterus. It is a muscular tube about 12 cm long situated in the mesosalpinx, which is the upper free bor-

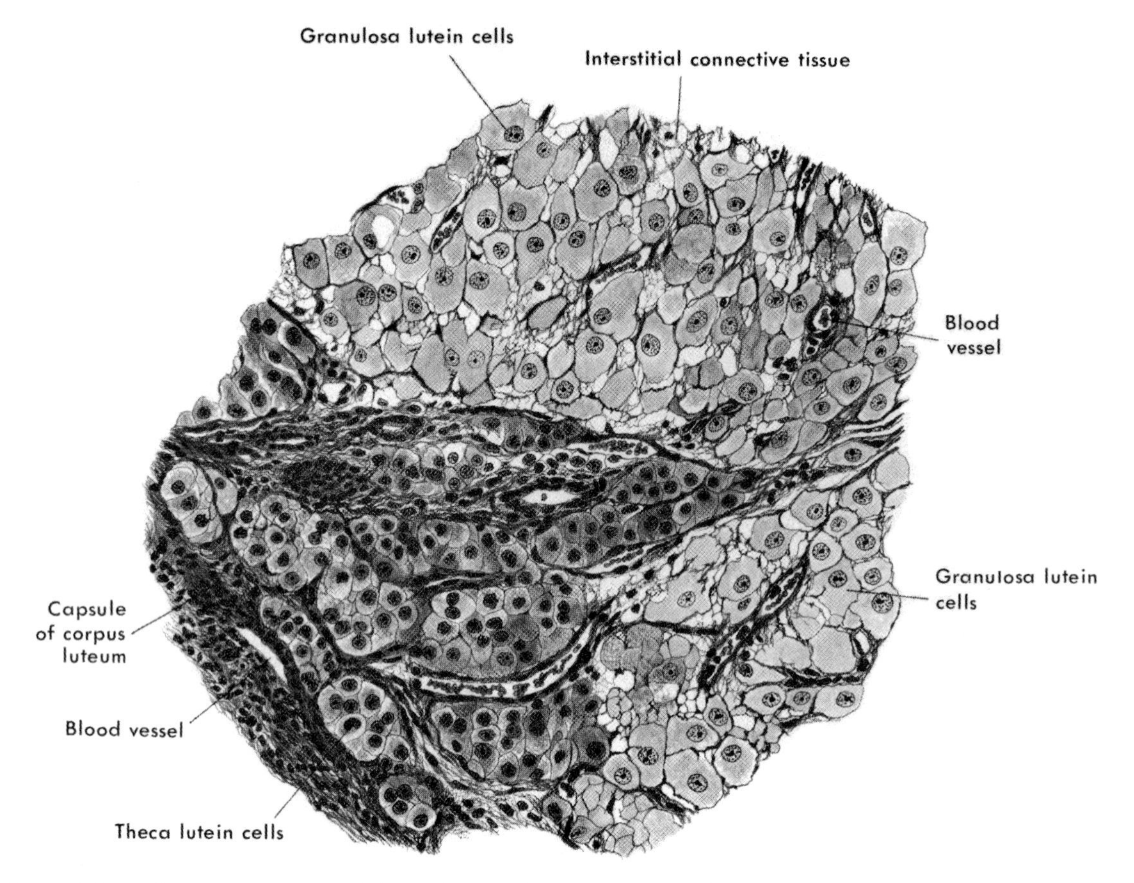

Figure 32–18. Drawing of an area at the periphery of a corpus luteum of pregnancy showing the large pale-staining granulosa lutein cells and the smaller darker-staining theca lutein cells.

der of the broad ligament of the uterus. Its lumen is open to the peritoneal cavity at its upper end and it opens into the uterine cavity at the other end. The funnel-shaped abdominal end is called the *infundibulum* of the oviduct. Its margins are drawn out into numerous tapering, fringe-like processes, the *fimbriae*. An expanded intermediate segment, below the infundibulum, is the *ampulla* and the slender medial third near the uterine wall is the *isthmus* of the oviduct (Fig. 32–22).

HISTOLOGICAL ORGANIZATION

The wall of the oviduct consists of an outer serous layer, a muscular coat, and the mucosa. In the ampulla, the mucosa is relatively thick and forms numerous elaborately branched longitudinal folds or folia. Therefore, in cross section, the lumen appears as a labyrinthine system of narrow spaces between branching folia that are covered by epithelium (Figs. 32–23C and 32–24). In the isthmus, the folds are much lower and less highly branched (Fig. 32–23B), and in the interstitial segment, they are reduced to low ridges (Fig. 32–23A).

The oviduct is lined by simple columnar epithelium in which the cells are tallest on the fimbria, in the infundibulum, and ampulla, and diminish in height nearer the uterus. The cells are of two types, ciliated and nonciliated. These were formerly thought to be simply different functional phases of the same cell type, but the nonciliated cells are now regarded as secretory. The need for cells with a secretory function at the site of fertilization is evident. Of the enormous numbers of sperm in the ejaculate, relatively few reach the ampulla of the oviduct, where they await the ovum. The epithelium of the oviduct must maintain an environment containing the necessary gases and nutrients to sustain their motility and to permit them to undergo *capacitation*, a series of biochemical changes by which they attain their full capacity for fertilization. Passage of the ovum through the tube also involves a delay during which the fertilized

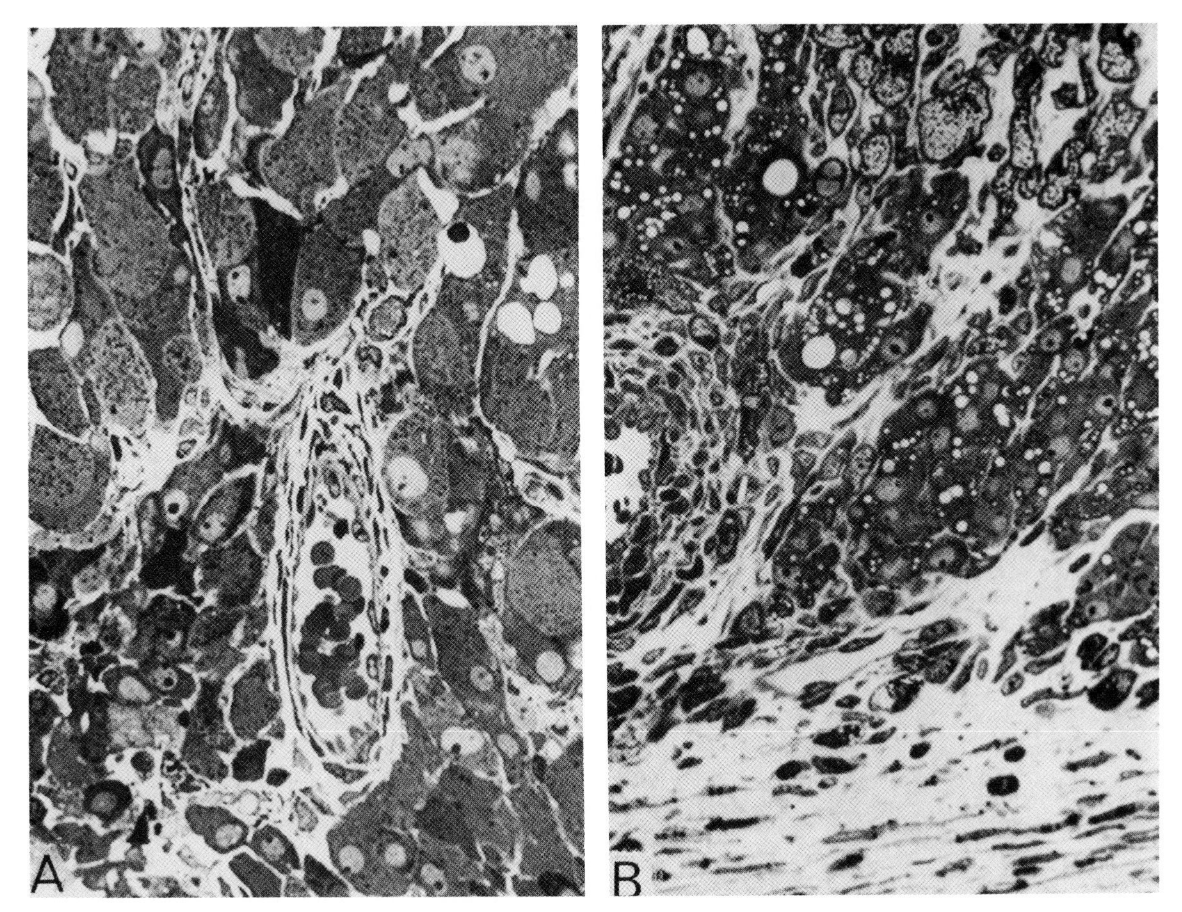

Figure 32–19. (A) Photomicrograph of the periphery of a human corpus luteum at 9 weeks gestation. The larger cells, above, are granulosa lutein cells and the smaller cells ones, below, are theca lutein cells, derived from the theca interna. (B) Corpus luteum of about 1 day after ovulation. Cells of the theca interna have luteinized and are invading the corpus luteum. (Photomicrographs courtesy of Crisp, T.M. et al. 1970. Am. J. Anat. 127:37.)

ovum progresses to the blastocyst stage capable of implantation in the endometrium of the uterus.

This early development no doubt requires a special environment. The nature of the secretory products of the oviductal mucosa is still largely unknown. In rodents, the nonciliated cells have been found to secrete a 200 kD glycoprotein that infiltrates the zona pellucida of the ovum, but what role, if any, it plays in fertilization or nutrition of the ovum is unclear. There are significant species differences in oviductal function and the occurrence of this glycoprotein has not yet been demonstrated in primates. In the rabbit, an albuminous coat is added to the ovum, and in monotremes and some marsupials, a thin shell, as well as an albuminous coat, is formed around the ovum during its passage through the oviduct.

In primates, the epithelium of the oviduct undergoes cyclic changes along with those of the uterine mucosa. These have been most thoroughly studied in the rhesus monkey, but similar changes occur in the human Fallopian tube. The relative numbers of ciliated and nonciliated cells are under endocrine control (Fig. 32–25). Cyclic changes are most marked on the fimbriae, in the infundibulum, and upper ampulla, and diminish toward the isthmus. The cells of the epithelium enlarge and begin ciliogenesis early in the follicular phase of the cycle. Cytological evidence of increased activity is also detectable in the secretory cells of the epithelium. These changes reach their peak at midcycle and are reversed in the luteal phase of the cycle. In the preovulatory phase, the mean percentage of ciliated cells on the fimbriae is 48% and declines to about 4% in the late luteal phase. Dedifferentiation of the ciliated cells on the fimbriae is so complete that it is difficult to distinguish them from the

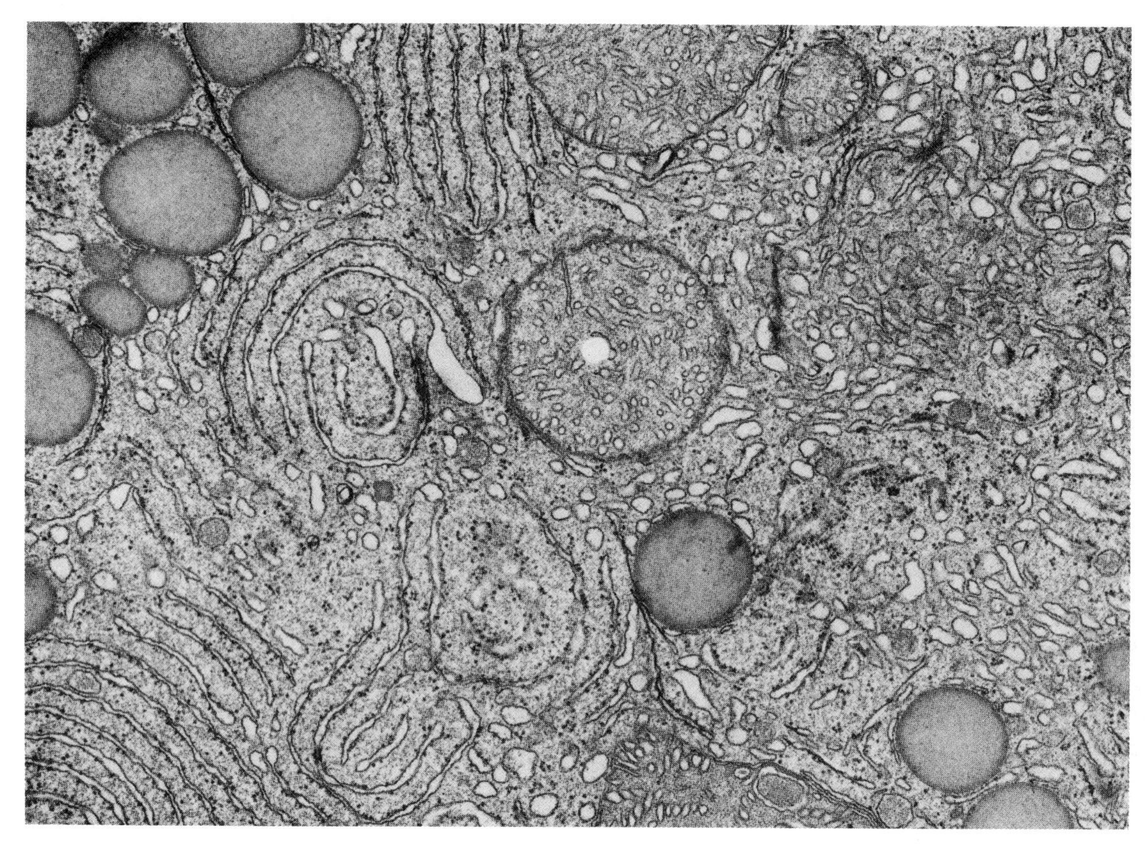

Figure 32–20. Electron micrograph of an area of cytoplasm from a human granulosa lutein cell at 9 weeks gestation. As in other steroid-secreting cells, there is an extensive smooth endoplasmic reticulum consisting of closely packed, branching and anastomosing tubules. Granular reticulum is also present in limited amount. (From Crisp, T.M. et al. 1970. Am. J. Anat. 127:37.)

relatively inactive secretory cells. The cyclic changes are only slightly less dramatic in the ampulla. There is little change in the epithelium of the isthmus, suggesting that this segment is less estrogen dependent. After ovariectomy, the oviductal epithelium dedifferentiates and the fimbriae are almost completely deciliated (Fig. 32–26A). Regression is less evident in the ampulla where some cells retain their cilia. Within 1 week after administration of estradiol, there is a remarkable recovery, with restoration of cilia and evidence of secretory activity.(Fig. 32–26B). Ciliated epithelia in other parts of the body are completely indifferent to circulating estrogens.

Hormones also appear to influence the rate of ciliary beat. In the rabbit, a significant increase in beat frequency is reported to occur 48 h after copulation. A similar increase occurs in the estrogen-primed oviduct of the monkey after administration of progesterone. Thus, estrogen appears to prepare the oviduct for ovum transport, and progesterone accelerates ciliary beat at the time when the ovum would be expected to be in transit. Later in the cycle, progesterone favors loss of cilia.

The lamina propria of the oviductal mucosa consists of fibroblast-like cells and limited numbers of lymphocytes and monocytes in a network of reticular fibers. The fusiform cells seem to have the same developmental potentialities as some of those in the submucosa of the uterus because in rare instances of tubal pregnancy, they differentiate into typical decidual cells. A muscularis mucosae is lacking, and the mucosa rests directly on the underlying muscularis. The smooth muscle does not form distinct layers differing in their fiber orientation. The innermost bundles of smooth muscle are circular, but toward the periphery, longitudinal bundles appear in increasing number and, near the surface of the oviduct, bundles with this orientation predominate. A few smooth muscle cells extend from the wall of the tube into the broad ligament. The narrow spaces between the bundles of smooth muscle are occupied by loose connective tissue.

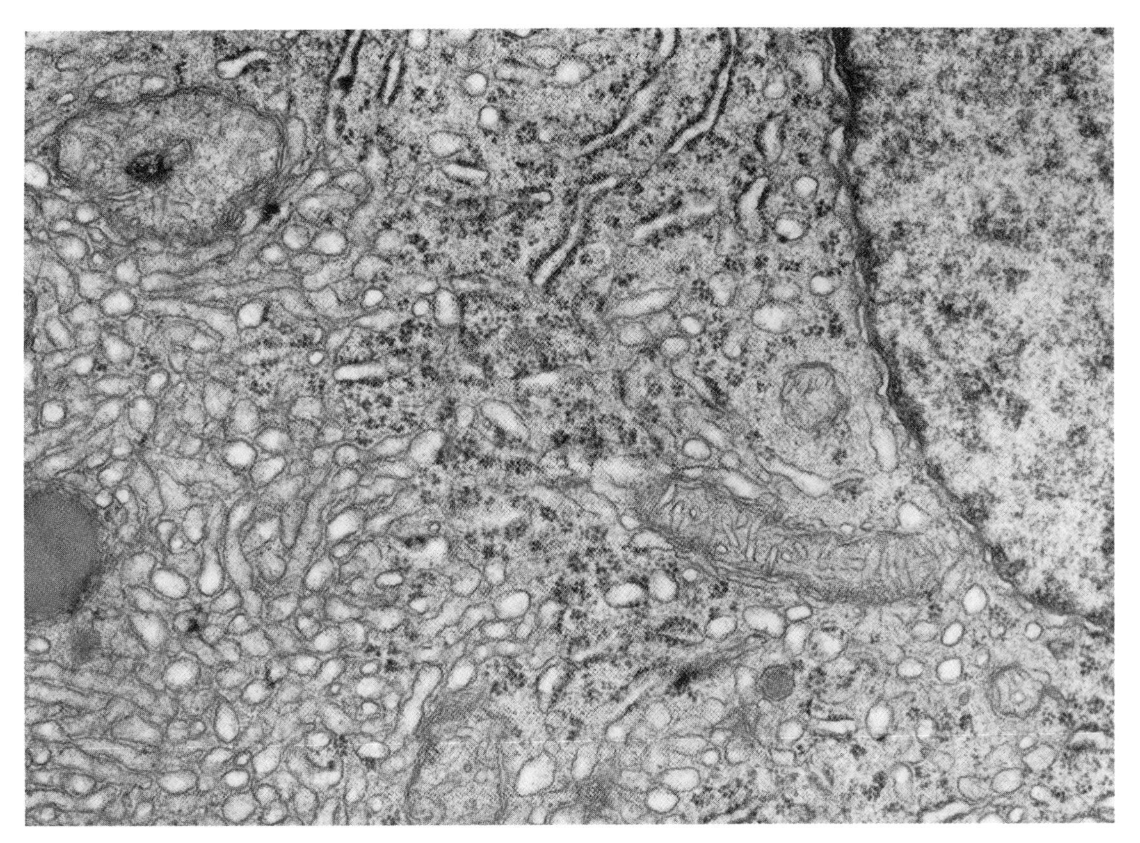

Figure 32–21. Electron micrograph of an area of cytoplasm from a theca lutein cell of a human corpus luteum at 9 weeks gestation. Lipid droplets are numerous and both rough and smooth endoplasmic reticulum are abundant. The mitochondria are highly variable in size and have tubular cristae. These cytological features are typical of cells secreting steroids. (From Crisp, T.M. et al. 1970. Am. J. Anat. 127:37.)

Beneath the mucosa of the ampulla and infundibulum and extending into the fimbriae, there are rather large blood vessels, predominantly veins. At the time of ovulation, contraction of smooth muscle bundles between these vessels has an effect comparable to that seen in erectile tissue. With outflow restricted, the veins become engorged, resulting in enlargement and turgescence of the fimbriae. This, combined with contraction of their intrinsic smooth muscle and that of the infundibulum, brings the ostium of the oviduct into contact with the surface of the ovary, favoring entry of the ovum. At the same time, rhythmic waves of contraction begin to sweep along the oviduct from the infundibulum toward the isthmus. These contractions, together with the beating of the cilia toward the isthmus, achieve the transport of the ovum to the uterus.

BLOOD VESSELS, LYMPHATICS, AND NERVES

There are many blood vessels under the serosa of the oviduct and in the mucosa that are continuations of the uterine and ovarian vessels. In histological sections, lymphatics in the core of the mucosal folds appear as long clefts that might be misinterpreted as artifacts, but closer inspection reveals their thin endothelial lining. During the period of vascular engorgement in midcycle, these lymphatics are distended with lymph and this no doubt contributes to increased turgor that erects the mucosal folds.

Large bundles of nerves accompany the blood vessels in the serosa and in the outer portion of the muscularis. The oviduct receives both sympathetic and parasympathetic innervation. There is a plexus in the inner portion of the muscularis that provides branches to the muscle and to the mucosa. The innervation of the oviduct has not been extensively studied.

UTERUS

The human uterus is a pear-shaped organ with a thick muscular wall that is continuous,

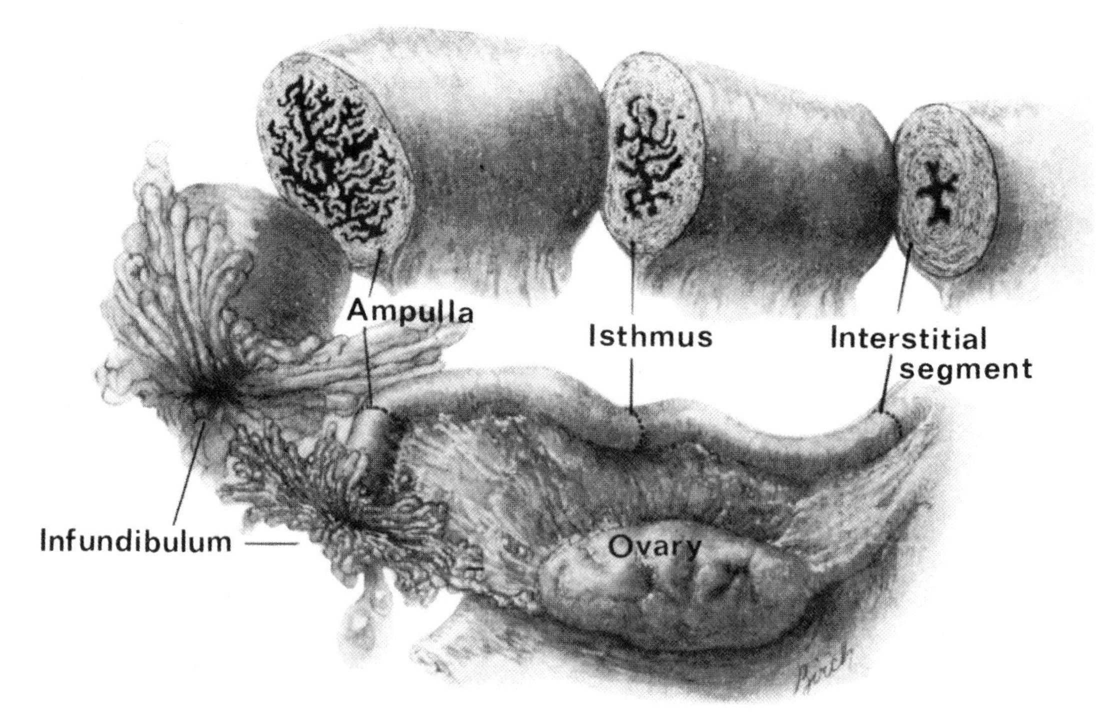

Figure 32–22. Drawing illustrating the mucosal pattern of successive segments of the human oviduct, and the topographical relation of the oviduct to the ovary. (From Eastman, M.J. and L.M. Hellman, eds. 1961. William's Obstetrics, 13th ed. New York, Appleton, Century, Crofts. Labeling added.)

on either side of its broad upper portion, with the wall of the two Fallopian tubes. It is slightly flattened and normally tipped forward so that its broad surfaces are dorsal and ventral. It is about 7 cm long, 4 cm across at its widest, and 2.5 cm thick. The peritoneum covering its dorsal and ventral surfaces continues from the sides of the organ to the wall of the pelvis, forming the two leaves of the *broad ligaments* which support the organ. The rounded upper portion of the uterus above a line joining the openings of the oviducts is referred to as the *fundus*. The wide upper two-thirds of the organ is the *corpus uteri* or *body* and a slightly narrower portion below this is the *isthmus*. A cylindrical lower segment is the *cervix* and the portion of the cervix that protrudes into the upper end of the vagina is its *portio vaginalis*. There is a flattened uterine cavity, triangular in outline, with its two upper corners continuous with the lumina of the oviducts and the lower corner continuous with the slender *cervical canal* which opens into the vagina at the *external os of the uterus*. The greater part of the thick uterine wall is smooth muscle of the *myometrium* and its cavity is lined by a glandular mucosa called the *endometrium* (Fig. 32–27).

The uterus receives the products of conception from one of the oviducts and its endometrium undergoes elaborate cytological changes and vascular modifications to provide sustenance to the embryo throughout its development. The myometrium, quiescent throughout most of gestation, later hypertrophies in preparation for expulsion of the fetus at birth.

MYOMETRIUM

The myometrium is 1.25 cm in thickness and made up of flat or cylindrical bundles of smooth muscle that interlace in all directions but four more-or-less distinct layers can be discerned. Immediate below the endometrium there is a thin layer called the *stratum submucosum* with bundles predominantly longitudinal, but with some admixture of oblique bundles. Around the intramural portion of the oviducts, this layer forms circumferential rings that may have a sphincter-like action. Outside of the stratum submucosum is the *stratum vasculare*, so named because it contains many blood vessels that give it a spongy appearance in section. Longitudinal bundles of smooth muscle predominate in this layer. In the next peripheral layer, the *stratum supravasculare*, the bundles are mainly circular but

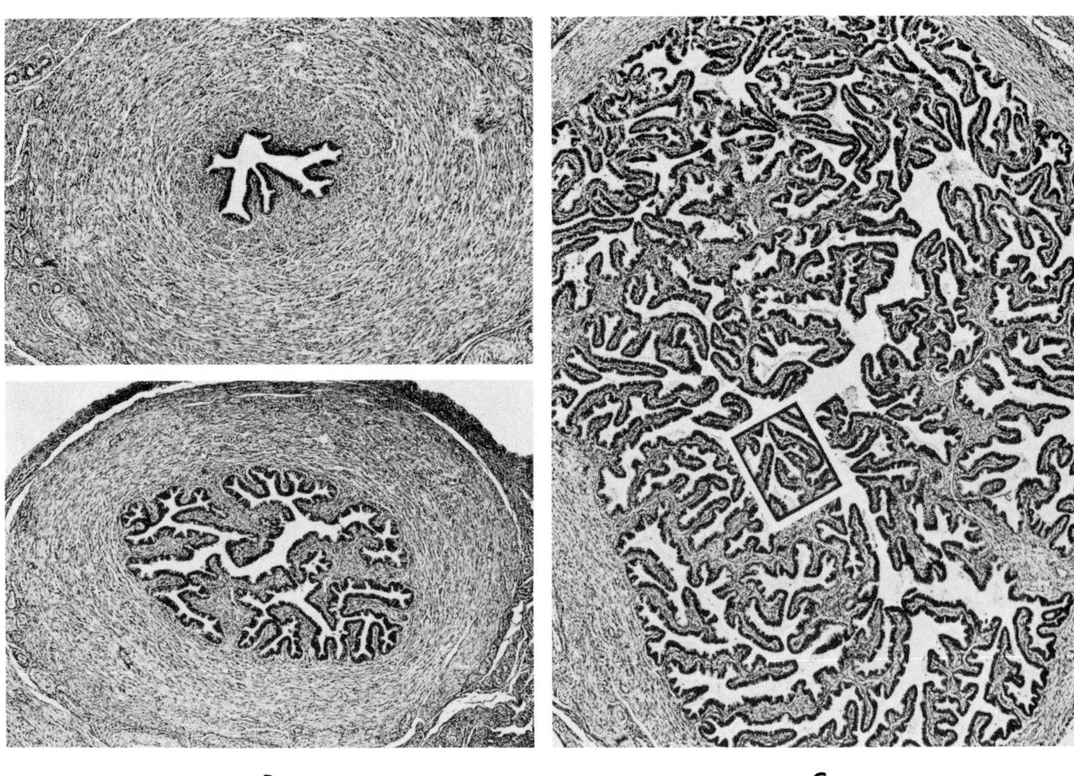

Figure 32–23. Photomicrographs of the Fallopian tube of a 23-year-old woman. (A) Pars interstitialis; (B) the isthmus; (C) the outer portion of the ampulla. Area enclosed in the rectangle is shown at higher magnification in Fig. 32–24.

some longitudinal bundles are found among them. The outermost layer, the *stratum subserosum,* is a relatively thin layer of longitudinally oriented fiber bundles. The two most superficial layers are continuous with the smooth muscle layers of the oviducts and send a few bundles laterally into the round and broad ligaments. At the isthmus of the uterus, smooth muscle decreases while fibrous tissue increases, and the cervix consists almost entirely of dense collagenous connective tissue with some admixture of elastic fibers.

HISTOPHYSIOLOGY OF THE MYOMETRIUM

The size of cells in the myometrium is dependent on estrogens secreted by the ovary. The length of the smooth muscle cells varies from 40 to 90 μm in different phases of the menstrual cycle, with fibers being shortest immediately after menstruation. In the absence of estrogen, the uterine smooth muscle atrophies. The high levels of hormone secreted during pregnancy result in a 10-fold increase in length of the fibers and a 24-fold increase in the volume of the uterus as a whole. Hypertrophy of smooth muscle cells accounts for most of the increase in size of the gravid uterus, but there also appears to be some increase in cell number as well. Whether this is attributable to cell division or to differentiation of smooth muscle cells from mesenchymal cells in the connective tissue between muscle bundles is still debated. The growth of the uterus also involves some increase in its connective tissue. This is verified by analyses showing a fourfold increase in total uterine collagen. In the return of the uterus to normal size after pregnancy, the size of the smooth muscle cells rapidly decreases and some of them may undergo apoptosis, programmed cell death.

In the nonpregnant uterus, there are intermittent shallow contractions that are not attended by any subjective sensation. More forceful contractions may occur during sexual

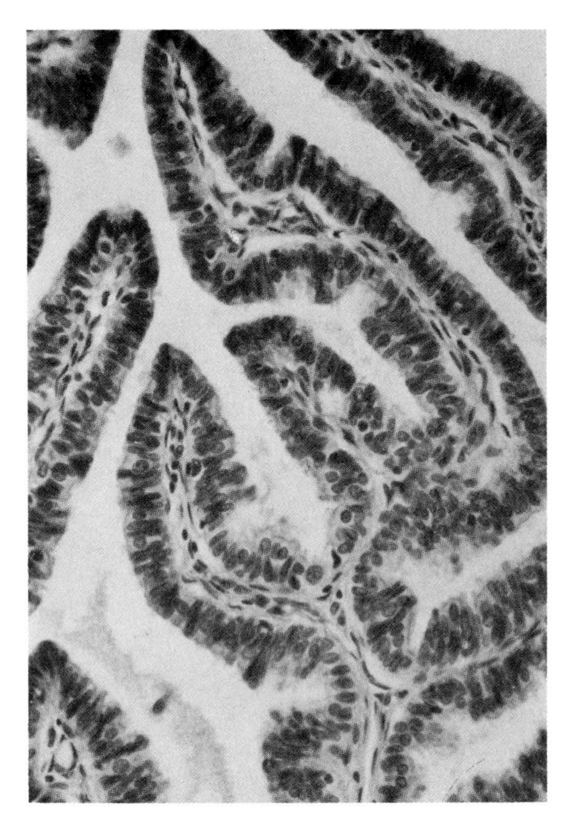

Figure 32–24. Photomicrograph of branching folds of the human tubal mucosa. For orientation, see Fig. 32–23.

stimulation and during menstruation, resulting in cramp-like abdominal pain. The factors controlling these contractions are poorly understood.

The spontaneous contractile activity of the myometrium is greatly reduced during pregnancy. Early animal experiments suggested that contraction was inhibited in the gravid uterus by progesterone secreted by the corpus luteum of pregnancy and that uterine contractions in labor were initiated by withdrawal of this inhibition. This interpretation has now fallen into disfavor for lack of unequivocal evidence for an inhibiting effect of progesterone on human uterine muscle. Cross-circulation experiments between pregnant and nonpregnant animals have, however, clearly demonstrated that there is some blood-borne substance that is inhibitory. This is now believed to be the peptide hormone *relaxin*, mentioned earlier in the chapter as a secretory product of the corpus luteum of pregnancy. The hormone *oxytocin*, secreted by the neurohypophysis, is a powerful stimulant of uterine contraction late in pregnancy. It is often used by obstetricians to initiate labor.

Parturition is a very complex physiological process that we do not completely understand. It is apparent that a cooperative interplay of the fetal and maternal endocrine systems is necessary for termination of gestation. Increased production of estrogens by the placenta and activation of the fetal adrenal gland to release corticotrophic hormone appear to be involved and these lead to production of *prostaglandins* in the fetal membranes and myometrium that initiate uterine contractions. After rupture of the fetal membranes and evacuation of the amniotic fluid, irritation and distension of the cervix by the fetal head is a further stimulus to uterine contractions. Secretion of oxytocin by the posterior pituitary increases the expulsive force of contractions in the second stage of labor, and, after delivery, it continues to promote contraction of the uterus to minimize blood loss after placental detachment.

ENDOMETRIUM

Endometrium is the term descriptive for the mucosa lining the cavity of the uterus. It is 4–5 mm in thickness, at the height of its development, and consists of a simple columnar epithelium from which tubular glands extend downward into a thick lamina propria commonly called the *endometrial stroma*. The principal functions of the endometrium are to prepare for reception of the blastocyst, to participate in its implantation and nutrition, and to form the maternal portion of the placenta. From puberty until menopause, the endometrium goes through monthly cyclic changes in its structure, in response to the fluctuating levels of blood-born ovarian hormones. At the end of each cycle, in which no ovum was fertilized, the greater part of the thickness of the endometrium sloughs off, accompanied by extravasation of blood from the vessels in its stroma. The products of these degenerative changes appear as a bloody vaginal discharge, the *menstrual flow*, which continues for 3–5 days.

There are two zones in the endometrium: The *functionalis* is the upper half to two-thirds that will be sloughed off at the next menstruation, and the *basalis* is a deeper portion that remains and regenerates the functionalis during the first half of the next cycle. Gynecological pathologists define four zones of the endo-

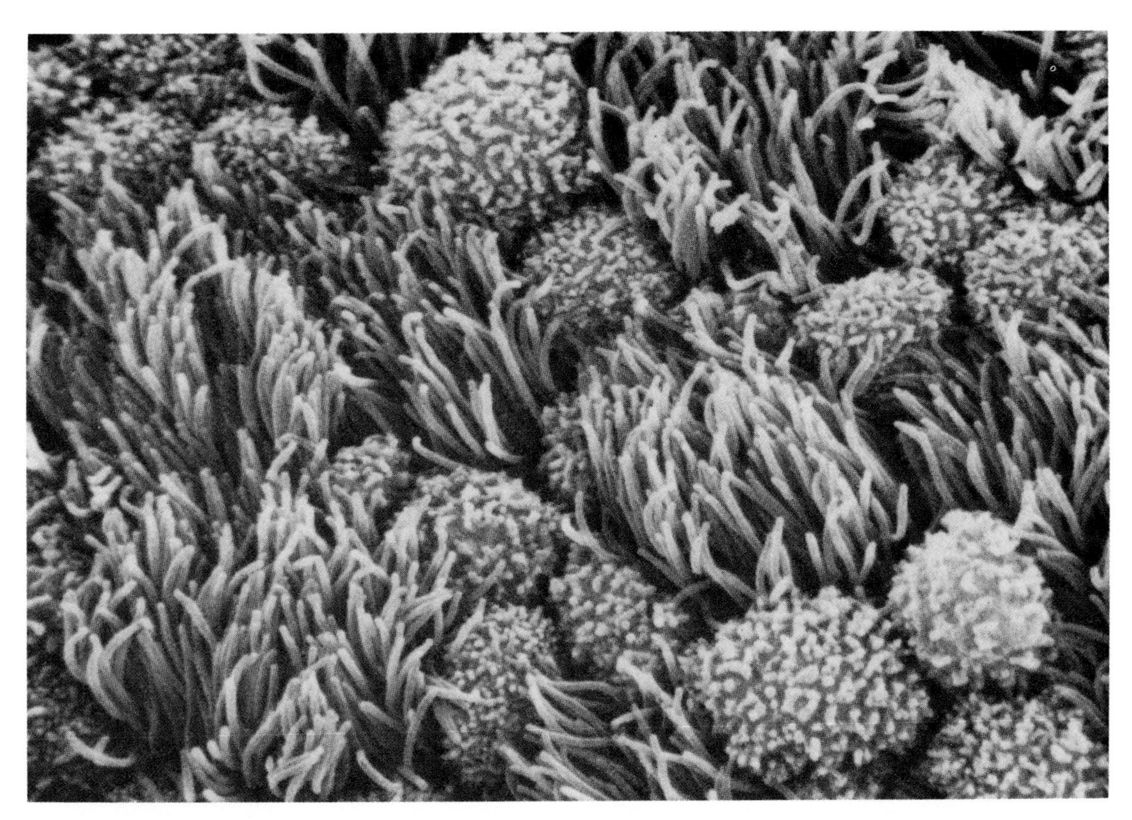

Figure 32–25. Scanning electron micrograph of the surface of the epithelium on a fimbria of a rabbit oviduct, in the postovulatory period, showing the numerous ciliated cells and the short microvilli on the convex apices of the secretory cells. (From Rumery, R.E. and E.M. Eddy. 1974. Anat. Rec. 178:83.)

metrium at successive levels from the free surface to its base. The functionalis is divided into *zone I* consisting of the surface epithelium and the subjacent stroma; and *zone II* which includes the straight upper segments of the uterine glands. The basalis is divided into *zone III* containing the branching lower segments of the glands, and *zone IV*, the bottoms of the glands and their associated stroma. This zonation is useful in their examination of endometrial biopsies to establish the stage of the cycle, but it has little to offer in our general description of the endometrium.

To understand the changes occurring at menstruation and in placentation, it is necessary to have some knowledge of the specialized blood supply of the endometrium. The *uterine arteries* course longitudinally along the sides of the uterus, in the broad ligament. On either side, several branches of these arteries penetrate the myometrium to its stratum vasculare. There, *arcuate arteries* take a circumferential course in the myometrium to the midline, where they anastomose with corresponding arteries from the other side. Branches of the arcuate arteries pass through the stratum submucosum of the myometrium to reach the endometrium. At the endometrial–myometrial boundary, they give off *basal arteries* supplying the basalis. Continuing upward toward the functionalis, they are unbranched but become very tortuous and are called the *spiral arteries*. In the lower portion of the functionalis, they give rise to arterioles that go on to supply a dense capillary network immediately beneath the epithelium at the surface of the endometrium. At all levels of the endometrium, there is a network of thin-walled veins with sinusoidal expansions.

Throughout the greater portion of the menstrual cycle, the spiral arteries constrict and dilate rhythmically, so that the endometrium, viewed with the naked eye, is alternately blanched and suffused with blood. Late in the cycle, there is a prostaglandin-mediated spasm of the spiral arteries that results in necrotic changes in the functionalis that culminate in menstruation.

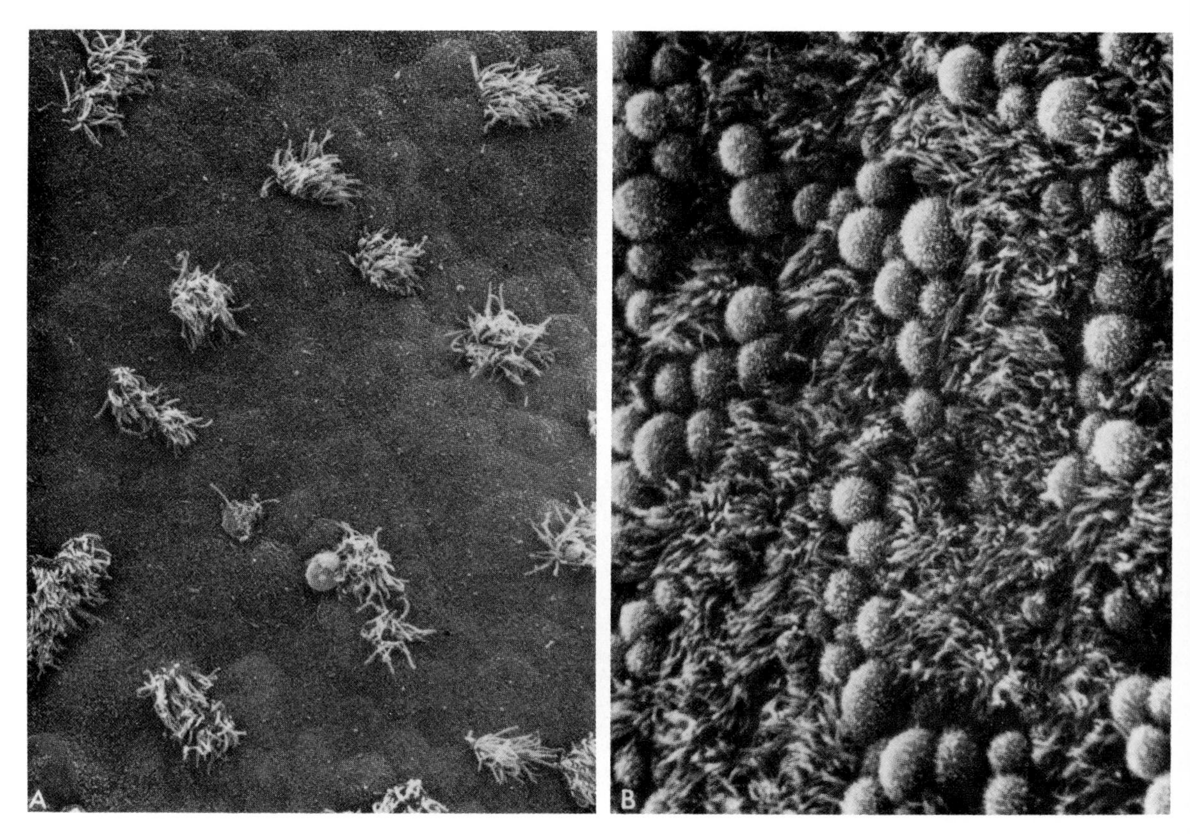

Figure 32–26 Scanning electron micrographs illustrating the dependence of the cytological differentiation of the oviductal epithelium on ovarian hormones. (A) Epithelium on a fimbria of rabbit oviduct, 16 months after ovariectomy. The surface is flat and smooth with only occasional ciliated cells. (B) Epithelium of the other oviduct, of the same rabbit, after 10 days of estrogen replacement. (From Rumery, R.E. and E.M. Eddy. 1974. Anat. Rec. 178:83.)

CYCLIC CHANGES IN THE ENDOMETRIUM

In a normal menstrual cycle, the endometrium goes through a continuous sequence of histological changes, but for descriptive purposes the cycle is divided into three stages: the *proliferative*, the *secretory*, and the *menstrual* phases. These are correlated with the endocrine functions of the developing ovarian follicles. The proliferative phase coincides with the secretion of estrogens by the growing follicles. The secretory phase is the period during which a functional corpus luteum is secreting progesterone, and the menstrual phase is a period of degeneration associated with a rapid decline in stimulation of the endometrium by ovarian hormones (Fig. 32–28).

Proliferative Phase (Follicular Phase)

Beginning at the end of menstrual flow and continuing for 12–14 days, there is a three- to fourfold increase in the thickness of the endometrium. Many cells are found in mitosis, both in the epithelium and in the stroma, as the surface epithelium is being restored and the tubular glands are increasing in length (Fig. 32–29A). The spiral arteries, shortened in the sloughing of the functionalis, are growing in length but do not yet extend into the subsurface stroma, and they are only moderately coiled. As the glands lengthen, they become sinuous and their columnar epithelial cells begin to accumulate glycogen. The proliferative activity continues until midcycle and then declines over the 24 h following ovulation on day 14 of an ideal 28-day cycle. By that time, the regenerated endometrium is again richly vascularized with newly formed capillaries and there may be some diapedesis of erythrocytes into the stroma immediately beneath the surface epithelium. Traces of blood may leak from superficial capillaries, may enter the uterine lumen, and may reach the vagina. Such intermenstrual bleeding is very rare in humans, but midcycle bleeding is common in the dog. During the proliferative

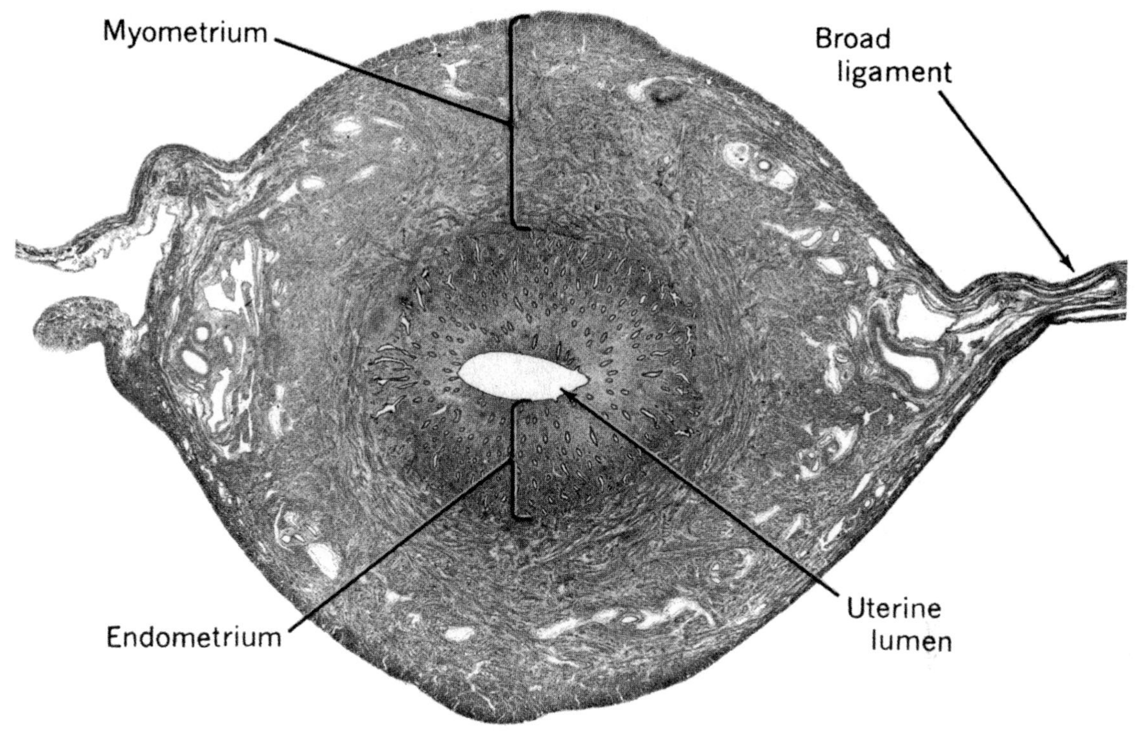

Figure 32–27. Photomicrograph of a cross section of the macaque uterus illustrating the thick myometrium and the endometrium in a late proliferative stage of the cycle. (Courtesy of H. Mizoguchi.)

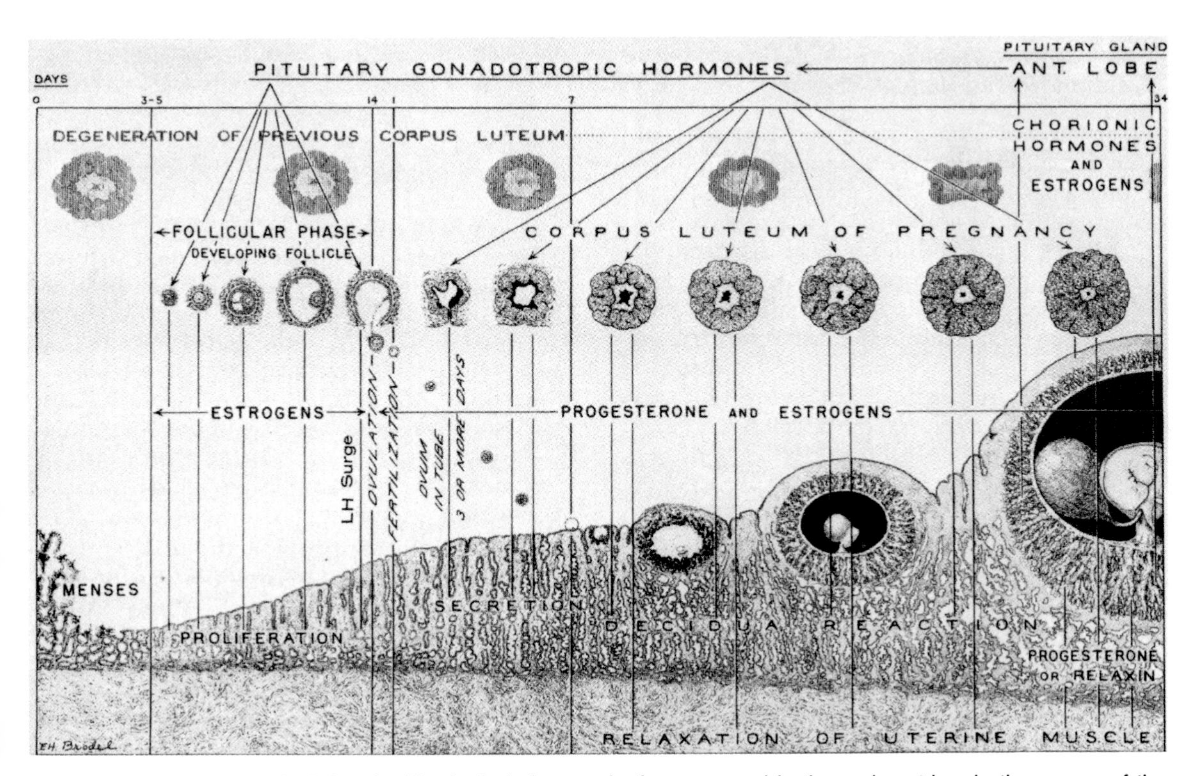

Figure 32–28. Drawing depicting the histological changes in the ovary and in the endometrium in the course of the menstrual cycle, and the hormones controlling these changes. (From Eastman, N.J. ed. 1956. William's Obstetrics, 11th ed. Englewood Cliffs, NJ, Appleton-Century-Crofts.)

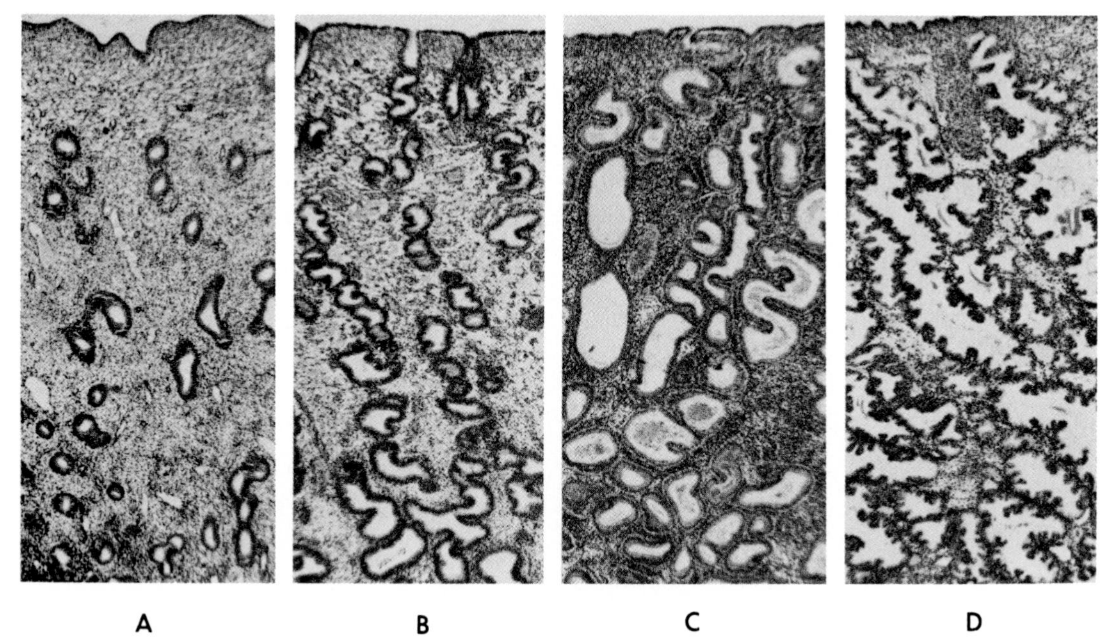

Figure 32–29. Photomicrographs of human endometrium in different phases of the menstrual cycle and early pregnancy. (A) Proliferative endometrium of the ninth day; (B) early secretory endometrium, 15th day; (C) later secretory endometrium, 19th day; (D) gestational hyperplasia, 12th day of pregnancy. (Courtesy of A.T. Hertig.)

phase of the cycle, the endometrium has increased from a postmenstrual thickness of 0.5 mm to 2–3 mm.

Secretory Phase (Luteal Phase)

Early in this phase there may be some further thickening of the endometrium, but this is due mainly to edema of the stroma and accumulation of secretion in the glands. The nucleus of the glandular cells is displaced toward their apex by accumulation of glycogen in the basal cytoplasm, but this is transitory and is not seen after active secretion begins. The glands in the functionalis continue to grow, becoming tortuous and showing lateral sacculations that give them a relatively large lumen of irregular outline (Fig. 32–29B and 32–29C). The glands in the basalis remain more slender and their walls relatively straight. The lumen of the glands is filled with a carbohydrate-rich secretion. Elongation and convolution of the spiral arteries continues and, as they extend into the stroma near the surface, they become more prominent in sections due to thickening of their adventitia by epithelioid stromal cells that form a cuff around them. Edema of the stroma increases and the endometrium reaches its maximum thickness of about 5 mm by the 22nd day of the cycle. Increasing numbers of stromal cells take on an epithelioid appearance and become concentrated in the upper part of the endometrium where they form a *stratum compactum* distinct from the *stratum spongiosum* in the lower portion where the stromal cells do not undergo this cytological change.

Menstrual Phase

In a cycle in which an ovum is not fertilized, marked vascular changes occur in the endometrium about 2 weeks after ovulation. The endometrium is blanched for hours at a time, owing to constriction of the spiral arteries that deprives the functionalis of oxygenated blood. The endometrium stains more deeply and appears more cellular because it has lost much of its interstitial fluid. The glands cease to secrete and the stroma is invaded by large numbers of leukocytes. After about 2 days of intermittent interruption of blood flow to the upper two-thirds of the endometrium, constriction of the spiral arteries becomes continuous, resulting in ischemia of the functionalis, while blood continues to flow in the basalis. Necrotic changes in the functionalis progress. Hours later, the constricted arteries reopen, permitting blood to flow through vessels that have been damaged by ischemia. Vessel walls rupture and blood escapes into the stroma and soon breaks out into the uterine lumen.

Clumps of blood-soaked necrotic endometrium break away leaving the torn ends of glands and open ends of blood vessels exposed at a new surface. Blood continues to ooze from the open ends of veins, contributing to the menstrual flow. Normally, this blood does not clot. The average loss of blood is 35 ml, but greater losses are common. By the third or fourth day of menstruation, the entire functionalis has sloughed off.

The basalis of the endometrium remains intact and viable, and before menstrual flow has entirely ceased, epithelial cells begin to proliferate and migrate from the open ends of the glands to restore a surface epithelium. New blood vessels sprout from those at the base and the stromal cells proliferate and secrete the fibrous and amorphous components of an abundant extracellular matrix. With the onset of these regeneratative activities, the proliferative phase of a new cycle begins.

REVIEW

The changes in the endometrium in the course of a normal menstrual cycle are so consistent that an experienced histologist or pathologist can quite accurately determine the day of the cycle by examining a biopsy of the endometrium (Fig. 32–30). By carrying out such a procedure, in the second half of the cycle, it is also possible to establish whether a woman is having an ovulatory, or an anovulatory, cycle. Endometrial biopsies are essential for investigating disorders of the menstrual cycle and the cause of infertility. Because of their clinical importance, it may be useful to review here the criteria for recognizing the phases of the endometrial cycle. *Proliferative phase*: endometrium 1–4 mm thick; glands straight and narrow; mitoses numerous in all layers; no coiled arteries in upper third. *Secretory phase*: endometrium 4–6 mm thick; glands wide, sinuous, and sacculated; epithelial cells tall with surface blebs; superficial stroma edematous; mitoses confined to coiled arteries which extend to near the surface. *Premenstrual phase*: endometrium 4–5 mm thick; lumen of glands wide and irregular in outline; arteries highly coiled; stroma relatively dense and infiltrated with leukocytes. *Menstrual phase*: endometrium 0.5–3 mm thick and denuded of surface epithelium; glands collapsed and short; extravasated blood in a dense superficial stroma; arteries short and relatively straight.

Sporadic reference has been made earlier in the chapter to the effects of hormones on the uterus and ovaries, but the endocrine functions of the hypothalamus, pituitary gland, and ovaries are so basic to an understanding of the physiology of reproduction that it may be helpful to review these before going on to describe the changes in the tract that are associated with pregnancy.

Neurones in the hypothalamus release gonadotrophin releasing hormones (GnRH) that control the release of gonadotrophins (FSH and LH) by the anterior pituitary. Secretion of follicle-stimulating hormone (FSH) stimulated growth of follicles in the ovary. The developing follicles, in turn, secrete estradiol that stimulates endometrial growth and differentiation during the proliferative phase of the menstrual cycle. Estradiol reaching its peak level as midcycle approaches acts back on the hypothalamus, resulting a pulse of GnRH which results in a midcycle surge of luteinizing hormone (LH) that triggers ovulation and transformation of the collapsed follicle into a corpus luteum (Fig. 32–31). Secretion of progesterone by the corpus luteum, in the secretory phase of the cycle, induces further changes in the endometrium, preparing it for implantation and nutrition of the blastocyst developing from the fertilized ovum during transport through the oviduct. If the cycle is anovulatory, or the ovum is not fertilized, the endometrium breaks down after about 2 weeks, followed by menstruation.

In most mammals, the peak of circulating estrogens shortly before ovulation affects certain centers in the brain, making the female receptive to the male in a *period of heat* or *estrus*. Although the hormonal changes in the menstrual cycle of the human are basically the same as those of the estrus cycle in other species, in women, there is no subjective or behavioral indication that ovulation has occurred or is imminent.

The feedback of excess ovarian hormones to the hypothalamus to diminish the release of GnRH is the basis of a common method of conception control in which orally administered analogues of ovarian steroids act on the hypothalamus to suppress the surge of LH that is necessary for ovulation.

In a cycle in which an ovum is fertilized, the endometrium is invaded, on about the seventh day after ovulation, by the *trophoblast* of the implanting blastocyst. As trophoblast proliferates in developing the *placenta*, it becomes a major source of hormones essential for the

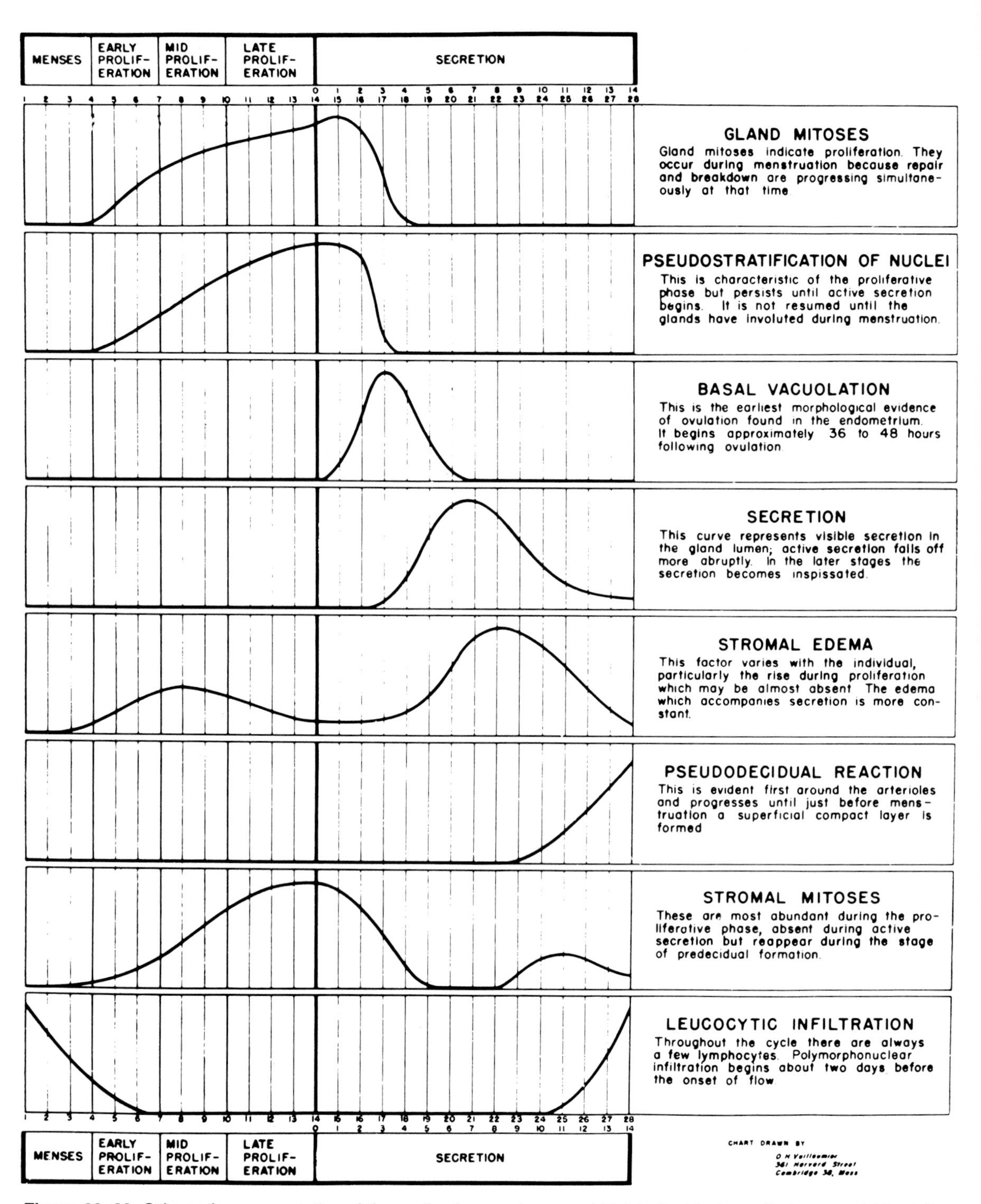

Figure 32–30. Schematic representation of the cyclic changes in several histological features that are useful in dating endometrial biopsies. (From Noyes, R.W., A.T. Hertig, and J. Rock. 1950. Fertil. Steril. 1:3.)

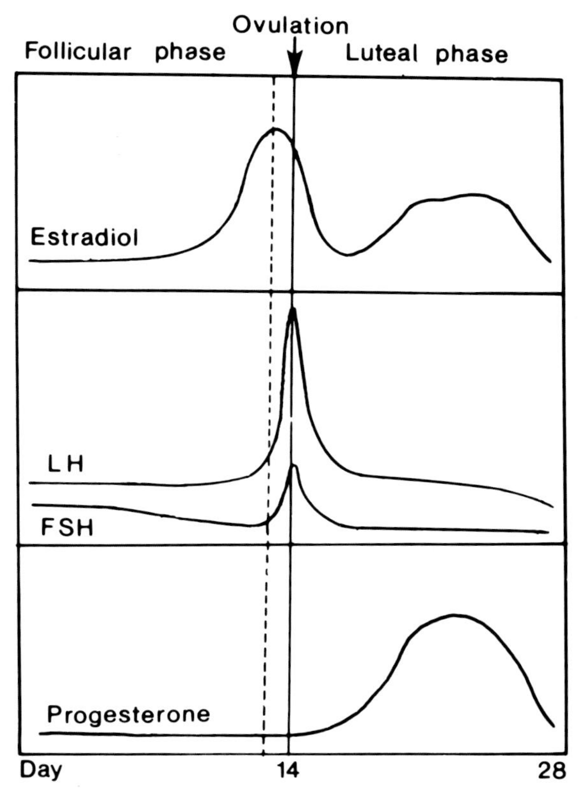

Figure 32–31. Illustration of changes in the levels of ovarian and hypophyseal hormones in the course of an ideal 28-day menstrual cycle. Estrogen, reaching a peak late in the follicular phase, acts back on the hypothalamus, inducing release of GnRH which results in a surge of LH that triggers ovulation. Secretion of progesterone by the corpus luteum rises in the luteal phase and then falls if the ovum is not fertilized.

maintenance of pregnancy. Secretion of the hormone *human chorionic gonadotrophin* (HCG) begins as early as 8 days after ovulation, and its detection is the basis of a common pregnancy test. HCG acts on the ovary to maintain the corpus luteum of pregnancy and, thus, insure the continued secretion of progesterone until this function is taken over by the placenta a few weeks later in gestation. Progesterone stimulates the secretory endometrium and suppresses menstruation for the duration of pregnancy. Progesterone also binds to receptors on uterine smooth muscle, inhibiting contraction and ensuring myometrial quiescence throughout gestation. There is suggestive evidence that progesterone blocks a T-lymphocyte-mediated immune response that might tend to reject the fetus as an antigenic foreign body.

IMPLANTATION

As it passes down the Fallopian tube, the fertilized ovum divides repeatedly, forming a small spherical mass of cells called the *morula*. After this reaches the uterine lumen, on about the fourth day, a central cavity appears in its interior and it then consists of many cells forming a hollow sphere, called the *blastocyst* (Fig. 32–32 and 32–34). It remains free in the lumen for a day or two and then attaches to the surface of the secretory endometrium. The endometrium responds by transformation of its fusiform, or stellate, stromal cells into large, polyhedral, pale-staining *decidual cells* that contain large stores of glycogen and lipid in their cytoplasm. The function of the decidual cells is debated, but they apparently create a favorable milieu for nutrition of the early embryo, and, much later, they form a distinct layer that facilitates dehiscence of the placenta at the termination of pregnancy. Although the normal stimulus for the *decidual reaction* of the endometrium is the implantation of a blastocyst, traumatization, or introduction of any foreign body into the progesterone-primed endometrium, will result in a local accumulation of these cells forming a *deciduoma*.

At the time of implantation, there is a cluster of cells at one pole of the blastocyst, called the *inner cell mass*, which is destined to form the embryo proper, whereas the remainder of the hollow sphere consists of *trophoblast cells* that will form the placenta. Rapid proliferation of the trophoblast cells gives rise to an inner layer of *cytotrophoblast*, composed of separate cells, and a thick outer layer, the *syncytial trophoblast* which is a continuous multinucleate layer of protoplasm in which no cell boundaries are discernible (Figs. 32–33 and 32–35). The cytotrophoblast is mitotically active and continuously forms new cells that fuse with, and are incorporated into, the growing syncytiotrophoblast.

The syncytiotrophoblast actively erodes the endometrium, enabling the blastocyst, as a whole, to sink deeper into it. By the 11th day, it is entirely within the endometrium, and surrounded by thick trophoblastic syncytium. The discontinuity created in the surface of the endometrium is covered by cellular debris in a fibrin clot until the epithelium regenerates over the implantation site. This type of implantation, in which, the blastocyst becomes completely embedded in, and encapsulated by, endometrium is called *interstitial implanta-*

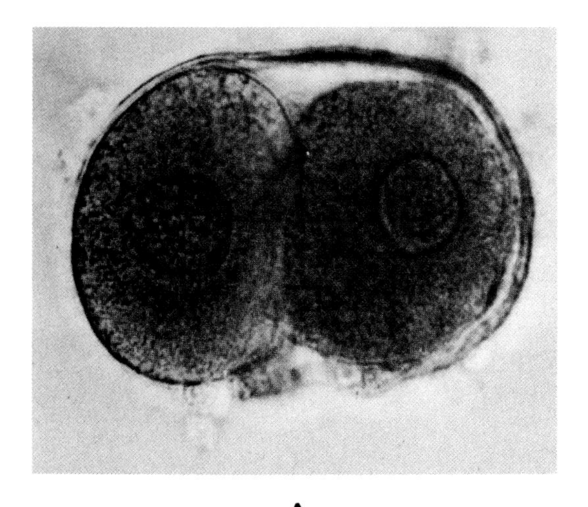

A

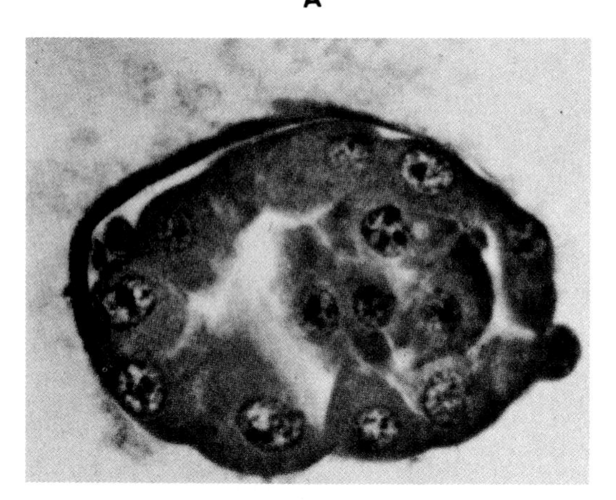

B

C

Figure 32–32. Photomicrographs of early human ova. (A) Two-cell stage recovered from Fallopian tube (age 1–2.5 days). (B) Free 58-cell intrauterine blastocyst. Zona pellucida disappearing. (C) Free 107-cell human blastocyst, recovered from uterine cavity (age 4.5 days). Inner cell mass is at the right. (From Hertig, A., J. Rock, and E. Adams. 1956. Am. J. Anat. 98:435.)

tion and is characteristic of the human and other primates. As the expanding layer of syncytiotrophoblast around the blastocyst continues to invade the surrounding endometrium, it becomes permeated by a labyrinthine system of intercommunicating lacunae filled with blood liberated from blood vessels it has eroded (Fig. 32–35). This blood is the initial source of nourishment for the embryo, and its liberation from endometrial vessels is the first step toward establishment the utero-placental circulation on which the growth of the fetus will later depend.

At 11 days postovulation, the embryo proper is a bilaminar disc consisting of a thick plate of columnar epithelial cells, the *ectoderm*, and a thinner layer of squamous or cuboidal cells, the *endoderm*. The ectodermal plate is continuous at its margins with a layer of squamous cells that enclose a small *amniotic cavity*. The endoderm is continuous at its margins with a sheet of cells that encloses the *yolk sac*. A wide space, the *exocoelom*, between these derivatives of the inner-cell mass and the trophoblastic shell is traversed by thin strands of *extraembryonic mesenchyme*. The broad peripheral zone of trophoblast is henceforth called the *chorion*.

PLACENTA

From the 11th to the 16th day, the products of conception continue to enlarge at the expense of the surrounding endometrium. Erosion of endometrial blood vessels becomes more extensive with many communications forming between the endometrial venous sinuses and the lacunae within the syncytiotrophoblast. From the 15th day onward, cords of trophoblast grow outward from the trophoblastic shell forming the *primary chorionic villi*. These are soon invaded at their base by mesenchyme that advances to their tips, converting the primary villi into *secondary chorionic villi* (Fig. 32–36), consisting of an outer layer of syncytial trophoblast and an inner layer of cytotrophoblast around a core of mesenchyme (Fig. 32–40). They are bathed in maternal blood that flows sluggishly through a system of intercommunicating vascular channels that collectively form the *intervillous space*.

From the ends of some of the secondary chorionic villi, cords of cells, the *cytotrophoblastic cell columns*, grow across the intervillous space. On reaching the opposite wall, they spread laterally along it, coalescing with simi-

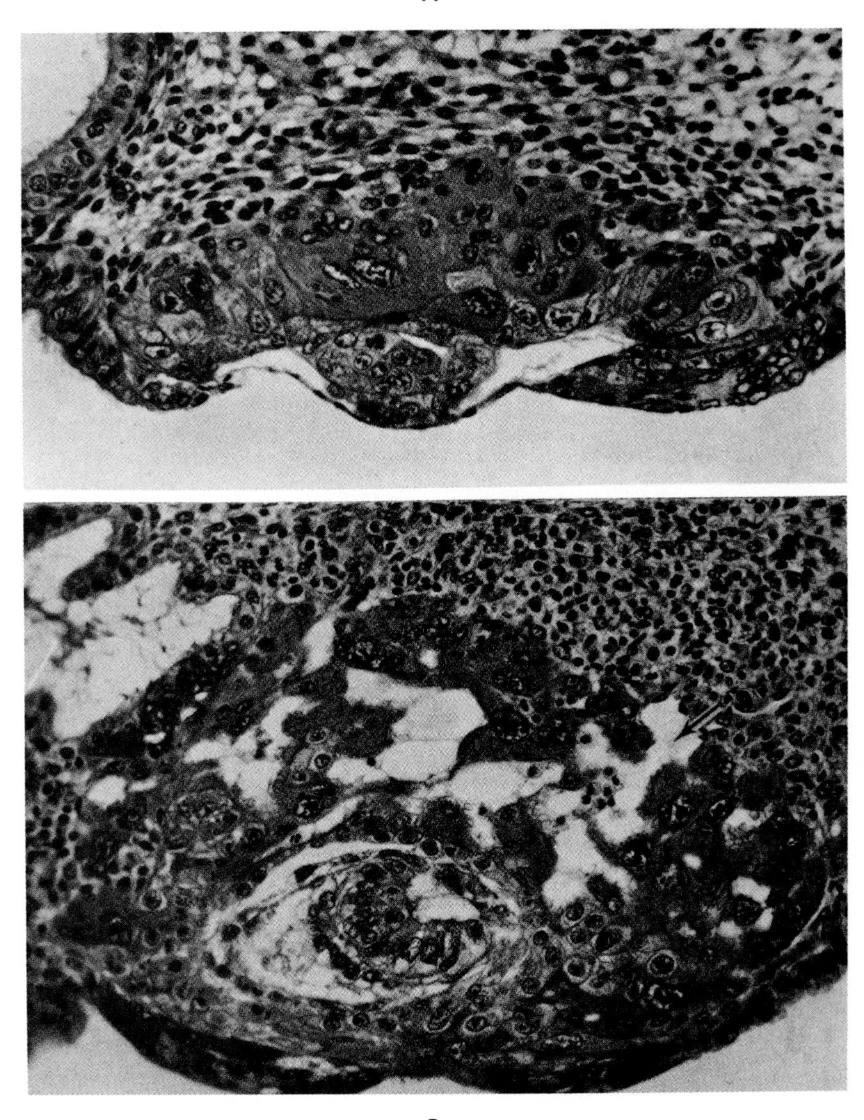

Figure 32–33. Photomicrographs of early human implantation sites. (A) At seven days, the embryo is a simple bilaminar disc. Development of the amniotic cavity is beginning and there is a sizable plaque of syncytio- and cytotrophoblast. (B) At nine days, the embryo is a bilaminar disc. The syncytiotrophoblast now shows prominent lacunae. Note (at arrow) maternal blood sinus communicating with a lacuna. (After Hertig, A. and J. Rock. Carnegie Contrib. to Embryol. No 125:1. 1941. Courtesy of Carnegie Institution of Washington.)

lar outgrowths from neighboring villi to form a continuous *trophoblastic shell* that is interrupted only at sites of communication of maternal blood vessels with the intervillous space. Vigorous mitotic activity within this layer provides for rapid circumferential growth and enlargement of the intervillous space. Throughout the remainder of gestation, the intervillous space is lined by trophoblast and traversed by villi that are fixed to the maternal tissue via their continuity with the trophoblastic shell. The placental villi absorb nutrients from the maternal blood in the intervillous space and excrete wastes into it. The efficiency of this exchange is greatly enhanced after development of the fetal vascular system.

In the vascularization of the mesenchymal cores of the villi, discontinuous endothelium-lined spaces first develop and these subsequently coalesce to form continuous blood vessels. These establish connections with other

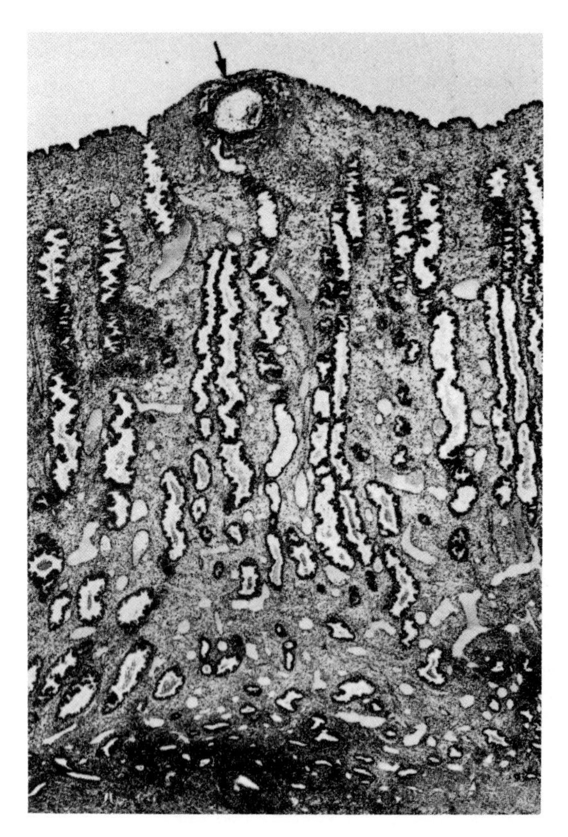

Figure 32–34. Human gestational endometrium with an 11-day implantation (at arrow). The entire thickness of the endometrium is shown. The glands are secretory and the stroma edematous. (After Hertig, A. and J. Rock. Carnegie Contrib. to Embryol. No 125:1. 1941. Carnegie Institution of Washington.)

vessels developing concurrently in the mesenchyme of the deeper portion of the chorion and in the *body stalk* that will later become the umbilical cord. By the 22nd day, fetal blood begins to circulate through the vessels in the placental villi. Thereafter, the villi are referred to as the *tertiary villi* or *definitive villi.* At this stage, villi radiate from the entire periphery of the chorion. Later in development of the placenta, those that extend across the intervillous space to the trophoblastic shell give rise to many lateral branches that float free in the blood circulating in the intervillous space.

As placental development progresses, descriptive terms for its parts proliferate. The villi that arise from the chorionic plate are usually called *stem villi* (Figs. 32–37 and 32–38); those that cross the intervillous space and join the cytotrophoblastic shell are called *anchoring villi*; and those with free ends projecting into the blood are called *terminal villi* (Fig. 32–39). The stem villi have up to 15 generations of branching. The very slender tips of the terminal villi are no doubt moved about by blood flow in the intervillous space, and small portions may break off, forming the so-called *trophoblastic knots.* The majority of these remain enmeshed among the villi, but a few may be swept into the maternal circulation as emboli that become lodged in small vessels of the maternal lungs. The very great number of highly branched placental villi presents a very large surface area for exchange of nutrients and metabolites with the blood. In the mature human placenta, the villous surface is estimated to be about 10 m^2. The additional surface amplification achieved by the microvilli on the syncytial trophoblast probably brings the total surface area to nearly 90 m^2.

Because not all areas of the endometrium are intimately associated with the products of conception, it is convenient to have separate descriptive terms for its different regions. Early in pregnancy, the endometrium modified by the decidual reaction is called the *decidua*, and within it the portion that underlies the products of conception is the *decidua basalis.* This portion will later form the maternal portion of the definitive placenta. The thinner superficial layer over the adluminal side of the embryo and its trophoblastic shell is the *decidua capsularis*, and that portion lining the remainder of the uterus is called the *decidua vera.*

Villi are equally numerous around the entire circumference of the chorion, during the first 8 weeks, but as pregnancy advances, the villi associated with the decidua basalis rapidly increase in number and length, whereas those associated with the decidua capsularis degenerate, so that by the third month, this surface of the chorion is smooth and relatively avascular. Henceforth, this region is called the *chorion laeve*, whereas the portion associated with the decidua basalis retains its villi and is called the *chorion frondosum.* This discoid basal area of the chorion will go on to form the fetal portion of the definitive placenta.

As the volume of the conceptus increases and it bulges further into the uterine lumen, the overlying decidua capsularis becomes greatly attenuated, and when its blood supply is finally jeopardized, it degenerates. By four and half months, the uterine lumen is largely obliterated (Figs. 32–41 and 32–42), the decidua capsularis is no longer present and the chorion laeve has fused with the decidua vera

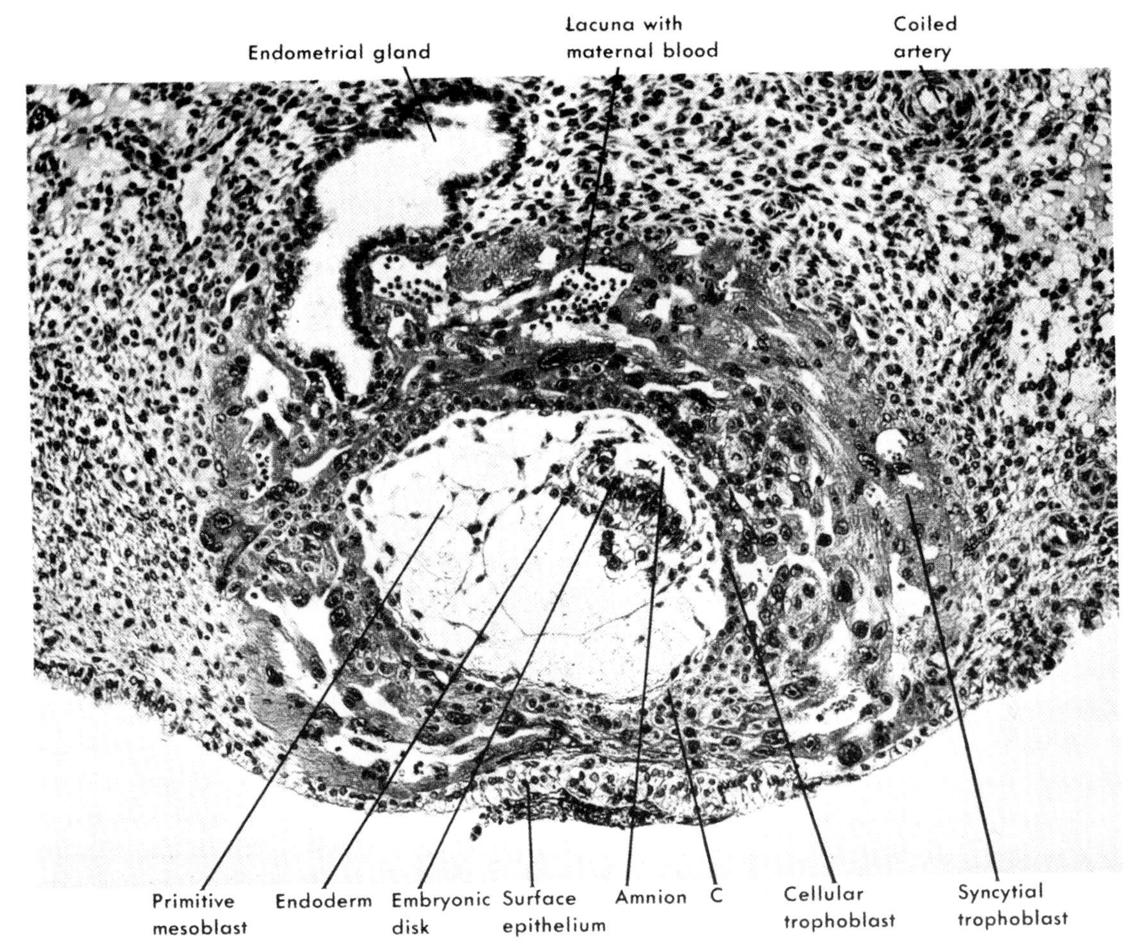

Figure 32–35. Photomicrograph from the same section as in Fig. 32–34, at higher magnification. The bulk of the implanted ovum consists of syncytial trophoblast invading the endometrium. Inside of the syncytium, cytotrophoblast forms a simple epithelium with obvious cell boundaries. The cytotrophoblast immediately surrounds the loosely organized cells of the primitive chorionic mesoblast. The embryonic disc is evident within the mesoblast. (After Hertig, A. and J. Rock. Carnegie Contrib. to Embryol. No 125:1. 1941. Courtesy of Carnegie Institution of Washington.)

on the opposite side of the uterine lumen. In the subsequent development of the placenta, there is a steady increase in number and length of the villi of the chorion frondosum and an expansion of the intervillous space. During the fifth month, incomplete septa grow into the intervillous space from the underlying decidual basalis, partitioning the placenta into 10–15 subunits called *cotyledons.*

ULTRASTRUCTURE OF THE TROPHOBLAST

The cytotrophoblast consists of relatively undifferentiated cells with a euchromatic nucleus and pale-staining cytoplasm, containing few organelles. They are attached to one another and to the overlying syncytium by desmosomes. The cytoplasm is rich in free ribosomes, but there is very little rough endoplasmic reticulum. Although they have been shown to be capable of steroid synthesis in vitro, they contain little or no smooth endoplasmic reticulum in vivo. The mitochondria are somewhat larger than those of the syncytium. In the first 2 months of pregnancy, they store glycogen but contain little thereafter. The cells of the cytotrophoblast serve as stem cells for the expanding syncytiotrophoblast. They progressively decrease in number and from the fifth month onward, they show little mitotic activity, and no longer form a continuous layer.

The free surface of the syncytial trophoblast is irregular in outline and is provided with

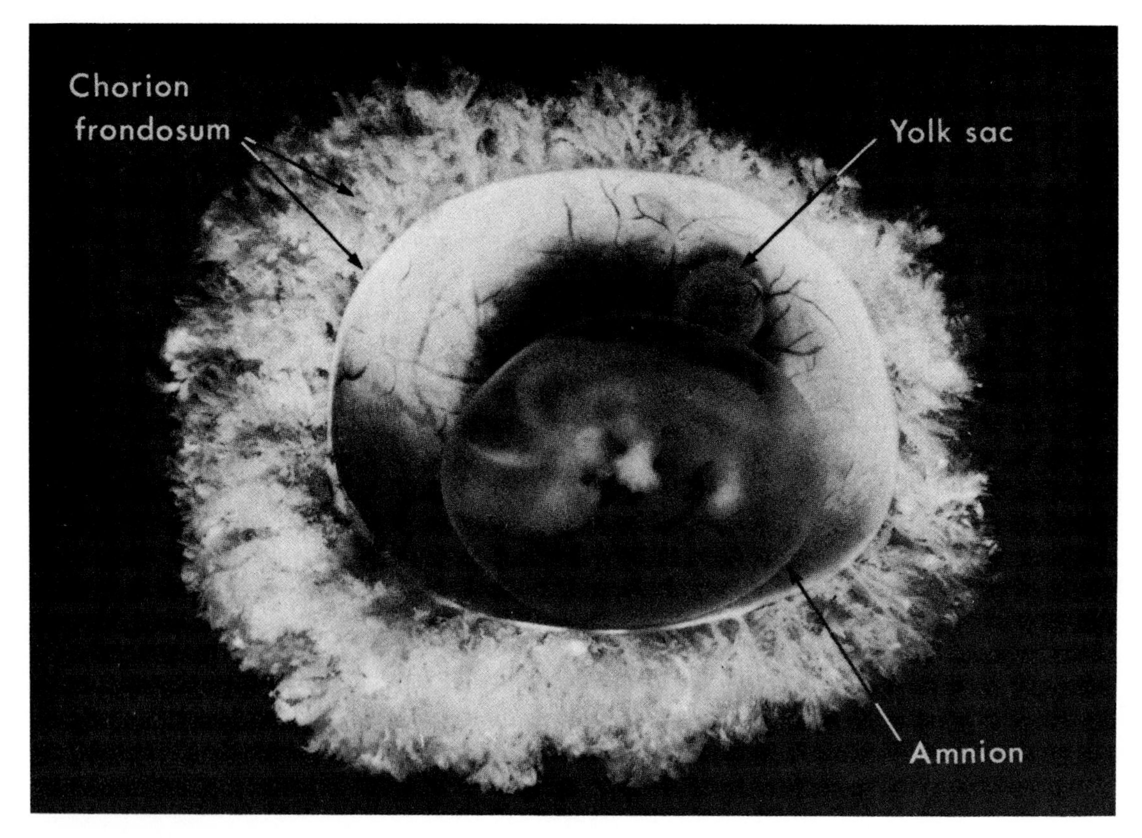

Figure 32–36. Photograph of a 40-day-old human embryo (Carnegie No. 8537) showing the myriad placental villi projecting from the entire surface of the chorion. (McKay, D.G. and M.V. Richardson. 1955. Am. J. Obs. Gyn. 69:735. Courtesy of Carnegie Institution of Washington.)

very numerous microvilli. Between the bases of the microvilli, there are many coated vesicles engaged in receptor-mediated endocytosis, and vesicles are abundant in the apical cytoplasm. The nuclei of the syncytium tend to gather in groups. Multiple Golgi complexes are widely distributed in the cytoplasm and there is an extensive rough endoplasmic reticulum and many free ribosomes, but there is very little smooth endoplasmic reticulum, an organelle usually associated with steroid secretion. The long mitochondria have both foliate and tubular cristae. The form of the mitochondrial cristae and presence of numerous cholesterol-containing lipid droplets is consistent with steroidogenesis by the syncytium, but the virtual absence of smooth endoplasmic reticulum is puzzling. One must assume that, in this case, the enzymes of the biosynthetic pathway for steroids reside in the membrane of the rough endoplasmic reticulum.

As pregnancy progresses, the syncytial trophoblast comes to vary greatly in thickness. Thick areas containing clusters of nuclei alternate with very thin areas devoid of nuclei. Dilated capillaries in the core of the villi are closely applied to the attenuated areas of the syncytium so that the barrier between the maternal and fetal blood is little more than 2 μm, a relationship reminiscent of the thin blood-air diffusion barrier in the lungs.

PLACENTAL CIRCULATION

Blood, poor in oxygen, is carried from the fetus to the placenta by the *umbilical arteries* in the umbilical cord. At the junction of the cord with the placenta, the umbilical arteries divide into several radially disposed placental arteries that branch repeatedly in the chorionic plate. Numerous branches from these pass into the stem villi and ramify into their numerous branches, forming capillary networks that extend into the terminal villi where gas exchange takes place. The oxygen-rich venous blood, collecting in thin-walled veins in the villi, returns through veins of increasing size that fol-

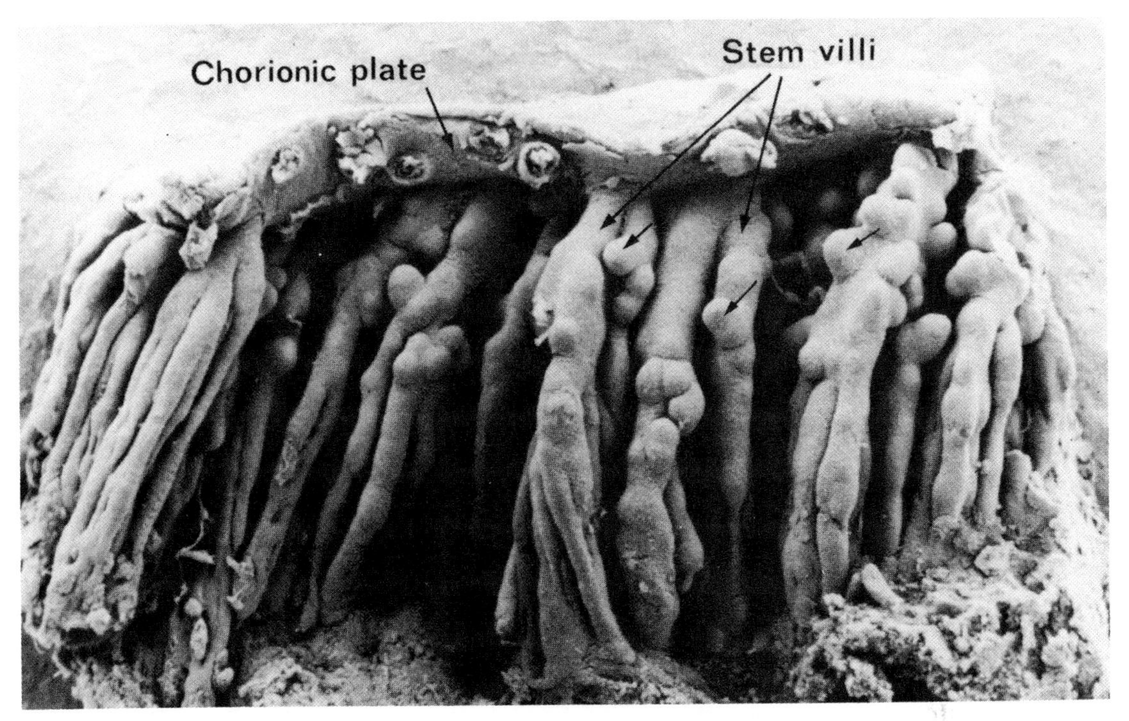

Figure 32–37. Scanning micrograph of a portion of the placenta of a macaque at 22 days gestation. Side branches from the stem villi are just beginning to appear (small arrows). (From King, B. 1982. Anat. Embryol. 165:361.)

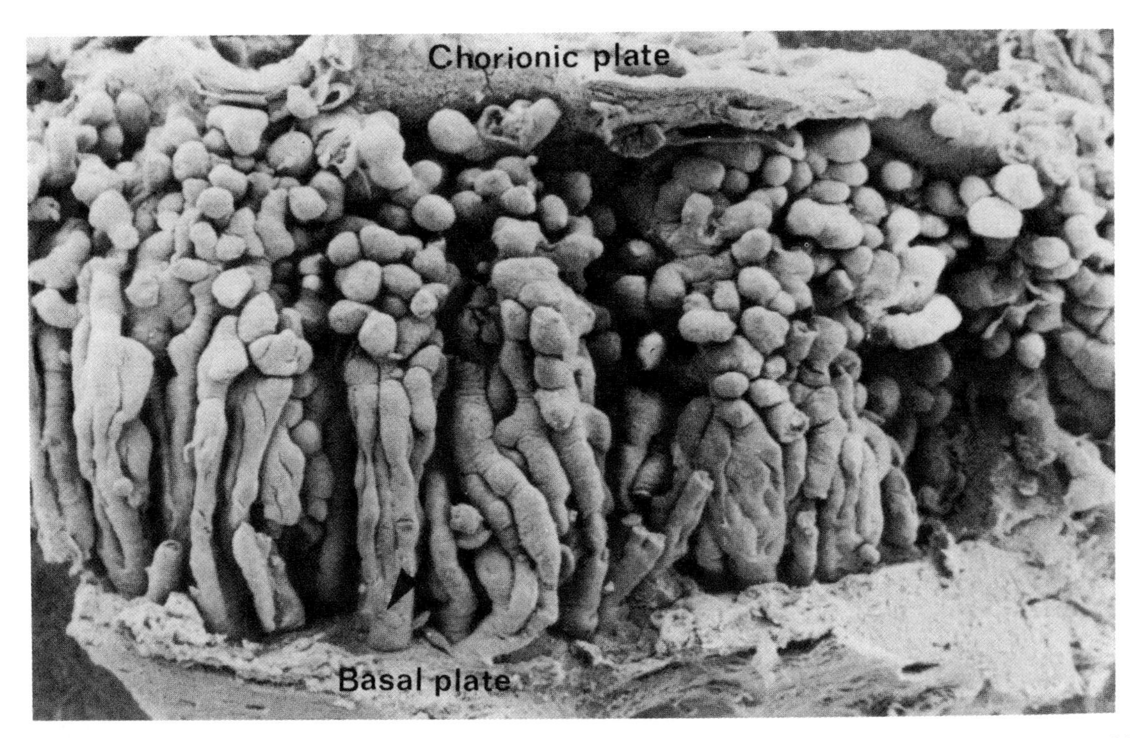

Figure 32–38. Scanning micrograph of a portion of the placental disc of a macaque at 31 days of gestation. Villous side branches have continued to develop near the chorionic plate. (From King, B. 1982. Anat. Embryol. 165:361.)

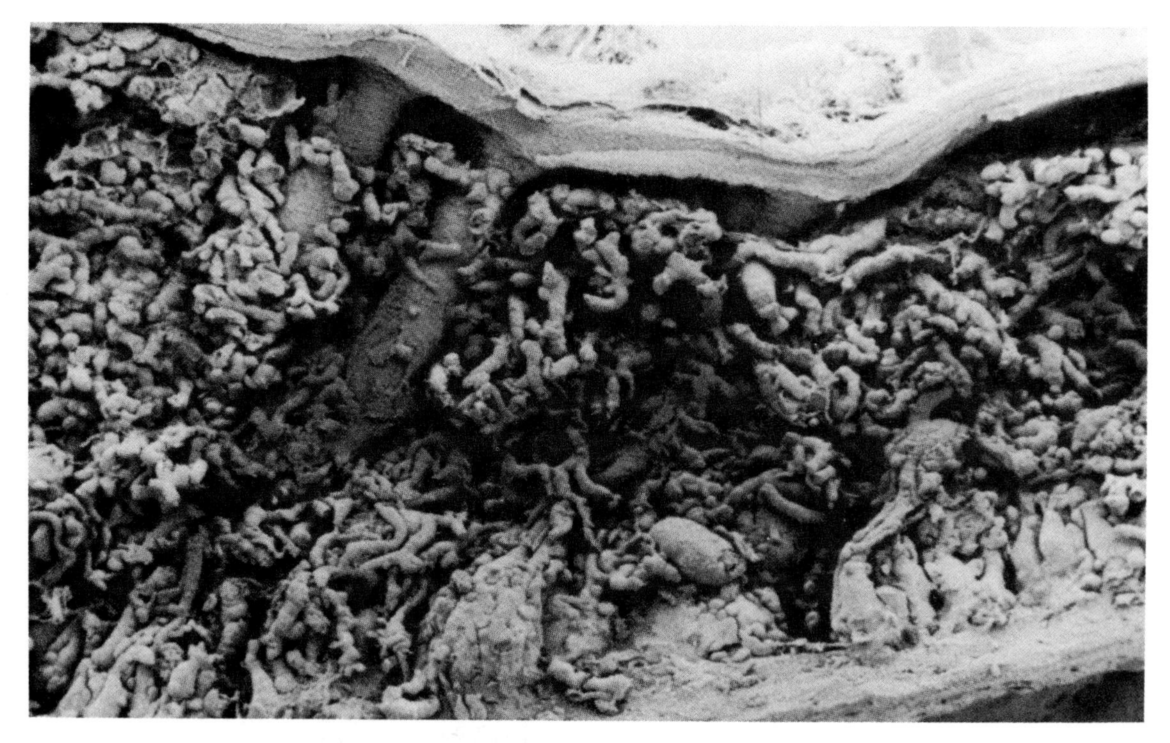

Figure 32–39. Scanning micrograph of a portion of the placenta of a macaque at 60 days of gestation. Large stem villi can be seen at the upper left, but most of the placenta now consists of slender branching terminal villi. (From King, B. 1982. Anat. Embryol. 165:361.)

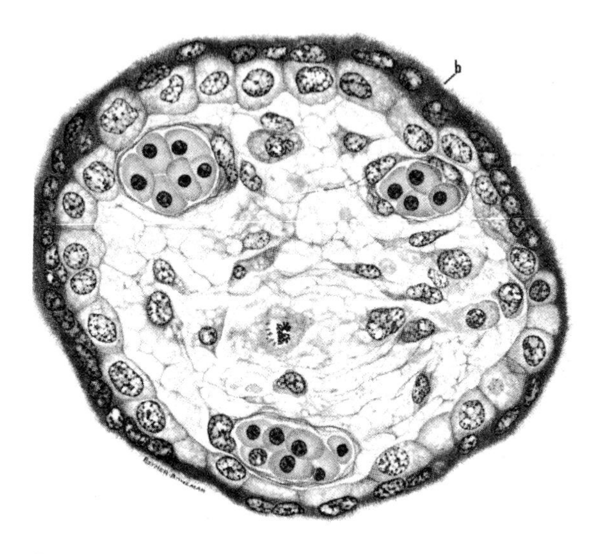

Figure 32–40. Drawing of a section through a placental villus from a 2 cm human embryo. The syncytial trophoblast is on the outside, and a layer of cytotrophoblast beneath it. Vessels in the mesenchyme of the core are filled with nucleated primitive erythroblasts.

low the course of the arteries to the chorionic plate. There, they are confluent with larger veins that converge to form a single, large *umbilical vein* that carries the blood from the placenta, through the umbilical cord, to the ductus venosus, which enters the fetal vena cava near the right atrium of the heart.

On the maternal side of the circulation, blood from arcuate branches of the uterine artery is carried in the coiled arteries of the decidua through openings in the basal plate of the placenta into the intervillous space. Flow from these vessels is pulsatile and is ejected at a pressure considerably higher than that prevailing in the space. Therefore, it spurts in jets deep into the intervillous space, and as its pressure is dissipated, it flows back more slowly over the surface of the placental villi, permitting exchange of metabolites (Fig. 32–43). In the hemochorial placenta of the human, the syncytial trophoblast is exposed directly to the maternal blood and the diffusion barrier between maternal and fetal blood is very thin. The pressure of the inflowing blood, and its fountain-like expulsion, tend to force the blood against the opposite wall and back toward the basal plate, where it is drained

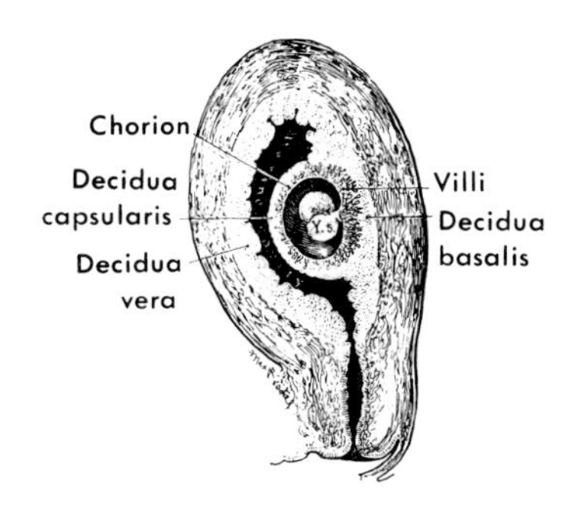

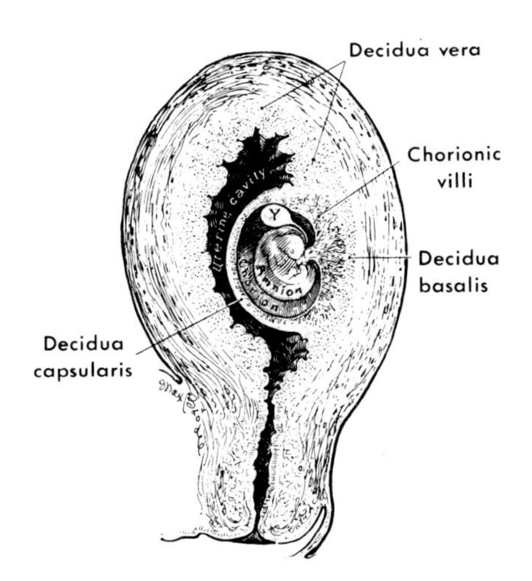

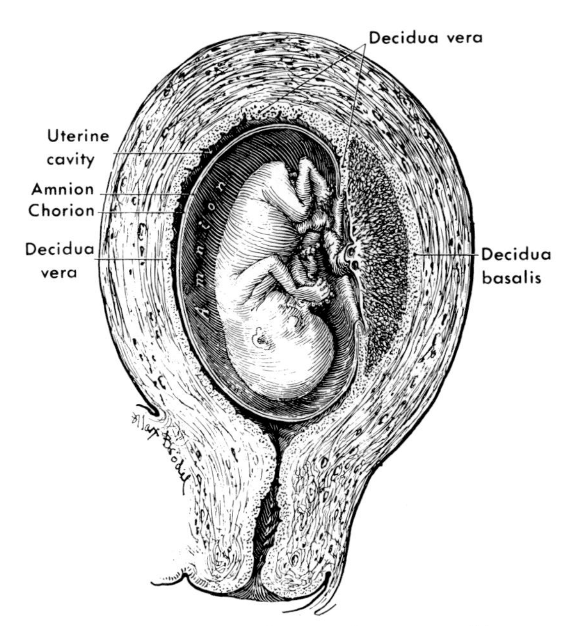

Figure 32–41. Drawings of successive stages of human pregnancy showing the gradual obliteration of the uterine lumen, disappearance of the decidua capsularis, and establishment of the definitive discoid placenta. (Drawing by M. Brödel, from Williams, J. 1927. Am. J. Obs. Gyn. 13:1.)

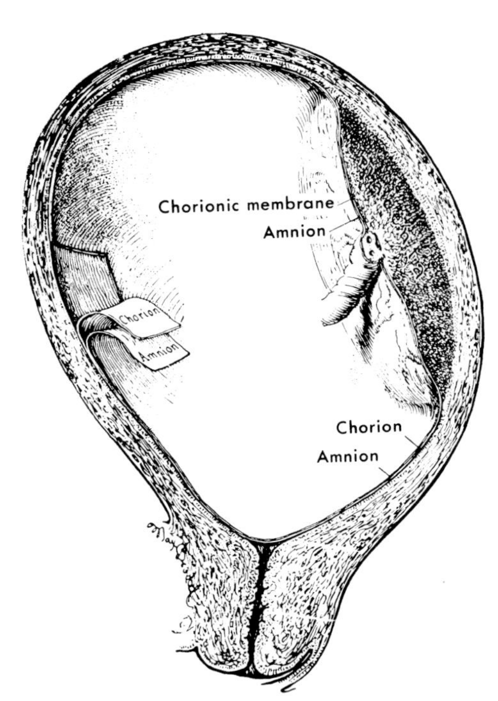

Figure 32–42. Drawing of the disposition of the fetal membranes in the later months of pregnancy. The amnion and chorion have come into contact and have adhered to each other and to the decidua vera. (Drawing by M. Brödel, from Williams, J. 1927. Am. J. Obs. Gyn. 13:1.)

away through the numerous communications between the intervillous space and dilated veins in the decidua basalis, from where it flows to the uterine veins.

HISTOPHYSIOLOGY OF THE PLACENTA

The maternal and fetal blood are brought into close proximity in the placenta for exchange of gases, nutrients, and waste products. Owing to the syncytial nature of the trophoblast, substances cannot traverse it via a paracellular route. All substances entering or leaving the fetal blood must pass through the syncytiotrophoblast. Oxygen, carbon dioxide, fatty acids, steroids, and electrolytes can traverse it by *passive diffusion*. Glucose and certain other substances cross it more rapidly than would be expected from passive diffusion and it is likely that carrier molecules are involved in *facilitated diffusion*. The fetus synthesizes its own proteins from amino acids that cross the placental barrier by active transport. The membrane of the syncytium contains receptors for insulin, transferrin, and the Fc por-

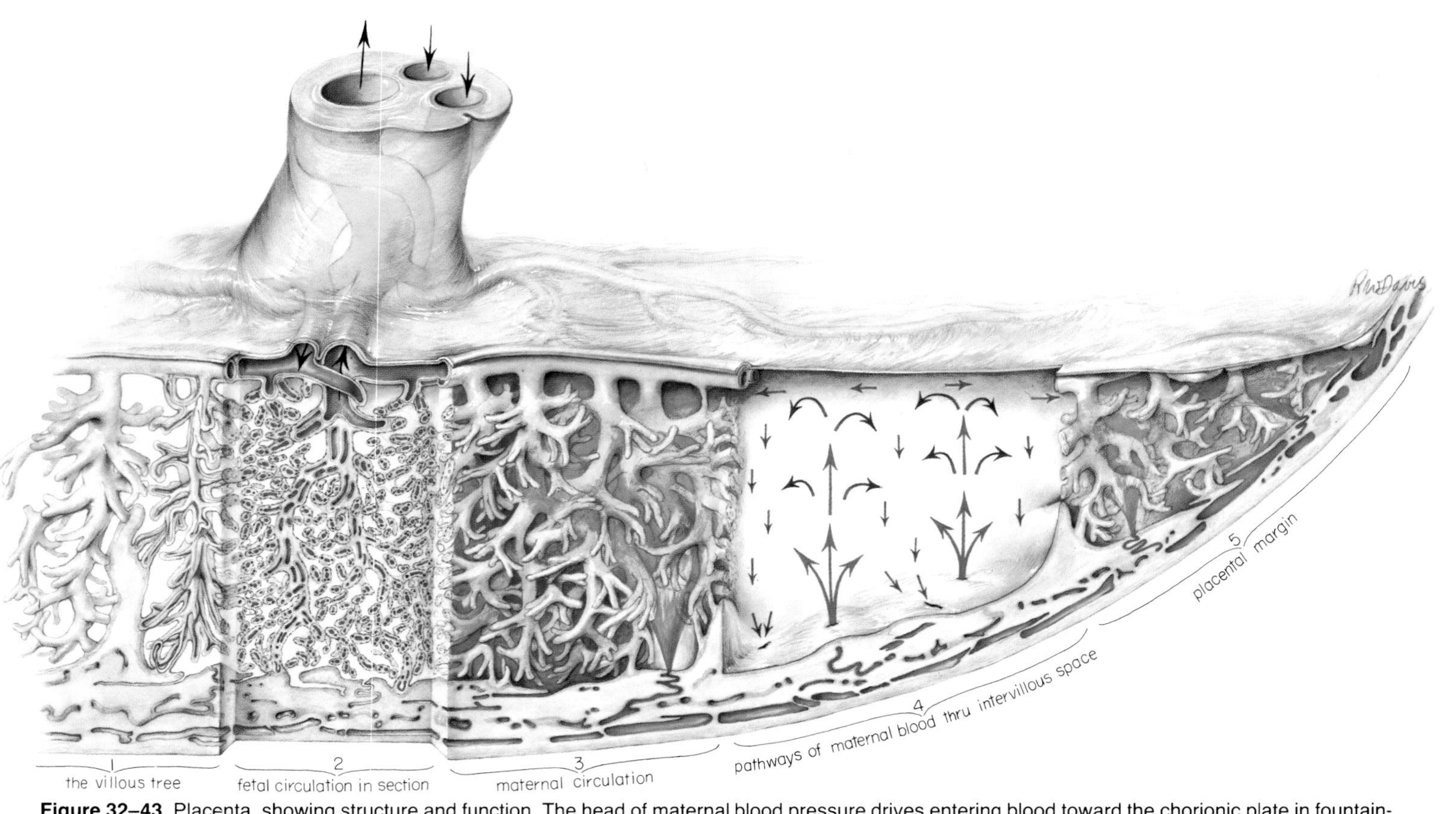

Figure 32–43. Placenta, showing structure and function. The head of maternal blood pressure drives entering blood toward the chorionic plate in fountain-like spurts. As the head of pressure is dissipated, lateral dispersion of blood occurs. Inflowing arterial blood pushes venous blood out into the endometrial veins. (After Ramsey, E.M. and J.W. Harris. 1966. Contrib. Embryol. 38 Carnegie Contr. to Embryol. No 261. Vol. 38:61. Courtesy of the Carnegie Institution of Washington. Drawing by Ranice Crosby.)

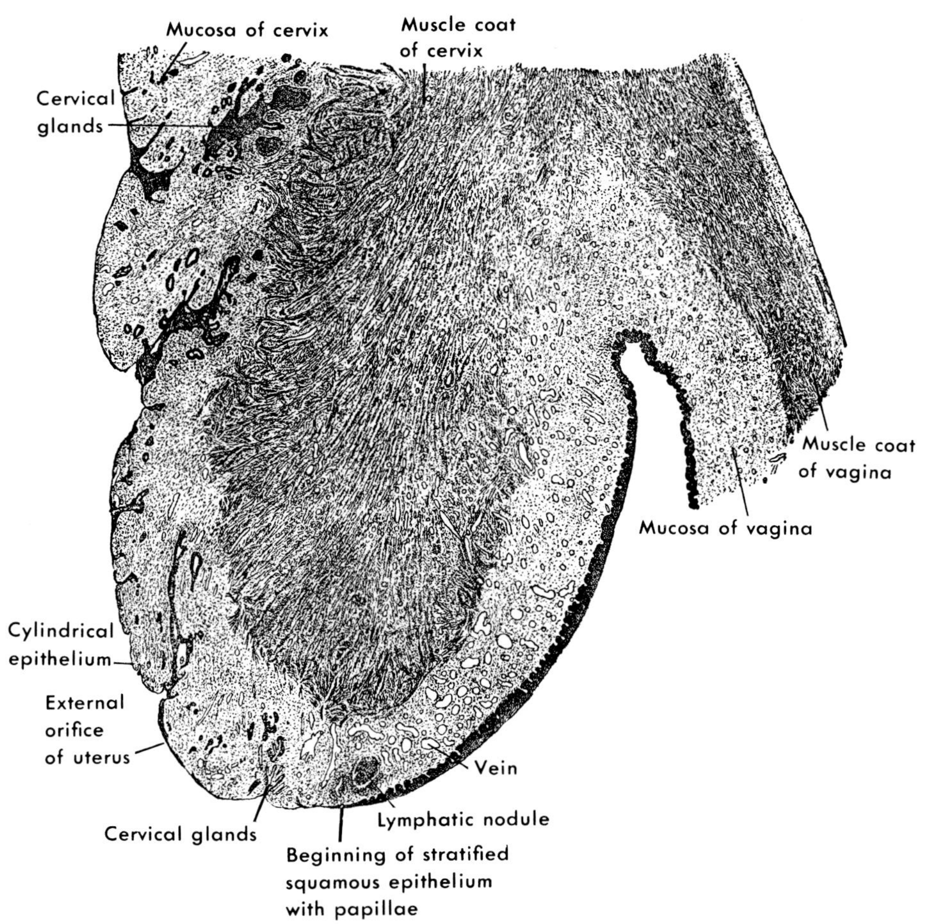

Figure 32–44. Sagittal section through the posterior half of the portio vaginalis of the cervix, and the vaginal fornix of a young woman. (After von Ebner, 1902 in 6th ed. A. von Kölliber's Handbuch der Gewebelehre.)

tion of immunoglobulins and other macromolecules that are taken up by *receptor-mediated endocytosis* and moved across the epithelium in transport vesicles. Exocytosis by the syncytium is involved in release of hormones into the maternal blood.

The placenta is a major endocrine organ producing hormones that are essential for the maintenance of pregnancy. One of the first to be secreted by the trophoblast is *human chorionic gonadotrophin* (hCG) which can be detected in the maternal blood 6–8 d after fertilization and increases rapidly up to the fifth month of pregnancy. This glycoprotein hormone resembles luteinizing hormone in its chemical structure and is similar in function. It maintains the corpus luteum of pregnancy and stimulates its secretion of progesterone.

The placenta also secretes progesterone and estrogens that have a paracrine effect on the endometrium, stimulating proliferation and differentiation of the decidual cells to maintain a favorable uterine environment for fetal development. Progesterone is released into the maternal blood and, by full term, it reaches five times the level found in the luteal phase of a normal menstrual cycle. It binds to receptors on smooth muscle of the myometrium and inhibits uterine contraction for the duration of pregnancy. As suggested earlier in the chapter, it may also favor continuation of pregnancy by inhibiting cell-mediated responses of T-lymphocytes that are involved in rejection of grafts of foreign tissue.

The trophoblast has little capacity for production of cholesterol as a precursor in the synthesis of progesterone. It is dependent on receptor-mediated uptake of cholesterol in low-density lipoprotein (LDL) from the maternal blood. Its inability to synthesize cholesterol from acetate may be related to the absence of extensive smooth endoplasmic reticulum in the syncytial trophoblast noted above.

The production of estrogens by the syncytiotrophoblast is also unusual in that it lacks the enzyme necessary for conversion of progesterone to estrogen and relies on androgens produced in the maternal and fetal adrenal glands, as precursors for estrogen synthesis. The principal estrogen produced is *estriol* rather than estradiol. The maternal urinary estriol level becomes nearly a thousand times the level of this hormone in the nonpregnant state. The functional significance of such high levels of maternal estrogens is poorly understood.

The placenta also produces the polypeptide hormone *placental lactogen*. Its chemical structure is related to that of the growth hormone, somatotrophin. It has a lactogenic action in some species, but no effect on the mammary gland has been demonstrated in the human and it is now more commonly referred to as *somatomammotrophin*. It has some growth-promoting action, but probably more significant are its effects on maternal carbohydrate and fat metabolism. It appears to diminish maternal glucose utilization and to stimulate lipolysis, making more glucose and fatty acids available to the fetus.

Less attention has been directed to the fetal membranes other than the placenta. The fetus is surrounded by amniotic fluid which steadily increases in volume from a few milliliters early in gestation to 700–1000 ml near full term. This fluid is isotonic with maternal and fetal extracellular fluid until near term when it becomes hypertonic. The fetal urethra becomes patent at 8–9 weeks and, thereafter, the fetus urinates into the amniotic fluid about once an hour. At term, the volume of urine passed is about 650 ml per day. The fetus also swallows the amniotic fluid. The composition and osmolarity of the fluid are effectively controlled. In experiments in which 25% of the amniotic fluid was replaced with an isotonic solution, the composition of the fluid returned to normal in a few hours. The permeability of the amnion has been shown to be influenced by hormones, especially prolactin from the fetal pituitary and cortisol from the fetal adrenal.

CERVIX UTERI

The cervix of the uterus surrounds a fusiform *cervical canal* about 3 cm in length. It is continuous, above, with the uterine cavity through a constriction called the *internal os* and with the vagina, below, through the *external os*. The canal is lined by a mucosa with a highly irregular surface elevated into branching ridges or folds called the *plicae palmatae*. The mucosa is 2–3 mm in thickness and is very different from that lining the body of the uterus. It is lined by a tall columnar epithelium in which the greater part of the cytoplasm is occupied by droplets of mucus displacing the nucleus to the cell base. The glands are less numerous than in the endometrium and they are oriented oblique to the axis of the cervical canal, which is usually filled with mucus. The glands are extensively branched and their epithelium is similar to that on the surface. Isolated ciliated cells may be found among the mucus-secreting cells. The necks of one or two glands may become occluded, resulting in the accumulation of mucus within their lumen, transforming them to cysts up to 6 mm in diameter, called *Nabothian cysts*. These are pathological, but they are very common.

Near the external os, there is an abrupt transition from the simple columnar epithelium lining the canal to a stratified squamous epithelium that continues over the surface of the portio vaginalis that projects into the vagina. The cells of several of the superficial layers of this stratified epithelium are filled with glycogen. After childbearing, patches of columnar epithelium may extend from the endocervix onto the portio vaginalis. These tend to become sites of mild inflammation and are a common cause of increased vaginal discharge (leukorrhea). These areas of ectopic columnar epithelium are inappropriately called *cervical erosions*. It is believed that, if not treated, they predispose to cervical cancer, which accounts for 10% of all cancer deaths in women. The superficial squamous cells of the cervical epithelium are constantly being exfoliated into the vaginal fluid and can be examined in "vaginal smears." This technique is widely used to search for abnormal cells that may permit a very early diagnosis of cancer.

The mucosa of the endocervix does not undergo cyclic changes comparable to those of the endometrium, but the quantity and physical properties of its secretion are influenced by the circulating levels of hormones. The glands secrete about 60 mg of mucus a day throughout the greater part of the cycle, but there is a nearly 10-fold increase in their rate of secretion at midcycle. There is also a marked change in its consistency, from a very viscous mucus to a more highly hydrated less viscous fluid around the time of ovulation. This change has significance for fertility because the more viscous mucus prevailing though much of the cycle seems to be a hostile environment for spermatozoa and a serious impediment to their progress toward the site of fertilization. The changes occurring at midcycle favor their migration up the reproductive tract. In pregnancy, the cervical glands hypertrophy and accumulate secretion to such an extent that the stroma between them is reduced to thin septa.

The wall of the cervix is composed mainly of dense connective tissue, with smooth muscle accounting for only 15% of its mass. Smooth muscle is entirely absent from the portio vaginalis. Very late in pregnancy, changes take place in the fibrous and amorphous components of the extracellular matrix that make the cervix softer and more pliable, facilitating its dilatation by the advancing head of the near-term fetus.

The mucus secreted by the endocervix contains the enzyme *lysozyme* which cleaves the proteoglycans of bacterial cell walls. It is believed to contribute to the local defenses against the bacterial flora of the lower reproductive tract. In experimental animals, lysozyme production seems to be influenced by hormones because its intracellular concentration is highest during estrus. Although not yet demonstrated, the same may be true of women in midcycle.

VAGINA

The vagina is a distensible fibromuscular tube, 8–9 cm in length, extending from the vestibule of the female external genitalia to the cervix of the uterus. In the virgin, the opening of the vagina is partially closed by a crescentic transverse fold or fenestrated membrane, called the *hymen*. After its disruption remanents persist as small rounded elevations around the orifice, called the *carunculae hymenales*. The wall of the vagina consists of the mucosa, the muscular coat, and adventitial connective tissue. The adventitia is a thin layer of dense connective tissue which gives way peripherally to loose connective tissue that joins the vagina to the urethra and bladder anteriorly and to the rectum and anal canal posteriorly. This layer contains an extensive venous plexus and the vaginal plexus of nerves derived from the splanchnic nerve plexus of the pelvis.

The muscular coat is composed of interlacing bundles of smooth muscle cells arranged both longitudinally and circumferentially. The longitudinal bundles greatly predominate in the outer half of the coat. A thin circumferential band of striated muscle fibers, called the *bulbospongeosus muscle*, is found in the muscle layer around the ostium of the vagina.

The vaginal mucosa consists of a typical stratified squamous epithelium and an underlying lamina propria. The epithelium is 150–200 μm in thickness and does not undergo the striking cyclic changes commonly observed in this epithelium in many other species. It is made up of about 45 layers of cells in the follicular phase of the cycle and about 30 in the luteal phase. The superficial cells may contain keratohyalin granules, but they retain stainable nuclei and undergo little keratinization. Their cytoplasm is filled with glycogen in midcycle, which diminishes in amount later in the cycle. In electron micrographs, the cells are joined by numerous desmosomes and occasional gap junctions. The latter are most numerous in the basal layers. Tight junctions of limited extent and lamellar intercellular deposits of a lipid material are found near the surface of the epithelium. These appear to constitute a permeability barrier to large water-soluble molecules. Electron-opaque tracers readily infiltrate the intercellular spaces from the base of the epithelium but do not penetrate the intercellular clefts in the superficial layers.

The vagina is devoid of glands and the fluid that lubricates its surface is believed to be contributed, in large measure, by glands in the cervix of the uterus. It is generally agreed that the vaginal fluid increases in amount during sexual stimulation. This was formerly attributed to transudation from capillaries in the lamina propria and movement through the intercellular channels of the epithelium to the lumen. The obvious discrepency between this interpretation and the demonstration of a permeability barrier to electron-opaque tracers has not been fully resolved.

The intercellular spaces of the epithelium are accessible to mononuclear leukocytes from the blood. Lymphocytes breach the basal lamina and invade enlarged intercellular spaces. They are normally present in considerable numbers in the basal region of the epithelium and there may rarely be lymphoid nodules in the lamina propria. As in the skin, Langerhans cells are present in the basal and intermediate layers, where they are assumed to participate

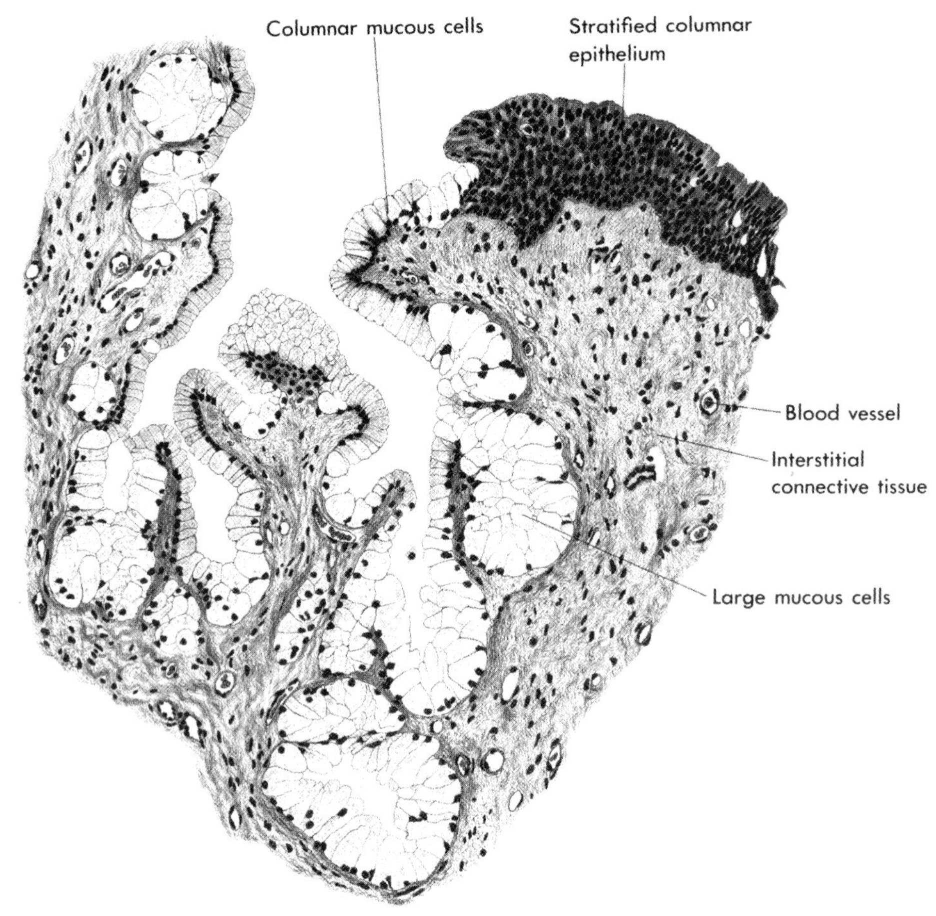

Figure 32–45. Section of Bartholin gland. A large duct with patches of stratified columnar epithelium gives off smaller branches, lined with columnar mucous cells, and continuing into tubuloalveolar terminal portions, which are lined with large mucous cells.

in antigen presentation and to cooperate with T-lymphocytes in immune surveillance of the vaginal epithelium.

The superficial cells of the vaginal mucosa are continuously shed throughout the cycle, but this desquamation is greater late in the luteal phase and during menstruation. Glycogen from the exfoliated cells is a rich substrate for certain members of the bacterial flora, which break it down to lactic acid, lowering the pH of the vagina. Because the amount of glycogen in the epithelium is controlled by estrogens, the pH of the vaginal fluid is lowest at midcycle. With less estrogen being secreted in the luteal phase of the cycle, less glycogen is formed and the pH of the vagina rises, favoring growth of the protozoan parasite, *Trichomonas vaginalis*. Thus, administration of estrogen is a useful adjunct to antimicrobial therapy for this and other vaginal infections.

EXTERNAL GENITALIA

The external genital organs of the female are the *clitoris, labia minora, labia majora,* and certain glands that open into the *vestibule*, the space flanked by the labia minora. In its embryological development, the clitoris corresponds to the dorsal portion of the penis in the male. It consists of two small erectile, corpora cavernosa, ending in a rudimentary *glans clitoridis*. The vestibule, between the labia minora, is lined with stratified squamous epithelium, and into it, open the urethra and the vagina. Around the opening of the urethra and on the body of the clitoris are several small *vestibular glands (glandulae vestibulares minores)* that contain mucus-secreting cells and resemble the glands of Littré in the male urethra. Two larger glands, the *glands of Bartholin (glandulae vestibulares majores)*, each about 1 cm in diameter, are located in the lateral walls of the vestibule and open onto the inner or medial surface of the labia minora. They are tubuloalveolar glands, corresponding in structure to the bulbourethral glands of the male and secreting a similar lubricating mucus (Fig. 32–45).

The labia minor are covered with stratified squamous epithelium which contains some pigment in its deeper layers and has a thin keratinized layer at the surface. The labia have a core of spongy connective tissue permeated by networks of fine elastic fibers. Adipose cells are lacking in the core of the labia minora. Blood vessels are abundant in their connective tissue. There are no hairs on these labia, but they have numerous large sebaceous glands.

The labia majora are plump folds of skin containing a large amount of subcutaneous adipose tissue and a thin layer of smooth muscle that corresponds to the tunica dartos of the scrotum in the male. The outer surface of the labia majora bears hair in varying amount, whereas the inner surface is smooth and hairless. Sebaceous and sweat glands are numerous on both surfaces.

The external genital organs are richly supplied with sensory nerve endings. Meissner's corpuscles are found in the papillae at the base of the epithelium and genital corpuscles are present in the subpapillary layer. Pacinian corpuscles have been reported in the deeper parts of the connective tissue of the labia majora and in the cavernous bodies of the clitoris.

BIBLIOGRAPHY

GENERAL

Austin, C.R. and R.V. Short, eds. 1972–76. Reproduction in Mammals, Vols. 1–6. London, Cambridge University Press.

Finn, C.A. and D.G. Porter. 1974. The Uterus. Handbooks of Reproductive Biology. London, Paul Elek, Ltd.

Greep, R.O., ed. 1975. Handbook of Physiology, Sect. 7, Endocrinology, Vol. II: Female Reproductive System. Washington, DC, American Physiological Society.

Yen, S.S. and R.B. Jaffe. 1986. Reproductive Endocrinology, Physiology, Pathophysiology, and Clinical Management, 2nd ed. Philadelphia, W.B. Saunders Co.

OVARY

Baker, T.G. and L.L. Franchi. 1967. The fine structure of oogonia and oocytes in human ovary. J. Cell Sci. 2:213.

Coutts, J.R.T., ed. 1981. The Functional Morphology of the Human Ovary. Lancaster, England, MTP Press.

Crisp, T.M., D.A. Dessouky, and F.R. Denys. 1970. The fine structure of the human corpus luteum of early pregnancy and during the progestational phase of the menstrual cycle. Am. J. Anat. 127:37.

Enders, A.C. 1962. Observations on the fine structure of lutein cells. J. Cell Biol. 12:101.

Gillim, S.W., A.K. Christensen, and C.E. McLennan. 1969. Fine structure of human granulosa and theca lutein cells at the stage of maximum progesterone secretion during the menstrual cycle. Anat. Rec. 163:189.

Jones, R.E., ed. 1978. The Vertebrate Ovary: Comparative Biology and Evolution. New York, Plenum Press.

Long, J.A. 1973. Corpus luteum of pregnancy in the rat, ultrastructural and cytochemical observations. Biol. Reprod. 8:87.

Mathieu, P., J. Rahier, and K. Thomas. 1981. Localization of relaxin in human gestational corpus luteum. Cell Tissue. Res. 219:213.

Mossman, M.H., M.J. Keoring, and D. Ferry. 1964. Cyclic changes of interstitial gland tissue of the human ovary. Am. J. Anat. 115:235.

Murakami, T., Y. Ikebuchi, A. Ohtsuka, A. Kikuta, T. Taguchi, and O. Ohtani. 1988. Blood vascular wreath of rat ovarian follicle, with special reference to its changes in ovulation and luteinization. Arch. Histol. Cytol. 51:299.

Osvaldo-Decima, L. 1970. Smooth muscle in the ovary of rat and monkey. J. Ultrastr. Res. 29:283.

Peters, H. and K.P. McNatty. 1980. The Ovary. Berkeley, CA, University of California Press.

Sawyer, H.R., C.L. Moeller, and G.P. Kozlowski. 1985. Immunocytochemical localization of neurophysin and oxytocin in ovine corpora lutea. Biol. Reprod. 34:543.

Wolgemuth, D.J., J. Celenza, D.S. Bundman, and B.S. Dunbar. 1984. Formation of the rabbit zona pellucida and its relationship to ovarian follicular development. Develop. Biol. 106:1.

OVULATION AND FERTILIZATION

Blandau, R.J. 1955. Ovulation in the living albino rat. Fertil. Steril. 6:391.

Decker, A. 1951. Culdescopic observations on the tubo-ovarian mechanism of ovum reception. Fertil. Steril. 2:253.

Wassarman, P.M. 1987. The biology and chemistry of fertilization. Science 235:553.

OVIDUCT

Abe, H. and T. Oikawa. 1991. Immunocytochemical localization of an oviductal zona pellucida glycoprotein in the oviductal epithelium of the golden hamster. Anat. Rec. 229:305.

Brenner, R.M. 1967. Electron microscopy of estrogen effects on ciliogenesis and secretory cell growth in rhesus monkey oviduct. Anat. Rec. 157:218.

Kan, W.K., E. Roux, S. St-Jaques, and G. Bleau. 1990. Demonstration by lectin-gold cytochemistry of transfer of glycoconjugates of oviductal origin to the zona pellucida of oocytes after ovulation in hamsters. Anat. Rec. 226:37.

Odor, D.L., P. Gaddum-Rosse, R.E. Rummery, and R.J. Blandau. 1980. Cyclic variations in the oviductal ciliated cells during the menstrual cycle and after estrogen treatment in the Macaque. Anat. Rec. 198:59.

Oura, C. and K. Toshimori. 1990. Ultrastructural studies of the fertilization of mammalian gametes. Internat. Rev. Cytol. 122:105.

Rummery, R.E. and E.M. Eddy. 1974. Scanning electron

microscopy of the fimbriae and ampulla of rabbit oviducts. Anat. Rec. 178:83.

UTERUS

Bartelmez, G.W., G.W. Corner, and C.G. Hartman. 1951. Cyclic changes in the endometrium of the rhesus monkey. Contrib. Embryol. Carnegie Inst. 34:99.

Bartelmez, G.W. 1957. The phases of the menstrual cycle and their interpretation in terms of the pregnancy cycle. Am. J. Obs. Gyn. 74:931.

Garfield, R.E., D. Merret, and A.K. Gorver. 1980. Gap junction formation and regulation in the myometrium. Am. J. Physiol. 239:213.

Kaiserman-Abramof, I.R. and H. Padykula. 1989. Ultrastructural epithelial zonationof the primate endometrium. Am. J. Anat. 184:13.

Markee, J.E. 1950. The morphological and endocrine basis of menstrual bleeding. Progr. Gynecol. 2:63.

Noyes, R.W., A.T. Hertig, and J. Rock. 1950. Dating the endometrial biopsy. Fertil. Steril. 1:3.

Padykula, H.A., L.G. Coles, J.A. McCracken, and I.R. Kaiserman-Abramof. 1984. A zonal pattern of cell proliferation and differentiation in the rhesus endometrium during the estrogen surge. Biol. Reprod. 31:1103.

CERVIX

Blandau, R.J. and K. Moghissu. 1973. The Biology of the Cervix. Chicago, IL, University of Chicago Press.

Flukman, C.F. 1958. The glandular structures of the cervix uteri. Surg. Gyn. Obst. 106:515.

Mogissi, K.S. 1972. The function of the cervix in fertility. Fertil. Steril. 23:295.

Nicosia, S.V. and J.M. Sowinsk. 1984. Ultrastructural immunocytochemical localization of lysozyme in the mucociliary epithelium of the endocervix in different hormonal states. Anat. Rec. 209:469.

Vickery, B.H. and J.P. Bennett. 1968. The cervix and its secretion in mammals. Physiol. Rev. 48:135.

IMPLANTATION AND PLACENTATION

Amoroso, E.C. 1952. *In* A.S. Parkes, ed. Marshall's Physiology of Reproduction, Vol. 2, Chap. 15. London, Longmans Green & Co, Ltd.

Amoroso, E.C. 1961. Histology of the placenta. Br. Med Bull. 17:81.

Boyd, J.D. and W.J. Hamilton. 1970. The Human Placenta. Cambridge, England, W. Heffer and Sons, Ltd.

Enders, A.C. 1965. Formation of the syncytium from cytotrophoblast in the human placenta. Obst. Gynecol. 25:378.

Enders, A.C. 1968. Fine structure of anchoring villi of the human placenta. Am. J. Anat. 122:419.

Hamilton, W.J. and J.D. Boyd. 1960. Development of the human placenta in the first three months of gestation. J. Anat. 94:297.

Hertig, A.T. and J. Rock. 1954. Two human ova of the previllous stage, having a development age of about seven and nine days respectively. Contrib. Embryol. Carnegie Inst. 31:67.

Hertig, A.T., J. Rock, and E.C. Adams. 1956. A description of 34 human ova within the first 17 days of development. Am. J. Anat. 98:435.

King, B.F. and D.N. Menton. 1975. Scanning electron microscopy of human placental villi from early and late gestation. Am. J. Obs. Gyn. 122:824.

Mossman, H.W. 1937. Comparative morphogenesis of the fetal membranes and accessory uterine structures. Contrib. Embryol. Carnegie Inst. 29:129.

Nelson, D.M., A.C. Enders, and B.F. King. 1978. Cytological events in involved in protein synthesis in cellular and syncytial trophoblast of human placenta. J. Cell Biol. 76:400.

Wislocki, G.B. and H.S. Bennett. 1943. The histology and cytology of the human and monkey placenta, with special reference to the trophoblast. Am J. Anat. 73:335.

VAGINA

Burgos, M.H. and C.E. Roig de Vargas-Linares. 1970. Cell junctions in the human vaginal epithelium. Am. J. Obs. Gyn. 108:565.

Gregoire, A.T. and P.F. Parakkal. 1972. Glycogen content in the vaginal tissue of normal cycling and estrogen and progesterone treated rhesus monkeys. Biol. Reprod. 7:9.

King, B.F. 1983. Ultrastructure of the non-human primate vaginal epithelium: a freeze–fracture and tracer perfusion study. J. Ultrastr. Res. 83:99.

Young, W.G. et al. 1985. The effect of atrophy, hyperplasia and keratinization accompanying the estrus cycle on Langerhans cells in mouse vaginal epithelium. Am. J. Anat. 174:173.

33 MAMMARY GLAND

The mammary glands are specialized accessory glands that have evolved in mammals to provide for the nourishment of their offspring. They are paired glands that are initiated in the embryo along two *mammary lines* that extend from the axilla to the groin on the ventral aspect of the thorax and abdomen, on either side of the midline. Mammary glands may arise anywhere along these lines in various species. In the human, only two normally develop on the thorax, but additional accessory nipples or small glands are not uncommon.

The differentiation of mammary glands in the embryo is similar in the two sexes. In the male, little additional development occurs in postnatal life, but in the female, the glands undergo extensive structural changes associated with puberty, pregnancy, and menopause. The female breast reaches its greatest development in about the 20th year. Atrophic changes appear by the 40th year and become marked after menopause. In addition to these long-term changes, related to age, the breasts undergo slight variations in size in the course of each menstrual cycle, and very striking changes in size and in the functional activity of the glandular tissue during pregnancy and lactation.

NIPPLE AND AREOLA

The nipple is located in the center of a circular pigmented area of the skin, called the *areola*. Here, the base of the stratified squamous epithelium of the epidermis is invaded by unusually long dermal papillae containing capillaries that bring blood close to the surface, imparting a pinkish color to this region in children and in blonde individuals. At puberty, the epidermis becomes pigmented and this pigmentation greatly increases during pregnancy.

Fifteen to twenty *lactiferous ducts* that open onto the tip of the nipple are the excretory ducts of the separate lobes of the mammary gland. Between them are large sebaceous glands, some of which open onto the skin, whereas others may open into the terminal portions of the ducts (Fig. 33–1). This portion of the ducts is lined by keratinized squamous epithelium continuous with that on the skin of the nipple. Desquamated squamous cells may accumulate and occlude the ducts of the inactive gland. Most of the substance of the nipple is dense connective tissue that contains many elastic fibers that attach to the skin on the sides of the nipple. Similar elastic fibers are abundant in the connective tissue beneath the areola and are responsible for the fine wrinkling of the overlying skin. There are circularly oriented smooth muscle fibers around the base of the nipple and other bundles radiating from it into the tissue beneath the areola. Contraction of these results in wrinkling of the skin of the areola and erection of the nipple in response to cold and tactile or emotional stimulation. At other times, the nipple is relatively flat. In the areola, there are the *areolar glands of Montgomery* which have a structure intermediate between sweat glands and true mammary glands. At the margin of the areola, there are large sweat glands and sebaceous glands without associated hairs.

The skin at the tip of the nipple is richly innervated by free nerve endings and there are also sensory organs, such as Meissner's corpuscles, in the dermal papillae. There are similar superficial nerves and end organs on the sides of the nipple and in the areola. Pacinian corpuscles may also be found deep in the dermis and in the glandular tissue. The sensory innervation of the nipple and areola are important because their stimulation, by a suckling infant, initiates the sequence of neural and neurohumoral events that result in ejection of milk. Stimulation also helps to maintain secretion of prolactin by the pituitary which is essential for continued lactation.

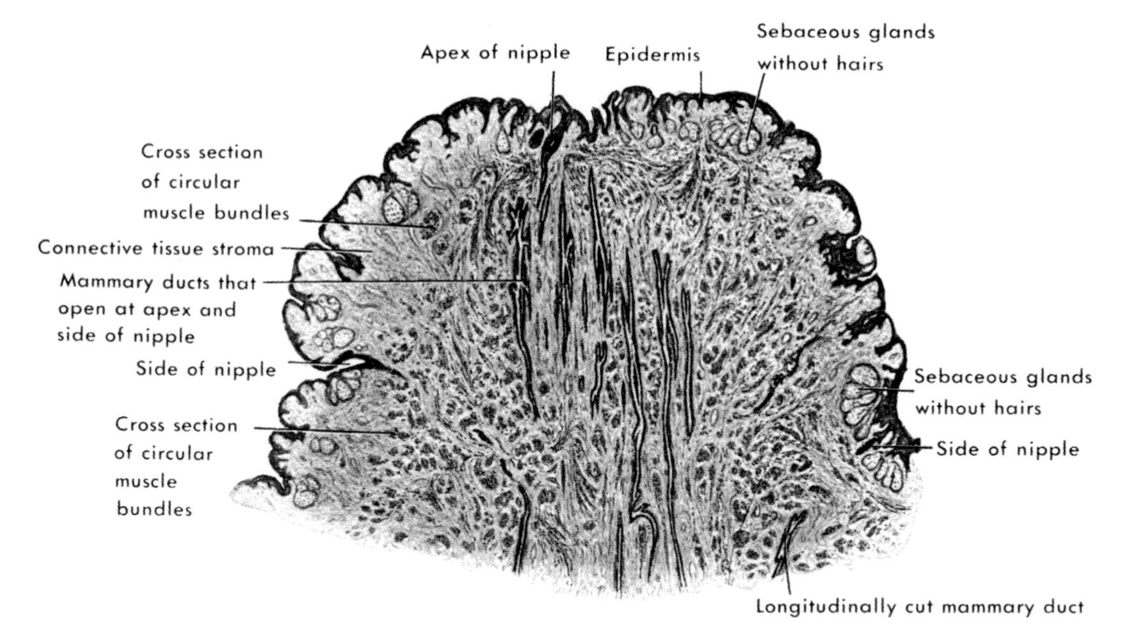

Figure 33–1. Longitudinal section of the nipple of a female breast. (After Schaffer, J., Lehrbuch der Histologie und Histogenese. Verlag von W. Engelmann, Leipzig, 1922.

RESTING MAMMARY GLAND

The mammary gland is a compound tubulo-alveolar gland consisting of 15–20 lobes drained by the same number of *lactiferous ducts* that open on the tip of the *nipple* (*mammary papilla*). The lobes radiate from the nipple and areola and are separated by connective tissue and adipose tissue. The lactiferous duct of each lobe goes through several orders of branching, to drain multiple small lobules, each consisting of a group of alveoli around one of the terminal branches of that lactiferous duct. Thus, unlike other major glands, which have a single large duct, the mammary gland is a conglomerate made up of a variable number of independent units, each having its own excurrent duct. Beneath the areola, each of the lactiferous ducts is slightly dilated to form a *lactiferous sinus*, where a small amount of milk may accumulate in the active gland. Distal to this, the duct narrows again and continues to its opening at the tip of the nipple. The larger elements of the duct system are lined by cuboidal epithelium two cells thick which become stratified squamous epithelium a short distance below the opening of the duct. The smaller ducts are lined by simple columnar epithelium.

In the mature gland, the smallest lobules consist of an *alveolar duct* from which project small saccular evaginations, the *alveoli* (Fig. 33–2). At birth, the gland consists only of branching lactiferous ducts with no alveoli. As puberty approaches, the duct system elongates under the influence of ovarian hormones, and small, solid, spheroidal masses of polygonal epithelial cells appear on the ends and sides of the smallest ducts. These have no lumen but are capable of developing into alveoli, after appropriate hormonal stimulation. Myoepithelial cells between the epithelium and the basal lamina are spindle shaped and oriented longitudinally on the smallest ducts. As alveoli develop, their associated myoepithelial cells become stellate in shape and their radiating processes form a wide-meshed network around each alveolus (Fig. 33–3). True secreting alveoli do not appear until pregnancy occurs.

The mammary gland does not have a capsule. Interlobar connective tissue septa extend inward from the subcutaneous tissue surrounding the gland. A looser more cellular connective tissue which contains less collagen extends inward from the interlobar septa and surrounds the lobules. This loose stroma is believed to permit greater distensibility when the epithelial portions of the gland hypertrophy during pregnancy and lactation. Adipose cells tend to accumulate in the interlobar septa but not in the intralobular stroma. Individual

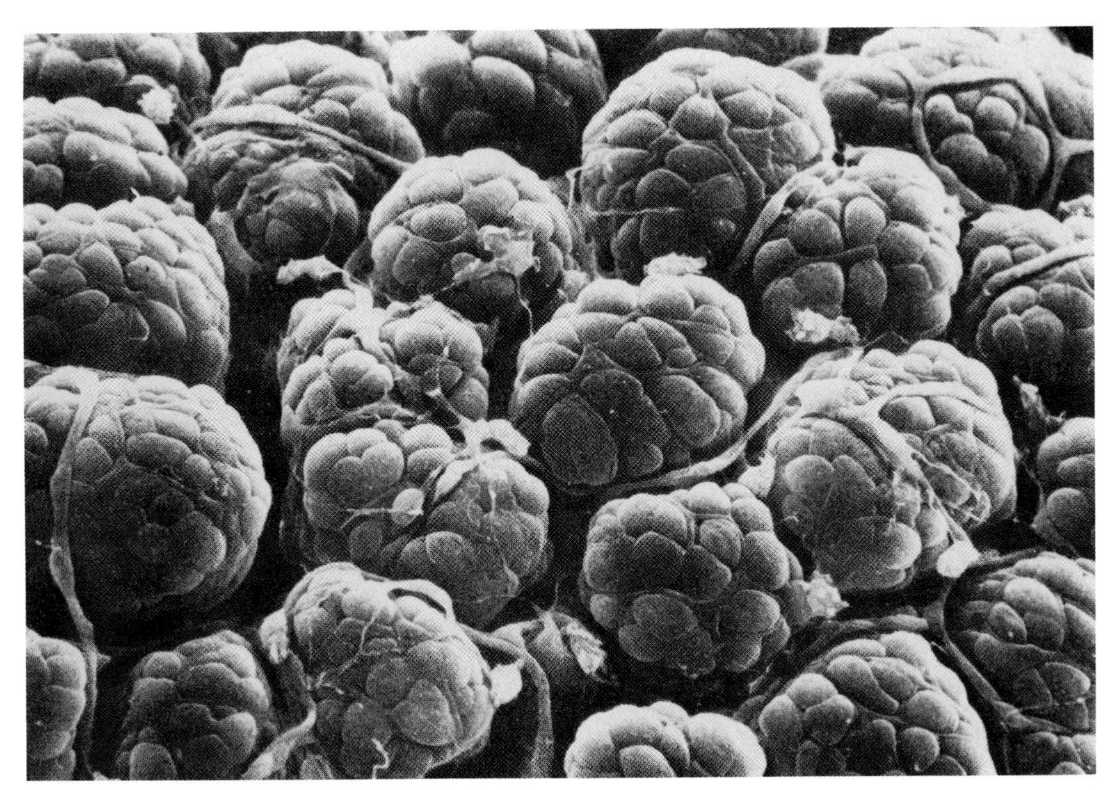

Figure 33–2. Scanning electron micrograph of the alveoli of a rodent mammary gland. The tissue was exposed to enzymes, during preparation, to digest away the collagen fibers, extracellular matrix, and basal lamina, thus exposing the bases of the epithelial cells and the myoepithelial cells. (Micrograph from Nagato, T., 1980. Cell Tissue Res. 209:1.)

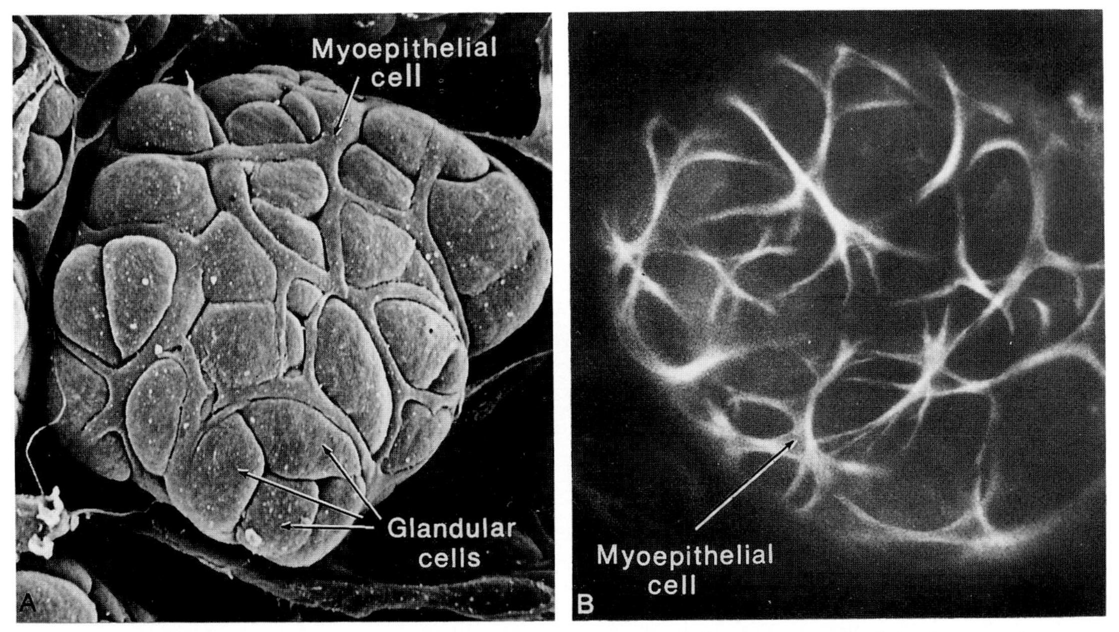

Figure 33–3. (A) Scanning micrograph of an acinus of the mammary gland showing myoepithelial cells occupying grooves between the bases of the secretory cells. (Micrograph courtesy of Nagato, T., 1980. Cell Tissue Res. 209:1.) (B) Acinus of a mammary gland stained with a fluorescent probe for actin. (Micrograph courtesy of Emerman, J. and W. Vogl. 1986. Anat. Rec. 216:405.)

variation in the amount of adipose tissue is largely responsible for the differences in breast size.

There has been disagreement as to whether there are significant changes in the mammary gland during the menstrual cycle. This is due, in part, to the rarity of opportunities to obtain normal human breast tissue for study at known stages. Early in the cycle, the cells seem to form more-or-less solid cords and it is not easy to distinguish alveolar ducts from alveoli, in histological sections. Later in the cycle, the cells are reported to become cuboidal, or low columnar, and a lumen may be detectable. From the few studies available, it is probably safe to conclude that there are microscopically detectable cyclic changes in the epithelial portion of the mammary gland, but these are relatively slight. In addition, the surrounding connective tissue appears more highly vascular at midcycle. The obvious changes in breast size and the sense of engorgement experienced by some women around midcycle are attributable mainly to increased blood flow and some associated edema of the connective tissue of the breast.

In the male, the mammary gland consists of a rudimentary duct system with no development of alveoli. The duct system is, however, somewhat responsive to hormonal stimulation and may undergo some transient proliferation during puberty. In a common congenital disorder, Klinefelder's syndrome, which includes testicular hypoplasia, and in patients with testicular tumors that produce estrogens, there may be considerable development of mammary glands, a condition described as *gynecomastia*.

THE ACTIVE MAMMARY GLAND

The elevated levels of circulating estrogens and progesterone in pregnancy bring about major changes in the mammary glands. There is a rapid growth in length and branching of the duct system and proliferation of alveoli. This growth of the epithelial components of the gland takes place, in part, at the expense of the adipose tissue of the breast which regresses concurrently with the growth of the glandular tissue. During this period of growth, there is also an increasing infiltration of the stroma with lymphocytes, plasma cells, and eosinophils. In the later months of pregnancy, hyperplasia of the glandular tissue slows down and the continuing enlargement of the breasts is due mainly to enlargement of the parenchymal cells and distension of the alveoli and ducts with a secretion rich in lactoproteins but poor in lipid. This constitutes the *colostrum*, the first secretory product that comes from the breasts after birth. It has special laxative properties and contains immunoglobulins that provide the newborn with some measure of passive immunity. In the first few days after parturition, infiltration of the mammary stroma by lymphocytes diminishes. The postpartum reduction in blood levels of estrogen and progesterone appear to stimulate the pituitary to secrete *prolactin*. The secretion of colostrum then gives way to copious secretion of true milk rich in lipids.

The histological appearance of different regions of the active mammary gland varies considerably, suggesting that not all areas are in the same functional state at the same time. In some areas the walls of dilated alveolar ducts and acini are thin and the wide lumen is filled with milk. In other areas, the lumen is narrow and the epithelium relatively thick (Figs. 33–4 and 33–5). The shape of the epithelial cells varies from flat to low columnar. Where the cells are tall, their apices are often separated and project into the lumen as rounded protrusions. If the cells are short, the free surface of the epithelium is usually more-or-less smooth. The cells are generally acidophilic but may have some basophilia of their basal cytoplasm. Droplets of lipid accumulate in the cytoplasm and some may be very large and project into the lumen. In the preparation of histological sections, the lipid is extracted and large clear vacuoles are found in place of the lipid droplets. Small proteinaceous secretory granules are also found in the apical cytoplasm.

In electron micrographs, the areas of cytoplasm that were basophilic in histological sections contain numerous parallel arrays of granular endoplasmic reticulum. There is a large supranuclear Golgi complex, a moderate number of mitochondria, and a few lysosomes. Two distinct secretory products are evident in these cells: lipid droplets and protein-containing granules. These are released by different mechanisms. The protein is synthesized in the endoplasmic reticulum and first becomes visible as multiple dense spherical granules about 400 μm in diameter in vesicles associated with the trans-face of the Golgi complex. These vesicles move to the apex of the cell and fuse with the plasmalemma, discharging their content into the lumen of the

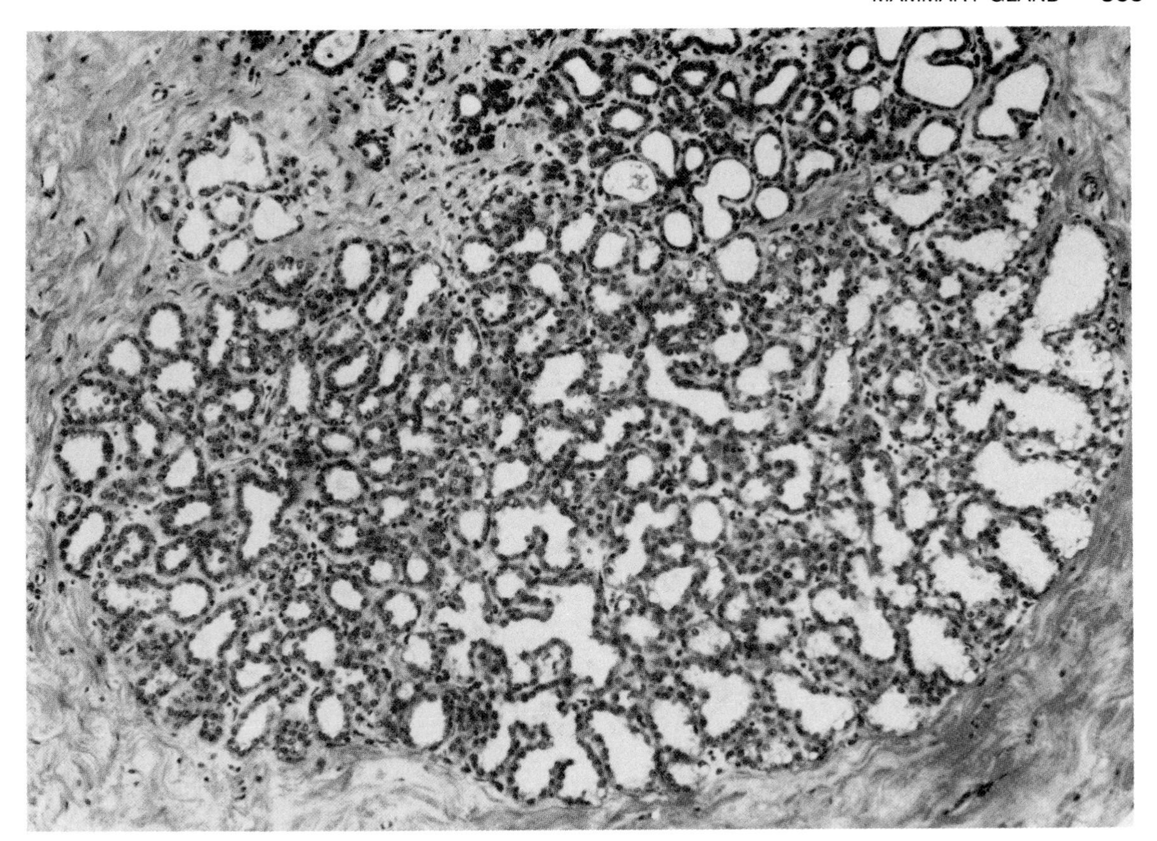

Figure 33–4. Photomicrograph of a small area of human mammary gland at 8 months of pregnancy. The gland is prepared for lactation, but there is no secretion in the lumen of the alveoli.

acinus (Figs. 33–6 and 33–7). Thus, the synthesis of the protein component of milk is much the same as that of other protein-secreting cells, and its mode of secretion is classified as *merocrine*.

The synthesis of the lipid component of milk apparently does not involve the reticulum or the Golgi complex. Small lipid droplets arise free in the cytoplasmic matrix and these fuse with one another to form lipid droplets of increasing size. The largest of these come to project into the lumen, covered on that side, only by the cell membrane (Figs. 33–8 and 33–9). As they protrude further into the lumen, they are ultimately pinched off, surrounded by a detached portion of the plasmalemma. This mode of release can be considered *apocrine* in the sense that it involves loss of some of the apical membrane of the cell, and in some instances a thin film of cytoplasm, but the amount of the cell that is lost is far less than was envisioned by classical cytologists who introduced the concept of apocrine secretion.

Lymphocytes are occasionally found between the epithelial cells of the alveoli. Also, between the epithelial cells or between them and the basal lamina are occasional cells with a pale cytoplasm, containing numerous small lipid droplets and vacuoles with a granular or membranous content. These were formerly interpreted as degenerating epithelial cells, but it seems more likely that they are macrophages. The long, slender branching processes of the myoepithelial cells occupy recesses between or beneath the bases of the secretory cells. The form and relationships of these cells are best seen in scanning electron micrographs of glands that have been exposed to collagenase during specimen preparation to remove the basal lamina and the collagen fibers of the surrounding connective tissue (Fig. 33–2). In glands examined during pregnancy or lactation, the myoepithelial cells are filled with closely packed actin filaments. If intact alveoli are stained with a highly specific fluorescent probe for actin, the myoepithelial cells and their branching processes fluoresce brilliantly. In transmission electron micrographs of thin sections, there are spindle-

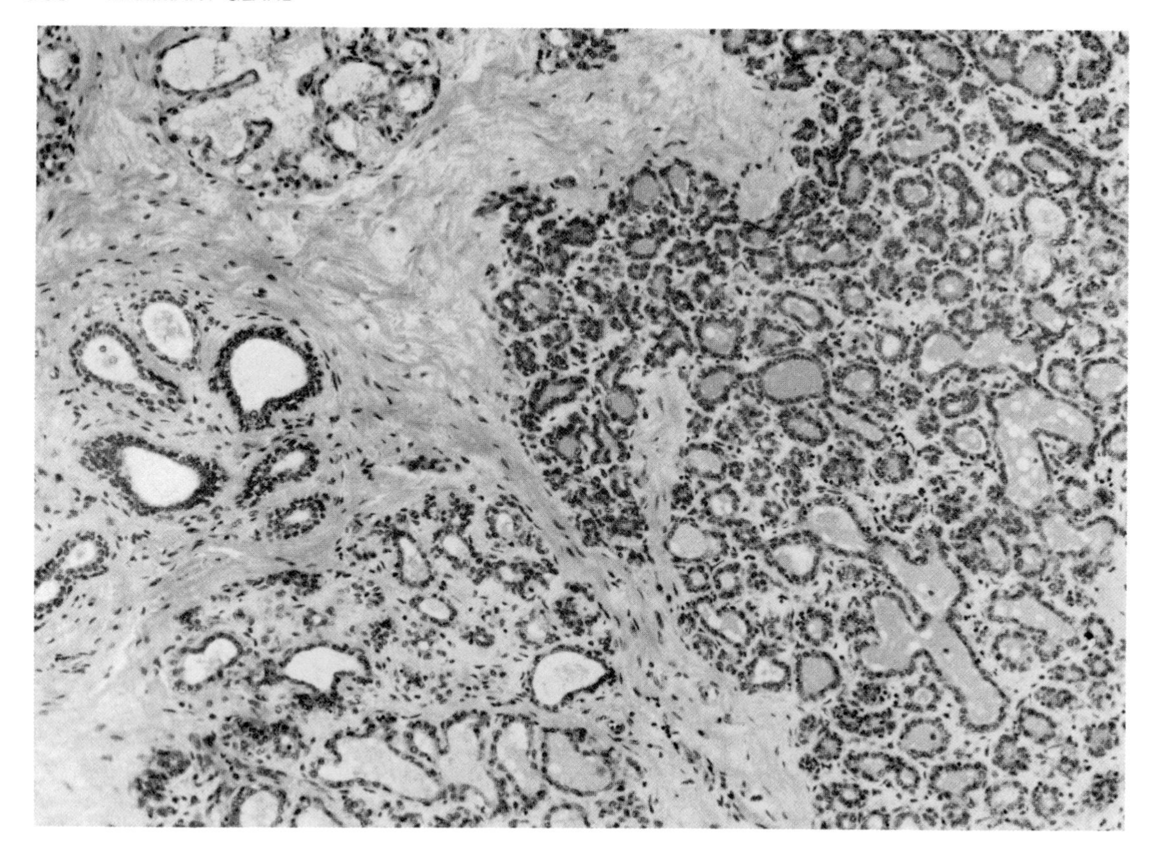

Figure 33–5. Photomicrograph of a lactating human mammary gland. Note the milk in the lumen of the alveoli and the local variations in activity. In some areas, the alveoli have a wide lumen containing abundant secretion, whereas in other areas, the lumen is quite small.

shaped densities among bundles of actin filaments, like those found in smooth muscle cells. The organelles of the myoepithelial cells are concentrated in the perinuclear region, but occasional mitochondria and profiles of endoplasmic reticulum extend into the cell processes.

At the termination of lactation, the secretory cells undergo involution with a very striking decrease in their size and numerous lysosomes and residual bodies appear in their cytoplasm. Changes of this kind are not observed in the myoepithelial cells, but their processes are partially retracted so that they are more plump with the bulk of their cytoplasm around the nucleus.

HISTOPHYSIOLOGY OF THE MAMMARY GLAND

Complex neural and endocrine mechanisms are involved in development of the mammary gland, in initiation of milk production and in milk ejection from the active gland. Some of the endocrine events have been mentioned earlier but at the risk of some redundancy, they will be summarized here. The growth of the duct system, initiated at puberty, is due mainly to estrogens secreted by the ovary, and prolactin secreted by the pituitary. Maximal development of the ducts also seems to require the hypophyseal hormone somatotrophin and glucocorticoids from the adrenal cortex. Stimulation by these hormones also leads to the increase in connective tissue and adipose tissue that is responsible for the visible enlargement of the breasts at puberty.

The resting mammary gland of the adult female has a well-developed duct system and a few rudimentary alveoli, but the cells contain very little rough endoplasmic reticulum and clearly are not yet fully differentiated for production of milk. In the early weeks of pregnancy, elevated levels of estrogen, progesterone, prolactin, and glucocorticoids stimulate further growth and differentiation of alveoli,

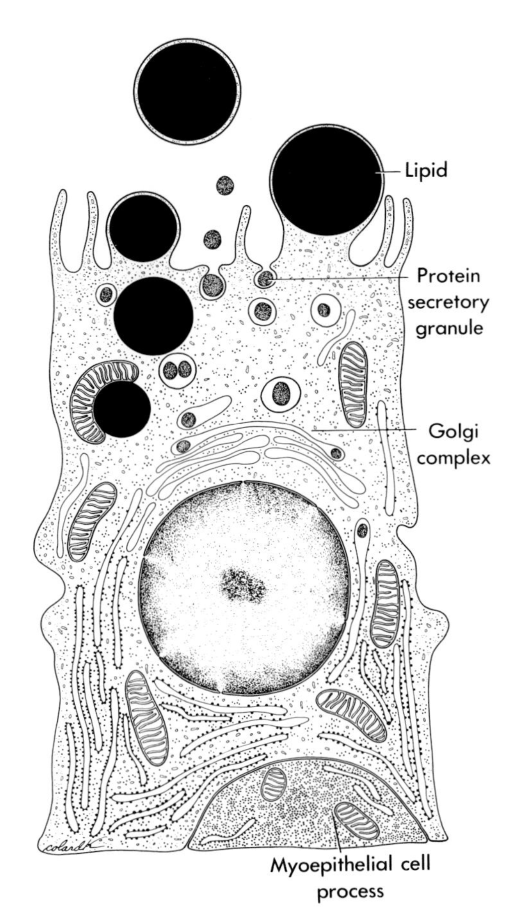

Figure 33–6. Drawing of a cell from a lactating mammary gland showing differing modes of secretion of the protein and lipid components of the milk. Lipid droplets are extruded, enveloped in plasma membrane and a thin layer of cytoplasm, whereas protein-secretory granules are released by fusion of their limiting membrane with the plasmalemma. (Drawing based on observations of Bargmann, W., and A. Knoop. 1959. Zeitschr. Zellforsch. 49:344.)

and this continues after the placenta becomes the dominant source of estrogen, progesterone, and placental lactogen. The hormone-dependent differentiation of the mammary epithelium also requires its interaction with the surrounding stroma and with components of the basal lamina. The abundant adipose tissue of the breast is not there simply for cosmetic purposes. In vitro studies have shown that co-culture of mammary tissue with adipocytes greatly promotes growth and differentiation of mammary epithelium. Components of the basal lamina also have a significant effect on the expression of tissue-specific genes for the synthesis of casein and lactalbumin. Inhibition of basal lamina formation, in vivo, disrupts duct elongation, branching, and alveolar development. Mammary epithelial cells, in vitro, can acquire function only when they deposit a basal lamina. Addition to cultures of a gel containing components of basal lamina (laminin, type-IV collagen, heparan sulfate proteoglycans) induces a 70–100-fold increase in synthesis of casein and lactalbumin. Thus, interaction of mammary epithelium with components of the extracellular matrix and with adipose cells seems to play an important role in regulation of epithelial function. Actual secretion of milk does not occur until after the birth of the baby. After delivery of the placenta, there is a precipitous drop in hormones that had inhibited milk secretion by the prepared mammary gland. In the absence of this inhibition, prolactin, secreted by the pituitary, is a powerful lactogenic stimulus for the mammary epithelium and full lactation is established within a few days.

Once lactation is initiated, the cells synthesize their products continuously, but the release of milk is episodic. In the intervals between breast feedings, most of the milk secreted is stored within the lumen of the alve-

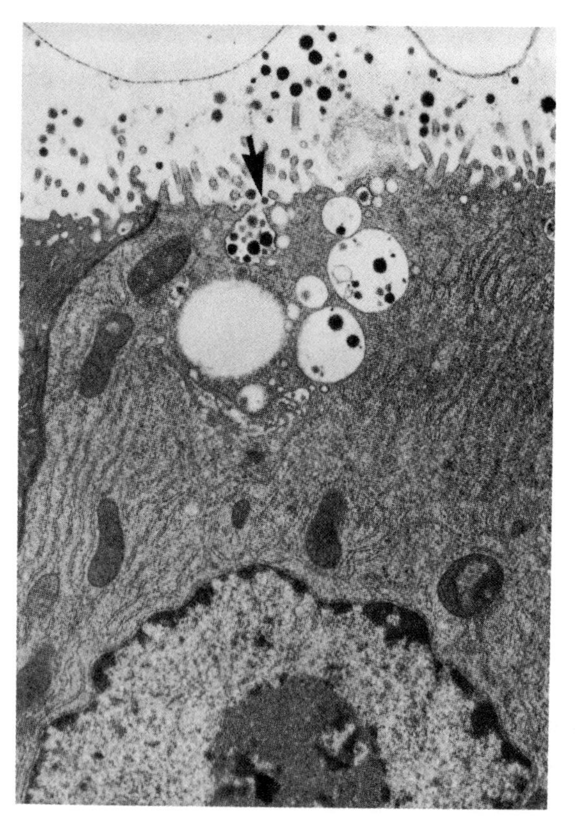

Figure 33–7. Electron micrograph of a mammary epithelial cell showing several vesicles containing multiple granules of milk protein. One is in the process of exocytosis (at arrow). (Micrograph courtesy of A. Ichikawa.)

oli and small ducts. At feeding time, the visual and tactile stimuli associated with handling the baby in anticipation of nursing are relayed via the hypothalamus to the pituitary, resulting in release of a surge of prolactin from the anterior lobe and *oxytocin* from its posterior lobe. Prolactin, rising briefly to 10-fold the basal level, is carried in the blood to the mammary gland, where it causes increased secretion of milk into the alveoli. Oxytocin causes contraction of the myoepithelial cells around the alveoli and small ducts, resulting in "milk letdown," an expulsion of the accumulated milk. When these complex mechanisms all proceed smoothly, the average milk production of a mother breast-feeding one infant is in excess of 1100 ml/24h, for the first 6 months of lactation, and a mother of twins may produce over 2100 ml/24h.

Milk has many components. It contains water (~88%), protein (~1.3%), carbohydrate (~6.5%), and lipid (~3.3%). In addition, there are electrolytes (Na^+, K^+ Cl^-), minerals (Fe^{++} Mg^{++} and Ca^{++}), and immunoglobulins (IgE and IgA). The principal protein of milk is *casein* and the principal carbohydrate is *lactose*. If lipid is not adequately represented in the maternal diet, it can be drawn from reserves in her adipose tissue. The demand for calcium may considerably exceed the dietary intake, and to meet this need, the parathyroid glands enlarge during lactation, and secrete parathormone to mobilize calcium from her bones. It has recently been found that the lactating mammary gland also produces a 16 kD peptide hormone very similar to parathormone in its amino-acid sequence. This hormone is believed to play a role in mobilization of calcium from bone and its incorporation into milk.

The immunoglobulin of milk is synthesized by plasma cells in the connective tissue of the gland. These are believed to differentiate from lymphocytes previously exposed to enteric pathogens in the submucosa of the mothers intestines. IgA is taken up by receptor-mediated endocytosis at the basolateral sur-

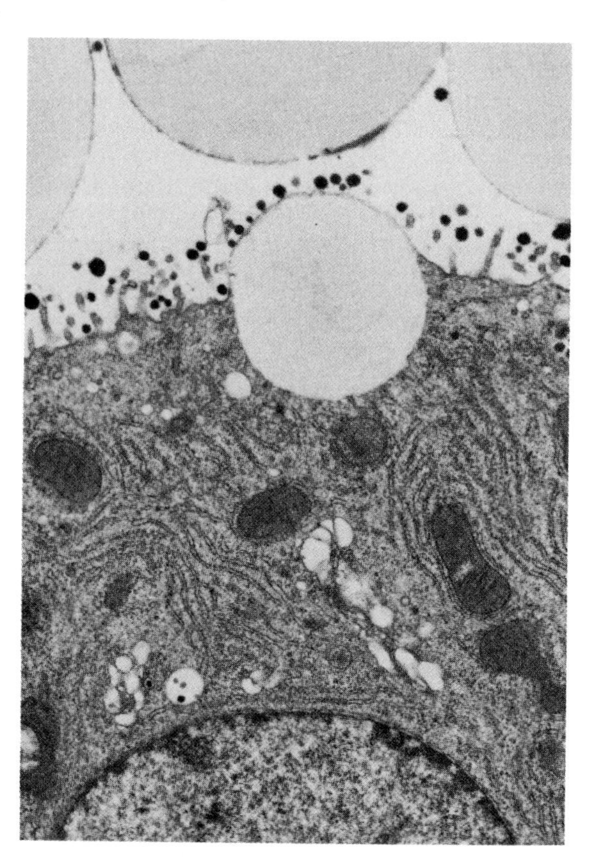

Figure 33–8. Micrograph of a mammary epithelial cell with a lipid droplet protruding into the lumen, covered by a portion of the apical plasma membrane. Secreted lipid droplets and granules of milk protein can be seen in the lumen.(Micrograph courtesy of A. Ichikawa.)

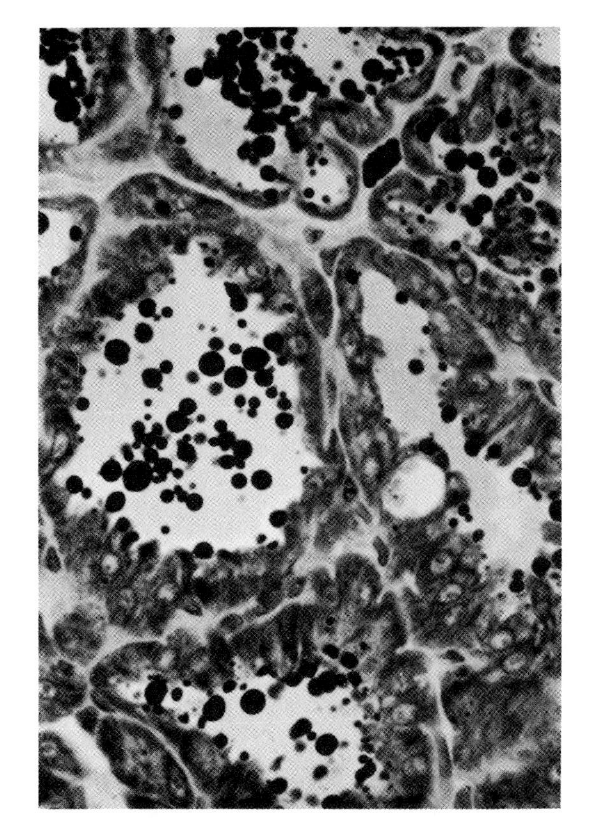

Figure 33–9. Photomicrograph of lactating mammary gland of mouse, fixed in osmium tetroxide. Large droplets of lipid are preserved both in the apex of the cells and in the lumen of the alveoli. The smaller protein granules are not visible at this magnification. (Preparation by N. Feder.)

face of the mammary epithelial cells, transported in small vesicles to the cell apex and discharged into the lumen (Fig. 33–10). In the fourth and fifth month of lactation, a mother may be secreting, in her milk, as much as 0.5 g of immunoglobulin a day. The antibodies reaching the lumen of the baby's intestine resist enteric infections which are a common cause of infant mortality. Early weaning and bottle-feeding deprive the infant of this passive immunity.

The periodic surges of prolactin release, associated with nursing, are necessary to sustain lactation. The tendency of mothers in developed countries to prolong the intervals between feedings and to abandon nighttime feedings, as soon as possible, contributes to their poor lactational performance. In contrast, women in primitive societies, whose babies are always with them and are fed on demand day or night, are able to continue breast-feeding for up to three and a half years.

In women who are breast-feeding a baby, there is usually a concurrent suppression of the menstrual cycle and ovulation, referred to as *lactational amenorrhea*. Its mechanism is poorly understood, but it is speculated that the neural inputs to the hypothalamus generated by suckling, stimulate the release of β-endorphin, which, in turn, suppresses the release of gonadotrophin releasing hormone (GnRH). The resulting depression of luteinizing hormone secretion by the pituitary is probably the cause of failure of these women to ovulate. Prolonged lactation is the only form of contraception practiced by the majority of women in developing countries.

REGRESSION OF THE MAMMARY GLAND

With regular suckling, lactation can be maintained for many months, but if milk is

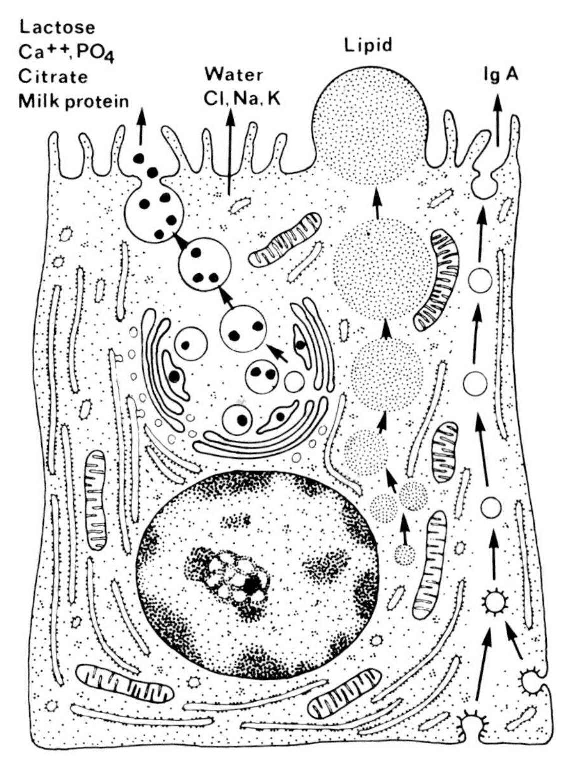

Figure 33–10. Diagram of the transcellular pathways involved in milk secretion. Casein, lactate, calcium, and citrate are packaged in the Golgi and released by exocytosis. Lipid droplets, enveloped in portions of the cell membrane, are released in a unique form of apocrine secretion. Water and ions freely diffuse through the membrane. Immunoglobulins, taken up by receptor-mediated endocytosis at the basolateral region of the cell, are transported in small vesicles and released at the cell apex. (Redrawn and modified after Neville, M.C. et al. 1983. *In* Lactation: Physiology, Metabolism, and Breast-Feeding. New York, Plenum Press.)

not removed, the glands become greatly distended and milk production soon ceases. This is due, in part, to interruption of the neurohormonal mechanism for maintenance of prolactin secretion by the pituitary, but the engorgement of the unemptied breasts may also compress the blood vessels, reducing access of oxytocin to the myoepithelial cells. After a few days, the secretion remaining in the alveolar spaces and ducts is absorbed and the glands gradually return to a resting state. They do not return completely to their pregravid state, however, because remanents of secretion may persist for some time and many of the alveoli that formed during pregnancy do not entirely disappear.

The process of mammary gland involution has been studied mainly in experimental animals, but the changes in the human gland are no doubt quite similar. One of the early changes after weaning is the synthesis and secretion, at the cell base, of matrix-degrading enzymes (gelatinase, stromolysin) that cause dissolution of the basal lamina, which, as previously stated, is essential for maintenance of epithelial cells function. Messenger RNA for casein synthesis declines and the cells rapidly dedifferentiate. A few days after weaning, the epithelium is flat, due to distension of the alveoli with retained milk. As this is resorbed, there is a gradual collapse of the alveoli, and a concomitant increase in perialveolar connective tissue and adipose cells. Macrophages in the vicinity of the alveoli are greatly increased, but there is no true inflammatory reaction. By 15–20 days after weaning, the glandular tissue has been largely replaced by connective tissue and adipose tissue, and the remaining alveoli and small ducts have been reduced to solid cords of inactive epithelial cells.

Early in the process of regression, electron micrographs reveal an accumulation of intracellular secretory protein in large vacuoles in the alveolar cells, and an increase in the number and size of autophagic vacuoles containing mitochondria and other organelles. There is a progressive increase in the number of macrophages that have invaded the epithelium, and these show abundant evidence of heterophagic activity. Because some of the heterophagic vacuoles contain organelles and secretory granules, it seems likely that these have been taken up from degenerating epithelial cells. In later stages of regression, some degenerating epithelial cells slough off into the lumen and are disposed of there by macrophages.

Concomitant with the increase of autophagic and heterophagic vacuoles in electron micrographs, histochemical and biochemical studies show that there is an increase in the lysosomal enzymes aryl sulfatase, cathepsin-D, and acid phosphatase, even though the activity of nonlysosomal enzymes is rapidly declining. Thus, the removal of cellular material during regression of the glands is due to synthesis and activation of lysosomal enzymes in the early stages of the process. Despite this widespread autophagic activity, viable epithelial cells persist in the solid alveoli and terminal ducts of the resting gland, and in a subsequent pregnancy, the process of growth and differentiation into a functioning gland is repeated.

In old age, the mammary gland undergoes gradual involution, with atrophy of the solid alveoli and terminal portions of the duct system so that it reverts to the prepubertal condition. Equally striking changes occur in the connective tissue, which becomes less cellular and contains much less collagen and few adipose cells. The breast as a whole becomes very soft and flat to the chest.

The mammary epithelium is often a site of pathological changes. The disorder called chronic cystic disease of the breast is quite common in women between 30 and 50 years of age. Some of the terminal ducts lose their continuity with the rest of the duct system and may form fluid-filled cysts of varying size. The breast is also the most common site of cancer in women. About 1 in 17 newborn girls will develop breast cancer at some time in her life—an incidence three times that of cancer of the colon, which is the second most common malignancy.

BLOOD AND LYMPHATIC VESSELS

The arteries to the mammary gland arise from the internal mammary artery, thoracic branches of the axillary artery, and the intercostal arteries. They course along the larger ducts and give rise to dense capillary networks around the alveoli of the gland. The veins drain into the axillary and anterior thoracic veins.

Lymphatic capillaries abound in the connective tissue around the alveoli. These collect along the course of the mammary ducts into a subpapillary plexus. From there, several larger vessels conduct the lymph to lymph nodes in the axilla and in the subclavicular region, but they also have connections with lymphatics that penetrate the intercostal spaces to reach parasternal lymph nodes within the thorax. An understanding of the principal pathways of lymphatic drainage is of clinical importance owing to the necessity of removing the regional lymph nodes during radical mastectomy for breast cancer.

INNERVATION

The nerves to the breast are from anterior and cutaneous branches of the fourth, fifth, and sixth thoracic nerves. They are sympathetic nerves and their norepinephrine containing endings can be found among the smooth muscle cells of the nipple and between the muscularis and adventitia of the arteries. There is no evidence that cholinergic nerves supply any portion of the gland. A few sensory fibers leave the perivascular networks and lie near the walls of the ducts. There is no evidence of a nerve supply to the myoepithelial cells or to the secretory cells. The activation of the latter is dependent on hormones from the ovaries and pituitary. There is a dense nerve plexus in and around the nipple supplying encapsulated end organs and giving rise to free endings. These sensory endings are responsible for the afferent impulses that signal suckling by the baby and activate neurons in the hypothalamus to induce release of oxytocin by the posterior pituitary resulting in let down of the milk.

BIBLIOGRAPHY

Banarjee, M.R. 1976. Responses of the mammary gland to hormones. Internat. Rev. Cytol. 47:1.

Blum, J.L., M.E. Ziegler, and M.S. Wicha. 1987. Regulation of rat mammary gene expression by extracellular components. Exp. Cell Res. 173:322.

Emerman, J.T. and A.W. Vogl. 1986. Cell size and shape changes in the myoepithelial cells of the mammary gland during differentiation. Anat. Rec. 216:405.

Forsyth, I.A. 1982. Growth and differentiation of mammary glands. Oxford Rev. Reprod. Biol. 4:47.

Hebb, C. and J.L. Linzell. 1970. Innervation of the mammary gland. A histochemical study in the rabbit. Histochem. J. 2:491.

Helminen, H.J. and J.L.E. Ericsson. 1968. Studies on mammary gland involution. I. On the ultrastructure of the lactating mammary gland. J. Ultrastr. Res. 25:193.

Helminen, H.J. and J.L.E. Ericsson. 1968. Studies on mammary gland involution. II. Ultrastructural evidence for auto- and heterophagocytosis. J. Ultrastr. Res. 25:214.

Kurosumi, K., Y. Kobayashi, and N. Baba. 1968. The fine structure of mammary glands of lactating rats with special reference to the apocrine secretion. Exp. Cell Res. 50:177.

Levine, J.F. and F.E. Stockdale. 1985. Cell–cell interactions promote epithelial cell differentiation. J. Cell Biol. 100:1415.

Linzell, J.L. and M. Peaker. 1971. Mechanism of milk secretion. Physiol. Rev. 51:564.

Martinez-Hernandez, A., L.M. Fink, and G.B. Pierce. 1976. Removal of the basement membrane in the involuting breast. Lab. Investig. 31:455.

Miller, M.R. and M. Kasahara. 1959. Cutaneous innervation of the female breast. Anat. Rec. 135:153.

Mills, E.S. and Y.J. Topper. 1970. Some ultrastructural effects of insulin, hydrocortisone, and prolactin on mammary gland explants. J. Cell. Biol. 44:310.

Mostov, K.E., J.P. Krackenbuhl, and G. Blobel. 1980. Receptor-mediated transcellular transport of immunoglobulin: synthesis of secretory component as multiple and transcellular forms. Proc. Nat. Acad. Sci. USA 77:7257.

Nagato, T.H., H. Yoshida and Y. Uehara. 1980. A scanning electron microscope study of myoepithelial cells in eccrine glands. Cell Tissue Res. 209:1.

Nemanic, M.K. and D.R. Pitelka. 1971. A scanning electron microscope study of the lactating mammary gland. J. Cell Biol. 48:411.

Pitelka, D.R. and S.T. Hamamoto. 1983. Ultrastructure of the mammary secretory cell. *In* T.D. Mepham, ed. Biochemistry of Lactation. New York, Elsevier Biomedical Press.

Radnor, C.J.P. 1972. Myoepithelium in the involuting mammary gland of the rat. J. Anat. 112:355.

Richards, R.J. and G.K. Benson. 1971. Ultrastructural changes accompanying involution of the mammary gland of the rat. J. Endocrinol. 51:127.

Sekhri, K.K., D.R. Pitelka, and K.B. DeOme. 1967. Studies of mouse mammary glands. I. Cytomorphosis of the normal mammary gland. J. Nat. Cancer Inst. 39:495.

Short, R.V. 1984. Breast feeding. Sci. Am. 250:23.

Stirling, J.W., and J.A. Chandlet, 1977. The fine structure of the normal resting terminal ductal-lobular unit of the female breast. Virchow's Arch. Path. Anat. Histol. 372:205.

Stirling, J.W., and J.A. Chandler, 1976. The fine structure of ducts and subareolar ducts in the resting gland of the female breast. Virchow's Arch. Path. Anat. Histol. 373:119.

Talhouk, R.S., M.J. Bissell, and Z. Werb. 1992. Coordinated espression of extracellular matrix-degrading proteinases and their inhibitors regulates mammary epithelial function during involution. J. Cell Biol. 118:1271.

Thapa, S., R. Short, and M. Potts, 1988. Breast-feeding, birth spacing and their effects on child survival. Nature 335:679.

Thiede, M.A. and G.A. Rodan. 1988. Expression of a calcium mobilizing parathyroid hormone-like peptide in lactating mammary gland. Science 242:278.

Topper, Y.S. and C.S. Freeman. 1980. Multiple hormone interactions in the developmental biology of the mammary gland. Physiol. Rev. 60:1049.

Vorherr, H., ed. 1979. Human Lactation. New York, Grune and Stratton.

Wicha, C.J., C.H. Knight, C.V.P. Addey, D.M. Blatchford, M. Travers, C.N. Bennett, and M. Peaker. 1990. Effects of inhibition of basement membrane collagen deposition on rat mammary gland development. Develop. Biol. 80:253.

34
THE EYE

Elio Raviola

The ability to react to light is a widespread property of living matter. Plants use solar energy for photosynthesis and exhibit phototropic responses. Primitive invertebrates have scattered photoreceptor cells that detect varying intensities of light and enable them to position themselves favorably with respect to light or darkness. Vertebrates have evolved eyes—more efficient organs with a *cornea* and a *lens* to concentrate light and focus an image on closely packed photoreceptors in a *retina*, which detects light and encodes the various parameters of the image for transmission to the brain. The eyes of most vertebrates are placed on the sides of the head, where they provide a nearly complete panoramic view of the environment. *Panoramic vision*, together with the evolution of muscles and reflexes for rotation of the eyes, provided early warning against predators. On the other hand, in many predatory mammals and birds, the orbits gradually moved forward so that the uniocular fields of vision came to overlap in varying degree and the sector of the environment in front of the animal was seen by both eyes. Complex neural mechanisms developed to coordinate and fuse the slightly different images, thus achieving *binocular vision* and, in some instances, stereoscopic vision with perception of depth in a three-dimensional view of the environment essential to successful pursuit of prey. Acquisition of stereoscopic vision, evolution of a large brain to process the information, and freeing of the hands from a locomotor function enabled our hominoid ancestors to develop the manipulative skills that contributed to the ascendancy of humans.

STRUCTURE OF THE EYE IN GENERAL

The anterior segment of the eye, the *cornea*, is transparent, permitting the rays of light to enter. The rest of the wall of the eye is opaque, and possesses a darkly pigmented inner surface which absorbs light rays. The posterior segment of the eye is, to a great extent, lined with photosensitive nervous tissue, the *retina*, which develops as an outgrowth of the brain. The cavity of the eyeball is filled with transparent media arranged in separate bodies which, together with the cornea, act as a system of convex lenses. These produce, on the photosensitive layer of the retina, an inverted and reduced image of the objects in the environment.

The wall of the eyeball is composed of three layers: the tough, fibrous *corneoscleral coat*; the middle, vascular coat or *uvea*; and the innermost layer, the photosensitive *retina*. The thick fibrous layer protects the delicate inner structures of the eye and, together with the intraocular fluid pressure, serves to maintain the shape and turgor of the eyeball. It is divided into a large opaque posterior segment, the *sclera*, and a smaller transparent anterior segment, the *cornea*. The uvea is concerned with the nutrition of the retina and production of aqueous humor. It also provides mechanisms for visual accommodation and control of the amount of light entering the eye. Its three regional differentiations are the *choroid*, the *ciliary body*, and the *iris*. The choroid is the highly vascular portion of the uvea that underlies the photosensitive retina. Extending forward from the scalloped anterior margin of the retina, called the *ora serrata*, to the corneoscleral junction is the *ciliary body*. It forms a belt 5–6 mm wide around the interior of the eyeball and contains the smooth muscle that makes this structure the instrument of *accommodation*, acting on the lens to bring light rays from nearby objects to focus on the retina. The iris is a thin continuation of the ciliary body projecting over the anterior surface of the lens, with its free edge outlining the *pupil*. The diameter of the iris is approximately 12 mm. Its opening, the pupil, can be reduced or expanded through the contraction or relaxation of the *constrictor* and *dilator muscles* of the pupil. In this way, the iris functions as

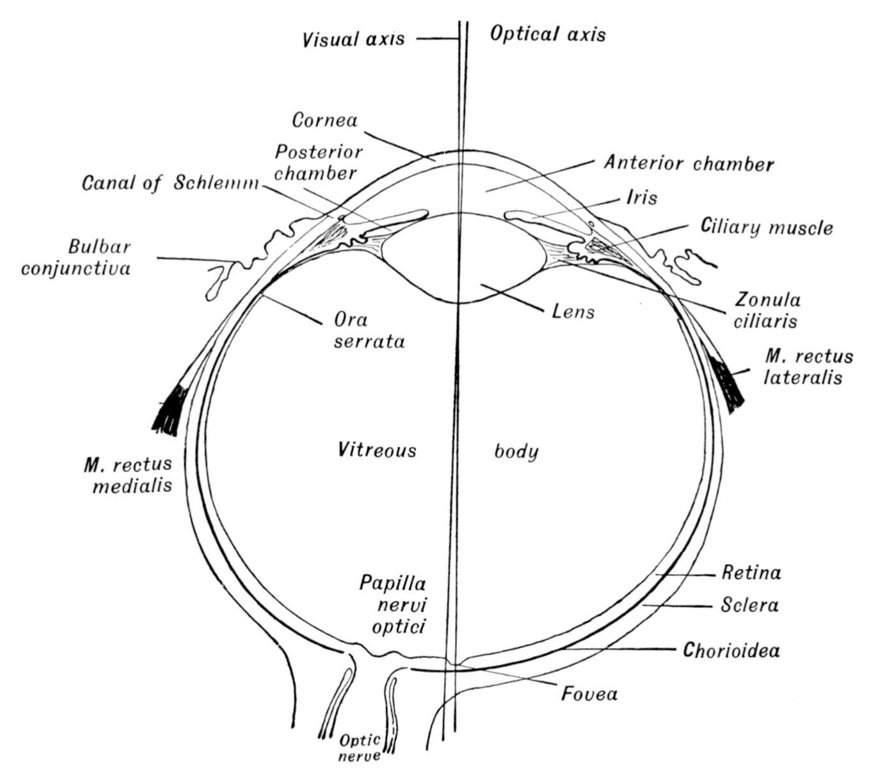

Figure 34–1. Diagram of a horizontal meridional section through the right eye of man.

an adjustable optic diaphragm regulating the amount of light entering the eye (Figs. 34–1 and 34–2).

The innermost layer, the retina, contains, in its sensory part, the receptors for light and the complex neural networks that encode the visual information and send impulses through the *optic nerve* to the brain. The spot where the nerve leaves the eyeball, the *papilla* of the optic nerve, is a pink disc approximately 1.4 mm in diameter located about 3 mm medial to the posterior pole of the eye. The portion of the retina anterior to the ora serrata and lining the inner surface of the ciliary muscle (*ciliary portion* of the retina) and that lining the posterior surface of the iris (*iridial portion* of the retina) are not photosensitive. These will be discussed with the uvea and iris.

The transparent *dioptric media* include the cornea and the contents of the cavity enclosed by the tunics of the eye. Because of the considerable difference between the index of refraction of the cornea and that of the surrounding air, the cornea is the chief refractive element of the eye. Of the enclosed transparent media, the most anterior is the *aqueous humor*. It is contained in the *anterior chamber*, a small cavity bounded in front by the cornea and in back by the iris and the central portion of the anterior surface of the lens. The *posterior chamber*, also filled with aqueous humor, is a narrow annular space enclosed anteriorly by the iris and the ciliary body and posteriorly by the lens and its suspensory ligament (Figs. 34–1 and 34–2).

The next of the transparent media is the *crystalline lens*. This is an elastic, biconvex body suspended from the inner surface of the ciliary body by a circular ligament, the *ciliary zonule*. It is placed directly behind the pupil between the aqueous humor and the vitreous body posteriorly. The lens is second in importance to the cornea as a refractive element of the eye, and is the dioptric organ of accommodation.

The greater portion of the cavity of the eye, situated between the posterior surface of the lens and the ciliary body anteriorly, and the retina posteriorly, is the *vitreal cavity*, filled with a viscous transparent substance, the *vitreous body*. It permits light to pass freely from the lens to the photoreceptors.

The retina is transparent in the living state. Only its outermost layer, the *pigment epithelium*, is opaque and forms the first barrier to the rays of light. The inner surface of the

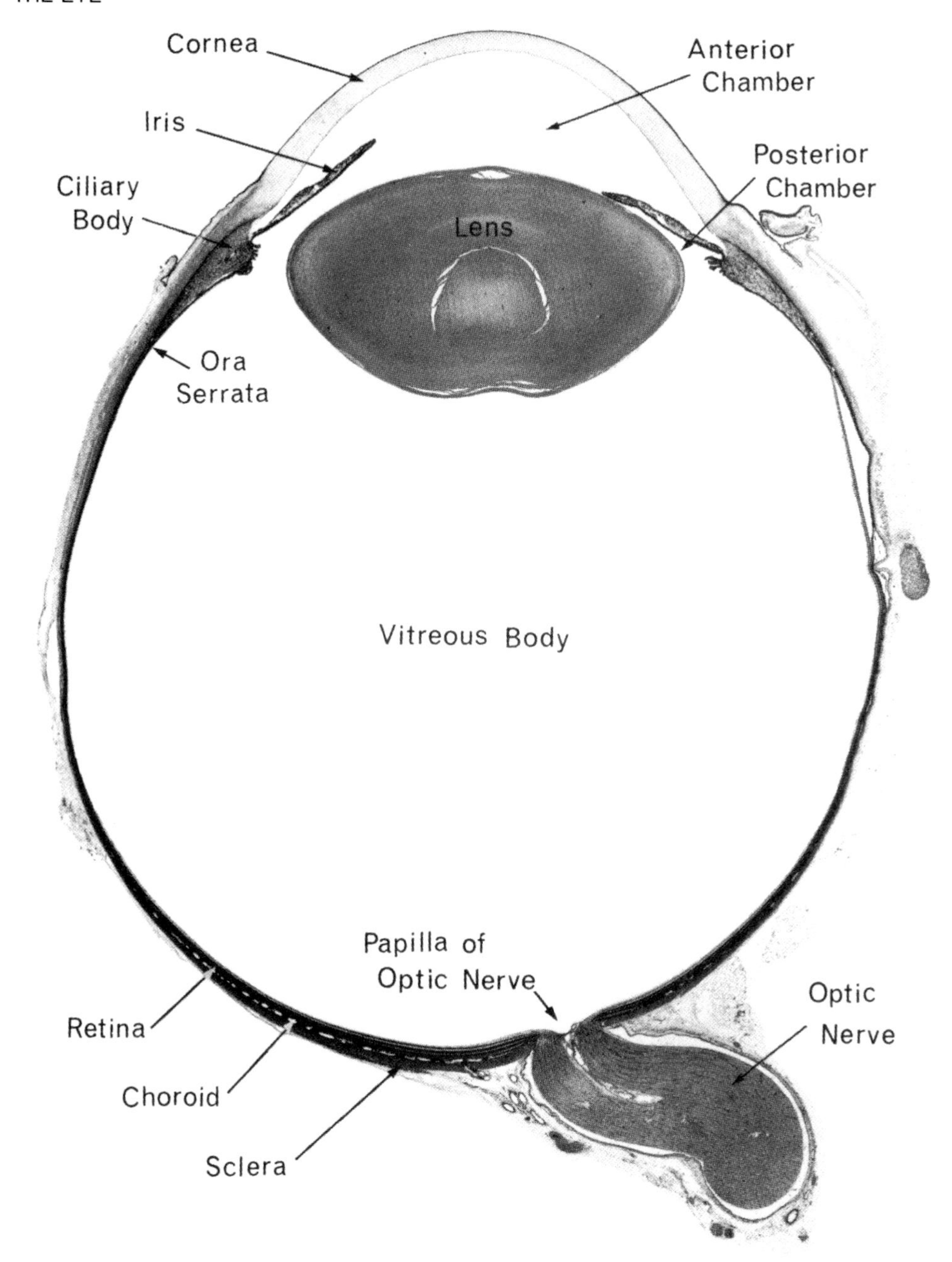

Figure 34–2. Photomicrograph of a meridional section of the eye of a rhesus monkey. (Courtesy of H. Mizoguchi.)

retina as seen with the ophthalmoscope is called the *fundus*.

DIMENSIONS, AXES, PLANES OF REFERENCE

The adult human eyeball is a roughly spherical body about 24 mm in diameter and weighing 6–8 g. The center of the cornea is the *anterior pole*; the posterior pole is located between the optic disc and the *fovea*, a thin depression in the retina providing the most distinct vision. The line connecting the two poles is the *anatomical axis*. The *visual axis* is the line drawn from the center of the fovea to the apparent center of the pupil (Fig. 34–1). The *equatorial plane* is vertical and perpendicular to the visual axis, passing through the greatest width of the eyeball, the *equator*. The planes passing through the axis determine the *meridians* of the eye. The two most important are the vertical and horizontal medians. The vertical passes through the fovea and divides the eyeball, including the retina, into nasal and temporal halves. The plane of the horizontal meridian divides the eyeball and the retina into an upper and a lower half. These two planes divide the eyeball and the retina into four quadrants: an upper nasal, an upper temporal, a lower nasal, and a lower temporal.

The *anteroposterior diameter* along the axis of the eye is 24 mm, or a little more. The *inner axis*, the distance between the inner surface of the cornea and the inner surface of the retina, at the posterior pole, is a little less than 22 mm. The *optical axis* passes through the optical centers of the refractive media and is almost identical with the anatomical axis. The visual axis, where it touches the retina, is from 4° to 7° lateral and 3.5° below the optical axis.

The *radius of curvature* of the larger posterior segment measures somewhat less than 13 mm, and gradually decreases toward the corneoscleral junction. The cornea has the smallest radius of curvature, approximately 7.8 mm (outer corneal surface).

The eyeball is lodged in a soft tissue cushion filling the bony orbit of the skull and made up of loose connective tissue and fatty tissue, muscles, fasciae, blood and lymphatic vessels, nerves, and a gland. This soft tissue cushion permits the eye to move freely around its *center of rotation*. The eye is connected to the general integument by the *conjunctiva*, which lines the lids and continues over the eyeball to the margins of the cornea. The lids are a mechanical protection against external noxious agents.

SCLERA

The sclera is 1 mm thick at the posterior pole, 0.4–0.3 mm at the equator, and 0.6 mm toward the edge of the cornea. It consists of flat bundles of type-I collagen fibrils that run in various directions parallel to the surface. Between these bundles are networks of elastic fibers. The cells of the sclera are flat, elongated fibroblasts. Melanocytes can also be found in the deeper layers, especially in the vicinity of the entrance of the optic nerve.

The tendons of the eye muscles are attached to the outer surface of the sclera, which, in turn, is connected with a dense layer of connective tissue—the *fascial sheath* of the eye or *capsule of Tenon*—by an exceedingly loose system of thin collagenous membranes separated by clefts—the *episcleral space* or *space of Tenon*. The eyeball and the capsule of Tenon rotate together in all directions on a bed of orbital fat.

Between the sclera and the choroid is a layer of loose connective tissue with elastic networks and numerous melanocytes and fibroblasts. When these two tunics are separated, part of this loose tissue adheres to the choroid and part to the sclera as its *suprachoroid lamina*.

CORNEA

The cornea is slightly thicker than the sclera, measuring 0.8–0.9 mm in the center and 1.1 mm at the periphery. In the human, the refractive power of the cornea, which is a function of the index of refraction of its tissue (1.376) and of the radius of curvature of its surface (7.8 mm), is twice as high as that of the lens.

In a cross section through the cornea, the following layers can be seen: (1) the corneal epithelium, (2) the membrane of Bowman, (3) the stroma, or substantia propria, (4) the membrane of Descemet, and (5) the endothelium (Fig. 34–3).

CORNEAL EPITHELIUM

The epithelium is stratified squamous, with an average thickness of 50 μm. It consists, as a rule, of five to seven layers of cells. The outer surface is composed of large squamous cells, connected to one another by zonulae occludentes and provided with microvilli and a system of apical ridges or microplicae. As in other types of stratified squamous epithelium, the cells are connected with one another by many short interdigitating processes that adhere at desmosomes. The cytoplasm contains numerous mitochondria and scattered profiles of granular endoplasmic reticulum in a cytoplasmic matrix filled with randomly oriented intermediate (cytokeratin) filaments.

The epithelium of the cornea is extremely sensitive and contains numerous free nerve endings. It is endowed with a remarkable capacity for wound healing. Minor injuries heal rapidly by a gliding movement of the adjacent epithelial cells to fill the defect. Mitoses appear later and may be found at considerable distance from the wound because it is thought that the renewal of the epithelium is ensured by stem cells that reside in the basal epithelial layer at the limbus. A few mitoses, however,

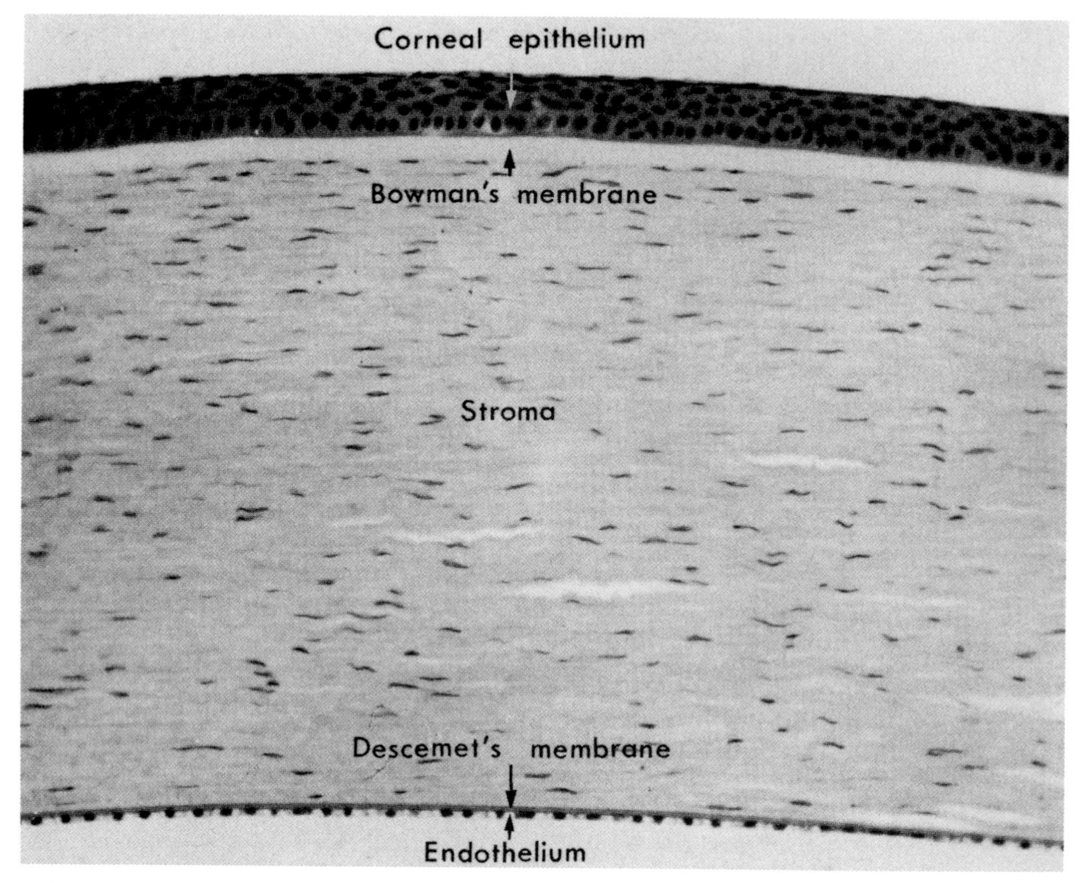

Figure 34–3. Photomicrograph of a section of human cornea. (After Kuwabara, T. 1966. *In* R.O. Greep, ed. Histology, 2nd ed. New York, McGraw-Hill Book Co.)

can be found in the basal cell layer under normal conditions.

BOWMAN'S MEMBRANE

The corneal epithelium rests on a faintly fibrillar lamina 6–9 μm thick. This structure is not actually a membrane, as its name suggests, but is the outer layer of the substantial propria of the cornea, from which it cannot be separated. It is nevertheless distinguishable with the optical microscope because its fibers are not so well ordered. With the electron microscope, it is seen to consist of a feltwork of randomly arranged type-I collagen fibrils, about 18 nm in diameter, which may show a periodic banding. It does not contain elastin and ends abruptly at the margin of the cornea. Bowman's membrane is not present in all mammals; in rabbits, the cornea epithelium rests on a simple basal lamina.

STROMA OR SUBSTANTIA PROPRIA

This layer forms about 90% of the thickness of the cornea (Fig. 34–3). It is a transparent regular connective tissue whose bundles of collagen form thin lamellae arranged in many layers. In each layer, the direction of the bundles changes and those in successive layers cross at various angles (Figs. 34–3 and 34–4). The lamellae everywhere interchange fibers and, thus, are kept tightly together. The fibrils are somewhat thicker than those of Bowman's membrane, measuring about 28 nm on the average, and consist of collagens type-I and type-V. They are regularly spaced at a distance of 55 nm from one another, and the spaces between them, as well as those between bundles and lamellae, are occupied by a ground substance largely consisting of the proteoglycans chondroitin and keratan sulfate. As a whole, the composition of the stroma is 78% water, 1% salts, and 21% macromolecules. Of these, 15% is collagen in the

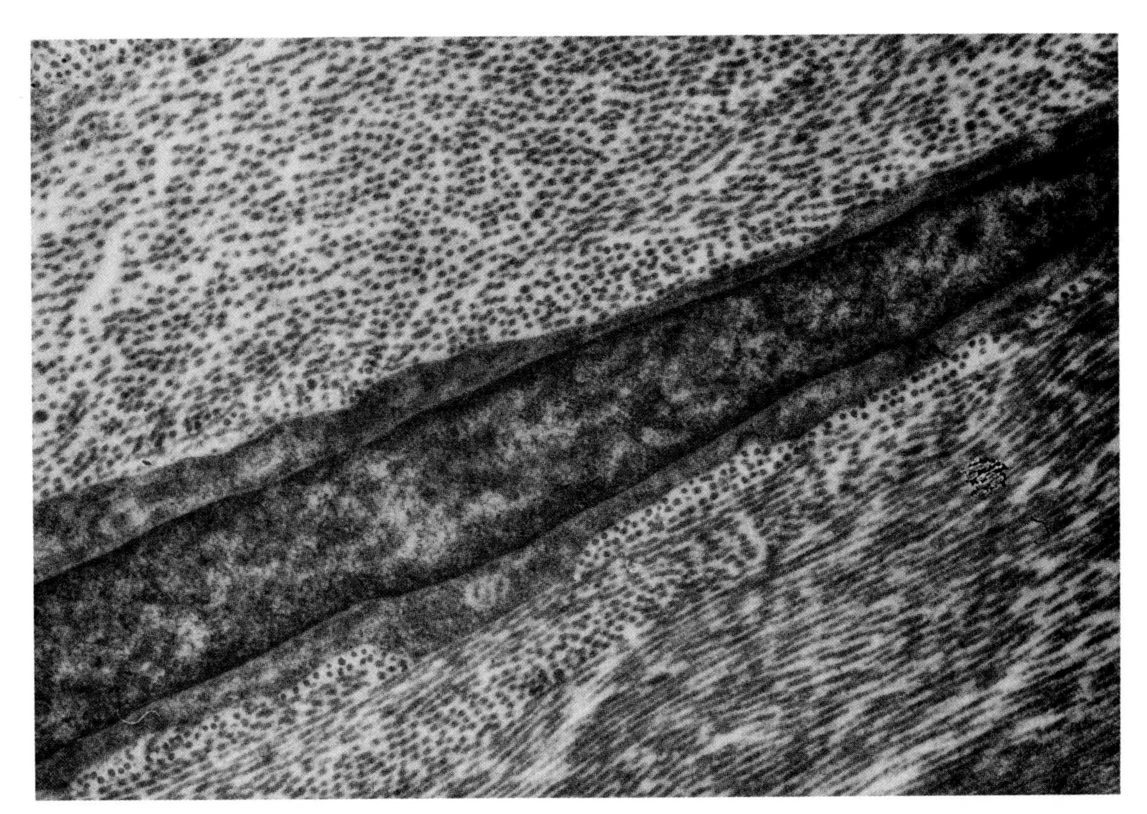

Figure 34–4. Electron micrograph of a part of a keratocyte in the cornea, and the surrounding layers of collagen fibrils, oriented at right angles to one another (Micrograph courtesy of M. Jakus.)

form of fibrils, 5% other proteins, 0.7% keratan sulfate, and 0.3% chondroitin sulfate. The cells of the stroma are long, slender fibroblasts (keratocytes) lodged in narrow clefts among the parallel bundles of collagen fibrils. In addition, the stroma always contains a number of lymphocytes which migrate from the blood vessels of the corneal limbus. In inflammation, enormous numbers of neutrophilic leukocytes and lymphocytes penetrate between the lamellae.

DESCEMET'S MEMBRANE AND CORNEAL ENDOTHELIUM

This homogeneous-appearing lamella, 5–10 μm thick, can be isolated from the posterior surface of the substantia propria. At the periphery of the cornea, Descemet's membrane continues as a thin layer on the surface of the trabeculae of the limbus. In its structure, it is essentially a very thick basal lamina elaborated by the corneal endothelium, which rests on it (Figs. 34–3 and 34–5). It appears homogeneous under the light microscope, but when examined with the electron microscope, Descemet's membrane of older individuals may show an apparent cross-striation, with bands about 107 nm apart connected by filaments less than 10 nm in width and about 27 nm apart (Fig. 34–6A). Tangential sections reveal a two-dimensional array of nodes, about 107 nm apart and connected by filaments to form hexagonal figures (Fig. 34–6B). The diagram in Fig. 34–7 shows the relationship between the images seen in the two planes. Histochemical data, chemical analyses, and X-ray diffraction studies support the conclusion that the filaments forming this hexagonal array consist of type-VIII collagen molecules, polymerized through end-to-end interactions. In young individuals, Descemet's membrane is more homogeneous in appearance. It is suggested that the hexagonal pattern of fibers forms with advancing age by aggregation of collagen that is normally dispersed in the amorphous ground substance. This and other atypical forms of collagen occur in the membrane at the periphery of the cornea, where randomly oriented fibrous bands with a 100-nm periodicity are frequently encountered. These are

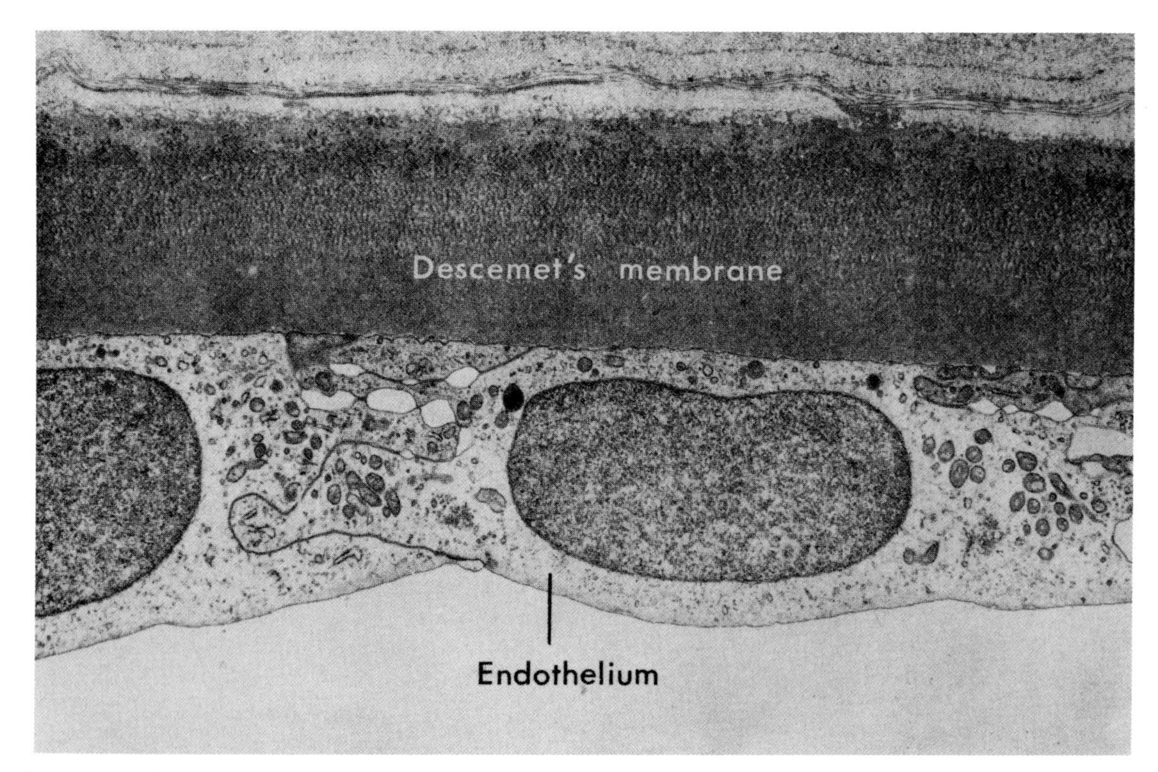

Figure 34–5. Electron micrograph of the endothelium and underlying Descemet's membrane from a human eye. (Courtesy of T. Kuwabara.)

particularly common in *Hassall–Henle bodies* or *warts*, dome-shaped protrusions from the periphery of Descemet's membrane into the anterior chamber, which occur with increasing frequency in human eyes after the age of 20.

The inner surface of the membrane of Descemet is covered by a layer of large squamous cells connected by incomplete zonulae occludentes (Fig. 34–5); thus, the intercellular spaces between these endothelial cells permit free exchange of fluid between corneal stroma and anterior chamber.

HISTOPHYSIOLOGY OF THE CORNEA

The transparency of the cornea is great although less than that of the aqueous humor. It is due to its thinness, to the fact that collagen fibers are poor light scatterers, and, finally, to the uniform diameter and regular spacing of the fibrils, so that scattered waves cancel each other by destructive interference. How the regular spacing of the fibrils is maintained is still a matter of speculation. One hypothesis holds that the proteoglycans exert a swelling pressure which is opposed by links that limit the separation between the fibrils. Type-XII collagen molecules may represent such links that prevent bundles and lamellae from falling apart. Thus, the orderly arrangement of the fibrils may result from the turgor of the interfibrillar matrix, coupled to the uniform length of the inextensible interfibrillar type-XII collagen bridges. An increase in the amount of interfibrillar fluid, such as occurs in swelling, causes cloudiness of the cornea.

The cornea is avascular, and its central region depends on diffusion from the aqueous humor for its nourishment. The blood vessels of the limbus supply the peripheral cornea by diffusion, and account for the presence, in the corneal stroma, of leukocytes and substances that are excluded from the aqueous humor. Oxygen for the corneal epithelium comes directly from the atmosphere. The contribution of tears to corneal nourishment seems to be negligible.

The cornea is one of the few organs that can be successfully transplanted into allogeneic recipients. One explanation for this phenomenon is that the lack of blood vessels protects the transplanted cornea from the host's immune system.

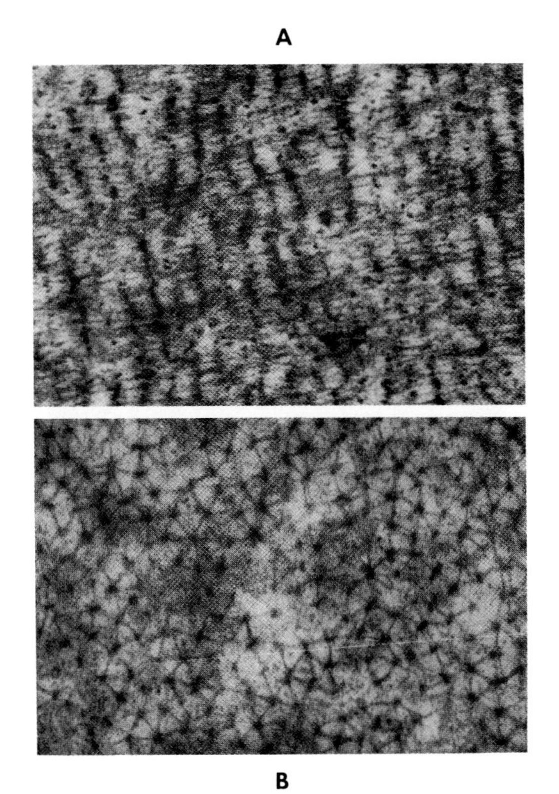

Figure 34–6. Electron micrographs of Descemets's membrane showing the unusual configuration of collagen characteristic of this layer. (A) Cross section illustrating a striated appearance; (B) tangential section illustrating the hexagonal arrangement of nodes connected by filaments. (Courtesy of M. Jakus.)

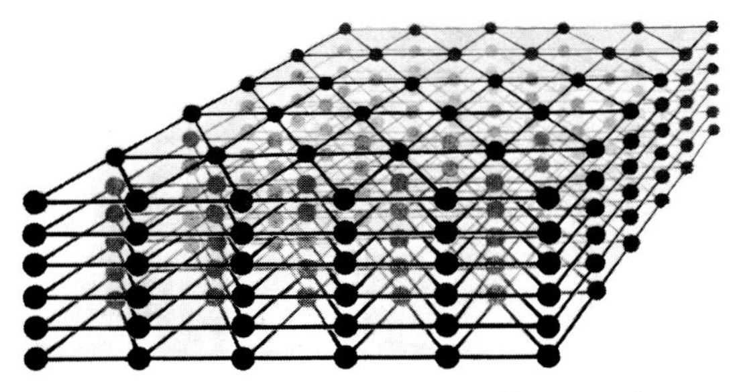

Figure 34–7. Diagram of the structure of Descemet's membrane based on electron micrographs. (Courtesy of M. Jakus.)

THE LIMBUS

The *limbus* or sclerocorneal junction is an important region of the eye because it represents a valuable landmark for the ophthalmologist and contains the apparatus for the outflow of the aqueous humor (Figs. 34–8 and 34–9). About 1.5–2 mm wide, its outer surface displays an outer depression called the *external scleral sulcus*, where the gently curving sclera is continuous with the more convex cornea. On its inner aspect, the sclerocorneal stroma is marked by a circular depression, the *internal scleral sulcus*, which is filled in by the *trabecular meshwork* and the *canal of Schlemm*, specialized tissues constituting the outflow system for the aqueous humor. On the posterior lip of the internal scleral sulcus, the scleral stroma projects toward the interior of the eye, forming a small circular ridge, the *scleral spur*. This affords attachment to the trabecular meshwork anteriorly and to the ciliary muscle posteriorly.

At the limbus, there is a gradual transition of the corneal epithelium into that of the conjunctiva of the bulb (Fig. 34–8). The membrane of Bowman terminates and is replaced by the conjunctival stroma and the anterior margin of the capsule of Tenon. In the connective tissue underlying the epithelium, the conjunctival vessels form arcades that extend radially into the cornea for about 0.5 mm beyond the limbal edge. These vessels nourish the periphery of the cornea and are the source of the occasional lymphocytes found in the corneal stroma. The blood vessels that invade the corneal stroma in chronic inflammation arise from these loops. When the limbus is examined in a living subject with the slit-lamp microscope, *aqueous veins*, veins containing aqueous humor instead of blood, may be seen emerging from the limbal stroma and contributing to the plexus of episcleral veins. At the limbus, the collagenous sclera gradually continues into the corneal stroma and its collagenous bundles progressively acquire the uniform small diameter and orderly arrangement typical of the cornea. Deep to the stroma of the limbus, Descemet's membrane ends and gives way to the spongy tissue of the *trabecular meshwork*, situated between the anterior chamber, the root of the iris, the limbal stroma, and the scleral spur (Figs. 34–9 and 34–10). The trabecular meshwork is composed of a large number of flattened, fenestrated connective tissue sheets and branching and anastomosing beams or trabeculae. These are completely invested by an attenuated endothelium, continuous with the corneal endothelium (Fig. 34–11). They bound a labyrinthine system of minute passages, the intertrabecular spaces, which communicate with the anterior chamber and are filled with aqueous humor.

Interposed between the trabecular meshwork and the limbal stroma is the *canal of Schlemm*, a flattened vessel that extends

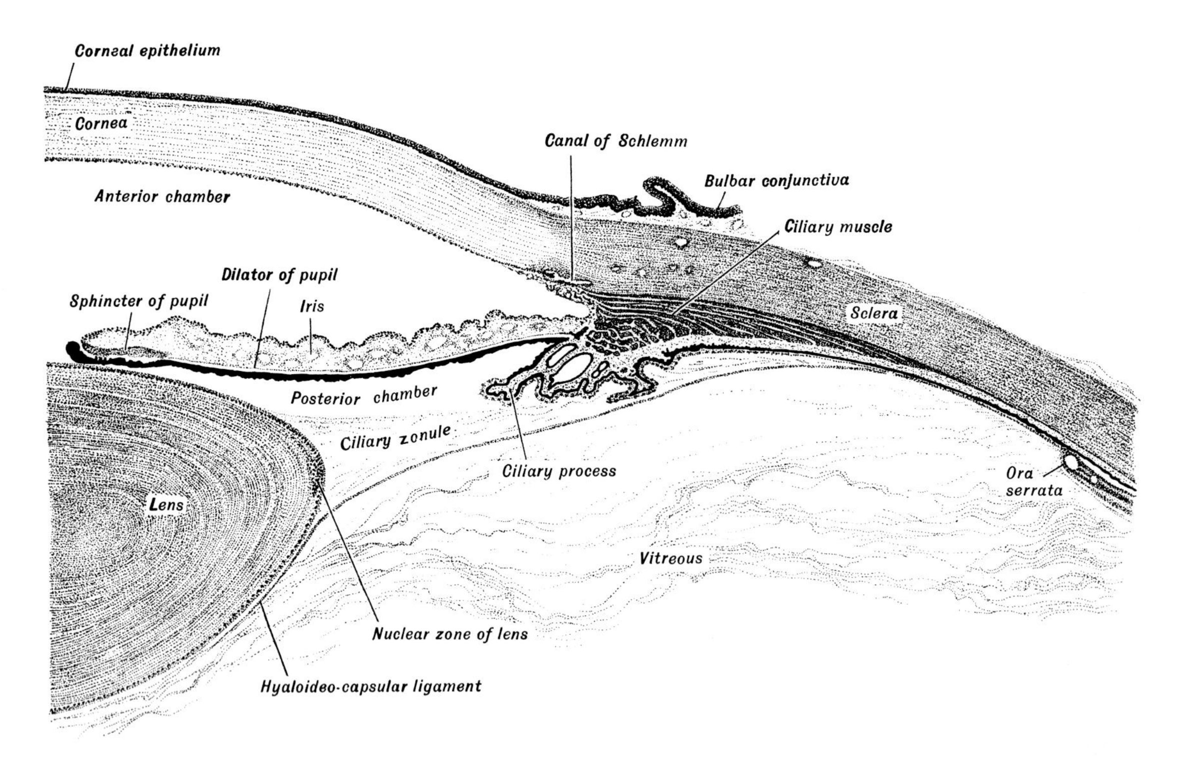

Figure 34–8. Diagram of a meridional section of human eye showing the location of the ciliary body. (Modified after Schaffer, J. Lehrbuch der Histologie und Histogenes. Verlag von W. Engelmann, Leipzig. 1922.)

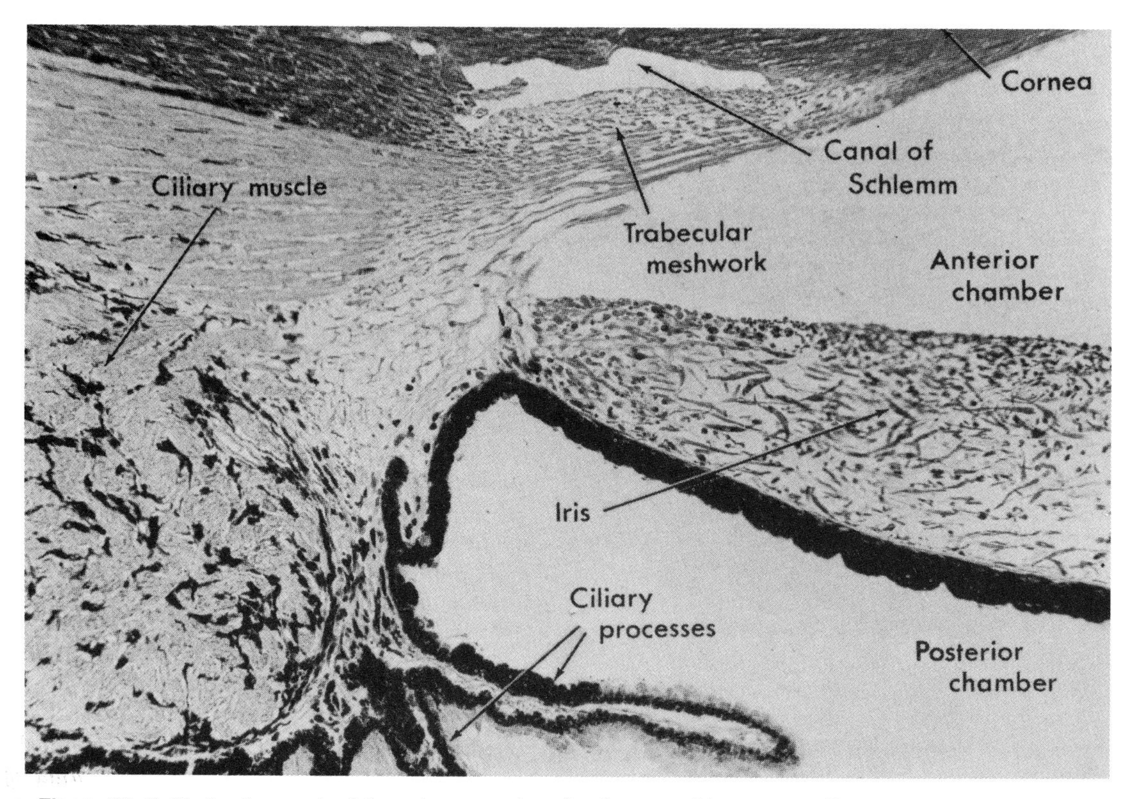

Figure 34–9. Photomicrograph of the sclerocorneal angle of a normal human eye (Courtesy of T. Kuwabara.)

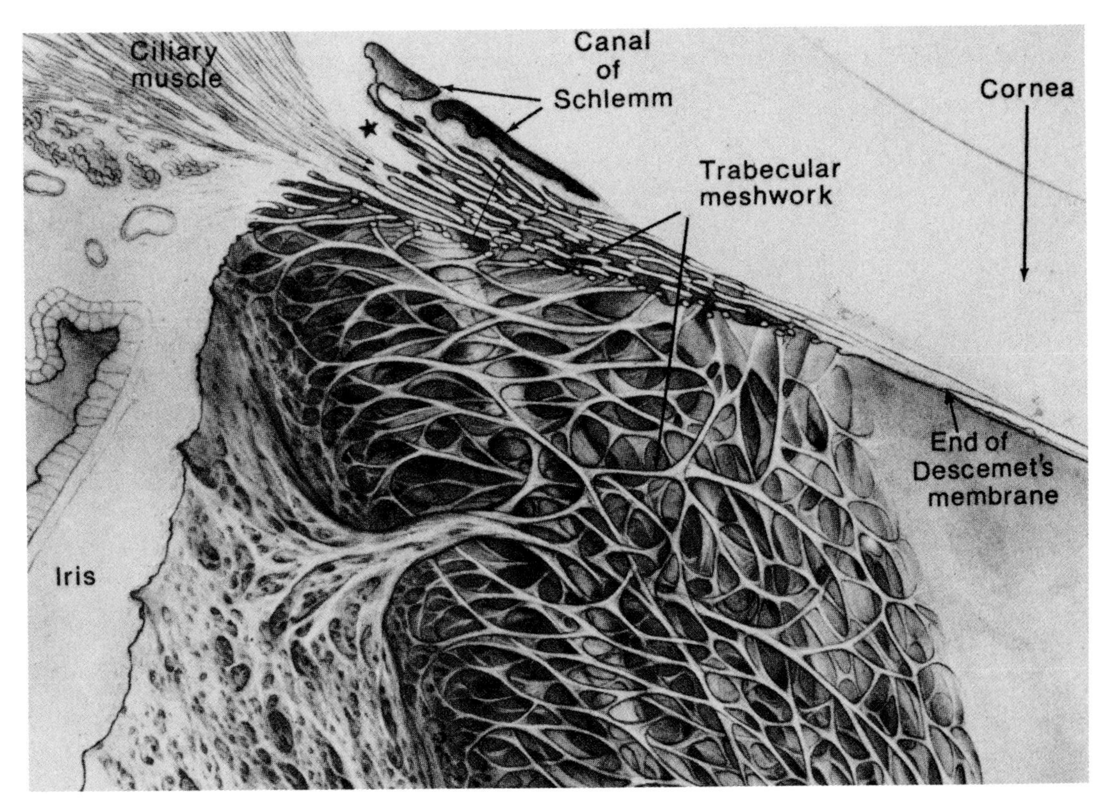

Figure 34–10. Drawing of the components of the outflow system of the aqueous humor. The star indicates the so-called spur. (After Hogan, M.Y., J.A. Alvarado, and J.E. Weddell. 1971. Histology of the Human Eye. Philadelphia, W.W. Saunders Co.)

around the entire circumference of the limbus. The canal of Schlemm has a varicose outline and in places breaks up into irregular branches that coalesce again. The wall of the canal consists of endothelium, a discontinuous basal lamina, and a thin layer of connective tissue. On the outer wall of the canal, that is, toward the limbal stroma, the endothelium is extremely attenuated (Fig. 34–12); on the inner wall of the canal, toward the trabecular meshwork, the endothelium varies greatly in thickness with different techniques of specimen preparation and may display large intracellular or intercellular vacuoles. Great importance has been attributed to these "giant vacuoles," because it is believed that they are involved in the process of aqueous humor reabsorption from the anterior chamber.

The lumen of the canal does not communicate directly with the spaces of the trabecular meshwork but is separated from them by the following layers: (1) the endothelium that invests the internal wall of the canal; (2) the connective tissue adventitia of the canal, which here becomes especially rich in stromal cells and is usually referred to as juxtacanalicular connective tissue; and (3) the endothelial lining of the trabecular spaces.

From the outer wall of the canal, 25–35 *collector channels* arise, which join the deep veins of the limbus; these, in turn, pass to the surface of the limbal stroma and empty into the episcleral veins.

Aqueous humor contained in the anterior chamber permeates the maze of minute intercommunicating passages of the trabecular meshwork; then, it reaches the lumen of the canal of Schlemm and is finally drained by the episcleral veins. The precise pathway followed by the aqueous humor from the intertrabecular spaces to the lumen of the Schlemm canal is poorly understood. The Schlemm canal usually contains aqueous humor, but it may rarely fill with blood when there is stasis and back pressure in the venous system. Obstruction to the filtration of aqueous humor through the intertrabecular spaces or to its drainage via the canal of Schlemm results in the rise of intraocular pressure characteristic of the serious eye disease *glaucoma*.

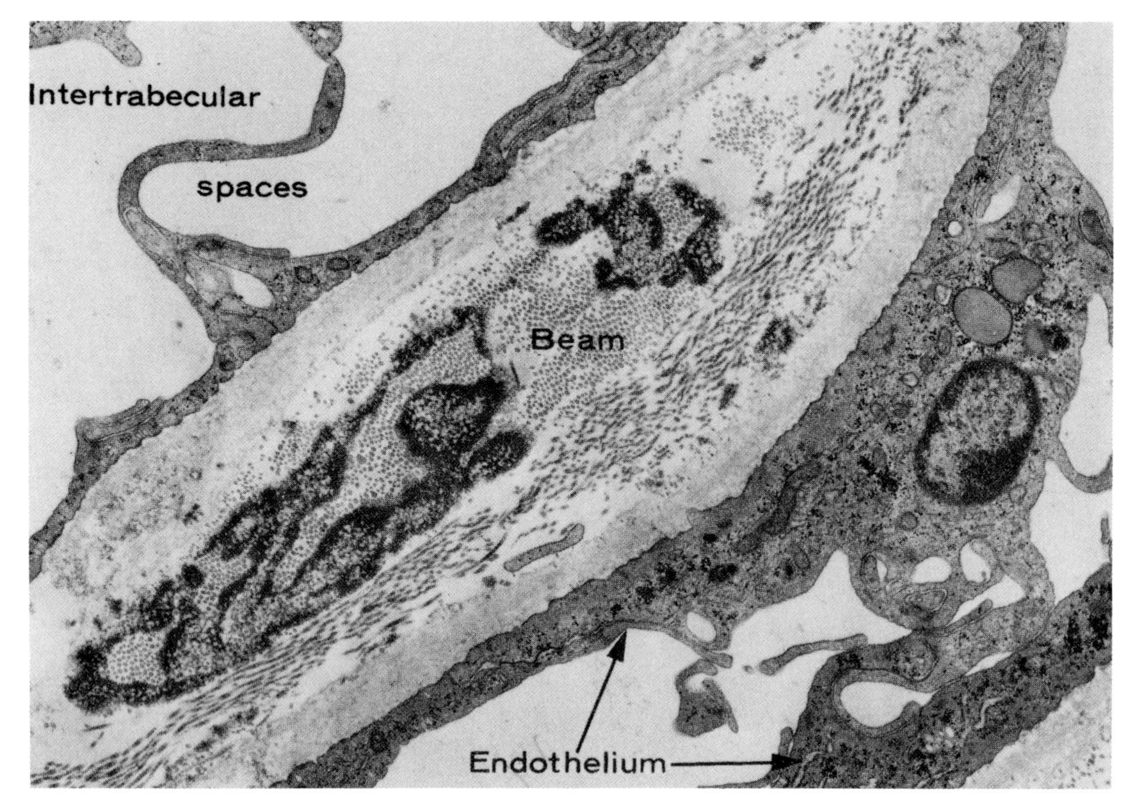

Figure 34–11. Electron micrograph of a beam of the trabecular meshwork in a monkey eye. A thick basal lamina separates the connective tissue core of the beam from the investing endothelial cells. (From Raviola, G. 1974. Investig. Ophthalmol. 13:828.)

THE UVEA OR VASCULAR TUNIC

CHOROID

The choroid is a thin soft brown layer adjacent to the inner surface of the sclera. Between the sclera and choroid is a potential cleft, the *perichoroidal space* which is traversed by thin lamellae that run obliquely from the choroid to the sclera and form a loose pigmented tissue layer, the *suprachoroidal lamina*. This is composed of fine transparent sheets, with fibroblasts on their surface and with a rich network of elastic fibers. Large, flat melanocytes are scattered everywhere between, and within, the connective tissue lamellae. In the suprachoroid, as in the rest of the uvea, there are also scattered macrophages. The lamellae of the suprachoroid pass without a distinct boundary into the substance of the choroid proper. This tunic can be subdivided into three main layers: from outside inward, they are (1) the vessel layer, (2) the choriocapillary layer, and (3) the glassy membrane, or *Bruch's membrane* (Fig. 34–13).

Vessel Layer

This consists of a multitude of large and medium-sized arteries and veins. The spaces between the vessels are filled with loose connective tissue rich in melanocytes. The lamellar arrangement here is much less distinct than in the suprachoroid. According to some, the vessel layer contains strands of smooth muscle that are independent of the walls of blood vessels.

Choriocapillary Layer

This is a capillary network arranged in one plane. In places, this layer is connected with the vessel layer. The individual capillaries have large and rather irregular caliber; toward Bruch's membrane, their endothelium is fenestrated. The layer is thicker and the

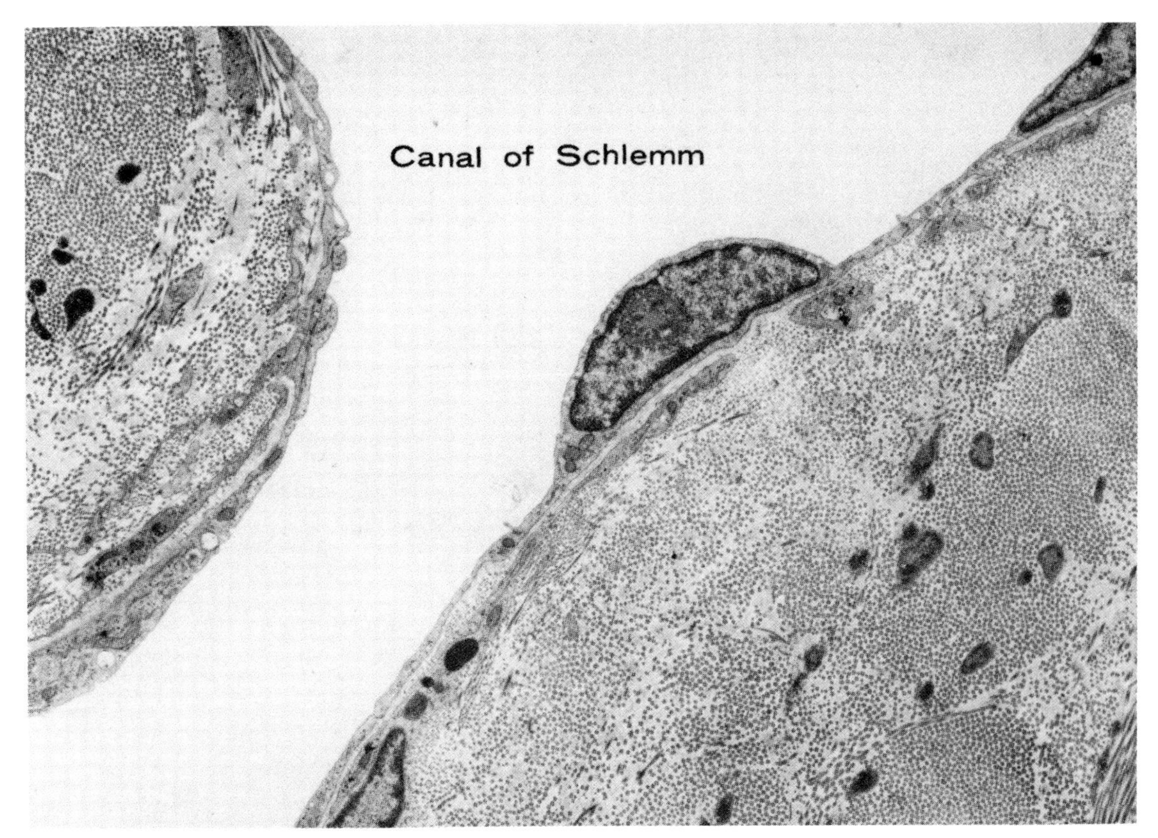

Figure 34–12. Canal of Schlemm in a monkey eye. The external wall of the canal consists of an attenuated endothelium, a discontinuous basal lamina, and an adventitial layer of flattened fibroblasts. These are surrounded by collagen fibers of the stroma of the limbus, seen here in cross section. (From Raviola, G. 1974. Investig. Ophthalmol. 13:828.)

capillary network denser in the region underlying the fovea. Anteriorly, it ends near the ora serrata.

Bruch's Membrane (Glassy Membrane)

This is a refractile layer 1–4 μm thick between the choroid and the pigment epithelium of the retina. The electron microscope has shown that this so-called membrane is not a homogeneous structure but consists of five different components: (1) the basal lamina of the endothelium of the capillaries of the choriocapillary layer; (2) a first layer of collagen fibers; (3) a network of elastic fibers: (4) a second layer of collagen fibers; and (5) the basal lamina of the pigment epithelium of the retina.

CILIARY BODY

If the eyeball is cut across along its equator, and its anterior half is inspected from within after removal of the vitreous, a sharply outlined, dentate border is seen running around the inner surface of the wall in front of the equator (Fig. 34–14). This is the *ora serrata* or *ora terminalis* of the photosensitive retina. The zone between the ora and the edge of the lens is the *ciliary body*, a thickening of the vascular tunic. Its surface is covered by the darkly pigmented, nonphotosensitive ciliary portion of the retina. In a meridional section through the eye bulb, the ciliary body appears as a thin triangle with its small base facing the anterior chamber of the eye and attached by its anterior and outer angle to the scleral spur. The long, narrow posterior angle of its triangular section extends backward and merges with the choroid (Fig. 34–8). The inner aspect of the ciliary body is divided into a narrow anterior zone, the *ciliary crown*, and a broader posterior zone, the *ciliary ring*. Seen in surface view, the inner surface of the ring has shallow grooves, *ciliary striae*, which run forward from the teeth of the ora serrata. On its inner surface, the ciliary crown has 70 radially arranged ridges,

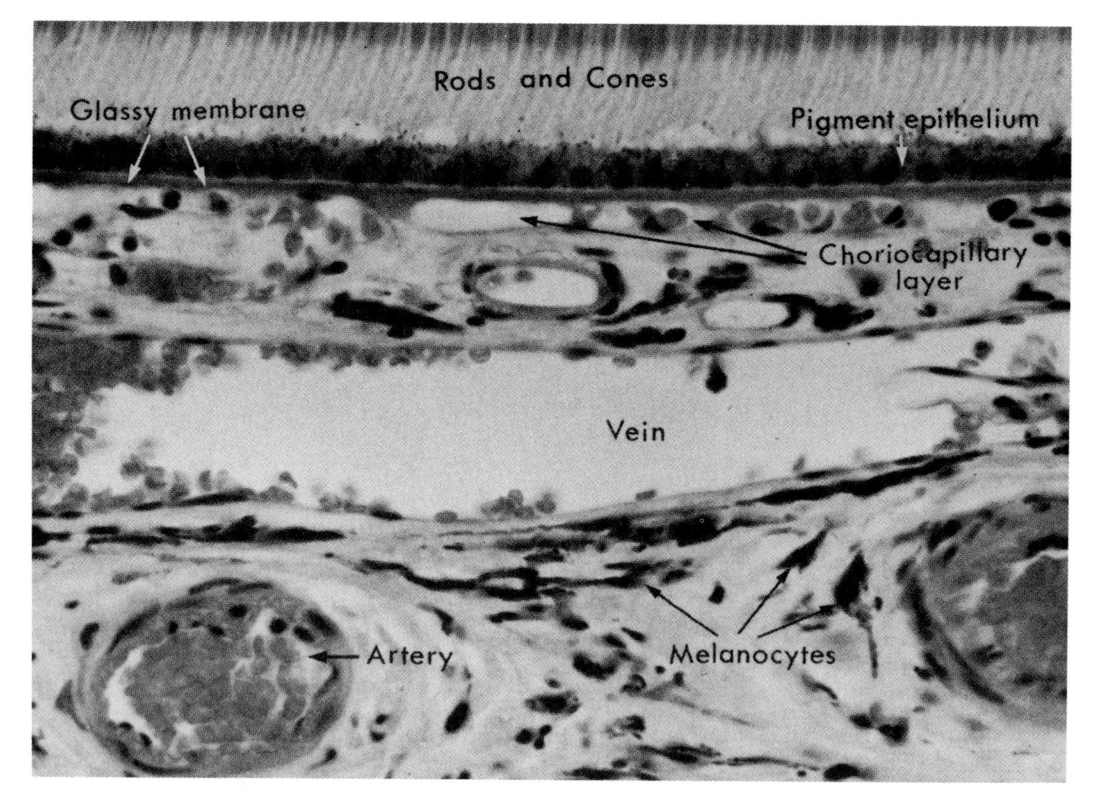

Figure 34–13. Photomicrograph of the choroid and the outermost layers of the retina (top). (After Kuwabara, T. 1966. *In* R.O. Greep, ed. Histology, 2nd ed. New York, McGraw-Hill Book Co.)

the *ciliary processes* (Fig. 34–8, 34–9, and 34–14).

The bulk of the ciliary body, exclusive of the ciliary processes, consists of the muscle of accommodation, the *ciliary muscle*. It is smooth muscle and is composed of three portions. Closest to the sclera is the *muscle of Brücke* whose bundles are deployed chiefly in the meridional direction. This outer part of the ciliary muscle stretches the choroid and is also

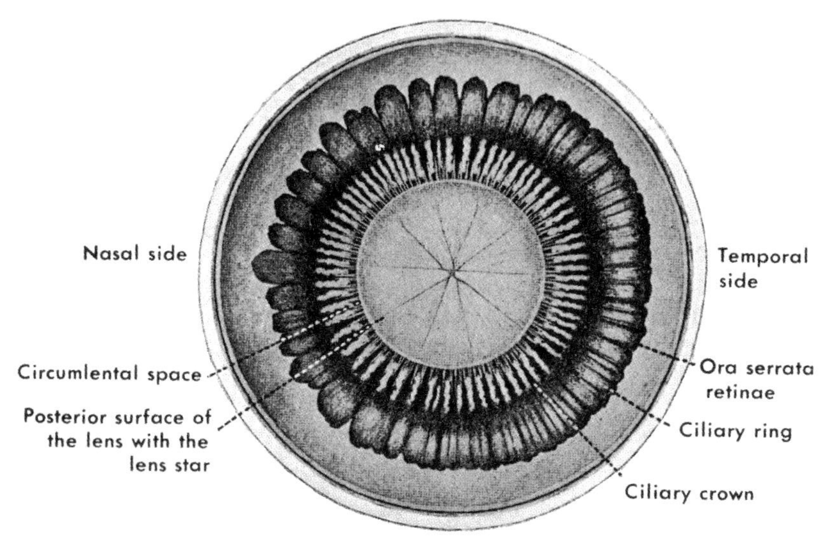

Figure 34–14. Drawing of the anterior half of the eye, seen from within. The ora serrata and ciliary crown are clearly depicted. (After Salzmann, M. 1912. Anatomie und Histologie des menschlich Augapfels in Normal-Zustande, Leipzig.)

called the *tensor muscle of the choroid.* In the next inward portion of the ciliary muscle, the bundles of muscle cells radiate fanlike from the region of the scleral spur toward the cavity of the eyeball. This is the *radial* or *reticular portion* of the ciliary muscle. The third, or *circular portion* of the ciliary muscle (Müller's muscle), is usually absent in the newborn, appearing in the course of the second or third year. The contraction of this portion relaxes the tension on the lens and, thus, is important in accommodation for near vision. The classical subdivision of the ciliary muscle into three portions has been challenged as too schematic because, in fact, the muscle fibers seem to be interwoven in a tridimensional network, but with regions where fibers of meridional, radial, and circular orientation predominate. The interstices between the muscular bundles are filled with a small amount of connective tissue containing abundant elastic fibers and melanocytes (Fig. 34–9). The latter become especially numerous toward the sclera.

The inner, *vascular layer* of the ciliary body consists of connective tissue and numerous blood vessels. In the ciliary ring, it is the direct continuation of the same layer of the choroid. In the region of the ciliary crown, it covers the inner surface of the ciliary muscle and forms the core of the ciliary processes. The vessels are almost exclusively capillaries and veins of varying caliber. The corresponding arteries ramify in the peripheral layers of the ciliary body. The capillary endothelium is fenestrated and freely permeable to plasma proteins. The connective tissue is dense, especially near the root of the iris, and contains abundant elastic fibers. In old age, it often shows hyaline degeneration.

The ciliary portion of the retina continues forward beyond the ora serrata as the *ciliary epithelium* investing the inner surface of the ciliary body. Its function is the production of the aqueous humor. The ciliary epithelium consists of two layers of cells, an inner layer of nonpigmented elements bounding the posterior chamber and an outer pigmented layer which rests on the stroma of the ciliary body (Fig. 34–15). Toward the root of the iris, the cells of the inner epithelial layer gradually accumulate pigment granules. Because of the embryonal origin of the ciliary epithelium from the edge of the double-walled optic cup, the pole of the nonpigmented cells directed toward the interior of the eye is usually referred to as the cell base, whereas the base of the pigmented cells is the end that adjoins the stroma of the ciliary body. Thus, the apices of the pigmented and nonpigmented epithelial cells face each other. At intervals, they are separated by discontinuous intercellular spaces called *ciliary channels.*

A basal lamina invests both surfaces of the ciliary epithelium: that toward the stroma of the ciliary body is continuous with the basal lamina of the pigment epithelium of the retina; the other is continuous with the inner limiting membrane of the retina.

The basal and lateral regions of the nonpigmented cells are occupied by a labyrinth of interdigitating processes formerly describes as "membrane infoldings" (Fig. 34–16). In this respect, the nonpigmented cells resemble other epithelia actively engaged in transport of ions and water. Between the central nucleus and the cell apex is the cell center, consisting of a well-developed Golgi complex, a centriole, and occasionally a cilium, which protrudes from the cell surface in a channel bounded by the plasma membrane. The cytoplasm is permeated by cisternae of the granular endoplasmic reticulum, tubules of agranular reticulum, and bundles of filaments radiating from the desmosomes that join adjacent cells. The mitochondria are not especially numerous, nor do they appear to be arranged in an orderly manner with respect to the plasmalemmal invaginations, as is the case for the convoluted tubules of the kidney, or the striated ducts of the salivary glands. Especially prominent in the pigmented epithelial cells are the melanin granules, which completely fill the cytoplasm, leaving but little space for a moderate number of mitochondria and thin bundles of filaments. The nucleus is located toward the apex of the cell, being separated from it by a small Golgi complex. The plasma membrane at the base of the cell is repeatedly invaginated, but the basal labyrinth is not as complex as in nonpigmented cells.

The ciliary epithelium is exceptional among actively transporting epithelia because it consists of two layers of cells, both provided with a basal labyrinth of interdigitating processes. These structural specializations suggest that the ciliary epithelium represents a unique biological device, consisting of two pumps working in series. This might result in a considerable amplification of the transport efficiency, but it requires accurate synchronization of the cells' activity. Gap junctions probably ensure such a precise coordination of the function of the myriad independent cell units; they connect adjacent pigmented cells. Furthermore,

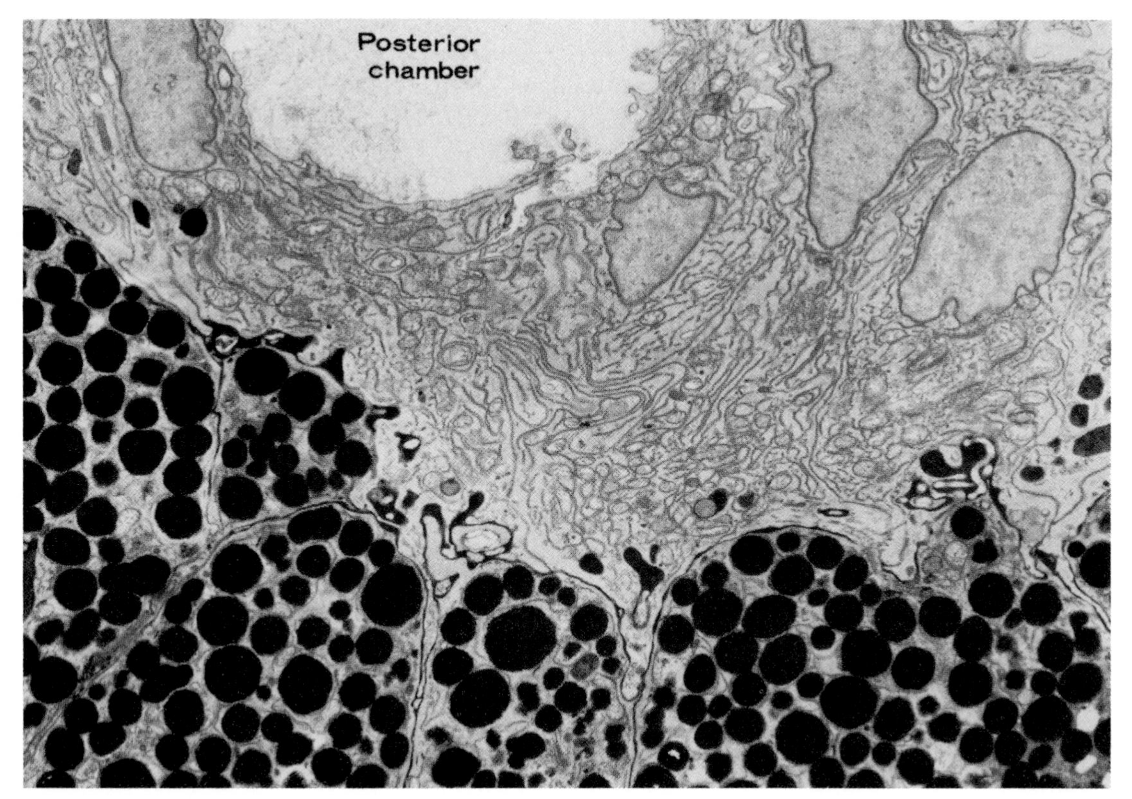

Figure 34–15. Low-power micrograph of the ciliary epithelium of a monkey that was injected intravenously with horseradish peroxidase. The ciliary epithelium consists of two cell layers, one nonpigmented (top), which bounds the posterior chamber, and the other which is pigmented (bottom) rests on the stroma of the ciliary body. The tracer has escaped through the permeable walls of the vessels of the ciliary body and has permeated the intercellular clefts between pigmented and nonpigmented cells; its further progression toward the posterior chamber has been blocked by the tight junctions which connect the apices of the nonpigmented cells. (From Raviola, G. 1974. Investig. Ophthlamol. 13:828.)

the lateral surfaces of the nonpigmented cells are connected to each other by an elaborate zonula occludens, a zonula adherens and a few desmosomes.

Aqueous Humor and the Blood-Aqueous Barrier

Proper eye functioning requires a precise spatial arrangement of the retina with respect to the refractive media and a special chemical composition of the intraocular fluids, optimally adjusted to the metabolic needs of the retina, lens, and cornea. The aqueous humor subserves both of these functions. An accurate balance between its rates of production and reabsorption is responsible for maintenance of the intraocular pressure, which confers mechanical stability on the ocular structures. Its specific composition, different from plasma, and somewhat resembling cerebrospinal fluid, cooperates with the blood-retinal barrier in generating an extracellular environment best suited to the functional requirements of the cells of the retina, lens, and cornea. Finally, it nourishes the lens which lacks a blood supply.

The aqueous fluid is a clear, watery fluid of slightly alkaline reaction with an index of refraction of 1.33, contained in the anterior and posterior chambers of the eye. In its chemical composition, the aqueous humor differs from blood plasma in its lower content of proteins; higher content of ascorbate, pyruvate and lactate; and lower content of urea and glucose. Also, its electrolyte content is slightly different from that of plasma. Continuously secreted by the ciliary epithelium, probably through a process of active transport, it fills the posterior chamber, nourishes the lens, and permeates the vitreous body. From the posterior chamber, it flows into the anterior chamber through the pupil and is finally drained through the trabecular meshwork and canal of Schlemm. The flow of the

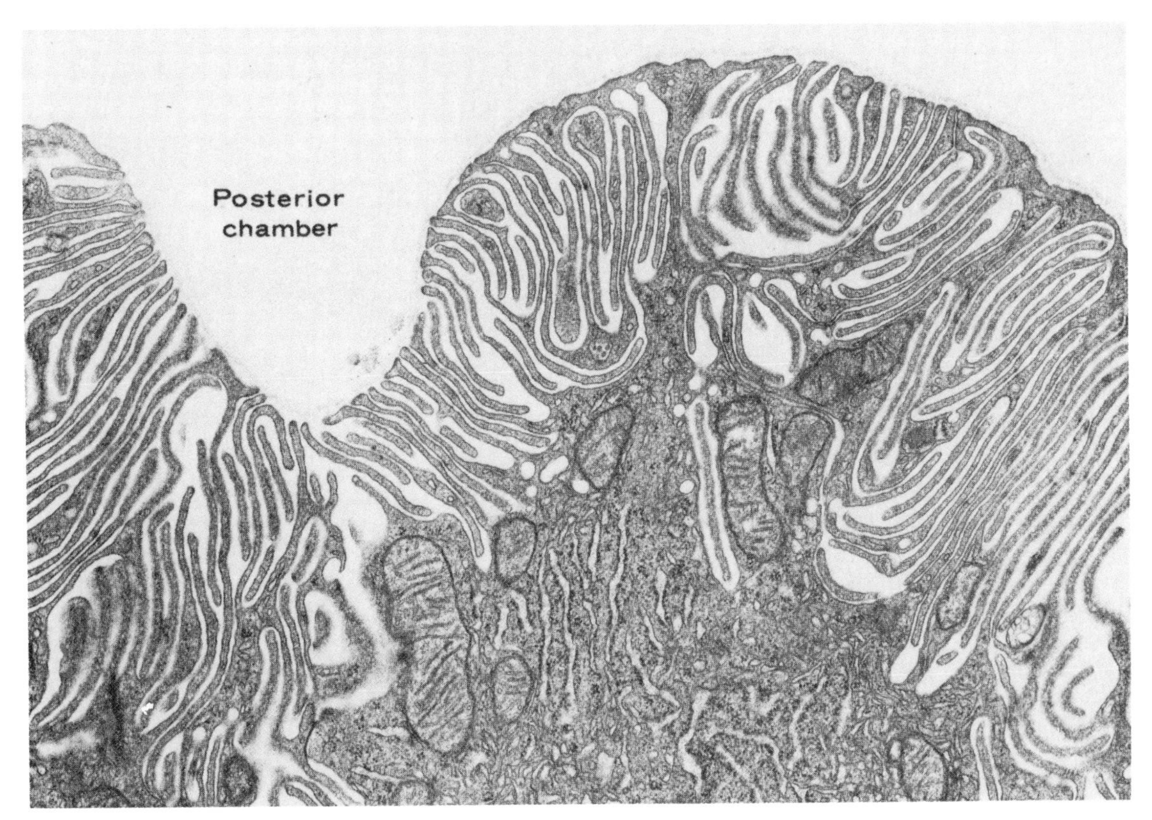

Figure 34–16. Electron micrograph of the ciliary epithelium of a rabbit. The base of the nonpigmented cells, shown here, consists of a complex labyrinth of slender interdigitating processes. (Courtesy of G. Raviola).

aqueous humor is determined by the difference in pressure between the fluids within the eye (about 20 mm Hg) and the pressure in the episcleral veins (about 13 mm Hg). In turn, the intraocular pressure is generated by an accurate adjustment of the rate of aqueous humor secretion by the ciliary epithelium and its rate of reabsorption at the limbus. When this balance is disrupted, as in glaucoma, the intraocular pressure increases, with devastating effects on the function of the eye.

Secretion of a fluid, such as the aqueous humor, with a composition different from that of plasma is possible only if free diffusion of solutes between the blood and the chambers of the eye is prevented. This is the role of the so-called *blood-aqueous barrier*, the peculiar physiological mechanism that limits the exchange of materials between the vascular compartment and the interior of the eye. When an ultrastructural tracer, such as horseradish peroxidase, is injected into the bloodstream, it rapidly diffuses across the permeable walls of the vessels of the ciliary body, permeates the stroma underlying the ciliary epithelium, and is finally blocked by the tight junctions that connect the apices of the nonpigmented cells (Fig. 34–15). These junctions, which limit free movement of molecules between ciliary body stroma and posterior chamber, are, therefore, believed to represent the major anatomical site of the blood-aqueous barrier.

IRIS

The posterior surface of the iris, near the pupil, rests on the anterior surface of the lens; in this way, the iris separates the anterior chamber from the posterior chamber. The margin of the iris connected with the ciliary body is called the *ciliary margin*, or the root of the iris. The pupil is surrounded by the *pupillary margin of the iris*. The iris diminishes in thickness toward both margins. Besides its individually varying color, the anterior surface of the iris presents certain distinct markings. About 1.5 mm from the pupil, a jagged line, concentric with the pupillary margin, separates the anterior surface into a *pupillary*

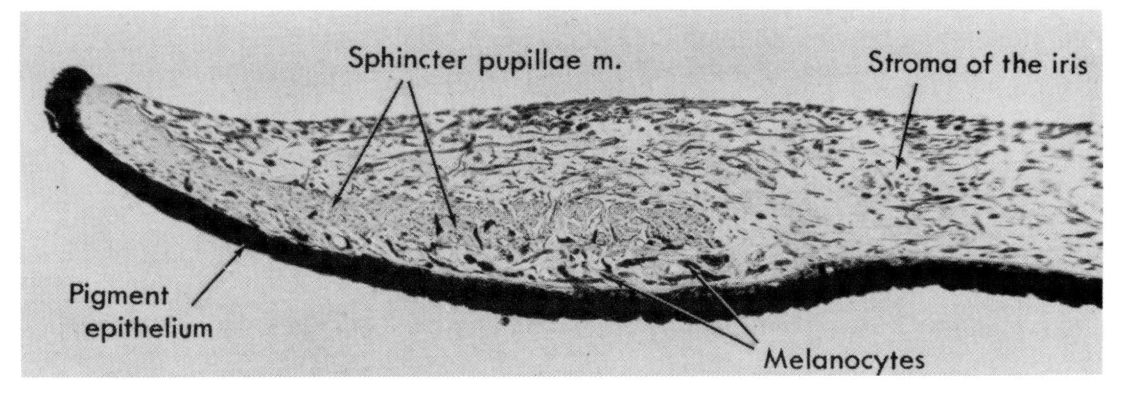

Figure 34–17. Photomicrograph of a section through the human iris. (Courtesy of T. Kuwabara.)

zone and a wider *ciliary zone*. Near the pupillary and ciliary margins, the anterior surface has many irregular excavations, the *crypts*, which may extend deep into the tissue. In addition, there are oblique, irregularly arranged contraction furrows, which are especially marked when the pupil is dilated.

The main mass of the iris consists of a loose, pigmented, highly vascular connective tissue. The anterior surface of the stroma is lined with a discontinuous layer of fibroblasts and melanocytes. A thin layer of stroma immediately beneath this cell investment, the *anterior stromal sheet* or lamella, is devoid of blood vessels. Deep to this is a layer containing numerous vessels; their walls consist of endothelium, pericytes, and an unusually thick connective tissue adventitia. The posterior surface of the iris is covered with a double layer of heavily pigmented epithelium, the iridial extension of the retina (Figs. 34–9 and 34–17).

The anterior stromal sheet or lamella contains a few collagenous fibers and many fibroblasts and melanocytes in a homogeneous ground substance. The color of the iris depends on the quantity and the arrangement of the pigment and on the thickness of the lamella. If this layer is thin and its cells contain little or no pigment, the black pigment epithelium on the posterior surface, as seen through the colorless tissue, gives the iris a blue color (Fig. 34–18). An increasing amount of pigment brings about the varying shades of gray and greenish hues. Large amounts of dark pigment cause the brown color of the iris. In albinos, the pigment is absent or scanty, and the iris is pink owing to its rich vascularity.

The epithelial pigment layer on the posterior surface of the iris is a direct continuation of the ciliary portion of the retina and, like it, originally consists of two layers of epithelium. The inner nonpigmented layer of the ciliary portion of the retina becomes heavily pigmented in the iridial region with dark brown melanin granules that obscure the cell outlines. The posterior or inner surface is covered by the *limiting membrane of the iris*, a typical basal lamina. The outer or anterior pigmented layer becomes less pigmented. These outer epithelial cells, derived from the outer wall of the embryonic optic cup, undergo a remarkable transformation into contractile elements, the *myoepithelium of the dilator pupillae*.

Being an adjustable diaphragm, the iris contains two muscles that keep the membrane stretched and hold it against the surface of the lens. The contraction of the circular *sphincter of the pupil* reduces the diameter of the pupil. It is a thin, flat ring surrounding the margin of the pupil. Its breadth changes, according to the degree of contraction of the iris, from 0.6 to 1.2 mm. Its smooth msucle fibers are arranged in thin, circumferentially oriented bundles (Fig. 34–17). The *dilator of the pupil* opens the pupil and consists of radially arranged myoepithelial elements, which form a thin membrane between the vessel layer and the pigment epithelium (Fig. 34–19).

The innervation of the two muscles is quite different. The dilator is innervated by sympathetic postganglionic neurons located in the superior cervical ganglion. Their axons pass to the trigeminal ganglion, then into the ophthalmic branch of the latter, and finally reach the dilator muscle through the long ciliary nerves. The sphincter muscle is innervated by parasympathetic fibers from postganglionic neurons located in the ciliary ganglion, and their axons reach the sphincter with the short ciliary nerves. The sympathetic and parasympathetic divisions of the automatic nervous

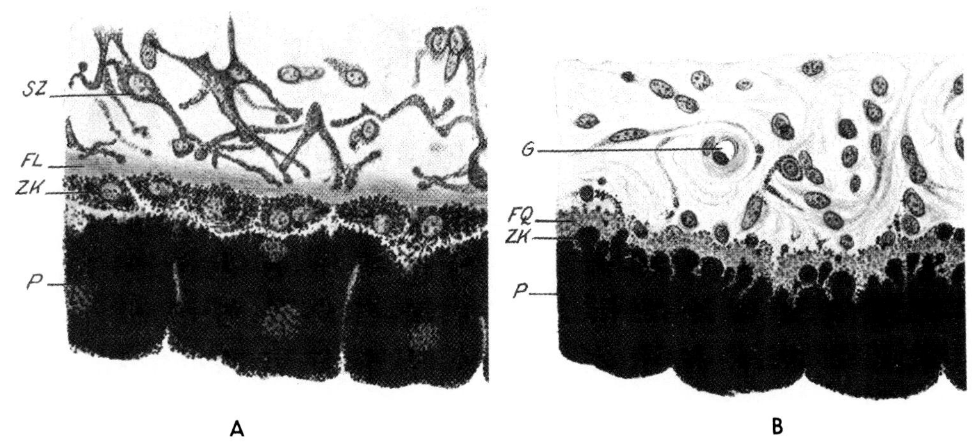

Figure 34–18. Drawing of sections of the human iris. (A) Posterior part of a radial section of a dark iris, from an enucleated eye. FL, fibrillae of the dilator muscle in longitudinal section; P, pigment epithelium of the inner layer of the iridial portion of the retina; SZ, melanocytes of the vascular layer; ZK, pigment-containing cell bodies of the dilator muscle (anterior layer of the iridial portion of the retina). (B) Section of a light human iris. FQ, fibers of the dilator muscle, in cross section; G, blood vessel of the stroma. Other symbols, as in (A). (After Schaffer, J., 1922. Lehrbuch der Histologie und Histogenese, Verlag von W. Engelmann, Leipzig.)

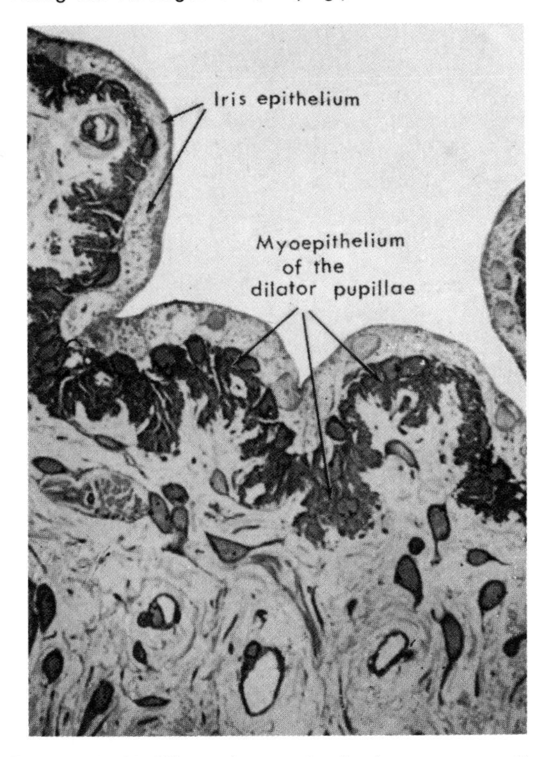

Figure 34–19. Photomicrograph of a transverse section through the posterior surface of albino rabbit iris showing the pale cuboidal iris epithelium and the underlying dark-staining myoepithelium of the dilator pupillae muscle (After Richardson, K.C. 1964. Am. J. Anat. 114:173.)

system, thus, have opposite effects on the pupil. On the other hand, the sphincter and the ciliary muscles, which are both innervated by the short ciliary nerves, work in concert. When the eye accommodates for near vision by contraction of the ciliary muscle, there is a simultaneous contraction of the pupillary sphincter.

In electron micrographs, the axons among the contractile elements of the sphincter pupillae are seen to be packed with synaptic vesicles typical of cholinergic axons. Axons associated with the dilator muscle contain a mixture of adrenergic sympathetic nerve fibers.

An accurate adjustment of the size of the pupil modifies the amount of light entering the eye, thus permitting useful vision over a wide range of light intensities. Furthermore, as the pupil constricts, in brilliant light, the depth of focus of the dioptric media is increased and aberrations are minimized.

The blood vessels of the iris in the rhesus monkey, and possibly in the human, are unusual in that their walls have the same structure irrespective of their diameter and cannot be classified according to the traditional morphological criteria for distinguishing arterioles, capillaries, and venules (Fig. 34–20). No smooth msucle is found in any of these vessels. Their wall consist of a continuous layer of endothelium on a thin basal lamina, pericytes enclosed between two layers of the basal lamina, and an adventitia of fibroblasts, melanocytes, and occasional macrophages. The intercellular clefts of the endothelium are closed by tight junctions that prevent paracellular escape of macromolecules from the blood, and plasmalemmal vesicles do not transport any significant amount of blood-borne peroxidase across the endothelium. However, if this

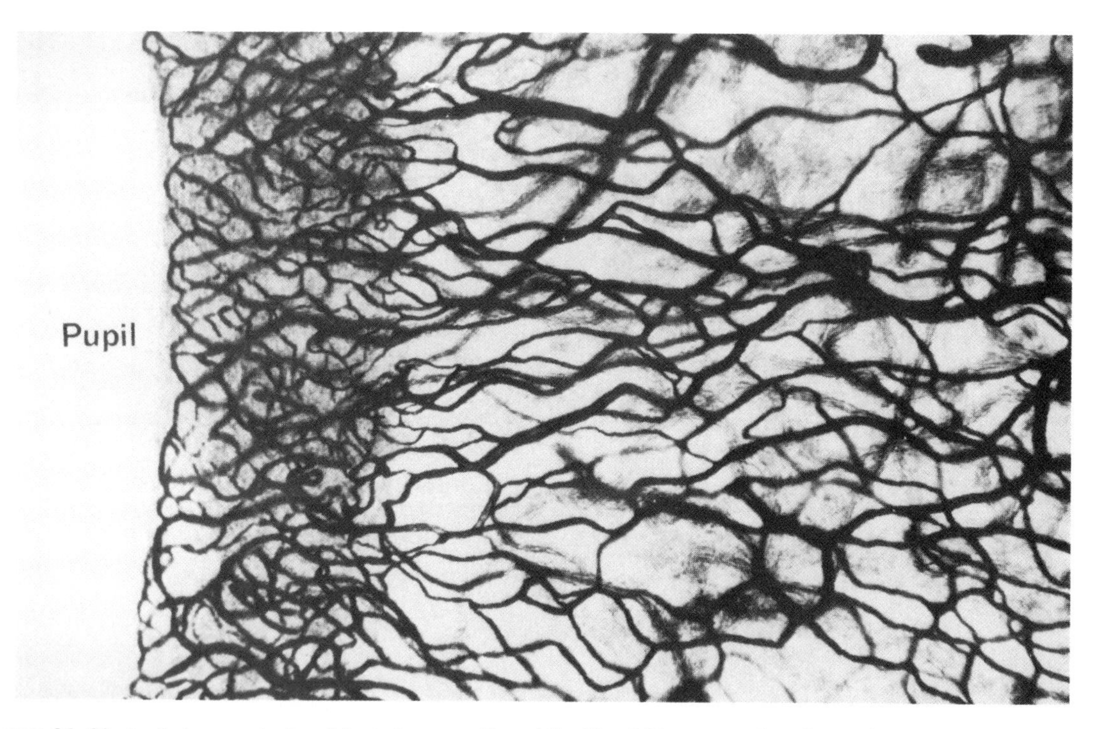

Figure 34–20. A whole mount of an injected preparation of the iris of *Macaca mulatta* in moderate mydriasis. A series of large radial vessels give rise to a complex network of intermediate and small vessels throughout the iris. A continuous arcade of small vessels is seen at the pupillary margin. (Photomicrograph from Freddo, T. and G. Raviola. 1982. Investig. Ophthalmol. Vis. Sci. 22:279.)

tracer is perfused through the anterior chamber, it freely enters the iridial stroma and reaches the lumen of the vessels by transcellular vesicular transport. The lumenal and ablumenal plasma membranes of the endothelium seem to bear a different electrical charge because anionic molecules are readily transported to the lumen, but cationic substances are excluded. It is suggested that in the iridial vessels there is a unidirectional vesicular transport that selectively moves anionic organic substances from the anterior chamber to the bloodstream. The importance of this pathway in aqueous humor dynamics has yet to be evaluated.

REFRACTIVE MEDIA OF THE EYE

The cornea and the anterior and posterior chambers of the eye have been described. The other components of the refractive apparatus of the eye are the crystalline lens and the vitreous body.

LENS

The lens is a transparent, biconvex body situated immediately behind the pupil. Its shape changes during the process of accommodation. Its outer form varies somewhat in different persons and also with age. Its diameter ranges from 7 mm in the newborn to 10 mm in the adult. Its thickness is approximately 3.7–4 mm, increasing during accommodation to 4.5 mm and more. The posterior surface is more convex than the anterior, the respective radii of curvature being 6.9 and 10 mm. The lens weighs 0.2 g and is slightly yellow.

The lens is covered with a homogeneous, highly refractile *capsule*, an 11–18 μm coating that is essentially an exceedingly thick basal lamina. It contains type-IV collagen, laminin, entactin, heparan sulfate proteoglycan, and fibronectin. Anteriorly, the capsule invests the outer surface of the layer of cuboidal cells that make up the epithelium of the lens (Figs. 34–21 and 34–22). The cells of the lens epithelium are cuboidal, with a height of 10 μm and a width of 13 μm. Their cytoplasm contains the usual complement of organelles and a cytoskeleton that is especially well developed under the cell surface. The apices of the lens epithelial cells are directed posteriorly and interface with the surface of the lens fibers. Unlike most other epithelia, the lens epithelium is essentially devoid of tight junctions; adjacent

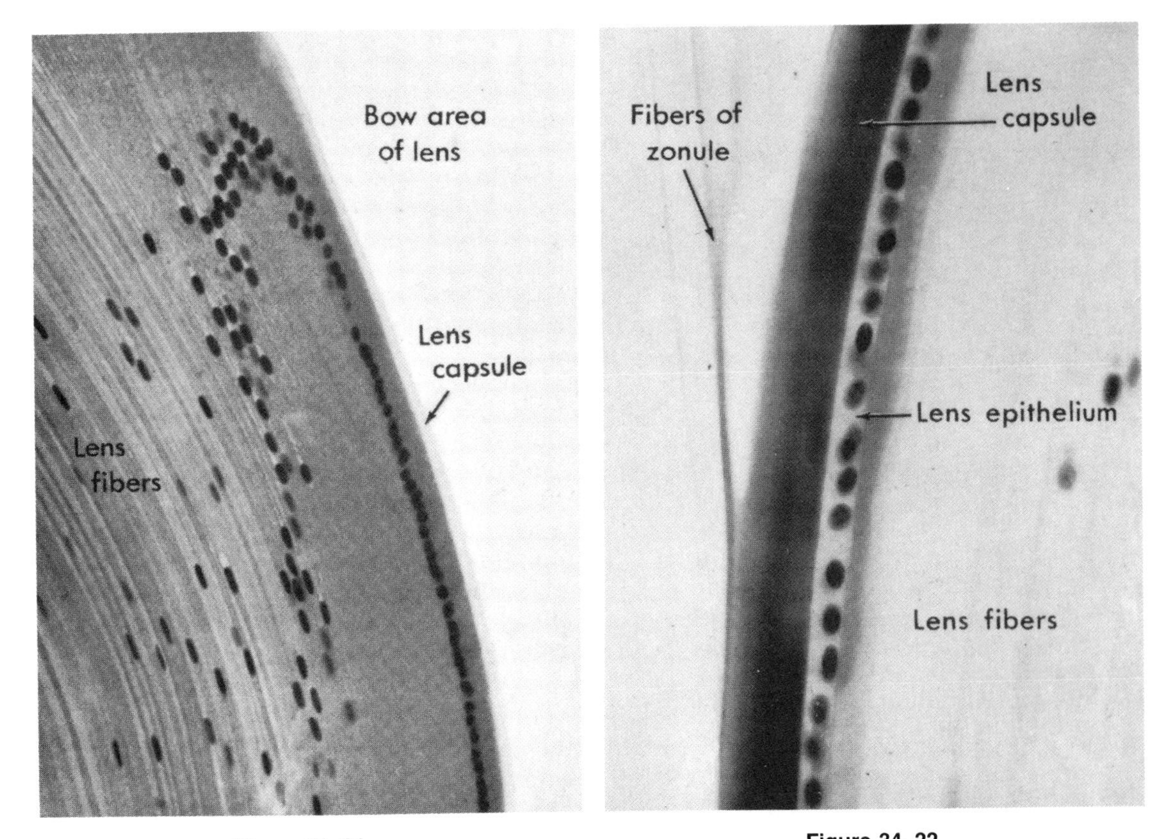

Figure 34–21

Figure 34–22

Figure 34–21. Photomicrograph of the bow area of the human lens, where the epithelial cells become greatly elongated to form lens fibers (Courtesy of T. Kuwabara.)

Figure 34–22. Higher-magnification photomicrograph of human lens stained with the periodic-acid–Schiff reaction. The lens capsule over the epithelium stains strongly for carbohydrates. Zonule fibers are shown merging with the capsule. (Courtesy of T. Kuwabara.)

cells are interconnected by desmosomes and gap junctions. Fewer gap junctions are observed between lens epithelial cells and lens fibers.

Toward the equator, the lens epithelial cells approach a columnar form and become arranged in meridional rows. Becoming progressively elongated, the cells at the equator are transformed into *lens fibers* that constitute the bulk of the substance of the lens. In this transitional, or *nuclear zone*, the cells have a characteristic arrangement.

The posterior surface of the lens is occupied by lens fibers, directly invested by the capsule. In the human lens, each lens fiber is a six-sided prism 7–10 mm long, 8–12 μm wide, and only 2 μm thick (Fig. 34–23). In the region of the nucleus, the thickness may reach 5 μm. The prismatic fibers of the cortical zone of the lens are hexagonal in cross section. The cell surfaces are about 15 nm apart and attached by numerous gap junctions. The cells of the lens epithelium and the fibers of the equatorial region both exhibit complex interdigitations of their surfaces. This is particularly marked at the "sutures," where cortical fibers from opposite sectors of the lens converge (Fig. 34–23). Because these interdigitations occur principally in the anterior curvature, periaxial zone, and equator—those regions that undergo the greatest dimensional changes—it has been suggested that their presence may be associated with changes in fiber shape in the mechanism of intracapsular accommodation.

The lens fibers have a finely granular cytoplasm, with a few small vesicles scattered through the ectoplasmic region of the cell and occasional mitochondria in the vicinity of the sutures, but, in general, the organelles and inclusions are exceedingly sparse. The principal components of the cytosol of the lens fibers

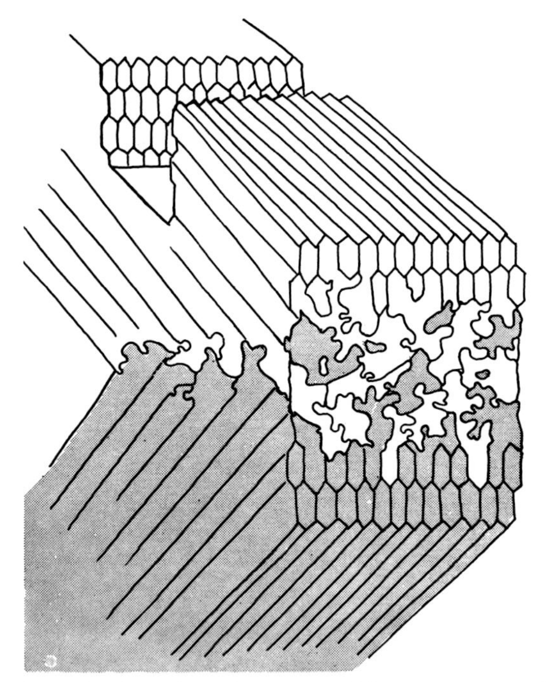

Figure 34–23. Schematic drawing of the arrangement of the lens fibers. They occur in rows and have a prevailing hexagonal cross section, except in the suture area where there may be considerable irregularity and interdigitation of the fibers converging from opposite sides of the lens. (After Wanko, T. and M. Gavin. 1961. The Structure of the Eye. New York, Academic Press.)

are proteins called *crystallins*, and a cytoskeleton mainly consisting of actin and abundant intermediate filaments of vimentin (Fig. 34–24). The protein content of the lens fibers is 60%, the highest of any cell in the body, and this confers on the lens its high refractive index. The crystallins are the most abundant and typical lens proteins; they belong to two unrelated families, the α- and the $\beta\gamma$-crystallins, which together account for 90% of the total lens proteins. Crystallins are related to proteins that have different functions in the rest of the body but are used in the lens for the sole purpose of increasing its refractive index. Faced with the task of filling the cytoplasm of lens fiber with protein, evolution has probably selected genes that encode thermodynamically stable proteins that can survive for the entire life of the individual.

The lens serves as a dioptric medium that cooperates with the cornea in focusing light rays from distant objects onto the photoreceptor layer of the retina. In addition, its power can be varied, so that the eye can also focus on nearby objects (accommodation). The lens can be optically active because it is transparent: This property is due to the fact that its fiber's microscopic fluctuations in index of refraction of the cytoplasm are minimal and there is no extracellular matrix between the fibers. In addition, the biological lens is far superior to those made by man because its spherical and chromatic aberrations are minimized by a gradual increase in the refractive index from the periphery (1.38) to the center (1.50). This gradient exists because the concentration of crystallins increases from 15% in the cortical fibers to 70% in the central ones.

The lens is held in position by a system of fibers constituting the *ciliary zonule*. The zonule fibers (Fig. 34–8) arise from the epithelium of the ciliary portion of the retina. Near the ciliary crown, they fuse into thicker fibers and finally form about 140 bundles. At the anterior margin of the ciliary processes, they leave the surface of the ciliary body and radiate toward the equator of the lens. The larger ones are straight and reach the capsule in front of the equator of the lens (*anterior zonular sheet*). The thinner fibers assume a slightly curved course and are attached to the posterior surface of the lens (*posterior zonular sheet*). All zonular fibers break up into a multitude of finer fibers, which fuse with the substance of the outermost layer of the lens capsule (Fig. 34–22). With the electron microscope, the zonular fibers appear as bundles or sheets of exceedingly fine filaments, 11–12 nm in diameter, which have a hollow appearance in cross section (Fig. 34–25). They are digested with elastase, but not by collagenase, and have an amino-acid composition different from collagen. They are identical to the microfibrils embedded in the elastic fibers of other organs. Where the vitreous body touches the lens capsule, it forms the *hyaloideocapsular ligament*.

The radii of curvature of the surfaces of the several dioptric media of the normal eye, especially of the lens and their indices of refraction, are such that light rays coming from a remote point form an inverted, and real, image of the object in the layer of the photoreceptor cones and rods of the retina. If the object is approaching, the light rays diverge more and more and the image moves backward in the retina. A change in position of an object from infinite distance to about 5 m causes the image to shift about 60 μm backward in the retina. Because this image is still within the outer segments of the rods and cones, accommodation is not needed. For nearer distances, accommodation is necessary.

In a camera, the focusing of objects that

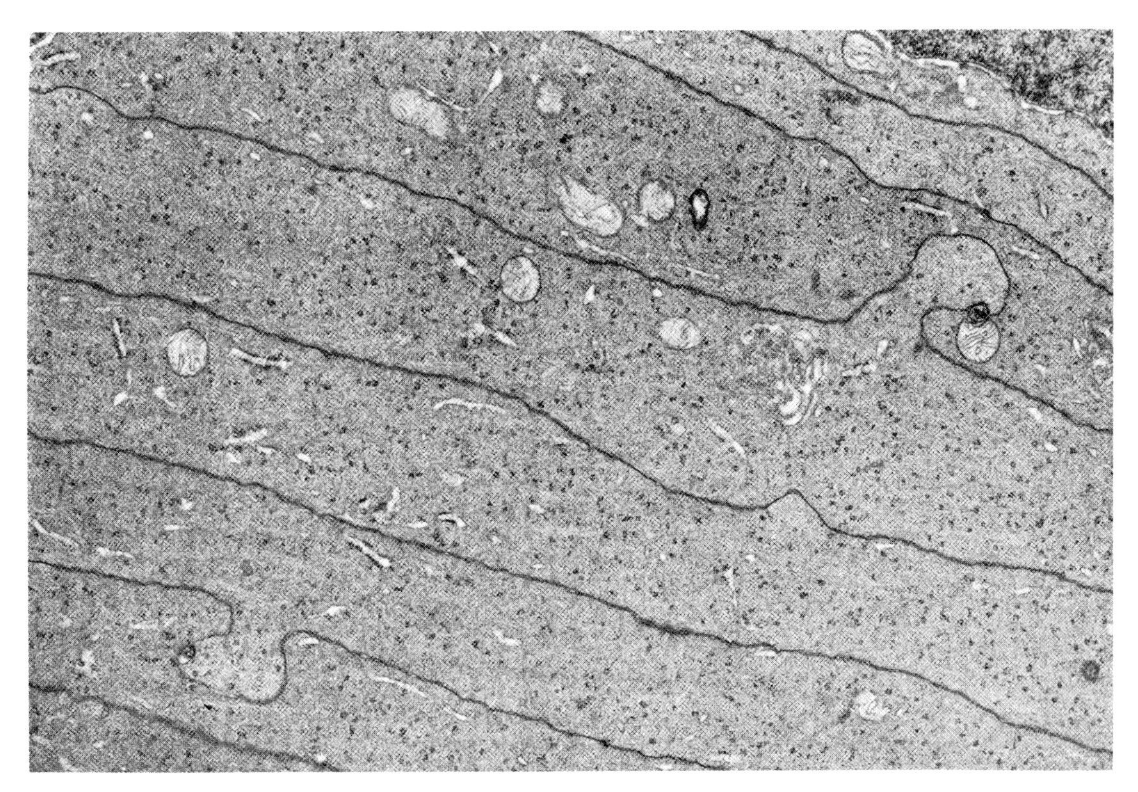

Figure 34–24. Electron micrograph of cortical fibers of the human lens. A few profiles of granular endoplasmic reticulum, occasional mitochondria, and numerous polysomes are distributed in an otherwise homogeneous cytoplasm. (Courtesy of T. Kuwabara.)

move nearer to the lens is effected by moving the ground-glass plate away from the lens. In the higher vertebrates, and in the human, the curvature of the lens is changed. When the eye is at rest, the lens is kept stretched by the ciliary zonule in the plane vertical to the optical axis. When the eye has to focus on a near object, the ciliary muscle contracts—its meridional fibers pull the choroid and the ciliary body forward, whereas its circular fibers, acting as a sphincter, move the ciliary body toward the axis of the eye. This relieves the tension on the zonule; the lens gets thicker and its surface, especially at the anterior pole, becomes more convex. This increases the refractive power of the lens and keeps the focus within the photoreceptor layer.

VITREOUS BODY

The vitreous body fills the vitreous cavity between the lens and the retina. It adheres everywhere to the optical portion of the retina, and the connection is especially firm at the ora serrata. Farther forward, it gradually recedes from the surface of the ciliary portion of the retina.

The fresh vitreous body is a colorless, structureless, gelatinous mass with a glass-like transparency. Its index of refraction is 1.334. Nearly 99% of the vitreous body consists of water. A liquid and a solid phase can be distinguished in it; the liquid phase contains hyaluronic acid in the form of long coiled molecules enclosing large amounts of water; the solid phase is collagen in the form of thin fibrils that lack the usual 64-nm periodicity and are arranged in a random network; these fibrils are heteropolymers of type-II and type-XI collagens like the fibrils of hyaline cartilage. The hyaluronate of the liquid phase is joined to the collagen network by weak bonds. The peripheral region of the vitreous body, or cortex, has more collagen fibrils and hyaluronate than the central region and contains cells, called *hyalocytes*, which may be concerned with the synthesis of collagen and hyaluronic acid. Macrophages are also occasionally found.

Extending through the vitreous body from the papilla of the optic nerve to the posterior surface of the lens is the *hyaloid canal* (canal

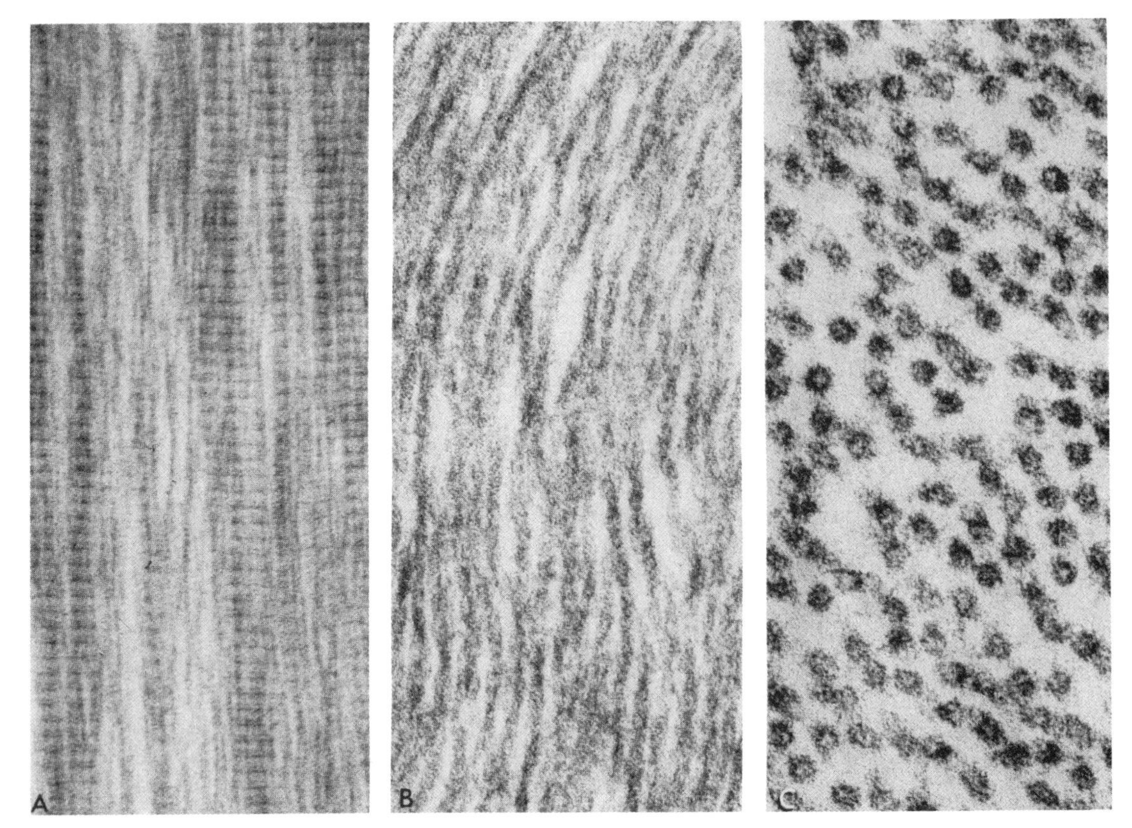

Figure 34–25. Electron micrographs of the ciliary zonule in the monkey eye. (A) and (B) High magnification of the zonular fibers which are made up of exceedingly fine fibrils, 11–12 nm in diameter. When the fibrils are tightly packed, as in (A), the zonular fibers appear cross striated. (C) In cross section, the fibrils have a hollow appearance. (From Raviola, G. 1971. Investig. Ophthalmol. 10:851.)

of Cloquet). It is a residue remaining after the resorption of the embryonic hyaloid artery. It has a diameter of 1 mm and is filled with liquid. In the living, especially in young persons, it is visible with the help of the slit-lamp microscope.

THE RETINA

The retina is the innermost of the three coats of the eyeball and is the photoreceptor organ. It arises in early embryonic development by a bilateral evagination of the prosencephalon, the *primary optic vesicle*. Later it is transformed by local invagination into the *secondary optic vesicle*. Each optic cup remains connected with the brain by a stalk, the future optic nerve. In the adult, the derivatives of the bilaminar secondary optic vesicle consist of an outer pigmented epithelial layer, the *pigment epithelium*, and an inner sheet, the *neural retina* or the *retina proper*. The latter contains elements similar to those of the brain, and it may be considered to be a specially differentiated part of the brain.

The *optical*, or functioning, portion of the retina lines the inner surface of the choroid and extends from the papilla of the optic nerve to the ora serrata anteriorly. At the papilla, where the retina is continuous with the tissue of the nerve, and at the ora serrata, the retina is firmly connected with the choroid. In the retina, exclusive of the fovea, the papilla, and the ora serrata, 10 parallel layers can be distinguished from outside inward (Figs. 34–26 and 34–27): (1) the pigment epithelium; (2) the layer of rods and cones; (3) the outer limiting membrane; (4) the outer nuclear layer; (5) the outer plexiform layer; (6) the inner nuclear layer; (7) the inner plexiform layer; (8) the layer of ganglion cells; (9) the layer of optic nerve fibers; and (10) the inner limiting membrane. About 2.5 mm lateral to the border of the optic papilla, the inner surface of the retina shows a shallow, round depression, the *fovea* (Figs. 34–26 and 34–45). This is surrounded by the *central area*,

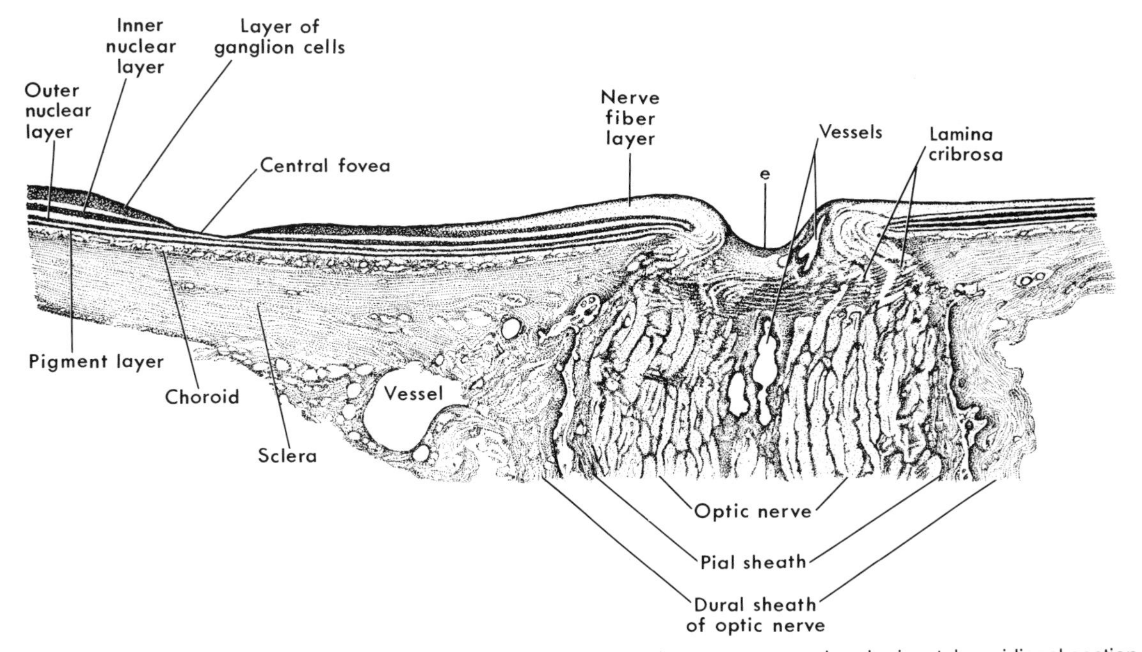

Figure 34–26. Drawing of the central fovea and entrance of the optic nerve as seen in a horizontal meridional section of an enucleated human eye. (Redrawn and slightly modified from Schaffer, U. 1922. J. Lehrbuch der Histologie und Histogenese. Verlag von W. Engelmann, Leipzig.)

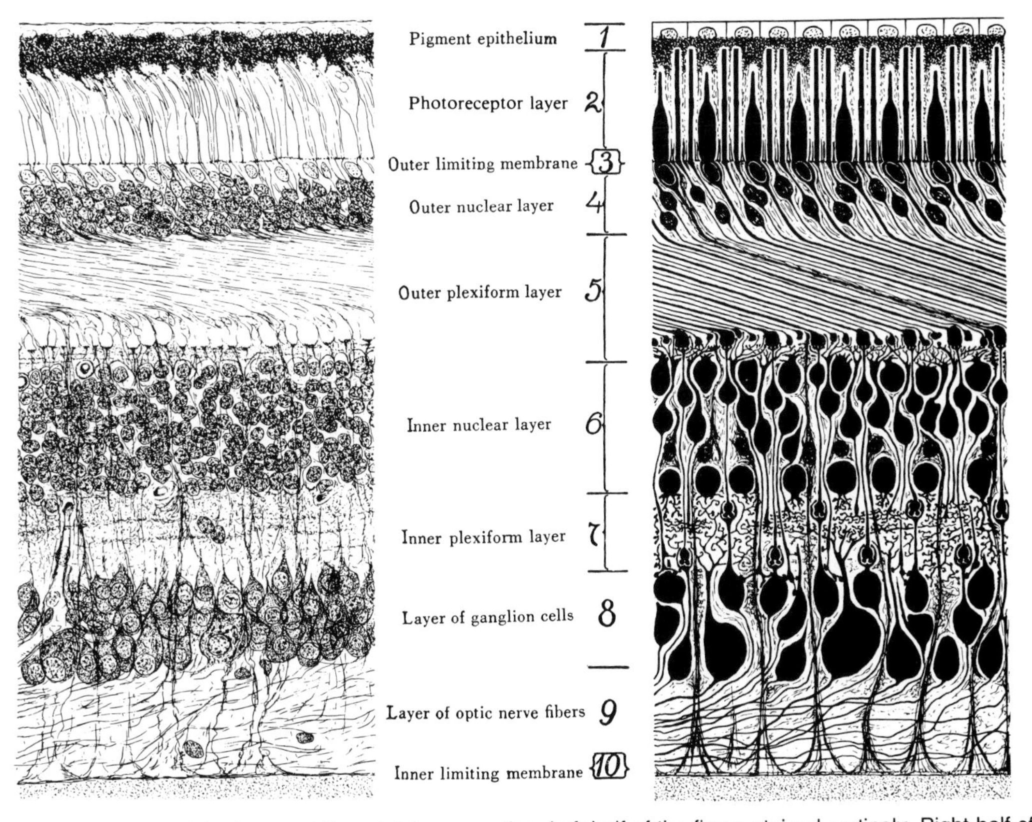

Figure 34–27. Drawing of the layers of the adult human retina. Left half of the figure stained routinely. Right half of the figure, a schematic reconstruction from sections stained with Golgi's method. (Slightly modified from Polyak, S. 1941. The Retina. University of Chicago Press, Chicago.)

distinguished by the great number of ganglion cells and by the general refinement and even distribution of the structural elements, especially of the rods and cones. The smallest and most precisely ordered sensory elements of the retina are in the fovea, where they are accumulated in greatest numbers. In the retinal periphery, the elements are fewer, larger, and less evenly distributed.

When detached from the pigment epithelium, the fresh retina is almost perfectly transparent. It has a distinctly red color because of the presence in its rod cells of *visual purple* or *rhodopsin*. Light rapidly bleaches the visual purple; in darkness, the color gradually reappears. The fovea and its immediate vicinity contain yellow pigment and are called the *macula lutea*. Large blood vessels circle above and below the central fovea, whereas only fine arteries, veins, and capillaries are present in it. In the very center of the fovea, in an area measuring 0.5 mm across, even the capillaries are absent, greatly increasing its transparency.

Only the portion of the image of an external object that falls on the fovea is seen sharply. Accordingly, the eyes are moved so as to bring the object of special attention into this central part of the visual field. Photoreceptors are absent from the optic papilla. This is the "blind spot" of the visual field.

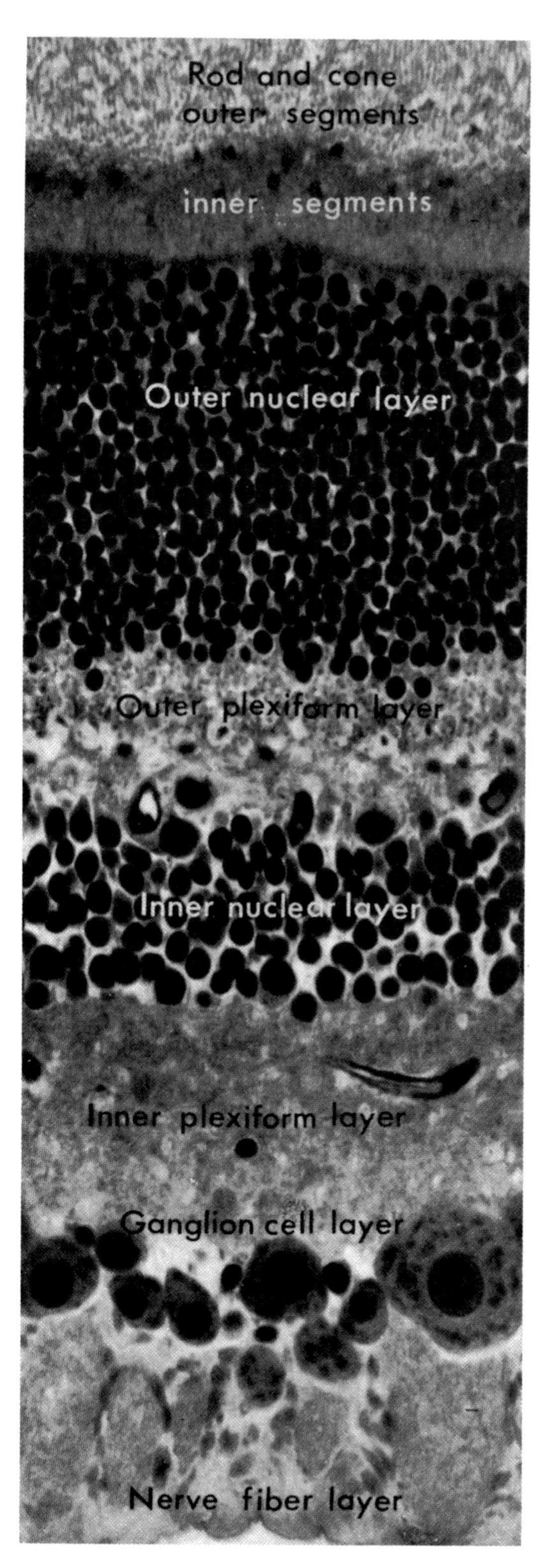

Figure 34–28. Photomicrograph of the retina of a cat's eye. (Courtesy of A.J. Ladman.)

PIGMENT EPITHELIUM

This sheet of heavily pigmented epithelial cells is derived from the outer layer of the cup-like outgrowth of the embryonic nervous system that gives rise to the retina, and it has traditionally been included as one of the layers of the retina (Figs. 34–26 and 34–29). Bruch's membrane, on the other hand, has been considered part of the choroid. The demonstration that this latter structure includes the basal lamina of the pigment epithelium makes it illogical to assign the pigment epithelium to the retina and its basal lamina to the choroid. Some authors, therefore, prefer to consider the pigment epithelium as a component of the choroid. Although the cells of this layer extend processes that interdigitate with the retinal rods and cones, there is no actual anatomical connection between the photosensitive and the pigmented layers, except at the head of the optic nerve and at the ora serrata. An artifactitious separation is found between the two layers in most histological preparations. Also, in the "retinal detachment" that

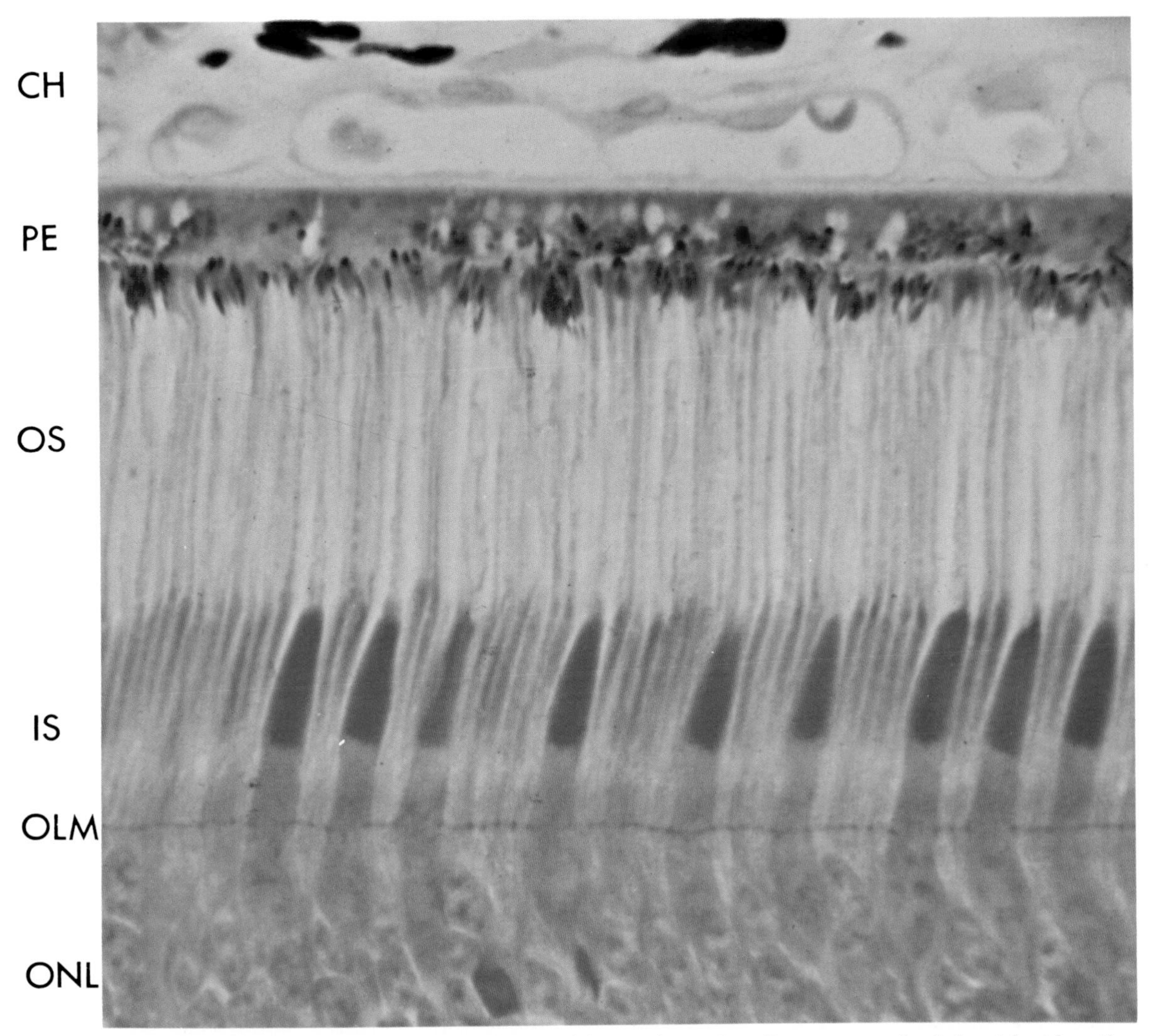

Figure 34–29. Photomicrograph of the outermost layers of the monkey retina. Cones are easily distinguished from the rods because their inner segment is larger and the ellipsoid is heavily stained. CH, choroid; PE, pigment epithelium; OS, outer segments; IS, inner segments; OLM, outer limiting membrane; ONL, outer nuclear layer. (Courtesy of J. Rostgaard.)

is a common cause of partial blindness, the separation occurs along this plane of cleavage between the photosensitive elements of the retina and the pigment epithelium.

Pigment epithelial cells have a remarkably regular shape, appearing as hexagonal prisms about 14 μm wide and 10–14 μm tall; toward the ora serrata, they increase in diameter. The cell base, which rests on Bruch's membrane, displays the labyrinth of interdigitating processes typical of actively transporting epithelia, whereas the lateral cell surface has only a slightly undulating course. Adjacent cells are connected to each other by a junctional complex consisting of apical gap junctions, followed by an elaborate tight junction and a zonula adherens. The cell apex which faces the rods and cones gives rise to two sorts of processes: cylindrical sheaths, which invest the tips of the photoreceptor outer segments, and slender microvilli, which occupy the interstices between the photoreceptors. The cell nucleus is displaced toward the cell base, and numerous mitochondria intervene between the nucleus and the basal labyrinth of interdigitating processes. The most prominent feature of the apical cytoplasm is the presence of numerous melanin granules, elliptical or rounded in shape. A second important component of the apical cytoplasm consists of residual bodies filled with lamellar debris, which represents the partially digested residue of the phagocytized tips of the rod outer segments. Another prominent feature of the cytoplasm of these cells is a highly developed agranular endoplasmic reticulum in the form of a rich network of branching and anastomosing tubules that permeate the interstices among the melanin granules and residual bodies. Cisternae of the granular endoplasmic reticulum and a supranuclear Golgi apparatus complete the list of cytoplasmic organelles.

The pigment epithelium has many important functions. The tight junctions that seal the intercellular spaces between adjoining epithelial cells protect the retina proper from undesirable metabolites that may be present in the stroma of the choroid. The pigment granules absorb light after it has traversed the photoreceptor layer, thus preventing its reflection from the external ocular tunics. In retinas of lower vertebrates, it has been shown that the pigment granules migrate along cell processes among the photoreceptors on illumination, thus effectively screening scattered light, and they return to the cell body in the dark.

The pigment epithelium participates in the continuous renewal of the underlying photoreceptors. This activity will become clearer after reading the following section on the structure of the rod cells. It will suffice here to say that membranous discs are continuously being exfoliated from the tips of the outer segment of the rods, which are surrounded by processes of the pigment epithelium. Thousands of these discs are phagocytized by the pigment epithelium every day. Although phagocytosis by macrophages has been extensively studied, phagocytosis by epithelial cells is rare. Macrophages bind and ingest damaged cells, bacteria, and other particulates whose surface is coated with antibody or complement. Studies on the pigment epithelial cells, grown in culture and exposed to fragments of rod outer segments, erythrocytes, or bacteria, have shown that they ingest 900 times more rod outer segment fragments than they do erythrocytes. Thus, phagocytosis by these cells has been shown to be a highly specific process.

Regeneration of rhodospin after exposure to light occurs only if photoreceptors maintain an intimate relationship with the pigment epithelium. In fact, the pigment epithelium participates in the visual cycle by reducing *all-trans-retinal*, a product of the degradation of the photoreceptor pigments by light, to *all-trans-retinol*, (vitamin A), followed by isomerization of the vitamin and finally by regeneration of *11-cis-retinal*, which is the chromophore of the visual pigment. During the visual cycle, the vitamin-A derivatives move to the pigment epithelium in the course of light adaptation and return to the photoreceptors during dark adaptation. Because vitamin-A derivatives are fat-soluble hydrocarbons, they can pass from cell to cell when bound to a special transport protein. In the pigment epithelial cells, they may be stored in the membranes of the agranular endoplasmic reticulum.

The retina proper contains six types of neurons: (1) *photoreceptor cells*, (2) *horizontal cells*, (3) *bipolar cells*, (4) *amacrine cells*, (5) *interplexiform cells*, and (6) *ganglion cells*. Photoreceptor, horizontal, and bipolar cells synapse with each other in the *outer plexiform layer*; bipolar, amacrine, and ganglion cells synapse with each other in the *inner plexiform layer*. Interplexiform cells provide a centrifugal pathway for transfer of signals from the inner to the outer plexiform layer. The axons of the ganglion cells leave the retina to become fibers of the optic nerve. The retinal neurons are supported by neuroglial elements called *radial cells of Müller*.

PHOTORECEPTORS

There are two kinds of photoreceptor cells, the *rod cells* and the *cone cells*. Their outer segments are the parts sensitive to light, and the light rays, before reaching them, must first penetrate most of the retina. The rods mediate vision in dim light but are incapable of signaling in bright light. Daylight vision is mediated by the cones, which also sense colors. At the ends of the rods and cones farthest from the lens is the cell region which absorbs light and generates signals. At the proximal end of the cell is a synaptic ending that relays the signals to other neurons in the retina by releasing a chemical neurotransmitter. The outer segment of the rods presents to the light a very large area of photosensitive membrane containing the reddish pigment *rhodopsin*. The rods are exquisitely sensitive, being able to produce a detectable signal on absorption of a single photon of light. The cones are of three kinds, each containing a pigment that absorbs strongly in short-, medium-, or long-wavelength regions of the visible spectrum. The differences in absorption of the three cone pigments provide the basis for color vision.

Rod Cells

The rods are long, slender, highly specialized cells closely packed in parallel array and oriented with their outer portions perpendicular to the layers of the retina (Figs 34–26 and 34–29). The straight, outer, cylindrical region of the cell, or rod proper, extends from the pigment epithelium to the so-called *outer limiting membrane*. Beneath this, the rod proper continues into a thin process, the *outer fiber* which expands into the cell body to accommodate the nucleus. From the cell body, the *inner fiber*, a slender process 1 μm or less in diameter, extends through the outer nuclear layer and into the *outer plexiform layer* where it terminates in a pear-shaped *rod spherule* which is the site of synaptic contact of the rod inner fiber with the processes of *bipolar* and *horizontal cells* (Figs. 34–39 and 34–41).

The cylindrical outer portion of the rod cell consists of an *outer segment* connected to an *inner segment* by a slender stalk. In the fresh condition, the outer segment appears homogeneous and highly refractile under the microscope and is birefringent in polarized light. The structure of the rod cells has been greatly clarified by electron microscopy. In longitudinal section, the outer segment is seen to be composed of hundreds of parallel lamellae oriented transverse to its long axis (Figs. 34–32A and 34–33). Each lamella is, in fact, an invagination of the plasmalemma that became separated from the cell surface and was, thus, transformed into a flat disc, approximately 2 μm in diameter and 14 nm thick. In section, each disc appears as a pair of parallel membranes separated by a space 8 nm wide which is closed at both ends. The membranes of these flat sacs contain the visual pigment *rhodospin* which can be seen as intramembranous particles in freeze–fracture preparations (Fig. 34–34). The rhodospin molecules react to light by undergoing a conformational change that results in generation of a signal that propagates along the cell to the spherules, where it causes release of neurotransmitter at the synapse.

The outer segment of the rod is joined to the inner segment by a slender stalk which contains nine longitudinally oriented doublet microtubules that arise from a basal body in the distal end of the inner segment (Fig. 34–32A). Thus, in transverse section, the stalk has the appearance of a defective cilium possessing the nine peripheral doublets but lacking the central pair of microtubules. Studies on the development of the photoreceptors in the embryo have shown that the outer segments of the rods and cones do, in fact, arise by modification of a cilium.

The outer portion of the inner segment is commonly called the *ellipsoid* and its inner portion, the *myoid*. The ellipsoid contains the basal body of the cilium, an adjacent centriole, and a large number of mitochondria. A few cross-striated rootlets, originating from the basal body, extend inward among the mitochondria. The myoid contains the Golgi complex, cisternae of granular and agranular reticulum, free ribosomes, and numerous microtubules.

In the cell body, the rod nucleus is smaller than that of the cones and its chromatin is more condensed. Rod nuclei make up the majority of the nuclei in the outer nuclear layer of the retina in all regions except in the fovea, where rods are few, and in its center, where they are absent. In the outer plexiform layer, the rod inner fibers, rich in microtubules, assume a slanting-to-horizontal course in the central region of the retina (Fig. 34–42), but they are vertical in more peripheral regions. The rods also show some regional variation in their dimensions. The thickness of their inner segments in the central area is 1.8–2.0 μm gradually increasing to 2.5 or 3.0 μm near the ora serrata. Their length decreases from approximately 60 μm, near the fovea, to 40 μm in the far periphery. Their highest density is 170,000 rods/mm^2 and their total number, in the human retina, is approximately 92 million. Nocturnal species of mammals have large numbers of rods and relatively few cones. Species active in the daytime have retinas especially rich in cones.

The outer segments of the rods extend into deep recesses in the overlying pigment epithelium. As previously stated, their tips are continually being exfoliated and phagocytized by the cells of the pigment epithelium. The length of the rods is maintained by protein synthesis in the endoplasmic reticulum and Golgi of the myoid region and the assembly of new discs at the inner end of the outer segment (Fig. 34–35). The newly formed discs are slowly displaced toward the tip of the rod as additional discs are formed behind them. Complete renewal of the rod outer segment, in the rat, takes about 10 days.

Cone Cells

These neural cells are made up of essentially the same parts as the rod cells, but they

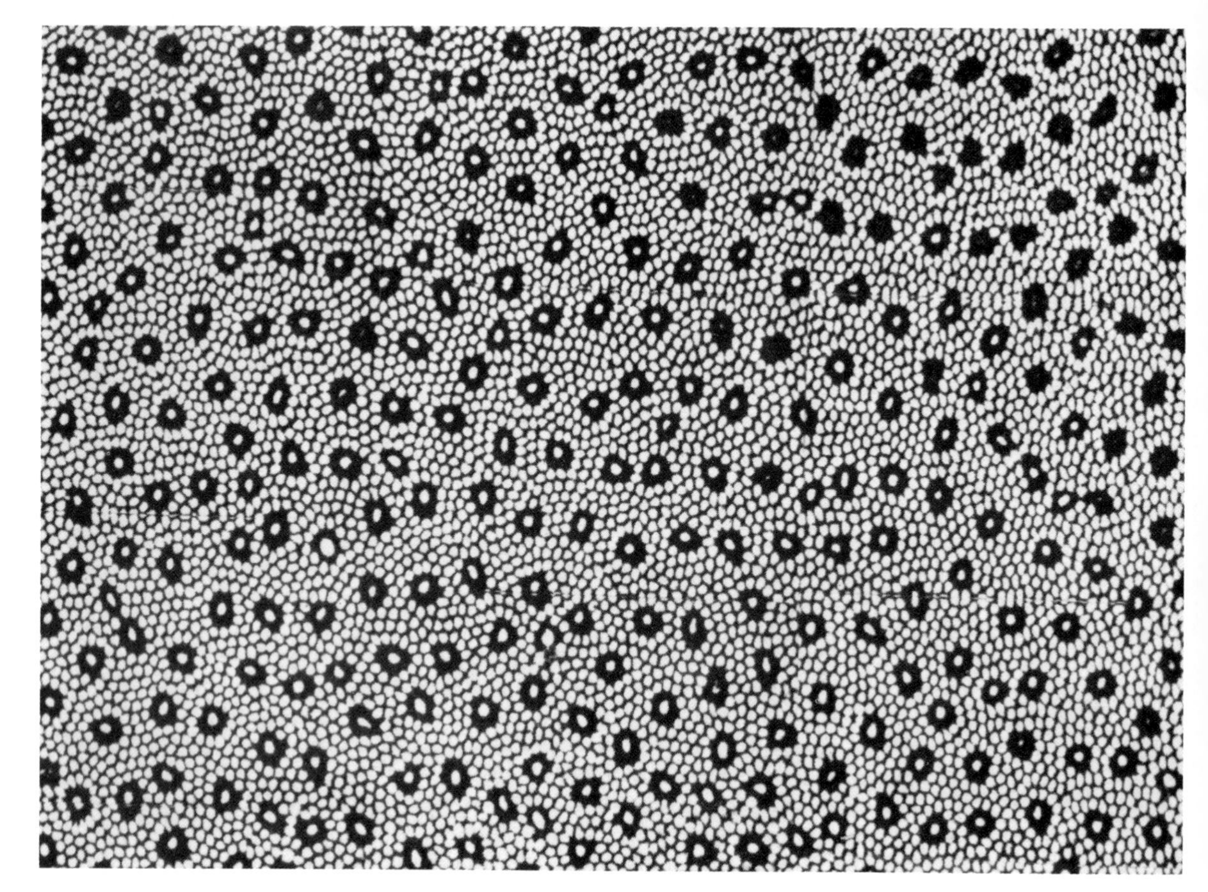

Figure 34–30. Negative image of a light micrograph of a cross-section through the outer segments of the photoreceptor cells in the periphery of the monkey retina. The large diameter of the cone inner segments keeps the rods at a distance from the cone outer segments. (Courtesy of E. Raviola).

differ in certain details (Figs. 34–29, 34–31, and 34–32). There is no visual purple in the cones, but instead, there are pigments sensitive to blue, green, and red light. Instead of a slender cylinder, the outer segment of the cone is a long conical structure, considerably wider than a rod, at its base, and tapering down to a blunt rounded tip. As in the rod, the outer segment is made up of a large number of discs stacked one above the other, but in contrast to rods, the membranes of the discs retain their continuity with the plasma membrane so that their narrow cleft is open to the extracellular space (Fig. 34–30B). In primate foveal cones, however, the outer segments have the same disc structure as in rods.

The cone outer segment is also connected to the inner segment by an eccentrically placed modified cilium, arising from a basal body set in the distal end of the inner segment. The other member of the diplosome is usually oriented at a right angle to the basal body, and striated rootlets extend downward among the longitudinally oriented mitochondria that crowd the ellipsoid. Cone inner segments are very similar in their fine structure to those of the rod cells (Figs. 34–36 and 34–37).

The cones vary considerably in different regions of the retina. In the central fovea, they measure 75 μm or more in length and their inner segment is 1.6–2.2 μm in diameter. Their length gradually decreases to 45 μm at the periphery. The relative length of the outer and the inner segment is usually 3 : 4. In the fovea, the two segments are approximately the same length.

In contrast to rods, the turnover of cone outer segments does not involve continuous movement of the discs toward the pigment epithelium because proteins synthesized in the inner segment are inserted randomly into the disc membranes throughout the outer segment. As in rods, however, cone outer segments grow in length and their tips are shed

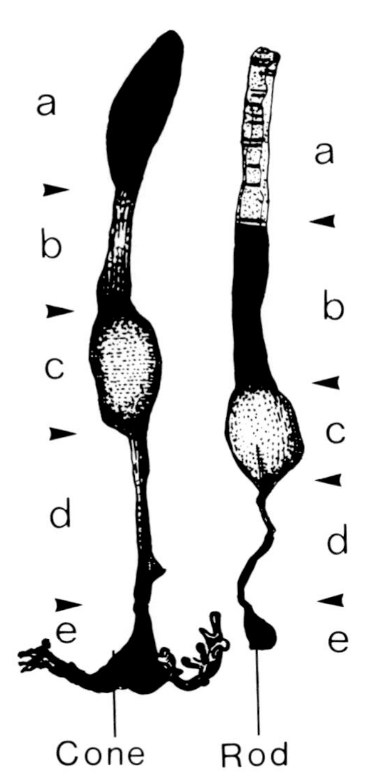

Figure 34–31. A cone cell and rod cell from a rabbit retina, stained with the Golgi technique and drawn with a camera lucida. (a) outer segment, (b) inner segment, (c) cell body, (d) inner fiber, (e) synaptic ending (pedicle in the cone, spherule in the rod). (Courtesy of G. Sacchi and E. Raviola.)

and phagocytized by the pigment epithelial cells.

Proximal to the outer limiting membrane, the inner cone segment merges with its body containing a nucleus, which is larger and paler staining than the rod nucleus. The bodies and nuclei of the cones, in contrast to those of the rods, are arranged in a single row immediately beneath the outer limiting membrane. Exceptional in this regard are the cones of the outer fovea, whose nuclei are accumulated in several rows. Only in this region do the cones have an *outer fiber*. But, from the body of all cones, a stout, smooth *inner fiber* descends to the middle zone of the outer plexiform layer, where it terminates with a thick triangular or club-shaped synaptic ending, the *cone pedicle*. Up to a dozen short, barb-like processes emanate from the base of each pedicle, except in the fovea, where there are usually none. These outgrowths are deployed horizontally in the outer plexiform layer. The length and course of the inner cone fibers may vary considerably, depending on the region, the longest (600 μm) and most nearly horizontal, being those in the central area, where the inner rod and cone fibers form a thick fiber layer at the boundary between the outer nuclear and outer plexiform layers, called the *outer fiber layer of Henle*. The inner cone fibers have all the characteristics of an axon, whereas the cone pedicle has those of a synaptic ending of a neuron and makes synapses with bipolar and horizontal cells.

The number of cones in the human retina is estimated at 4 to 5 million. Attempts at identifying the different chromatic types of cones have been only partially successful. Human cone pigments absorb photons in three regions of the light spectrum: 419 nm (blue), and 531 nm (green), and 558 nm (red). Blue cones have been identified in primates by labeling with monoclonal antibodies to blue opsin; they represent 10% of the total cone population and they are absent in the most central region of the fovea. The discrimination of red from green cones has not yet been possible because their opsin sequences are very similar. Recent psychophysical studies indicate that red cones outnumber the green ones 2 : 1.

The relative number and distribution of the rods and cones in different vertebrates present great variations, depending on their mode of life. In diurnal birds, the cones are more numerous than the rods. In most diurnal reptiles, rods are exceedingly rare. In many nocturnal vertebrates, only rods are present, although in others, a few rudimentary cones can be found among numerous rods. On similar comparative data, M. Schultze (1866) based his assumptions that there was a difference in function of the two kinds of photoreceptors.

OUTER LIMITING MEMBRANE

The dense-staining line, traditionally called the *outer limiting membrane*, is not a membrane at all. Instead, it is found, in electron micrographs, to be a row of zonulae adherentes where the photoreceptor cells are attached to the Müller cells which surround and support all of the neural elements (Fig. 34–38). Distal to this row of junctions, tufts of microvilli project from the free surface of the Muller cells into the interstices between the rod and cone inner segments.

HORIZONTAL CELLS

These cells are typical neurons whose bodies form the uppermost one or two rows of the inner nuclear layer. From the scleral end

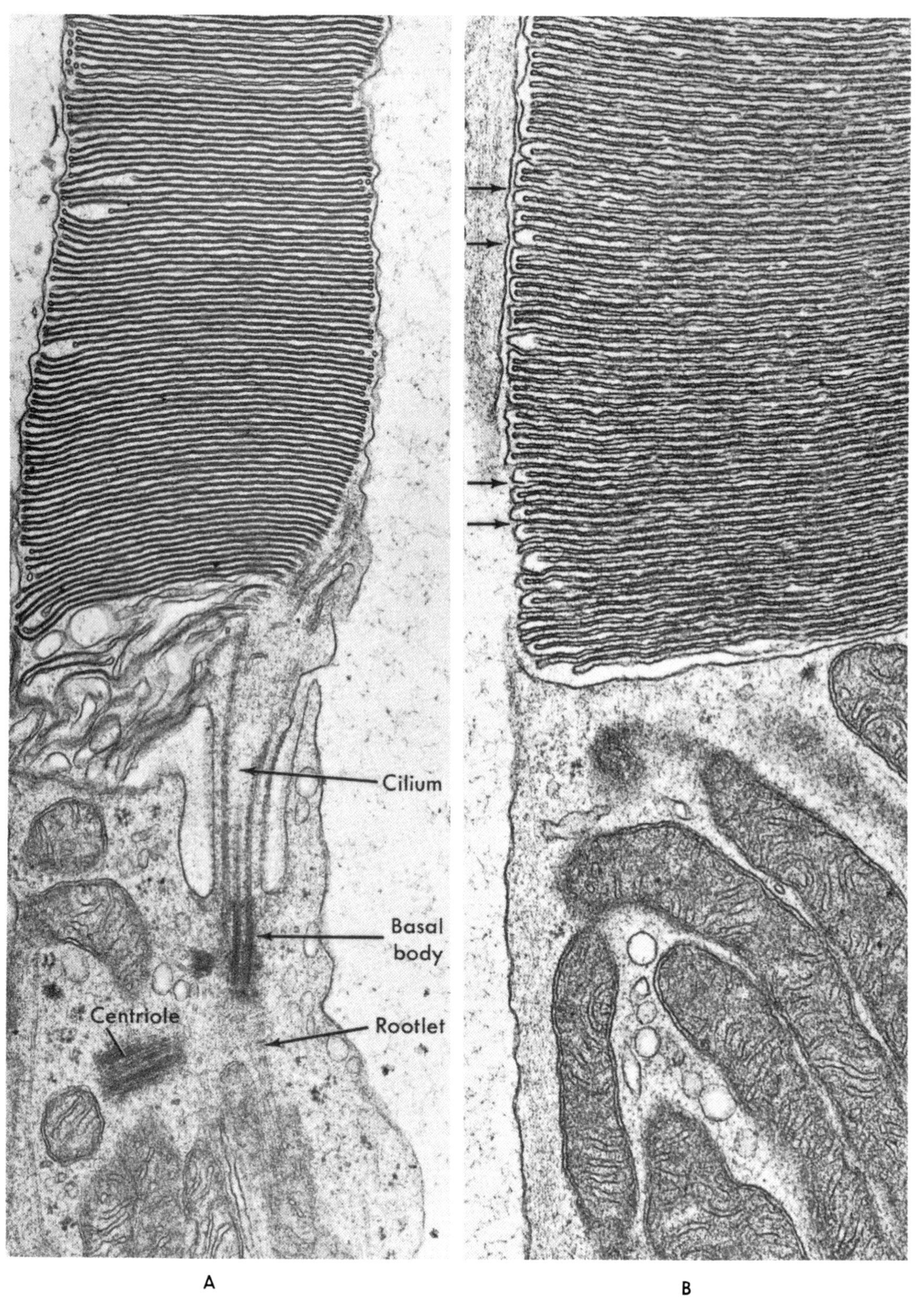

Figure 34–32. (A) Electron micrograph of a portion of the outer and inner segment of a rod, showing the connection of the two by a modified cilium. (B) Corresponding region of a cone. Note that some of the discs of the latter are open to the extracellular space (arrows). (Courtesy of T. Kuwabara.)

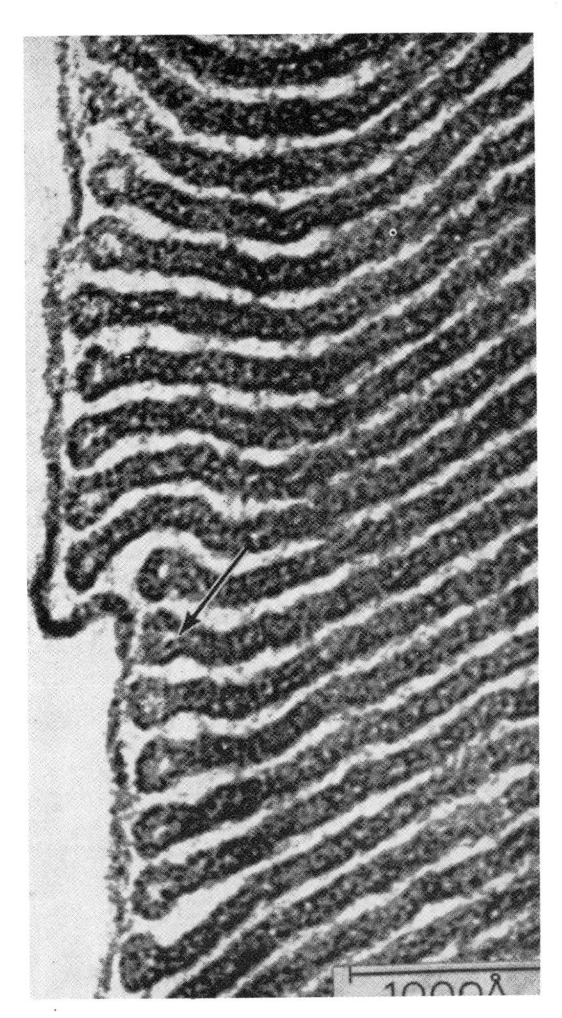

Figure 34–33. High-magnification electron micrograph showing profiles of the membranous discs of the outer segment of a rod cell from frog retina. They show a compact granular fine structure. (Courtesy of H. Fernandez-Moran.)

of the body, arise short dendritic twigs, which form several tufts deployed in the outer plexiform layer. Each dendritic tuft is connected to a single cone pedicle. According to the destination of their axon, two kinds of horizontal cells are distinguished in the human retina: H-I horizontal cells have an axon that takes a horizontal course in the outer plexiform layer and its terminal twigs come into contact with rod spherules. In H-II horizontal cells, the axon is connected to cones. In mammals, such as the cat and rabbit, the horizontal cells that are homologous to human HII cells do not have an axon (Fig. 34–39).

BIPOLAR CELLS

These neurons extend from the outer to the inner plexiform layer and, therefore, stand approximately upright with respect to the retinal layers (Figs. 34–39 and 34–40). Their body is located in the inner nuclear layer and gives rise to one or more primary dendrites, which ascend to the outer plexiform layer, where they branch and connect with the photoreceptor cell terminals. The single, inwardly directed axon of the bipolar cells ramifies in the inner plexiform layer, where it is synaptically related to ganglion and amacrine cells. Many types of bipolar cells have been described in the primate retina: *rod bipolar cells* are exclusively connected to rods, whereas *cone bipolar cells* are connected to cones. There is only one type of rod bipolar that forms *invaginating synapses* (see below) with rod spherules. Cone bipolars are divided into *midget cone bipolars* which contact a single red

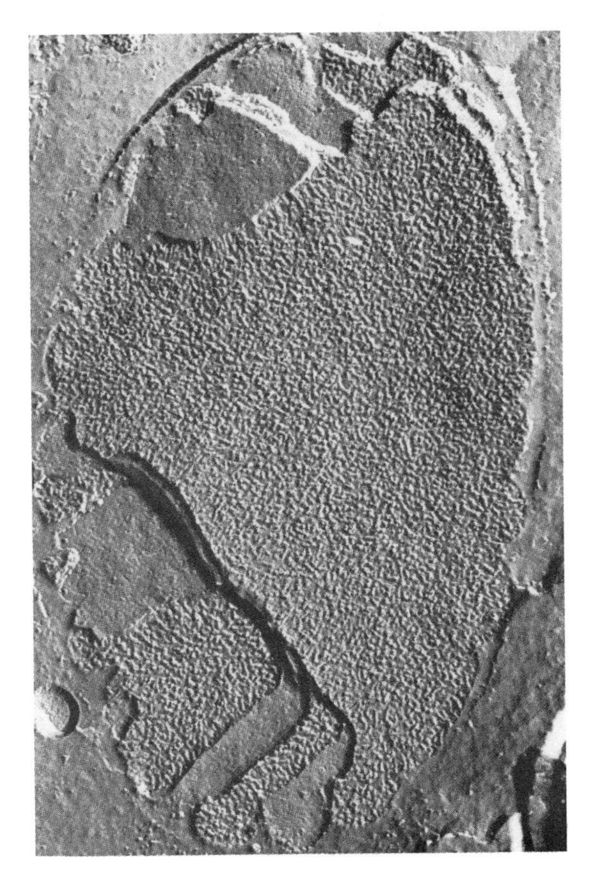

Figure 34–34. Freeze–fracture appearance of a disc from a rod outer segment. The membranes contain a large number of particles, which are probably rhodopsin. (Courtesy of E. Raviola.)

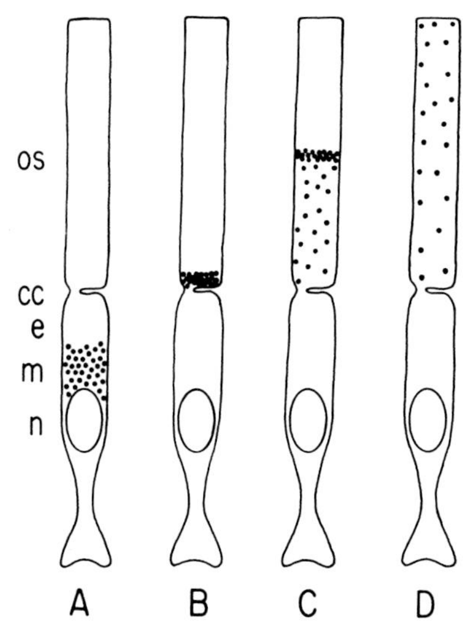

Figure 34–35. Diagram illustrating the turnover of rod outer segments. After injection of radioactive amino acid, the label is first concentrated in the myoid of the rod cells, where the ribosomes and Golgi are present (A); later, labeled protein moves to the membranous discs at the base of the outer segment (B); and ascends progressively toward the tip of the rods (C); finally, it disappears from the rods (D), but can be found in residual bodies of the pigment epithelial cells (not shown). (From Young, R.W. and D. Bok, 1969. J. Cell Biol. 42:392.)

or green cone; *blue cone bipolars* that contact one to three blue cones; and *diffuse cone bipolars* which contact six to seven cones without showing any spectral preference. Both midget and diffuse bipolars are, in turn, subdivided into *flat* and *invaginating* varieties according to the type of synapses made with cone pedicles (see below).

OUTER PLEXIFORM LAYER

This is the region of synaptic interplay between photoreceptor, bipolar, and horizontal cells. The synaptic terminals of cone cells, or pedicles, are large pyramidal endings containing synaptic vesicles and mitochondria. Their flattened base is invaginated at many points to enclose the tips of the dendrites of the horizontal and invaginating bipolar cells (midget and diffuse). The remaining free surface of the base of the pedicle makes hundreds of superficial or basal contacts with the dendrites of the flat midget and flat diffuse cone bipolars. With a high degree of consistency and geometric order, each of the 12–25 synaptic invaginations of a cone pedicle contains the tip of two horizontal cell dendrites and one dendrite of an invaginating bipolar cell (a *triad*). The horizontal cell dendrites may contain synaptic vesicles, are deeply inserted, and lie on either side of a wedge-shaped projection of the pedicle called the *synaptic ridge*. The dendrite of the invaginating bipolar cell lies centrally and more superficially, separated from the apex of the ridge by the cleft intervening between adjoining horizontal cell dendrites. The synaptic ridge is bisected by a dense lamella, or synaptic ribbon, surrounded by a halo of synaptic vesicles; the ribbon sits at a right angle to the apex of the ridge, separated from the pedicle membrane by a trough-shaped body, the arciform density (Fig. 34–41B). The significance of the synaptic ribbon is poorly understood, but it is probably instrumental in capturing synaptic vesicles and positioning them near the plasma membrane. The superficial, or basal contacts, of cone pedicles do not display prominent junctional specializations; the synaptic cleft is slightly enlarged and the adjoining membranes of the pedicle and bipolar dendrites bear a layer of fluffy cytoplasmic material.

Rod spherules have a single synaptic invagination and no basal contacts. In their invaginated synapse, two deeply inserted axonal ending of H-I horizontal cells lie on either side of a ridge containing a ribbon and vesicles (Fig. 34–41A) The tips of one to four dendrites belonging to the rod bipolar cells lie centrally and less deeply inserted. The axonal endings of the horizontal cells often contain synaptic vesicles.

Using Golgi's chromo-argentic impregnation and electron microscopy, the neural interconnections in the outer plexiform layer of the primate retina have been worked out in great detail. Both invaginating and flat midget bipolars are "private" cone bipolars; that is, each of them is contacted by a single cone pedicle. The invaginating variety, however, sends its dendrites to the invaginating synapses, whereas the flat variety makes basal contacts with the cone pedicles. The diffuse cone bipolars, on the other hand, touch about six cone pedicles at invaginating or superficial contacts. The rod bipolar cells connect exclusively with rod cells; their dendritic terminals end as slightly inserted processes in the invaginations of numerous spherules. HI horizontal cells contact cone cells with their dendrites and rod cells with their axon; both dendritic and axonal terminals of these cells end as deeply inserted processes in the invaginating synapses (Fig. 34–42). Primate HII horizontal

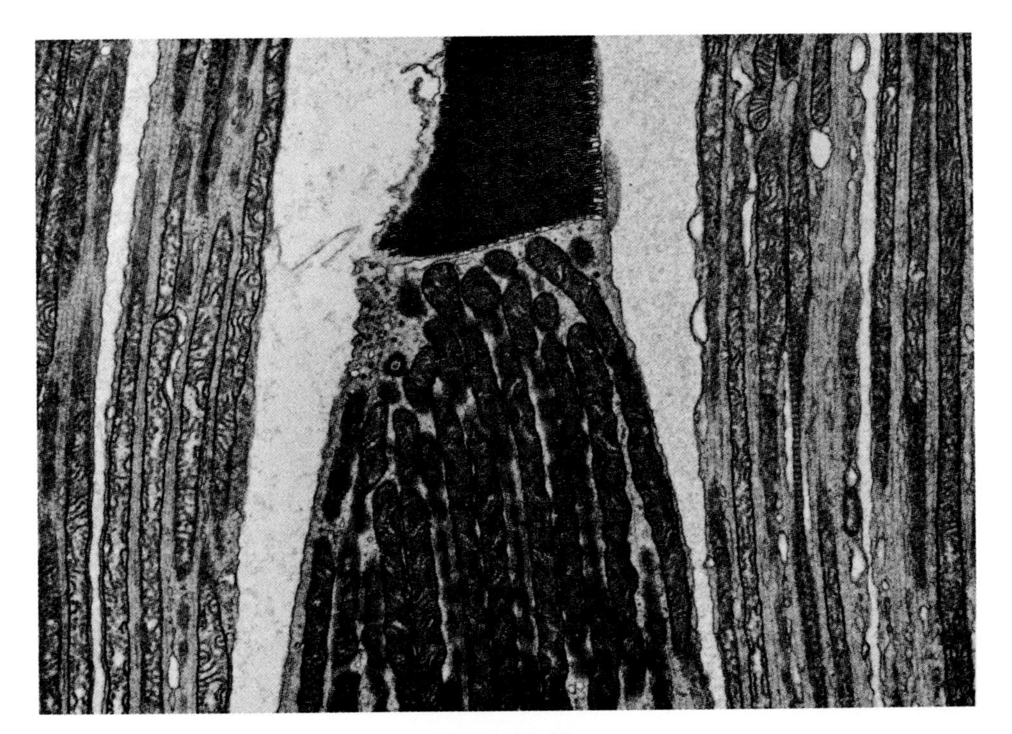

Figure 34–36

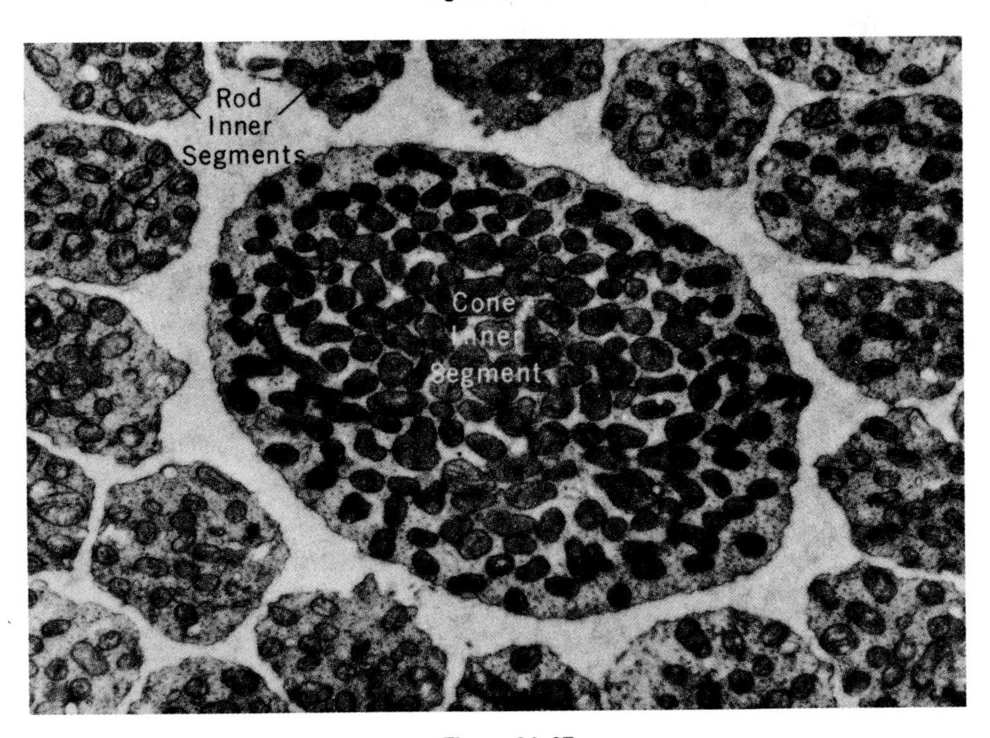

Figure 34–37

Figure 34–36. Vertical section of the inner segments of a cone and several adjacent rods in the human retina showing the larger size of the cone and the high concentration of longitudinally oriented mitochondria in the ellipsoid. (Micrograph courtesy of T. Kuwabara.)

Figure 34–37. Horizontal section through the inner segments of a cone and several rods in the rat retina. (After Marchesi, V.T., M.L. Sears, and R.J. Barnett. 1964. Investig. Ophthalmol. 3:1.)

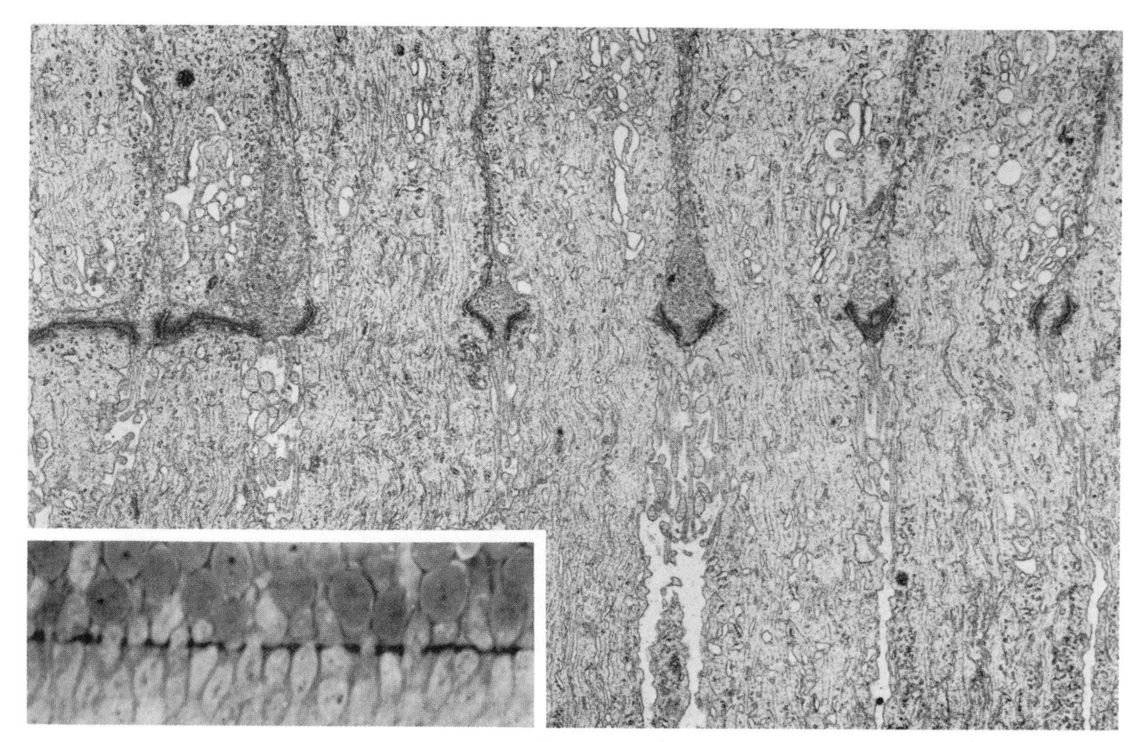

Figure 34–38. Electron micrograph of the region of the "outer limiting membrane" of the retina showing that it is not a membrane, as it appears to be with the light microscope (inset), but a row of zonulae adherentes between the rod and cone cells and the surrounding Muller cells (Micrograph courtesy of T. Kuwabara.)

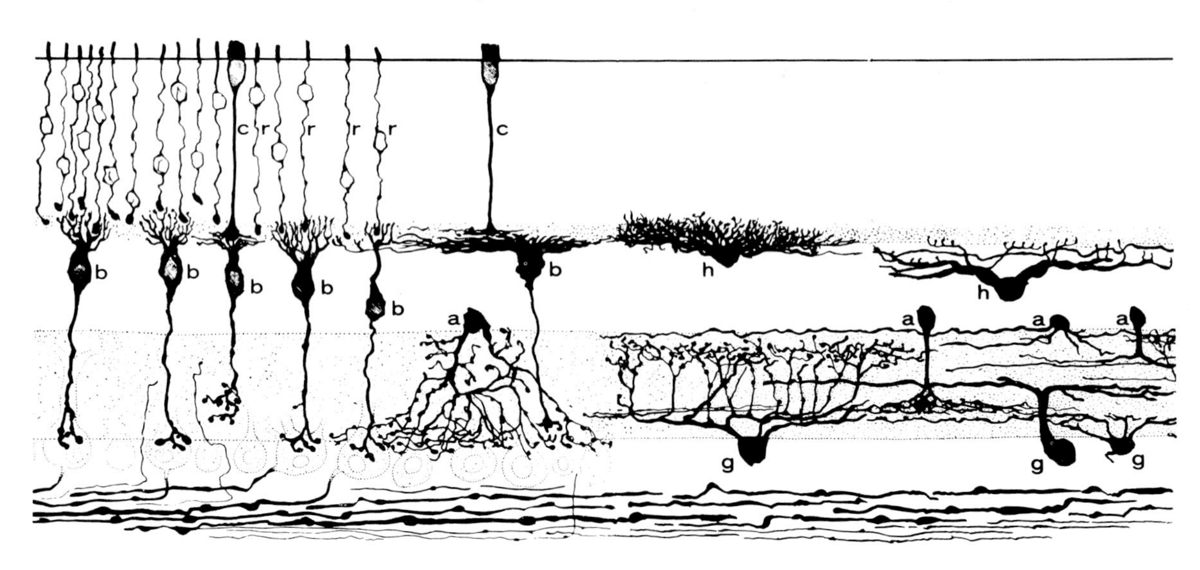

Figure 34–39. Neuronal types in the retina of mammals as they appear with the light microscope after Golgi chromargentic impregnation. (r) Rod cells (dog); (c) cone cells (dog); (b) bipolar cells (dog); (h) horizontal cells (dog); (a) amacrine cells (dog and ox); (g) ganglion cells (ox). In rod and cone cells, the photoreceptor proper is not represented. (Modified, after Cajal, R., 1893, Manual de Histologie Normal, Madrid.)

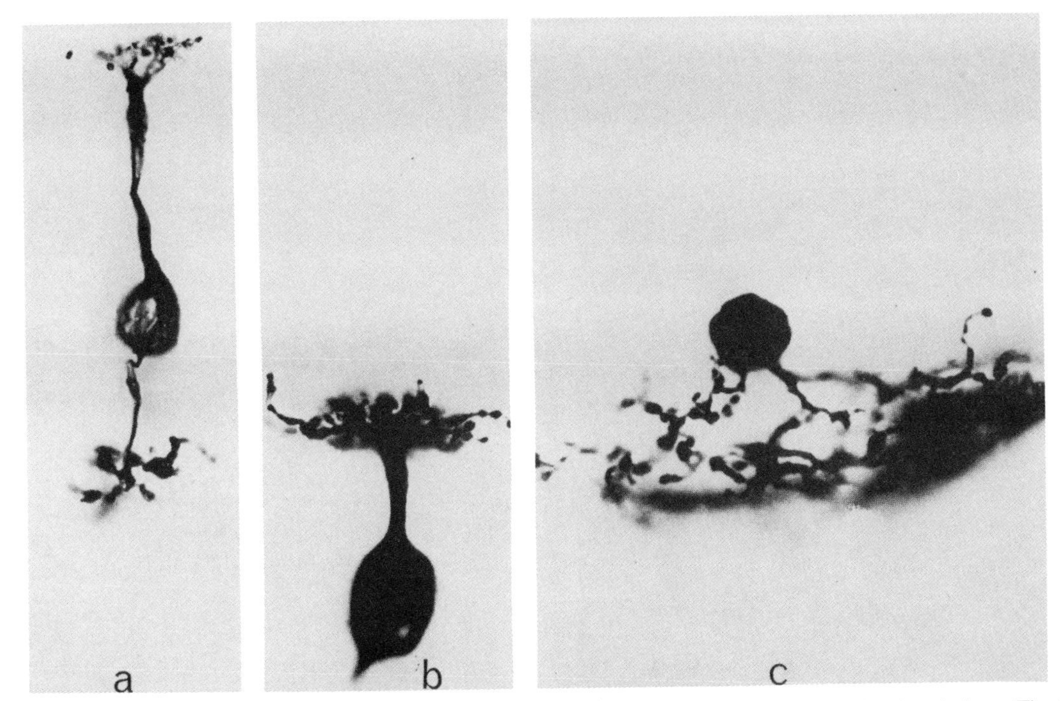

Figure 34–40. (a) Bipolar cell; (b) ganglion cell; (c) amacrine cell, all impregnated with the Golgi technique. The bipolar and ganglion cells are from the retina of *Macacca mulatta*; the amacrine cell is from the rabbit. (Photomicrograph courtesy of E. Raviola.)

cells, and axonless horizontal cells of nonprimate mammals, exclusively contact cones as lateral elements of invaginating synapses.

Amacrine Cells

Most of these neurons have numerous dendrites but lack an axon (Figs. 34–39 and 34–40C). Their body lies in the vitreal part of the inner nuclear layer or among the bodies of ganglion cells (displaced amacrines), and their dendrites spread in the inner plexiform layer. They connect with each other, with the axonal endings of the bipolar cells, and with the dendrites of the ganglion cells. The primate retina contains numerous varieties of amacrine cells; these are classified as *diffuse* and *stratified*. Diffuse amacrine cells send their dendritic branches throughout the thickness of the inner plexiform layer, whereas the ramifications of the stratified amacrine cells are confined to different sublaminae of the inner plexiform layer.

Interplexiform Cells

Interplexiform cells have their perikaryon in the inner nuclear layer and send their processes to both plexiform layers. In the inner plexiform layer, their processes are both presynaptic and postsynaptic to amacrine cell dendrites. In the outer plexiform layer, their processes are exclusively presynaptic to horizontal and bipolar cells. Thus, the input to these cells is confined to the inner plexiform layer, whereas their output is in both plexiform layers.

Ganglion Cells

Ganglion cells represent the terminal link of the neural networks of the retina. With their dendrites, they connect with bipolar endings and amacrine dendrites in the inner plexiform layer; their body is located in the ganglion cell layer; their axon, which becomes a fiber of the optic nerve, conducts to the brain the results of the complex neural activity that takes place in the retina. The primate retina contains numerous varieties of ganglion cells, classified according to the shape of their dendritic tree and the mode of distribution of their dendritic branches in the inner plexiform layer.

Polyak classified primate ganglion cells according to both their size and the shape of their dendritic tree. *Midget ganglion cells* are

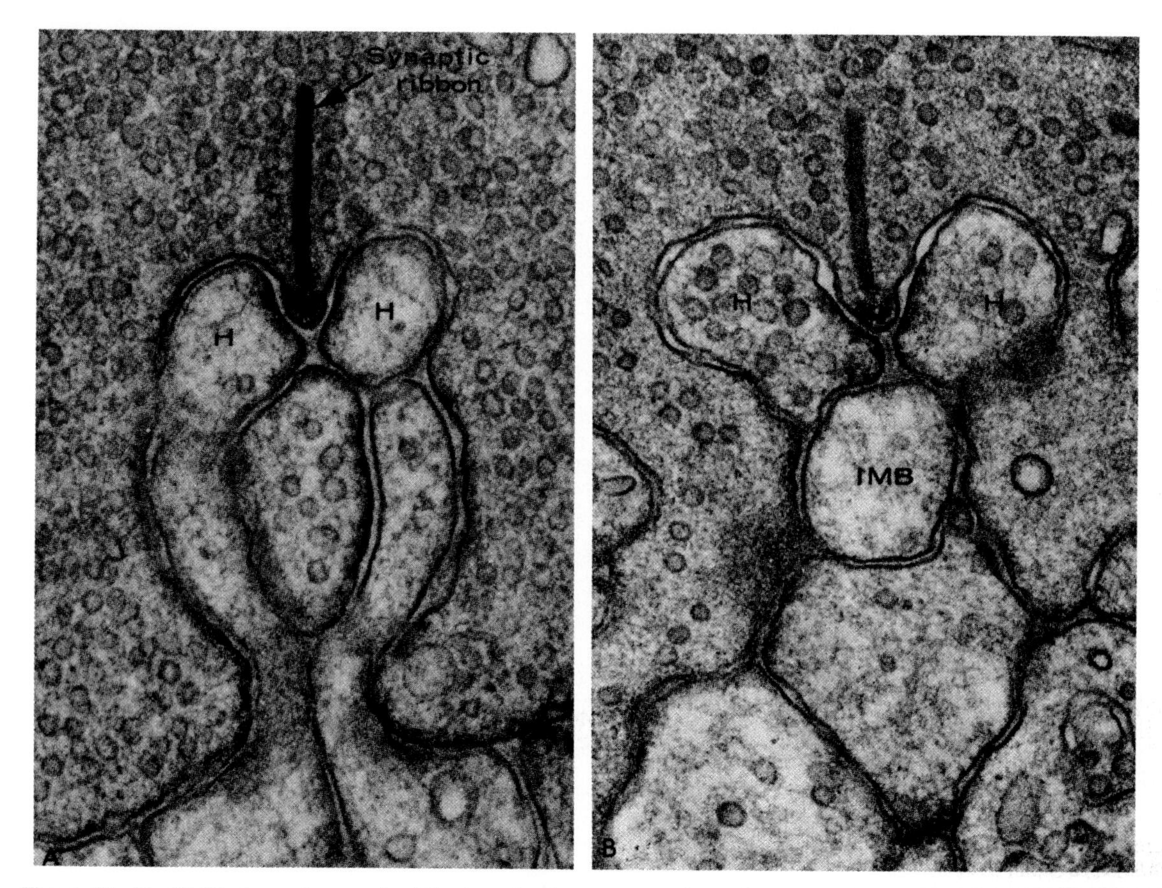

Figure 34–41. (A) Electron micrograph of the invaginating synapse of a rod spherule in the rabbit retina. Two deeply inserted processes (H), probably arising from the axon of horizontal cells, lie on either side of a wedge-shaped projection of the spherule (synaptic ridge), which contains the synaptic ribbon, surrounded by a halo of synaptic vesicles, and the arciform density. The dendrites of the rod bipolar cells cannot be identified in this micrograph. (B) Invaginating synapse of a cone pedicle in the retina of a monkey. A typical "triad" consists of two deeply invaginated dendrites of the horizontal cells (H) and a slightly inserted, centrally positioned dendrite of an invaginating midget bipolar cell (IMB). Note the synaptic vesicles in the horizontal cell dendrites. (Micrograph courtesy of E. Raviola.)

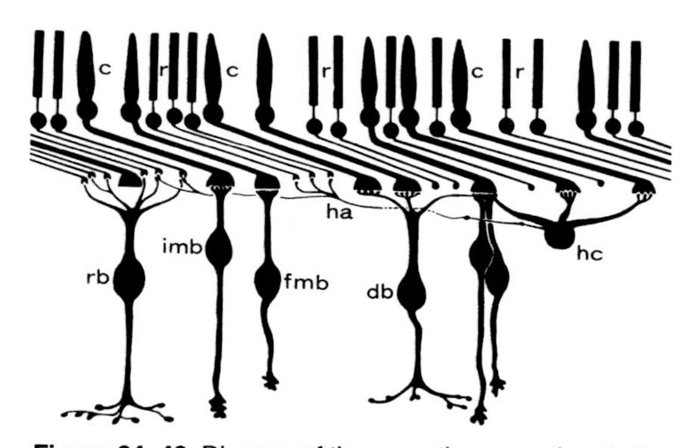

Figure 34–42. Diagram of the synaptic connections in the outer plexiform layer of the primate retina. For explanation, see text. (c) Cone cells; (r) rod cells; (rb) rod bipolar cells; (imb) invaginating midget bipolar cell; (fmb) flat midget bipolar; (db) diffuse cone bipolar cell; (ha) horizontal cell axon; (hc) horizontal cell. (From Kolb, H. 1970. Phil. Trans. Roy. Soc. London B 258:261.)

small neurons with a single, thin, apical process that ascends into the inner plexiform layer, where it gives rise to a small number of short dendrites gathered into an extremely limited arbor. These dendrites receive most of their ribbon synaptic input from a single midget bipolar cell and can, therefore, be regarded as a conduit for transfer to the brain of the signals arising from each individual cone. The axon of the midget ganglion cells terminates in the parvicellular portion of the lateral geniculate nucleus; for this reason, midget ganglion cells are referred to as *P-cells* by visual physiologists. *Parasol ganglion cells* have bodies larger than midget ganglion cells; they give rise to one or several apical dendrites, which ascend into the inner plexiform layer and spread into a flat arbor consistently largely than the dendritic tree of midget ganglion cells. The synaptic connections of para-

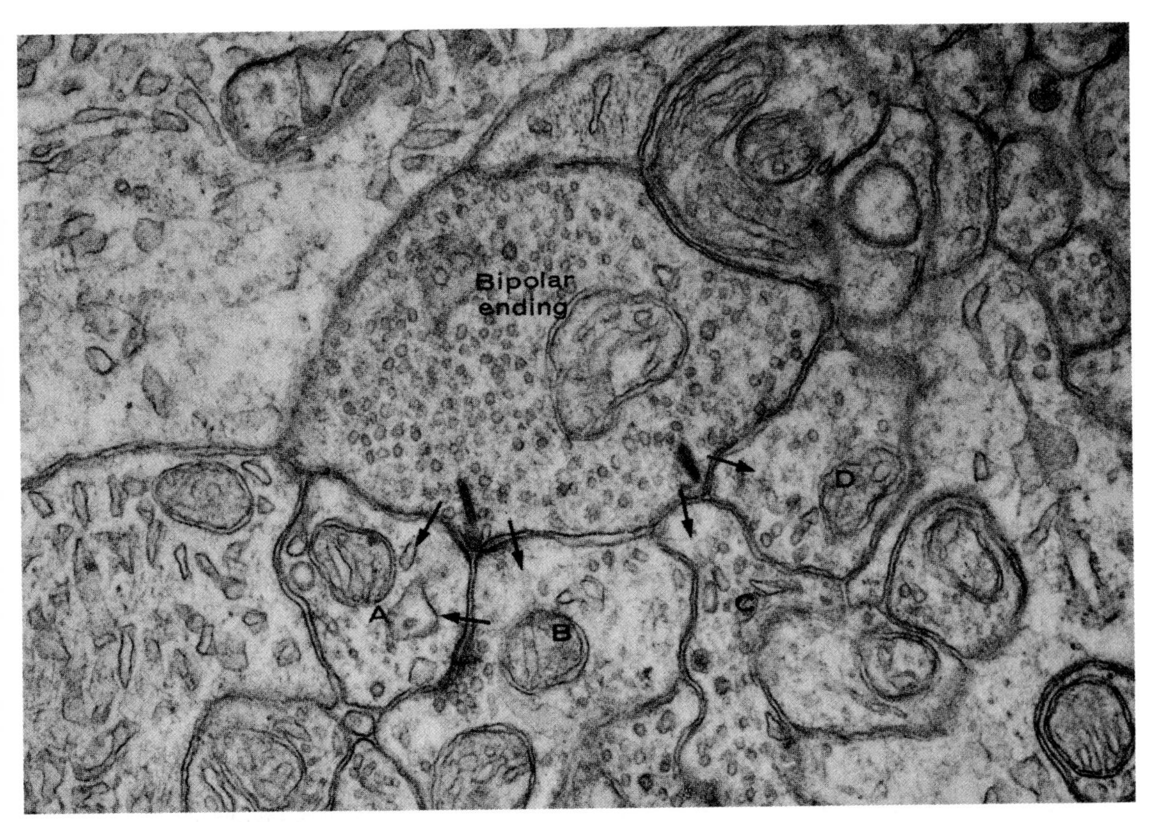

Figure 34–43. Electron micrograph of a portion of the inner plexiform layer in monkey retina. An axonal ending of a bipolar cell makes two ribbon synapses with four processes (labeled A, B, C, and D). Processes B, C, and D contain synaptic vesicles and may represent dendrites of amacrine cells. Process B makes a conventional type of synaptic contact with process A, whose identity is unknown. Arrows indicate the direction of synaptic influences (Courtesy of E. Raviola.)

sol ganglion cells with bipolar and amacrine cells are not known. The axon of parasol ganglion cells terminates in the magnocellular portion of the lateral geniculate nucleus, and for this reason, these neurons are called *M-cells*. Further types of primate ganglion cells were described by Polyak as shrub, small diffuse, garland, and giant cells; neither the connections nor the function of these cells are known.

INNER PLEXIFORM LAYER

This is the region of synaptic interplay between bipolar, amacrine, and ganglion cells. Two types of synaptic contacts are found in this layer, the ribbon synapse, and a more conventional type of synaptic contact, which lacks the ribbon and is characterized by clustering of the synaptic vesicles against the presynaptic membrane (Fig 34–43). At ribbon synapses, the axon endings of the bipolar cells are presynaptic to amacrine and ganglion cell dendrites. Amacrine dendrites, in turn, make conventional synapses with bipolar endings, ganglion cell dendrites, and dendrites of other amacrine cells. Reciprocal synapses between bipolar terminals and amacrine dendrites frequently occur in this layer, with the bipolar contacting the amacrine cell as the presynaptic element of a ribbon synapse, and the amacrine cell returning a conventional feedback synapse onto the bipolar. Thus, amacrine cell dendrites have the unusual property of containing synaptic vesicles and behaving as presynaptic elements of *dendroaxonic* and *dendrodendritic* synapses. The existence of dendrodentritic synapses has also been described in the olfactory bulb, where the granule cells, which lack an axon, establish reciprocal dendrodendritic synapses with the dendrites of the mitral cells.

The precise pattern of neural interconnections in the inner plexiform layer is presently the subject of active investigations. Sublayers can be distinguished within it, for the axonal arborizations of the bipolar cells and the den-

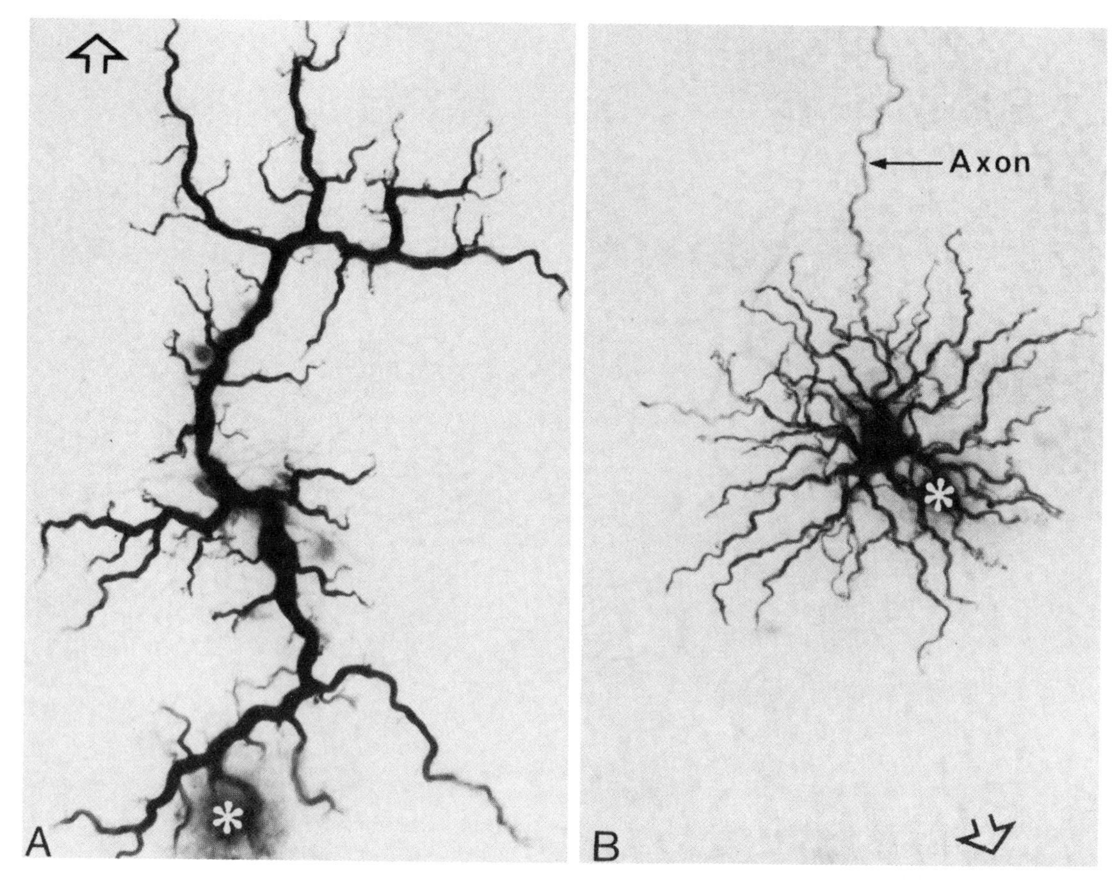

Figure 34–44. Horizontal cells of rabbit retina. (A) An axonless horizontal cell injected with horseradish peroxidase. The cell has a small number of stout, tortuous dendrites, which branch sparsely and have minute terminal branchlets. At the asterisk, a Müller cell has been stained with peroxidase that leaked from the electrode during penetration. (B) The somatic end of an axon-bearing horizontal cell. The cell has numerous wavy dendrites radiating in all directions. These have clusters of small terminal branchlets. The site of electrode penetration is marked by an asterisk. The open arrows indicate the direction to the optic nerve head. (From Dacheux, R.F., and E. Raviola. 1982. J. Neurosci. 2:1486.)

dritic expansions of the stratified amacrine and ganglion cells are distributed at different levels within the layer. This, and recent findings in nonprimate retinas, suggest that the various types of bipolar, amacrine, and ganglion cells establish specific synaptic connections with each other. However, the details of their "wiring" have not yet been worked out for the human retina.

OPTIC NERVE FIBERS

The optic nerve fibers have a special course owing to the presence of the centrally placed fovea. In general, they converge radially toward the optic papilla. However, those originating in the upper temporal quadrant of the retina circle above the central area, whereas those originating in the lower temporal quadrant circle below it on their way to the papilla. They follow the larger retinal vessels fairly closely. A line connecting the fovea with the temporal circumference of the retina separates the optic nerve fibers of the upper from those of the lower temporal quadrant. This separation is preserved along the central visual pathway as far as the cortex.

In primates, each retina is divided into two halves along the vertical meridian passing through the center of the fovea. The fibers from the nasal half cross in the optic chiasma and pass to the optic tract of the opposite side; those from the temporal half enter the tract on the same side. Each optic tract is, therefore, composed of fibers from the temporal half of the retina of the same side and the nasal half of the retina of the opposite eye. This arrangement remains in the visual radiation in the occipital lobes of the brain. It accounts for the blindness in the opposite halves of the two fields of view (homonymous hemianopsia) when the optic tract or the visual radiation of one side is interrupted.

INNER LIMITING MEMBRANE

This traditional term is no longer appropriate because the electron microscope has revealed that it is not a membrane but merely the basal lamina of the Müller cells. It separates their inner conical ends from the vitreous body.

NEUROGLIAL ELEMENTS OF THE RETINA

Being a modified part of the brain, the retina contains supporting elements of neuroglial character. The most important of these are the radial cells of Müller. These are present throughout the central area, including the fovea, as well as in the periphery. Their oval nuclei lie in the middle zone of the inner nuclear layer. The cell body is a slender pillar that extends radially from the outer to the inner limiting membrane. In the two plexiform layers, the radial pillars give off many branches, which form a dense neuroglial network in whose meshes are lodged the ramifications of the neurons described earlier. In the nuclear layers, the Müller cells have deep excavations that envelop the bodies of the retinal neurons.

At the limit between the outer nuclear layer and the layer of rods and cones, Müller cells have prominent zonulae adherentes that form the linear density formerly interpreted as an outer limiting membrane.

CENTRAL AREA AND FOVEA

The place of most distinct vision is slightly lateral to the papilla. This region, the *central area* (macula lutea), is characterized by the presence of cones and other neural elements in numbers greater than elsewhere, and by their structural specialization and synaptic perfection. In the center of this area, the layers inward from the outer nuclear layer are displaced laterally, producing a shallow depression on the vitreal surface of the retina, called the *central fovea*.

The fovea is a very shallow bowl with its concavity toward the vitreous (Fig. 34–45). It is located in the middle of the central area, 2–2.5 mm on the temporal side of the papilla. In its center, a *floor* or *fundus* can be distinguished, together with the *slopes* and a *margin of the fovea*. The width of the entire foveal depression measures 1.5 mm. Because the retina is much thinner in the foveal floor, it is exclusively nourished by the choroidal circulation. Thus, retinal blood vessels stop at the very edge of the foveal floor or 275 μm from the very center. The *avascular central territory* is almost as large as the rodless area (450–500 μm). Because of the absence of blood vessels, images can reach the foveal photoreceptors free of optical distortions.

In the fundus of the fovea, the cones are thinner and longer than elsewhere in the retina. The central *rod-free* area, where only cones are present, measures 500–550 μm in diameter and contains up to 30,000 cones.

HISTOPHYSIOLOGY OF THE RETINA

The eye is essentially a camera obscura provided with dioptric media: the cornea, aqueous humor, the adjustable crystalline lens, and the vitreous body. The inner surface of this dark chamber is lined with the photosensitive retina. The rays of light emanating from each point of an illuminated object impinging on the cornea are refracted by it and converge on the lens. In the lens, the rays are further refracted and focused in the photosensitive layer of the retina. In relation to the object, the retinal image is inverted (because of the crossing of the rays in the pupil's aperture); it is a real image and is very much reduced in size.

In the retina, the quanta of incident light are converted, or transduced, by the photoreceptor cells into nerve signals; these are elaborated by the networks of retinal neurons and finally translated into a code of nerve impulses, which is conducted to the brain by the fibers of the optic nerve.

The transduction process can be conveniently subdivided into primary and secondary steps. The primary step is a photochemical reaction and consists in the absorption of a quantum of light by one of the visual pigments contained in the discs of the photoreceptor outer segments, and a subsequent configurational change in the absorbing molecule. The secondary step consists of changes in the con-

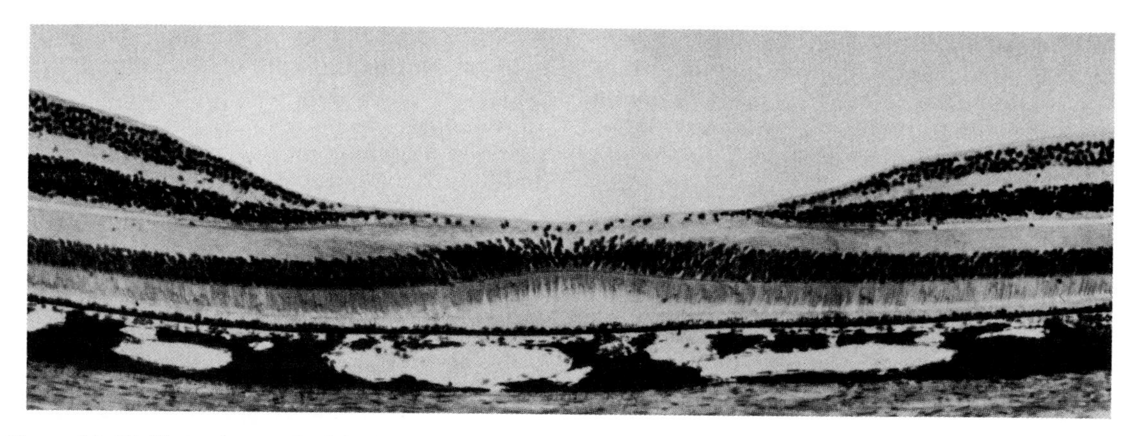

Figure 34–45. Photomicrograph of the fovea of a macaque retina showing the marked reduction in thickness in this area of maximal visual acuity. (Courtesy of H. Mizoguchi.)

centration of internal transmitters within the cytoplasm of the outer segments, which influence the ionic permeability of the plasma membrane and cause the hyperpolarization of the photoreceptor cell.

Rod and cone cells differ in their sensitivity to intensity and wavelength of light. Rod cells are active in dim illumination (scotopic vision) and contain a single visual pigment, rhodopsin, which absorbs light of various wavelengths but is most efficient in the blue-green. In the human retina, there are three types of cones, containing different visual pigments that absorb maximally red, blue, or green light; cone cells are active under the conditions of diurnal illumination (photopic vision).

Visual pigments consist of a combination of vitamin-A aldehyde, known as *retinal*, with a protein of the class called *opsins*. Opsins are hydrophobic proteins with one retinal group per molecule, a carbohydrate side-chain, no phospholipid, and a molecular weight of about 27,000 daltons. They are buried within the membrane of the discs of the photoreceptor outer segments. When retinal is combined with opsin in the dark-adapted retina, it has a bent and twisted form (*11-cis*). When the pigment molecule absorbs a quantum of light, the shape of the retinal becomes straight (*all-trans*) and separates from opsin, which, in turn, undergoes a conformational change. This leads to activation of various enzymes and the lowering of the concentration of cGMP in the outer segment. cGMP represents the internal transmitter that regulates the patency of the ion channels in the plasma membrane. In the dark, sodium ions are continuously pumped out of the cell in the inner segment and reenter the cell through sodium channels located in the plasma membrane of the outer segment. Light diminishes or suppresses this "dark current" by blocking the sodium channels of the outer segment, and, thus, causes the hyperpolarization of the photoreceptor cell. Meanwhile, photoreceptor and pigmented epithelial cells cooperate in regenerating 11-cis-retinal and recombining it with opsin into the light-absorbing form of the pigment molecule.

Most of our present knowledge on the electrophysiology of retinal neurons stems from intracellular recordings in nonprimate retinas. Stripped of many important details, the complex story of the interneuronal relationships in the retina is as follows. Most retinal neurons generate slow, graded potentials; spikes first appear in amacrine cells and are especially typical of the ganglion cell response. The photosensitive rod and cone cells are depolarized and release transmitter in the dark; the light-induced hyperpolarization decreases the output of transmitter by their synaptic endings. In cold-blooded vertebrates, there are two physiological classes of horizontal cells: *luminosity* horizontal cells which respond to illumination of the photoreceptors by hyperpolarization; and *chromaticity* horizontal cells, which may hyperpolarize or depolarize, depending on the wavelength of the stimulating light. In the retina of the turtle, the hyperpolarization of luminosity horizontal cells causes depolarization of the cone cells; it has, therefore, been suggested that cones receive, from horizontal cells, a feedback synapse. In all vertebrates, there are two physiological classes of bipolar cells, one depolarizing and the other hyperpolarizing on stimulation by light. Bipolar cells are the first elements in the chain of retinal neurons that show a "center-and-surround" organization of their receptive field; that is, the cell response to stimulation of neighboring photoreceptors is antagonized by the stimulation of distant photoreceptors. Furthermore, some bipolars are color-coded; that is, they respond to light of specific wavelength. The response of bipolars to stimulation of the photoreceptors in the center of their receptive field may be mediated by a photoreceptor-to-bipolar synapse. The "surround effect" is probably due to the activity of the horizontal cells, which are activated by distant photoreceptors and, in turn, antagonize the center response of the bipolar cells by exerting an inhibitory feedback onto the photoreceptors that are presynaptic to the bipolar. Thus, the function of the synapses in the outer plexiform layer is to signal the intensity and color of the retinal image and, at the same time, to accentuate its contrast through the activation of the horizontal cells.

The signals of bipolar cells are further processed in the inner plexiform layer by the amacrine and ganglion cells before their conduction to the brain in the form of changes in frequency of the nerve impulses traveling along the fibers of the optic nerve.

The function of the amacrine cells is poorly understood; there are many varieties of them, both morphological and physiological, and they modulate the transfer of signals from bipolar to ganglion cells. In the monkey retina, two main types of ganglion cells were identified by intracellular recordings, one responding to the onset and the other to the cessation of a light stimulus applied to the center of their receptive field. Among the on-center cells, some are not color-coded and phasic—that is, they discharge transiently to sustained stimuli of any wavelength (M-cells); others are color-coded and tonic—that is, they discharge continuously to sustained stimuli of either green or red light (P-cells). It has been speculated that the neural interactions in the inner plexiform layer may be concerned with codification of the dynamic or temporal aspects of the visual image, but much work remains to be done before the significance of the synaptic interactions among bipolar, amacrine, and ganglion cells is fully elucidated.

BLOOD VESSELS OF THE EYE

These arise from the ophthalmic artery and can be subdivided into two groups, which are almost completely independent and anastomose with each other only in the region of the entrance of the optic nerve. The first group, the *retinal system*, represented by the central artery and vein, supplies a part of the optic nerve and the inner retina. The second, the *ciliary system*, is destined for the uveal tunic; through the uvea, it provides for nourishment of the outer retina. Like the brain, the retina is protected from circulating macromolecules by a *blood-retina barrier*; its structural basis is mainly the zonulae occludentes that seal the intercellular spaces between the cells of the pigment epithelium and those between the endothelial cells of the retinal blood vessels.

LYMPH SPACES OF THE EYE

True lymph capillaries and larger lymph vessels are present only in the scleral conjunctiva. In the eyeball, they are absent. Certain potential spaces do exist within the eye. A fluid injected into the space between the choroid and sclera penetrates along the walls of the vortex veins into the space of Tenon. The latter continues as the *supravaginal space* along the outer surface of the dural sheath of the optic nerve to the optic foramen. From the anterior chamber, injected liquid passes into the posterior chamber and also into Schlemm's canal. All of these spaces cannot, however, be regarded as belonging to the lymphatic system.

NERVES OF THE EYE

The nerves of the eye are the optic nerve, originating from the retina, and the ciliary nerves, supplying the eyeball with motor, sensory, and sympathetic fibers.

The optic nerve arises in the embryo as an evagination of the prosencephalon and is not a peripheral nerve like the other cranial nerves but is a tract of the central nervous system. It consists of about 1200 bundles of nerve fibers whose myelin sheaths are produced by oligodendroglial cells.

The meninges and the intermeningeal spaces of the brain continue into the optic nerve. The outer sheath of the nerve is formed by the dura, which continues toward the eyeball and fuses with the sclera. The intermediate sheath is formed by the arachnoid and the inner sheath, by the pia mater. The pia mater forms a connective tissue layer that is closely adherent to the surface of the nerve and fuses with the sclera at the entrance of the optic nerve. This pial layer sends connective tissue partitions and blood vessels into the nerve. Inflammatory processes can extend from the eyeball toward the meningeal spaces of the brain through the spaces between the sheaths.

The optic nerve leaves the posterior pole of the eyeball in a slightly oblique direction and continues into the entrance canal of the optic nerve. Just after leaving the eye through the opening in the lamina cribrosa, the fibers acquire their myelin sheaths. The central artery and central vein reach the eyeball through the optic nerve; they penetrate the nerve on its lower side at a distance from the eyeball varying from 5–20 mm, but usually 6–8 mm.

EYELIDS AND ACCESSORY ORGANS OF THE EYE

The eyelids form during embryonic development as folds of skin that advance to overlie the anterior surface of the eyeball. Thus, the lids are covered on their outside by the stratified squamous epithelium of the skin. At the lid margins, this epithelium and its lamina propria continue, with some modification, onto the inner surface of the lids as the *palpebral conjunctiva* and this is reflected onto the eyeball as the *bulbar conjunctiva*. The potential space between the lids and the eyeball is the *conjunctival sac*, and the deep recesses where the palpebral conjunctiva of the upper and lower lids becomes continuous with the bulbar conjunctive are called the *superior* and *inferior fornices*.

The thin skin of the eyelids is provided with sweat glands, many fine hairs, and associated sebaceous glands (Fig. 34–46). The dermis is much thinner than that of skin elsewhere and has few papillae. It becomes somewhat thicker near the margins of the lids. It may contain a few pigment cells. The thin layer of underlying connective tissue is rich in elastic fibers and is devoid of fat cells.

The *eyelashes* are large hairs set obliquely in three or four rows along the edge of the lids. Their follicles penetrate deeply into the underlying connective tissue. Their associated sebaceous glands are small, and arrector pili muscles are absent. The eyelashes are replaced about every 100 to 150 days. Between the follicles of the eyelashes are modified sweat glands, called the *glands of Moll*. Unlike sweat glands elsewhere, their terminal portion is not highly coiled. The lining epithelium consists of pyramidal apocrine cells and these are surrounded by a myoepithelial layer. The lumen of the glands may be considerably dilated. The ducts generally open into the follicles of the lashes and are lined by an epithelium consisting of two layers of cells. The nature and function of the secretion of these glands is unknown.

Beneath the subcutaneous tissue of the lids there is a thin layer of striated muscle that is the palpebral portion of a facial muscle, the *orbicularis oculi* (Fig. 34–46). The portion immediately adjacent to the follicles of the eyelashes is also called the *ciliary muscle*. The upper lid is more mobile than the lower lid and, in opening the eye, it is raised by the *levator palpebrae superioris*. A continuation of the tendon of this muscle, the *palpebral fascia*, is attached to the anterior surface of the *superior tarsus*—a curved plate of dense connective tissue that forms a stiffening component maintaining a curvature of the lid that conforms to the curvature of the eyeball. In the upper lid, there are also strands of smooth muscle comprising the *superior tarsal muscle* that extends from the aponeurosis of the levator palpebrae muscle to the upper edge of the superior tarsus. A less well-defined layer of smooth muscle is also found in the lower lid inserting into the much smaller *inferior tarsus*.

Embedded in the substance of the tarsus of both lids are the *Meibomian glands*, of which there are about 25 in the upper lid and 20 in the lower. They are elongated and parallel to one another with their ducts opening, in a single row, on the free edge of the lids at the line of transition from the skin to the conjunctiva. They are lobulated, alveolar, sebaceous glands drained by short ducts into a long central excretory duct lined by stratified squamous epithelium

At the margin of the lids, there is a transition from the stratified squamous epidermis to the stratified epithelium of the conjunctiva. The number of layers in this epithelium becomes fewer and the superficial cells become low cuboidal. Scattered among these cells are mucus-secreting goblet cells (Fig. 34–47). In the conjunctiva of the fornix, the epithelium is thicker and goblet cells much more numerous. The secretion of these cells is important because it spreads over the surface of the conjunctiva and cornea as a major component of the *tear film* that lubricates and protects the

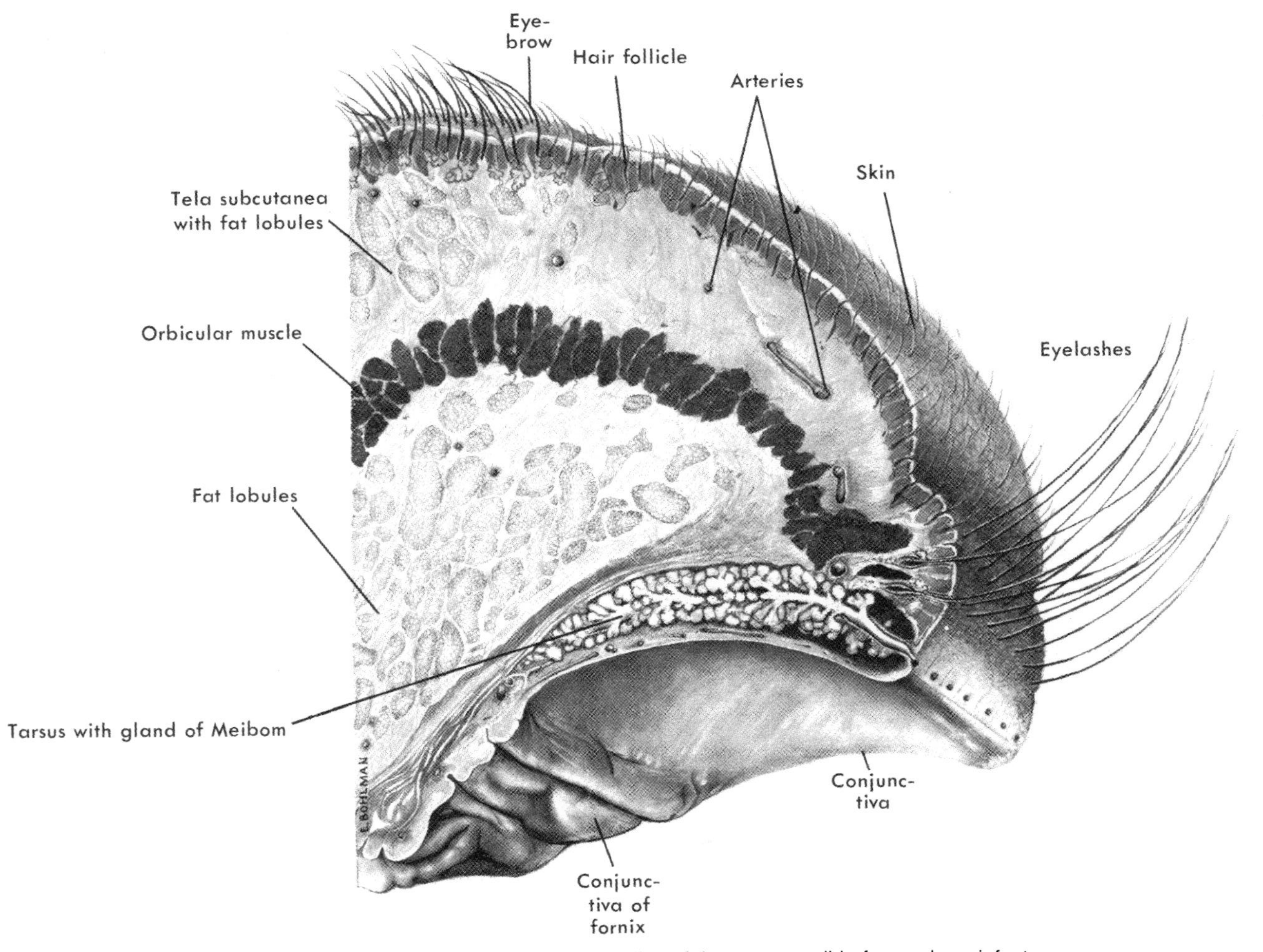

Figure 34–46. Camera lucida drawing of a slice of the upper eyelid of a newborn infant.

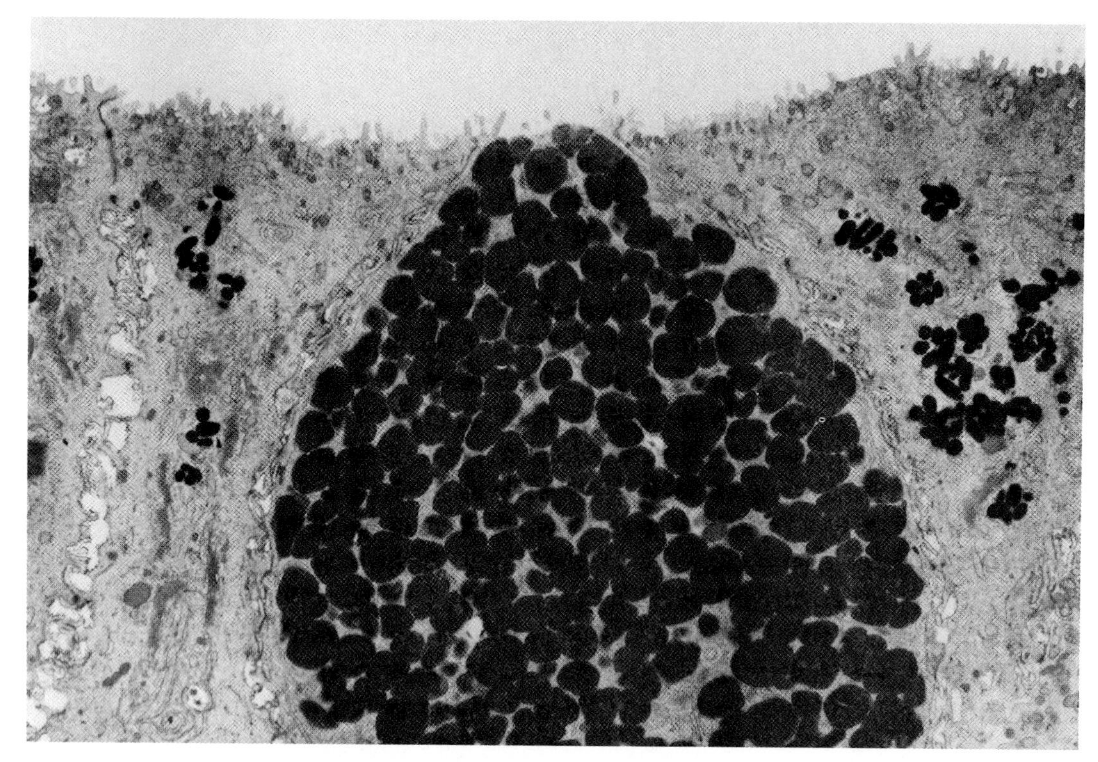

Figure 34–47. Electron micrograph of the superficial portion of the conjunctival epithelium of *Macaca mulatta* showing a goblet cell and clusters of melanosomes in the neighboring epithelial cells. (Micrograph courtesy of E. Raviola.)

underlying epithelia. The significance of this mucus layer has not been fully appreciated because it is not adequately preserved with routine methods of specimen preparation. However, when the mucus is chemically stabilized by exposure to quaternary ammonium compounds and then examined by electron microscopy after freeze-substitution, it is found to form a layer 1.5–2 μm thick on the bulbar conjunctiva (Fig. 34–48). Over the cornea, it is 0.4–1 μm thick and somewhat more dense. At high magnifications, the mucus layer appears as a meshwork of very thin cross-linked glycoprotein filaments, resembling those of the glycocalyx on the short microvilli of the underlying conjunctival epithelial cells. This layer, thus, appears to be a major component of the tear film which consists of a thin outer layer of lipid and an intermediate aqueous layer, in addition to the relatively thick inner coat of mucus. Over the cornea, this trilaminar film is the first component that refracts light entering the eye and it is essential for normal vision, and for protection against keratitis and conjunctivitis.

Over the corneoscleral junction, the conjunctival epithelium assumes a stratified squamous character and continues as such over the cornea. At the inner palpebral commissure, the conjunctiva forms a semilunar fold which is a rudimentary homologue of the nictitating membrane, or third eyelid, of lower vertebrates. Some smooth muscle is found in the connective tissue of this fold.

LACRIMAL GLAND

A number of glands secrete into the conjunctival sac, moistening and lubricating the surfaces of the eyeball and the lids. Of these glands, only the *lacrimal gland* reaches a degree of development that makes it readily visible. It has the size and shape of an almond and is lodged beneath the conjunctiva at the upper lateral side of the eyeball. It consists of a number of glandular lobules and has 6 to 12 excretory ducts that open along the upper and lateral quadrant of the superior conjunctival fornix.

The lacrimal gland is a tubuloalveolar gland. Its terminal portions have a relatively

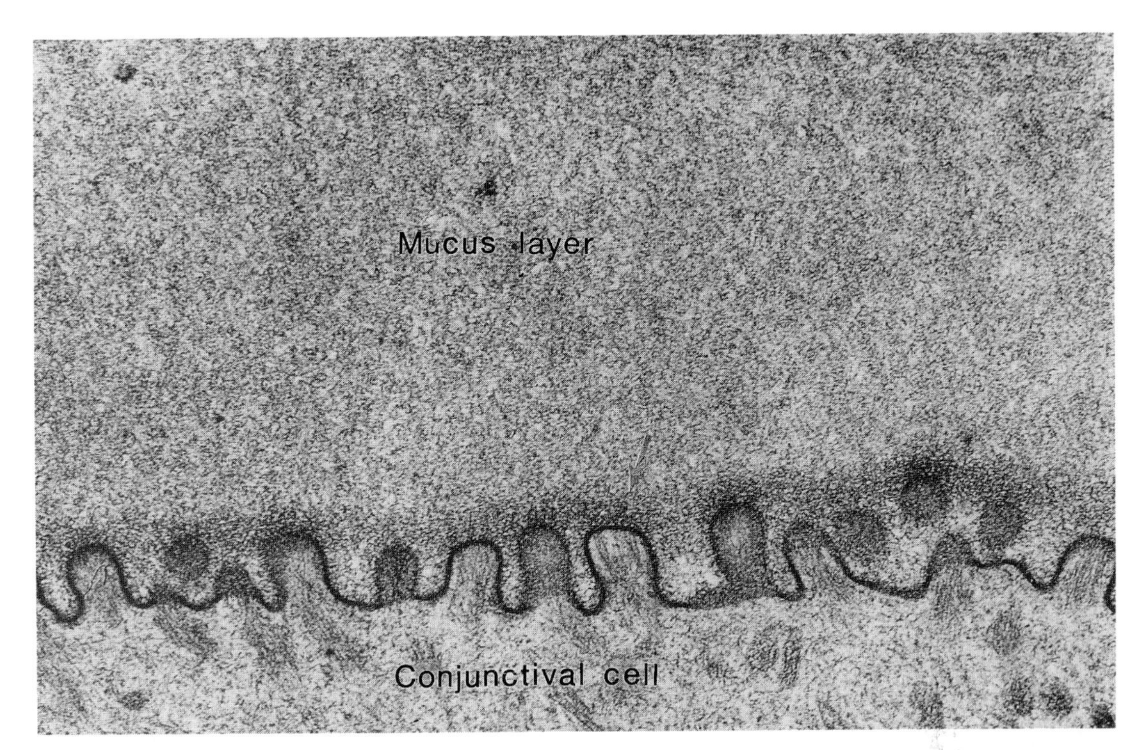

Figure 34–48. Electron micrograph of the apical portion of a conjunctival epithelial cell and the overlying mucus which constitutes the innermost layer of the protective and lubricating tear film. (Micrograph courtesy of Nichols, B. 1985. Investig. Ophthalmol. Vis. Sci. 26:464.)

large lumen, with irregular saccular out-pocketings. The glandular cells rest on a distinct basal lamina and resemble those of the serous salivary glands. However, they have a narrower columnar shape and contain small lipid droplets and large pale secretion granules. There are secretory canaliculi between the cells, and there are conspicuous myoepithelial cells between their base and the basal lamina. The larger intralobular ducts have a two-layered epithelium.

On the inner surface of the lids, especially near the upper edge of the tarsus of the upper lid, there are varying numbers of small accessory lacrimal glands—the *tarsal lacrimal glands*.

From the conjunctival cavity, tears reach the region of the inner palpebral commissure (internal canthus). Here the two eyelids are separated by a triangular space, referred to as the *lacrimal lake*, in which secretion accumulates temporarily. From here, it passes through two tiny orifices, called *lacrimal points*, one on the margin of each eyelid, and into two *lacrimal ducts*. These converge medially into the *lacrimal sac*, from where the *nasolacrimal duct* leads downward into the inferior meatus of the nasal cavity.

The wall of the excretory lacrimal passages is made up of connective tissue and lined by epithelium. That of the lacrimal ducts is stratified squamous epithelium. The lacrimal sac and nasolacrimal duct are lined by a tall pseudostratified columnar epithelium.

From the bottom of the lacrimal lake, between the two lacrimal ducts, there is a small, soft, mass of tissue that bulges forward. This is the *lacrimal caruncle*. Its top is covered by a thick stratified squamous epithelium, in which the uppermost layers of cells are flattened but not keratinized. This epithelium contains some mucous cells and it gradually merges with the conjunctival epithelium. The lamina propria contains bundles of striated muscle, sweat glands, abortive lacrimal glands, and tiny hairs with sebaceous glands. These latter are the source of the whitish secretion that often collects in the region of the inner palpebral commissure.

BIBLIOGRAPHY

GENERAL

Davson, H. 1972. The Physiology of the Eye. New York, Academic Press.

Fine, B.S. and M. Yanoff. 1972. Ocular Histology. New York, Harper and Row.

Hogan, M.J., J.A. Alvarado, and J.E. Weddell. 1971. Histology of the Human Eye. Philadelphia, W.B. Saunders Co.

CORNEA

Hay, E.D. 1980. Development of the vertebrate cornea. Internat. Rev. Cytol. 63:263.

Jakus, M.A. 1956. Studies on the cornea. II. The fine structure of Descemet's membrane. J. Biophys. Biochem. Cytol. (Suppl.) 2:243.

Mishima, S. 1965. Some physiological aspects of the precorneal tear film. Arch. Ophthalmol. 73:233.

Nichols, B.A., M.L. Chiappino, and C.R. Dawson. 1985. Demonstration of the mucous layer of the tear film by electron microscopy. Investig. Ophthalmol. Vis. Sci. 26:464.

IRIS

Freddo, T.F. and G. Raviola. 1982. Homogeneous structure of the blood vessels in the vascular tree of *Macacca mulatta* iris. Investig. Ophthalmol. Vis. Sci. 22:279.

Gregersen, E. 1958. The spongy structure of the human iris. Acta Ophthalmol. 36:522.

Raviola, G. and J.M. Butler. 1984. Unidirectional transport mechanism of horseradish peroxidase in the vessels of the iris. Investig. Ophthalmol. Vis. Sci. 25:827.

Richardson, K.C. 1964. The fine structure of the albino rabbit iris with special reference to the identification of adrenergic and cholinergic nerves and nerve endings in its intrinsic muscles. Am. J. Anat. 114:172.

CILIARY BODY

Fine, B.S. 1966. Structure of the trabecular meshwork and the canal of Schlemm. Trans. Am Acad. Ophthalmol. Otolaryngol. 70:777.

Inomata, H., A. Bill, and G.H. Smelser. 1972. Aqueous humor pathways through the trabecular meshwork and into Schlemm's canal in the cynomologus monkey (Macacca iris). Am. J. Ophthalmol. 78:760.

Ishikawa, T. 1962. The fine structure of the human ciliary muscle. Investig. Ophthalmol. 1:587.

Raviola, G. 1977. The structural basis of the blood-ocular barriers. Exp. Eye Res. (Suppl.) 25:27.

Raviola, G. 1971. The fine structure of the ciliary zonule and ciliary epithelium. Investig. Ophthalmol. 10:851.

Raviola, G. and E. Raviola. 1978. Intercellular junctions in the ciliary epithelium. Investig. Ophthalmol. Vis. Sci. 10:958.

Raviola, G. and E. Raviola. 1981. Paracellular route of aqueous outflow in the trabecular meshwork and Schlemm's canal. Investig. Ophthalmol. 21:52.

Toates, F.M. 1972. Accommodation function of the human eye. Physiol. Rev. 52:828.

Tormey, J. McD. 1963. Fine structure of the cviliary epithelium of the rabbit with particular reference to "infolded membranes," "vesicles," and the effects of Diamox. J. Cell Biol. 17:641.

LENS AND VITREOUS BODY

Farnsworth, P.N., S.C. Fu, P.A. Burke, and I. Bahia. 1974. Ultrastructure of the rat eye lens fibers. Investig. Ophthalmol. 13:274.

Swann, D.A. 1980. Chemistry and biology of the vitreous body. Internat. Rev. Exp. Pathol. 22:2.

Wank, T. and M.A. Gavin. 1959. Electron microscopic study of lens fibers. J. Biophys. Biochem. Cytol. 6:97.

RETINA

Bok, D. 1985. Retinal photoreceptor-pigment epithelium interactions. Investig. Ophthalmol. Vis. Sci. 26:1659.

Borwein, E. 1983. Scanning electron microscopy of monkey foveal photoreceptors. Anat. Rec. 205:363.

Dacheux, R.F. and E. Raviola. 1982. Horizontal cells in the retina of the rabbit. J. Neurosci. 2:1486.

Dowling, J.E. 1970. Organization of vertebrate retinas. Investig. Ophthalmol. 9:665.

Masland, R.H. 1986. The functional architecture of the retina. Sci. Am. 255 (6):102.

Mayerson, P.L. and M.O. Hall. 1986. Rat retinal pigment epithelial cells show specificity of phagocytosis in vitro. J. Cell Biol. 103:299.

Polyak, S. 1941. The Retina. Chicago, IL, University of Chicago Press.

Raviola, E. 1976. Intercellular junctions in the outer plexiform layer of the retina. Investig. Ophthalmol. 15:881.

Raviola, E. and N.B. Gilula. 1975. Intramembrane organization of specialized contacts in the outer plexiform layer of the retina. J. Cell. Biol. 65:192.

Raviola, G. and E. Raviola. 1967. Light and electron microscopic observations on the inner plexiform layer of the rabbit retina. Am. J. Anat. 120:403.

Rodieck, R.W. 1973. The Vertebrate Retina. San Francisco, W.H. Freeman.

Schwartz, E.A. 1982. First events in vision: the generation of responses in vertebrate rods. J. Cell Biol. 90:271.

Steinberg, R.H., S.K. Fisher, and D.H. Anderson. 1980. Disc morphogenesis in vertebrate photoreceptors. J. Comp. Neurol. 190:501.

Young, R.W. 1976. Visual cells and the concept of renewal. Investig. Ophthalmol. 15:700.

Young, R.W. and D. Bok. 1969. Participation of the retinal pigment epithelium in the outer segment renewal process. J. Cell Biol. 42:392.

35

THE EAR

The ear is a remarkably sensitive sensory organ that receives and translates sound, between 16 and 20,000 cycles/s, into nerve impulses that are interpreted in the auditory centers of the brain. The organ of hearing consists of three parts: the *external ear* that receives the sound waves, the *middle ear* where the waves are transformed by three minute auditory ossicles into mechanical vibrations that are transmitted to the fluid of the *internal ear*. The movement of the fluid results in vibrations of a thin membrane which are sensed by specialized epithelial cells that stimulate associated endings of the auditory nerve. In addition to the organs for perception and analysis of sound, the inner ear contains *vestibular organs* that sense linear or rotational acceleration of the head and generate nerve impulses that serve to maintain the body's equilibrium.

EXTERNAL EAR

AURICLE

The *auricle* or *pinna* consists of an irregularly shaped plate of elastic cartilage, 0.5–1 mm in thickness, overlain by a perichondrium containing abundant elastic fibers. The skin covering the cartilage has a distinct subcutaneous layer only on the posterior of the auricle. It is provided with a few short hairs and associated sebaceous glands. In old men, scattered large stiff hairs develop on the edge of the auricle and on the ear lobe. Sweat glands are rare and, when present, they are small.

EXTERNAL ACOUSTIC MEATUS

The *acoustic meatus* is the canal extending from the auricle inward to the tympanic membrane (ear drum) and is about 2.5 cm long. Its outer third is a continuation of auricular cartilage and the inner two-thirds is a canal in the temporal bone (Fig. 35–1). The skin lining the meatus is thin and firmly attached to the underlying perichondrium and periosteum. There are numerous coarse hairs projecting into the outer third of the meatus and these become more prominent in old age. The sebaceous glands associated with the hair follicles are exceptionally large. The skin in this segment also contains *cerumenous glands* which are a special form of coiled, tubular, apocrine sweat glands that secrete *cerumen*, a brown waxy secretion. Each glandular tubule is surrounded by a thin network of myoepithelial cells. In the resting state, the gland lumen is large and the lining epithelium is cuboidal, but in the active state, the cells are columnar and the lumen constricted. The ducts of the cerumenous glands open either onto the free surface of the skin or into the necks of the hair follicles. The cerumen is believed to provide a kind of waterproofing for the skin lining the meatus and, together with the coarse hairs, it is believed to discourage the entry of insects.

MIDDLE EAR

The middle ear includes the *tympanic cavity* and its contents, the *auditory ossicles*; the *eustachian tube*; and the *tympanic membrane* or eardrum, which closes the tympanic cavity externally (Fig. 35–1).

The tympanic cavity is an irregularly shaped, air-filled space about 6–15 mm in diameter, within the temporal bone. Its lateral wall is formed largely by the tympanic membrane and its medial wall by the bony wall of the internal ear (Fig. 35–1). Posteriorly, it is continuous with the air-filled cavities of the mastoid process of the temporal bone, and anteriorly, it continues into the *auditory tube* (eustachian tube) which is the communication between the tympanic cavity and the nasopharynx. The cavity contains the three *auditory ossicles* and the *tensor tympani* and *stapedius* muscles that are connected with the ossicles. The cavity is lined by squamous epithelium,

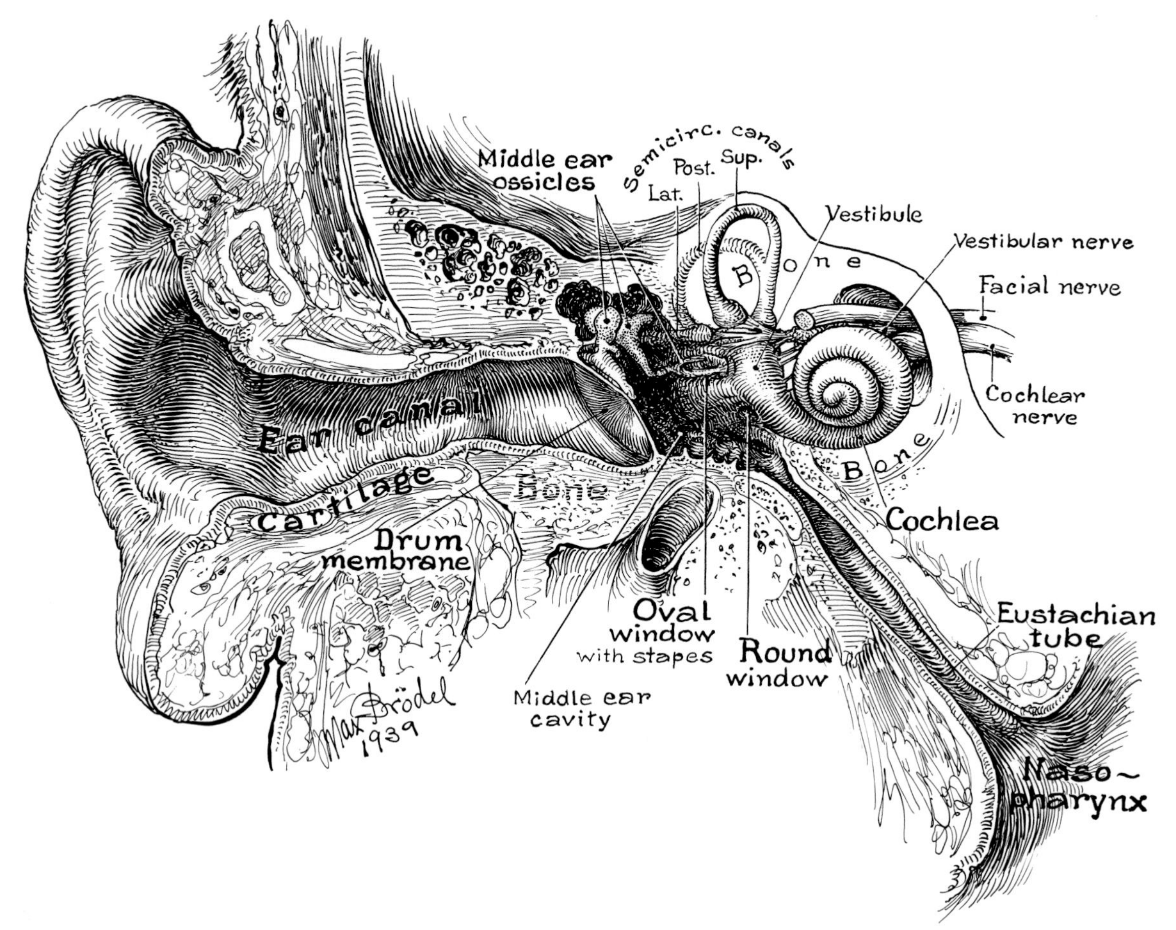

Figure 35–1. Schematic representation of the anatomical relations of the various components of the human ear. (Brödel, M. 1946. *In* Malone, J., Guild, M. and B. Crowe, eds. Three Unpublished Drawings of the Human Ear. Philadelphia, W.B. Saunders Co.

but near the opening of the auditory tube and near the edge of the tympanic membrane, it is cuboidal and may be provided with cilia. The lining contains no glands.

AUDITORY OSSICLES

Three small articulated bones, the *malleus, incus*, and *stapes*, extend across the cavity from the attachment of the malleus to the tympanic membrane to the medial wall, where the foot-plate of the stapes fits into the *fenestra vestibuli* or *oval window*, an opening in the bony labyrinth of the inner ear (Fig. 35–1). The foot-plate of the stapes is held in the oval window by an annular fibrous ligament. The three bones are connected by typical diarthrodial joints and are supported in the cavity by tiny ligaments. The lining of the tympanic cavity is reflected over the ossicles and is firmly bound to their periosteum. The function of the ossicles is to transfer the energy of the relatively weak sound pressure waves of the air in the external auditory meatus into more forceful vibrations of the fluid in the inner ear. The chain of ossicles acts rather like a hydraulic press, with the piston-like action of the foot-plate of the stapes transforming the small pressure on the surface of the eardrum into a 20-fold greater pressure on the fluid of the inner ear.

TYMPANIC MEMBRANE

The oval, semitransparent tympanic membrane takes the form of a very flat cone with its apex directed medially (Fig. 35–1). Its conical form is maintained by the insertion, on its

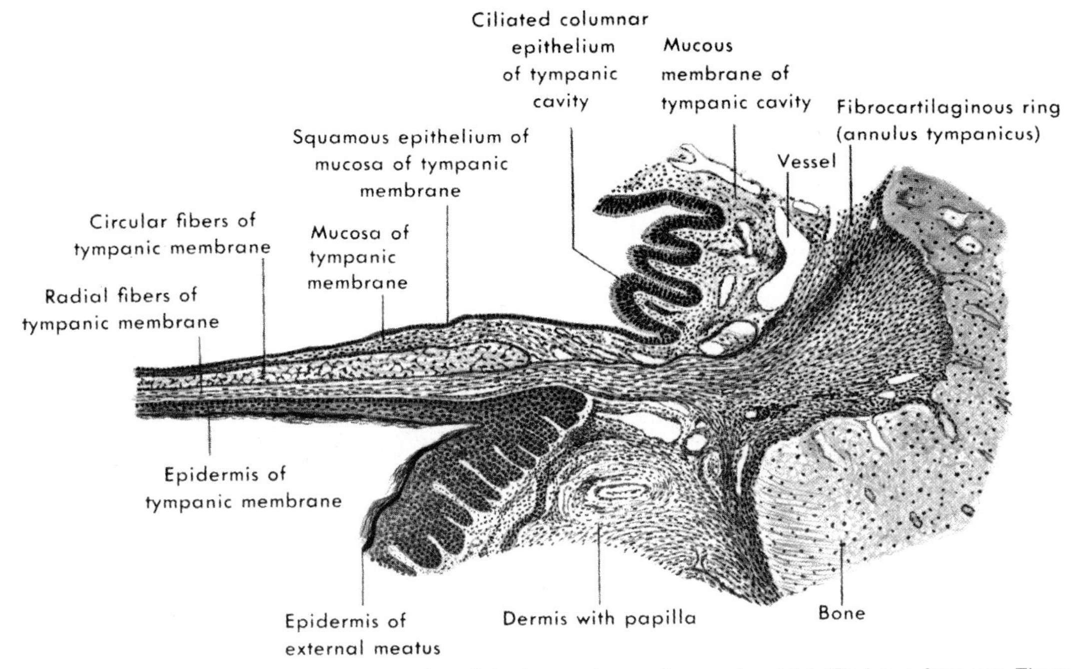

Figure 35–2. Cross section of the outer edge of the tympanic membrane of a child. (Redrawn from von Ebner.)

medial surface, of the manubrium of the malleus, which tends to draw the center of the membrane medially. The membrane is made up of two layers of collagenous fibers and fibroblasts. In the outer layer, the collagenous fibers are oriented radially, whereas those of the inner layer have a circular disposition (Fig. 35–2). There are also thin networks of elastic fibers. In rodents, the fine fibers of the tympanic membrane lack the cross-striations characteristic of collagen, and it has been suggested that they are a distinct protein specialized for the unique function of this membrane. However, in the human, they are reported to be thin fibers of typical collagen. The fibers are taut throughout the greater part of the membrane, constituting its *pars tensa*, but in its anterosuperior quadrant, there is a small triangular area, the *pars flaccida* (Schrapnell's membrane), that is lax and virtually devoid of collagen fibers. The outer surface of the tympanic membrane is covered by a very thin (50–60 μm) layer of skin with no hair or glands. Its inner surface is lined by the mucosa of the tympanic cavity, here only 20–40 μm in thickness and consisting of squamous epithelium and a thin lamina propria containing sparse collagen fibers and capillaries. The vessels and nerves reach the center of the membrane via the subepithelial connective tissue overlying the manubrium of the malleus.

AUDITORY TUBE (EUSTACHIAN TUBE)

From the anterior wall of the tympanic cavity, the *auditory tube* courses anteromedially and inferiorly for about 4 cm to open on the posterodorsal wall of the nasopharynx. The first third, near the tympanic cavity, is supported by bone and the remainder is supported medially by cartilage and laterally by fibrous tissue. In cross sections of the auditory tube, the cartilage supporting it medially and superiorly has a hook-like configuration (Fig. 35–3). The cartilage is elastic throughout most of its length but loses its elastic fibers and becomes hyaline cartilage near its pharyngeal end. The diameter of the tube is somewhat constricted at the junction of its cartilaginous and bony segments and this portion is referred to as the *isthmus*. The lumen of the tube is flattened in the vertical plane and lined by a mucosa that is plicated into rugae at both the pharyngeal and tympanic ends. In the bony portion of the tube, it is relatively thin and composed of low, columnar, ciliated epithelium, resting on a thin lamina propria that is firmly bound to the periosteum. In the cartilaginous portion of the tube, the epithelium is pseudostratified and composed of tall columnar cells many of which are ciliated. The underlying lamina propria, in this segment, contains many compound, tubuloalveolar glands that secrete mucus via ducts opening

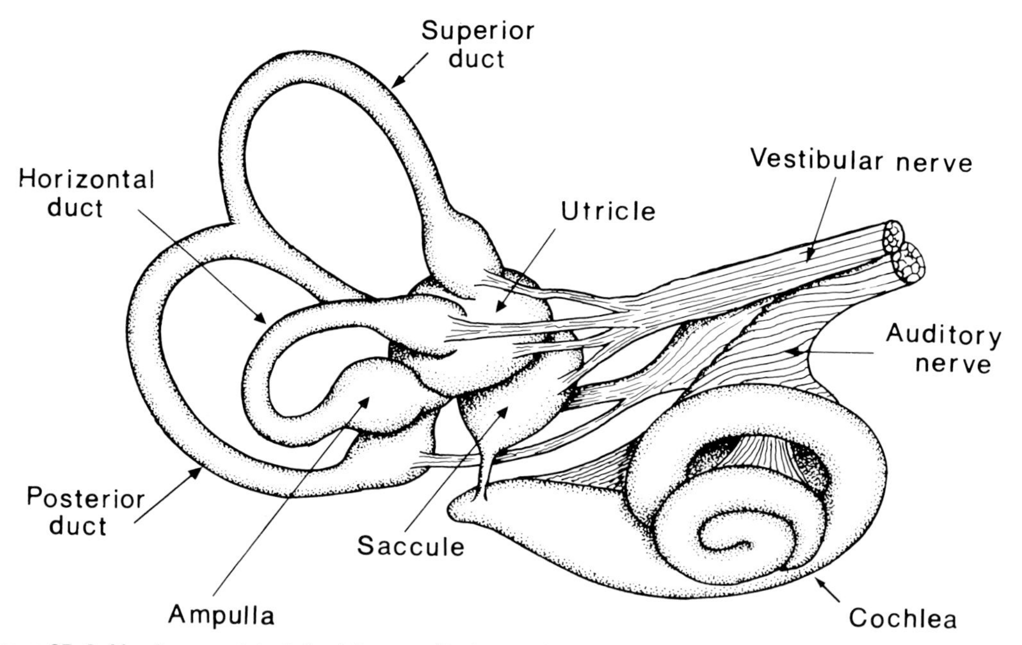

Figure 35–3. Membranous labyrinth of the ear. (Redrawn after D.E. Parker, *Scientific American* 243:120, 1980.)

into the tubule lumen. In this region, near the pharynx, goblet cells are interspersed among the columnar epithelial cells.

There is considerable individual variation in the number and distribution of ciliated and goblet cells, and in the degree of development of the glandular elements. Throughout the lamina propria, in both segments of the tube, a great many lymphocytes can be found, the number varying with age and from one individual to another. Near the pharyngeal opening, there are often discrete collections of lymphoid tissue forming the so-called *tubal tonsils*. The auditory tube is usually closed, but during the act of swallowing or yawning, it is briefly opened by contraction of neighboring palatine muscles, allowing pressure in the tympanic cavity to equalize with that outside.

INTERNAL EAR

The several components of the internal ear occupy a series of communicating cavities in the petrous portion of the temporal bone that collectively compose the *osseous labyrinth*. Within these cavities is the *membranous labyrinth*, consisting of two small sacs, the *utricle* and the *saccule*, three *semicircular ducts* (anterior, posterior, and lateral) emanating from the utricle, and the *cochlear duct* occupying a spiral bony canal of the osseous labyrinth (Fig. 35–3). All portions of the continuous membranous labyrinth contain a fluid called the *endolymph*. Its wall is separated from the wall of the osseous labyrinth by a *perilymphatic space* containing a fluid of different composition, called the *perilymph*. The central portion of the osseous labyrinth, containing the utricle and saccule is referred to as the *vestibule*.

THE SEMICIRCULAR DUCTS

During sudden changes in orientation, sensory receptors in the semicircular ducts and vestibular organs respond to acceleration of the head to generate nerve impulses to the brain that initiate reflexes which tend to restore normal body position.

The sensory receptors of the semicircular ducts are located in small dilatations of each, called *ampullae*. These are situated near the junction of the ducts with the utricle. In the floor of each ampulla, there is a transverse ridge, the *crista ampullaris*. The orientation of the ridge ensures that it is affected by any movement of the ridge with respect to the endolymph within the semicircular duct. The sensory epithelium over the top of the crista consists of two cell types, *hair cells* and *supporting cells*. The hair cells do not extend down to the basal lamina but occupy rounded recesses between the apices of the surrounding sup-

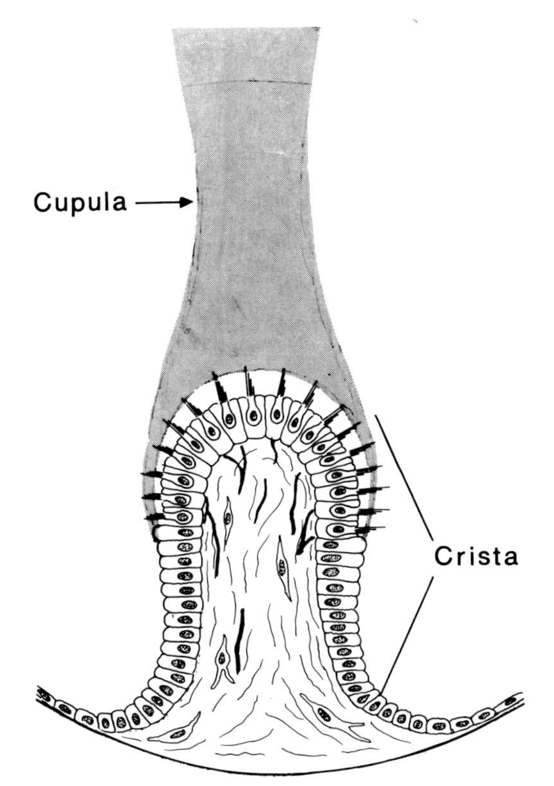

Figure 35–4. The crista ampullaris of a semicircular duct (Redrawn after D.E. Parker, *Scientific American* 243:120, 1980.)

porting cells. On their free surface, they have a single kinocilium and a cluster of specialized stereocilia ("hairs") that extend upward into the base of a gelatinous structure, called the *cupula*, which projects into the lumen of the ampulla (Fig. 35–4). In vivo, the protein-polysaccharide of the cupula is a firm gel, but it is soluble in the fixatives commonly used, and it is seldom preserved in histological preparations.

Two types of hair cells are recognized. *Type-I hair cells* are plump, flask-shaped cells with a rounded base and a narrower neck region. The nucleus is locate basally and surrounded by mitochondria. There is a supranuclear Golgi complex, occasional cisternae of rough endoplasmic reticulum, and many small vesicles (Fig 35–5). The 50–100 stereocilia on the free surface vary in length in a stepwise fashion, so that the bundle, as a whole, has a beveled appearance, with the tallest hairs (10 μm) near the kinocilium and the shortest (1 μm) on the opposite side. Each stereocilium, or hair, is limited by the plasma membrane and contains a bundle of several hundred actin filaments spaced about 10 nm apart and extensively cross-linked by minute strands of the protein *fimbrin* (Fig. 35–6). The cross-linking of the actin filaments makes the stereocilia unusually rigid. Each stereocilium is isodiametric along most of its length, but near its base it tapers down to a narrower segment containing as few as 20 actin filaments. These continue downward into the cytoplasm as a slender rootlet whose filaments mingle with those of an unusually dense terminal web, or cuticular plate, traversing the apical cytoplasm immediately beneath the plasma membrane. When pressure is applied to the stereocilia they bend only at their narrow neck region.

The *type-II hair cells* are more columnar in form and their kinocilium, stereocilia, and cytoplasmic organelles are similar to those of the type-I cells, but the Golgi complex is somewhat larger and small vesicles are found in greater number throughout the cytoplasm. The distinction between the two types of hair-cells depends more on the configuration of their innervation than on their cytological differences.

In the case of the type-I hair cells, nerves penetrate between the supporting cells and form a chalice-like ending completely investing their rounded base (Fig. 35–5). At one or more sites in the peripheral cytoplasm of the rounded base of the hair-cell, there is a dense band oriented perpendicular to the plasmalemma and surrounded by a halo of small vesicles. These structures resemble the so-called *synaptic ribbons* found in sensory cells of the retina. They are thought to be specializations characteristic of chemical synapses. In addition to these, there are areas where the presynaptic and postsynaptic membranes are only 5 nm apart. These areas resemble low-resistance contacts found in certain electrical synapses, but, at present, there is no physiological evidence to support their identification, as such, in the hair cells.

The nerves to the type-II hair cells do not form a calyx but end in a number of relatively small terminal boutons (Fig. 35–5). Synaptic ribbons are also found in the peripheral cytoplasm of the type-II hair cells opposite the thickened plasmalemma of certain of the terminal boutons. Some of the endings contain clear synaptic vesicles (non-granulated vesicles), and others contain dense-cored vesicles (granulated vesicles). The former are associated with afferent nerves that carry information to the brain. The latter are thought to be endings of efferent nerves that carry impulses modulating the sensitivity of the type-II hair

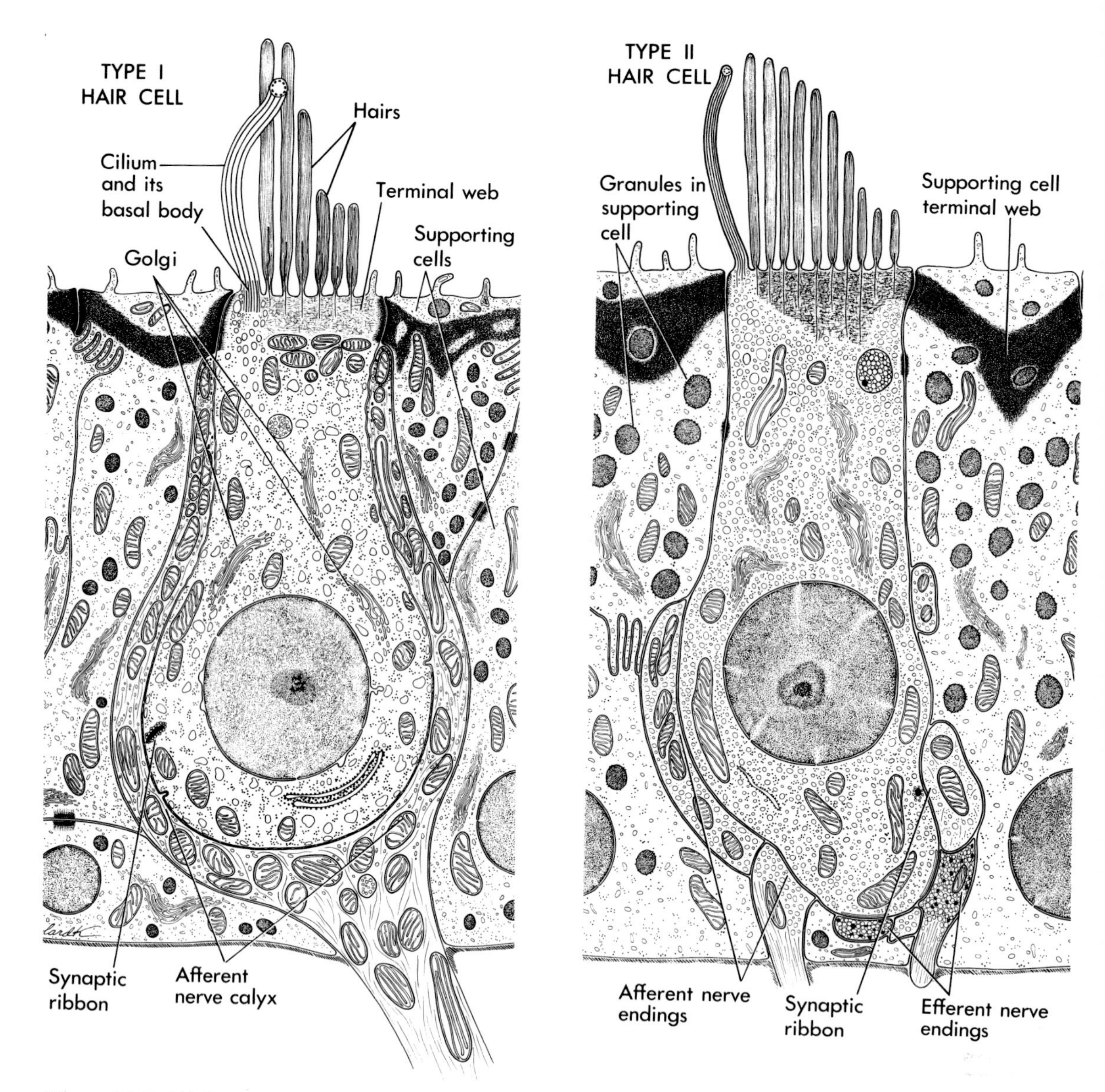

Figure 35–5. (A) Drawing of the principal ultrastructural features of the type-I vestibular hair cell. (B) A comparable depiction of the type-II hair cell which lacks a nerve calyx. (Drawn by Sylvia Collard Keene.)

cells to stimuli, but this has not been firmly established. It is clear that the synaptic relationships are far more complicated than was imagined before the advent of electron microscopy, and their exact nature remains unsettled.

The supporting cells of the epithelium of the crista ampullaris have attracted less investigative attention than the hair cells. They have a few microvilli on their free surface and are bound to each other and to the adjacent hair cells by typical junctional complexes. The cell body is often somewhat contorted so that the full length of any given cell can seldom be seen in a single section. The nucleus is basal and the cytoplasm contains microtubules running vertically from the basal cytoplasm to a dense terminal web which is thicker than that of the hair cells. There is a well-developed Golgi complex and what appear to be secretory granules are associated with it. Little is known about possible functions of these cells, other than support of the hair cells. The presence of putative secretory granules in their cytoplasm suggests that they may either contribute to the nutrition of the hair cells or may

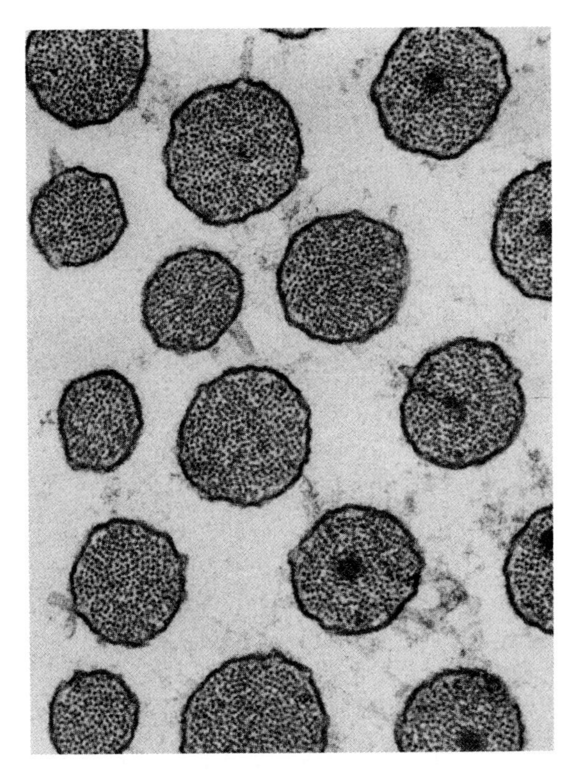

Figure 35–6. Electron micrograph of a cross section of the stereocilia of a guinea pig hair cell showing the large number of filaments in their interior. (Micrograph courtesy of H. Engström.)

be involved in the production of the endolymph.

When the head is quickly rotated, the endolymph in the semicircular ducts, which has considerable inertia, tends to remain stationary while the wall of the ducts move. There is, therefore, a slight relative movement of the endolymph in the ducts in a direction opposite to that of the rotation of the head. The cupulae of the cristae ampullaris projecting into the fluid are moved slightly, bending the stereocilia of the hair cells. These cells act as minute strain-gauges responding to bending of their stereocilia toward the kinocilium by increasing the frequency of afferent nerve impulses. The brain responds by activating muscles influencing the position of the eyes, and other muscle groups that tend to correct any disturbance of equilibrium.

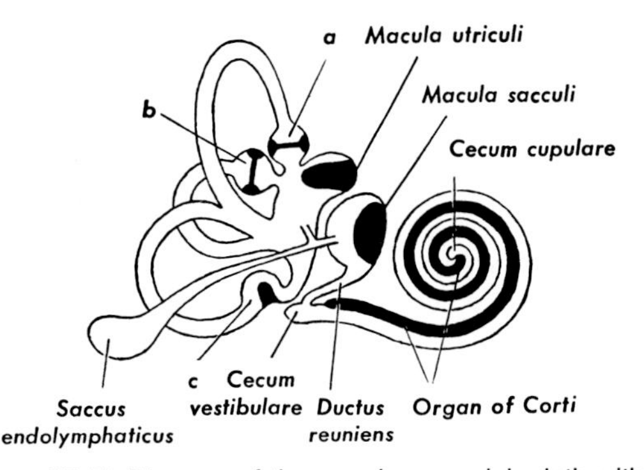

Figure 35–7. Diagram of the membranous labyrinth with the neuroepithelial receptor areas indicated in black. (a), (b), and (c) are the ampullae of the superior, lateral, and posterior semicircular ducts, respectively. (Modified from von Ebner.)

The anterior (or superior) semicircular duct and the posterior semicircular duct are oriented approximately vertically, at an angle to one another, and the lateral duct is nearly horizontal. The ends of the three semicircular ducts are continuous with the wall of the utricle. The medial end of the anterior duct and the upper end of the posterior duct become confluent so that there are only five orifices of semicircular ducts opening into the utricle.

UTRICLE

The wall of the utricle and saccule consists of an outer fibrous layer, an intermediate layer of delicate vascular connective tissue and an inner layer of epithelium that varies from squamous to low cuboidal, except in specialized receptor regions where it becomes columnar and more complex in its organization. *Dark* and *light* cells are distinguishable in the unspecialized regions of the epithelium. The light cells have sparse microvilli on their apical surface and occasional micropinocytosis vesicles. Their cytoplasm contains small numbers of ribosomes and relatively few mitochondria. The dark cells have nuclei that are highly irregular in outline and are often located near the apical surface. The apical cytoplasm contains abundant coated vesicles, larger smooth vesicles, and occasional lipid droplets. The basal cytoplasm contains many long mitochondria that occupy slender compartments limited by infolding of the basal plasma membrane. The respective functions of the dark and light cells are poorly understood. However, owing to the ultrastructural similarity of the dark cells to ion-transporting cells elsewhere in the body, it is speculated that these cells may play a role in control of the ionic composition of the endolymph.

In the floor of the utricle, there is a thickened area of specialized sensory epithelium, 2 to 3 mm in diameter, called the *macula utri-*

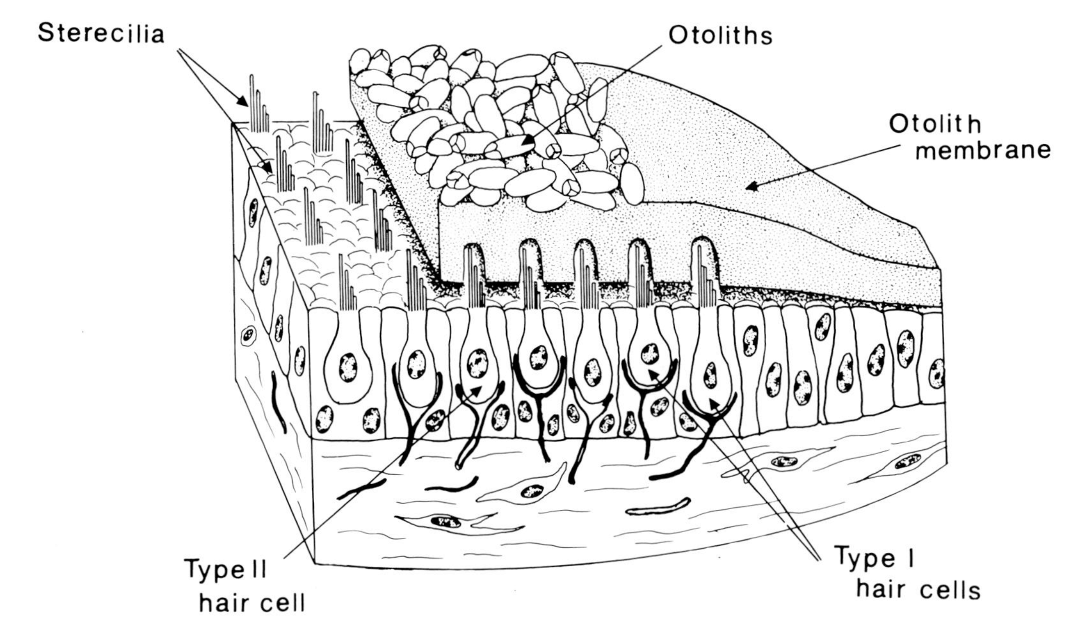

Figure 35–8. Drawing of a portion of the macula utriculae showing the relation of the otolithic membrane to the hair cells. The membrane is cut away, at the left, to show the stereocilia on the rows of hair cells. (Redrawn after D.E. Parker, *Scientific American* 243:125, 1980.)

culi. It consists of *hair cells* and *supporting cells*. The epithelium of the macula is essentially identical to that of the cristae ampullaris, consisting of supporting cells and two types of hair cells. The kinocilium and stereocilia of the hair cells project into the under side of the so-called *otolithic membrane*. Despite its traditional name, this structure is not a membrane, but a moderately thick layer of gelatinous material like that forming the cupula of the crista ampullaris. It differs, however, in that it contains a multitude of minute (3–5 μm) crystalline bodies, the *otoliths* (or *otoconia*) partially embedded in its upper surface (Fig. 35–8). These consist of protein and calcium carbonate and are thought to provide additional inertia that resists displacement of the membrane by external force. Thus, when a linear acceleration is applied to the head, the otolith membrane tends to remain stationary while the hair cells beneath it slide slightly, bending the hairs backward. Bending of the hairs triggers changes in the frequency of nerve impulses reaching the brain.

SACCULE

The utricle communicates with the saccule through a narrow *ductus utriculosaccularis*. In the anterior wall of the globular saccule there is an ovoid thickening of the wall called the *macula of the saccule* which is virtually identical in its organization to the macula of the utricle. Because the macula of the saccule is in the vertical anterior wall, its hair cells respond to movement that is at a right angle to movement that activates the macula of the utricle, which is horizontal when the head is in the upright position. Thus, in different positions of the head, different hair cells are stimulated, and this provides the brain with information as to the position of the head with respect to the pull of gravity.

Small ducts from the utricle and saccule join to form the *endolymphatic duct* that courses downward in the vestibular aqueduct in the petrous portion of the temporal bone to end in a small dilatation, the *endolymphatic sac*, situated between the layers of the meninges. The duct is lined by a squamous to cuboidal epithelium like that lining the rest of the membranous labyrinth. However, near the end of the duct there is a transition to tall columnar cells. These are of two types, dark and light cells. The darker cells have a large irregularly shaped nucleus and a free surface that is relatively smooth, but the cell base has some shallow infoldings of the membrane. The free surface of the light cells bears a profusion of long microvilli. Between the bases of the microvilli there are numerous micropinocytotic invaginations of the membrane. There are also sizable clear vacuoles in the apical cytoplasm. The plasma membrane at the cell base is relatively smooth but the lateral membranes extensively interdigitate with those of neighboring cells. The ultrastructure of the light cells suggests that they are specialized for absorption. There is supporting evidence that the endolymphatic sac is a site of active absorption of endolymph. Neutrophils and macrophages from the surrounding connective tissue can also cross the epithelium to phagocytize cellular debris and other particulates that may accumulate in the lumen of the endolymphatic sac.

In addition to the endolymphatic duct, there is a short tube, the *ductus reuniens* that runs downward from the lower part of the saccule to the basal end of the cochlear duct.

COCHLEA

The cochlea is the portion of the osseous labyrinth anteromedial to the vestibule. It is a spiral bony canal about 35 mm in length that makes two and three-quarter turns around a conical pillar of spongy bone, called the *modiolus*. At its base, there is an opening into the tympanic cavity, the *fenestra vestibuli* that is closed by the foot-plate of the *stapes*, which transmits sound vibrations from the tympanic membrane to the *organ of Corti*, the organ of hearing located in the *cochlear duct*. A spiral ridge or ledge, the *spiral lamina*, projects from the modiolus into the cochlear canal. From its thin edge, a sheet of connective tissue, the *basilar membrane*, extends across the canal to its opposite wall to join the *spiral ligament of the cochlea*, a thickening of the periosteum. A second partition, the *vestibular membrane*, arising from a soft tissue ridge on the upper surface of the spiral lamina, diverges from the basilar membrane and joins the spiral ligament (Fig. 35–10). The lumen of the cochlear canal is, thus, partitioned into three spiral chambers: the *scala vestibuli* (above), the *scala tympani* (below) and, between these, the *scala media*. The scala media, or cochlear duct, is triangular in cross section with its apex at the limbus. Its roof is the vestibular membrane and its floor is formed by the spiral lamina and the basilar membrane. The scala media contains endolymph, and the scala vestibuli and scala tympani are perilymphatic spaces, and they communicate, at the apex of the cochlea, through a small opening, the *helicotrema*.

On the outer surface of the vestibular membrane (Reissner's membrane), toward the scala vestibuli, there is a layer of squamous perilymphatic cells so thin that it is scarcely detectable with the light microscope. The surface, toward the scala media, is lined by squamous cells that bear, on their free surface, many short clavate microvilli, resembling those found on the cells of the choroid plexus. Lateral cell processes interdigitate extensively with those of neighboring cells, and the basal surface is highly infolded, suggesting that this epithelium may have a role in water and electrolyte transport.

Stria Vascularis

At the wall of the cochlea, the epithelium on the inner side of the vestibular membrane is continuous with a band of stratified epithelium, called the *stria vascularis*, which contains an intraepithelial plexus of capillaries (Fig. 35–10). In this epithelium, it is possible to distinguish two types of cells—a layer of light-staining *basal cells* and a superficial layer of darker-staining *marginal cells*. A third cell type, *intermediate cells*, has been described by some investigators. Although the latter are intermediate between basal and marginal cells in location, they are difficult to distinguish from basal cells by their ultrastructure or staining properties. The convex free surface of the marginal cells is covered with microvilli and their dense cytoplasm contains many small vesicles and mitochondria. The basal portion of the cell consists of a labyrinthine system of narrow cell processes occupied by long mitochondria (Fig. 35–11). The lighter intermediate and basal cells contain relatively few mitochondria but have radiating processes that interdigitate with the processes of other intermediate cells and with those of the marginal cells. The basal cells also have ascending processes that may form cup-like structures that surround, and partially isolate, the bases of the marginal cells. The intraepithelial capillaries are closely enveloped by descending processes of the marginal cells and ascending processes of the basal and intermediate cells.

On the lateral wall of the cochlear duct, the stria vascularis extends from the vestibular membrane, superiorly, to the *spiral prominence*, inferiorly. There, its basal layer is continuous with a thin layer of cells over the prominence, which is a highly vascular thickening of the periosteum that follows a spiral course on the lateral wall of the cochlear duct for its entire

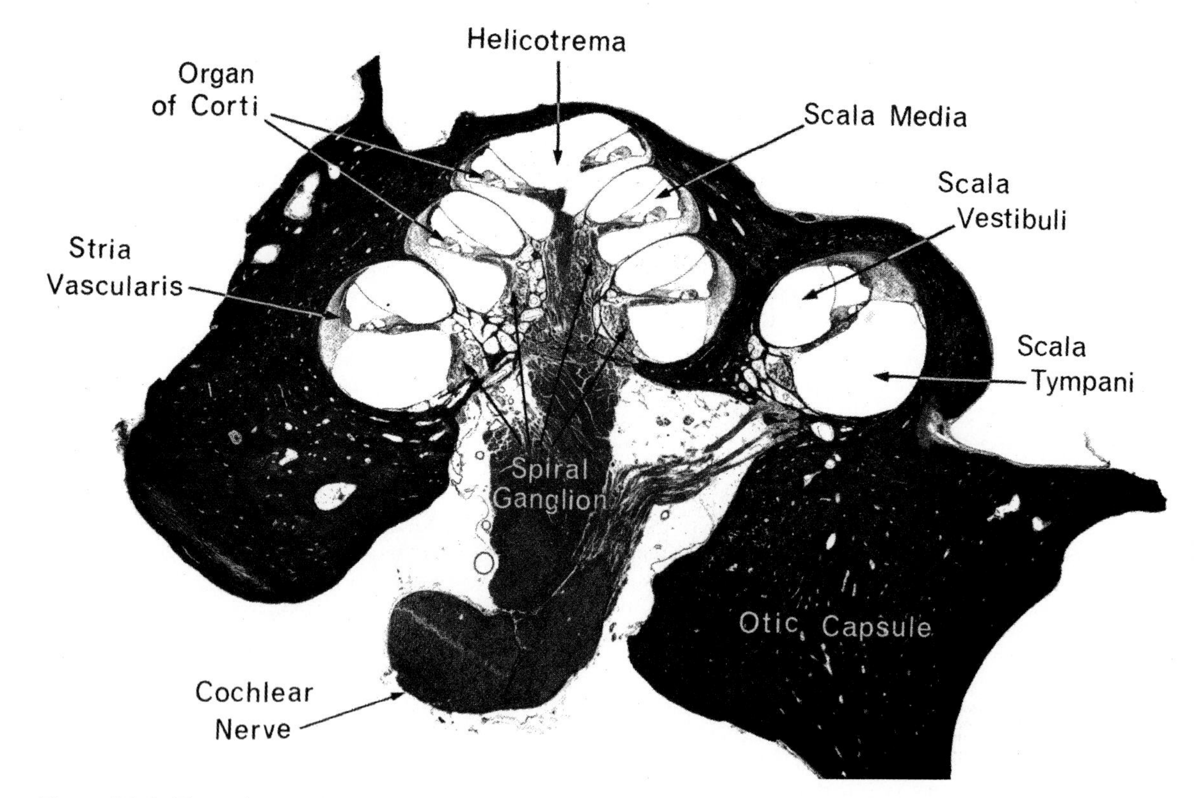

Figure 35–9. Photomicrograph of a section through the axis of the cochlea showing the organ of Corti on the basilar membrane, and the scala vestibuli, scala media, and scala tympani. (Courtesy of H. Mizoguchi.)

length. Below the spiral prominence, the epithelium lines the *external spiral sulcus* and then is reflected onto the basilar lamina. The cells in the sulcus take on a cuboidal shape, and those continuing onto the basilar membrane are known as the *cells of Claudius*. In the basal coil of the cochlea, but not elsewhere, small groups of polyhedral *cells of Boettcher* are interposed between the cells of Claudius and the basilar membrane. These cells have large spherical nuclei and their cytoplasm is denser than that of the adjoining cells of Claudius. The plasma membrane over their lower half has small villi that interdigitate with adjacent cells or project into intercellular spaces. Their function is not known.

In electron micrographs, the elaborate basal compartmentation of the marginal cells of the stria vascularis resembles that of other cells in the body that are involved in electrolyte transport. This suggested that this specialized epithelium might be important in maintaining the unique ionic composition of the endolymph. This is borne out by explorations with microelectrodes which indicate that the stria vascularis is the source of the large positive endocochlear electrical potential (see below).

Spiral Limbus

Where the vestibular membrane and the basilar membrane converge at the inner angle of the scala media, the periosteal connective tissue over the osseous spiral lamina bulges into the scala media, forming the *limbus of the spiral lamina* (Fig. 35–10). Its tapering upper edge projects laterally over a recess called the *internal spiral sulcus* (or tunnel) (Fig. 35–12), bounded above by the vestibular lip, and below by the tympanic lip of the limbus, which is continuous with the basilar membrane (Figs. 35–12 and 35–13). Within the body of the limbus, the collagen fiber bundles are oriented vertically, forming distinctive markings, inappropriately called the *auditory teeth.* Between these bundles are stellate fibroblasts. Uniformly spaced along the upper surface of the limbus, between the auditory teeth, are the so-called *interdental cells* that secrete the *tectorial membrane*, which extends laterally over the hair cells of the organ of Corti. The bases of the interdental cells are firmly embedded in the connective tissue of the limbus, and their apices spread out over the surface of the limbus where they interdigitate and are joined

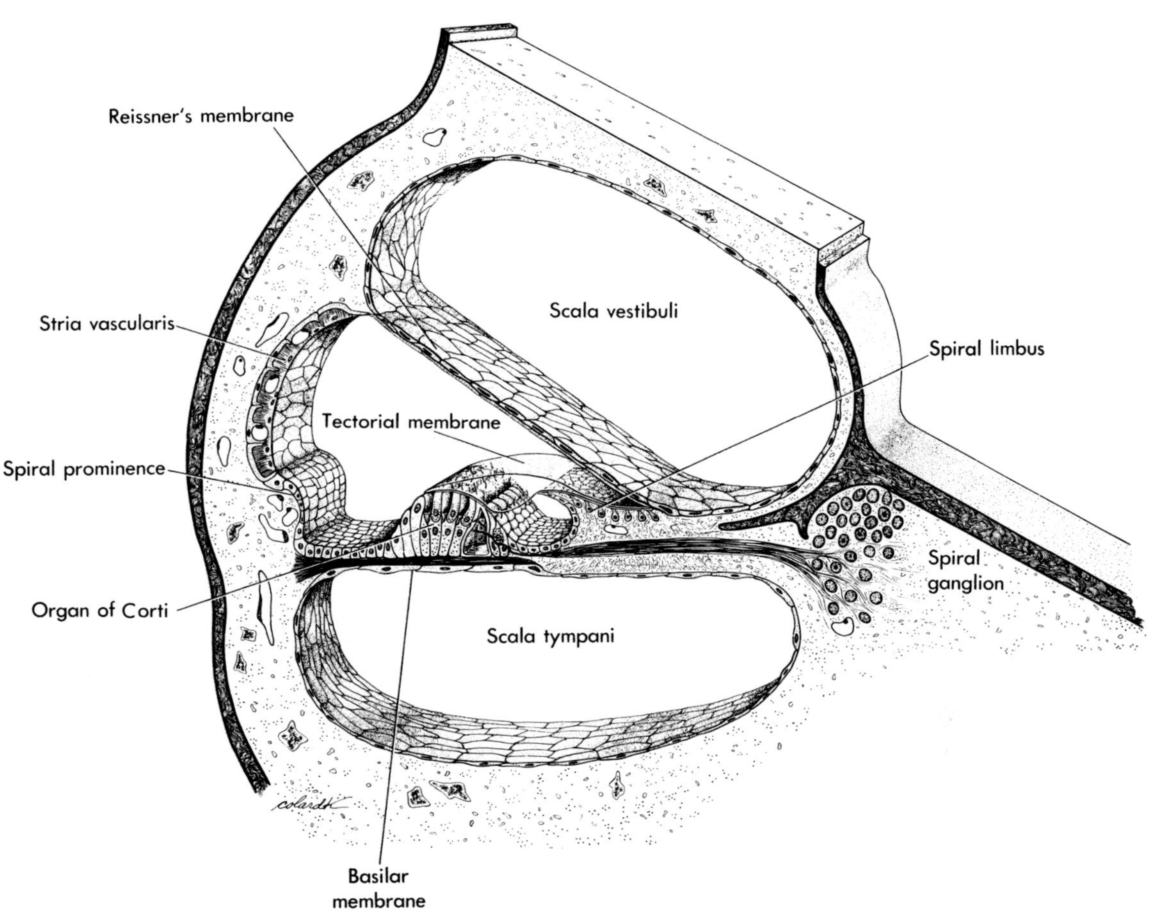

Figure 35–10. Schematic representation of a section through one of the turns of the cochlea showing the principal structures in the scala media. (Drawing by Silvia Collard Keene.)

by junctional complexes to form a continuous sheet over the limbus.

Tectorial Membrane

The tectorial membrane, secreted at the upper surface of the interdental cells, forms a cuticular layer over these cells and extends laterally, beyond the vestibular lip of the limbus, to cover the organ of Corti (Fig. 35–13). The tips of the longer hair cells of this organ are embedded in, or bound to, the under side of the tectorial membrane. The space commonly seen between the membrane and the hair cells, in electron micrographs, is now thought to be artifactitious. The tectorial membrane is composed of fine filaments embedded in a gelatinous matrix rich in mucopolysaccharides. Its fibers consist of a protein believed to be similar to epidermal keratin.

Basilar Membrane

The basilar membrane extends across the cochlear canal from the spiral lamina on the modiolus to the spiral ligament on its lateral wall. It separates the scala media from the scala tympani and supports the organ of Corti. It is about 0.25 mm across and 35 mm long, extending from the base of the cochlea to its apex. It has two zones: a thin *zona arcuata* between its medial attachment and the base of outermost cells of the organ of Corti; and a thicker outer portion, the *zona pectinata*, from there to the spiral ligament. The zona arcuata that supports the organ of Corti is made up of radially oriented 10-nm collagen-like fibrils. The zona pectinata is a trilaminar structure. The upper layer is a meshwork of fibers, mainly transverse in their orientation. The lower layer consists of longitudinal fibers, and between these is a structureless intermediate layer containing a few fibroblast-like cells.

The width of the basilar membrane gradually increases from 0.20 mm in the basal turn of the cochlea to 0.36 mm at the apex, and the diameter of its component fibers gradually decreases. As a result of these dimensional

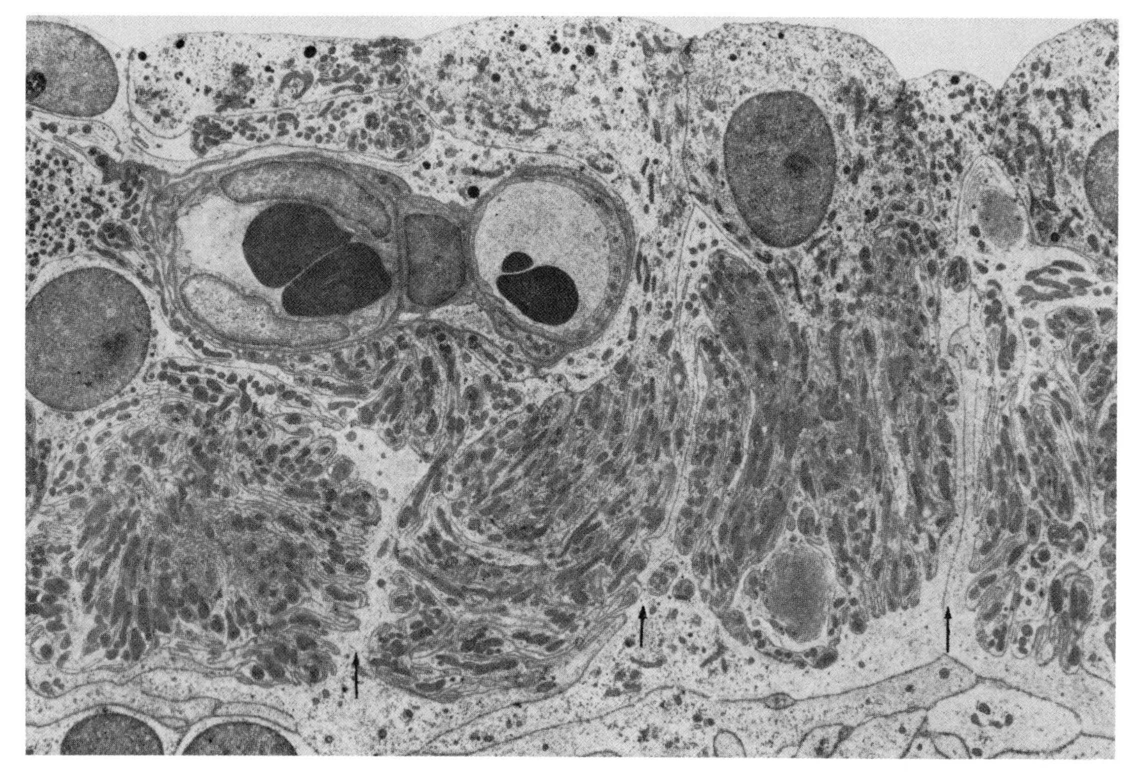

Figure 35–11. Electron micrograph of the stria vascularis of the cat inner ear illustrating the intraepithelial capillaries, the ascending processes of the basal cells (at arrows), and the dark-staining, elaborately infolded bases of the marginal cells. (From Hinojosa, R. and E. Rodriguez-Eschandia. 1966. Am. J. Anat. 118:631.)

and ultrastructural differences along the length of the basilar membrane, it is believed to vibrate at a higher frequency near the base, and at a lower frequency, near the helicotrema. These differences in resonance along the length of the basilar membrane are important in the discrimination of the frequency, or pitch, of sounds.

Organ of Corti

In the epithelium covering the basilar membrane, the cells become tall columnar at the lateral border of the internal spiral sulcus and form the complex sensory *organ of Corti,* the receptor for auditory stimuli (Figs. 35–12 and 35–13). This highly specialized epithelium is composed of hair cells and several kinds of supporting cells.

The supporting cells have certain characteristics in common. They are tall slender cells extending from the basilar membrane to the free surface of the organ of Corti and they contain conspicuous bundles of microtubules and filaments. Although the bodies of some of these cells are separated by wide intercellular spaces, their apical portions are in contact with each other, and with the hair cells, to form a highly ordered continuous free surface of the organ of Corti, referred to as the *reticular lamina* (Figs. 35–14 and 35–15). The several types of supporting cells include *inner* and *outer pillar cells, inner* and *outer phalangeal cells, border cells,* and the *cells of Hensen.*

The *inner pillar cells* have a broad base resting on the basilar membrane and a slender conical body extending upward. The segment of the cell body containing the nucleus is situated basally, at the inner angle of a wide triangular intercellular space, called the *inner tunnel* (Fig. 35–13). This space is continuous throughout the length of the cochlea and is bounded below by thin lateral extensions of the base of the pillar cells that rest on the basilar membrane. It is bounded above by the converging cylindrical bodies of the inner and outer pillar cells. The most distinctive feature of the inner pillar cells, viewed with the light microscope, is a large, dark-staining bundle of filaments that courses from the cell base, upward through the slender cell body to end at the apex, where the cell widens into a thin

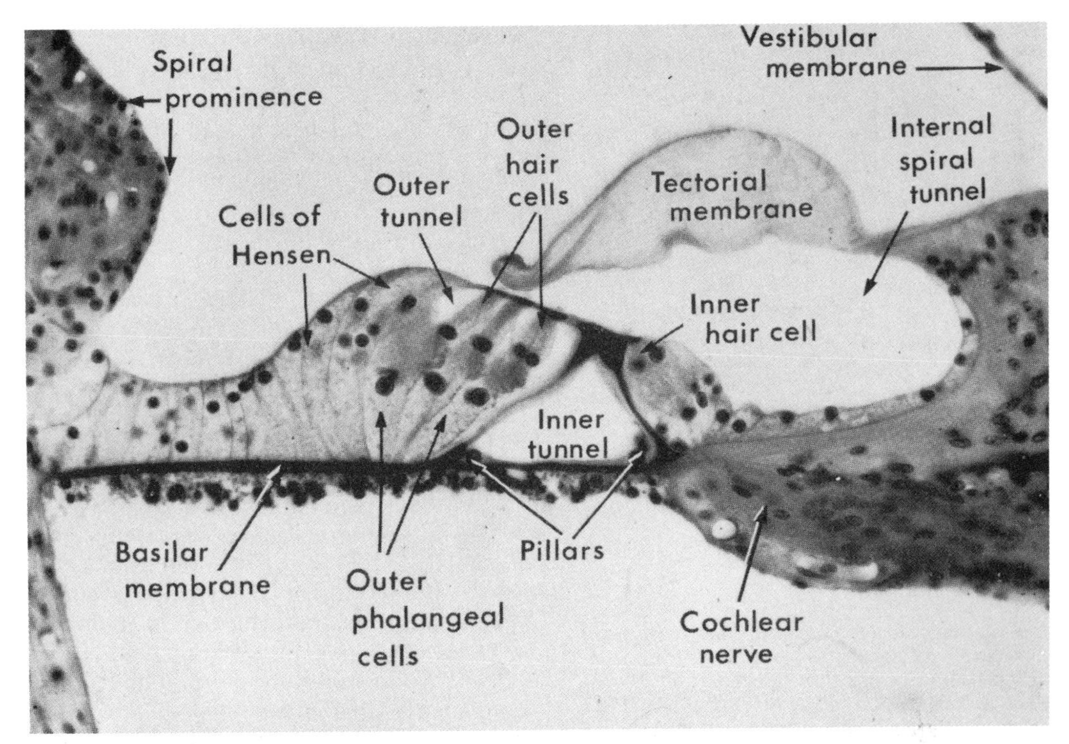

Figure 35–12. Photomicrograph of the organ of Corti of a cat. The tectorial membrane has been lifted off of the hair cells during specimen preparation. (Micrograph courtesy of H. Engström.)

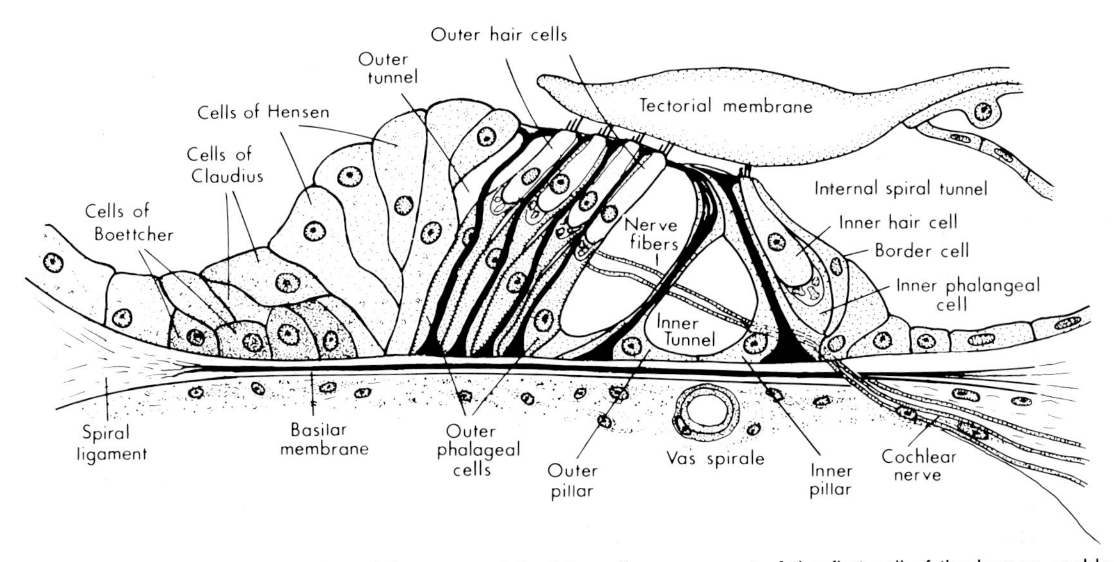

Figure 35–13. Drawing of a section of the organ of Corti from the upper part of the first coil of the human cochlea. (Redrawn and slightly modified after Held, J. 1908. Untersuchungen über der feineren Bau des Ohrlabyrinthes der Wierbeltiere Vol. I & II. Teubner, Leipzig.)

horizontal plate that contacts neighboring pillar cells and the inner hair cells (Fig. 35–16). What appeared, in histological sections, to be a bundle of tonofibrils is found in electron micrographs to be a bundle of closely spaced parallel microtubules, with 6-nm microfilaments interspersed among them (Fig. 35–17).

The *outer pillar cells* are longer and more oblique in their orientation, leaning toward the inner pillars. They have a broad thin base

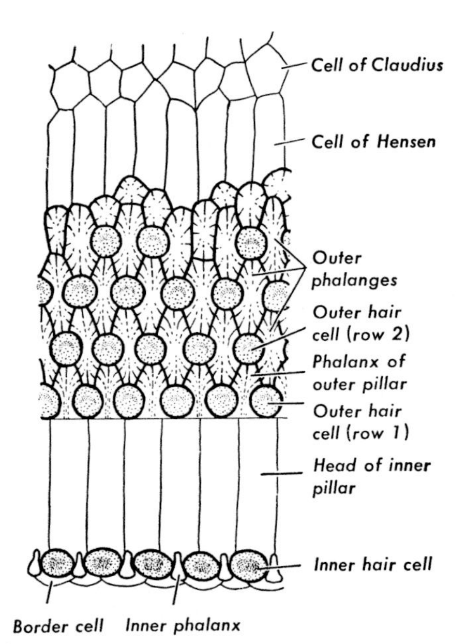

Figure 35–14. Diagram of the organ of Corti viewed from above showing the relationship of the heads of the phalangeal cell processes to the hair cells. (Modified from Kolmer, W. 1907. Arch. f. mikr. Anat. 74:259 and Schaffer, J. 1922. Lehrbuch der Histologie und Histogenese Verlag von W. Engelmann, Leipzig.)

adjoining that of the inner pillar cells. The cell body is similar, but its expanded upper end has a somewhat different shape. It abuts the underside of the flat head of the inner pillar cell. From lower down on the cell body, it also sends out a phalangeal process with a flat head that forms junctions, in the reticular lamina, with the hair cells and the expanded head of the phalangeal processes of the outer phalangeal cells, located between the rows of hair cells. The inner pillar cells number about 5600 and the outer pillars 3800. On average, the heads of three inner pillars abut the heads of two outer pillars. The area of contact between them is quite large, ensuring that they form a sound support for the hair cells.

The *outer phalangeal cells* (cells of Deiters) are the supporting cells for the three or four rows of outer hair cells. Their base is columnar with a cup-shaped upper end occupied by the inferior third of a hair cell. Thus, they surround the base of the hair cell and also the bundles of afferent and efferent nerves traveling to the hair cell (Fig. 35–18). The apex of these cells does not reach the free surface of the organ of Corti, but a slender phalangeal process projecting from the side of the cell does reach the reticular lamina (Figs. 35–19 and 35–20). This process is internally reinforced by a bundle of microtubules and filaments and its expanded distal end forms a flat plate joined, at its edges, to the hair cell it is supporting, and to the hair cell in the next row. The upper two-thirds of the hair cells is not immediately surrounded by other cells but is exposed within a fluid-filled *space of Nuel* which communicates with the inner tunnel through clefts between the pillar cells. The fluid that bathes the hair cells and occupies the space of Nuel and the tunnel is apparently sealed off from the endolymphatic space and, thus, may have a composition differing from that of either the endolymph or perilymph.

The *inner phalangeal cells* are arranged in a row on the inner side of the inner pillar cells. In contrast to the outer phalangeal cells, there are no large intercellular spaces between these supporting cells and the inner hair cells; indeed, they completely surround them. The relationship between the two is analogous to that between the supporting cells and hair cells of the vestibular system. The inner phalangeal cells are contiguous with a row of slender cells, termed *border cells*, which mark the inner boundary of the organ of Corti (Fig. 35–13). There is a gradual transition in height from these cells to the low cuboidal or squamous cells that line the internal spiral sulcus. The outer border of the organ of Corti is delimited by the tall *cells of Hensen* adjacent to the last row of outer phalangeal cells. These are arranged in several rows decreasing rapidly in height to become continuous laterally with the cells of Claudius.

There are two types of hair cells in the cochlea. The *inner hair cells* are arranged in a single row along the entire length of the organ of Corti. The *outer hair cells* form three rows and are lodged between the outer pillar cells and the outer phalangeal cells. In the human, a fourth, and sometimes a fifth, row may be found near the apex of the cochlea.

Inner hair cells resemble the type-I cells of the vestibular labyrinth in many respects. They are relatively short cells with a slightly narrowed neck region. The specializations of their free surface include 50–60 stereocilia (hairs) distributed on the cell surface in a U-shaped pattern. As in vestibular hair cells, the stereocilia have a core of actin filaments arranged in a paracrystalline array. The core is stabilized by cross-links of fimbrin between the actin filaments and these contribute to the stiffness of the shaft. The core is connected to the inner surface of the plasmalemma of the stereocilium by small densities about 4 nm

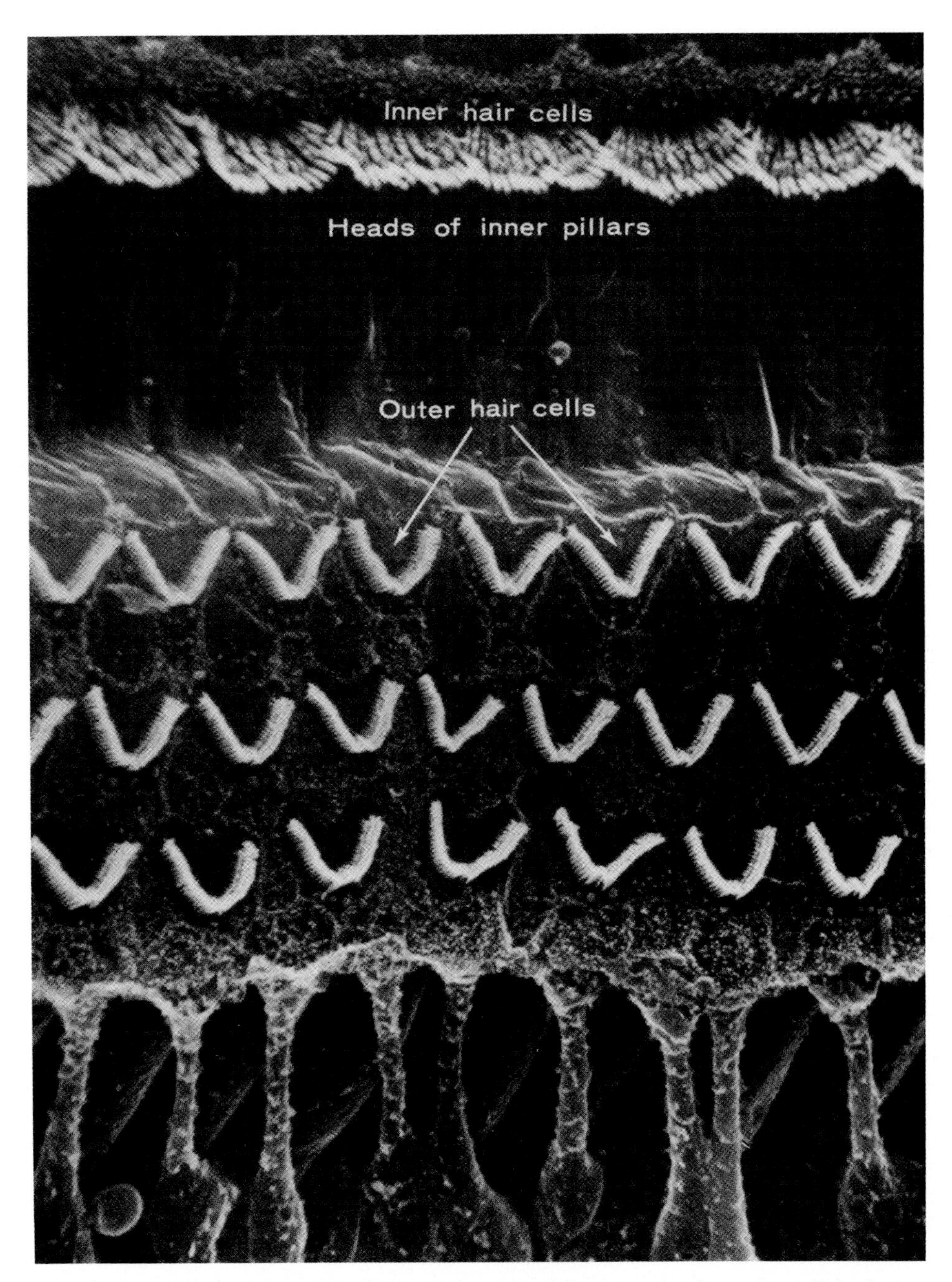

Figure 35–15. Scanning electron micrograph of guinea pig organ of Corti as seen from above. This view corresponds to that diagrammed in Fig. 35–14. (Micrograph courtesy of H. Engström.)

in diameter. Similar connections radiate from the slender portion of the core where the base of the stereocilium is continuous with the apical plasma membrane. The stereocilia of the inner hair cells gradually increase in length from the base to the apex of the cochlea.

It has recently been shown that minute filaments extend from the upper end of each shorter stereocilium to the membrane of the nearest taller stereocilium (Fig 35–21). These so-called *tip links* are not preserved after long exposure to the osmium tetroxide used as a fixative for electron microscopy, and they were only revealed recently. Since their discovery, they have aroused great interest as a component of the postulated *tension-gated transducer channels* responsible for depolarization of the cells on bending of the stereocilia.

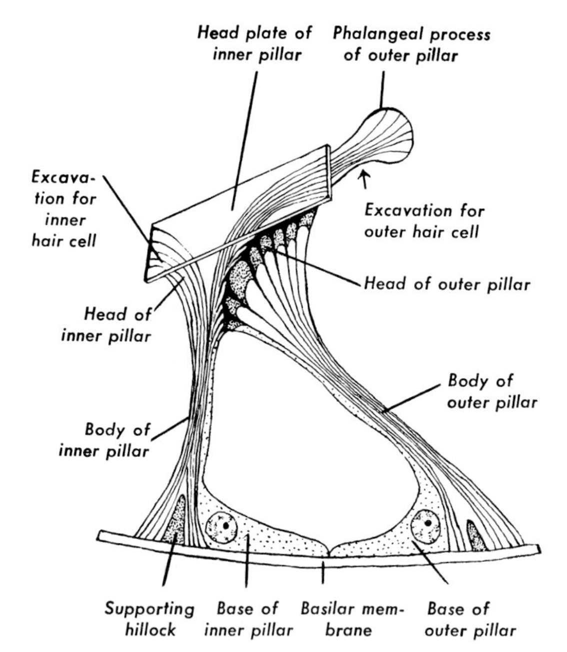

Figure 35–16. Diagram of the inner and outer pillars of the organ of Corti. (Modified from Kolmer, W. 1907. Arch. f. mikr. Anat. 74:259.)

A kinocilium is lacking but is represented by a basal body and associated centriole beneath the apical plasma membrane. The rootlets of the hairs extend downward into, and sometimes through, a thick terminal web, or cuticular plate, that traverses the apex of the cell and ends in the junctional complexes with adjacent supporting cells. Actin filaments of various orientation form the web across the cell apex, and others course parallel, forming a circumferential ring at the level of the zonula adherens. The nucleus is located in the central region of the cell. The cytoplasm contains abundant mitochondria aggregated beneath the terminal web and scattered elsewhere in the cell. There are also profiles of rough and smooth endoplasmic reticulum, occasional lysosomes, and many small vesicles. Microtubules are present in small numbers, mainly in the basal cytoplasm.

The synaptic area of the cell extends from the base to the level of the nucleus. The majority of the endings contacting the inner hair cells are sparsely vesiculated and are considered to be afferent endings of the cochlear nerve. Although some of these run along the side of the cell up to the level of the nucleus, not all of the area of contact is synaptic. The sites of afferent synaptic transmission are recognized by presynaptic and postsynaptic membrane thickening and by the presence of synaptic ribbons in the adjacent cytoplasm of the hair cell. Ninety-five percent of the afferent fibers of the cochlea are associated with the inner hair cells. In addition to these, there are occasional small endings containing large numbers of synaptic vesicles, of which some have dense cores. Although these heavily vesiculated endings rarely contact the hair cell, they often make contact with the afferent nerve fibers just before these make contact with the inner hair cell.

Outer hair cells differ significantly from inner hair cells in their ultrastructure and this has led to the assumption that the two cell types have quite different functions. They are long cylindrical cells with a basally placed euchromatic nucleus. The hairs on their free surface are distributed in a distinctive W-shaped pattern, and there are more rows of hairs than on the inner hair cells (Fig. 35–22). Up to 100 hairs have been counted and the stepwise gradation in their length is more apparent than in inner hair cells. A kinocilium is lacking, but a basal body is present beneath the base of the W. Deep to the terminal web, dense lipid-like inclusions are interspersed among highly convoluted elements of the granular endoplasmic reticulum. Mitochondria are generally located in the basal cytoplasm, but some are aligned parallel to the lateral cell membranes. There are extensive cisternae of the endoplasmic reticulum in the peripheral cytoplasm, parallel to the lateral cell membranes. Unlike the supporting cells, hair cells do not have a cytoskeleton of intermediate filaments nor do they have desmosomes to which such filaments normally attach. However, outer hair cells do have a thin *cortical lattice* about 25 nm beneath the lateral cell membrane. In isolated cells, this cytoskeletal lattice maintains the cell shape and resists mechanical deformation even after removal of the plasmalemma by detergents. It consists of many closely spaced circumferential filaments 5–7 nm in diameter, cross-linked at regular intervals by thinner longitudinal filaments. In the portion of the cell above the level of the nucleus, the plasmalemma overlying this lattice has a unique structure. In etched freeze–fracture preparations, it contains large intramembrane particles, closely packed at a density of about 2500 particles per square micrometer. Such dense arrays of intramembrane particles are not found in comparable preparations of inner hair cells. Short, dense *pillars* are reported to link these particles to the circumferential filaments of the cortical lattice.

The base of the outer hair cell is set in a

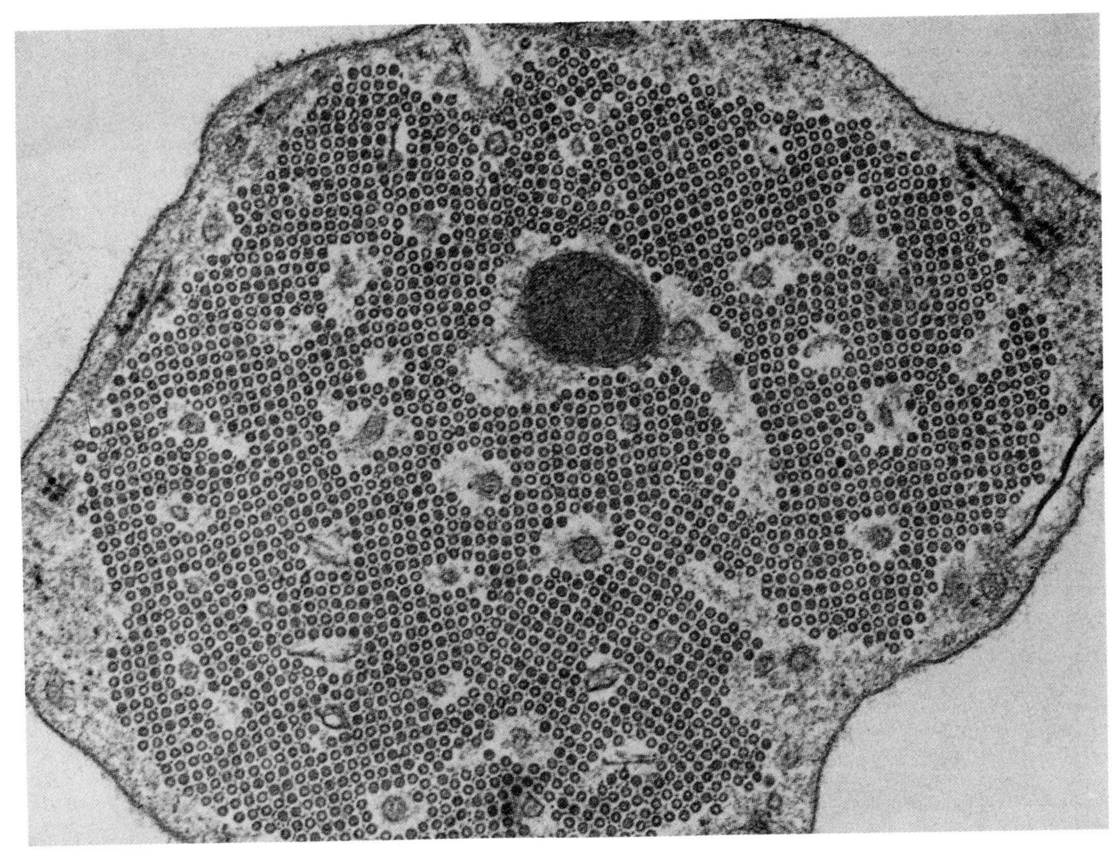

Figure 35–17. Electron micrograph of a cross section through an inner pillar cell showing the highly ordered bundle of microtubules and filaments, interrupted by rather uniformly spaced tubular elements of the endoplasmic reticulum. (Micrograph courtesy of H. Engström.)

cup-like depression in the upper end of its supporting phalangeal cell body. Both afferent and efferent nerve endings are in contact with the hair cell in this region. The efferent endings on the outer hair cells are larger than those of the afferent fibers and contain many densely packed vesicles. A single flat cisterna, the *subsynaptic cisterna*, is found in the cytoplasm parallel to the plasmalemma for the entire length of the efferent synapse.

The hair cells are evenly distributed in rows and their apices are fixed in position in the rather rigid *reticular lamina* which is a mosaic of the apical ends of the hair cells, surrounded by the flat, plate-like heads of the outer phalangeal cell processes (Fig. 35–14). Owing to the bundles of microtubules in the inner and outer pillar cells, which attach to the junctional complexes in their heads, and the comparable microtubule bundles of the phalangeal cell processes, the basilar membrane, the pillar cells, and the reticular lamina are believed to move together as a unit. Thus, during vibration of the basilar membrane, a rocking motion of the reticular membrane is believed to result in a shearing motion of the hair cells with respect to the tectorial membrane with which they are in contact. The resulting deflection of the stereocilia and depolarization of the hair cells generates a stimulus to the afferent nerve fibers in synaptic contact with their base.

Millions of people suffer from hearing loss attributable to loss or damage to hair cells. In cold-blooded animals, hair cells are produced throughout life and damaged cells are replaced, but it has long been assumed that in humans, and other mammals, hair cells are formed only in the embryo and that their loss in adult life due to aging, trauma, or aminoglycoside antibiotics will inevitably result in permanent deafness. There has been some modification of this pessimistic view due to recent ultrastructural studies which have shown that, in guinea pigs, vestibular hair cells destroyed by gramicidin can be regenerated. Other studies on vestibular sensory epithelia of guinea pigs, and humans, cultivated in vitro, after destruction of hair cells with antibiotics, have demonstrated a limited capacity of

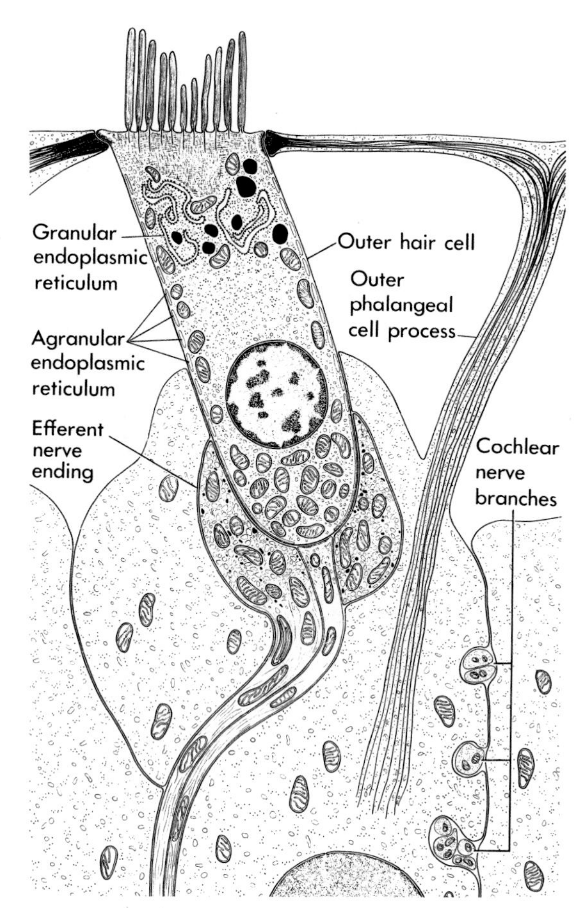

Figure 35–18. Schematic representation of the relationship between an outer hair cell and the head of the process of its supporting phalangeal cell. Note the termination of the bundle of microtubules of the phalangeal cell process in the junctional complex with the hair cell. (Drawing by Sylvia Collard Keene.)

the supporting cells to proliferate and differentiate into hair cells.

HISTOPHYSIOLOGY OF THE INNER EAR

The foregoing description of the highly complex structure of the inner ear may not have conveyed a coherent explanation of how it works. It may, therefore, be helpful to review briefly the traditional interpretation of the function of its several sensory components.

As previously stated, the vestibular apparatus responds to acceleration of the head during any sudden disturbance of equilibrium by generating nerve impulses to the brain that initiate reflexes which restore the body to its normal position. The vestibular receptor for *linear acceleration* of the head is the horizontally oriented *macula* in the fluid-filled utricle. The stereocilia of its hair cells project upward into the *otolith membrane* which contains crystals of calcium carbonate called otoliths or otoconia. These are thought to provide added inertia that resists displacement of the membrane by external forces. When the head undergoes linear acceleration, the membrane tends to remain relatively stationary, whereas the hair cells beneath it move slightly with the wall of the utricle. This causes a deflection of the hairs in a direction opposite to that of the head movement. This, in turn, triggers nerve impulses that relay this information to the brain initiating corrective reflexes. The orientation of the macula of the saccule is nearly vertical and it responds to head movements at a right angle to those that activate the macula of the utricle.

The receptors that detect *angular acceleration* of the head are situated in the *ampullae* of the three semicircular canals. Here, the hair cells are on the surface of the *crista ampullaris* and their stereocilia project into the *cupula.* Angular acceleration of the head causes motion of the wall of the canal, relative to the endolymph in its lumen. As the cupula is displaced by this movement, the stereocilia are flexed in the opposite direction, resulting in depolarization of the hair cells and an increase in the rate of transmission of impulses to the brain.

Sound waves produce vibrations of the *tympanic membrane* that are transmitted via the incus, malleus, and stapes to the fluid in the cochlear canal. These bones of the middle ear have an amplifying effect, transforming a very small pressure on the eardrum to a 20-fold greater pressure on the fluid in the cochlea. The foot-plate of the stapes acts like a piston alternately compressing and easing pressure on the fluid. The resulting vibrations of the basilar membrane cause a rocking motion of the organ of Corti and the resulting shearing forces move the stereocilia of the hair cells, with respect to the overlying tectorial membrane. Deflection of the stereocilia toward the tall side of the hair bundle causes depolarization of the hair cells generating impulses in the associated afferent nerves.

The ability of the ear to distinguish the frequency, or pitch, of the sound has long been attributed to differences in the width of the basilar membrane along its length and to differences in the length of the stereocilia on the

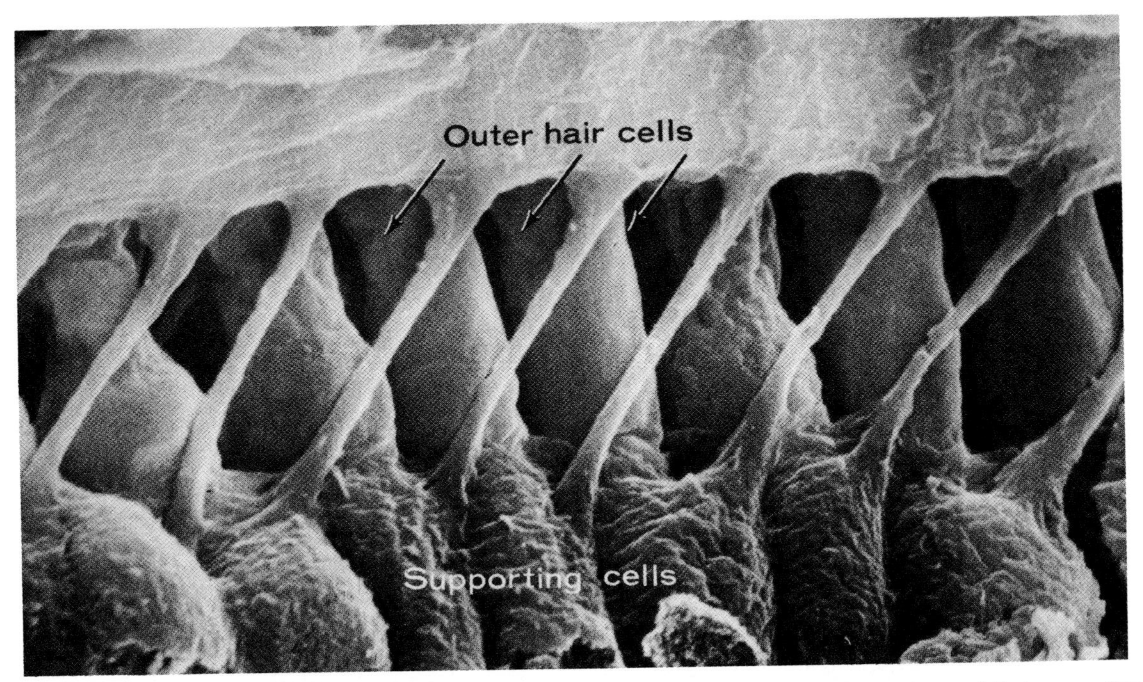

Figure 35–19. Scanning electron micrograph of outer hair cells and the slender lateral processes of their supporting phalangeal cells (cells of Deiters). (Micrograph courtesy of H. Engström.)

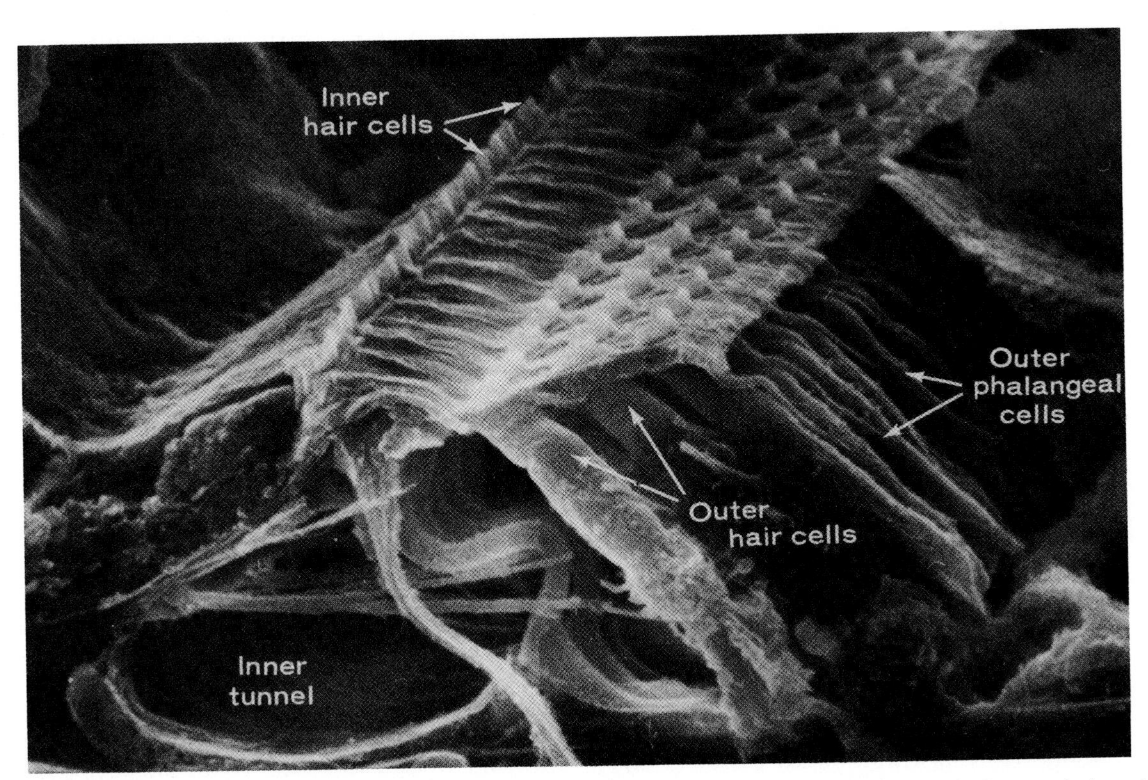

Figure 35–20. Scanning electron micrograph of a guinea pig organ of Corti, cut transversely, in front and viewed longitudinally. Note the rows of hairs (top) and the outer phalangeal cells (at the right). (Micrograph courtesy of H. Engström.)

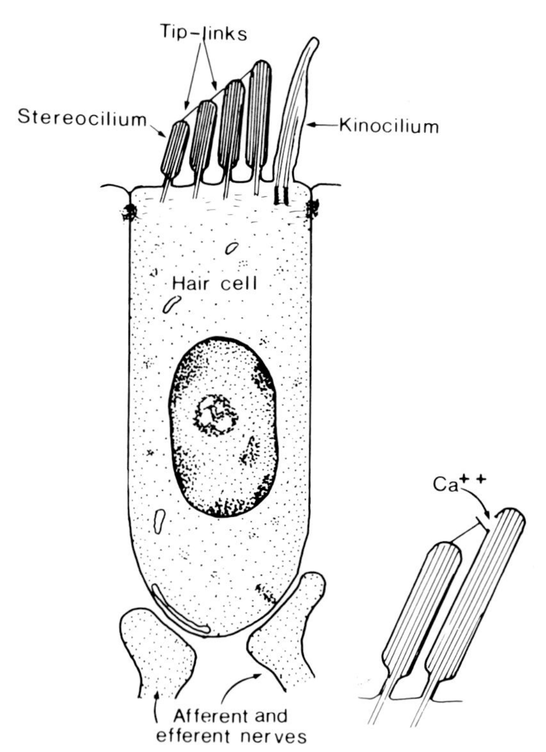

Figure 35–21. Drawing of a vestibular hair cell showing its kinocilium, stereocilia, and tip links. (Redrawn after Corwin, J.T. and M.E. Warchol. 1991. Annu. Rev. Neurosci. 14:301.)

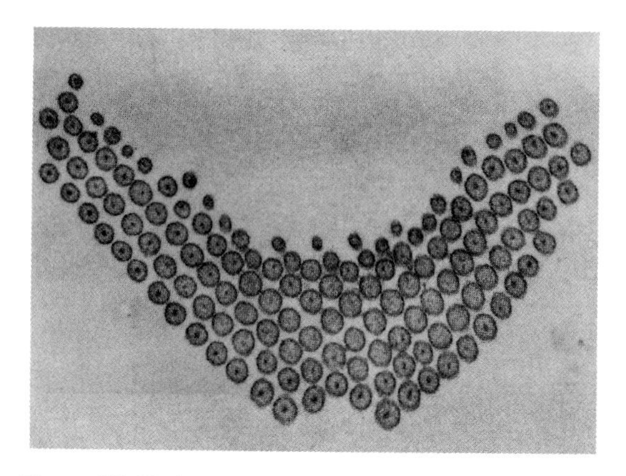

Figure 35–22. Low-power electron micrograph of a cross section of the stereocilia on a hair cell of the human organ of Corti, showing their W-like configuration. (Courtesy of R. Kimura.)

hair cells. Each tone was believed to produce maximal amplitude of vibration in a different region of the membrane, with sounds of high frequency having the greatest effect on the membrane near the base of the cochlea, and sounds of low frequency producing maximal vibration near the helicotrema. Nerve fibers from each level along the membrane are thought to conduct impulses to an area of the brain where there are neurones that are activated by specific frequencies.

Buried within the temporal bone, the inner ear was long inaccessible to experimentation, but in the past two decades, it has become possible to remove its receptor organs, and even single hair cells, and to maintain them for some time, in vitro, in fluid of appropriate electrolyte composition. By mechanically stimulating these isolated elements and recording the resulting electrical responses, much additional information has been gained to fill the gaps in the broad outline of inner ear function outlined above.

The hair cells are found to have a negative intracellular potential of −150mV with respect to the endolymph bathing their free surface. This is a higher resting potential than is found in any other cells in the body and this probably increases their sensitivity to very slight movements of their hairs. Their displacement toward the tall side of the bundle opens channels, permitting influx of cations that depolarize the cell by tens of millivolts. A deflexion of the tips of the hairs by 50–120 nm results in a near maximal response of the hair cells. A deflection of only about + 3 nm is the threshold for hearing. This is said to be comparable to displacement of the top of the Eiffel tower by a thumbs breadth. There are no more than 100 transduction channels per cell, and although they have not yet been isolated, they are estimated to be at least 0.7 nm in diameter. They are relatively nonselective, but potassium (K^+), which is present in high concentration in the endolymph, is the cation that carries most of the transduction current but calcium is also involved. The time course of ion-channel opening is so short that it is unlikely that a second messenger is involved. The mechanism of opening of the channels has now been clarified by the discovery of the *tip links.* These are so situated that they would be stretched by deflection of the hairs toward the tall side of the bundle and would, thus, act as gating springs opening the ion channels. Their orientation is also consistent with the greater sensitivity of the hair cells to displacement of the hairs toward the tall side of the bundle.

There have also been interesting new findings relating to the mechanism of sound-frequency selectivity within the cochlea. The passive mechanism, based on differing width of the basilar membrane along its length, still

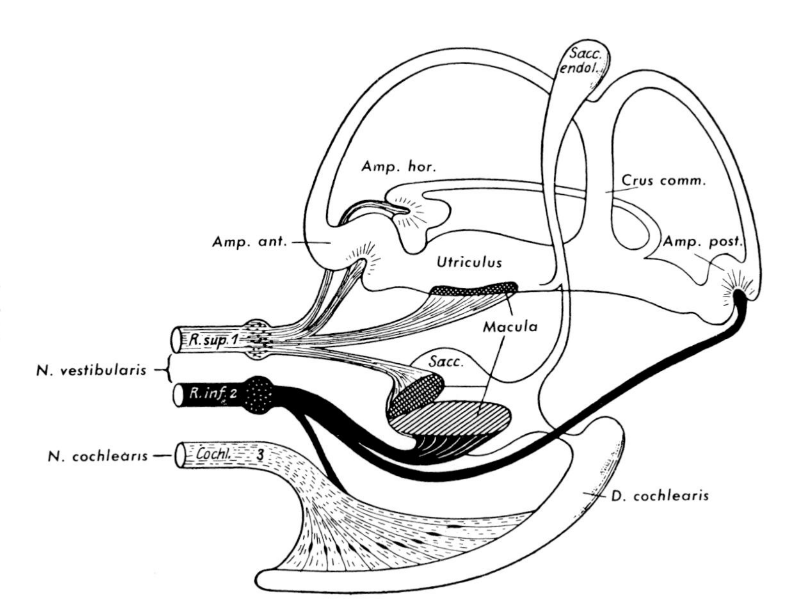

Figure 35–23. Diagram of the distribution of nerves to the membranous labyrinth of the rabbit. (After Kolmer, W. 1909. Arch. f. mikr. Anat. 74:259.)

holds, but there is new evidence for an active fine-tuning of frequency selectivity by motor activity of the hair cells. The outer hair cells normally vary in length from 20–50 μm, near the base of the cochlea, to 75–90 μm, near its apex. Isolated outer hair cells in the absence of the basilar membrane have been found to respond to mechanical or electrical stimulation with a slight change in their length. Long cells respond best to low frequencies, and short cells to high frequencies. The best frequency for inducing a motor response in a given cell is correlated with the length of the cell and its original position in the cochlea. When depolarized, outer hair cells can contract about 10% of their normal length over a time span of 30–60 s. This is described as their *slow motility*. When stimulated with an AC voltage the cells respond with a lengthwise oscillation of about 4% of the their length. This is referred to as their *fast motility*. The mechanism of these motor responses of the hair cells is a subject of debate. There is no ultrastructural evidence for actin-myosin interaction. Ingenious experiments, involving observations on a small area of the lateral cell membrane inside the tip of a patch electrode, suggest that the motor is not in the cytoplasm but in the specialized region of the lateral cell membrane above the level of the nucleus. An increase in membrane area was observed in response to hyperpolarization and a decrease in response to depolarization. The changes in cell length would then be secondary to changes in the total area of the cell membrane. It was suggested that the increase and decrease in membrane area result from voltage-dependent conformational changes in the large intramembrane particles, in this region, that are connected to the circumferential filaments of the cortical lattice. Other possible mechanisms have been suggested, and this problem has yet to be solved to the satisfaction of all investigators.

THE PERILYMPHATIC LABYRINTH

As previously indicated, the membranous labyrinth is a closed system of thin-walled channels which communicate freely with one another. It includes the utricle and saccule in the vestibule, the semicircular ducts, and the cochlear duct. All portions of the membranous labyrinth are filled with the viscous fluid called *endolymph*. The spaces surrounding the membranous labyrinth constitute the *perilymphatic labyrinth*. It includes the narrow space between the wall of the utricle and saccule and the surrounding bone, and the wider scalae vestibuli and tympani that flank the cochlear duct. It contains cells, fibers, and the fluid called *perilymph*.

Where the space is narrow, the perilymphatic tissue is a very loose reticulum made up primarily of the highly attenuated processes of many stellate perilymphatic cells, with very few associated extracellular fibers. In the wider parts of the perilymphatic labyrinth, more fibers are formed and may make up a relatively dense sheath 1–2 μm thick. In some species, the fibers associated with the perilymphatic cells differ from any other known extracellular fiber. They occur in bundles composed of a variable number of dense 10-nm filaments which have been shown to be made up of four 5-nm subunits helically wound around one another and embedded in an amorphous matrix. The cells that line the scala vestibuli and scala tympani are not stellate but are very thin squamous cells except in the vicinity of the basilar membrane where they may become cuboidal. They have no distinctive ultrastructural features.

The fluids in the perilymphatic labyrinth and the membranous labyrinth are strikingly different in their chemical composition. The perilymph is quite similar to extracellular fluid, in general, whereas the endolymph resembles intracellular fluid in its ionic composition, being rich in K^+ and low in Na^+. The source of the perilymph is still in debated. Some believe it is an ultrafiltrate of blood plasma, whereas others think it is derived from cerebrospinal fluid. It is generally agreed that endolymph is a product of secretion, but the site of its production remains unclear. The cells of the stria vascularis, those of the spiral prominence in the cochlea, and the cells around the maculae and cristae in the vestibule have been considered likely candidates, and electron micrographs reveal that all of these cells have a structure consistent with a secretory function. In autoradiographic studies, cells of the planum semilunatum, adjacent to the vestibular receptor sites, have been implicated in elaboration of sulfated mucopolysaccharides. Measurements with microelectrodes have suggested that the high potential of the scala media results from ion secretion by the stria vascularis, but the origin of the endolymph is still shrouded in uncertainty.

NERVES OF THE LABYRINTH

The sensory areas of the labyrinth are supplied by the eighth cranial nerve. It consists of two parts, the *vestibular* and the *cochlear nerves*, which differ in their function and central connections. Each is composed of primary afferent fibers from the sensory areas, and efferent feedback fibers from the central nervous system. The cell bodies of the afferent fibers are bipolar cells located in the *spiral ganglion* (cochlear ganglion) in the modiolus, and in the *vestibular ganglion* (Scarpa's ganglion) in the internal auditory meatus of the temporal bone.

The vestibular nerve divides into a superior and an inferior branch. The superior branch supplies the horizontal crista ampullaris, the superior crista ampullaris, the macula utriculi, and a small part of the macula sacculi. The inferior branch supplies the posterior crista ampullaris and the major portion of the macula sacculi. It also sends a small branch to the cochlear nerve.

The bipolar cell bodies, both in the vestibular ganglion and in the cochlear ganglion, are invested by a thin layer of myelin and this continues onto the axons. The axons of the cochlear nerve lose their myelin as they run through the openings of the osseous spiral lamina beneath the inner hair cells. Myelin persists in the vestibular nerve until the nerve enters the sensory area.

The cochlear nerve contains two morphological kinds of afferent nerve fibers. The more numerous kind radiates from the spiral ganglion in parallel bundles to the nearest segments of the organ of Corti. Because of their course, they are called the *radial acoustic fibers*. The second category of fibers, usually fewer and thicker than the first, are also arranged radially at the outset, but after reaching the outer hair cells of the organ of Corti, they turn sharply and follow a spiral course. These are called the *spiral fibers* (Fig. 35–23). The functional implications of these differing patterns of distribution are unclear. The relationship between the peripheral receptors and acoustic neurons is not as individualized as the monosynaptic relationship of the foveal cones in the retina, but it is sufficiently restricted to permit the reception of stimuli localized to small segments along the length of the cochlea.

The vestibular nerve terminates centrally in the reflex centers of the medulla oblongata and cerebellum. Its cortical connections are unknown, but it mediates reflex movements of the eyes through its thalamic connections. The cochlear nerve synapses in the cochlear nucleus, from which fibers ascend in the lateral lemniscus to the medial geniculate body of the thalamus and then to the temporal gyri of the cortex.

Both the vestibular and the cochlear divisions of the eighth cranial nerve contain appreciable numbers of efferent fibers that originate bilaterally from the vicinity of the superior olive. Initially, these fibers travel in the vestibular nerve, but within the internal auditory meatus, some efferent fibers reach the cochlear nerve via the anastomosis between the vestibular and cochlear nerve. The peripheral terminations of the efferent component are presumably at the hair cells, but incontrovertible evidence for the position and mode of ending of these fibers is still lacking. Stimulation of the efferent bundle results in suppression of auditory nerve activity, and anatomical evidence derived from sectioning the bundle indicates that the "granulated" endings are efferent because they apparently degenerate after sectioning.

BLOOD VESSELS OF THE LABYRINTH

The labyrinthine artery is a branch of the inferior cerebellar artery. It enters the internal auditory meatus and divides into the *vestibular artery* and the *common cochlear artery*. The latter divides into the *vestibulocochlear artery* and the *cochlear artery proper*. The vestibular artery supplies the upper and lateral parts of the utricle and saccule and parts of the superior and lateral semicircular ducts. It forms dense networks of capillaries in the region of the maculae. The vestibulocochlear artery supplies, with its vestibular branch, the lower and medial parts of the utricle and saccule, the crus commune, and the posterior semicircular duct. Its cochlear branch supplies the lowest part of the first cochlear coil.

The cochlear artery proper penetrates the cavities of the modiolus, where its tortuous branches run spirally to the apex. This is the so-called *spiral modiolar artery*. From it, branches go to the spiral ganglion and through the periosteum of the scala vestibuli and the osseous spiral lamina to the inner parts of the basilar membrane. Here, the capillaries are arranged in arcades in the tympanic covering layer under the tunnel and the limbus. The stria vascularis and spiral crest receive their blood through branches of the spiral modiolar artery, which run in the roof of the scala vestibuli. They do not form connections with the vessels of the basilar membrane. The lower wall of the scala tympani receives its own small arteries from the same source.

The course of the veins of the labyrinth is quite different from that of the arteries. There are three main venous drainage channels. In the cochlea, veins originate in the region of the spiral prominence and run downward and inward through the periosteum of the scala tympani to the spiral vein, which is found under the spiral ganglion. Above the spiral vein is the small vein of the spiral lamina, which receives a part of the blood from the spiral lamina and spiral ganglion and is connected by anastomoses with the spiral vein. These cochlear veins form a plexus in the modiolus, which empties partly into the internal auditory vein and partly into the vein of the cochlear aqueduct, which drains into the jugular vein. The veins of the vestibule empty into the veins of vestibular and cochlear aqueducts.

This arrangement of the vessels in the internal ear seems to ensure the best possible protection of the sound receptors from the arterial pulse wave. The arteries are arranged, for the most part, in the wall of the scala vestibuli, whereas the wall of the scala tympani contains the veins. The course of the spiral arteries in the modiolus probably also contributes to the damping of pulsations.

True lymphatics are absent from the labyrinth. Instead, fluid is drained into the perilymphatic spaces which are connected with the subarachnoid space. A certain amount of drainage may also be effected through perivascular and perineural connective tissue sheaths.

BIBLIOGRAPHY

GENERAL

Bast, T.H., and B.J. Anson. 1949. The Temporal Bone and the Ear. Springfield, IL, Charles C Thomas.

Bekesy, G. von. 1960. Experiments in Hearing. New York, McGraw-Hill Book Co.

Davis, H. 1968. Mechanisms of the inner ear. Ann. Otol. 77:644.

Engstrom, H., H. Ades, and A. Anderson. 1966. Structural Pattern of the Organ of Corti. Stockholm, Almquist and Wicksell.

Iurato, S., ed. 1967. Submicroscopic Structure of the Inner Ear. New York, Pergamon Press.

EXTERNAL EAR

Perry, E.T. 1957. The Human Ear Canal. Springfield, IL, Charles C Thomas.

Sophian, L.H. and B.H. Senturia. 1954. Anatomy and histology of the external ear in relation to the histogenesis of external otitis. Laryngoscope 64:772.

EUSTACHIAN TUBE

Graves, G.O. and L.F. Edwards. 1944. The eustachian tube. A Review of its descriptive, microscopic, topographic anatomy, and clinical anatomy. Arch. Otolaryngol. 39:359.

Ladman, A.J. and A.J. Mitchell. 1955. The topographical relations and histological characteristics of the tubuloacinar glands of the eustachian tube of mice. Anat. Rec. 121:167.

VESTIBULAR ORGANS

Citron, L., D. Exley, and C.S. Hallspike. 1956. Formation, circulation, and chemical properties of the labrinthine fluids. Br. Med. Bull. 12:101.

Flock, A. 1964. The ultrastructure of the macula utriculi with special reference to directional interplay of sensory responses as revealed by morphological polarization. J. Cell Biol. 22:413.

Guild, S.R. 1927. Observations on the structural and normal contents of the ductus and saccus endolymphaticus in the guinea pig. Am. J. Anat. 39:1.

Guild, S.R. 1927. Circulation of the endolymph. Am. J. Anat. 39:57.

Kimura, R.S., P.G. Lundquist, and J. Wersall. 1964. Secretory epithelial linings in the ampullae of the guinea pig labyrinth. Acta Otolaryngol. 57:517.

Lundquist, P.G. 1965. The endolymphatic duct and sac in the guinea pig. Acta Otolaryngol. (Suppl.) 201:1.

Ormerod, F.C. 1960. The physiology of the endolymph. J. Laryngol. Otol. 74:659.

Osborne, M.P., S.D. Comis, and J.O. Pickles. 1984. Morphology and cross-linkage of stereocilia in the guinea pig labyrinth examined without the use of osmium as a fixative. Cell Tissue Res. 237:43.

Wersall, J. and A. Flock. 1963. Physiological aspects on the structure of reticular end organs. Acta Otolaryngol. (Suppl.) 192:85.

Wersall, J. 1956. Studies on the structure and innervation of the sensory epithelium of the cristae ampullares in the guinea pig. Acta Otolaryngol. (Suppl.) 126:5

COCHLEA

Bredberg, G. 1968. Cellular pattern and nerve supply of the human organ of Corti. Acta Otolaryngol. (Suppl.) 236:1.

Brownell, W.E., C.R. Bader, D. Bertrand, and Y. de Ribaupierre. 1985. Evoked mechanical responses of isolated cochlear outer hair cells. Science 227:194.

Brundin, L., A. Flock, and B. Canlon. 1989. Sound-induced motility of isolated cochlear outer hair cells is frequency specific. Nature 342:814.

Dallos, P., B.N. Evans, and R. Hallworth. 1991. Nature of the motor element in electrokinetic shape changes of cochlear outer hair cells. Nature 350:155.

Engstrom, H., H. Ades, and J. Hawkins. 1962. Structure and function of the sensory hair cells of the inner ear. J. Acoust. Soc. Am. 34:1356.

Fernandez, E. 1951. The innervation of the cochlea (guinea pig). Laryngoscope 51:1152.

Flock, A. 1971. Transduction in hair cells. *In* W.R. Lowenstein, ed. Handbook of Sensory Physiology I. Principles of Receptor Physiology. Berlin, Springer-Verlag.

Forge, A., L. Li, J.T. Corwin, and G. Nevill. 1993. Ultrastructural evidence for hair cell regeneration in the mammalian inner ear. Science 259:1616.

Hudspeth, A.J. 1983. The hair cells of the inner ear. Sci. Am. 248:54.

Hudspeth, A.J. 1985. The cellular basis of hearing. The biophysics of hair cells. Science 230:745.

Kalinec, F., M.C. Holley, K.H. Iwasa, D.J. Lim, and B. Kachar. 1992. A membrane-based force generation mechanism in auditory sensory cells. Proc. Nat. Acad. Sci. USA 89:8671.

Kimura, R.S. 1966. Hairs of the cochlear sensory cells and their attachment to the tectorial membrane. Acta Otolaryngol. 61:55.

Kimura, R.S., H.F. Schuknecht, and I. Sundo. 1965. Fine morphology of the sensory cells of the organ of Corti in man. Acta Otolaryngol. 58:390.

Rodriguez-Echandia, E.L. and M.H. Burgos. 1965. The fine structure of the stria vascularis of the guinea pig inner ear. Zeitschr. Zellforsch. 67:600.

Index

A

B

C

D

E

F

G

H

I

J

K

L

M

N

O

P

R

S

T

U

V

W

X

Y

Z